KIDNEY TRANSPLANTATION: PRINCIPLES AND PRACTICE

SEVENTH EDITION

Sir Peter J. Morris, MD, PhD, FRS, FRCS
Emeritus Nuffield Professor of Surgery,
University of Oxford;
Honorary Professor,
University of London;
Director,
Centre for Evidence in Transplantation,
Royal College of Surgeons of England,
London, UK

Stuart J. Knechtle, MD, FACS
Clinical Director;
Professor of Surgery and Pediatrics;
Mason Chair of Transplant Surgery,
Emory Transplant Center,
Atlanta, GA, USA

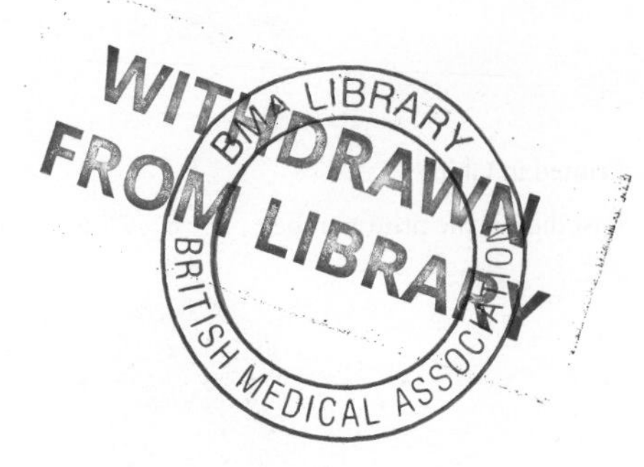

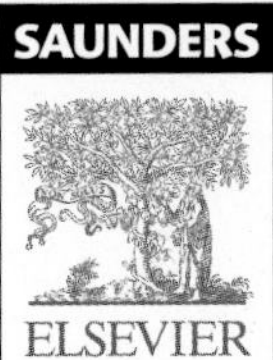

Edinburgh London New York Oxford Philadelphia St Louis Sydney Toronto 2014

ELSEVIER
SAUNDERS

First edition 1979
Second edition 1984
Third edition 1988
Fourth edition 1994
Fifth edition 2001
Sixth edition 2008

Notices

Knowledge and best practice in this field are constantly changing. As new research and experience broaden our understanding, changes in research methods, professional practices, or medical treatment may become necessary.

Practitioners and researchers must always rely on their own experience and knowledge in evaluating and using any information, methods, compounds, or experiments described herein. In using such information or methods they should be mindful of their own safety and the safety of others, including parties for whom they have a professional responsibility.

With respect to any drug or pharmaceutical products identified, readers are advised to check the most current information provided (i) on procedures featured or (ii) by the manufacturer of each product to be administered, to verify the recommended dose or formula, the method and duration of administration, and contraindications. It is the responsibility of practitioners, relying on their own experience and knowledge of their patients, to make diagnoses, to determine dosages and the best treatment for each individual patient, and to take all appropriate safety precautions.

To the fullest extent of the law, neither the Publisher nor the authors, contributors, or editors, assume any liability for any injury and/or damage to persons or property as a matter of products liability, negligence or otherwise, or from any use or operation of any methods, products, instructions, or ideas contained in the material herein.

A catalogue record for this book is held in the British Library.

ISBN: 9781455740963

Ebook ISBN: 9781455774050

Printed in China

Last digit is the print number: 9 8 7 6 5 4 3 2 1

KIDNEY TRANSPLANTATION

Executive Content Strategist: Michael Houston
Content Development Specialists: Rachael Harrison and Alexandra Mortimer
Project Manager: Sukanthi Sukumar
Designer: Christian Bilbow
Illustration Manager: Jennifer Rose
Illustrator: Antbits Ltd
Marketing Manager: Abigail Swartz

CONTENTS

VIDEO TABLE OF CONTENTS

Access all videos online at expertconsult.com. See inside front cover for activation code.

PREFACE TO THE FIRST EDITION

Renal transplantation is now an accepted treatment of patients in end-stage renal failure. A successful transplant restores not merely life but an acceptable quality of life to such patients. The number of patients in end-stage renal failure in the Western World who might be treated by hemodialysis and transplantation is considerable and comprises some 30-50 new patients/million of population. Unfortunately in most, if not all, countries the supply of kidneys for transplantation is insufficient to meet the demand. Furthermore, hemodialysis facilities are usually inadequate to make up this deficit so that many patients are still dying of renal disease who could be restored to a useful and productive life. Nevertheless, few of us would have imagined even 10 years ago that transplantation of the kidney would have become such a relatively common procedure as is the case today, and indeed well over 30,000 kidney transplantations have been performed throughout the world.

Transplantation of the kidney for the treatment of renal failure has been an attractive concept for many years. As long ago as 1945, three young surgeons at the Peter Bent Brigham Hospital in Boston, Charles Hufnagel, Ernest Landsteiner and David Hume, joined the vessels of a cadaver kidney to the brachial vessels of a young woman who was comatose from acute renal failure due to septicemia. The kidney functioned for several days before it was removed, and the woman regained consciousness. Shortly afterwards, the woman's own kidneys began to function and she made a full recovery. The advent of the artificial kidney at that time meant that this approach to the treatment of acute renal failure was no longer necessary, but attention was soon given to the possibility of transplanting kidneys to patients with end-stage renal failure who were requiring dialysis on the newly developed artificial kidney to stay alive.

Although the first experimental kidney transplants in animals were reported first in Vienna by Dr. Emerich Ulmann in 1902 and then in 1905 by Dr. Alexis Carrel in the United States, the problem of rejection was not mentioned by either author. Later in 1910, Carrel did discuss the possible differences between an autograft and a homograft. The vascular techniques developed by Carrel for the anastomosis of the renal vessels to the recipient vessels are still used today. But in 1923, Dr. Carl Williamson of the Mayo Clinic clearly defined the difference between an autografted and homografted kidney and even published histological pictures of a rejecting kidney. Furthermore, he predicted the future use of tissue matching in renal transplantation.

> *It is unfortunate that the lower animals, such as the dog, do not possess a blood grouping like that of man. In the future it may be possible to work out a satisfactory way of determining the reaction of the recipient's blood serum or tissues to those of the donor and the reverse; perhaps in this way we can obtain more light on this as yet relatively dark side of biology.*

The recognition that allogeneic tissues would be rejected was further established in later years by Drs. Gibson and Medawar, who treated burn patients with homografts in Glasgow during the Second World War. Indeed, it was the crash of a bomber behind the Medawars' house in Oxford during the early years of the war that first stimulated his interest in transplantation, especially of skin.

In his address at the opening of the new Oxford Transplant Unit in 1977, Sir Peter Medawar recounted this event.

> *Early in the war, an R.A.F. Whitley bomber crashed into a house in North Oxford with much serious injury and loss of life. Among the injured was a young man with a third degree burn extending over about 60% of his body. People burned as severely as this never raised a medical problem before: they always died; but the blood transfusion services and the control of infection made possible by the topical use of sulphonamide drugs now made it possible for them to stay alive. Dr. John F. Barnes, a colleague of mine in Professor H. W. Florey's School of Pathology, asked me to see this patient in the hope that being an experimental biologist I might have some ideas for treatment. With more than half his body surface quite raw, this poor young man was a deeply shocking sight; I thought of and tried out a number of ingenious methods, none of which worked, for ekeing out his own skin for grafting, trying to make one piece of skin do the work of ten or more. The obvious solution was to use skin grafts from a relative or voluntary donor, but this was not possible then and it is not possible now.*
>
> *I believe I saw it as my metier to find out why it was not possible to graft skin from one human being to another, and what could be done about it. I accordingly began research on the subject with the Burns Unit of the Glasgow Royal Infirmary, and subsequently in the Zoology Department in Oxford. If anybody had then told me that one day, in Oxford, kidneys would be transplanted from one human being to another, not as a perilous surgical venture, but as something more in the common run of things, I should have dismissed it as science fiction; yet it is just this that has come about, thanks to the enterprise of Professor Morris and his colleagues.*

Nevertheless in 1951, David Hume in Boston embarked on a series of cadaver kidney transplants in which the kidney was placed in the thigh of the recipient. All but one of these kidneys were rejected within a matter of days or weeks, the one exception being a patient in whom the kidney functioned for nearly 6 months and enabled the patient to leave the hospital! This event provided hope for the future as no immunosuppressive therapy had been used in this patient. At this time, the problems of rejection of kidney allografts in the dog were being clearly defined by Dr. Morton Simonsen in Copenhagen and Dr. William Dempster in London, but in 1953, a major boost to transplantation research was provided by the demonstration, by Drs. Rupert Billingham, Lesley Brent and Peter Medawar, that tolerance to an allogeneic skin graft in an adult animal could be produced by injecting the fetus with donor strain tissue, thus confirming experimentally the clonal selection hypothesis of Burnet and Fenner in the recognition of self and non-self. The induction of specific unresponsiveness of a host to a tissue allograft has remained the ultimate goal of transplant immunologists ever since.

Then in 1954, the first kidney transplant between identical twins was carried out successfully at the Peter Bent Brigham Hospital which led to a number of further successful identical twin transplants in Boston and elsewhere in the world over the next few years.

There still remained the apparently almost insoluble problem of rejection of any kidney other than an identical-twin kidney. The first attempts to suppress the immune response to a kidney allograft employed total body irradiation of the recipient and were carried out by Dr. Merril's group in Boston, two groups in Paris under the direction of Drs. Kuss and Hamburger, respectively, and by Professor Shackman's group in London. Rejection of a graft could be suppressed by irradiation, but the complications of the irradiation were such that this was really an unacceptable approach, although an occasional relatively long-term acceptance of a graft provided encouragement for the future.

Then came the discovery by Drs. Schwartz and Dameshek in 1959 that 6-mercaptopurine could suppress the immune response of rabbits to human serum albumin. Shortly afterwards, they showed that the survival of skin allografts in rabbits was significantly prolonged by the same drug. This event ushered in the present era of renal transplantation, for very quickly Roy Calne in London and Charles Zukoski working with David Hume in Virginia showed that this same drug markedly prolonged the survival of kidney allografts in dogs. And indeed, 6-mercaptopurine was first used in a patient in Boston in 1960. Elion and Hitchings of the Burroughs Wellcome Research Laboratories in New York State then developed azathioprine, which quickly replaced 6-mercaptopurine in clinical practice as it was less toxic. With the addition of steroids, the standard immunosuppressive therapy of today was introduced to the practice of renal transplantation in the early sixties.

Not that this meant the solution of the problems of renal transplantation for this combination of drugs was dangerous and mortality was high in those early years. But there was a significant number of long-term successful transplants, and as experience grew, the results of renal transplantation improved. Another major area of endeavor in renal transplantation at that time was directed at the study of methods of matching donor and recipient for histocompatibility antigens with the aim of lessening the immune response to the graft and so perhaps allowing a decrease in the immunosuppressive drug therapy. Although this aim has only been achieved to any great extent in siblings who are HLA identical, tissue typing has made a significant contribution to renal transplantation, perhaps best illustrated by the recognition in the late sixties that the performance of a transplant in the presence of donor-specific presensitization in the recipient leads to hyperacute or accelerated rejection of the graft in most instances. Nevertheless, the more recent description of the Ia-like system in man (HLA-DR) may have an important impact on tissue typing in renal transplantation. The present decade also has seen an enormous effort directed at immunological monitoring in renal transplantation and at attempts to induce experimental specific immunosuppression. We have solved most of the technical problems of renal transplantation; we have been left with the problem of rejection and the complications arising from the drug therapy given to prevent rejection.

Although the contributions in this book cover all aspects of renal transplantation, certain subjects, as for example immunological monitoring before transplantation, transplantation in children and cancer after renal transplantation, have received considerable emphasis as they do represent developing areas of great interest, and I must take responsibility for this emphasis. For in the seventies we have seen many of the principles and practice of renal transplantation become established and the areas of future investigation become more clearly defined. With an ever-increasing demand for renal transplantation, more and more people in many different disciplines, doctors (surgeons, physicians, pathologists, virologists, immunologists), nurses, scientists and ancillary staff are becoming involved in renal transplantation either in the clinic or in the laboratory. It is to these people I hope this book will be of value.

Sir Peter J. Morris
Oxford, UK
November 1978

PREFACE TO THE SEVENTH EDITION

It is amazing, at least from our point to view, to realise that it is 35 years (1978) since the first edition of Kidney Transplantation: Principles and Practice was published. In 1954, the first successful kidney transplant was performed by the late Joseph Murray at the Peter Bent Brigham Hospital in Boston. Thus as we look back on the first edition it certainly made us realise how far we have come. Although at times people working in kidney transplantation feel a little despondent that we are not making sufficient progress, progress, as always, continues to be made, which is certainly evident if you review the past six editions of this book.

In this edition we have a number of new authors and have added some additional chapters. For example the new immunosuppressive agent that has appeared on the screen is Belatacept (a fusion protein which inhibits co stimulation) and as there are a considerable number of well conducted randomised controlled trials of this new biological agent all showing considerable promise, we felt it was worthy of a chapter by itself, at least in this edition. We also have added a chapter on paired exchange programmes for living donors which has become widespread now throughout the world. Finally we have added a chapter on evidence in transplantation where it becomes increasingly apparent that we do need to have a better basis of evidence for what we do. The remaining chapters cover much the same topics as in the previous editions but of course in many of those areas there have been considerable changes and so a lot of updating has been necessary. One might ask why we have a chapter on azathioprine alone? This is really because it is a good and safe agent, perhaps discarded a little early, but as it was the first immunosuppressive agent available way back in the 1960's then if for no other reason than a historical one, it deserves a brief chapter.

Patient and graft survival continued to improve in the short and medium term and in most units good risk patients can achieve one year graft survival of 90% or better at one year, but the long term survival of kidney grafts has not improved all that much despite the various new immunosuppressive agents. Chronic allograft nephropathy remains a major problem. Again in the preservation area hypothermic machine preservation is being revaluated with promising results now available and this is extensively discussed on the chapter on preservation. There is a separate chapter on steroids, but now concentrating on steroid avoidance or sparing. For the first time we have now an electronic edition in keeping with changes in media presentation, and added video clips to more thoroughly illustrate the principles related to our field.

Renal transplantation is an exciting area and we have to be grateful to the scientists and clinicians that made the current results possible and to the thousands of patients who have participated in this evolution of renal transplantation over the last 50 years.

Sir Peter J. Morris
London, UK

Stuart Knechtle
Atlanta, GA, USA

LIST OF CONTRIBUTORS

Richard D.M. Allen, MBBS, FRACS
Professor of Transplantation Surgery, University of Sydney; Director of Transplantation Services, Royal Prince Alfred Hospital, Sydney, Australia
Ch 28 Vascular and Lymphatic Complications after Kidney Transplantation

Frederike Ambagtsheer, MSc, LLM
Scientific Researcher, Erasmus MC University Hospital, Department of Internal Medicine, Kidney Transplantation Section, Rotterdam, The Netherlands
Ch 41 Ethical and Legal Aspects of Kidney Donation

Amit Basu, MD, FACS, FRCS(Edin)
Attending Transplant Surgeon, Transplant Center, North Shore Long Island Jewish Health System, Manhasset, New York, USA
Ch 17 Calcineurin Inhibitors

Simon Ball, MA, PhD, FRCP
Consultant Nephrologist, Queen Elizabeth Hospital Birmingham, Birmingham, UK
Ch 02 Immunology of Graft Rejection

Adam D. Barlow, MBBS, MRCS, MD
Specialist Registrar in Transplantation, Transplant Group, Department of Infection, Immunity and Inflammation, University of Leicester, Leicester, UK
Ch 05 Access for Renal Replacement Therapy;
Ch 05 Clip 01 Laparoscopic: Peritoneal Dialysis - Catheter Insertion Techniques

Rolf N. Barth, MD
Associate Professor of Surgery, Division of Transplantation, University of Maryland School of Medicine, Baltimore, MD, USA
Ch 08 Donor Nephrectomy;
Ch 08 clip 01 Laparoendoscopic single site (LESS) donor nephrectomy: technique and outcomes

J. Andrew Bradley, PhD, FRCS, FMedSci
Professor of Surgery, University of Cambridge; Honorary Consultant Surgeon, Addenbrooke's Hospital, Cambridge, UK
Ch 19 mTor Inhibitors: Sirolimus and Everolimus

Jeremy R. Chapman, MD, MB, BChir, FRACP, FRCP
Clinical Professor of Renal Medicine, Centre for Transplant and Renal Research, University of Sydney, Sydney, Australia; Westmead Hospital, Westmead, Australia
Ch 04 The Recipient of a Kidney Transplant

Robert B. Colvin, MD
Massachusetts General Hospital and Harvard Medical School, Boston, MA, USA
Ch 26 Pathology of Kidney Transplantation

Lynn D. Cornell, MD
Consultant, Division of Anatomic Pathology; Associate Professor of Laboratory Medicine and Pathology, Mayo Clinic College of Medicine, Mayo Clinic, Rochester, MI, USA
Ch 26 Pathology of Kidney Transplantation

Fiona J. Culley, PhD
National Heart and Lung Institute, Imperial College London, London, UK
Ch 02 clip 02 3-D rotational image of immune synapses

Margaret J. Dallman, DPhil
Professor of Immunology and Principal, Faculty of Natural Sciences, Department of Life Sciences, Imperial College London, London, UK
Ch 02 Immunology of Graft Rejection

Andrew Davenport, MD
Consultant Renal Physician, UCL Centre for Nephrology, Royal Free Hospital, London, UK
Ch 03 Chronic Kidney Failure: Renal Replacement Therapy

Dan Davis, PhD
Department of Life Sciences, Imperial College London, London, UK
Ch 02 clip 01 Formation of an immune synapse;
Ch 02 clip 03 An NK cell killing its target

Alton B. Farris, III, MD
Department of Pathology, Emory University Hospital, Atlanta, GA, USA
Ch 26 Pathology of Kidney Transplantation

Jay A. Fishman, MD
Profesor of Medicine; Director, Transplant Infectious Disease and Compromised Host Program, Harvard Medical School and Massachusetts General Hospital, Boston, MA, USA
Ch 31 Infection in Kidney Transplant Recipients

Andria L. Ford, MD, MSCI
Assistant Professor in Neurology, Washington University in St. Louis School of Medicine; Attending Physician, Barnes-Jewish Hospital, St. Louis, MO, USA
Ch 33 Neurological Complications after Kidney Transplantation

Julie Franc-Guimond, MD
Associate Professor, University of Montreal, Montreal, Quebec, Canada
Ch 12 Transplantation and the Abnormal Bladder

Patricia M. Franklin, MSc, BSc(Hons), RGN
Kidney Patient Advisor – Psychologist, Oxford Renal Medicine and Transplant Centre, The Churchill Hospital, Oxford, UK
Ch 40 Psychological Aspects of Kidney Transplantation and Organ Donation

Peter J. Friend, MA, MB, BCHIR, FRCS, MD
Professor of Transplantation, University of Oxford; Consultant Surgeon Oxford University NHS Trust Oxford Transplant Centre, Nuffield Department of Surgical Sciences, Oxford, UK
Ch 9 Kidney Preservation;
Ch 11 Surgical Techniques of Kidney Transplantation

Susan V. Fuggle, BSc(Hons), MSc, DPhil, FRCPath
Reader in Transplant Immunology, University of Oxford; Director of Clinical Transplant Immunology, Transplant Immunology and Immunogenetics, Oxford Transplant Centre, Churchill Hospital, Oxford, UK
Ch 10 Histocompatibility in Kidney Transplantation

Robert S. Gaston, MD
Robert G. Luke Chair in Transplant Nephrology; Medical Director of Kidney and Pancreas Transplantation; Co-Director, Comprehensive Transplant Institute, University of Alabama at Birmingham, Birmingham, AL, USA
Ch 18 Mycophenolates

Sommer E. Gentry, PhD
Associate Professor of Mathematics, Department of Mathematics, United States Naval Academy, Annapolis, MD; Department of Surgery Johns Hopkins University School of Medicine, Baltimore, MD, USA
Ch 25 Kidney Paired Donation Programs for Living Donors

Ricardo González, MD
Auf der Bult Youth and Children's Hospital, Hannover Medical School, Hannover, Germany; Charité University Medicine Berlin, Berlin, Germany
Ch 12 Transplantation and the Abnormal Bladder

Angelika C. Gruessner, MS, PhD
Professor of Public Health and Research, University of Arizona; Chief Information Officer, Cancer Center Division, University of Arizona College of Medicine, Tucson, AZ, USA
Ch 36 Pancreas and Kidney Transplantation for Diabetic Nephropathy

Rainer W.G. Gruessner, MD
Professor of Surgery and Immunobiology; Chair, Department of Surgery, University of Arizona College of Medicine, Tucson, AZ, USA
Ch 36 Pancreas and Kidney Transplantation for Diabetic Nephropathy

David Hamilton, PhD, FRCS
Honorary Senior Lecturer, Bute Medical School, St Andrews University, St Andrews, Scotland
Ch 01 Kidney Transplantation: A History

James P. Hunter, BSc(Hons), MBChB, MRCS
Senior Clinical Research Fellow, Transplant Group, Department of Infection, Immunity and Inflammation, University of Leicester, Leicester, UK
Ch 05 Access for Renal Replacement Therapy;
Ch 05 Clip 01 Laparoscopic: Peritoneal Dialysis - Catheter Insertion Techniques

Alan G. Jardine, BSc, MD, FRCP
Professor of Renal Medicine, University of Glasgow, Glasgow, Scotland
Ch 30 Cardiovascular Disease in Renal Transplantation

Sasha Nicole Jenkins, MD, MPH
Emory Department of Dermatology Chief Resident, Emory University, Department of Dermatology Atlanta, GA, USA
Ch 34 Non-malignant and Malignant Skin Lesions in Kidney Transplant Patients

Juan Antonio Jiménez, MD, PhD
Resident Physician, Glickman Urological and Kidney Institute, Cleveland Clinic Foundation, Cleveland, OH, USA
Ch 29 Urological Complications after Kidney Transplantation

Laura S. Johnson, MD
Department of Surgical Critical Care/Trauma/ Acute Care Surgery, Washington Hospital Center, Washington, DC, USA
Ch 06 Brain Death and Cardiac Death: Donor Criteria and Care of Deceased Donor;
Ch 06 clip 01 Brain Death Examination

Allan D. Kirk, MD, PhD, FACS
Professor of Surgery and Pediatrics, Emory University; Scientific Director, Emory Transplant Center, Emory University Hospital, Atlanta, GA, USA
Ch 20 Antilymphocyte Globulin, Monoclonal Antibodies, and Fusion Proteins;
Ch 21 Belatacept

Stuart J. Knechtle, MD, FACS
Clinical Director; Professor of Surgery and Pediatrics; Mason Chair of Transplant Surgery, Emory Transplant Center, Atlanta, GA, USA
Ch 14 Early Course of the Patient with a Kidney Transplantation;
Ch 39 Results of Renal Transplantation

Simon R. Knight, MChir, MA, MB, FRCS
Deputy Director, Centre for Evidence in Transplantation, Clinical Effectiveness Unit, Royal College of Surgeons of England, London, UK; Academic Clinical Lecturer in Transplant Surgery, Nuffield Department of Surgical Sciences, University of Oxford, Oxford, UK
Ch 16 Steroids;
Ch 42 Evidence in Transplantation

Aoife Lally, MD, FRCPI
Consultant Dermatologist, Department of Dermatology, St Vincent's University Hospital, Dublin, Ireland
Ch 34 Non-malignant and Malignant Skin Lesions in Kidney Transplant Patients

Christian P. Larsen, MD, PhD
Dean, Emory University School of Medicine; Vice President For Health Center Integration, Emory University, Atlanta, GA, USA
Ch 21 Belatacept

Jin-Moo Lee, MD, PhD
Professor of Neurology, Radiology and Biomedical Engineering; Director, Cerebrovascular Disease Section, Department of Neurology, Washington University School of Medicine; Attending Physician, Barnes-Jewish Hospital, St. Louis, MO, USA
Ch 33 Neurological Complications after Kidney Transplantation

Henri G.D. Leuvenink, MD, PhD
Associate Professor, Department of Surgery, University of Groningen, Surgical Research Laboratory, University Medical Center Groningen, Groningen, The Netherlands
Ch 09 Kidney Preservation

Michael R. Lucey, MD
Professor of Medicine; Chief, Division of Gastroenterology and Hepatology, Department of Medicine, University of Wisconsin School of Medicine and Public Health, Madison, Wisconsin
Ch 32 Liver Disease among Renal Transplant Recipients

Barbara Ludwikowski, MD
Auf der Bult Youth and Children's Hospital, Hannover, Germany
Ch 12 Transplantation and the Abnormal Bladder

Malcolm P. MacConmara, MB, BCh, BAO
Associate in Surgery, Fellow Abdominal Organ Transplantation, Emory Transplant Center, Emory University, Atlanta, GA, USA
Ch 07 Medical Evaluation of the Living Donor

Chantal Mathieu, MD, PHD
Professor of Endocrinology, University of Leuven, Leuven, Belgium
Ch 22 Other Forms of Immunosuppression

Emily P McQuarrie, BSc, MD, MRCP
Specialist Trainee and Clinical Research Fellow in Renal Medicine, Institute of Cardiovascular and Medical Sciences, University of Glasgow, Glasgow, UK
Ch 30 Cardiovascular Disease in Renal Transplantation

Juan C. Mejia, MD
Transplant Surgery Fellow, Starzl Transplant Institute, University of Pittsburgh Medical Center, Pittsburgh, PA, USA
Ch 17 Calcineurin Inhibitors

M. Rafique Moosa, MB, ChB, FCP, MD, FRCP
Professor and Head, Department of Medicine, Faculty of Health Sciences, Stellenbosch University, Cape Town, South Africa
Ch 38 Kidney Transplantation in Developing Countries

Sir Peter J. Morris, MD, PhD, FRS, FRCS
Emeritus Nuffield Professor of Surgery, University of Oxford; Honorary Professor, University of London; Director, Centre for Evidence in Transplantation, Royal College of Surgeons of England, London, UK
Ch 15 Azathioprine;
Ch 42 Evidence in Transplantation

Brian J. Nankivell, MD, PhD, FRACP
Transplant Physician, Department of Renal Medicine, Westmead Hospital, Sydney, Australia
Ch 27 Chronic Allograft Failure

Kenneth A. Newell, MD, PhD
Professor of Surgery, Division of Transplantation, Department of Surgery, Emory University School of Medicine; Director, Living Donor Kidney Program, Emory Transplant Center, Atlanta, GA, USA
Ch 07 Medical Evaluation of the Living Donor

Claus U. Niemann, MD
Professor of Anesthesia and Surgery, Department of Anesthesia and Perioperative Care, Department of Surgery, Division of Transplantation, University of California San Francisco, San Francisco, CA, USA
Ch 13 Perioperative Care of Patients Undergoing Kidney Transplantation

Michael L. Nicholson, MD, DSc, FRCS
Professor of Transplant Surgery, Transplant Group, Department of Infection, Immunity and Inflammation University of Leicester, Leicester, UK
Ch 05 Access for Renal Replacement Therapy;
Ch 05 Clip 01 Laparoscopic: Peritoneal Dialysis - Catheter Insertion Techniques

John O'Callaghan, MBBS, MRCS
Specialist Registrar in Transplant Surgery, Oxford Transplant Unit, Churchill Hospital, Oxford, UK
Ch 09 Kidney Preservation

Stephen Pastan, MD
Associate Professor of Medicine; Medical Director, Kidney and Pancreas Transplant Program, Emory Transplant Center, Emory University School of Medicine, Atlanta, GA, USA
Ch 14 Early Course of the Patient with a Kidney Transplantation

Rachel E. Patzer, MD, PhD
Assistant Professor, Department of Renal Medicine, Emory University School of Medicine, Department of Surgery, Division of Transplantation, Rollins School of Public Health, Department of Epidemiology, Atlanta, GA, USA
Ch 39 Results of Renal Transplantation

Thomas C. Pearson, MD, DPhil
Livingston Professor of Surgery, Department of Surgery, Emory University, Atlanta, GA, USA
Ch 21 Belatacept

Liset H.M. Pengel, PhD
Chief Executive Officer and Senior Research Associate, Centre for Evidence in Transplantation, The Royal College of Surgeons of England, London, UK
Ch 42 Evidence in Transplantation;
Ch 42 clip 01 The Transplant Library on OvidSP;
Ch 42 clip 02 The Transplant Library on Evidentia

Jacques Pirenne, MD, MSc, PhD
Chief, Abdominal Transplant Surgery; Professor of Surgery, University Leuven (KUL), Leuven, Belgium
Ch 22 Other Forms of Immunosuppression

Nicholas Byron Pitts, MD
St. Vincent Emergency Physicians, Inc., Indianapolis, IN, USA
Ch 06 clip 01 Brain Death Examination

Rutger J. Ploeg, MA, BA, MD, PHD, FRCS
Professor of Transplant Biology; Consultant Surgeon, Clinical and Translational Research, Nuffield Department of Surgical Sciences, Oxford Transplant Centre, University of Oxford, Oxford, UK
Ch 09 Kidney Preservation

John P. Rice, MD
Division of Gastroenterology and Hepatology, Department of Medicine, University of Wisconsin School of Medicine and Public Health, Madison, WI, USA
Ch 32 Liver Disease among Renal Transplant Recipients

Nasia Safdar, MD, PhD
Associate Professor of Medicine, Division of Infectious Diseases, Department of Medicine, University of Wisconsin School of Medicine and Public Health, Madison, WI, USA; Associate Chief of Staff for Research, VAMC
Ch 32 Liver Disease among Renal Transplant Recipients

Adnan Said, MD, MS
Associate Professor of Medicine, Division of Gastroenterology and Hepatology, University of Wisconsin School of Medicine and Public Health; Chief, Gastroenterology and Hepatology, Wm. S. Middleton VAMC, Madison, WI, USA; Program Director, Transplant Hepatology
Ch 32 Liver Disease among Renal Transplant Recipients

Blayne A. Sayed, MD, PhD
Resident, Department of Surgery, Emory University, Atlanta, GA, USA
Ch 21 Belatacept

Dorry L. Segev, MD, PhD
Professor of Surgery, Epidemiology, and Biostatistics, Department of Surgery, Johns Hopkins University School of Medicine, Department of Epidemiology, Johns Hopkins Bloomberg School of Public Health, Baltimore, MD, USA
Ch 25 Kidney Paired Donation Programs for Living Donors

Ron Shapiro, MD
Professor of Surgery, Robert J. Corry Chair in Transplantation Surgery, Thomas E. Starzl Transplantation Institute, University of Pittsburgh, Pittsburgh, PA, USA
Ch 17 Calcineurin Inhibitors

Daniel Shoskes, MD
Professor of Surgery (Urology), Glickman Urological and Kidney Institute, Cleveland Clinic Foundation, Cleveland, OH, USA
Ch 29 Urological Complications after Kidney Transplantation

Ben Sprangers, MD, PhD
Professor of Nephrology and Transplant Immunology, University of Leuven, Leuven, Belgium
Ch 22 Other Forms of Immunosuppression

Mark D. Stegall, MD
Professor of Surgery and Immunology, Mayo Clinic College of Medicine, Mayo Clinic, Rochester, MI, USA
Ch 24 Transplantation in the Sensitized Recipient and Across ABO Blood Groups

Ram M. Subramanian, MD
Intensivist and Hepatologist, Departments of Medicine and Surgery, Emory University School of Medicine, Atlanta, GA, USA
Ch 06 Brain Death and Cardiac Death: Donor Criteria and Care of Deceased Donor;
Ch 06 clip 01 Brain Death Examination

Craig J. Taylor, PhD, FRCPath
Consultant Clinical Scientist; Director of Histocompatibility Immunogenetics, Tissue Typing Laboratory, Cambridge University Hospitals NHS Foundation Trust, Cambridge, UK
Ch 10 Histocompatibility in Kidney Transplantation

John F. Thompson, MD, FRACS, FACS
Executive Director, Melanoma Institute Australia; Professor of Surgery (Melanoma and Surgical Oncology), The University of Sydney; Head of Department of Melanoma and Surgical Oncology, Royal Prince Alfred Hospital, Sydney, NSW, Australia
Ch 35 Cancer in Dialysis and Kidney Transplant Patients

Katie D. Vo, MD
Associate Professor in Radiology; Director, Diagnostic Neuroradiology Fellowship; Director, Cerebrovascular Imaging, Washington University in St. Louis Medical Center, Barnes-Jewish Hospital, St. Louis, MI, USA
Ch 33 Neurological Complications after Kidney Transplantation

Mark Waer, MD, PhD
Professor of Nephrology and Transplant Immunology, University of Leuven, Leuven, Belgium
Ch 22 Other Forms of Immunosuppression

Barry Warshaw, MD
Associate Professor of Pediatrics, Emory University School of Medicine; Medical Director, Pediatric Renal Transplant Program Children's Healthcare of Atlanta, Atlanta, GA, USA
Ch 37 Renal Transplantation in Children

Christopher J.E. Watson, MD, FRCS
Professor of Transplantation, University of Cambridge; Honorary Consultant Surgeon, Addenbrooke's Hospital, Cambridge, UK
Ch 11 Surgical Techniques of Kidney Transplantation; Ch 19 mTor Inhibitors: Sirolimus and Everolimus

Angela C. Webster, MBBS MM(Clin Epi), PhD, FRCP(UK), FRACP
Associate Professor, Clinical Epidemiology and Nephrologist, University of Sydney and Westmead Hospital, Sydney, NSW, Australia
Ch 35 Cancer in Dialysis and Kidney Transplant Patients

Willem Weimar, MD, PhD
Professor of Internal Medicine, Erasmus MC University Hospital, Department of Internal Medicine, Nephrology and Transplantation Section, Rotterdam, The Netherlands
Ch 41 Ethical and Legal Aspects of Kidney Donation

Jennifer T. Wells, MD
Consultant Hepatologist, Baylor University Medical Center, Dallas, TX, USA
Ch 32 Liver Disease among Renal Transplant Recipients

Pamela Winterberg, MD
Assistant Professor of Pediatrics, Division of Nephrology, Emory University School of Medicine and Children's Healthcare of Atlanta, Atlanta, GA, USA
Ch37 Renal Transplantation in Children

Kathryn J. Wood, DPhil
Transplantation Research Immunology Group, Professor of Immunology, Nuffield Department of Surgical Sciences, John Radcliffe Hospital, University of Oxford, Oxford, UK
Ch 23 Approaches to the Induction of Tolerance

C. Spencer Yost, MD
Professor of Anesthesia, Department of Anesthesia and Perioperative Care, Department of Surgery, Division of Transplantation, University of California San Francisco, San Francisco, CA, USA
Ch 13 Perioperative Care of Patients Undergoing Kidney Transplantation

Fiona Zwald, MD, MRCPI
Assistant Professor of Dermatology, Emory Transplant Dermatology Clinic, Mohs Micrographic Surgery, Dept of Dermatology, Emory University School of Medicine, Atlanta, GA, USA
Ch 34 Nonmalignant and Malignant Skin Lesions in Kidney Transplant Patients

CHAPTER 1

KIDNEY TRANSPLANTATION: A HISTORY

David Hamilton

CHAPTER OUTLINE

The modern period of transplantation began in the late 1950s, but two earlier periods of interest in clinical and experimental transplantation were the early 1950s and the first two decades of the 20th century. Hamilton[22] provides a bibliography of the history of organ transplantation. Table 1-1 summarizes landmarks in kidney transplantation.

EARLY EXPERIMENTS

Interest in transplantation developed in the early part of the 20th century because experimental and clinical surgical skills were rapidly advancing, and many of the pioneering surgeons took an interest in vascular surgical techniques as part of their broad familiarity with the advance of all aspects of surgery. Payr's demonstration of the first workable, although cumbersome, stent method of vascular suturing led to widespread interest in organ transplantation in Europe. Many centers were involved, notably Vienna, Bucharest, and Lyon. The first successful experimental organ transplant was reported by Ullmann in 1902. Emerich Ullmann (1861–1937) (Figure 1-1) had studied under Edward Albert before obtaining a position at the Vienna Medical School, which was then at its height. Ullmann's article shows that he managed to autotransplant a dog kidney from its normal position to the vessels of the neck, which resulted in some urine flow. The animal was presented to a Vienna medical society on March 1, 1902, and caused considerable comment.[55] At this time, Ullmann was Chief Surgeon to the Spital der Baumhertigen Schwestern, and his experimental work was done in the Vienna Physiology Institute under Hofrath Exner. Exner's son Alfred had already tried such a transplant without success. In the same year, another Vienna physician, Alfred von Decastello, physician assistant at the Second Medical Clinic, carried out dog-to-dog kidney transplants at the Institute of Experimental Pathology.[15]

Ullmann and von Decastello had used Payr's method, and later in 1902 Ullmann demonstrated a dog-to-goat kidney transplant that, to his surprise, passed a little urine for a while. Neither Ullmann nor von Decastello continued with this work, although von Decastello was noted for his work on blood groups, and Ullmann published extensively on bowel and biliary surgery.

In Lyon, the department headed by Mathieu Jaboulay (1860–1913) had a major influence (Figure 1-2). In his research laboratories, his assistants Carrel, Briau, and Villard worked on improved methods of vascular suturing, leading to Carrel's famous article credited with establishing the modern method of suturing.[9] Carrel left to work in the United States, and in the next 10 years he published extensively on organ grafting, successfully carrying out autografts of kidneys in cats and dogs and showing that allografts eventually failed after functioning briefly. He was awarded a Nobel Prize for this work in 1912.

HUMAN KIDNEY TRANSPLANTS

Jaboulay, Carrel's teacher, had carried out the first recorded human kidney transplant in 1906,[28] although Ullmann later claimed an earlier attempt in 1902.[56] Jaboulay was later to be better known for his work on thyroid and urological surgery, but, doubtless encouraged by the success of Carrel and others in his laboratory, he carried out two xenograft kidney transplants using a pig and goat as donors, transplanting the organ to the arm or thigh of patients with chronic renal failure. Each kidney worked for only 1 hour. This choice of an animal donor

TABLE 1-1 **Landmarks in Kidney Transplantation**

1902	First successful experimental kidney transplant[55]
1906	First human kidney transplant – xenograft[28]
1933	First human kidney transplant – allograft[54]
1950	Revival of experimental kidney transplantation[16,49]
1950–1953	Human kidney allografts without immunosuppression, in Paris[17,32,48] and Boston[27]
1953	First use of live related donor, Paris[34]
1954	First transplant between identical twins, Boston[40]
1958	First description of leukocyte antigen Mac[13]
1959–1962	Radiation used for immunosuppression, in Boston[39] and Paris[20,30]
1960	Effectiveness of 6-mercaptopurine (6-MP) in dog kidney transplants[5,62]
1960	Prolonged graft survival in patient given 6-MP after irradiation[31]
1962	First use of tissue matching to select a donor and recipient[14,31,53]
1966	Recognition that positive crossmatching leads to hyperacute rejection[29,53]
1967	Creation of Eurotransplant[45]
1967	Development of kidney preservation
1973	Description of the transfusion effect[4]
1978	First clinical use of cyclosporine[8]
1978	Application of matching for HLA-DR in renal transplantation[5]
1987	First of new wave of immunosuppressive agents appears (tacrolimus)
1997	Transgenic pigs produced

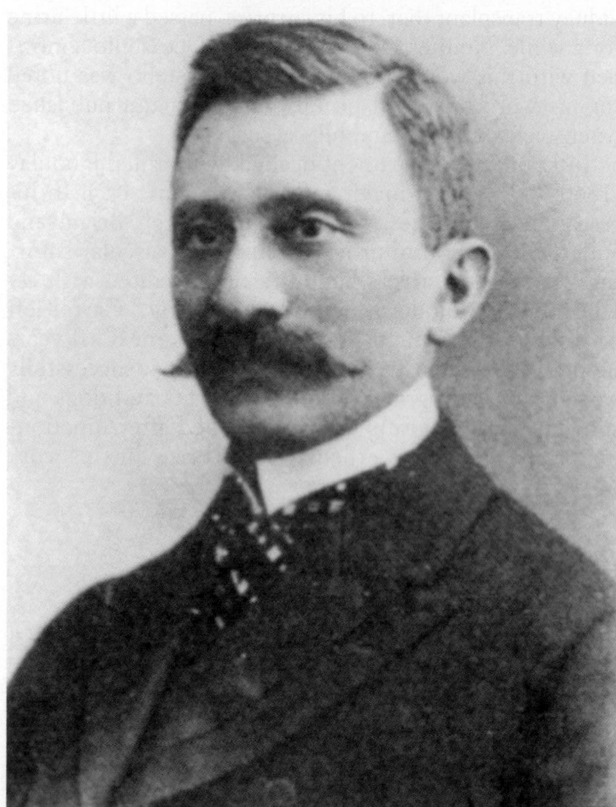

FIGURE 1-1 ■ Emerich Ullmann (1861–1937) carried out the first experimental kidney transplants in dogs in 1902. (Courtesy of the Vienna University, Institute for the History of Medicine.)

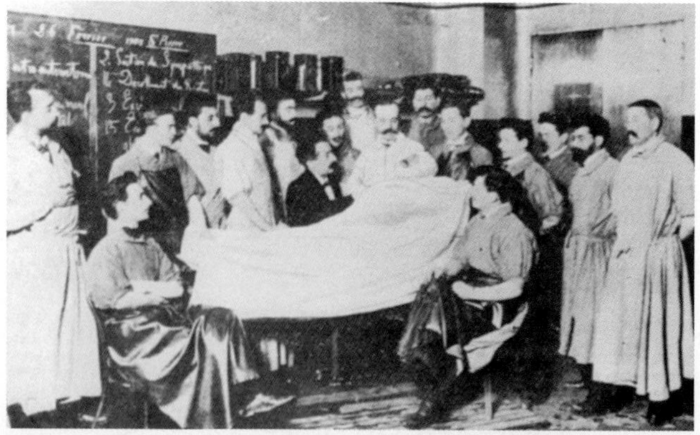

FIGURE 1-2 ■ Mathieu Jaboulay (1860–1913) and his surgical team at Lyon in 1903. Until his death in a rail accident, Jaboulay made numerous surgical contributions and encouraged Alexis Carrel's work on vascular anastomosis. In 1906, Jaboulay reported the first attempt at human kidney transplantation.

was acceptable at that time in view of the many claims in the surgical literature for success with xenograft skin, cornea, or bone.

More is known of the second and third attempts at human kidney transplantation. Ernst Unger (1875–1938) (Figure 1-3) had a thorough training in experimental work and set up his own clinic in 1905 in Berlin, being joined there by distinguished colleagues. He continued with experimental work and by 1909 reported successful transplantation of the kidneys en masse from a fox terrier to a boxer dog. The urine output continued for 14 days, and the animal was presented to two medical societies. By 1910, Unger had performed more than 100

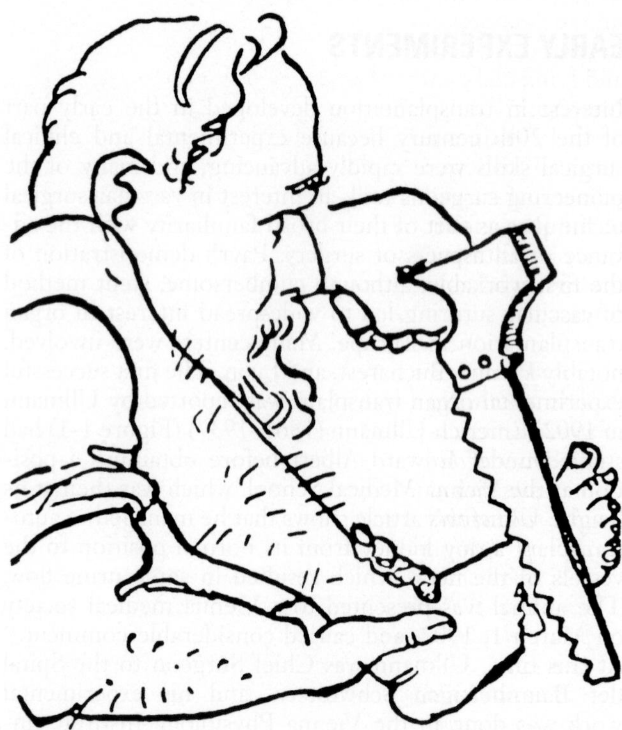

FIGURE 1-3 ■ A contemporary cartoon of Ernst Unger (1875–1938) at work at the Rudolf Virchow Hospital, Berlin. (Courtesy of the Rudolf Virchow Hospital.)

experimental kidney transplants. On December 10, 1909, Unger attempted a transplant using a stillborn child's kidney grafted to a baboon. No urine was produced. The animal died shortly after the operation, but postmortem examination showed that the vascular anastomosis had been successful. This success and the new knowledge that monkeys and humans were serologically similar led Unger to attempt, later in the same month, a monkey-to-human transplant.[57] The patient was a young girl dying of renal failure, and the kidney from an ape was sutured to the thigh vessels. No urine was produced. Unger's report concluded that there was a biochemical barrier to transplantation, a view mistakenly advocated by the basic science of the day; his main contributions thereafter were in esophageal surgery. (For a biography of Unger, see Winkler.[61])

These early experiments established that kidney transplants were technically possible. Methods of study of renal function were primitive then; without routine measurement of blood urea and without any radiological methods, subtle studies of transplant function were impossible. This impossibility plus the uncertainty of the mechanism of allograft rejection led to a diminished interest in organ transplantation after about 10 years of activity. By the start of World War I, interest in organ transplantation had almost ceased and was not resumed in the European departments of surgery after the war. Carrel had switched his attention to studies of tissue culture. Interest elsewhere also was low; in Britain and the United States, scarce research funds were being applied to fundamental biochemistry and physiology, rather than applied projects of clinical relevance. Transplantation immunology faded away after the bright start in the capable surgical hands of Carrel, Murphy's sound grasp of immunosuppression, and Landsteiner's awareness of the serological detection of human antigens. Carrel, Murphy, and Landsteiner all worked at the Rockefeller Institute in New York.

In 1914, in a remarkable lecture to the International Surgical Society, Carrel did anticipate the future development of transplantation. His colleague, J. B. Murphy, at the Rockefeller Institute, had found that radiation or benzol treatment would increase the "take" of tumor grafts in rats, and Carrel realized the potential of these findings:

> *It is too soon to draw any definite conclusions from these experiments. Nevertheless it is certain that a very important point has been acquired with Dr. Murphy's discovery that the power of the organism to eliminate foreign tissue was due to organs such as the spleen or bone marrow, and that when the action of these organs is less active a foreign tissue can develop rapidly after it has been grafted.*
>
> *It is not possible to foresee whether or not the present experiments of Dr. Murphy will lead directly to the practical solution of the problem in which we are interested.*
>
> *The surgical side of the transplantation of organs is now completed, as we are now able to perform transplantations of organs with perfect ease and with excellent results from an anatomical standpoint. But as yet the methods cannot be applied to human surgery, for the reason that homoplastic transplantations are almost always unsuccessful from the standpoint of the functioning of the organs. All our efforts must now be directed toward the biological methods which will prevent the reaction of the organism against foreign tissue and allow the adapting of homoplastic grafts to their hosts.*[10]

THE MIDDLE YEARS

Until the revival of interest in transplantation in the 1950s, the 1930s and 1940s were a stagnant period in clinical science. The great European surgical centers had declined; in North America, only at the Mayo Clinic was there a cautious program of experimental transplantation without building on Carrel's work, notably failing to make attempts at immunosuppression. In transplantation circles, such as they were, there was not even the confidence to counter the vivid claims of Voronoff to rejuvenate human patients via monkey gland grafts, and the endless reports of successful human skin homografts were not examined critically.

The main event of this period was an isolated and little-known event – the first human kidney allograft. It was performed in the Ukraine by the Soviet surgeon Yu Yu Voronoy.[58] Voronoy was an experienced investigator, and he eventually performed six such transplants up to 1949. Voronoy (1895–1961) trained in surgery at Kiev under Professor V. N. Shamov and obtained experience there with serological methods of blood transfusion, then in their developmental stage. He used these methods to detect complement-fixing antibodies after testis slice transplants, and later he had some success with the same methods applied to kidney grafts (Figure 1-4). In 1933, Voronoy transplanted a human kidney of blood group B to a patient of blood group O with acute renal failure as a result of mercuric chloride poisoning. The donor kidney was obtained from a patient dying as a result of a head injury and was transplanted to the thigh vessels under local anesthetic; the warm time for the kidney was about 6 hours. There was a major mismatch for blood groups, and despite a modest exchange transfusion, the kidney never worked. The patient died 2 days later; at postmortem, the donor vessels were patent. By 1949, Voronoy reported six such transplants, although no substantial function

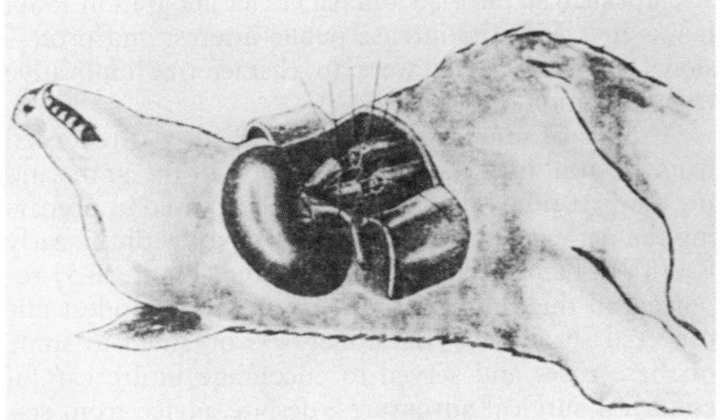

FIGURE 1-4 ■ Yu Yu Voronoy (1895–1961) had experience with dog allografts before carrying out the first human kidney allograft in 1933 at Kherson in the Ukraine. His experimental animal model is shown here.

had occurred in any. (For a biography of Voronoy, see Hamilton and Reid[23] and Matevossian and colleagues.[33])

POST WORLD WAR II

The sounder basis of transplantation immunology, which followed Medawar's pioneer studies during World War II, led to a new interest in human transplantation. In 1946, a human allograft kidney transplant to arm vessels under local anesthetic was attempted by Hufnagel, Hume, and Landsteiner at the Peter Bent Brigham Hospital in Boston. The brief period of function of the kidney may have helped the patient's recovery from acute renal failure; it marked the beginning of that hospital's major interest in transplantation and dialysis.[35]

In the early 1950s, interest in experimental and clinical kidney transplantation increased. With a growing certainty that immunological mechanisms were involved, the destruction of kidney allografts could be reinvestigated. Simonsen, then an intern in Ålborg in Denmark, persuaded his surgical seniors to teach him some vascular surgery; using dog kidney transplants, he reported on the mechanism of kidney rejection.[49] Dempster in London also re-examined this question.[16] Both workers found, like Küss in Paris, that the pelvic position of the kidney was preferable to a superficial site, and both concluded that an immunological mechanism was responsible for failure. Dempster found that radiation, but not cortisone, delayed rejection. Both workers considered that a humoral mechanism of rejection was likely.

In the early 1950s, two groups simultaneously started human kidney transplantation. In Paris, with encouragement from the nephrologist Jean Hamburger, the surgeons Küss (five cases),[32] Servelle (one case),[48] and Dubost (one case)[17] reported on kidney allografts without immunosuppression in human patients, placing the graft in the now-familiar pelvic position. The Paris series included a case reported by Hamburger of the first live-related kidney transplant, the donor being the mother of a boy whose solitary kidney had been damaged in a fall from a height. The kidney functioned immediately, but was rejected abruptly on the 22nd day.[34] In the United States, the Chicago surgeon Lawler had been the first to attempt such an intra-abdominal kidney allograft in 1950; it was met with the intense public interest and professional skepticism that were to characterize innovative transplantation thereafter.

A series of nine cases, closely studied, was recorded from Boston, using the thigh position of the graft, and for the first time hemodialysis had been used in preparing the patients, employing Merrill's skill with the early Kolff/Brigham machine. David Hume (Figure 1-5) reported on this Boston experience in 1953. Modest unexpected survival of the kidney was obtained in some of these cases and served to encourage future careful empirical surgical adventures, despite advice from scientists to wait for elegant immunological solutions. Although small doses of adrenocorticotropic hormone or cortisone were used, it was thought that the endogenous immunosuppression of uremia was responsible

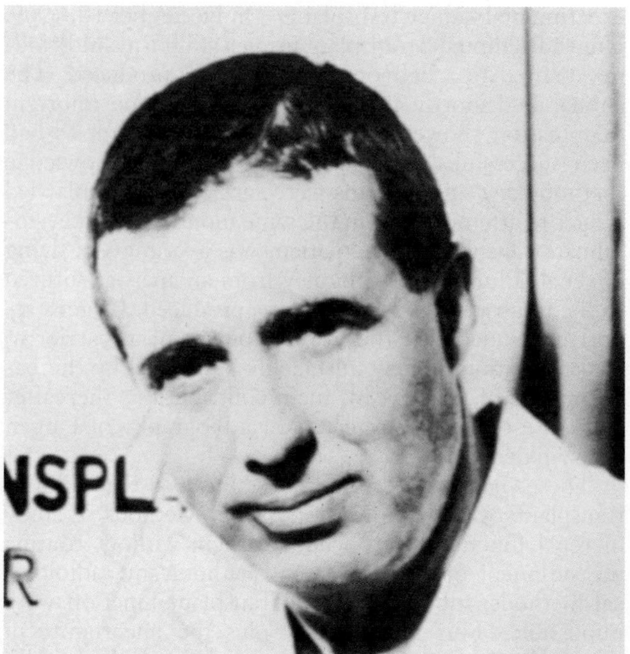

FIGURE 1-5 ■ David M. Hume (1917–1973) pioneered human kidney transplantation at the Peter Bent Brigham Hospital, Boston, and the Medical College of Virginia. He died in an air crash at the age of 55.

for these results, rather than the drug regimen. Many of Hume's tentative conclusions from this short series were confirmed later, notably that prior blood transfusion might be beneficial, that blood group matching of graft and donor might be necessary, and that host bilateral nephrectomy was necessary for control of post-transplant blood pressure.[27] The first observation of recurrent disease in a graft was made, and accelerated arteriosclerosis in the graft vessels was noted at postmortem. Other cases were reported from Chicago, Toronto, and Cleveland in the early 1950s, but because no sustained function was achieved, interest in clinical and experimental renal allograft transplantation waned, despite increasing knowledge of basic immunological mechanisms in the laboratory.

The technical lessons learned from the human allograft attempts of the early 1950s allowed confidence in the surgical methods, and in Boston, on December 23, 1954, the first transplant of a kidney from one twin to another with renal failure was performed. From then on, many such transplantations were performed successfully in Boston.[40] Although sometimes seen now merely as a technical triumph, valuable new findings emerged from this series. Some workers had predicted that, in the short term, the activity of the inactive bladder could not be restored, and that in the long term, human kidney grafts would decline in vitality as a result of denervation or ureteric reflux. Other workers were convinced that a single kidney graft could not restore biochemical normality to an adult, and that in any case the existing changes caused by chronic renal failure were irreversible. All of these gloomy predictions were neutralized by the success of the twin kidney transplants, and the greatest triumph came when one such recipient became pregnant and had a normal infant, delivered cautiously by cesarean section, with the anxious transplanters in attendance. Many of the twin recipients are still alive today, although the good results were tempered by failures caused by the prompt return of glomerulonephritis in some transplanted kidneys. This complication was later much reduced by immunosuppression. Other lessons learned were that the hazard of multiple donor renal arteries provided a need for pretransplant angiography of the kidneys in living donors, although it still was not thought necessary to perfuse or cool the donor organ. Lastly, there was the first airing of the legal aspects of organ donation, particularly the problem of consent in young, highly motivated related donors. (For an account of this period, see Murray and colleagues.[42])

IMMUNOSUPPRESSION AND THE MODERN ERA

In 1948, the first patients crippled with rheumatoid arthritis were given the Merck Company's Cortone (cortisone) at the Mayo Clinic, and intense worldwide interest in the pharmacological actions of adrenal cortical hormones followed. Careful studies by Medawar's group in the early 1950s suggested a modest immunosuppressive effect of cortisone, but when Medawar shortly afterward showed profound, specific, and long-lasting graft acceptance via the induction of tolerance, the weak steroid effect was understandably sidelined and thought to be of no clinical interest. Induction of tolerance in adult animals (rather than newborns) was accomplished by lethal irradiation and bone marrow infusion, and with this strong lead from the laboratory, it was natural that the first attempts at human immunosuppression for organ transplants were with preliminary total-body irradiation and allograft bone marrow rescue. These procedures were carried out in Paris, Boston, and elsewhere in the late 1950s.

This regimen was too difficult to control, and graft-versus-host disease was inevitable. It was found unexpectedly that sublethal irradiation alone in human patients was quite immunosuppressive, however, and this approach was used until 1962, the year of the first general availability of azathioprine (Imuran). In Boston, 12 patients were treated in this way, but with only one long-term survival in a man receiving his transplant from his non-identical twin.[39] In Paris, similar success was obtained with sibling grafts.[20,30] These isolated kidney survivals after a single dose of radiation gave further hope and showed again that the immunology of humans, dogs, and mice is different. These cases also showed that if a human organ could survive the initial crucial rejection period, it could be protected or adapted to the host in some way, possibly shielded by new endothelium, by enhancement, or, as suggested later, by microchimeric tolerance induced by mobile cells in the graft.

CHEMICAL IMMUNOSUPPRESSION

In 1958, at the New England Medical Center, attempts were made at human bone marrow transplantation for aplastic anemia and leukemia. To enable the marrow grafts to succeed, irradiation of the recipient was used. Results were poor, and mortality was high. Schwartz and Dameshek[47] looked for alternatives to irradiation and reasoned that an anticancer drug, such as 6-mercaptopurine (6-MP) or methotrexate, might be of use for immunosuppression in their patients. (For an account of this period, see Schwartz.[46]) Their important paper in 1959, showing a poor immune response to foreign protein in rabbits treated with 6-MP,[47] was noticed by Roy Calne, then a surgeon in training at the Royal Free Hospital, London, and David Hume, new Chairman of Surgery at the Medical College of Virginia. Calne had been disappointed at the failure of irradiation to prolong kidney allograft survival in dogs and, like others looking for an alternative, he found that 6-MP was successful.[5] Zukoski and colleagues[63] in Richmond found the same effect.

In 1960, Calne visited Boston for a period of research with Murray, and Hitchings and Elion of Burroughs Wellcome, then at Tuckahoe, provided him with new derivatives of 6-MP.[6] Of these, BW57-322 (later known as azathioprine (Imuran)) proved to be more successful in dog kidney transplants and less toxic than 6-MP.[7]

In 1960–1961, 6-MP was used in many human kidney transplants. In London at the Royal Free Hospital, three cases were managed in this way, but without success, although one patient receiving a live related transplant died of tuberculosis rather than rejection.[24] In Boston, no lasting human kidney function was obtained, but in Paris, Küss and associates[31] reported one prolonged survival of a kidney from a non-related donor when 6-MP was used with intermittent prednisone in a recipient who also had received irradiation as the main immunosuppressive agent (Figure 1-6). This case was the first success for chemical immunosuppression.

This change in approach, giving lifelong, risky medication with toxic drugs, although an obvious development in retrospect, was accepted with reluctance because it meant leaving aside, at least in the short term, the hopes from the work of the transplantation immunologists for the elegant, specific, one-shot, non-toxic tolerance regimen. Many workers thought that entry into this new paradigm was only a temporary diversion.

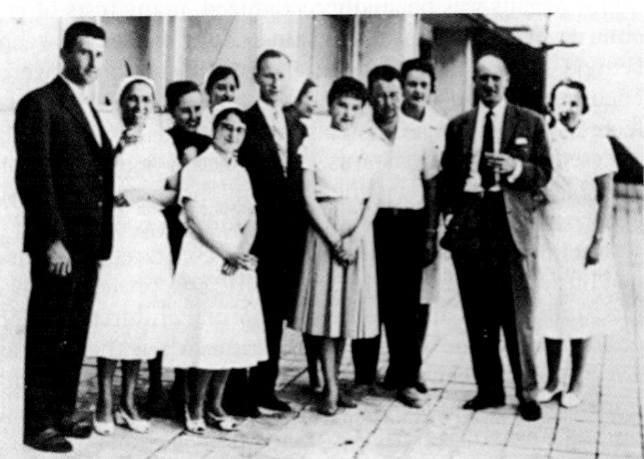

FIGURE 1-6 ■ R. Küss (right) and M. Legrain (center) in 1960 with their first long-term kidney transplant survivor. The patient and her brother-in-law donor (center right) are shown with the staff of the unit at the Hôpital Foch. Immunosuppression with irradiation and mercaptopurine was used. (Courtesy of Prof. M. Legrain.)

In 1961, azathioprine became available for human use; the dosage was difficult to judge at first. The first two Boston cases using the drug did not show prolonged survival of the grafts, but in April 1962 the first extended successes with human kidney allografts were obtained.[41] Shortly afterward, at the bedside rather than in the laboratory, it was discovered that steroids, notably prednisolone, when given with azathioprine had a powerful synergistic effect. The regular use of both together became a standard regimen after reports by Starzl and colleagues[51] and Goodwin and coworkers,[19] and this combined therapy continued to be the routine immunosuppressive method despite many other suggested alternatives, until azathioprine was displaced by cyclosporine much later. Use of the combined immunosuppression and the increasing use of live related donors (rather than occasional twin or free or cadaver kidneys), along with the remarkably good results reported in 1963 from Denver[51] and Richmond,[26] greatly encouraged the practice of transplantation. (For an account of this period, see Starzl.[50])

A TIME OF OPTIMISM

The mid-1960s was a period of great optimism. The rapid improvement in results seemed to indicate that routine success was at hand. Looking to the future, calculations were made that suggested that enough donor organs would be available in the future if all large hospitals cooperated, and such donations did start to come from outside the transplantation pioneer hospitals. Transplantation societies were set up, and specialist journals were started. The improvements in regular dialysis treatment meant an increasing pool of patients in good health suitable for transplantation, and this allowed for better and planned preparation for transplantation. With a return to dialysis being possible, heroic efforts to save a rejected kidney were no longer necessary. Management of patients improved in many aspects, and the expected steroid long-term effects were met and managed (primarily by the demonstration that low-dose steroids were as effective as high-dose steroids). The need for cooling of donor organs was belatedly recognized, many tests of viability were announced, and transport of organs between centers began. Bone disease and exotic infections were encountered and treated, but the kidney units were affected by a hepatitis B epidemic in the mid-1960s, which affected morale and status. The narrow age limit for transplantation was widened, and in Richmond the first experience with kidney grafts in children was obtained.

Recipients of kidney transplants re-entered the normal business of life and became politicians, professors, pilots, and fathers and mothers of normal children. Other good news in the United States came when the federal government accepted the costs of regular dialysis and transplantation in 1968. There were always unexpected findings, usually reported from the pioneer units with the longest survivors. Cautiously, second kidney transplants were performed at Richmond when a first had failed; these did well, and the matter became routine. Chronic rejection and malignancy first were reported in kidney transplant recipients from Denver. As a result of the optimism, experimental heart transplantation started, the first human livers were grafted, and there was a revival of interest in xenotransplantation. Although the attempts of Reemtsma and coworkers,[44] Hume,[25] and Starzl[50] at transplantation with chimpanzee or baboon kidneys ultimately failed, rejection did not occur immediately, and the cases were studied closely and described.

In the search for better immunosuppression, there was great excitement when laboratory studies by Woodruff and Medawar produced a powerful immunosuppressive antilymphocyte serum, and production of versions suitable for human use started.[62] Initial results were favorable, but the whole antilymphocyte serum had an unspectacular role thereafter, added to from 1975 onward by the use of monoclonal antibody versions. Hopes for another biological solution to transplantation were raised in 1969 when French and Batchelor[18] found an enhancing serum effect in the new experimental model of rat kidney transplantation made possible by the development of microsurgical methods, but it proved impossible to mimic the effect in humans.

TISSUE TYPING

The greatest hopes resided in the evolution of tissue-typing methods, which entered routine use in 1962 (Figure 1-7).[14,21] The increasing identification of the antigens of the HLA system seemed to promise excellent clinical results in the future from close matching made possible when choosing from a large pool of patients. Sharing of kidneys in Europe started in 1967 at van Rood's suggestion,[45] and in North America, Amos and Terasaki set up similar sharing schemes on both coasts of the United States. Others followed throughout the world, and these organizations not only improved the service but also soon gathered excellent data on kidney transplant survival. The need to transport kidneys within these schemes encouraged construction of perfusion pumps designed to increase the survival of organs and the distance they could be transported.[1] Much work on perfusion fluids was done until the intracellular type of fluid devised by Collins et al. in 1969 allowed a simple flush

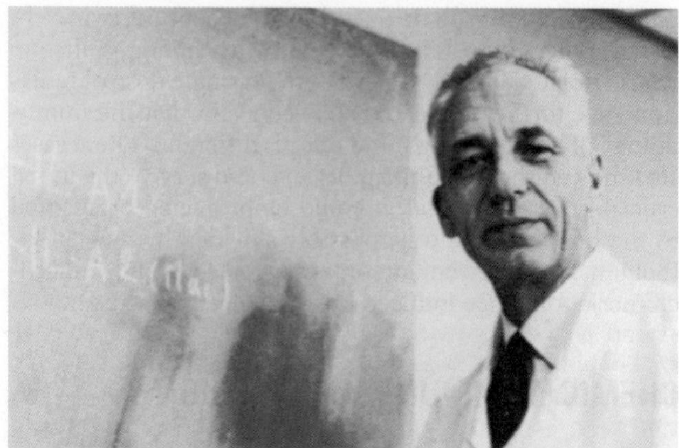

FIGURE 1-7 ■ Jean Dausset first described an antigen MAC, later known as HLA-2, defined by numerous antisera from multi-transfused patients, and which later was shown to be part of the major histocompatibility complex in humans (HLA).

and chill to suffice for prolonged storage.[11] Although the hopes for typing were not fully realized, such schemes had other benefits in obtaining kidneys when urgently required for patients with rarer blood groups, for children, or for highly sensitized patients. Such patients had been recognized by the new lymphocytotoxicity testing using a crossmatch between donor cells and recipient serum. First noted by Terasaki and associates[53] and described in more detail by Kissmeyer-Nielsen and colleagues[29] in 1966 and Williams and colleagues,[60] such pretransplant testing explained cases of sudden failure and led to a marked diminution in hyperacute rejection.

THE 1970s PLATEAU

The 1970s was a period of consolidation, of improvements in data collection such as the valuable European Dialysis and Transplant Association surveys, and increased sophistication in HLA typing methods and organ-sharing schemes. Cadaver organ procurement generally increased as a result of wider involvement of the public and medical profession, although the number of patients waiting for transplantation persistently exceeded the organs available, and donation declined transiently during times of public concern over transplantation issues. Governments took initiatives to increase donations; in the United Kingdom, the Kidney Donor Card was introduced in 1971, becoming a multidonor card 10 years later. In hospital practice, methods of resuscitation and intensive care improved, and the concept of brain death was established to prevent prolonged, pointless ventilation, although its immediate application to transplantation provoked controversy. Despite many new claims for successful methods of immunosuppression, such as trials of splenectomy, thymectomy, and thoracic duct drainage, as well as a new look at cyclophosphamide, no agent except antithymocyte globulin became established in routine use.

Although patient survival after kidney transplantation continued to increase, the 1970s did not show the expected increase in cadaver graft survival. Some groups reported decreased survival figures; this paradox was solved partly by the demonstration that blood transfusion during regular dialysis, which had been discouraged because of the risk of sensitization, was beneficial to the outcome of kidney transplantation,[43] an observation made some years earlier by Morris and coworkers.[37]

The 1970s ended with two innovations that revived hopes of reaching the goal of routine, safe, and successful kidney transplantation. Ting and Morris[54] reported the successful clinical application of HLA-DR matching, and Calne and associates[8] revived memories of the excitement of the early days of the use of azathioprine by introducing into clinical practice the first serious rival to it in 20 years, cyclosporine, which had been discovered to be a powerful immunosuppressive agent by Borel.[3] Cyclosporine replaced the earlier drug regimens and was the dominant agent in use until the 1990s. Transplantation had grown to a sufficiently large clinical service that it was worth the attention of the pharmaceutical companies, and in the 1990s steady production of new agents occurred – tacrolimus, mycophenolate mofetil, rapamycin, FTY720, brequinar, and others. Any drug with promise was marketed aggressively, and sponsored trials became a routine part of clinical life.

The improved results of transplantation meant that the procurement of organs became a more dominant issue. Comparisons of transplantation practice throughout the world showed remarkable differences in attitudes to use of live related donors and cadaver organs, depending on religion and cultural traditions. Kidney transplantation had started as a difficult surgical and scientific challenge confined to a few academic centers in the developed world, but its success had led to the technique becoming a routine service in all parts of the world.[4] In some nations not sharing western attitudes, the donor shortage meant the appearance of undesirable commercial developments in renal transplantation, such as the purchase of kidneys from living unrelated donors (discussed in more detail in Chapter 38).[36]

WAITING FOR XENOGRAFTS

As the demand for kidney transplants continued to exceed supply, other initiatives appeared and included study of nations and areas with high donation rates (e.g., Spain), the regulated use of properly motivated unrelated individuals, and a return to the use of marginal cadaver kidneys, notably from non-heart-beating donors. As all attempts to increase donor supply fell short of the ever-rising target, the radical alternative of the use of animal organs was examined afresh. Profound immunosuppression alone was ineffective and, at first, methods of removing natural antibody from recipient plasma were tried to deal with the hyperacute phase of xenograft organ rejection. Although the traditional hopes for xenografting of human patients had assumed that "concordant" species such as the monkey would be used, a new strategy using genetic engineering methods first used a line of transgenic pigs, a distant species discordant with humans, with a modified endothelium that reduced the complement-mediated immediate reaction.[2] Hopes continue that these early developments will evolve into a sophisticated successful routine.[12] Meanwhile, the kidney transplanters can only watch, with detached interest, the emergence of stem cell use in cellular transplantation.

These new hopes for xenografts raised old fears among the public and legislators, notably regarding disease transmission. Although this had been a familiar problem in human-to-human transplantation and had been met regularly and dealt with, governments required reassurances about xenotransplantation with the added threat of retrovirus transmission.

CONCLUSION

Kidney transplantation was the first of the organ transplant procedures to develop because of availability of live donors and the crucial backup of dialysis. When radical new ideas are to be tested, pioneers still turn to kidney transplantation. Kidney transplantation is where it all started, with good reason, and it will always be a test bed for major innovation.

In the early 1990s, Murray[38] was awarded the Nobel Prize in Medicine for his pioneer work in renal transplantation and in the development of many new immunosuppressive agents, including drugs and monoclonal antibodies. The future promises to be exciting. Nowhere is the excitement of the past reflected better than in the recollections of 35 of the pioneers of transplantation gathered together by Terasaki.[52]

REFERENCES

1. Belzer FO, Ashby BS, Dunphy JS. 24-Hour and 72-hour preservation of canine kidneys. Lancet 1967;2:536.
2. van den Bogaerde J, White DJG. Xenogeneic transplantation. Br Med Bull 1997;53:904.
3. Borel JF. Comparative study of in vitro and in vivo drug effects on cell mediated cytotoxicity. Immunology 1976;31:631.
4. Burdick JF, DeMeester J, Koyama I. Understanding organ procurement and the transplant bureaucracy. In: Ginns LC, Cosimi AB, Morris PJ, editors. Transplantation. Boston: Blackwell; 1999. p. 875–94.
5. Calne RY. The rejection of renal homografts: inhibition in dogs by 6-mercaptopurine. Lancet 1960;1:417.
6. Calne RY. The development of immunosuppressive therapy. Transplant Proc 1981;13:44.
7. Calne RY, Alexandre GPJ, Murray JE. The development of immunosuppressive therapy. Ann N Y Acad Sci 1962;99:743.
8. Calne RY, White DJG, Thiru S, et al. Cyclosporin A in patients receiving renal allografts from cadaver donors. Lancet 1978;2:1323.
9. Carrel A. La technique operatoire des anastomoses vasculaires et la transplantation des viscères. Lyon Med 1902;98:859.
10. Carrel A. The transplantation of organs. New York Times April 14, 1914.
11. Collins GM, Bravo-Shugarman M, Terasaki PI. Kidney preservation for transportation: initial perfusion and 30 hours' ice storage. Lancet 1969;2:1219.
12. D'Apice A, Cowan PJ. Gene-modified pigs. Xenotransplantation 2008;15:87.
13. Dausset J. Iso-leuco-anticorps. Acta Haematol (Basel) 1958;20:156.
14. Dausset J. The challenge of the early days of human histocompatibility. Immunogenetics 1980;10:1.
15. von Decastello A. Experimentelle nierentransplantation. Wien Klin Wochenschr 1902;15:317.
16. Dempster WJ. The homotransplantation of kidneys in dogs. Br J Surg 1953;40:447.
17. Dubost C, Oeconomos N, Vaysse J, et al. Resultats d'une tentative de greffe rénale. Bull Soc Med Hop Paris 1951;67:1372.
18. French ME, Batchelor JR. Immunological enhancement of rat kidney grafts. Lancet 1969;2:1103.
19. Goodwin WE, Mims MM, Kaufman JJ. Human renal transplant, III: technical problems encountered in six cases of kidney homotransplantation. Trans Am Assoc Genitourin Surg 1962;54:116.
20. Hamburger J, Vaysse J, Crosnier J, et al. Transplantation of a kidney between non-monozygotic twins after irradiation of the receiver: good function at the fourth month. Presse Med 1959;67:1771.
21. Hamburger J, Vaysse J, Crosnier J, et al. Renal homotransplantation in man after radiation of the recipient. Am J Med 1962;32:854.
22. Hamilton D. Organ transplantation: a history. Pittsburgh: Pittsburgh University Press; 2012.
23. Hamilton D, Reid WA. Yu Yu Voronoy and the first human kidney allograft. Surg Gynecol Obstet 1984;159:289.
24. Hopewell J, Calne RY, Beswick I. Three clinical cases of renal transplantation. BMJ 1964;1:411.
25. Hume DM. Discussion. Ann Surg 1964;160:409.
26. Hume DM, Magee JH, Kauffman HM, et al. Renal homotransplantation in man in modified recipients. Ann Surg 1963;158:608.
27. Hume DM, Merrill JP, Miller BF, et al. Experiences with renal homotransplantation in the human: report of nine cases. J Clin Invest 1955;34:327.
28. Jaboulay M. Greffe de reins au pli du coude par soudure arte. Bull Lyon Med 1906;107:575 [For a biography of Jaboulay, see Biogr Med Paris 10:257, 1936.].
29. Kissmeyer-Nielsen F, Olsen S, Peterson VP, et al. Hyperacute rejection of kidney allografts. Lancet 1966;2:662.
30. Küss R, Legraine M, Mathe G, et al. Prémices d'une homotransplantation rénale de soeur à frère non jumeaux. Presse Med 1960;68:755.
31. Küss R, Legraine M, Mathe G, et al. Homologous human kidney transplantation. Postgrad Med J 1962;38:528.
32. Küss R, Teinturier J, Milliez P. Quelques essais de greffe du rein chez l'homme. Mem Acad Chir 1951;77:755.
33. Matevossian E, Kern H, Hüser N, et al. Surgeon Yurii Voronoy (1895–1961) – a pioneer in the history of clinical transplantation. Transpl Int 2009;22:1132.
34. Michon L, Hamburger J, Oeconomos N, et al. Une tentative de transplantation rénale chez l'homme. Presse Med 1953;61:1419.
35. Moore FD. Give and take: the development of tissue transplantation. Philadelphia: WB Saunders; 1964.
36. Morris PJ. Problems facing the society today. Transplant Proc 1987;19:16.
37. Morris PJ, Ting A, Stocker J. Leucocyte antigens in renal transplantation, I: the paradox of blood transfusions in renal transplantation. Med J Aust 1968;2:1088.
38. Murray JE. Human organ transplantation: background and consequences. Science 1992;256:1411.
39. Murray JE, Merrill JP, Dammin GJ, et al. Study of transplantation immunity after total body irradiation: clinical and experimental investigation. Surgery 1960;48:272.
40. Murray JE, Merrill JP, Harrison JH. Kidney transplantation between seven pairs of identical twins. Ann Surg 1958;148:343.
41. Murray JE, Merrill JP, Harrison JH, et al. Prolonged survival of human kidney homografts by immunosuppressive drug therapy. N Engl J Med 1963;268:1315.
42. Murray JE, Tilney NL, Wilson RE. Renal transplantation: a twenty-five year experience. Ann Surg 1976;184:565.
43. Opelz G, Sengar DPS, Mickey MR, et al. Effect of blood transfusions on subsequent kidney transplants. Transplant Proc 1973;5:253.
44. Reemtsma K, McCracken BH, Schlegel JU, et al. Renal heterotransplantation in man. Ann Surg 1964;160:384.
45. van Rood JJ. Histocompatibility testing. Copenhagen: Munkgaard; 1967.
46. Schwartz RS. Perspectives on immunosuppression. In: Hitchings GH, editor. Design and achievements in chemotherapy. Research Triangle Park, Durham, NC: Burroughs Wellcome; 1976. p. 39–41.
47. Schwartz R, Dameshek W. Drug-induced immunological tolerance. Nature 1959;183:1682.
48. Servelle M, Soulié P, Rougeulle J, et al. Greffe d'une reine de supplicie à une malade avec rein unique congénital, atteinte de nephrite chronique hypertensive azotémique. Bull Soc Med Hop Paris 1951;67:99.
49. Simonsen M. Biological incompatibility in kidney transplantation in dogs: serological investigations. Acta Pathol Microbiol Scand 1953;32:1.
50. Starzl TE. Personal reflections in transplantation. Surg Clin North Am 1978;58:879.
51. Starzl TE, Marchioro TL, Waddell WR. The reversal of rejection in human renal homografts with subsequent development of homograft tolerance. Surg Gynecol Obstet 1963;117:385.
52. Terasaki PI. History of transplantation: thirty-five recollections. Los Angeles: UCLA Tissue Typing Laboratory; 1991.
53. Terasaki PI, Marchioro TL, Starzl TE. In: Amos DB, van Rood JJ, editors. Histocompatibility testing. Washington, DC: National Academy of Sciences; 1965. p. 83.
54. Ting A, Morris PJ. Matching for B-cell antigens of the HLA-DR (D-related) series in cadaver renal transplantation. Lancet 1978;1:575.
55. Ullmann E. Experimentelle nierentransplantation. Wien Klin Wochenschr 1902;15:281 [For a biography of Ullmann, see Lesky E. Die erste Nierentransplantation: Emerich Ullmann (1861-1937). Munch Med Wochenschr 116:1081, 1974.].
56. Ullmann E. Tissue and organ transplantation. Ann Surg 1914;60:195.
57. Unger E. Nierentransplantation. Berl Klin Wochenschr 1909;1:1057.

58. Voronoy Yu Yu. Sobre el bloqueo del aparato reticulo-endothelial. Siglo Med 1936;97:296.
59. White OJG, Langford A, Cozzi EE, et al. Production of pigs transgenic for human DAF. Xenotransplantation 1995;2:213.
60. Williams GM, Hume DM, Hudson RP, et al. Hyperacute renal-homograft rejection in man. N Engl J Med 1968;279:611.
61. Winkler FA. Ernst Unger: a pioneer in modern surgery. J Hist Med Allied Sci 1982;37:269.
62. Wolstenholme GEW, O'Connor M, editors. Antilymphocytic serum. London: J&A Churchill; 1967.
63. Zukoski CF, Lee HM, Hume DM. The effect of 6-mercaptopurine on renal homograft survival in the dog. Surg Forum 1960;11:47.

CHAPTER 2

IMMUNOLOGY OF GRAFT REJECTION

Simon Ball • Margaret J. Dallman

CHAPTER OUTLINE

Transplantation is the optimal treatment for many people with advanced kidney failure. In most instances this involves a donor who is genetically and therefore antigenically distinct from the recipient, the consequence of which is an immune response termed rejection. An inflammatory response is initiated by physiological stress in the donor, organ harvesting, storage, implantation, and reperfusion. This non-specific response provides the context from which emerges specific immune recognition of antigenic differences between the donor and recipient. The cumulative effect of these events causes destruction of the transplant, as originally described by Little and Tyzer in animal models of susceptibility to tumors.[210] The immunological basis of transplant rejection was then proposed by Gorer[104] and defined by Medawar using evidence that rejection displays specificity and memory for donor tissue and is consequent upon infiltration by leukocytes.[97,244–246] Our understanding of the immune system has evolved considerably, and we are able to describe in detail many of the molecular and cellular events that contribute to rejection. This has contributed to the development of a range of biological agents that target specific aspects of the immune response, with a view to optimizing the risk–benefit ratio of immunosuppression. This might be further developed by cell-based therapies now being explored, which aim to actively regulate alloantigen-specific responses.

Those therapeutic agents currently used in clinical practice have resulted in an impressively low incidence of acute rejection, particularly if the recipient is unsensitized. A description of the immunology of graft rejection relevant to current clinical practice must therefore inform an understanding of the immune contribution to chronic allograft injury, barriers to transplantation in those with donor-specific humoral immunity, and the penalties associated with intensified non-specific immunosuppression. In this context sits a need for biomarkers that offer not only prognostic information prior to graft injury but also diagnostic information prior to immutable programming of injurious alloimmune memory. Indeed, targeting

TABLE 2-1 **Transplant Terminology**

Autograft (autologous transplant)	Transplantation of an individual's own tissue to another site (e.g., the use of a patient's own skin to cover third-degree burns or a saphenous vein femoropopliteal graft)
Isograft (syngeneic or isogeneic transplant)	Transplantation of tissue between genetically identical members of the same species (e.g., kidney transplant between identical twins or grafts between mice of the same inbred strain)
Allograft (allogeneic transplant)	Transplantation of tissue between genetically non-identical members of the same species (e.g., cadaver renal transplant or graft between mice of different inbred strains)
Xenograft (xenogeneic transplant)	Transplantation of tissue between members of different species (e.g., baboon kidney into a human)

immunosuppressive agents to those patients most likely to benefit and away from those most likely to be harmed could have more beneficial potential than developing any single novel therapy. Although this goal, a form of personalized medicine, remains elusive, it is perhaps most immediately susceptible to incremental developments in our understanding of the immune system and to sophisticated analyses of large datasets.

This chapter describes the molecular and cellular events of the immune response, as currently understood. It assumes a basic level of knowledge of the immune system. The reader is referred to other books for general descriptions of the immune system.[268,294] See Table 2-1 for terminology.

INITIATION OF ALLOIMMUNITY BY THE INNATE IMMUNE SYSTEM

The Trauma of Transplantation

The immune response to a solid-organ transplant can be understood in a series of relatively well-defined stages (Figure 2-1), the first being the trauma to which a graft is subjected during harvesting and implantation. In the case of deceased donors this is preceded by hemodynamic and neuroendocrine responses to brainstem death, which alone may result in activation of the innate immune system. Harvesting and subsequent storage involve cooling the kidney, perfusion with preservation solution, and storage for potentially long periods before transplantation. These events sensitize the organ to reperfusion injury on revascularization. The constituents of preservation solutions and various experimental approaches, including normothermic preperfusion,[140] remote ischemic preconditioning and pharmacological interventions, aim to reduce these effects on the kidney (see Chapter 9). There remain, however, inevitable changes to cell membranes and the concentrations of intracellular ions, adenosine nucleotides, uric acid, and reactive oxygen species. These are in varying degrees cytopathic and activate inflammasomes (see below), resulting in cytokine generation.[340] Cell membrane injury and other stress responses result in activation of complement and coagulation cascades and generation of mediators such as heat shock proteins (HSPs) and high-mobility group B-1 (HMGB-1) that engages Toll-like receptors (TLRs). There is upregulation of cell surface molecules such as P-selectin and integrins and further amplification and diversification of chemokine and cytokine cascades. All these changes promote dendritic cell (DC), monocyte, and lymphocyte migration in and out of the graft, with inevitable consequences for adaptive immunity. The importance of these various influences on the immune response is suggested by the superior outcome of live donor transplants even in the face of significant major histocompatibility complex (MHC) mismatch,[226] the importance of cold ischemia time in graft outcome,[260,306] and reportedly higher rates of rejection observed in individuals with delayed graft function.[306,307]

Indeed, in experimental models of ischemia-reperfusion injury (IRI), there is evidence of T-lymphocyte infiltration[7] and subsequent histology reminiscent of chronic allograft injury.[388] It may be that such responses account for the observation that in the untransplanted population chronic kidney disease may arise following acute kidney injury that initially recovers.[212]

Innate Immunity

The cells and mediators involved in early non-antigen-specific responses are derived from the innate immune system, which provides a first-line defense against tissue damage and invading pathogens. Activation of vascular endothelium and the induction of various proinflammatory cytokines such as interleukin (IL)-1, IL-6, and tumor necrosis factor (TNF-α) can be demonstrated early posttransplantation. The upregulation of proinflammatory cytokines combined with increased expression of adhesion molecules[177] results in an early infiltrate of inflammatory cells, including macrophages.[243] This early inflammatory response also triggers the egress of graft tissue-resident, bone marrow-derived DCs.[192,193] These early events in themselves do not constitute graft rejection being observed in syngeneic grafts.[58] The severity of the initial injury and the nature of the subsequent inflammatory infiltrate are however central to the generation of alloantigen-specific immunity: a maximally damaged organ generates a maximal "danger signal,"[238] which promotes adaptive immunity, manifest as rejection when donor and recipient are antigenically distinct.

Receptors of the Innate Immune System

The innate immune system recognizes and responds to molecules expressed by pathogens (pathogen-associated molecular patterns (PAMP)), for example, specific carbohydrates, lipopolysaccharide, flagellin, lipoteichoic acid, and double-stranded RNA; or molecules generated by damaged tissue (damage-associated molecular patterns (DAMP)), for example, extracellular adenosine triphosphate (ATP),[235] hyaluronan,[416] falling intracellular potassium,[157] oxidative stress,[425] and the release of HSPs and HMGB-1.[267] These pattern recognition receptors

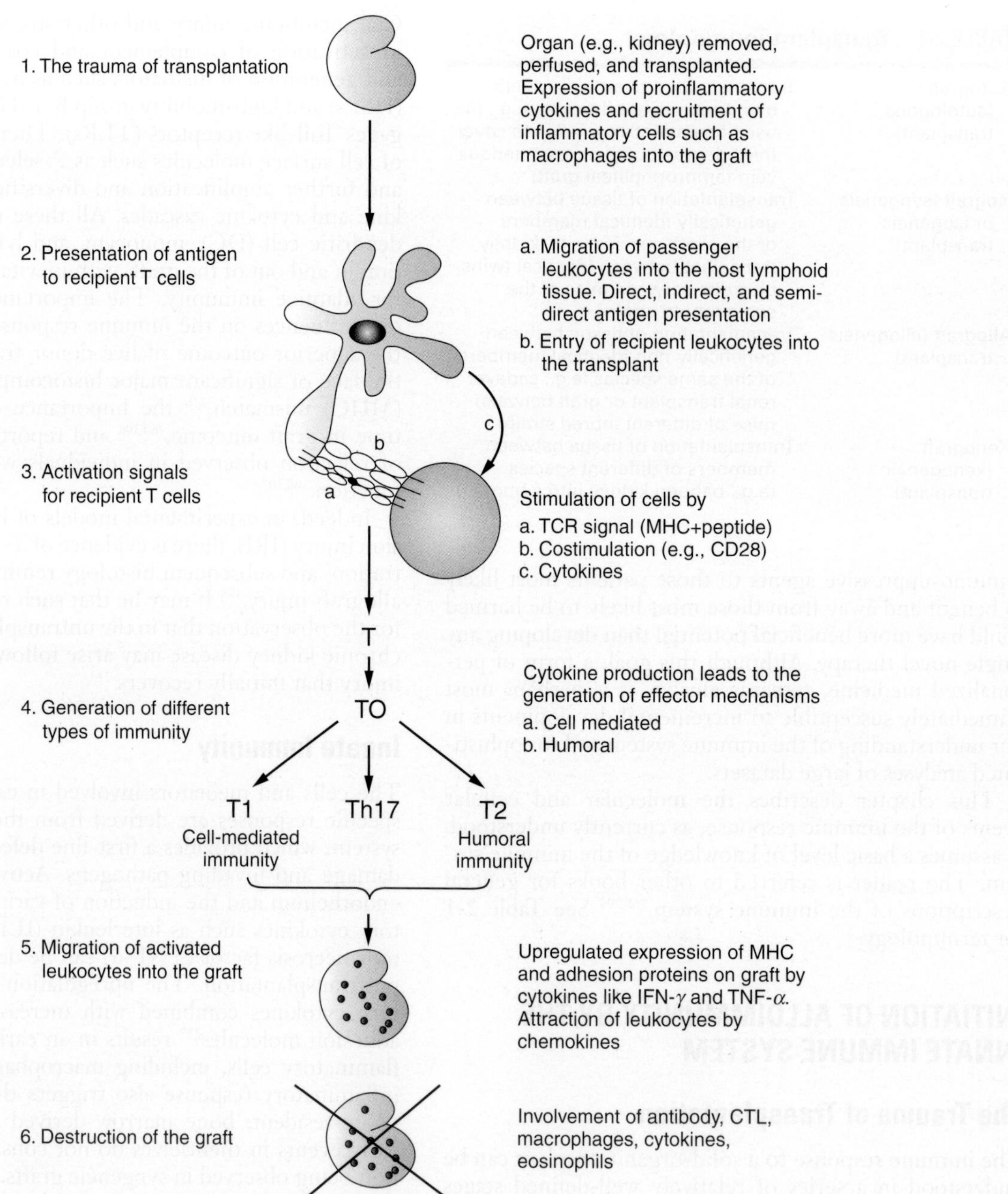

FIGURE 2-1 ■ The evolution of the immune response after kidney transplantation. CTL, cytotoxic T cell; IFN, interferon; MHC, major histocompatibility complex; TCR, T-cell receptor; TNF, tumor necrosis factor.

include soluble molecules such as C-reactive protein, ficolins, and mannan-binding lectin [312] and cell-associated molecules such as TLRs,[282] retinoic acid inducible gene-1 like receptors,[272] and Nod-like receptors.[298]

Cells of the innate immune system, such as macrophages and DCs, are activated by these ligands directly through cell surface receptors or indirectly via products such as soluble complement components (Figure 2-2).[312] There is resulting enhanced cytocidal and antigen-presenting capacity together with phenotypic changes (such as cytokine production) that subsequently influence polarization of adaptive immunity.[328] The role of these elements in the initiation of adaptive immune responses in the context of transplantation remains to be fully described; nevertheless it is apparent that endogenous ligands released after tissue damage are generated in the context of transplantation. These are particularly associated with donor brain death, exemplified by recent studies of HMGB-1 expression and its binding to TLR-4.[181] It may also be that brain death is associated with intestinal bacterial translocation and therefore activation of PAMPs as well as DAMPs.[179] Experimentally, manipulation of the adaptor molecules associated with PAMPs and DAMPs, such as MyD88 and TRIF, results in less effective immunity to transplantation antigens and this in turn can result in indefinite allograft survival.[101] However, this finding depends on the absence of the adaptor protein from both donor and recipient and is greatly diminished in donor–recipient pairs that are mismatched beyond a single minor antigen.[242,380]

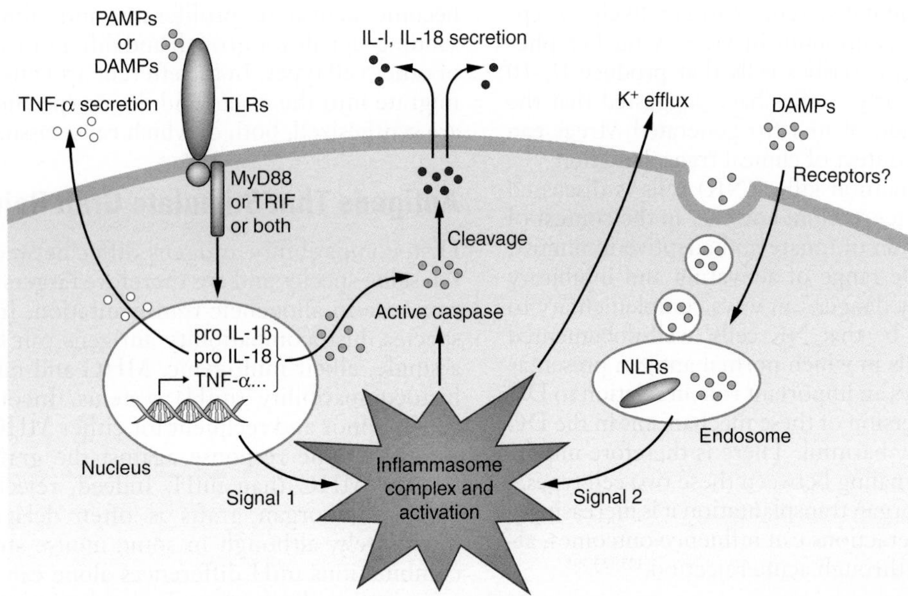

FIGURE 2-2 ■ Activation of the inflammasome. Following infection the innate immune system becomes rapidly activated. Over the past decade or so, we have begun to define the germline-encoded receptor systems (pattern recognition receptors) which, through their recognition of pathogen-associated molecular patterns (PAMPs), are involved in this process. Such receptors may be found at the cell surface of innate immune cells (e.g., Toll-like receptors, TLRs; C-type lectin receptors) or in the cytoplasm (e.g., Nod-like receptors, NLRs; Rig-I-like receptors). These receptors are coupled to signaling pathways which result in transcriptional activation and expression of proinflammatory cytokines. More recently, it has become clear that some of these receptors are also activated by endogenous and/or non-pathogen-associated compounds, the danger-associated molecular patterns (DAMPs, e.g., nucleic acids, adenosine triphosphate (ATP) and uric acid crystals), and it is likely that such molecules play a role in the activation of the innate immune system following transplantation. The combination of signaling through TLRs (signal 1) and other receptors (signal 2) can lead to inflammasome activation. The inflammasome is a large, multiprotein complex which is critical in the production of active interleukin (IL)-1β and IL-18, two proinflammatory cytokines known to be produced following transplantation and often found in transplants with chronic graft dysfunction. Both cytokines are produced in a precursor form (pro IL-1β and pro IL-18), which requires cleavage by caspase-1. It is the inflammasome complex which activates caspase-1 from its own precursor, pro-caspase-1. The inflammasome complex is becoming increasingly well characterized and indeed is an attractive target for intervention in a variety of inflammatory diseases. TNF, tumor necrosis factor.

Cells at the Intersection of Innate and Adaptive Immunity

The innate immune system involves a range of protective mechanisms, which were built on by adaptive immunity in jawed vertebrates. The innate immune system also plays a crucial role in shaping adaptive immune responses according to the context in which antigen is encountered. This detection and communication of context plays a role in self-tolerance and in the polarization of immune responses reflected in patterns of cytokine production and associated cellular and effector mechanisms. These have evolved to ensure optimal targeting of different effector mechanisms against viruses, bacteria of various sorts, fungi, protozoa, and multicellular parasites.[332]

The antigen specificity of this interaction between innate and adaptive immunity relies on the fact that innate immune cells of the monocyte lineage present antigen to T cells. This involves cell contact, thereby conferring specificity on a range of costimulatory and paracrine interactions. Indeed, the DC is specialized to such an extent that its primary role is to integrate these various danger signals and instruct antigen-specific naive lymphocytes. This role is bidirectional: antigen-specific T cells may themselves influence the DC phenotype, thereby polarizing the DC response in the presence of antigen not only on the basis of the current environment in which the antigen is delivered but also the previous context, information held in the phenotype of T memory cells. Indeed, these interactions play an important role not only in productive immunity but also in immune tolerance. DCs play an important role in mediating the effects of T-regulatory cells (Tregs), as discussed in a later section.

A similar set of considerations can be applied to monocytes and tissue-resident macrophages, which play roles as effector cells augmented by stimuli from both the innate and adaptive immune systems. They can also play a role in antigen presentation and in association with this receive and transmit information that confers particular patterns of polarization. Thus monocyte phenotype can be polarized, similarly to T cells, into M1 and M2 by various treatments, including interferon-γ (IFN-γ) and IL-4 or IL-10 respectively. The M1 phenotype produces high levels of reactive oxygen species with other cytotoxic intermediates and proinflammatory cytokines, such as IL-1β and TNF-α, whereas M2 monocytes express IL-10 and IL-1 receptor antagonist, high levels of scavenger receptors, and are involved in tissue remodeling. This apparent polarization described in experimental systems is in fact likely to represent a phenotypic continuum in vivo. A further phenotype, called Mreg, describes cells that produce IL-10 but not IL-12, and early studies have suggested that the therapeutic application of in vitro-generated Mregs can be beneficial in the context of clinical transplantation.[143]

The function of natural killer (NK) cells is discussed in more detail in a later section; however in the context of cells at the intersection of innate and adaptive immunity, they integrate a wide range of activating and inhibitory signals that "quantify danger," in ways complementary to DCs.[119] It may also be that NK cells' well-documented role in surveying cells in which normal antigen presentation is subverted plays an important role in relation to DC function, since subversion of these mechanisms in the DC would be particularly harmful. There is therefore important bidirectional signaling between these two cell types.

In the context of organ transplantation it is increasingly evident that NK interactions can influence outcomes, although perhaps not through acute rejection.[123,124,392]

Complement

The complement system is a well-defined series of soluble proteins, enzymes, and receptors that act as a cascade to mediate a wide range of effector functions. Although normally activated by infection, complement can also be activated by a variety of endogenous signals, including hypoxia and tissue injury.[398,399] The significance of proximal complement components in mediating many aspects of the response to transplanted organs is now well recognized, above and beyond simple generation of the final membrane attack complex: C5–9.

As mentioned above, activation of complement contributes to IRI. Evidence for this includes experiments involving mice in which genes for complement components are silenced. Importantly, these experiments identify local complement production by the donor organ rather than serum complement as being of most importance to IRI and subsequent rejection.[303,424] Inhibiting the action of soluble mediators arising from complement activation, for example C5a, has been shown to antagonize early posttransplantation events such as monocyte influx, through mechanisms acting directly on infiltrating cells but also acting on renal endothelium and epithelium.[8,205]

In addition to this role in mediating innate responses to tissue damage, there is increasing evidence that soluble products of complement components influence adaptive immune responses, both acting directly and via altered antigen-presenting cell (APC) function. T-lymphocyte effector function, differentiation, and indeed expansion and contraction are influenced, particularly by local production of complement. Nevertheless it is possible that in the early posttransplantation highly dysregulated environment, remote complement activation plays a role.

STIMULATION OF ADAPTIVE ALLOIMMUNITY

The antigen-specific or adaptive immune response to a graft occurs in two main stages. In the afferent arm, donor antigens stimulate recipient lymphocytes, which become activated, proliferate, and differentiate while sending signals for growth and differentiation to a variety of other cell types. In the efferent arm effector leukocytes migrate into the organ and donor-specific alloantibodies are synthesized, both of which cause tissue damage.

Antigens That Stimulate Graft Rejection

Histocompatibility antigens differ between members of the same species and are therefore targets of the immune response in allogeneic transplantation. In all vertebrate species, histocompatibility antigens can be divided into a single, albeit multigenic, MHC and numerous minor histocompatibility (miH) systems. Incompatibility between donor and recipient for either MHC or miH leads to an immune response against the graft, more vigorous for MHC than miH. Indeed, rejection of MHC-compatible organ grafts is often delayed, sometimes indefinitely, although in some mouse strain and organ combinations miH differences alone can result in acute rejection similar to that observed across full MHC mismatch.[297] On the other hand the outcomes of allogeneic stem cell transplantation between human leukocyte antigen (HLA)-identical siblings can be very significantly affected by miH mismatches, causing graft-versus-host disease.[90]

Major Histocompatibility Antigens

There is substantial similarity between the MHC in different species with respect to immunogenetics and protein structure. The genes within the MHC are divided into class I, II, and III.[34] The human MHC (HLA) is described more fully in Chapter 10.

MHC class I proteins (Figure 2-3) are cell surface glycoproteins composed of two chains – the alpha chain (molecular weight approximately 45 kD), which is highly polymorphic and encoded within the MHC by a class I gene, and a non-variable β_2-microglobulin chain (molecular weight approximately 12 kD) encoded elsewhere. In contrast to the heavy chain, β_2-microglobulin is not anchored in the membrane (Figure 2-3A), so that it may be exchanged for, or stabilized by, β_2-microglobulin in solution. MHC class I proteins are expressed on most nucleated cells, albeit at variable levels, and are generally responsible for activating T cells bearing the CD8 surface protein (CD8$^+$ cells).

MHC class II proteins are encoded entirely within the MHC and are composed of two membrane-anchored glycoproteins (Figure 2-3A) of similar molecular weight (alpha chain, 35 kD; beta chain, 28 kD). These proteins primarily stimulate T cells bearing the CD4 surface protein (CD4$^+$ cells). The tissue distribution of MHC class II proteins is far more restricted than that of class I, being expressed constitutively only by B lymphocytes, DCs, and some endothelial cells (particularly in humans). During an immune or inflammatory response, many other cell types may be induced to express MHC class II proteins.[59,73,88,92,236]

MHC class I and II proteins form a similar three-dimensional structure at the cell surface (see Figure 2-3B and C for ribbon diagrams of HLA-A2). Within this

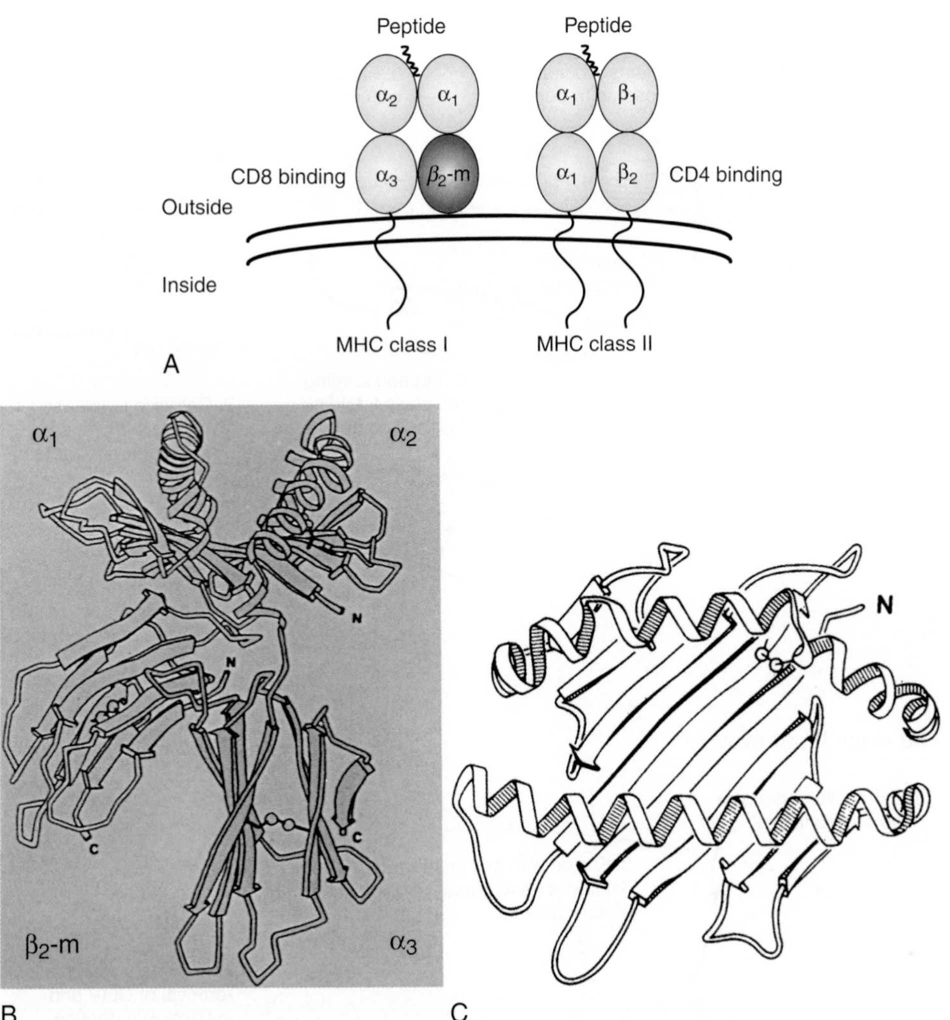

FIGURE 2-3 ■ Stick diagrams of major histocompatibility complex (MHC) class I and II and ribbon diagrams of human leukocyte antigen (HLA)-A2. (A) Stick diagram showing MHC class I and II as associated with the cell membrane. The MHC class I-associated molecule, β_2-microglobulin (β_2-m), is not membrane-inserted. (B and C) The structure of the human MHC complex class I antigen HLA-A2. The peptide groove is clearly visible lying between the two alpha helices. (B) Side view. (C) Bird's eye, or the T cell's, view. MHC class II proteins have a similar structure, although the ends of the groove are less closely associated, allowing the peptide to extend beyond the constraints of the groove.

structure is a groove, flanked by two alpha helices, and the amino acids in this groove are those that are most highly polymorphic. During the synthesis and transport of MHC class I and II proteins to the cell surface, they become associated with small peptides that fit into the groove. The groove of MHC class I has a closed structure, allowing peptides no longer than about 8–10 amino acids in size to be accommodated, whereas that of MHC class II has a more open structure, permitting the ends of the peptides to flop out of the groove, allowing it to accommodate peptides of at least 13 – and often many more – amino acids.

A major difference between proteins of the two MHC classes is in the origin of these peptides. They are largely acquired from the intracellular environment in the case of class I and the extracellular environment in the case of class II (Figure 2-4). Nevertheless, so-called cross-presentation between these pathways may occur, particularly in the context of specialized antigen presentation by DCs.[19,381]

A combination of MHC and peptide forms a compound epitope that is engaged by the antigen-specific receptor T-cell receptor (TCR). The peptide-binding groove is usually occupied by many different peptides, derived from self proteins (often those from the MHC) which, during infection, are replaced by those derived from pathogens.[40] The TCR repertoire is subject to negative thymic selection so that autoreactive cells are purged and to positive thymic selection for TCR that engage with peptides presented by autologous MHC. When a pathogen invades, MHC proteins become loaded with foreign peptides that are engaged by TCR in a self-restricted immune response. The extraction and sequencing of peptides bound within MHC proteins,[309,324] along with the three-dimensional structure of the MHC, have generated computable rules by which it is possible to predict sequences likely to bind in the groove and to interpret patterns of antigenicity.[28,82,351,373]

Several other proteins encoded within the MHC aid the assembly and loading of class I and II proteins

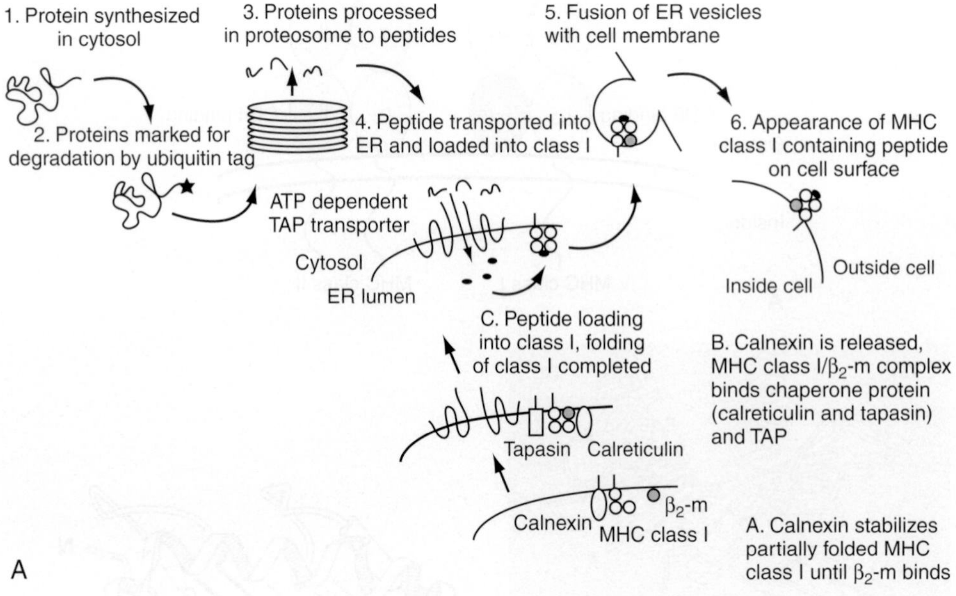

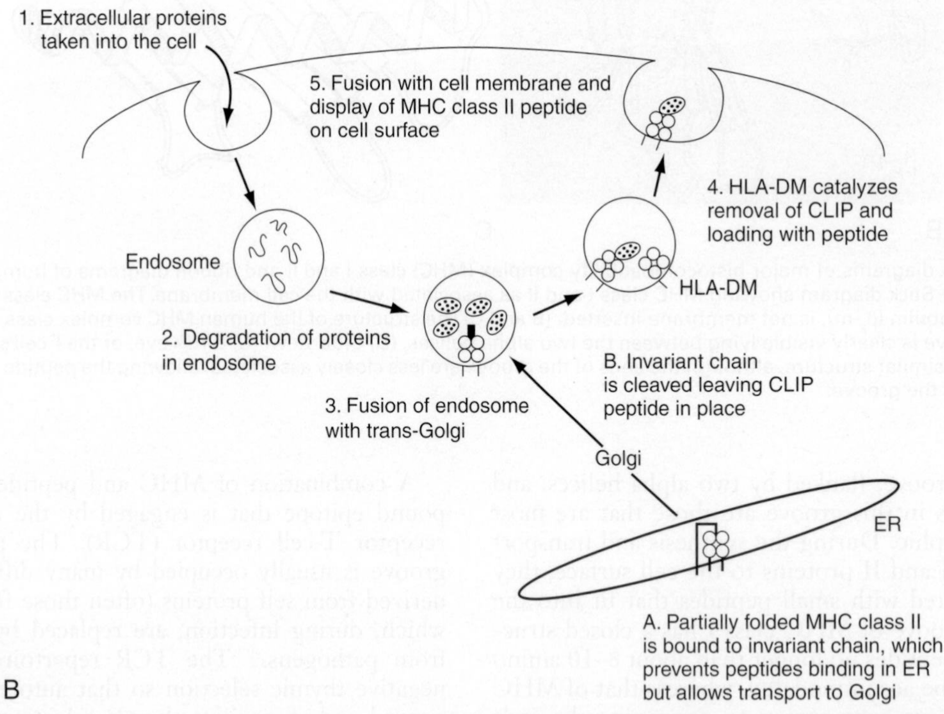

FIGURE 2-4 ■ Antigen processing and presentation in the major histocompatibility complex (MHC) class I and II pathways. (A) Processing of endogenous antigens occurs primarily by way of the class I pathway. Peptides are produced and loaded into MHC class I proteins, as shown in steps 1 through 4. During the synthesis of MHC class I proteins (steps A through C), the alpha chain is stabilized by calnexin before β_2-microglobulin (β_2-m) binds. Folding of the MHC class I/β_2-m remains incomplete, but the complex is released by calnexin to bind with the chaperone proteins, tapasin and calreticulin. Only when the transporter associated with antigen processing (TAP) delivers peptide to the MHC class I/β_2-m can folding of this complex be completed and transport to the cell membrane occur (steps 5 and 6). (B) Processing of exogenous antigens occurs primarily by way of the class II pathway. Antigens are taken up into intracellular vesicles where acidification aids their degradation into peptide fragments (steps 1 and 2). Vesicles containing peptides fuse with trans-Golgi-containing class II-associated invariant chain peptide (CLIP)–MHC class II complexes (step 3). DM aids removal of CLIP and loading of peptide before the class II peptide complex is displayed on the cell surface (steps 4 and 5). MHC class II proteins are synthesized in the endoplasmic reticulum (ER), where peptide binding is prevented by invariant chain. Invariant chain is cleaved, leaving the CLIP peptide still in place (steps A and B), before fusing with acidified vesicles containing peptide. In B lymphocytes and epithelial cells of the thymus, an atypical class II protein, HLA-DO, is expressed that is a dimer of HLA-DOα and HLA-DOβ. Similar to HLA-DM, it is not expressed at the cell surface and inhibits the action of HLA-DM. Its precise role is unknown. ATP, adenosine triphosphate; HLA, human leukocyte antigen.

with peptides (Figure 2-4). One type of class II protein, HLA-DM, does not appear on the cell surface, but plays a role in exchanging the class II-associated invariant chain peptide for the antigenic peptide in class II proteins before they emigrate to the cell surface.[317] The LMP (proteosome components) and transporters associated with antigen processing (TAP) genes also lie within the MHC and are involved in processing and loading of peptides for presentation. The understanding of antigen processing and presentation pathways has increased greatly and is of particular importance in studying responses to infectious agents, autoantigens, and tumor antigens.[53,200,255–257,264,316,354,405]

The structural resolution of MHC proteins (Figure 2-2), their engagement with TCR proteins,[21,27,95] along with an understanding of the mechanisms of antigen processing and presentation represent some of the most important advances in immunology over the last 20 years.[325] They also provide insight into the structural basis whereby MHC antigens, evolved to respond to fight infection, play such a significant role in transplantation.

It is the specific role of MHC class I and II molecules in presenting antigenic peptide to the TCR that underlies their significance as barriers to transplantation. Firstly, MHC antigens are highly polymorphic. This is likely to have evolved in response to their role as restriction elements in the response to pathogen-derived peptides. Certain cohorts of animals within species that have limited polymorphism at MHC loci have been devastated by infections that are cleared without difficulty in closely related species with polymorphic MHC.[284] This polymorphism is an important driver to humoral sensitization stimulated by pregnancy, blood transfusion, and prior transplantation. The immune mechanisms involved in these responses are not however fundamentally different to those involved with any other antigen. The cellular immune response to alloantigen is however fundamentally different at least in magnitude, because MHC molecules bind a diverse range of endogenous peptides, which are therefore normally presented at the cell surface. Allogeneic MHC generate a correspondingly wide range of compound epitopes distinct from the repertoire generated by syngeneic MHC. These are therefore recognized as foreign and engaged by the TCR in the so-called direct alloimmune response. The cellular immune response to MHC alloantigens is consequently unique in its diversity and therefore the number of T cells that can be recruited to an immune response.[81,87]

MHC Antigens in Experimental Models of Transplantation

Data from experiments performed between congenic strains of animals in which only MHC class I or II antigens differ in donor and recipient show that both contribute to graft rejection, although frequently grafts with only MHC class I disparities reject more slowly than grafts with class II or both class I and II differences.[175,320] Mice in which either MHC class I (class $I^{-/-}$ mice) or MHC class II (class $II^{-/-}$ mice) are disrupted have been used as both donor and recipient in experimental transplantation. The literature regarding this work is complex. In many studies lack of class I or II antigens on donor tissue alone has little effect on graft survival.[9,75,206,232] In other experiments, graft survival may be prolonged or permanent when donor tissue lacks either class I[70,131] or class II only[35] or both class I and II antigens.[35,232,287] It is clear from all of this work that results vary when different types of grafts are used, probably reflecting a greater or lesser involvement of different T-cell subsets.[35,131] In summary, the extensive underlying literature indicates that it is likely that cellular alloimmunity directed at both classes I and II plays a significant role in rejection but arguably the class II restricted $CD4^+$ T-cell response which interacts with diverse effector mechanisms is of greatest significance.

Non-Classical MHC Antigens

As described earlier, several genes within the class I and II regions do not encode classic MHC proteins. In addition to those involved in antigen processing, others encode non-classic MHC proteins that are similar in structure to classic MHC proteins but are non-polymorphic. These may have antigen-presenting capacity for specialized antigens, such as lipids (e.g., mycolic acid and lipoarabinomannan from *Mycobacterium*) or peptides of different sequence but with common characteristics (e.g., with *N*-formylated amino termini). Others such as HLA-G play a role in immune regulation,[37] particularly at the feto–maternal barrier.[71]

The class III region of the MHC is large and contains genes encoding proteins with a wide range of functions, including many with roles in the immune system, such as TNF-α and TNF-β.[251] Polymorphisms that determine the production of such cytokines have also been linked to certain immune responses, including transplant rejection.[390]

Minor Histocompatibility Antigens

Although the highest degree of genetic polymorphism within a species lies within the MHC, many other loci encode proteins with a lower degree of variability. It is clear from genetic studies that these proteins can act as transplantation antigens; they are miH antigens. Their structure and distribution were for many years elusive. Although T cells could recognize and respond to cells from MHC-identical individuals, it was almost impossible to raise antibodies against the antigens involved, making biochemical characterization difficult. The knowledge that T cells recognize small peptides, together with the application of molecular genetic techniques, allowed the characterization of the prototypic miH antigen, the male antigen or H-Y.[345,403] From such work, it is clear that miH antigens generally represent peptides from low-polymorphic proteins presented in the MHC groove, in the same way as a conventional antigen derived from infectious agents. The so-called H-Y antigen is actually derived from a group of such proteins encoded on the Y chromosome.[108,345,346,403] The first observation explains why it has been difficult to raise antibodies to miH antigens: the combination of autologous MHC with allogeneic peptide constitutes a relatively poor conformational determinant for antibody binding, whilst being an adequate determinant for TCR engagement.

miH antigens can play a prominent role in rejection in a recipient who is given an MHC-compatible graft but in whom pre-existing sensitization to miH antigens exists. This situation can be shown in the rat and mouse[83,372] and probably explains the occurrence of rejection episodes (which rarely result in graft loss) in renal transplants performed between HLA-identical siblings. Multiple miH differences have been shown to represent an immunogenic stimulus equivalent to that of the MHC in a non-sensitized recipient of a cardiac allograft in the mouse[372] but it is difficult to gather similar data in clinical transplantation. Tissue-specific polymorphic protein antigens have also been described, for example in mouse skin[368] and rat kidney.[127] An endothelial-monocyte antigenic system has been shown in humans, and it has been suggested that cells sensitized to these antigens can cause graft damage. This area has been reviewed by other authors.[105,318,355]

Donor Dendritic Cells and Direct Antigen Presentation

Immunization with MHC antigen in the form of a soluble membrane extract or liposomes may not produce an immune response, whereas integrated cell surface MHC proteins are generally highly immunogenic. Presentation of MHC class I antigen on cells that do not express class II antigens (e.g., red blood cells in rodents or platelets) does not produce a good primary immune response, suggesting that MHC class II antigens must be present on the immunizing cells for an optimal cellular immune response to be generated. In some cases, presentation of incompatible class I antigens in the absence of class II antigen not only may fail to evoke a primary immune response but also may initiate a state of tolerance (see Chapter 23).

The level of immunogenicity of MHC proteins varies considerably with the cell type on which they are found. DCs of various types are found throughout the body in both non-lymphoid and lymphoid tissues.[54,126] As previously stated, these cells rapidly migrate out of the transplanted organ to the recipient lymphoid system, where they are able to interact with and stimulate the host immune response.[192,193] On migration these tissue-resident immature DCs[310] mature rapidly into APCs that are highly potent in their ability to stimulate T lymphocytes.[149,364,366] Mature DCs express a high level of MHC class I and II antigens together with a range of costimulatory proteins and cytokines (see below) and as such are able to stimulate CD4+ and CD8+ T lymphocytes efficiently.[367] They are uniquely powerful in stimulating naive T cells, earning them the title of professional APCs. It is generally accepted that such cells, derived from the transplant, are a major stimulus for adaptive immunity in the recipient.

Direct Antigen Presentation (Figure 2-5A)

Allogeneic MHC on DCs derived from the graft will be occupied by a wide range of different endogenous peptides derived from donor tissue, both from non-polymorphic proteins[324] but also from MHC proteins themselves.[99,289]

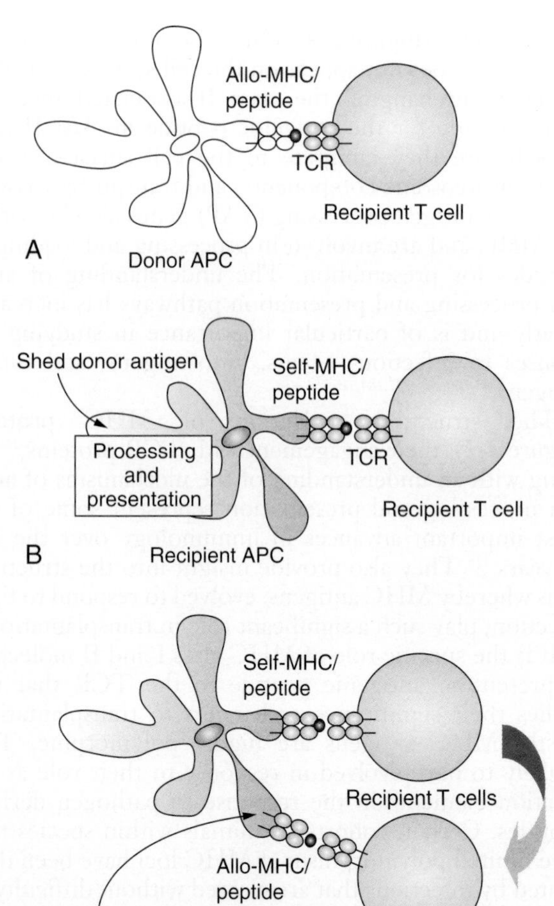

FIGURE 2-5 ■ (A–C) Direct, indirect, and semidirect pathways of antigen presentation. Sensitization of the recipient can occur by antigen presentation delivered through passenger leukocytes or dendritic cells of donor origin (direct antigen presentation) (A) or recipient origin (indirect or semidirect antigen presentation) (B and C). APC, antigen-presenting cell; MHC, major histocompatibility complex; TCR, T-cell receptor.

These combinations of peptide and MHC generate a range of compound epitopes that can be engaged by recipient TCR. They differ from self as a consequence of both different structural conformations and different peptides that are presented due to structural differences in the peptide binding groove.[262] The T-cell response to allogeneic MHC occurs at a remarkably high frequency: in the order of 1 in 100. This relates in part to the wide range of endogenous peptides that occupy the MHC groove, generating an equivalent number of compound epitopes. It has recently been shown that this is also consequent upon the capacity of the TCR to recognize multiple distinct ligands, that is, polyspecificity is a feature of TCR engagement.[87,262] These observations were predicated by observations of cross-reactivity between different alloantigens and between infectious organism-derived peptide with self and alloantigen (unsurprisingly, given the high frequency of response).[1,121,214] Allen and colleagues have recently presented data to suggest that alloreactivity is primarily limited by the range of peptides within the groove rather than any other structural feature of the MHC protein.[262]

These observations not only apply to naive cells but also to recall antigens (although there may be some selection for higher TCR affinity). As most experimental studies of transplantation, and in particular tolerance induction, use naive rodents raised in a sterile environment, these are unlikely to reflect accurately the alloresponse observed clinically. In clinical transplantation a substantial component of the allogeneic response is made by memory cells. It is perhaps not surprising therefore that strategies to induce transplantation tolerance which succeed in the naive animal are unsuccessful in previously infected animals.[1,25]

Indirect Antigen Presentation (Figure 2-5B)

Alloantigens can themselves be processed conventionally by the recipient immune system, that is, can be processed and presented by recipient APCs in a self-restricted fashion. This is termed indirect antigen presentation (Figure 2-5B). From what we understand about antigen processing and presentation (Figure 2-4), it seems likely that most allogeneic MHC peptides are presented in the context of class II MHC antigens because it is this pathway that deals with proteins exogenous to the cell. Mechanisms of cross-presentation do however allow peptides derived from cytosolic proteins to bind MHC class II and exogenous proteins to appear in the context of MHC class I.

The indirect pathway accounts for the fact that, in animal models, elimination of passenger leukocytes from the graft does not abolish – although it may alleviate – rejection. Its significance was demonstrated more than 20 years ago; Fangmann and coworkers showed that peptides derived from rat class I antigens were able to immunize animals via the indirect pathway and prime rejection of a subsequent skin graft carrying the class I antigens from which the peptides were derived.[86] Subsequent experiments showed skin grafts from class $II^{-/-}$ mice transplanted on to normal mice were rejected in a $CD4^+$ T-cell-dependent manner.[410] The interpretation of these experiments was that this was consequent upon self class II restricted presentation of exogenous alloantigen, that is, stimulation through the indirect pathway.[9,197,198] Other animal models demonstrated that, whilst rejection may be relatively insensitive to costimulation deficiency in the donor, this was not true of the recipient – data interpreted as indicating that costimulation provided by recipient APCs is more important in the initiation of graft rejection than is the costimulation provided by donor APCs.[227] The simplest interpretation again is that indirect presentation plays a more important role than direct presentation in such models, although the possibility that costimulation provided by recipient APCs is important, rather than antigen presentation and costimulation, cannot be discounted.

In clinical transplantation and in particular in the context of chronic allograft dysfunction, evidence for the role of indirect allorecognition has been presented in various reports using as antigen peptides derived from polymorphic regions of MHC antigens[271,301] or using cytoplasmic membrane protein preparations.[13,139] These studies need careful interpretation however, since such assays present particular difficulties for reproducibility and standardization in an outbred population.[356,397]

It has been considered that the direct allogeneic response dominates acute rejection and indirect allogeneic response allows for ongoing class II restricted responses following the loss of donor DCs.[52,352,415] This is however almost certainly an oversimplification,[18,269] particularly in the setting of a mature immune system with a diverse repertoire of memory cells. Nevertheless, the role of indirect allorecognition in providing cognate help to B-cell alloantibody formation[48,334] and the significant risk for graft loss associated with non-donor-specific as well as donor-specific antibody,[142,185] has been interpreted as support for the importance of indirect allorecognition. This is likely to apply to both acute and chronic rejection mediated through various effector mechanisms, both humoral and cellular.[15,377]

Semidirect Antigen Presentation (Figure 2-5C)

If host T cells are stimulated by recipient-derived DCs via indirect antigen presentation, the MHC restriction of the effector cell population is to the recipient rather than the donor. Naive T cells are primed most efficiently by DCs; however donor-derived DCs are rapidly lost following transplantation so that the opportunity for such stimulation via the direct pathway may only be short-lived.

If the effector arm of the immune response is not MHC-restricted (for example, in delayed-type hypersensitivity (DTH)), this is not such an issue. However, if this is the case (for example, in the case of cytotoxic T cells), then this may prevent alloimmune priming. Also, there is some experimental evidence to suggest that even if direct allogeneic $CD8^+$ T-cell priming can occur, then it requires T-cell help, that is, it requires $CD4^+$ T-cell help mediated via the indirect pathway.[197] There are various potential mechanisms to explain these findings, one being that donor class I and recipient class II colocate on the recipient DC. This is supported by evidence that intact proteins can be exchanged between cells in cell culture systems, that MHC proteins transfer in vivo,[133] and that transferred MHC stimulates allogeneic responses in vitro.[17,125,133,326] The importance of this semidirect pathway of antigen presentation to transplant outcomes remains to be clearly established.

A corollary to this discussion is that such pathways may also be relevant to the clearance of viral infection in the transplanted organ. This is dependent upon a repertoire selected on self MHC that includes specificity for viral antigen presented in the context of donor MHC. Deficiency in either may contribute to the emergence of viral infection in a transplanted kidney. This could contribute to the relative restriction of some infections to the transplanted organ, independently of the immunosuppressive load, a feature of BK nephropathy.[56]

Activation and Types of Dendritic Cell

So far this chapter has concentrated on the role that DCs (or other APCs) play in activating T lymphocytes. The role of DCs is however wide-ranging, playing a crucial role in immunological tolerance[285] and tuning adaptive immunity to ensure different effector mechanisms are used efficiently. DC subsets can be defined on the basis of their localization, morphology, cell surface, and functional phenotypes. A detailed description of their different roles is beyond the scope of this chapter; however other aspects of their functions will be discussed.

Classical DCs exhibit a so-called immature phenotype characterized by a high level of antigen uptake but relatively low levels of cell surface MHC and costimulatory molecule expression. Their subsequent maturation is accompanied by upregulation of these cell surface molecules, migration to secondary lymphoid organs and, generally, secretion of proinflammatory cytokines. This maturation process is stimulated by engagement of PAMPs and DAMPs.[365,387] Under certain circumstances maturation can be altered, with cytokine production diverted to promotion of tolerance, for example, increased IL-10 production.[153]

Pattern recognition by DCs seems not simply to involve the detection of "danger" but also "safety" (under non-inflamed conditions); they integrate a range of signals that maintain an immature, tolerogenic phenotype. These pathways and associated intracellular signaling[230] are only now being explored; they seem to involve molecules such as ILT3 and ILT4, Fc receptors (which can be activating (FcγRIII) or inhibitory (FcγRIIB)) and C-type lectins (which also can be activating or inhibitory). Other factors identified as promoting a tolerogenic DC phenotype include vitamin D_3, prostaglandin E_2, IL-10, and transforming growth factor-β (TGF-β).[288]

DCs with an immature or partly mature phenotype, that can present antigen and migrate to secondary lymphoid sites but deliver tolerogenic rather than activating signals, play a crucial role in the induction of Tregs, T-cell anergy, and deletion.[224,365] These effects are mediated by secretion of cytokines such as IL-10 and TGF-β which promote the emergence of Treg cells and through expression of negative costimulatory molecules such as PDL1/2, ICOS-L, ILT3/4, and Fas ligand. Equally, Tregs, and indeed other cell types, including macrophages and NK T cells, interact reciprocally in maintaining the tolerogenic phenotype of DCs. These mechanisms also involve the secretion of cytokines such as IL-10 as well as CTLA-4-B7 engagement that upregulates DC expression of indoleamine 2,3-dioxygenase (IDO).

This reciprocity between DCs and other cells is not limited to the maintenance of tolerance but applies also to productive immunity, that is, effector T cells can contribute to DC maturation[353] and functional phenotype.[314] For example, ligation of CD40 on DCs by CD154 (CD40 ligand) on the T cell results in upregulation of B7 proteins, which in turn can promote T-cell priming. This type of positive feedback is likely also to extend to the functional polarization of antigen-specific responses.[304] These interrelationships are necessary for the stability of tolerance and immunological memory. They also account for the particular difficulties in reprogramming alloimmune responses in the context of a mature immune system with a substantial memory response.

Other forms of DC do not necessarily arise from the same developmental pathways as classical DCs; for example, Langerhans cells are DCs that reside in the epidermis and in the adult constitute an apparently self-renewing population of cells. Plasmacytoid DCs reside primarily in bone marrow and the periphery; they are relatively long-lived and seem to play a role in the initial response to viral infection. Both these cell types can also present antigen to T cells and therefore play a role integrating signals to direct adaptive immunity, directly through interactions with lymphocytes but also through interactions with classical DCs.

ACTIVATION OF CELLULAR IMMUNITY

Location of T-Cell Activation

After small-bowel transplantation, recipient-derived leukocytes, including T lymphocytes, migrate in large numbers into the mesenteric lymph nodes and Peyer's patches of the graft, generating a marked cytokine response within 24 hours of grafting.[147,167,385,386] This likely results from normal homing of such cells because the small bowel is so rich in lymphoid tissue. It is likely that these T cells, if not already activated, may become so within the allograft, which is rich in mature DCs.

Naive lymphocytes are thought normally to recirculate from blood into lymphoid tissues without entering peripheral tissues and as such might be unlikely to become activated in grafts which are not so rich in lymphoid tissue. The extent to which naive T cells enter transplants other than small bowel and become activated in situ is therefore less clear – the cells do not express the adhesion proteins and chemokine receptors normally associated with homing to peripheral tissues, nor are the DCs within the graft mature. It is evident, however, that naive cells can recirculate in small numbers through peripheral tissues,[49,50] although the extent to which they can become activated within such peripheral sites is unclear. Indeed, in mice bearing the aly mutation, which lack secondary lymphoid tissue, graft rejection is abrogated.[187,188] However, the aly mutation affects not only the formation of secondary lymphoid tissue, but also TCR and CD28 signaling and this may explain the finding that splenectomized mice lacking either lymphotoxin (LT)-α or LT-β (which also do not have lymph nodes or Peyer's patches) are able to reject grafts, albeit in an attenuated fashion.[423] Further evidence suggests that, whilst direct antigen presentation may occur within a graft, indirect presentation occurs in the draining lymphoid tissue.[16]

In certain chronic inflammatory situations, lymphoid neogenesis or ectopic accumulations of lymphoid cells develop within peripheral tissues, and can provide an environment in which naive cells can become activated. The possibility that lymphoid neogenesis also occurs and is important in the context of transplantation has been suggested by studies in a mouse cardiac transplant model in which the presence of such accumulations occurred in a high proportion of grafts undergoing chronic rejection.[10]

During acute graft rejection of organs other than small bowel, it would seem that T cells are most likely to become activated in draining or local lymphoid tissue where they can interact in an optimal fashion with optimally activated donor or host-derived DCs. The contribution of naive T-cell recirculation to acute graft rejection is probably minor, although its role in the longer term may become more important. The possibility that naive cells recirculate through peripheral tissues for the purposes of tolerance induction rather than activation[49] is interesting and should be considered in the context of longer-term graft function and survival.

Immune Synapse

T-lymphocyte activation absolutely requires TCR engagement and signaling through the CD3 complex; however it is evident that a great deal more is involved when MHC peptide is engaged at another cell's surface. An immune synapse is formed in which the TCR and coreceptors (CD4 and CD8), adhesion receptors, costimulatory and coinhibitory molecules assemble into supramolecular activation complexes (SMACs) within the lipid bilayer, followed by the assembly of intracellular signaling complexes, in particular involving the linker for activation of T cells (LAT).[65,78,106] There are associated changes in cytoskeletal proteins, which may be involved in signal transduction directly and indirectly through effects on TCR-binding kinetics. Initial models of the synapse derived from experiments using antigen-presenting lipid bilayers involved the formation of a central (c) SMAC into which TCR move, closely associated with CD28. This is surrounded by the lymphocyte function-associated antigen (LFA)-1-rich peripheral (p) SMAC and CD45-rich distal SMAC. In DCs it seems similar structures are formed, albeit with perhaps multiple cSMAC structures.

T-Cell Receptor Signals

The TCR has no catalytic activity of its own. It forms a complex with six CD3 subunits ($\gamma\delta\varepsilon_2\zeta_2$) containing immunoreceptor tyrosine-based activation motifs (ITAMs).[215] Lck phosphorylates these ITAMs following TCR ligation, resulting in association with the ζ-chain-associated protein kinase, ZAP70.[402] The precise mechanism by which TCR ligation translates into phosphorylation is unclear but activation may involve TCR dimerization and CD45 which dephosphorylates and activates LCK (although subsequent exclusion of CD45 from the synapse may underlie increases in ITAM phosphorylation). ZAP70 recruitment results in phosphorylation of the adapter proteins SLP76 and LAT. LAT facilitates the formation of multiprotein complexes that drive T-cell activation pathways, including phospholipase Cγ activation of calcium signaling, diacylglycerol activation of protein kinase Cθ, Ras-MAP kinase signaling through SH2 containing proteins such as GRB2 and SOS, and cytoskeletal interactions involving a wide range of molecules.[14] This results in de novo expression of a wide range of genes encoding cytokines and cell surface proteins. These signaling pathways are increasingly characterized; they are the targets of established and novel immunosuppressive medication and are described in detail elsewhere.[14,89,159,215,402,414]

Second or Costimulatory Signals

Antigen-specific receptors (the TCR and B-cell receptor (BCR)) underlie adaptive immunity. Their engagement (with the relevant coreceptor, for T cells CD4 or CD8) initiates clonal activation. However this alone does not determine the fate of the response; rather it is engagement of a wide range of other cell surface receptors. These costimulatory molecules determine and mediate short-term function and long-term fate during priming, expansion, and death of T cells and B cells. There are many families of costimulatory molecules, including those of the of immunoglobulin superfamily (e.g., B7), TNF family (e.g., CD154), G protein-coupled receptors (e.g., C3a and C5a receptors) and lectin receptors (e.g., DC-SIGN). As increasing numbers of molecules have been described, it has become evident that these interactions are highly complex, involving paracrine as well as cell contact-dependent mechanisms.

Through these and other interactions, the APC acts as an integrator of danger signals that fundamentally inform T-cell activation and are themselves informed by interaction with T cells. The need for this dialogue to be antigen-specific places interactions between cell surface molecules on the APC and T cell at the heart of the immune response. At a clonal level these interactions can be activating[382] or inhibitory,[401] whilst at a system or polyclonal level they result in different cell fates, including differentiation into effector, memory, or regulatory phenotypes.[409] Indeed, recent data suggest these interactions are likely to generate considerable functional heterogeneity within the antigen-stimulated T-cell compartment.[278]

This sophisticated understanding has evolved from a two-signal model that remains extremely influential in conceptualizing T-lymphocyte activation.[26,186] It identified that non-antigen-specific interactions could determine short-term and long-term consequences of TCR engagement manifest as T-cell clonal activation (proliferation and IL-2 production) or proliferative non-responsiveness followed by stable non-responsiveness, even in the face of an adequate second signal: anergy.[151,152,189,343,344] Anergic cells can inhibit the activation of neighboring T cells,[36,91,213] that is, manifest regulatory activity.[45]

The molecular basis for the costimulatory or "second" signal for naive T-cell activation was defined as that between CD28 and the B7 family molecule, now known as CD80.[207] These costimulatory interactions were not only the first to be described but also the first to be manipulated in the setting of clinical transplantation[5,74] and are therefore described in more detail in the next section.

CD28–B7 Interaction

The cell surface protein CD28 is now known to be a member of a family of similar proteins.[42,109,313] Activation of downstream signaling via CD28 results from ligation with B7 family proteins, CD80 or CD86. These proteins are expressed by APCs such as DCs and are readily able to engage CD28 during antigen presentation. Signaling through CD28 in the context of TCR ligation results in an increase in glucose metabolism and high levels of cytokine and chemokine expression. High levels of IL-2 are produced; T cells proliferate and resist apoptosis.

The requirement for CD28 signals for CD8+ T cells or for primed CD4+ T cells is less clear. The prevailing view for CD4+ cells is that if they have not been stimulated very recently by antigen, they require costimulation for reactivation, but even recently activated cells can be shown to be costimulation-dependent.[118,233] Experimentally, it can be shown that, in certain situations virus-reactive CD8+ cells are independent of CD28.[184,428] On occasion even CD4+ cells may exhibit CD28 independence, in the face of a strong TCR stimulus. To become activated in the absence of costimulation probably requires prolonged TCR engagement in the presence of a large antigenic load, which may occur in association with viral infections and occasionally in other situations. If the amount and duration of initial antigen exposure are limited, however, then even CD8+ memory T cells may require costimulation for activation. A memory response is generally less dependent upon CD28. This is an important finding in the context of clinical transplantation, where a large proportion of the alloreactive pool has previously been antigen-activated as a result of its cross-reactivity with pathogen-derived peptides (see earlier). Certainly CD28 blockade is unlikely to drive tolerance induction in a previously primed system. This provides one possible explanation for the finding that targeting this costimulatory pathway is less effective in attenuating transplantation responses in humans than would have been predicted from rodent studies.

Mice with a disrupted cd28 gene have impaired immune responses but can reject skin grafts, albeit in a delayed fashion[164]; this is likely due to other costimulatory proteins that can substitute the action of CD28.[42,313,350] Blocking the CD28 pathway in normal animals inhibits the alloimmune response and results in prolonged graft survival or tolerance.[203,295,389] The most widely used reagent for this purpose has been CTLA-4-Ig. This blocks B7 engagement of both CD28 and CTLA-4, the latter of which could be counterproductive because CTLA-4 acts primarily as a coinhibitory molecule counterbalancing the effects of CD28. This is evident in the severe phenotype of CTLA-4$^{-/-}$ mice, in which animals die from lymphoproliferative disorder within a few weeks of birth. Similar in structure to CD28, CTLA-4 inhibits the earliest events in T-cell activation. CTLA-4 has a higher affinity for CD80 and CD86 than does CD28[47,342] and its engagement with CD80 induces a lattice structure at the cell surface consisting of alternating CTLA-4 and CD80 homodimers. These properties of CTLA-4 may limit the ability of CD80 to interact with and cluster CD28 at the immune synapse, potentially explaining the finding that low levels of CTLA-4 can be effective at inhibiting immune responses. CTLA-4 may also deliver a negative intracellular signal[85] independent of its effect on CD28 that halts cell cycle progression and IL-2 production[182] or affects TCR engagement.[339] The actions of CTLA-4 may be even more complex at a polyclonal level since CTLA-4 engagement may promote Treg function in vivo.[148,408]

Other Costimulatory Molecules

Since the role of CD28 engagement was defined other members of this family of molecules have been identified; bound by various ligands they generate effects that can broadly be termed costimulatory – ICOS, DNAM, and CRTAM – or coinhibitory – CTLA-4, PD-1, BTLA, LAG-3, TIM-3, TIGIT, and LAIR-1.

A second major family of costimulatory molecules on the T-cell surface is the TNF superfamily, including CD27, CD134 (OX40), and CD137 (4-1BB), which interact with a range of TNF receptor family members. On the T-cell surface the TNF receptor family member CD154 (CD40 ligand, gp39) itself interacts with CD40 on B cells, DCs, and monocytes. Larsen and coworkers showed that blocking this interaction could prolong graft survival in a mouse cardiac transplant model.[190] Even more impressive, however, were data that combined CD28 and CD40 blockade-induced permanent survival of allogeneic skin grafts in mice with no long-term deterioration of graft integrity.[191] Tolerance to graft antigens could not be shown in these mice, despite the excellent survival of the transplant itself. In a large-animal setting, kidney graft rejection in monkeys can be prevented completely with antibodies to CD154[170]; however its clinical application is limited by thromboembolic events associated with its expression on platelets. Alternative approaches using non-depleting antibodies to CD40 are therefore now being explored.[12]

The significance of the many different interactions with costimulatory molecules, cytokines, and other soluble ligands are now understood to be responsible for T-cell differentiation that is highly diverse, even within a population with identical antigen specificities. The experimental basis of this understanding follows the development of new flow cytometric techniques which allow multiparameter phenotyping of cells.[278] A more complete description of these various costimulatory pathways and their multifaceted actions can be found in various reviews.[208,350,426]

An understanding that memory T cells are an important barrier to successful engraftment in the presence of immunosuppression and to tolerance induction, combined with the fact that they may be relatively resistant to CD28 inhibition, has directed interest toward identifying molecular targets in T-memory cells. The expression of CD2 on T-effector memory cells,[211,406] of LFA-1 on T-memory cells[11] and even expression of a specific potassium channel on T-effector memory cells[110] have been investigated. These approaches require further assessment and are not without potential competing risks.[22,66]

The Generation of Effector Immunity and Cytokine Production

The consequences of TCR engagement and costimulation are proliferation and differentiation of the T cells into effector phenotypes and concomitant production of cytokines required by other cell types. The prototypic helper role – the production of cytokines and involvement in cellular interactions to promote different effector mechanisms – was recognized to be a highly important function of CD4+ cells. CD8+ cells may sometimes contribute to this role and emerge independently of CD4+ T-cell help.[63,180,219,232,319–321,337,360,383] These dependencies can now be seen in a wider context of cross-talk between a wide range of different cell types. Nevertheless CD4+

cells remain important to the initiation of graft rejection, a fact demonstrated by workers in diverse experimental systems.[59,113,115,216,218]

Subsets of T-helper cells develop following repeated antigen stimulation; they are characterized by the production of particular cytokines that direct elements of the immune response and target different effector mechanisms against viruses, bacteria of various sorts, fungi, protozoa, and multicellular parasites.[332] The prototypical pattern of polarization based on cytokine production was that between Th1 or Th2 cells (Figure 2-6). Th1 cells mainly produce IFN-γ; they are involved in cell-mediated inflammation and immunoglobulin class switching to IgG antibodies, whereas Th2 cells produce IL-4, IL-5, and IL-13, and are involved in IgE class switching and eosinophil recruitment.

Cytotoxic T-cell populations may also diverge in their cytokine production, so T1 and T2 populations can be referred to. More recently, a discrete population of T cells has been described, characterized by the production of IL-17, which seems to play an important role in the clearance of extracellular pathogens and in autoimmune pathology. Th17 differentiation seems to require TGF-β with IL-6 or with IL-21. IL-23 stabilizes this differentiation. More recently, IL-1 and IL-2 have been reported as playing a role in determining the production of IL-10 and IFN-γ by Th17 cells.[427] In the context of transplantation it is evident that Th17 cells can mediate an alloimmune response that translates into a form of acute rejection; however, the extent to which this depends upon IL-17A production and its significance in a fully competent immune system remain to be determined.[2]

The significance of different patterns of response in their determination of graft outcome is highly dependent upon the model used, that is, the particular outcomes and timeframes studied and competing factors involved. Many groups have found that tolerance or reduced donor-directed reactivity was associated with decrease in the prolonged expression of the T1-associated cytokines IL-2 and IFN-γ.[29,30,61,254,376] There is some evidence that the expression of T2 cytokines is preserved during the development of so-called tolerance[57,103,336,376]; however clones of T lymphocyte that have T2-like properties are capable of initiating graft rejection in other models.[395,421] Furthermore in robust models of tolerance (rather than prolonged allograft survival), rapid shutdown of cytokines rather than preferential T2 cytokine production has been observed.[160,295]

The role of different cytokines in allograft rejection has been approached by manipulating experimental systems in various different ways, including the use of neutralizing antibodies and the assessment of mouse strains in which genes for specific cytokines have been genetically manipulated. Importantly, the interpretation of these experiments requires due consideration: firstly, whether absence of the cytokine in question could have influenced maturation of the immune system under investigation; secondly, because there is considerable degeneracy in the action of different cytokines; and thirdly, because the same cytokine may have apparently opposing actions depending upon the context of engagement with its receptor.

This is illustrated by studies of IL-2$^{-/-}$ or IFN-γ$^{-/-}$ mice which demonstrated that neither were required for rejection.[331,363] IL-15 can, for example, substitute many of the actions of IL-2 and IL-15 transcripts are found in grafts placed in IL-2$^{-/-}$ mice. Subsequent studies demonstrated that, whilst neither IL-2 nor IFN-γ was required for rejection, both were required for tolerance induction.[55] This suggested non-redundant functions for both IL-2[225,329] and IFN-γ[335,404,413] in Treg function.

The conclusion from all of these studies is that an effector immune response driven by either T1 or T2 cells is damaging, although in some cases the response driven

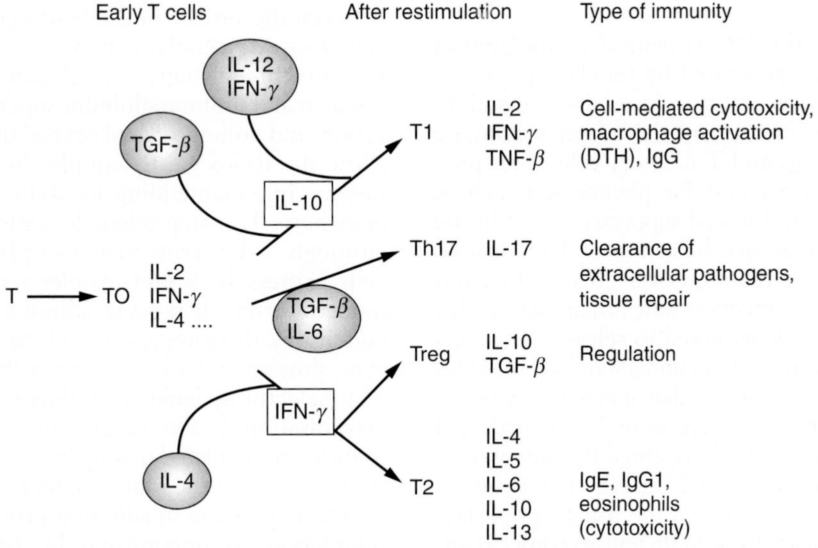

FIGURE 2-6 ■ T1/T2/Th17 cell differentiation and immunity. Cytokines produced by T cells and that influence their divergence to T1, T2, and Th17 subsets are shown, defining the effector immunity generated. Cytokines that may positively (in circles) or negatively (in squares) regulate divergence of the T1, T2, and Th17 cells are shown. Cells with a regulatory or suppressive function (Treg) also may be generated de novo during an immune response, likely diverging from the T2 pathway. Such cells differ from naturally occurring Tregs, which have a CD25^{+} cell surface phenotype, but nevertheless function in a similar fashion to control immunity. DTH, delayed-type hypersensitivity; IFN, interferon; Ig, immunoglobulin; IL, interleukin; TGF, transforming growth factor; TNF, tumor necrosis factor.

by T2 cells may be not as immediately detrimental as that driven by T1 cells. T2 cells may though drive immune mechanisms that act over a longer time period. The individual actions of certain cytokines still are not fully understood, but it would seem, given the data on IL-2 and IFN-γ, that such cytokines may assume different functions depending on the timing or perhaps location and origin of their production. The involvement of Th17 cells in protective immunity and immune-mediated pathology is an area of intense investigation and the precise role of such cells in transplantation remains uncertain. As well as a potential role in mediating alloantigen-specific inflammation there are some data to suggest that Th17 responses may play a role in autoimmune responses in the setting of transplantation[275]; however this too remains unproven.

T-Regulatory Cells

A healthy immune system is subject to checks and balances that prevent autoimmunity and ensure proportionate, timely, and efficient response to infectious agents. This involves control of immune responses by cells with regulatory function, including both naturally occurring CD4+ CD25+ Tregs of thymic origin and induced CD4+ CD25+ Tregs generated in the periphery. These cells modulate productive immunity through various mechanisms, including the production of cytokines such as IL-10, TGF-β, and IL-35,[3] adenosine production,[67] downregulation of DC costimulation and upregulation of IDO.[45] Tregs may also have more direct actions on effector cell viability through mechanisms that involve granzyme B.[102]

Cells with alternative phenotypes have also been defined as contributing to immune regulation, including IL-10-secreting Tr-1 cells,[93] CD28− CD8+ cells that appear to have specificity for Qa-1 (equivalent to HLA-E in humans)[154,396,418] and, more recently, B cells with regulatory function.[240]

It is thought that the DC is central to integration of many of the signals generated by regulatory mechanisms that impinge upon adaptive immunity,[290] distilling information from the innate and the adaptive immune systems, including Tregs and T-memory cells. This provides a mechanism to account for phenomena such as infectious tolerance[305] and linked suppression.[45,174] In the context of these observations the action of Tregs can be seen as promoting Treg function over effector function and in the presence of infection and inflammation this metastable state becomes disrupted to release the generation of effector immunity. This understanding provides a background to the conclusion that mechanisms of action of Tregs are inevitably closely related to induction of Tregs and maintenance of a tolerogenic DC phenotype.

The phenotype of CD4+ CD25+ Treg cells is highly dependent upon the expression of the transcription factor FoxP3, which appears to be sufficient to confer regulatory activity, including suppression of IL-2 and IFN-γ production, expression of CTLA-4 and GITR. FoxP3 is therefore an important marker of Treg activity although, at least in the case of inducible Tregs, it is not clear that their phenotype remains stable in all circumstances.[422] CTLA-4 appears to play an important role in Treg function.[148,384] The mechanism of action of CTLA-4 in this setting seems to involve CD80/86 engagement on DC associated with modulation of IDO expression,[45,111] although this seems unlikely to be the sole mechanism of action and requires further experimental assessment.

There is ample evidence for the importance of Tregs in many models of experimental transplantation tolerance,[155,196,338] well illustrated in models using donor-specific transfusion and non-depleting anti-CD4 antibody in which Treg function seems to play a crucial mechanistic role.[31] In particular there seems to be an important role for self-restricted cells that therefore recognize antigen through the indirect pathway.[33,172] Perhaps more importantly, recent evidence in humanized animal models suggests that the infusion of non-specifically expanded Tregs can abrogate the acquisition of transplant arteriosclerosis, opening potential translation into the clinical setting.[79,138,270,378]

MECHANISMS OF GRAFT INJURY

Migration of Activated Cells into the Graft

To enter a site of inflammation or immune response, leukocytes must migrate across the vascular endothelium. This migration process is controlled by the elaboration of cell attractants or chemokines and by cell–cell interactions between the leukocyte and the endothelium.[369] Activated and memory cells bear adhesion proteins, chemokine receptors, and addressins, which allow homing to and migration into peripheral tissues.[221,222]

Cell–Cell Interactions

The adhesion of leukocytes to the endothelium is a complex multistep process that involves a series of interactions between the surface of the leukocyte and the endothelial cell or its extracellular matrix.[169,369] The proteins involved fall into three groups: the selectins and members of the integrin and immunoglobulin superfamilies. Initial interaction and rolling of leukocytes along the endothelium allow the leukocyte to sample the endothelial environment, while maintaining its ability to detach and travel elsewhere. This step is largely controlled by the selectins, although α_4 integrins may also play a role. Endothelial cells express IL-8 and platelet-activating factor, which induces strong leukocyte adhesion. Under the correct conditions, this interaction leads to signaling to the leukocyte, slowing and arresting the rolling process. Shedding of L-selectin by leukocytes allows their detachment and extravasation.[241] The latter stages of leukocyte transmigration are regulated mainly by the β_2 integrins and adhesion proteins of the immunoglobulin superfamily.

The expression of adhesion proteins involved in these interactions is upregulated by proinflammatory cytokines. Ischemic damage alone results in increased expression of several cytokines and, of these, IL-1 upregulates the expression of members of the selectin family.[50,300] Other adhesion proteins, such as intercellular adhesion molecule (ICAM)-1 and vascular cell adhesion molecule

(VCAM)-1 of the immunoglobulin superfamily and endothelial-specific selectin (E-selectin), are upregulated by cytokines induced by donor brain death[194] and implantation. Therefore before an immune response has been generated, the graft becomes attractive to circulating leukocytes. Although naive lymphocytes tend not to home into non-lymphoid sites, in clinical transplantation a significant proportion of the response is constituted by memory cells, which may do so. Antigen-activated lymphocytes have an altered recirculation pattern and migrate into extralymphoid sites.[32,221,299] They may show tissue-selective homing and preference for sites in which they are most likely to re-encounter their specific antigen.[333] This process may be facilitated further by cognate recognition by the T cell of MHC class II–peptide complexes on the vascular endothelium,[234] which likely results in the accumulation of antigen-specific lymphocytes within the site of inflammation, in this case the graft.

One practical aspect with respect to transplantation is that it may be possible to hide or block the expression of the proteins involved in leukocyte extravasation, slowing or preventing the rejection process. Blocking the adhesion proteins by using antibodies or by inhibiting their expression has been attempted in experimental and clinical transplantation settings.[51,60,128,141] In general, cocktails of antibodies are more potent than single antibodies,[417] although the results vary (in one case a combination of antibodies to ICAM-1 and LFA-1 was shown to result in accelerated rejection of rat cardiac allografts[261]). Antisense oligonucleotides have been used in an attempt to prevent the expression of ICAM-1 and have been effective in prolonging graft survival in experimental models.[370] Small-molecule inhibitors also may effectively interrupt the interactions required for leukocyte adhesion and extravasation.[277] The possibility that these types of reagent may simultaneously be effective in blocking IRI and in controlling the rejection process[371] is an attractive one, which remains under investigation.

Chemokines

Chemokines are chemotactic cytokines: small proteins that play a crucial role in leukocyte trafficking under both normal conditions and in the setting of inflammation. There are more than 40 different chemokines that in the main map to two major structural families: CC or β chemokines (e.g., MIP-1α/β, RANTES, and MCP-1) which attract T cells, monocyte/macrophages, DCs, NK cells, and some polymorphs, and CXC or α chemokines (e.g., IL-8 and IFN-γ-inducible protein) which primarily attract neutrophils and T cells.[120,122,250,286,323] There is a correspondingly wide range of chemokine receptors, although homeostatic chemokines tend to be relatively restricted in their pattern of usage whilst inflammatory chemokines are more promiscuous in their utilization of different receptors.

The role of chemokine production by vascular endothelium following reperfusion has already been discussed.[120,204] Inevitably, chemokines play an important role in any response that involves inflammatory cell infiltration, including acute rejection[72,84,107,120,122] and chronic rejection. For example, in animal models $CCR1^{-/-}$ mice accept MHC class II mismatched grafts without immunosuppression and MHC class I and II mismatched grafts with only low-dose immunosuppression[94]; long-term surviving grafts do not appear to show signs of chronic dysfunction. Although $CXCL10^{-/-}$ recipients show normal rejection kinetics of a $CXCL10^{-/-}$ graft, $CXCL10^{-/-}$ grafts placed in normal recipients show prolonged survival.[121] This important role in cell trafficking and function has led to inevitable interest in therapeutic manipulation of the chemokine network in transplantation,[283] albeit that simple inhibitory strategies are likely to be limited by the aforementioned cross-talk between receptors and ligands.

Mechanisms of Cytotoxicity

The immune system generates many different effector mechanisms depending on the challenge it meets. In certain infections, a single mechanism seems to be essential for the clearance of the causative organism, and the absence of that mechanism renders the host susceptible to disease. In the clearance of lymphocytic choriomeningitis virus infections in mice, cytotoxic cells are absolutely required, and disabling this arm of immunity by disrupting the perforin gene leads to the death of infected animals.[162] Most known effector mechanisms of the immune system are capable of damaging a graft such that the obliteration of any single effector mechanism has little beneficial effect on graft survival. This is one reason why it is difficult to prevent graft rejection without disabling the central components of the immune system and why multiple immunosuppressive medications are required in clinical transplantation. It likely accounts for the fact that, once established, the rejection response is so difficult to control, particularly in the long term.

Specificity of Cellular Immune Responses in Rejection

The nature of tissue destruction during rejection reveals a lot about the processes involved. For example, graft destruction can show fine specificity for cells carrying donor alloantigens. The elegant studies of Mintz and Silvers show the potential for exquisite specificity of donor cell lysis in experiments using allophenic mice as tissue donors.[252,253] Allophenic or tetraparental mice are bred by fusing embryos from mice of two different genetic origins. The tissues of the resulting mosaic offspring are composed of patches of cells from each parental type. Mintz and Silvers performed experiments using mice with different coat colors, and when skin from an allophenic donor was grafted to mice of either parental origin, only the cells of non-identical type were rejected, leaving cells of recipient type intact and capable of hair growth. These studies have been repeated and extended in experiments performed by Rosenberg and Singer.[321] In this work, an initial large inflammatory/immune response was observed but this resolved, remarkably leaving cells only of the recipient genotype in place. In a different type of experiment, Sutton and colleagues[374] showed that transplantation of an intimate mixture of allogeneic and syngeneic pancreatic islets resulted in destruction only of the allogeneic cells, with no evidence of bystander damage to the syngeneic islets.

It is difficult to imagine how an essentially non-specific effector mechanism, such as that involved in DTH lesions, could mediate graft rejection that is so specific. Bystander destruction of tissue is however observed in other experimental systems. For example, Snider and Steinmuller[358] showed that destruction of bystander tissue may occur in the immune response to miH antigens. In their experiments, cytotoxic T-cell clones reactive with a variety of minor antigens (e.g., H-Y and Epa-1 antigens) were injected intradermally together with their specific antigen into a syngeneic animal, which did not express that antigen. As a result, ulcerating skin lesions developed that were radiosensitive, suggesting the involvement of a non-specific, host-derived effector mechanism in the tissue destruction. In the experiments described earlier using donor tissue from tetraparental animals, if most cells in the graft were allogeneic to the recipient, the overwhelming inflammatory response leads to destruction of the entire tissue.

These experiments demonstrate that both antigen-specific and non-antigen-specific effector mechanisms may be involved in graft destruction. In both types of experiment, the initial damage was mediated in a specific fashion; however, if there is a massive inflammatory response then tissue destruction can be non-specific. Its extent reflects the proportion of allogeneic cells present and their location, since vascular endothelial damage can result in tissue ischemia and rapid generation of non-specific danger signals. The vascular endothelium is therefore arguably the most important target in kidney transplantation. An appreciation of these subtle differences in specificity is of particular importance in understanding the immunopathology of viral diseases such as BK nephropathy and their relationship to mechanisms of rejection.[4,76]

Cytotoxic T-Cell Responses

In cell culture systems, MHC-mismatched lymphocytes proliferate and produce cytokines in response to one another in the mixed lymphocyte reaction. The resulting cytokine production allows the differentiation of precursor cytotoxic T lymphocytes (CTLs) into effector cells that lyse target cells bearing the mismatched MHC antigens.[129,137] The fact that a powerful yet antigen-specific response is generated rapidly in mixed lymphocyte reaction has made the CTL a prime suspect as the central effector mechanism of acute graft rejection.

Considerable evidence suggests that CTLs may be involved in graft rejection. First, CTLs may be recovered from allografts that are undergoing rejection, but they are present only at low levels in grafts of animals that have been treated with cyclosporine to prevent rejection.[24,237] Second, cloned populations of CTLs are capable of causing the type of tissue damage associated with rejection. Third, most MHC class I antigen-directed CTLs express the CD8 protein, and graft rejection often may be delayed after the depletion of $CD8^+$ cells.[46,218,223,297,383]

Conversely, graft destruction may occur in the absence of demonstrable CTL activity, and the presence of such cells within a graft may not always lead to graft destruction.[6,62] Rats given a donor-specific preoperative blood transfusion may retain a subsequent renal allograft indefinitely, but cells extracted from such grafts show high and persistent donor-specific CTL activity. The simple conclusion from these studies is that CTLs cannot always reject grafts, although the possibility that the action of these CTLs may be blocked in the graft itself, or that the activity of CTLs in cell culture does not accurately reflect their potential in the animal, must be considered. These results remain intriguing, however, and provide direct evidence of the presence of cytotoxic effector cells within an organ graft that is not ultimately rejected.

CTLs are able to kill their targets through the elaboration of perforins, granzymes, and granulysin through activation of the Fas death pathway, or through secretion of the cytokine TNF-α. Their involvement in graft rejection has been questioned further by the finding that mice deficient in perforin (perforin knockouts) are able to reject tumor,[400] skin,[348] and organ grafts,[341] even when the grafts are resistant to Fas-mediated and TNF-α-mediated killing.[400] In the experiments of Schulz and colleagues,[341] grafts mismatched only at the MHC class I are rejected more slowly in perforin knockout mice, however, indicating that, in this situation at least, cytotoxic cells are important in rejection.

As alluded to earlier, even if CTLs themselves do not mediate the tissue damage that ultimately results in graft loss, they still may be important in generating the destructive response to the graft. Through the elaboration of high levels of IFN-γ and other cytokines or chemokines, they are able to recruit and activate cells involved in DTH lesions, initiating acute or chronic rejection.

Alloantibody and Alloantigen-Specific B cells

The target antigens for damaging allogeneic antibodies are primarily MHC class I, MHC class II,[41] MICA,[429] and the ABO blood group antigens.[327] Minor alloantigens are potential targets; however they are rarely defined in clinical transplantation. H-Y antibodies have been reported to portend acute rejection, although any long-term consequence to H-Y mismatch is evidently small. Similarly, autoimmunity to antigens, including the angiotensin II type I receptor[77] (expressed by vascular smooth-muscle cells), is a rare but important complication of kidney transplantation. Other autoantigens to which antibody responses emerge in allogeneic transplantation, such as vimentin[161] and collagen,[150] have mostly been analyzed in cardiothoracic transplantation, although there is increasing interest in the potential contribution of autoimmune responses to chronic rejection in other settings.[165,275,347]

Donor-specific antibody may cause damage in different ways, most notably through complement activation. This is the dominant mechanism in hyperacute rejection due to preformed antibody[176] and has recently been specifically targeted using the C5 specific monoclonal antibody eculizumab.[362] The major target antigens for such preformed antibodies are firstly ABO blood group antigens. These widely expressed antigens are defined by the presence of specific trisaccharides present on glycoproteins and glycolipids. Antibodies to them are formed in the neonatal period, it is thought following exposure to gut flora. The second group of target antigens for preformed antibodies are the highly polymorphic MHC antigens to which the recipient may be exposed through prior transplantation, blood transfusions, or pregnancy.[64,173,263,291,407] Indeed, this serological definition of HLA arose prior to its recognition as the MHC: the target for cellular alloimmunity and the restriction element for T-cell immunity in general. In the 1960s recognition of the importance of donor–recipient blood group compatibility[361] and development of a test to screen for preformed anti-HLA antibodies using the lymphocytotoxic cross-match[291] fundamentally changed the short-term outcomes of transplantation.

It may also be that antibody-mediated complement activation can play a role in later rejection events. Complement component 4d (C4d) can be detected by immunostaining of biopsies suffering chronic rejection.[239] This usually occurs in the presence of anti-HLA antibody. On the other hand the precise significance of this finding needs to be considered in light of its frequent detection following planned ABO-incompatible transplantation, without a clear-cut relationship to adverse events.[114,168] Donor-directed antibody may also cause tissue damage through antibody-dependent cellular cytotoxicity, where antibody acts as a bridge between the target tissue and the effector cell, activating lytic machinery and causing tissue damage.[296] Indeed, there is emerging evidence that NK cell transcripts are a feature of chronic antibody-mediated rejection.[134]

The effects of donor-specific antibody need not be a sole consequence of immediate cytotoxicity. Anti-HLA antibody binding activates endothelial cells.[199] Through interactions of HLA with transmembrane proteins of various sorts this results in mTOR/Akt,[158] protein kinase A, and MAP kinase signaling which drive proliferation,[276] adhesion molecule and coagulation factor upregulation[311] and secretion of cytokines and chemokines.[311] All these factors may be implicated in the structural changes associated with chronic rejection.

Conversely antibody binding to vascular endothelium without cytotoxicity may protect against subsequent circumstances in which cytotoxicity would have been expected to prevail. This may occur if antigen-specific antibody levels are initially low or there is a period of protection from complement-mediated damage. The process is termed accommodation and is poorly understood.[68,69,330] It is likely to involve multiple mechanisms, including: reduced antigen density, endothelial cell resistance to antibody-mediated injury via upregulation of antiapoptotic and complement regulatory proteins and downregulation of procoagulant factor production.[156,274,330,359] There is some evidence that antibodies with different antigen specificities, such as for ABO blood group antigens or HLA, may activate different pathways that contribute to accommodation.[149,195] An understanding of these mechanisms may in part explain differential long-term outcomes in blood group-incompatible compared to HLA-incompatible transplantation[258] and define potential cytoprotective pathways.

The significantly worse outcomes observed in transplant recipients in whom anti-HLA antibodies are detected may also reflect the wider role of B cells in the immune response. In particular HLA-specific B cells are important APCs due to their ability to expand clonally and efficiently take up antigen via the BCR. They therefore stimulate HLA (indirect pathway)-specific T cells and play an important role in the optimal activation, generation, and maintenance of T-cell memory.[279,281] In addition to antigen presentation and costimulation, B cells secrete a range of cytokines that play a role in T-cell activation and indeed regulation. There is now evidence that B cells contribute to regulating immune responses. This has primarily been reported as consequent upon the production of IL-10; however other potential mechanisms have been implicated involving both soluble factors and cell contact. This has important implications for therapeutic strategies that involve the depletion or manipulation of the B-cell population.[240]

The molecular pathways that support B-cell proliferation and differentiation have been increasingly defined and are now emerging as potential targets in autoimmunity. These are therefore likely to be adapted to alloimmunity as alternatives to the depleting strategies already tried with agents such as rituximab (an anti-CD20 monoclonal antibody).[44,391] Since antibody production primarily derives from plasma cells, targeting B cells alone is likely to have relatively little efficacy in reversing humoral allosensitization; however, modulation of B-cell activation and survival may influence the generation of alloantibody and B-cell support for cellular immunity. Potential targets on the B cell include costimulatory receptors CD19, CD21, the inhibitory receptors CD22 and FcγRIIB and soluble B-cell-activating factors such as BAFF and TACI.[43] Some of these are present on later-stage B-cell lineage and may therefore affect antibody production. However it is likely that other strategies will be required in those with significant pre-existing humoral immunity.

Natural Killer Cells

NK cells play a role as effector cells, lysing sensitive targets according to the presence or absence of specific target antigens. For example, the activating receptor NKG2D is engaged by MICA and MICB, that are induced in allografts during acute and chronic rejection.[171] The binding of these ligands to NKG2D activates NK cells to enhance effector functions, whereas the engagement of killer immunoglobulin-like receptors (KIRs) by KIR ligands such as HLA-C (KIR2DL1 and KIR2DL2) and HLA-Bw4 (KIR3DL1) generally inhibits function. Inhibitory receptor function underlies the phenomenon of responses to "missing self",[163,209] which contributes to tumor immunity,[132] the killing of stem cells,[20] and hybrid resistance in experimental models of transplantation.[392]

Although the importance of NK cells in bone marrow transplantation has been long established,[265,266] their role in solid-organ transplantation has taken longer to be recognized. Several laboratories using different experimental models found that grafts survive indefinitely in the presence of demonstrable NK effector activity,[6,24] although more recently CD28-independent rejection in mouse models of transplantation has been shown to be NK-dependent and sensitive to blockade of NKG2D.[166] The role of NK cells in the afferent arm of immunity via interaction with DCs[112,123] and production of high levels of IL-12 and IFN-γ has prompted a re-evaluation of their role. There is now evidence that, whilst insufficient alone to cause acute rejection, NK cells contribute significantly to the alloimmune response. For example, genetic studies of donor and recipient HLA-C type (grouped as C1 and C2 depending upon polymorphisms at positions 77 and 80 and which seem to exhibit differential NK cell inhibition) suggest that long-term outcomes may be influenced by donor or recipient interaction with KIRs.[123,124] This has also been observed when KIR HLA mismatches are analyzed in HLA-compatible transplantation.[394] Recently NK transcripts have been found in association with late alloantibody-associated rejection[134] and in animal models NK cells have been found to contribute to alloantibody-mediated chronic allograft vasculopathy,[135] leading to a re-evaluation of NK-mediated antibody-dependent cytotoxicity and other potential mechanisms of NK-mediated injury.

Macrophages and Delayed-Type Hypersensitivity Reactions

T cells initiate a DTH reaction,[203] which involves an essentially non-specific effector phase (as described by Koch in 1891 in the tuberculin skin reaction[9]), characterized by an infiltrate of lymphocytes and cells of the monocyte/macrophage lineage. Damage occurs in a tissue during a DTH reaction through the elaboration of various noxious substances, including reactive nitrogen and oxygen intermediates and TNF-α. Support for the involvement of DTH, which is likely mediated by M1 macrophages, in graft rejection comes from situations in which CTL responses are not detectable (e.g., in irradiated rats reconstituted with CD4+ cells).[217]

The high level of inflammatory mediators and the type of changes within grafts undergoing chronic rejection suggest a role for activated M1 macrophages also in this process.[39,130,292,293] Cytokines such as IL-1, TNF-α, TGF-β, and platelet-derived growth factor lead to smooth-muscle proliferation; TGF-β and platelet-derived growth factor result in an increased synthesis of extracellular matrix proteins. These cytokines are products of activated macrophages and may result in the atherosclerotic and fibrotic changes associated with chronic graft failure.

Although, as illustrated above, the macrophage has largely been implicated as an agent of destruction and damage in transplantation, new knowledge about the contribution of M2 macrophages to injury repair, together with the identification of the Mreg macrophage, suggests that a re-evaluation of macrophage activity in transplants is timely.[38,231] Reagents to analyze the presence of the different macrophage populations, together with experiments that directly test the ability of different populations to damage or repair tissue, will be important in redefining the role of macrophages following transplantation.

Cytokines

The primary role of cytokines in an immune response to a graft is to initiate proliferation, differentiation, and homing of leukocytes in the generation of immunity. However, certain cytokines also may directly damage tissue acutely or chronically. As described earlier, TNF-α, produced by CTLs and macrophages, may damage a graft, and blocking the effects of TNF with neutralizing antibodies can prolong organ graft survival.[23,144–146] The minimal effects of these antibodies suggest, however, that the TNFs may not contribute centrally to graft rejection, or that when neutralized other effector mechanisms take over. Islets seem to be particularly susceptible to damage mediated by proinflammatory cytokines, indicating that these may be a more important component in the rejection of islet transplants.[228,229,308,411]

Eosinophils

It has been recognized for years that episodes of acute and chronic kidney allograft rejection are associated with various levels of eosinophilia,[178,180,280] and that this may be associated with vascular rejection,[247] but an implication of such cells in graft destruction has been more difficult to accumulate. In an experimental model of acute mouse cardiac allograft rejection in which the depletion of CD8+ T lymphocytes results in a dominant T2 response, rejection seems to be mediated by eosinophils.[380] In another model, in which acute rejection of MHC class II disparate mouse skin grafts was studied, IL-5-dependent infiltration with eosinophils was observed. In this model, when Fas/FasL interactions were absent, neutralizing antibodies to IL-5 blocked eosinophilia and rejection, implicating the eosinophil as an effector cell in this system.[202] In another experimental model of skin allograft rejection, the same group showed a role for IL-5 and eosinophilia in chronic rejection, but in this system, not all of the pathology could be attributed to eosinophils.[201] In situations in which classic pathways of graft rejection are absent or are dominated by a T2-type response, the eosinophil seems to be crucial in graft destruction.[100]

Target Cells of Destructive Immunity

The relative importance of specific target cells in alloimmunity is likely to vary between specific organs and indeed between individuals with different histories of sensitization.

Renal parenchymal cells may be targets for tissue destruction, and in the kidney, tubular cells elaborate cytokines and chemokines that can attract and activate T cells.[315,412] The kidney is a highly vascular organ, and the medulla constantly at the limit of tissue hypoxia. In humans vascular endothelium expresses both MHC class I and MHC class II and blood vessels are a major target of the inflammatory response in acute rejection.[98] Indeed, vascular involvement, often associated with the presence of alloantibodies, seems to be associated with a significantly worse outcome.[220] These two factors are independently associated with long-term graft loss. This prognostic difference between cellular and vascular rejection may reflect fundamentally different origins and effector mechanisms; however it is possible that vascular involvement simply drives greater tissue hypoxia, and therefore further amplification of danger signals, with adverse consequences for the evolving adaptive immune response. This may be as true of microvascular changes as those seen in large blood vessels.

Chronic Rejection

The subject of chronic rejection and chronic allograft injury in general is discussed in detail in Chapter 27. It is however clear that the immune system plays an important role in chronic allograft damage and ultimately in determining allograft survival. In recent years the prominent role of calcineurin inhibitor toxicity[273] in paradigms of chronic allograft injury has been revised[116,357] but should not be dismissed.[259,349] The pathophysiology of chronic rejection remains incompletely understood despite application of a wide range of approaches to assess kidney histology,[248] protein and gene expression,[80,117] as well as peripheral blood representation of humoral[142,185,379] and cellular alloimmunity.[18,301,356] The reason for this incomplete understanding is likely to be a reflection of the heterogeneous processes that can result in similar clinical and indeed histological endpoints,[183,357] a situation exacerbated by the temporal separation between cause and effect (at least determined in clinically indisputable terms such as graft survival, or substantial changes in renal function).

Thus chronic allograft injury may arise from ongoing alloimmune responses; it may be consequent upon ongoing autoimmunity initiated by alloimmune-mediated damage[165,347,393] or dysregulated repair mechanisms arising from the particular pattern of damage produced by initial alloimmunity. In any case non-specific mechanisms in which low-grade endothelial damage results in platelet deposition on the arterial wall and growth factor production can cause proliferation of smooth-muscle cells in the media of the arterial wall and their subsequent invasion of the intima.[130] This response-to-injury hypothesis, first proposed for atherosclerosis,[322] has been tested in an experimental transplant model in the rat using an aortic allograft.[249] These grafts undergo an initial acute inflammatory reaction in the adventitia, which subsides and is followed by gradual migration of proliferating muscle cells from the vascular media to the intima and the appearance of intimal fibrosis. When induced, this allograft arteriosclerosis is not reversible by transplanting the aortic allograft back into a syngeneic recipient. The development of these chronic arterial lesion is associated with cytokines (IL-1, IL-6, TNF, IFN-γ), growth factors (platelet-derived growth factor, TGF-β), and lipid mediators of inflammation (eicosanoids and platelet activation factor). This is evidence for the latter response to injury mechanism of chronic allograft injury, which may of course be exacerbated not only by immune mechanisms but also by calcineurin inhibitor toxicity,[357] hypertension,[302] chronic renal dysfunction,[375] and other vascular risk factors.[419] It may therefore be the case that interventions that maintain endothelial health and minimize dysregulated repair could have broad utility.

The role of alloimmunity in progressive graft loss is suggested particularly by studies in which the presence of donor-specific anti-HLA antibodies are associated with worse outcome. In principle this antibody response could be a secondary phenomenon consequent upon damage. Interestingly, non-donor-specific antibody is also a risk factor for graft loss and this has been interpreted as evidence of the significance of non-humoral donor-specific alloimmunity that is associated with humoral non-donor-specific alloimmunity.[377] Since non-donor-specific alloimmunity is unlikely to arise secondary to damage, this suggests that alloimmunity precedes graft damage. Even then it does not prove that ongoing alloimmune-mediated damage is a necessary feature of chronic rejection.

A range of animal models suggest that immune mechanisms contribute to the ongoing progression of chronic transplant vasculopathy. Histological changes resembling those in clinical transplantation can be induced by the passive transfer of donor-reactive antibody, through a mechanism that does not seem to require complement fixation[136] (a finding with important implications for the therapeutic use of inhibitors of complement activation to prevent complement-mediated hyperacute or acute rejection[362]). Antibody binding to vascular endothelium alone may be sufficient for chronic transplant vasculopathy, as discussed above; however it is possible that other as yet unexplored mechanisms may be important. For example, a recent experimental model suggests that NK cells contribute significantly to a lesion resembling chronic transplant vasculopathy in a manner that is Fc receptor-dependent.[135] These studies support those in clinical transplantation that chronic rejection is associated with the presence of donor-specific antibodies. On the other hand a parallel range of experimental models that generate similar histological abnormalities can be observed in which cellular mechanisms predominate.[96,420] In all these analyses it should be borne in mind that, in all but the most highly controlled experimental systems, it is likely that multiple immune mechanisms contribute to allograft injury; equally, simply because a lesion that resembles transplant vasculopathy can be induced through a particular immune mechanism does not require it to be clinically significant.[420]

SUMMARY

The immune response to an allogeneic organ is highly complex. The MHC generates a uniquely diverse set of antigens, the responses to which in a mature immune system cross-react on established memory. This range of antigens can then stimulate immune responses via an array of effector mechanisms, modified but rarely abolished by the use of immunosuppressive medications. Over the course of the last decade the importance of the innate immune system in the initiation and polarization of immune responses following transplantation has been increasingly recognized. This is linked to a central role of DCs of both donor and recipient origin in stimulating productive immunity but also potentially in promoting immune-regulatory mechanisms in appropriate circumstances. A greater understanding of immune-regulatory mechanisms may in the future allow for intervention in which inhibition of alloantigen-specific responses could improve the risk–benefit ratio of therapies, to prevent rejection. Similarly, better understanding and an ability to assay alloantigen-specific effector immunity may allow better targeting of non-specific immunosuppression. These strategies are of particular importance in managing long-term outcomes since this is when most transplants are now lost, although this clearly poses a particular challenge to approaches to our understanding of the immune mechanisms involved.

REFERENCES

1. Adams AB, Williams MA, Jones TR, et al. Heterologous immunity provides a potent barrier to transplantation tolerance. J Clin Invest 2003;111:1887–95.
2. Agorogiannis EI, Regateiro FS, Howie D, et al. Th17 cells induce a distinct graft rejection response that does not require IL-17A. Am J Transplant 2012;12:835–45.
3. Akdis M, Burgler S, Crameri R, et al. Interleukins, from 1 to 37, and interferon-gamma: receptors, functions, and roles in diseases. J Allergy Clin Immunol 2011;127:701–21, e1-70.
4. Albrecht JA, Dong Y, Wang J, et al. Adaptive immunity rather than viral cytopathology mediates polyomavirus-associated nephropathy in mice. Am J Transplant 2012;12:1359–60.
5. Archdeacon P, Dixon C, Belen O, et al. Summary of the US FDA approval of belatacept. Am J Transplant 2012;12:554–62.
6. Armstrong HE, Bolton EM, McMillan I, et al. Prolonged survival of actively enhanced rat renal allografts despite accelerated cellular infiltration and rapid induction of both class I and class II MHC antigens. J Exp Med 1987;165:891–907.
7. Ascon M, Ascon DB, Liu M, et al. Renal ischemia-reperfusion leads to long term infiltration of activated and effector-memory T lymphocytes. Kidney Int 2009;75:526–35.
8. Asgari E, Zhou W, Sacks S. Complement in organ transplantation. Curr Opin Organ Transplant 2010;15:486–91.
9. Auchincloss Jr H, Lee R, Shea S, et al. The role of "indirect" recognition in initiating rejection of skin grafts from major histocompatibility complex class II-deficient mice. Proc Natl Acad Sci U S A 1993;90:3373–7.
10. Baddoura FK, Nasr IW, Wrobel B, et al. Lymphoid neogenesis in murine cardiac allografts undergoing chronic rejection. Am J Transplant 2005;5:510–6.
11. Badell IR, Russell MC, Thompson PW, et al. LFA-1-specific therapy prolongs allograft survival in rhesus macaques. J Clin Invest 2010;120:4520–31.
12. Badell IR, Thompson PW, Turner AP, et al. Nondepleting anti-CD40-based therapy prolongs allograft survival in nonhuman primates. Am J Transplant 2012;12:126–35.
13. Baker RJ, Hernandez-Fuentes MP, Brookes PA, et al. Loss of direct and maintenance of indirect alloresponses in renal allograft recipients: implications for the pathogenesis of chronic allograft nephropathy. J Immunol 2001;167:7199–206.
14. Balagopalan L, Coussens NP, Sherman E, et al. The LAT story: a tale of cooperativity, coordination, and choreography. Cold Spring Harbor Perspect Biol 2010;2:a005512.
15. Ballet C, Renaudin K, Degauque N, et al. Indirect CD4+ TH1 response, antidonor antibodies and diffuse C4d graft deposits in long-term recipients conditioned by donor antigens priming. Am J Transplant 2009;9:697–708.
16. Baratin M, Bonin K, Daniel C. Frontline: peripheral priming of alloreactive T cells by the direct pathway of allorecognition. Eur J Immunol 2004;34:3305–14.
17. Bedford P, Garner K, Knight SC. MHC class II molecules transferred between allogeneic dendritic cells stimulate primary mixed leukocyte reactions. Int Immunol 1999;11:1739–44.
18. Bestard O, Nickel P, Cruzado JM, et al. Circulating alloreactive T cells correlate with graft function in longstanding renal transplant recipients. J Am Soc Nephrol 2008;19:1419–29.
19. Bevan MJ. Cross-priming for a secondary cytotoxic response to minor H antigens with H-2 congenic cells which do not cross-react in the cytotoxic assay. J Exp Med 1976;143:1283–8.
20. Bix M, Liao NS, Zijlstra M, et al. Rejection of class I MHC-deficient haemopoietic cells by irradiated MHC-matched mice. Nature 1991;349:329–31.
21. Bjorkman PJ, Saper MA, Samraoni B, et al. Structure of the human class I histocompatibility antigen, HLA-A2. Nature 1987;329:506–12.
22. Bloomgren G, Richman S, Hotermans C, et al. Risk of natalizumab-associated progressive multifocal leukoencephalopathy. N Engl J Med 2012;366:1870–80.
23. Bolling S, Kunkel SL, Lin H. Prolongation of cardiac allograft survival in rats by anti-TNF and cyclosporin combination therapy. Transplantation 1992;53:283–6.
24. Bradley JA, Mason DW, Morris PJ. Evidence that rat renal allografts are rejected by cytotoxic T cells and not by nonspecific effectors. Transplantation 1985;39:169–75.
25. Brehm MA, Markees TG, Daniels KA, et al. Direct visualization of cross-reactive effector and memory allo-specific CD8 T cells generated in response to viral infections. J Immunol 2003;170:4077–86.
26. Bretscher P, Cohn M. A theory of self-nonself discrimination. Science 1970;169:1042–9.
27. Brown JH, Jardetzky TS, Gorga JC, et al. Three-dimensional structure of the human class II histocompatibility antigen HLA-DR1. Nature 1993;364:33–9.
28. Brusic V, Bajic VB, Petrovsky N. Computational methods for prediction of T-cell epitopes – a framework for modelling, testing, and applications. Methods 2004;34:436–43.
29. Bugeon L, Cuturi M-C, Hallet M-M, et al. Peripheral tolerance of an allograft in adult rats – characterization by low interleukin-2 and interferon-γ mRNA levels and by strong accumulation of major histocompatibility complex transcripts in the graft. Transplantation 1992;54:219–25.
30. Burdick JF, Clow LW. Rejection of primarily vascularized heart grafts. III Depression of the interleukin 2 mechanism early after grafting. Transplantation 1990;50:476–81.
31. Bushell A, Jones E, Gallimore A, et al. The generation of CD25+ CD4+ regulatory T cells that prevent allograft rejection does not compromise immunity to a viral pathogen. J Immunol 2005;174:3290–7.
32. Butcher EC. The regulation of lymphocyte traffic. Curr Top Microbiol Immunol 1986;128:85–122.
33. Callaghan CJ, Rouhani FJ, Negus MC, et al. Abrogation of antibody-mediated allograft rejection by regulatory CD4 T cells with indirect allospecificity. J Immunol 2007;178:2221–8.
34. Campbell RD, Trowsdale J. Map of the human major histocompatibility complex. Immunol Today 1993;14:349–52.
35. Campos L, Naji A, Deli BC, et al. Survival of MHC-deficient mouse heterotopic cardiac allografts. Transplantation 1995;59:187–91.
36. Carlin LM, Yanagi K, Verhoef A, et al. Secretion of IFN-gamma and not IL-2 by anergic human T cells correlates with assembly of an immature immune synapse. Blood 2005;106:3874–9.
37. Carosella ED, Gregori S, LeMaoult J. The tolerogenic interplay(s) among HLA-G, myeloid APCs, and regulatory cells. Blood 2011;118:6499–505.
38. Chadban SJ, Wu H, Hughes J. Macrophages and kidney transplantation. Semin Nephrol 2010;30:278–89.
39. Chen J, Myllarniemi M, Akyurek LM, et al. Identification of differentially expressed genes in rat aortic allograft vasculopathy. Am J Pathol 1996;149:597–611.
40. Chicz RM, Urban RG, Lane WS, et al. Predominant naturally processed peptides bound to HLA-DR1 are derived from MHC-related molecules and are heterogeneous in size. Nature 1992;358:764–8.
41. Claas FH. HLA antibody testing: a tool to facilitate not to prevent organ transplantation. Int J Immunogenet 2008;35:275–7.
42. Clarkson MR, Sayegh MH. T-cell costimulatory pathways in allograft rejection and tolerance. Transplantation 2005; 80:555–63.
43. Clatworthy MR. Targeting B cells and antibody in transplantation. Am J Transplant 2011;11:1359–67.
44. Clatworthy MR, Watson CJ, Plotnek G, et al. B-cell-depleting induction therapy and acute cellular rejection. N Engl J Med 2009;360:2683–5.
45. Cobbold SP, Adams E, Nolan KF, et al. Connecting the mechanisms of T-cell regulation: dendritic cells as the missing link. Immunol Rev 2010;236:203–18.
46. Cobbold SP, Jayasuriya A, Nash A, et al. Therapy with monoclonal antibodies by elimination of T cell subsets in vivo. Nature 1984;312:548–51.
47. Collins AV, Brodie DW, Gilbert RJ, et al. The interaction properties of costimulatory molecules revisited. Immunity 2002;17:201–10.
48. Conlon TM, Saeb-Parsy K, Cole JL, et al. Germinal center alloantibody responses are mediated exclusively by indirect-pathway CD4 T follicular helper cells. J Immunol 2012;188:2643–52.
49. Cose S. T-cell migration: a naive paradigm? Immunology 2007;120:1–7.
50. Cose S, Brammer C, Khanna KM, et al. Evidence that a significant number of naive T cells enter non-lymphoid organs as part of a normal migratory pathway. Eur J Immunol 2006;36:1423–33.

51. Cosimi AB, Conti D, Delmonico FL, et al. In vivo effects of monoclonal antibody to ICAM-1 (CD54) in nonhuman primates with renal allografts. J Immunol 1990;144:4604–12.
52. Cramer DV, Qian S, Harnaha J, et al. Cardiac transplantation in the rat I. The effect of histocompatibility differences on graft arteriosclerosis. Transplantation 1989;47:414–9.
53. Cresswell P. Assembly, transport and function of MHC class II molecules. Annu Rev Immunol 1994;12:259–93.
54. Daar AS, Fuggle SV, Hart DNJ, et al. Demonstration and phenotypic characterisation of HLA-DR positive interstitial dendritic cells widely distributed in human connective tissue. Transplant Proc 1983;XV(Suppl. 1):311–5.
55. Dai Z, Lakkis FG. The role of cytokines, CTLA-4 and costimulation in transplant tolerance and rejection. Curr Opin Immunol 1999;11:504–8.
56. Dall A, Hariharan S. BK virus nephritis after renal transplantation. Clin J Am Soc Nephrol 2008;3(Suppl. 2):S68–75.
57. Dallman MJ. Cytokines as mediators of organ graft rejection and tolerance. Curr Opin Immunol 1993;5:788–93.
58. Dallman MJ, Larsen CP, Morris CP. Cytokine gene transcription in vascularised organ grafts–analysis using semiquantitative polymerase chain reaction. J Exp Med 1991;174:493–6.
59. Dallman MJ, Mason DW, Webb M. Induction of Ia antigens on murine epidermal cells during the rejection of skin allografts. Eur J Immunol 1982;12:511–8.
60. Dallman MJ, Porter ACG, Larsen CP, et al. Lymphokine production in allografts–analysis of RNA by northern blotting. Transplant Proc 1989;20:296–8.
61. Dallman MJ, Shiho O, Page TH, et al. Peripheral tolerance to alloantigen results from altered regulation of the interleukin 2 pathway. J Exp Med 1991;173:79–87.
62. Dallman MJ, Wood KJ, Morris PJ. Specific cytotoxic T cells are found in the nonrejected kidneys of blood-transfused rats. J Exp Med 1987;165:566–71.
63. Dalloul AH, Chmouzis E, Ngo K, et al. Adoptively transferred CD4+ lymphocytes from CD8–/– mice are sufficient to mediate rejection of MHC class II or class I disparate skin grafts. J Immunol 1996;156:411–4.
64. Dankers MK, Roelen DL, Korfage N, et al. Differential immunogenicity of paternal HLA class I antigens in pregnant women. Hum Immunol 2003;64:600–6.
65. Davis DM, Dustin ML. What is the importance of the immunological synapse? Trends Immunol 2004;25:323–7.
66. De Jager PL, Baecher-Allan C, Maier LM, et al. The role of the CD58 locus in multiple sclerosis. Proc Natl Acad Sci U S A 2009;106:5264–9.
67. Deaglio S, Dwyer KM, Gao W, et al. Adenosine generation catalyzed by CD39 and CD73 expressed on regulatory T cells mediates immune suppression. J Exp Med 2007;204:1257–65.
68. Delikouras A, Dorling A. Transplant accommodation. Am J Transplant 2003;3:917–8.
69. Delikouras A, Fairbanks LD, Simmonds AH, et al. Endothelial cell cytoprotection induced in vitro by allo- or xenoreactive antibodies is mediated by signaling through adenosine A2 receptors. Eur J Immunol 2003;33:3127–35.
70. Desai NM, Bassiri H, Kim J, et al. Islet allograft, islet xenograft and skin allograft survival in CD8+ T lymphocyte-deficient mice. Transplantation 1993;55:718–22.
71. Deschaseaux F, Delgado D, Pistoia V, et al. HLA-G in organ transplantation: towards clinical applications. Cell Mol Life Sci 2011;68:397–404.
72. DeVries ME, Ran L, Kelvin D. On the edge: the physiological and pathophysiological role of chemokines during inflammatory and immunological responses. Semin Immunol 1999;11:95–104.
73. de Waal RMW, Bogman MJJ, Mass CN, et al. Variable expression of Ia antigens on the vascular endothelium of mouse skin allografts. Nature 1983;303:426–9.
74. Dharnidharka VR. Costimulation blockade with belatacept in renal transplantation. N Engl J Med 2005;353:2085–6.
75. Dierich A, Chan SH, Benoist C, et al. Graft rejection by T cells not restricted by conventional major histocompatibility complex molecules. Eur J Immunol 1993;23:2725–8.
76. Drachenberg CB, Papadimitriou JC, Mann D, et al. Negative impact of human leukocyte antigen matching in the outcome of polyomavirus nephropathy. Transplantation 2005;80:276–8.
77. Dragun D, Muller DN, Brasen JH, et al. Angiotensin II type 1-receptor activating antibodies in renal-allograft rejection. N Engl J Med 2005;352:558–69.
78. Dustin ML, Depoil D. New insights into the T cell synapse from single molecule techniques. Nat Rev Immunol 2011;11:672–84.
79. Edinger M, Hoffmann P. Regulatory T cells in stem cell transplantation: strategies and first clinical experiences. Curr Opin Immunol 2011;23:679–84.
80. Einecke G, Reeve J, Sis B, et al. A molecular classifier for predicting future graft loss in late kidney transplant biopsies. J Clin Invest 2010;120:1862–72.
81. Ely LK, Burrows SR, Purcell AW, et al. T-cells behaving badly: structural insights into alloreactivity and autoimmunity. Curr Opin Immunol 2008;20:575–80.
82. Engelhard VH, Altrich-Vanlith M, Ostankovitch M, et al. Post-translational modifications of naturally processed MHC-binding epitopes. Curr Opin Immunol 2006;18:92–7.
83. Fabre JW, Morris PJ. Studies on the specific suppression of renal allograft rejection in presensitised rats. Transplantation 1975;19:121–33.
84. Fairchild RL, VanBuskirk AM, Kondo T, et al. Expression of chemokine genes during rejection and long-term acceptance of cardiac allografts. Transplantation 1997;63:1807–12.
85. Fallarino F, Fields PE, Gajewski TF. B7-1 engagement of cytotoxic T lymphocyte antigen 4 inhibits T cell activation in the absence of CD28. J Exp Med 1998;188:205–10.
86. Fangmann J, Dalchau R, Fabre JW. Rejection of skin allografts by indirect allorecognition of donor class I major histocompatibility complex peptides. J Exp Med 1992;175:1521–9.
87. Felix NJ, Donermeyer DL, Horvath S, et al. Alloreactive T cells respond specifically to multiple distinct peptide–MHC complexes. Nat Immunol 2007;8:388–97.
88. Fellous M, Nir U, Wallach D, et al. Interferon-dependent induction of mRNA for the major histocompatibility antigens in human fibroblasts and lymphoblastoid cells. Proc Natl Acad Sci U S A 1982;79:3082–6.
89. Fernandes RA, Yu C, Carmo AM, et al. What controls T cell receptor phosphorylation? Cell 2010;142:668–9.
90. Flowers ME, Inamoto Y, Carpenter PA, et al. Comparative analysis of risk factors for acute graft-versus-host disease and for chronic graft-versus-host disease according to National Institutes of Health consensus criteria. Blood 2011;117:3214–9.
91. Frasca L, Carmichael P, Lechler R, et al. Anergic T cells effect linked suppression. Eur J Immunol 1997;27:3191–7.
92. Fuggle SV, McWhinnie D, Morris PJ. Precise specificity of induced tubular class II antigens in renal allografts. Transplantation 1987;44:214–20.
93. Fujio K, Okamura T, Yamamoto K. The family of IL-10-secreting CD4+ T cells. Adv Immunol 2010;105:99–130.
94. Gao W, Topham PS, King JA, et al. Targeting of the chemokine receptor CCR1 suppresses development of acute and chronic cardiac allograft rejection. J Clin Invest 2000;105:35–44.
95. Garcia KC, Degano M, Stanfield RL, et al. An ab T cell receptor structure at 2.5Å and its orientation in the TCR-MHC complex. Science 1996;274:209–19.
96. Gasser M, Waaga-Gasser AM, Kist-van Holthe JE, et al. Chronic rejection: insights from a novel immunosuppressive-free model of kidney transplantation. J Am Soc Nephrol 2004;15:687–94.
97. Gibson JM, Medawar PB. The fate of skin homografts in man. J Anat 1943;77:299–310.
98. Glotz D, Lucchiari N, Pegaz-Fiornet B, et al. Endothelial cells as targets of allograft rejection. Transplantation 2006;82(Suppl.): S19–21.
99. Golding H, Singer A. Role of accessory cell processing and presentation of shed H-2 alloantigens in allospecific cytotoxic T lymphocyte responses. J Immunol 1984;133:597–605.
100. Goldman M, Le Moine A, Braun M, et al. A role for eosinophils in transplant rejection. Trends Immunol 2001;22:247–51.
101. Goldstein DR, Tesar BM, Akira S, et al. Critical role of the Toll-like receptor signal adaptor protein MyD88 in acute allograft rejection. J Clin Invest 2003;111:1571–8.
102. Gondek DC, Lu LF, Quezada SA, et al. Cutting edge: contact-mediated suppression by CD4+CD25+ regulatory cells involves a granzyme B-dependent, perforin-independent mechanism. J Immunol 2005;174:1783–6.

103. Gorczynski RM. Immunosuppression induced by hepatic portal venous immunization spares reactivity in IL-4 producing T lymphocytes. Immunol Lett 1992;33:67–78.
104. Gorer PA. The antigenic basis of tumour transplantation. J Pathol Bacteriol 1938;47:231–52.
105. Goulmy E. Minor histocompatibility antigens: from transplantation problems to therapy of cancer. Hum Immunol 2006;67:433–8.
106. Grakoui A, Bromley SK, Sumen C, et al. The immunological synapse: a molecular machine controlling T cell activation. Science 1999;285:221–7.
107. Grandaliano G, Gesualdo L, Ranieri E, et al. Monocyte chemotactic peptide-1 expression and monocyte infiltration in acute renal transplant rejection. Transplantation 1997;63:414–20.
108. Greenfield A, Scott D, Pennisi D, et al. An H-YDb epitope is encoded by a novel mouse Y chromosome gene. Nat Genet 1996;14:474–8.
109. Greenwald RJ, Freeman GJ, Sharpe AH. The B7 family revisited. Annu Rev Immunol 2005;23:515–48.
110. Grgic I, Wulff H, Eichler I, et al. Blockade of T-lymphocyte KCa3.1 and Kv1.3 channels as novel immunosuppression strategy to prevent kidney allograft rejection. Transplant Proc 2009;41:2601–6.
111. Grohmann U, Orabona C, Fallarino F, et al. CTLA-4-Ig regulates tryptophan catabolism in vivo. Nat Immunol 2002;3:1097–101.
112. Guan H, Moretto M, Bzik DJ, et al. NK cells enhance dendritic cell response against parasite antigens via NKG2D pathway. J Immunol 2007;179:590–6.
113. Gurley KE, Lowry RP, Clarke-Forbes RD. Immune mechanisms in organ allograft rejection: II. T helper cells, delayed type hypersensitivity and rejection of renal allografts. Transplantation 1983;36:401–5.
114. Haas M, Segev DL, Racusen LC, et al. C4d deposition without rejection correlates with reduced early scarring in ABO-incompatible renal allografts. J Am Soc Nephrol 2009;20:197–204.
115. Hall BM, DeSaxe I, Dorsch SE. The cellular basis of allograft rejection in vivo: restoration of first set rejection of heart grafts by T helper cells in irradiated rats. Transplantation 1983;36:700–5.
116. Halloran PF, de Freitas DG, Einecke G, et al. An integrated view of molecular changes, histopathology and outcomes in kidney transplants. Am J Transplant 2010;10:2223–30.
117. Halloran PF, de Freitas DG, Einecke G, et al. The molecular phenotype of kidney transplants. Am J Transplant 2010;10:2215–22.
118. Hamel ME, Noteboom E, Kruisbeek AM. Non-responsiveness of antigen-experienced CD4 T cells reflects more stringent co-stimulatory requirements. Immunology 1998;93:366–75.
119. Hamerman JA, Ogasawara K, Lanier LL. NK cells in innate immunity. Curr Opin Immunol 2005;17:29–35.
120. Hancock WW. Chemokines and transplant immunobiology. J Am Soc Nephrol 2002;13:821–4.
121. Hancock WW, Gao W, Csizmadia V, et al. Donor-derived IP-10 initiates development of acute allograft rejection. J Exp Med 2001;193:975–80.
122. Hancock WW, Wang L, Ye Q, et al. Chemokines and their receptors as markers of allograft rejection and targets for immunosuppression. Curr Opin Immunol 2003;15:479–86.
123. Hanvesakul R, Kubal C, Moore J, et al. KIR and HLA-C interactions promote differential dendritic cell maturation and is a major determinant of graft failure following kidney transplantation. PLoS One 2011;6:e23631.
124. Hanvesakul R, Spencer N, Cook M, et al. Donor HLA-C genotype has a profound impact on the clinical outcome following liver transplantation. Am J Transplant 2008;8:1931–41.
125. Harshyne LA, Watkins SC, Gambotto A, et al. Dendritic cells acquire antigens from live cells for cross-presentation to CTL. J Immunol 2001;166:3717–23.
126. Hart DN, Fabre JW. Demonstration and characterisation of Ia positive dendritic cells in the interstitial connective tissues of the rat heart and other tissues, but not brain. J Exp Med 1981;154:347–61.
127. Hart DN, Fabre JW. Kidney-specific alloantigen system in the rat. Characterisation and role in transplantation. J Exp Med 1980;151:651–66.
128. Haug CE, Colvin RB, Delmonico FL, et al. A phase I trial of immunosuppression with anti-ICAM-1 (CD54) mAb in renal allograft recipients. Transplantation 1993;55:766–73.
129. Hayry P, Defendi V. Mixed lymphocyte cultures produce effector cells: model in vitro for allograft rejection. Science 1970;168:133–5.
130. Hayry P, Mennander A, Raisanen-Sokolowski A, et al. Pathophysiology of vascular wall changes in chronic allograft rejection. Transplant Rev 1993;7:1–20.
131. Henretta J, Araneda D, Pittman K, et al. Marked prolongation of incompatible class I deficient heart allografts: paradoxical effects between primarily and secondarily vascularized allografts. Transplant Proc 1995;27:1303–4.
132. Herberman RB, Djeu JY, Kay HD, et al. Natural killer cells: characteristics and regulation of activity. Immunol Rev 1979;44:43–70.
133. Herrera OB, Golshayan D, Tibbott R, et al. A novel pathway of alloantigen presentation by dendritic cells. J Immunol 2004;173:4828–37.
134. Hidalgo LG, Sellares J, Sis B, et al. Interpreting NK cell transcripts versus T cell transcripts in renal transplant biopsies. Am J Transplant 2012;12:1180–91.
135. Hirohashi T, Chase CM, Della Pelle P, et al. A novel pathway of chronic allograft rejection mediated by NK cells and alloantibody. Am J Transplant 2012;12:313–21.
136. Hirohashi T, Uehara S, Chase CM, et al. Complement independent antibody-mediated endarteritis and transplant arteriopathy in mice. Am J Transplant 2010;10:510–7.
137. Hodes RJ, Svedmyr EA. Specific cytotoxicity of H-2-incompatible mouse lymphocytes following mixed culture in vitro. Transplantation 1970;9:470–7.
138. Hoffmann P, Eder R, Edinger M. Polyclonal expansion of human CD4(+)CD25(+) regulatory T cells. Methods Mol Biol 2011;677:15–30.
139. Hornick PI, Mason PD, Baker RJ, et al. Significant frequencies of T cells with indirect anti-donor specificity in heart graft recipients with chronic rejection. Circulation 2000;101:2405–10.
140. Hosgood SA, Barlow AD, Yates PJ, et al. A pilot study assessing the feasibility of a short period of normothermic preservation in an experimental model of non heart beating donor kidneys. J Surg Res 2011;171:283–90.
141. Hourmant M, Bedrossian J, Durand D, et al. A randomized multicenter trial comparing leukocyte function-associated antigen-1 monoclonal antibody with rabbit antithymocyte globulin as induction treatment in first kidney transplantations. Transplantation 1996;62:1565–70.
142. Hourmant M, Cesbron-Gautier A, Terasaki PI, et al. Frequency and clinical implications of development of donor-specific and non-donor-specific HLA antibodies after kidney transplantation. J Am Soc Nephrol 2005;16:2804–12.
143. Hutchinson JA, Riquelme P, Sawitzki B, et al. Cutting edge: immunological consequences and trafficking of human regulatory macrophages administered to renal transplant recipients. J Immunol 2011;187:2072–8.
144. Imagawa DK, Millis JM, Olthoff KM, et al. The role of tumor necrosis factor in allograft rejection II. Evidence that antibody therapy against tumor necrosis factor-alpha and lymphotoxin enhances cardiac survival in rats. Transplantation 1990;50:189–93.
145. Imagawa DK, Millis JM, Olthoff KM, et al. The role of tumor necrosis factor in allograft rejection I. Evidence that elevated levels of tumor necrosis factor-alpha predict rejection following orthotopic liver transplantation. Transplantation 1990;50:219–25.
146. Imagawa DK, Millis JM, Seu P, et al. The role of tumor necrosis factor in allograft rejection. III. Evidence that anti-TNF antibody therapy prolongs allograft survival in rats with acute rejection. Transplantation 1991;51:57–62.
147. Ingham-Clark CL, Cunningham AJ, Crane PW, et al. Lymphocyte infiltration patterns in rat small-bowel transplants. Transplant Proc 1990;22:2460.
148. Ise W, Kohyama M, Nutsch KM, et al. CTLA-4 suppresses the pathogenicity of self antigen-specific T cells by cell-intrinsic and cell-extrinsic mechanisms. Nat Immunol 2010;11:129–35.
149. Iwasaki K, Miwa Y, Ogawa H, et al. Comparative study on signal transduction in endothelial cells after anti-a/b and human leukocyte antigen antibody reaction: implication of accommodation. Transplantation 2012;93:390–7.
150. Iwata T, Philipovskiy A, Fisher AJ, et al. Anti-type V collagen humoral immunity in lung transplant primary graft dysfunction. J Immunol 2008;181:5738–47.

151. Jenkins MK, Pardoll DM, Mizuguchi J, et al. Molecular events in the induction of a nonresponsive state in interleukin 2-producing helper T-lymphocyte clones. Proc Natl Acad Sci U S A 1987;84:5409–13.
152. Jenkins MK, Schwartz RH. Antigen presentation by chemically modified splenocytes induces antigen-specific T cell unresponsiveness in vitro and in vivo. J Exp Med 1987;165:302–19.
153. Jiang A, Bloom O, Ono S, et al. Disruption of E-cadherin-mediated adhesion induces a functionally distinct pathway of dendritic cell maturation. Immunity 2007;27:610–24.
154. Jiang H, Canfield SM, Gallagher MP, et al. HLA-E-restricted regulatory CD8(+) T cells are involved in development and control of human autoimmune type 1 diabetes. J Clin Invest 2010;120:3641–50.
155. Jiang S, Lechler RI. Regulatory T cells in the control of transplantation tolerance and autoimmunity. Am J Transplant 2003;3(5):516–24.
156. Jin YP, Fishbein MC, Said JW, et al. Anti-HLA class I antibody-mediated activation of the PI3K/Akt signaling pathway and induction of Bcl-2 and Bcl-xL expression in endothelial cells. Hum Immunol 2004;65:291–302.
157. Jin C, Flavell RA. Molecular mechanism of NLRP3 inflammasome activation. J Clin Immunol 2010;30:628–31.
158. Jindra PT, Jin YP, Rozengurt E, et al. HLA class I antibody-mediated endothelial cell proliferation via the mTOR pathway. J Immunol 2008;180:2357–66.
159. Jordan MS, Koretzky GA. Coordination of receptor signaling in multiple hematopoietic cell lineages by the adaptor protein SLP-76. Cold Spring Harbor Perspect Biol 2010;2:a002501.
160. Josien R, Pannetier C, Douillard P, et al. Graft-infiltrating T helper cells, CD45RC phenotype, and Th1/Th2-related cytokines in donor-specific transfusion-induced tolerance in adult rats. Transplantation 1995;60:1131–9.
161. Jurcevic S, Ainsworth ME, Pomerance A, et al. Antivimentin antibodies are an independent predictor of transplant-associated coronary artery disease after cardiac transplantation. Transplantation 2001;71:886–92.
162. Kagi D, Seiler P, Pavlovic J, et al. The roles of perforin- and Fas-dependent cytotoxicity in protection against cytopathic and non-cytopathic viruses. Eur J Immunol 1995;25:3256–62.
163. Karre K. NK cells, MHC class I molecules and the missing self. Scand J Immunol 2002;55:221–8.
164. Kawai K, Shahinian A, Mak TW, et al. Skin allograft rejection in CD28-deficient mice. Transplantation 1996;61:352–5.
165. Keller MR, Burlingham WJ. Loss of tolerance to self after transplant. Semin Immunopathol 2011;33:105–10.
166. Kim J, Chang CK, Hayden T, et al. The activating immunoreceptor NKG2D and its ligands are involved in allograft transplant rejection. J Immunol 2007;179:6416–20.
167. Kim PC, Levy GA, Koh I, et al. Immunologic basis of small intestinal allograft rejection. Transplant Proc 1991;23:830.
168. King KE, Warren DS, Samaniego-Picota M, et al. Antibody, complement and accommodation in ABO-incompatible transplants. Curr Opin Immunol 2004;16:545–9.
169. Kirby JA. Function of leucocyte adhesion molecules during allograft rejection. In: Tilney NL, Strom TB, Paul LC, editors. Transplantation biology: cellular and molecular aspects. Philadelphia: Lippincott-Raven; 1996.
170. Kirk AD, Burkly LC, Batty DS, et al. Treatment with humanized monoclonal antibody against CD154 prevents acute renal allograft rejection in nonhuman primates. Nat Med 1999;5:686–93.
171. Kirwan SE, Burshtyn DN. Regulation of natural killer cell activity. Curr Opin Immunol 2007;19:46–54.
172. Kishimoto K, Yuan X, Auchincloss Jr H, et al. Mechanism of action of donor-specific transfusion in inducing tolerance: role of donor MHC molecules, donor co-stimulatory molecules, and indirect antigen presentation. J Am Soc Nephrol 2004;15:2423–8.
173. Kissmeyer-Nielsen F, Olsen S, Petersen VP, et al. Hyperacute rejection of kidney allografts associated with pre-existing humoral antibodies against donor cells. Lancet 1966;2:662–5.
174. Kleijwegt FS, Laban S, Duinkerken G, et al. Transfer of regulatory properties from tolerogenic to proinflammatory dendritic cells via induced autoreactive regulatory T cells. J Immunol 2011;187:6357–64.
175. Klein J, Chiang CL, Hauptfeld V. Histocompatibility antigens controlled by the I region of the murine H-2 complex. J Exp Med 1977;145:450–4.
176. Knechtle SJ, Halperin EC, Murphy CE, et al. The effect of cyclosporine, total lymphoid irradiation, and cobra venom factor on hyperacute rejection. J Heart Transplant 1985;4:541–5.
177. Koo DD, Welsh KI, Roake JR, et al. Ischemia/reperfusion injury in human kidney transplantation: an immunohistochemical analysis of changes after reperfusion. Am J Pathol 1998;153:557–66.
178. Kormendi F, Amend WJC. The importance of eosinophil cells in kidney allograft rejection. Transplantation 1988;45:537–9.
179. Koudstaal LG, Ottens PJ, Uges DR, et al. Increased intestinal permeability in deceased brain dead rats. Transplantation 2009;88:444–6.
180. Krieger NR, Yin DP, Fathman CG. CD4+ but not CD8+ cells are essential for allorejection. J Exp Med 1996;184:2013–8.
181. Kruger B, Krick S, Dhillon N, et al. Donor Toll-like receptor 4 contributes to ischemia and reperfusion injury following human kidney transplantation. Proc Natl Acad Sci U S A 2009;106:3390–5.
182. Krummel MF, Allison JP. CTLA-4 engagement inhibits IL-2 accumulation and cell cycle progression upon activation of resting T cells. J Exp Med 1996;183:2533–40.
183. Kubal C, Cockwell P, Gunson B, et al. Chronic kidney disease after nonrenal solid organ transplantation: a histological assessment and utility of chronic allograft damage index scoring. Transplantation 2012;93:406–11.
184. Kundig TM, Shahinian A, Kawai K, et al. Duration of TCR stimulation determines costimulatory requirement of T cells. Immunity 1996;5:41–52.
185. Lachmann N, Terasaki PI, Budde K, et al. Anti-human leukocyte antigen and donor-specific antibodies detected by luminex posttransplant serve as biomarkers for chronic rejection of renal allografts. Transplantation 2009;87:1505–13.
186. Lafferty KJ, Bootes A, Dart G, et al. Effect of organ culture on the survival of thyroid allografts in mice. Transplantation 1976;22:138–49.
187. Lakkis FG. Where is the alloimmune response initiated? Am J Transplant 2003;3:241–2.
188. Lakkis FG, Arakelov A, Konieczny BT, et al. Immunologic “ignorance” of vascularized organ transplants in the absence of secondary lymphoid tissue. Nat Med 2000;6:686–8.
189. Lamb JR, Skidmore BJ, Green JM, et al. Induction of tolerance in influenza virus-immune T lymphocyte clones with synthetic peptides of influenza haemagglutinin. J Exp Med 1983;157:1434–47.
190. Larsen CP, Alexander DZ, Hollenbaugh D, et al. CD40-gp39 Interactions play a critical role during allograft rejection: suppression of allograft rejection by blockade of the CD40-gp39 pathway. Transplantation 1996;61:4–9.
191. Larsen CP, Elwood ET, Alexander DZ, et al. Long term acceptance of skin and cardiac allografts after blocking CD40 and CD28 pathways. Nature 1996;381:434–8.
192. Larsen CP, Morris PJ, Austyn JM. Migration of dendritic leukocytes from cardiac allografts into host spleens. A novel pathway for initiation of rejection. J Exp Med 1990;171:307–14.
193. Larsen CP, Steinman RM, Witmer-Pack M, et al. Migration and maturation of Langerhans cells in skin transplants and explants. J Exp Med 1990;172:1483–93.
194. Laskowski I, Pratschke J, Wilhelm MJ, et al. Molecular and cellular events associated with ischemia/reperfusion injury. Ann Transplant 2000;5:29–35.
195. Le Bas-Bernardet S, Blancho G. Antibodies directed against AB blood antigens or human leukocyte antigen molecules activate different intracellular pathways explaining their differential effects toward accommodation. Transplantation 2012;93:354–5.
196. Lechler RI, Garden OA, Turka LA. The complementary roles of deletion and regulation in transplantation tolerance. Nat Rev Immunol 2003;3(2):147–58.
197. Lee RS, Grusby MJ, Glimcher LH, et al. Indirect recognition by helper cells can induce donor-specific cytotoxic T lymphocytes in vivo. J Exp Med 1994;179:865–72.
198. Lee RS, Grusby MJ, Laufer TM, et al. CD8+ effector cells responding to residual class I antigens, with help from CD4+ cells stimulated indirectly, cause rejection of “major histocompatibility complex-deficient” skin grafts. Transplantation 1997;63:1123–33.
199. Lee CY, Lotfi-Emran S, Erdinc M, et al. The involvement of FcR mechanisms in antibody-mediated rejection. Transplantation 2007;84:1324–34.
200. Lehner PJ, Cresswell P. Recent developments in MHC-class-I-mediated antigen presentation. Curr Opin Immunol 2004;16:82–9.

201. Le-Moine A, Flamand V, Demoor FX, et al. Critical roles for IL-4, IL-5 and eosinophils in chronic skin allograft rejection. J Clin Invest 1999;103:1659–67.
202. Le-Moine A, Surquin M, Demoor FX, et al. IL-5 mediates eosinophilic rejection of MHC class II-disparate skin allografts in mice. J Immunol 1999;163:3778.
203. Lenschow DJ, Herold KC, Rhee L, et al. CD28/B7 regulation of Th1 and Th2 subsets in the development of autoimmune diabetes. Immunity 1996;5:285–93.
204. Lentsch AB, Yoshidome H, Cheadle WG, et al. Chemokine involvement in hepatic ischemia/reperfusion injury in mice: roles for macrophage inflammatory protein-2 and KC. [corrected and republished article, originally printed in Hepatology 1998;27:507–512] Hepatology 1998;27:1172–7.
205. Li K, Fazekasova H, Wang N, et al. Functional modulation of human monocytes derived DCs by anaphylatoxins C3a and C5a. Immunobiology 2012;217:65–73.
206. Li X, Faustman D. Use of donor beta 2-microglobulin-deficient transgenic mouse liver cells for isografts, allografts and xenografts. Transplantation 1993;55:940–6.
207. Linsley PS, Clark EA, Ledbetter JA. T-cell antigen CD28 mediates adhesion with B cells by interacting with activation antigen B7/BB-1. Proc Natl Acad Sci U S A 1990;87:5031–5.
208. Linterman MA, Vinuesa CG. Signals that influence T follicular helper cell differentiation and function. Semin Immunopathol 2010;32:183–96.
209. Ljunggren HG, Karre K. In search of the "missing self": MHC molecules and NK cell recognition. Immunol Today 1990;11:237–44.
210. Little CC, Tyzer EE. Further experimental studies on the inheritance of susceptibility to a transplantable tumour carcinoma (JWA) of the Japanese Waltzing mouse. J Med Res 1916;33:393–453.
211. Lo DJ, Weaver TA, Stempora L, et al. Selective targeting of human alloresponsive CD8+ effector memory T cells based on CD2 expression. Am J Transplant 2011;11:22–33.
212. Lo LJ, Go AS, Chertow GM, et al. Dialysis-requiring acute renal failure increases the risk of progressive chronic kidney disease. Kidney Int 2009;76:893–9.
213. Lombardi G, Sidhu S, Batchelor R, et al. Anergic T cells as suppressor cells in vitro. Science 1994;264:1587–9.
214. Lombardi G, Sidhu S, Daly M, et al. Are primary alloresponses truly primary? Int Immunol 1990;2:9–13.
215. Love PE, Hayes SM. ITAM-mediated signaling by the T-cell antigen receptor. Cold Spring Harbor Perspect Biol 2010;2:a002485.
216. Loveland BE, Hogarth PM, Ceredig R, et al. Delayed type hypersensitivity and allograft rejection in the mouse: correlation of effector cell phenotype. J Exp Med 1981;153:1044–57.
217. Lowry RP, Blais D. Tumour necrosis factor alpha in rejecting rat cardiac allografts. Transplant Proc 1988;20:245–7.
218. Lowry RP, Gurley KE, Forbes RD. Immune mechanisms in organ allograft rejection. I. Delayed-type hypersensitivity and lymphocytotoxicity in heart graft rejection. Transplantation 1983;36:391–401.
219. Lunsford KE, Horne PH, Koester MA, et al. Activation and maturation of alloreactive CD4-independent, CD8 cytolytic T cells. Am J Transplant 2006;6:2268–81.
220. Macdonald FI, Ashraf S, Picton M, et al. Banff criteria as predictors of outcome following acute renal allograft rejection. Nephrol Dial Transplant 1999;14:1692–7.
221. Mackay CR. Homing of naive, memory and effector lymphocytes. Curr Opin Immunol 1993;5:423–7.
222. Mackay CR. Immunological memory. Adv Immunol 1993;53:217–65.
223. Madsen JC, Peugh WN, Wood KJ, et al. The effect of anti-L3T4 monoclonal antibody treatment on first-set rejection of murine cardiac allografts. Transplantation 1987;44:849–52.
224. Mahnke K, Enk AH. Dendritic cells: key cells for the induction of regulatory T cells? Curr Top Microbiol Immunol 2005;293:133–50.
225. Maloy KJ, Powrie F. Fueling regulation: IL-2 keeps CD4+ Treg cells fit. Nat Immunol 2005;6:1071–2.
226. Mandal AK, Snyder JJ, Gilbertson DT, et al. Does cadaveric donor renal transplantation ever provide better outcomes than live-donor renal transplantation? Transplantation 2003;75:494–500.
227. Mandelbrot DA, Furukawa Y, McAdam AJ, et al. Expression of B7 molecules in recipient, not donor, mice determines the survival of cardiac allografts. J Immunol 1999;163:3753–7.
228. Mandrup-Poulsen T, Bendtzen K, Nerup J. Affinity-purified human interleukin I is cytotoxic to isolated islets of Langerhans. Diabetologia 1986;29:63–7.
229. Mandrup-Poulsen T, Helqvist S, Molvig J, et al. Cytokines as immune effector molecules in autoimmune endocrine diseases with special reference to insulin-dependent diabetes mellitus. Autoimmunity 1989;4:191–218.
230. Manicassamy S, Reizis B, Ravindran R, et al. Activation of beta-catenin in dendritic cells regulates immunity versus tolerance in the intestine. Science 2010;329:849–53.
231. Mannon RB. Macrophages: contributors to allograft dysfunction, repair, or innocent bystanders? Curr Opin Organ Transplant 2012;17:20–5.
232. Mannon RB, Nataraj C, Kotzin BL, et al. Rejection of kidney allografts by MHC class 1-deficient mice. Transplantation 1995;59:746–55.
233. Marelli-Berg FM, Barroso-Herrera O, Lechler RI. Recently activated T cells are costimulation-dependent in vitro. Cell Immunol 1999;195:18–27.
234. Marelli-Berg FM, Frasca L, Weng L, et al. Antigen recognition influences transendothelial migration of CD4+ T cells. J Immunol 1999;162:696–703.
235. Mariathasan S, Weiss DS, Newton K, et al. Cryopyrin activates the inflammasome in response to toxins and ATP. Nature 2006;440:228–32.
236. Mason DW, Dallman MJ, Barclay AN. Graft-versus-host disease induces expression of Ia antigen in rat epidermal cells and gut epithelium. Nature 1981;293:150–1.
237. Mason DW, Morris PJ. Inhibition of the accumulation, in rat kidney allografts, of specific – but not nonspecific – cytotoxic cells by cyclosporine. Transplantation 1984;37(1):46–51.
238. Matzinger P. Tolerance, danger, and the extended family. Annu Rev Immunol 1994;12:991–1045.
239. Mauiyyedi S, Pelle PD, Saidman S, et al. Chronic humoral rejection: identification of antibody-mediated chronic renal allograft rejection by C4d deposits in peritubular capillaries. J Am Soc Nephrol 2001;12:574–82.
240. Mauri C, Bosma A. Immune regulatory function of B cells. Annu Rev Immunol 2012;30:221–41.
241. McEver RP, Beckstead JH, Moore KL, et al. GMP-140, a platelet alpha-granule membrane protein, is also synthesized by vascular endothelial cells and is localized in Weibel-Palade bodies. J Clin Invest 1989;84:92–9.
242. McKay D, Shigeoka A, Rubinstein M, et al. Simultaneous deletion of MyD88 and Trif delays major histocompatibility and minor antigen mismatch allograft rejection. Eur J Immunol 2006;36:1994–2002.
243. McLean AG, Hughes D, Welsh KI, et al. Patterns of graft infiltration and cytokine gene expression during the first 10 days of kidney transplantion. Transplantation 1997;63:374–80.
244. Medawar PB. Behaviour and fate of skin autografts and skin homografts in rabbits. J Anat 1944;78:176–99.
245. Medawar PB. A second study of the behaviour and fate of skin homografts in rabbits. J Anat 1945;79:157–76.
246. Medawar PB. Immunity to homologous grafted skin. III. The fate of skin homografts transplanted to the brain, to subcutaneous tissue and to the anterior chamber of the eye. Br J Exp Pathol 1948;29:58–69.
247. Meleg-Smith S, Gauthier PM. Abundance of interstitial eosinophils in renal allografts is associated with vascular rejection. Transplantation 2005;79:444–50.
248. Mengel M, Sis B, Haas M, et al. Banff 2011 meeting report: new concepts in antibody-mediated rejection. Am J Transplant 2012;12:563–70.
249. Mennander A, Tisala S, Paavonen T, et al. Chronic rejection of rat aortic allograft. II. Administration of cyclosporine induces accelerated allograft arteriosclerosis. Transpl Int 1991;4:173–9.
250. Merani S, Truong WW, Hancock W, et al. Chemokines and their receptors in islet allograft rejection and as targets for tolerance induction. Cell Transplant 2006;15:295–309.
251. Milner CM, Campbell RD. Genetic organization of the human MHC class III region. Front Biosci 2001;6:D914–26.

252. Mintz B, Silvers WK. Histocompatibility antigens on melanoblasts and hair follicle cells. Cell-localized homograft rejection in allophenic skin grafts. Transplantation 1970;9:497–505.
253. Mintz B, Silvers WK. "Intrinsic" immunological tolerance in allophenic mice. Science 1967;158:1484–6.
254. Mohler KM, Streilein JW. Lymphokine production by MLR-reactive reaction lymphocytes obtained from normal mice and mice rendered tolerant of class II MHC antigens. Transplantation 1989;47:625–33.
255. Monaco JJ. Major histocompatibility complex-linked transport proteins and antigen processing. Immunol Res 1992;11:125–32.
256. Monaco JJ. Pathways for the processing and presentation of antigens to T cells. J Leukoc Biol 1995;57:543–7.
257. Monaco JJ. Structure and function of genes in the MHC class II region. Curr Opin Immunol 1993;5:17–20.
258. Montgomery JR, Berger JC, Warren DS, et al. Outcomes of ABO-incompatible kidney transplantation in the United States. Transplantation 2012;93:603–9.
259. Moore J, Middleton L, Cockwell P, et al. Calcineurin inhibitor sparing with mycophenolate in kidney transplantation: a systematic review and meta-analysis. Transplantation 2009;87:591–605.
260. Moore J, Tan K, Cockwell P, et al. Predicting early renal allograft function using clinical variables. Nephrol Dial Transplant 2007;22:2669–77.
261. Morikawa M, Tamatani T, Miyasaka M, et al. Cardiac allografts in rat recipients with simultaneous use of anti-ICAM-1 and anti-LFA-1 monoclonal antibodies leads to accelerated graft loss. Immunopharmacology 1994;28:171–82.
262. Morris GP, Ni PP, Allen PM. Alloreactivity is limited by the endogenous peptide repertoire. Proc Natl Acad Sci U S A 2011;108:3695–700.
263. Morris PJ, Ting A. Studies of HLA-DR with relevance to renal transplantation. Immunol Rev 1982;66:103–31.
264. Moss CX, Tree TI, Watts C. Reconstruction of a pathway of antigen processing and class II MHC peptide capture. EMBO J 2007;26:2137–47.
265. Murphy WJ, Kumar V, Bennett M. Acute rejection of murine bone marrow allografts by natural killer cells and T cells. Differences in kinetics and target antigens recognized. J Exp Med 1987;166:1499–509.
266. Murphy WJ, Kumar V, Bennett M. Rejection of bone marrow allografts by mice with severe combined immune deficiency (SCID): evidence that NK cells can mediate the specificity of marrow graft rejection. J Exp Med 1987;165:1212–7.
267. Murphy SP, Porrett PM, Turka LA. Innate immunity in transplant tolerance and rejection. Immunol Rev 2011;241:39–48.
268. Murphy KP, Travers P, Walport M. Janeway's immunobiology. 8th edn. New York: Taylor & Francis; 2011.
269. Nadazdin O, Boskovic S, Wee SL, et al. Contributions of direct and indirect alloresponses to chronic rejection of kidney allografts in nonhuman primates. J Immunol 2011;187:4589–97.
270. Nadig SN, Wieckiewicz J, Wu DC, et al. In vivo prevention of transplant arteriosclerosis by ex vivo-expanded human regulatory T cells. Nat Med 2010;16:809–13.
271. Najafian N, Salama AD, Fedoseyeva EV, et al. Enzyme-linked immunosorbent spot assay analysis of peripheral blood lymphocyte reactivity to donor HLA-DR peptides: potential novel assay for prediction of outcomes for renal transplant recipients. J Am Soc Nephrol 2002;13:252–9.
272. Nakhaei P, Genin P, Civas A, et al. RIG-I-like receptors: sensing and responding to RNA virus infection. Semin Immunol 2009;21:215–22.
273. Nankivell BJ, Borrows RJ, Fung CL, et al. The natural history of chronic allograft nephropathy. N Engl J Med 2003;349:2326–33.
274. Narayanan K, Jaramillo A, Phelan DL, et al. Pre-exposure to sub-saturating concentrations of HLA class I antibodies confers resistance to endothelial cells against antibody complement-mediated lysis by regulating Bad through the phosphatidylinositol 3-kinase/Akt pathway. Eur J Immunol 2004;34:2303–12.
275. Nath DS, Basha HI, Mohanakumar T. Antihuman leukocyte antigen antibody-induced autoimmunity: role in chronic rejection. Curr Opin Organ Transplant 2010;15:16–20.
276. Nath N, Bian H, Reed EF, et al. HLA class I-mediated induction of cell proliferation involves cyclin E-mediated inactivation of Rb function and induction of E2F activity. J Immunol 1999;162:5351–8.
277. Nemoto T, Burne MJ, Daniels F, et al. Small molecule selectin ligand inhibition improves outcome in ischemic acute renal failure. Kidney Int 2001;60:2205–14.
278. Newell EW, Sigal N, Bendall SC, et al. Cytometry by time-of-flight shows combinatorial cytokine expression and virus-specific cell niches within a continuum of CD8+ T cell phenotypes. Immunity 2012;36:142–52.
279. Ng YH, Oberbarnscheidt MH, Chandramoorthy HC, et al. B cells help alloreactive T cells differentiate into memory T cells. Am J Transplant 2010;10:1970–80.
280. Nolan CR, Saenz KP, Thomas CA, et al. Role of eosinophils in chronic vascular rejection in renal allografts. Am J Kidney Dis 1995;26:634–42.
281. Noorchashm H, Reed AJ, Rostami SY, et al. B cell-mediated antigen presentation is required for the pathogenesis of acute cardiac allograft rejection. J Immunol 2006;177:7715–22.
282. Obhrai J, Goldstein DR. The role of Toll-like receptors in solid organ transplantation. Transplantation 2006;81:497–502.
283. O'Boyle G, Ali S, Kirby JA. Chemokines in transplantation: what can atypical receptors teach us about anti-inflammatory therapy? Transplant Rev (Orlando) 2011;25:136–44.
284. O'Brien SJ, Roelke ME, Marker L, et al. Genetic basis for species vunerability in the cheetah. Science 1985;227:1428–34.
285. Ohnmacht C, Pullner A, King SB, et al. Constitutive ablation of dendritic cells breaks self-tolerance of CD4 T cells and results in spontaneous fatal autoimmunity. J Exp Med 2009;206:549–59.
286. Oppenheim JJ, Wang JM, Chertov O, et al. The role of chemokines in transplantation. In: Tilney NL, Strom TB, Paul LC, editors. Transplantation biology: cellular and molecular aspects. Philadelphia: Lippincott-Raven; 1996. p. 187–200.
287. Osorio RW, Ascher NL, Jaenisch R, et al. Major histocompatibility complex class 1 deficiency prolongs islet allograft survival. Diabetes 1993;42:1520–7.
288. Palomares O, O'Mahony L, Akdis CA. The many routes of dendritic cells to ensure immune regulation. J Allergy Clin Immunol 2011;127:1541–2.
289. Parham P, Clayberger C, Zorn SL, et al. Inhibition of alloreactive cytotoxic T lymphocytes by peptides from the OL2 domain of HLA-A2. Nature 1987;325:625–8.
290. Palomares O, O'Mahony L, Akdis CA. The many routes of dendritic cells to ensure immune regulation. J Allergy Clin Immunol 2011;127:1541–2.
291. Patel R, Terasaki PI. Significance of the positive crossmatch test in kidney transplantation. N Engl J Med 1969;280:735–9.
292. Paul LC, Benediktsson H. Chronic transplant rejection: magnitude of the problem and pathogenetic mechanisms. Transplant Rev 1993;7:96–113.
293. Paul LC, Saito K, Davidoff A, et al. Growth factor transcripts in rat renal transplants. Am J Kidney Dis 1996;28:441–50.
294. Paul WE. Fundamental immunology. 6th ed. Philadelphia: Wolters Kluwer/Lippincott Williams & Wilkins; 2008.
295. Pearson TC, Alexander DZ, Winn KJ, et al. Transplantation tolerance induced by CTLA-4 Ig. Transplantation 1994;57:1701–6.
296. Perlmann P, Holm G. Cytotoxic effects of lymphoid cells in vitro. Adv Immunol 1969;11:117–93.
297. Peugh WN, Superina RA, Wood KJ, et al. The role of H-2 and non-H-2 antigens and genes in the rejection of murine cardiac allografts. Immunogenetics 1986;23:30–7.
298. Philpott DJ, Girardin SE. Nod-like receptors: sentinels at host membranes. Curr Opin Immunol 2010;22:428–34.
299. Picker LJ, Butcher EC. Physiological and molecular mechanisms of lymphocyte homing. Annu Rev Immunol 1992;10:561–91.
300. Pober JS, Gimbrone Jr MA, Lapierre LA, et al. Overlapping patterns of activation of human endothelial cells by interleukin 1, tumour necrosis factor and immune interferon. J Immunol 1986;137:1893–6.
301. Poggio ED, Clemente M, Riley J, et al. Alloreactivity in renal transplant recipients with and without chronic allograft nephropathy. J Am Soc Nephrol 2004;15:1952–60.
302. Pratschke J, Paz D, Wilhelm MJ, et al. Donor hypertension increases graft immunogenicity and intensifies chronic changes in long-surviving renal allografts. Transplantation 2004;77:43–8.
303. Pratt JR, Basheer SA, Sacks SH. Local synthesis of complement component C3 regulates acute renal transplant rejection. Nat Med 2002;8:582–7.

304. Pulendran B, Tang H, Manicassamy S. Programming dendritic cells to induce T(H)2 and tolerogenic responses. Nat Immunol 2010;11:647–55.
305. Qin S, Cobbold SP, Pope H, et al. "Infectious" transplantation tolerance. Science 1993;259:974–7.
306. Quiroga I, McShane P, Koo DD, et al. Major effects of delayed graft function and cold ischaemia time on renal allograft survival. Nephrol Dial Transplant 2006;21:1689–96.
307. Qureshi F, Rabb H, Kasiske BL. Silent acute rejection during prolonged delayed graft function reduces kidney allograft survival. Transplantation 2002;74:1400–4.
308. Rabinovitch A, Pukel C, Baquerizo H. Interleukin-1 inhibits glucose-modulated insulin and glucagon secretion in rat islet monolayer cultures. Endocrinology 1988;122:2393–8.
309. Rammensee H-G, Falk K, Rotzschke O. Peptides naturally presented by MHC class I molecules. Annu Rev Immunol 1993;11:213–44.
310. Reis e Sousa C, Stahl PD, Austyn JM. Phagocytosis of antigens by Langerhans cells in vitro. J Exp Med 1993;178:509–19.
311. Reyes-Vargas E, Pavlov IY, Martins TB, et al. Binding of anti-HLA class I antibody to endothelial cells produce an inflammatory cytokine secretory pattern. J Clin Lab Anal 2009;23:157–60.
312. Ricklin D, Hajishengallis G, Yang K, et al. Complement: a key system for immune surveillance and homeostasis. Nat Immunol 2010;11:785–97.
313. Riley JL, June CH. The CD28 family: a T-cell rheostat for therapeutic control of T-cell activation. Blood 2005;105:13–21.
314. Rissoan M-C, Soumelis V, Kadowaki N, et al. Reciprocal control of T helper cell and dendritic cell differentiation. Science 1999;283:1183–6.
315. Robertson H, Wong WK, Talbot D, et al. Tubulitis after renal transplantation: demonstration of an association between CD103+ T cells, transforming growth factor beta1 expression and rejection grade. Transplantation 2001;71:306–13.
316. Robinson JH, Delvig AA. Diversity in MHC class II antigen presentation. Immunology 2002;105:252–62.
317. Roche PA. HLA-DM: an in vivo facilitator of MHC class II peptide loading. Immunity 1995;3:259–62.
318. Roopenian D, Choi EY, Brown A. The immunogenomics of minor histocompatibility antigens. Immunol Rev 2002;190:86–94.
319. Rosenberg AS. The T, cell populations mediating rejection of MHC class I disparate skin grafts in mice. Transpl Immunol 1993;2:93–9.
320. Rosenberg AS, Mizuochi T, Singer A. Analysis of T cell subsets in rejection of K^b mutant skin allografts differing at class I MHC. Nature 1986;322:829–31.
321. Rosenberg AS, Singer A. Cellular basis of skin allograft rejection: an in vivo model of immune-mediated tissue destruction. Annu Rev Immunol 1992;10:333–58.
322. Ross R, Glomset JA. The pathogenesis of atherosclerosis. N Engl J Med 1976;295:369–77.
323. Rossi D, Zlotnik A. The biology of chemokines and their receptors. Annu Rev Immunol 2000;18:217–42.
324. Rotschke O, Falk K, Faath S, et al. On the nature of peptides involved in T cell alloreactivity. J Exp Med 1991;174:1059–71.
325. Rudolph MG, Stanfield RL, Wilson IA. How TCRs bind MHCs, peptides, and coreceptors. Annu Rev Immunol 2006;24:419–66.
326. Russo V, Zhou D, Sartirana C, et al. Acquisition of intact allogeneic human leukocyte antigen molecules by human dendritic cells. Blood 2000;95:3473–7.
327. Rydberg L. ABO-incompatibility in solid organ transplantation. Transfus Med 2001;11:325–42.
328. Sacks SH. Complement fragments C3a and C5a: the salt and pepper of the immune response. Eur J Immunol 2010;40:668–70.
329. Sakaguchi S, Ono M, Setoguchi R, et al. Foxp3+ CD25+ CD4+ natural regulatory T cells in dominant self-tolerance and autoimmune disease. Immunol Rev 2006;212:8–27.
330. Salama AD, Delikouras A, Pusey CD, et al. Transplant accommodation in highly sensitized patients: a potential role for Bcl-xL and alloantibody. Am J Transplant 2001;1:260–9.
331. Saleem S, Konieczny BT, Lowry RP, et al. Acute rejection of vascularized heart allografts in the absence of IFNγ. Transplantation 1996;62:1908–11.
332. Sallusto F, Lanzavecchia A. Heterogeneity of CD4+ memory T cells: functional modules for tailored immunity. Eur J Immunol 2009;39:2076–82.
333. Santamaria-Babi LF, Moser R, Perez-Soler MT, et al. Migration of skin-homing T cells across cytokine-activated human endothial cell layers involves interaction of the cutaneous lymphocyte-associated antigen (CLA), the very late antigen-4 (VLA-4) and the lymphocyte function-associated antigen-1 (LFA-1). J Immunol 1995;154:1543–50.
334. Sauve D, Baratin M, Leduc C, et al. Alloantibody production is regulated by CD4+ T cells' alloreactive pathway, rather than precursor frequency or Th1/Th2 differentiation. Am J Transplant 2004;4:1237–45.
335. Sawitzki B, Kingsley CI, Oliveira V, et al. IFN-gamma production by alloantigen-reactive regulatory T cells is important for their regulatory function in vivo. J Exp Med 2005;201:1925–35.
336. Sayegh MH, Akalin E, Hancock WW, et al. CD28-B7 blockade after alloantigenic challenge in vivo inhibits Th1 cytokines but spares Th2. J Exp Med 1995;181:1869–74.
337. Schilham MW, Fung-Leung WP, Rahemtulla A, et al. Alloreactive cytotoxic T cells can develop and function in mice lacking both CD4 and CD8. Eur J Immunol 1993;23:1299–304.
338. Schliesser U, Streitz M, Sawitzki B. Tregs: application for solid-organ transplantation. Curr Opin Organ Transplant 2012;17(1):34–41.
339. Schneider H, Downey J, Smith A, et al. Reversal of the TCR stop signal by CTLA-4. Science 2006;313:1972–5.
340. Schroder K, Tschopp J. The inflammasomes. Cell 2010;140:821–32.
341. Schulz M, Schuurman HJ, Joergensen J, et al. Acute rejection of vascular heart allografts by perforin-deficient mice. Eur J Immunol 1995;25:474–80.
342. Schwartz JC, Zhang X, Nathenson SG, et al. Structural mechanisms of costimulation. Nat Immunol 2002;3:427–34.
343. Schwartz RH. A cell culture model for T lymphocyte clonal anergy. Science 1990;248:1349–56.
344. Schwartz RH. T cell clonal anergy. Curr Opin Immunol 1997;9:351–7.
345. Scott DM, Ehrmann IE, Ellis PS, et al. Identification of a mouse male-specific transplantation antigen, H-Y. Nature 1995;376:695–8.
346. Scott DM, Ehrmann IE, Ellis PS, et al. Why do some females reject males? The molecular basis for male-specific graft rejection. J Mol Med 1997;75:103–14.
347. Seetharam A, Tiriveedhi V, Mohanakumar T. Alloimmunity and autoimmunity in chronic rejection. Curr Opin Organ Transplant 2010;15:531–6.
348. Selvaggi G, Ricordi C, Podack ER, et al. The role of the perforin and Fas pathways of cytotoxicity in skin graft rejection. Transplantation 1996;62:1912–5.
349. Sharif A, Shabir S, Chand S, et al. Meta-analysis of calcineurin-inhibitor-sparing regimens in kidney transplantation. J Am Soc Nephrol 2011;22:2107–18.
350. Sharpe AH, Abbas AK. T-cell costimulation – biology, therapeutic potential, and challenges. N Engl J Med 2006;355:973–5.
351. Shastri N, Cardinaud S, Schwab SR, et al. All the peptides that fit: the beginning, the middle, and the end of the MHC class I antigen-processing pathway. Immunol Rev 2005;207:31–41.
352. Shirwan H. Chronic allograft rejection. Do the Th2 cells preferentially induced by indirect alloantigen recognition play a dominant role? Transplantation 1999;68:715–26.
353. Shreeder V, Moodycliffe AM, Ullrich SE, et al. Dendritic cells require T cells for functional maturation in vivo. Immunity 1999;11:625–36.
354. Simitsek PD, Campbell DG, Lanzavecchia A, et al. Modulation of antigen processing by bound antibodies can boost or suppress class II major histocompatibility complex presentation of different T cell determinants. J Exp Med 1995;181:1957–63.
355. Simpson E, Roopenian D, Goulmy E. Much ado about minor histocompatibility antigens. Immunol Today 1998;19:108–12.
356. Smith HJ, Hanvesakul R, Bentall A, et al. T lymphocyte responses to nonpolymorphic HLA-derived peptides are associated with chronic renal allograft dysfunction. Transplantation 2011;91:279–86.
357. Snanoudj R, Royal V, Elie C, et al. Specificity of histological markers of long-term CNI nephrotoxicity in kidney-transplant recipients under low-dose cyclosporine therapy. Am J Transplant 2011;11:2635–46.
358. Snider ME, Steinmuller D. Nonspecific tissue destruction as a consequence of cytotoxic T lymphocyte interaction with antigen-specific target cells. Transplant Proc 1987;19:421–3.

359. Soares MP, Lin Y, Anrather J, et al. Expression of heme oxygenase-1 can determine cardiac xenograft survival. Nat Med 1998;4:1073–7.
360. Sprent J, Schaeffer M, Lo D, et al. Properties of purified T cell subsets II. In vivo class I vs class II H-2 differences. J Exp Med 1986;163:998–1011.
361. Starzl TE, Marchioro TL, Holmes JH, et al. Renal homografts in patients with major donor-recipient blood group incompatibilities. Surgery 1964;55:195–200.
362. Stegall MD, Diwan T, Raghavaiah S, et al. Terminal complement inhibition decreases antibody-mediated rejection in sensitized renal transplant recipients. Am J Transplant 2011;11:2405–13.
363. Steiger J, Nickerson PW, Steurer W, et al. IL-2 knockout recipient mice reject islet cell allografts. J Immunol 1995;155:489–98.
364. Steinman RM, Gutchinov B, Witmer MD, et al. Dendritic cells are the peripheral stimulators of the primary mixed leukocyte reaction in mice. J Exp Med 1983;157:613–27.
365. Steinman RM, Hawiger D, Nussenzweig MC. Tolerogenic dendritic cells. Annu Rev Immunol 2003;21:685–711.
366. Steinman RM, Hemmi H. Dendritic cells: translating innate to adaptive immunity. Curr Top Microbiol Immunol 2006;311:17–58.
367. Steinman RM, Witmer MD. Lymphoid dendritic cells are potent stimulations of the primary mixed leucocyte reaction in mice. Proc Natl Acad Sci U S A 1978;75:5132–6.
368. Steinmuller D, Wachtal SS. Passenger leukocytes and induction of allograft immunity. Transplant Proc 1980;12:100–6.
369. Stepkowski SM. Therapeutic potential for adhesion antagonists in organ transplantation. Curr Opin Organ Transplant 2002;7:366–72.
370. Stepkowski SM, Chen W, Geary R, et al. An oral formulation for intracellular adhesion molecules-1 antisense oligonucleotides. Transplant Proc 2001;33:3271.
371. Subramanian S, Bowyer MW, Egan JC, et al. Attenuation of renal ischemia-reperfusion injury with selectin inhibition in a rabbit model. Am J Surg 1999;178:573–6.
372. Superina RA, Peugh WN, Wood KJ, et al. Assessment of primarily vascularized cardiac allografts in mice. Transplantation 1986;42:226–7.
373. Suri A, Lovitch SB, Unanue ER. The wide diversity and complexity of peptides bound to class II MHC molecules. Curr Opin Immunol 2006;18:70–7.
374. Sutton R, Gray DW, McShane P, et al. The specificity of rejection and the absence of susceptibility of pancreatic islet beta cells to nonspecific immune destruction in mixed strain islets grafted beneath the renal capsule in the rat. J Exp Med 1989;170:751–62.
375. Taal MW, Zandi-Nejad K, Weening B, et al. Proinflammatory gene expression and macrophage recruitment in the rat remnant kidney. Kidney Int 2000;58:1664–76.
376. Takeuchi T, Lowry RP, Konieczny B. Heart allografts in murine systems. Transplantation 1992;53:1281–94.
377. Tambur AR, Bray RA, Takemoto SK, et al. Flow cytometric detection of HLA-specific antibodies as a predictor of heart allograft rejection. Transplantation 2000;70:1055–9.
378. Tang Q, Bluestone JA, Kang SM. CD4(+)Foxp3(+) regulatory T cell therapy in transplantation. J Mol Cell Biol 2012;4:11–21.
379. Terasaki PI, Ozawa M. Predictive value of HLA antibodies and serum creatinine in chronic rejection: results of a 2-year prospective trial. Transplantation 2005;80:1194–7.
380. Tesar BM, Zhang J, Li Q, et al. TH1 immune responses to fully MHC mismatched allografts are diminished in the absence of MyD88, a Toll-like receptor signal adaptor protein. Am J Transplant 2004;4:1429–39.
381. Tewari MK, Sinnathamby G, Rajagopal D, et al. A cytosolic pathway for MHC class II-restricted antigen processing that is proteasome and TAP dependent. Nat Immunol 2005;6:287–94.
382. Thompson CB, Lindsten T, Ledbetter JA, et al. CD28 activation pathway regulates the production of multiple T-cell-derived lymphokines/cytokines. Proc Natl Acad Sci U S A 1989;86:1333–7.
383. Tilney NL, Kupiec-Weglinski JW, Heidecke CD, et al. Mechanisms of rejection and prolongation of vascularized organ allografts. Immunol Rev 1984;77:185–216.
384. Tivol EA, Borriello F, Schweitzer AN, et al. Loss of CTLA-4 leads to massive lymphoproliferation and fatal multiorgan tissue destruction, revealing a critical negative regulatory role of CTLA-4. Immunity 1995;3:541–7.
385. Toogood GJ, Rankin AM, Tam PKH, et al. The immune response following small bowel transplantation I. An unusual pattern of cytokine expression. Transplantation 1996;62:851–5.
386. Toogood GJ, Rankin AM, Tam PKH, et al. The immune response following small bowel transplantation II: a very early cytokine response in the gut associated lymphoid tissue. Transplantation 1997;63:1118–23.
387. Trombetta ES, Mellman I. Cell biology of antigen processing in vitro and in vivo. Annu Rev Immunol 2005;23:975–1028.
388. Tullius SG, Heemann UW, Azuma H, et al. Alloantigen-independent factors lead to signs of chronic rejection in long-term kidney isografts. Transpl Int 1994;7(Suppl. 1):S306–7.
389. Turka LA, Linsley PS, Lin H, et al. T-cell activation by the CD28 ligand B7 is required for cardiac allograft rejection in vivo. Proc Natl Acad Sci U S A 1992;89:11102–5.
390. Turner D, Grant SC, Yonan N, et al. Cytokine gene polymorphism and heart transplant rejection. Transplantation 1997;64:776–9.
391. Tyden G, Genberg H, Tollemar J, et al. A randomized, doubleblind, placebo-controlled, study of single-dose rituximab as induction in renal transplantation. Transplantation 2009;87:1325–9.
392. Uehara S, Chase CM, Kitchens WH, et al. NK cells can trigger allograft vasculopathy: the role of hybrid resistance in solid organ allografts. J Immunol 2005;175:3424–30.
393. Valujskikh A, Fedoseyeva E, Benichou G, et al. Development of autoimmunity after skin graft rejection via an indirect alloresponse. Transplantation 2002;73:1130–7.
394. van Bergen J, Thompson A, Haasnoot GW, et al. KIR-ligand mismatches are associated with reduced long-term graft survival in HLA-compatible kidney transplantation. Am J Transplant 2011;11:1959–64.
395. Van Buskirk AM, Wakely ME, Orosz CG. Transfusion of polarized TH2-like cell populations into SCID mouse cardiac allograft recipients results in acute allograft rejection. Transplantation 1996;62:229–38.
396. Van Kaer L. Comeback kids: CD8(+) suppressor T cells are back in the game. J Clin Invest 2010;120:3432–4.
397. Waanders MM, Heidt S, Koekkoek KM, et al. Monitoring of indirect allorecognition: wishful thinking or solid data? Tissue Antigens 2008;71:1–15.
398. Walport MJ. Complement. First of two parts. N Engl J Med 2001;344:1058–66.
399. Walport MJ. Complement. Second of two parts. N Engl J Med 2001;344:1140–4.
400. Walsh CM, Hayashi F, Saffron DC, et al. Cell-mediated cytotoxicity results from, but may not be critical for, primary allograft rejection. J Immunol 1996;156:1436–41.
401. Walunas TL, Lenschow DJ, Bakker CY, et al. CTLA-4 can function as a negative regulator of T cell activation. Immunity 1994;1:405–14.
402. Wang H, Kadlecek TA, Au-Yeung BB, et al. ZAP-70: an essential kinase in T-cell signaling. Cold Spring Harbor Perspect Biol 2010;2:a002279.
403. Wang W, Meadows LR, den Haan JMM, et al. Human H-Y: a male-specific histocompatibility antigen derived from the SMCY protein. Science 1995;269:1588–90.
404. Warnecke G, Feng G, Goto R, et al. CD4+ regulatory T cells generated in vitro with IFN-γ and allogeneic APC inhibit transplant arteriosclerosis. Am J Pathol 2010;177:464–72.
405. Watts C, Moss CX, Mazzeo D, et al. Creation versus destruction of T cell epitopes in the class II MHC pathway. Ann N Y Acad Sci 2003;987:9–14.
406. Weaver TA, Charafeddine AH, Agarwal A, et al. Alefacept promotes co-stimulation blockade based allograft survival in nonhuman primates. Nat Med 2009;15:746–9.
407. Williams GM, Hume DM, Hudson Jr RP, et al. "Hyperacute" renal-homograft rejection in man. N Engl J Med 1968;279:611–8.
408. Wing K, Onishi Y, Prieto-Martin P, et al. CTLA-4 control over Foxp3+ regulatory T cell function. Science 2008;322:271–5.
409. Wing K, Yamaguchi T, Sakaguchi S. Cell-autonomous and -non-autonomous roles of CTLA-4 in immune regulation. Trends Immunol 2011;32:428–33.
410. Wise M, Zelenika D, Bemelman F, et al. CD4 T cells can reject major histocompatibility complex class I-incompatible skin grafts. Eur J Immunol 1999;29:156–67.
411. Wolf BA, Hughes JH, Florholmen J, et al. Interleukin-1 inhibits glucose-induced Ca^{2+} uptake by islets of Langerhans. FEBS Lett 1989;248:35.

412. Wong WK, Robertson H, Carroll HP, et al. Tubulitis in renal allograft rejection: role of transforming growth factor-beta and interleukin-15 in development and maintenance of CD103+ intraepithelial T cells. Transplantation 2003;75:505–14.
413. Wood KJ, Sawitzki B. Interferon gamma: a crucial role in the function of induced regulatory T cells in vivo. Trends Immunol 2006;27:183–7.
414. Wucherpfennig KW, Gagnon E, Call MJ, et al. Structural biology of the T-cell receptor: insights into receptor assembly, ligand recognition, and initiation of signaling. Cold Spring Harbor Perspect Biol 2010;2:a005140.
415. Yamada A, Laufer TM, Gerth AJ, et al. Further analysis of the T-cell subsets and pathways of murine cardiac allograft rejection. Am J Transplant 2003;3:23–7.
416. Yamasaki K, Muto J, Taylor KR, et al. NLRP3/cryopyrin is necessary for interleukin-1beta (IL-1beta) release in response to hyaluronan, an endogenous trigger of inflammation in response to injury. J Biol Chem 2009;284:12762–71.
417. Yang HC, McElroy RJ, Kreider JW, et al. In situ expression of platelet-derived growth factor (PDGF-beta) during chronic rejection is abolished by retransplantation. J Surg Res 1995;59:205–10.
418. Yu Y, Zitzner JR, Houlihan J, et al. Common gamma chain cytokines promote rapid in vitro expansion of allo-specific human CD8+ suppressor T cells. PLoS One 2011;6:e28948.
419. Zaki AM, Hirsch GM, Lee TD. Contribution of pre-existing vascular disease to allograft vasculopathy in a murine model. Transpl Immunol 2009;22:93–8.
420. Zecher D, Li Q, Williams AL, et al. Innate immunity alone is not sufficient for chronic rejection but predisposes healed allografts to T cell-mediated pathology. Transpl Immunol 2012;26:113–8.
421. Zelenika D, Adams E, Mellor A, et al. Rejection of H-Y disparate skin grafts by monospecific CD4+ Th1 and Th2 cells: no requirement for CD8+ T cells or B cells. J Immunol 1998;161:1868–74.
422. Zhou X, Bailey-Bucktrout SL, Jeker LT, et al. Instability of the transcription factor Foxp3 leads to the generation of pathogenic memory T cells in vivo. Nat Immunol 2009;10:1000–7.
423. Zhou P, Hwang KW, Palucki D, et al. Secondary lymphoid organs are important but not absolutely required for allograft responses. Am J Transplant 2003;3:259–66.
424. Zhou W, Patel H, Li K, et al. Macrophages from C3-deficient mice have impaired potency to stimulate alloreactive T cells. Blood 2006;107:2461–9.
425. Zhou R, Tardivel A, Thorens B, et al. Thioredoxin-interacting protein links oxidative stress to inflammasome activation. Nat Immunol 2010;11:136–40.
426. Zhu Y, Yao S, Chen L. Cell surface signaling molecules in the control of immune responses: a tide model. Immunity 2011;34:466–78.
427. Zielinski CE, Mele F, Aschenbrenner D, et al. Pathogen-induced human TH17 cells produce IFN-gamma or IL-10 and are regulated by IL-1beta. Nature 2012;484:514–8.
428. Zimmerman C, Seiler P, Lane P, et al. Antiviral immune responses in CTLA4 transgenic mice. J Virol 1997;71:1802–7.
429. Zou Y, Stastny P, Susal C, et al. Antibodies against MICA antigens and kidney-transplant rejection. N Engl J Med 2007;357:1293–300.

CHAPTER 3

Chronic Kidney Failure: Renal Replacement Therapy

Andrew Davenport

CHAPTER OUTLINE

INTRODUCTION

Renal replacement therapy (RRT) is a general term encompassing a range of different treatment modalities for patients with what was formally termed acute renal failure and end-stage kidney disease, which are now called acute kidney injury stage 3 (AKI-3)[32] and chronic kidney disease stage 5 (CKD5),[20] respectively (Table 3-1). RRT includes various forms of dialysis (hemodialysis, hemodiafiltration, and peritoneal dialysis), hemofiltration, and renal transplantation. Dialysis has rapidly expanded from a treatment restricted for AKI in teaching hospitals in the 1960s to now a routine treatment for hundred of thousands of patients with CKD worldwide. However all types of RRT are incomplete solutions for CKD, with a 5-year life expectancy for a dialysis patient in the United Kingdom of around 45%, somewhere between that of patients with ovarian and bowel cancer (www.renalreg.com).

The management of patients with CKD centers on trying to slow down the progression of underlying kidney disease and reducing cardiovascular risk factors, as many more patients will die of cardiovascular disease compared to those who progress to dialysis (CKD5d).[18] Uncontrolled hypertension is the major risk factor for progression followed by proteinuria. Angiotensin-converting enzyme inhibitors and angiotensin receptor blockers are the preferred antihypertensives, aiming for blood pressure targets of 130–40/80–90 mmHg, depending upon the age of the patient. In a minority of cases specific management strategies may be appropriate to halt progression, such as immunosuppression for patients with renal vasculitis or lupus nephritis. Thereafter management is directed to control the complications of progressive kidney disease, hypervolemia, anemia, acidosis, and renal bone disease.[19] In progressive CKD then patient education is vital, so that patients can make an informed decision about whether to have RRT or opt for a conservative non-dialysis approach, accepting that they will die of azotemia. For those patients opting for RRT, it is important to plan ahead, asking about potential live organ donors, creating vascular access for those choosing hemodialysis, and considering embedding a peritoneal dialysis catheter, which can be readily superficialized when peritoneal dialysis is required.

RRT programs continue to expand (Table 3-2), and, although <0.04% of the UK population have CKD requiring RRT, this consumes 2–3% of the overall UK health budget. The challenge for nephrologists and transplant surgeons is to provide the most appropriate RRT of the highest quality for the individual patient at the lowest possible cost. Quality standards and clinical practice guidelines have been developed by both national and international organizations (e.g., British Transplantation Society, Renal Association, European Dialysis and Transplant Association, Kidney Disease Improving Global Outcomes).

DEFINITION AND TIMING REFERRAL

The estimate of glomerular filtration rate (eGFR) system (Table 3-1A) was introduced into the United Kingdom to alert non-renal specialists that patients with what appeared to be high normal or mildly elevated serum creatinine had CKD, and therefore are more at risk from nephrotoxic drugs. Unfortunately, serum creatinine is not linearly associated with glomerular filtration rate and is affected by diet, exercise, and drugs (Table 3-2). Patients with CKD stage 3 can be managed by primary care physicians unless they have rapidly progressive kidney disease, or proteinuria or hematuria, whereas those in stage 4 and 5 should be under the care of specialist nephrologists. However, there is still a relatively high number of avoidable late referrals of patients with CKD5.[31] In some cases, this situation is unavoidable – the patients may have had a truly silent illness or an acute presentation of an irreversible renal injury (e.g., myeloma, antiglomerular basement membrane disease, or renal vasculitis).

TABLE 3-1A Staging for Chronic Kidney Disease*

CKD Stage	eGFR (mL/min/1.73 m²)
Stage 1	>90
Stage 2	60–90
Stage 3a	45–60
Stage 3b	30–44
Stage 4	15–29
Stage 5	<15 mL/min
Stage 5d	Dialysis

*Staging for chronic kidney disease (CKD), based on an estimate of glomerular filtration rate (eGFR) following the modification of diet in renal disease (MDRD) 4 value equation. The suffix (p) can be used to denote the presence of proteinuria as defined by a spot urinary albumin:creatinine ratio of ≥30 mg/mmol, which is approximately equivalent to a protein:creatinine ratio of ≥50 mg/mmol (≥0.5 g/24 h).

TABLE 3-1B Staging for Acute Kidney Injury*

Stage	Serum Creatinine Criteria	Urine Criteria
1	↑ SCreat ≥0.3 mg/dL or 27 µmol/L above baseline within 48 h or ↑ SCreat ≥1.5–1.9× above baseline within 7 days	< 0.5 mL/kg/h for >6 h
2	↑ SCreat 2.0–2.9× above baseline within 7 days	< 0.5 mL/kg/h for >2 h
3	SCreat 3× above baseline or SCreat ≥4.0 mg/dL (350 µmol/L) or RRT within 7 days	< 0.3 mL/kg/h for 24 h or anuria for 12 h

*The baseline serum creatinine (SCreat) measurement should be the admission serum creatinine after resuscitation, or a recent clinic value. The change in serum creatinine should occur within 7 days. All patients who are treated by renal replacement therapy are staged as stage 3.

TABLE 3-2 Examples of Non-Renal Factors Which Affect Serum Creatinine Measurements, Without Changing Renal Function

Factor		Effect on Serum Creatinine
General factors	Age	Decreased
	Female sex	Decreased
Ethnicity compared to caucasoids	Black	Increased
	Asian	Decreased
Body habitus	Muscular	Increased
	Obese	Decreased
Chronic illness	Cirrhosis	Reduced
	Cancer	Reduced
	Heart failure	Reduced
Endocrine diseases	Hypothyroidism	Increased
Diet	Vegetarian	Reduced
	Meat stews	Increased
Drugs	Antibiotics	Trimethoprim
	Gastro-protection	Cimetidine
	Diuretics	Amiloride
		Spironolactone

The consequences for patients of late presentation are many, ranging from increased risk of infection due to the use of temporary central venous access catheters to the psychological impact of suddenly requiring dialysis, with major changes in lifestyle (dietary and fluid restriction, loss of employment). Not surprisingly, these unplanned starters have a worse prognosis,[5] incur greater healthcare costs,[2] and are less likely to activate on the renal transplant waiting list.

PREVALENCE AND INCIDENCE

The point prevalence of CKD is unknown as most patients are asymptomatic and unaware of its presence. Referral patterns increased in the United Kingdom following the introduction of the eGFR reporting system, due to the alerts sent back from pathology laboratories to primary care physicians.[15] Similarly, the prevalence of CKD increases as populations increase in body habitus and prevalence of diabetes.[14] In the latest UK renal registry report the prevalence of CKDd is 794 pmp, but varies within the United Kingdom, being higher in inner-city ethnic populations, and lower in predominantly affluent caucasoid suburbs, with the incidence varying between 88 and 120 pmp (http://www.renalreg.com/Reports/2010.html).

The differences in incidence and prevalence of CKD requiring RRT (Table 3-3) depend both upon patient factors, such as the incidence of diabets and hypertension in the population studied, and heathcare spending.[13] In 2009, the highest incidence of CKD5d reported came from Morelos in Mexico, followed by Jalisco (Mexico), United States, Taiwan, and Japan, whereas Brazil, Iceland, Philippines, Russia, and Bangladesh reported<100 000 per million (www.usrds.org/2011/). However it must be recognized that there is a difference between the incidence of the disease and the incidence of patients starting RRT, as more affluent countries will start more elderly patients with additional comorbidities,[12] and the incidence of CKD increases exponentially with age, whereas less affluent countries tend to restrict RRT to younger patients with fewer comorbidities. Similarly, transplantation rates also differ between countries, and although this is dependent upon the provision and access to dialysis, it can also be affected by cultural and religious practices which limit cadaveric transplantation.

The numbers of patients on RRT worldwide have yet to reach a steady state, particularly in developing economies. This will only occur when the number of new patients accepted into programs is balanced by the number of deaths.

ETIOLOGY

As RRT is an expensive supportive treatment, the key goal would be to prevent or limit the progression of CKD. Unfortunately only a minority of conditions can be halted, and even then only if treated early, such as withdrawal of nephrotoxic analgesics and lithium and appropriate treatment of infections, such as tuberculosis, inflammatory conditions, including sarcoid, and autoimmune diseases, most commonly vasculitis and systemic lupus erythematosus, and more recently, enzyme replacement therapy for conditions such as Fabry's disease. The incidence of diseases that cause CKD change with age, such that childhood CKD may be associated with congenital abnormalities, including urethral valves, prune-belly syndrome, vesicoureteric reflux, whereas patients older than age 65 are more likely to have renovascular disease, hypertensive nephropathy, myeloma, and prostatic obstruction.

The prevalence of inherited diseases, such as polycystic kidney disease, appears to be similar in different ethnic populations; however diabetic nephropathy tends to follow the rate of diabetes in the underlying population. In addition some forms of interstitial nephritis have distinctive geographical patterns or predilection for particular ethnic groups, such as Balkan nephropathy, Chinese herbal nephropathy, associated with ingestion of Aristolochic herbs, and South Asian interstitial nephropathy.

Screening programs, coupled with prompt treatment and investigation of urosepsis, have reduced the number of children with vesicoureteric reflux progressing to CKD5d. However these causes comprise only a minority of cases, with the vast majority of patients developing progressive CKD due to small-vessel disease in

TABLE 3-3 Incidence and Prevalence of Chronic Kidney Disease Treated by Dialysis, and Transplantation Prevalence of Functioning Grafts and Transplant Rate (Rates Expressed per Million Population)

	Dialysis	***Dialysis***	***Dialysis***	***Dialysis***	***Transplant***	***Transplant***
Year	**2004**	**2006**	**2009**	**2009**	**2009**	**2009**
Country	Incidence	Incidence	Incidence	Prevalence	Prevalence	Rate
Argentina	137	141	151	634		35.3
Australia	97	118	107	834	361	26.4
Bangladesh	7	8	13	140		0.6
Brazil	107	185	99	481		22.2
Chile	157	144	151	1109	191	15.1
Denmark	131	119	125	838	303	40.3
France	140	140	149	1094	509	43.5
Israel	189	191	193	1087	383	28.6
Japan	267	275	287	2205		
Korea Republic	175	186	174	1114	225	24.5
Mexico Jalisco	346	346	419	1314	458	41.7
Mexico Morelos		553	597	978	32	
Netherlands	106	113	123	895	508	50
New Zealand	113	119	132	858	325	28
Philippines	75	80	87	110	5	7.1
Russia	17	28	35	173	38	5.9
Spain	175	128	129	1034	495	49.8
Taiwan	405	418	317	2447		
UK (England and Wales)	100	116	110	793	375	38.5
USA	347	365	374	1811	562	57.7

association with hypertension and diabetes. Such health screening programs have centered on the measurement of eGFR to establish an earlier diagnosis of CKD, and then active treatment of cardiovascular risk factors, as hypertension and proteinuria are the key risk factors for progression.[19] As angiotensin-converting enzyme inhibitors and angiotensin receptor blockers are potent antihypertensive agents, and also appear to have an additional effect in terms of reducing proteinuria, these agents are preferentially prescribed. As patients develop progressive CKD, appetite declines, so patients tend to self-restrict protein, and protein-restricted diets do not appear to have any additional benefit, provided that blood pressure is adequately controlled.[16]

For most patients, establishing the cause of CKD can be determined by history, physical examination, simple urine dipstick testing, coupled with specific biochemical and immunological investigations and renal imaging. Patients may have a family history of adult polycystic kidney disease, glomerulonephritis, reflux nephropathy, and hypertension. Physical examination may reveal femoral arterial bruits and signs of cholesterol embolization in renovascular disease, or skin and joint changes in vasculitis and autoimmune diseases. Patients with glomerular hematuria and proteinuria require renal biospy as glomerulonephritis or systemic disease may be amenable to specific therapies.

Transplant surgeons prefer to know the cause of CKD in potential kidney transplant recipients, as some conditions can recur posttransplantation, including some forms of focal segmental glomerular sclerosis, hemolytic uremic syndrome and dense deposit disease, a form of membranoproliferative glomerulonephritis. Similarly, other renal conditions may be inherited, and need to be screened in family members volunteering as living donors. In addition, patients with urogenital malformations or recurrent urosepsis may require surgical reconstruction or nephrectomy prior to transplantation to reduce the risk of subsequent infections.

TREATMENT OF CKD5

Ideally patients with CKD5 should be involved in the decision to choose a form of RRT, whether conservative management or dialysis. In practice, economic and cultural pressures, the limit in kidney donor supply, and medical prejudices often dictate what treatment patients receive. This is particularly the case for patients who have had no or minimal predialysis nephrological care, who by default typically start hemodialysis using a central venous access catheter.

As life expectancy and quality of life are typically greater with transplantation, then transplantation should be considered for all patients with an expected 5-year survival or greater. Pre-emptive transplantation is an option for CKD patients attending nephrological care if a suitable living donor is available; otherwise patients opting for dialysis should be allowed to choose between hemodialysis and peritoneal dialysis, so that vascular access can be created prior to initaion of hemodialysis, and for peritoneal dialysis, embedding a peritoneal dialysis catheter is also an option. Home dialysis should be encouraged for patients with appropriate home circumstances, especially if patients have partners who can act as helpers, as home hemodialysis provides patients with an option for more frequent or longer overnight dialysis sessions. Although in-center hemodialysis may be the default option, ideally hemodialysis patients should dialyse close to home, in local hospital satellite or free-standing self-care centers, to minimize traveling time.

Apart from Mexico (Table 3-4), and some South-East Asian countries which have a peritoneal dialysis first policy, hemodialysis remains the most common mode of RRT worldwide. The differences between countries are at times difficult to understand and are due to the balance between medical and financial resources, reimbursement, and patient locality. For example, in New Zealand many patients live in rural environments distant from hospitals, and as such home-based therapies, peritoneal dialysis, and home hemodialysis are more favored. Likewise, in Australia, center hemodialysis resources are somewhat limited, so favoring home-based therapies. On the other hand countries such as Japan and the United States, which offer greater financial reimbursement for hemodialysis, typically have greater center-based hemodialysis programs.

Dialysis

General Aspects

The aims of dialysis are to maintain homeostasis, in terms of electrolyte, acid–base, volume status, and removal of the products of nitrogen metabolism that accumulate in CKD. Dialysis adequacy is typically measured by urea

TABLE 3-4 **Proportion (%) of Chronic Kidney Disease Patients Treated by Different Dialysis Modalities in 2009**

Country	Hemodialysis	Home Hemodialysis	Peritoneal Dialysis
Argentina	95.9	0	4.1
Australia	69.6	9.4	21.1
Bangladesh	98.6	0	1.4
Brazil	92.3	0	7.7
Chile	95.3	0	4.7
Denmark	73.4	4.9	21.7
France	88.4	1.1	10.5
Israel	93.3	0	6.7
Japan	96.7	0.1	3.2
Korea Republic	83.1	0	16.9
Mexico Jalisco	41.5	0	58.5
Mexico Morelos	42.4	0	57.6
Netherlands	79.7	2.5	17.9
New Zealand	48.7	16.3	35
Philippines	93.3	0	6.7
Russia	91.3	0	8.7
Spain	90.6	0.2	9.2
Taiwan	89.7	0	10.3
UK (England and Wales)	82.2	2.5	15.1
USA	91.9	1.1	6.9

clearance, although urea itself is only one of many azotemic toxins that accumulate in CKD5d patients as a consequence of nitrogen turnover. The original National Co-operative Dialysis Study[24] showed that there was a minimal amount of urea clearance that patients required to sustain wellbeing. To correct for different patient sizes, urea clearance was normalized and expressed as a dimensionless formula, termed Kt/V_{urea}, where for hemodialysis K is the dialyzer urea clearance, and for peritoneal dialysis the combination of urinary and peritoneal urea clearances, t the time, and V_{urea} the volume of urea distribution in the body. For hemodialysis Kt/V_{urea} is expressed per dialysis session, whereas for peritoneal dialysis it is expressed per week. Over time the target Kt/V_{urea} value for adequate dialysis has increased from 1.0 to 1.4 for thrice-weekly hemodialysis treatments,[28] and a minimum weekly value of 1.7 for peritoneal dialysis.[35] Whereas peritoneal dialysis is a continuous therapy, hemodialysis is typically an intermittent treatment with three sessions of 4 hours' duration, scheduled either Monday, Wednesday, Friday or Tuesday, Thursday, Saturday.

However it should be recognized that what is considered to be adequate dialysis provides the equivalent of only 6–10 mL/min of glomerular filtration rate so that there are many consequences of CKD for which additional measures are needed.

Hypertension and Fluid and Electrolyte Balance

Hypertension is common in CKD patients both prior to starting and when also treated by dialysis, and is usually associated with expansion of the extracellular fluid volume caused by positive sodium and water balance. Hemodialysis patients find it difficult to stick to target dry weights and frequently gain 2 kg or more between hemodialysis sessions. Dietary sodium restriction is essential, but most patients also require ultrafiltration with dialysis, unless they have good residual renal function. Excessive water intake can lead to dilutional hyponatremia. Longer-acting antihypertensive drugs are preferred as short-acting vasodilators may exacerbate intradialytic hypotension when the rate of ultrafiltration during dialysis exceeds that of plasma refilling from the extracellular space. Although there are target blood pressures for the general population, there are no agreed targets for hemodialysis patients, as blood pressure typically falls with hemodialysis, as excessive sodium and fluid is removed, and blood pressure measurements taken immediately prior to dialysis do not correspond to 24-hour ambulatory blood pressure recordings during the interdialytic interval.

Dialysis only removes around 60 mmol of potassium a day so that dietary restriction is essential. Hyperkalemia has effects on cardiac muscle (arrhythmias) and on skeletal muscle (weakness and ultimately paralysis). More hemodialysis patients die towards the end of the 2-day interval between dialysis sessions, just prior to the first dialysis session of the week, at a time when they are most likely to be most volume-overloaded and hyperkalemic. A persistent metabolic acidosis usually indicates insufficient dialysis and the need for an increase in hours of hemodialysis or the daily volume of peritoneal dialysis fluid.

Hematopoiesis and Immunity

Erythropoiesis is reduced in patients with CKD, who also have higher iron requirements than the general population due to increased hepcidin, which reduces gastrointestinal iron absorption and iron release from the reticuloendothelial system. The introduction of erythropoietin-stimulating agents (ESAs) has been one of the major advances in the management of patients with CKD5. Hemoglobin targets have been reduced recently (www.kdigo.org), due to the report of increased risk of stroke in patients with higher hematocrit, with most clincial guidelines now advocating a target of 10–12.0 g/dL.[26] Patients who fail to respond to ESAs adequately are usually found to be iron-deficient or have active bleeding or to have foci of infection and inflammation. Oral iron supplements are typically inadequate and most patients require intravenous iron preparations. Too rapid an increase in hematocrit can lead to uncontrolled hypertension and seizures; high hematocrits are associated with increased risk of vascular access thrombosis, particularly arteriovenous grafts, and occasional hyperkalemia. Since the introduction of ESAs, blood transfusion requirements have generally reduced, which may reduce third-party HLA sensitization. Platelet counts are normal in CKD, but their function is abnormal (see under Hemostasis).

Infections are the second major cause of death in CKD5 patients. Cell-mediated immunity is depressed in chronic renal failure, which explains the failure to clear hepatitis B infection and the higher risk of reactivating tuberculosis and varicella-zoster, and reduced response to hepatitis B and other vaccinations.

Calcium, Phosphate, and the Skeleton

Changes in calcium and phosphate homeostasis occur early in the course of progressive CKD as a result of reduced renal phosphate clearance, despite an increase in phosphotonins, such as fibroblast factor 23 and reduced production of the active form of vitamin D, 1,25-dihydroxycholecalciferol, which depends on 1α-hydroxylation in the kidney. Phosphate retention and relative deficiency of 1,25-dihydroxycholecalciferol cause an increase in the secretion of parathyroid hormone (PTH) by the parathyroid glands, which eventually become hyperplastic and then autonomous. Although the increased concentration of PTH enhances phosphate excretion, it increases bone turnover by disturbing the balance between osteoblast and osteoclast activity, so disorganizing bone structure, with Loozer's zones, microfractures, and increased risk of tendon rupture. As such, most CKDd patients require supplemental 1-hydroxycholecalciferol to control hyperparathyoidism. Hyperphosphatemia needs to be controlled by taking agents designed to bind phosphate in the gastrointestinal tract. These phosphate binders may contain elemental calcium or the rare earth lanthanum, or an inert plastic-based ion exchange resin. Patients with CKD are prone to soft-tissue calcification, typically medial arterial calcification, which can lead to soft-tissue calcinosis with skin and fat ischemia and necrosis in severe cases. This typically occurs in the setting of inflammation with an increased serum calcium phosphate product, in patients with vitamin K (often secondary to warfarin therapy) or 25-hydroxy-vitamin D_3 deficiency, and either oversuppressed or very overactive parathyroid glands.

Nutrition and Metabolism

Malnutrition is common in dialysis patients and is caused by inappropriate dietary restrictions, anorexia due to reduction in orexigeni hormones acyl-ghrelin with corresponding increased leptin, acidosis, and insulin resistance, and is aggravated by intercurrent infections, and reduced sense of taste and smell. In addition appetite may be further suppressed in peritoneal dialysis patients due to acid reflux and constipation. Such patients may have simple malnutrition, which responds to enteral feeding, or in more severe cases protein energy wasting, with loss of muscle mass and hypoalbuminemia. Thus dialysis patients are recommended to eat 1.2 g protein/kg/day. Hypercholesterolemia is more common with peritoneal dialysis patients due to absorption of glucose from the dialysate and hypertriglyceridemia from heparin administration with hemodialysis.

Hemostasis

Untreated CKD5 patients have a bleeding diathesis, which is, in part, a consequence of abnormal platelet function, with prolonged bleeding times. However once patients are adequately dialysed, they are more at risk of thrombosis.

Skin

Itching is a common symptom in dialysis patients and is aggravated by dry skin, secondary to reduced apocrine function, heat, and stress. In some cases itching is due to deposition of calcium phosphate crystals secondary to a high calcium (Ca) inorganic phosphate (P_i) product (>6.25 mmol^2/L^2, >70 mg^2/dL^2), or similarly high magnesium, or due to abnormal demyelinated nerve fiber ending sensitivity. Treatment with antihistamines and moisturizing skin lotions with menthol sometimes helps, but in cases of neuropathy patients often require trials of oral gabapentin, ondansetron, or naltrexone to downregulate pain receptor sensitivity and local treatments with capsaicin cream or ultraviolet B phototherapy.

More recently, the widespread use of gadolinium chelates as contrast agents for magnetic resonance (MR) scans has led to gadolinium deposition in the skin and other tissues, causing nephrogenic systemic fibrosis. There is no current treatment, and therefore gadolinium-enhanced MR scans should be limited in CKDd patients, and as the risk currently appears to be less with macrocyclic gadolinium chelates, these agents are to be preferred.[36]

Neurological and Musculoskeletal Manifestations

Uremic encephalopathy usually manifests as subtle cognitive impairment and is an indication for increasing dialysis dose. Coma and seizures are rare, except in non-compliant patients who skip treatments. An asymmetrical distal polyneuropathy is common in patients with CKD5. The symptoms are those of dysesthesia – a prickling or burning sensation and, rarely, footdrop. Restless legs, especially at night, are a nuisance and may respond to low-dose dopamine agonists, including premipexole and carbergoline at night. An autonomic neuropathy is variable in its effects – manifesting mostly as sexual dysfunction and sluggish cardiovascular reflexes during hemodialysis, with increased risk of intradialytic hypotension. Median nerve compression in the carpal tunnel, caused by β_2-microglobulin amyloid deposition, is a specific form of uremic mononeuropathy, typically affecting the arm with an arteriovenous fistula or graft. This complication is declining with the introduction of ultra-pure-quality dialysates and high-flux hemodialyzers. Gout and pseudogout due to pyrophosphate crystals cause a painful crystal arthropathy. Aluminum toxicity due to contaminated dialysate or occasionally following consumption of large numbers of aluminum-based medications can rarely cause a pseudoparkinsonian syndrome, coma, and even death.

Endocrine Abnormalities

There are diverse abnormalities in hormone production, control, protein binding, catabolism, and tissue effects in dialysis patients. The most obvious examples are those of the vitamin D–PTH axis and erythropoietin due to loss of renal function, but thyroid hormone, growth hormone, and both prolactin and sex hormones are also affected. Women usually are infertile, and men often have erectile dysfunction. Sildenafil and other phosphodiesterase-5 inhibitors have proved effective but should be used with caution in patients with heart disease and avoided in patients prescribed nitrates for angina. However, many of these "apparent" endocrine abnormalities are reversed by more frequent and longer hemodialysis sessions, suggesting that they are consequent upon inadequate delivery of RRT. Indeed, greater RRT dosing restores female fertility, and with daily hemodialysis treatments pregnancies can be sustained and intrauterine growth retardation minimized.

Psychological Problems

The psychological problems of dialysis patients, usually anxiety and depression, are the predictable and understandable consequences of loss of health, control, and pleasure. Depression is more common in unplanned dialysis starters compared to those who have been counseled in predialysis nephrological clinics. For average patients dialysis dictates their lifestyle, and, not surprisingly, depressed patients have increased mortality.[7]

Initiation of Dialysis

When should dialysis be started in a patient with CKD? Symptomatic patients, those who are losing weight, and patients with volume overload, uncontrolled acidosis, or hyperkalemia should initiate dialysis (Table 3-5). However, recent studies have shown that there is no advantage to starting the apparently stable asymptomatic patient who is maintaining weight, not fluid-overloaded, with controlled biochemistry (not acidotic or hyperkalemic) on dialysis until the glomerular filtration rate falls to around 5 mL/min.[8]

TABLE 3-5 **Indications to Initiate Dialysis in Patients with Chronic Kidney Disease**

Biochemical indications	Refractory hyperkalemia >6.5 mmol/L Serum urea >50 mmol/L not due to hypovolemia Refractory metabolic acidosis pH≤7.1
Clinical indications	End-organ damage: pericarditis, encephalopathy, neuropathy, myopathy, uremic bleeding, weight loss Refractory volume overload

Hemodialysis

During hemodialysis, water-soluble solutes that are small enough to pass through the pores of a semipermeable dialyzer membrane diffuse move down a concentration gradient. In addition the application of a pressure gradient across the semipermeable membrane leads to ultrafiltration or convection due to a bulk water movement across the membrane; this leads not only to water loss, but also to a convective loss of those water-soluble solutes that are able to pass through the membrane pores. In routine practice, this requires a dialysis membrane with a surface area of 1.0–2.0 m^2 (now conveniently packaged as single-use sterilized hollow-fiber dialyzers), a blood flow of 200–350 mL/min, and a countercurrent flow of dialysate, generated by a proportioning machine, of 500–800 mL/min. The dialysis machine generates the dialysate by adding concentrated electrolytes and sodium bicarbonate to dialysis water, warming it, checking its conductivity, and pumping it through the dialyzer membrane and then to waste. The machine pumps the blood from the patient through the dialyzer membane and returns it via a venous bubble trap with an air detector alarm to prevent air embolism. Anticoagulation can be achieved by a single bolus of low-molecular-weight heparin or by a bolus of unfractionated heparin followed by a continuous infusion. Modern dialysis machines can be programmed to remove fluid gained in the interdialytic interval, and by altering the dialysate sodium concentration, temperature, and the rate of ultrafiltration, reduce the risk of intradialytic hypotension. Dialysis prescription can be altered by choice of dialyzer membrane, surface area, blood and dialysate flow rates, dialysate composition and temperature, and frequency and duration of the dialysis session.

Hemodialysis treatments traditionally used low-flux dialyzers, which effectively cleared small-sized solutes, such as urea, but were not effective in clearing middle-sized solutes such as β_2-microglobulin. As such dialyzer membranes were developed with larger pore sizes designed to remove more middle-sized solutes, termed high-flux, and studies have suggested a survival advantage for high-flux dialysis.[6,23] Hemodiafiltration, which involves the ultrafiltration of fluid across a high-flux dialyzer with compensatory reinfusion of ultrapure dialysate, increases middle-sized molecule clearances further. This approach is often tolerated better by patients with unstable cardiovascular systems, with less frequent intradialytic hypotension.[22]

The key to adequate hemodialysis is reliable vascular access (see Chapter 5). Poorly functioning access inevitably leads to poor dialysis and increases morbidity. Reliance on central venous access exposes patients to increased risk of bacterial infection, venous thrombosis, and stenoses.

The organization and management of hemodialysis units are major exercises. The aim is to use the capital equipment and staff in the most economical way. Dialysis units generally should have not less than 10 stations running two, preferably three, shifts a day, 6 days a week, with one nurse or dialysis technician being responsible for 4–6 dialysis patients at a time. An important consideration is the production of large volumes of water in the generation of dialysate. Tap water is purified by filtration to remove bacteria, softening to remove calcium, carbon filtration to remove small organic compounds such as chloramines, and reverse osmosis to remove other contaminating substances, including metals and nitrites. The water system should run 24 hours a day to prevent stagnation and biofilm deposition, with ideally multiple passes through the reverse osmosis system to improve final water quality to achieve ultrapure water, which is essential if high-flux and hemodiafiltration treatments are used. Water ring-mains require regular cleaning and disinfection.

Patients who are hepatitis B antigen-positive should be dialyzed in isolation and on dedicated dialysis machines. Hepatitis B vaccinations are recommended and are most effective if administered before CKD5 develops. Universal precautions are said to be sufficient to prevent spread of human immunodeficiency virus and hepatitis C, but many centers cohort these patients to prevent nosocomial transmission.

Complications

Hypotension occurs in up to 30% of dialysis sessions and most commonly is secondary to intravascular hypovolemia. It is more common when large volumes of fluid have to be removed during a short hemodialysis session after excessive gains between dialyses. It also occurs more often if patients eat during dialysis. Hypotension usually responds to laying the patient flat or head-down, stopping ultrafiltration, or giving a volume of normal saline or hypertonic glucose. Muscle cramps (approximately 5–20% of dialyses) often accompany hypotension, an excessively low target weight, or the use of a low-sodium dialysate. Correction of these or the administration of a hypertonic solution (saline or glucose) usually is effective treatment. Regular sufferers may be helped by prophylactic quinine sulfate. Nausea, vomiting, and headache also are fairly common during hemodialysis. Mild chest and back pains may be related to complement activation by the dialysis membrane and are less common with biocompatible membranes. Some patients may have allergic reactions to heparins, or some of the organic chemicals which are released from the glues in the dialyzer cap, or from the plastic polymers used in the blood lines, particularly if there has been minimal rinsing of the dialysis circuit. Pyrogen or microbial contamination of the dialysate occasionally may occur. Patients developing fever and/or rigors on dialysis must be examined carefully for evidence of infection of dialysis access; blood cultures should be taken, and patients empirically treated with broad-spectrum antibiotics whilst awaiting cultures.

Peritoneal Dialysis

Peritoneal dialysis is the process by which solutes, buffer, waste products, and fluid are exchanged between the blood in the peritoneal capillaries and the solution infused into the peritoneal cavity. This exchange takes place across the peritoneal barrier, which comprises the capillary wall, interstitial matrix, the visceral mesothelial cells and overlying glycocalyx, but considerable absorption of solutes and water also occurs via the peritoneal lymphatics. The efficiency of solutes cleared depends on the vascularity and surface area of the peritoneum, the blood flow, the permeability of the barrier, the volume and frequency of the dialysate instilled, and the osmotic or oncotic gradient generated by glucose, glucose polymer, or amino acid content of the dialysate.

Dialysis Adequacy

The efficacy of peritoneal dialysis can be altered only by changes in the volume and frequency of exchanges. Weekly creatinine clearance and urea clearance (measured using the weekly *Kt/V*) are used to assess adequacy of peritoneal dialysis.[35] The CANUSA study prospectively followed 680 patients after starting continuous ambulatory peritoneal dialysis (CAPD).[3] Although patient survival was related to Kt/V_{urea} (5% increase in relative risk of death for every 0.1 decrease in Kt/V_{urea}), this reduced over time as a result of the loss of residual renal function with no change in peritoneal dialysis clearance. A larger study also found a correlation with residual function but not peritoneal dialysis clearance, and currently there is no evidence that increasing peritoneal dialysis dose reduces morbidity or mortality.[27] Most circumstantial data suggest that more dialysis is better, and the current consensus is that the target should be above a combined Kt/V_{urea} (dialysis and residual renal function) of 1.7 per week. *V* is estimated from height, weight, age, and sex, but the ideal body weight should be used to avoid inaccuracies in obese or fluid-overloaded patients. A creatinine clearance of 50 L/1.73 m^2 also has been suggested as a target. As residual renal function reduces, it may become impossible to achieve target clearance, even with larger and more frequent exchanges, especially for larger patients, and transfer to hemodialysis is necessary.

Dialysis Transport

After infections, the next common cause of peritoneal dialysis treatment failure is loss of ultrafiltration. Transport status should be assessed by a standard 4-hour dwell with a 2.0-L exchange, and ultrafiltration failure defined as <200 mL net ultrafiltrate with a 3.86% or greater glucose concentration, or net zero ultrafiltration with a 2.27% glucose exchange. Patients differ in the speed at which creatinine moves from capillary blood to dialysate and corresponding loss of the glucose from the dialysate to the patient (Figure 3-1). On the one hand fast transporters clear small water-soluble uremic toxins faster than slow transporters, but as they also lose the glucose osmotic gradient, are more likely to have problems with maintaining ultrafiltration, and at risk of becoming volume-overloaded.

Automated Peritoneal Dialysis

Automated peritoneal dialysis (APD) is an increasingly popular form of peritoneal dialysis. Patients connect themselves to a peritoneal dialysis machine for a series of overnight cycling exchanges. The duration of therapy is typically between 7 and 10 hours, with 4–7 cycles of 1.5–3.0 L. Slow transporters require longer treatment times, with fewer larger-volume cycles, whereas faster transporters may have shorter treatment times, and more frequent lower-volume cycles. If patients do not have adequate residual renal function for solute clearance or volume control, then they may also require one long daytime exchange, sometimes termed continuous cycling peritoneal dialysis, or even two daytime additional exchanges, opti-choice peritoneal dialysis.

APD is a good treatment for children and the elderly because it can be set up at home by a relative or caregiver and allowed to run automatically overnight, and also for patients who are active and working, by freeing them from daytime exchanges.

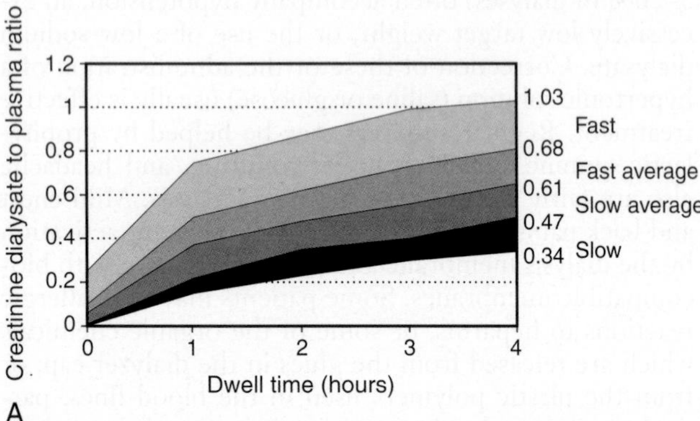

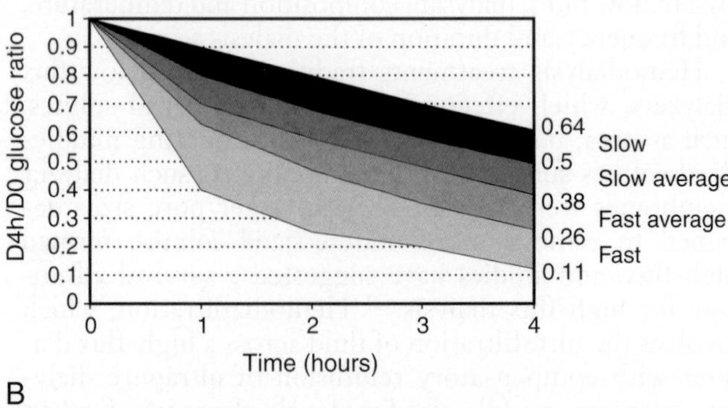

FIGURE 3-1 ■ Changes in creatinine (A) and glucose (B) during a standard 2-L peritoneal dialysis exchange during a 4-hour dwell are used to categorize patients in terms of transporter status. Although fast transporters have higher creatinine clearances, as the glucose gradient falls quicker, they are prone to sodium retention due to reduced osmotically driven ultrafiltration. D0 refers to the initial glucose concentration; otherwise dialysate concentrations refer to 4-hour drain.

Continuous Ambulatory Peritoneal Dialysis

CAPD is the most widely used form of peritoneal dialysis worldwide and relies on the prolonged dwell phase to make up for the lower frequency of exchanges. Dialysis is continuous, exchanges following one another, usually without interruption. To deliver sufficient dialysis, three to five 1.5–3-L exchanges are performed every 24 hours. The usual routine starts in the morning with the drainage of the overnight dialysis fluid and is followed by the installation of the first bag of dialysate of the day. The next change is before lunch, the next late afternoon, and the last immediately before bed. Each exchange typically takes 30–40 minutes to complete. If patients have a tendency to absorb fluid from the overnight exchange, they should drain out and cap off the catheter overnight and start dialysis on a dry peritoneum in the morning. The volume of dialysate instilled depends on the abdominal capacity of the patient (1.5 L for small adults and children, 2 L for regular-sized adults, and 3 L for large men). The glucose concentration depends on the amount of ultrafiltration required to keep the extracellular fluid volume constant. To generate a higher volume, strong bags of 2.27% and even 3.86% glucose are provided, usually as the first exchange of the day and only overnight in slow transporters. However, 7.5% icodextrin dialysate solutions can be used to replace hypertonic glucose (2.27% or 3.86%) for a long daytime or overnight dwell, and are particularly useful for fast transporters. Icodextrin exerts an oncotic pressure and has a more gradual and sustained effect on ultrafiltration than glucose-based dialysates.

Practical Considerations

For all types of peritoneal dialysis, a properly placed peritoneal dialysis catheter is required (see Chapter 5). The intraperitoneal tip should be in the pelvis, free from the omentum. The internal cuff must be watertight and sewn outside the peritoneum. The track should be diagonal, and the catheter should emerge away from the belt line with the external cuff 2 cm from the skin exit site. The major dialyzer companies provide a selection of peritoneal dialysis solutions, varying in volume, osmotic strength, pH, and calcium concentration.

The key issue in peritoneal dialysis is the avoidance of infection introduced at the time of connection of the dialysis bag to the transfer set, which is attached to the peritoneal dialysis catheter. Originally the connection was made by spiking the port of the peritoneal dialysis bag, and was associated with increased risk of introducing infection. Improvements in connectology have led to the introduction of the flush-before-fill technique, when about 30 mL of sterile fresh dialysate from the new dialysate bag at the beginning of each exchange is flushed to the waste effluent dialysate bag and not infused into the peritoneal cavity, so that bacteria introduced at the time of the connection of the new bag is rinsed away. In addition skin microorganisms can migrate along the catheter track, and thus exit site care is important to limit skin colonization. Chlorhexidine or alcohol-based antiseptic wipes are typically used in combination with antiseptic or antibiotics creams.

Indications for and Advantages of Peritoneal Dialysis

Peritoneal dialysis has some major advantages over hemodialysis, but there are equally many limitations and drawbacks. In the basic CAPD mode, peritoneal dialysis is at least 25% cheaper than hemodialysis in that it does not require an expensive dialysis machine and large numbers of technically expert trained nursing staff. As peritoneal dialysis is a home-based therapy patients are not constrained by their dialysis slots. However peritoneal dialysis becomes expensive if beset by complications, such as peritonitis, that require hospital admission. CAPD is particularly useful in patients experiencing practical difficulties with hemodialysis, for example, vascular access problems or cardiovascular instability. It has social advantages for children and mothers of young children.

The disadvantages include peritonitis, exit site infections, ultrafiltration failure, the absorption of glucose leading to weight gain, and the amount of time required to go through the disciplined exercise of performing an aseptic exchange. Thus patients without accommodation or ready access to clean running water, or those unable or unwilling to perform asepetic exchanges are not suitable candidates for peritoneal dialysis. However peritoneal dialysis can be successfully performed in the favelas of Brazil. Some patients, particularly young women, refuse peritoneal dialysis, due to embarrassment with the catheter and an aesthetic dislike of the discomfort and appearance of a distended abdomen.

Posttransplantation

After transplantation, provided that graft function is adequate, the peritoneal dialysis catheter can be capped off and left. The catheter exit site should be dressed as per usual, and the catheter typically removed after 3 months, when the transplant function is stable. If the graft fails within 3 months, the catheter needs to be flushed to remove debris and fibrin. Infection occasionally is introduced at this first exchange after a break (see also subsequent section on Dialysis posttransplant).

Complications

Loss of Ultrafiltration

A proportion of patients (10–30% by 5 years but increasing with time) retain fluid after more than 4 hours' dwell and have poor ultrafiltration, even with more hypertonic fluid. It occurs transiently after peritonitis and is more likely to become a chronic problem after multiple attacks. Patients present with hypertension and fluid overload, and it is important to exclude constipation, loss of residual renal function, or poor compliance with dialysis or excessive fluid intake. Ultrafiltration failure due to fast transport status is referred to as type 1 failure. Low ultrafiltration associated with slow transport is termed type 2 failure, and is associated with loss of surface area, usually as a result of encapsulating peritoneal sclerosis (EPS).

In the early stages, reduced ultrafiltration can be managed by using shorter dwell times and leaving the peritoneum dry overnight. The use of an overnight solution of 7.5% icodextrin (a glucose polymer) that is oncotically active but too large to be rapidly absorbed is an alternative strategy. When fluid retention occurs during daytime exchanges, even with medium or strong bags, the only option to avoid abandoning peritoneal dialysis is to convert from CAPD to APD, sometimes with an additional daytime icodextrin exchange.

Peritonitis

Peritonitis is a potentially serious problem and one of the most common complications of peritoneal dialysis. Its average incidence is one episode per 24–36 patient months. The incidence of peritonitis is reduced by using the flush-before-fill technique, and some reports suggest that using antibiotic exit site creams can further reduce the risk of peritonitis.

Around 57% of cases are due to Gram-positive organisms, 18% due to Gram-negative organisms, and about 15% are culture-negative. Coagulase-negative staphylococci are the most common cause of peritonitis, and typically cause a relatively mild symptomatic peritonitis, which usually responds promptly to treatment, but can relapse due to penetration of organisms into the catheter biofilm. *Staphylococcus aureus* usually causes a severe peritonitis with marked systemic features, including high fever and hypotension. Response to antibiotics is less good, and the catheter is more likely to be removed for a non-resolving infection. *Pseudomonas* accounts for approximately 5% of cases and also tends to invade the catheter biofilm, often necessitating catheter removal, as infections often recur.

Peritonitis usually presents as cloudy bags (apparent with >50 leukocytes/μL) and abdominal pain, but the latter may precede the former by one exchange or 1–2 days. There may be fever (more common in children), nausea and vomiting (approximately 30%) and, when severe, hypotension. Abdominal tenderness with peritonism is the major clinical finding. The effluent peritoneal fluid following a 4-hour dwell contains greater than 100 leukocytes (>50% neutrophils) per μL (normally <10/μL, although the number may be higher after a dry period, for example, during the day in patients on APD).[21] Peritonitis may be present with lower cell counts, particularly with short dwells. Cloudy bags are occasionally due to macrophages and/or eosinophils and are not associated with peritonitis.

The diagnosis is made in the presence of any two of the following: abdominal pain, cloudy bags, or the presence of bacteria on Gram stain. The differential diagnosis includes intraperitoneal infections, including appendicitis, cholecystitis, diveriticular disease, pancreatitis, and bowel perforations. Typically intra-abdominal pathology is accompanied by increased peritoneal effluent, red blood cells as well as leukocytes, whereas PD peritonitis has very few red blood cells, despite increased leukocytes. In cases of clinical doubt, or in cases failing to respond promptly to therapy, a computed tomography (CT) abdominal scan should be performed to exclude additional intra-abdominal pathology, before proceeding to catheter removal in refractory cases.

A variety of regimens are successful, for example, intraperitoneal vancomycin, 2 g (1 g if <60 kg), left to dwell for 4–6 hours and repeated after 7 days, and oral ciprofloxacin, or antibiotics injected into each CAPD exchange (gentamicin loading dose 8 mg/L then 4 mg/L, and first- or second-generation cephalosporin 250 mg/L loading dose then 125 mg/L). Patients treated by APD can convert to CAPD until the pathologic organism is identifed with antibiotic specificities, or patients can be treated with vancomycin and ciprofloxacin as above, or given intraperitoneal antibiotics in a single daytime exchange (gentamicin 0.4 mg/kg/day then adjusted according to antibiotic levels in combination with a first- or second-generation cephalosporin 1.5 g/day). In centers with a high risk of fungal peritonitis, antifungal prophylaxis with fluconazole should be co-administered either at 50 mg daily, or 200 mg for 3 days.

Unless patients are ill, they are generally treated as outpatients (approximately 80%). Depending upon the results of the microbiology cultures, one or both antibiotics are continued, or new antibiotics started in cases of resistance, and in cases of no bacterial growth both antibiotics are continued. If the patient fails to respond within 48 hours and is unwell, microbacteriology advice should be sought. Further delay in response should raise the possibility of fungal peritonitis. Occasionally (<5%), peritonitis is secondary to intra-abdominal disease, such as diverticulitis, appendicitis, or perforated viscus, and if suspected, laparotomy is indicated.

Patients with recurrent episodes of peritonitis from the same organism may have persistent infection of the catheter or its track or it may be due to the buildup of a biofilm on the catheter that provides protection for bacteria from antibiotics. This buildup can be treated by removal of the peritoneal dialysis catheter with a rest on hemodialysis and later placement of a fresh catheter or by removal and replacement at the same operation. Recurrent peritonitis may be due to poor technique, and this should be reassessed carefully.

Exit Site and Tunnel Infection

Nearly half of all exit sites are colonized by skin bacteria. *S. aureus* colonization of the exit site is usually associated with nasal carriage, and used to account for more than 50% of all exit site infections. Prevention is the best strategy; peritoneal catheters should be placed so that the peritoneal dialysis catheter exits preferably vertically downwards or laterally to aid drainage of the subcutaneous tunnel, and the exit site is positioned to avoid mechanical damage from skirt or pant waist bands and belts. Patients should be educated about the importance of daily washing, drying, avoiding forceful removal of scabs, and avoiding tugging the catheter by careful tethering.

Exit site infections can be further reduced by using antiseptic creams and gels; more recently, topical antibiotics, such as mupirocin, have been introduced, as these reduce Gram-positive organism colonization, and proportionately more infections with Gram-negative organisms, in particular *Pseudomonas*, are now being reported. Although this approach is recommended by the International Society of Peritoneal Dialysis,[29] some centers have not followed this advice due to concerns of introducing antibiotic resistance.

Exit site infections should be guided by advice on local microbiology; because staphylococci are common, 2 weeks of flucloxacillin is typically first-line treatment. Recurrence may be treated effectively by adding rifampicin to flucloxacillin. Sometimes the outer cuff extrudes, and shaving this may solve the problem, but catheter replacement may be necessary, especially if there is evidence of a tunnel infection or recurrent peritonitis.

Anatomical Complications

Abdominal fluid increases intra-abdominal pressure and predisposes to the development of hernias, which are relatively common (10–15% of all peritoneal dialysis patients and higher in patients with polycystic kidneys). Although often asymptomatic, prompt repair is essential because they inevitably enlarge, and there is the risk of obstruction and/or strangulation. Acid reflux, indigestion, and a feeling of fullness also are more common than in patients on hemodialysis. Hernias can be confirmed by performing a CT peritoneogram.

Infusion pain on draining fluid into the abdomen is relatively common early on but usually settles. This pain can be reduced by using neutral pH dialysate at body temperature and may be improved by slowing the inflow rate. Drain pain at the end of a cycle is more common with cyclers. It may improve by treating constipation; if not, then clamping the line after the fast drain has finished and starting the next cycle usually resolves pain. If air is introduced into the system, it relocates under the diaphragm, causing severe pleuritic pain referred to the shoulder.

Scrotal or labial edema occurs when fluid leaks from the peritoneum to subcutaneous tissues. This condition usually occurs soon after insertion of the Tenckhoff catheter and spontaneously settles after resting for a few weeks. Occasionally, patients have a congenital communication between the pleura (usually right side) and peritoneum, resulting in a hydrothorax. As these leaks tend to be small, diagnosis can be difficult as biochemical analysis of the pleural fluid is typically equivocal – neither peritoneal dialysate nor serum – with no leak demonstrated on CT peritoneogram. However, if 2 L of 7.5% icodextrin is instilled, then sampling the pleural fluid 4 hours later, and checking for a starch reaction with iodine, which will confirm that the fluid is dialysate, is the most reliable diagnostic test.

Other problems include back pain due to the change in posture secondary to large-volume daytime exchanges.

Encapsulating Peritoneal Sclerosis

Repeated exposure to peritoneal dialysis fluids causes changes to the peritoneuem, typified by increased interstitial matrix deposited in the parietal peritoneum, and browning discoloration due to deposition of advanced glycosylation end-products. As the peritoneeum thickens, numerous small capillaries and lymphatics develop, which increase the effective vascular surface area, and patients become faster transporters. In addition to this natural thickening of the peritoneum, some patients develop an inflammatory reaction, which can lead to deposition of a cocoon-like fibrosis around the small bowel, with tethering leading to small-bowel obstruction, malabsorption, and 50% mortality in severe cases. EPS can occur many years after switching modalities from peritoneal dialysis to hemodialysis, and also after transplantation, with patients presenting with signs of small-bowel obstruction. Although EPS can be precipitated by severe peritonitis, the only common factor linked to its development is the duration of peritoneal dialysis therapy, with an incidence of 3% at 5 years, then rapidly rising to around 15% at 10 years. Diagnosis is often made at laparotomy, but CT scan appearances may show small-bowel tethering, small-bowel dilatation with septation, and calcification of the mesentery. Tamoxifen and steroids may have a role during the inflammatory phase, but not once fibrosis is established, then total parenteral nutrition and surgery in specialized centers may be required.[11]

Metabolic Complications

The peritoneal fluid contains high concentrations of glucose. It has been estimated that 200 g of glucose (more with many high-concentration bags and during peritonitis) may be absorbed daily, equivalent to 800 kcal. This absorption may cause obesity, hyperglycemia, and hyperinsulinemia. The glucose load stimulates fat synthesis, and hypertriglyceridemia is common. Cholesterol levels also rise during the first year on CAPD. Albumin levels often are low. The explanation is multifactorial, including simple dilution due to volume expansion, losses in the fluid and malnutrition because of poor appetite, especially during and after peritonitis.

About 25% of CAPD patients are hypokalemic, and they may need potassium-sparing diuretics or supplements. A few need a stringent low-potassium diet. Some patients using 2.5–3-L lactate-based exchanges run high bicarbonate levels, which usually settle when switched to neutral pH bicarbonate solutions. Alkalosis has been associated with lethargy, nausea, and headaches.

CHOICE AND PLANNING FOR THE INDIVIDUAL PATIENT

Patients with CKD are never cured, and often change RRT modality during their lifetime. This requirement for different modalities of RRT, each with its own limitations and risks, calls for a coordinated and multidisciplinary approach.

As renal transplantation offers better survival and quality of life, patients should first be assessed for their suitability. There are few absolute contraindications, and the decision has to be based on an overall assessment of the patient's current fitness and ability to withstand surgery and immunosuppression, and subjective assessment of compliance and estimated life expectancy. Availability of kidneys may also influence selection policy.

The best first option is a pre-emptive transplant from a living related or living donor because this avoids the need for an initial period of dialysis and the creation of permanent vascular access. It also enables planning of transplantation, such that blood group and even HLA-mismatched donors can also be considered. Planning can avoid major disruption to the life of young patients at a crucial stage in their education or career. Nephrologists should emphasize the much longer survival of living donor transplants, the lower morbidity, and the reduced doses of immunosuppression. Although it must be acknowledged that the transplants ultimately may fail, families of young patients should be reminded of the benefits of 10 years of dialysis-free life in the early years after the development of CKDd, which would allow completion of education, establishment of a career, and having a family.

If living donor transplantation is not possible, the next best option is to put the patient forward for a pre-emptive cadaver donor transplant, if possible. Apart from avoiding dialysis, this option allows the patient to spend a longer period in the recipient pool; because there is less urgency, the patient can wait for a better-matched kidney. However, some nephrologists object to this policy on the grounds that it is unfair to patients already on dialysis who may have waited a long time for a transplant. Given the shortage of cadaver kidneys and the superior survival of well-matched grafts, this objection can be rejected. It always has to be accepted that pre-emptive transplantation cannot be guaranteed success, and patients should be counseled that they may need dialysis postoperatively for hyperkalemia, or in cases of delayed graft function and graft failure.

If dialysis is necessary before transplantation can be performed, then the best holding treatment depends on the length of time waiting for a graft. If the patient is physically fit, not sensitized, and has a potential living donor available, then peritoneal dialysis is a good holding treatment because it avoids the need for creating permanent or temporary vascular access. Occasionally, such patients would be held on hemodialysis using a temporary internal jugular venous catheter, but this should only be considered a short-term option and discouraged because of the risks of infection and the development of venous stenoses, which may exclude the arm from future arteriovenous fistula formation. If the wait for a transplant is indeterminate, then patients should go down the local patient pathways for creating vascular access for those opting for hemodialysis, and for peritoneal dialysis either elective insertion of an embedded peritoneal dialysis catheter, or timely catheter insertion closer to the time of dialysis initiation.

DIALYSIS POSTTRANSPLANT

The need for dialysis after transplantation is determined by early graft function, which in turn depends on many factors related to the donor organ (see Chapter 14). During any period when graft function is absent or compromised, it is essential to modify doses of drugs for which the predominant route of excretion is the kidney. Particular care is required for aminoglycoside antibiotics (see Chapter 31), certain muscle relaxants (see Chapter 13), and opiates, the active metabolites of which accumulate in CKD5. Important examples are listed in Table 3-6.[1]

TABLE 3-6 **Drugs that Require Dose Reduction or Avoidance in Patients with Chronic Kidney Disease Stage 5d**

Drug Class and Specific Drugs	Comment
Antimicrobial	
Aminoglycosides	Reduce dose, ototoxic
Acyclovir	Reduce dose
Cephalosporins	Reduce dose
Co-trimoxazole	Reduce dose, increases creatinine
Ethambutol	Reduce dose, retinal toxicity
Ganciclovir	Reduce dose
Nitrofurantoin	Avoid, neuropathy
Penicillins	Avoid high doses, fits
Vancomycin	Reduce dose, ototoxic
Anesthetic	
Pancuronium	Avoid, prolonged paralysis
Gallamine	Avoid, prolonged paralysis
Opiates	Reduce dose, prolonged effect
Suxamethonium	Increases plasma potassium concentrations
Analgesics	
Non-steroidal inflammatories	Avoid, risk losing residual renal function
Opiates	Reduce dose and frequency as metabolites accumulate, causing toxicity. Less likely with fentanyl and oxycodone
Gastrointestinal	
Metoclopramide	Be aware of extrapyramidal effects
H_2 antagonists	Reduce dose
Magnesium salts	Monitor magnesium concentration
Cardiac	
Digoxin	Reduce dose and frequency
β-Blockers	May need to reduce dose
Spironolactone	Avoid, hyperkalemia
ACE inhibitors	Monitor creatinine and potassium
Clofibrate	Avoid, muscle injury
Oral hypoglycemics	
Chlorpropamide	Avoid, hypoglycemia
Tolbutamide	Reduce dose
Biguanides	Avoid, lactic acidosis

ACE, angiotensin-converting enzyme.

Hemodialysis

Hemodialysis should be performed as for any postoperative patient (i.e., as remote from the surgical procedure as is safe for the control of potassium and fluid balance). In practice, this is usually more than 24 hours after the operation. The main risk is hemorrhage from the operation wound and biopsy sites, but in practice the risks are small with short daily dialyses, coupled with regular predialyzer saline flushing (100 mL every 30 minutes) and citrate-based dialysate (Citrasate), which removes the need for systemic anticoagulation. For the patient with an unstable cardiovascular system, hemofiltration or hemodiafiltration is preferable, with higher dialysate sodium concentration (5 mmol/L above serum sodium up to 145 mmol/L) and dialysate cooled to 35°C.[33] The usual vascular access should be used for intermittent hemodialysis treatments, but fistulae should not be used for continuous forms of RRT.

Vascular access should be monitored in the postoperative phase. Periods of hypotension predispose to collapse and thrombosis of fistulae and arteriovenous grafts, especially those with pre-existing stenoses. The accesses must be explored and flow restored as soon as possible, not only for their immediate use, but also for the long term should the graft fail. Rehabilitation of patients with failed renal transplants is prolonged greatly if they lose their vascular access as well.

Postoperatively, due to the inflammatory reaction initiated by the transplanted kidney, capillary endothelial leak leads to patients being several kilograms above their dialysis target weight, as intravenous fluids are administered to maintain systemic blood pressure and central venous pressure. It is reasonable to dialyze patients to above their so-called pretransplant dry weight in the postoperative period. This approach minimizes the risk of intradialytic hypotension which may delay the graft opening up and even predispose to thrombosis of the anastomosis. However it must be recognized that some of the anti-T-cell agents predispose to an acute pulmonary leak, leading to pulmonary edema, which can be life-threatening in volume-overloaded patients (see Chapter 20).

Continuous Ambulatory Peritoneal Dialysis

Peritoneal dialysis can be performed safely after the transplant procedure, provided that the peritoneum has not been breached; the risk can be minimized by draining the peritoneum before surgery. However, due to inflammatory milieu posttransplantation, many patients behave as fast transporters, requiring shorter dwell times and higher glucose dialysates to prevent further volume loading.

If clear fluid is observed leaking from the transplant wound, measuring the glucose concentration will confirm peritoneal dialysate, in which case dialysis should be stopped immediately, the peritoneum should be drained, and hemodialysis used to support the patient. Peritoneal dialysis can be reinstituted at about 7 days but should be with low volumes or preferably using a cycling machine that allows small volumes and short dwell times. Patients should not be transplanted during an episode of peritonitis.

RETURN TO DIALYSIS AFTER TRANSPLANT FAILURE

The return to dialysis after transplantation is a difficult period for the patient and the nephrologist. Not only are there understandable emotional difficulties, but also there are frequently physical problems. Early graft failure is less traumatic for the patient who has not enjoyed independence from dialysis. Immunosuppression, particularly steroid doses, should be reduced rapidly and the patient returned to the usual dialysis schedule. Grafts that fail early usually are removed surgically, but the need for this often is precipitated by the reduction in immunosuppression. It has long been recognized that patient survival is affected adversely by graft failure.

Patients whose long-term grafts have failed present more complex problems. The temptation to maintain a failing graft should be resisted because it is better for the patient to be established on dialysis than to suffer the continual effects of uremia and immunosuppression.[4] The physician has to discuss with the patient the appropriate modality, which may be different from that employed before transplantation. Time spent on peritoneal dialysis pretransplantation should be taken into account when estimating the risk of EPS. If the graft is failing slowly, then the appropriate patient pathway for establishing vascular or peritoneal access should be followed.

Patients frequently have many side effects from immunosuppression, such as osteoporosis, skin atrophy and malignancy, hyperglycemia, hypertension, and secondary hyperparathyroidism. Although prednisolone should be withdrawn gradually, this needs to be done cautiously over a 3–4-month period. Even then the patient is at risk of hypoadrenalism and should be warned that he or she will require an increased dose of steroids to cover any intercurrent illness. It is reasonable to perform a short Synacthen test if there is doubt about the adrenal status to ensure that withdrawal has been effected safely.

Patients with failing grafts should have the same nephrological care as CKD4 patients in terms of volume, blood pressure, cardiovascular risk factor, phosphate control, and renal bone disease and renal anemia management, with appropriate dietary advice.[19]

RRT MODALITY AND SURVIVAL

Although the overall survival for patients receiving transplants is greater than for those remaining on dialysis, it must be recognized that there is a selection bias of the younger fitter patients for transplantation; for example, unadjusted 2009 US Renal Data Survey (USRDS) mortality per 1000 patients days was greatest for hemodialysis (197), compared to 150 for peritoneal dialysis and 33.3 for transplantation. Even so, comparisons show improved survival for transplant recipients compared to those who remain active on the transplant waiting list but continue on dialysis. Wolfe and colleagues reported that long-term mortality was 48–82% lower among transplant recipients than among patients on the waiting list,[34] and a later analysis showed better 5- and 10-year survival for transplanted patients who had dialysis for 6 months (78% and 63% respectively) or less compared to those who had dialyzed for 2 years (58% and 28% respectively).[25]

Again, selection bias has to be considered when interpreting survival for different dialysis modes. For example, the 5-year adjusted survival for RRT patients reported in the USRDS 2010 report showed 73% for transplant recipients, 40% for peritoneal dialysis, and 34% for hemodialysis. However there have been very few studies actually randomizing patients to either peritoneal dialysis and hemodialysis, and the largest study (NECOSADS) did not show major difference between standard dialysis modes.[17] Home hemodialysis patients have better survival; this may be due not only to patient selection, but also because they have access to better-quality dialysis in terms of more frequent and longer dialysis sessions.

Survival on dialysis depends not only on patient factors, but also on acceptance criteria and transplantation rates. In the United Kingdom and other countries there is an increasing trend towards offering elderly comorbid patients conservative or palliative care (no dialysis). This can then confound dialysis survival data, from countries such as Germany, which do not have conservative management programs. As expected, age has the greatest effect on survival; for example the UK Renal Registry reported 1- and 10-year survival for patients aged 18–64 of 85.9% and 44.3% respectively, which fell to 64.2% and 3.8% for those aged >65 years (http://www.renalreg.com/Reports/2010.html). Thereafter additional comorbidities, in particular diabetes, reduce life expectancy, as with the general population. However, despite advances in medicine and dialysis technology, the overall 5-year survival of RRT patients lies between that of ovarian and bowel cancer, which reinforces the need to improve RRT and tackle the causes of accelerated cardiovascular disease in CKD patients.

QUALITY OF LIFE

Whereas mortality is a hard end point, patients also want information about expected quality of life when trying to decide upon treatment modalities. Unfortunately, quality of life is difficult to quantitate, especially because there are major differences in the ages and other circumstances of patients being managed by the various modalities. Employment is an important criterion by which the quality of life or outcome of RRT can be judged, and in this respect transplant recipients are at a major advantage. There is no doubt that the quality of life of a transplant patient with minimal complications is far greater than that of even the most well-adjusted hemodialysis patient.[10] Despite the initiation of dialysis, many patients continue to have multiple symptoms, with pain, fatigue, pruritus, and constipation present in more than 50%. Potentially treatable symptoms include bone and joint pains, insomnia, mood disturbance, sexual dysfunction, parasthesia, and nausea.

The advantages are less clear cut if comparison is made between an independent home hemodialysis patient and a transplant patient who suffers major complications of immunosuppression. The ANZDATA Registry is one of the few to examine the issue of quality of life systematically. The 1998 report showed that 85% of transplant recipients were judged to have a normal quality of life in that they were able to carry on normal activities with only minor symptoms.[9] Only 44% of dialysis patients were in this category; however, 83% of dialysis patients were self-caring; 9% required considerable or special assistance. However more recent reports did not show any difference, but this again may be biased by RRT acceptance criteria.[30]

REFERENCES

1. Ashley C, Currie A, editors. The renal drug handbook. 3rd ed. Oxford: Radcliffe Publishing; 2009.
2. Black C, Sharma P, Scotland G, et al. Early referral strategies for management of people with markers of renal disease: a systematic review of the evidence of clinical effectiveness, cost-effectiveness and economic analysis. Health Technol Assess 2010;14(21):1–184.
3. Canada-USA (CANUSA) Peritoneal Dialysis Study Group. Adequacy of dialysis and nutrition in continuous peritoneal dialysis: association with clinical outcomes. J Am Soc Nephrol 1996;7:198.
4. Cattran DC, Fenton SS. Contemporary management of renal failure: outcome of the failed allograft recipient. Kidney Int 1993;41(Suppl.):S36.
5. Chan KE, Maddux FW, Tolkoff-Rubin N, et al. Early outcomes among those initiating chronic dialysis in the United States. Clin J Am Soc Nephrol 2011;6(11):2642–9.
6. Cheung AK, Rocco MV, Yan G, et al. Serum beta-2 microglobulin levels predict mortality in dialysis patients: results of the HEMO study. J Am Soc Nephrol 2006;17(2):546–55.
7. Chilcot J, Davenport A, Wellsted D, et al. An association between depressive symptoms and survival in incident dialysis patients. Nephrol Dial Transplant 2011;26(5):1628–34.
8. Cooper BA, Branley P, Bulfone L, et al. A randomized, controlled trial of early versus late initiation of dialysis. N Engl J Med 2010;363(7):609–19.
9. Disney APS, Russ GR, Walker R, et al., editors. ANZDATA registry report 1998. Adelaide, South Australia: Australia and New Zealand Dialysis and Transplant Registry; 1998.
10. Griva K, Stygall J, Ng JH, et al. Prospective changes in health-related quality of life and emotional outcomes in kidney transplantation over 6 years. J Transplant 2011;2011:671571.
11. Habib SM, Betjes MG, Fieren MW, et al. Management of encapsulating peritoneal sclerosis: a guideline on optimal and uniform treatment. Neth J Med 2011;69(11):500–7.
12. Hobbs H, Stevens P, Klebe B, et al. Referral patterns to renal services: what has changed in the past 4 years? Nephrol Dial Transplant 2009;24(11):3411–9.
13. Hossain MP, Palmer D, Goyder E, et al. Social deprivation and prevalence of chronic kidney disease in the UK: workload implications for primary care. QJM 2012;105(2):167–75.
14. Juutilainen A, Kastarinen H, Antikainen R, et al. Trends in estimated kidney function: the FINRISK surveys. Eur J Epidemiol 2012;27:305–13.
15. Kagoma YK, Weir MA, Iansavichus AV, et al. Impact of estimated GFR reporting on patients, clinicians, and health-care systems: a systematic review. Am J Kidney Dis 2011;57(4):592–601.
16. Klahr S, Levey AS, Beck GJ, et al. The effects of dietary protein restriction and blood-pressure control on the progression of chronic renal disease: modification of diet in Renal Disease Study Group. N Engl J Med 1994;330:877.
17. Korevaar JC, Feith GW, Dekker FW, et al. Effect of starting with hemodialysis compared with peritoneal dialysis in patients new on dialysis treatment: a randomized controlled trial. Kidney Int 2003;64(6):2222–8.
18. Levey AS, Atkins R, Coresh J, et al. Chronic kidney disease as a global public health problem: approaches and initiatives – a position statement from kidney disease improving global outcomes. Kidney Int 2007;72(3):247–59.
19. Levey AS, Coresh J. Chronic kidney disease. Lancet 2012;379(9811):165–80.
20. Levey AS, Eckardt KU, Tsukamoto Y, et al. Definition and classification of chronic kidney disease: a position statement from kidney disease: improving global outcomes (KDIGO). Kidney Int 2005;67(6):2089–100.
21. Li PK, Szeto CC, Piraino B, et al. Peritoneal dialysis-related infections recommendations: 2010 update. Perit Dial Int 2010;30(4):393–423.
22. Locatelli F, Altieri P, Andrulli S, et al. Hemofiltration and hemodiafiltration reduce intradialytic hypotension in ESRD. J Am Soc Nephrol 2010;21(10):1798–807.

23. Locatelli F, Martin-Malo A, Hannedouche T, et al. Effect of membrane permeability on survival of hemodialysis patients. J Am Soc Nephrol 2009;20(3):645–54.
24. Lowrie EG, Laird NM, Parker TF, et al. Effect of haemodialysis prescription on patient morbidity: report from the National Cooperative Dialysis Study. N Engl J Med 1981;305:1176.
25. Meier-Kriesche HU, Kaplan B. Waiting time on dialysis as the strongest modifiable risk factor for renal transplant outcomes: a paired donor kidney analysis. Transplantation 2002;74:1377–81.
26. Mikhail A, Srivastora R, Richardson R. Anaemia. Renal Association clinical guidelines 5th version 2010. Available online at: www.renal.org/clinical/guidelinessection/AnaemiaInCKD.aspx.
27. Paniagua R, Amato D, Vonesh E, et al. Effects of increased peritoneal clearances on mortality rates in peritoneal dialysis: ADEMEX, a prospective, randomized, controlled trial. J Am Soc Nephrol 2002;13(5):1307–20.
28. Parker 3rd TF, Husni L, Huang W, et al. Survival of haemodialysis patients in the United States is improved with a greater quantity of dialysis. Am J Kidney Dis 1994;23:670–80.
29. Piraino B, Bernardini J, Brown E, et al. ISPD position statement on reducing the risks of peritoneal dialysis-related infections. Perit Dial Int 2011;31(6):614–30.
30. Sayin A, Mutluay R, Sindel S. Quality of life in hemodialysis, peritoneal dialysis, and transplantation patients. Transplant Proc 2007;39:3047–53.
31. Smart NA, Titus TT. Outcomes of early versus late nephrology referral in chronic kidney disease: a systematic review. Am J Med 2011;124(11):1073–80.
32. Srisawat N, Hoste EE, Kellum JA. Modern classification of acute kidney injury. Blood Purif 2010;29(3):300–7.
33. Vinsonneau C, Camus C, Combes A, et al. Continuous venovenous haemodiafiltration versus intermittent haemodialysis for acute renal failure in patients with multiple-organ dysfunction syndrome: a multicentre randomised trial. Lancet 2006;368(9533):379–85.
34. Wolfe RA, Ashby VB, Milford EL, et al. Comparison of mortality in all patients on dialysis, patients on dialysis awaiting transplantation, and recipients of a first cadaveric transplant [see comments]. N Engl J Med 1999;341:1725.
35. Woodrow G, Davies S. Peritoneal Dialysis Renal Association clinical guidelines 5th version 2010. Available online at: www.renal.org/clinical/guidelinessection/peritoneal.
36. Zou Z, Zhang HL, Roditi GH, et al. Nephrogenic systemic fibrosis: review of 370 biopsy-confirmed cases. JACC Cardiovasc Imaging 2011;4(11):1206–16.

USEFUL WEBSITES

Acute Dialysis Quality Initiative, www.adqi.net.

Australia and New Zealand Renal Registry, www.anzdata.org.au/v1/report_2010.html.

British Transplant Society clinical guidelines, www.bts.org.uk.

European Dialysis and Transplantation clinical practice guidelines, www.ndt-educational.org/guidelines.asp.

International Society for Peritoneal Dialysis clinical guidelines, www.ispd.org.

Kidney Disease Improving Global Outcomes, www.kdigo.org.

National Institute for Health and Clinical Excellence, www2.evidence.nhs.uk.

Renal Association clinical guidelines, www.renal.org/clinical/guidelinessection/.

UK Renal Registry, http://www.renalreg.com/Reports/2010.html.

United States of America Renal Data Survey, www.usrds.org/2011/.

CHAPTER 4

THE RECIPIENT OF A KIDNEY TRANSPLANT

Jeremy R. Chapman

CHAPTER OUTLINE

THE PATIENT WITH CHRONIC KIDNEY DISEASE

Most patients with chronic kidney disease (CKD) in developed economies of the world are first seen by medical services with time to plan transition to end-stage renal failure therapy. The insidious nature of uremia deludes many into failing to take the opportunity to understand their disease, learn about their dialysis, transplant and palliative care options, and plan their future. It is probably the relatively asymptomatic decline in renal function that accounts for why so many ignore the warnings and fail to return for follow-up until they are brought into the emergency department hyperkalemic, acidotic, and confused. The physician's primary aim is thus often to ensure that the patient and family understand the prognosis and their need to make longer-term decisions, while at the same time managing treatable problems and retarding the progression of CKD. Intelligent and financially stable members of the community tend to be better prepared for the onset of end-stage kidney disease, while at the other extreme the poorly educated, frightened, or non-compliant tread a hazardous course to dialysis and, all too often, to an earlier death.

It is not surprising that those who plan their treatment well and receive a living donor transplant pre-emptively before the requirement for dialysis tend to have the best outcomes.[19,69] It should also not be surprising that access to pre-emptive living donor transplantation is better for

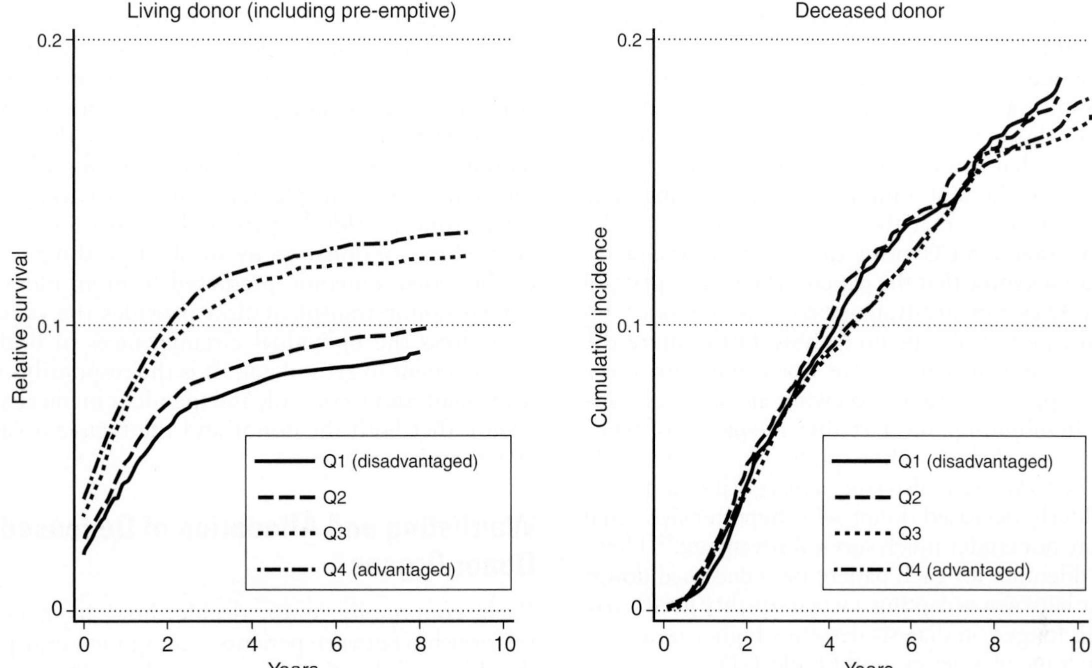

FIGURE 4-1 ■ The role of socioeconomic status in access to living and deceased donor transplantation in Australia. Q, quartile of socioeconomic disadvantage. (From Grace BS, Clayton PA, Cass A, et al. Transplantation rates for living- but not deceased-donor kidneys vary with socioeconomic status in Australia. Kidney Int 2013; 83: 138–145.)

patients with higher socioeconomic status[40] (Figure 4-1). Most people are however treated by hemodialysis or peritoneal dialysis for weeks, months, or years before finally being transplanted. There are some benefits to pretransplant dialysis, especially if the patient is chronically debilitated by CKD, or if time is needed to enable a family member to understand the benefits of offering a kidney. For some the experience of dialysis provides an important demonstration of life without a kidney transplant, which usually strengthens their resolve both to undergo the operation and accept the long-term consequences of immunosuppression. This chapter attempts to identify the issues that patients, their family, and the community must consider before deciding to have a kidney transplant.

GENERAL CONCEPTS

Fitness to Transplant

The patient has, in principle, only one simple question to consider: will the quality and quantity of life be better after a transplant than on dialysis? For many people the answer is clear and unequivocal – either because the alternative of long-term dialysis treatment is either not available or unaffordable (www.who.int/transplantation/knowledgebase/en) or because transplantation is the obvious solution since they are young and otherwise fit. For some people, however, the answer is clouded in uncertainty because of the relative unavailability of organs for transplantation, or because they have comorbid conditions that will be exacerbated by the operation or the ensuing immunosuppression.

Quality of life is perhaps the single most important issue for most people and yet the field has found the social sciences difficult to grasp and there are few studies comparing quality of life on dialysis and after transplantation. Most clinicians find it hard to identify living individuals with a lower quality of life after a successful transplant than they had or would have had on dialysis, and thus find it easy to advocate for transplantation. This approach discounts the patient deaths and graft failures, and the diminished quality of life for those who struggle with the consequences of immune deficiency, infections, and malignancies. Transplant programs tend to substitute graft survival data for true quality of life data and use it as a surrogate, but objective, measure of the success that each individual might expect[97] instead of a measured comparison of quantity of life.[76,115] In countries without sufficient dialysis capacity, the decision to receive a kidney transplant is obvious for almost all patients, since transplantation is the only alternative to a slow death from uremia. This does assume access to both immunosuppressant drugs and lifelong specialist medical follow-up, either of which may not be available and without which transplantation becomes a futile delusion. The understanding by a patient and family of the lifelong commitment needed for a transplant is an important factor. Patient survival rates are substantially impacted by compliance with follow-up, and that is dependent on patients' expectations. Transplantation has been promoted as a cure, when it is actually a complicated treatment requiring regular follow-up by specialists working in sophisticated medical centers using expensive drugs. If the patient and family fail to understand the costs, level of follow-up, and compliance that will be required of them, then it is likely that the published statistics of average survival will not apply to them.

Predicting the success rate after transplantation relies on characteristics of both the recipient and the donor. Probably the most comprehensive studies comparing transplant recipients with those remaining on dialysis come from the United States where it has been possible to track the outcomes of all individuals entered on to the transplant waiting list and compare those who were transplanted with those who remained on dialysis.[76,115] These studies show that transplantation carries the greater risk of death for the first 3 months or so, reversing after that point in time so that the risk of death is equal by 6–9 months, thereafter favoring the transplant recipient. Similar analyses show that the patient who is transplanted pre-emptively carries an advantage compared to one who has needed a period of time on dialysis; furthermore the longer the period of dialysis, the worse the outcome.[19] These data apply to patients receiving an "average" donor graft, highlighting the fact that recipients of well-matched young living donor grafts do substantially better.[75] The converse is also true: a marginal donor graft from an elderly deceased donor with hypertensive renal damage may not confer much survival advantage.[86] There remains a dilemma for each patient on a deceased donor waiting list between accepting a worse-quality graft early and waiting longer on dialysis despite a higher mortality rate, in the hope of a better graft (Table 4-1).

The patients' expectations from a successful transplant are to die in old age with a perfectly functioning kidney. The reality is that they will die much earlier than an age- and sex-matched individual without renal disease, and more than half will have lost their graft before they die.[16,74] From the patient's perspective, graft failure before death represents failure, but from the community's perspective premature death with a functioning graft could be seen to represent wasted years of graft function that could have been applied to someone with a better prognosis.

Appropriateness to Transplant

There are two ways to examine this question, which can be considered either from the view of the recipient or the donor. These are not the same and it is important to understand that these perspectives may lead to different decisions about the appropriateness of a particular transplant. To illustrate the difference: consider a father or mother in their late 60s without any comorbid conditions, deciding whether or not to accept a donation from a 30-year-old son or daughter. The son or daughter may consider it appropriate to offer a kidney to the parent, acknowledging the small but real immediate and possible, but unknown, long-term risks to him- or herself. The parent may consider it highly inappropriate to place his or her offspring at even the slightest risk to provide a few years of better quality of life. In the reverse situation it may be considered appropriate for a 20-year-old recipient to be transplanted, but not to accept a donor offer from an elderly parent, both because of the increased risk of donation by an older person and because of the worse outcome predicted from an older kidney. Living donor transplantation provides the opportunity to address the individual circumstances of both donor and recipient in great detail. It is the responsibility of the transplant unit to provide independent medical advice to ensure that both the donor and the recipient can arrive at a considered decision.

TABLE 4-1 **Survival Advantage in Australia**

	Dialysis Mortality	*Transplant Mortality*
Age	**Rate (per 100 patient years)**	**Rate (per 100 patient years)**
<25	1.13 (0.28–4.51)	0.30 (0.13–0.67)
25–44	4.64 (3.55–6.06)	0.43 (0.29–0.63)
45–64	9.79 (8.89–10.79)	1.46 (1.22–1.74)
65–84	17.61 (16.50–18.81)	3.00 (2.30–3.91)
≥85	30.37 (25.43–36.26)	–

Data courtesy of ANZDATA 2011: McDonald S, Hurst K, editors. Registry Report 2011. Adelaide, South Australia: Australia and New Zealand Dialysis and Transplant Registry.

Waitlisting and Allocation of Deceased Donor Organs

Each community must decide how to manage the relationship between patients waiting for a transplant and the deceased donor kidney offers. In most countries national, regional, or local waiting lists provide access to the offer, although in some places, where deceased donors are rare, selection may be ad hoc. The percentage of dialysis patients actively listed for transplantation varies quite surprisingly, with 24% in the United States and 55% in the United Kingdom (http://www.organdonation.nhs.uk/ukt/statistics/transplant_activity_report/transplant_activity_report.asp).[71] There are not only barriers due to age and comorbidities but also from demographic, geographical, and socioeconomic factors. The community – when asked – almost always defines "equity of access" as the most important factor, but the reality is a complex balance of medical utility and sometimes conflicting notions of equity. Healthcare professionals are far from agreed on what should constitute the criteria for medical eligibility and whether or not it is appropriate to include consideration of social and lifestyle factors, ability to understand and adhere to treatment, as well as medical estimates of prognosis.

There are many published guidelines on assessment for transplant waiting lists, which have been reviewed in 2012.[5] The stated aim of almost all of these guidelines is to provide objective and explicit advice to the clinician faced with an individual patient assessment. Most achieve a comprehensive perspective, but there are substantial differences over the methodology behind each recommendation. There is a largely consistent approach to the required level of renal impairment and medical comorbidities, with most also providing broad statements on age criteria, life expectancy, and both psychological and social factors. The impact of high body mass index (BMI) is interpreted as both a criterion for surgical acceptability and a medical criterion predicting cardiovascular and other morbidity and mortality, but advice is based on expert opinion rather than hard evidence. Shortage of donor organs in most environments leaves a tension between maximizing utility on the one hand and equity on the other. In resolving this tension, most guidelines attempt to promote a transparent decision-making process in the absence of a robust formula that is universally applicable to each individual.

Once a list of eligible recipients has been created, explicit algorithms are required for allocation of a particular donor offer. These must take into account medical issues such as blood group, histocompatibility, and crossmatching, and may also consider sociodemographic criteria such as waiting times and comparative donor and recipient ages.[62,70,71] Most developed countries have well-organized computer algorithms determined by committees including both medical and lay representatives, with audit of compliance. In allocation systems where this does not happen, it is hard to see how either fairness or utility can be served, and the appropriateness of organ allocation demonstrated to the community. Corrupt practices are undoubtedly the outcome in some countries.

COUNSELING

What the Patient Needs to Know

The transplant unit has the responsibility to provide each patient with advice based on his or her own medical conditions and education about the options for long-term treatment. The starting point for such education is thus in many countries a comprehensive evaluation of the suitability, availability, and financial cost of dialysis options. The quality of physical and emotional wellbeing provided by dialysis therapy usually becomes abundantly clear to most patients, either through meeting other patients already on dialysis, or through dialysis education programs, and finally, definitively, through direct personal experience, except in that small minority able to undergo pre-emptive transplantation.

A comprehensive evaluation needs to be provided by the transplant unit of each individual's medical risks if the patient were to undergo a kidney transplant.[52] Much of the rest of this chapter details the medical assessment, but a checklist is provided in Table 4-2. This list includes those issues that impact upon the individual patient's technical transplantability as well as the short- and long-term factors that influence hard outcomes. In assessing the patient's suitability for a transplant operation the physician will be focused on the heart and lungs, the surgeon on the blood vessels and bladder. The surgeon will need to discuss the various complications and risks of the surgical procedure, while the physician discussion should revolve around the drugs, long-term risks, and follow-up protocols. Providing patients with sufficient knowledge on organ allocation processes, the pros and cons of particular donor kidney offers, and on the financial costs that they will be expected to bear is easily left out of a traditional medical consultation. Most established transplant programs thus have additional formal education sessions provided by a range of specialized coordinators, social workers, and pharmacists. The internet and social media increasingly provide a wide range of both good and bad information which patients will certainly access extensively (http://www.kidney.org/transplantation/, http://www.kidney.org.au, http://www.umm.edu/transplant/patient/index.html). A guide to the better material and warnings against the bad sources of information must also play a part in the advice provided by the transplant program.

TABLE 4-2 Checklist for Pretransplant Education of the Patient and Family

1. Medical condition
   - General cardiorespiratory fitness for operation
   - Impact of obesity
   - Vascular system suitability for operation
     - Urological complications
     - Risks of recurrent renal disease
2. Fitness for lifelong immunosuppression
   - Infections
   - Malignancies, especially skin cancers
   - Cardiovascular risk factors
3. Histocompatibility and organ donor source: impact on outcomes
4. Waiting times and allocation systems on the deceased organ donor waiting list
5. Availability and donor outcomes of living donor procedures
6. Financial costs and specific risks of the donor and transplant procedures, including disease transmission from the donor
7. Financial and adverse event costs of prophylactic immunosuppressive and anti-infective drugs
8. Long-term follow-up protocol
9. Short- and long-term risks of graft failure and death after transplantation
10. Consideration of acceptance of extended criteria donor organs
11. Patient-specific issues, e.g., options for pancreas transplantation in diabetics and liver/kidney in primary oxalosis

Consent

It is, of course, normal practice to seek written informed consent just prior to undergoing any surgical procedure and all transplant operations are preceded by such a ritual signing of a legalistically phrased document. Somewhere amongst this scant and hastily signed documentation will be the expectation that individuals have accepted all the risks of transplantation, from transmission of serious disease from the donor through to the side effects of every drug that they will be given. Many patients will also be presented with a dazzling array of research protocols to sign up to, with patient information sheets of many pages of closely typed and densely constructed language designed to protect the researcher, hospital, and pharmaceutical company more than inform the patient. This documentation of "consent" often takes place under pressure of time and in the middle of the night, even sometimes on the telephone. It is hard to see how anything provided by the patient in the haste of the anesthetic workup, no matter what it is written on, can be argued to be informed consent. Legal opinions have been given that suggest that no reliance can be placed upon a patient's decision taken under the pressure of an immediate pretransplant consent, unless backed by extensive prior education and information. In constructing education programs, it would be wise for the transplant unit to consider the traditional "operation consent form" a legally valueless protection.

What the Potential Living Donor Needs to Know

A potential living donor usually needs to be provided information on both the recipient outcomes and the donor operation, with its attendant risks, in order to decide on whether or not to proceed.

Donors who expect, for the recipient, only a successful outcome from their donation have a reasonable chance of being badly disappointed. It is thus essential that the best estimates of the risks of death and graft failure are clearly laid before the donor.[54,55] It is also important for most donors to appreciate the dialysis alternatives available to the patient, as well as the deceased donor waiting list times. In countries with substantial waiting lists and long waiting times, living donation clearly offers huge advantages that are not so clearly apparent where deceased donor waiting times are short. In countries with high deceased donor rates, the advantages of providing a better kidney with better long-term survival may be less obvious, but just as real.

A living donor must provide fully informed consent to a surgeon with no conflicts of interest through their care of the potential recipient.[24] In addition it is relevant for donors to appreciate their blood group and histocompatibility match with the recipient, as well as any concerns that there might be about the crossmatching data. A general overview of the risks that the recipient faces will help to ensure that the small percentages of procedures that end in disaster are not followed by endless recrimination and litigation. More importantly, a well-prepared donor is better able psychologically to face the future after a failed transplant or even the death of the recipient.

What the Family Needs to Know

The families of pediatric patients are best regarded as if they were the patient, with respect to the information and counseling (see Chapter 40) that they require, though there are special considerations that young age brings to bear on the decision making in kidney transplantation. The family of the adult patient is in a special situation compared to other areas of medicine, since the family represent a potential source of organ donation and cannot simply be thought of as emotionally involved onlookers and supporters for the patient. Transplant units vary in the way in which information is provided about the potential to donate a kidney, with some distributing information packs directly to all known family members, while others await specific approaches before providing information on living related donation. In countries with low deceased organ donation rates, the increasing attention being placed upon living donation creates the ambience for routine dissemination of information to family members and friends.[96] Accurate provision of specific relevant information is dependent upon the consent of the recipient to release his or her private medical details. Asking the question: "Is there anyone in the family who would donate you a kidney?" elicits some interesting insights into the dynamics of families with members with serious chronic illness. Some patients refuse to consider a discussion of their illness with their family, while others are glad that an independent person is prepared to raise awareness in their family of the seriousness of their illness.

Lack of information is almost always the starting point for a breakdown in trust and communication between patients, their family, and their medical attendants. For this reason it is important that even the most distant of families are aware of the possibility of a poor outcome from transplantation and the importance of compliance with medication and follow-up to the long-term success of the transplant.

SPECIFIC MEDICAL CONSIDERATIONS

Cardiac (see Chapter 30)

The first consideration of any patient undergoing a major operation is the state of that patient's heart. Dialysis patients, and especially diabetic dialysis patients, have high incidences of both symptomatic and asymptomatic ischemic heart disease and thus a careful evaluation of the heart is essential.[63] Evidence-based agreement on how to perform that assessment is lacking and thus highly dependent upon local expertise and opinion.

All patients need a careful clinical history and examination, including an electrocardiogram and usually also an echocardiogram to assess left ventricular function and a stressed echocardiogram or myocardial perfusion study to exclude significant ischemic heart disease. While CKD itself is the strongest risk factor for coronary artery disease, it is also important to assess obesity, family history, lipid profile, blood pressure, smoking history, and diabetes.[52] Attitudes to smoking history vary amongst transplant units from outright refusal to transplant those patients who continue to smoke through to more liberal approaches.[20]

Some transplant programs require routine coronary angiography prior to acceptance on to a waiting list. There is certainly a rationale for such an approach given the high levels of coronary disease uncovered by such a strategy.[29] The only randomized trial of surgical or medical intervention in this situation (diabetics with CKD) was so unequivocal about the value of intervention that the trial was halted and the non-intervention arm offered surgery or angioplasty.[65] The weaknesses of this study (it only assessed diabetics and optimum medical therapy would not be considered optimum today) and the lack of alternative randomized studies leave the field with uncertainties, but also a very clear view that diabetic patients need comprehensive cardiac evaluation.

A lesser strategy is to use a non-invasive test such as a stressed dopamine echocardiogram[103] or stressed nuclear study[18] or, more recently, computed tomography (CT) coronary angiography[84] as a screening method for asymptomatic and low-risk patients, thus reserving coronary angiography for those with symptoms, significant risk factors, or a positive screening test. This is not foolproof and relies upon the negative predictive value of the screening test, so that the occasional patient with ischemic heart disease will still be transplanted unknowingly and without the consideration of prior treatment of the cardiac disease. Patients will also be operated on knowingly with minor abnormalities in the screening tests reflecting disease in minor coronary branches and leading sometimes to postoperative chest pain, troponin leakage into the blood, and only minor cardiovascular instability.

Proceeding to transplantation in patients with normal left ventricular function and normal coronary vasculature is the easy decision. The more complex issue is deciding who to transplant despite known cardiac disease, which needs to be considered not only on its own merits, but also because of the implications that it carries for widespread vascular disease.[52] There is no evidence-based answer to this question as yet and clinicians must thus rely upon local opinion-based decisions, guided by some general principles:

- Treatable coronary and valvular disease is almost always worth treating before transplantation rather than afterwards, both because of the risks posed by the cardiac disease during the transplant procedure and because of the risks that cardiac interventional procedures carry in the presence of immunosuppression and a functioning transplant.[64]
- It is usually wiser to avoid transplantation if, despite treatment of coronary artery and/or valvular disease, there remains a substantial risk of infarction of a large area of myocardium, or there is substantial left ventricular dysfunction. Cardiac disease is the single largest cause of mortality in both the dialysis and transplant populations and there is little evidence that transplantation will beneficially alter the outcome of ischemic heart disease.[30] There is less certainty with respect to congestive cardiac failure, where poorly dialyzed patients may recover significant function when uremia and chronic fluid overload are corrected by transplantation.[9]
- In patients with severe and irreversible cardiac dysfunction, the remaining consideration is the option of combined heart and kidney transplantation, available to very limited numbers of young and otherwise healthy individuals transplanted in highly specialized centers.[43]

Vascular (see Chapter 28)

There is an absolute requirement for an available recipient artery for anastomosis of the transplant renal artery. Atheromatous iliac arteries that have been ossified through years of CKD management must thus be carefully assessed by the surgeon planning to perform the transplant. Absence of intermittent claudication and presence of palpable femoral and pedal pulses may be sufficient to confirm transplantability. There are however many potential recipients with a high risk of severe vascular disease, where duplex ultrasound scanning of the femoral and carotid vessels will identify those at significant risk of peripheral or cerebrovascular events either during or after transplantation.[82]

Selection of patients with known pre-existing peripheral vascular disease must include a general assessment of their prognosis as well as specific assessment of the vascular supply needed for the transplant operation. The largest numbers of patients commencing dialysis in most developed countries are elderly obese type 2 diabetics and many have severe peripheral vascular disease.[109] Only a very small proportion of such patients prove to be suitable for transplantation because of the combined effects of obesity, cardiac and vascular disease on their operative mortality and 3–5-year survival rates.[116] Two-thirds of dialysis patients requiring lower-limb amputations are dead within 2 years, implying that this group of patients has such a poor prognosis that only a very few highly selected patients could be accepted for transplantation.[28]

Symptomatic cerebrovascular disease presents a separate problem in selection for transplantation. A history of transient ischemic attacks obviously promotes a search for a cardiac or carotid vascular cause, which, if diagnosed and resolved or treated, need not contraindicate subsequent transplantation.[25] The complication that warfarin anticoagulation of patients with atrial fibrillation provides the transplant unit can usually be overcome with a rapid anticoagulant reversal protocol and then use of heparin in the posttransplant period before re-anticoagulation (Table 4-3). Warfarin therapy is thus not an absolute contraindication to acceptance for a deceased donor transplant. Completed stroke and severe carotid disease, however, often place the patient in the same category as those with severe cardiac or peripheral vascular disease with respect to their general prognosis and the futility of transplantation. A major consideration is the propensity for the use of double antiplatelet therapy with both aspirin and Persantin or clopidogrel after intervention – see section on coagulation disorders, below.

One group of patients who need particular attention are those with adult polycystic kidney disease, especially if they have a personal or family history of cerebral aneurysm.[47] Evaluation of such high-risk patients requires cerebral vascular imaging such as cerebral CT angiography or a magnetic resonance image angiogram to exclude berry aneurysms, before proceeding to transplantation.

Respiratory

Assessment of respiratory disease in the potential transplant candidate has two purposes: to identify patients at risk from the anesthetic; and to identify patients who will be at risk of life-threatening infection in the long

TABLE 4-3 **Anticoagulant Reversal Protocol Prior to Transplant Surgery**

A patient on warfarin who requires surgery within the next 8 hours should receive:

1. 1 unit of fresh frozen plasma (FFP)
2. 5 mg intravenous vitamin K
3. Prothrombinex (human prothrombin complex): dose adjusted for international normalized ratio (INR) and patient weight
   - INR 2–3.9: 25 units/kg
   - INR 4–5.9: 35 units/kg
   - INR >6.0: 50 units/kg
   - Prothrombinex (1000 units/vial) – calculate to the nearest 1000 units
4. Check prothrombin time (PT)/activated partial thromboplastin time (APTT) prior to surgery and 4–8 hours later if surgery is delayed
5. If surgery is to occur >8 hours from reversal, FFP is not required but PT/APTT needs to be rechecked before surgery to confirm adequate reversal

term as the result of immunosuppression. The former is thus based around assessment of smoking and both acute reversible and chronic obstructive airways disease. It is no different to the assessment that must be made before any elective operation.[49] The latter is a more complex decision and remains largely subjective. The diseases of importance are bronchiectasis, tuberculosis, and prior fungal infections, all of which may quickly become uncontrollable under the influence of immunosuppression. Formal evaluation of the degree of respiratory compromise and the frequency and severity of infective exacerbations will determine the advisability of transplantation of the patient with bronchiectasis.

Active pulmonary tuberculosis must be identified from routine chest X-ray and effectively treated before consideration of transplantation.[3] Patients at high risk of reactivation of tuberculosis after transplantation include those from areas with high endemic rates.[100] History of exposure, calcified lesions on chest X-ray or elsewhere, and a positive skin test to purified protein derivative (PPD) all provide evidence of past exposure and risk of disease, but a negative PPD test cannot be relied upon to exclude disease in the anergic dialysis population, leading to exploration of the Quantiferon Gold test as an alternative.[56] BCG vaccination is not safe after transplantation,[50] thus transplant units in endemic areas tend to advise high-risk patients to have a full treatment course for tuberculosis after transplantation. In developed countries, based on slender evidence,[3] management usually involves adding a prophylactic course of isoniazid for 6 months.[94]

Hepatic Disease (see Chapter 32)

Hepatitis B

The majority of dialysis patients with past or current hepatitis B will have been identified through routine testing of serum for hepatitis B surface antigen (HBsAg) and antibodies to hepatitis B core and surface antigens. Many dialysis programs have a routine hepatitis vaccination policy to improve protection from cross-infection, even though vaccination is much more effective if administered before the need for dialysis.[53] Thus most patients being assessed for transplantation have been screened for prior exposure to hepatitis B.

Data from transplantation of chronically infected HBsAg-positive patients, predominantly gained in the 1980s and 1990s, demonstrate worse outcomes than for HBsAg-negative patients.[31]

Knowledge of the status of the liver histology is important in predicting outcomes after kidney transplantation, with poor medium- to long-term results with pre-existing chronic active hepatitis and with cirrhosis.[33] It is now clear that use of posttransplant lamivudine therapy has not carried the survival benefits hoped for, at least in one carefully evaluated Korean study.[89] Choice of immunosuppression after transplantation may influence the progression of hepatitis, with concern expressed about steroids, azathioprine, and cyclosporine reactivating hepatitis B in the chronic carrier.[21] Hepatitis B is not a contraindication to kidney transplantation, but established cirrhosis raises the option of combined liver and kidney transplantation.[81] Data at present indicate that a survival advantage is conferred by combined renal and liver transplantation in those patients on dialysis as a result of CKD prior to the requirement for liver transplantation, and is far from predictable in patients with liver failure and either hepatorenal syndrome or other forms of acute kidney injury.[46]

Hepatitis C

Hepatitis C represents different challenges to transplant programs in different countries, with high prevalence in dialysis programs with reuse of dialysis consumables and in patients transfused in the 1980s. The natural history of hepatitis C infection leads to high proportions of patients eventually developing significant liver disease.[60] Treatment of patients with hepatitis C infection is made complex – if not impossible – by renal failure and requirement for dialysis since therapeutic agents are poorly tolerated by dialysis patients.[23] Hepatitis C genotypes 2 and 3 are more responsive to therapy than genotype 1 and thus it is warranted to attempt to treat patients before the onset of dialysis, though the genotype may not affect posttransplant outcomes.[83] Assessment of patients for the transplant waiting list should include hepatitis C antibody routinely, and if that test is positive, also hepatitis C RNA testing and assessment of viral load, as well as genotyping. Most units rely on liver histology to assess the severity of hepatitis in potential transplant recipients, with advanced disease providing a relative contraindication to kidney transplantation. One recent study demonstrated that age and albumin levels correlated significantly with outcome but that cirrhosis did not statistically impact outcome based on small numbers.[88] Hepatitis C-infected patients without significant liver disease certainly survive better if transplanted than if they remain on dialysis,[91] but do not fare as well as those without hepatitis C. The shortage of donor organs has raised the question, in most jurisdictions, of use of hepatitis C-positive kidneys in hepatitis C-positive recipients, especially those positive for hepatitis C RNA with genotype 1. It has been long established that there is no justification for the use of a hepatitis C-positive kidney in a patient who has never been infected or who has cleared virus, i.e., is hepatitis C antibody-positive, but RNA-negative.[92]

Other Liver Disease

Potential kidney transplant recipients may suffer from other causes of significant liver disease, such as alcoholic liver disease, polycystic liver in association with polycystic kidney disease, or cholelithiasis. It is thus important and relatively simple to assess both liver function and appearance of the liver on ultrasound. Fatty infiltration of the liver is the commonest finding of such screening protocols and may be associated with diabetes but is not in itself a contraindication to transplantation. Severe liver disease, no matter what the cause, inhibits acceptance for kidney transplantation of most patients. There is diversity of opinion on the role of prophylactic cholecystectomy in dialysis patients with known gallstones, with the larger studies not supporting this approach,[42] but others advocating routine pretransplant screening and surgery for known gallstones.[101]

Infectious Disease (see Chapter 31)

Vaccination Strategies

General community protection from infectious disease will, in most countries, have led to routine childhood vaccination against measles, mumps, polio, rubella, diphtheria, tetanus, pertussis, *Haemophilus influenzae* B, and varicella-zoster, and, more recently, human papillomavirus which has been added to the list. Pneumococcal and hepatitis B vaccination programs, though widespread, are far from universal. It is especially important in pediatric practice to ensure that vaccination has not been forgotten amongst the problems of pediatric renal failure.[36,93] In adult practice it is also important to understand each patient's vaccination history and to remedy deficiencies as soon as possible since the responses to vaccines are generally impaired in the dialysis population.[59]

Vaccination of patients after transplantation is either dangerous and thus contraindicated with live vaccines, or may fail with killed antigen vaccines, since the medication used to prevent allograft rejection is well designed to suppress production of an antibody response to a viral antigen. Mycophenolate mofetil, for example, is especially capable of preventing antibody production after vaccination.[104] Live vaccines are absolutely contraindicated after transplantation, with the commonest errors being the use of yellow fever vaccination in travelers to South America and chickenpox vaccination with attenuated virus, leading to life-threatening disseminated pox virus infection in transplant recipients.

Human Immunodeficiency Virus

Transplantation of individuals with human immunodeficiency virus (HIV) was contraindicated until the recent era of antiretroviral therapy. The consequences of immunosuppressing a patient who was infected with HIV but untreated were discovered during the 1980s in patients infected before transplantation or when the virus was unwittingly transmitted through organ donation.[98] Expertise has however developed in a number of centers for managing HIV-positive patients after transplantation, with acceptable results.[79,90,107] It is universal practice to test both recipients and donors for antibodies to HIV and for antigen using a nucleotide antigen test, with the decision to transplant the positive recipient dependent upon a CD4 count greater than 200 cells/mL and the concomitant availability of highly active antiretroviral therapy and local expertise in the transplant center. In South Africa, the use of HIV-positive donors for HIV-infected patients has been an interesting side effect of the very high prevalence of HIV in that country.

Other Viral Infections – CMV, EBV, HHV6/7, HHV8

Knowledge of a recipient's status with respect to all herpesviruses has become increasingly relevant because of the impact of these viruses after transplantation.

Chemoprophylaxis for cytomegalovirus (CMV), which also protects recipients for human herpesvirus (HHV) 6 and HHV7, is usually based upon knowledge of the donor and recipient CMV serological status. Transplantation of an Epstein–Barr virus (EBV)-positive organ into an EBV-negative recipient carries an increased risk of active EBV infection after transplantation and also of development of posttransplant lymphoproliferative disease. All patients should thus be tested for antibody status with respect to each of the herpesviruses. The Transplantation Society Guidelines on CMV provide a useful basis for understanding the alternative testing and therapeutic options available.[58]

Dental

The traditional approach to evaluation of the transplant recipient includes ensuring adequate dental hygiene and review of dentition prior to acceptance for transplantation. It is certainly true that gingival hypertrophy was a consequence of higher doses of cyclosporine, especially when combined with nifedipine, and that infected dentition may cause problems after transplantation. This has been ameliorated with use of tacrolimus and alternative antihypertensives and it would now be an unusual candidate in whom the dentition provides a risk of transplantation sufficient to outweigh the risk of continued dialysis compared to transplantation, though it is certainly important to avoid bacterial endocarditis through prophylactic antibiotics.

Miscellaneous Infections – Syphilis, Strongyloides, *Toxoplasmosis,* Trypanosoma

Transplant programs must pay heed to the particular infectious risks that are both endemic and prevalent in their geographical region, in order to evaluate properly the posttransplant risks for their transplant recipients.[67] *Trypanasoma cruzi*, the causative organism of Chagas' disease, is for example prevalent in South and Central America. It may be transmitted by donation and reactivated by immunosuppression, requiring serology and blood polymerase chain reaction surveillance and early treatment.[92]

Syphilis, *Strongyloides*, and toxoplasmosis have all been reported as opportunistic reactivations after transplantation. In most areas of the world transplant programs require a heightened awareness and lower threshold for suspicion of these diseases, rather than specific strategies for these uncommon problems. Testing for syphilis serology is still practiced by many programs, but is not seen as essential in recipients from most developed countries. It is good practice to check the patient's eosinophil count and pursue a diagnosis of infection in anyone with a raised count.

Malignancy (see Chapter 35)

There is a clear and defined additional risk of malignancy in patients with CKD and especially after transplantation. This increased risk is assumed to be due to an effect of immunosuppression either on normal mechanisms for control of neoplastic cells or more likely the impact on viral carcinogenesis.[110] This knowledge has been translated to a reluctance to transplant patients who have had a prior cancer, for fear that immunosuppression will allow recurrence that might otherwise not happen.

Australian data question this set of assumptions. Firstly, a number of cancers are increased in CKD patients and in patients on dialysis, as well as after transplantation.[111] Secondly, the increased risk is restricted to a number of types of cancer, such as skin and lip cancers, renal tract cancers, and those for which a viral etiology is either established or suspected. The implication for the potential transplant recipient is that cancers which are now understood to occur at the same rate as in the normal population should probably be considered differently to those where the risk is increased.

It has been standard advice not to transplant a patient within 2–5 years of diagnosis and definitive treatment of cancer, depending upon which cancer is under consideration. Most guidelines suggest careful screening for cancers in patients on the transplant waiting list.[5] Unfortunately such blanket rules, though easy to apply, do not take into consideration the variability of the biology of the different cancers and especially do not consider the individual risks of recurrence. Table 4-4 gives a list of cancer types that are known to be increased in dialysis and transplant patients and should thus be viewed with considerable caution in patients being assessed for transplantation. Melanoma, for example, is known to respond to T-cell immunotherapy and has a substantially increased risk after transplantation. It is known to recur in normal individuals and to metastasize aggressively. Melanoma has also been observed to recur after transplantation with long disease-free intervals pretransplantation and must thus be approached very conservatively. Breast and prostate cancer, on the other hand, do not seem to be increased in dialysis and transplant patients, but have substantial metastatic potential. To avoid transplanting a patient who will succumb to metastatic cancer soon after transplantation, it is thus prudent to advise a waiting period of at least 2 years, depending to a certain extent on the predicted risk of spread in any given individual.

Common cancers occur commonly in dialysis and transplant patients. It is important not to shift the clinical emphasis from common cancers to rare cancers, such as Kaposi's sarcoma, just because these rare cancers occur with a greatly increased risk compared to the general population. The common cancers in the Australian data include kidney, bladder, colon, lung, melanoma, breast, and prostate (Table 4-4). There is no specific guideline for cancer screening prior to listing a dialysis patient for transplantation. It would, however, be reasonable at least to ensure that screening guidelines recommended in the general population for cervical, breast, and bowel screening have been undertaken.

TABLE 4-4 **Suggested Disease-Free Time Intervals Before Transplantation of Patients with Prior Cancers**

Site (ICD-10 Codes)	
CKD-Associated Cancer	
Kidney (C64)	>2 years
Renal pelvis (C65)	>2 years
Ureter (C66)	>2 years
Bladder (C67)	>2 years
Other urinary organs (C68)	>2 years
Non-CKD-Associated	
Non-melanoma skin	(Local treatment)
Lip (C00)	(Local treatment)
Tongue (C01–C02)	>2 years
Mouth (C03–C06)	>2 years
Salivary gland (C07–C08)	>2 years
Esophagus (C15)	>2 years
Stomach (C16)	>2 years
Small intestine (C17)	>2 years
Colon (C18)	>2 years
Rectum (C19–C20)	>2 years
Anus (C21)	>2 years
Liver (C22)	(Contraindicated without liver transplant)
Gallbladder (C23–C24)	>2 years
Pancreas (C25)	>2 years
Larynx (C32)	>2 years
Trachea; bronchus and lung (C33–C34)	>2 years
Melanoma (C43)	>5 years – assess risk of metastasis
Mesothelioma (C45)	>2 years
Kaposi sarcoma (C46)	>2 years – use TORi immunosuppression
Connective and other soft tissue (C47–C49)	>2 years
Breast (C50)	>5 years
Vulva (C51)	>2 years
Cervix uteri (C53)	>2 years
Corpus uteri (C54)	>2 years
Ovary (C56)	>2 years
Penis (C60)	>2 years
Prostate (C61)	>2 years
Testis (C62)	>2 years
Eye (C69)	>2 years
Brain (C71)	>2 years
Thyroid (C73)	>2 years
Hodgkin disease (C81)	>5 years
Non-Hodgkin lymphoma (C82–C85)	>5 years
Leukemia (C91–C95)	>5 years

CKD, chronic kidney disease; TORi, target of rapamycin inhibitors.

Duration before considering transplantation = the period after apparent successful cure of the individual cancer when transplantation may be considered if investigations substantiate cure of the cancer. Note also comments for individual cancers.

Recurrence of cancer has been recorded despite disease-free periods exceeding those suggested here. Each individual patient must be assessed individually and these intervals may be too long or too short for individual circumstances. (Data from reference 110.)

Multiple myeloma needs specific consideration of prior bone marrow transplantation.

Psychiatric Disease and Drug Dependency

Compliance after transplantation and the patient's responses to the psychological stresses of transplantation should be uppermost in the minds of clinical teams evaluating recipients. Non-compliance with both medication and clinical follow-up is amongst the most distressing and devastating causes of loss of grafts. Prevention of this problem starts with understanding the patient before transplantation and responding to the different risks for non-compliance.[15] It is clear that the majority of non-compliant patients do not have a psychiatric disorder, but many with a psychiatric disorder are at risk of poor compliance.

There are two dominant reasons for careful evaluation of the psychiatric state of potential recipients: their ability to understand and consent to the transplant procedure; and the impact of psychiatric disease after transplantation. Formal psychological testing and psychiatric assessment may be required to evaluate a given individual's capacity to provide properly informed consent. Alcohol and drug abuse raise many practical, medical, ethical, and moral questions which also have to be evaluated carefully in each individual. Abstinence from chemical dependency would be regarded as essential for acceptance to the transplant waiting list by most transplant programs, but it is difficult to assure and monitor in practice.

Bone

Renal bone disease status and the degree of control of the calcium phosphate product are both important indicators of bone disease and vascular risk after transplantation.[78] In children the additional consideration of growth potential and the impact of uremia on the one hand and corticosteroids on the other are relevant considerations.

The past few years have seen an explosion in available therapies for renal bone disease and the exact status of hyperparathyroidism at the time of transplantation is less critical than it has been in the past.[87] It is important to optimize control of the features of renal bone disease, with special attention to attempting to normalize the calcium phosphate product in order to minimize hyperparathyroidism, osteoporosis, and vascular calcification after transplantation.

Gastrointestinal Tract

Perforation of a peptic ulcer has led to many transplant recipient deaths in the era of high corticosteroid use and before routine introduction of H_2 receptor blockers and more recently the proton pump inhibitors after transplantation. The incidence of untreated *Helicobacter pylori*/peptic ulcer disease is now quite low and many units use either low-dose or complete avoidance of steroids combined with omeprazole or a similar proton pump inhibitor to prevent peptic ulceration, despite the potential for interaction with immunosuppressant drug absorption.[32] Gastroesophageal reflux, malabsorption syndromes, celiac disease, diverticulosis, and cholelithiasis may all present issues for specific consideration in individual patients. It is hard to justify routine screening for peptic ulcer disease or cholelithiasis, but there are protagonists for both strategies.

Diabetes

Recipients with diabetes require special consideration with different issues in patients with type 1 and type 2 diabetes. Transplantation rates of diabetic patients fluctuate markedly by era and by transplant program, driven by the observed mortality rates, development, and availability of simultaneous pancreas and kidney transplantation (SPK), and the comorbid conditions experienced in many diabetics with nephropathy.[82]

Type 1 Diabetes Mellitus

The first decision for patients with type 1 diabetes is whether or not to seek a SPK transplant.[48] In countries where this expertise is available the two options that provide the best patient survival are pre-emptive living related kidney transplantation and SPK transplantation (Figure 4-2). Acceptance criteria for SPK transplantation usually include a rather stricter age cutoff than for kidney transplants and almost all units use routine invasive cardiac investigation. SPK is a realistic therapy for approximately half of the potential type 1 recipients with end-stage renal failure and compares with living donor kidney transplantation for patient and kidney outcomes.[117] Selection of patients for SPK transplants is focused even more on vascular and cardiac operative risks, but is otherwise similar to selection for kidney transplantation. The procedure is more demanding on both surgeon and patient; it takes longer and involves the additional risk of pancreas exocrine drainage either into the bladder or, more commonly, into the bowel. Postoperative recovery takes longer because of the ileus induced by the bowel surgery and immunosuppression is on the whole more intense than for a simple kidney transplant. Against these issues, the patient must set the benefits of good glucose control without exogenous insulin administration, reduced

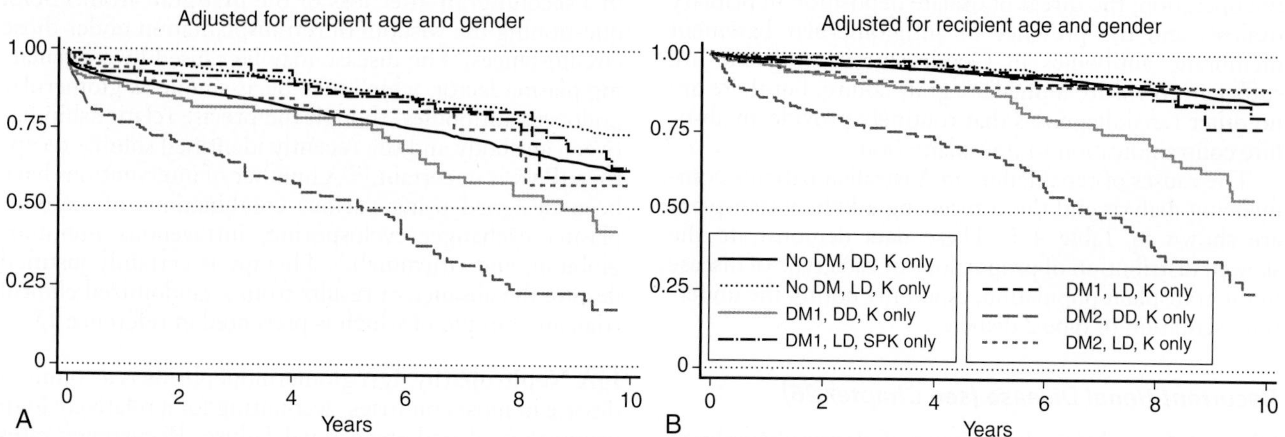

FIGURE 4-2 ■ The outcome of renal transplantation based on diabetes status, type of kidney, and presence of a simultaneous pancreas transplant. (A) Kidney graft survival. (B) Patient survival. DM1, type 1 diabetes mellitus; DM2, type 2 diabetes mellitus; LD, living donor transplant; DD, deceased donor transplant; K, kidney alone; SPK, simultaneous pancreas kidney. (Data courtesy of Australian National Pancreas Transplant Registry Report 2012. Sydney, Australia: ANPTR.)

long-term complications of diabetes, and improved survival compared to a deceased donor kidney alone.[117]

Detailed consideration of SPK transplantation is beyond the scope of this chapter, but it is undoubtedly a good solution for type 1 diabetics suitable for kidney transplantation and without a living donor or with severe secondary complications.[44] The role of islet transplantation is still evolving such that consideration of islet transplantation before, after, or with a simultaneous kidney remains the subject of formal clinical trials in a limited number of centers globally. While the results in those specialized centers are encouraging, there is still insufficient evidence to lead to widespread adoption of islet transplants outside clinical trials.[38]

Type 2 Diabetes Mellitus

Transplantation of the majority of patients with end-stage renal failure due to type 2 diabetes represents a challenge to both surgical and medical expertise, since the epidemic of type 2 diabetes that is sweeping both the developed and developing world involves predominantly obese, older patients with significant comorbid vascular disease. The disease is treacherous for both patients and physicians, since the neuropathy that so often accompanies the nephropathy leads to underestimation of the severity of symptoms, especially ischemic heart disease, and to exacerbation of the clinical impact of comorbid peripheral vascular disease. Only a small proportion of type 2 diabetics are suitable for transplantation because of the impact of age, obesity, and these comorbid conditions, and transplant units need to have specific policies for the evaluation of cardiac and vascular disease of those deemed suitable otherwise; a small minority may be helped by SPK transplantation, but this is not widely adopted as a therapy.[114]

Renal Disease

The range of underlying renal diseases of patients on dialysis and those accepted for transplant waiting lists are similar, since few diseases actually prevent successful kidney transplantation. The physical size of the kidneys in patients with adult polycystic kidney disease may impede the operation; the threat of oxalate deposition in primary oxalosis and the presence of antiglomerular basement membrane antibodies in Goodpasture's syndrome are sufficient to ensure immediate graft failure, but there are no other renal diagnoses that routinely provide an absolute contraindication to transplantation.

The causes of renal failure in Australian patients commencing dialysis and those receiving a kidney transplant are shown in Table 4-5. These data demonstrate the skewed distribution of proportions of each type of disease in the transplant population, especially noting the underrepresentation of type 2 diabetes.

TABLE 4-5 **Causes of Renal Failure in Patients Commencing End-Stage Renal Disease Therapy and Receiving a Renal Transplant in Australia 2010**

Diagnosis	Dialysis Patients (%)	Transplant Recipients (%)
Glomerulonephritis	22	46
Analgesic nephropathy	2	1
Polycystic kidney	7	13
Reflux nephropathy	3	6
Hypertensive nephropathy	14	6
Diabetes mellitus	35	12
Miscellaneous	12	2
Unknown	6	4

Data courtesy of ANZDATA 2011: McDonald S, Hurst K, editors. Registry Report 2011. Adelaide, South Australia: Australia and New Zealand Dialysis and Transplant Registry.

Recurrent Renal Disease (see Chapter 26)

Glomerulonephritis. Recurrence of glomerulonephritis in the kidney transplant is an issue that needs routine discussion with patients who have a diagnosis of focal and segmental glomerular sclerosis, IgA nephropathy and, to a lesser extent, other immune-mediated glomerular diseases. It is important to distinguish between the risk of recurrence and the risk of graft failure due to recurrence and, while the risk is real, it is seldom sufficient to contraindicate transplantation. A seminal analysis of the ANZDATA database demonstrated, however, that it is a significant cause of late graft loss, causing twice as many losses over a 10-year period as acute rejection, but half as many as chronic allograft nephropathy or death with a functioning graft.[10] There have been many attempts, over the years, to summarize the risks for different diseases,[10,13,52,57,68,95] and a further attempt is shown in Table 4-6, in which the risks of disease recurrence and graft failure are presented from general literature review.

Focal Segmental Glomerulosclerosis (FSGS). Recurrence of primary FSGS is one of the more difficult issues that must be addressed by transplant units. Risk factors for recurrence include: young age of the recipient, the duration of native disease from onset to development of end-stage renal failure, mesangial proliferative pathology, and the possibility that the risk is higher in related donor grafts.[73,106] There is a very high risk of recurrence in a second graft after loss of the first graft from FSGS, questioning the wisdom of retransplantation under those circumstances. The disease may be caused by a circulating plasma factor, which may be as simple as glomerular podocyte antibodies, though the precise relationship between antibody and the recently identified soluble receptor suPAR is uncertain.[112] A number of interventions have been designed using various combinations of steroids, plasma exchange, cyclosporine, intravenous immunoglobulin, and rituximab.[13] Therapy is certainly justified despite the absence of results from a randomized clinical trial, an example of which is presented in reference 13.

IgA Nephropathy. IgA glomerulonephritis is a common disease in most countries, accounting for a relatively high proportion of end-stage renal failure. Recurrence rates are high, especially if sought in renal biopsies after transplantation using specific identification of IgA deposits in the glomeruli.[7] IgA is thus amongst the commonest of

TABLE 4-6 **The Risks of Recurrence of Renal Disease After Transplantation and the Risks of Graft Loss as a Result of Recurrence, Derived from Literature Review**

Disease	Risk of Recurrence (%)	10-Year Risk of Graft Loss From Recurrence (%)
Glomerulonephritis		
Focal segmental sclerosis	20–30	8–15
IgA nephropathy	40–50	5–15
Henoch–Schönlein purpura	10–20	5–10
Mesangiocapillary type I	20–30	10–15
Mesangiocapillary type II	80–90	5–10
Membranous	10–20	10–25
Hemolytic uremic syndrome	10–30	10–15
ANCA-positive vasculitis	10–15	5
Pauci-immune	10–20	5–10
Goodpasture's syndrome (antibody-positive)	100	80
Systemic lupus erythematosus	1	1
Metabolic and Other Diseases		
Diabetic nephropathy	100	Low
Amyloidosis	30	Low
Oxalosis	90–100	80
Cystinosis	0	0
Fabry's disease	100	0
Alport's syndrome*	3–4	2
Light-chain nephropathy	10–25	10–30
Mixed essential cryoglobulinemia	50	40
Scleroderma	20	5–10

ANCA, antineutrophil cytoplasmic antibody.
*The risk of de novo antiglomerular basement membrane antibody-mediated Goodpasture's syndrome.

recurrent diseases, but is generally slow to cause renal impairment and graft loss.[73] It is commoner after living related donor grafts, but recurrence doesn't seem to impact on early or medium-term graft survival and thus should not restrain use of living donors, though use of steroid-free regimens may increase recurrence rates.[17] Assessment of the family donor, however, needs to include consideration of the possibility that IgA may be familial disease and thus also affect the potential donor.

Henoch-Schönlein Purpura. This is a predominantly pediatric disease with a previously reported high recurrence rate and graft loss.[77] A recent analysis has challenged this view through data on 43 patients across six transplant units in Europe with recurrence rates of 11.5% and graft loss rates of 7.5% at 10 years.[51] It is common practice not to transplant during active clinical disease but to await quiescence, but the data supporting this practice are not substantial.

Membranous Nephropathy. Membranous glomerulonephritis may occur as either de novo or recurrent disease after transplantation. It is becoming clear that de novo appearance of membranous histology is related to chronic alloimmune antibody-mediated rejection, but that autoantibodies specific for the phospholipase A_2 receptor are present in the majority of patients with recurrent membranous glomerulonephritis.[22]

Mesangiocapillary Glomerulonephritis. Type 1, 2, and 3 mesangiocapillary glomerulonephritides are all uncommon diseases with quite high recurrence rates after transplantation.[2,13] Recent evidence that recurrence of type 3 – dense deposit disease – may be treated by eculizumab offers hope for what is otherwise a disease conferring a high risk of graft failure.[72]

Antiglomerular Basement Membrane Disease. There is very little recent experience of recurrence of Goodpasture's syndrome after transplantation because of the early and convincing reports of recurrence in the presence of circulating antibody and advice to await clearance before transplantation.[12,113] It is thus essential to ensure a negative antiglomerular basement membrane antibody test before transplantation.

One of the minutiae of information that somehow all medical students can recall is that, because patients with Alport's syndrome have abnormal basement membrane antigens, they have been reported to produce antibodies in response to the normal basement membrane of a transplanted kidney, producing the unusual appearance of allogeneic antiglomerular basement membrane disease in a small percentage of patients.[39]

Recurrent Vasculitis. Antineutrophil cytoplasmic antibodies (ANCA) were discounted as a cause of recurrent crescentic glomerulonephritis in 127 patients in whom the incidence of recurrence was 17%, but with no association with presence of ANCA.[80] A more recent publication has, however, demonstrated a much lower recurrence rate of 0.02% per patient year.[34] Current data thus support transplantation of this group of patients without the need to resolve circulating antibody levels, but there are data to suggest that delaying transplantation until vasculitis is quiescent improves patient outcomes. Recurrence has been treated traditionally with cyclophosphamide, but more recently with rituximab.[35,85]

Hereditary Disease. Primary oxalosis has a high recurrence rate after transplantation and is now usually successfully treated by combined kidney and liver transplantation, correcting the metabolic abnormality simultaneously. The condition has been mimicked by long-term high-dose vitamin C administration in a dialysis-dependent patient, leading to widespread secondary deposition of oxalate throughout the body, giving the appearance of pseudogout.

Fabry's disease and cystinosis are both inherited enzyme deficiencies which cause renal disease through accumulated glycosphingolipid and cystine respectively. The former leads to recurrent disease in the transplant but the latter only to extrarenal deposition of cystine. Both are, to a certain extent, treatable, and recurrent disease should be preventable with recombinant alpha-galactosidase A enzyme replacement and oral analogs of cysteamine respectively.[61,66]

Tuberous sclerosis, while not leading to recurrent disease, deserves special consideration because of the high lifetime risk of developing renal cell carcinoma in the native kidneys. The risk of tumor can be managed either by bilateral nephrectomy or through regular screening by CT. The known responsiveness of the angiomyolipomata of tuberose sclerosis to the mTOR inhibitors is significant and warrants selection of one or other of these agents in the immunosuppression protocol.[45]

Urogenital Tract Abnormalities (see Chapter 12)

Bladder. Recognition of the patient with bladder dysfunction is important and sometimes obvious but sometimes subtle. Patients with the triad syndrome or other congenital obstructive uropathy, spina bifida, and diabetics are at easily recognizable risk of poor bladder function based on careful history taking and investigation with urodynamic studies. The more subtle problems that may be encountered include asymptomatic prostatic enlargement in an anuric dialysis-dependent patient and the very small-capacity bladder that will be encountered in long-term dialysis patients who have been anuric for many years. Creation of alternative bladder conduits is less popular than it has been, both because of the morbidity of the surgical procedures required and the long-term risks of carcinoma if a bladder reconstruction has been achieved using bowel. Self-catheterization is an easier and safer option than major abdominal surgery for the majority of patients with bladder dysfunction.[11]

Reflux Nephropathy. Recurrent urinary tract infection and reflux nephropathy seldom lead to life-threatening septicemia before transplantation, but when the experience of an individual demonstrates otherwise, bilateral nephrectomy can be justified if antibiotic prophylaxis fails to ameliorate the risk. Recurrent urinary sepsis is much more common after transplantation despite prophylactic measures and may threaten both the graft and the patient. Bilateral native nephrectomy thus becomes the lesser risk in a few patients after transplantation.

Polycystic Kidney Disease. The size of the polycystic kidneys must be evaluated before transplant surgery, preferably by the surgeon who will be implanting the new kidney. CT can provide an excellent view of the anatomical challenge that will face the surgeon when the patient is horizontal on the operating table, but will underplay the space available for the transplant when the patient stands up. Unilateral nephrectomy may be needed between the onset of dialysis therapy and a kidney transplant precluding pre-emptive transplantation. The native polycystic nephrectomy is, however, too large a procedure to add to the kidney transplant and should not be contemplated for the sake of 4 weeks of dialysis treatment.

Coagulation Disorders

Hemorrhage during the transplant and coagulation of the graft or other vital vascular conduit after the operation require careful prediction and management. Coagulation disorders and the risk of thrombosis are much more predictable today through screening tests (Table 4-7). Use of heparin starting soon after transplantation in those identified as having a possible thrombotic tendency seems to reduce the risk of thrombosis.[13]

The risk of hemorrhage is usually easily identified from the medical history and from a careful review of the medication list. Iatrogenic hemorrhage is much more common than inherited disorder such as hemophilia, especially with the widespread use of anticoagulation for atrial fibrillation and after vascular stenting.[11] Each transplant unit thus requires a protocol for the rapid reversal of anticoagulation, usually involving small doses of vitamin K, together with fresh frozen plasma replacement (Table 4-3). Double antiplatelet anticoagulation for patients with cardiac or dialysis fistula stents has led to concern over postoperative bleeding, especially in combination with prophylactic postoperative heparin.

Obesity

Increasing BMI, in the most recent large cohort analysis, is not associated with increased risks of death or graft loss but is associated with new-onset posttransplant diabetes mellitus.[1,108] The depth of abdominal fat certainly challenges the surgeon and without careful management can lead to increased risk of wound infection and other problems. The data now suggest that low BMI is the greater concern, with malnourished patients having higher mortality rates. The problem that both physician and patient face is the task of reducing weight in the very obese and increasing weight in the malnourished before transplantation. In patients treated by peritoneal dialysis it is especially hard to change the body habitus derived from the high carbohydrate intake from peritoneal dialysis fluids, such that a switch to hemodialysis may be the only option. Lifestyle changes are sometimes achievable when kidney transplantation is the goal.

TABLE 4-7 Risks of Thrombosis and Coagulation Disorder

Medication
Dual antiplatelet therapy
Aspirin
Warfarin
Heparin
Low-molecular-weight heparins
Coagulation
Medical history of thrombosis
Coagulation tests: prothrombin time, activated partial thromboplastin time
Factor V Leiden, protein C, protein S, antithrombin III deficiency
Antiphospholipid antibodies
Full blood count: polycythemia
Hemostasis
Medication history (warfarin, aspirin, clopidogrel, dipyridamole)
Medical history of bleeding
Medical history of liver disease
Coagulation tests: skin bleeding time, activated partial thromboplastin time, and congenital factor deficiencies

Psychosocial Factors

Smoking provides serious cardiovascular and pulmonary risks before, during, and after transplant surgery and is heavily discouraged by all programs.[8] The unanswered question remains whether or not it is appropriate to transplant patients who continue to smoke. Many in both the lay and professional communities argue that it is not appropriate for the community to provide access to the scarce resource of a donated kidney if the patient continues to self-harm through smoking.

Recreational drug abuse is often a more covert, but equally important, risk factor for success after transplantation.[99] It is clearly important to wean patients from drug dependency, testing compliance and assessing the possibility of recent hepatitis or HIV infection before activating them on the transplant waiting list. Psychiatric evaluation and treatment are often an essential component of preparation for transplantation in drug dependency, but may be rejected or unsuccessful. Families may be the harshest critics of such individuals and thus not offer living kidney donation, leaving transplant programs with the decision of whether or not it is appropriate to provide access to a deceased donor kidney. Documented abstinence for 6 months and determination of likely compliance after transplantation provide a non-judgmental approach to resolving this dilemma, but are in themselves complex assessments.

Alcohol dependency leads to very similar challenges to those provided by other recreational chemicals. Alcoholism may be well hidden and needs an enquiring and suspicious clinical evaluation, including an understanding of the impact on the liver as well as the psychological state of the patient. Compliance and reliability for follow-up after transplantation are important factors which will influence patient and graft outcomes.

Mental illness requires formal evaluation and treatment, with the important additional need to determine the patient's ability to understand and consent to kidney transplantation. There is a small cluster of patients whose renal failure results from chronic lithium toxicity used in the treatment of bipolar depression; additionally patients with a variety of psychiatric diseases are not immune from also developing renal failure. There is no substitute for an independent psychiatric evaluation of fitness to consent and ensure optimal pre- and postoperative psychiatric treatment.[26]

Sensitization and Transfusion Status (see Chapters 10 and 24)

Good knowledge of the anti-HLA antibody status and both the patient and donor's HLA type is critical to success but outside the scope of this chapter.

Previous Transplantation

Previous kidney transplants provide both visible and invisible barriers to the next transplant, both of which need to be considered carefully. Retransplantation is usually even less successful than the first transplant procedure was and requires very careful assessment of the patient's immunological reactivity. The total number of individuals with chronic graft loss is increasing in most countries, as is the number of patients with non-renal organ transplants requiring a kidney transplant as a result of nephrotoxicity or other cause of chronic renal failure.[105]

The clinician's decision to offer retransplantation is sometimes hard. Should a patient who has lost a first graft due to non-compliance with medication be offered the chance to destroy another priceless donation the same way? Perhaps the older, wiser, and now experienced individual will be a model of compliance the second time around? Assessment of the medical suitability for transplantation needs to be just as rigorous the second time as it was the first time, noting especially that infective, malignant, and cardiovascular disease are all more common in the previously transplanted than in the dialysis patient.

Opinion and practices have varied with respect to the management of a failed graft,[6,27] but the evidence is hardening in favor of early graft nephrectomy.[4,102] Transplant nephrectomy is a reasonably low-risk procedure that removes an ongoing source of foreign antigenic stimulation and allows for discontinuation of immunosuppression without risk of incurring a rejection response. Nephrectomy is always carried out in cases of early acute graft failure from whatever cause, but may not be in chronic graft failure.

PREPARATION FOR TRANSPLANTATION

To Join and Remain on the Deceased Donor Waiting List

The majority of this chapter has defined the issues of importance for assessment, selection, and preparation of candidates for the transplant waiting lists. Table 4-8 provides a list of issues that should be considered for every patient. Acceptance should then lead to histocompatibility testing and entry on to the transplant waiting list. The initial evaluation may be performed many years before the kidney becomes available and thus repeated reassessment is also required over the years that a patient may be on the waiting list. Compliance with the needs of the transplant waiting list and, in particular, providing a current blood sample for crossmatching may sort out the willing and motivated patients from the non-compliant. Most programs maintain serum screening protocols to identify patients who are sensitized, both to predict the chances of receiving a transplant and in order to evaluate better donor T- and B-cell crossmatch results obtained after working hours.

Maintaining a current record of clinical events and relevant serology for infectious disease (HIV, hepatitis B and C especially) should be the province of the dialysis unit responsible for the patient's treatment. Ensuring that all this information is available to the transplant program in the middle of the night remains challenging and likely to fail without a good information system. In the final analysis there is little alternative but to ensure that those who are managing the patient on a daily basis are always contacted when a kidney offer is made.

An additional issue that has been raised by the dearth of donors and the burgeoning waiting lists has been prior consent to receive offers for donors outside the standard

TABLE 4-8 **Screening Tests that Should be Routinely Considered Prior to a Living Donor Transplant or Acceptance on to a Transplant Waiting List**

General History and Physical Examination	
Diagnosis of Cause of Renal Disease, with Specific Tests as Required	
Virus Exposure	
HIV antibody	HIV-1 and HIV-2
Hepatitis B	HBsAg, HBcAb, HBsAb
Hepatitis C	HCVAb (HCV RNA if HCVAb positive)
Cytomegalovirus	CMV IgG
Herpesvirus	Herpes simplex IgG, herpes varicella-zoster IgG, HHV6 and HHV7 IgG
Epstein–Barr virus	EBV IgG
Other Infectious Disease	
In endemic areas	PPD skin testing
	Trypanosoma cruzi serology
	Coccidioides serology
	Strongyloides serology
	West Nile virus serology
	HTLV I and II serology
	HHV8 serology
Toxoplasma screening	
Syphilis screening	
Chest X-ray with follow-up tests as required if abnormal	
Other Disease	
Electrocardiogram	
Echocardiogram/stressed cardiac test with follow-up tests as required if abnormal	
Abdominal ultrasound (kidneys, gallbladder, liver, spleen)	
Vascular duplex ultrasound (femoral/carotid)	

HIV, human immunodeficiency virus; HBsAg, hepatitis B surface antigen; HBcAb, hepatitis B core antibody; HBsAb, hepatitis B surface antibody; HCVAb, hepatitis C virus antibody; CMV, cytomegalovirus; IgG, immunoglobulin G; HHV, human herpesvirus; EBV, Epstein–Barr virus; PPD, purified protein derivative; HTLV, human T-lymphotropic virus.

donor criteria. It is unreasonable to expect the patient to consent meaningfully in the middle of the night to a complex offer of an older donor kidney or one infected with hepatitis C. Thus many programs have special categories of prior consent which permit individuals to choose to receive a kidney from an extended criteria donor,[41] an old donor,[37] or one infected with the same virus that they carry – be it hepatitis B or C or HIV.[14]

To Undergo Elective Living Donor Transplantation

The assessment of the recipient of a living donor graft is, by contrast to the deceased donor recipient, a more orderly and planned affair. Despite this the focus is often more on the suitability of the donor and less on the recipient. Ensuring that the donor and recipient are assessed by different nephrologists and different surgeons brings attention back to the recipient. Providing that there is good communication between the two teams, it is possible to manage the interface between donor and recipient issues smoothly and effectively. It is just as important for the donor to understand the risks of a poor outcome in the recipient as it is for the recipient to understand them. A donor unaware of the possibility of recurrent disease in a patient with FSGS, for example, will reasonably ask why he or she was not informed before the donation. The risk of death at operation for a particular recipient may be acceptable to that individual, but not to the donor, who may be unprepared for that possibility. The opposite situation may also occur. A donor may undertake risky behavior, such as intravenous drug abuse or unprotected high-risk intercourse, which the recipient may know more about than either the donor or recipient's medical teams. Understanding the level and nature of the risk is paramount for the recipient.

To Undergo Deceased Donor Transplantation

A transplant team will receive the news that a kidney is available for a particular patient only a few hours before the operation needs to be performed. All too often, the allocation takes place in the middle of the night and the news is passed through a transplant coordinator and junior doctors. The patient and family will not be in contact with the individuals who have assessed them and who care for their dialysis. Their questions and uncertainties will be carried away in a rush of investigations, including a chest X-ray, an electrocardiogram, routine blood tests, bowel preparation, shower, anesthetic evaluation, immunosuppressive medication, and perhaps also preoperative hemodialysis. Despite this rush of activity, the pressure to reduce cold ischemia time for the kidney and to meet the deadlines and timetables of operating suites tends to overshadow the needs for discussion and informed consent. This emphasizes the need for full education and information during the workup for acceptance on to the transplant waiting list.

REFERENCES

1. Aalten J, Christiaans MH, de Fijter H, et al. The influence of obesity on short- and long-term graft and patient survival after renal transplantation. Transpl Int 2006;19(11):901.
2. Andresdottir MB, Assmann KJM, Hoitsma AJ, et al. Renal transplantation in patients with dense deposit disease: morphological characteristics of recurrent disease and clinical outcome. Nephrol Dial Transplant 1999;14:1723.
3. Apaydin S, Altiparmak MR, Serdengecti K, et al. *Mycobacterium tuberculosis* infections after renal transplantation. Scand J Infect Dis 2000;32:501.
4. Ayus JC, Achinger SG, Lee S, et al. Transplant nephrectomy improves survival following a failed renal allograft. J Am Soc Nephrol 2010;21(2):374–80.
5. Batabyal P, Chapman JR, Wong G, et al. Clinical practice guidelines on wait-listing for kidney transplantation: consistent and equitable? Transplantation 2012;94:703–13.
6. Bennett WM. The failed renal transplant: in or out? Semin Dial 2005;18(3):188.
7. Berger J. Recurrence of IgA nephropathy in renal allografts. Am J Kidney Dis 1988;12:371.
8. Bluman LG, Mosca L, Newman N, et al. Preoperative smoking habits and postoperative pulmonary complications. Chest 1998;113:883.
9. Borentain M, Le Feuvre C, Helft G, et al. Long-term outcome after coronary angioplasty in renal transplant and hemodialysis patients. J Interv Cardiol 2005;18(5):331.
10. Briganti EM, Russ GR, McNeil JJ, et al. Risk of renal allograft loss from recurrent glomerulonephritis. N Engl J Med 2002;347(2):103.

11. Cabello BR, Quicios DC, López ML, et al. The candidate for renal transplantation work up: medical, urological and oncological evaluation. Arch Esp Urol 2011;64(5):441–60.
12. Cameron JS. Glomerulonephritis in renal transplants. Transplantation 1982;34:237.
13. Canaud G, Audard V, Kofman T, et al. Recurrence from primary and secondary glomerulopathy after renal transplant. Transpl Int 2012;25(8):812–24.
14. Carbone M, Cockwell P, Neuberger J. Hepatitis C and kidney transplantation. Int J Nephrol 2011;2011:593291.
15. Chapman JR. Compliance: the patient, the doctor, and the medication? Transplantation 2004;77(5):782–6.
16. Chapman JR, O'Connell PJ, Nankivell BJ. Chronic renal allograft dysfunction. J Am Soc Nephrol 2005;16(10):3015.
17. Clayton P, McDonald S, Chadban S. Steroids and recurrent IgA nephropathy after kidney transplantation. Am J Transplant 2011;11(8):1645–9.
18. Cortigiani L, Desideri A, Gigli G, et al. Clinical, resting echo and dipyridamole stress echocardiography findings for the screening of renal transplant candidates. Int J Cardiol 2005;103(2):168.
19. Cosio FG, Alamir A, Yim S, et al. Patient survival after renal transplantation: I. The impact of dialysis pre-transplant. Kidney Int 1998;53:767.
20. Cosio FG, Falkenhain MF, Pesavento TE, et al. Patient survival after renal transplantation II: the impact of smoking. Clin Transplant 1999;13:336.
21. David-Neto E, Americo da Fonseca J, Jota de Paula F, et al. The impact of azathioprine on chronic viral hepatitis in renal transplantation: a long-term single-centre, prospective study on azathioprine withdrawal. Transplantation 1999;68:976.
22. Debiec H, Martin L, Jouanneau C, et al. Autoantibodies specific for the phospholipase A_2 receptor in recurrent and de novo membranous nephropathy. Am J Transplant 2011;11(10):2144–52.
23. Degos F, Pol S, Chaix ML, et al. The tolerance and efficacy of interferon-alpha in haemodialysis patients with HCV infection: a multicentre, prospective study. Nephrol Dial Transplant 2001;16:1017.
24. Delmonico F, Council of the Transplantation Society. A report of the Amsterdam forum on the care of the live kidney donor: data and medical guidelines. Transplantation 2005;79(Suppl. 6):S53.
25. de Mattos AM, Prather J, Olyaei AJ, et al. Cardiovascular events following renal transplantation: role of traditional and transplant-specific risk factors. Kidney Int 2006;70(4):757.
26. DiMartini A, Crone C, Fireman M, et al. Psychiatric aspects of organ transplantation in critical care. Crit Care Clin 2008;24(4):949–53.
27. Douzdjian V, Rice JC, Carson RW, et al. Renal retransplants: effect of primary allograft nephrectomy on early function, acute rejection and outcome. Clin Transplant 1996;203(2):203.
28. Eggers PW, Gohdes D, Pugh J. Nontraumatic lower limb extremity amputations in the Medicare end-stage renal disease population. Kidney Int 1999;56:1524.
29. Feringa HH, Bax JJ, Schouten O, et al. Ischemic heart disease in renal transplant candidates: towards non-invasive approaches for preoperative risk stratification. Eur J Echocardiogr 2005; 6(5):313.
30. Foley RN, Murray AM, Li S, et al. Chronic kidney disease and the risk for cardiovascular disease, renal replacement, and death in the United States Medicare population, 1998 to 1999. J Am Soc Nephrol 2005;16(2):489.
31. Fornairon S, Pol S, Legendre C, et al. The long-term virologic and pathologic impact of renal transplantation on chronic hepatitis B virus infection. Transplantation 1996;62:297.
32. Gabardi S, Olyaei A. Evaluation of potential interactions between mycophenolic acid derivatives and proton pump inhibitors. Ann Pharmacother 2012;46(7–8):1054–64.
33. Gane E, Pilmore H. Management of chronic viral hepatitis before and after renal transplantation. Transplantation 2002;74:427.
34. Geetha D, Eirin A, True K, et al. Renal transplantation in antineutrophil cytoplasmic antibody-associated vasculitis: a multicenter experience. Transplantation 2011;91(12):1370–5.
35. Geetha D, Seo P, Specks U, et al. Successful induction of remission with rituximab for relapse of ANCA-associated vasculitis post-kidney transplant: report of two cases. Am J Transplant 2007;7(12):2821–5.
36. Genc G, Ozkaya O, Aygun C, et al. Vaccination status of children considered for renal transplants: missed opportunities for vaccine preventable diseases. Exp Clin Transplant 2012;10(4):314–8.
37. Giessing M, Fuller TF, Friedersdorff F, et al. Outcomes of transplanting deceased-donor kidneys between elderly donors and recipients. J Am Soc Nephrol 2009;20(1):37–40.
38. Gill RG, Bishop NH. Clinical islet transplantation: where immunity and metabolism intersect? Curr Opin Endocrinol Diabetes Obes 2012;19(4):249–54.
39. Gobel J, Olbricht CJ, Offner G, et al. Kidney transplantation in Alport's syndrome: long-term outcome and allograft anti-GBM nephritis. Clin Nephrol 1992;38:299.
40. Grace BS, Clayton PA, Cass A, et al. Transplantation rates for living- but not deceased-donor kidneys vary with socioeconomic status in Australia. Kidney Int 2012 Aug 15;.
41. Grams ME, Womer KL, Ugarte RM, et al. Listing for expanded criteria donor kidneys in older adults and those with predicted benefit. Am J Transplant 2010;10(4):802–9.
42. Greenstein SM, Katz S, Sun S, et al. Prevalence of asymptomatic cholelithiasis and risk of acute cholecystitis after kidney transplantation. Transplantation 1997;63:1030.
43. Groetzner J, Kaczmarek I, Mueller M, et al. Freedom from graft vessel disease in heart and combined heart- and kidney-transplanted patients treated with tacrolimus-based immunosuppression. J Heart Lung Transplant 2005;24(11):1787.
44. Gruessner AC, Sutherland DE, Gruessner RW. Long-term outcome after pancreas transplantation. Curr Opin Organ Transplant 2012;17(1):100–5.
45. Haidinger M, Werzowa J, Weichhart T, et al. Targeting the dysregulated mammalian target of rapamycin pathway in organ transplantation: killing 2 birds with 1 stone. Transplant Rev (Orlando) 2011;25:145–53.
46. Hibi T, Sageshima J, Molina E, et al. Predisposing factors of diminished survival in simultaneous liver/kidney transplantation. Am J Transplant 2012;12:2966–73.
47. Hughes PD, Becker GJ. Screening for intracranial aneurysms in autosomal dominant polycystic kidney disease. Nephrology (Carlton) 2003;8(4):163.
48. Isla PP, Moncho VJ, Guasch AO, et al. Impact of simultaneous pancreas-kidney transplantation: patients' perspectives. Patient Prefer Adherence 2012;6:597–603.
49. Johnson CP, Kuhn EM, Hariharan S, et al. Pre-transplant identification of risk factors that adversely affect length of stay and charges for renal transplantation. Clin Transplant 1999; 13(2):168.
50. Joint statement by the Advisory Council for the Elimination of Tuberculosis and the Advisory Committee on Immunization Practices. The role of BCG vaccine in the prevention and control of tuberculosis in the United States. MMWR Morb Mortal Wkly Rep 1996;45:1.
51. Kanaan N, Mourad G, Thervet E, et al. Recurrence and graft loss after kidney transplantation for Henoch-Schönlein purpura nephritis: a multicenter analysis. Clin J Am Soc Nephrol 2011 Jul;6(7):1768–72.
52. Kasiske BL, Cangro CB, Hariharan S, et al. The evaluation of renal transplant candidates: clinical practice guidelines. Am J Transplant 2001;1(Suppl. 2):7.
53. Kasiske BL, Vazquez MA, Harmon WE, et al. Recommendations for the outpatient surveillance of renal transplant recipients: American Society of Transplantation. J Am Soc Nephrol 2000;4:S1.
54. Kayler LK, Rasmussen CS, Dykstra DM, et al. Gender imbalance and outcomes in living donor renal transplantation in the United States. Am J Transplant 2003;3(4):452.
55. Kennedy SE, Mackie FE, Rosenberg AR, et al. Waiting time and outcome of kidney transplantation in adolescents. Transplantation 2006;82(8):1046.
56. Kirsch S, Sester M. Tuberculosis in transplantation: diagnosis, prevention, and treatment. Curr Infect Dis Rep 2012;14:650–7.
57. Kotanko P, Pusey CD, Levy JB. Recurrent glomerulonephritis following renal transplantation. Transplantation 1997;63:1045.
58. Kotton CN, Kumar D, Caliendo AM, et al. International consensus guidelines on the management of cytomegalovirus in solid organ transplantation. Transplantation Society International CMV Consensus Group. Transplantation 2010;89(7):779–95.
59. Kruger S, Seyfarth M, Sack K, et al. Defective immune response to tetanus toxoid in haemodialysis patients and its association with diphtheria vaccination. Vaccine 1999;17:1145.

60. Lauer GM, Walker BD. Hepatitis C virus infection. N Engl J Med 2001;345:41.
61. Lidove O, Joly D, Barbey F, et al. Clinical results of enzyme replacement therapy in fabry disease: a comprehensive review of literature. Int J Clin Pract 2007;61(2):293.
62. Lim WH, McDonald SP, Russ GR. Effect on graft and patient survival between shipped and locally transplanted well-matched cadaveric renal allografts in Australia over a 10-year period. Nephrology (Carlton) 2006;11(1):73.
63. Lin K, Stewart D, Cooper S, et al. Pre-transplant cardiac testing for kidney-pancreas transplant candidates and association with cardiac outcomes. Clin Transplant 2001;15(4):269.
64. Manske CL, Nelluri S, Thomas W, et al. Outcome of coronary artery bypass surgery in diabetic transplant candidates. Clin Transplant 1998;12(2):73.
65. Manske CL, Wang Y, Rector T, et al. Coronary revascularisation in insulin-dependent diabetic patients with chronic renal failure. Lancet 1992;340(8826):998.
66. Markello TC, Bernardini IM, Gahi WA. Improved renal function in children with cystinosis treated with cysteamine. N Engl J Med 1993;328:1157.
67. Martín-Dávila P, Fortún J, López-Vélez R, et al. Transmission of tropical and geographically restricted infections during solid-organ transplantation. Clin Microbiol Rev 2008;21(1):60–96.
68. Mathew TH. Recurrent disease after renal transplantation. Transplant Rev 1991;5:31.
69. Mathew TH, McDonald SP, Russ GR. Donor and recipient risk factors and choice of immunosuppression determine long-term outcome in renal transplantation. Transplant Proc 2001;33(7-8):3400.
70. Mayer G, Persijn GG. Eurotransplant kidney allocation system (ETKAS): rationale and implementation. Nephrol Dial Transplant 2006;21(1):2.
71. McBride MA, Harper AM, Taranto SE. The OPTN waiting list, 1988–2002. Clin Transplant 2003;2003:53.
72. McCaughan JA, O'Rourke DM, Courtney AE. Recurrent dense deposit disease after renal transplantation: an emerging role for complementary therapies. Am J Transplant 2012;12(4):1046–51.
73. McDonald SP, Russ GR. Recurrence of IgA nephropathy among renal allograft recipients from living donors is greater among those with zero HLA mismatches. Transplantation 2006;82(6):759.
74. McDonald SP, Russ GR. Survival of recipients of cadaveric kidney transplants compared with those receiving dialysis treatment in Australia and New Zealand 1991–2001. Nephrol Dial Transplant 2002;17(12):2212.
75. Meier-Kriesche HU, Cibrik DM, Ojo AO, et al. Interaction between donor and recipient age in determining the risk of chronic renal allograft failure. J Am Geriatr Soc 2002;50(1):14.
76. Merion RM, Ashby VB, Wolfe RA, et al. Deceased-donor characteristics and the survival benefit of kidney transplantation. JAMA 2005;294(21):2726.
77. Meulders Q, Pirson Y, Cosyns J-P, et al. Course of Henoch–Schönlein nephritis after renal transplantation. Report on ten patients and review of the literature. Transplantation 1994;58:1179.
78. Morales E, Gutierrez E, Andres A. Treatment with calcimimetics in kidney transplantation. Transplant Rev (Orlando) 2010;24(2):79–88.
79. Muller E, Barday Z, Mendelson M, et al. Renal transplantation between HIV-positive donors and recipients justified. S Afr Med J 2012;102(6):497–8.
80. Nachman PH, Segelmark M, Westman K, et al. Recurrent ANCA-associated small vessel vasculitis after transplantation: a pooled analysis. Kidney Int 1999;56:1544.
81. Nadim MK, Sung RS, Davis CL, et al. Simultaneous liver–kidney transplantation summit: current state and future directions. Am J Transplant 2012;12:2901–8.
82. Nankivell BJ, Lau S-G, Chapman JR, et al. Progression of macrovascular disease after transplantation. Transplantation 2000;69:574.
83. Natov SN, Lau JY, Ruthazer R, et al. Hepatitis C virus genotype does not affect patient survival among renal transplant candidates. The New England Organ Bank Hepatitis C Study Group. Kidney Int 1999;56:700.
84. Norby GE, Günther A, Mjøen G, et al. Prevalence and risk factors for coronary artery calcification following kidney transplantation for systemic lupus erythematosus. Rheumatology (Oxford) 2011 Sep;50(9):1659–64.
85. Nyberg G, Akesson P, Norden G, et al. Systemic vasculitis in a kidney transplant population. Transplantation 1997;63:1273.
86. Ojo AO. Expanded criteria donors: process and outcomes. Semin Dial 2005;18(6):463.
87. Palmer SC, Strippoli GF, McGregor DO. Interventions for preventing bone disease in kidney transplant recipients: a systematic review of randomized controlled trials. Am J Kidney Dis 2005;45(4):638.
88. Paramesh AS, Davis JY, Mallikarjun C, et al. Kidney transplantation alone in ESRD patients with hepatitis C cirrhosis. Transplantation 2012;94(3):250–4.
89. Park S, Yang S, Han J, et al. Long-term impact of prophylactic antiviral treatment in hepatitis B surface antigen positive renal allograft recipients. Clin Nephrol 2012;78:303–11.
90. Pelletier SJ, Norman SP, Christensen LL, et al. Review of transplantation of HIV patients during the HAART era. Clin Transplant 2004;63.
91. Pereira BJ, Natov SN, Bouthot BA, et al. Effects of hepatitis C infection and renal transplantation on survival in end-stage renal disease. The New England Organ Bank Hepatitis C Study Group. Kidney Int 1998;53:1374.
92. Pereira BJ, Wright TL, Schmid CH, et al. A controlled study of hepatitis C transmission by organ transplantation. The New England Organ Bank Hepatitis C Study Group. Lancet 1995;345:484.
93. Prelog M, Pohl M, Ermisch B, et al. Demand for evaluation of vaccination antibody titers in children considered for renal transplantation. Pediatr Transplant 2007;11(1):73–6.
94. Ramos EL, Kasiske BL, Alexander SR, et al. The evaluation of candidates for renal transplantation: the current practice of US transplant centers. Transplantation 1994;57:490.
95. Ramos EL, Tisher CC. Recurrent diseases in the kidney transplant. Am J Kidney Dis 1994;24:142.
96. Rodriguez JR, Cornell DL, Lin JK, et al. Increasing live donor kidney transplantation: a randomized controlled trial of a home-based educational intervention. Am J Transplant 2007;7(2):394.
97. Rosenberger J, van Dijk JP, Nagyova I, et al. Predictors of perceived health status in patients after kidney transplantation. Transplantation 2006;81(9):1306.
98. Rubin H, Jenkins RL, Shaw BW, et al. The acquired immunodeficiency syndrome and transplantation. Transplantation 1987;44:1.
99. Rundell JR, Hall RC. Psychiatric characteristics of consecutively evaluated outpatient renal transplant candidates and comparisons with consultation – liaison inpatients. Psychosomatics 1997;38:269.
100. Sakhuja V, Jha V, Varma PP, et al. The high incidence of tuberculosis among renal transplant recipients in India. Transplantation 1996;61:211.
101. Sarkio S, Salmela K, Kyllönen L, et al. Complications of gallstone disease in kidney transplantation patients. Nephrol Dial Transplant 2007;22(3):886–90.
102. Sener A, Khakhar AK, Nguan CY, et al. Early but not late allograft nephrectomy reduces allosensitization after transplant failure. Can Urol Assoc J 2011;5(6):E142–7.
103. Sharma R, Pellerin D, Gaze DC, et al. Dobutamine stress echocardiography and cardiac troponin T for the detection of significant coronary artery disease and predicting outcome in renal transplant candidates. Eur J Echocardiogr 2005;6(5):327.
104. Smith KG, Isbel NM, Catton MG, et al. Suppression of the humoral immune response by mycophenolate mofetil. Nephrol Dial Transplant 1998;13(1):160.
105. Srinivas TR, Stephany BR, Budev M, et al. An emerging population: kidney transplant candidates who are placed on the waiting list after liver, heart, and lung transplantation. Clin J Am Soc Nephrol 2010;5(10):1881–6.
106. Stephanian E, Matas AJ, Mauer SM, et al. Recurrence of disease in patients re-transplanted for focal segmental glomerulosclerosis. Transplantation 1992;53:755.
107. Stock PG, Barin B, Murphy B, et al. Outcomes of kidney transplantation in HIV-infected recipients. N Engl J Med 2010;363(21):2004–14.
108. Strejar E, Molnar MK, Kovesdy CP, et al. Associations of pretransplant weight and muscle mass with mortality in renal transplant recipients. Clin J Am Soc Nephrol 2011;6(6):1463–73.

109. The ESRD Incidence Study Group. Divergent trends in the incidence of end-stage renal disease due to type 1 and type 2 diabetes in Europe, Canada and Australia during 1998–2002. Diabet Med 2006;23(12):1364.
110. Vajdic CM, McDonald SP, McCredie MR, et al. Cancer incidence before and after kidney transplantation. JAMA 2006; 296(23):2823.
111. van Leeuwen MT, Webster AC, McCredie MRE, et al. Effect of reduced immunosuppression after kidney transplant failure on risk of cancer: population based retrospective cohort study. BMJ 2010;340:c570.
112. Wei C, El Hindi S, Li J, et al. Circulating urokinase receptor as a cause of focal segmental glomerulosclerosis. Nat Med 2011;17(8):952–60.
113. Wilson CB, Dixon FJ. Antiglomerular basement membrane antibody induced glomerulonephritis. Kidney Int 1973;3:74.
114. Wiseman AC, Gralla J. Simultaneous pancreas kidney transplant versus other kidney transplant options in patients with type 2 diabetes. Clin J Am Soc Nephrol 2012;7(4):656–64.
115. Wolfe RA, Ashby VB, Milford EL, et al. Comparison of mortality in all patients on dialysis, patients on dialysis awaiting transplantation and recipients of a first cadaveric transplant. N Engl J Med 1999;341:1725.
116. Wong G, Howard K, Chapman JR, et al. Comparative survival and economic benefits of deceased donor kidney transplantation and dialysis in people with varying ages and co-morbidities. PLoS One 2012;7(1):e29591.
117. Young BY, Gill J, Huang E, et al. Living donor kidney versus simultaneous pancreas-kidney transplant in type I diabetics: an analysis of the OPTN/UNOS database. Clin J Am Soc Nephrol 2009;4(4):845–52.

CHAPTER 5

ACCESS FOR RENAL REPLACEMENT THERAPY

James P. Hunter • Adam D. Barlow • Michael L. Nicholson

CHAPTER OUTLINE

INTRODUCTION

The expanding population of dialysis patients in the United Kingdom is leading to increasing numbers of patients beginning renal replacement therapy (RRT).[27] Many patients have multiple comorbid conditions, such as diabetes and ischemic heart disease, and many are obese. Long-term access for RRT through either arteriovenous fistulas (AVF) or peritoneal dialysis (PD) catheters is increasingly challenging and over the past decade has expanded into a multispecialty discipline. Many patients have undergone multiple previous access procedures, have arteriosclerosis, and are unsuitable for transplantation. Such patients require careful access planning involving liaison between nephrologists, radiologists, and surgeons. Vascular access surgery with an increasing volume of patients has become part of the vascular surgeon's caseload. Furthermore, PD catheter insertion has broadened to include nephrologists, largely as a result of the advent of peritoneoscopic catheter insertion under local anesthetic. Complex grafts, including axillary loop and thigh loop grafts, are becoming more commonplace and AVF surveillance and maintenance of fistula patency are now roles of the interventional radiologist.

VASCULAR ACCESS CATHETERS

Temporary Vascular Access

Central venous catheters (CVC) for vascular access are an essential temporizing measure in a select group of patients who require immediate or emergent hemodialysis.

TABLE 5-1 Indications for Tunneled Hemodialysis Catheters

During maturation of autogenous arteriovenous fistulas
During maturation of continuous ambulatory peritoneal dialysis
Patients awaiting a living donor transplant
Dialysis bridge following failure of current access to permit planning and imaging for long-term access
Permanent access – all other sites exhausted, severe cardiac dysfunction, or patient choice

About 40% of new end-stage renal failure patients present acutely and require short-term vascular access. In the United States the number of patients initiating hemodialysis who have a temporary catheter is as high as 70%.[6,27] The indications for CVC insertion are displayed in Table 5-1. The ideal properties of a CVC are a biologically neutral material that does not induce catheter lumen thrombosis or perivascular reaction and subsequent venous thrombosis. The catheter should be soft and compliant, easy to insert and durable, and should be coated with an agent that reduces bacterial proliferation and biofilm formation. Furthermore it should be inexpensive and permit blood flow of >350 mL/min to facilitate efficient dialysis. A nephrologist or radiologist usually inserts cuffed, tunneled catheters that provide immediate access to the circulatory system using the Seldinger technique. Uncuffed, non-tunneled catheter can be inserted at the bedside and used immediately but can only be used for a maximum of 3 weeks.

The three commonest locations of choice for temporary vascular access are the internal jugular vein (IJV), subclavian vein, and common femoral vein. Historically the subclavian vein was the preferred initial location because of the discretion of the line position and convenience for the patient. Unlike with catheter placement in the femoral vein, the patient with a subclavian catheter can be ambulatory. However, the incidence of stenosis is reportedly as high as 50% following subclavian vein cannulation, although there are values as low as 18% in the literature.[58,76] Figure 5-1 shows an example of a right arm venogram in a patient with a subclavian vein stenosis. The high risk of central stenosis highlights the importance of avoiding the subclavian vein for temporary venous access unless there are no other options.

Currently the favored site for temporary venous access is the IJV, in particular the right IJV. Although some patients find the visibility of the catheter in the neck above the collar unsightly, its placement in the IJV has certain advantages. In particular the direct route into the superior vena cava (SVC) leads to higher patency rates and fewer complications.[11] The left IJV can also be used but is less desirable because the course of the catheter through the brachiocephalic vein into the SVC is more tortuous and the tip of the catheter can abut the caval wall. Overall, with more refined catheter placement, judicious use of sites other than IJV, reduction in catheter duration, and the advent of soft Silastic catheters, the complication rates of central venous access have been reduced.[14]

IJV catheter placement can be performed either surgically, using a cut-down at the medial border of sternocleidomastoid, or via the Seldinger technique, using ultrasound to guide the needle into the vessel. The tip of the catheter should be at the junction of the SVC and right atrium as this affords the most optimal blood flow through the catheter. Temporary access catheters provide the clinician with time to investigate the most appropriate long-term access. This usually involves imaging of the venous anatomy to decide on the most appropriate native vein for AVF formation. However, tunneled catheters can provide access for months and even years, particularly in those patients in whom native venous conduits for AVF formation have been exhausted. Indeed, in such patients, tunneled catheter placement is becoming more adventurous, with reports of transhepatic, translumbar, and even transmediastinal approaches being used as last-resort procedures.[65,70,86]

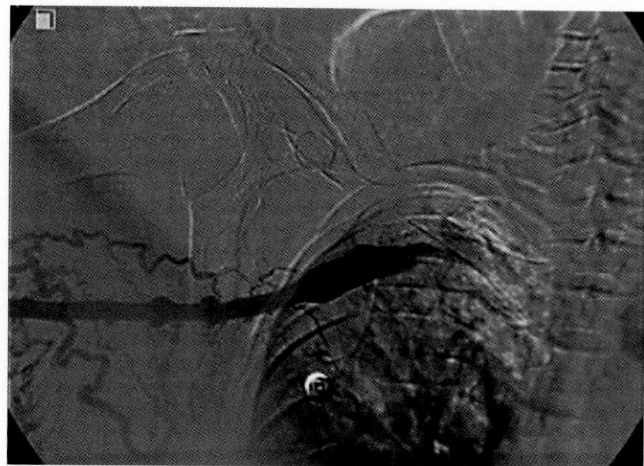

FIGURE 5-1 ■ Venographic image following injection of contrast into a forearm vein, illustrating a right-sided subclavian vein stenosis. Note the tapering of the contrast and the absence of contrast in the brachiocephalic vein, which filled slowly on later images. Note also the thready, tortuous collateral vessels visible in the upper arm and axilla as a result of the stenosis.

Catheter Insertion Techniques

Traditionally tunneled dialysis catheters were inserted by surgeons using a cut-down method. Increasingly nephrologists and radiologists are using Seldinger techniques under ultrasound guidance to place dialysis catheters percutaneously. Under ultrasound guidance the Seldinger procedure is comparable to surgical insertion with high rates of first-pass success in cannulation.[111] It is essential to place catheters under fluoroscopic control, whichever method is used, to ensure that the tip of the catheter is placed in the SVC. The malposition rate of catheters when placed without fluoroscopic control has been shown to be as high as 29%.[17] Catheters within the right atrium minimize recirculation and there is some evidence they have higher patency rates.[103] However there is a small risk of atrial perforation and catheter-induced arrhythmias. Furthermore the risk of local thrombus formation, alongside catheter thrombosis, outweighs the benefit of right atrium placement and it is largely avoided. As such, the junction of the SVC and right atrium is generally considered the most favorable location for the catheter tip. A list of complications associated with CVC insertion is displayed in Table 5-2.

TABLE 5-2 **Complications of Central Venous Catheter Insertion**
Arterial puncture
Bleeding
Pneumothorax
Hemothorax
Hemomediastinum
Atrial perforation
Air embolus
Arrhythmias
Primary failure

Complications of Hemodialysis Catheters

Catheter Dysfunction

Catheter dysfunction, also called catheter malfunction, was historically defined as "failure to attain and maintain adequate extracorporeal blood flow sufficient to perform dialysis in a timely fashion." A recent collaboration of transplant surgeons and physicians, the North American Vascular Access Consortium, introduced a new definition in an attempt to create a uniform standard. Dysfunction was defined as the first occurrence of: (1) peak blood flow of 200 mL/min or less for 30 minutes during a dialysis treatment; (2) mean blood flow of 250 mL/min or less during two consecutive dialysis treatments; or (3) inability to initiate dialysis owing to inadequate blood flow, after attempts to restore patency have been attempted.

Dysfunction accounts for 17–33% of all catheter removals and can be either early or late.[101] Early dysfunction is due to technical error such as kinking of the catheter in the subcutaneous tunnel or catheter malpositioning. Late dysfunction is due to central vein occlusion, catheter thrombosis, and fibrin sheath formation. Catheter thrombosis has an estimated frequency of 0.5–3 episodes per 1000 days and an incidence of 46% and is the major cause of catheter dysfunction.[48] Antifibrinolytic therapy introduced via the catheter is the treatment of choice and first-line therapy is usually 5000 IU/mL of urokinase of sufficient volume to fill the lumen. This can be repeated immediately and, if bolus dosing fails, can be followed by a systemic infusion of 20 000 IU/mL/h over 6 hours or a continuous infusion during dialysis of 250 000 IU.[15] A recent double-blind placebo-controlled randomized trial of tenecteplase versus placebo in patients with catheter dysfunction demonstrated that patients treated with tenecteplase had significantly increased flow rates (>300 mL/min). Patients within the study with <1 day of catheter dysfunction had the greatest benefit, with 35% of tenecteplase-treated patients gaining adequate dialysis flow rates compared to 8% in the placebo group.[114]

If, following attempted thrombolysis, catheter dysfunction persists then imaging of the catheter to obtain further information is indicated. Direct injection of contrast via the arterial port can help to elucidate the presence of a fibrin sheath. Features such as a filling defect or retrograde flow of contrast along the sheath are sometimes present, although the signs are often subtle. Hoshal et al. examined 55 patients at autopsy and demonstrated that a fibrin sheath was present in 100%.[44] The ubiquitous nature of the fibrin sheath is not always clinically evident. Indeed, dysfunction due to the presence of a fibrin sheath has been estimated at 13–57%, which means that more than half of catheters are without dysfunction, even with a fibrin sheath present.[107] Treatment of a fibrin sheath usually involves replacement of the catheter at a new location but there is evidence to support mechanical stripping, which is carried out using a snare around the catheter, inserted via the femoral vein. Some studies report success rates of up to 100% following mechanical stripping but other studies demonstrate poor success, with catheter dysfunction returning by the fifth dialysis session.[40,46] Even though mechanical stripping has acceptable complication rates, there are documented cases of clinically evident pulmonary embolism.[127]

Central Vein Occlusion

The presence of occlusive thrombus in the central veins, in particular the SVC, is asymptomatic in about 30% of cases. Although it can manifest as catheter dysfunction, the presence of arm and facial edema or prominent superficial vessels should raise suspicion of central venous occlusion or stenosis. Thrombus is usually detected by angiography either from instillation of contrast via the catheter or through a peripheral vein. However transesophageal Doppler and contrast-enhanced cross-sectional imaging are also useful diagnostic tools. The treatment of central vein thrombus depends upon the chronicity of the thrombus. Acute thrombus may respond to fibrinolytic therapy, such as recombinant tissue plasminogen activator, as detailed above. However fibrinolytic therapy will not have any effect on older, organized thrombus. Percutaneous angioplasty and stenting have an increasing role in maintaining CVC patency and recanalization of stenosed or occluded vessels.[14,67]

Infection

Septic complications from CVC are well documented and the longevity of modern cuffed and tunneled catheters is still limited by infection. Catheter-related bacteremia rates for cuffed, tunneled catheters ranges from 0.016 to 0.29 per 100 days, whereas for uncuffed, non-tunneled catheters these values rise to 0.16–0.86 per 100 days.[15] Catheter-related infections include exit site infection, tunnel infections, and catheter-associated bacteremia. Sepsis is the most significant cause of catheter-associated morbidity and mortality and usually results from catheter-associated bacteremia. Catheter infection is responsible for between 6% and 28% of catheter failure.[62] Gram-positive skin-dwelling bacteria, in particular *Staphylococcus* species, are the major culprits, although *Pseudomonas*, a Gram-negative organism, has been isolated in up to 16% of patients.[58] *Staphylococcus aureus* is the commonest causative organism and is found in up to 43% of catheter-associated bacteremia. Methicillin-resistant *S. aureus* (MRSA) infection has been reported in 12–38% of cases of bacteremia and has the worst prognosis and highest mortality.[62] The route of infection is twofold, either tracking along the external surface of the catheter or via the lumen. Bacteria track from the skin, usually prior to healing of the exit site wound, along the external surface of the catheter along a biofilm. A biofilm is a matrix produced by the bacteria that protects them from antibiotic therapy and cannot be eradicated. Although a significant proportion of catheters will be colonized with pathogenic bacteria, infection only occurs once a certain quantitative threshold of bacteria has been reached. Intraluminal spread of infection is due to transfer of organisms from skin or surrounding clothing directly on to the catheter and is usually attributable to persons handling the catheter, typically healthcare workers. Strategies to prevent catheter infection begin with the patient and should include anybody handling the catheter. The National Kidney Foundation Kidney Disease Outcomes Quality Initiative (KDOQI) guidelines recommend that dialysis staff wear protective facemasks and sterile gloves and use chlorhexidine or a suitable alternative to clean the catheter.[1]

Exit site infections present with localized erythema with or without discharge and often respond to topical or oral antibiotics. Unresponsive infections or those with discharge, no signs of systemic sepsis, and no bacterial growth on blood culture should be treated with parenteral antibiotic therapy. If these measures fail and the infection is persistent or there are signs of systemic sepsis then the catheter should be replaced using a different tract and ideally at a distant site. Catheter-associated bacteremia can initially be treated with parenteral antibiotics and the KDOQI guidelines recommend treatment for 3 weeks.[1] However, if the patient is hemodynamically unstable or fails to improve following 36 hours of parenteral antibiotics, with bactericidal serum levels of an appropriate antibiotic, the catheter should be removed. Serious complications from catheter-associated infections occur in 3–44% of cases and include endocarditis, osteomyelitis, thrombophlebitis, septic arthritis, spinal epidural abscess, and large atrial thrombi. Mortality from catheter-associated infections is greatest when *S. aureus* is the culprit, with a reported rate of up to 30% in some units. MRSA has three to five times higher mortality compared with methicillin-sensitive strains and is considerably more costly to treat and manage.[62]

FISTULAS AND SYNTHETIC GRAFTS

AVFs using native venous conduits are associated with high long-term patency and low complications rates and should be the vascular access of choice for patients requiring long-term hemodialysis. These advantages are offset by relatively high primary failure rates (up to 37%), and the duration required for the fistula to mature, which can be in excess of 6 weeks for radiocephalic AVF.[98] Synthetic grafts have lower rates of primary failure and can be used for dialysis earlier; indeed, some new synthetic grafts can be needled as early as 12 hours following formation.[12] However the complication rates are considerably higher and the long-term patency is significantly lower than native AVF. Furthermore the KDOQI guidelines are that 80% of hemodialysis patients should have a native AVF for dialysis access.[1]

Historical Development of Vascular Access Surgery

In 1960 Quinton, Dillard, and Scribner described the first arteriovenous shunt, which was a synthetic tube that remained external to the skin following anastomosis to the radial artery and cephalic vein (Figure 5-2). This innovation permitted repeated dialysis and was the catalyst for early vascular access surgeons to develop more refined techniques. The Scribner shunt had significant disadvantages, including high rates of infection and thrombosis, requiring multiple revision procedures. Arguably the biggest advance in AVF surgery was the Brescia-Cimino radiocephalic fistula in 1966, which was a side-to-side anastomosis of the radial artery and cephalic vein at the wrist (Figure 5-3). As the first autogenous fistula, it solved many of the problems associated with an external shunt and it remains the initial procedure of choice today.

AVF surgery evolved through the 1970s as a result of either the failing of wrist AVF or inadequacy of forearm vessels, to include various elbow fistulas, including brachiocephalic and brachiobasilic AVF. Cascardo described the first brachiocephalic AVF in 1970, which was an end-of-vein to side-of-artery anastomosis. Subsequently synthetic grafts became available and were typically used following the exhaustion of native veins.

Planning Vascular Access

Patients on long-term dialysis are living longer and may need to be maintained on dialysis for many years. The key to achieving the greatest utility from native AVF includes carefully planned access procedures and protecting the veins. Medical and nursing staff involved in the care of renal patients are usually well educated in the importance of protecting forearm and anticubital fossa veins from intravenous cannulation and venepuncture. The dorsum of the hand should be used for access to the venous system if at all possible and the importance of this should be emphasized to patients so that they can have some responsibility for the care of their veins. Further to this the central veins should also be preserved, in particular the subclavian vein, which has high rates of stenosis. Minimizing CVCs by careful access planning and pre-emptive AVF formation is an important way of avoiding temporary venous

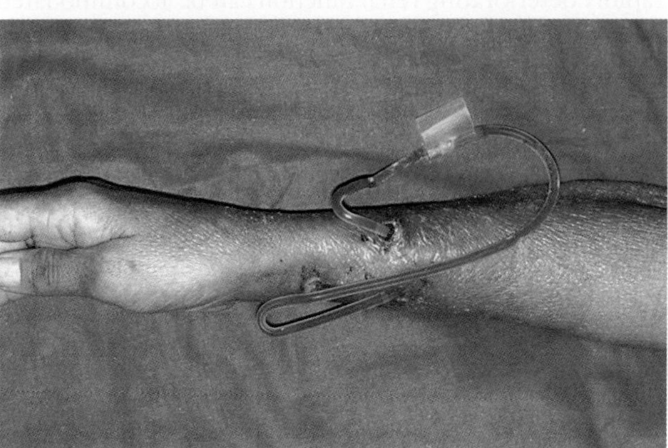

FIGURE 5-2 ■ Scribner shunt.

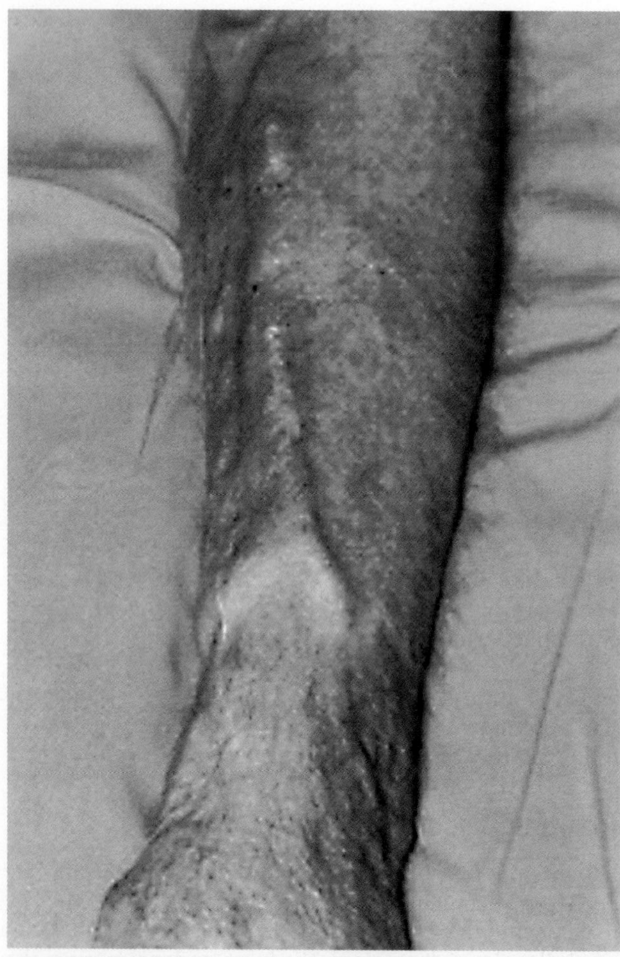

FIGURE 5-3 ■ Brescia-Cimino radiocephalic arteriovenous fistula.

catheters. There are a few general principles that are important in the planning of vascular access. The upper limb should be used in preference to the lower limb and distal sites should be used before proximal sites. This permits the maximum use from a particular vessel and preserves proximal sites for future use. It is also preferential to use the non-dominant arm ahead of the dominant arm and this is particularly important in patients who needle their own fistula at home. The formation of pre-emptive AVF requires liaison between nephrologist and surgeon and flexibility in theater list planning to ensure patients with rapidly deteriorating renal function can be accommodated before reaching end-stage disease.

Requirements of Arteriovenous Fistulas for Hemodialysis

The veins of the arm can be catheterized easily and repeatedly, but their blood flow is too low to support hemodialysis. The creation of an AVF produces an arterialized venous channel, which yields the combined advantage of large diameter and high blood flow. The ideal AVF has the following features:

1. A blood flow of at least 300 mL/min
2. A large diameter, which facilitates venepuncture
3. Sufficient length to allow two dialysis needles to be inserted
4. Creation by a simple and quick operation, preferably under local anesthetic
5. A good long-term patency rate.

Preoperative Assessment

The three requirements for a successful AVF are:

1. Good arterial supply – inflow
2. Adequate vein – conduit
3. Patent central veins – outflow.

Adequacy of the inflow to the arm can usually be assessed clinically with palpation of the brachial, ulnar, and radial pulses. Pulse volume and the quality of the arteries can be assessed and Allen's test can be used to determine patency of the palmar arch and the dominance of radial or ulnar artery in supplying the hand. This involves the patient elevating the hand and making a fist for about 30 seconds; the ulnar and radial arteries are then occluded. Ulnar pressure is released and the color should return to the blanched hand within a few seconds. If color does not return the test is considered positive and the ulnar artery supply to the hand is not sufficient.

If the patient has clinically questionable vessels then duplex imaging can be undertaken to aid in decision making. Suitability of arm veins can also usually be determined clinically using a tourniquet placed proximally on the arm. The cephalic vein can usually be traced from the anatomical snuffbox along the lateral aspect of the forearm into the cubital fossa. It can have many tributaries in the forearm, which may reduce AVF success, and it must be patent to the elbow and be greater than 3 mm to stand a good chance of success.[90] In thin patients the basilic vein can usually be palpated at the elbow and on the medial aspect of the distal arm but is usually impalpable once it runs underneath the deep fascia. Outflow can only be assessed using imaging techniques such as duplex and venography. Venography is usually favored and, although imaging is not required in all patients, it is advisable in those in whom vascular access is problematic or in patients who have had CVCs.

Anesthesia

The majority of upper-limb AVFs can be performed under local anesthetic, in particular wrist and elbow fistulas. The anesthetic choice is surgeon-dependent but 1% lidocaine with 1:200 000 epinephrine injected subdermally provides an instant anesthetic effect and minimizes bleeding. For more extensive procedures such as transposition of the basilic vein and forearm loop grafts, a regional block with local infiltration may suffice. Regional anesthesia has the added advantage of blocking sympathetic nerves as well as sensory nerves, which reduces vasospasm. In prolonged operations or if the patient is intolerant of the procedure, the anesthetist can administer a short-acting sedative to avoid a general anesthetic (GA). This is advantageous as many patients with renal failure have significant cardiovascular disease and other comorbid conditions, making a GA high risk. Surgical procedures in the axilla and lower limb usually require GA.

Surgical Technique

Vascular access surgery requires adherence to the basic principles of vascular anastomosis. The vessels are anastomosed using a fine, continuous, non-absorbable, monofilament suture with eversion of the edges to ensure a smooth transition between two intimal surfaces. There must be no tension between the anastomosed vessels and the sutures must include all layers of the arterial wall to avoid the creation of a subintimal flap. Suture placement is crucial and as such optical magnification using surgical telescopes is an advantage. Technical precision is important and this is aided by the availability of good-quality microvascular instruments.

Autogenous Arteriovenous Fistulas

Wrist Fistula

The initial procedure of choice, in patients with suitable vessels, is a radiocephalic AVF at the wrist. The operation is performed under local anesthetic as a day case procedure and has the advantage of low complication rates and high long-term patency. The original Brescia-Cimino AVF involved a side-to-side radial artery-to-cephalic vein anastomosis, although more recently an end of cephalic vein to side of radial artery has come into favor. The original Brescia-Cimino AVF often led to venous hypertension in the hand (Figure 5-4) whereas the end-to-side variation does not. Once established, the radiocephalic AVF remains relatively free of complications and has 2-year patency rates as high as 75%, although up to 37% will fail to mature. [23,30,90,98]

The surgical technique for formation of radiocephalic fistulas follows. The cephalic vein and radial artery are exposed via a longitudinal, oblique, or S-shaped incision depending upon the proximity of the vessels and the preference of the surgeon. The cephalic vein is mobilized for 3 cm from beneath the lateral skin flap, ensuring preservation of the sensory dorsal branch of the radial nerve. The artery is located lateral to the tendon of flexor carpi radialis and lies underneath the fibers of the deep fascia, which must be divided. Between 2 and 3 cm of artery should be mobilized and branches of the vessel can be ligated and divided. The vein and artery are controlled proximally and distally with vascular slings and microvascular clamps. In an end-to-side anastomosis the cephalic vein is ligated distally and divided obliquely to leave a spatulated end for anastomosis. An arteriotomy is then performed on the anterolateral surface of the radial artery. In a side-to-side anastomosis an arteriotomy (1–1.5 cm) is performed on the lateral aspect of the vessel; following this, a venotomy of equal length is performed on the medial side of the cephalic vein. A 7/0 non-absorbable, monofilament suture with two needles is then used to perform a continuous anastomosis. Once the anastomosis has been completed and in the presence of an acceptable thrill within the vein, the distal cephalic artery can be ligated and divided.

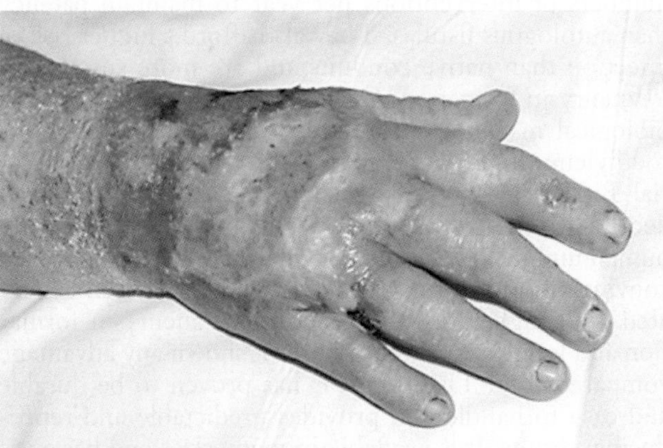

FIGURE 5-4 ■ Venous ulceration on the dorsum of the right hand as a result of venous hypertension in a patient with multiple previous arm fistulas and a functioning brachial artery-to-basilic vein loop graft. Radiological imaging demonstrated retrograde flow in the main draining vein driving the venous hypertension. The vein was successfully embolized with a coil inserted via percutaneous procedure. The hypertension improved and the ulcer healed.

In a successful procedure there should be a thrill present once the clamps have been released and the slings loosened. In the absence of a thrill one must ensure the patient is not hypotensive, there are no adventitial bands constricting the vein, and there are no errors, such as an intimal flap or twisting of the vein.

Elbow Fistulas

In the presence of failed radiocephalic fistulas or inadequate forearm vessels an autogenous elbow fistula should be the next procedure of choice. A brachiocephalic AVF is usually the first procedure of choice at the elbow and is a straightforward procedure performed under local anesthetic.

Brachiocephalic Arteriovenous Fistulas. The original brachiocephalic AVF was described as an end-to-side anastomosis of the cephalic vein to the brachial artery (Figure 5-5). As with radiocephalic AVF, if the elbow vessels are small, then a side-to-side configuration can

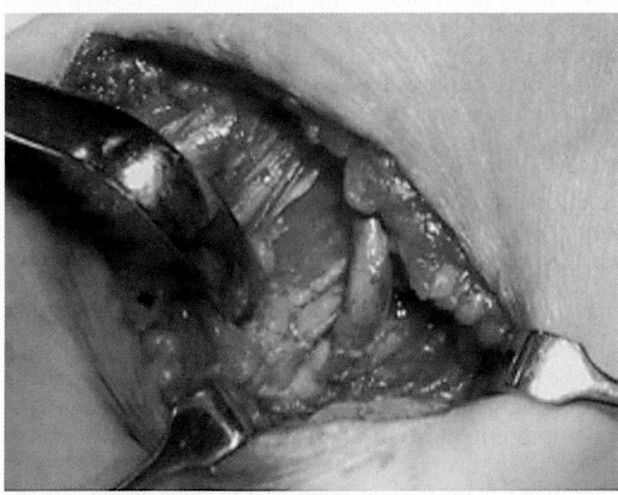

FIGURE 5-5 ■ Operative photographic image of completed brachiocephalic arteriovenous fistula, illustrating an end-of-cephalic vein to side-of-brachial artery anastomosis.

also be used. The main disadvantage of a brachiocephalic AVF is the relatively short length of vein that is present in the arm for needling. Furthermore the cephalic vein at the elbow is often used for venepuncture and can be sclerosed and unsuitable for use. The median cubital vein often drains into the cephalic vein and can also be used for anastomosis to the brachial artery. The venous anatomy in the cubital fossa is variable and it is important to establish how the veins are related before deciding upon which vessel to use. The surgical technique for the brachiocephalic fistula is the same in principle as for the radiocephalic at the wrist. The main advantage of brachiocephalic AVF is the excellent secondary patency rate, which is up to 80% at 3 years and 70% at 4 years.[22,54] Unlike with radiocephalic fistulas, there can be a significant increase in flow rates in brachiocephalic fistulas, which can lead to high-output cardiac failure and steal syndrome. Such complications may be avoided by ensuring the arteriotomy does not exceed 75% of the diameter of the artery.

Brachiobasilic Arteriovenous Fistula. The basilic vein originates on the medial aspect of the forearm at the wrist from the dorsal venous network of the hand. It runs superficially in the forearm and usually communicates with the cephalic vein via the median cubital vein at the elbow. It only remains superficial for a short distance in the arm before coursing beneath the deep fascia to run up the medial aspect of the arm alongside the medial cutaneous nerve of the forearm. Broadly, brachiobasilic fistula formation can be split into one-stage and two-stage procedures. A one-stage procedure is usually performed under GA and requires an extensive incision from the cubital fossa running longitudinally along the medial aspect of the arm towards the axilla. The basilic vein is mobilized from beneath the deep fascia and all tributaries are ligated and divided. Once an appropriate length has been exposed, the vein is divided and placed superficial to the medial cutaneous nerve of the forearm. The vein can then either be tunneled subcutaneously, or, as is preferred in our unit, the lateral skin flap can be undermined and the vein placed in a suitable position for needling. The vein can then be anastomosed to the brachial artery in an end-to-side disposition. The deep fascia is then closed beneath the vein to ensure that it remains superficial. The advantages of a one-stage procedure are that it only requires one operation and a single hospital stay and the fistula can be used more quickly. The disadvantage is that, if the fistula fails, the patient has undergone a significant procedure, with a substantial incision, usually under GA (Figure 5-6). A two-stage procedure comprises a first stage, during which the basilic vein is anastomosed to the brachial artery under local anesthetic, through a small cubital fossa incision. The fistula is then assessed for maturation 4–6 weeks following formation and, if deemed adequate, the more extensive second stage can be performed. The second-stage procedure is usually performed under GA, although a regional block with local anesthetic infiltration can be used. The incision is as described above in the one-stage procedure. The vein is mobilized from its bed beneath the deep fascia, all the branches are ligated, and it is then transposed as described above. If the medial cutaneous nerve of the forearm is

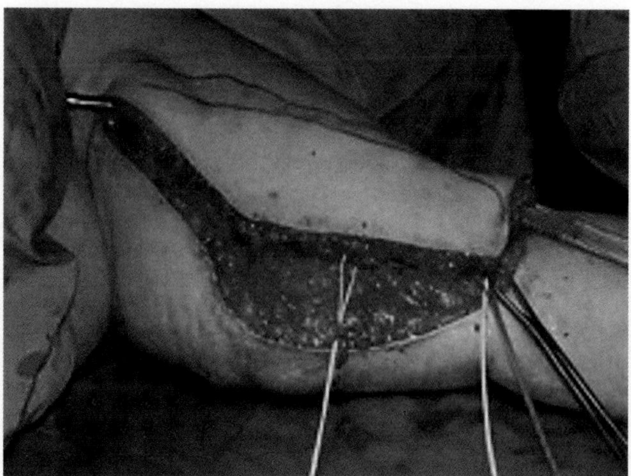

FIGURE 5-6 ■ Operative photographic image of the extensive incision required for exposure of the basilic vein to enable the vein to be transposed in a brachiobasilic arteriovenous fistula.

coursing across the fistula and at risk of damage during needling, then the fistula should be divided, positioned superficial to the nerve, and reanastomosed. Recent data support the use of brachiobasilic AVF ahead of prosthetic grafts, demonstrating improved long-term patency and a lower frequency of intervention.[61,71] The patency rates at 2 years range from 50% to 80%, with one randomized study yielding patency rates of 70% at 3 years.[54] Brachiobasilic fistulas do however have higher wound complication rates due to the extensive incision required. One recent study demonstrated that the two-stage procedure had more favorable patency rates than a one-stage procedure at 1 year (34% versus 88%; P=0.047).[92]

Graft Arteriovenous Fistulas

Prosthetic grafts are typically reserved for patients who have exhausted native venous access, although in the United States they are used as primary procedures. Grafts have lower long-term patency rates and higher numbers of interventions per year to maintain patency than autologous fistulas. They also afford a higher risk of infection than native conduits and are more susceptible to aneurysm formation. Grafts can be either synthetic or biological in composition, and expanded polytetrafluoroethylene (ePTFE) is the most commonly used material. Biological grafts have included bovine carotid artery, decellularized bovine ureter, bovine mesenteric vein, and human umbilical vein, but they have all failed to produce convincing long-term results.[108] They have been associated with high rates of infection and aneurysm formation and long-term patency has not shown any advantage compared to ePTFE. ePTFE has proven to be durable and easy to handle and provides predictable and reproducible results. It is available in many sizes and has a variety of "funnels" at the venous end to aid patency and accommodate surgeon preference. A prosthetic graft can be anastomosed to any suitable artery and vein, in an end-to-side disposition, and then tunneled subcutaneously. It can be performed under local anesthetic but usually requires GA. Early grafts were typically fashioned in a straight orientation, originated at the radial artery, and were anastomosed to a suitable vein in the cubital fossa. Grafts in a "j" disposition and "loop" grafts have become increasingly popular and prosthetic material can also be used as an interposition graft either to replace a section of a fistula that is beyond salvage or to bypass a location that has an adequate distal arterial supply but no adjacent vein. Brachioaxillary grafts provided a straightforward secondary procedure in the presence of an adequate brachial artery but absence of suitable cephalic and basilic veins at the elbow (Figure 5-7). To date, in the literature, loop grafts have been constructed in the forearm and arm; on the chest wall; in the thigh; and as a necklace, from one axilla to the other. More elaborate procedures have also been undertaken, including brachiojugular grafts,[87] and a straight graft has successfully been fashioned from the axillary artery to the external iliac vein.[25]

The advantage of prosthetic grafts is their versatility and use in salvage procedures in complex patients. However the disadvantages are the side effect profile, in particular the infection rates and high incidence of thrombosis. Infection rates are between 11% and 35%, compared to about 2% for autologous fistulas.[4] Long-term patency is reported at about 60% at 2 years and rates of thrombosis are 10-fold higher than autologous AVF.[7,68] Stenosis is also a problem, which is thought to be due to the graft stimulating neoepithelialization, intimal hyperplasia, and subsequent stenosis. Furthermore, ePTFE grafts are not self-sealing and thus rely on the subsequent fibrotic response of the surrounding tissue for hemostasis before the graft can be safely punctured. This process typically takes about 4 weeks and, although grafts can be needled earlier, there is an increased risk of infection and hematoma formation. There are new self-sealing grafts on the market that have shown promising results and can be cannulated within 72 hours of surgery.[12]

Fistula Maturation and Venepuncture

Historically fistulas were allowed to mature for 6 weeks to enable the vein to arterialize and dilate to a size appropriate for needling. Fistula maturation is dependent on the size and quality of the vessels and the individual, and some fistulas are ready to be used within a couple of weeks. Early needling of immature fistulas can lead to hematoma and thrombosis and therefore all AVFs should be assessed clinically and be deemed mature enough before needling is attempted. If, after 6–8 weeks of maturation, the fistula still appears immature, then one should consider duplex imaging to ensure there is no structural reason, such as a stenosis that is impairing maturation.

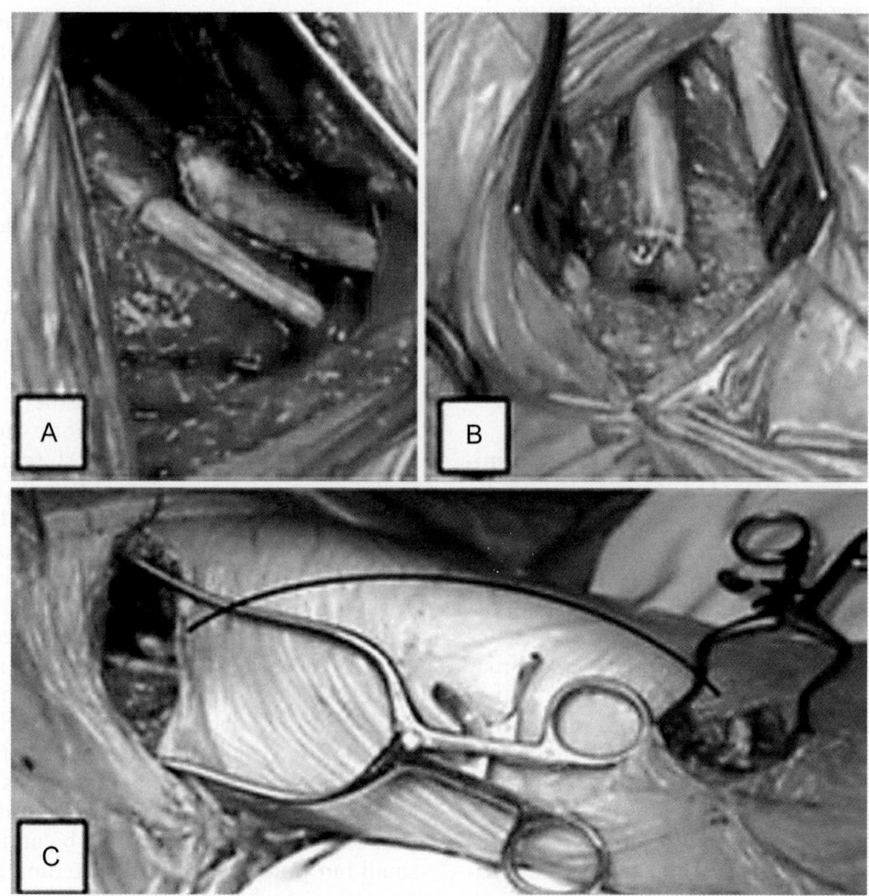

FIGURE 5-7 ■ Operative photographic images of an expanded polytetrafluroethylene (ePTFE) brachioaxillary prosthetic graft. (A) Proximal limb of 6mm ePTFE graft with an end-to-side anastomosis of graft with axillary vein (median nerve is the tubular-looking structure adjacent to the graft). (B) Distal limb of 6mm ePTFE graft with an end-to-side anastomosis of graft with brachial artery. (C) Broad operative view of the procedure demonstrating exposure of axillary vein and brachial artery graft anastomoses. The graft runs through a subcutaneous tunnel, represented by the line on the photograph.

Once needling begins, the site at which this occurs is at the discretion of the dialysis staff. Rotating needling sites is advisable as repetitively using the same site – so-called "button-holing" – can lead to damage to the vessel wall, resulting in aneurysm and pseudoaneurysm formation. Alongside nursing preference, for the ease of needling at the same site, there may also be pressure from the patient as the skin becomes devoid of nerve endings within the scar tissue at the site of repetitive needling and is therefore less painful. Rotating needling sites in prosthetic grafts is particularly important, as the skin at the needling site is at risk of necrosis, leaving the graft exposed and highly susceptible to infection.

Complications of Arteriovenous Fistulas

Hemorrhage

Bleeding from an AVF can be categorized as early, which is within the first 24 hours, or late, which is any time thereafter. Early bleeding is due to technical error within the anastomosis or slipping of a ligature. The need to return to theater for exploration of bleeding is uncommon as hematoma formation is usually due to generalized oozing as a result of uremic platelet dysfunction.[91] Late hemorrhage from an AVF is usually from a needling site immediately following dialysis and often occurs in patients who are anticoagulated. Direct pressure on the site of venepuncture will usually stop the bleeding and reversal of anticoagulation is not often necessary. Bleeding from aneurysms or at needling sites as a result of infection can be catastrophic and very frightening for the patient. Although direct pressure may be sufficient to control hemorrhage, surgical exploration is often required and may result in ligation of the fistula, for which the patient must agree consent. Exploration of a late bleed from a fistula should be performed under GA as an extensive incision is often required to gain proximal control of the vessels and it can be extremely unsettling for the patient.

Thrombosis

Thrombosis of an AVF can occur at any time from immediately following completion of the anastomosis to decades later. Early thrombosis may be as a result of patient factors such as hypotension, either as a result of fluid depletion following dialysis or cardiac failure, and is a poor prognostic sign both in terms of thrombosis risk and fistula maturation. Immediate thrombosis in the presence of adequate-quality and appropriate-sized vessels may be due to technical error. Early thrombectomy with a Fogarty catheter and refashioning of the anastomosis may salvage the fistula. Late thrombosis is usually due to the presence of a gradually progressive stenosis secondary to neointimal hyperplasia, and these account for about 85% of all stenoses.[7] Treatment of fistula thrombosis has progressed from primarily a surgical problem into the territory of interventional radiology. Radiologists now carry out the majority of interventions percutaneously to retain long-term AVF patency. As such the initial management of a patient with late AVF thrombosis is imaging of the fistula, using either duplex ultrasound or venography. The advantage of interventional radiology is that, following percutaneous thrombectomy, the culpable stenosis can be identified by angiography and treated with balloon angioplasty in a dual procedure. Furthermore the central veins can be imaged simultaneously to ensure that an occult central stenosis is not contributing to the fistula dysfunction. A recent comprehensive review of percutaneous intervention for thrombosed vascular access demonstrated an 80% success rate in retaining patency and avoiding temporary access catheters.[8] Percutaneous balloon angioplasty should be the first-line treatment for stenosis and, if that is unsuccessful, then surgical thrombectomy should be considered.[7] Fistulas that are unsuitable for percutaneous intervention often require revision due to anastomotic or perianastomotic strictures that cannot be treated by angioplasty. Standard Fogarty vascular thrombectomy catheters are usually sufficient to clear early, soft thrombus but are not designed to penetrate mature thrombus. Fistulas that require surgical revision must retain enough length to accommodate two dialysis needles following revision.

Infection

Vascular access surgery is classed as "clean surgery" and the surgeon and theater team should be scrupulous about asepsis in renal patients. Although the procedure is "clean," infection rates in renal patients are higher because of the relative immunocompromised state uremia produces. Uremia affects the immune system by inhibiting the bactericidal, phagocytic, and chemotactic action of neutrophils and by suppressing both B-cell and T-cell responses.[38] Furthermore, renal patients are more readily colonized by *Staphylococcus aureus* compared with the general population, with an incidence of up to 70% upper respiratory tract colonization compared to 15% respectively.[130] *S. aureus* is the leading culprit in infective complications of vascular access conduits and is often resistant to first-line antibiotics. Routine use of antibiotics for autologous AVF formation is not universal. However in any procedure in which prosthetic material is used, a second-line intravenous antibiotic such as vancomycin or teicoplanin should be given. Uremia-induced platelet dysfunction predisposes renal failure patients to bleeding and meticulous hemostasis is essential to reduce postoperative hematoma formation, which is a risk factor for infection. Wound infection rates are as low as 2–3%[4] following autologous AVF formation and usually respond well to standard wound care measures. Drainage of any collections either by liberal suture removal or formal evacuation and irrigation under anesthesia alongside antibiotic therapy resolves the majority of infections. If there is concern about the severity of the infection or if MRSA is isolated and the infection is not responding to antibiotic therapy then surgical debridement and inspection of the anastomosis should be undertaken. There is a small but potentially life-threatening risk of hemorrhage from an infected fistula and ligation of the fistula may be required. Superficial wound infection in a patient with underlying prosthetic material should always be treated seriously. Aggressive, early antibiotic therapy should be employed to treat the infection and reduce the risk of graft infection. Superficial infection can often be treated successfully but if there is a purulent infection or the graft is proven to be infected it must be removed.

Aneurysm Formation

Vascular access conduits are at risk of both true and false aneurysm formation. False aneurysm (also termed pseudoaneurysm) formation usually occurs at an overused needling site. The incidence of false aneurysm is about 10% in prosthetic grafts and 2% in autologous AVF.[131] Treatment can be radiological or surgical, with the latter being the conventional method. Surgical repair usually involves over-sewing the defect or removing the damaged section of graft and restoring the AVF either by direct end-to-end anastomosis or by using an interposition graft. Increasingly interventional radiological methods are employed first; direct injection of thrombin into the defect is usually sufficient if the defect is less than 1 cm and percutaneous deployment of a covered stent can also be used to exclude the aneurysm from the circulation. True aneurysms are relatively common in upper limb fistulas and older fistulas are more likely to become aneurysmal (Figure 5-8). Aside from the fistula being unsightly, most aneurysms are uncomplicated and at extremely low risk of rupture. However, aneurysms that are rapidly increasing in size, or have thin skin or infection present should be surgically corrected or ligated.

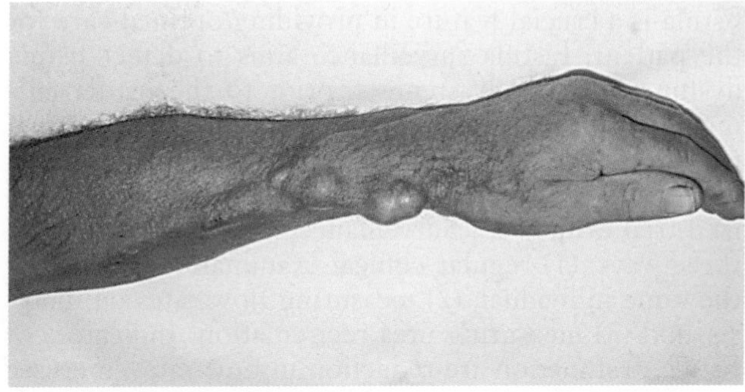

FIGURE 5-8 ■ True aneurysm of arteriovenous fistula.

Steal Syndrome

Steal syndrome is diagnosed when there is hypoperfusion of the limb distal to the arteriovenous anastomosis; it is uncommon and reportedly only present in 1–8% of patients.[28] Steal syndrome is most common in the upper limb in procedures involving the brachial artery and patients with arteriosclerosis and diabetes are particularly at risk. The presence of a small brachial artery (less than 5 mm) at the time of surgery should alert the surgeon to the possibility of steal syndrome and limiting the arteriotomy to 75% of the vessel diameter may reduce the overall risk. Symptoms of steal syndrome range from mild ones, such as a cold hand, through to severe ischemia with rest pain, neurological deficit, and tissue loss. Mild steal syndrome usually improves with conservative management and the improvement is due to increase in collateral flow around the elbow. Duplex imaging will establish whether there is reversal of flow distal to the anastomosis, which is characteristic of steal syndrome. If symptoms are severe or there is critical ischemia due to the steal syndrome then surgical intervention is indicated. The simplest intervention is ligation of the fistula, which almost invariably ameliorates the symptoms, but the fistula is then lost. A more complex but elegant approach is the distal revascularization interval ligation (DRIL). This procedure utilizes either saphenous vein or ePTFE to bypass the anastomosis, following which the brachial artery is ligated distal to the original arteriovenous anastomosis (Figure 5-9).[97] This ingenious procedure permits blood flow to the distal arm via the newly anastomosed bypass graft prior to flow into the fistula and, although performed uncommonly, has excellent results, with medium-term patency rates of 83–100%.[28]

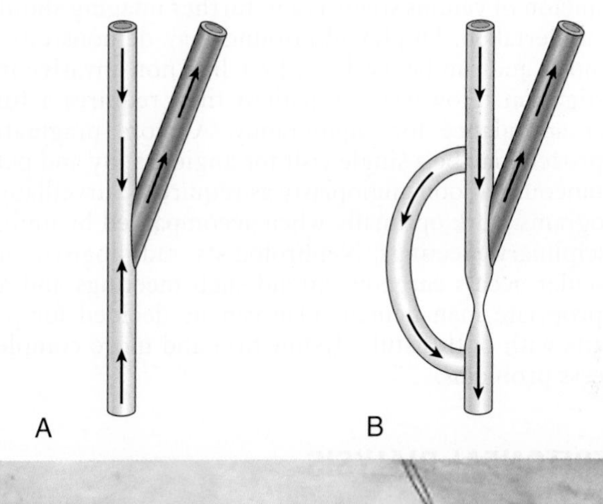

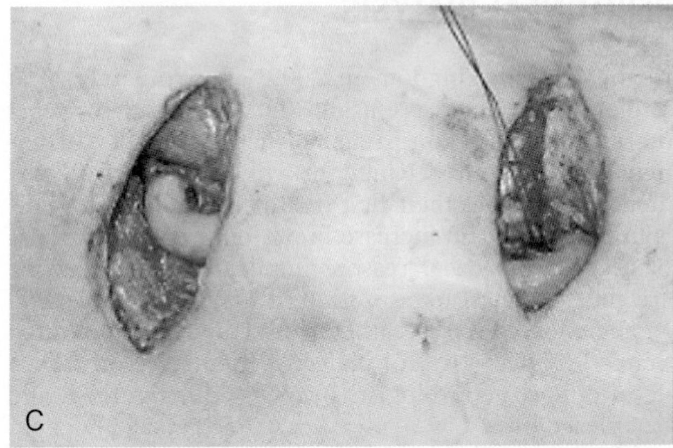

FIGURE 5-9 ■ (A) Diagram of an arteriovenous fistula (AVF) demonstrating steal syndrome. (B) Diagram illustrating distal revascularization interval ligation procedure (DRIL). (C) Operative photographic image of DRIL procedure. (A) An AVF with blood flow direction characteristic of vascular steal syndrome. Note the reversal of flow distal to the anastomosis in the artery. (B) DRIL procedure, during which a bypass graft is anastomosed to the artery proximal and distal to the AVF. Following this the artery is then ligated distal to the AVF, allowing blood to flow into both the distal artery and the AVF. (C) Surgical exposure of the brachial artery proximal and distal to the AVF; the bypass graft used was a bovine ureter. The ligature around the artery highlights the position at which the artery was ligated.

Arteriovenous Fistula Surveillance

Hemodialysis patients have often been receiving healthcare for many years, may have had previous kidney transplants, and are familiar with the complexities of managing a chronic disease. An AVF is a lifeline enabling the patient to dialyze and preserving the fistula is a crucial feature in providing optimal care for the patient. Fistula surveillance aims to detect fistula dysfunction, usually stenosis, prior to the fistula failing.[99] Fistula surveillance programs have been shown to reduce the incidence of thrombosis and improve long-term patency, although there is no large randomized trial evidence.[57] Surveillance can be carried out in three ways: (1) regular clinical examination, ideally by the same individual; (2) measuring flow rates on dialysis; and (3) measuring urea recirculation. Indicators of fistula dysfunction are reduction in flow rates, increase in pressure, poor urea excretion, and reduction in palpable thrill. Flow rates of <500 mL/min should raise suspicion of venous stenosis and further imaging should be undertaken. Duplex ultrasound may demonstrate a stenosis and can be used as a first-line non-invasive investigation. However the patient then requires a further attendance for angiography. A more pragmatic approach may be a single visit for angiography and percutaneous balloon angioplasty as required. Surveillance programs work optimally when accompanied by multidisciplinary meetings. Nephrologists, radiologists, and vascular access surgeons attend such meetings and an appropriate management plan can be decided for patients with both fistula dysfunction and more complex access problems.

PERITONEAL DIALYSIS

In the United Kingdom in 2009, approximately 15% of dialysis patients were using PD.[110] Over recent years there has been a consistent fall in the number of patients in the United Kingdom with renal failure commenced on PD as their first treatment modality.[110] This is in part due to an increase in pre-emptive renal transplantation, but other reasons implicated in the decline are the structural organization of dialysis facilities and arrangements for PD catheter insertion. In the United States less than 10% of dialysis patients are on PD,[117] despite most nephrologists believing this figure should be at least 40%.[59]

The concept behind PD is straightforward. The peritoneum, with a total surface area of 2 m^2, is composed of endothelium, interstitium, and mesothelium and can act as an efficient semipermeable membrane. Infusing a hypertonic dialysate fluid into the peritoneal cavity allows ultrafiltration of solutes and electrolytes.

PD does have certain advantages over hemodialysis. Recent studies have described improved survival in PD patients, particularly in the first 1–2 years after commencing RRT.[41,123] However, after 1.5–2 years on dialysis, the risk of death in PD patients becomes equivalent to that in hemodialysis patients. The reasons for this improved survival have yet to be clarified, although maintenance of residual renal function may be a factor, as this is better preserved in PD patients as compared to those on hemodialysis.[74] PD patients usually report greater satisfaction than those on hemodialysis,[26,95] which may relate to the greater autonomy afforded by PD. Furthermore, the cost of PD per patient per year is approximately one-third less than that of hemodialysis.[117]

However, the major drawback of PD is technique failure, which remains high. A recent multicenter prospective study found that 25% of PD patients transferred to hemodialysis, 70% within the first 2 years after commencing PD.[45] Despite reductions in peritonitis, infection remains the primary cause of technique failure.

Peritoneal Dialysis Delivery Systems and Catheters

PD is a closed-loop system comprising dialysate fluid, a delivery system, and an indwelling peritoneal catheter. Fluid is infused under gravity from a reservoir of dialysate. Luer-Lok or rotating self-lock devices have been devised to connect the dialysate bag with the delivery system for ease of connection and sterility. The Y delivery systems are the most commonly used (Figure 5-10). The single branch of the Y is connected to the indwelling peritoneal catheter via an inert titanium connector and the upper two branches are connected to the dialysate reservoir and an empty bag. This configuration allows complete drainage of any contaminating dialysate fluid before infusion of sterile, fresh fluid through the indwelling catheter. Several randomized controlled trials have shown the superiority of various Y systems over conventional PD systems in reducing the incidence of infective complications.[16]

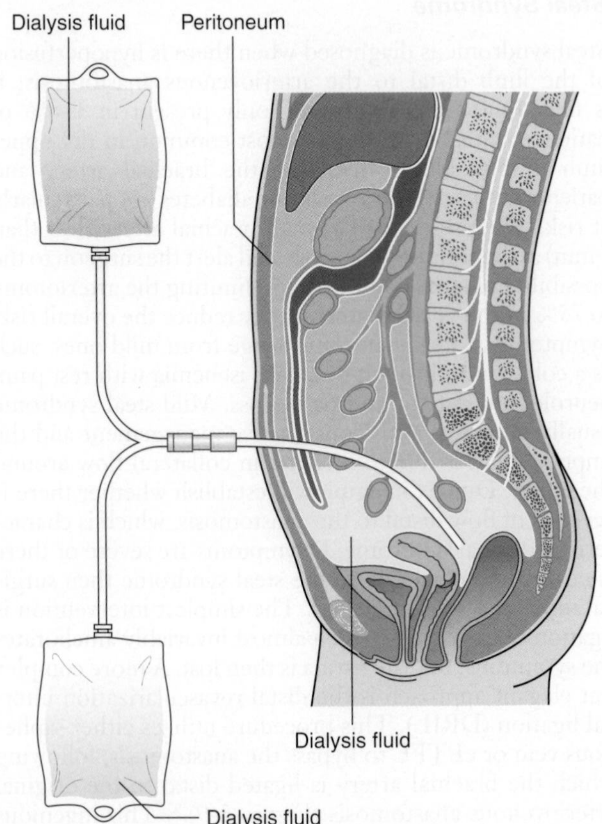

FIGURE 5-10 ■ Sagittal section demonstrating the optimal position for a peritoneal dialysis tube located in the pouch of Douglas. The diagram also illustrates a Y-delivery system for peritoneal dialysis fluid.

Catheter Selection

PD catheters should be soft, flexible, atraumatic, radiopaque and relatively inert. Several different catheters are available, but the Tenckhoff catheter is the most popular. The original Silastic Tenckhoff design was a straight, 5-mm external diameter tube, with two Dacron cuffs and a perforated intraperitoneal segment. Many variations of the Tenckhoff device exist, including catheters with single cuffs and coiled intraperitoneal ends. A number of randomized trials have compared straight versus coiled PD catheters,[2,20,21,66,78,96,129] with a meta-analysis demonstrating no significant difference in the risk of peritonitis, exit site or tunnel infection, or catheter removal.[106] A further meta-analysis did demonstrate an increased risk of catheter tip migration with coiled catheters, but this was not associated with an increased risk of catheter failure.[129] A single randomized trial has compared single- versus double-cuffed catheters and again shown no significant difference in the risk of peritonitis, exit site or tunnel infection, or catheter removal.[19] However, a large comparative study based on Canadian registry data did show a reduced risk of *Staphylococcus aureus* peritonitis in patients with double-cuffed catheters.[78]

Catheter Insertion

Not all patients are suitable for PD. Severe peritoneal adhesions, inflammatory bowel disease, and previous encapsulating peritoneal sclerosis (EPS) are absolute contraindications. Obesity, advanced age, abdominal hernias, stomas, and chronic obstructive pulmonary disease are relative contraindications. Severe colonic diverticulosis may increase the translocation of gut organisms, and there is a strong association between diverticular disease and Gram-negative PD peritonitis. Although PD can be performed in patients with stomas, there is a predisposition to infection. Abdominal wall hernias may enlarge in patients receiving PD and should, if possible, be repaired prior to or at the time of catheter insertion. Table 5-3 lists the relative and absolute contraindications to PD catheter insertion.

A variety of techniques for catheter insertion have been described, including open surgical, percutaneous, peritoneoscopic, and laparoscopic.

In the open technique, the catheter is introduced via a small vertical infraumbilical incision placed in the midline or paramedian position, with the preperitoneal cuff positioned in the rectus abdominis muscle. Before positioning the catheter should be flushed and immersed in saline as wet cuffs stimulate more rapid tissue ingrowth. A small incision is made in the peritoneum, and the tube is inserted using blunt forceps with or without a metal stylet within the catheter lumen. The tube tip must be placed in the rectovesical pouch in men and the rectovaginal pouch of Douglas in women. The peritoneum is closed with an absorbable suture around the cuff to create a watertight seal, and the linea alba or rectus sheath closed with a non-absorbable suture. The extraperitoneal segment of the catheter is tunneled subcutaneously and brought out at a conveniently placed lateral exit site. At the end of the procedure, the catheter should be flushed to ensure free inward and outward flow of dialysate fluid. Two randomized control trials have compared a midline versus lateral insertion site for PD catheters,[18,96] with a meta-analysis showing no significant difference in risk of peritonitis, exit or tunnel site infection, or mortality.[106] Catheter removal was reported in one trial and shown to be significantly reduced with midline insertion.

Over recent years, laparoscopic insertion of PD catheters has superseded the open surgical technique in a number of centers. Laparoscopy provides the ability to assess and address anatomical problems that may result in mechanical obstruction, such as adhesions, and allows placement of the catheter in the correct position in the pelvis under direct vision. There are a number of techniques for laparoscopic PD catheter insertion described in the literature. The principles are as follows. A 5- or 10-mm camera port is placed in either the left or right upper quadrant so as not to interfere with the catheter insertion site. The tunnel for the catheter can be created using either a further 5-mm port or specific kits containing a needle with an expandable plastic sheath and serial dilators (Figure 5-11). A further port can be inserted to allow manipulation of the catheter into the pelvis if required. Once the catheter is in a suitable position the pneumoperitoneum is released and the subcutaneous tunnel created.

The percutaneous and peritoneoscopic techniques are both variations on the Seldinger technique and utilize a similar kit to that described above for use in the laparoscopic technique. In the percutaneous technique, ultrasound guidance can be used to determine a safe puncture site where there is maximum separation between bowel and the anterior abdominal wall. Following puncture, the position within the peritoneum can be confirmed by injecting contrast under fluoroscopic control. A guidewire is then placed and serial dilators passed to create a tunnel. A peel-away sheath is then introduced into the peritoneal cavity, through which the catheter is passed, before the sheath is removed and the catheter tunneled subcutaneously. In the peritoneoscopic technique, rather than using fluoroscopic guidance, the position within the peritoneal cavity is confirmed using a 2.2-mm telescope introduced down the peel-away sheath.

TABLE 5-3 Contraindications to Peritoneal Dialysis

Absolute Contraindications	Relative Contraindications
Encapsulating peritoneal sclerosis Inflammatory bowel disease Large irreparable abdominal hernia	Severe obesity Severe peritoneal adhesions Large abdominal wall hernias Abdominal stomas Chronic obstructive airways disease Psychosocial factors likely to result in poor compliance Physical disability Learning disability

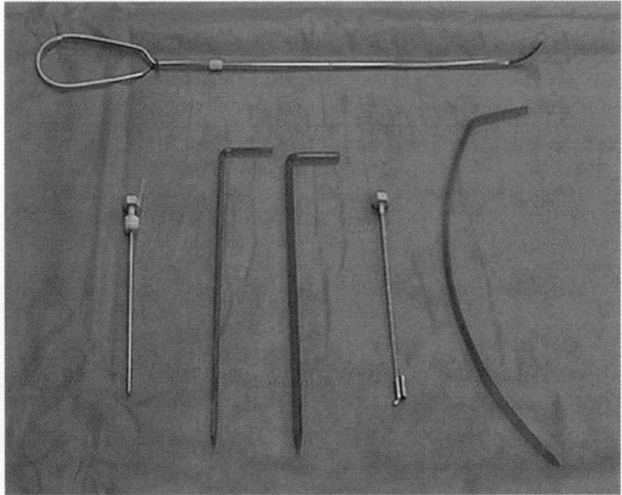

FIGURE 5-11 ■ YTec insertion kit. The components of the kit include, from left to right: insertion trocar with plastic sheath; medium and large-sized tract dilators; cuff insertion device and subcutaneous tunneling device. The single-cuff peritoneal dialysis tube with metal insert is at the top.

Three randomized controlled trials have compared laparoscopic with open insertion of PD catheters[31,47,113] and one peritoneoscopic with open.[128] A meta-analysis of three of these trials showed no significant differences in risk of mortality, peritonitis, exit site or tunnel infection, catheter removal, or technique failure.[106] A further multicenter randomized controlled trial is ongoing.[39]

No randomized controlled trials have been conducted to compare percutaneous techniques with other techniques. Two comparative studies of percutaneous versus open surgical insertion of PD catheters have been reported: one demonstrated no difference between the techniques,[82] whereas the other reported a significantly higher early leak rate in the percutaneous group.[94]

Complications Associated with Peritoneal Dialysis Catheters

Bleeding

Bloody fluid is a common finding, occurring in 30% of patients for the first few catheter exchanges after insertion. The bleeding most often arises from small vessels on the peritoneal surface at the catheter entry site and usually stops within 24 hours. If bleeding does occur, frequent flushing of the catheter or, if possible, low-volume exchanges reduce the rate of catheter obstruction by clots.[32] Bleeding long after insertion may occur with EPS.

Pain

The first attempts at dialysate infusion can produce discomfort. This is more common with straight catheters when infusion pressure is greatest. With coiled catheters pain is less likely because dialysate flows through the side perforations. The pain is usually temporary and resolves within a few weeks. Slower infusion rates and incomplete drainage may alleviate symptoms.

Cuff Extrusion

The most important factor for cuff extrusion is the depth at which the subcutaneous cuff is implanted; at least 2 cm below the skin is required. Tension on the extraperitoneal portion of the catheter, such as during bag exchange, can bring a poorly implanted cuff to the surface, or it may relate to an exit site or tunnel infection.

Catheter Obstruction

This is usually due to outflow obstruction, which can be extrinsic or related to catheter positioning. Clotted blood may collect in the distal portion of the catheter shortly after surgery; this can be treated effectively with a per-catheter infusion of heparin, streptokinase, or urokinase.[102,132]

Extrinisic compression causing obstruction can be due to bladder distension, an impacted sigmoid colon, or uterine fibroids. Constipation is a very common cause of catheter malfunction and laxatives should always be used for the initial management of poor drainage, even if there is no history or radiological evidence of constipation. Omental wrapping remains the commonest cause of refractory catheter obstruction (Figure 5-12), responsible in 35–80% of cases. All of the above causes may result in catheter tip migration out of the pelvis. However, not all migrated catheters become obstructed and conversely catheters well positioned in the pelvis may still become obstructed. Approximately half of all catheters migrate to some extent over time, but only 20% of migrated catheters malfunction.[24]

Persisting catheter obstruction after treatment for constipation is an indication for manipulation, either fluoroscopically using a stiff guidewire or surgically. Initial success rates for guidewire manipulation have been reported between 78% and 85%.[75,84,104] However, this improvement in catheter patency is temporary and patency rates after 30 days are in the range of 29% and 85%; this is probably because the underlying problem, be it omental wrapping or adhesions, has not been addressed. Failure

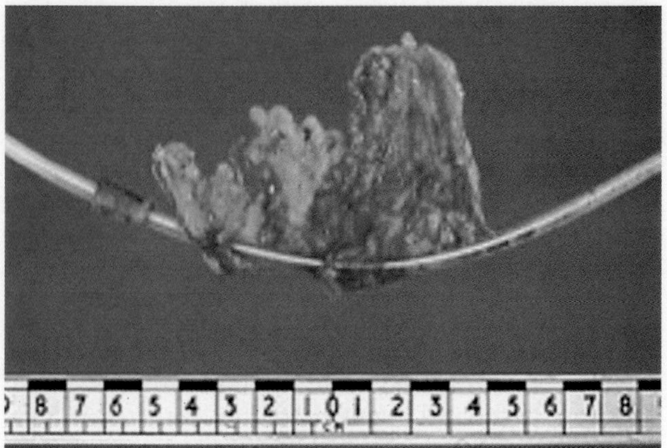

FIGURE 5-12 ■ Omentum attached to peritoneal dialysis tube.

of guidewire manipulation to restore catheter function is an indication for laparoscopic intervention. This allows direct visualization of the cause of catheter obstruction and definitive treatment, including catheter repositioning, adhesiolysis, omentectomy, or omentopexy.

Pericatheter Leak

Any variable that predisposes to poor wound healing (e.g., steroids, obesity, malnutrition, diabetes) may culminate in pericatheter leakage, rates of which have been reported between 7% and 24%. Choice of surgical technique may determine leak rates; leaks are said to be more common with midline catheter insertion compared with lateral insertion,[21] but this is not our experience. Pericatheter leakage allows fluid extravasation around the catheter or accumulation in the lower abdominal wall.

Some investigators suggest leak localization with computed tomography combined with peritoneal contrast enhancement[115] or magnetic resonance peritoneography.[3,89] When an early postoperative leak develops, dialysate exchange should be stopped for 2–4 weeks, necessitating a temporary switch to hemodialysis. Late-onset leaks usually require catheter replacement. Pericatheter leaks associated with herniation should be treated by catheter removal and hernia repair. Only after allowing for adequate healing (e.g., 2–3 months) should further catheter insertion be attempted.

Hernias

The increased intra-abdominal pressures after infusion of dialysate can enlarge pre-existing hernias, so it is best to repair these pre-emptively before commencement of PD. The reported prevalence of de novo abdominal hernias in PD patients is 2.5–25%.[77,79,124] One study showed 32% of all hernias occur at the site of catheter insertion, 18% are inguinal, 27% are epigastric or umbilical, and 23% are incisional.[79] The pressure of dialysate can cause recanalization of a patent processus vaginalis, which manifests as scrotal or labial edema, shortly after full dialysate exchanges are begun. Surgical ligation is necessary, with a postoperative regimen of low-volume, high-frequency dialysate exchanges until healing has occurred or temporary conversion to hemodialysis.

The repair of hernias that occur once PD has been established is controversial. Ideally the repair should avoid a breach of the peritoneal membrane. Use of polypropylene mesh in incisional hernia repair, attached to the deep aponeurosis without opening the peritoneum, allows immediate use of PD.[37]

Some surgeons withhold PD for many weeks after inguinal hernia repair, fearing fluid leak or recurrence. PD can be safely commenced immediately with low-volume, high-frequency exchanges.[72]

Exit Site and Tunnel Infections

As lone entities, exit site and tunnel infections pose little risk, but the possibility of developing PD peritonitis demands careful attention to the infections; PD peritonitis occurs in approximately 12% of patients with exit site or tunnel infections.

An exit site infection is defined by the presence of purulent drainage, with or without erythema of the skin.[60] Reported rates of exit site infections range from 0.05 to 1.02 episodes per patient per year.[66,84,120] Erythema at the exit site without purulent drainage can be an early indication of infection but can also be a simple skin reaction, particularly in newly inserted catheters. A positive culture from an exit site in the absence of purulent drainage represents colonization rather than infection and is not an indication for treatment. A tunnel infection may present with erythema, edema, or tenderness over the subcutaneous portion of the catheter; however it is often clinically occult and only detectable on ultrasound scanning.[85] The majority of exit site and tunnel infections are caused by *Staphylococcus aureus* and *Pseudomonas aeruginosa*[60]: nasal carriage of *S. aureus* increases the risk of exit site infection fourfold. Table 5-4 summarizes the recommended management of exit site problems and infections. Following catheter removal, simultaneous reinsertion is feasible, albeit with a new exit site on the contralateral side and under antibiotic coverage.[63,88]

Peritoneal Dialysis Peritonitis

Peritonitis is the most significant complication of PD and is the second commonest cause of mortality in PD patients. Incidence from large audits ranges from 0.2 to 0.6 episodes per patient per year.[33,36,49] The International Society for Peritoneal Dialysis (ISPD) guidelines give an acceptable peritonitis rate of no more than one episode every 18 months.[60] Although less than 4% of peritonitis episodes result in death, peritonitis is a contributory factor in 16% of deaths in PD patients.[60] At least a quarter of episodes culminate in catheter removal.[33,49] The most common portal of entry for infection is the exit site prior to wound healing.

The first indication of peritonitis is the presence of cloudy effluent containing >100 × 10^6/L leukocytes. Abdominal pain usually follows and abdominal tenderness is typically generalized and often associated with

TABLE 5-4 Treatment of Exit Site Problems and Infections

Problem	Treatment
Erythema alone, no discharge	Topical chlorhexidine, mupirocin, hydrogen peroxide
Overgranulation	Silver nitrate cauterization
Gram-positive infection	Flucloxacillin, co-amoxiclav, vancomycin, rifampicin, cephalosporins
Gram-negative infection	Ciprofloxacin, gentamicin
Pseudomonas infection	Ciprofloxacin plus another agent (e.g., cephalosporin) and catheter removal
Fungal infection	Catheter removal with systemic antifungal agent

rebound tenderness. Other signs include pyrexia, nausea and vomiting, and diarrhea. Localized pain or tenderness should raise suspicions of surgical pathology such as appendicitis or cholecystitis.

The causative organisms in PD peritonitis generally differ from the organisms causing "surgical" peritonitis. In the latter case, infections are usually polymicrobial, consisting of aerobic and anaerobic bacteria, whereas a single microorganism is usually isolated in primary PD peritonitis. *S. aureus, S. epidermidis* and *Streptococcus* species account for 60–80% of cases, with coagulase-negative staphylococci constituting 30–40% and streptococci constituting 10–15%. Yeast, such as *Candida*, are the most common cause of fungal peritonitis, entering via the catheter or commonly per vaginam.

Dialysate samples for microbiological examination should be taken from the first cloudy bag, for culture and antibiotic sensitivities. Cultures can be negative in half of patients, however, even with signs of PD peritonitis.[121] Nevertheless, ISPD guidelines state that no more than 20% of PD peritonitis cases should be culture-negative,[60] and if this is not the case the process of specimen testing should be re-evaluated. Other investigations include abdominal and chest radiographs to check for catheter position and air under the diaphragm, although pneumoperitoneum is not attributable to perforation in all patients on PD.

To prevent delay in treatment, antibiotic therapy should be commenced as soon as cloudy effluent is seen and dialysate has been sent for culture. Empiric therapy must cover both Gram-negative and positive organisms. Regimens tend to be center-specific dependent on local antibiotic sensitivities, but should include Gram-negative cover by a third-generation cephalosporin or aminoglycoside and Gram-positive cover by vancomycin or a cephalosporin.[60] Intraperitoneal administration is superior to intravenous dosing.[125] Once culture and sensitivity results are available, antibiotic therapy can be adjusted to narrow-spectrum agents as appropriate. In polymicrobial peritonitis, particularly in association with anerobic bacteria, the risk of death is increased and an urgent surgical evaluation should be sought, as early laparotomy may reduce mortality.[116,122]

The majority of episodes of PD peritonitis will respond to antibiotic therapy and, in mild cases, patients do not require hospital admission. However, there are circumstances where catheter removal is required, as outlined in Table 5-4. The majority of patients undergo laparotomy and catheter removal, with concomitant peritoneal washout. Laparoscopic removal and washout have been shown to be as effective as the open technique, but associated with less postoperative pain and bowel dysfunction.[5]

Refractory peritonitis is defined as failure of the effluent to clear after 5 days of appropriate antibiotic therapy. Prolonged attempts to treat refractory peritonitis medically are associated with extended hospital stay, peritoneal membrane damage, increased risk of fungal peritonitis, and death.[13] Relapsing peritonitis is defined as an episode with the same organism that occurs within 4 weeks of completion of therapy and is more likely to require catheter removal than uncomplicated PD peritonitis.[10] Fungal peritonitis is often serious with a high mortality, and catheter removal is indicated immediately after fungi are identified by microscopy or culture.[73] *Mycobacterium* infection is a particular problem in at-risk cohorts. Diagnosis can be difficult, but should be suspected in the presence of persistently elevated mononuclear cell counts with negative cultures. Acid-fast bacilli smears of dialysate fluid may be negative in 90% of cases, but formal cultures are usually positive.[64] Treatment consists of long-term antituberculous therapy. Catheter removal is usually undertaken, although it is not considered necessary for cure. Mortality attributed to tuberculous peritonitis is around 15%, and much of this may relate to treatment delay.[109]

After a severe episode of PD peritonitis necessitating catheter removal, less than half of patients are able to return to PD, and only a third will remain on PD for over 1 year.[112] Reasons for technique failure include adhesions and permanent membrane failure.

Encapsulating Peritoneal Sclerosis

EPS is a rare, but potentially life-threatening complication of PD. The definition of EPS is signs of intermittent and persistent or recurrent gastrointestinal obstruction, with macroscopic and/or radiological evidence of sclerosis, calcification, peritoneal thickening, or encapsulation of the intestines.[50]

The prevalence of EPS is between 0.5% and 2.5%[9,51,52,93] and its incidence increases with the duration of PD.[50] Reported mortality rates are high (25–55%), especially during the first year after diagnosis, and also increase with the duration of PD.[9,51,52,93] Patients may present with abdominal pain, a decline in net ultrafiltration, ascites, bloody effluent (7–50%[93]), bowel obstruction, vomiting, malnutrition, or an abdominal mass.

The pathogenesis involves loss of the mesothelial layer of the peritoneum with submesothelial thickening as a result of sclerosis and fibrosis.[43,69,126] A number of factors have been implicated in the development of EPS, including duration of PD, composition of dialysate solutions, peritonitis episodes, and genetic predisposition.[55]

The diagnosis is confirmed by radiological studies. Ultrasonography may reveal bowel wall thickening, a thick-walled mass containing bowel loops, loculated ascites, and fibrous adhesions.[42] Computed tomography demonstrates peritoneal enhancement, thickening and calcification, associated with adhesions, bowel obstruction, fluid loculations, and a cocoon of bowel (Figure 5-13).[105,119]

The mainstay of treatment for patients with EPS should be supportive care with enteral or parenteral nutrition. Surgery to remove all fibrotic tissue and free the bowel is a major undertaking, with a mean operative time of 7 hours and a mortality of around 7%.[53] However, bowel function is restored in 96% of patients, although 25% of patients will require repeat surgery. To try and prevent recurrence patients are treated with immunosuppressive agents postoperatively, most commonly corticosteroids. Other drug treatments utilized in the treatment of EPS include tamoxifen and angiotensin-converting enzyme inhibitors, although strong evidence for their benefit is lacking.

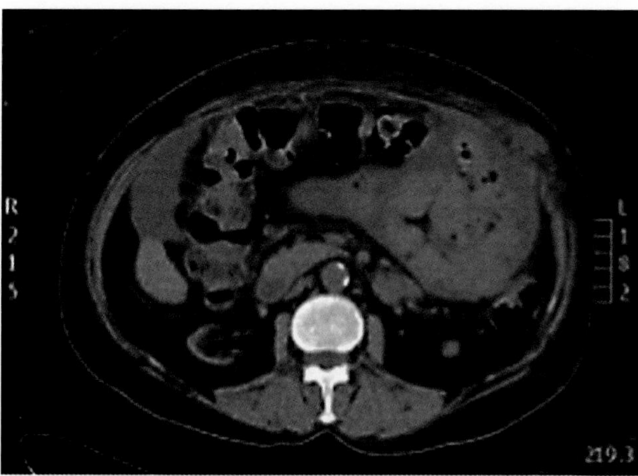

FIGURE 5-13 ■ Computed tomography image illustrating the characteristic radiological finding in encapsulating peritoneal sclerosis. Note the cocoon of small bowel in the left iliac fossa.

RENAL TRANSPLANT ISSUES WITH PERITONEAL DIALYSIS

When a PD patient receives a successful renal transplant, the PD catheter can be removed, but the timing of this requires careful judgment. In most cases the catheter is removed during the first 6 weeks posttransplant. Earlier removal is feasible when good allograft function is predicted, such as after a live donor transplant. Removal should be delayed in the presence of delayed graft function. Every effort must be made not to breach the peritoneum at the time of transplantation to avoid a PD leak and the need for temporary hemodialysis. There is also a risk of peritransplant infection if dialysate leaks into the transplant bed.

Active PD peritonitis is an absolute contraindication to transplantation, but it may be safe to proceed if the patient has had recent infections but several days of intraperitoneal antibiotics and the effluent is clear. Previous studies have highlighted the risks of infection after renal transplantation. The incidence of peritonitis can be 35%,[80] but it is not usually life-threatening. Patients receiving PD at the time of transplantation have significantly higher infection rates compared to those on hemodialysis, but this is reduced when patients convert to hemodialysis just prior to transplantation.[81]

Some studies have demonstrated a high incidence of posttransplantation EPS, typically developing within 1 year of the procedure.[29,56] Whether this is related to discontinuing PD or to the transplantation process remains unclear.

A few studies have shown less delayed graft function after renal transplant in patients on PD compared with those on hemodialysis,[35,118] which may relate to volume status at the time of transplantation or residual native renal function. A further study has also demonstrated a significantly lower all-cause mortality in transplanted patients on PD compared with those on hemodialysis.[100]

CONCLUSION

The importance of efficacious, complication-free dialysis for the overall wellbeing of patients undergoing peritoneal and hemodialysis cannot be understated.

Optimal physical and psychological health for the dialysis patient can be achieved by multidisciplinary care and central to this is effective dialysis access. Early planning of access procedures permits a smooth transition from predialysis to dialysis and minimizes the use of temporary venous catheters. Furthermore, effective dialysis access provides a lifeline for an ever-increasing group of patients in whom transplantation is deemed unsuitable.

REFERENCES

1. NKF-DOQI clinical practice guidelines for vascular access. Am J Kidney Dis 1997;30:S150–91.
2. Akyol AM, Porteous C, Brown MW. A comparison of two types of catheters for continuous ambulatory peritoneal dialysis (CAPD). Perit Dial Int 1990;10:63–6.
3. Arbeiter KM, Aufricht C, Mueller T, et al. MRI in the diagnosis of a peritoneal leak in continuous ambulatory peritoneal dialysis. Pediatr Radiol 2001;31:745–7.
4. Bachleda P, Utikal P, Kalinova L, et al. Infectious complications of arteriovenous ePTFE grafts for haemodialysis. Biomed Pap Med Fac Univ Palacky Olomouc Czech Repub 2010;154:13–9.
5. Barlow AD, Yates PJ, Hosgood SA, et al. Case-control comparison of laparoscopic and open washout for peritoneal dialysis-associated peritonitis. Br J Surg 2008;95:1416–9.
6. Beathard GA. Strategy for maximizing the use of arteriovenous fistulae. Semin Dial 2000;13:291–6.
7. Bent CL, Sahni VA, Matson MB. The radiological management of the thrombosed arteriovenous dialysis fistula. Clin Radiol 2011;66:1–12.
8. Bittl JA. Catheter interventions for haemodialysis fistulas and grafts. JACC Cardiovasc Interv 2010;3:1–11.
9. Brown MC, Simpson K, Kerssens JJ, et al. Encapsulating peritoneal sclerosis in the new millennium: a national cohort study. Clin J Am Soc Nephrol 2009;4:1222–9.
10. Burke M, Hawley CM, Badve SV, et al. Relapsing and recurrent peritoneal dialysis-associated peritonitis: a multicenter registry study. Am J Kidney Dis 2011;58:429–36.
11. Canaud B, Beraud JJ, Joyeux H, et al. Internal jugular vein cannulation using 2 silastic catheters. A new, simple and safe long-term vascular access for extracorporeal treatment. Nephron 1986;43:133–8.
12. Chemla ES, Nelson S, Morsy M. Early cannulation grafts in straight axillo-axillary angioaccesses avoid central catheter insertions. Semin Dial 2011;24:456–9.
13. Choi P, Nemati E, Banerjee A, et al. Peritoneal dialysis catheter removal for acute peritonitis: a retrospective analysis of factors associated with catheter removal and prolonged postoperative hospitalization. Am J Kidney Dis 2004;43:103–11.
14. Cimochowski GE, Worley E, Rutherford WE, et al. Superiority of the internal jugular over the subclavian access for temporary dialysis. Nephron 1990;54:154–61.
15. Conlon PJ, Schwab SJ, Nicholson ML, editors. Hemodialysis vascular access: practice and problems. Eastbourne, UK: Oxford University Press; 2007.
16. Daly CD, Campbell MK, MacLeod AM, et al. Do the Y-set and double-bag systems reduce the incidence of CAPD peritonitis? a systematic review of randomized controlled trials. Nephrol Dial Transplant 2001;16:341–7.
17. Deitel M, McIntyre JA. Radiographic confirmation of site of central venous pressure catheters. Can J Surg 1971;14:42–52.
18. Ejlersen E, Steven K, Lokkegaard H. Paramedian versus midline incision for the insertion of permanent peritoneal dialysis catheters. A randomized clinical trial. Scand J Urol Nephrol 1990;24:151–4.
19. Eklund B, Honkanen E, Kyllonen L, et al. Peritoneal dialysis access: prospective randomized comparison of single-cuff and double-cuff straight Tenckhoff catheters. Nephrol Dial Transplant 1997;12:2664–6.

20. Eklund BH, Honkanen EO, Kala AR, et al. Peritoneal dialysis access: prospective randomized comparison of the swan neck and Tenckhoff catheters. Perit Dial Int 1995;15:353–6.
21. Eklund BH, Honkanen EO, Kala AR, et al. Catheter configuration and outcome in patients on continuous ambulatory peritoneal dialysis: a prospective comparison of two catheters. Perit Dial Int 1994;14:70–4.
22. Elcheroth J, de Pauw L, Kinnaert P. Elbow arteriovenous fistulas for chronic haemodialysis. Br J Surg 1994;81:982–4.
23. Enzler MA, Rajmon T, Lachat M, et al. Long-term function of vascular access for haemodialysis. Clin Transplant 1996;10:511–5.
24. Ersoy FF, Twardowski ZJ, Satalowich RJ, et al. A retrospective analysis of catheter position and function in 91 CAPD patients. Perit Dial Int 1994;14:409–10.
25. Evans DC, Upton EC, Lawson JH. Axillary to common iliac arteriovenous graft for haemodialysis access: case report and review of "exotic" axillary-based grafts. J Vasc Access 2005;6:192–5.
26. Fadem SZ, Walker DR, Abbott G, et al. Satisfaction with renal replacement therapy and education: the American Association of Kidney Patients Survey. Clin J Am Soc Nephrol 2011;6:605–12.
27. Feest TG, Rajamahesh J, Byrne C, et al. Trends in adult renal replacement therapy in the UK: 1982–2002. QJM 2005;98:21–8.
28. Field M, Blackwell J, Jaipersad A, et al. Distal revascularisation with interval ligation (DRIL): an experience. Ann R Coll Surg Engl 2009;91:394–8.
29. Fieren MW, Betjes MG, Korte MR, et al. Posttransplant encapsulating peritoneal sclerosis: a worrying new trend? Perit Dial Int 2007;27:619–24.
30. Fokou M, Ashuntantang G, Teyang A, et al. Patients' characteristics and outcome of 518 arteriovenous fistulas for hemodialysis in a sub-Saharan African setting. Ann Vasc Surg 2012;26:674–9.
31. Gadallah MF, Pervez A, el-Shahawy MA, et al. Peritoneoscopic versus surgical placement of peritoneal dialysis catheters: a prospective randomized study on outcome. Am J Kidney Dis 1999;33:118–22.
32. Gadallah MF, Torres-Rivera C, Ramdeen G, et al. Relationship between intraperitoneal bleeding, adhesions, and peritoneal dialysis catheter failure: a method of prevention. Adv Perit Dial 2001;17:127–9.
33. Ghali JR, Bannister KM, Brown FG, et al. Microbiology and outcomes of peritonitis in Australian peritoneal dialysis patients. Perit Dial Int 2011;31:651–62.
34. Glass C, Maevsky V, Massey T, et al. Subclavian vein to right atrial appendage bypass without sternotomy to maintain arteriovenous access in patients with complete central vein occlusion, a new approach. Ann Vasc Surg 2009;23:465–8.
35. Goldfarb-Rumyantzev AS, Hurdle JF, Scandling JD, et al. The role of pretransplantation renal replacement therapy modality in kidney allograft and recipient survival. Am J Kidney Dis 2005;46:537–49.
36. Golper TA, Brier ME, Bunke M, et al. Risk factors for peritonitis in long-term peritoneal dialysis: the Network 9 peritonitis and catheter survival studies. Academic Subcommittee of the Steering Committee of the Network 9 Peritonitis and Catheter Survival Studies. Am J Kidney Dis 1996;28:428–36.
37. Guzman-Valdivia G, Zaga I. Abdominal wall hernia repair in patients with chronic renal failure and a dialysis catheter. Hernia 2001;5:9–11.
38. Haag-Weber M, Horl WH. Uremia and infection: mechanisms of impaired cellular host defense. Nephron 1993;63:125–31.
39. Hagen SM, van Alphen AM, Ijzermans JN, et al. Laparoscopic versus open peritoneal dialysis catheter insertion, LOCI-trial: a study protocol. BMC Surg 2011;11:35.
40. Haskal ZJ, Leen VH, Thomas-Hawkins C, et al. Transvenous removal of fibrin sheaths from tunneled haemodialysis catheters. J Vasc Interv Radiol 1996;7:513–7.
41. Heaf JG, Lokkegaard H, Madsen M. Initial survival advantage of peritoneal dialysis relative to haemodialysis. Nephrol Dial Transplant 2002;17:112–7.
42. Hollman AS, McMillan MA, Briggs JD, et al. Ultrasound changes in sclerosing peritonitis following continuous ambulatory peritoneal dialysis. Clin Radiol 1991;43:176–9.
43. Honda K, Nitta K, Horita S, et al. Morphological changes in the peritoneal vasculature of patients on CAPD with ultrafiltration failure. Nephron 1996;72:171–6.
44. Hoshal Jr VL, Ause RG, Hoskins PA. Fibrin sleeve formation on indwelling subclavian central venous catheters. Arch Surg 1971;102:353–8.
45. Jaar BG, Plantinga LC, Crews DC, et al. Timing, causes, predictors and prognosis of switching from peritoneal dialysis to haemodialysis: a prospective study. BMC Nephrol 2009;10:3.
46. Janne d'Othee B, Tham JC, Sheiman RG. Restoration of patency in failing tunneled haemodialysis catheters: a comparison of catheter exchange, exchange and balloon disruption of the fibrin sheath, and femoral stripping. J Vasc Interv Radiol 2006;17:1011–5.
47. Jwo SC, Chen KS, Lee CC, et al. Prospective randomized study for comparison of open surgery with laparoscopic-assisted placement of Tenckhoff peritoneal dialysis catheter – a single center experience and literature review. J Surg Res 2010;159:489–96.
48. Kakkos SK, Haddad GK, Haddad RK, et al. Effectiveness of a new tunneled catheter in preventing catheter malfunction: a comparative study. J Vasc Interv Radiol 2008;19:1018–26.
49. Kavanagh D, Prescott GJ, Mactier RA. Peritoneal dialysis-associated peritonitis in Scotland (1999–2002). Nephrol Dial Transplant 2004;19:2584–91.
50. Kawaguchi Y, Kawanishi H, Mujais S, et al. Encapsulating peritoneal sclerosis: definition, etiology, diagnosis, and treatment. International Society for Peritoneal Dialysis Ad Hoc Committee on Ultrafiltration Management in Peritoneal Dialysis. Perit Dial Int 2000;20(Suppl. 4):S43–55.
51. Kawanishi H, Kawaguchi Y, Fukui H, et al. Encapsulating peritoneal sclerosis in Japan: a prospective, controlled, multicenter study. Am J Kidney Dis 2004;44:729–37.
52. Kawanishi H, Long-Term Peritoneal Dialysis Study Group. Encapsulating peritoneal sclerosis in Japan: prospective multicenter controlled study. Perit Dial Int 2001;21(Suppl. 3):S67–71.
53. Kawanishi H, Moriishi M, Ide K, et al. Recommendation of the surgical option for treatment of encapsulating peritoneal sclerosis. Perit Dial Int 2008;28(Suppl. 3):S205–10.
54. Koksoy C, Demirci RK, Balci D, et al. Brachiobasilic versus brachiocephalic arteriovenous fistula: a prospective randomized study. J Vasc Surg 2009;49:171–7.
55. Korte MR, Sampimon DE, Betjes MG, et al. Encapsulating peritoneal sclerosis: the state of affairs. Nat Rev Nephrol 2011;7:528–38.
56. Korte MR, Yo M, Betjes MG, et al. Increasing incidence of severe encapsulating peritoneal sclerosis after kidney transplantation. Nephrol Dial Transplant 2007;22:2412–4.
57. Kumbar L, Karim J, Besarab A. Surveillance and monitoring of dialysis access. Int J Nephrol 2012;2012:649–735.
58. Leblanc M, Bosc JY, Paganini EP, et al. Central venous dialysis catheter dysfunction. Adv Ren Replace Ther 1997;4:377–89.
59. Ledebo I, Ronco C. The best dialysis therapy? Results from an international survey among nephrology professionals. NDT Plus 2008;1:403–8.
60. Li PK, Szeto CC, Piraino B, et al. Peritoneal dialysis-related infections recommendations: 2010 update. Perit Dial Int 2010;30:393–423.
61. Lioupis C, Mistry H, Rix T, et al. Comparison among transposed brachiobasilic, brachiobrachial arteriovenous fistulas and Flixene vascular graft. J Vasc Access 2011;12:36–44.
62. Lok CE, Mokrzycki MH. Prevention and management of catheter-related infection in haemodialysis patients. Kidney Int 2011;79:587–98.
63. Lui SL, Li FK, Lo CY, et al. Simultaneous removal and reinsertion of Tenckhoff catheters for the treatment of refractory exit-site infection. Adv Perit Dial 2000;16:195–7.
64. Lui SL, Lo CY, Choy BY, et al. Optimal treatment and long-term outcome of tuberculous peritonitis complicating continuous ambulatory peritoneal dialysis. Am J Kidney Dis 1996;28:747–51.
65. Lund GB, Trerotola SO, Scheel Jr PJ. Percutaneous translumbar inferior vena cava cannulation for haemodialysis. Am J Kidney Dis 1995;25:732–7.
66. Lye WC, Kour NW, van der Straaten JC, et al. A prospective randomized comparison of the swan neck, coiled, and straight Tenckhoff catheters in patients on CAPD. Perit Dial Int 1996;16(Suppl. 1):S333–5.
67. Mansour M, Kamper L, Altenburg A, et al. Radiological central vein treatment in vascular access. J Vasc Access 2008;9:85–101.
68. Marx AB, Landmann J, Harder FH. Surgery for vascular access. Curr Probl Surg 1990;27:1–48.

69. Mateijsen MA, van der Wal AC, Hendriks PM, et al. Vascular and interstitial changes in the peritoneum of CAPD patients with peritoneal sclerosis. Perit Dial Int 1999;19:517–25.
70. Matsuura J, Dietrich A, Steuben S, et al. Mediastinal approach to the placement of tunneled haemodialysis catheters in patients with central vein occlusion in an outpatient access center. J Vasc Access 2011;12:258–61.
71. Maya ID, O'Neal JC, Young CJ, et al. Outcomes of brachiocephalic fistulas, transposed brachiobasilic fistulas, and upper arm grafts. Clin J Am Soc Nephrol 2009;4:86–92.
72. Mettang T, Stoeltzing H, Alscher DM, et al. Sustaining continuous ambulatory peritoneal dialysis after herniotomy. Adv Perit Dial 2001;17:84–7.
73. Miles R, Hawley CM, McDonald SP, et al. Predictors and outcomes of fungal peritonitis in peritoneal dialysis patients. Kidney Int 2009;76:622–8.
74. Moist LM, Port FK, Orzol SM, et al. Predictors of loss of residual renal function among new dialysis patients. J Am Soc Nephrol 2000;11:556–64.
75. Moss JS, Minda SA, Newman GE, et al. Malpositioned peritoneal dialysis catheters: a critical reappraisal of correction by stiff-wire manipulation. Am J Kidney Dis 1990;15:305–8.
76. Naroienejad M, Saedi D, Rezvani A. Prevalence of central vein stenosis following catheterization in patients with end-stage renal disease. Saudi J Kidney Dis Transpl 2010;21:975–8.
77. Nelson H, Lindner M, Schuman ES, et al. Abdominal wall hernias as a complication of peritoneal dialysis. Surg Gynecol Obstet 1983;157:541–4.
78. Nielsen PK, Hemmingsen C, Friis SU, et al. Comparison of straight and curled Tenckhoff peritoneal dialysis catheters implanted by percutaneous technique: a prospective randomized study. Perit Dial Int 1995;15:18–21.
79. O'Connor JP, Rigby RJ, Hardie IR, et al. Abdominal hernias complicating continuous ambulatory peritoneal dialysis. Am J Nephrol 1986;6:271–4.
80. O'Donoghue D, Manos J, Pearson R, et al. Continuous ambulatory peritoneal dialysis and renal transplantation: a ten-year experience in a single center. Perit Dial Int 1992;12:242, 245-9.
81. Passalacqua JA, Wiland AM, Fink JC, et al. Increased incidence of postoperative infections associated with peritoneal dialysis in renal transplant recipients. Transplantation 1999;68:535–40.
82. Perakis KE, Stylianou KG, Kyriazis JP, et al. Long-term complication rates and survival of peritoneal dialysis catheters: the role of percutaneous versus surgical placement. Semin Dial 2009;22:569–75.
83. Piraino B. Management of catheter-related infections. Am J Kidney Dis 1996;27:754–8.
84. Plaza MM, Rivas MC, Dominguez-Viguera L. Fluoroscopic manipulation is also useful for malfunctioning swan-neck peritoneal catheters. Perit Dial Int 2001;21(2):193–6.
85. Plum J, Sudkamp S, Grabensee B. Results of ultrasound-assisted diagnosis of tunnel infections in continuous ambulatory peritoneal dialysis. Am J Kidney Dis 1994;23:99–104.
86. Po CL, Koolpe HA, Allen S, et al. Transhepatic PermCath for haemodialysis. Am J Kidney Dis 1994;24:590–1.
87. Polo JR, Sanabia J, Garcia-Sabrido JL, et al. Brachial-jugular polytetrafluoroethylene fistulas for haemodialysis. Am J Kidney Dis 1990;16:465–8.
88. Posthuma N, Borgstein PJ, Eijsbouts Q, et al. Simultaneous peritoneal dialysis catheter insertion and removal in catheter-related infections without interruption of peritoneal dialysis. Nephrol Dial Transplant 1998;13:700–3.
89. Prokesch RW, Schima W, Schober E, et al. Complications of continuous ambulatory peritoneal dialysis: findings on MR peritoneography. AJR Am J Roentgenol 2000;174:987–91.
90. Reilly DT, Wood RF, Bell PR. Prospective study of dialysis fistulas: problem patients and their treatment. Br J Surg 1982;69:549–53.
91. Remuzzi G. Bleeding in renal failure. Lancet 1988;1:1205–8.
92. Reynolds TS, Zayed M, Kim KM, et al. A comparison between one- and two-stage brachiobasilic arteriovenous fistulas. J Vasc Surg 2011;1632–8, discussion 1639.
93. Rigby RJ, Hawley CM. Sclerosing peritonitis: the experience in Australia. Nephrol Dial Transplant 1998;13:154–9.
94. Rosenthal MA, Yang PS, Liu IL, et al. Comparison of outcomes of peritoneal dialysis catheters placed by the fluoroscopically guided percutaneous method versus directly visualized surgical method. J Vasc Interv Radiol 2008;19:1202–7.
95. Rubin HR, Fink NE, Plantinga LC, et al. Patient ratings of dialysis care with peritoneal dialysis vs haemodialysis. JAMA 2004;291:697–703.
96. Rubin J, Didlake R, Raju S, et al. A prospective randomized evaluation of chronic peritoneal catheters. Insertion site and intraperitoneal segment. ASAIO Trans 1990;36:M497–500.
97. Schanzer H, Skladany M, Haimov M. Treatment of angioaccess-induced ischemia by revascularization. J Vasc Surg 1992;16:861–4, discussion 864-866.
98. Schinstock CA, Albright RC, Williams AW, et al. Outcomes of arteriovenous fistula creation after the fistula first initiative. Clin J Am Soc Nephrol 2011;6:1996–2002.
99. Schwab SJ, Quarles LD, Middleton JP, et al. Hemodialysis-associated subclavian vein stenosis. Kidney Int 1988;33:1156–9.
100. Schwenger V, Dohler B, Morath C, et al. The role of pretransplant dialysis modality on renal allograft outcome. Nephrol Dial Transplant 2011;26:3761–6.
101. Shaffer D. Catheter-related sepsis complicating long-term, tunneled central venous dialysis catheters: management by guidewire exchange. Am J Kidney Dis 1995;25:593–6.
102. Shea M, Hmiel SP, Beck AM. Use of tissue plasminogen activator for thrombolysis in occluded peritoneal dialysis catheters in children. Adv Perit Dial 2001;17:249–52.
103. Shusterman NH, Kloss K, Mullen JL. Successful use of double-lumen, silicone rubber catheters for permanent haemodialysis access. Kidney Int 1989;35:887–90.
104. Simons ME, Pron G, Voros M, et al. Fluoroscopically-guided manipulation of malfunctioning peritoneal dialysis catheters. Perit Dial Int 1999;19:544–9.
105. Stafford-Johnson DB, Wilson TE, Francis IR, et al. CT appearance of sclerosing peritonitis in patients on chronic ambulatory peritoneal dialysis. J Comput Assist Tomogr 1998;22:295–9.
106. Strippoli GF, Tong A, Johnson D, et al. Catheter type, placement and insertion techniques for preventing peritonitis in peritoneal dialysis patients. Cochrane Database Syst Rev 2004;(4) CD004680.
107. Suhocki PV, Conlon Jr PJ, Knelson MH, et al. Silastic cuffed catheters for haemodialysis vascular access: thrombolytic and mechanical correction of malfunction. Am J Kidney Dis 1996;28:379–86.
108. Tahami VB, Hakki H, Reber PU, et al. Polytetrafluoroethylene and bovine mesenterial vein grafts for haemodialysis access: a comparative study. J Vasc Access 2007;8:17–20.
109. Talwani R, Horvath JA. Tuberculous peritonitis in patients undergoing continuous ambulatory peritoneal dialysis: case report and review. Clin Infect Dis 2000;31:70–5.
110. The Renal Association. UK renal registry rhirteenth rnnual report. Bristol, UK: UK Renal Registry; 2010.
111. Trerotola SO, Johnson MS, Harris VJ, et al. Outcome of tunneled haemodialysis catheters placed via the right internal jugular vein by interventional radiologists. Radiology 1997;203:489–95.
112. Troidle L, Gorban-Brennan N, Finkelstein FO. Outcome of patients on chronic peritoneal dialysis undergoing peritoneal catheter removal because of peritonitis. Adv Perit Dial 2005;21:98–101.
113. Tsimoyiannis EC, Siakas P, Glantzounis G, et al. Laparoscopic placement of the Tenckhoff catheter for peritoneal dialysis. Surg Laparosc Endosc Percutan Tech 2000;10:218–21.
114. Tumlin J, Goldman J, Spiegel DM, et al. A phase III, randomized, double-blind, placebo-controlled study of tenecteplase for improvement of haemodialysis catheter function: TROPICS 3. Clin J Am Soc Nephrol 2010;5:631–6.
115. Twardowski ZJ, Tully RJ, Ersoy FF, et al. Computerized tomography with and without intraperitoneal contrast for determination of intraabdominal fluid distribution and diagnosis of complications in peritoneal dialysis patients. ASAIO Trans 1990;36:95–103.
116. Tzamaloukas AH, Obermiller LE, Gibel LJ, et al. Peritonitis associated with intra-abdominal pathology in continuous ambulatory peritoneal dialysis patients. Perit Dial Int 1993;13(Suppl. 2):S335–7.
117. U.S. Renal Data System. USRDS 2009 Annual data report: atlas of chronic kidney disease and end-stage renal disease in the United States, 2009. Bethesda, MD: National Institutes of Health, National Institute of Diabetes and Digestive and Kidney Diseases; 2012.

118. Vanholder R, Heering P, Loo AV, et al. Reduced incidence of acute renal graft failure in patients treated with peritoneal dialysis compared with haemodialysis. Am J Kidney Dis 1999;33:934–40.
119. Vlijm A, Stoker J, Bipat S, et al. Computed tomographic findings characteristic for encapsulating peritoneal sclerosis: a case-control study. Perit Dial Int 2009;29:517–22.
120. Vogt K, Binswanger U, Buchmann P, et al. Catheter-related complications during continuous ambulatory peritoneal dialysis (CAPD): a retrospective study on sixty-two double-cuff Tenckhoff catheters. Am J Kidney Dis 1987;10:47–51.
121. von Graevenitz A, Amsterdam D. Microbiological aspects of peritonitis associated with continuous ambulatory peritoneal dialysis. Clin Microbiol Rev 1992;5:36–48.
122. Wakeen MJ, Zimmerman SW, Bidwell D. Viscus perforation in peritoneal dialysis patients: diagnosis and outcome. Perit Dial Int 1994;14:371–7.
123. Weinhandl ED, Foley RN, Gilbertson DT, et al. Propensity-matched mortality comparison of incident haemodialysis and peritoneal dialysis patients. J Am Soc Nephrol 2010;21:499–506.
124. Wetherington GM, Leapman SB, Robison RJ, et al. Abdominal wall and inguinal hernias in continuous ambulatory peritoneal dialysis patients. Am J Surg 1985;150:357–60.
125. Wiggins KJ, Craig JC, Johnson DW, et al. Treatment for peritoneal dialysis-associated peritonitis. Cochrane Database Syst Rev 2008;(1) CD005284.
126. Williams JD, Craig KJ, von Ruhland C, et al. The natural course of peritoneal membrane biology during peritoneal dialysis. Kidney Int Suppl 2003;(88)S43–9.
127. Winn MP, McDermott VG, Schwab SJ, et al. Dialysis catheter "fibrin-sheath stripping": a cautionary tale! Nephrol Dial Transplant 1997;12:1048–50.
128. Wright MJ, Bel'eed K, Johnson BF, et al. Randomized prospective comparison of laparoscopic and open peritoneal dialysis catheter insertion. Perit Dial Int 1999;19:372–5.
129. Xie J, Kiryluk K, Ren H, et al. Coiled versus straight peritoneal dialysis catheters: a randomized controlled trial and meta-analysis. Am J Kidney Dis 2011;58:946–55.
130. Yu VL, Goetz A, Wagener M, et al. *Staphylococcus aureus* nasal carriage and infection in patients on haemodialysis. Efficacy of antibiotic prophylaxis. N Engl J Med 1986;315:91–6.
131. Zibari GB, Rohr MS, Landreneau MD, et al. Complications from permanent haemodialysis vascular access. Surgery 1988;104:681–6.
132. Zorzanello MM, Fleming WJ, Prowant BE. Use of tissue plasminogen activator in peritoneal dialysis catheters: a literature review and one center's experience. Nephrol Nurs J 2004;31:534–7.

CHAPTER 6

Brain Death and Cardiac Death: Donor Criteria and Care of Deceased Donor

Laura S. Johnson • Ram M. Subramanian 

CHAPTER OUTLINE

INTRODUCTION

As the number of people awaiting organ transplantation grows yearly, the relative scarcity of available organs increasingly requires a standardized, evidence-based approach to the management of each donor. From the initial diagnosis of brain death or imminent cardiac death to the optimization of donor physiology prior to removal of organs, the intensivist plays an integral role in this first portion of the transplantation process.

BRAIN DEATH

Incidence and Causes

In the United States, just over 53 000 people die of traumatic brain injuries (TBI) each year.[12] These occur primarily from firearm-related events, motor vehicle-related events, and fall-related events. Firearm-related events remain the most prevalent causes of TBI, with 75% of deaths from self-inflicted injuries and 40% of deaths from assaults coming from brain injury.[12] Homicide-related deaths have increased over the last decade in people 20–24 years of age.[12] Motorcyclists are also at risk for TBI. Deaths from brain injury in this population have actually doubled over the last decade despite adoption in some states of universal helmet laws. While implementation of helmet laws can decrease motorcyclist mortality, the lack of a nationwide universal helmet law limits the effectiveness of this protective measure.[12] However, in the overall population of people who would constitute donor candidates, the death rate has decreased significantly, attributable primarily to increased safety measures aimed at motor vehicle drivers.

Physiologic Response

Brain tissue ischemia, the root source of brain death, triggers a series of well-defined effects as the damage progresses from the cerebral cortex through the brainstem. These effects proceed in a consistent sequence. Ischemia of the cerebral cortex and upper brainstem (the midbrain) results in a predominance of parasympathetic activity. Clinically, this manifests as hypotension and bradycardia. Subsequently, brainstem ischemia at the level of the pons triggers elevations of norepinephrine and epinephrine well above normal physiologic levels, while leaving some functional parasympathetic nuclei. This results in the "Cushing's reflex," characterized by significant hypertension due to an increase in systemic vascular resistance (SVR), and a concomitant bradycardia as the still functional parasympathetic reflex arc attempts to compensate. As the ischemia progresses through the pontine region to the medulla, the parasympathetic nuclei can no longer function, leaving unopposed sympathetic input throughout the body. This is the period referred to as the "autonomic storm." Finally, complete brainstem ischemia results in a decrease in sympathetic output and complete cardiovascular collapse, similar to the vasodilatory shock that occurs after a high spinal cord injury. These changes have very specific effects throughout the body, which are best considered by organ system.

Cardiac

Multiple levels of cardiac dysfunction are seen after brain death, ranging from histologic changes consistent with patchy myocardiocyte ischemia and necrosis, to more structural changes associated with ventricular dysfunction. In addition, there are well-characterized electrocardiographic changes. While the mechanisms associated with these observations are not completely understood, the physiologic impact of the autonomic storm can be tied to a number of these changes.

Hemodynamic changes follow the level of brainstem injury, with an initial catecholamine surge resulting in significant elevations in SVR.[46] Since cardiac output is influenced inversely by the resistance of the vascular beds it pumps against, this elevation in SVR results in a decrease in cardiac output. Pressure transmission results in an increase in left atrial pressure, often above mean pulmonary artery pressure (see Pulmonary section). Subsequent decreases in sympathetic input lead to a decrease in SVR, often below baseline values, a decrease in myocardial contractility, and venodilation. Intravascular volume is thus relatively low, and this decrease in preload with accompanying hypotension results in decreased coronary perfusion. Myocardial contractility is then further impacted by ischemia. Despite these hemodynamic changes, gross echocardiographic changes vary, with just under 50% of brain-injured patients having left ventricular systolic dysfunction, most with evidence of segmental wall motion abnormality.[17] The electrocardiographic changes progress in a similar fashion from parasympathetic overload (sinus bradycardia and occasional complete heart block) to sympathetic overload (sinus tachycardia, progressing to ventricular tachycardia). Eventually, there is a return to normal sinus rhythm, with eventual resolution of the acute ischemic changes that initially appear.[46]

Pulmonary

The cardiac dysfunction during the autonomic storm directly contributes to pulmonary dysfunction in brain-dead patients. The intense increase in SVR results in left atrial pressures often in excess of pulmonary artery pressures. This significantly alters intravascular hydrostatic pressure. In addition, increased blood return to the right atrium with systemic shunting increases pulmonary blood flow. Both of these changes result in destruction of pulmonary capillary integrity, and cause pulmonary edema, and alveolar and interstitial hemorrhage.[49] Also, evidence suggests that the catecholamine storm can directly stimulate pulmonary capillary permeability due to interactions with the alpha-adrenoceptor.[74]

Inflammation-mediated acute lung injury also contributes to pulmonary dysfunction after brain injury. Brain death initiates an inflammatory response that subsequently leads to additional non-cardiogenic pulmonary edema. Lavage samples from donors have demonstrated significant increases in inflammatory markers relative to non-brain-dead controls.[19] In this setting, additional damage to the lung from ventilator-induced injury represents the second insult in a "double-hit" model of pulmonary injury.[31]

Renal

Kidneys also demonstrate decreased survival when obtained from brain-dead donors. This has been attributed to both inflammatory infiltrates in renal grafts and ischemia reperfusion injury that occurs as the period of autonomic storm waxes and wanes.[6,45] The kidneys are also affected by posterior pituitary failure and the cessation in production of arginine vasopressin (AVP). This results in central diabetes insipidus, a common occurrence in brain-dead patients, occurring in up to 78% of patients.[23] Inappropriately dilute urine output increases rapidly, leading to hypovolemia and hypernatremia. The hypovolemia can worsen the already precarious hemodynamic status of the brain-dead donor, while the resulting hypernatremia has a significant negative impact on renal and hepatic graft function.

Hepatic

While the liver is tolerant of prolonged periods of ischemia, it nevertheless is impacted by both brain death-related inflammation and prolonged hypernatremia. The direct effects of inflammation have yet to be elucidated, but biopsies after brain death demonstrate increases in inflammatory cells, which can potentially increase the risk of primary non-function and acute rejection.[27,77]

Hypernatremia, defined as a plasma sodium level >155 mmol/L, has also been associated with poor outcomes after transplant. Presumably, the hyperosmolar cellular milieu established in hepatocytes while the donor is hypernatremic results in osmotic injury when the liver is transplanted into a non-hypernatremic recipient.[70]

Endocrine

Pituitary failure is the primary source of endocrine abnormalities associated with brain death. However, not all hormones decrease to the same amount. Novitzky et al. demonstrated in animal studies that, while AVP drops to undetectable levels by 6 hours, and free triiodothyronine (T_3) concentrations dropped to 50% of baseline within an hour of injury and were undetectable by 9 hours after injury, adrenocorticotropic hormone (ACTH) and thyroid-stimulating hormone (TSH) were not significantly lower when measured at 16 hours after injury.[48] While other animal studies have shown less dramatic thyroid hormone responses, they have nevertheless demonstrated differential responses of other pituitary hormones to brain death.[23] Human studies suggest that these differences can be attributed to anatomic differences between the anterior and posterior pituitary: while posterior pituitary hormones (antidiuretic hormone, or AVP) decrease rapidly after brain death, anterior pituitary hormone (ACTH, TSH) changes are less predictable. The exact mechanisms for this difference are yet to be fully elucidated.

Inflammatory

There are two triggers of inflammatory response to brain death. The first is direct neural tissue damage, which results in inflammation of the central nervous system. The second is in response to ischemia-reperfusion injury that occurs during the period of supranormal SVR in response to pontine ischemia. Release of inflammatory cytokines has been demonstrated locally in response to brain injury.[41] Cytokine profiles in donor groups have also been studied given the observation that graft function is better after living donor transplantation.[68] However, future work is necessary to identify ways to blunt these responses and improve donor graft function (Figure 6-1).

Diagnosis

The diagnosis of brain death is a clinical diagnosis based on the presence or absence of a set of responses to neurologic stimuli. In the half century since the Harvard Committee first reported on "irreversible coma" as a new criterion for death, numerous variations on the determination of brain death have been proposed.[1] However, after the President's Commission for the Study of Ethical Problems in Medicine equated cardiac death and brain death in 1981,[24] the modern criteria for brain death determination were set. These were then expounded upon by the American Academy of Neurology in 1995,[56] and more recently reviewed and revalidated by Wijdicks and colleagues in 2010.[80] Ranging from electroencephalograms to neuropathologic examination,[78] none of the ancillary tests have proven as consistently reliable as a clinical examination done by a physician experienced in performing these tests.

Several prerequisites have to be met prior to initiation of a brain death examination. First, there needs to be evidence of a catastrophic brain injury that is compatible with a possible diagnosis of brain death. This can be established either clinically (evidence of gross head trauma) or using basic neuroimaging (computed tomography (CT)). However, it is important to remember that CT findings are not themselves confirmatory for brain death, and may be misleading. Complicating medical conditions that may interfere with clinical assessment have to be addressed and resolved (Table 6-1). Note here that severe facial and ocular trauma will interfere with many of the brain death tests, making it difficult to

TABLE 6-1 Confounding Conditions and Exclusions in the Diagnosis of Brain Death

Hypothermia
Diagnosis of brain death requires core temperature >32°C
Absence of brainstem reflexes when core temperature <28°C
Drug intoxications
Barbiturates
Tricyclics
Alcohol
Narcotics
Benzodiazepines
Antipsychotics
Antiepileptics
Antihistamines
Acute metabolic endocrine derangements
Electrolyte, acid–base derangements
Uremia
Hepatic coma
Hypoglycemia
Hypothyroid
Neurological diseases
Persistent vegetative state
Locked-in syndrome
Akinetic mutism

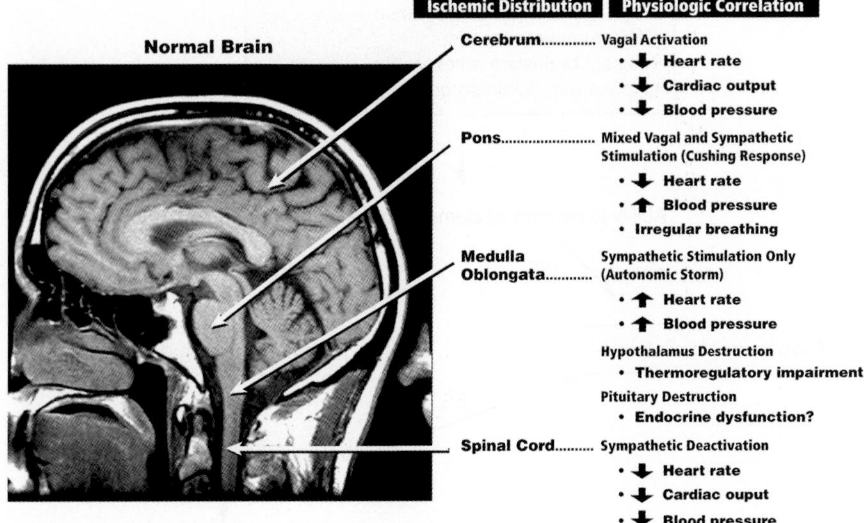

FIGURE 6-1 ■ The distribution and pathophysiological correlation of the rostral–caudal progression of cerebral-spinal ischemia termed coning, which eventuates in herniation and brain death. (Courtesy of Kenneth E. Wood, DO.)

make a definitive clinical diagnosis if they are present. However, in addition to traumatic injuries, severe electrolyte disturbances (hyper- or hyponatremia, hyper- or hypoglycemia), severe acid–base disturbances (profound acidosis), and endocrine dysfunctions (profound cortisol depletion or hypothyroidism) must be identified and corrected. No drug intoxication or evidence of poisoning can be present. This requires performing a drug screen, and waiting for clearance of any alcohol to below the legal limit for driving (0.08%). In addition, it is necessary to identify any medications given in the hospital that could result in central nervous system depression; these need to have cleared the patient's system prior to proceeding with testing. An appropriate time has been suggested at five times a drug's half-life, assuming normal hepatic and renal function. Reversal agents are appropriate where available (opiates and benzodiazepines). Finally, the patient must at least have a core body temperature >32 °C prior to starting the brain death exam. Severe hypothermia, defined as core body temperature <32 °C, impacts papillary light response, with complete loss of brainstem reflexes at core temperatures <28 °C. While rewarming techniques are beyond the scope of this chapter, for most patients a warming blanket should be sufficient to obtain appropriate temperatures prior to starting the examination.

Once these prerequisites have been met, the brain death examination can proceed (Figure 6-2). There are three major findings that need to be identified and documented to confirm brain death. These are: (1) coma or unresponsiveness; (2) absence of brainstem reflexes; and (3) apnea.

1. Coma or unresponsiveness. This component requires that there is no motor response or eye movement to noxious stimuli, typically described as nail bed pressure or supraorbital pressure. Often, this can be the most difficult part of the examination for practitioners, as a wide range of spontaneous or reflex movements have been described in the literature. These include everything from isolated jerks of the upper extremities to cremasteric and abdominal muscle reflexes to respiratory-like movements.[11,66] More extreme reflexes have elicited more fanciful descriptions, including the "Lazarus sign," where a combination of shoulder, neck, and extremity movements makes patients appear to rise from the bed.[66] Clinical expertise is necessary to differentiate between these movements, and central and cerebral motor responses to pain. Ultimately, these movements do not invalidate the diagnosis of brain death, but it is important for the clinician to be aware of these responses so as to counsel family members appropriately.

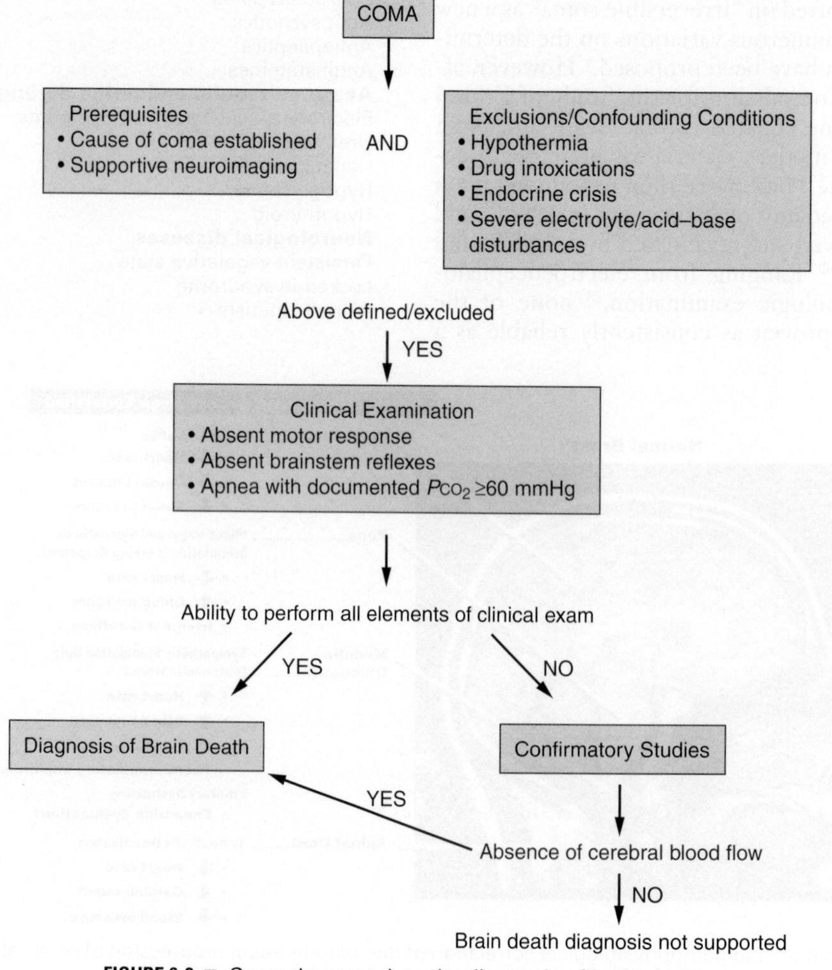

FIGURE 6-2 ■ General approach to the diagnosis of brain death.

2. Absence of brainstem reflexes[56,80]
   a. Pupillary reflex (cranial nerve (CN) II and III)
      i. Pupils are round or oval, typically of mid-range size (4 mm), though some can be as dilated as 9 mm
      ii. Pupils show no response to light
   b. Ocular movement (CN III, VI, and VIII)
      i. Oculocephalic reflex. Otherwise known as the "doll's eye" sign, in brain death the pupils will not show any movement as the head is turned rapidly to one side or the other. Caution: This test is not to be utilized in patients who have a suspicion of spine instability or fracture.
      ii. Vestibulo-ocular reflex. Also known as the "caloric reflex test," this test requires confirmation of a clear external auditory canal and elevation of the head to 30° prior to starting. Each external auditory canal is irrigated (separately, with an interval of at least 5 minutes) with approximately 50 mL of ice water. In the presence of brain death, no eye movement will be seen during the 1-minute observation period, regardless of the ear irrigated.
   c. Facial sensation and facial motor response (CN V and VII)
      i. Absence of a corneal reflex (eyelid movement/"blink reflex" – CN V_1 and VII). While many texts describe performing this test with a cotton swab, some centers have moved towards stimulation with a puff of air from an empty 10-cc syringe. This decreases the risk of corneal damage from direct contact, while still providing a sufficient stimulus to potentially evoke a response.
      ii. Absence of a jaw reflex (masseter reflex – CN V_3). For this test, the mandible is tapped at a downward angle just below the lips. A positive test would result in the upwards movement of the mandible in response. Usually, this reflex is very slight.
      iii. Absence of facial movement to noxious stimuli (CN V_3 and VII). Deep pressure on the supraorbital ridge or mandibular condyles at the temporomandibular joint should not result in any facial muscle movement (grimacing).
   d. Pharyngeal and tracheal reflexes (CN IX and X)
      i. Pharyngeal reflex ("gag reflex" – CN IX and X). Posterior pharyngeal stimulation with a tongue blade or hard suction catheter should not elicit a response. Note that this is separate from the tracheal reflex.
      ii. Tracheal reflex ("cough reflex" – CN X). Tracheal stimulation, usually achieved by suctioning the endotracheal tube, should not elicit a response over multiple passes.
3. Apnea. The absence of a drive to breathe is the final test in the clinical evaluation of brain death. Normally, an elevation in CO_2 above a critical level (in the United States defined as >60 mmHg)[24] will stimulate the respiratory center in the brainstem (medulla), which then signals the respiratory muscles to breathe. The apnea test is designed to provoke this response in an effort to establish whether the medulla (the lowest anatomic segment of the brainstem) is alive.
   a. Prerequisites
      i. Normotension (systolic blood pressure ≥90 mmHg)
      ii. Normothermia (core temperature >36 °C)
      iii. Euvolemia
      iv. Eucapnea ($PaCO_2$ 35–45 mmHg)
      v. Absence of hypoxia
      vi. No prior history of CO_2 retention (no history of chronic obstructive pulmonary disease or obstructive sleep apnea)
   b. Preparation
      i. Preoxygenate the patient with 100% O_2 prior to the test; target is a PaO_2 > 200 mmHg
      ii. Reduce the ventilation frequency to 10–12 breaths/min to achieve eucapnea
      iii. Measure arterial PO_2, PCO_2, and pH after these preparatory steps prior to starting the test
   c. Testing
      i. Disconnect the patient from the ventilator
      ii. Continue to deliver 100% FiO_2 at the level of the carina through a suction catheter or straight nasal cannula placed through the endotracheal tube
      iii. Observe closely for respiratory movements (abdominal, chest, neck) that could produce adequate tidal volumes
      iv. Continue the test as long as the patient remains stable. If, at the completion of 8–10 minutes, the patient remains stable, another 1–2 minutes can be taken prior to drawing an arterial blood gas. If the patient becomes hypotensive (systolic blood pressure <90 mmHg), hypoxic (O_2 sat <85%), or develops cardiac arrhythmias, at any time prior to a full 8–10 minutes, an arterial blood gas needs to be drawn immediately and the ventilator needs to be reconnected
   d. Result interpretation
      i. If respiratory movements are observed, the test is negative and the patient is not brain-dead
      ii. If respiratory movements are not observed, and the $PaCO_2$ is >60 mmHg or >20 mmHg above baseline normal $PaCO_2$, the test is positive and the patient is clinically brain-dead
      iii. If respiratory movements are not observed, but the test was halted early for hemodynamic instability and the $PaCO_2$ parameters were not met, the test is indeterminate and additional testing should be considered.

This test cannot be performed on every patient; approximately 10% of patients will be hemodynamically unstable at the time testing could occur, or prior to the conclusion of testing, requiring a premature stop.[79] In these circumstances, other tests may be utilized.

Additional testing is not required by the American Association of Neurology guidelines, as brain death is a clinical examination. However, in patients for whom

TABLE 6-2 Confirmatory Studies

Cerebral angiography
Contrast agent injected under high pressure into anterior and posterior circulations
Absence of cerebral filling at carotid and vertebral entrance into skull
Potential for contrast-induced nephrotoxicity
Rarely performed
Cerebral scintigraphy (technetium ^{99m}Tc-HMPAO)
Can be performed at bedside in brief time
Good correlation with conventional angiography
Isotope angiography
Albumin labeled with technetium 99m
Can be performed at bedside
Delayed filling of sagittal and transverse sinuses
Posterior cerebral circulation not visualized
Transcranial Doppler ultrasound
Middle cerebral artery through temporal bone above zygomatic arch and vertebral or basilar arteries through suboccipital transcranial windows bilaterally
Lack of transcranial Doppler signals should not be interpreted as confirmatory because 10% of patients may not have temporal windows
May not be diagnostic with intratentorial lesions
Electroencephalogram
No electrical activity for 30 minutes
Complex technical requirements

a complete examination cannot be performed, ancillary testing can be useful.[24,80] Certain hospital or state guidelines on the declaration of brain death may also require an additional test, and therefore the practitioner is encouraged to review hospital and state-specific requirements (Table 6-2).

CARDIAC DEATH

With less than 1% of deaths in the United States occurring from brain death, it has become a priority in the transplantation community to expand available sources for organs to transplant. One way this has been done is to re-evaluate donor criteria and designate so-called "expanded criteria" donors based on age and comorbidities. Another way this has been achieved has been to redefine "standard" donor criteria based on scientific evidence; this has been most successful in the arena of lung transplantation.[76]

Finally, the most recent method has been to revisit donation after circulatory death (DCD). Historically, the first transplants were done using organs from asystolic donors, but with professional acceptance of brain death following the 1968 Ad Hoc Committee of Harvard Medical School review of the issue,[1] and evidence of improved outcomes from donors whose hearts continue to beat, DCD faded into obscurity. However, with new evidence that organs can tolerate short periods of warm ischemia with successful outcomes, DCD is being revived by the transplant community.[7,8,43,50] Often this option is possible for patients who have suffered a significant head injury requiring full cardiopulmonary support, but who are not able to undergo brain death testing.[38] Less frequently patients who have had cardiac arrests or suffer from terminal respiratory diseases may be good candidates for DCD.[38]

Diagnosis

Deceased circulatory death is categorized using the modified Maastricht classification.[30] While the possibility for acute retrieval from an uncontrolled DCD does exist, for the purposes of this chapter only controlled DCD will be discussed (Table 6-3).

Controlled DCD takes place when a planned withdrawal of cardiorespiratory support has been determined to be the best course for a particular patient. Naturally, this necessitates ongoing discussions with the family about the patient's wishes and plans of care. After families express the desire to proceed with withdrawal, a representative from the organ procurement organization can present the option of DCD. Determining who will be a good candidate, or in other words, which patients will die within an acceptable warm ischemia time, is difficult. Suntharalingam et al. have shown that younger age, high FiO_2, and mode of mandatory ventilation (pressure support versus pressure control/volume control versus synchronized intermittent mandatory ventilation) were independently associated with shorter times to death.[71] More recently published scoring systems have shown some promise in determining who will die within 60 minutes, but with 20–25% of patients not correctly identified, it is still useful to offer this option to all families who request withdrawal of care.[13,57,81]

Once DCD has been authorized, every attempt is made to keep the patient medically stable until treatment is withdrawn. A short period of time is necessary to allow for organ allocation, but this process should not be extended over several days out of respect for the patient and family. Once arrangements have been made, the patient is transported to the operating room, at which point the family is allowed to pay their respects. The medical

TABLE 6-3 Maastritch Criteria for Deceased Cardiac Donation

Maastricht Classification	Presentation of Death		Organs Procurable
I	Dead on arrival	Uncontrolled	Tissue (heart valves/ corneas)
II	Unsuccessful resuscitation	Uncontrolled	Kidney
III	Anticipated cardiac arrest	Controlled	All organs except heart
IV	Cardiac arrest in a brain-dead donor	Controlled	
V	Unexpected cardiac arrest in a hospital inpatient	Uncontrolled	

team responsible for the patient in the intensive care setting then proceeds with withdrawal of care, and after a period of 5 minutes of continuous asystole (monitoring with an electrocardiograph and arterial line), the patient is declared dead.[38,58] Stiegler and colleagues have shown recently in an animal model that there is no return of brainstem function after 5 minutes of asystole, even if cardiopulmonary resuscitation is started at 5 minutes.[69] At this point, the transplant team can proceed with organ recovery (Figure 6-3).

Clearly, this process has significant ethical implications, and has raised questions around the world regarding the nature of death and organ donation. Until the ethicists decide otherwise, the most important role the medical team can play in a DCD is to enforce the "dead donor rule," wherein patients can only become donors after they are dead, and recovery of organs cannot cause a donor's death. There is some thought that premortem interventions, such as obtaining blood samples and maintaining life-sustaining therapy while organ allocation processes take place, are acceptable, as the overall goal is to respect the patient's final wish for organ donation.[38,58] However, procedures that can cause serious harm, such as systemic heparinization, or cause pain, such as femoral cannulation, are not permitted until the patient has been declared clinically dead.[38] It is also important to note that the transplantation team can have absolutely no involvement in patient management until after death has been declared, to avoid a conflict of interest. Critical care physicians should be familiar with their hospital's policy on DCD, as they are often the individuals declaring death in these situations.

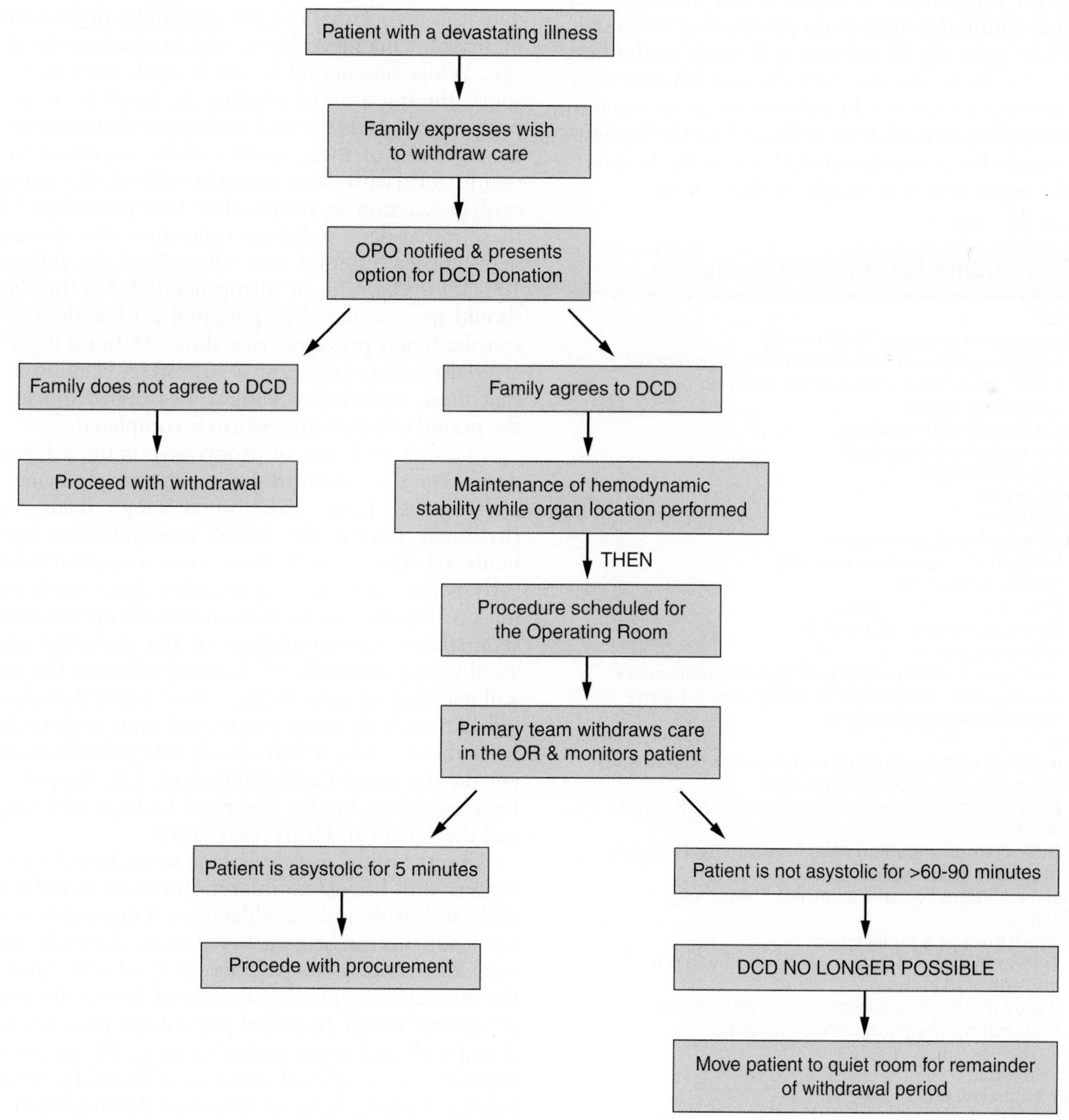

FIGURE 6-3 ■ General approach to the diagnosis of brain death. OPO, organ procurement organization; DCD, donation after circulatory death; OR, operating room.

DONOR MANAGEMENT

The management of organ donor candidates falls under the purview of the critical care physician. As such, the same systematic approach employed when managing other patients in the intensive care unit should be used in the management of potential organ donors. Approaches to organ donor management following a protocol have been shown to improve the overall number of organs transplanted, with no detrimental effects on graft function.[37,61,65] As a result, various international groups have endorsed standardized pathways for the management of potential organ donors.[67,84] Donor management guidelines are constantly undergoing re-evaluation and updating as the science of critical care advances; the guidelines laid out in Table 6-4 represent the current recommendations in the management of organ donation. For the context of this section, it is important to remember that the smooth integration of organ donor management techniques within the context of a pre-existing systematic approach to critically ill patients will result in the best outcomes for these patients, regardless of whether they proceed to organ donation. In addition, strict attention to donor management guidelines will result in the highest-quality organs for procurement, and ensure the best outcomes for organ donation recipients (Table 6-4).

TABLE 6-4 Donor Management Guidelines

- Cardiac
  - Mean arterial pressure 70–90 mmHg
    - Treat hypertension with short-acting beta-blocker
    - Treat hypotension with volume, followed by vasoactive agents
  - Heart rate 60–120 beats/min
  - Urine output 0.5–3 mL/kg/h
  - Hemoglobin 8 g/dL
  - $Scvo_2$ >70%
- Respiratory
  - Mechanical ventilation goals
    - Fraction of inspired oxygen 0.40
    - Normal arterial pH
    - Tidal volumes 8–10 mL/kg
    - Plateau pressure <35 cm H_2O
  - Fluid management
    - Judicious fluid administration to avoid pulmonary edema, with diuresis as necessary after the early resuscitative phase of care
- Renal
  - Euvolemia with appropriate end-organ perfusion and oxygen delivery (UOP 0.5–3 mL/kg/h)
    - Early recognition and correction of DI (UOP >4 mL/kg/h)
    - DDAVP 8 ng/kg loading dose followed by 4 ng/kg/h titrated to urine output <3 mL/kg/h
  - Plasma sodium concentration 140–155 mmol/L
- Endocrine
  - Thyroid hormone replacement
    - Triiodothyronine 4 μg bolus followed by 3 μg/h infusion × 10 hours
    - If only thyroxine is available, start 20 μg bolus followed by 10 μg/h infusion × 10 hours
  - Euglycemia
- Miscellaneous
  - Normothermia

$Scvo_2$, central venous oxygen saturation; UOP, urine output; DI, diabetes insipidus; DDAVP, desmopressin.

Cardiac

As described previously, the cardiovascular system is subject to rapid changes over the course of brain death. A proactive approach to management of these patients can decrease the percentage of donors who suffer a cardiac arrest in the predonation period, typically reported as 5–10% of all potential donors.[40] Overall, the hemodynamic goals for a potential organ donor are the same as for any other patient in the intensive care unit: to optimize cardiac output so as to achieve organ perfusion with minimal vasoactive support. Linking the physiology of brain death to effects on cardiac status can better direct therapy to this end.

The earliest impact of brain death on cardiac function is during the autonomic storm, during which time catecholamine concentrations reach supraphysiologic levels. This can result in one or several of the following: increased heart rate, increased blood pressure, increased cardiac output, and increased SVR. All of these result in a deficit in myocardial oxygen availability in the setting of increased demand, and can result in anatomic heart damage. While this period is self-limited, and can be quite short, the question of whether it should be treated has been raised. Audibert and colleagues demonstrated that management of these initial cardiac responses to autonomic storm with short-acting beta-blockade can improve cardiac function in hearts after transplantation.[4] Given these initial data, judicious utilization of a short-acting beta-blocker (esmolol 100–500 μg/kg bolus followed by 100–300 μg/kg/min, or nitroprusside 0.5–5.0 μg/kg/min) should be considered in potential cardiac donors when systolic blood pressures rise above 160 mmHg or mean arterial pressures rise above 90 mmHg, keeping in mind that these medications should be stopped quickly once the period of autonomic storm is completed.[67]

The first 48 hours of progressive brain ischemia and death are characterized by an increased incidence of arrhythmias. Early arrhythmias range from tachyarrhythmias during the initial catecholamine surge to bradyarrhythmias as the heart tries to accommodate the early period of severe hypertension; later bradyarrhythmias will occur due to vagus nerve disruption and parasympathetic overstimulation of the sinoatrial node or atrial ventricular node.[70,82] As many as one in five patients will manifest an arrhythmia.[16] Strict control of electrolye imbalances, body temperature, and acidosis can help mitigate these issues, which should otherwise be treated as per the Advanced Cardiopulmonary Life Support guidelines published by the American College of Cardiology and the American Heart Association.

After the initial catecholamine surge, loss of vasomotor centers with brainstem infarction results in reduction of SVR and profound vasodilatation. Often, this is a time when patients can become hypotensive due to the physiology of distributive shock. This can also further destabilize the myocardium, previously injured during the period of autonomic storm. Standard physiologic parameters associated with end-organ perfusion should be targeted, and include a mean arterial pressure >70 mmHg, urine output 0.5–3 mL/kg/h, heart rate of 60–120 beats/min, and a hemoglobin >8 g/dL.[40,84] Acidosis needs to be corrected, targeting a pH 7.40–7.45. Volume expansion is the initial therapy of choice, using isotonic fluids or colloids (blood or albumin), with a target of euvolemia at the end of resuscitation. Fluid choice should be tailored depending on potential organs to be harvested, as crystalloid administration in excess can decrease the chances of successful lung harvest.

If volume alone is insufficient to attain these goals quickly, as may be the case in up to 80% of donors, vasoactive agent support is required.[83] The use of vasoactive agents has been shown to improve organ viability by stabilizing the donor. If a vasopressor is necessary, the role of norepinephrine in the treatment of another form of vasodilatory shock (septic shock) has been extrapolated to the management of organ donors.[60] Norepinephrine, in comparison to dopamine, has been shown to have equivalent outcome results with fewer side effects, and while some animal data have suggested significant delay in primary graft function when norepinephrine is utilized, this has to date not been repeated in the human population.[22,60] As a result, norepinephrine has become the vasoactive agent of choice in the treatment of vasodilatory shock, bearing in mind that early and aggressive volume resuscitation decreases the overall need for any vasoactive agent, and promotes early titration and removal of any vasoactive agent that is initiated.[60] Arginine Vasopressin (AVP) (0.04 U/min) may also be an appropriate choice in the early periods of vasodilatory shock.[84] Vasopressin has also been shown to improve outcomes after kidney transplant, a result that is ascribed to a decrease in microvascular thombotic events after "pretreating" the endothelium. It is therefore another useful vasoactive agent in the treatment of vasodilatory shock after brain death. If an inotrope is required, it is important to realize that the vasodilatory effects of dobutamine, especially in the setting of hypovolemia, may provoke additional hypotension and tachycardia. However, at low doses (5 μg/kg/min), dobutamine has been shown to have some protective effects in animal models of renal transplant.[22] If the donor is tachycardic at baseline, milrinone is a better first-line inotropic agent.

Aside from standard physiologic monitoring, invasive markers of volume status can be very useful, especially when donors may have confounding factors impacting their urine output (mannitol, diabetes insipidus). Central venous pressure (CVP) has been the traditional parameter of choice, with a target range of 4–12 mmHg.[84] However, in the setting of mechanical ventilation, this measure has significant limitations due to alterations in intrathoracic pressure. CVP monitoring does allow measurement of central venous oxygen saturation ($ScvO_2$), a marker of organ perfusion and delivery. Regardless of whether this parameter is checked intermittently or continuously, the target range is still a $ScvO_2$ >70%.[84] It should be noted that there are no prospective randomized studies looking at brain-dead patients and $ScvO_2$ values; potentially higher $ScvO_2$ could reflect a "new normal" as the brain is no longer consuming oxygen.[55] However, this value still represents a useful target for end-organ oxygen delivery and consumption. If there is a concern for myocardial depression, either pre-existing in the donor or as a result of brain death itself, additional monitoring can be used. While pulmonary artery catheters have been used to optimize cardiac output in the past, more recent data suggest that echocardiography can provide equivalent information.[44] In addition, the use of dynamic indices of cardiac function, such as pulse pressure variation and stroke volume variation, has been promoted in the intensive care literature as a more accurate measure of preload than static indices such as CVP or pulmonary capillary wedge pressure. A large randomized control trial of the use of these markers in the transplant population to maximize organ harvest through early goal-directed donor management is currently underway. Regardless of the modality used to evaluate cardiac function, the recommended targets are a cardiac index >2.4 L/min/m^2 and a mean arterial pressure of >70 mmHg.[84]

It is important to remember that donor management techniques also increase the potential for the heart transplantation as an end in itself. After stabilizing the donor and reaching standard physiologic norms, initial evaluation of the heart should be performed using echocardiography, evaluating for structural heart disease, left ventricular ejection fraction, and gross wall motion abnormalities.[84] However, it should be noted that while single-use echocardiography is helpful in screening for anatomic abnormalities, it is not sufficient for the evaluation of physiologic suitability. Given evidence that young hearts with left ventricular dysfunction can recover from the initial insult of autonomic storm, serial evaluation of cardiac function after optimizing volume status and repleting hormone deficiencies (discussed later) provides the best data for determining suitability for transplant. Cardiac catheterization is reserved for the assessment of potential donor hearts from patients 45 years of age or older, or at the particular request of the transplant center.

Respiratory

Perhaps nowhere has the adoption of a standardized protocol made as much impact for organ recovery as in the management of potential lung donors. Historically, lung procurement has been as low as 7% from all available organ donors, and hovers optimally around 16%, with multiple factors contributing to this rate.[76] These include acute lung injury after brain death, atelectasis, aspiration, and pneumonia. While previous work demonstrated that a standardized protocol could improve recovery, implementation of the San Antonio Lung Transplant donor management protocol, developed by Luis Angel and colleagues, has demonstrably doubled their ability to identify and transplant lungs from donors at their institution.[3] Following in the footsteps of previous work that suggested marginal lung donor candidates could actually produce adequate lungs for transplant recipients, Angel et al. were able to show not only an increase in the number of "poor" donors optimized to ideal or extended criteria donors with implementation of their protocol, but also that no significant 30-day or 1-year mortality differences were observed between groups.[3]

Lung-protective ventilation, the strategy to prevent ventilator-associated lung trauma from a combination of overstretch of lung parenchyma and oxygen toxicity (as defined as a delivered FiO_2 greater than 0.60 for greater than 48 hours), is helpful in managing potential lung donors. However, active alveolar recruitment maneuvers to improve oxygenation take precedence, as PaO_2/FiO_2 ratios are the major determining criteria for transplantation. The San Antonio group describes alveolar recruitment for all patients with a PaO_2/FiO_2 ratio less than 300, or when pulmonary infiltrates on chest X-ray were consistent with pulmonary edema or atelectasis.[3] The technique used was 2 hours of pressure-controlled ventilation, set with a positive end-expiratory pressure of 15 cmH_2O and an inspiratory pressure of 25 cm H_2O. Patients were then switched back to conventional volume-controlled ventilation for 30 minutes, and a chest X-ray was rechecked. If both the chest X-ray and the PaO_2/FiO_2 ratio were improved, recruitment was considered a success. However, baseline targets of oxygenation and ventilation (PO_2 >80 mmHg and PCO_2 30–35 mmHg) need to be met, even if patients are not candidates for lung donation, in order to maintain appropriate oxygen delivery to the other organs.[84] Lung recruitment strategies need to be balanced with appropriate peak and plateau airway pressures to avoid negative effects on patient hemodynamics.

Strict monitoring of volume status is the next important component of lung management in the donor population. Cardiac instability during the autonomic storm causes significant shifts in blood pressure, and, without strict parameters, can result in significant volume overload. With direct catecholamine impact on alveolar permeability, fluid can redistribute into the pulmonary interstitium. In addition, an increase in the left atrial pressure due to increased SVR can result in functional heart failure and cardiogenic pulmonary edema. Several studies have demonstrated that pulmonary edema decreases the potential for lung transplantation.[59,75] Judicious fluid administration and administering diuretics as tolerated are parts of the overall strategy for decreasing pulmonary edema and optimizing oxygenation prior to donation.

Standard intensive care unit management for the prevention of ventilator-associated pneumonia and aspiration pneumonitis should be continued. This includes elevating the head of the bed at least 30° at all times, administration of deep vein thrombosis prophylaxis (mechanical and chemical methods), and administration of a proton pump inhibitor for the prevention of gastritis. If, after lung recruitment measures, infiltrates or contusions persist on chest X-ray, bronchoscopy with bilateral lavage can be performed to evaluate those areas.

The most important concept in the management of donors for lung transplantation is to remember that every donor should be considered a potential lung donor, since standardized attention to a few basic management principles can result in optimization of initially poor-quality organs.

Renal

Most considerations relative to donor renal function have been mentioned already in the section on cardiovascular management. Euvolemia with appropriate end-organ perfusion and oxygen delivery is the goal of intensive donor management. It is important to mention here that, in the process of managing the brain injury prior to brain death, the donor is likely to have been exposed to a number of agents with diuretic properties (mannitol, hypertonic saline). These agents can complicate both the hemodynamic stability of an already hypovolemic patient, and impact the diagnosis of renal-specific processes associated with brain injury. It is important for these agents to be carefully documented and considered when evaluating urine output.

The target for urine output, as previously mentioned, is the same as for any other patient in the intensive care unit – approximately 0.5–1 mL/kg/h. However, up to 2.5–3 mL/kg/h can be considered normal in donors as they equilibrate from fluid repletion during periods of hemodynamic instability.[67] It is important to avoid an excessively positive fluid balance – there is a significant body of literature in critical care suggesting that this can lead to end-organ dysfunction, and in fact fluid-restrictive strategies have demonstrated improvement in the numbers of lungs transplanted. [3,5]

If urine output targets exceed 4 mL/kg/h, diabetes insipidus should be suspected. The hypothalamic–posterior pituitary neuronal connections become hypoxic with the progression of brain death, and production of AVP ceases. As a result, despite relative hypotension in the setting of loss of sympathetic tone, the kidneys continue to secrete large volumes of dilute urine until the patient becomes profoundly hypovolemic and oliguric. This is also associated with hypernatremia, known to be detrimental for potential liver donors. Treatment is aimed at restoring intravascular volume, at the same time supplementing the loss of AVP. Supplementation can be done either with desmopressin (DDAVP 8 ng/kg loading dose followed by 4 ng/kg/h titrated to urine output), or with continuous infusion of AVP (1 U bolus followed by 0.01–0.04 U/min).[34,84] Desmopressin is a more selective vasopressin receptor agonist, targeting V2 receptors, and therefore has significant antidiuretic properties without the concomitant vasopressor activity of AVP.[34,82] It can therefore be used without increasing organ vasoconstriction and causing posttransplant impairment. However, if the patient is requiring vasopressor support in addition to volume repletion, AVP is a better choice.

Hypernatremia, a side effect of diabetes insipidus, has been associated with increased rates of liver graft loss, and possibly renal graft function.[18,29,72,73] Serum sodium levels should be kept between 140 and 155 mmol/L, in an effort to decrease osmotic gradients between donor liver and recipient vasculature upon reanastomosis.[52] In addition, a balanced nutritional approach using dextrose-based solutions is helpful for maintaining hepatic glycogen stores; however, this cannot be done at the expense of glycemic control.[52]

Endocrine

Hormonal resuscitation is a concept in organ donor management aimed at addressing the three endocrine deficiencies of brain death that can impact outcomes.

The first of these is thyroid hormone (thyroxine (T_4) and triiodothyronine (T_3)) depletion. The exact mechanism of thyroid hormone function is as yet not fully elucidated, but several studies have implicated low levels of thyroid hormone as a contributory factor to the hemodynamic instability following brain death. Novitzky and colleagues were able to demonstrate in a series of animal and human studies that the administration of T_3 improved cardiac function, decreased hemodynamic instability, and transitioned brain-dead donors from anaerobic metabolism to aerobic metabolism.[47,48] Additional work by other authors has confirmed these findings while using T_4, and suggested that the use of thyroid hormone replacement can increase the overall number of organs harvested from a single donor.[61,63,64] Rosendale et al. looked at recipient outcomes, and were able to demonstrate that, for cardiac recipients, 1-month survival was improved with a 50% decrease in early graft dysfunction, although this improvement occurred in conjunction with the use of steroids.[62] Overall, current recommendations call for thyroid hormone supplementation, preferably with T_3 due to its more rapid onset and decreased susceptibility to influence by exogenous factors.[84] T_3 can be dosed at 4 μg bolus followed by 3 μg/h infusion for 10 hours.[34] If T_3 is unavailable, T_4 can be used at 20 μg bolus followed by a 10 μg/h infusion for 10 hours.[82]

Vasopressin, as mentioned above, is a pharmacologic agent in both brain death-related peripheral vasodilatation and diabetes insipidus. Again, treatment is aimed at restoring intravascular volume, while at the same time supplementing the loss of AVP. Corticosteroid administration is the third component of hormone resuscitation, and is based on two possible mechanisms of function. The first is the attenuation of the inflammatory process associated with brain death. Two studies looking at posttransplant liver rejection markers, inflammatory markers, and posttransplant cardiac function demonstrated improvement in both parameters when steroid therapy was given to the donor.[32,62] In addition, lung procurement was demonstrated to be directly tied to the administration of steroids, which was related to increased oxygenation.[20] However, more recent work has suggested that, while suppression of the inflammatory state does occur, the incidence of rejection in liver and kidney recipients was not improved with steroid pretreatment.[2,28] The second physiologic derangement for which steroid administration is useful is for adrenal insufficiency, which can make hemodynamic management a challenge. However, this therapeutic use is often empiric, as diagnosis studies can take a significant period of time, and so the real incidence of adrenal insufficiency is unknown. Current guidelines still endorse the use of methylprednisolone (15 mg/kg bolus) as part of hormone resuscitation.[84]

Finally, while not part of hormone resuscitation, glycemic control is an important ongoing component of intensive care management of the donor. Between stress-related insulin resistance after brain injury and the replacement of free water deficits during diabetes insipidus with free water solutions that contain dextrose, donors can become quite hyperglycemic.[42] While strict glycemic control has not been studied in this population, continuing to manage severe hyperglycemia (glucose >180 mg/dL) is suggested to help mitigate the inflammatory response and prevent infection.[51] Evidence suggests that renal function over the course of donor management worsens significantly in the setting of persistent hyperglycemia and significant glycemic shifts[9]; this of course would impact renal transplant recipients. In addition, pancreas function in the recipient is impacted by donor glucose levels, with normoglycemia improving outcomes.[21] An insulin infusion therapy can be titrated for this effect.

Infectious Disease

While donor to recipient infection transmission is well documented and can result in serious, and potentially fatal, outcomes, most donor infections independently are not contraindications to transplantation.[54] Those that are listed in Table 6-5.[15] Effective treatment of pre-existing donor infections can result in successful transplantation, as can transplantation of a donor organ exposed to a chronic viral infection to a recipient with the same exposure history.[35] It is important to recognize infections in donors and treat them quickly and efficiently so as to keep the donation process moving forward. Treatment starts with good prevention – standard intensive care unit policies for the prevention of hospital-acquired infections (pneumonias, central line-associated blood stream infections, and urinary tract infections) should be maintained even after the focus of care has transitioned.

A high index of suspicion for infection is the next step. There are many reasons why a donor will not mount a standard response to infection – loss of thermoregulation preventing fevers, pre-existing leukocytosis secondary to the inciting injury, massive blood transfusions, or use of steroids resulting in immunosuppression. Therefore, it is important to pay attention to other clinical markers, including the skin examination, sputum characteristics, chest X-ray findings, and urinalysis results. Choice and interpretation of cultures, as well as guidelines for surveillance cultures when no infection is obvious, are at the discretion of the Organ Procurement Agency;

TABLE 6-5 Infection Diagnoses that Exclude Transplantation

- Active fungal, parasitic, viral, or bacterial meningitis or encephalitis
- Bacterial
  - Tuberculosis
  - Gangrenous bowel or perforated bowel or intra-abdominal sepsis
- Viral
  - Active hepatitis B or C
  - Rabies
  - Retroviral infections, including HIV, HTLV-I/II
  - Active herpes simplex, EBV, varicella, or CMV viremia, or pneumonia
  - West Nile virus
- Fungal
  - Active infection with *Cryptococcus, Aspergillus, Histoplasma, Coccidioides*
  - Active candidemia or invasive yeast
- Parasites
  - Active infection with *Trypanosoma cruzi* (Chagas), *Leishmania, Strongyloides*, or *Plasmodium* sp. (malaria)
- Prion
  - Creutzfeldt–Jakob disease

HIV, human immunodeficiency virus; HTLV, human T-lymphotropic virus; EBV, Epstein–Barr virus ; CMV, cytomegalovirus.

however, it is always useful to obtain a Gram stain of the initial specimen to allow early antibiotic tailoring.[54] Antibiotic choice is also a regional matter, as local sensitivities will change regularly. However, it is important to tailor broad empiric therapy as soon as culture results are available. In the presence of renal or hepatic dysfunction, extended criteria donors (age), and obesity, it is important to adjust antibiotic dosing.[54]

Hematology

Anemia should be avoided in organ donors in order to optimize oxygen delivery to various organs. Recommendations are currently to target a hemoglobin level of 8 g/dL, in an effort to limit potential immunosuppressive effects while maximizing hemodynamic stability and oxygen delivery.

Coagulopathy can occur for a variety of reasons in the donor. Donors may have pre-existing conditions that can result in coagulopathy, including cardiac arrhythmias, for which they are treated with anticoagulation. Iatrogenic causes need to be ruled out, including dilutional coagulopathy, acidosis, and hypothermia. The loss of hypothalamic thermoregulation in the brain-dead donor, in addition to the inability to vasoconstrict or shiver, results in a poikilothermic donor.[42] Close attention needs to be paid to environmental control of temperature and the temperature of infusing fluids in order to prevent the adverse effects of hypothermia. Core temperature should be maintained above 34 °C with the use of warming blankets, fluid warmers, and ventilator heating units for inhaled gases.

Additionally, the release of cerebral proteins into the circulation with brain death can trigger a consumptive coagulopathy (disseminated intravascular coagulopathy) or a hypercoaguable state.[33] Any evidence of coagulopathy should be identified early and treated based on bleeding risk. Pre-existing coagulopathies (secondary to medication) should be identified and reversed if at all possible. Donor acidosis and hypothermia should be corrected, and consideration should be given to a 1:1:1 ratio of packed red blood cells, fresh frozen plasma, and platelet resuscitation model for patients who are bleeding (similar to trauma resuscitation), as this has been shown to decrease both time to hemodynamic stability and coagulopathy.[14] If available, thromboelastography can augment traditional measures of coagulopathy, and potentially indicate patients at risk for hypercoaguable states early in their management.[53] Standard intensive care unit protocol for the prevention of deep vein thrombosis should be continued.

OTHER TOPICS IN DONOR MANAGEMENT

Ethics

The ethical ramifications of organ transplantation, and the responsibilities inherent in maintaining the spirit in which a donation is made, are never far from the surface in the management of organ donors. With an increasing focus on the concept of first-person authorization for donation, wherein the designation as "donor" of a given individual is held as a mandate for the care team to facilitate donation in appropriate circumstances, comes increasing scrutiny of the field of organ transplantation. Recently, several vocal criticisms of the system could be seen in the mainstream media, focused primarily on remuneration for donation and the allocation process.[25,39] It is part of the responsibility of the care team to continue to educate patients, family members, and the community about both the process through which donation happens, and the importance of the act of donation for the donor and the recipient. Only through education and transparency will the transplantation community continue to engender patient support, and ensure an ongoing stream of willing donors.

Future Technologies

With the current shortage of available organs for transplantation, much work is being done to extend the donor pool and optimize the organs that are available for transplantation. Approaches range from the microcellular – chemical and electrical modulation of the inflammatory cascade brought on by brain death – to the macrocellular, using normothermic organ management to decrease the differential effects of warm ischemia and cold perfusion. [10,26,48] There has even been a resurgence of interest in using extracorporeal membrane oxygenation for DCD preservation during the period of organ optimization.[36] This is an exciting time to be involved in the field of organ donation, as new technologies bring new possibilities for donor management.

CONCLUSION

In conclusion, the field of organ donor management continues to evolve. The application of both critical care best practices and organ transplantation research to the clinical management of organ donors has allowed for improvements in both the number and quality of organs recovered. Now known as donor management guidelines, these best practices will allow practitioners to continue to provide optimal medical care to both the donor and eventually the recipient.

REFERENCES

1. Ad Hoc Comittee of the Harvard Medical School to Examine the Definition of Brain Death. A definition of irreversible coma. JAMA 1968;205:337–49.
2. Amatschek S, Wilflingseder J, Pones M, et al. The effect of steroid pretreatment of deceased organ donors on liver allograft function: a blinded randomized placebo-controlled trial. J Hepatol 2012;56:1305–9.
3. Angel LF. Impact of a lung transplantation donor-management protocol on lung donation and recipient outcomes. Am J Respir Crit Care Med 2006;174:710–6.
4. Audibert G, Charpentier C, Seguin-Devaux C, et al. Improvement of donor myocardial function after treatment of autonomic storm during brain death. Transplantation 2006;82:1031–6.
5. Bagshaw SM, Bellomo R. The influence of volume management on outcome. Curr Opin Crit Care 2007;13:541–8.
6. Barklin A. Systemic inflammation in the brain-dead organ donor. Acta Anaesthesiol Scand 2009;53:425–35.

7. Barlow AD, Metcalfe MS, Johari Y, et al. Case-matched comparison of long-term results of non-heart beating and heart-beating donor renal transplants. Br J Surg 2009;96:685–91.
8. Bellingham JM, Santhanakrishnan C, Neidlinger N, et al. Donation after cardiac death: a 29-year experience. Surgery 2011;150:692–702.
9. Blasi-Ibanez A, Hirose R, Feiner J, et al. Predictors associated with terminal renal function in deceased organ donors in the intensive care unit. Anesthesiology 2009;110:333–41.
10. Brockmann J, Reddy S, Coussios C, et al. Normothermic perfusion: a new paradigm for organ preservation. Ann Surg 2009;250:1–6.
11. Conci F, Procaccio F, Arosio M, et al. Viscero-somatic and viscero-visceral reflexes in brain death. J Neurol Neurosurg Psychiatry 1986;49:695–8.
12. Coronado VG, Xu L, Basavaraju SV, et al. Surveillance for traumatic brain injury-related deaths – United States, 1997–2007. Morb Mortal Wkly Rep Surveill Summ 2011;60:1–32.
13. de Groot YJ, Lingsma HF, Bakker J, et al. External validation of a prognostic model predicting time of death after withdrawal of life support in neurocritical patients. Crit Care Med 2012;40:233–8.
14. Dente CJ, Shaz BH, Nicholas JM, et al. Improvements in early mortality and coagulopathy are sustained better in patients with blunt trauma after institution of a massive transfusion protocol in a civilian level I trauma center. J Trauma 2009;66:1616–24.
15. Domínguez-Gil B, Delmonico FL, Shaheen FAM, et al. The critical pathway for deceased donation: reportable uniformity in the approach to deceased donation. Transpl Int 2011;24:373–8.
16. Dosemeci L, Yilmaz M, Cengiz M, et al. Brain death and donor management in the intensive care unit: experiences over the last 3 years. Transplant Proc 2004;36:20–1.
17. Dujardin KS, McCully RB, Wijdicks EF, et al. Myocardial dysfunction associated with brain death: clinical, echocardiographic, and pathologic features. J Heart Lung Transplant 2001;20:350–7.
18. Figueras J, Busquets J, Grande L, et al. The deleterious effect of donor high plasma sodium and extended preservation in liver transplantation. A multivariate analysis. Transplantation 1996;61:410–3.
19. Fisher AJ, Donnelly SC, Hirani N, et al. Enhanced pulmonary inflammation in organ donors following fatal non-traumatic brain injury. Lancet 1999;353:1412–3.
20. Follette DM, Rudich SM, Babcock WD. Improved oxygenation and increased lung donor recovery with high-dose steroid administration after brain death. J Heart Lung Transplant 1998;17:423–9.
21. Gores PF, Gillingham KJ, Dunn DL, et al. Donor hyperglycemia as a minor risk factor and immunologic variables as major risk factors for pancreas allograft loss in a multivariate analysis of a single institution's experience. Ann Surg 1992;215:217–30.
22. Gottmann U, Brinkkoetter PT, Bechtler M, et al. Effect of pre-treatment with catecholamines on cold preservation and ischemia/reperfusion-injury in rats. Kidney Int 2006;70:321–8.
23. Gramm H-J, Meinhold H, Bickel U, et al. Acute endocrine failure after brain death? Transplantation 1992;54:851–7.
24. Guidelines for the determination of death: report of the medical consultants on the diagnosis of death to the President's Commission for the study of ethical problems in medicine and biochemical and behavioral research. JAMA 1981;246:3.
25. Hensley S. The ethics of compensating organ donors. Available online at: http://www.npr.org/2012/05/22/153293669/the-ethics-of-compensating-organ-donors.
26. Hoeger S, Bergstraesser C, Selhorst J, et al. Modulation of brain dead induced inflammation by vagus nerve stimulation. Am J Transplant 2010;10:477–89.
27. Jassem W, Koo DD, Cerundolo L, et al. Leukocyte infiltration and inflammatory antigen expression in cadaveric and living-donor livers before transplant. Transplantation 2003;75:2001–7.
28. Kainz A, Wilflingseder J, Mitterbauer C, et al. Steroid pretreatment of organ donors to prevent postischemic renal allograft failure: a randomized, controlled trial. Ann Intern Med 2010;153:222–30.
29. Kazemeyni SM, Esfahani F. Influence of hypernatremia and polyuria of brain-dead donors before organ procurement on kidney allograft function. Urol J 2008;5:173–7.
30. Kootstra G, Daemen JH, Oomen AP. Categories of non-heart-beating donors. Transplant Proc 1995;27:2893–4.
31. Kosleradzki M, Lisik W, Rowinski W, et al. Progress in abdominal organ transplantation. Med Sci Monit 2011;17:RA282–91.
32. Kotsch K, Ulrich F, Reutzel-Selke A, et al. Methylprednisolone therapy in deceased donors reduces inflammation in the donor liver and improves outcome after liver transplantation: a prospective randomized controlled trial. Ann Surg 2008;248:1042–50.
33. Laroche M, Kutcher ME, Huang MC, et al. Coagulopathy after traumatic brain injury. Neurosurgery 2012;70:1334–45.
34. Linos K, Fraser J, Freeman WD, et al. Care of the brain-dead organ donor. Curr Anaesth Crit Care 2007;18:284–94.
35. Lumbreras C, Sanz F, Gonzalez A, et al. Clinical significance of donor-unrecognized bacteremia in the outcome of solid-organ transplant recipients. Clin Infect Dis 2001;33:722–6.
36. Magliocca JF, Magee JC, Rowe SA, et al. Extracorporeal support for organ donation after cardiac death effectively expands the donor pool. J Trauma 2005;58:1095–102.
37. Malinoski DJ, Daly MC, Patel MS, et al. Achieving donor management goals before deceased donor procurement is associated with more organs transplanted per donor. J Trauma 2011;71:990–6.
38. Manara AR, Murphy PG, O'Callaghan G. Donation after circulatory death. Br J Anaesth 2011;108:i108–21.
39. Marchione M. Dick Cheney's heart transplant reopens debate over age. Huffington Post 2012 Mar 25.
40. Mascia L, Mastromauro I, Viberti S, et al. Management to optimize organ procurement in brain dead donors. Minerva Anestesiol 2009;75:125–33.
41. McKeating EG, Andrews PJ, Signorini DF, et al. Transcranial cytokine gradients in patients requiring intensive care after acute brain injury. Br J Anaesth 1997;78:520–3.
42. Marvin MR, Morton V. Glycemic control and organ transplantation. J Diabetes Sci Technol 2009;3:1365–72.
43. Monbaliu D, Pirenne J, Talbot D. Liver transplantation using donation after cardiac death donors. J Hepatol 2012;56:474–85.
44. Murthi SB, Hess JR, Hess A, et al. Focused rapid echocardiographic evaluation versus vascular cather-based assessment of cardiac output and function in critically ill trauma patients. J Trauma 2012;72:1158–64.
45. Nagareda T, Kinoshita Y, Tanaka A, et al. Clinicopathology of kidneys from brain-dead patients treated with vasopressin and epinephrine. Kidney Int 1993;43:1363–70.
46. Novitzky D. Detrimental effects of brain death on the organ donor. Transplant Proc 1997;29:3770–2.
47. Novitzky D. Novel actions of thyroid hormone: the role of triiodothyronine in cardiac transplantation. Thyroid 1996;6:531–6.
48. Novitzky D, Cooper DKC, Rosendale JD, et al. Hormonal therapy of the brain-dead organ donor: experimental and clinical studies. Transplantation 2006;82:1396–401.
49. Novitzky D, Wicomb WN, Rose AG, et al. Pathophysiology of pulmonary edema following experimental brain death in the chacma baboon. Ann Thorac Surg 1987;43:288–94.
50. Oto T. Lung transplantation from donation after cardiac death (non-heart-beating) donors. Gen Thorac Cardiovasc Surg 2008;56:533–8.
51. Powner D. Donor care before pancreatic tissue transplantation. Prog Transplant 2005;15:129–37.
52. Powner D. Factors during donor care that may impact liver transplant outcomes. Prog Transplant 2004;14:241–9.
53. Powner D. Thromboelastography during adult donor care. Prog Transplant 2010;20:163–8.
54. Powner D, Allison TA. Bacterial infection during adult donor care. Prog Transplant 2007;17:266–74.
55. Powner D, Doshi PB. Central venous oxygen saturation monitoring: role in adult donor care? Prog Transplant 2010;20:401–6.
56. Quality Standards Subcommittee of the American Academy of Neurology. Practice parameters for determining brain death in adults. Neurology 1995;45:1012–4.
57. Rabinstein AA, Yee AH, Mandrekar J, et al. Prediction of potential for organ donation after cardiac death in patients in neurocritical state: a prospective observational study. Lancet Neurol 2012;11:414–9.
58. Reich DJ, Mulligan DC, Abt PL, et al. ASTS recommended practice guidelines for controlled donation after cardiac death organ procurement and transplantation. Am J Transplant 2009;9:2004–11.

59. Reilly PM, Grossman M, Rosengard BR, et al. Lung procurement from solid organ donors: role of fluid resuscitation in procurement failures. Chest 1996;110:220S–7S.
60. Rivers EP, Katranji M, Jaehne KA, et al. Early interventions in severe sepsis and septic shock: a review of the evidence one decade later. Minerva Anestesiol 2012;78:712–24.
61. Rosendale JD, Chabalewski FL, McBride MA, et al. Increased transplanted organs from the use of a standardized donor management protocol. Am J Transplant 2002;2:761–8.
62. Rosendale JD, Kauffman HM, McBride MA, et al. Hormonal resuscitation yields more transplanted hearts, with improved early function1. Transplantation 2003;75:1336–41.
63. Salim A, Martin M, Brown C, et al. Using thyroid hormone in brain-dead donors to maximize the number of organs available for transplantation. Clin Transplant 2007;21:405–9.
64. Salim A, Vassiliu P, Velmahos GC, et al. The role of thyroid hormone administration in potential organ donors. Arch Surg 2001;136:1377–80.
65. Salim A, Velmahos GC, Brown C, et al. Aggressive organ donor management significantly increases the number of organs available for transplantation. J Trauma 2005;58:991–4.
66. Saposnik G, Basile VS, Young GB. Movements in brain death: a systematic review. Can J Neurol Sci 2009;36:154–60.
67. Shemie SD. Organ donor management in Canada: recommendations of the forum on medical management to optimize donor organ potential. Can Med Assoc J 2006;174:S13–30.
68. Stangl M, Zerkaulen T, Theodorakis J, et al. Influence of brain death on cytokine release in organ donors and renal transplants. Transplant Proc 2001;33:1284–5.
69. Stiegler P, Sereinigg M, Puntschart A, et al. A 10 min "no-touch" time – is it enough in DCD? A DCD animal study. Transpl Int 2012;25:481–92.
70. Subramanian A, Brown D. Management of the brain-dead organ donor. Contemp Crit Care 2010;8:1–12.
71. Suntharalingam C, Sharples L, Dudley C, et al. Time to cardiac death after withdrawal of life-sustaining treatment in potential organ donors. Am J Transplant 2009;9:2157–65.
72. Totsuka E, Fung U, Hakamada K, et al. Analysis of clinical variables of donors and recipients with respect to short-term graft outcome in human liver transplantation. Transplant Proc 2004;36:2215–8.
73. Totsuka E, Fung JJ, Ishii T, et al. Influence of donor condition on postoperative graft survival and function in human liver transplantation. Transplant Proc 2000;32:322–6.
74. van der Zee H, Malik AB, Lee BC, et al. Lung fluid and protein exchange during intracranial hypertension and role of sympathetic mechanisms. J Appl Physiol 1980;48:273–80.
75. Venkateswaran RV, Patchell VB, Wilson IC, et al. Early donor management increases the retrieval rate of lungs for transplantation. Ann Thorac Surg 2008;85:278–86.
76. Weill D. Donor criteria in lung transplantation: an issue revisited. Chest 2002;121:2029–31.
77. Weiss S, Kotsch K, Francuski M, et al. Brain death activates donor organs and is associated with a worse I/R injury after liver transplantation. Am J Transplant 2007;7:1584–93.
78. Wijdicks EF, Pfeifer EA. Neuropathology of brain death in the modern transplant era. Neurology 2008;70:1234–7.
79. Wijdicks EF, Rabinstein AA, Manno EM, et al. Pronouncing brain death: contemporary practice and safety of the apnea test. Neurology 2008;71:1240–4.
80. Wijdicks EF, Varelas PN, Gronseth GS, et al. Evidence-based guideline update: determining brain death in adults. Report of the Quality Standards Subcommittee of the American Academy of Neurology. Neurology 2010;74:1911–8.
81. Wind J, Snoeijs MGJ, Brugman CA, et al. Prediction of time of death after withdrawal of life-sustaining treatment in potential donors after cardiac death. Crit Care Med 2012;40:766–9.
82. Wood KE, Becker BN, McCartney JG, et al. Care of the potential organ donor. N Engl J Med 2004;351:2730–9.
83. Wood KE, Coursin DB. Intensivists and organ donor management. Curr Opin Anaesthesiol 2007;20:97–9.
84. Zaroff JG, Rosengard BR, Armstrong WF, et al. Consensus conference report: maximizing use of organs recovered from the cadaver donor: cardiac recommendations, March 28–29, 2001, Crystal City, VA. Circulation 2002;106:836–41.

CHAPTER 7

MEDICAL EVALUATION OF THE LIVING DONOR

Malcolm P. MacConmara • Kenneth A. Newell

CHAPTER OUTLINE

INTRODUCTION

There are over 90 000 patients with end-stage renal disease (ESRD) currently on the transplant waiting list and for most of them the optimal treatment is to receive a kidney from a living donor.[38] Despite the substantial increase in live donor kidney transplant procedures over the past 20 years, the number of patients awaiting transplantation continues to rise. This increased need for transplant organs has driven the trend towards increased utilization of kidneys from live donors with complex medical conditions.[32] The evaluation of the living donor must be continuously scrutinized and carefully regulated in order to maintain donor safety during this unique and extraordinary act of altruism. The key challenge to evaluating potential living donors remains unchanged and is to select suitable donors efficiently while, most importantly, minimizing their risk.

HISTORICAL PERSPECTIVE AND CURRENT STATUS

The first organ transplant to result in long-term success was a living donor kidney transplant performed at the Peter Bent Brigham Hospital (now Brigham and Women's Hospital) in Boston in 1954.[23] A surgical team led by Nobel Laureate Joseph Murray transplanted a kidney removed from Ronald Herrick into his identical twin brother Richard. This procedure was truly life-saving as it was performed prior to the advent of effective dialysis. The preoperative evaluation included a lengthy assessment of the donor as well as detailed ethical discussions. The investigations included fingerprint analysis and a review of obstetric reports to confirm monozygotic twins, together with skin grafting to test donor and recipient compatibility.[24] The nephrectomy went without difficulty and the donor lived a further 56 years without sequelae.[23]

Prior to the advent of potent immunosuppressive regimes, transplantation of organs from living related donors offered individuals with ESRD the greatest opportunity for successful transplantation. Consensus among medical and ethical experts led to the legal acceptance of brainstem death criteria in late 1970s.[1] This new legislation, together with the introduction of new immunosuppressive agents such as cyclosporine and OKT3 in the 1980s, prompted an upsurge in the use of deceased donor organs and relative decline in the percentage of organ transplants performed using organs from living donors. Live donation re-emerged in the 1990s as an important source for kidney transplants and has risen considerably in number over the past two decades. The explanations for the dramatic escalation in the utilization of living donors are likely multiple, including: (1) the ever-increasing waiting times for organs from deceased donors; (2) the demonstration of a survival benefit associated with kidneys from living donors as compared to kidneys from deceased organ donors; and (3) the shift to publicly preferred minimally invasive procedures. The first laparoscopic donor nephrectomy was described by Ratner et al. in 1995.[30] The minimally invasive technique was demonstrated to lessen postoperative pain and to result in shorter hospital stays and recovery periods when compared with open donor nephrectomy.[31,40] The technique quickly gained support and has become the favored approach to donor nephrectomy.

A total of 80 347 live donor nephrectomies were completed between 1994 and 2009 in the United States and living donors currently represent 34% of all kidney transplants.[13,33] Since reaching a peak in 2004, the number of living donor transplants has plateaued and even declined slightly in recent years. The factors influencing these variations are likely complex; however, changing economic stability is likely to play a role. In addition, changes in organ allocation that occurred with the implementation of the Share 35 rule, which mandated that children under the age of 18 receive priority for organs from donors younger than 35 years of age, have significantly reduced waiting times for pediatric patients. An unintended consequence of this change in policy is that the number children receiving kidneys from living donors has declined.[2] There has been a significant increase in unrelated living donor transplants and these now account for 14% of all kidney transplants.[17] Differences in donation patterns can also be attributed to program-specific activities, as well as geographical location. Longer waiting times seen in the north-east and west of the United States have prompted increased utilization of live donors in these regions.

Caucasian donors comprise approximately 70% of living donors while accounting for 34% of the national renal transplant waiting list. African Americans account for 11–13% of living donors. Ethnic minorities remain disproportionately underrepresented when percentages of patients with ESRD are compared to living donor procedures.[7] The profile of potential donors has seen a dramatic change, with trends toward donors who are older, increasingly obese, and with increasingly complex medical conditions. The proportion of living donors aged over 50 has increased from 13.9% in 1994 to 22.8% in 2008.[33] Similarly, the median body mass index (BMI) of donors has risen to 26.4 while a BMI of greater than 30, previously viewed as a contraindication to donation, is present in as many as 30% of live donors.[15,25]

The process of donor evaluation has evolved since the first donor nephrectomy in 1954. Transplant centers remain under intense scrutiny and their activities are held to the highest levels of clinical, ethical, and legal standards. Reflecting the desire to obtain the best possible outcomes, the evaluation process has become increasingly complex using biochemical, immunologic, and genetic testing as well as advanced imaging technologies to evaluate the donor more accurately. This progressively detailed workup must be balanced against prohibitive cost, as well as the impact of incidental findings on donor health and future wellbeing. The changing demographics and increasing complexity of living donors will require further modifications of evaluation standards, specifically in the area of surveillance of long-term donor outcome in these complex patients, to ensure that the donor risk is minimized.

RATIONALE FOR LIVE KIDNEY DONATION

Patients who receive living donor grafts have superior long-term survival, as well as shorter waiting times. In addition, live donation allows elective planning with optimization of the recipient's health status. Living donor renal transplantation provides the only realistic opportunity for most recipients of undergoing transplantation prior to the initiation of dialysis. This is particularly important, as pre-emptive transplantation has been shown to confer a significant benefit with respect to increased survival of the transplanted kidney.[21]

Life expectancy for kidney transplant recipients far exceeds that for similar patients treated using dialysis.[41] Importantly, kidneys from living donors offer substantial additional benefits compared to kidneys from deceased organ donors. The living donor kidney is thoroughly evaluated in an elective setting with an array of screening tools and the health of the kidney carefully estimated. The recipient can be counseled with increased certainty of graft quality, risk of infection, or cancer transmission. Early graft function is significantly better for kidneys from living versus deceased donors. The primary non-function rates for deceased and living kidney donors are 2.7% and 1.4% while the rates of delayed graft function are 23.5% and 3.4% respectively.[27] More importantly, the benefits of living donor kidneys extend to long-term outcomes. The survival rates of kidneys from deceased and living donors at 10 years are 42.7% and 59.6% respectively. The conditional half-lives of kidneys from deceased and living donors are 14.7 and 26.6 years in the current era.[27] It is striking that the half-life of a living donor kidney in 1991 (15.8 years) exceeds that of a kidney from a deceased donor in 2007 (14.7 years). The individual benefit in graft longevity also translates into a significant benefit for patients on the deceased donor waitlist since fewer patients will require relisting and retransplantation.

While transplantation using kidneys from deceased organ donors is associated with significant benefits for most patients with ESRD relative to continued dialysis, it is well recognized that the time from listing to transplantation is steadily increasing. The median time to transplantation for waitlisted patients increased from 2.61 years in 1998 to 3.37 years in 2006.[27] Wait time is significantly influenced by recipient race and ethnicity, panel-reactive antibody, and geographic region. It is important to note that these median wait times do not reflect patients who died while on the waitlist or those removed from the waitlist due to the development of medical conditions thought to preclude transplantation. The progressively longer waiting time for a deceased donor kidney exposes patients to the cumulative risk of renal failure, dialysis, and associated comorbidities, most importantly cardiovascular disease.[21]

Although it is not possible to determine the waiting time for patients undergoing living donor renal transplantation with certainty, it is undoubtedly shorter than the waiting time for organs from deceased donors. This shorter average waiting time for living donor kidney from initial donor screening to transplantation confers significant advantages. The recipient operation can be planned and the recipient optimized. Ideally, the recipient can undergo transplantation prior to requiring dialysis. Recipients of living donor kidneys are also more likely to complete full rehabilitation as measured by return to employment.[11] In addition reducing recipient time on dialysis has been shown to halt the progression of cardiovascular disease.[22] Finally, the shorter wait time for recipients of kidneys from living donors is associated with a decreased risk of immunologic sensitization, which can further prolong waiting times and negatively influence the outcome of transplantation. Current data demonstrate that 67.9% of recipients undergoing living donor transplantation are unsensitized relative to 59.7% of individuals undergoing deceased donor renal transplantation.[27] Early rehabilitation, shorter hospital stays, and reduced readmissions are all important benefits of living donor transplantation. From the societal perspective the reduced time on dialysis associated with living donor renal transplantation may reduce healthcare costs related to dialysis.

RISKS OF LIVE KIDNEY DONATION

Donor nephrectomy is generally a safe procedure with very low risk of morbidity or mortality. Nonetheless any complication must be seen in the context of harm to a healthy individual. Current legislation mandates that transplant centers report all donor deaths occurring within 6 weeks of donation or during the period of time before the donor is discharged from surgical care. Based on this reporting the estimated surgical mortality from donor nephrectomy is approximately 3 per 10 000 cases. The surgical mortality rate has remained unchanged notwithstanding the trend towards older and increasingly complex donors. This risk is consistent with a recent report documenting 14 operative deaths, as determined by center reporting and review of the Social Security Master Death File, out of 51 153 individuals who were kidney donors between October 1999 and December 2008.[9] Nonfatal complications, including hemorrhage requiring transfusion and the need for reoperation, complicate 2% and less than 1% of donor nephrectomies respectively.[27] Incisional hernias and bowel obstruction have an incidence of 1%. Reports indicate that the need to convert from a minimally invasive approach to an open procedure is equally rare. Table 7-1 outlines common short- and long-term complications of donor nephrectomy.

TABLE 7-1 **Donor Complications**

	Risk (Percent of Donations Unless Stated)
Mortality	0.02–0.03
Major Complication	
Bleeding	2.2
Bowel obstruction	1.0
Vascular injury	0.2
Open conversion	0.7–1.1
Reoperation	0.2
Blood transfusion	0.4
Wound infection	2.1
Urinary tract infection	4.5
Readmission (including nausea, vomiting, gastroenteritis, abdominal pain, ileus, bowel obstruction)	0.9–2.0
Hernia repair	0.8
End-stage renal failure	180 per million/year (average 260 per million/year in US population) Additional risk in obese, elderly, and African American donors
Hypertension	15–25

Sources: OPTN/SRTR 2010 Annual Data Report. Rockville, MD: Department of Health and Human Services, Health Resources and Services Administration, Healthcare Systems Bureau, 2011; Davis CL, Cooper M. The state of U.S. living kidney donors. Clin J Am Soc Nephrol 2010;5:1873–80; Ibrahim HN, Foley R, Tan LP, et al. Long-term consequences of kidney donation. N Engl J Med 2009;360:459–69; Segev DL, Muzaale AD, Caffo BS, et al. Perioperative mortality and long-term survival following live kidney donation. JAMA 2010;303:959–66.

THE EVALUATION PROCESS

The process of donor evaluation, as with the donation procedure itself, must maintain non-maleficence as the primary objective. The medical screening process should promptly identify potentially acceptable donors, quantify the risk to donor and recipient, and exclude unsuitable donors with minimal harm. The rapid determination of unsuitable donors allows new potential donors to be identified. The process should be efficient and cost-effective. The order in which various investigations are undertaken will vary between centers and be influenced by specific medical issues related to donor comorbidities, personal or family history. Further practical considerations such as proximity to the transplant center and availability of the donor to attend evaluation will also influence the order of testing. There have been increasing efforts to standardize and legislate the evaluation processes. The Organ Procurement and Transplant Network (OPTN) was given mandate by the Secretary of Health and Human Services to develop policies and to oversee living kidney donation in 2002. In addition, the transplant organizations continue to expand self-regulatory processes and guidelines to ensure the welfare of the donor. The core components of the evaluation process include: (1) education, counseling, and consent of the donor; (2) psychosocial evaluation; (3) medical evaluation; and (4) review of all results at a multidisciplinary meeting.

Education, Counseling, and Consent of the Potential Donor

Consent should first be given to undergo the evaluation process since this process represents a potential risk to the donor. Invasive medical investigations carry complications such as allergic reactions to injected contrast agents. Information derived from the evaluation may be harmful to or unwanted by the donor, e.g., knowledge gained about unsuspected infections or malignancy. Blood group and human leukocyte antigen (HLA) typing information may uncover misconceptions about family relationships.[42] Potential donors should be carefully educated about all aspects of the evaluation and must understand that they are free to withdraw from the process at any time. The program should be supportive of the donor and defend the confidentiality of donor findings and donor decisions.

The act of obtaining consent for kidney donation is not an event but rather a process. Educating potential living kidney donors about the risks, both operative and long-term, should involve all of the members of the living donor team, including the surgeon, nephrologist, social worker, mental health expert, and living donor advocate. The consenting process should occur over some period of time in order to give the potential donor adequate time to reflect upon these risks and ask questions. It is important to confirm that the donor understands the process clearly and the ability to consent is demonstrated. In this regard it is concerning that a recent study demonstrated that, while 90% of living kidney donors indicated that they understood the impact of living donor transplantation on the recipient's health, the components of the evaluation process, and the short-term risks associated with living kidney donation, a much smaller percentage understood the psychological risks (69%), long-term risks (52%), and financial risks (32%).[39] It is equally concerning that 40% expressed feeling some pressure to donate. Finally it is important to remember that beyond addressing the general issues related to living kidney donation that apply equally to all potential donors, the details of informed consent should be tailored to each individual donor with discussion of how older age, higher BMI, and other comorbidities may be associated with increased risk of early surgical complications or later renal dysfunction. In addition to providing potential donors with national outcome data, transplant programs should provide donors with their own current center-specific outcomes data.

A recent significant change to the process of evaluating potential living kidney donors is the introduction of an independent living donor advocate (ILDA). The inclusion of an ILDA in the evaluation of potential living donors resulted from the recommendations of a group of individuals representing the transplant community who met in 2000. They proposed that all transplant programs performing living donor renal transplants should identify an individual with expertise in transplantation who is not involved in the evaluation of potential recipients and "whose sole focus is on the best interest of the donor." In 2007 the Department of Health and Human Services and the United Network for Organ Sharing (UNOS) issued a joint statement mandating the inclusion of an ILDA as a component of the living donor evaluation process and providing some guidance related to the definition and responsibilities of this position. However there is considerable variability between different programs in the education, training, relationship to the transplant program, and self-identified roles and responsibilities of ILDAs. While variability in the role of the ILDA exists, commonly agreed-upon responsibilities of the ILDA include advocating, protecting, and promoting the interests of the donor, educating the donor, and evaluating the willingness and emotional stability of the donor.[35]

Psychosocial Evaluation

The psychosocial evaluation should be carried out by a trained psychiatrist, psychologist, or social worker with a particular interest and expertise in transplantation. Within the assessment the mental health worker should conduct: (1) a psychological assessment with identification of active mental health problems; (2) a social assessment including high-risk behaviors; and (3) an assessment of the ability of the donor to consent ensuring that the donor's decision is free of inducement or coercion. Information should be gathered from interactions with each member of the evaluation team.

Medical Screening Process

The medical evaluation should include: (1) history and physical examination with specific focus on renal disease and family history of renal disease; (2) laboratory testing to evaluate renal function and determine immunological compatibility; (3) identification of transmissible infectious disease; (4) evaluation of renal anatomy with cross-sectional imaging; and (5) completion of an age-appropriate health screening including cancer screening.[19,26,28]

Components of the evaluation may be carried out at a health center convenient to the potential donor. A detailed history and examination concentrates on symptoms and signs of renal disease, as well as personal and familial risk factors for future problems (Table 7-2). Comorbidities, including hypertension, diabetes, cardiovascular or cerebrovascular disease, must be sought and quantified. Multiple blood pressure readings should be taken and basic laboratory studies performed, including a complete blood count, a comprehensive metabolic profile, a lipid profile, urinalysis, and coagulation studies. A 24-hour urine collection is essential to quantify renal function (creatinine clearance) and assess for proteinuria. Patients with a history of renal stones should undergo appropriate metabolic testing to determine whether they have a physiologic condition that predisposes them to developing recurrent calculi. Further evaluation of diabetes in high-risk donors should include oral glucose tolerance testing and hemoglobin A_{1c} measurement. Similarly, a 24-hour blood pressure study should be completed in those at increased risk of hypertension.

Assessment of the immunologic compatibility of the donor and recipient requires determination of the donor and recipient ABO type as well as performing a crossmatch to detect the presence of donor-specific antibodies in the recipient. Screening of recipients to determine their panel-reactive antibody and assign specificities to antibodies if detected is routinely performed and is critical for interpreting the results of the crossmatch in equivocal cases or when the autologous crossmatch is positive. Similarly, HLA typing of the donor is important for interpreting the results of any positive crossmatch and may be useful in choosing between donors in those cases where there

TABLE 7-2 Components of the Evaluation

History and Physical Examination
Initial interview with specific focus on renal disease and family history of renal disease*
Completion of a detailed health questionnaire*
Donor education and completion of evaluation of consent*
Detailed history and physical examinations by transplant nephrologists and surgeons
Multiple complete vital signs
Detailed evaluation by mental health expert
Interview with independent living donor advocate

Laboratory Testing to Evaluate Renal Function and Determine Immunological Compatibility
Blood pressure – three separate measurements*
Additional 24-hour blood pressure monitoring study as indicated*
24-hour urine collection to quantify creatinine clearance and measure proteinuria*
Oral glucose tolerance test and HbA_{1C} if indicated*
Metabolic workup if previous renal stones*
Donor ABO typing*
Complete blood count with platelet count and differential
Comprehensive metabolic panel to include fasting serum glucose and measurement of transaminases
Fasting lipid profile
Coagulation studies to include the prothrombin time, international normalized ratio, and partial thromboplastin time
Urinalysis and culture
Electrocardiograph
Chest X-ray
Crossmatch performed*
Human leukocyte antigen (HLA) typing of the donor may be done at this time

Identify Transmissible Infectious Disease
Human immunodeficiency virus, hepatitis B and C
Rapid plasma reagin
Testing for tuberculosis (TB) –TB skin testing or QuantiFERON-TB Gold
Testing for *Strongyloides, Trypanosoma cruzi*, and West Nile virus for donors from endemic areas

Evaluation of Renal Anatomy with Cross-Sectional Imaging
Abdominal imaging using computed tomography angiography or magnetic resonance angiography

Age-Appropriate Health Screening, Including Cancer Screening
Prostate-specific antigen (recommendations based on donor age and family history)
Gynecologic examination with Papanicolaou smear
Colonoscopy
Mammogram
Pregnancy test if indicated
Echocardiography and cardiac stress testing as indicated
Pulmonary function studies and computed tomography scanning of the chest as indicated

*May be completed by donor at local hospital before visit to transplant center.

are multiple potential donors. In cases where a donor is determined to be immunologically incompatible with the recipient, alternatives include identifying additional living donors, waiting for a kidney from a deceased organ donor, or considering paired donation and/or desensitization.

The donor must also be evaluated for communicable diseases. Serologic testing for hepatitis B and C as well as human immunodeficiency virus is mandatory. Potential donors who test positive for hepatitis B core antibody and test negative for hepatitis B surface antigen should be tested for evidence of infection by polymerase chain reaction (PCR). If the PCR study shows no evidence of infection and the recipient is immune to hepatitis B, transplantation may proceed after appropriate counseling of the donor and recipient. Screening for tuberculosis (TB) using TB skin testing or an interferon-gamma release assay such as QuantiFERON-TB Gold, although not mandated, is highly recommended, especially in at-risk populations. Donors with a positive test for TB should be treated for 6–9 months before proceeding with kidney donation. In those cases where this delay would pose a significant risk to the recipient or overly complicate the logistics of living kidney donation, proceeding with transplantation and simultaneous treatment of both the donor and recipient is possible, although treatment may complicate the management of the recipient due to the effects of isoniazid on the metabolism of some immunosuppressive drugs. Potential donors should also be screened for syphilis using the rapid plasma reagin test. Donors from Central or South America, individuals who have recently traveled there, or those who previously spent significant amounts of time in these regions should be screened for Chagas' disease. Finally, donors who proceed with donation in spring, summer, or fall months should be screened for acute infection by West Nile virus.

Abdominal imaging is typically performed later in the donor evaluation to reduce cost and minimize the risks of radiation exposure and contrast reactions. The optimal imaging modality remains a source of debate. Angiography, once the mainstay for defining renal anatomy, is now rarely used. In its place computed tomographic angiography (CTA) or magnetic resonance angiography (MRA) is used to evaluate the donor kidneys, define vascular anatomy, and assess donors for other abdominal anomalies or pathology. These imaging modalities are particularly important for assessing anatomic variations affecting the renal arteries, veins, or ureters that are important considerations in determining the suitability of an individual for living kidney donation (Figures 7-1 to 7-4). While magnetic resonance imaging (MRI/MRA) and computer-assisted tomography are thought to be equally accurate for defining renal anatomy and detecting incidental findings that may influence the decision about an individual's suitability to be a living kidney donor, MRA has the advantage of avoiding ionizing radiation and potentially nephrotoxic contrast agents but is much less sensitive for detecting small renal or ureteral stones. In the end the choice of the optimal imaging modality should probably be made based on considerations of local imaging expertise.[12]

Individuals whose test results are compatible with living kidney donation undergo further diagnostic studies and imaging. All donors should be evaluated for cardiovascular disease. Young donors with no significant medical history may require no more than an electrocardiogram. Potential donors greater than 50 years of age or those over 40 with risk factors for coronary artery disease such as tobacco use, hypertension, an abnormal electrocardiogram, or a strong family history of early coronary disease should undergo cardiac stress testing. Potential donors found to have a murmur should undergo echocardiography. Donors with a history of syncope, dizziness,

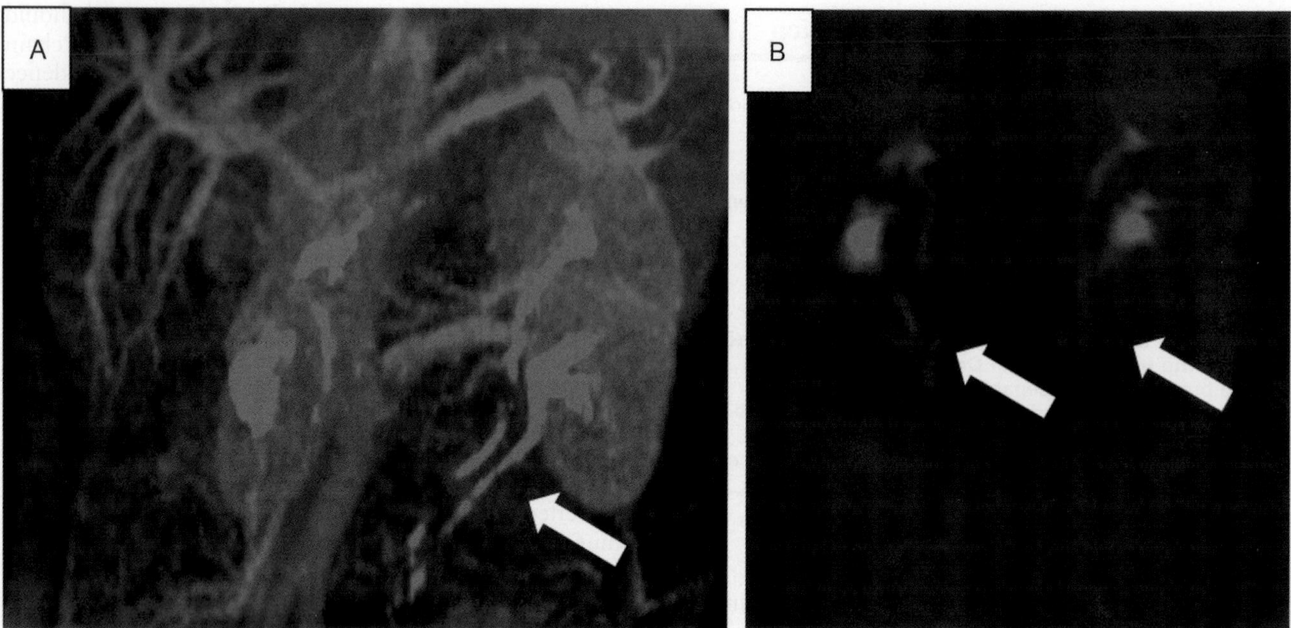

FIGURE 7-1 ■ Duplication of the renal collecting system. (A) Image from a computed tomography angiogram demonstrating a left kidney with duplicated ureters. (B) Magnetic resonance imaging demonstrating duplication of the collecting systems of both the right and left kidneys. Arrows in each panel identify the duplicated ureters.

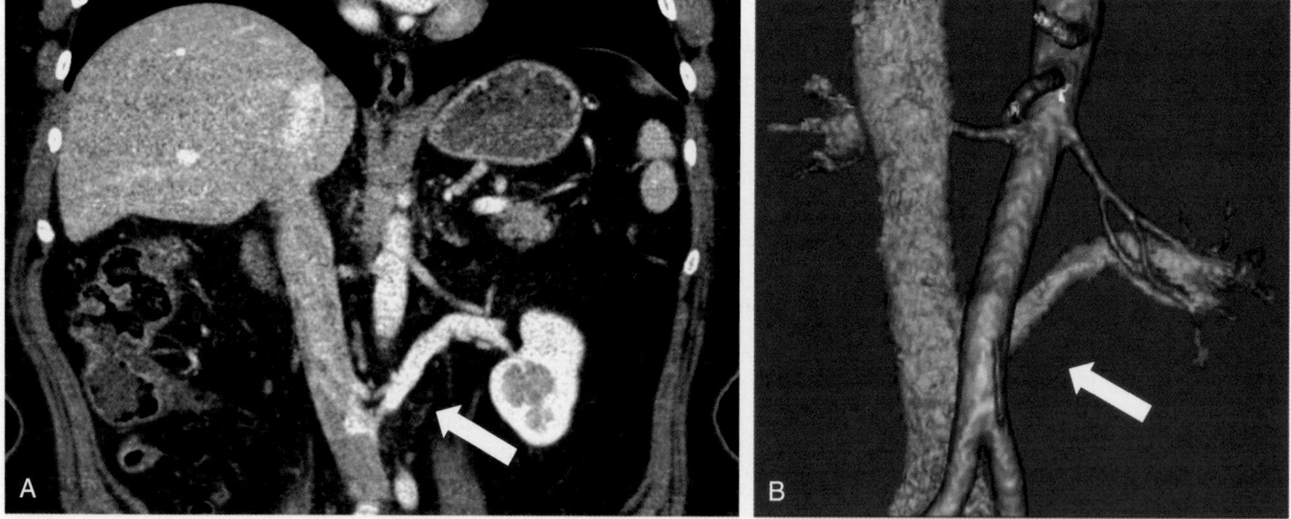

FIGURE 7-2 ■ Renal venous anomalies – retroaortic left renal vein. (A) Image from a computed tomography angiogram demonstrating a retroaortic left renal vein (arrow identifies the retroaortic left renal vein). Note the characteristic inferior course of the retroaortic left renal vein relative to the left renal artery. (B) Reconstructed image clearly demonstrating the left renal vein coursing posterior to the aorta.

or palpitations should undergo both an echocardiogram and Holter monitoring. All potential donors should have a chest X-ray. Those with a history of cigarette smoking or an abnormal chest X-ray may require pulmonary function testing or a chest CT for further evaluation. Cancer screening is completed in accordance with the American Cancer Society guidelines.[34]

Review of All Results at a Multidisciplinary Meeting

Review of the results from the living kidney donor evaluation is completed by a multidisciplinary evaluation committee. This panel should include a nephrologist, surgeon, living donor coordinator, an ILDA, social worker, and/or mental health expert with knowledge about kidney transplantation and donation. This team should be independent of the recipient evaluation to prevent possible conflict of interest. Table 7-3 lists those conditions generally thought to represent absolute and relative contraindications to living kidney donation.

Special Considerations in the Evaluation and Selection of Living Kidney Donors

The goal of the extensive testing that comprises the donor evaluation is to identify any physical or mental health conditions that could potentially increase the

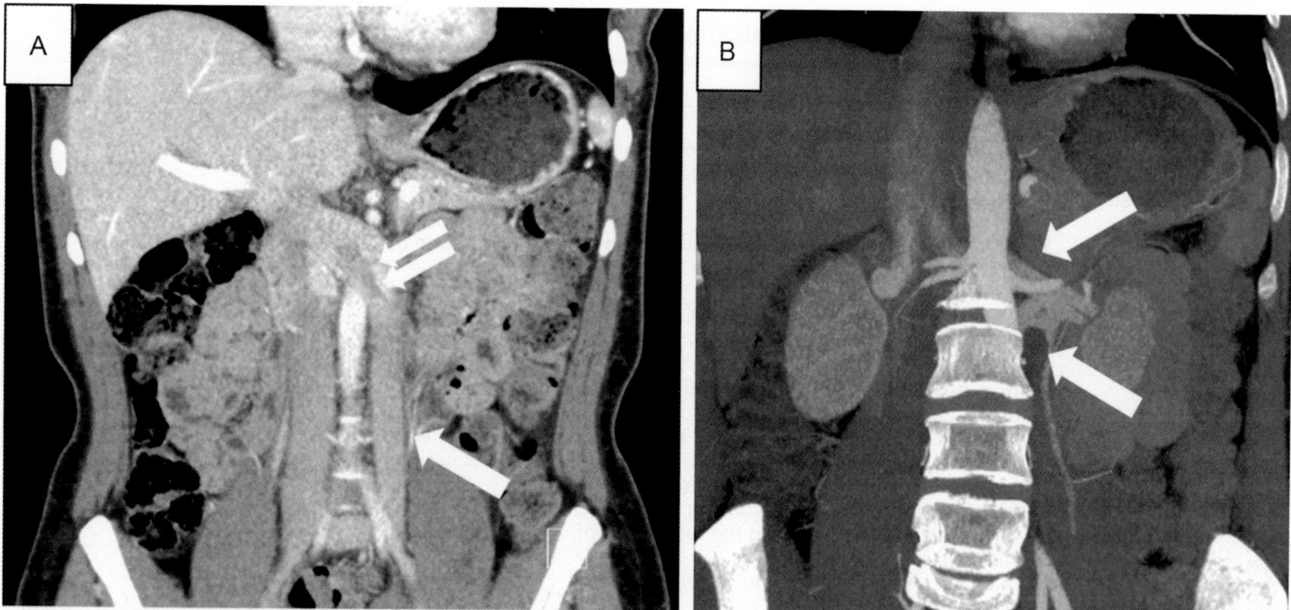

FIGURE 7-3 ■ Renal venous anomalies – duplication of the inferior vena cava and circumaortic left renal vein. (A) Duplication of the inferior vena cava (arrow identifies the duplicated, left-sided inferior vena cava and double arrow demonstrates the left-sided inferior vena cava crossing the aorta to join the main, right-sided inferior vena cava). (B) Circumaortic left renal vein (arrows indicate the component of the left renal vein that cross anterior and posterior to the aorta and the relationship to the left renal artery).

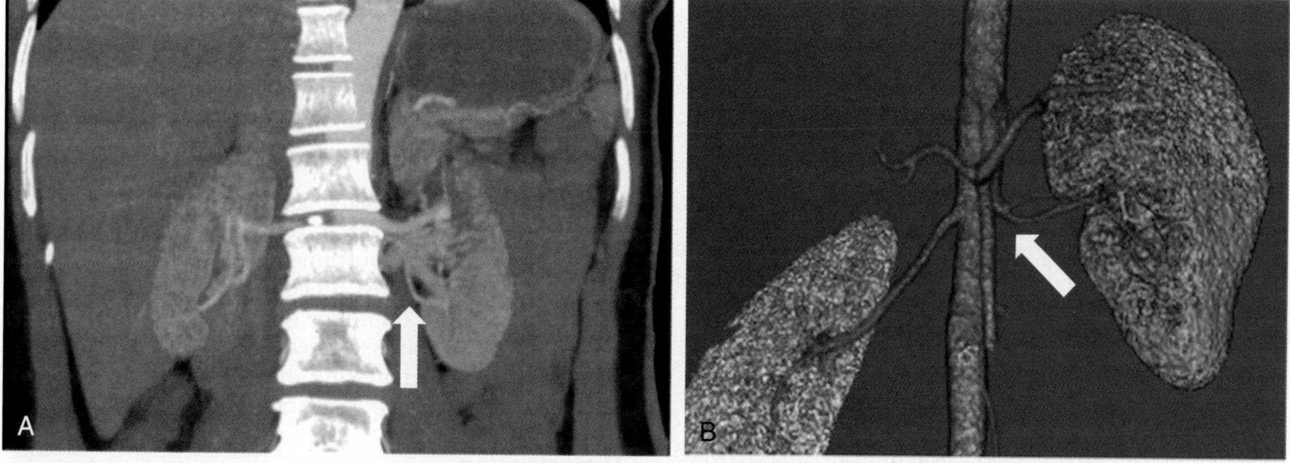

FIGURE 7-4 ■ Anatomic abnormalities of the renal arteries. (A) Left kidney with two renal arteries with a small-caliber lower pole artery arising from the aorta immediately inferior to the main left renal artery (arrow indicates the position of the two renal arteries). (B) Reconstructed image from a computed tomography angiogram demonstrating a left renal artery with an early bifurcation (arrow indicates the larger, superior and smaller, inferior branches of the left renal artery).

operative or long-term risks to the potential living kidney donor or potentially harm the recipient through the transmission of infectious or neoplastic diseases. The often-heard statement is that living kidney donors must be "perfectly healthy" individuals. However, those familiar with living kidney donation realize that this phrase embodies an idealized notion rather than the practical realities of assessing potential living kidney donors. It has been reported that 24.2% of living kidney donors in the United States in the current era have some form of medical abnormality that places them at increased risk of cardiovascular or renal disease in the future.[32] In this study factors that were used to define medically complex donors included obesity (12.8% of donors), hypertension (10.3% of donors), and an estimated glomerular filtration rate (eGFR) of $<60\,mL/min/1.73\,m^2$ (4.2% of donors). Multiple criteria for medical complexity were present in 2.7% of all donors. Interestingly, the proportion of medically complex donors was greatest at large transplant centers and those at which living donor transplants represented a higher proportion of the total transplants performed. This trend toward the use of more medically complex living kidney donors raises the obvious concern that estimates of risk derived from the study of past cohorts, who may have been generally more healthy than donors in the current era, may no longer be accurate. Factors most commonly encountered that contribute to the medical complexity of living kidney donors are: (1) age; (2) hypertension; (3) obesity; (4) impaired glucose tolerance; (5) reduced renal function or previous renal stones; and (6) heritable diseases associated with renal disease.

TABLE 7-3 **Absolute and Relative Contraindications**

	Absolute	Relative
Age	Less than 18 years	Over 65 excluded from many programs
Informed consent	Impaired ability to make an autonomous decision due to mental or psychiatric condition	
Substance abuse	Active substance abuse	Abstinence from substance abuse with documented completion of rehabilitation
Hypertension	Multiple agents or high doses of single agents for control End-organ injury Additional strong risk factors for cardiovascular disease	Borderline or control with single agents
Diabetes	Diabetes mellitus	Impaired glucose tolerance
Obesity	Morbid obesity (BMI >35) or obesity (BMI >30) with comorbid conditions	Obesity
Renal disease	Evidence of renal disease including a reduced creatinine clearance (GFR <80 mL/min), proteinuria (>250 mg), or hematuria	Borderline creatinine clearance, microscopic hematuria
Renal stones	Multiple or recurrent renal calculi of a metabolic condition that predisposes to the recurrence of renal calculi	Single renal stone
Inherited renal disease	ADPKD, SLE, Alport's syndrome, IgA nephropathy	TBMD, mutations in APOL1
Infection	HIV, hepatitis B, hepatitis C, West Nile virus, Chagas' disease	Hepatitis B core antibody
Cancer	Cancer current or treated but at significant risk for recurrence	
Cardiovascular disease	Coronary or peripheral vascular disease Valvular heart disease	
Renal anatomic abnormalities	Significant discrepancy in the kidney sizes	Vascular anomalies (Figures 7-1 to 7-4)

BMI, body mass index; GFR, glomerular filtration rate; ADPKD, adult polycystic kidney disease; SLE, systemic lupus erythematosus; IgA, immunoglobulin A; TBMD, thin basement membrane disease; HIV, human immunodeficiency virus.

Donor Age

While virtually all programs exclude individuals less than 18 years of age from donating, a survey of 132 transplant centers in the United States revealed that 60% of the programs had no upper age limit for living kidney donors. This survey also revealed that only 21% excluded donors over 65 years of age.[19] Consistent with these data, there is a clear trend toward the acceptance of older individuals as living kidney donors. Registry data indicate that between 2000 and 2009 the mean age of living kidney donors increased from 39.6 to 41.3 years of age while the percentage of living kidney donors in the 50–64-year-old age range increased from 18.1% to 25% and the percentage of donors between 18 and 34 years of age declined from 33.2% to 30.3%.[27] These changes may be the result of the increasing age of the recipient population and the effect of this on their pool of potential living donors. In addition there is an increasing caution on the part of many programs related to kidney donation by very young individuals.[19] This caution may arise from concerns about the maturity of these young donors and their ability to make decisions about organ donation autonomously as well as concerns related to their longer expected survival relative to older individuals who may be more mature and who have had more time to demonstrate the stability of their health. With respect to the impact of increasing donor age on the potential complications, despite the intuitive sense that older living kidney donors might be at increased risk, several groups have reported that the perioperative risk is not increased in older living donors.[3,5,10] Similarly, kidney donation does not seem to impact renal function or life expectancy disproportionately in older as compared to younger living donors. In contrast to the lack of effect that donor age has on donor outcomes, advanced donor age does seem to be associated with reduced graft function and survival, suggesting the need to consider donor age when weighing different transplant options.

Hypertension

In the past hypertension was considered an absolute contraindication to kidney donation by most transplant programs. A survey of transplant programs performed in 1995 indicated that 54% of programs would exclude a donor with persistent borderline blood pressures and that 64% would exclude a donor who required a single antihypertensive agent to achieve a normal blood pressure.[6] In contrast, a repeat survey conducted in 2007 indicated that only 36% and 47% of programs excluded donors with persistent borderline blood pressures and one-drug hypertension respectively.[19] While in 1995 no programs indicated that they would consider hypertensive individuals requiring two drugs for control of hypertension, the 2007 survey indicated that a significant number of programs would consider carefully screened individuals taking two medications for hypertension as potential living kidney donors. Most programs that now allow hypertensive individuals to proceed with kidney donation restrict kidney donation in the setting of hypertension to donors older than 45–50 years of age, Caucasian individuals, and those without evidence of end-organ disease as reflected by findings such as left ventricular hypertrophy, proteinuria, or retinopathy. Similarly, hypertensive individuals with additional risk factors for cardiovascular disease such as obesity, smoking, hyperlipidemia, or a strong family history of coronary artery disease should be counseled against proceeding with living kidney donation. Similar considerations are applied by many programs when considering individuals with a history of pre-eclampsia or eclampsia as potential living kidney donors. A further important consideration in this group is the desire to have additional children in the future. The greater flexibility in considering hypertensive individuals for kidney donation is based on the finding that with short- to intermediate-term follow-up well-controlled hypertension in appropriately selected donors has not been shown to worsen blood pressure control after kidney donation or adversely impact renal function relative to non-hypertensive living donors.[36,37]

Obesity

It is well recognized that the prevalence of obesity has been increasing in the United States over the last three decades. Reflecting this trend, the BMI of living kidney donors is increasing. In 2000 14.4% of all living kidney donors were considered obese (BMI >30) whereas by 2008 obesity was noted in 19.5% of living donors.[9] Contrary to the noted trend toward increasing obesity in living kidney donors, there appears to be a greater awareness about the risks of obesity and kidney donation on the part of transplant programs. Data from a 1995 survey revealed that only 16% of programs excluded donors for "moderate" obesity. Similar data from a 2007 survey noted that 52% of programs excluded donors with a BMI >35 and 10% excluded donors with a BMI of >30. The rationale for excluding obese individuals from living kidney donation has less to do with the technical difficulties related to the surgery or perioperative risk and more to do with the long-term potential risks associated with a unilateral nephrectomy in an obese individual. Extensive data suggest an association between obesity and kidney disease, particularly glomerular diseases. Analysis of the Kaiser Permanente database demonstrates an association between increasing degrees of obesity and a time-dependent increase in the risk of developing ESRD.[14] This risk may be increased or accelerated in obese individuals undergoing unilateral nephrectomy for indications other than kidney donation as reflected by an increase in the prevalence of proteinuria and a declining eGFR in individuals with a BMI >30.[29]

Diabetes and Impaired Glucose Tolerance

The American Diabetes Association defines diabetes as a fasting plasma glucose of >126 mg/dL, a plasma glucose of >200 mg/dL 2 hours after a 75 g oral glucose challenge, or a hemoglobin A_{1c} of >6.5. While virtually all transplant programs exclude potential donors with overt diabetes from living kidney donation, the definition of impaired glucose tolerance and the thresholds for excluding donors with abnormal glucose homeostasis are more variable.[19] In the setting of uncertainty or if risk factors for the development of diabetes are present, such as African American race, individuals with a BMI >27, first-degree family members with diabetes, a history of gestational diabetes, or delivery of a child with a birth weight >9 lb (4 kg), many programs obtain a 2-hour oral glucose tolerance test to provide more information about the future risk of developing diabetes. Additional studies considered useful by some centers include measurement of hemoglobin A_{1c} and anti-islet antibodies in potential donors with a strong family history of diabetes. Careful attention to the fasting lipid profile is also very helpful. While hyperlipidemia as an isolated abnormality is rarely considered to be an exclusion criterion for living kidney donation, dyslipidemia in the setting of impaired glucose tolerance and obesity constitutes the metabolic syndrome and is associated with an increased risk of developing overt diabetes and cardiovascular disease in the future. While there is no definitive evidence linking living kidney donation to an increase in the future morbidity and mortality of individuals with the metabolic syndrome, it is reasonable to exclude these individuals from living kidney donation based on the known health risks associated with the metabolic syndrome in the general population.

Reduced Renal Function

Somewhat surprisingly, a retrospective review of data collected by the organ procurement and transplantation network demonstrated that 4.2% of all living kidney donors had an eGFR of <60 mL/min/1.73 m^2.[32] It is not obvious how this can be reconciled with the survey data indicating that the majority of programs exclude donors with a GFR of <80 mL/min/1.73 m^2.[19] One possibility is that the concordance of the eGFR and the measured GFR is less than perfect. The majority of programs (approximately 90%) make use of a 24-hour urine collection in order to determine the GFR, with most of the rest of the programs using methods based upon either radioactive isotopes or iodinated tracers. Increasingly, programs are adopting more stringent criteria related to the renal function of potential living kidney donors, with some programs utilizing 90 mL/min/1.73 m^2 in order to preclude living kidney donation by individuals with stage II chronic kidney disease, defined as a GFR of 60–89 mL/min/1.73 m^2, while other programs require that living kidney donors have a GFR within two standard deviations of the mean GFR for age-matched individuals. Regardless of the methodology used, determination of GFR is somewhat imprecise, with repeated measures frequently yielding significantly different results. It is therefore important to consider other important findings that may be associated with or predictive of renal diseases. Proteinuria is perhaps one of the best predictors for the development of kidney disease. Significant proteinuria, defined as excretion of >180 mg of protein per day, requires further evaluation. In this setting determination of the albumin to creatinine ratio on a spot urine sample may be useful in distinguishing significant from non-significant proteinuria. Excretion of >250 mg of protein per day in the urine is almost always considered significant and excludes living kidney donation in all except those with a documented benign cause of proteinuria such as postural proteinuria. Hematuria is another finding that may indicate significant underlying renal pathology. The finding of hematuria, defined as >3–5 red blood cells per high-power field, requires further evaluation. Excluding females who are menstruating, first steps in the evaluation of hematuria should include a urine culture and abdominal imaging to assess for the presence of an occult urinary tract infection or renal calculus. A history of frequent urinary tract infections should prompt a urologic evaluation to include urodynamic studies and cystoscopy in order to exclude an anatomic factor that predisposes the potential donor to recurrent urinary tract infections. Most programs now allow individuals with a history of kidney stones to proceed with organ donation, assuming that stones are not currently present and that the workup for metabolic conditions that predispose to the formation of stones is negative. Extra caution is warranted in individuals with a history of multiple episodes of kidney stones. In patients who do not have evidence of a urinary tract infection or kidney stone as the cause of persistent hematuria, cystoscopy and a renal biopsy would be indicated. Many programs now consider individuals with persistent microscopic hematuria to be acceptable candidates for kidney donation if the urologic evaluation and renal biopsy do not reveal a significant underlying disease. Finally, in those potential renal donors with borderline low renal function, abdominal imaging is very important to assess the appearance of the kidneys. Significant discrepancy in the sizes of the kidneys, evidence of cortical atrophy, the presence of numerous renal cysts, or vascular abnormalities such as renal artery stenosis or fibromuscular dysplasia would all be indicative of underlying disease processes that would preclude living kidney donation.

Heritable Diseases Associated with Renal Pathology

In cases where the intended recipient of a kidney from a closely related living donor has a known heritable condition as the cause of ESRD or for those potential living donors with a strong family history of kidney diseases or failure, the possibility that the donor may also have a heritable disease that could result in kidney injury or failure must be considered. In this setting it may be necessary to perform genetic testing and a renal biopsy in addition to the standard elements of the living donor evaluation to exclude the presence of a heritable disease that could result in renal injury. Relatively common renal diseases with a genetic component include adult polycystic kidney disease (ADPKD), systemic lupus erythematosus (SLE), thin basement membrane disease (TBMD), Alport's syndrome, and IgA nephropathy.

ADPKD is the most common of the heritable renal diseases and is the fourth leading cause of ESRD. It exists in two forms resulting from two distinct genetic mutations. PKD1 accounts for 85% of all individuals with ADPKD and is a consequence of a mutation in chromosome 16. PKD2 is less common, affecting 15% of individuals with ADPKD; it may manifest itself later in life, and results from a mutation in chromosome 4. ADPKD may be excluded in individuals greater than 30 years of age if high-resolution cross-sectional abdominal imaging does not demonstrate cysts within the kidneys. For individuals less than 30 who are considering living kidney donation and have a family history of ADPKD, genetic testing is required. This is greatly facilitated by knowing the mutation responsible for ADPKD in the affected relative(s).

SLE may develop in approximately 12% of individuals with an affected first-degree relative. Evaluation of potential living kidney donors with a first-degree relative with known SLE should include studies to detect antinuclear antibodies, antiphospholipid antibodies, and measurement of complement levels. Potential donors in whom the results of these studies suggest a risk for the development of SLE should be educated about this risk and counseled that they are not appropriate candidates for living kidney donation.

Heritable kidney diseases that manifest themselves through hematuria include IgA nephropathy, Alport's syndrome, and TBMD. IgA nephropathy usually presents with episodic gross hematuria that may or may not be associated with persistent microscopic hematuria. A renal biopsy demonstrating meningeal proliferation and IgA deposits is diagnostic and would be cause to exclude the affected individual from living kidney donation given the 25–30% incidence of eventual progression to ESRD. Alport's syndrome results from mutations in genes related to collagen biosynthesis. Alterations in type IV collagen result in characteristic findings affecting the eye, cochlea, and kidney and include cataracts and retinal lesions, sensorineural hearing loss, and hematuria. Although there are different modes of inheritance, most are X-linked, making the disease more severe in males by virtue of their single X chromosome. Males in affected families who are over the age of 20 years of age and have none of the manifestations of Alport's syndrome may proceed to kidney donation, as may females with normal urinary studies. TBMD is another cause of asymptomatic hematuria. Unlike hematuria related to IgA nephropathy and Alport's syndrome, TBMD is not usually associated with progressive renal dysfunction. If the diagnoses of IgA nephropathy and Alport's syndrome can be excluded, individuals who have microscopic hematuria without evidence of severe thinning of their basement membranes on renal biopsy can be considered as acceptable kidney donors, although they should be counseled that the long-term consequences of kidney donation in the setting of TBMD remain incompletely understood.

The incidence of ESRD following living kidney donation is rare in all racial and ethnic groups but is more common in African American donors as compared to Caucasian donors.[16] This raises the possibility that genetic variations may contribute to the risk of developing ESRD following living kidney donation. Consistent with this hypothesis, mutations in a gene on chromosome 22 that encodes APOL1 have been associated with an increased risk of focal segmental glomerulosclerosis in African Americans. Mutant forms of the APOL1 gene, termed G1 and G2, occur in nearly one-third of all African Americans without known kidney disease and two-thirds of those with chronic kidney disease. Evolutionary pressures that select for this gene are related to the protective effects of a single copy of the gene against fatal infections by the *Trypanosoma* parasite responsible for "sleeping sickness." However, two mutated copies of the at-risk mutations result in a twofold increase in the risk of ESRD. Based upon the frequency of these mutations in the African American population and their strong association with ESRD, some practitioners and programs now recommend prospective screening of all potential African American living kidney donors.[8] However, given the lack of data demonstrating the impact of this mutation on the outcomes of living kidney donors as well as the potential implications for an already disadvantaged group, many transplant professionals counsel further study before recommending the widespread adoption of routine screening for APOL1 mutations as an exclusion criterion for potential living kidney donors.

Special Considerations Pertaining to Non-directed Living Kidney Donors and Donors Participating in Paired Donor Exchange Programs

While the absolute contraindications to living kidney donation apply equally to all potential donors, the relative contraindications must be considered in light of the relative "benefit" to the donor. The observation that an increasing percentage of living kidney donors are not related to their recipients raises the possibility that the emotional benefit associated with living donation may be reduced for these more distantly or even unrelated donors. This may be particularly true for non-directed, altruistic donors who may never meet their recipient. Each of these factors needs to be considered in discussing the risk-to-benefit ratio with prospective living donors. Based on considerations of this nature many programs apply the selection criteria more stringently to non-directed donors in comparison to donors who are closely related to their intended recipient. Similarly, the growth of transplants performed in the setting of desensitization programs or paired donor exchange (PDE) programs may significantly alter the anticipated outcomes of living donor kidney transplantation. Recipients who undergo desensitization are generally at increased risk of immune-mediated graft injury and complications related to the desensitization regimen and the intensified immunosuppression required. In some circumstances it may be expected that the intermediate and long-term graft survival of recipients undergoing desensitization will be inferior to that of recipients without pre-existing sensitization to the donor.[4,20] While difficult to quantify in an absolute sense on an individual basis, potential donors should be educated about the potential to obtain an inferior result so that they can make an informed decision about whether or not they wish to proceed. Participation in PDE programs also poses some unique considerations for educating and evaluating potential living donors. The unique considerations related to participation in PDE programs relate primarily to logistic and organizational issues. In the setting of traditional living donor kidney transplantation the donor and recipient are free to choose a date that best fits their medical need but also takes into consideration other factors such as those related to employment, travel, and family commitments. In the setting of transplants performed through PDE programs the wishes and needs of the other donor/recipient pairs may limit the freedom to choose a preferred date for surgery. In practice, exchange transplants are usually scheduled for the earliest logistically feasible date, giving donors and their recipients less time to make arrangements with their employers, family, and friends who will provide support during their convalescence. Finally, as donors and recipients remain unknown to each other in PDE programs there may be concerns on the part of some individuals related to the incomplete knowledge of the other participating pair(s). Specifically, uncertainty may exist with respect to the other pair's medical histories and the equivalency of the kidneys being exchanged. PDE offers a significant benefit to recipients whose only potential donors are incompatible but does require that the transplant team fully educate the donor and recipient about these types of unique considerations.

Long-term Follow-up of Living Kidney Donors

Living donor kidney transplantation has been practiced for nearly six decades and the number of individuals who have donated a kidney for transplantation is estimated to exceed 120000. Thus it would seem obvious that the risks and consequences of living kidney donation would be known in exacting detail. This is generally true for the operative risks associated with living kidney donation due to the mandatory reporting of living donor deaths and major complications requiring surgical intervention in the early postoperative period. However, there is substantially more uncertainty with respect to the long-term impact of living kidney donation on the donor's medical, psychosocial, and fiscal health. Several recent reports suggest that living kidney donation is not associated with a measurable increase in the risks of death, renal disease, or renal failure compared to the general population or cohorts of self-identified healthy individuals matched for variables such as age, gender, race, and ethnicity.[15,16,33] However, many of the studies cited as evidence that living kidney donation is associated with extremely low long-term risks to the donor are by necessity examining patients who donated in the relatively distant past. As already discussed, the medical complexity of living kidney donors has increased significantly and continues to increase relative to donors from previous eras. Furthermore, the introduction of new surgical techniques such as robotic donor nephrectomy and laparoendoscopic single-site donor nephrectomy may be associated with operative risks that are qualitatively or quantitatively different. The only means of providing potential living kidney donors with an accurate prediction of the operative and long-term risks of living donation is to consider the long-term follow-up of living donors to be a critical component of the living kidney donation.

Despite the reassurance provided by the numerous studies reporting the generally excellent long-term health of living kidney donors, it must be acknowledged that all studies to date suffer from the lack of a control population that accurately mirrors the excellent health status of living kidney donors. Perhaps the best approach to assessing the impact of living kidney donation on long-term donor health would be to compare medically suitable individuals who were approved to donate but did not proceed with donation to approved individuals who proceeded with kidney donation. While this approach has obvious merit, studies employing this design have proven difficult for a variety of reasons. Additional challenges to studies aimed at defining the long-term risks of living kidney donation are related to the very low incidence of major, donation-related adverse events and the observation that the adverse consequences of living kidney donation usually occur years to decades after donor nephrectomy. Consequently, to be informative, studies of the long-term risks of living kidney donation would need to follow large numbers of individuals over a period of 20–30 years.

Irrespective of the logistic and financial barriers, numerous studies aimed at defining the risks of living kidney donation are in progress.[18] Several of these major initiatives are summarized below.

1. Assessing Long-Term Outcomes of Living kidney Donation (ALTOLD) – an eight-center, 36-month study of renal, cardiovascular, and bone mineral outcomes in 200 living donors and 200 matched control individuals.
2. Renal and Lung Living Donors Evaluation (RELIVE) – a study of 8951 living kidney donors utilizing national databases to assess vital status, occurrence of ESRD, and death. Subsets of patients will be examined to quantify renal function and determine the presence of cardiovascular disease.
3. Kidney Donor Outcomes Cohort (KDOC) study (ClinicalTrials.gov identifier NCT01427452) – a seven-center, 24-month study of surgical, medical, functional, and psychological outcomes in 280 living kidney donors, 280 recipients of living donor kidneys, and 160 healthy individuals for comparison.
4. Long-term Effects of Becoming a Living Kidney Donor study (ClinicalTrials.gov identifier NCT00936078) – a study conducted largely in Canada of 600 individuals, including previous living kidney donors and healthy comparison subjects identified by the donor. These groups will be compared with respect to long-term medical, psychosocial, and financial conditions.
5. Live Kidney Donor Study – Cross-Sectional and Historical Cohort Study (ClinicalTrials.gov identifier NCT00951977) – a study utilizing national databases to compare 7864 previous living kidney donors to 2500 control subjects. Variables to be assessed include the incidence of hypertension, proteinuria, renal disease, anemia, cardiovascular disease, and stroke. Quality of life and insurance status will also be assessed.

Regardless of the barriers to collecting reliable and complete outcomes following living kidney donation, the benefits in terms of providing those considering living kidney donation adequate information upon which to base their decision is intuitively obvious. While many question the mechanism(s) by which these data are to be obtained, none question the need to gather this information or the moral imperative of the transplant community to participate vigorously in this effort. Consistent with this sense of responsibility, the UNOS Board of Directors recently accepted a series of recommendations from the Living Donor Committee to mandate that transplant centers must collect and report selected clinical and laboratory data for living kidney donors at 6, 12, and 24 months following donation. The board of directors also accepted recommendations that set acceptable thresholds for data completeness and reporting in order to be in compliance.

SUMMARY

Although much has changed in living kidney donation, the primary goals of ensuring donor health and wellness while still affording recipients the benefit of living donor renal transplantation remain unchanged. The changing health status of the donor population together with the continued evolution of the processes and procedures of living donation provide new challenges that require that the transplant community continually reassess the risks of living kidney donation and develop new policies and procedures to safeguard living donors. Central to the process of minimizing the risk to living kidney donors is the thoroughness of the medical and psychosocial evaluation and the rigor of the process to insure informed consent by the donor. To this end the donor evaluation process is increasingly complex as the medical, demographic, and psychosocial features of living donors change. Despite these challenges the careful evaluation of potential living donors continues to provide patients with ESRD the benefits of living donor renal transplantation while simultaneously exposing the donor to low risks.

REFERENCES

1. Ad Hoc Committee. A definition of irreversible coma. Report of the Ad Hoc committee of the Harvard medical school to examine the definition of brain death. JAMA 1968;205:337–40.
2. Axelrod DA, McCullough KP, Brewer ED, et al. Kidney and pancreas transplantation in the United States, 1999–2008: the changing face of living donation. Am J Transplant 2010;10:987–1002.
3. Balachandran VP, Aull MJ, Charlton M, et al. Kidneys from older living donors provide excellent intermediate-term outcomes after transplantation. Transplantation 2012;94:499–505.
4. Bentall A, Cornell LD, Gloor JM, et al. Five-year outcomes in living donor kidney transplants with a positive crossmatch. Am J Transplant 2013;13:76–85.
5. Berger JC, Muzaale AD, James N, et al. Living kidney donors ages 70 and older: recipient and donor outcomes. Clin J Am Soc Nephrol 2011;6:2887–93.
6. Bia MJ, Ramos EL, Danovitch GM, et al. Evaluation of living renal donors. The current practice of US transplant centers. Transplantation 1995;60:322–7.
7. Bratton C, Chavin K, Baliga P. Racial disparities in organ donation and why. Curr Opin Organ Transplant 2011;16:243–9.
8. Cohen DM, Mittalhenkle A, Scott DL, et al. African American living-kidney donors should be screened for APOL1 risk alleles. Transplantation 2011;92:722–5.
9. Davis CL, Cooper M. The state of U.S. living kidney donors. Clin J Am Soc Nephrol 2010;5:1873–80.
10. Dols LFC, Kok NFM, Roodnat JI, et al. Living kidney donors: impact of age on long-term safety. Am J Transplant 2011;11:737–42.
11. Eng M, Zhang J, Cambon A, et al. Employment outcomes following successful renal transplantation. Clin Transplant 2012;26:242–6.
12. Gluecker TM, Mayr M, Schwarz J, et al. Comparison of CT angiography with MR angiography in the preoperative assessment of living kidney donors. Transplantation 2008;86:1249–56.

13. Gordon EJ. Informed consent for living donation: a review of key empirical studies, ethical challenges and future research. Am J Transplant 2012;12:2273–80.
14. Hsu CY, McCulloch CE, Iribarren C, et al. Body mass index and risk for end-stage renal disease. Ann Intern Med 2006;144:21–8.
15. Ibrahim HN, Foley R, Tan LP, et al. Long-term consequences of kidney donation. N Engl J Med 2009;360:459–69.
16. Lentine KL, Schnitzler MA, Xiao H, et al. Racial variation in medical outcomes among living kidney donors. N Engl J Med 2010;363:724–32.
17. Levey AS, Danovitch G, Hou S. Living donor kidney transplantation in the United States – looking back, looking forward. Am J Kidney Dis 2011;58:343–8.
18. Living Kidney Donor Follow-Up Conference Writing Group. Living kidney donor follow-up: state-of-the-art and future directions, conference summary and recommendations. Am J Transplant 2011;11:2561–8.
19. Mandelbrot DA, Pavlakis M, Danovitch GM, et al. The medical evaluation of living kidney donors: a survey of US transplant centers. Am J Transplant 2007;7:2333–43.
20. Marfo K, Lu A, Ling M, et al. Desensitization protocols and their outcome. Clin J Am Soc Nephrol 2011;6:922–36.
21. Meier-Kriesche HU, Kaplan B. Waiting time on dialysis as the strongest modifiable risk factor for renal transplant outcomes: a paired donor kidney analysis. Transplantation 2002;74:1377–81.
22. Meier-Kriesche HU, Schold JD, Srinivas TR, et al. Kidney transplantation halts cardiovascular disease progression in patients with end-stage renal disease. Am J Transplant 2004;4:1662–8.
23. Murray JE. Ronald Lee Herrick Memorial: June 15, 1931–December 27, 2010. Am J Transplant 2011;11:419.
24. Murray JE. Surgery of the soul: reflections on a curious career. Boston, MA: Boston Medical Library; 2001.
25. Nogueira JM, Weir MR, Jacobs S, et al. A study of renal outcomes in obese living kidney donors. Transplantation 2010;90:993–9.
26. OPTN Guidance for the Development of Program-specific Living Donor Medical Evaluation Protocols. Available online at http://optn.transplant.hrsa.gov/ContentDocuments/Guidance_ProgramSpecificLivingKidneyDonorMedEvalProtocols.pdf.
27. OPTN/SRTR 2010 annual data report. Rockville, MD: Department of Health and Human Services, Health Resources and Services Administration, Healthcare Systems Bureau; 2011.
28. Pham PC, Wilkinson AH, Pham PT. Evaluation of the potential living kidney donor. Am J Kidney Dis 2007;50:1043–51.
29. Praga M, Hernandez E, Herrero JC, et al. Influence of obesity on the appearance of proteinuria and renal insufficiency after unilateral nephrectomy. Kidney Int 2000;58:2111–8.
30. Ratner LE, Ciseck LJ, Moore RG, et al. Laparoscopic live donor nephrectomy. Transplantation 1995;60:1047–9.
31. Ratner LE, Kavoussi LR, Schulam PG, et al. Comparison of laparoscopic live donor nephrectomy versus the standard open approach. Transplant Proc 1997;29:138–9.
32. Reese PP, Feldman HI, McBride MA, et al. Substantial variation in the acceptance of medically complex live kidney donors across US renal transplant centers. Am J Transplant 2008;8:2062–70.
33. Segev DL, Muzaale AD, Caffo BS, et al. Perioperative mortality and long-term survival following live kidney donation. JAMA 2010;303:959–66.
34. Smith RA, Cokkinides V, Brawley OW. Cancer screening in the United States, 2012: a review of current American Cancer Society guidelines and current issues in cancer screening. CA Cancer J Clin 2012;62:129–42.
35. Steel J, Dunlavy A, Friday M, et al. A national survey of independent living donor advocates: the need for practice guidelines. Am J Transplant 2012;12:2141–9.
36. Tent H, Sanders JFS, Rook M, et al. Effects of preexistent hypertension on blood pressure and residual renal function after donor nephrectomy. Transplantation 2012;93:412–7.
37. Textor S, Taler S. Expanding criteria for living kidney donors: what are the limits? Transplant Rev 2008;22:187–91.
38. US Department of Health and Human Services. Organ procurement and transplantation network; 2012. Available online at: http://optn.transplant.hrsa.gov/ [accessed 12.01.12].
39. Valapour M, Kahn JP, Bailey RF, et al. Assessing elements of informed consent among living donors. Clin Transplant 2011;25:185–90.
40. Wolf Jr JS, Merion RM, Leichtman AB, et al. Randomized controlled trial of hand-assisted laparoscopic versus open surgical live donor nephrectomy. Transplantation 2001;72:284–90.
41. Wolfe RA, Ashby VB, Milford EL, et al. Comparison of mortality in all patients on dialysis, patients on dialysis awaiting transplantation, and recipients of a first cadaveric transplant. N Engl J Med 1999;341:1725–30.
42. Young A, Kim SH, Gibney EM, et al. Discovering misattributed paternity in living kidney donation: prevalence, preference, and practice. Transplantation 2009;87:1429–35.

CHAPTER 8

DONOR NEPHRECTOMY

 Rolf N. Barth

CHAPTER OUTLINE

DECEASED DONOR NEPHRECTOMY

Deceased donor renal donation remains the predominant source of transplantable kidneys. In the United States, deceased donors provide approximately 12 000 kidneys per year or two-thirds of the available pool of transplantable kidneys (Figure 8-1).[27] Deceased donors are divided into subgroups of donation after brain death (DBD) and donation after cardiac death (DCD). DBD donors are pronounced dead by both clinical and radiological evaluations that vary by institution. The operations from these donors are conducted in controlled settings with careful physiologic monitoring to ensure optimal organ perfusion and oxygenation until perfusion and cooling of donor organs. DBD donors accounted for 88% of donors in 2009 and, while total numbers have increased over the last decade, the proportion of DBD donors decreased from 2000 when DBD donors provided 97% of deceased donor kidneys.[27] Both DBD and DCD kidneys are further differentiated as either standard criteria donors (SCD) or extended criteria donors (ECD) depending if the donor is either 60 years old or older, or if a donor is 50–59 years old with the presence of at least two of the following: hypertension, death from cerebrovascular accident, or terminal creatinine higher than 1.5 mg/dL. While total proportions of SCD and ECD donors have remained fairly stable over the last decade, the contribution of DCD donors has become increasingly important (Figure 8-2).

DONATION AFTER BRAIN DEATH

Kidneys from DBD donors are usually recovered in conjunction with recovery of other abdominal and thoracic organs and require coordination of the surgical teams performing different roles (Figure 8-3). The abdominal cavity is opened and isolation and control of the infra-abdominal aorta are accomplished. In cases where the liver is recovered, isolation of either the inferior mesenteric vein or portal vein can also be achieved. The aorta is cannulated after administering heparin, and in appropriate cases venous cannulation is performed. In coordination with thoracic recovery, perfusion is initiated, the aorta is clamped in a supraceliac location, and either the inferior vena cava or right atrium is transected and suction or drainage devices are placed to facilitate perfusion. The abdominal organs are packed with ice for cooling while flushing and recovery of other organs are performed. Mobilization of the ascending and descending colon can be performed to allow for direct exposure of the kidneys to ice. Recovery of thoracic organs, liver, and pancreas generally precedes recovery of the kidneys.

Recovery of the kidneys can be performed either individually or en bloc. Individual recovery of the kidneys is performed by transecting the left renal vein at the vena cava. The aorta and vena cava can both be transected inferiorly at the level of cannulation (usually just superior to bifurcation) and at a superior level of the superior mesenteric artery (SMA) and right renal vein. Division of the aorta should be performed by incising the base of the SMA and with an oblique angle entering the aorta superior to identify renal arteries as they often enter close to this level. Superior transection of the aorta should be performed to ideally preserve a Carrel patch on both the right and left renal arteries. The right renal vein should be identified prior to transection of the vena cava to preserve a superior cuff that can be used to reconstruct a venous extension when necessary.

Individual recovery starts with either side by isolating the ureter and gonadal vein and transecting distally. Care should be taken to leave tissue around the ureter with sharp dissection, so as to minimize the risk of devascularizing the ureter by stripping it of adjacent tissues. The anterior wall of the aorta can be longitudinally sharply

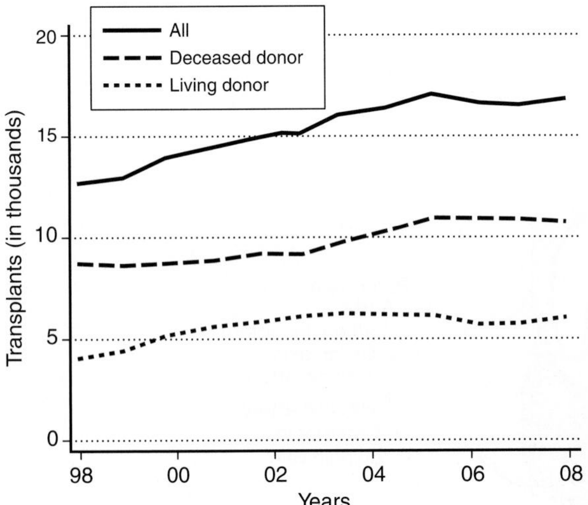

FIGURE 8-1 ■ Transplanted kidneys in the United States, 1998–2009. Increases in total numbers of both deceased and living donor kidneys have been recognized. Living donor kidney numbers have been stable in more recent years compared to an increased number of deceased donor organs, especially from donation after cardiac death (DCD) donors. (From Organ Procurement and Transplantation Network (OPTN) and Scientific Registry of Transplant Recipients (SRTR). OPTN / SRTR 2010 Annual Data Report. Rockville, MD: Department of Health and Human Services, Health Resources and Services Administration, Healthcare Systems Bureau, Division of Transplantation; 2011.)

transected, followed by division of the posterior wall and with care taken to identify single or multiple renal arteries and leave sufficient tissue for Carrel patches around each vessel. From an inferior approach working from the midline and posterior to the aorta, all tissues can be sharply divided with attention to the location of the ureter to avoid inadvertent injury. Working both superiorly and laterally the vasculature and kidneys can be separated from the abdominal and retroperitoneal attachments. Preference to more posterior dissection in the psoas muscle will minimize the risk of injuring renal arteries. Regardless of extent, Gerota's fascia should be removed with the kidneys to be separated at a later time. The right kidney should be removed with all remaining vena cava to preserve a conduit for venous extension grafts when necessary.

En bloc recovery of the kidneys is performed without longitudinal transection of the aorta or division of the renal vein. Inferior to superior dissection is performed posterior to the aorta and vena cava, and with initial isolation of the ureters to avoid injury. Separation of the kidneys is then performed after removal with the similar goals of leaving aortic cuff for all renal arteries and the vena cava with the right kidney.

If concerns exist for the quality of perfusion based on the appearance of the kidneys, direct cannulation and perfusion of the right and left renal arteries can be performed on the back table. While this step is not always necessary, concern regarding poor perfusion or mottled appearance of the kidneys can direct additional flushing.

DONATION AFTER CARDIAC DEATH

While in total numbers DBD donors account for the majority of recovered and transplanted kidneys, DCD has become an increasingly common source of deceased donor kidneys in recent years. In the United States in 2009, DCD donors yielded more kidneys per donor (1.9) than either SCD (1.8) or ECD (1.6).[27]

Recovery of kidneys from DCD donors is performed in a similar manner to brain-dead donors with few modifications. Individual hospitals and organ procurement organizations set specific guidelines for time limits for recovery to be performed after withdrawal of life support that vary between 60 and 120 minutes. These waiting periods occur either in a preoperative setting or in the operating room. According to local practice, patients are declared deceased after cessation of pulse,

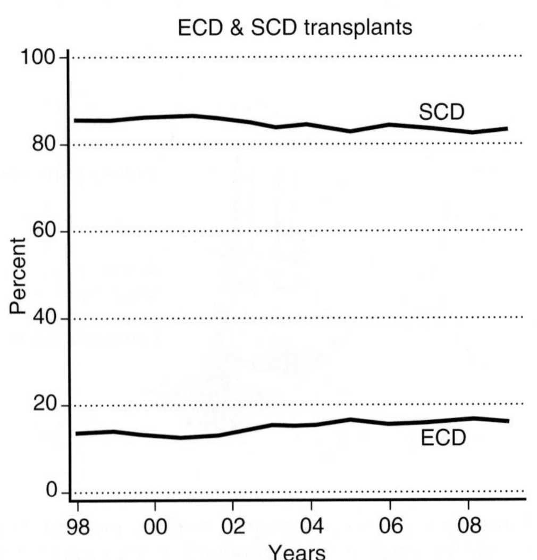

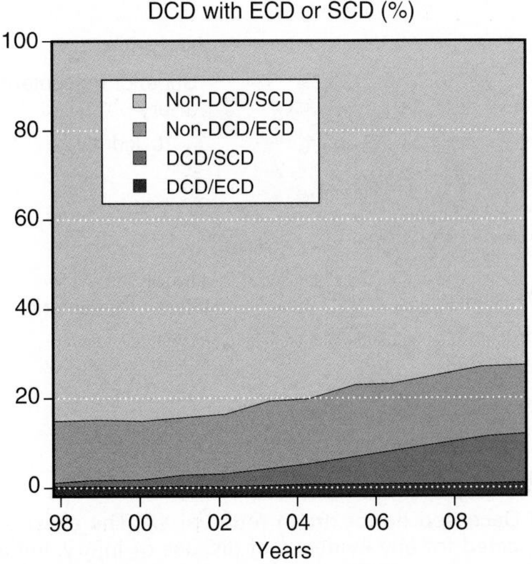

FIGURE 8-2 ■ Kidneys transplants by donor type, 1998–2009. The ratio of transplanted kidneys from standard criteria donors (SCDs) and extended criteria donors (ECDs) have demonstrated little change since 2000 (left); however, the contribution of donation after cardiac death (DCD) donors has become an increasing source of transplantable kidneys, accounting for over 10% of deceased donor kidneys. (From Organ Procurement and Transplantation Network (OPTN) and Scientific Registry of Transplant Recipients (SRTR). OPTN/SRTR 2010 Annual Data Report. Rockville, MD: Department of Health and Human Services, Health Resources and Services Administration, Healthcare Systems Bureau, Division of Transplantation; 2011.)

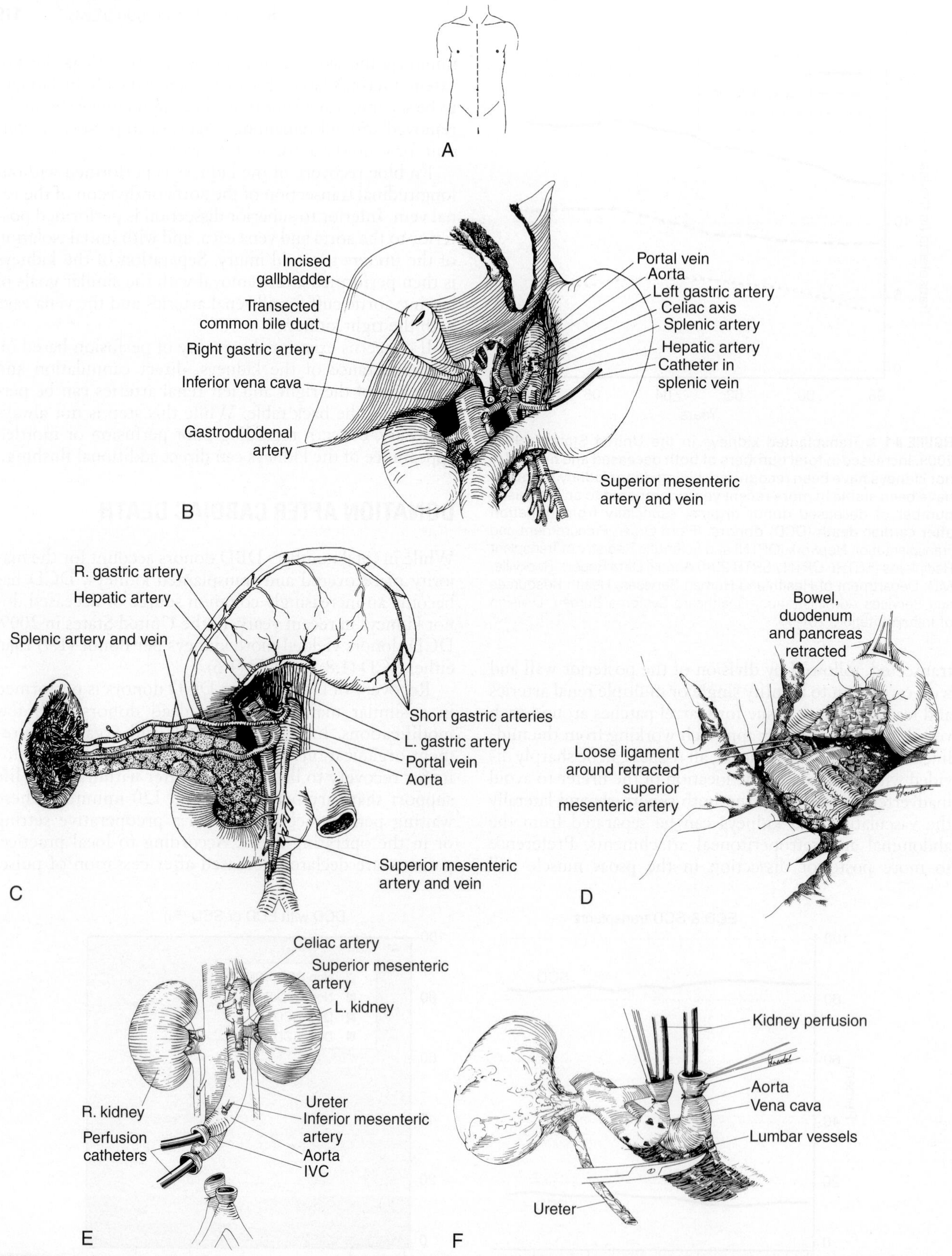

FIGURE 8-3 ■ Deceased donor organ retrieval. (A) The chest and abdomen are opened through a midline incision. The abdominal cavity is inspected for any evidence of disease or injury. Initial control of the distal aorta is obtained in the case that urgent flushing becomes necessary. (B) The splenic vein is catheterized through the inferior mesenteric vein for portal perfusion. Limited portal dissection with distal ligation of the common bile duct and incision and flushing of the gallbladder. (C) Pancreas dissection can be performed by division of the short gastric vessels and medial visceral rotation of the spleen and pancreas in a plane posterior to the splenic vein and artery. (D) The duodenum should be widely mobilized allowing for access to the superior mesenteric artery and infrahepatic vena cava. (E) The distal aorta is cannulated with a perfusion catheter after heparinization and drainage devices may be placed in the distal vena cava. IVC, inferior vena cava. (F) Aortic crossclamp is performed in the supraceliac location and perfusion and cooling with ice are performed. After removal of thoracic organs, liver, and pancreas, kidney dissection is commenced. Additional attention should be directed to preserving ureteral length and aortic cuff around the origin of single or multiple renal arteries. Kidneys can be recovered individually or en bloc.

cardiac rhythm, or electrical activity. The cessation of all pulseless electrical activity has not been deemed necessary as a criterion for declaration in the absence of pulse pressure.[3] An additional waiting period of between 2 and 5 minutes occurs before initiation of organ recovery.

The period of warm ischemia time between withdrawal of life support and the initiation of cooling and perfusion with organ preservation solutions contributes to the increased rates of delayed graft function and organ dysfunction seen with DCD organs. Thus, the surgical procedure needs to be performed in an expedited fashion to cool and perfuse organs as soon as possible. A midline incision from sternal notch to pubis is rapidly performed and, using combinations of sharp and blunt dissection, the abdominal cavity is entered and the distal aorta is cannulated with a perfusion catheter with or without isolated control. Immediate perfusion should commence at this point. Transection of the distal inferior vena cava and placement of drainage device or suction catheter can be performed to facilitate perfusion. Depending on recovery of the liver or thoracic organs, the aorta can be clamped at the level of the descending thoracic aorta after opening the chest. DCD recoveries for kidneys alone can avoid opening the chest and clamping of the aorta should occur at the supraceliac level. The abdominal cavity should then be packed with ice during perfusion. Rapid surgical technique to obtain crossclamp and removal of the organs from the abdominal cavity into cool solution on the back table may improve outcomes, as has been reported with other organs.[34] Modified technical approaches, including balloon catheter placement for in situ preservation or use of extracorporeal support after death, have not achieved substantial impact in improving results.[24,36]

While infusion of the preservation solution is completing, surgical recovery of the kidneys can be performed with a similar technique to recovery in DBD donors. While expedient technique is important, precision remains paramount in these circumstances to prevent the higher rates of surgical damage and organ discard that have been reported.[1] After removal of the kidneys from the abdominal cavity, additional perfusion can be performed once the kidneys are in cold solution depending on either preference or concerns regarding the quality of intra-abdominal perfusion. While supportive data exist regarding the ability of hypothermic pulsatile perfusion to improve outcomes for DCD kidneys, conflicting data still exist and thus this conclusion is not uniform.[16,35]

LIVING DONOR NEPHRECTOMY

Kidneys from living donors provide an invaluable resource in both quantity and quality. In the United States approximately 6000 kidneys annually, or one-third of transplantable kidneys, are provided by living donors. The number of living donors almost equals the number of deceased donors when comparing the total number of patients and is of central importance for renal transplantation. The quality of living donor kidneys is likewise superior in every objective measurement, including immediate graft function rates, graft half-life, and life-years gained for recipients. The available pool of donors has remained relatively stable over recent years, although demographics increasingly represent unrelated, altruistic, and even elderly donors (Figure 8-1). The primary responsibility of the donor surgeon is patient safety, and this overarching concern must be involved in every pre-, intra-, and postoperative decision. The reliably safe outcomes with donor nephrectomy and good long-term renal function of donors are paramount to preserve the justification for removing a kidney from a healthy donor.

ANESTHETIC MANAGEMENT

Communication with anesthesia is important to ensure that good urine output is achieved throughout the case. Pneumoperitoneum has been demonstrated to impair venous return influencing renal perfusion, and volume expansion has been demonstrated as the primary intervention to counteract this effect.[23] Patients will often require greater than 5 L of crystalloid to achieve a robust urine output. Mannitol can be administered in divided doses of 12.5 g to augment urine output. Low urine output should be monitored for and addressed aggressively by administering additional intravenous fluids and decreasing or eliminating pneumoperitoneum until good urine output is achieved.

While inadequate volume resuscitation is the most likely factor, identifying other confounding factors for low urine output, including relative hypotension, inability to tolerate pneumoperitoneum, or other physiologic events, is important to determine whether the case should proceed. While rare, our practice is not to proceed with surgery if adequate urine output cannot be achieved.

Also of obvious importance is achieving adequate relaxation, which is necessary for pneumoperitoneum to provide abdominal domain to perform surgery. Diminishing abdominal domain will result from patients who are inadequately paralyzed and will result in difficulty making surgical progress. This may be realized at midpoints of the case as initial paralytic agents may require redosing.

We do not routinely administer heparin prior to division of the renal vessels and have not observed complications from this practice. Some surgeons will administer low-dose intravenous heparin (3000 units intravenously) prior to vascular division with reversal by administering protamine after removal of the kidney.

Regardless of the technical approach, control of postoperative pain should be initiated during the operative case. Intraoperative administration of narcotics provides transient pain control. The use of local anesthetics and systemic non-steroidal agents can minimize postoperative pain and narcotic requirements. We routinely inject 0.5% bupivacaine into port and extraction sites and consider the use of intravenous ketorolac for most patients. Additionally, initiating regularly scheduled oral narcotics soon after surgery can prevent intense pain spikes as local agents diminish.

OPEN DONOR NEPHRECTOMY

Open donor nephrectomy continues to be increasingly replaced by minimally invasive surgical techniques. In fact, surgeons trained in recent eras may have little or no experience with standard or mini-open techniques. Nonetheless, these techniques may be employed by select centers and surgeons based upon indication or preference. Relative indications may include the presence of complicated vascular anatomy, prior operations that complicate laparoscopic approaches, or right nephrectomy. While these techniques deserve an appropriate place in the arsenal of living donor nephrectomy, laparoscopic techniques can be successfully utilized in almost all cases. Despite reduced invasiveness of mini-open incisions, laparoscopic techniques still result in comparatively decreased pain, faster return to work, and higher patient satisfaction.[19,28]

Standard open techniques depend on the division of muscle and possible rib resection compared to mini-open approaches that are muscle sparing and avoid rib resection. The mini-open techniques have been reported to improve donor outcomes compared to standard open techniques.[38] After the induction of general anesthesia, patients are positioned in a flexed lateral decubitus orientation on the operative table. The patient is prepped and draped from the inferior rib margin to the superior iliac spine. A lateral oblique incision is performed inferior to the 12th rib with division or separation of the oblique and transverse musculature. Segmental resection of the inferior rib may be necessary to improve exposure to the upper pole of the kidney. Combinations of manual and electrocautery dissection are performed around Gerota's fascia to permit retractor placement. The peritoneal cavity is swept anteromedially as planes are created to the level of the renal vein and artery. Retractors can be placed either on fixated platforms or by handheld techniques. Retroperitoneal dissection is continued around the kidney and inferiorly to identify and isolate the ureter and gonadal vessels. The ureter should be dissected close to the level of the iliac vessels to ensure adequate length. Complete mobilization of the kidney is performed and the artery and vein are isolated proximal to insertion in the aorta or vena cava. The adrenal gland can be separated from the parenchyma of the kidney lateral to medial. The adrenal vein on the left side may be divided between ligatures or clips to maximize renal vein length. Lumbar veins posterior to the renal vein should be divided to also maximize renal vein length. This can be performed between vascular clamps, surgical clips, or stapling devices. After complete isolation of the vascular pedicle, division of the ureter and renal vessels proceeds. The ureter and gonadal vein are divided distally with ligatures, clips, or stapling devices. The renal artery or arteries are then divided. This can be performed by ligation with or without suture or stapling device. Finally, the renal vein can be divided in a similar technique. Vascular clamps can be utilized to maximize vessel length with subsequent ligation and suturing of vessels after removal of the kidney. The presence of multiple vessels requires planning for the order of division. Placement of multiple vascular clamps may prove difficult with limited space, thus stapling devices may be preferred. Transfixing techniques with either sutures or staples should be used for the renal artery and vein stumps to minimize bleeding risk.

Inspection for good hemostasis with or without placement of hemostatic adjuncts is then performed. Abdominal wall closure is performed in multiple layers and with preference for absorbable suture. Local anesthetic can be injected to provide local pain control and minimize systemic requirements. Similarly, intravenous non-steroidals may be used to provide pain relief and minimize narcotic requirements. These should be discontinued after 48 hours. Postoperatively, patients can receive intravenous and oral narcotics, and can be normalized on diet and activity.

LAPAROSCOPIC DONOR NEPHRECTOMY

Initial reports in 1991 were made of a laparoscopic approach of a nephrectomy for tumor with morcellation and extraction.[6] In 1995, this approach had been successfully applied to living donor nephrectomy, as Ratner et al. made the first report of laparoscopic nephrectomy for transplantation with immediate graft function.[29] Initial comparisons of open and laparoscopic approaches reported substantial improvements in donor recovery.[7] These donor benefits were confirmed in subsequent studies.[26,37] Recent randomized controlled trials have demonstrated improved donor satisfaction, less morbidity, and equivalent graft outcomes.[32] Early large series reported concerns regarding complications, especially with regard to the ureter, with the laparoscopic technique that decreased as progressive technical experience was achieved.[14] The improved patient recovery and minimally invasive approach have even permitted discharge for select patients on the first postoperative day.[21] Additionally, the advent of laparoscopic donor nephrectomy was associated with increased living donation rates and overall volumes providing important recipient benefit.[30]

In the United States, as of 2009, almost all living donor nephrectomies are performed by a laparoscopic approach, with twice as many performed with a hand-assisted approach (Figure 8-4). The minority of cases performed via an open approach has continued to decrease over the last 5 years with less than 5% of donated kidneys performed via open retroperitoneal (3.9%) or transabdominal (1.1%) approaches (Figure 8-4).[27]

Hand-Assisted Technique

Hand-assisted techniques are the preferred approach for many groups and allow for combinations of manual dissection and retraction with laparoscopic visualization and energy devices. Most series report improved speed with hand-assisted techniques as compared to other laparoscopic approaches.[33] The intra-abdominal presence of a hand may also be perceived as an improved safety benefit for manual control of bleeding or other injury that may occur. While large series do not specifically support these concepts, most surgeons are comfortable with open techniques providing direct manual control. The hand port site is also generally used as the extraction site and does not add morbidity, although its location is generally in

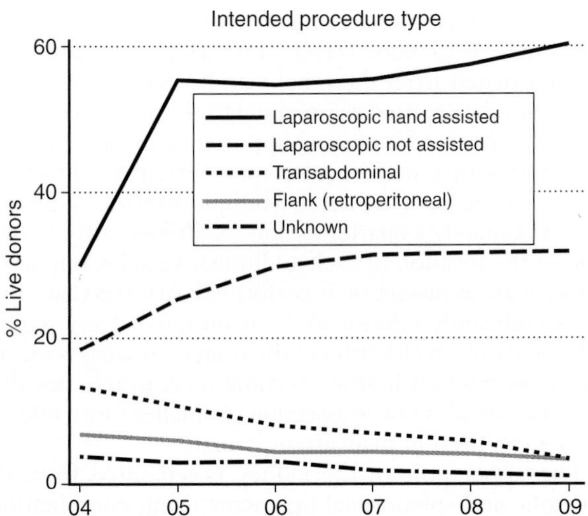

FIGURE 8-4 ■ Technical approach for living donor kidney recovery in the United States. Laparoscopic techniques have been widely adopted and account for 95% of the technical approaches with a majority performing hand-assisted techniques. Open surgical techniques continue to demonstrate diminishing contribution.

an upper midline location and thus more visible than alternate extraction sites. The technical steps for recovery are similar to the total laparoscopic approach (see below) with the obvious addition of a hand to assist.

Total Laparoscopic Approach

Total laparoscopic approach for donor nephrectomy is performed with the donor in either a total or modified lateral position with flexion of the operative table to open the space between the iliac crest and ribs (Figure 8-5). After sterile preparation and draping of the abdomen, a Veress needle can be placed in the left lower quadrant and used to insufflate the abdomen to 15 mmHg pressure. Our preference is to utilize camera visualization through the first port that is placed with subsequent direct visualization of each additional port. Combinations of 5 mm and 12 mm ports are placed in periumbilical, superior and inferior mid-abdominal and lateral locations. A 12 mm port placement in the periumbilical location allows for interchange of dissecting and stapling devices.

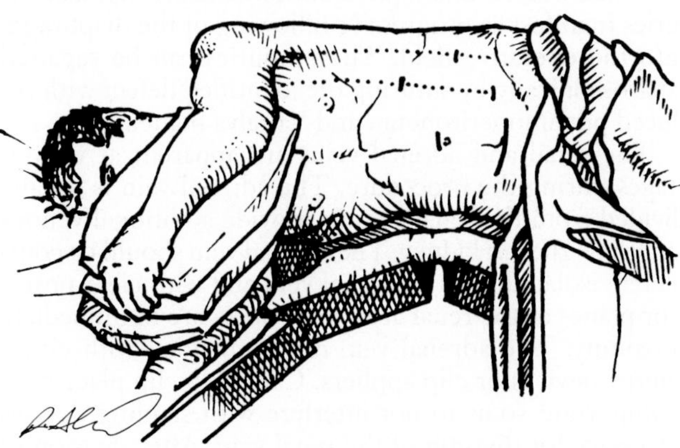

FIGURE 8-5 ■ Positioning and incision placement for laparoscopic left donor nephrectomy. The donor is positioned in a right lateral decubitus position with flexion opening the space between costal margin and iliac crest. A 12 mm port is placed periumbilically and options for 5–12 mm ports in superior and inferior midclavicular and lateral mid-axillary positions. Extraction can be performed through a transverse Pfannenstiel incision.

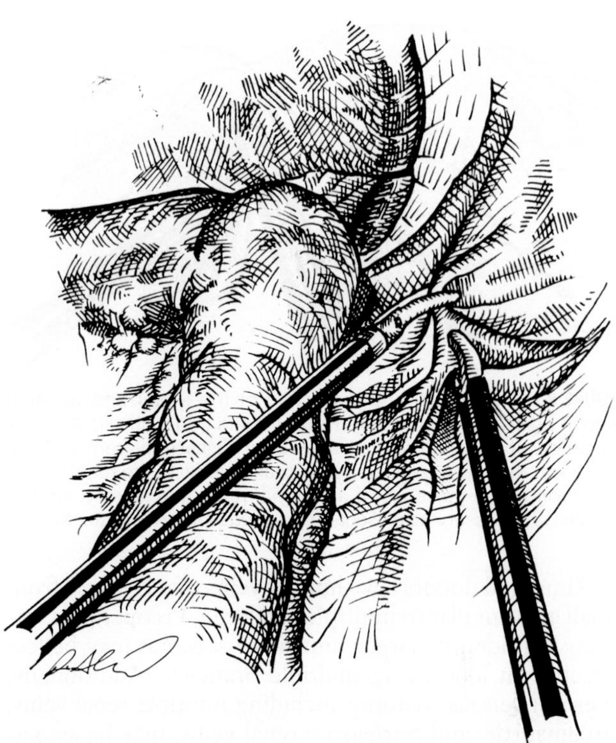

FIGURE 8-6 ■ Mobilization of colon. The line of Toldt and splenocolic ligament are divided with an energy device (i.e., harmonic scalpel) and the colon and mesentery are swept medially. Care must be taken to avoid or identify a mesenteric defect during medial mobilization of the colon and mesentery.

The left colon is mobilized along the line of Toldt by dividing this line with the harmonic scalpel or other energy device (Figure 8-6). The colon and mesentery should be swept medially, taking care not to cause a mesenteric defect or injure mesenteric vessels. If a mesenteric defect is identified this should be repaired with suture or clips and the completion of the case to avoid the potential for internal hernia formation. After the mesentery has been swept medially off the psoas and kidney, the ureter and gonadal vein are identified. The ureter can be identified just superior to the iliac vessels or near the inferior pole of the kidney. Care should be taken not to directly grasp the ureter or use energy devices in direct proximity given the potential for unrecognized injury. A plane should be created under the ureter and gonadal vein that can then be elevated while remaining tissues are dissected (Figure 8-7). Our preference is to use an energy device as small vessels can be present in some of these tissue planes. Dissection should be carried distally to a level immediately superior to the iliac vessels to provide adequate recipient length. Proximal to the kidney, elevation of the ureter and gonadal vein is performed as lymphatics and vessels are identified and divided. We generally do not divide the gonadal vein, although in certain cases this may provide additional exposure to the renal artery and vein.

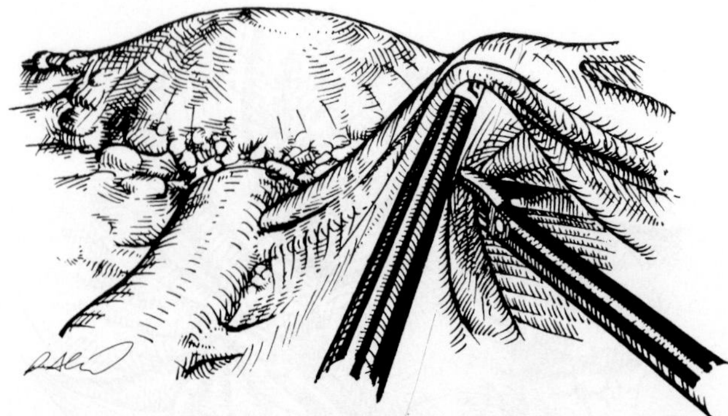

FIGURE 8-7 ■ Elevation and dissection of the ureter and gonadal vein. A plane is created under the ureter and gonadal vein. Anterior elevation of these structures allows for dissection from a distal level near the iliac vessels to a proximal location of the renal hilum. Attention to the presence of additional renal arteries and lumbar vessels is necessary as dissection proceeds superior to the hilum.

Almost all donors have lumbar veins that can vary from small and singular to multiple and large. Preoperative imaging will identify larger lumbar vessels, but may be less effective in identifying multiple branches. Additionally, aberrant venous anatomy, including multiple renal veins, circumaortic, and retroaortic renal veins, may be associated with variants in lumbar venous anatomy. Smaller lumbar veins can be divided with energy devices. Larger lumbar vessels (>6 mm to over 10 mm) should be divided with either clip appliers or stapling devices (Figure 8-8). Judgment as to the possible interference of metallic clips with subsequent stapling devices needed to divide renal artery and vein is important, as clips can interfere with proper closing and stapling. Vascular staples, in contrast, do not generally interfere with the ability to place stapling devices over or in close proximity.

Elevation of the kidney from the lower pole can then reveal the renal artery and vein. Lymphatics are present in varying amounts and density around the vessels, and require dissection, isolation, and division. Division of the periaortic lymphatics demands precision with energy devices as the risk of injury and bleeding exists if these devices come into contact with blood vessels. The artery should be completely isolated from the renal vein by careful dissection, and should be exposed as proximal to the aorta as safely as possibly. This is of increased importance in early branching arteries that may require more extensive dissection down to the level of the aorta. Multiple arteries are present in approximately a quarter of donors. Preoperative knowledge of the location of each additional vessel is important to anticipate as dissection is performed. Arteries that originate significantly inferior to the main renal artery require additional care in elevation of the ureter, gonadal vein, and kidney, as traction injuries become increasingly possible. Likewise, avoiding overdissection of smaller more inferior arteries can prevent inadvertent injury.

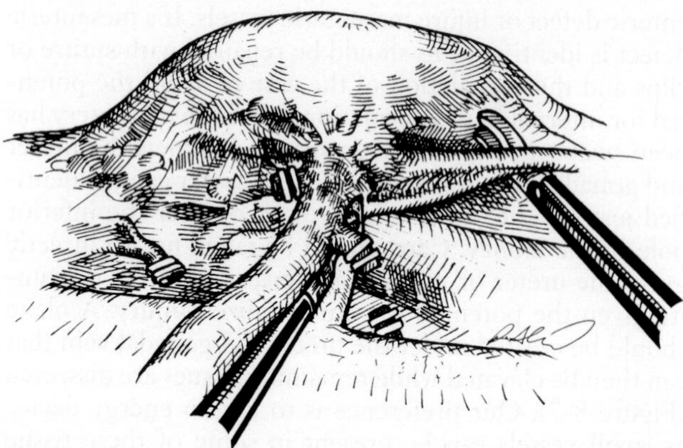

FIGURE 8-8 ■ Division of the adrenal and lumbar veins. As the kidney is elevated with instruments, dissection of the lumbar vein from surrounding lymphatics can be performed. Smaller adrenal and lumbar veins can be divided with energy devices; larger vessels should either be clipped and divided or divided with a stapling device. Consideration of likely division sites of the renal artery and vein should be performed to avoid interference of clips with stapling devices.

The upper pole of the kidney is separated from the renocolic and splenorenal ligaments using combinations of blunt dissection and energy devices. The spleen can be retracted medially in combination with lateral retraction of the kidney to open this space. Retraction of the spleen and surrounding tissues can also be a potentially hazardous maneuver and should be done with blunt instruments or graspers to avoid injury to the spleen. As this space is developed, the adrenal gland requires separation from the upper pole of the kidney. The adrenal gland is often identifiable and can be gently positioned with a grasper as dissection is performed immediately lateral to the gland. In obese donors, it may be difficult to identify the adrenal gland, and dissection along separate tissue planes that belong either medially with the adrenal gland or laterally with Gerota's fascia is performed in potentially ambiguous territory. Upper pole vessels often occupy the space between the adrenal gland and kidney; therefore, closer proximity to the adrenal gland and away from the renal hilum is preferred. Dissection of the upper pole of the kidney should be carried down to the level of the psoas muscle and superior to the diaphragm. We perform separation of Gerota's fascia from the diaphragm and psoas with energy devices to minimize even small amounts of venous bleeding. Care needs to be taken with dissection around the diaphragm so as to not inadvertently injure or perforate with resultant pneumothorax. Unrecognized injuries manifest as progressive billowing of the diaphragm into the operative field. These injuries can be repaired laparoscopically by suturing the identified defect with reduced pneumoperitoneum and Valsalva maneuvers.

The renal and adrenal veins are apparent at various stages during the procedure. The adrenal vein is usually divided from the renal vein to provide additional venous length on the left kidney. The adrenal vein should be completely isolated from the renal vein and with clear posterior planes as the renal artery and aorta are in immediate proximity. The adrenal vein can be divided with either energy devices or clip appliers. Care with clip placement is important so as to not interfere with stapling devices necessary for division of the renal vein. After division of the adrenal vein, the renal artery is easier to identify and dissection can be completed of the periaortic lymphatics. Tissues can be swept medially off the anterior surface of the renal vein to provide maximal length. Elevation of the renal vein with a blunt instrument and clearance of a posterior plane can also be completed.

We generally perform separation of the kidney from retroperitoneal attachments as a final step. If the kidney is mobilized too early in the case, the kidney can inadvertently rotate medially and complicate vascular dissection. The ureter and gonadal vein are identified and a lateral window is created with an energy device. This window is opened superiorly as the kidney is progressively retracted medially. This likewise will lead to immediate proximity with the diaphragm at the upper pole of the kidney and requires additional attention to avoid injury. We leave Gerota's fascia intact with the kidney as we perform this dissection. Separation of the kidney from the Gerota's fascia, even when extensive, can be difficult with densely adherent fat that may risk capsular injury to the kidney. As the kidney is completely mobilized medially, the psoas muscle and origin of the renal artery become apparent. Dissection of the posterior and superior aspects of the renal artery can sometimes be facilitated with the kidney in a medial location. Likewise, lumbar vessels may sometimes be easier to identify and divide with the kidney medially rotated.

Extraction can be performed via either a Pfannenstiel or lower midline incision. Through either approach, the rectus is exposed and a 15 mm port is inserted to accommodate a large endocatch bag for retrieval. Alternately, the Endo Catch bag can be directly placed through a small defect in the peritoneum. Care needs to be taken not to have an uncontrolled violation of the peritoneal cavity, otherwise pneumoperitoneum will not be maintained during vascular stapling.

Division of the ureter and gonadal vein is performed first with a vascular staple load. This is performed distally with direct observation of the distal stapler to confirm that the iliac vessels are not in proximity. The renal arteries are then divided next with the kidney elevated to maximal height. If multiple arteries exist and are separated by more than 5–10 mm, we divide the inferior vessel first, followed by new staple loads for superior arteries. If arteries are in close proximity they can be taken with a single staple load. After arteries are divided, the kidney is retracted to a maximal lateral extent and a stapler is placed on the renal vein as proximal to the vena cava as safely possible.

Stapling requires care and attention to the stapling device and staple loads. An experienced scrub nurse or technician should be familiar with expedient reloading of the stapler. Concerns regarding the function or proper reloading of the device justify replacement with a new stapling device that should be immediately available in the operating room. Prior to firing the stapling device, direct visualization of proper alignment of the stapler, including the distal extent of the device and proper position of the staple cartridge, should be confirmed by the surgical team (Figure 8-9). This includes care not to close the stapler across metal clips which can cause misfire. Stapler misfires are very infrequent with limited reports; however, they can be catastrophic and require expedient management.[12] The most significant danger is for improper stapling prior to division of the vessel with a cutting device. A transected bleeding artery or vein should be controlled directly with a laparoscopic instrument or hand if possible. If the vessel can be controlled determination can be made whether the vessel can be restapled, clipped, or oversewn with laparoscopic techniques. If this is not possible, direct pressure should be attempted while a midline laparotomy incision is made for direct exposure and repair. Non-cutting stapling devices may offer advantages when preserving early bifurcations because of a decreased width of the device. Additional non-cutting devices allow for confirmation of the correct placement of staples before subsequently dividing the vessel with endoscopic scissors. Plastic or metallic clips should not be used to ligate main renal vessels and the US Food and Drug Administration issued a specific alert in 2011 that updated 2006 warnings regarding the use of Weck Hem-o-lok ligating clip for renal artery ligation in living kidney donors secondary to risk of postoperative dislodgement and hemorrhage.[8] Additional recommendations have been made, which are broadly adhered to, that transfixion of tissue is the only acceptable method for renal artery division in living donor nephrectomy.

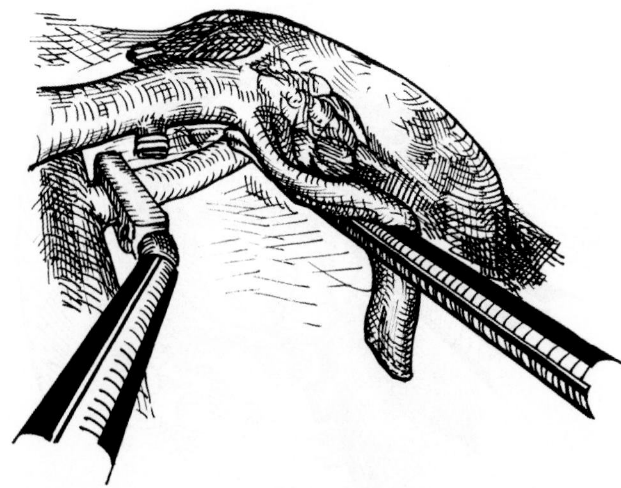

FIGURE 8-9 ■ Division of the renal artery. The kidney can be retracted lateral and anterior with instruments as a vascular stapling device is placed just beyond the origin of the renal artery. Cutting or non-cutting staplers can be used, but attention to the distal location of the stapler is important to avoid clips or other improper positioning.

After all vessels have been transected, the kidney should be confirmed to be free of all retroperitoneal attachments. Residual attachments can be divided with energy devices or additional staple loads if present. The Endo Catch bag is directly deployed under the kidney and the kidney and ureter are placed completely in the bag under direct visualization (Figure 8-10). The bag should also be closed under direct visualization as injury to the kidney or ureter can occur if they are not contained within the bag. Rarely, a kidney may be unable to be placed in the bag because of size or other technical issues. Manual retrieval should then be performed quickly and if possible while retaining pneumoperitoneum to aid in the identification and control of the kidneys. The rectus can be opened in either a vertical or transverse direction as the kidney is retrieved from the abdominal cavity.

The kidney is immediately placed on ice and brought to the back table for preparation. Staple lines should be transected and direct cannulation and flushing of all renal arteries are performed until clear effluent is achieved.

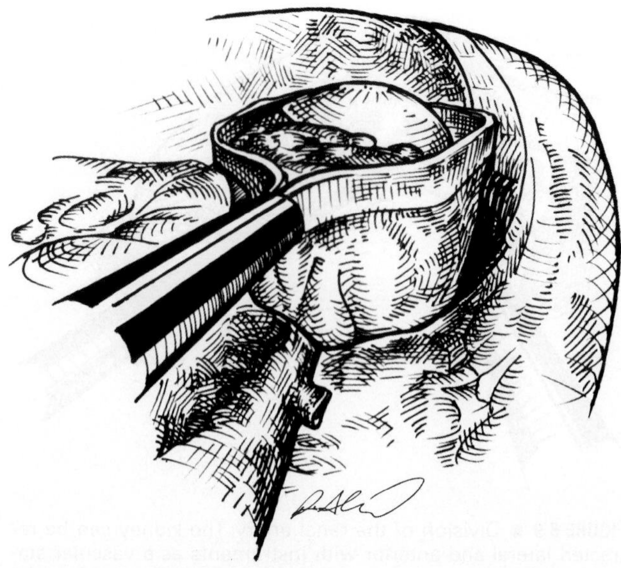

FIGURE 8-10 ■ Placement of the kidney into an Endo Catch bag. After division of ureter and vascular structures the kidney and entire ureter should be placed into an Endo Catch bag under direct visualization. Once all structures are inside the bag, it can be closed and extracted through the selected incision site.

The extraction can be closed with either running or absorbable (PDS or Maxon) #1 sutures. After closure of the extraction incision, pneumoperitoneum is re-established and confirmation of good hemostasis at all dissection and vascular division sites is performed. Occasionally, gonadal vessels will require additional clip placement at the level of the ureteral division. Renal artery and vein should be directly observed. Blood is aspirated from the retroperitoneal space and near the spleen to confirm no unidentified bleeding. Hemostatic agents are not generally required, but can be placed as adjunction to hemostatic maneuvers when necessary. Mesenteric defects can be repaired at this point if identified (as discussed above). Challenging bleeding sources include adrenal, splenic, and lumbar venous sources. If adrenal or splenic bleeding cannot be confirmed to be controlled, consideration for removal should be given. Lumbar venous bleeding can be difficult to manage and, if direct control and sealing with energy device or clip placement cannot be achieved, attempt to oversew should be made. The procedure should never be completed if there is continued bleeding and drains are almost never indicated.

Ports can be removed under direct visualization. Larger port (12 and 15 mm) sites can be closed as practiced per routine of the surgical team. The extraction and skin incisions are anesthetized with injectable agents (lidocaine or Marcaine) and closed with absorbable subcuticular sutures. Ketorolac can be used per physician discretion to minimize postoperative discomfort and narcotic use.

RIGHT DONOR NEPHRECTOMY

Laparoscopic right donor nephrectomy is performed in the overwhelming minority of cases, with rates between 1% and 4% at large US centers. Initial challenges with laparoscopic right nephrectomy resulted in increased vascular complications compared to left kidneys. Modifications in donor techniques to preserve donor vein length and in the recipient to mobilize the iliac venous system can improve these outcomes.[25] Nonetheless, multiple renal arteries and anomalous renal venous anatomy are not contraindications for left donor nephrectomy. The presence of stones, cysts, or lesions within the right kidney is a strong indication for right nephrectomy.

The operative approach is modified by the requirement of liver retraction. After the peritoneum has been incised with partial mobilization of the right liver lobe, one instrument is positioned to elevate the liver over the superior pole of the right kidney. The operation is further modified by the requirement for division of the right gonadal vein that inserts directly into the vena cava. The right adrenal vein does not need to be divided as it is separate from the renal vein. The shorter right renal vein also requires extra attention to stapling with either cutting or non-cutting vascular stapling devices. Maximum retraction of the kidney and exposure of the vena cava are performed to allow placement of the stapling device for maximum vein length.

SINGLE-PORT DONOR NEPHRECTOMY

The possibility to reduce donor morbidity and/or improve patient satisfaction through new techniques has been attempted with the introduction of laparoendoscopic single-site surgery and supporting devices. The operation can allow for the entire procedure and extraction incision to be concealed within the umbilicus of the donor and a very small residual scar once healed (Figure 8-11). The technique was first described in 2008 as a feasible approach with good outcomes.[9] Some

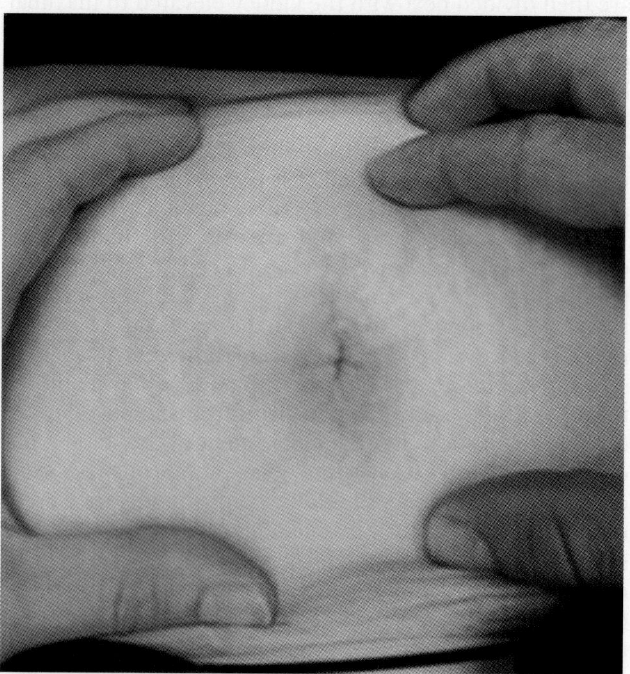

FIGURE 8-11 ■ Cosmetic result of single-port donor nephrectomy 2 years postdonation. Single-port donor nephrectomy performed through the umbilicus with transumbilical extraction allows for minimization of the apparent incision length with minimal residual scar.

supportive evidence exists that this approach offers improved recovery in comparison to standard laparoscopic techniques.[5] Our center has utilized this approach since 2009 as the routine approach for over 200 kidney donors and has reported on equivalent safety with improved patient satisfaction as compared to multiport laparoscopy.[2]

The single-port devices commercially available allow for entry of three, four, or more instruments (Figure 8-12). The differences in hand maneuvers necessary to perform the surgery through a single site are not substantially different and can be reasonably achieved through techniques of either port minimization with standard laparoscopic techniques or initiation of procedures through a single port with additional port placement as indicated. Commitment to early placement of additional ports has allowed for equivalent safety in our experience. The most critical maneuvers in laparoscopic donor nephrectomy are the vascular dissection around the vein and artery and subsequent stapling. These maneuvers involve fine movements that we have found not to be limited by a single-port approach.

We found four techniques were important to mastery of the single-port approach and normalization of operative times with total laparoscopic approaches. First, ventilation of smoke and vapor through the single-port device is important and has been incorporated into later designs of available devices. Second, elevation of the lower pole of the kidney anterior and medially allows for opening of the space between the renal artery and vein for dissection. Third, retraction of the upper pole inferiorly and laterally provides separation of the kidney from splenic and adrenal attachments, and facilitates dissection of the renal artery from a superior approach. Finally, a plan should be determined for extraction of the kidney after division of the vasculature. Depending on the device utilized, the skin and fascial incisions require extension to safely deliver the kidney without significant trauma. Removal through too small a fascial or skin incision can injure the kidney and should not be aggressively attempted.

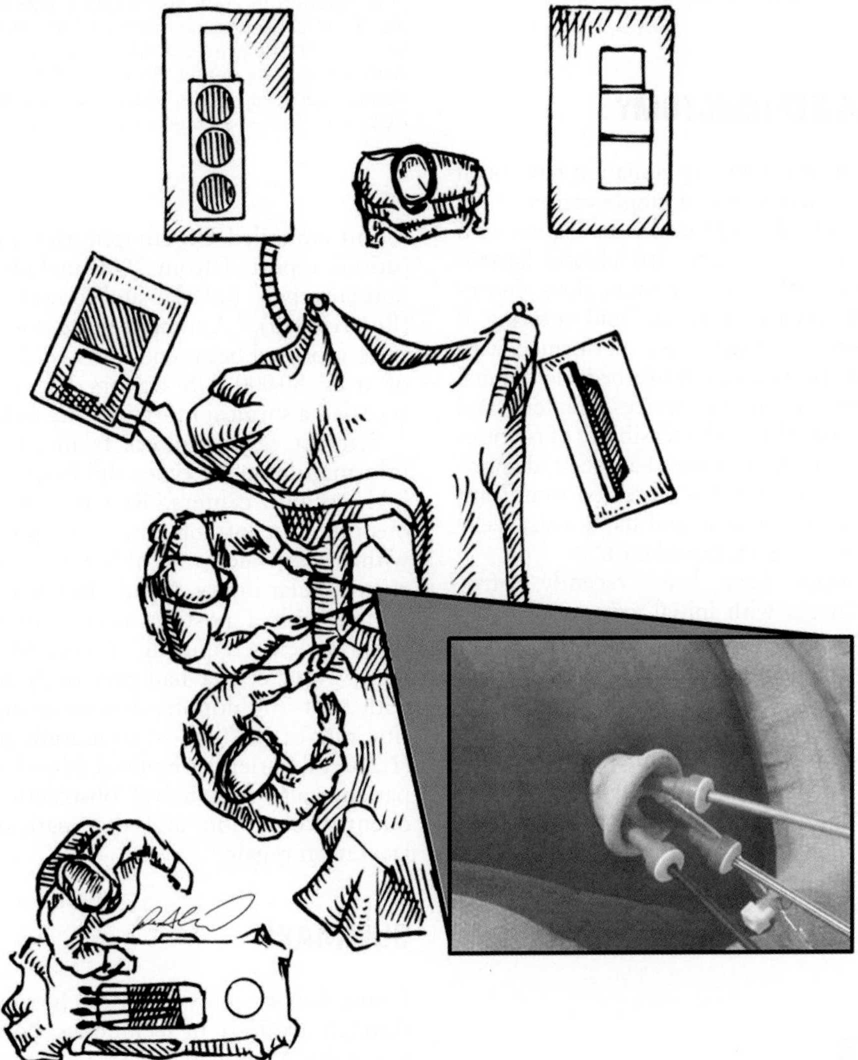

FIGURE 8-12 ■ Single-port donor nephrectomy. Patient position and operating room setup are similar to standard laparoscopic nephrectomy. Surgeon and assistant are in close proximity as multiple instruments and camera are inserted through the umbilical port. The assistant operating the camera and/or additional instrument must pay attention to avoiding interference with the primary surgeon's instruments.

The procedure can be performed with standard laparoscopic instrumentation and cameras, although articulating cameras and instruments have been introduced that may facilitate the procedure with experience. The substitution of the single-port device for multiple ports required in either hand-assisted or total laparoscopic approaches does not demonstrate substantial cost differences.

We have reported on normalization of our operative times and ability to perform right and left nephrectomies with single or multiple arteries and veins. We do experience approximately 10% rate of additional port placement, most commonly in obese donors. While complication rates are similar to other techniques, concern for umbilical hernia necessitates careful attention to proper technique for closure of the fascia. This technique continues to be our preferred approach for all living kidney donors and fits into an algorithm of preferred approaches, being single-port laparoscopy, multiport laparoscopy, hand-assisted laparoscopy, and open techniques. The improved cosmesis and potential other benefits of this technique may also translate to increased interest in living kidney donation with a further slight reduction in the invasiveness of the surgery.

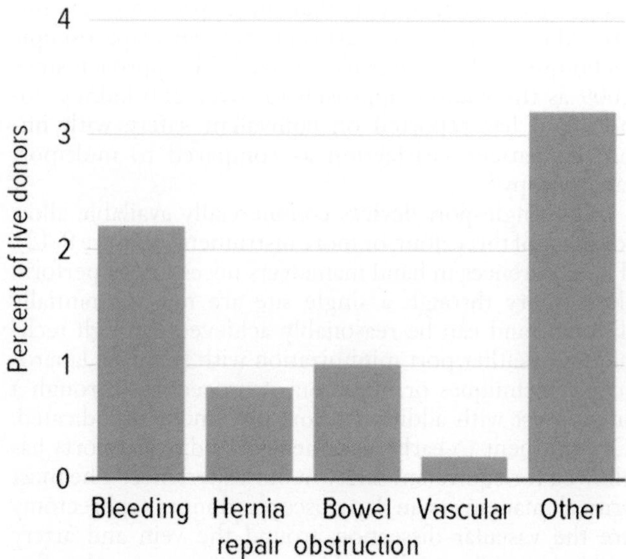

FIGURE 8-13 ■ Complication rates from donor nephrectomies in the United States. Bleeding was the most common complication reported in 2008, followed by bowel obstruction and hernia. (From Organ Procurement and Transplantation Network (OPTN) and Scientific Registry of Transplant Recipients (SRTR). OPTN/SRTR 2010 Annual Data Report. Rockville, MD: Department of Health and Human Services, Health Resources and Services Administration, Healthcare Systems Bureau, Division of Transplantation; 2011.)

ROBOTIC DONOR NEPHRECTOMY

Robotic approaches in living kidney donation have been reported, with largest series out of single centers.[10,11,13] Potential advantages include improved visualization with three-dimensional camera systems, articulating laparoscopic instrumentation allowing for meticulous dissection of complicated vascular anatomy, and suturing if necessary. The robotic approaches are performed with multiple laparoscopic ports and require bedside manual assistant ports for use of energy devices, staplers, and eventually for extraction. While the feasibility of robotic-assisted laparoscopic nephrectomies has been demonstrated, early reports have not demonstrated significant advantages over total laparoscopic and hand-assist techniques, while demonstrating increased cost.[4]

Single-port platforms have been recently introduced for robotic devices with initial experience being gained predominantly with laparoendoscopic single-site cholecystectomy.[20] Application of these new devices for donor nephrectomy has not been reported; however, urologic and cadaveric studies have revealed the possible application for renal surgery.[17,18] The great potential for robotic approaches to overcome limitations of single-port surgery may allow for wider application of both techniques; however, current instrumentation does not allow for articulation or use of energy devices. Continued technologic advancement may improve the ability of robotic approaches to add significant advantages to the donor surgery.

COMPLICATIONS

The 2010 report from the Organ Procurement and Transplantation Network (OPTN) and Scientific Registry of Transplant Recipients (SRTR) revealed most recent compiled US complication rates. Major complications reported from 2008 included bleeding (2.2%), hernia repair (0.8%), and bowel obstruction (1.0%) (Figure 8-13).[27] A total of three donation-related deaths were reported between 2005 and 2009. Further analysis of over 80 000 US donors between 1994 and 2009 revealed a surgical mortality rate of 0.03%.[31]

Largest series reports from single centers provide information on the types and frequencies of events from high-volume centers. Reports on 1200 donors demonstrated an intraoperative complication rate of 1.6% with a conversion rate of 0.92%, most commonly from renovascular injury. An additional 4.0% of patients presented with a postoperative complication, with only three patients requiring surgery for internal hernia or ileus.[22] Our center had previously reported experience with over 700 donors, demonstrating an open conversion rate of 1.6%, most commonly from vascular injury (1.2% of patients required blood transfusion).[15] Five patients also had bowel obstruction requiring subsequent exploration and one patient required splenic laceration repair.

SUMMARY

Living donor nephrectomy can be successfully performed through a variety of techniques, both open and laparoscopically. Minimally invasive techniques have been associated with decreased morbidity and improved recovery courses of patients and should be viewed as the preferred approach for the majority of patients. Nonetheless, the key principle of donor safety should be used to make final decisions regarding donation techniques. Different centers and surgeons may have a variety of approaches that result in good and safe outcomes. Thus, surgeon experience becomes an important consideration in determining the specific approach that is best for each patient.

Acknowledgment

Acknowledgment is made to Phil Brazio, MD, for illustrating the technique of laparoscopic donor nephrectomy accompanying this chapter.

REFERENCES

1. Ausania F, White SA, Pocock P, et al. Kidney damage during organ recovery in donation after circulatory death donors: data from UK national transplant database. Am J Transplant 2012;12:932–6.
2. Barth RN, Phelan M, Goldschen LE, et al. Single-port donor nephrectomy provides improved patient satisfaction and equivalent outcomes. Ann Surg 2012 Sep 10.
3. Bernat JL, D'Alessandro AM, Port FK, et al. Report of a national conference on donation after cardiac death. Am J Transplant 2006;6:281–91.
4. Boger M, Lucas SM, Popp SC, et al. Comparison of robot-assisted nephrectomy with laparoscopic and hand-assisted laparoscopic nephrectomy. JSLS 2010;14:374–80.
5. Canes D, Berger A, Aron M, et al. Laparo-endoscopic single site (LESS) versus standard laparoscopic left donor nephrectomy: matched-pair comparison. Eur Urol 2010;57:95–101.
6. Clayman RV, Kavoussi LR, Soper NJ, et al. Laparoscopic nephrectomy: initial case report. J Urol 1991;146:278–82.
7. Flowers JL, Jacobs S, Cho E, et al. Comparison of open and laparoscopic live donor nephrectomy. Ann Surg 1997;226:483–9.
8. Friedman AL, Peters TG, Ratner LE. Regulatory failure contributing to deaths of live kidney donors. Am J Transplant 2012;12:829–34.
9. Gill IS, Canes D, Aron M, et al. Single port transumbilical (E-NOTES) donor nephrectomy. J Urol 2008;180:637–41.
10. Gorodner V, Horgan S, Galvani C, et al. Routine left robotic-assisted laparoscopic donor nephrectomy is safe and effective regardless of the presence of vascular anomalies. Transpl Int 2006;19:636–40.
11. Horgan S, Vanuno D, Sileri P, et al. Robotic-assisted laparoscopic donor nephrectomy for kidney transplantation. Transplantation 2002;73:1474–9.
12. Hsi RS, Ojogho ON, Baldwin DD. Analysis of techniques to secure the renal hilum during laparoscopic donor nephrectomy: review of the FDA database. Urology 2009;74:142–7.
13. Hubert J, Renoult E, Mourey E, et al. Complete robotic-assistance during laparoscopic living donor nephrectomies: an evaluation of 38 procedures at a single site. Int J Urol 2007;14:986–9.
14. Jacobs SC, Cho E, Dunkin BJ, et al. Laparoscopic live donor nephrectomy: the University of Maryland 3-year experience. J Urol 2000;164:1494–9.
15. Jacobs SC, Cho E, Foster C, et al. Laparoscopic donor nephrectomy: the University of Maryland 6-year experience. J Urol 2004;171:47–51.
16. Jochmans I, Moers C, Smits JM, et al. Machine perfusion versus cold storage for the preservation of kidneys donated after cardiac death: a multicenter, randomized, controlled trial. Ann Surg 2010;252:756–64.
17. Kaouk JH, Autorino R, Laydner H, et al. Robotic single-site kidney surgery: evaluation of second-generation instruments in a cadaver model. Urology 2012;79:975–9.
18. Khanna R, Stein RJ, White MA, et al. Single institution experience with robot-assisted laparoendoscopic single-site renal procedures. J Endourol 2012;26:230–4.
19. Kok NF, Lind MY, Hansson BM, et al. Comparison of laparoscopic and mini incision open donor nephrectomy: single blind, randomised controlled clinical trial. BMJ 2006;333:221.
20. Konstantinidis KM, Hirides P, Hirides S, et al. Cholecystectomy using a novel single-site robotic platform: early experience from 45 consecutive cases. Surg Endosc 2012;26:2687–94.
21. Kuo PC, Johnson LB, Sitzmann JV. Laparoscopic donor nephrectomy with a 23-hour stay: a new standard for transplantation surgery. Ann Surg 2000;231:772–9.
22. Leventhal JR, Paunescu S, Baker TB, et al. A decade of minimally invasive donation: experience with more than 1200 laparoscopic donor nephrectomies at a single institution. Clin Transplant 2010;24:169–74.
23. London ET, Ho HS, Neuhaus AM, et al. Effect of intravascular volume expansion on renal function during prolonged CO_2 pneumoperitoneum. Ann Surg 2000;231:195–201.
24. Magliocca JF, Magee JC, Rowe SA, et al. Extracorporeal support for organ donation after cardiac death effectively expands the donor pool. J Trauma 2005;58:1095–101.
25. Mandal AK, Cohen C, Montgomery RA, et al. Should the indications for laparascopic live donor nephrectomy of the right kidney be the same as for the open procedure? Anomalous left renal vasculature is not a contraindiction to laparoscopic left donor nephrectomy. Transplantation 2001;71:660–4.
26. Nogueira JM, Cangro CB, Fink JC, et al. A comparison of recipient renal outcomes with laparoscopic versus open live donor nephrectomy. Transplantation 1999;67:722–8.
27. Organ Procurement and Transplantation Network (OPTN) and Scientific Registry of Transplant Recipients (SRTR). OPTN/SRTR 2010 annual data report. Rockville, MD: Department of Health and Human Services, Health Resources and Services Administration, Healthcare Systems Bureau, Division of Transplantation; 2011.
28. Perry KT, Freedland SJ, Hu JC, et al. Quality of life, pain and return to normal activities following laparoscopic donor nephrectomy versus open mini-incision donor nephrectomy. J Urol 2003;169:2018–21.
29. Ratner LE, Ciseck LJ, Moore RG, et al. Laparoscopic live donor nephrectomy. Transplantation 1995;60:1047–9.
30. Schweitzer EJ, Wilson J, Jacobs S, et al. Increased rates of donation with laparoscopic donor nephrectomy. Ann Surg 2000;232:392–400.
31. Segev DL, Muzaale AD, Caffo BS, et al. Perioperative mortality and long-term survival following live kidney donation. JAMA 2010;303:959–66.
32. Simforoosh N, Basiri A, Tabibi A, et al. Comparison of laparoscopic and open donor nephrectomy: a randomized controlled trial. BJU Int 2005;95:851–5.
33. Slakey DP, Wood JC, Hender D, et al. Laparoscopic living donor nephrectomy: advantages of the hand-assisted method. Transplantation 1999;68:581–3.
34. Taner CB, Bulatao IG, Willingham DL, et al. Events in procurement as risk factors for ischemic cholangiopathy in liver transplantation using donation after cardiac death donors. Liver Transpl 2012;18:100–11.
35. Watson CJ, Wells AC, Roberts RJ, et al. Cold machine perfusion versus static cold storage of kidneys donated after cardiac death: a UK multicenter randomized controlled trial. Am J Transplant 2010;10:1991–9.
36. Wind J, Snoeijs MG, van der Vliet JA, et al. Preservation of kidneys from controlled donors after cardiac death. Br J Surg 2011;98:1260–6.
37. Wolf Jr JS, Merion RM, Leichtman AB, et al. Randomized controlled trial of hand-assisted laparoscopic versus open surgical live donor nephrectomy. Transplantation 2001;72:284–90.
38. Yang SL, Harkaway R, Badosa F, et al. Minimal incision living donor nephrectomy: improvement in patient outcome. Urology 2002;59:673–7.

CHAPTER 9

KIDNEY PRESERVATION

John O'Callaghan • Henri G.D. Leuvenink • Peter J. Friend • Rutger J. Ploeg

CHAPTER OUTLINE

TOWARDS "TAILORED" PRESERVATION STRATEGIES

To date, donor kidneys are very different from those retrieved two decades ago. To maintain quality and increase viability different donor types and kidneys procured for transplantation require different preservation strategies using more adjusted methods and solutions.

Transplant waiting lists have universally lengthened since their creation, and at a greater rate than the availability of donors. The classical donor type was that of the deceased, heart-beating donor, or donation after brain death (DBD). These were typically younger people suffering irreversible brain damage during motor vehicle accidents, referred to as standard criteria donors (SCD). Declining numbers of this donor type are available due to a combination of improved neurosurgery and road safety. Transplant programs are therefore increasingly turning to expanded criteria donation (ECD) and donation after circulatory death (DCD) to meet the shortfall. Each donor type is associated with risk factors that could affect the outcome of the transplant and therefore the methods of preservation are crucial. Many organ donors are now complex, with comorbidities and an associated cascade of injury to the donor organs such that the applied preservation strategies become even more important.

ECD was established as a defined donor group based upon the association of certain factors with reduced graft survival. Historically ECD were known as "marginal" or "expanded" donors but are now more appropriately referred to as "higher risk." They are defined as donors over 60 years old, or aged 50–59 years, with at least two of the following conditions: cerebrovascular cause of death, serum creatinine over 1.5 mg/dL, hypertension.[102] Transplantation of an ECD kidney gives a substantial survival advantage over maintenance on dialysis from 18 months posttransplant, despite the negative comparison with kidneys from SCD.[96] Graft survival for ECD kidneys is, by definition, inferior to that for SCD. The relative risk of graft loss for ECD kidneys is greater than 1.7 times that of SCD kidneys.[102] Absolute differences in graft survival show a 15% and 16% reduction at 1 and 3 years.[83]

The use of ECD kidneys has risen in many countries.[65,98] In the United States the number of ECD kidneys rose by 36% between the years 1999 and 2005, while SCD rose by approximately 13%.[98] ECD contributed 22% of the kidneys transplanted in the United States in 2009.[32]

DCD has also been explored in order to meet the demands of transplant waiting lists. The different types of DCD may be categorized using the Maastricht criteria[70] (Table 9-1). Typically, DCD donors are those who have suffered massive brain injury but do not meet the criteria for brain death. A decision to withdraw supportive treatment is made independently of donor status (so-called "controlled DCD" or Maastricht category III) and organs from these patients undergo a period of warm ischemia as well as the inflammatory processes of brain death. Patients who have circulatory arrest in relatively uncontrolled situations may also become cardiac death donors. These so-called "uncontrolled DCD," or Maastricht

TABLE 9-1 Maastricht Categories of Donation after Circulatory Death

Category	Description
I	Dead on arrival at the hospital
II	Unsuccessful resuscitation at the hospital
III	Withdrawal of supportive treatment
IV	Cardiac arrest following establishment of brain death

categories I and II, do not undergo brain death but experience a longer period of warm ischemia than controlled DCD. Kidneys from DCD have a higher risk of delayed graft function (DGF) and primary non-function (PNF) than kidneys from DBD.[68,116] Despite effects on the early graft function, kidneys from DCD have equivalent long-term graft survival to DBD kidneys in large reviews and meta-analysis.[68,116,121] DCD kidneys also confer a survival advantage compared to remaining on dialysis whilst awaiting a DBD transplant.[15]

Following declining numbers of suitable brain-death donors, the use of kidneys from DCD has increased in many countries. In the United Kingdom, for example, the use of DCD kidneys has rocketed from 3% of deceased donor transplants in 2000 to 32% in 2009.[121] In the Eurotransplant region the use of DCD kidneys has permitted a 44% increase in available kidneys for transplantation, and they have outnumbered the grafts recovered from DBD since 2001.[116] Despite support from the Institute of Medicine, the use of DCD kidneys in the United States has not increased at such a rate: DCD accounted for approximately 13% of deceased donor kidneys in the United States in 2009[32] and there is considerable variation by region[32,56] (Figure 9-1).

Not only has the age of DBD donors increased, but also the spectrum of cause of death has shifted. Increasingly, cerebrovascular accident is the leading cause of death.[121] Brain injury and ischemia lead to inflammatory processes that can injure kidneys prior to retrieval and lead

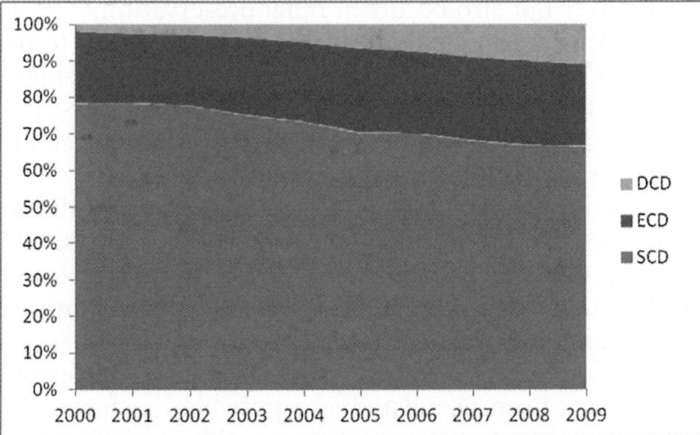

FIGURE 9-1 ■ In recent years the use of kidneys from donation after circulatory death (DCD) has increased in the United States. Percentage is of all deceased donor kidneys retrieved. ECD, expanded criteria donation; SCD, standard criteria donors. (Based on Organ Procurement and Transplantation Network/Scientific Registry of Transplant Recipients data as of October 1, 2010.)

to subsequent injury at reperfusion.[16,93] Cerebral ischemia results in hemodynamic instability, hypothermia, coagulopathy, and electrolyte disturbances.[29,30,33] A surge in circulating catecholamines and a subsequent drop in their levels causes tachycardia, arrhythmias, and then hypotension.[30,33] Following brain injury renal tubules are therefore exposed to an inflammatory and metabolic milieu that can result in increased urinary sodium excretion[46,57] and fibrous proliferation of the arterial intima.[91] There is evidence that brain death increases the immunogenicity of transplanted organs,[69] associated with a higher rejection rate than organs from live donors.[103] Cerebrovascular accident as the cause of donor death is independently associated with an increased risk of graft loss.[102]

The risk factors associated with prolonged warm ischemia time, the inflammatory processes set in motion by brain death and the agonal phase, require different strategies in organ preservation that are more complex than we are used to with SCD. Due to recent developments in the spectrum of donors required to address transplant waiting lists, hypothermic machine perfusion (HMP) and normothermic techniques are therefore being evaluated. To date, however, the majority of donor kidneys have been stored by hypothermic preservation to maintain viability and prevent further injury.

PRINCIPLES OF COLD STORAGE PRESERVATION

After circulatory arrest, tissue metabolism continues for some time; however, the absence of oxygen and nutrients will rapidly lead to major metabolic problems within renal cells. The suppression of metabolism is therefore essential to maintain organ viability during the preservation period. Reduction of the core temperature of the kidney below 4°C will result in a reduction of metabolism to 5–8% in the majority of cells and will diminish enzyme activity.[117] Calne et al. showed that simple cooling of kidneys in ice water preserved renal function for 12 hours.[23] The development of preservation solutions that targeted harmful pathways during cold preservation enabled longer storage times and preservation quality improved.[81] Despite the beneficial concept of hypothermia, unwanted side effects in the preserved organ still occur. These effects can only be partly counteracted by preservation solutions (Figure 9-2).

Harmful effects of hypothermic preservation include:

- Cell swelling
- Acidosis
- Altered enzyme activity
- Calcium accumulation
- Production of reactive oxygen species (ROS).

Energy and Acidosis

Tissue hypoxia during organ preservation results in a rapid fall in intracellular adenosine triphosphate (ATP) levels. Even at temperatures as low as 0–4°C, cellular ATP content is rapidly depleted and cells switch to anaerobic

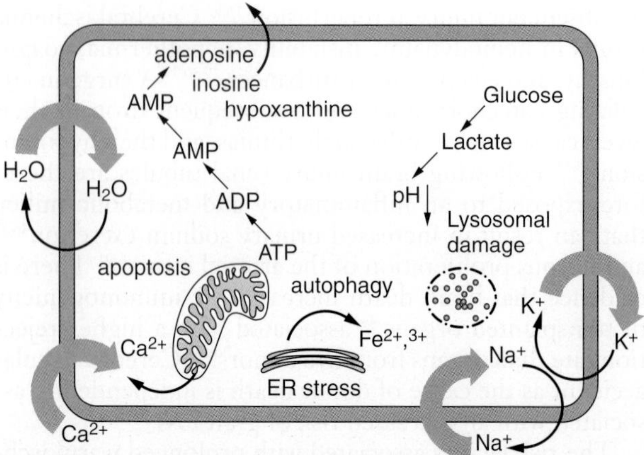

FIGURE 9-2 ■ Negative effects of cold ischemia are breakdown of adenosine triphosphate (ATP), acidosis, release of lysosomal enzymes, endoplasmic reticulum (ER) stress, increased Na^+ and Ca^{2+} influx to the cell, and subsequent cell swelling. AMP, adenosine monophosphate; ADP, adenosine diphosphate.

metabolism to support cellular processes. This leads to a much less efficient production of ATP, but also to the production of lactic acid and acidosis.[45,78] The contribution of acidosis to ischemic injury is pH-dependent. Severe acidosis activates phospholipases and proteases, causing lysosomal damage and eventually cell death.[15] Mild acidosis (pH 6.9–7.0), however, has been suggested to have a protective effect by inhibiting phosphofructokinase as the rate-limiting step in glycolysis.[15,49] Adequate control of pH is therefore an important function of preservation solutions.

Cell Swelling

Changes in cellular structures observed during preservation are cell swelling and formation of protruding pockets.[61] The mechanism underlying these changes is the impaired activity of the Na^+/K^+-ATP-dependent pump. As a result, sodium excretion is reduced and sodium passively enters the cell, attracted by the negative charge of cytoplasmic proteins. This creates a hyperosmolar intracellular environment and subsequently an influx of water. To re-establish the disturbed Donnan equilibrium and to prevent cell swelling, impermeants and colloids are added to preservation solutions.

Effective impermeants are saccharides and non-saccharide anions. Molecular size determines the success of extracellular impermeants in preservation solutions, with larger molecules being most successful.[48,120,129] Colloids such as starches are large molecules that are retained in the vascular compartment.

Reactive Oxygen Species

ROS are generated by several processes in ischemic and postischemic reperfused organs.[82] An extensively studied generator of ROS is xanthine oxidase, which simultaneously produces hydrogen peroxide (H_2O_2) and the superoxide anion (O^{2-}).[72,112] The subsequent reduction of H_2O_2, catalyzed by iron, leads to hydroxyl radical formation (OH^-). ROS react rapidly with other molecules, which results in severe damage to lipids, nucleic acids, and proteins during reperfusion – the ischemia-reperfusion injury (IRI).[22,71] In addition to xanthine oxidase, which in human renal transplantation may be of minor importance, since it is not abundant in human cells, in contrast to rodents,[114] several other sources of ROS are important. Infiltration of leukocytes in the graft after reperfusion results in production of mainly superoxides (known as the respiratory burst).

Mitochondrial malfunctioning resulting from partial reduction of the respiratory chain is an important contributor to ROS formation after reperfusion. The formation of ROS has long been considered to contribute to cellular injury during the reperfusion phase but not during cold preservation.[22,71] However, some reports suggest that oxygen radicals are formed during reperfusion as well as during cold preservation.[109,110]

Calcium

During normal circumstances a large difference in free calcium concentration exists between the intracellular and extracellular space fluid. This difference is maintained by active transport of Ca^{2+} by several ATP-dependent processes, including Ca^{2+}-ATPase and Na^+/Ca^{2+} exchanger.[10] During cold preservation, cellular ATP concentrations fall, leading to increased intracellular Ca^{2+}. Accumulation of Ca^{2+} in the cold phase will lead to activation of calcium-dependent processes such as calpain activation and protein kinase C signaling. Calpain activation leads to loss of cell structure by breakdown of the cytoskeletal spectrin.[43] Calpain activity has been shown to be increased in cold-stored hepatocytes, and further increased during rewarming.[67]

Enzymes

Intracellular proteases are involved in the breakdown of proteins during preservation, most likely due to the absence of oxygen. Also, matrix metalloproteinases (MMPs) may be activated during cold preservation, leading to detachment of endothelial cells from the underlying matrix. This phenomenon has been predominantly studied in the liver but also occurs in renal preservation.[123,126] To reduce this detrimental effect by blocking MMPs (especially MMP 2 and 9), the addition of the often-disputed colloid, hydroxyethylene starch (HES), in University of Wisconsin (UW) solution has been shown to play an important role.[126]

Another relevant family of enzymes activated during cold preservation is the apoptosis-related caspases.[25,34,94] During prolonged preservation, free iron is released from cytochrome P-450.[58] The release of free iron will, in combination with hydrogen peroxide, lead to severe production of ROS.[104,134] Recently, changes in autophagy fluxes have been postulated as a possible mechanism of increasing injury with increasing cold ischemia times (CIT). Although most studied in the liver,[44,75] preclinical work indicates that autophagy may also be important in kidneys.[125] In relation to this, Minor et al.[77,85] have also postulated that endoplasmic reticulum stress might be involved in cold ischemia-induced injury. This was subsequently confirmed by Peralta et al.[100]

As described above, during cold preservation, cellular homeostasis is no longer sustained. Major derangements are shifts in electrolytes, changes in pH, intracellular enzymes and proteins, and increase in intracellular water. Preservation solutions are therefore composed to counteract these processes. We have chosen to concentrate on the clinically used preservation solutions.

COMPOSITION OF CLINICALLY USED SOLUTIONS

Numerous preservation solutions have been evaluated for the static cold storage of kidneys for transplantation.[95] They differ considerably in terms of their chemical composition (Table 9-2). A few examples of the most important solutions in international clinical practice are described below.

Eurocollins Solution

The first static cold storage solution was developed by Collins in the late 1960s.[28] A minor modification by the Eurotransplant Foundation in 1976, eliminating magnesium, resulted in the Eurocollins (EC) solution which was used mainly in the era before the UW solution was developed.

EC is a simple intracellular-like preservation solution. Phosphate was used for pH buffering and glucose served as the osmotic agent. Since glucose is able to cross the cell membrane, it is a source for ATP and lactate in an anaerobic environment, reducing its impermeant effectiveness.[90] Since the introduction of UW, most centers have been using this solution. A randomized clinical trial comparing EC with UW showed that DGF was significantly lower in the UW group (23% versus 33%). Also, 1-year graft survival was found to be significantly higher in the UW group.[101] As a result of this study, EC was no longer the preferred solution for kidney preservation in Europe.

University of Wisconsin Solution

Continuous and systematic research by Belzer and Southard in the 1980s led to the development of the UW solution and its clinical introduction in 1987. Metabolically inert substrates such as lactobionate and raffinose served as osmotic agents (Table 9-2). HES is used as a colloid. The colloids were originally added to hypothermic machine preservation solutions to prevent tissue edema due to hydrostatic pressure. Belzer and Southard used diafiltrated HES in UW as they originally aimed at developing one solution suitable for both cold storage and HMP. The feasibility of HES as a colloid in UW has been extensively debated. HES prevents interstitial edema and has a beneficial effect on MMPs, but increases viscosity.[101,128] Analyzing the effect of HES on red blood cells, several authors have shown an increased red blood cell aggregation when large molecular-sized HES is present.[89,128] This effect could partially explain the slower washout of blood and initially patchy reperfusion of organs when UW is used.[122] In UW, the compounds allopurinol and glutathione (GSH) are included to prevent formation of ROS. Allopurinol inhibits xanthine oxidase, which improves kidney preservation, while liver or pancreas preservation is almost unaffected.[12]

GSH is a tripeptide which has free radical-trapping properties. This important antioxidant is oxidized to glutathione disulfide together with converting peroxides. Experimental studies have shown the importance of GSH in models of both renal tubular injury and isolated

TABLE 9-2 Composition of Preservation Solutions

		EC	UW	HTK	HOC	Celsior	IGL-1
Buffers (mM)	K_2HPO_4	15	–	–	–	–	–
	KH_2PO_4	43	25	–	–	–	25
	$NaHCO_3$	10	–	–	10	–	–
	Histidine	–	–	198	–	30	–
Impermeants (mM)	Glucose	195	–	–	–	–	–
	Lactobionate	–	100	–	–	80	100
	Citrate	–	–	–	80	–	–
	Mannitol	–	–	38	185	60	–
	Raffinose	–	30	–	–	–	30
Electrolytes (mM)	Chloride	15	20	32	–	42	20
	Calcium	–	–	0.0015	–	0.25	–
	Magnesium	–	5	4	40	13	5
	Potassium	115	120	9	84	15	25
	Sodium	10	30	15	84	100	120
ROS scavengers (mM)	Allopurinol	–	1	–	–	–	1
	Glutathione	–	3	–	–	3	3
	Tryptophan	–	–	2	–	–	–
Nutrients (mM)	Adenosine	–	5	–	–	–	5
	Glutamate	–	–	–	–	20	–
	Ketoglutarate	–	–	1	–	–	–
Colloids (mM)	HES	–	0.25	–	–	–	–
	PEG	–	–	–	–	–	0.03
Osmolality (mOsm)		406	320	310	400	255	320

EC, Eurocollins; HES, hydroxyethylene starch; HOC, hyperosmolar citrate; HTK, histidine-tryptophan-ketoglutarate; IGL-1, Institut Georges Lopez-1; PEG, polyethylene glycol; ROS, reactive oxygen species; UW, University of Wisconsin.

perfused liver.[60,132] In the absence of GSH, less ATP was generated and more lactate dehydrogenase was released.[60,131] Subsequent studies have shown the benefit of GSH after kidney transplantation and that GSH is especially important in long-term liver preservation.[17]

To date, UW is considered the gold-standard preservation solution for kidney, liver, pancreas, and small bowel.[13,26,31,35,41,62,101]

Histidine-Tryptophan-Ketoglutarate Solution

Histidine-tryptophan-ketoglutarate solution (HTK) was initially introduced as a cardioplegic solution in open-heart surgery by Bretschneider in the 1970s.[20] The basic design of the solution consists of a very potent buffer, histidine, combined with two amino acids (Table 9-2). Tryptophan serves as a membrane stabilizer and antioxidant while ketoglutarate acts as a substrate for anaerobic metabolism during preservation.[90] Mannitol is a slightly larger monosaccharide than glucose but, unlike glucose, it cannot be metabolized and does not pass the cell membrane easily. Furthermore, it is added for its beneficial effect as a free radical scavenger. In addition to mannitol, tryptophan protects the organs against ROS-mediated damage. Tryptophan acts as an antioxidant through its oxidative metabolites in the kyunerine pathway, such as 5-hydroxytryptophan.[27,37] In a cultured rat hepatocyte experiment, the amount of thiobarbituric acid-reactive substances (TBARS) as a marker for ROS-mediated injury was measured. After 24 hours' preservation TBARS were significantly higher in HTK-preserved hepatocytes compared to UW, suggesting superior antioxidant capacity of UW due to the combination of GSH and allopurinol.[105]

HTK has a low viscosity and, to achieve complete tissue equilibration according to Bretschneider, high volumes (~15 L) have to be rinsed through the organs at low flow rates. A multicenter randomized prospective trial comparing UW with HTK in kidney preservation showed equal results in terms of the incidence of DGF (33% versus 33%).[31] For prolonged cold storage times with HTK (>24 hours), however, few data are available. One single-center study reported a significantly higher incidence of DGF with HTK than UW (50% versus 24%) when CIT was over 24 hours.[107] The opposite was reported in a more recent study, with much higher DGF rate associated with UW than with HTK (56% versus 16%).[2] Direct comparison of these conflicting findings is impossible due to a different definition of DGF in the two studies.

Hyperosmolar Citrate Solution

Hyperosmolar citrate (HOC, also known as Marshall's solution) is used for renal transplantation primarily in the United Kingdom and Australia.[79,92] HOC is a citrate/$NaHCO_3$ buffered solution with mannitol as the impermeant. Due to its composition as a hypertonic solution, HOC prevents the entry of fluid into cells[3] and has been shown to be effective in experimental kidney preservation.[108] A recent evaluation revealed no major differences in transplant outcome in the United Kingdom between HOC and UW or HOC and Celsior,[14] although recent work by Kay and colleagues in experimental transplantation showed more edema in kidneys flushed with HOC compared with UW.[66]

Celsior Solution

Celsior solution was developed initially for cardiac preservation in the early 1990s. It is similar to UW in composition and it has since proven to be of use in the preservation of kidneys, liver, and pancreas.[13,26,99] Unlike UW, it has a high sodium content (100 mM) and low potassium content (15 mM), and is relatively low in viscosity, as it does not contain HES. It combines the inert osmotic agent philosophy of UW together with the strong buffering capacity of HTK. Furthermore, Celsior solution contains lactobionate and mannitol as impermeants, along with reduced GSH as an antioxidant.

Institut Georges Lopez-1 Solution

The HES controversy initiated a search for other colloids, e.g., dextran and polyethylene glycol (PEG).[1,11,24] Besides the high viscosity associated with HES, its tendency to cause red cell aggregation in animal experimental models,[128] and in vitro,[9,89] justified the search for alternatives such as PEG. PEG is a neutral, water-soluble, non-toxic polymer. Although chemically not a true colloid, it acts like a colloid by the binding of water. In addition, PEG can bind to cell membranes and create layers of "structured water," preventing the approach of cells. This induces a type of immune camouflage by interfering with identification of the graft as foreign by cells of the immune system.[36] PEG prevents the activation of reperfusion-induced inflammation, which can have a long-term effect on graft outcome, particularly through interference with danger signal production.[57] Several studies, both experimental and clinical, have now confirmed the efficacy of PEG for liver but also for kidney, pancreas, small bowel, and heart preservation.[8,59,132,136]

A recent systematic review and meta-analysis compared evidence from randomized controlled trials (RCTs) and prospective controlled trials of preservation fluids.[95] The authors concluded that there was good evidence that UW and HTK reduced DGF in comparison with EC solution. The comparisons included of UW with HTK were limited to one adequately sized study of DBD kidneys that demonstrated no difference in outcome.[31] There were three RCTs that compared UW to Celsior: two were small and one had a large number of dropouts. No difference in DGF was demonstrated by these three studies individually or in meta-analysis.[95]

HYPOTHERMIC MACHINE PERFUSION REVISITED

HMP was the original method of renal preservation during the early years of renal transplantation.[7] Following the development of preservation fluids that achieved equivalent results to HMP in a static setting, and hence with reduced costs, static storage overtook HMP as the prevalent method of renal graft preservation. Changes in the donor pool have recently prompted a return to the

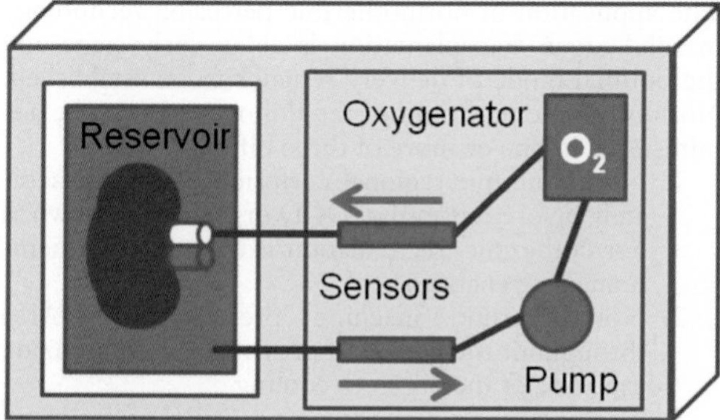

FIGURE 9-3 ■ Hypothermic machine perfusion devices maintain the stored kidney in a bath of preservation solution surrounded by ice. The same solution is withdrawn from the bath and pumped (via an oxygenator in some cases) through the renal artery of the kidney. Temperature and flow dynamics can be monitored.

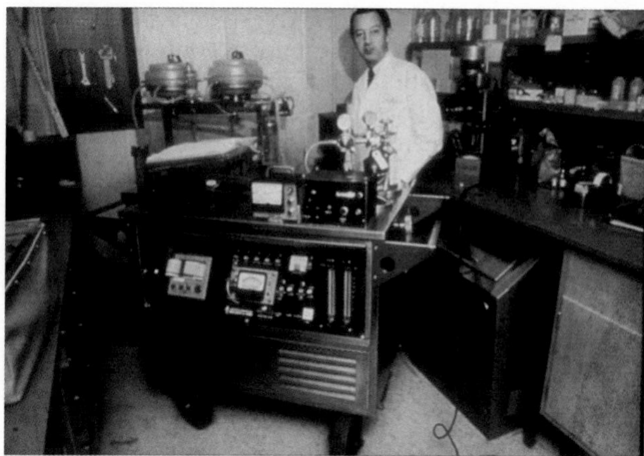

FIGURE 9-4 ■ Professor F. O. Belzer with the first "transportable" machine perfusion system.

use of HMP. It has demonstrated beneficial effects for DBD,[87] but in particular DCD[63] and ECD,[124] where the potential to reduce DGF and PNF rates, and improve graft survival, is greater.

For HMP the retrieved kidney is placed within a reservoir chamber filled with chilled preservation solution surrounded by an ice box (Figure 9-3). The renal artery is cannulated and a recirculating pump is used to generate a pulsatile or continuous flow of preservation solution. The fluid exits the renal vein and enters the reservoir from where the pump collects it again to continue the process. The pump can be pressure- or flow-targeted and allows the monitoring of the renal resistance to flow. The flow of preservation fluid ensures uniform renal cooling and allows constant flush-out of metabolites. The preservation fluid can be oxygenated if required. In early years HMP was associated with tissue edema due to the relatively high hydrostatic pressures involved and this prompted the development of perfusion fluids with strong oncotic effects to retain fluid within the vascular compartment. Human albumin solution was used initially, followed by human plasma derivatives. Currently, the synthetic perfusate, called the Belzer machine perfusion solution, is most widely used. Belzer machine perfusion solution is a high-sodium and low-potassium solution that incorporates HES. It differs from UW in that it contains gluconate instead of lactobionate as well as mannitol and the key buffer is HEPES (Figure 9-4).

A recent, large multicenter European RCT studied HMP in comparison with static cold storage.[87] Moers and the multinational group found that, across all donor types, rates of DGF could be lowered from approximately 27% to 21%. HMP was independently associated with a significantly reduced risk of DGF, with an odds ratio of 0.57, seen in DBD and DCD. When DGF did occur, it was also shorter following HMP (average 10 days versus 13 days). Both 1-year and 3-year graft survival was also significantly better for kidneys preserved by HMP. Of particular interest, in those kidneys that developed DGF, 1-year graft survival was better if preserved by HMP than static cold storage.[86] PNF was similarly low in both groups, at approximately 2% and 5%.

For DCD kidneys, where DGF rates are typically higher, there is a greater potential for improvement in outcomes. Results from a European RCT for DCD kidneys showed a large relative reduction in DGF, with rates dropping from approximately 70% to 54% when HMP was used.[63] A smaller RCT from the UK however did not find any benefit, with DGF rates equally low, at approximately 56% and 58%.[130] It should be noted that in the UK trial the DGF rate was lower to begin with and centers were free to commence HMP at any stage during preservation which resulted in significant shorter machine perfusion times than in the European RCT. One-year graft survival and PNF rates were the same for both modalities of preservation in both of these studies.

HMP has also been tested for ECD kidneys, where it may have more potential to improve upon transplant outcomes. In a large European RCT, HMP reduced PNF rates from 12% to 3%, although DGF rates were not statistically improved (30% to 22%, P=0.27). One-year graft survival was significantly improved following HMP (92% versus 80%).[124] Large database analyses have also shown a significant reduction in DGF with the use of HMP for ECD kidneys, but without such an impact on graft survival.[80,113,118]

A recent systematic review and meta-analysis has assessed the evidence from all RCTs comparing HMP with cold storage.[137] The authors concluded that HMP is associated with a reduction in DGF, with a relative risk between 0.70 and 0.92. The largest study included in the review demonstrated improved graft survival with HMP (European machine perfusion trial, described above).[87]

The evidence from registry data is somewhat conflicting and this may represent the inherent selection bias of these retrospective studies. Analysis of the Scientific Registry of Transplant Recipients (n=98 736 kidneys) found that HMP has been used more for diabetic, older, African-American donors or those with higher terminal creatinine and longer CIT.[113] Despite these associations, HMP was associated with reduced rates of DGF in this database (20% versus 28%). Data from the Collaborative Transplant Study (n=91 674 kidneys) found that HMP was associated with reduced graft survival compared to static cold storage, which may be due to the associations above.[97]

Some centers have concentrated on the additional monitoring and assessment that HMP allows. The renal resistance indices during perfusion have been extensively quoted as providing an opportunity to evaluate a marginal organ. The systematic bias in reviews of this technique and the discard of large numbers of kidneys has made it difficult to assess the relationship between renal resistance and graft outcome accurately. A large analysis of prospectively collected perfusion dynamics, which were not disclosed to transplant surgeons preoperatively, showed that renal resistance was an independent risk factor for DGF and graft loss.[64] However, it has poor predictive value and cannot be used as a stand-alone viability parameter.[64]

HMP also allows the collection and analysis of biomarkers in the perfusate during the preservation period. Six biomarkers were assessed during the European Machine Perfusion Trial.[88] These included: alanine aminopeptidase, aspartate aminotransferase, glutathione-*S*-transferase (GST), heart-type fatty acid-binding protein (H-FABP), lactate dehydrogenase, and *N*-acetyl-beta-D-glucosamine (NAG). Multivariate analysis of perfusates from the end of the preservation period showed that GST, H-FABP, and NAG were moderate, independent predictors of DGF.[88] None of the biomarkers were independently associated with PNF or decreased graft survival and should not be used as justification to discard a kidney.

NORMOTHERMIC PERFUSION

The term "normothermic perfusion" refers to the perfusion of an organ at normal physiological temperature. In the context of organ preservation this is clearly directly contrary to the basic scientific principle that has underpinned the whole of organ preservation since the start of clinical transplant programs, that of cold preservation.

Continued metabolism at hypothermic temperatures leads to the accumulation of metabolites, which form the substrates for subsequent IRI. HMP improves the situation, probably by removal of metabolic products, and this may be the basis of its proven benefit in more marginal organs.[63,87,124] HMP systems may also be configured to deliver oxygen, which has been shown experimentally to be beneficial.[84] However, the complex biological functions of mammalian cells are only effective within a narrow range of temperatures and the rationale of normothermic perfusion is, therefore, to maintain the organ within this range in order to minimize preservation injury.

Normothermic perfusion comprises:

- Oxygen delivery sufficient to maintain normal cellular ATP levels
- Physiological temperature to allow normal cellular functions
- Delivery of nutrition to prevent depletion of cellular energy substrates.

The purported advantages of normothermic perfusion are:

- Avoid cellular damage caused by cooling, independent of ischemia
- Minimize IRI by preventing the depletion of cellular ATP or by reversing this in organs that have previously been subjected to ischemia (as in DCD donors)
- Allow organ function to be assessed during storage in order to assess the viability of marginal donor organs.

The application of normothermic perfusion technology in solid-organ transplantation is at an early stage and the optimal mode of delivery remains to be established. Normothermic perfusion of the donor organ can be administered in one or more of three different ways:

1. Normothermic regional perfusion (NRP) immediately before retrieval of DCD organs (also known as normothermic recirculation/extracorporeal membrane oxygenation)
2. Normothermic machine preservation (NMP) throughout the period of preservation, minimizing exposure of the organ to cooling
3. Normothermic reconditioning (NRC) for a short period immediately prior to implantation.

Normothermic Regional Perfusion

In this technique the donor is attached to a cardiopulmonary bypass circuit soon after circulatory arrest. Cannulation of the donor's circulation is via the femoral, iliac, or intrathoracic vessels. It is essential to prevent reperfusion of the cerebral circulation during NRP and this is achieved by the use of an intra-aortic balloon (introduced via a femoral artery) or direct cross-clamping of the intrathoracic aorta.

There are good experimental data to show the benefit of NRP in models of DCD and increasing clinical use in a number of countries.[40] However, there is no formal RCT evidence as to the benefit of this approach in either controlled or uncontrolled DCD.

Increasing use of NRP has mirrored the increasing number of uncontrolled DCD donors in Spain and France. The kidney transplant center in Madrid, Spain, has successfully transplanted kidneys from Maastricht categories I, II, and IV DCD.[4,5,111] The 5-year graft survival is equal to DBD kidneys.[111] However, this success has been achieved at the price of a highly selective approach to donor acceptance and the discard rate for retrieved kidneys is very high in this setting (approximately 33%). The main reasons for discarding such organs are poor histology on biopsy, poor perfusion parameters, or positive viral serology.[5] The DGF rate is also high (68–80%), as is the PNF rate of 6%.[4,5] One center in Paris, France, has used the same approach for Maastricht category I and II DCD, accepting a longer warm ischemia time of up to 150 minutes, demonstrating higher rates of discard (43%) and DGF (92%), but a lower PNF rate (2%).[38] In a small series of Maastricht category II and IV donors in Barcelona, Spain, standard NRP was compared with hypothermic NRP and with in situ cold perfusion using EC solution.[127] The standard NRP group had lower rates of DGF (13%) compared to the other groups (55–75%) and less PNF than the in situ cold perfusion group (0% versus 22%).

There is little published experience of the use of NRP in controlled DCD. Theoretically it provides a means to reverse the acidosis and low oxygen levels that develop after the withdrawal of life support. Magliocca and the Michigan group report a case series (15 donors) with low rates of DGF (8%) and PNF (0%) in this setting.[76] A large cohort study from Taiwan demonstrated that NRP for kidneys from Maastricht categories II, III, and IV DCD could achieve 5-year graft survival rates comparable with kidneys from DBD.[73]

Normothermic Machine Perfusion

In this technique the kidney is placed within a chamber from which venous effluent can be collected and the urinary fluid can be drained from the ureter. The renal artery is cannulated to provide a recirculated blood flow. The system incorporates a centrifugal pump, oxygenator, and heat exchanger. Important early work in this area was performed by Brasile et al., who demonstrated in a canine model that very prolonged periods of warm ischemia could be tolerated successfully in organs that were preserved by NMP.[19,119] More recently a series of studies from the Leicester group of Nicholson and Hosgood have used a porcine kidney transplant model to demonstrate that normothermic perfusion with blood is a highly effective method to resuscitate kidneys that have been subjected to warm ischemia.[6,51] It is also a good platform for the delivery of other therapeutic strategies designed to minimize IRI, including carbon monoxide and hydrogen sulfide.[50,53] In parallel, studies in the porcine liver transplant model have corroborated these findings, showing that normothermic preservation can enable successful transplantation of organs following prolonged periods of warm ischemia.[21] The combination of NRP and NMP has been shown by the Barcelona group of Fondevila and Garcia-Valdecasas et al. to enable even greater tolerance of warm ischemia, again in a liver model,[39] suggesting that different normothermic perfusion strategies may be complementary.

Normothermic Reconditioning

The challenges of providing normothermic preservation from the time of retrieval to the time of implantation are considerable, not least because it requires the preservation device to be transportable from the donor hospital to the transplant unit, incurring logistic complexity and cost with respect to organ sharing and allocation. The use of normothermic perfusion for a shorter period immediately prior to transplantation is logistically a much simpler task, as it allows the process of retrieval and transport to be carried out using existing simpler and cheaper techniques.

The Leicester group has pioneered this approach both experimentally and clinically.[52] Using a porcine kidney reperfusion and transplant model, this group has demonstrated that a brief period of normothermic reconditioning (NRC) is effective in significantly improving the function of kidneys damaged by warm ischemia. These studies led on to the first clinical study which showed that, in a series of 20 ECD kidneys (including one DCD organ) treated with a short period of NRC, 19 organs functioned immediately.[54] Although this was a phase I study without a randomized control group, the result is striking in a group of patients with a predicted DGF rate of 30–40%.

Mechanism of Action

There is an increasing body of evidence that normothermic perfusion, whether delivered in the form of NRP, NMP, or NRC, is effective in improving the immediate function and survival rate of marginal donor organs, particularly those damaged by warm ischemia. The mechanism of benefit remains unclear, although a number of hypotheses are proposed and it is likely that a combination of mechanisms is involved.

NMP enables reperfusion of the organ and the establishment of normal cellular metabolism and energy stores in the absence of some of the key effector mechanisms of IRI. In experimental studies in which blood-based perfusion is used, there is evidence that depletion of leukocytes prior to perfusion reduces the reperfusion injury.[47] Leukocytes are an important component of IRI and this is, therefore, an unsurprising finding. Clinical studies are likely to use blood sourced from national blood transfusion services and therefore leukocyte-depleted.

This does not, however, provide an explanation for the beneficial effect of NRP, in which the organs are reperfused with the blood from the donor (the circuit is primed with crystalloid or colloid solution). In this situation, it is likely that the predominant mechanism of benefit is the immediate repletion of cellular energy stores prior to organ cooling and preservation – effectively converting the organ from one from a DCD donor to one from a DBD donor. There is evidence (Debabrata Roy, personal communication) that a 60-minute period of NRP protects the organ by ATP recovery and this directly correlates with recovery of mitochondrial function after reperfusion. In this context, the use of other pharmacological agents known to protect the mitochondrion may also be of clinical importance.

It has been suggested that a mechanism by which normothermic perfusion protects organs is that of ischemic preconditioning. This is a phenomenon whereby a brief period of cellular hypoxia followed by a period of recovery protects the cells from a subsequent more severe injury. The phenomenon is well documented in several systems (e.g., cardiac, neurological) and the mechanism involves the hypoxia-inducible factor pathway with a complex process of gene activation occurring as a consequence of hypoxia. This is part of the physiological response to hypoxia and greater understanding of this will open up new opportunities in organ protection.

Complement activation is known to be an important early event in IRI and experimental models of complement activation blockade have been shown to abrogate this injury.[135] It is likely, therefore, that the use of bank blood for NMP and NRC, with low levels of complement activity, is beneficial, although this has not been formally tested.

Cooling is known to be deleterious to organ function independent of preservation injury,[15,74] and it is likely that the avoidance of cooling (other than brief periods of cooling at retrieval and implantation) does contribute to the benefit of NMP. However, this hypothesis is difficult to test and there is no direct evidence to confirm or refute this.

All perfusion systems, both hypothermic and normothermic, provide continuous circulation of perfusate through the microcirculation. This removes metabolic products from the immediate environment, reducing the availability of xanthine and other molecules which act as substrates for the subsequent enzymatic processes that occur at reperfusion, producing superoxide radicals and other effectors of lipid peroxidation.[82]

Perfusion Fluid and Oxygen Carrier

Most groups developing normothermic perfusion have come to the conclusion that a specialized oxygen carrier is needed; this is based on the calculated continuing oxygen demand for normal metabolic function and the ability to deliver oxygen dissolved in solution. The large majority of normothermic perfusion studies have used blood as the oxygen carrier. Although red blood cells are highly evolved to provide oxygen to tissues, there are some disadvantages that have led some groups to investigate alternative oxygen carriers.

A number of compounds have been considered for use as an oxygen carrier in this context. These include naturally occurring molecules, such as Hemarina-M101, a large hemoglobin molecule derived from marine invertebrates (Nereididae worms),[29] modified bovine hemoglobin molecules, as incorporated in EMS solution,[18] and perfluorocarbon molecules.[55] The last of these has only been used clinically as an adjunct in cold preservation solutions and as part of the "two-layer" technique in pancreas preservation, but it has also been shown to be effective in an experimental model of kidney perfusion. Lifor, a solution incorporating a non-protein oxygen carrier, has been tested for short-term in situ normothermic preservation[106] and in a porcine model of subnormothermic renal perfusion.[42] Acellular fluids supplemented with hemoglobin could possibly resuscitate kidneys after a period of warm ischemia.[19]

Viability Assessment

An important potential advantage of NMP and NRC is the ability to measure biological parameters in the functioning organ before committing a patient to the risks of transplanting a marginal donor organ. A highly predictive means of testing viability would allow clinicians to use organs that had sustained a severe injury (typically kidneys from uncontrolled DCD donors) with a degree of confidence. The discard rate of kidneys from such donors is high and an effective method of viability assessment might improve the utilization of such organs greatly. For example, from a study in Spain in 2009, 105 kidneys were transplanted from uncontrolled DCD donors from a total of 154 recovered (68%).[33] Similar levels of discarded organs are seen in France, with a single center report of 54% utilization.[38] However, currently there is little consensus on what is the best method of viability assessment and this is an area where we may expect significant developments in future years.

FUTURE OUTLOOK

Future work in the field of renal preservation must establish which preservation strategies should be used when, and for which donors. Trials should target specific donor types and combine with an overall strategy to improve the outcome of kidney transplants from higher-risk donors. In Europe an integrated package of clinical trials to evaluate several targeted therapies proposed by the Consortium for Organ Preservation in Europe (COPE) and supported by an EU grant has been initiated. They will investigate the role of oxygenated HMP preservation and reconditioning will also be investigated in the preservation of ECD kidneys. In addition NRP prior to liver transplantation will be evaluated. Clinical trials must incorporate the collection and evaluation of both perfusate and tissue samples, which can be studied by modern molecular techniques in the search for biomarkers and in the development of suitable methods of viability assessment.

REFERENCES

1. Abdennebi HB, Steghens J-P, Hadj-Aïssa A, et al. A preservation solution with polyethylene glycol and calcium: a possible multiorgan liquid. Transpl Int 2002;15:348–54.
2. Agarwal A, Murdock P, Fridell JA. Comparison of histidine-tryptophan ketoglutarate solution and University of Wisconsin solution in prolonged cold preservation of kidney allografts. Transplantation 2006;81:480–2.
3. Ahmad N, Hostert L, Pratt JR, et al. A pathophysiologic study of the kidney tubule to optimize organ preservation solutions. Kidney Int 2004;66:77–90.
4. Alvarez J, del Barrio MR, Arias J, et al. Five years of experience with non-heart-beating donors coming from the streets. Transplant Proc 2002;34:2589–90.
5. Alvarez J, del Barrio R, Arias J, et al. Non-heart-beating donors from the streets: an increasing donor pool source. Transplantation 2000;70:314–7.
6. Bagul A, Hosgood SA, Kaushik M, et al. Experimental renal preservation by normothermic resuscitation perfusion with autologous blood. Br J Surg 2008;95:111–8.
7. Belzer FO, Ashby BS, Gulyassy PF, et al. Successful seventeen-hour preservation and transplantation of human-cadaver kidney. N Engl J Med 1968;278:608–10.
8. Ben Abdennebi H, El Rassi Z, Steghens JP, et al. Effective pig liver preservation with an extracellular-like UW solution containing the oncotic agent polyethylene glycol: a preliminary study. Transplant Proc 2002;34:762–3.
9. Ben Mosbah I, Saidane D, Peralta C, et al. Efficacy of polyethylene glycols in University of Wisconsin preservation solutions: a study of isolated perfused rat liver. Transplant Proc 2005;37:3948–50.
10. Bernardi P. Mithochondrial transport of cations: channels, exchangers, and permeability transition. Physiol Rev 1999;79:1127–55.
11. Bessems M, Doorschodt BM, Hooijschuur O, et al. Optimization of a new preservation solution for machine perfusion of the liver: which is the preferred colloid? Transplant Proc 2005;37:329–31.
12. Biguzas M, Jablonski P, Thomas AC, et al. Evaluation of UW solution in a rat kidney preservation model II. The effect of pharmacological additives. Transplantation 1990;49:1051–5.
13. Boggi U, Vistoli F, Del Chiaro M, et al. Pancreas preservation with University of Wisconsin and Celsior solutions: a single-centre, prospective, randomized study. Transplantation 2004;77:1186–90.
14. Bond M, Pitt M, Akoh J, et al. The effectiveness and cost-effectiveness of methods of storing donated kidneys from deceased donors: a systematic review and economic model. Health Technol Assess 2009;13:iii–iv, xi-xiv, 1-156.
15. Bonventre JV, Cheung JY. Effects of metabolic acidosis on viability of cells exposed to anoxia. Am J Physiol 1985;249:C149–59.
16. Bos EM, Leuvenink HGD, van Goor H, et al. Kidney grafts from brain dead donors: inferior quality or opportunity for improvement? Kidney Int 2007;72:797–805.
17. Boudjema K, van Gulik T, Lindell SL, et al. Effect of oxidized and reduced glutathione in liver preservation. Transplantation 1990;50:948–51.
18. Brasile L, Green E, Haisch C. Warm ex vivo perfusion prevents reperfusion injury in warm ischemically damaged kidneys. Transplant Proc 1997;29:3422–3.
19. Brasile L, Stubenitsky BM, Booster MH, et al. Overcoming severe renal ischemia: the role of ex vivo warm perfusion. Transplantation 2002;73:897–901.
20. Bretschneider HJ. Myocardial protection. Thorac Cardiovasc Surg 1980;28:295–302.

21. Brockmann J, Reddy S, Coussios C, et al. Normothermic perfusion: a new paradigm for organ preservation. Ann Surg 2009;250:1–6.
22. Byrne AT, Johnson AH. Lipid peroxidation. In: Grace P, Mathie R, editors. Ischaemia-reperfusion injury. Oxford: Blackwell Science; 1999. p. 148–56.
23. Calne RY, Pegg DE, Brown FL. Renal preservation by ice cooling. An experimental study relating to kidney transplantation from cadavers. Br Med J 1963;2:651–5.
24. Candinas D, Largiader F, Binswanger U, et al. A novel dextran 40-based preservation solution. Transpl Int 1996;9:32–7.
25. Castaneda MP, Swiatecka-Urban A, Mitsnefes MM, et al. Activation of mitochondrial apoptotic pathways in human renal allografts after ischemia-reperfusion injury. Transplantation 2003;76:50–4.
26. Cavallari A, Cillo U, Nardo B, et al. A multicenter pilot prospective study comparing Celsior and University of Wisconsin preserving solutions for use in liver transplantation. Liver Transpl 2003;9:814–21.
27. Christen S, Peterhans E, Stocker R. Antioxidant activities of some tryptophan metabolites: possible implication for inflammatory diseases. Proc Natl Acad Sci U S A 1990;87:2506–10.
28. Collins GM, Bravo-Shugarman M, Terasaki P. Kidney preservation for transportation. Initial perfusion and 30 hours' ice storage. Lancet 1969;294:1219–22.
29. Cooper DK, Novitsky D, Wicomb WN. The pathophysiological effects of brain death on potential donor organs, with particular reference to the heart. Ann R Coll Surg Engl 1989;71:261–6.
30. Darby JM, Stein K, Grenvik A, et al. Approach to management of the heartbeating "brain dead" organ donor. JAMA 1989;261:2222–8.
31. De Boer J, De Meester J, Smits JMA, et al. Eurotransplant randomized multicenter kidney graft preservation study comparing HTK with UW and Euro-Collins. Transpl Int 1999;12:447–53.
32. Department of Health and Human Services. HRaSA, Healthcare Systems Bureau, Division of Transplantation. Organ Procurement and Transplantation Network (OPTN) and Scientific Registry of Transplant Recipients (SRTR). OPTN/SRTR 2010. Annual Data Report; 2010.
33. Domínguez-Gil B, Haase-Kromwijk B, Van Leiden H, et al. Current situation of donation after circulatory death in European countries. Transpl Int 2011;24:676–86.
34. Duval M, Plin C, Elimadi A, et al. Implication of mitochondrial dysfunction and cell death in cold preservation- warm reperfusion-induced hepatocyte injury. Can J Physiol Pharmacol 2006;84:547–54.
35. Erhard J, Lange R, Scherer R, et al. Comparison of histidine-tryptophan-ketoglutarate (HTK) solution versus University of Wisconsin (UW) solution for organ preservation in human liver transplantation. Transpl Int 1994;7:177–81.
36. Eugene M. Polyethyleneglycols and immunocamouflage of the cells tissues and organs for transplantation. Cell Mol Biol (Noisy-le-Grand) 2004;50:209–15.
37. Feksa LR, Latini A, Rech VC, et al. Promotion of oxidative stress by L-tryptophan in cerebral cortex of rats. Neurochem Int 2006;49:87–93.
38. Fieux F, Losser M-R, Bourgeois E, et al. Kidney retrieval after sudden out of hospital refractory cardiac arrest: a cohort of uncontrolled non heart beating donors. Crit Care 2009;13:R141.
39. Fondevila C, Hessheimer AJ, Maathuis M-HJ, et al. Superior preservation of DCD livers with continuous normothermic perfusion. Ann Surg 2011;254:1000–7.
40. Fondevila C, Hessheimer AJ, Ruiz A, et al. Liver transplant using donors after unexpected cardiac death: novel preservation protocol and acceptance criteria. Am J Transplant 2007;7:1849–55.
41. Fridell JA, Agarwal A, Milgrom ML, et al. Comparison of histidine-tryptophan-ketoglutarate solution and University of Wisconsin solution for organ preservation in clinical pancreas transplantation. Transplantation 2004;77:1304–6.
42. Gage F, Leeser DB, Porterfield NK, et al. Room temperature pulsatile perfusion of renal allografts with Lifor compared with hypothermic machine pump solution. Transplant Proc 2009;41:3571–4.
43. Goll DE, Thompson VF, Li H, et al. The calpain system. Physiol Rev 2003;83:731–801.
44. Gotoh K, Lu Z, Morita M, et al. Participation of autophagy in the initiation of graft dysfunction after rat liver transplantation. Autophagy 2009;5:351–60.
45. Grace P. Ischaemia-reperfusion injury. Oxford: Blackwell Science; 1999.
46. Gramm HJ, Meinhold H, Bickel U, et al. Acute endocrine failure after brain death? Transplantation 1992;54:851–7.
47. Harper S, Hosgood S, Kay M, et al. Leucocyte depletion improves renal function during reperfusion using an experimental isolated haemoperfused organ preservation system. Br J Surg 2006;93:623–9.
48. Hart NA, Leuvenink HGD, Ploeg RJ. New solutions in organ preservation. Transplant Rev 2002;16:131–41.
49. Hochachka PW, Mommsen TP. Protons and anaerobiosis. Science 1983;219:1391–7.
50. Hosgood SA, Bagul A, Kaushik M, et al. Application of nitric oxide and carbon monoxide in a model of renal preservation. Br J Surg 2008;95:1060–7.
51. Hosgood SA, Barlow AD, Yates PJ, et al. A pilot study assessing the feasibility of a short period of normothermic preservation in an experimental model of non heart beating donor kidneys. J Surg Res 2011;171:283–90.
52. Hosgood SA, Nicholson ML. First in man renal transplantation after ex vivo normothermic perfusion. Transplantation 2011;92:735–8.
53. Hosgood SA, Nicholson ML. Hydrogen sulphide ameliorates ischaemia–reperfusion injury in an experimental model of non-heart-beating donor kidney transplantation. Br J Surg 2010;97:202–9.
54. Hosgood SA, Nicholson ML. The first clinical series of normothermic perfusion in marginal donor kidney transplantation. In: 15th Annual Congress of the British Transplantation Society; Glasgow; 2012. p. 80.
55. Hosgood S, Nicholson ML. The role of perfluorocarbon in organ preservation. Transplantation 2010;89:1169–75.
56. Howard RJ, Schold JD, Cornell DL. A 10-year analysis of organ donation after cardiac death in the United States. Transplantation 2005;80:564–8.
57. Howlett TA, Keogh AM, Perry L, et al. Anterior and posterior pituitary function in brain-stem-dead donors. A possible role for hormonal replacement therapy. Transplantation 1989;47:828–34.
58. Huang H, Salahudeen AK. Cold induces catalytic iron release of cytochrome P-450 origin: a critical step in cold storage-induced renal injury. Am J Transplant 2002;2:631–9.
59. Itasaka H, Burns W, Wicomb WN, et al. Modification of rejection by polyethylene glycol in small bowel transplantation. Transplantation 1994;57:645–8.
60. Jamieson NV, Lindell S, Sundberg R, et al. An analysis of the components in UW solution using the isolated perfused rabbit liver. Transplantation 1988;46:512–6.
61. Jamieson NV, Sundberg R, Lindell S, et al. Preservation of the canine liver for 24–48 hours using simple cold storage with UW solution. Transplantation 1988;46:517–22.
62. Janssen H, Janssen PH, Broelsch CE. Celsior solution compared with University of Wisconsin solution (UW) and histidine-tryptophan-ketoglutarate solution (HTK) in the protection of human hepatocytes against ischemia-reperfusion injury. Transpl Int 2003;16:515–22.
63. Jochmans I, Moers C, Smits JM, et al. Machine perfusion versus cold storage for the preservation of kidneys donated after cardiac death: a multicenter, randomized, controlled trial. Ann Surg 2010;252:756–62.
64. Jochmans I, Moers C, Smits J, et al. The prognostic value of renal resistance during hypothermic machine perfusion of deceased donor kidneys. Am J Transplant 2011;11:2214–20.
65. Kauffman HM, Bennett LE, McBride MA, et al. The expanded donor. Transplant Rev 1997;11:165–90.
66. Kay MD, Hosgood SA, Bagul A, et al. Comparison of preservation solutions in an experimental model of organ cooling in kidney transplantation. Br J Surg 2009;96:1215–21.
67. Kohli V, Gao W, Camargo CA, et al. Calpain is a mediator of preservation-reperfusion injury in rat liver transplantation. Proc Natl Acad Sci U S A 1997;94:9354–9.
68. Kokkinos C, Antcliffe D, Nanidis T, et al. Outcome of kidney transplantation from nonheart-beating versus heart-beating cadaveric donors. Transplantation 2007;83:1193–9.
69. Koo DDH, Welsh KI, McLaren AJ, et al. Cadaver versus living donor kidneys: impact of donor factors on antigen induction before transplantation. Kidney Int 1999;56:1551–9.

70. Kootstra G, Daemen JH, Oomen AP. Categories of nonheartbeating donors. Transplant Proc 1995;27:2893–4.
71. Kosieradzki M, Kuczynska J, Piwowarska J, et al. Prognostic significance of free radicals: mediated injury occurring in the kidney donor. Transplantation 2003;75:1221–7.
72. Kuppusamy P, Zweier JL. Characterization of free radical generation by xanthine oxidase. Evidence for hydroxyl radical generation. J Biol Chem 1989;264:9880–4.
73. Lee C-Y, Tsai M-K, Ko W-J, et al. Expanding the donor pool: use of renal transplants from non-heart-beating donors supported with extracorporeal membrane oxygenation. Clin Transplant 2005;19:383–90.
74. Levy MN. Oxygen consumption and blood flow in the hypothermic, perfused kidney. Am J Physiol 1959;197:1111–4.
75. Lu Z, Dono K, Gotoh K, et al. Participation of autophagy in the degeneration process of rat hepatocytes after transplantation following prolonged cold preservation. Arch Histol Cytol 2005;68:71–80.
76. Magliocca JF, Magee JC, Rowe SA, et al. Extracorporeal support for organ donation after cardiac death effectively expands the donor pool. J Trauma 2005;58:1095–101, discussion 1101–2.
77. Manekeller S, Schuppius A, Stegemann J, et al. Role of perfusion medium, oxygen and rheology for endoplasmic reticulum stress-induced cell death after hypothermic machine preservation of the liver. Transpl Int 2008;21:169–77.
78. Marshall VC. Preservation by simple hypothermia. In: Collins G, Dubernard JM, Land W, et al., editors. Kidney transplantation. Dordrecht: Kluwer Academic; 1997. p. 115–29.
79. Marshall VC. Renal preservation. In: Morris PJ, editor. Kidney transplantation: principles and practice. 5th ed. Saunders; 2001. p. 113–34.
80. Matsuoka L, Shah T, Aswad S, et al. Pulsatile perfusion reduces the incidence of delayed graft function in expanded criteria donor Kidney Transplantation. Am J Transplant 2006;6:1473–8.
81. McAnullty JF, Reid TW, Waller KR, et al. Successful six-day kidney prservation using trophic factor supplemented media and simple cold storage. Am J Transplant 2002;2:712–8.
82. McCord JM. Oxygen-derived free radicals in postischemic tissue injury. N Engl J Med 1985;312:159–63.
83. Metzger RA, Delmonico FL, Feng S, et al. Expanded criteria donors for kidney transplantation. Am J Transplant 2003;3 (Suppl. 4):114–25.
84. Minor T, Koetting M, Kaiser G, et al. Hypothermic reconditioning by gaseous oxygen improves survival after liver transplantation in the pig. Am J Transplant 2011;11:2627–34.
85. Minor T, Manekeller S, Sioutis M, et al. Endoplasmic and vascular surface activation during organ preservation: refining upon the benefits of machine perfusion. Am J Transplant 2006;6:1355–66.
86. Moers C, Pirenne J, Paul A, et al. Machine perfusion or cold storage in deceased-donor kidney transplantation. N Engl J Med 2012;366:770–1.
87. Moers C, Smits JM, Maathuis MHJ, et al. Machine perfusion or cold storage in deceased-donor kidney transplantation. N Engl J Med 2009;360:7–19.
88. Moers C, Varnav OC, van Heurn E, et al. The value of machine perfusion perfusate biomarkers for predicting kidney transplant outcome. Transplantation 2010;90:966–73.
89. Morariu AM, vd Plaats A, v Oeveren W, et al. Hyperaggregating effect of hydroxyethyl starch components and University of Wisconsin solution on human red blood cells: a risk of impaired graft perfusion in organ procurement? Transplantation 2003;76:37–43.
90. Mühlbacher F, Langer F, Mittermayer C. Preservation solutions for transplantation. Transplant Proc 1999;31:2069–70.
91. Nagareda T, Kinoshita Y, Tanaka A, et al. Clinicopathology of kidneys from brain-dead patients treated with vasopressin and epinephrine. Kidney Int 1993;43:1363–70.
92. Nicholson ML, Metcalfe MS, White SA, et al. A comparison of the results of renal transplantation from non-heart-beating, conventional cadaveric, and living donors. Kidney Int 2000;58(6):2585–91.
93. Nijboer WN, Schuurs TA, van der Hoeven JAB, et al. Effects of brain death on stress and inflammatory response in the human donor kidney. Transplant Proc 2005;37:367–9.
94. Oberbauer R, Rohrmoser M, Regele H, et al. Apoptosis of tubular epithelial cells in donor kidney biopsies predicts early renal allograft function. J Am Soc Nephrol 1999;10:2006–13.
95. O'Callaghan JM, Knight SR, Morgan RD, et al. Preservation solutions for static cold storage of kidney allografts: a systematic review and meta-analysis. Am J Transplant 2012;12:896–906.
96. Ojo AO, Hanson JA, Meier-Kriesche H, et al. Survival in recipients of marginal cadaveric donor kidneys compared with other recipients and wait-listed transplant candidates. J Am Soc Nephrol 2001;12:589–97.
97. Opelz G, Dohler B. Multicenter analysis of kidney preservation. Transplantation 2007;83:247–53.
98. Pascual J, Zamora J, Pirsch J. A systematic review of kidney transplantation from expanded criteria donors. Am J Kidney Dis 2008;52:553–86.
99. Pedotti P, Cardillo M, Rigotti P, et al. A comparative prospective study of two available solutions for kidney and liver preservation. Transplantation 2004;77:1540–5.
100. Peralta C, Brenner C. Endoplasmic reticulum stress inhibition enhances liver tolerance to ischemia/reperfusion. Curr Med Chem 2011;18:2016–24.
101. Ploeg RJ, van Bockel JH, Langendijk PT, et al. Effect of preservation solution on results of cadaveric kidney transplantation. The European Multicentre Study Group. Lancet 1992;340:129–37.
102. Port FK, Bragg-Gresham JL, Metzger RA, et al. Donor characteristics associated with reduced graft survival: an approach to expanding the pool of kidney donors. Transplantation 2002;74:1281–6.
103. Pratschke J, Wilhelm MJ, Kusaka M, et al. Accelerated rejection of renal allografts from brain-dead donors. Ann Surg 2000;232:263–71.
104. Rauen U, Petrat F, Li T, et al. Hypothermia injury/cold-induced apoptosis – evidence of an increase in chelatable iron causing oxidative injury in spite of low O_2-H_2O_2 formation. FASEB J 2000;14:1953–64.
105. Rauen U, Reuters I, Fuchs A, et al. Oxygen free radical mediated injury to cultured rat hepatocytes during cold incubation in preservation solutions. Hepatology 1997;26:351–7.
106. Regner KR, Nilakantan V, Ryan RP, et al. Protective effect of Lifor solution in experimental renal ischemia-reperfusion injury. J Surg Res 2010;164:e291–7.
107. Roels L, Coosemans W, Donck J, et al. Inferior outcome of cadaveric kidneys preserved for more than 24 hr in histidine-tryptophan-ketoglutarate solution. Leuven Collaborative Group for Transplantation. Transplantation 1998;66:1660–4.
108. Ross H, Marshall VC, Escott ML. 72-Hour canine kidney preservation using a new perfusate. Transplantation 1976;21:498.
109. Salahudeen AK. Cold ischemic injury of transplanted kidneys: new insights from experimental studies. Am J Physiol 2004;287:F181–7.
110. Salahudeen AK, Haider N, May W. Cold ischemia and the reduced long-term survival of cadaveric renal allografts. Kidney Int 2004;65:713–8.
111. Sanchez-Fructuoso AI, Prats D, Torrente J, et al. Renal transplantation from non-heart beating donors: a promising alternative to enlarge the donor pool. J Am Soc Nephrol 2000;11:350–8.
112. Schachter M, Foulds S. Free radicals and the xanthine oxidase pathway. In: Grace P, Mathie R, editors. Ischaemia-reperfusion injury. Oxford: Blackwell Science; 1999. p. 137–56.
113. Schold JD, Kaplan B, Howard RJ, et al. Are we frozen in time? Analysis of the utilization and efficacy of pulsatile perfusion in renal transplantation. Am J Transplant 2005;5:1681–8.
114. Simmonds HA, Goday A, Morris GS. Superoxide radicals, immunodeficiency and xanthine-oxidase activity – man is not a mouse. Clin Sci 1985;68:561–5.
115. Snoeijs MGJ, Schaubel DE, Hene R, et al. Kidneys from donors after cardiac death provide survival benefit. J Am Soc Nephrol 2010;21:1015–21.
116. Snoeijs MGJ, Winkens B, Heemskerk MBA, et al. Kidney transplantation from donors after cardiac death: a 25-year experience. Transplantation 2010;90:1106–12.
117. Southard JH, Belzer FO. Organ preservation. Annu Rev Med 1995;46:235–47.
118. Stratta RJ, Moore PS, Farney AC, et al. Influence of pulsatile perfusion preservation on outcomes in kidney transplantation from expanded criteria donors. J Am Coll Surg 2007;204:873–82, discussion 882–884.
119. Stubenitsky BM, Booster MH, Brasile L, et al. Exsanguinous metabolic support perfusion – a new strategy to improve graft function after kidney transplantation. Transplantation 2000;70:1254–8.

120. Sumimoto R, Jamieson NV, Kamada N. Examination of the role of the impermeants lactobionate and raffinose in a modified UW solution. Transplantation 1990;50:573–6.
121. Summers DM, Johnson RJ, Allen J, et al. Analysis of factors that affect outcome after transplantation of kidneys donated after cardiac death in the UK: a cohort study. Lancet 2010;376:1303–11.
122. t Hart NA, Van Der Plaats A, Leuvenink HGD, et al. Initial blood washout during organ procurement determines liver injury and function after preservation and reperfusion. Am J Transplant 2004;4:1836–44.
123. Topp SA, Upadhya GA, Strasberg SM. Cold preservation of isolated sinusoidal endothelial cells in MMP 9 knockout mice: effect on morphology and platelet adhesion. Liver Transpl 2004;10:1041–8.
124. Treckmann J, Moers C, Smits J, et al. Machine perfusion versus cold storage for preservation of kidneys from expanded criteria donors after brain death. Transpl Int 2011;24:548–54.
125. Turkmen K, Martin J, Akcay A, et al. Apoptosis and autophagy in cold preservation ischemia. Transplantation 2011;91:1192–7.
126. Upadhya GA, Strasberg SM. Glutathione, lactobionate, and histidine: cryptic inhibitors of matrix metalloproteinases contained in University of Wisconsin and histidine/tryptophan/ketoglutarate liver preservation solutions. Hepatology 2000;31:1115–22.
127. Valero R, Cabrer C, Oppenheimer F, et al. Normothermic recirculation reduces primary graft dysfunction of kidneys obtained from non-heart-beating donors. Transpl Int 2000;13:303–10.
128. van der Plaats A, t Hart NA, Morariu AM, et al. Effect of University of Wisconsin organ-preservation solution on haemorheology. Transpl Int 2004;17:227–33.
129. Wahlberg JA, Love R, Landegard L, et al. 72-hour preservation of the canine pancreas. Transplantation 1987;43:5–8.
130. Watson CJE, Wells AC, Roberts RJ, et al. Cold machine perfusion versus static cold storage of kidneys donated after cardiac death: a UK multicenter randomized controlled trial. Am J Transplant 2010;10:1991–9.
131. Weinberg JM, Davis JA, Abarzua M, et al. Cytoprotective effects of glycine and glutathione against hypoxic injury in renal tubules. J Clin Invest 1987;80:1446–54.
132. Wicomb WN, Hill JD, Avery J, et al. Optimal cardioplegia and 24-hour storage with simplified UW solution containing polyethylene glycol. Transplantation 1990;49:261–4.
133. Wijnen RMH, Linden CJ. Donor treatment after pronouncement of brain death: a neglected intensive care problem. Transpl Int 1991;4:186–90.
134. Wyllie S, Seu P, Gao FQ, et al. Deregulation of iron homeostasis and cold-preservation injury to rat liver stored in University of Wisconsin solution. Liver Transpl 2003;9:401–10.
135. Yang B, Hosgood SA, Bagul A, et al. Erythropoietin regulates apoptosis, inflammation and tissue remodelling via caspase-3 and IL-1β in isolated hemoperfused kidneys. Eur J Pharmacol 2011;660:420–30.
136. Zheng TL, Lanza RP, Soon-Shiong P. Prolonged pancreas preservation using a simplified UW solution containing polyethylene glycol. Transplantation 1991;51:63–6.
137. O'Callaghan JM, Morgan RD, Knight SR et al. Systematic review and meta-analysis of hypothermic machine perfusion versus static cold storage of kidney allografts on transplant outcomes. Br J Surg 2013;100:991–1001.

CHAPTER 10

HISTOCOMPATIBILITY IN KIDNEY TRANSPLANTATION

Susan V. Fuggle • Craig J. Taylor

CHAPTER OUTLINE

HISTORICAL BACKGROUND

In the 1960s the study of histocompatibility was stimulated as the early pioneers of clinical kidney transplantation realized that immunological mechanisms were responsible for allograft destruction. In 1961 the introduction of chemical immunosuppression using firstly 6-mercaptopurine followed soon after by azathioprine and steroids enabled short- and medium-term success, but 40–50% of deceased donor transplants were lost from immediate or early graft failure due to irreversible rejection in the first year and thereafter there was an insidious decline in graft function. These early experiences severely limited the success of human allotransplantation and led to the study of compatibility of transplanted tissue, which, over the following 40 years, gave rise to the specialty of histocompatibility and immunogenetics.

The first human leukocyte antigens (HLAs) were discovered in 1958 and subsequent years by Jean Dausset, Rose Payne, and Jon van Rood.[107] During the next few years many more HLAs were characterized using antibodies in sera obtained from multiparous women and from patients after multiple blood transfusions. Such antibodies were also demonstrated in patients after allograft rejection,[74] and antibodies present in recipient sera before kidney transplantation reactive with donor lymphocytes, either by leukoagglutination or by cytotoxicity, were associated with hyperacute rejection (HAR).[52,119] HLA was quickly recognized as the human equivalent of the major histocompatibility complex (MHC), previously identified in inbred rodents, the products of which control the recognition of self and foreign antigens.[40]

THE HLA SYSTEM

The HLA system encoded on the short arm of chromosome 6 is the most intensively studied region of the human genome. The region spans over 4 megabases and contains in excess of 250 expressed genes, making it the most gene-dense region characterized to date.[44] Of relevance to transplant clinicians and immunologists is that about 28% of these genes encode proteins with immune-related functions.

HLA has a central role in immune recognition for the defense against foreign pathogens and neoplasia, mediating T-cell signaling through presentation of self and foreign antigens in the form of short protein fragments (peptides) recognized by self-HLA-restricted T lymphocytes (see Chapter 1). Recognition of non-self peptides in the context of self HLA (i.e., altered self) is the function of the T-cell antigen receptor and elicits a powerful immune response. The extensive polymorphism of HLA has evolved to enable efficient binding of peptides from the vast array of potentially pathogenic organisms that invade and colonize our bodies. Therefore the evolutionary pressures to develop and maintain diversity vary with time and geographical area. As a consequence, HLA has adapted differently according to geographic region and ethnic group and HLA phenotypes differ across populations throughout the world.

HLA Genes and their Products

The HLA system is a complex multigene family consisting of more than 10 loci. HLA types are codominantly inherited on a maternal and paternal haplotype and transmitted as a single Mendelian trait (Figure 10-1); therefore an individual can express two alleles at each locus. The genes encoding HLA and their corresponding glycoprotein products are divided into two classes according to their biochemical and functional properties: HLA class I and HLA class II.

HLA Class I

HLA class I genes span 2 megabases at the telomeric end of the 6p21.3 region of chromosome 6. This region encodes the classical transplantation antigens (HLA-A, -B, and -C) that are expressed on virtually all nucleated cells.[19] Genes of the HLA class I loci encode the 44 kD heavy chains which associate with intracellular peptides present within the cytoplasm (Figure 10-2). The tertiary structure is stabilized on the cell surface by non-covalent association with β_2-microglobulin, a non-polymorphic 12 kD protein encoded on chromosome 15. The heavy chain consists of three extracellular immunoglobulin-like domains (α_1, α_2, α_3),

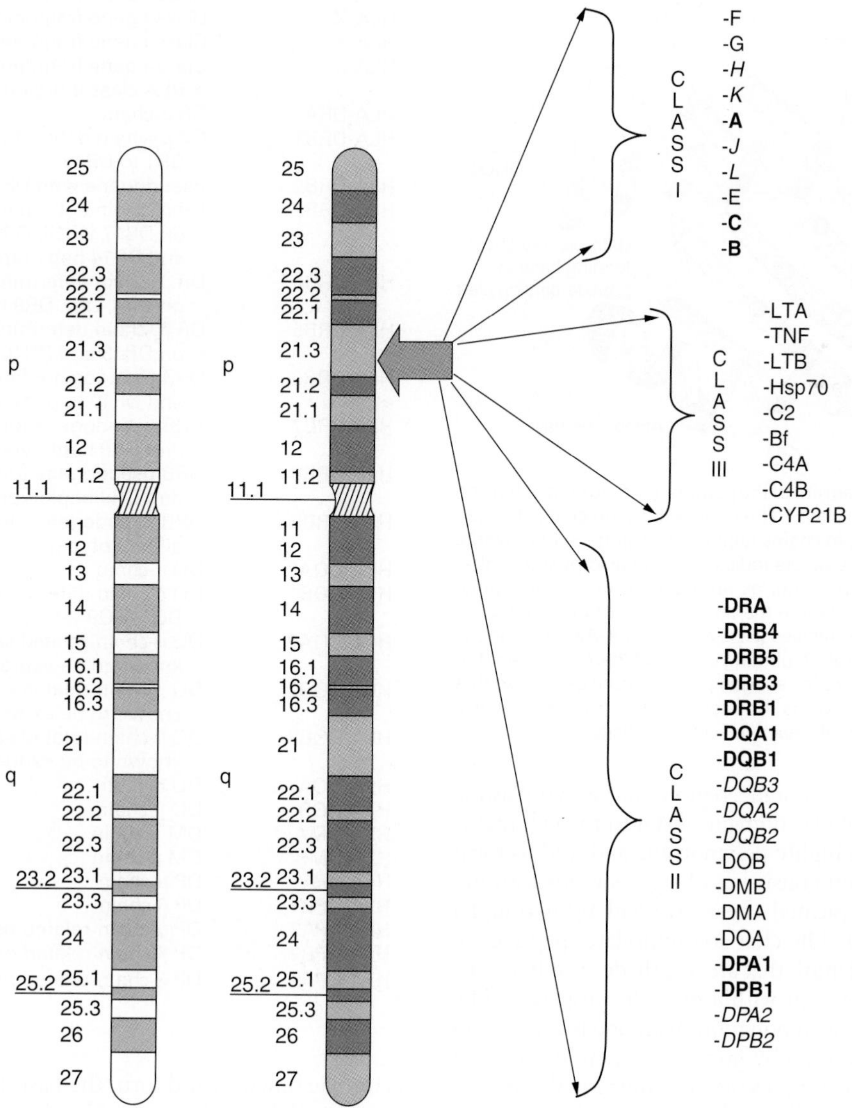

FIGURE 10-1 ■ Genomic organization of the human leukocyte antigen (HLA) region on chromosome 6. HLA antigens are codominantly inherited en bloc as a haplotype from maternal and paternal chromosomes. Italic type indicates pseudogenes. Normal type indicates "non-classical" HLA genes with no known role in clinical solid-organ transplantation. Bold type indicates genes encoding HLA products with clinical relevance to solid-organ transplantation.

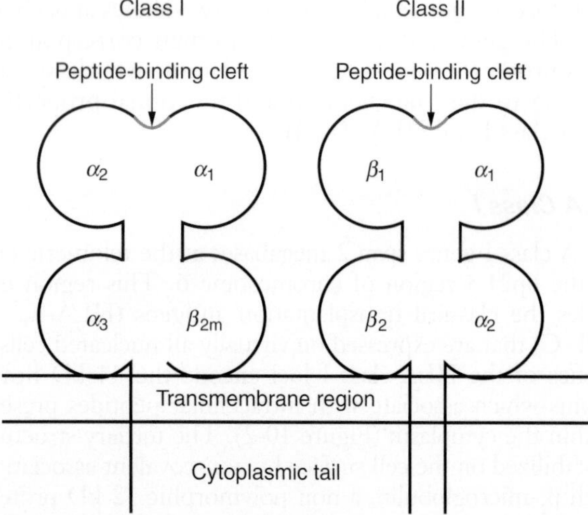

FIGURE 10-2 ■ Schematic representation of the domain structure of human leukocyte antigen (HLA) class I and II.

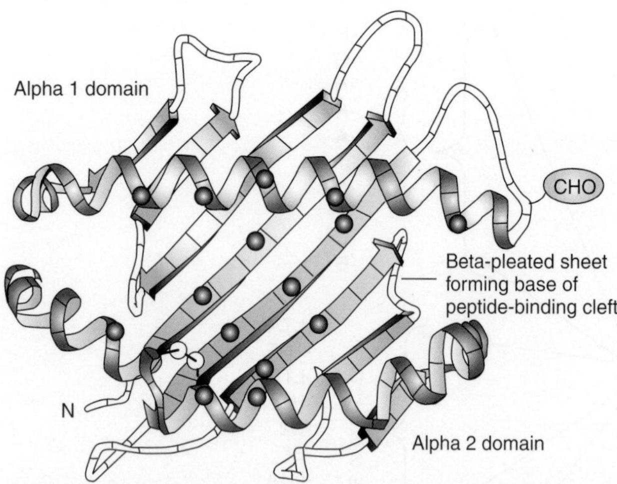

FIGURE 10-3 ■ Ribbon diagram of the peptide-binding cleft of human leukocyte antigen (HLA) class I. The peptide-binding cleft is formed by two alpha-helix protein chains (alpha 1 and alpha 2) that overlie a beta-pleated sheet. The boxes indicate amino acid positions that form the protein structure and, as an example of the HLA polymorphism, the red dots denote the amino acid residues that differ between two HLA-A specificities (HLA-A1 and HLA-A2) that line the base and sides of the peptide-binding cleft (and thereby govern the peptide-binding repertoire for antigen presentation) and those that face the outer surface towards the T-cell receptor (thereby governing the self-restricted or alloreactive T-cell specificity).

a hydrophobic transmembrane region, and a cytoplasmic tail. The two extracellular domains distal to the cell membrane (α_1 and α_2) are highly polymorphic and fold to form a peptide-binding cleft consisting of eight strands forming an antiparallel beta pleated sheet, overlaid by two alpha helices (Figure 10-3). The cleft accommodates peptides of 8–10 amino acids in length that are mostly derived from endogenous proteins present within the cell cytoplasm. The major areas of amino acid polymorphism line the sides and base of the cleft and thereby govern the peptide-binding repertoire of the HLA molecule. In contrast, the α_3 domain (proximal to the cell membrane) is highly conserved and acts as a ligand for CD8 expressed on T lymphocytes. This interaction confers HLA class I restriction on CD8-positive T lymphocytes which have a predominantly cytotoxic function and form the basis for cellular immunity to intracellular pathogens such as viruses.

TABLE 10-1 Human Leukocyte Antigen (HLA) Genes and their Products

Name	Molecular Characteristics
HLA-A	Class I α-chain
HLA-B	Class I α-chain
HLA-C	Class I α-chain
HLA-E	Associated with class I 6.2 kB Hind III fragment
HLA-F	Associated with class I 5.4 kB Hind III fragment
HLA-G	Associated with class I 6.0 kB Hind III fragment
HLA-H	Class I pseudogene
HLA-J	Class I pseudogene
HLA-K	Class I pseudogene
HLA-L	Class I pseudogene
HLA-N	Class I gene fragment
HLA-P	Class I gene fragment
HLA-S	Class I gene fragment
HLA-T	Class I gene fragment
HLA-U	Class I gene fragment
HLA-V	Class I gene fragment
HLA-W	Class I gene fragment
HLA-X	Class I gene fragment
HLA-Y	Class I gene fragment
HLA-Z	Class I gene fragment (located in the HLA class II region)
HLA-DRA	DR α-chain
HLA-DRB1	DR β_1-chain determining specificities DR1 to DR18
HLA-DRB2	Pseudogene with DR β-like sequences
HLA-DRB3	DR β_3-chain determining DR52 found on DR17, DR18, DR11, DR12, DR13, and DR14 haplotypes
HLA-DRB4	DR β_4-chain determining DR53 found on DR4, DR7, DR9 haplotypes
HLA-DRB5	DR β_5-chain determining DR51 found on DR15 and DR16 haplotypes
HLA-DRB6	DRB pseudogene found on DR1, DR2, and DR10 haplotypes
HLA-DRB7	DRB pseudogene found on DR4, DR7, and DR9 haplotypes
HLA-DRB8	DRB pseudogene found on DR4, DR7, and DR9 haplotypes
HLA-DRB9	DRB pseudogene, probably found on all haplotypes
HLA-DQA1	DQ α-chain
HLA-DQB1	DQ β-chain determining specificities DQ1–DQ9
HLA-DQA2	DQ α-chain-related sequence, not known to be expressed
HLA-DQB2	DQ β-chain-related sequence, not known to be expressed
HLA-DQB3	DQ β-chain-related sequence, not known to be expressed
HLA-DOA	DO α-chain
HLA-DOB	DO β-chain
HLA-DMA	DM α-chain
HLA-DMB	DM β-chain
HLA-DPA1	DP α-chain
HLA-DPB1	DP β-chain
HLA-DPA2	DP α-chain-related pseudogene
HLA-DPB2	DP β-chain-related pseudogene
HLA-DPA3	DP α-chain-related pseudogene

There are other class I loci and knowledge about their expression and function has emerged (Table 10-1). HLA-H, -J, -K, and -L are pseudogenes and HLA-N, -P, -S, -T,

-U, -V, -W, -X, -Y, and -Z are gene fragments that are not transcribed or translated. HLA-G is expressed on placental trophoblast cells, implicating a possible involvement in fetal–maternal development. HLA-E, -F, and -G have limited polymorphism and are known to act as ligands for natural killer (NK) cell inhibitory receptors (e.g., CD94). These loci may prove to be important in certain experimental xenograft models and in bone marrow transplantation (where NK cells are involved in the rejection process), but their clinical relevance in solid-organ transplantation has not yet been firmly established. There is, however, an emerging role for these molecules in innate immunity to persistent viruses such as cytomegalovirus and they may prove to have an important role in posttransplant viral defense.

HLA Class II

The HLA class II region consists of three main loci: HLA-DR, -DQ, and -DP. The glycoprotein products are heterodimers with non-covalently associated alpha and beta chains of molecular weight approximately 33 kD and 28 kD, respectively. Both chains have two extracellular immunoglobulin-like domains, a transmembrane region and a cytoplasmic tail (Figure 10-2). The membrane distal domains α_1 and α_1 form a peptide binding cleft similar to, but less rigid than, that of HLA class I, accommodating peptides of 10–20 amino acids that are derived predominantly from ingested (endocytosed or phagocytosed) extracellular (exogenous) proteins. The α_1 domains of HLA-DR, -DQ, and -DP are highly polymorphic and so govern the peptide binding repertoire. They are constitutively expressed on cells with immune function such as B lymphocytes, activated T lymphocytes, and antigen presenting cells (monocytes, macrophages, and cells of dendritic lineage). HLA class II expression can be induced on most cell types during inflammatory responses (including allograft rejection) by cytokines such as gamma-interferon and tumor necrosis factor-α.[19,35,36] The conserved membrane proximal domain associates with CD4 on T lymphocytes with predominantly helper/inducer function and thereby confers HLA class II restriction and forms the basis of cellular and humoral immunity to circulating pathogens such as bacteria.

HLA Polymorphism and Nomenclature. Early investigations into HLA polymorphism used relatively crude alloantisera able to distinguish only a limited number of antigens. Nearly half a century later, these simple techniques have been complemented by molecular methods capable of resolving HLA variants at the DNA sequence level and identifying single amino acid polymorphisms that are indistinguishable by serology. For example, there are currently 19 HLA-DR specificities defined by serological methods, compared to more than a thousand sequence variants (alleles) detected using DNA-based typing methods. The number of newly defined alleles identified is still increasing rapidly and has now surpassed even the highest expectations of the early pioneers.

Concomitant with the ever-increasing complexity of the HLA region, a nomenclature system has been developed to assign accurately HLA loci and their alleles.[64] This nomenclature system encompasses the methodology (serology, biochemistry, and DNA sequencing) and level to which the HLA genes and their products have been resolved. The nomenclature is complex and, to those outside the field, can appear confusing.

TABLE 10-2 **Resolution of Human Leukocyte Antigen (HLA)-Typing Methods and their Application to Renal Transplantation**

HLA-Typing Resolution	Method
HLA allele matching	High-resolution DNA sequence-based typing*
Split HLA specificity matching	Serology and low-resolution (generic) DNA typing†
Broad HLA specificity matching	Serology and low-resolution (generic) DNA typing
HLA-B, -DR matching	Serology and low-resolution (generic) DNA typing
Epitope matching	Serologically defined cross-reactive groups
	Serologically defined motifs/determinants
	Single amino acid residues
	Linear peptides and conformational epitopes
	Supertypic antigen matching
	Triplet amino acid mismatches (HLAMatchmaker)

*High-resolution DNA typing can be translated into low-resolution serological equivalents (allele families).

†Low-resolution HLA typing by polymerase chain reaction utilizes DNA primers designed to identify polymorphisms at a level comparable to serology.

Adapted from Taylor CJ, Dyer PA. Maximising the benefits of HLA matching for renal transplantation; alleles, specificities, CREGs, epitopes or residues? Transplantation 1999;68:1093–1094.

Resolution of HLA-Typing Methods. Serologically based HLA typing uses alloantisera and monoclonal antibodies that bind to tertiary epitopes of the cell surface HLA glycoproteins. There is a high degree of sequence homology between HLA specificities and identical amino acid sequence motifs (epitopes) are often shared between groups of antigens.[2,23,65]

The degree of HLA compatibility between transplant donors and recipients can be considered at many different levels of resolution, depending on the HLA-typing methodology (Table 10-2). This can range from single amino acid differences detected by high-resolution DNA sequence-based methods (allele matching) to serologically defined epitope matching. The influence of all levels of donor and recipient HLA compatibility has been considered in deceased donor kidney transplantation.[100] Although strongly implicated for negating graft-versus-host disease following unrelated bone marrow transplantation, a role for high-resolution allele matching in kidney transplantation has not been established. However, matching for serologically defined amino acids, epitopes, and specificities has been reported to benefit transplant outcome[53,96,112,121]

WHO Nomenclature for HLA. HLA genes and their polymorphic products have now been characterized and cloned and have been given official designations using the following principles. The genes are prefixed by the letters HLA followed by the locus or region, e.g., HLA-A, HLA-B, or HLA-D. The HLA-D region has several subregions denoted HLA-DR, -DQ, -DP, -DO, and -DM (Figure 10-1). These are followed by the letters A or B to define the gene encoding the alpha and beta chain gene product of that subregion, respectively (e.g., HLA-DRB genes code for the DR beta chain protein product). Where there is more than one A or B gene within a subregion, a corresponding number is given (e.g., HLA-DRB1; see Figure 10-1 and Table 10-1).

A new nomenclature system was launched by the World Health Organization (WHO) in 2010 to accommodate the growing number of HLA alleles being discovered.[64] In this system each allele is uniquely identified by up to four sets of digits separated by colons (termed fields), prefixed by an asterisk (*). The digits in the first field usually correlate with the serological specificity, for instance HLA-B*27 correlates with the serological specificity HLA-B27. However, for most serologically defined antigens there is further polymorphism detectable at the DNA and amino acid sequence level. The second field denotes the subtype, listed in the order the alleles were discovered. Alleles with different numbers at this level have nucleotide substitutions that alter the amino acid sequence, e.g., HLA-B*27:01, HLA-B*27:02, and so forth. The third field indicates synonymous substitutions within the coding region (i.e., there is no change in the amino acid sequence of the expressed protein) and the fourth field indicates polymorphism in non-coding regions.

Some alleles or genes contain sequence defects preventing normal antigen expression at the cell surface. Non-expressed alleles (null alleles) are indicated using the suffix "N" (e.g. HLA-DRB4*01:03:01N) whereas alleles with low expression or soluble (secreted) alleles carry the suffix "L" or "S" respectively. The suffix "C" indicates a protein detected within the cytoplasm and not on the cell surface, "A" aberrant expression, where there is doubt whether the protein is expressed, and "Q", questionable expression, where a given mutation has been previously shown to affect expression, but the level of expression has not been confirmed for the particular allele.

The HLA-DR and HLA-DP alpha chains are less polymorphic (DRA is diallelic) and therefore the HLA-DRB1 or -DPB1 allele (which code for the main polymorphic amino acid determinants present on the beta chain) is usually annotated alone. In contrast, both the HLA-DQ alpha and beta chains are polymorphic. To describe one of these alleles precisely, definition of both the A and B alleles may be required (e.g., HLA-DQA1*01:01 and DQB1*05:01). Although the alpha and beta chain protein products of the A and B gene pairs associate preferentially, there is also the possibility of the formation of novel hybrid molecules. A complete list of recognized HLA genes and their expressed products can be found at www.bmdw.org (Bone Marrow Donors Worldwide; HLA information).

Extended HLA Haplotypes. The HLA region displays strong linkage disequilibrium whereby certain HLA alleles are inherited together as a conserved HLA haplotype. Therefore extended HLA haplotypes involving HLA-A, -B, -C, -DR, and -DQ commonly exist within and between ethnic groups. This greatly improves the probability of locating an HLA-matched unrelated donor as common HLA haplotypes are frequently found within a population (e.g., HLA-A*01:01, -B*08:01, -C*07:01, -DRB1*03:01, -DRB3*01:01, -DQA1*05:01, -DQB1*02:01).[98] There is only relatively weak linkage centromeric to HLA-DQ because of a recombination "hot spot" between -DQ and -DP.

HLA on the Web

Information concerning the HLA system is rapidly expanding and articles such as this are always out of date by the time they go to print. However, there are a number of internet websites with useful links that are regularly updated. These provide contemporary articles and information concerning HLA genes, nomenclature, polymorphism, DNA, and amino acid sequences for both lay and professional readers:

www.anthonynolan.org.uk
www.ashi-hla.org/index.htm
www.bmdw.org
www.bshi.org.uk
www.efiweb.org
www.sanger.ac.uk.

HLA MATCHING

It was nearly 40 years ago that HLA matching between donor and recipient was associated with better transplant and patient survival.[67,74,83,111,113] Matching for the class I HLA-A and -B antigens influenced survival, but matching for the class II HLA-DR antigens was shown to have the most powerful effect.[113,114] Over the years there has been an overall improvement in transplant survival and a decrease in the survival advantage conferred by HLA matching.[13,67] The improvement can be attributed to a number of factors, but one of the most powerful is advancement in the potency of immunosuppression. This was clearly demonstrated in a local comparison of transplant survival in patients receiving azathioprine and prednisolone, cyclosporine and prednisolone, and triple therapy (cyclosporine, azathioprine, prednisolone) where 1-year transplant survival rates were 65%, 69%, and 81% respectively.[105] In this analysis HLA-DR compatibility still had a marked effect on the posttransplant clinical course, with an increased incidence of rejection in HLA-DR-mismatched grafts, the socioeconomic effects of which were increased use of immunosuppressive drugs, longer hospital stays, and higher 3-month creatinine levels.[97]

A beneficial effect of HLA matching can still be demonstrated in analyses of large datasets and national and international databases.[13,58,77] In solid-organ transplantation the effects of HLA matching reported are generally based on matching at the HLA-A, -B, and -DR loci, but the definition of a match may vary according to whether matching is considered only at the level of serological-equivalent specificities or whether the associated epitopes are also considered. There have been reports to suggest an additional benefit of matching at the amino acid sequence level and matching for HLA epitopes.[24,56,77] The effect of matching other HLA loci has been analyzed but demonstrating an independent effect is difficult due to linkage disequilibrium. Matching for HLA-DQ has been variously reported as having either a beneficial effect[117] or no effect on transplant outcome.[10,30] Registry analysis has shown that HLA-DPB matching has an effect on the transplant survival of regrafts, but not of first transplants[75] and a recent report has shown this effect to result from matching for certain immunogenic HLA-DPB epitopes.[57]

In analyzing the effect of HLA on transplant outcome, it is important that other factors known to have a strong influence on outcome are taken into account. In a rigorous multivariate analysis of factors influencing the outcome of primary deceased donor transplants in a cohort of transplants performed in the UK from 1986 to 1993, the year of transplant, donor and recipient age, waiting time to transplant, diabetes in the recipient, donor cause of death, exchange of kidneys, cold ischemia time, and HLA mismatching were found to influence transplant survival (death with function treated as failure). The best transplant survival was achieved in transplants that had no mismatches at HLA-A, -B, and -DR (000 mismatch grade). Other well-matched transplants, termed favorably matched transplants, with a maximum of one HLA-A and one HLA-B antigen mismatched in the absence of mismatches at HLA-DR (110, 100, 010 mismatch grades), had a significantly improved survival over transplants of all other match grades.[73] An analysis of factors influencing the long-term outcome of these transplants revealed that, for patients with transplants functioning after 6 years, only older donor age and diabetes had a significant detrimental influence on survival.

The influence of HLA mismatch on outcome of first deceased donor transplant has been investigated in a more recent cohort of patients in the United Kingdom, transplanted from 1995 to 2001. As a result of the allocation policy the recent transplants were significantly better matched than the previously analyzed cohort (1986–1993), where 46% of transplants were 0-DR mismatched and 10% had 2-DR mismatches, compared to 60% 0-DR mismatched and only 3% 2-DR mismatches in the 1995–2001 cohort. In a multivariate analysis there was no effect of HLA-A mismatching, but a significant effect of 2 mismatches at HLA-B and an incremental effect of mismatching at HLA-DR (Figure 10-4).[47,48]

There have been several recent publications from the Collaborative Transplant Study revealing associations between HLA-DR mismatching and a higher incidence of osteoporosis, hip fracture, increased hospitalization for infection, and increased death in the first 3 years posttransplant through infection.[78–80] These associations probably result from the higher levels of immunosuppression used in the management of poorly HLA-matched transplants.

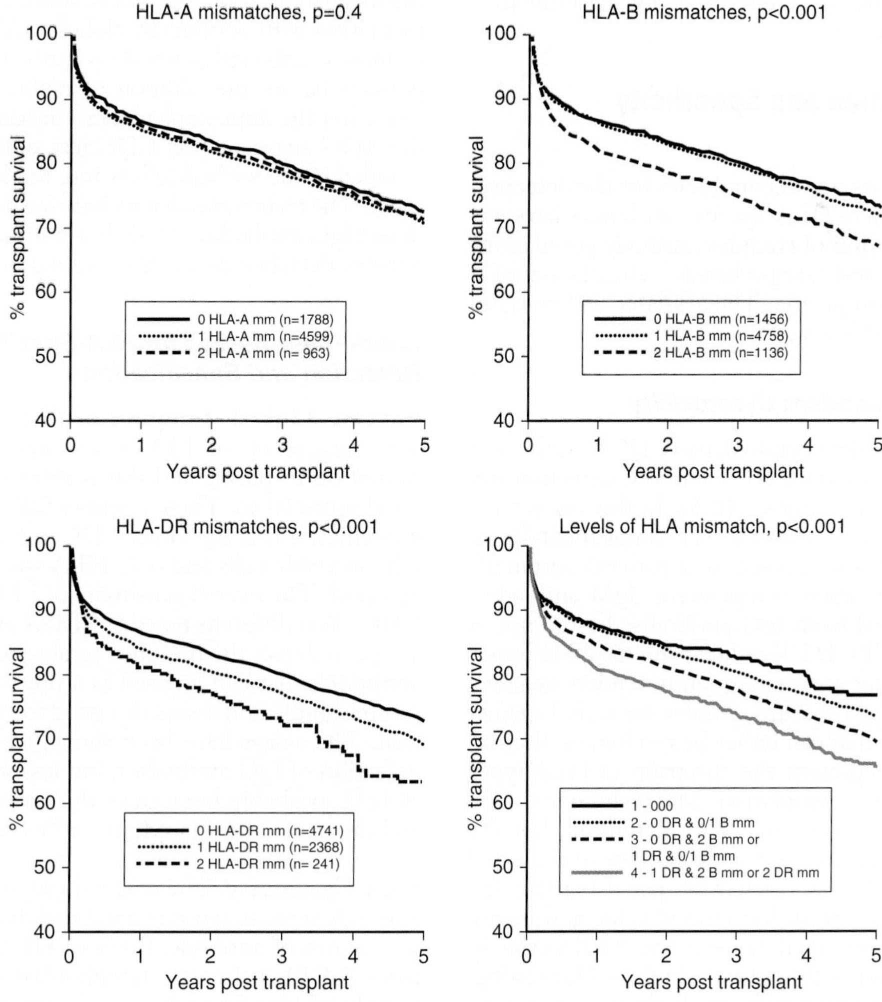

FIGURE 10-4 ■ (A–D) The influence of human leukocyte antigen (HLA)-A, -B, -DR mismatch on 5-year transplant survival. (Reproduced from Johnson RJ, Fuggle SV, O Neill J, et al. Factors influencing outcome after deceased heartbeating donor kidney transplantation in the UK: an evidence base for a new national kidney allocation policy. Transplantation 2010;89:379.)

HLA-SPECIFIC ALLOSENSITIZATION

Routes of Sensitization

An individual can become sensitized to HLA alloantigens as a result of blood transfusion, pregnancy, or previous organ transplantation. Transplantation of poorly HLA-matched kidneys can result in allosensitization to the mismatched donor HLA. Approximately 20% of pregnant women produce HLA-specific antibodies to paternally inherited fetal HLA antigens. The use of erythropoietin for the treatment of patients with anemia has decreased the use of blood transfusion in renal patients with a consequent decrease in the number of patients becoming sensitized by this route. It might be expected that the use of leukodepleted blood would prevent allosensitization, but there is evidence to suggest that this is not the case.[118] Furthermore, HLA-specific antibodies may be detected in patients who have not been exposed to these classical routes of sensitization. These idiopathic (natural) HLA-specific antibodies may result from cross-reactivity with infectious agents, which, in some cases, are reactive with specific epitopes expressed on denatured HLA proteins but absent on HLA proteins in their native form.[12] Such antibodies, however, do not react with native antigen in cell-based assays and are considered non-harmful to a transplanted kidney.[27,72,82]

Antibody Detection and Specificity Definition

Over the last 10 years new technologies for the detection and characterization of HLA-specific antibodies have enabled precise definition of complex antibody populations in serum samples and comprehensive elucidation of a patient's sensitization profile. The available technologies are briefly described below.

Complement-Dependent Cytotoxicity

Complement-dependent cytotoxicity (CDC) was the first technique routinely used for HLA antibody detection and for the crossmatch test (Figure 10-5). In this assay, lymphocyte target cells are used to detect complement-fixing IgG and IgM antibodies present in a patient's serum after the addition of rabbit complement. IgM antibodies can be differentiated from IgG antibodies by the use of dithiothreitol (DTT). DTT reduces the disulfide bonds in the IgM pentamer and consequently renders negative a reaction due to IgM. Serum samples are tested against lymphocyte panels that can either be random or alternatively selected to represent the spectrum of HLA types in the potential donor population. The technique can be used for limited antibody specificity definition, but the results are often expressed as the percentage of the panel to which the sample has reacted (% panel-reactive antibody: %PRA). This term has limited value and its use is now strongly discouraged, because the %PRA entirely depends on the composition of the panel used for testing. If a patient has a monospecific antibody to a specificity that is common in a population, and a random panel is used, then the %PRA will be high, but if the panel has been carefully selected to include rare and common specificities, the %PRA value for the same antibody may be low. Furthermore, %PRA values cannot be compared between panels or laboratories.

There are a number of other limitations of the CDC technique. Only complement-fixing antibodies are detected, and the sensitivity of the technique is dependent on viable target cells and the particular batch of rabbit complement used. Both HLA and non-HLA antibodies are detected. While the use of DTT can differentiate IgM from IgG antibodies, this does not indicate the specificity of the antibody and potentially clinically relevant weak IgG HLA-specific antibodies may also be rendered negative following the addition of DTT to patient serum. Reactivity resulting from an IgM HLA-specific antibody is indistinguishable from reactivity of an IgM autoreactive antibody. However, autoantibodies are frequently weak or non-reactive with lymphocytes from patients with B-cell chronic lymphatic leukemia (CLL) and therefore including these cells in a panel can be useful in elucidating a patient's antibody profile.[115] Alternatively serum samples can be preabsorbed with autologous cells to remove autoreactive antibodies, before screening for alloreactivity. There have been a number of approaches used to increase the sensitivity of the CDC test. These include increasing the incubation times, the wash (Amos) technique, and augmentation with antihuman globulin (AHG). In the Amos technique unbound antibody is washed from the cell suspension before the addition of rabbit complement, thus removing the anticomplementary factors in the serum. In the AHG augmentation CDC test, anti-kappa light chain is added to the washed cells before the addition of complement. The techniques that include wash steps preferentially detect IgG antibodies, as the lower-affinity IgM antibodies become detached during the washing process.

Solid-Phase Assays for HLA-Specific Antibody Detection and Specification

Enzyme-Linked Immunosorbent Assays (ELISA). The targets in an ELISA are soluble HLA proteins coated on to plastic and this is termed a solid-phase assay (Figure 10-6). These commercially available kits have immediate advantages over CDC in that the test does not rely on viable cells and only HLA-specific antibodies are detected. The overall sensitivity of ELISA is greater than CDC. Two different types of ELISA are routinely used – assays to detect the presence or absence of HLA-specific antibodies that can be used as a pre-screen of a patient's serum sample and assays designed for antibody specification. The assays have been shown to be reliable for the detection of IgG antibodies, but less so for the detection of IgM, probably because of the washing steps required and the lower affinity of IgM antibodies.

Flow Cytometry. The original use of flow cytometry in antibody screening was as a test to determine the presence or absence of antibody. Pools of HLA-typed target cells from B-CLL patients,[43] lymphoblastoid cell lines,[42,60] or peripheral blood lymphocytes,[91] constructed to cover the most frequent HLA specificities, have been used. Flow cytometry is more sensitive than CDC and primarily

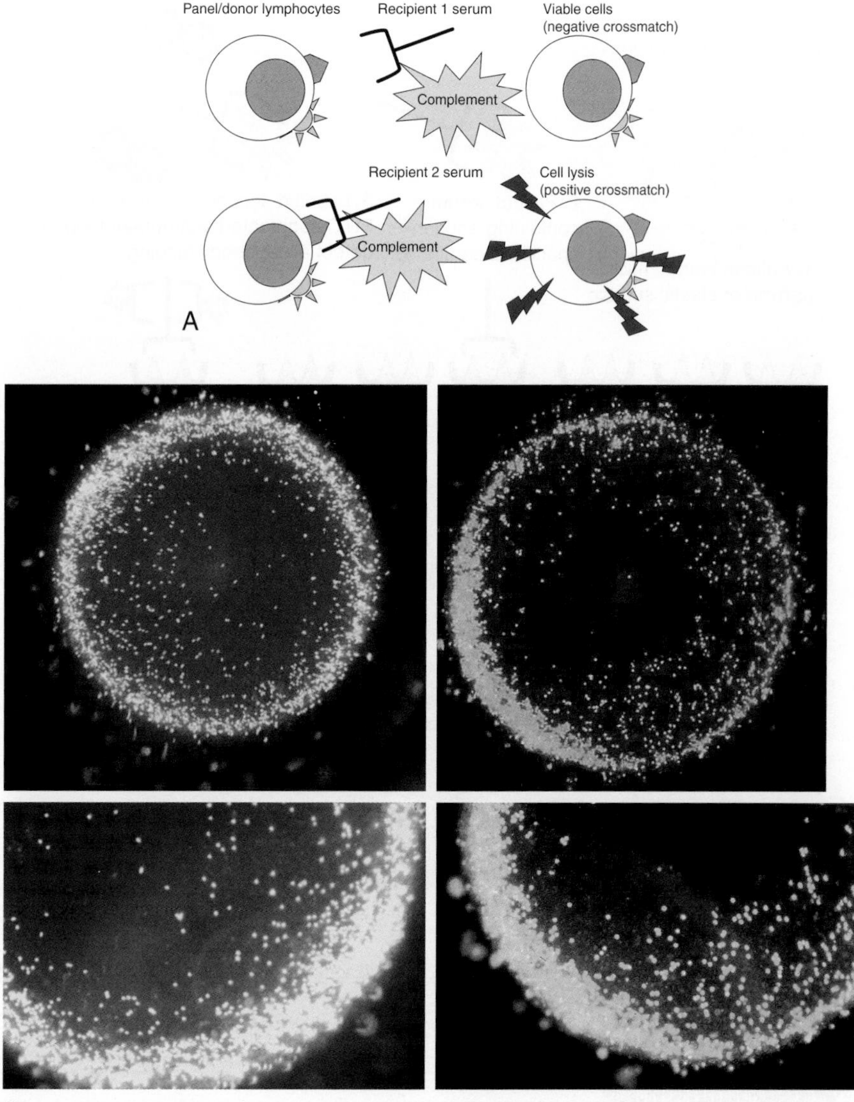

FIGURE 10-5 ■ (A) Lymphocytotoxic crossmatch test. Panel or donor lymphocytes are incubated with recipient serum in the wells of a microtiter (Terasaki) tray, followed by the addition of rabbit complement. After a second incubation period vital stains (e.g., acridine orange and ethidium bromide) are added and the wells are viewed using fluorescent (ultraviolet) microscopy to determine cell viability. (B) Lymphocytotoxic (complement-dependent cytotoxicity, CDC) crossmatch results. Left: viable lymphocytes take up acridine orange and appear a yellowy-orange color (negative crossmatch). Right: lysed cells (have pores in the lymphocyte cell membrane caused by antibody binding and complement activation) take up ethidium bromide and appear a brown color (positive crossmatch).

detects IgG antibodies. This offers the advantage that IgM autoreactive antibodies are not detected. However, although less frequent, IgG autoreactive antibodies will be detected by this method.

More recently, ELISA and conventional cell-based flow cytometry assays used for antibody screening have been largely superseded by more advanced commercial products for antibody detection and specification, with the development of antigen-coated polystyrene microbeads for use on a Luminex platform (Figure 10-6). The microbeads are impregnated with different ratios of two fluorescent dyes that enable differentiation of up to 100 different bead populations using a dedicated dual laser flow cytometer (Luminex platform). Each bead population is coated with purified protein molecules of multiple or single HLA class I or HLA class II alleles, which allow comprehensive detection and specification of HLA-A, -B, -C, and -DR, -DQ and -DP-specific antibodies respectively. The antigen-coated beads are incubated with patient serum and HLA-specific antibody binding is detected using a fluorescent labeled AHG antibody. The exquisite specificity of Luminex single antigen beads (SAB) enables rapid and simultaneous elucidation of multiple antibody populations in a patient's sera and, for the first time, facilitate accurate assessment of complex antibody profiles in highly sensitized patients (HSPs).[37,72] Although commercially available Luminex-based HLA-specific antibody detection and specification kits are currently licensed for qualitative use only, the semiquantitative readout (median fluorescence intensity) has been used to indicate antibody levels to help inform a pretransplant immunological risk assessment and enable real-time posttransplant monitoring for donor-specific antibody (DSA) to support the diagnosis and response to treatment of antibody-mediated rejection.[102] These assays are more sensitive than CDC and

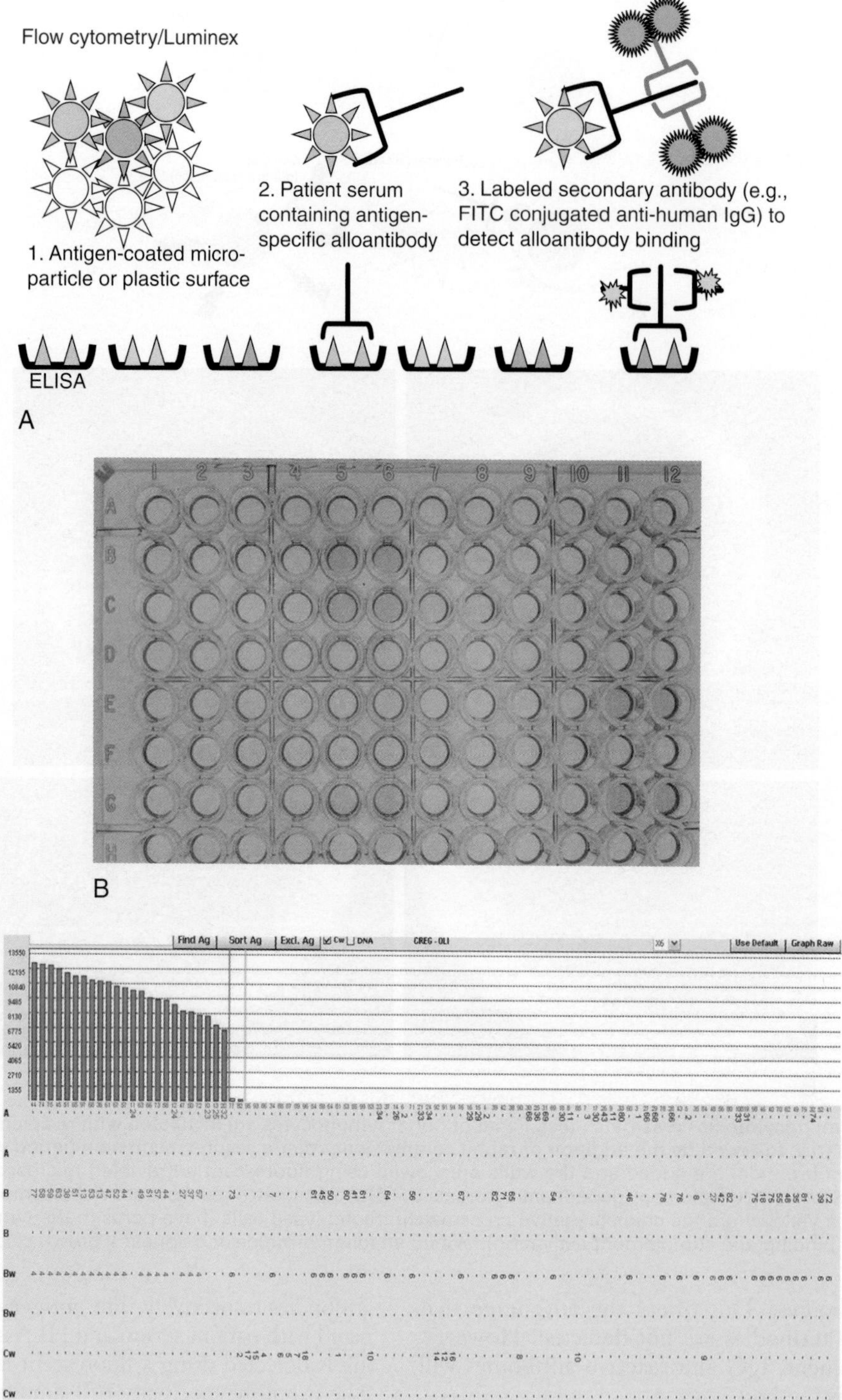

FIGURE 10-6 ■ (A) Schematic representation of antibody screening using solid-phase binding assays (enzyme-linked immunosorbent assay (ELISA) and flow cytometry/Luminex): 1. Purified human leukocyte antigen (HLA) proteins (either pooled HLA specificities or single antigen specificities) coated on to a solid phase (microtiter tray (ELISA) or microparticles (flow cytometry/Luminex)) are incubated with patient serum. 2. HLA-specific antibodies bind to the antigen-coated solid phase and non-specific antibodies are washed off. 3. IgG HLA-specific antibodies bound to the antigen-coated solid phase are detected using a conjugated (e.g., alkaline phosphatase (ELISA) or fluorescein isothiocyanate (FITC: flow cytometry/Luminex)) anti-human IgG secondary antibody and detected by colorimetric analysis (ELISA; e.g., using *p*-nitrophenyl phosphate) or fluorescent signal (flow cytometry/Luminex following excitation by a laser). (B) Example of HLA-specific antibody screening by ELISA. The plastic surface of each well in the microtiter tray is coated with pooled HLA specificities. Patient serum containing IgG HLA-specific antibodies is determined and quantified by colorimetric analysis (brown denotes a positive result). (C) An example of HLA-specific antibody specification using Luminex single antigen beads, illustrating binding to a common HLA epitope (HLA-Bw4) present on certain HLA-B antigens and HLA-A antigens HLA-A,23,24,25,32.

they primarily detect IgG, but can also be modified to detect IgM[51] and C1q/C4a complement-fixing antibodies.[15,93] Many laboratories are rapidly gaining experience with this technology, although the precise relationship between antibodies identified using such sensitive techniques compared to conventional methods and their clinical relevance have yet to be fully understood.[5]

Antibody-Screening Strategies. The aim of an antibody-screening strategy is to determine whether the patient has developed HLA-specific alloantibodies and, if so, the antibody level, immunoglobulin class, and specificity. The results facilitate the generation of a list of acceptable (antibody-negative or antibody levels below a predefined threshold) and unacceptable (antibody-positive) donor HLA mismatches for each patient to guide organ allocation and the selection of suitable (antibody-compatible) donor–recipient pairs. All laboratories supporting kidney transplantation have an antibody-screening strategy but may use different approaches and technologies. One common strategy, because many patients are non-sensitized, is to screen samples first with a sensitive methodology to detect the presence of HLA-specific antibody and then to perform further testing and analysis to determine the specificity of the antibodies in positive samples. In order to perform effective antibody screening, serum samples should be obtained regularly from patients on the transplant waiting list to provide a historical and contemporary assessment (within the last 3 months) of antibody specificity. Information about the nature and timing of potential sensitizing events is important in a patient's sensitization profile. If a potential sensitization event occurs, additional samples are required, e.g., 14 and 28 days following a transfusion with blood products.[8,45]

Patient Sensitization Profile and Definition of Unacceptable Specificities

The cumulative information obtained from an antibody-screening program, together with knowledge of the potential sensitizing events, enables the laboratory to develop a sensitization profile for patients on the transplant waiting list. The sensitization profile will be based on the complete sensitization history for the patient and includes the antibody priming event(s), timing of appearance/disappearance of antibody reactivity, the specificity, antibody level, and immunoglobulin class of HLA-specific antibodies and the presence/absence of non-HLA-specific (usually autoreactive) antibodies.

The comprehensive identification of HLA antibody specificities for a patient enables the definition of unacceptable HLA mismatches in a donor where DSA levels above a given threshold (i.e., likely to cause an IgG-positive donor lymphocyte crossmatch) are considered a veto to transplantation because of the concomitant risk of uncontrolled antibody-mediated rejection. The antibody level considered as unacceptable for a given donor HLA mismatch varies between patients and centers and is dependent on the clinically acceptable level of immunological risk, patient clinical status, donor type (i.e., live donor, donation after circulatory death, or donation after brain death), the likelihood of alternative (lower-risk) options, and the local clinical management policy for undertaking HLA-specific antibody-incompatible (HLAi) kidney transplantation. HLA mismatches from a previous transplant and mismatched paternal specificities in multiparous women may also be considered unacceptable. In countries or regions where there is exchange of kidneys, these unacceptable specificities are registered with the organ exchange organization, facilitating efficient allocation of organs and preventing unnecessary shipping of organs to patients where the crossmatch would be positive (termed virtual crossmatch).

All the information obtained through regular antibody screening of a patient awaiting transplantation is crucial in interpreting the results of a crossmatch test and in assessing the immunological risk of transplantation for a patient.

DONOR CROSSMATCH

Kidney transplantation in patients with high levels of IgG donor HLA-specific antibodies that are detected using the DTT modified CDC assay has a significant detrimental impact upon graft survival, with the majority of transplants succumbing to hyperacute or acute humoral rejection. Recipient antibodies against donor histocompatibility antigens bind to the vascular endothelium of the transplanted organ, which disrupts the intercellular junctions and causes release of cell surface heparin sulfate and loss of the antithrombotic state, thereby leading to rapid uncontrollable activation of the thrombotic and complement cascades. The resultant intravascular coagulation and interstitial hemorrhage can lead to graft destruction within minutes or hours after revascularization.

More recently, the clinical importance of low-level donor HLA-specific antibodies detectable using more sensitive Luminex-based assays and/or flow cytometric crossmatch (FC-XM) assay (but CDC-negative) has also become apparent as a cause of antibody-mediated rejection, but weak donor HLA-specific sensitization does not necessarily constitute a veto to transplantation, and instead informs an individualized immunological risk stratification. It is therefore necessary to consider the choice of crossmatch technique(s) used in conjunction with the antibody-screening strategy and patient's sensitization status.[101]

Crossmatch Techniques and their Clinical Relevance

Complement-Dependent Lymphocytotoxic Crossmatch

The donor lymphocytotoxic crossmatch test using CDC techniques was established in the 1960s and has remained a cornerstone for determining donor and recipient compatibility. The standard National Institutes of Health crossmatch technique involves the incubation of donor lymphocytes isolated from peripheral blood, lymph node, or spleen with recipient sera in the wells of a microtiter (Terasaki) tray, followed by the addition of rabbit serum as an exogenous source of complement

(Figure 10-5A). Recipient cytotoxic antibodies (predominantly IgM, IgG3, and IgG1) that bind donor cells cause activation of the classical complement pathway resulting in cell lysis, the extent of which can be quantified by the addition of vital stains and determination of viability by microscopy (Figure 10-5B). A high percentage of cell death above background levels is interpreted as a positive crossmatch, with the potential to damage a transplanted kidney. Ensuring a negative pretransplant lymphocytotoxic crossmatch using this basic technique has virtually eliminated HAR, but in its simplest form the CDC crossmatch carries several major drawbacks and has therefore been subject to many modifications.

During the 1970s it emerged that not all lymphocytotoxic antibodies causing a positive crossmatch are specific for donor histocompatibility antigens and some antibodies display autoreactivity, causing in vitro lysis of the patient's own cells in the CDC assay. It was demonstrated that transplantation could safely proceed in the presence of such antibodies.[116] Taylor and colleagues characterized these autoantibodies as polyreactive IgM, capable of low-affinity binding to multiple antigens due to weak electrostatic interactions.[104] Depending on antibody titer and/or affinity, they may display in vitro cytotoxicity to autologous and third-party (panel) B lymphocytes alone, or T and B lymphocytes and are often negative or only weakly reactive with B lymphocytes from patients with CLL.

The good sensitivity but poor specificity of the CDC assay in preventing HAR prompted a number of technical modifications. These included the Amos wash technique that removed non-damaging low-affinity IgM antibodies and anticomplementary immune complexes, extended postcomplement incubation times (increased from 1 hour to 2 hours) and the addition of AHG to enhance the detection of low-level IgG bound to donor cells. Although not conclusive, these modifications were perceived as beneficial, particularly in sensitized patients and regrafts, and were widely adopted in Europe and North America respectively.

B-Cell Crossmatch

Further advances came with the discovery by Ting and Morris in 1978[113] of the strong effect of HLA-DR matching on graft outcome, prompting investigators to consider the clinical relevance of HLA-DR-specific antibodies in rejection. Numerous studies were undertaken using separated donor B lymphocytes (that express both HLA class I and class II) as targets in the crossmatch test. The results of the analyses were contradictory and ranged from showing no effect, enhanced graft survival, and poor graft survival. These findings can now be explained by the heterogeneous antibodies that can cause a positive B-cell crossmatch. Most studies did not differentiate between non-damaging (autoreactive) and potentially harmful (HLA-specific) B-lymphocyte-reactive antibodies. The clinical interpretation of a B-cell crossmatch result is impossible without definition of the specificity of the antibody; indeed, d'Apice and Tait showed that most positive donor B-cell crossmatches are not caused by HLA-DR-specific antibodies.[20] In the studies where antibody specificity was defined, it was clear that the majority of positive B-cell crossmatches are caused by non-HLA-specific, usually B-cell autoreactive, antibodies that are not harmful to a transplant. A minority of positive B-cell crossmatches are caused by IgG HLA class II-specific antibodies that can be deleterious to transplant outcome, but are unlikely to cause HAR. The presence of unusually high-titer HLA-DR-specific antibodies can, however, cause HAR and such antibodies are more common in patients with previous graft rejection.[1,6,70,89]

The introduction of Luminex-based antibody screening has now enabled precise specification of donor HLA class II-specific antibodies. When applied together with the pretransplant donor B-cell crossmatch, this has confirmed the importance of HLA-DR, -DQ, and -DP antibodies and kidney allograft outcome.[7,22,26,49,81]

Crossmatch Serum Sample Selection (Timing)

An essential feature of the immune system is immunological memory and its ability to produce a rapid and vigorous secondary response on re-exposure to antigens to which an individual is already primed. To avert the risk of rejection caused by an anamnestic memory response, crossmatch regimens take account of serum samples obtained throughout a recipient's time on the transplant waiting list and are selected to represent peak periods of sensitization.

Immunoglobulin Class and Specificity

The findings of acceptable primary graft survival but poor regraft survival associated with a historic positive crossmatch prompted further modification of the CDC crossmatch assay to identify the immunoglobulin class and specificity of antibodies causing a positive crossmatch. Patient crossmatch serum was preincubated with a reducing agent (DTT) to distinguish IgM and IgG antibodies in the donor CDC crossmatch assay.[4,14] In addition, Taylor and colleagues[99] defined the antibody specificity (HLA-A, -B, -C, -DR, and -DQ) using a cytotoxicity inhibition assay to distinguish accurately between HLA class I, HLA class II, and non-HLA-specific antibodies causing a positive donor T- and/or B-cell crossmatch. The studies found acceptable primary and regraft survival associated with historic IgM HLA-specific sensitization but poor graft survival with historical IgG HLA-specific antibodies. These results indicated that past allosensitization events that only resulted in a transient primary response and IgM alloantibody production could be readily controlled by conventional cyclosporine-based immunosuppression whereas secondary responses (denoted as IgG-positive) that commonly occur after pregnancy and previous transplant rejection are indicative of immunological priming accompanied by T- and B-cell memory that is poorly controlled by immunosuppression. A number of studies provided corroborative evidence that historical DTT-resistant (IgG) CDC-positive crossmatches were immunologically high-risk whereas IgM alloantibodies could be safely ignored and the use of DTT has been widely adopted in the donor crossmatch assay.[106]

Flow Cytometric Crossmatch Test

While the CDC crossmatch was effective at averting HAR, it was apparent that a number of transplants still suffered primary non-function or delayed graft function and this was particularly prevalent in sensitized patients and regrafts. This indicated that early graft dysfunction in sensitized recipients may be caused by low levels of antibody, below the sensitivity threshold of the conventional CDC crossmatch. Garovoy and colleagues[38] addressed this question using a FC-XM test (Figure 10-7) capable of detecting weak IgG HLA-specific antibodies that were undetectable by CDC. In this retrospective study there was a higher incidence of delayed graft function and graft failure in the presence of a pretransplant flow cytometric-positive (but CDC-negative) donor crossmatch, indicating a pathogenic role for weak, sublytic, HLA-specific antibodies. Others quickly corroborated this finding, but a significant proportion of patients had an uneventful clinical course, despite a positive FC-XM. These data demonstrated a high sensitivity but lower specificity of a positive FC-XM in predicting early graft dysfunction caused by antibody-mediated rejection. Many centers were concerned that "false-positive" crossmatches would unnecessarily deny patients the opportunity of a transplant, and were deterred from adopting the technique in routine clinical practice.[59] Nevertheless, the predictive value of a positive result was high in sensitized patients and regrafts which carry an increased immunological risk of rejection and the increased assay sensitivity is widely used in such scenarios.[17,50] The specificity of the pretransplant T- and B-cell FC-XM test for predicting graft outcome has been further enhanced by the application of Luminex-based antibody screening; Couzi et al. showed that a positive donor FC-XM in patients with proven DSA determined using single-antigen HLA-specific antibody detection beads (Luminex-SAB) is associated with poor graft outcome compared to a negative FC-XM or a positive FC-XM in the absence of DSA.[18]

Crossmatch Policies and Clinical Interpretation

The purpose of a pretransplant donor crossmatch is to detect donor-specific sensitization that is predictive of hyperacute, acute, and chronic rejection (cellular and humoral) and to ensure appropriate therapeutic strategies are in place that are effective at controlling the ensuing rejection response. Therefore the crossmatch strategy must define the immunological risk by distinguishing antibodies that will be harmful, the type of rejection response that is likely to occur, and therapeutic strategies to treat and control the rejection response. Because of

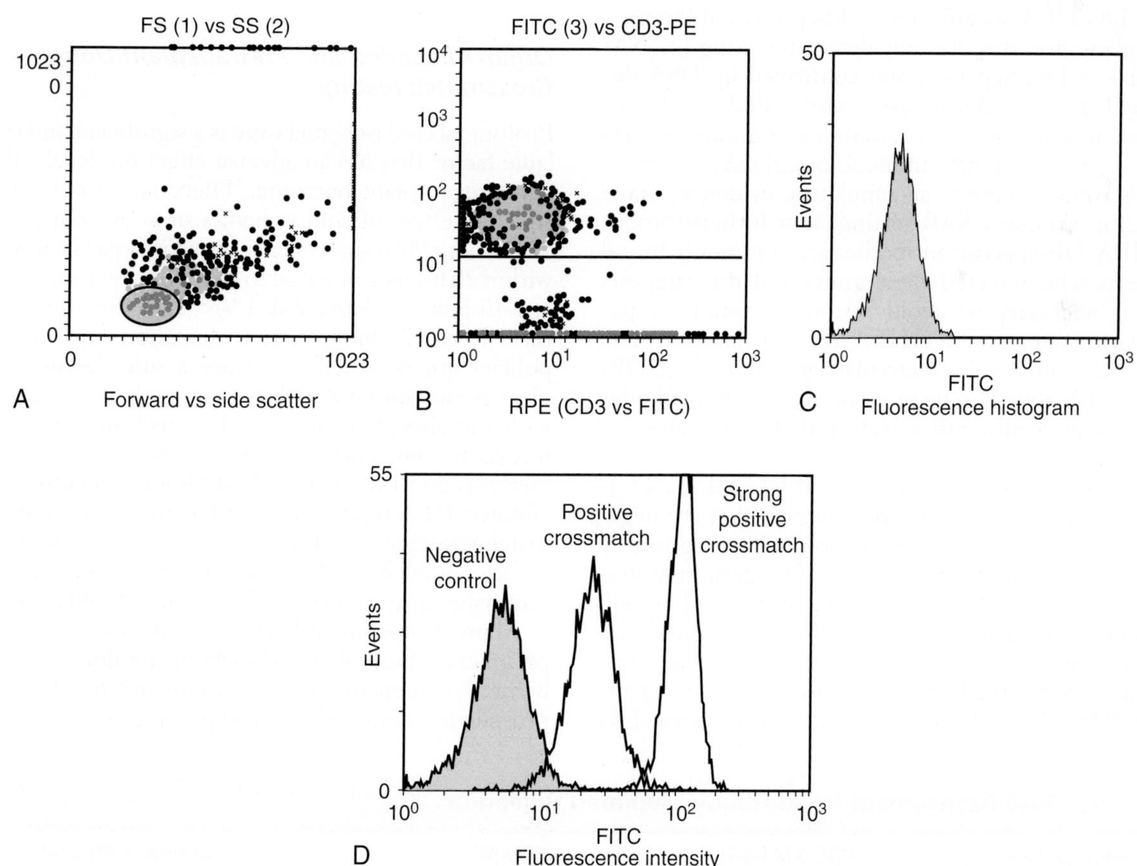

FIGURE 10-7 ■ Flow cytometric crossmatch test. (A) Cells pass through a laser beam and forward and side light scatter is detected by photomultiplier tubes. An "electronic gate" is used to select cells of morphological interest (in this case lymphocytes). (B) T lymphocytes are identified using a recombinant phycoerythrin (RPE)-labeled CD3-specific antibody and HLA-specific IgG bound to cells is identified with fluorescein isothiocyanate (FITC)-labeled antihuman IgG. (C) Light emission is detected and displayed as a fluorescence histogram. (D) Increased FITC fluorescence (a shift to the right on the fluorescence histogram) is a measure of HLA-specific IgG bound to T lymphocytes above that of the negative control, indicating a positive crossmatch.

the intricate relationship between this and the clinical program, crossmatch strategies vary widely between centers, depending on laboratory and clinical facilities and expertise.

The Crossmatch Veto: Which Antibodies are Harmful?

The two pretransplant crossmatch techniques described above (T- and B-cell CDC-XM and FC-XM), when applied together with information derived from antibody screening using lymphocyte panels (unmodified and DTT-modified CDC screening) and Luminex-SAB, provide an immunological risk stratification used to inform the decision whether to proceed or not to transplantation (immunological veto) and the level of acceptable risk required to guide clinical management. It is important to distinguish damaging from non-damaging antibodies and in this context the crossmatch can be viewed as a risk assessment for antibody-mediated rejection (Table 10-3). DSAs that are predictive of HAR (e.g., IgG CDC-XM positive or strong positive FC-XM detecting IgG HLA class I and class II specific antibodies present at the time of transplantation) in most cases constitute an absolute veto to transplantation unless pre-emptive antibody removal (desensitization) and posttransplant immunological monitoring programs are instigated (see Chapter 24). Weaker IgG HLA-specific antibodies present at the time of transplantation that are only detectable using FC-XM assays (i.e., CDC-negative) and confirmed by DSA detected by Luminex-SAB are associated with delayed graft function and acute humoral rejection and should be considered as an intermediate immunological risk.[26,34,86,102]

Furthermore, there is accumulating evidence, made possible by Luminex-SAB testing, that hitherto undefined HLA-DP-specific antibodies are commonly found in patients who rejected their grafts and this suggests that it is necessary to avoid retransplantation in patients with donor-reactive HLA-DP antibodies.[84] The presence of high levels of circulating donor HLA-DP-specific antibodies has been associated with antibody-mediated kidney allograft rejection that is refractory to treatment.[49]

The prognostic relevance of historic IgG HLA class I- and class II-specific positive crossmatches that are negative at the time of transplantation has not been rigorously addressed using the diverse armory of modern immunosuppressive options. In this scenario, although HAR will not occur, early acute humoral and/or accelerated cellular rejection that is refractory to treatment with conventional calcineurin-based immunosuppressive agents is likely.[14,99,106] It has been suggested that historical IgG alloantibodies act as a marker for T-cell priming and the presence of antigen-specific memory helper and cytotoxic T lymphocytes.[76,87] Such cells display cyclosporine resistance and their rapid reactivation upon repeat exposure to alloantigen elicits a powerful rejection response. Transplantation in patients with past high-level IgG donor HLA-specific sensitization is now undertaken in some specialist centers but this should be approached with caution and may require an augmented immunosuppressive therapy designed to control secondary (memory) T-cell and/or B-cell responses.[62]

There is no doubt that IgM non-HLA-specific lymphocytotoxic antibodies that cause a positive donor B-cell or T- and B-cell crossmatch are benign and have no harmful effect on transplant survival. In addition, good graft survival is reported with historic IgM donor HLA-specific positive crossmatches which can also be safely ignored.[88,99] Many centers believe this is also true for current IgM donor HLA-specific antibodies despite their potential to bind vascular alloantigens and activate complement. However, most IgM HLA-specific antibodies have low affinity and appear only transiently after blood transfusion, whereas persistent high-titer IgM HLA-specific antibodies with potential to cause HAR are rare. In practice, there are no confirmed cases of HAR caused by IgM donor HLA-specific antibodies and most centers do not attribute any clinical relevance to their presence.

Organ Allocation and Pretransplant Donor Crossmatch Testing

Prolonged cold ischemia time is a significant and controllable factor that has an adverse effect on deceased donor kidney transplant outcome. There is a progressive detrimental effect of cold ischemia time on transplant outcome, with 90% survival at 1 year for organs transplanted within 20 hours compared to 83% for organs transplanted at >30 hours (relative risk 1.9).[95] It is therefore essential that deceased donor organ allocation and crossmatch policies are designed to ensure a safe decision-making process and minimize delays in transplantation associated with the allocation process. The technical advances afforded by molecular (polymerase chain reaction-based) methods and Luminex-SAB antibody screening have facilitated HLA typing, organ allocation, and donor crossmatch strategies capable of identifying suitable recipients before completion of the organ retrieval operation, thus removing delays caused by histocompatibility testing.

Many histocompatibility laboratories receive donor peripheral blood obtained early in the donation process, before commencing the retrieval operation. This enables prospective donor HLA typing using a combination of

TABLE 10-3 **Risk Assessment for Antibody-Mediated Rejection**

Immunological Risk	CDC-XM (IgG)	FC-XM	Luminex-SAB DSA
High	Positive	Positive	Positive (MFI >5000)
Intermediate	Negative	Positive	Positive (MFI >2000)
Low	Negative	Negative	Positive (MFI 500–2000)

CDC-XM, complement-dependent cytotoxicity crossmatch; DSA, donor-specific antibody; FC-XM, flow cytometric crossmatch; IgG, immunoglobulin G; MFI, median fluorescence intensity; SAB, single antigen beads.

molecular and/or serological techniques and completion of local and national allocation algorithms to identify potential recipients before organ donation. In addition, modern cell separation techniques using immunomagnetic particles enable the recipient crossmatch to be performed using donor peripheral blood. In selected cases (e.g., non-sensitized patients with low immunological risk) archived sera collected within the last 3 months can be used in the crossmatch test, which can be completed before patient admission. In cases, however, where there have been recent allosensitization events and in patients undergoing repeat transplantation it is necessary to undertake a prospective pretransplant donor lymphocyte crossmatch using a current serum sample obtained within 24 hours before the transplant operation.

The Virtual Crossmatch

In selected cases where a patient's antibody profile has been completely characterized and comprehensive data concerning allosensitization events are known, deceased donor organ allocation can be undertaken based on knowledge of the donor HLA type and a negative virtual crossmatch. A negative virtual crossmatch is ascertained by comparing the HLA mismatches of a donor to the patient's recent and historical antibody-defined unacceptable mismatches, and when no donor HLA-specific antibodies are present, organs can be allocated to prospective recipients who have a high probability of a negative donor lymphocyte crossmatch. Such practice has been commonplace in the United Kingdom and Eurotransplant for many years and is effective at reducing the incidence of shipping deceased donor kidneys to patients who are subsequently found to have a positive crossmatch. The efficacy of this approach is, however, critically dependent on comprehensive donor HLA typing that includes a minimum resolution to define all clinically relevant HLA specificities to which a patient may develop antibodies. Donor HLA typing for HLA-C and -DQ loci is not routine in all countries and centers and under such circumstances a virtual crossmatch cannot be reliably performed.[9]

In carefully selected donor–recipient combinations where recipient sensitization is either absent or clearly defined low-level non-donor HLA-specific antibodies are present, a negative donor crossmatch can be predicted with sufficient confidence to omit the prospective pretransplant donor lymphocyte crossmatch and proceed directly to transplantation based on a negative virtual crossmatch.[103] The adoption and stringent adherence to these and similar crossmatch policies remove delays to the transplant operation associated with donor–recipient histocompatibility testing and is associated with reduced cold ischemia time and delayed graft function.[101]

Immunological Risk Stratification

Recent technological developments for the detection and characterization of donor HLA-specific antibodies together with the use of C4d to aid the histological diagnosis of humoral rejection has led to a new appreciation of the important role of antibodies in short- and long-term kidney allograft survival.[63,92] The role of histocompatibility laboratories has progressed from providing a simple binary decision to permit or veto transplantation to the development of immunological risk stratification policies that inform the clinical decision whether to proceed or not to transplantation and to selection of appropriate therapeutic options.

The antibody screening and donor crossmatch techniques described above (CDC, FC, and Luminex-SAB) provide different levels of sensitivity and specificity. This information, used together, can be used to inform an individualized pretransplant immunological risk assessment.[26] This ranges from: high immunological risk of HAR in the presence of current high-level IgG donor HLA-specific antibodies that constitute a veto to transplantation in the absence of effective antibody reduction therapy; intermediate immunological risk in which HAR is unlikely, but an increased incidence of humoral rejection necessitates proactive application of effective treatment strategies; and low immunological risk caused by low-level DSA associated with an increased incidence of rejection but little evidence of overall poor graft outcome. Such generalized risk stratification is not absolute because of additional factors such as immunological memory, peak antibody level, antibody priming source, and timing.

As a guide, Table 10-3 illustrates the level of immunological risk based on differences in sensitivity and specificity of the antibody screening and crossmatch techniques. CDC-XM detects only high levels of complement-fixing antibodies; FC-XM provides more sensitive assessment for the detection of low-level antibodies (below the threshold detectable by CDC); and Luminex-SAB provides the highest level of sensitivity for antibody detection, but when applied alone, provides the lowest level of specificity to predict graft rejection.

STRATEGIES FOR TRANSPLANTING SENSITIZED AND HIGHLY SENSITIZED PATIENTS

Patients with HLA antibodies reactive with a high proportion of a donor pool are clearly difficult to transplant and special strategies are required to find suitable kidneys for these patients. HSPs have been defined as patients with an IgG %PRA value of 85% or more, but a more meaningful definition may be patients who would have a positive crossmatch with >85% of available donors.

In order to find a crossmatch-negative kidney, HSPs need access to a large donor pool. A number of approaches have been adopted for transplanting HSPs. Eurotransplant introduced an Acceptable Mismatch Program for HSPs. In this program extensive antibody screening was performed to identify "windows" in the patient's immune repertoire. The HLA specificities of cells that do not react with the patient's serum were identified as windows or acceptable donor specificities to which the patient had not made antibodies. The Acceptable Mismatch Program includes minimal mismatching criteria of full HLA-DR compatibility or matching for one HLA-B and one HLA-DR specificity. In all, 43% of patients entered on to the program are transplanted within 6 months and 58% within 21 months.[16] When this system was first introduced the antibody screening was performed on carefully selected cells with only one mismatched antigen with the HSP. This approach was extremely labor-intensive and would only be possible in a laboratory with access to very large panels of HLA-typed cells. The advent of 002solid-phase assays with single antigen preparations, alternatively cell lines expressing single HLA antigens,[122] greatly expedites this type of approach. A computer algorithm, HLAMatchmaker, developed by Duquesnoy, may assist in defining acceptable mismatches.[23,25] In the algorithm each HLA specificity is represented as a string of amino acid triplets and it is possible to compare HLA specificities and thereby identify mismatched triplets. The theory is that if there are no triplets mismatched, then the specificity will not be recognized and an immune response will not be generated. Clearly HLA antigens are not linear sequences, nor are amino acids in a protein triplets; nevertheless the algorithm has been shown to assist in the process of specifying a patient's sensitization profile.[24,39,55]

In the United Kingdom, the approach has been different. In the national kidney allocation scheme implemented in 1998, HSPs were prioritized for well-matched transplants with no HLA-A, -B, or -DR mismatches between the donor and recipient (000 HLA-A, -B, -DR mismatch grade).[31] Sensitization data were also collected nationally and used for allocation purposes. The data collected were designed to capture an expert view of the patient's sensitization status, based on the patient's history, antibody-screening data, and the policy of the local transplant unit. Rather than reporting sensitization as PRA value, the key data registered were unacceptable specificities and HLA reactivity in a patient's serum that could not be accounted for from the unacceptable specificities defined. This was termed residual reaction frequency and, in HSPs if this figure was zero, i.e., the antibody profile had been completely specified, then the HSPs were also eligible for favorably matched transplants. These were transplants where there was a maximum of one HLA-A and one HLA-B mismatch in the absence of mismatches at HLA-DR (denoted 100, 010, 110 HLA-A, -B, -DR mismatches). This policy resulted in a threefold increase in the number of HSPs transplanted, with 62% of these transplants having a 000 mismatch grade.[32,34]

The basis for national kidney allocation in the UK changed in 2006 but the scheme retained both the priority given to HSPs for 000 mismatched transplants and access to other less well-matched kidneys for HSPs where the antibody profile is completely specified.[47]

One of the benefits of defining the antibody profile is to make it possible to estimate a patient's chance of receiving a transplant and inform decisions about the best therapeutic option for a patient. In the United Kingdom a calculated HLA antibody reaction frequency (%cRF) can be determined for patients on the transplant waiting list, by comparing a patient's unacceptable specificities and blood group against a file of 10000 UK donors. By including the patient's HLA type this can also be converted into a matchability score.[33] Patients with a high %cRF and low matchability score are likely to be difficult to transplant with an HLA antibody-compatible donor from the national deceased donor pool and therefore alternative approaches to immunological risk stratification and transplantation may be explored.

Antibody Removal (see Chapter 24)

There has been a recent resurgence of interest in using antibody removal techniques to reduce donor-specific HLA antibody prior to transplantation. In considering patients for antibody removal, it is important for the HLA antibody specificity and DSA titer to be determined prior to the commencement of antibody removal. This may help inform whether this approach is appropriate for a particular patient. Furthermore, during antibody removal it is important to monitor antibody levels to determine the effectiveness of the treatment regimen. Most centers use Luminex-SABs for antibody monitoring and advocate that a final crossmatch against the potential donor is performed. Following transplantation, antibody rebound usually occurs and monitoring antibody levels provides valuable information to indicate whether additional antibody removal is required. Experience in performing transplants following desensitization is mounting but because of the complexity in the management before and after transplantation, it may be that, in the longer term, patients for transplantation after antibody removal are referred to specialist centers.

Paired Exchange

Paired exchange, or living donor exchange, is another option for patients who have a potential living donor, but for reasons of HLA or ABO antibody incompatibility the transplant cannot proceed. In such schemes reciprocally compatible donors and recipients are paired through an allocation algorithm and exchange transplants are undertaken. Simple systems pair two recipients and their respective donors and the transplants occur simultaneously, but it is possible for multiple exchanges to be undertaken. When exchanges are undertaken simultaneously, although logistically complex, the process maximizes the chances that all transplants will proceed. There are other modifications of the process that facilitate chains of transplants. The first is domino paired donation, whereby a chain of simultaneous living donor transplants is initiated by a kidney from a non-directed altruistic donor and ends with transplantation of the last donor kidney into a recipient registered for a deceased donor transplant.[71] The second type of chain is termed non-simultaneous extended altruistic donor (NEAD) chain. In NEAD chains the transplants are not performed simultaneously and "bridge donors" are created, whose incompatible recipient is already transplanted and the donor waits to donate to another recipient. This process removes the requirement for complex logistics, but adds in a risk that the "bridge donor" may renege.[3] There are well-established kidney exchange programs in the United States and in Europe[21,46,90] (see Chapter 25). Of relevance to histocompatibility, in order to achieve efficient exchange it is crucial that patients' HLA antibody profiles are accurately defined to avoid positive crossmatches and disruption of planned exchanges. Most of the transplants have been performed where incompatibility has been avoided; nevertheless it is possible to combine antibody modulation and exchange to perform a more favorable antibody-incompatible transplant.

POSTTRANSPLANT MONITORING

There is an expanding literature on the role of pre-existing and de novo donor HLA-specific antibodies following kidney transplantation and consideration of these antibodies in conjunction with histopathological characterization of AMR in transplant biopsies through c4d staining. These factors are recognized as having an important role in transplant failure.[11,29,54,108] The proportion of recipients developing antibodies posttransplantation has been reported to range between 12% and 60%.[66] This figure will be influenced not only by the sensitivity of the assay system, but also by clinical factors such as the nature and degree of HLA mismatching between the donor and recipient and the immunosuppressive regimens.

The appearance of donor HLA-specific antibodies has been shown to be associated with a poorer outcome and with the occurrence of acute and chronic rejection and is now recognized as the leading pathology of graft attrition.[63] In recent reports where serial posttransplant serum samples were analyzed, donor-specific HLA antibodies were strongly predictive of allograft failure being detected before chronic rejection or transplant failure.[61,120] The results of a large international prospective trial that included over 4500 patients from 36 units also concluded that HLA antibody production precedes transplant failure.[110] The temporal relationship between the appearance of DSA and onset of graft dysfunction can, however, range from months to many years and it is not yet clear that clinical intervention is effective to attenuate the clinical outcome which is dependent on antibody level and specificity.[28,109]

Mismatched HLA antigens are important stimuli for an alloimmune response, but antibodies to non-classical polymorphic MHC antigens may also contribute. The MHC-related chain A and B antigens (MICA and MICB) are expressed on epithelia in response to cellular stress and on endothelium in vitro. In the kidney MICA and MICB expression has been reported on tubular epithelia.[41,85] Antibodies to MICA were first reported in the sera of transplant recipients,[94,126] but as the antigens are not expressed on lymphocytes,[124,125] MICA and MICB antibodies would remain undetected in standard antibody screening and crossmatch tests. In reports where MICA has been included as one of the targets studied transplant loss was greater in patients presensitized to MICA.[123] Other studies have demonstrated the presence of MICA antibodies in transplanted patients and a higher incidence of antibodies in patients whose transplants failed.[68,69]

CONCLUDING REMARKS

At the current time, HLA matching, definition of allosensitization, donor crossmatching, and posttransplant antibody monitoring make an important contribution to successful kidney transplant programs. Growing knowledge of immunological risk stratification together with accurate information about the availability and likelihood of alternative (lower-risk) donor options can guide the clinical decision to proceed or not to transplantation and initiate pre-emptive therapy to optimize posttransplant clinical course and long-term graft outcome. Rigid adherence to unacceptable HLA mismatches defined by Luminex-SAB alone may be unhelpful, but when applied together with CDC-XM and/or FC-XM, the information provides improved sensitivity and specificity to identify prospectively donor–recipient pairs with low, intermediate, and high risk of humoral rejection. High immunological risk usually constitutes a veto to transplantation, but low- and intermediate-risk HLAi transplantation should only be be avoided if alternative options are unlikely, and should only be undertaken with appropriate clinical caution. The immunological risk of proceeding to transplantation should be assessed together with the clinical risk of not proceeding and the patient remaining on dialysis.

The recent realization that donor HLA-specific alloantibodies are the leading cause of graft attrition has led to a re-examination of pre- and posttransplant allosensitization and the role of HLA matching. It is an exciting time as many of the traditional boundaries are being challenged to enable transplantation of patients who previously would have been unlikely to be transplanted.

Acknowledgment

CJT is supported by the NIHR Cambridge Biomedical Research Centre.

REFERENCES

1. Ahern AT, Artruc SB, DellaPelle P, et al. Hyperacute rejection of HLA-AB-identical renal allografts associated with B lymphocyte and endothelial reactive antibodies. Transplantation 1982;33:103.
2. Akkoc N, Scornik JC. Intramolecular specificity of anti-HLA alloantibodies. Hum Immunol 1991;30:91.
3. Aslagi I, Gichrist DS, Roth AE, et al. Non simultaneous chains and dominos in kidney paired donation – revisited. Am J Transplant 2011;11:984.
4. Ayoub GM, Terasaki PI, Tonai RJ. Improvements in detection of sensitization. Transplant Proc 1983;15:1202.
5. Badders JL, Houp JA, Sholander JT, et al. Considerations in interpreting solid phase antibody data. Hum Immunol 2010;71:18.
6. Berg B, Moller E. Immediate rejection of a HLA-A, B compatible, HLA-DR incompatible kidney with a positive donor-recipient B-cell crossmatch. Scand J Urol Nephrol Suppl 1980;54:36.
7. Billen EV, Christiaans MH, Doxiadis II, et al. HLA-DP antibodies before and after renal transplantation. Tissue Antigens 2010;75:278.
8. British Transplantation Society and British Society for Histocompatibility and Immunogenetics. Guidelines for the detection and characterisation of clinically relevant antibodies in solid organ transplantation, http://www.bts.org.uk/Documents/Guidelines/Active/A6.pdf.
9. Bryan CF, Luger AM, Smith JL, et al. Sharing kidneys across donor-service area boundaries with sensitized candidates can be influenced by HLA-C. Clin Transplant 2010;24:56.
10. Bushell A, Higgins RM, Wood KJ, et al. HLA-DQ mismatches between donor and recipient in the presence of HLA-DR compatibility do not influence the outcome of renal transplants. Hum Immunol 1989;26:179.
11. Cai J, Teraski PI. Humoral theory of transplantation – mechanism, prevention, and treatment. Hum Immunol 2005;66:334.

12. Cai J, Terasaki PI, Anderson N, et al. Intact HLA not β2m-free heavy chain-specific HLA class i antibodies are predictive of graft failure. Transplantation 2009;88:226.
13. Cecka JM. The UNOS scientific renal transplant registry – ten years of kidney transplants. In: Cecka M, Terasaki PI, editors. Clinical transplants 1997. Los Angeles: UCLA Tissue Typing Laboratory; 1998. p. 1–16.
14. Chapman JR, Taylor CJ, Ting A, et al. Immunoglobulin class and specificity of antibodies causing positive T cell crossmatches: relationship with renal transplant outcome. Transplantation 1986;42:608.
15. Chen G, Sequeira F, Tyan DBl. Novel C1q assay reveals a clinically relevant subset of human leukocyte antigen antibodies independent of immunoglobulin G strength on single antigen beads. Hum Immunol 2011;72:849.
16. Claas F, Witvliet MD, Duquesnoy RJ, et al. The acceptable mismatch program as a fast tool to transplant highly sensitised patients awaiting a post-mortal kidney: short waiting time and excellent graft outcome. Transplantation 2004;78:190.
17. Cook DJ, Terasaki PI, Iwaki Y, et al. The flow cytometry crossmatch in kidney transplantation. Clin Transpl 1987;409.
18. Couzi L, Araujo C, Guidicelli G, et al. Interpretation of positive flow cytometric crossmatch in the era of the single-antigen bead assay. Transplantation 2011;91:527.
19. Daar AS, Fuggle SV, Fabre JW, et al. The detailed distribution of MHC Class II antigens in normal human organs. Transplantation 1984;38:93–8.
20. d'Apice AJ, Tait BD. Most positive B cell crossmatches are not caused by anti-HLA-DR antibodies. Transplantation 1980;30:382.
21. De Klerk M, Kal-van Gestel JA, Haase-Kromwijk BD, et al. Eight years of the Dutch living donor kidney exchange program. Clin Transpl 2011;287.
22. Dunn TB, Noreen H, Gillingham K, et al. Revisiting traditional risk factors for rejection and graft loss after kidney transplantation. Am J Transplant 2011;11:2132.
23. Duquesnoy RJ. HLA matchmaker: a molecularly based algorithm for histocompatibility determination. I: description of the algorithm. Hum Immunol 2002;63:339.
24. Duquesnoy RJ, Takemoto S, de Lange P, et al. HLA-matchmaker: a molecularly based algorithm for histocompatibility determination. III. Effect of matching at the HLA-A, B amino acid triplet level on kidney transplant survival. Transplantation 2003;75:884.
25. Duquesnoy RJ, Witvliet M, Doxiadus II, et al. HLA-matchmaker based strategy to identify acceptable HLA class I mismatches for highly sensitised kidney transplant candidates. Transpl Int 2004;17:22.
26. Dyer PA, Claas FHJ, Doxiadis II, et al. Minimising the clinical impact of the alloimmune response through effective histocompatibility testing for organ transplantation. Transpl Immunol 2012;27:83–8.
27. El-Awar N, Terasaki PI, Nguygen A, et al. Epitopes of human leukocyte antigen class I antibodies found in sera of normal healthy males and cord blood. Hum Immunol 2009;70:844.
28. Everly MJ, Everly JJ, Arend LJ, et al. Reducing de novo donor-specific antibody levels during acute rejection diminishes renal allograft loss. Am J Transplant 2009;9:1063.
29. Feucht HE, Schneeberger H, Hillebrand G, et al. Capillary deposition of C4d complement fragment and early renal graft loss. Kidney Int 1993;43:1333.
30. Freedman BI, Thacker L, Heise ER, et al. HLA-DQ matching in cadaveric renal transplantation. Clin Transpl 1997;11:480.
31. Fuggle SV, Belger MA, Johnson RJ, et al. A new national scheme for the allocation of adult kidneys in the UK. In: Cecka JM, Terasaki P, editors. Clinical transplants 1998. Los Angeles: UCLA Tissue Typing Laboratory; 1999. p. 107–13.
32. Fuggle SV, Johnson RJ, Bradley JA, et al. Impact of the 1998 UK national allocation scheme for deceased heartbeating donor kidneys. Transplantation 2010;89:372.
33. Fuggle SV, Johnson RJ, Rudge CJ, et al. Human leukocyte antigen and the allocation of kidneys from cadaver donors in the United Kingdom. Transplantation 2004;77:618.
34. Fuggle SV, Martin S. Toward performing transplantation in highly sensitised patients. Transplantation 2004;78:186.
35. Fuggle SV, McWhinnie DL, Chapman JR, et al. Sequential analysis of HLA-class II antigen expression in human renal allografts. Induction of tubular class II antigens and correlation with clinical parameters. Transplantation 1986;42:144.
36. Fuggle SV, McWhinnie DL, Morris PJ. Precise specificity of induced tubular HLA-class II antigens in renal allografts. Transplantation 1987;44:214.
37. Fulton RJ, McDade RDC, Smith PL, et al. Advanced multiplexed analysis with the FlowMetrix system. Clin Chem 1997;43:1749.
38. Garovoy MR, Rheinschmidt MA, Bigos M, et al. Flow cytometric analysis: a high technology crossmatch technique facilitating transplantation. Transplant Proc 1983;15:1939.
39. Goodman RS, Taylor CJ, O'Rourke CM, et al. Utility of HLAMatchmaker and single-antigen HLA-antibody detection beads for identification of acceptable mismatches in highly sensitized patients awaiting kidney transplantation. Transplantation 2006;81:1331.
40. Gorer PA, Lyman S, Snell GD. Studies on the genetic and antigenic basis of tumour transplantation. Linkage between a histocompatibility gene and 'fused' in mice. Proc R Soc B 1948;151:57.
41. Hankey KG, Deachenberg CB, Papadimitriou JC, et al. MIC expression in renal and pancreatic allografts. Transplantation 2002;73:304.
42. Harmer AW, Heads AJ, Vaughan RW. Detection of HLA class I and class II specific antibodies by flow cytometry and PRA-STAT screening in renal transplant recipients. Transplantation 1997;63:1828.
43. Harmer AW, Sutton M, Bayne A, et al. A highly sensitive, rapid screening method for the detection of antibodies directed against HLA class I and class II antigens. Transpl Int 1993;6:277.
44. Horton R, Wilming L, Rand V, et al. Gene map of the extended human MHC. Nat Rev Genet 2004;5:889.
45. Howell M, Harmer A, Briggs D, et al. British Society for Histocompatibility and Immunogenetics and British Transplantation Society guidelines for the detection and characterisation of clinically relevant antibodies in allotransplantation. Int J Immunogenet 2010;37:435.
46. Johnson RJ, Allen JE, Fuggle SV, et al. Early experience of paired donation in the United Kingdom. Transplantation 2008;86:1672.
47. Johnson RJ, Fuggle SV, Mumford L, et al. A new UK (2006) national kidney allocation scheme (2006 NKAS) for deceased heartbeating donor kidneys. Transplantation 2010;89:387.
48. Johnson RJ, Fuggle SV, O Neill J, et al. Factors influencing outcome after deceased heartbeating donor kidney transplantation in the UK: an evidence base for a new national kidney allocation policy. Transplantation 2010;89:379.
49. Jolly EC, Key T, Rasheed H, et al. Pre-formed donor HLA-DP specific antibodies mediate acute and chronic antibody-mediated rejection following renal transplantation. Am J Transplant 2012;12:2845.
50. Karpinski M, Rush D, Jeffery J, et al. Flow cytometric crossmatching in primary renal transplant recipients with a negative anti-human globulin enhanced cytotoxicity crossmatch. J Am Soc Nephrol 2001;12:2807.
51. Khan N, Robson AJ, Worthington JE, et al. The detection and definition of IgM alloantibodies in the presence of IgM autoantibodies using flow PRA beads. Hum Immunol 2003;64:593.
52. Kissmeyer-Nielsen F, Olsen S, Petersen VP, et al. Hyperacute rejection of kidney allografts, associated with pre-existing humoral antibodies against donor cells. Lancet 1966;2:662.
53. Kobayashi T, Yokoyama I, Uchida K, et al. The significance of HLA-DRB1 matching in clinical renal transplantation. Transplantation 1992;54:238.
54. Koo DDH, Roberts ISD, Quiroga I, et al. C4d deposition in early renal allograft protocol biopsies. Transplantation 2004;78:398.
55. Kosmoliaptsis V, Bradley JA, Sharples LD, et al. Predicting the immunogenicity of HLA class I alloantigens using structural epitope analysis determined by HLAMatchmaker. Transplantation 2008;85:1817.
56. Kosmoliaptsis V, Sharples LD, Chaudhry A, et al. HLA class I amino acid sequence based matching following inter-locus subtraction and long-term outcome after deceased donor kidney transplantation. Hum Immunol 2010;71:851.
57. Laux G, Mansmann U, Deufel A, et al. A new epitope-based HLA-DPB matching approach for cadaver kidney retransplants. Transplantation 2003;75:1527.
58. Laux G, Opelz G. Immunological relevance of CREG matching in cadaver kidney transplantation. Transplantation 2004;78:442.

59. Lazda VA, Pollak R, Mozes MF, et al. The relationship between flow cytometer crossmatch results and subsequent rejection episodes in cadaver renal allograft recipients. Transplantation 1988;45:562.
60. Lederer SR, Scneeberger H, Albert E, et al. The role of preformed antibodies to DR-typed lymphoblastoid cell lines. Transplantation 1996;61:313.
61. Lee PC, Terasaki PI, Takemoto SK, et al. All chronic failures of kidney transplants were preceded by the development of HLA antibodies. Transplantation 2002;74:1192.
62. Lefaucheur C, Loupy A, Hill GS, et al. Preexisting donor-specific HLA antibodies predict outcome in kidney transplantation. J Am Soc Nephrol 2010;21:1398.
63. Loupy A, Hill GS, SuberBielle C, et al. Significance of C4d Banff scores in early protocol biopsies of kidney transplant recipients with pre-formed donor-specific antibodies (DSA). Am J Transplant 2011;11:56.
64. Marsh SGE, Albert ED, Bodmer WF, et al. Nomenclature for factors of the HLA system 2010. Tissue Antigens 2010;75:291–455.
65. Marsh SGE, Bodmer JG. HLA-DR and -DQ epitopes and monoclonal antibody specificity. Immunol Today 1989;10:305.
66. McKenna RM, Takemoto S, Terasaki PI. Anti-HLA antibodies after solid organ transplantation. Transplantation 2000;69:319.
67. Mickey MR. HLA matching in transplants from cadaver donors. In: Terasaki PI, editor. Clinical kidney transplants 1985. Los Angeles: UCLA Tissue Typing Laboratory; 1985. p. 45–56.
68. Mizutani K, Terasaki P, Bignon JD, et al. Association of kidney transplant failure and antibodies against MICA. Hum Immunol 2006;67:683.
69. Mizutani K, Teraski PI, Rosen A, et al. Serial ten year follow-up of HLA and MICA antibody production prior to graft failure. Am J Transplant 2005;5:2265.
70. Mohanakumar T, Rhodes C, Mendez-Picon G, et al. Renal allograft rejection associated with presensitization to HLA-DR antigens. Transplantation 1981;31:93.
71. Montgomery RA, Zachery AA, Ratner LE, et al. Domino aired kidney donation: a strategy to make best use of live nondirected donation. Lancet 2006;368:419.
72. Morales-Buenrostro LE, Terasaki PI, Marino-Vazquez LA, et al. "Natural" human leukocyte antigen antibodies found in nonalloimmunized healthy males. Transplantation 2008; 86:1111.
73. Morris PJ, Johnson RJ, Fuggle SV, et al. Analysis of factors that affect outcome of primary cadaveric renal transplantation in the UK. Lancet 1999;354:1147.
74. Morris PJ, Williams GM, Hume DM, et al. Serotyping for homotransplantation. XII. Occurrence of cytotoxic antibodies following kidney transplantation in man. Transplantation 1968;6:392.
75. Mytilineos J, Deufel A, Opelz G. Clinical relevance of HLA-DPB locus matching for cadaver kidney retransplants: a report of the Collaborative Transplant Study. Transplantation 1997;63:1351.
76. Oostingh GJ, Davies HFS, Bradley JA, et al. Comparison of allogeneic and xenogeneic in vitro T cell proliferative responses of sensitised patients awaiting kidney transplantation. Xenotransplantation 2003;10:545.
77. Opelz G. The importance of HLA antigen splits for kidney transplant matching. Lancet 1988;2:61.
78. Opelz G, Döhler B. Association of mismatches for HLA-DR with incidence of post-transplant hip fracture in kidney transplant recipients. Transplantation 2011;91:65.
79. Opelz G, Döhler B. Impact of HLA mismatching on incidence of post-transplant non-Hodgkin lymphoma after kidney transplantation. Transplantation 2010;89:567.
80. Opelz G, Döhler B. Pediatric kidney transplantation: analysis of donor age, HLA match and post-transplant non-Hodgkin lymphoma. Transplantation 2010;90:292.
81. Ottena HG, Verhaarb MC, Borsta HPE, et al. Pretransplant donor-specific HLA class-I and -II antibodies are associated with an increased risk for kidney graft failure. Am J Transplant 2012;12:1618.
82. Pereira S, Perkins S, Lee JH, et al. Donor-specific antibody against denatured HLA-A1: clinically nonsignificant? Hum Immunol 2011;72:492.
83. Persijn GG, Cohen B, Lansbergen Q, et al. Effect of HLA-A and -B matching on survival of grafts and recipients after renal transplantation. N Engl J Med 1982;307:905.
84. Qiu J, Cai J, Terasaki PI, et al. Detection of antibodies to HLA-DP in renal transplant recipients using single antigen beads. Transplantation 2005;80:1511.
85. Quiroga I, Salio M, Koo DDH, et al. Expression of MHC class I-related chain B (MICB) molecules on renal transplant biopsies. Transplantation 2005;81:1196.
86. Roelen DL, Doxiadis II, Claas FH. Detection and clinical relevance of donor specific HLA antibodies: a matter of debate. Transpl Int 2012;25:604.
87. Roelen DL, van Bree FP, Schanz U, et al. Differential inhibition of primed alloreactive CTLs in vitro by clinically used concentrations of cyclosporine and FK506. Transplantation 1993;56:190.
88. Roy R, Belles-Isles M, Pare M, et al. The importance of serum dithiothreitol treatment in crossmatching selection of presensitized kidney transplant recipients. Transplantation 1990;50:532.
89. Scornik JC, LeFor WM, Cicciarelli JC, et al. Hyperacute and acute kidney graft rejection due to antibodies against B cells. Transplantation 1992;54:61.
90. Segev DL, Genrty SE, Warren DS, et al. Kidney paired donation and optimizing the use of live donor organs. JAMA 2005;293:1883.
91. Shroyer TW, Deierhoi MH, Mink CA, et al. A rapid flow cytometry assay for HLA antibody detection using a pooled cell panel covering 14 serological crossreacting groups. Transplantation 1995;59:626.
92. Sis B, Jhangri GS, Bunnag S, et al. Endothelial gene expression in kidney transplants with alloantibody indicates antibody-mediated damage despite lack of C4d staining. Am J Transplant 2009;9:2312.
93. Smith JD, Hamour IM, Banner MR, et al. C4d fixing, Luminex binding antibodies – a new tool for prediction of graft failure after heart transplantation. Am J Transplant 2007;7:2809.
94. Sumitran-Holgersson SS, Wilczek HE, Holgersson J, et al. Identification of the nonclassical HLA molecules, MICA, as targets for humoral immunity associated with irreversible rejection of kidney allografts. Transplantation 2002;74:269.
95. Summers DM, Johnson RJ, Allen J, et al. Analysis of factors that determine outcome following transplantation with kidneys donated after cardiac death in the UK. Lancet 2010;376:1303.
96. Takemoto SK. HLA amino acid residue matching. Clin Transpl 1996;397.
97. Taylor CJ, Bayne AM, Welsh KI, et al. HLA-DR matching is effective in reducing post transplant costs in renal allograft recipients on triple therapy. Transplant Proc 1993;25:210.
98. Taylor CJ, Bolton EM, Pocock S, et al. Banking on human embryonic stem cells: estimating the number of donor cell lines needed for HLA matching. Lancet 2005;366:2019.
99. Taylor CJ, Chapman JR, Ting A, et al. Characterisation of lymphocytotoxic antibodies causing a positive crossmatch in renal transplantation: relationship to primary and regraft outcome. Transplantation 1989;48:953.
100. Taylor CJ, Dyer PA. Maximising the benefits of HLA matching for renal transplantation; alleles, specificities, CREGs, epitopes or residues? Transplantation 1999;68:1093.
101. Taylor CJ, Kosmoliaptsis V, Sharples LD, et al. Ten year experience of selective omission of the pre-transplant crossmatch test in deceased donor kidney transplantation. Transplantation 2010;89:185.
102. Taylor CJ, Kosmoliaptsis V, Summers DM, et al. Back to the future: application of contemporary technology to long-standing questions about the clinical relevance of HLA-specific alloantibodies in renal transplantation. Hum Immunol 2009;70:563.
103. Taylor CJ, Smith SI, Morgan CH, et al. Selective omission of the donor crossmatch before renal transplantation; efficacy, safety and effects on cold storage time. Transplantation 2000;69:719.
104. Taylor CJ, Ting A, Morris PJ. Production and characterisation of human monoclonal lymphocytotoxic autoantibodies from a renal dialysis patient. Tissue Antigens 1991;37:112.
105. Taylor CJ, Welsh KI, Gray CM, et al. Clinical and socio-economic benefits of serological HLA-DR matching for renal transplantation over three eras of immunosuppression regimens at a single unit. In: Terasaki PI, Cecka M, editors. Clinical transplants 1993. Los Angeles: UCLA Tissue Typing Laboratory; 1994. p. 233–41.

106. Ten Hoor GM, Coopmans M, Allebes WA. Specificity and Ig class of preformed alloantibodies causing a positive crossmatch in renal transplantation. The implications for graft survival. Transplantation 1993;56:298.
107. Terasaki PI, editor. History of HLA: ten recollections. Los Angeles, CA: UCLA Tissue Typing Laboratory; 1990.
108. Terasaki PI. Humoral theory of transplantation. Am J Transplant 2003;3:665.
109. Terasaki PI, Cai J. Human leukocyte antigen antibodies and chronic rejection: from association to causation. Transplantation 2008;86:377.
110. Terasaki PI, Ozawa M. Predicting kidney graft failure by HLA antibodies: a prospective trial. Am J Transplant 2004;4:438.
111. Terasaki PI, Thrasher DL, Hauber TH. Serotyping for homotransplantations: XIII. Immediate kidney rejection and associated pre-formed antibodies. In: Dausset J, Hamburger J, Mathe G, editors. Advances in transplantation. Copenhagen: Munksgaard; 1968. p. 225–9.
112. Thompson JS, Thacker LR. CREG matching for first cadaveric kidney transplants performed by SEOPF centers between October 1987 and September 1995. Southeastern Organ Procurement Foundation. Clin Transplant 1996;10:586.
113. Ting A, Morris PJ. Matching for the B-cell antigens of the HLA-DR series in cadaver renal transplantation. Lancet 1978;1:575.
114. Ting A, Morris PJ. Powerful effect of HLA-DR matching on survival of cadaveric renal allografts. Lancet 1980;2:282.
115. Ting A, Morris PJ. Reactivity of autolymphocytotoxic antibodies from dialysis patients with lymphocytes from chronic lymphocytic leukaemia (CLL) patients. Transplantation 1978;25:31.
116. Ting A, Morris PJ. Successful transplantation with a positive T and B cell crossmatch due to autoreactive antibodies. Tissue Antigens 1983;21:219.
117. Tong JY, Hsia S, Parris GL, et al. Molecular compatibility and renal graft survival – the HLA-DQB1 genotyping. Transplantation 1993;55:390.
118. Van den Watering L, Hermans J, Witvliet M, et al. HLA and red blood cell immunization after filtered and Buffy coat transfusion in cardiac surgery: a randomized controlled trial. Transfusion 2003;43:765.
119. Williams GM, Hume DM, Hudson Jr RP, et al. "Hyperacute" renal-homograft rejection in man. N Engl J Med 1968;279:611.
120. Worthington JE, Martin S, Al-Husseini DM, et al. Post-transplantation production of donor HLA-specific antibodies is a predictor of renal transplant outcome. Transplantation 2003;75:1034.
121. Wujciak T, Opelz G. Evaluation of HLA matching for CREG antigens in Europe. Transplantation 1999;68:1097.
122. Zoet YM, Eijsink C, Kardol MJ, et al. The single antigen expressing lines (SALs) concept: an excellent tool for the screening for HLA specific antibodies. Hum Immunol 2005;66:519.
123. Zou Y, Stastny P, Süsal C, et al. Antibodies against MICA antigens and kidney-transplant rejection. N Engl J Med 2007;357:1293.
124. Zwirner NW, Dole K, Stastny P. Differential surface expression of MICA by endothelial cells, fibroblasts, keratinocytes and monocytes. Hum Immunol 1999;60:323.
125. Zwirner NW, Fernandez-Vina MA, Stastny P. MICA, a new polymorphic HLA-related antigen, is expressed mainly by keratinocytes, endothelial cells, and monocytes. Immunogenetics 1998;47:139.
126. Zwirner NW, Marcos CY, Mirbaha F, et al. Identification of MICA as a new polymorphic alloantigen recognised by antibodies in sera of organ transplant recipients. Hum Immunol 2000;61:917.

CHAPTER 11

SURGICAL TECHNIQUES OF KIDNEY TRANSPLANTATION

Christopher J.E. Watson • Peter J. Friend

CHAPTER OUTLINE

Kidney transplantation is a major surgical procedure that involves both vascular and ureteric anastomoses, nowadays usually performed by a dedicated transplant surgeon, although in the past it was performed by urologists or vascular surgeons. Most recipients are already established on dialysis, although some may avoid dialysis by having the transplant pre-emptively, something that is particularly advantageous in children.[12,21] The recipients are frequently elderly, with other comorbidity (e.g., diabetes, cardiovascular disease, obesity), which increases the surgical and anesthetic challenges. In addition most have impaired platelet function through a combination of uremia and aspirin, and some will be on warfarin for previous thromboembolic disease or prosthetic heart valves. Thus this group of patients carry a relatively high operative risk.

PREPARATION OF RECIPIENT

The general preparation and selection of recipients for transplantation is discussed in Chapter 4. Potential kidney transplant recipients are carefully assessed before being placed on the waiting list and medical and surgical risk factors will have been identified and evaluated, and reassessed periodically while waiting. On admission for transplantation, a further careful history and physical examination are required to ensure that there is no immediate contraindication to major surgery, no changes since the patient was last assessed, and particular attention should be paid to the patient's fluid and electrolyte status. The patient may require dialysis before going to surgery because of fluid overload or a high serum potassium concentration; this will depend upon the nature of dialysis and when this was last carried out. Potassium often rises as a consequence of anesthesia, blood transfusion, and reperfusion of the kidney and it is essential to ensure that the patient has a normal serum potassium pretransplant. It is much easier, and safer, to dialyze a patient before transplant than immediately post transplant.

Immunosuppression may be commenced before the patient goes to surgery. Although there is no hard evidence that preoperative immunosuppression is necessary, many centers prefer a loading dose of a calcineurin inhibitor or antimetabolite to ensure a better blood level in the first hours post transplant. Induction agents (most typically basiliximab) are also started preoperatively. Where the recipient is receiving an antibody-mismatched graft (typically from a living donor), he or she will usually have received several days of preoperative immunosuppression in addition to undergoing antibody removal.

Although the transplant operation is a clean one, the patient will be immunosuppressed and is at high risk for wound infection. In addition it is possible for the deceased donor kidney to be contaminated in some way during retrieval, or to have a urinary tract infection as a consequence of the donor having a urethral catheter while on the intensive care unit before death. Infection in the vicinity of the vascular anastomosis may result in secondary hemorrhage which is an uncommon but catastrophic complication, resulting in loss of the kidney, compromise of distal circulation, and significant mortality. Therefore prophylactic antimicrobial therapy is usually given, with a spectrum to cover common skin organisms as well as possible urinary tract contaminants, although the evidence underpinning routine prophylaxis is poor.[11,18] Antimicrobial cover may also be required if the donor was known to be infected, such as donors dying from meningococcal meningitis; the advice of a specialist in microbiology is valuable in these situations.

After induction of anesthesia, a central venous catheter is inserted into the internal jugular vein (preferably under ultrasound guidance) to allow central venous pressure monitoring to ensure optimal fluid replacement and postoperative dialysis. Subclavian vein cannulation should be avoided if possible due to the risk of causing subclavian venous stenosis, which would prejudice future upper-limb vascular access when the kidney has failed. Other aspects of the induction of anesthesia and monitoring during the operative procedure are discussed in Chapter 13.

Once the patient is anesthetized, a urinary balloon catheter is aseptically inserted into the recipient's bladder (see later). The skin should be prepared carefully in the operating room; body hair is removed and the skin of the abdominal wall prepared with an antimicrobial agent, typically chlorhexidine gluconate in alcohol.[14] It is wise to prepare the entire abdomen from nipples to midthighs, especially in a recipient with vascular disease, because occasionally the original incision may need to be extended or abandoned and the opposite iliac fossa opened, or saphenous vein harvested to manage a vascular problem.

SITE

Although traditionally the right iliac fossa was used for implantation of the kidney,[30,37,46,47,63] in reality there is little to choose between sides. It has been suggested that the left kidney is best placed in the right iliac fossa and the right kidney in the left iliac fossa, an approach that places the pelvis and ureter medially to facilitate future ureteric reconstruction, should it be required. In contrast, placing the deceased donor kidney on the ipsilateral side with anastomoses to the external iliac vessels avoids crossing the renal artery and vein, and may facilitate the use of a subrectus pouch (see below); similarly, live donor kidneys implanted using the internal iliac artery may be placed contralaterally to avoid vessels crossing. In general, however, it is reasonable to use either iliac fossa for placement of the kidney.

Other factors which may dictate the optimal site of placement include the existence of previous abdominal incisions, particularly if placement of a transplant incision would result in devitalizing an area of abdominal wall. Previous venous thrombosis in one leg is an indication to use the opposite side lest the thrombus has obliterated the ipsilateral iliac veins. A history of venous cannulae in one leg is also a relative contraindication to use that side for fear of iliac venous thrombosis or partial thrombosis.

If a peritoneal dialysis catheter, colostomy, or ileostomy were emerging from one side of the abdomen, the contralateral side would usually be chosen, although it would be preferable to use the same side as an ileal conduit (urostomy) if this were to be used for ureteric implantation. In the presence of large polycystic kidneys, the side of the smaller polycystic kidney would be selected, assuming that there was room for the transplanted kidney below it. Occasionally the polycystic kidneys are too large to permit placement of a transplant. Such a situation should be picked up as part of the assessment process and one or both polycystic kidneys would be removed before the patient is activated on the transplant list to make room for a transplanted kidney, an operation best done through a midline incision to avoid later concerns regarding skin viability when performing the transplant incision.

In children, in whom the vascular anastomoses of the renal vessels may be to the aorta and vena cava because of the size of the kidney, the right side is preferred because the kidney is placed behind the cecum and ascending colon. Where combined pancreas and kidney transplantation is performed via a vertical midline transperitoneal approach, the pancreas is usually placed in the right iliac fossa and the kidney in the left iliac fossa. To prevent torsion of the renal pedicle the kidney is best placed in the retroperitoneal space, which is accessed by inserting an index finger into the prevesical space just lateral to the midline and developing the plane laterally.[67]

INCISION

There are two common incisions used to expose the external iliac vessels and bladder. The oblique Rutherford Morison or curvilinear incision is made in the right or left lower quadrant of the abdomen beginning almost in the midline 2 cm above the pubic tubercle and curving upward and 2 cm parallel to the inguinal ligament and ending just above the anterior superior iliac spine of the iliac crest. Caution is taken to avoid the lateral cutaneous nerve of the thigh, which emerges through external oblique 1 cm medial to the anterior superior iliac spine. In a child or small adult, this incision can be carried up to the costal margin to increase exposure (Figure 11-1).[40] The external oblique muscle and fascia are divided in the line of the incision and split to the lateral extent of the wound. This incision is carried medially on to the rectus sheath to permit retraction or division of part of the rectus muscle for later exposure of the bladder. To expose the peritoneum the internal oblique and transverse muscles are divided with cautery in the line of the incision.

The Alexandre or pararectal incision is slightly more vertical than that of Rutherford Morison. It starts 2 cm above the pubic symphysis and passes laterally and cranially along the edge of the rectus sheath, two finger

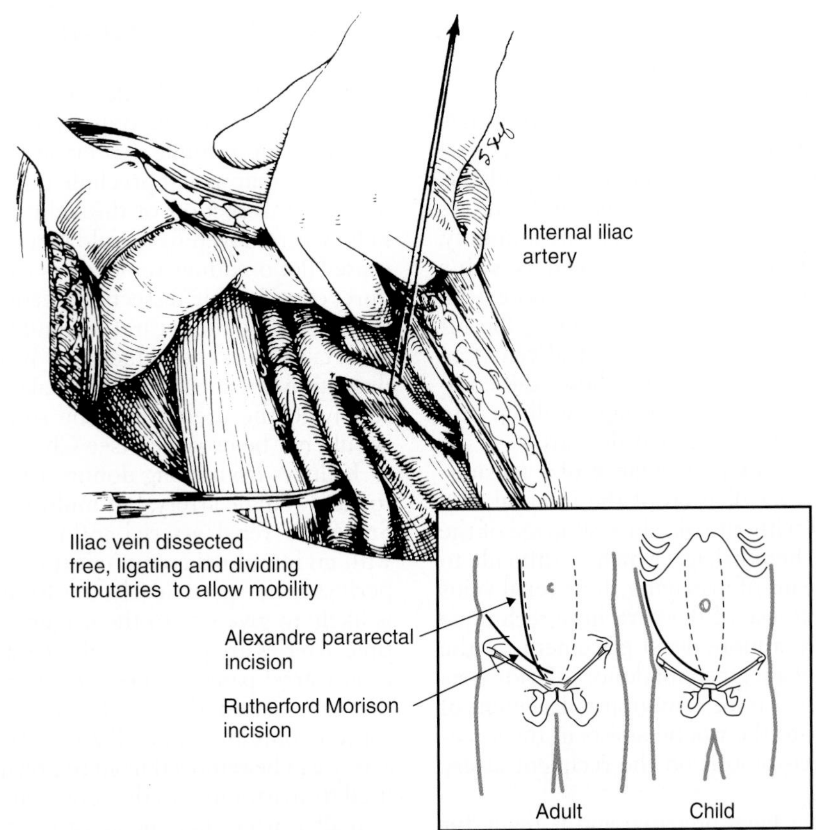

FIGURE 11-1 ■ **Iliac vessels dissected free. Inset, Incision for adult; incision for child.** (From Lee HM. Surgical techniques in renal transplantation. In: Morris PJ, editor. Kidney transplantation. London: Academic Press/Grune & Stratton; 1979. p. 146.)

breadths medial to the anterior superior iliac spine. The confluence of the oblique abdominal muscles just lateral to the rectus sheath (the spigelian fascia) is divided to expose peritoneum beneath.

Once the peritoneum is exposed the inferior epigastric vessels may be ligated and divided in order to improve access, but if there are multiple renal arteries, the inferior epigastric vessels should be preserved in the first instance in case the inferior epigastric artery is required for anastomosis to a lower polar renal artery. Also it may be wise to preserve this vascular supply to the rectus muscle if the muscle has been divided in previous surgery, for example, during a subcostal incision to remove an ipsilateral kidney, gallbladder, or spleen. Although division of the spermatic cord was advocated in early descriptions of the procedure and was common practice for many years, it should not be done and very rarely is required for adequate exposure. The spermatic cord may be freed laterally, which allows it to be retracted medially. In females the round ligament can be divided between ligatures.

PREPARATION OF OPERATIVE BED

After exposure of the transversalis fascia and peritoneum, the transversalis fascia is divided, and the peritoneum is reflected upward and medially to expose the psoas muscle and the iliac vessels. This is best done in a caudal to cranial direction. At this stage, a self-retaining retractor is inserted, such as a Bookwalter, an Omni-Tract, or a Turner Warwick ring; all have the advantage of providing good exposure while allowing the assistant to have both hands free to assist with the anastomosis. Depending on whether the internal iliac artery is to be anastomosed to the renal artery of the transplant kidney or whether the renal artery with a Carrel patch of aorta is to be anastomosed to the external iliac artery (the more usual technique), dissection proceeds in the first instance to expose the external, common, and internal iliac arteries. The lymphatics that course along the vessels are preserved where possible and separated from the artery without division. It has been suggested that lymphatics should be ligated and not divided, since this is said to prevent the later occurrence of a lymphocele, although what evidence there is does not support that (see Chapter 28).[19] The surgeon must be careful not to mistake the genitofemoral nerve for a lymph vessel. It lies on the medial edge of the psoas muscle, and a branch may cross the distal external iliac artery. If the internal iliac artery is to be used, it is important to mobilize a length of the common and external iliac arteries so that the internal iliac artery can be rotated laterally without kinking at its origin and so that the vascular clamps can be applied to the common and external iliac arteries when the internal iliac artery is short. Care is taken to inspect the origin of the internal iliac artery, if this is to be used, for any evidence of atheroma and, similarly, any atheromatous disease in the common or external iliac artery should be noted. If there are two or more renal arteries not on a Carrel patch of aorta, the dissection of the internal iliac artery is extended distally to expose the initial branches of the internal iliac artery, which may be suitable for anastomosis to individual renal arteries.

Having completed the exposure of the appropriate iliac arteries, dissection of the external iliac vein is performed. If a left kidney with a long renal vein is available, dissection of the external iliac vein alone generally allows a satisfactory anastomosis without tension. Uncommonly, if the kidney has a very short renal vein, such as with a right kidney or occasionally a left kidney whose vein has been shortened, or if the recipient is obese, the internal iliac vein and usually one or two gluteal veins can be ligated and divided. This technique allows the common and external iliac veins to be brought well up into the wound, particularly if the internal iliac artery is divided, and this facilitates the performance of a tension-free anastomosis. However division of the internal iliac and gluteal veins is not without risk, since slippage of the ligature may result in hemorrhage which is difficult to control. Alternative means of managing short renal veins are preferred, including: use of the parachute technique for venous anastomosis; a more distal placement on the external iliac vein; use of a segment of donor inferior vena cava to lengthen the renal vein. Temporary placement of the cold kidney graft into the wound assists in the selection of the sites for anastomosis on the recipient artery and vein.

When the kidney has been prepared and is ready for implantation, the vessels are now ready for clamping. Heparin may be administered in a modest dose (e.g., 30–60 IU/kg), although many surgeons simply cross-clamp the recipient vessels without heparinization in patients already on dialysis.

Vascular clamps are applied to the external iliac artery proximally and distally if an end-to-side anastomosis is to be performed; if the internal iliac artery is to be used, a vascular clamp is applied to the internal iliac artery close to its origin or to the common and external iliac arteries. The external iliac vein is clamped proximally and distally with vascular clamps or a Satinsky side clamp is used. After division of the internal iliac artery distally, the lumen is flushed out with heparinized saline. Similarly, if the external iliac artery or common iliac artery is to be used, an appropriate-sized arteriotomy is made and the lumen is flushed out again with heparinized saline; where the donor artery has no Carrel aortic patch, a hole punch is used to create a suitably sized hole for anastomosis. The venotomy similarly is flushed out with heparinized saline. Where possible the site of venotomy should be proximal or distal to a valve, and if a valve is present at the site of the venotomy, it should be removed carefully. Before making the arteriotomy or venotomy, the surgeon should mentally visualize the kidney in situ in its final resting place, as well as picturing the course that the renal artery and vein would take to ensure the optimal site for the anastomosis. Where the renal artery is much longer than the vein, it may either be electively anastomosed on the internal iliac artery or, more simply, the artery can be anastomosed to the external iliac artery but the kidney placed in a subrectus pouch fashioned by dissecting the peritoneum from the underside of the rectus muscle.[68] In such a position the longer artery tends to run a smooth course.

PREPARATION OF KIDNEY

The preparation of the deceased donor kidney should be done in advance of the transplant procedure in case some anomaly (for example, a previously unrecognized tumor) is present that would preclude transplantation. A varying degree of dissection of the kidney is required when the kidney is removed from cold storage. In the case of a deceased donor kidney removed as part of an en bloc procedure, considerable dissection needs to be performed, and this should be done carefully and with a good light on a back table with the kidney in a bowl of ice slush. In the dissection, great care must be taken to protect the blood supply to the ureter, and the so-called golden triangle should not be broached (see Chapter 29).

Kidneys from living donors are selected preferentially to have a single artery, but multiple arteries are common. Since the renal arterial inflow comprises end arteries with no intrarenal communication, all arteries need to be perfused, but particularly the lower-pole artery since it is likely to give rise to the ureteric blood supply. If multiple arteries are present and separate (i.e., not on a common Carrel patch), there are several surgical techniques that can be used: the vessels can be spatulated together to form a common trunk (Figure 11-2)[40]; the internal iliac artery can be removed from the recipient and its branches used to anastomose to the renal arteries on the back table; a smaller artery may be anastomosed end-to-side to the larger main renal artery; a small accessory artery can be anastomosed to the inferior epigastric artery; the renal arteries can be implanted separately into the external iliac artery. A small upper polar artery, if thought to be too small to anastomose safely to the major renal artery, may be ligated, provided that it supplies less than one-eighth of the kidney (this should be evident on perfusion of the kidney after removal).

A deceased donor kidney usually has a renal artery or arteries arising from a single aortic patch, and this patch should be trimmed to an appropriate size and used for anastomosis to the external iliac artery. If two renal arteries are widely separated on the aortic patch, the patch may be divided to allow separate implantation into the external iliac artery, or the two separate patches joined together to form a shorter patch, or one may be implanted end-to-side to the external iliac artery and the other to a branch of the internal iliac artery.

If there is more than one renal vein, smaller veins can be ligated, assuming that there is one large renal vein. If two renal veins are of equal size and are not arising from a single caval patch, there is a risk of subsequent venous infarction if one vein is ligated, and it is preferable to implant both veins separately or to join the veins to form a common trunk for a single anastomosis. A short right renal vein can be extended with donor inferior vena cava or external iliac vein.

The kidney should be kept cold during the implantation phase. This may be achieved in a number of ways, such as wrapping in a surgical gauze swab filled with crushed frozen saline. Another technique uses a surgical glove to contain the kidney together with crushed ice, the vessels being brought out through a small cut in the side of the glove. This technique not only keeps the kidney cool during the anastomosis,[55] but also facilitates handling the kidney.

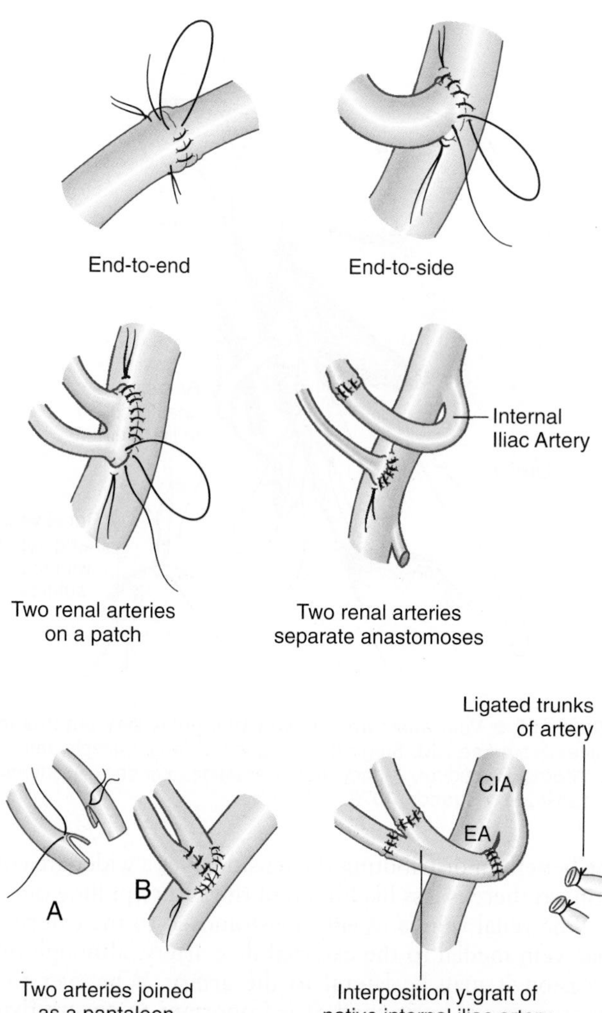

FIGURE 11-2 ■ Variations of renal artery anastomoses. (From Lee HM. Surgical techniques in renal transplantation. In: Morris PJ, editor. Kidney transplantation. London: Academic Press/Grune & Stratton; 1979. p. 150.)

REVASCULARIZATION

The question of whether the arterial anastomosis or the venous anastomosis should be done first depends on the final position of the kidney and the ease with which the second anastomosis may or may not be done. If the renal artery is to be anastomosed end-to-side – usually with a Carrel patch of aorta – to the external iliac artery, it is preferable to do the venous anastomosis first, then the end-to-side arterial anastomosis can be positioned correctly. If the renal artery is to be anastomosed to the internal iliac artery, the arterial anastomosis may be done first because this enables the renal vein to be positioned appropriately.

Arterial Anastomosis

The internal iliac artery is anastomosed end-to-end to the renal artery with 5-0 or 6-0 monofilament vascular suture using a three-point anastomosis technique, as described by Carrel in 1902,[10] or a two-point anastomosis (Figure 11-3)[40]; alternatively the parachute technique may be used, only tying the sutures after first placing all the sutures individually.

If there is a disparity between the renal artery and the internal iliac artery, the renal artery being considerably smaller in diameter, the renal artery may be spatulated along one side to broaden the anastomosis. If one side of the renal artery is spatulated, care should be taken to place the spatulation of the renal artery appropriately, taking into consideration the final curve of the internal iliac artery and the renal artery to avoid kinking when the kidney is placed in its final position (Figure 11-4).[40] If both arteries are small, the anastomosis should be performed with interrupted sutures to allow for expansion. In a child or a small adult with small arteries, the whole anastomosis should be performed with interrupted sutures.

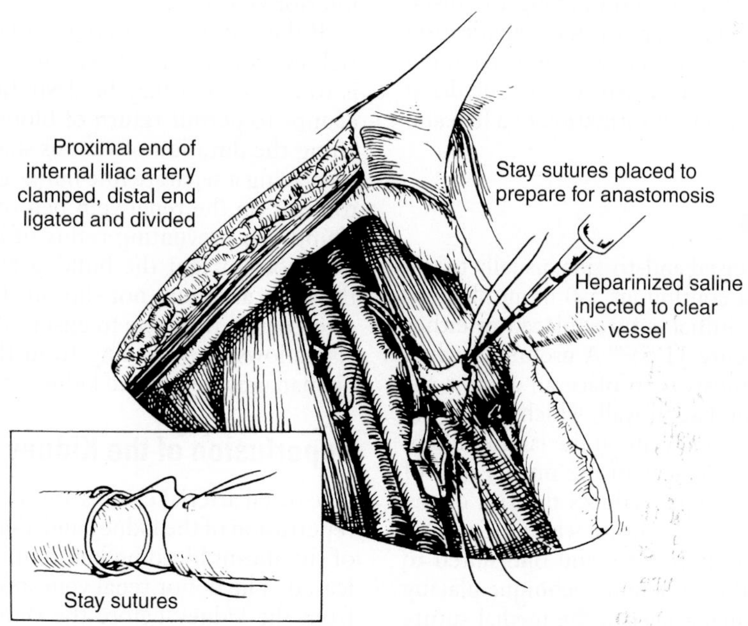

FIGURE 11-3 ■ Internal iliac (hypogastric) artery ligated and divided, the lumen flushed with heparinized saline. (From Lee HM. Surgical techniques of renal transplantation. In: Morris PJ, editor. Kidney transplantation. London: Academic Press/Grune & Stratton; 1979. p. 148.)

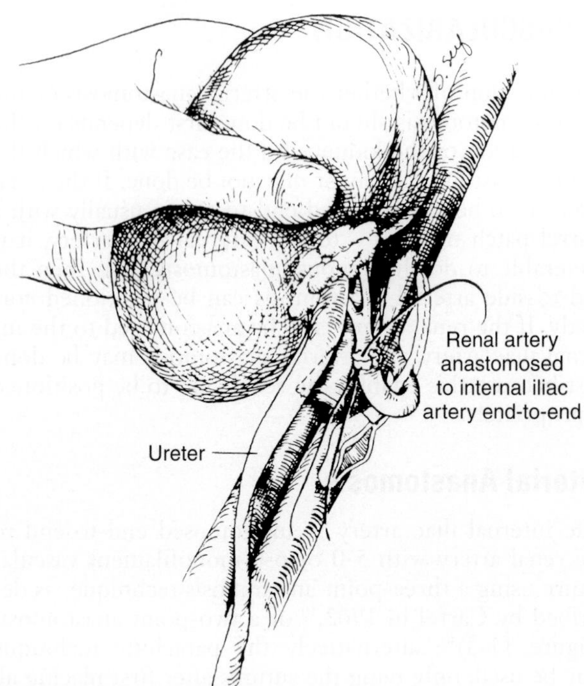

FIGURE 11-4 ■ Anastomosis of the renal artery to internal iliac artery. (From Lee HM. Surgical techniques of renal transplantation. In: Morris PJ, editor. Kidney transplantation. London: Academic Press/Grune & Stratton; 1979. p. 149.)

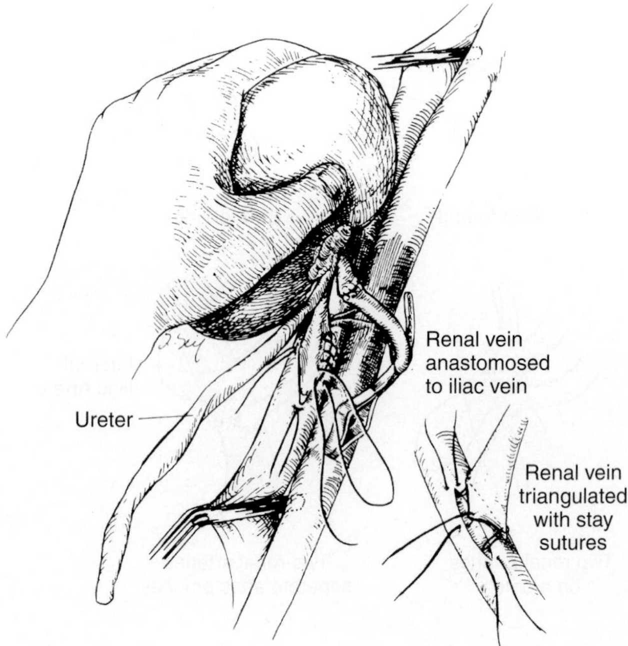

FIGURE 11-5 ■ Vein anastomosis with triangular stay sutures in place. (From Lee HM. Surgical techniques of renal transplantation. In: Morris PJ, editor. Kidney transplantation. London: Academic Press/Grune & Stratton; 1979. p. 151.)

An end-to-side anastomosis of the renal artery to the external iliac artery usually is performed using an appropriately trimmed cuff of aorta attached to the renal artery. An arteriotomy appropriately placed is performed in the external iliac artery, then the anastomosis is done with a continuous 5-0 or 6-0 monofilament vascular suture (Figure 11-2).[40] In older patients, and those who have been on dialysis some time, the intima may be calcified and be easily displaced from the wall of the artery. Particular care should be taken to ensure all the intima on the recipient artery is secured back in position during the anastomosis to prevent a dissection along the distal artery on reperfusion. In very severe cases of calcification of the recipient artery, it may be necessary to carry out a formal endarterectomy of the iliac artery, with the distal intima stitched in place to prevent formation of a flap and subsequent dissection.

Venous Anastomosis

The renal vein is anastomosed end-to-side, usually to the external iliac vein using a continuous 5-0 monofilament vascular suture, with the initial sutures placed at either end of the venotomy (Figure 11-5).[40] A useful aid when doing the venous anastomosis is to place an anchor suture at the midpoint of the lateral wall, which allows the external iliac vein and the renal vein on the lateral side of the anastomosis to be drawn clear of the medial wall of the anastomosis. This technique reduces the risk of the back wall being caught up in the suture while the medial wall is being sutured. An alternative, and one suited to larger patients, is to use the parachute technique placing several sutures at the cranial aspect of the medial suture line before parachuting the anastomosis down. This has the benefit of distributing the tension over a wider area of vein, so there is less likelihood of the suture pulling out.

The renal vein is usually anastomosed to the external iliac vein medial to the external iliac artery, although on occasion it may be lateral to the artery. Wherever the anastomosis is positioned, it is important to ensure that the renal vein is under no tension, and care should be taken that the vein is not twisted before starting the anastomosis. When a small child receives an adult kidney, it is sometimes necessary to shorten the renal vein to prevent kinking, especially when the vein is anastomosed to the inferior vena cava.

If the venous anastomosis is fashioned before the arterial anastomosis (such as when the external iliac artery is to be used), it may be desirable to remove the venous clamps to permit return of blood from the leg, so shortening the duration of venous stasis. This is best achieved by placing a separate fine bulldog clamp close to the anastomosis on the renal vein before removing the iliac vein clamps, so preventing reflux of blood into the kidney. It is important that the bulldog clamp is not traumatic to the vein, and does not slip off the vein – two clamps are often better than one to ensure the latter. This maneuver also allows any bleeding from the venous anstomosis to be managed before the kidney is revascularized.

Reperfusion of the Kidney

The distal arterial clamps are removed first, allowing slow reperfusion of the kidney and identification and correction of significant bleeding before the proximal clamps are released. The donor renal vein should be seen to fill rapidly from the kidney before the venous clamps are removed. Once the kidney is reperfused, attention should be paid to controlling significant bleeding points on the anastomoses and ligating any tributaries that were missed in the back table preparation. The quality of reperfusion is variable. Live donor kidneys and kidneys that have been subject to machine preservation reperfuse evenly and become pink very quickly. Deceased donor kidneys, particularly those with prolonged cold ischemia or those donated after circulatory death, tend to be patchy for some time. While this usually resolves over time, it is important to ensure:

- All the clamps have been removed
- The recipient has a good blood pressure
- There is no intimal dissection of the proximal recipient artery or the donor artery, the latter being a consequence of traction in the donor or extreme donor hypertension during coning.

Finally, if concern still exists, the Hume test can be reassuring. When the renal vein is occluded between finger and thumb, the kidney should swell and throb. When the vein is released the kidney palpably softens as the turgor goes.

RECONSTRUCTION OF THE URINARY TRACT

Once the kidney is perfused with recipient blood and hemostasis has been secured, reconstruction of the urinary tract is carried out. Transplantation of the left kidney into the right iliac fossa and the right kidney into the left iliac fossa reverses the normal anterior-to-posterior relationship of the vein, artery, and collecting system and positions the renal pelvis and ureter of the kidney transplant so that they are the most medial and superficial of the hilar structures.[46] This positioning simplifies primary (and secondary) urinary tract reconstruction, especially if pyeloureterostomy, ureteroureterostomy, or pyelovesicostomy is to be done. The factors that determine the type of urinary tract reconstruction are the length and condition of the donor ureter, the condition of the recipient's bladder or bladder substitute, the condition of the recipient's ureter, and the familiarity of the surgeon with the technique.

Suture material is an individual choice. Although urinary tract reconstruction with non-absorbable sutures has been described,[31,45] it leaves the recipient with the risk of stone formation. Modern synthetic absorbable monofilament sutures (e.g., polyglyconate and polydioxanone) have characteristics suitable for the immunocompromised kidney transplant recipient in whom delayed wound healing is possible.

Ureteroneocystostomy (Anastomosis of the Transplant Ureter Directly to the Bladder)

This is the usual form of urinary tract reconstruction. Its advantages are:

- It can be performed regardless of the quality or presence of the recipient ureter.
- It is several centimeters away from the vascular anastomoses.
- The native ureter remains untouched and therefore available for the treatment of ureteric complications.
- Native nephrectomy is unnecessary.

The goal is to anastomose the ureter to the mucosa of the bladder, with the distal ureter surrounded in a 2–3-cm tunnel so that, when the bladder contracts, there is a valve mechanism to prevent reflux of urine up the ureter.[41,50,51,64] The efficiency of this antireflux mechanism is variable.

The urinary catheter is connected to a Y connector with a bag filled with saline and an antibiotic and/or methylene blue dye on one line and a urinary collection bag on the other (Figure 11-6).[36] The use of an antibiotic in the solution reduces the risk of postoperative urinary infection,[56,57] while the dye reassures the surgeon it is the bladder that has been opened and not another viscus. With this system, the bladder can be filled, drained, and, if necessary, refilled during the procedure. It is especially helpful when the bladder is difficult to identify because of pelvic scar tissue, recipient obesity, or reduced capacity. After initially accommodating a small volume, the defunctioned bladder often accepts more fluid 1 or 2 hours into the transplantation procedure.[3]

Transvesical Ureteroneocystostomy

The traditional technique for transvesical ureteroneocystostomy is similar to that described by Merrill and colleagues[46] in the first successful kidney transplant from a twin (Figure 11-7).[40] The dome of the bladder is identified, and stay sutures or Babcock clamps are placed on either side of a proposed vertical midline incision. The urinary bladder is drained, and an incision is made through all layers of the anterior bladder wall. A retractor is placed into the dome of the bladder to expose the trigone. A point clear of the native ureter is

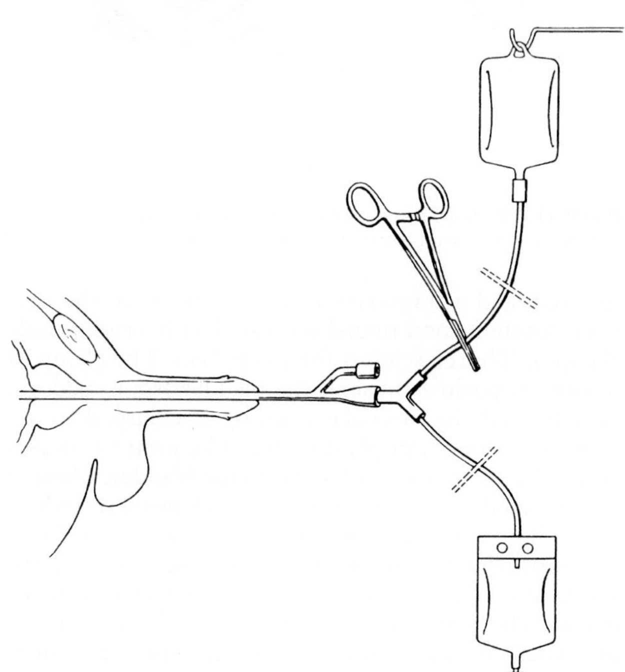

FIGURE 11-6 ■ **Y-tube system for rinsing, filling, and draining bladder or bladder substitute.** (From Kostra JW. Kidney transplantation. In: Kremer B, Broelsch CE, Henne-Bruns D, editors. Atlas of liver, pancreas, and kidney transplantation. Stuttgart: Georg Thieme Verlag; 1994. p. 128.)

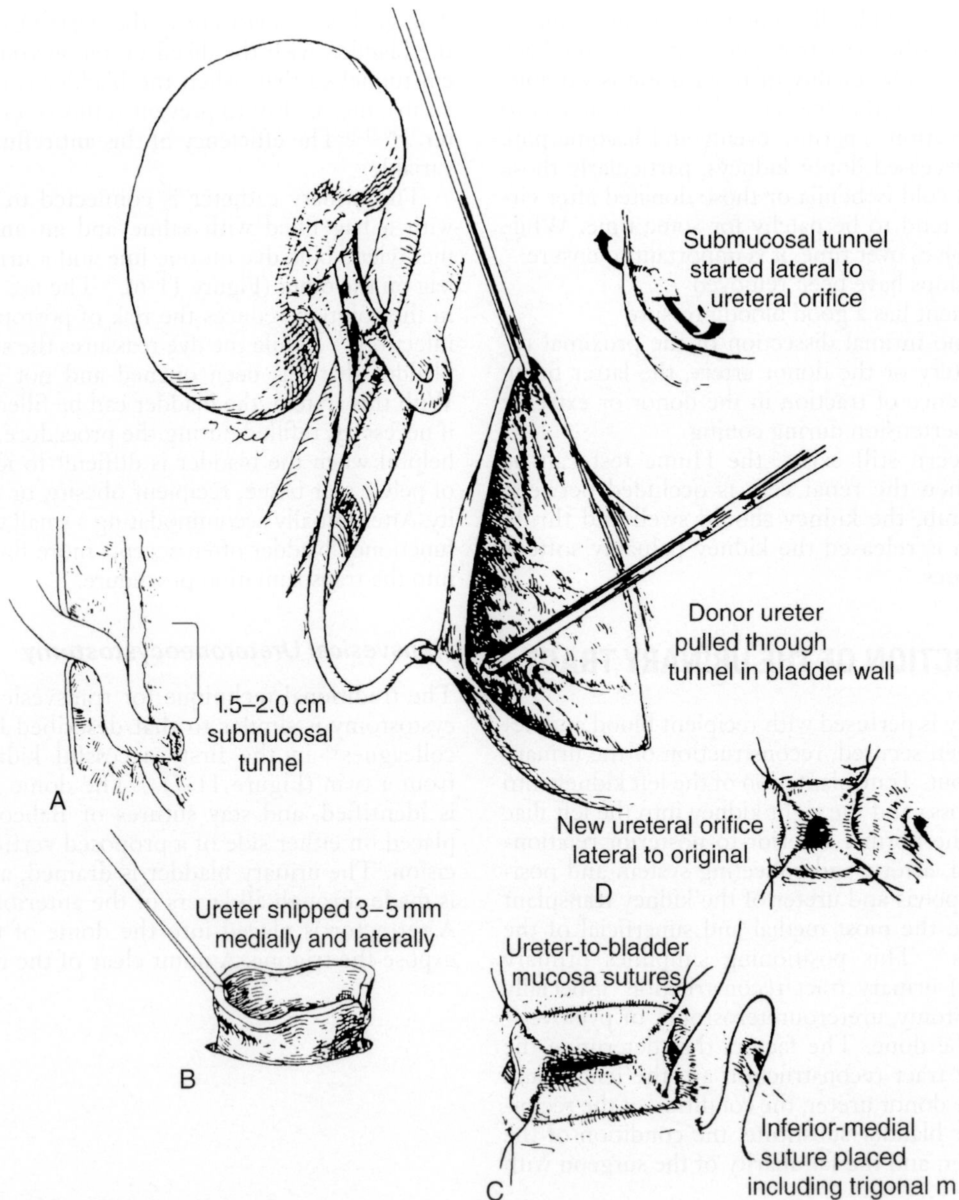

FIGURE 11-7 ■ (A–D) Transvesical ureteroneocystostomy. (From Lee DM. Surgical techniques of renal transplantation. In: Morris PJ, editor. Kidney transplantation. London: Academic Press/Grune & Stratton; 1979. p. 153.)

selected, and a transverse incision is made in the mucosa. A submucosal tunnel is created with a right-angle clamp or Thorek scissors for about 2 cm. The clamp or scissors is pushed through the bladder from inside to outside, and the muscular opening is enlarged to accept the kidney transplant ureter. The ureter is drawn under the spermatic cord and into the bladder, where it is transected at a length that prevents tension or redundancy. The cut end of the ureter is incised for 3–5 mm and approximated to the bladder mucosa with fine absorbable sutures. The inferior suture includes the bladder muscle to fix the ureter distally and to prevent its movement in the submucosal tunnel. The retractor is removed, and the cystotomy is closed with a single or double layer of 3-0 absorbable suture. The bladder can be refilled to check for leakage, and points of leakage can be repaired with interrupted sutures. Some surgeons use two bladder mucosal incisions about 2 cm apart[62]; when this technique is used, the proximal bladder mucosal incision is closed with a fine absorbable suture.

Extravesical Ureteroneocystostomy

This is the most common technique used. Although not producing such a "physiological" antireflux mechanism as the transvesical method, extravesical techniques are faster, do not require a separate cystotomy, and require less ureteric length (Figure 11-8). These factors should reduce operating time, bladder spasms, and hematuria. Extravesical techniques are based on the procedure described by Lich and colleagues.[41] Extravesical ureteroneocystostomy was adapted for renal transplantation by Woodruff in 1962,[70] and it is well illustrated by Konnak and colleagues (Figure 11-8).[35] A subsequent modification was the addition of a stitch to anchor the toe of the

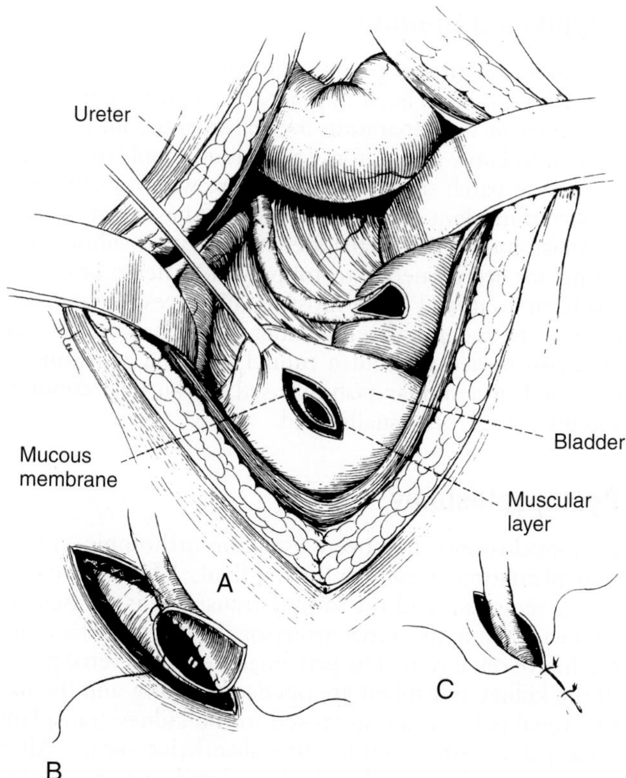

FIGURE 11-8 ■ (A–C) Extravesical ureteroneocystostomy. (From Konnak JW, Herwig KR, Turcotte JG. External ureteroneocystostomy in renal transplantation. J Urol 1972;108:380.)

spatulated ureter to the bladder to prevent proximal slippage of the ureter in the submucosal tunnel with loss of the antireflux valve and disruption of the ureteric anastomosis.[8,15]

A double-pigtail (double-J) ureteric stent reduces the incidence of leak and stenosis[7] and is widely used. This is passed retrograde up the donor ureter, after first cutting the ureter to a suitable length and spatulating its end. The bladder is distended with an antibiotic/dye solution through the urethral catheter. The lateral surface of the bladder is cleared of fat and the peritoneal reflection, a retractor is placed medially, another is placed inferolaterally, and a third retractor is placed cephalomedially to hold the peritoneum and its contents out of the way. Some authors recommend placing the ureter under the spermatic cord or round ligament, believing that this prevents posttransplant ureteric obstruction. A longitudinal oblique incision is made for approximately 3 cm until the bladder mucosa bulges into the incision. The bladder is partially drained via the urethral catheter, and the mucosa is dissected away from the muscularis on both sides to facilitate later creation of a submucosal tunnel for the ureter. The bladder mucosa is incised and 5/0 monofilament absorbable sutures (e.g., polydioxanone) placed through both ends of the incision. The ureter is brought up to the wound, and the mucosal sutures passed through the toe and heel of the spatulated end, and the ureter parachuted on to the bladder. The ureter is then anastomosed to the bladder mucosa with running sutures between the ureter and the mucosa of the bladder; some surgeons take a small amount of bladder muscle in

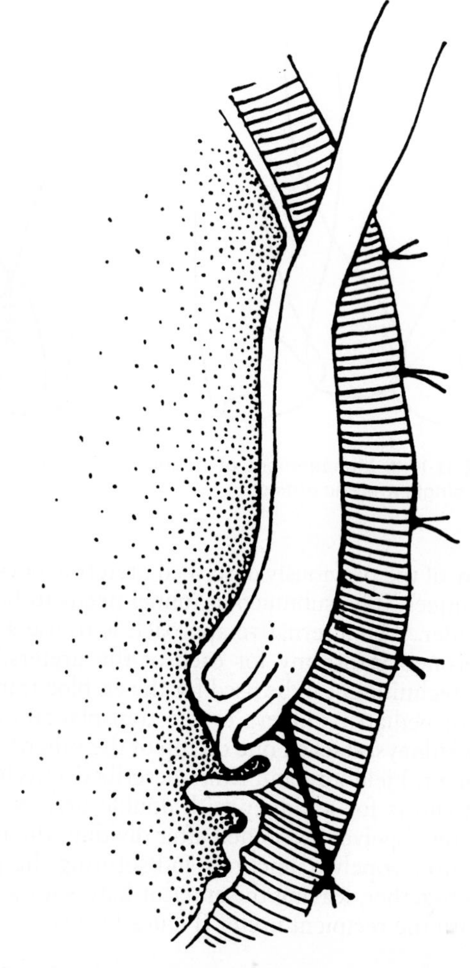

FIGURE 11-9 ■ One or two mattress sutures to anchor toe of transplant ureter to full-thickness bladder. This prevents ureteric slippage in the submucosal tunnel. (From Hinman F Jr. Ureteral reconstruction and excision. In: Hinman F Jr editor. Atlas of urologic surgery, 2nd ed. Philadelphia: WB Saunders; 1998. p. 799.)

the suture, whilst others suture to mucosa alone. Some authors recommend specifically anchoring the toe of the ureter with a horizontal or vertical mattress suture placed in the toe of the ureter and passed submucosally through the seromuscular layer of the bladder and tied about 5 mm distal to the cystotomy (Figure 11-9). When handling the ureter and bladder care should be taken to avoid crushing the delicate mucosa with forceps. Once the ureteric anastomosis is complete the seromuscular layer is closed over the ureter with interrupted absorbable sutures, care being taken to avoid narrowing the ureter in the process.

Double Ureters

Double ureters can be managed simply by leaving them in their common sheath, trimming them to appropriate length, spatulating them, and either anastomosing the medial edges together with a continuous or interrupted fine absorbable suture (Figure 11-10)[13,52] or joining them, one on top of the other, with a single stitch from the toe of the upper one to the heel of the lower one.[4] The conjoined ureters can be treated as a single ureter

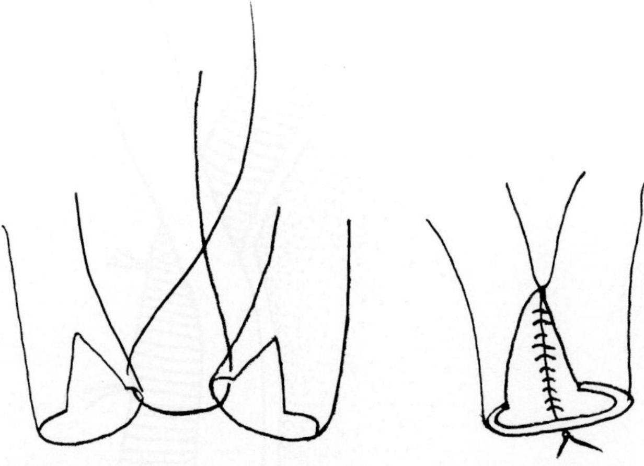

FIGURE 11-10 ■ Management of double ureters to make them into a single ureteric orifice.

by any of the previously described ureteroneocystostomy techniques. The submucosal tunnel needs to be made a bit wider. The alternative approach is to use a separate ureteroneocystostomy for each of the ureters.[66] These same techniques can be used for the en bloc transplantation of pediatric kidneys or the transplantation of two adult kidneys, stacked one on top of the other,[44] into one recipient. Fjeldborg and Kim[23] described a pyeloureteric anastomosis for a kidney with double ureters in which both renal pelves are joined after dividing the ureters at their ureteropelvic junctions and suturing the posterior walls together, leaving the anterior halves for anastomosis with the recipient ureter (Figure 11-11).[23]

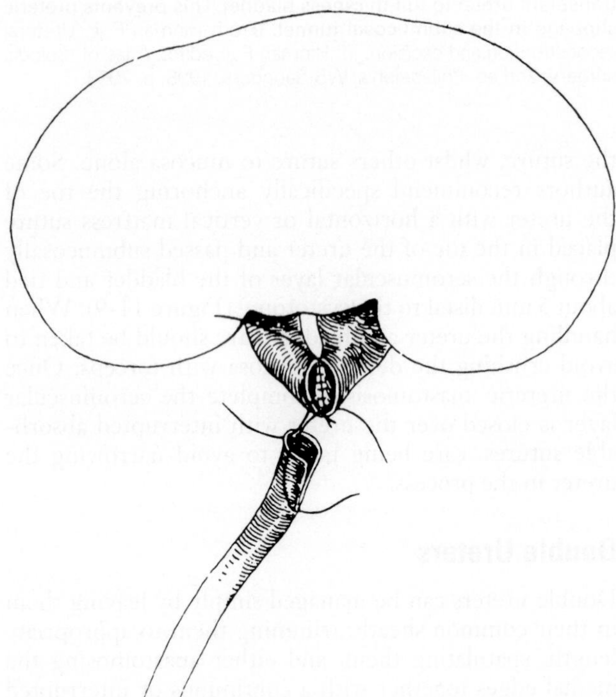

FIGURE 11-11 ■ Management of double ureters by pyelopyelostomy followed by conjoined pyeloureterostomy. (From Fjeldborg O, Kim CH. Double ureters in renal transplantation. J Urol 1972; 108:377.)

Augmented Bladder

In patients with congenital bladder abnormalities, the bladder may have been augmented as part of previous treatment or in preparation for transplantation. It is important to know the anatomy and blood supply of an augmentation patch so as not to interfere with it during the kidney transplant procedure. Ideally the ureter should be anastomosed to the bladder itself, with a submucosal tunnel for ureteroneocystostomy. Where ileum or cecum has been used, and is the most readily accessible component of the reconstructed bladder, the donor ureter may be anastomosed without a tunnel, and the anastomosis managed in a similar fashion used for an ileal conduit. Ureteric stents are usually used.

Pyelopyelostomy

Pyelopyelostomy has been used for orthotopic kidney transplantation, usually in the left flank.[24] The native kidney is removed, and the kidney transplant is revascularized with the native renal artery or the splenic artery and the native renal vein. The proximal ureter and renal pelvis of the kidney transplant are opened medially, and the native renal pelvis is anastomosed to the kidney transplant renal pelvis with a running fine absorbable suture. After completion of one wall, a double-pigtail ureteric stent is passed with or over a guidewire through the native ureter into the bladder, and the wire is withdrawn to allow the distal end to curl within the bladder. Its position in the bladder is confirmed by reflux of bladder irrigant up the stent. The proximal coil is placed in the renal pelvis of the kidney transplant, and the remaining half of the suture line is completed. Compared with ureteroneocystostomy, an advantage of urinary tract reconstruction with the native renal pelvis or ureter is the ease with which subsequent retrograde pyelography, stent placement, or ureteroscopy can be accomplished through the normally positioned ureteric orifice.

Pyeloureterostomy and Ureteroureterostomy

Pyeloureterostomy and ureteroureterostomy usually are done: when the transplant ureter's blood supply seems to be compromised; when the urinary bladder is difficult to identify because of pelvic scar; when the bladder does not distend enough for a ureteroneocystostomy; as a result of surgeon preference.[25,38,39] The techniques for ureteropyelostomy and ureteroureterostomy are similar (Figure 11-12). The posterior, or back wall, anastomosis is completed between the kidney transplant pelvis or ureter and the side or to the spatulated end of the native ureter; a double-pigtail ureteric stent is placed, and the anterior suture line is completed. The proximal native ureter is managed by:

- Leaving the native kidney in situ and using the side of the native ureter for the anastomosis
- Ipsilateral nephrectomy and proximal ureterectomy
- Ligation of the proximal ureter with the obstructed native kidney left in situ,[43,58] although this should not be done in the presence of urinary tract sepsis or where the recipient has previously undergone

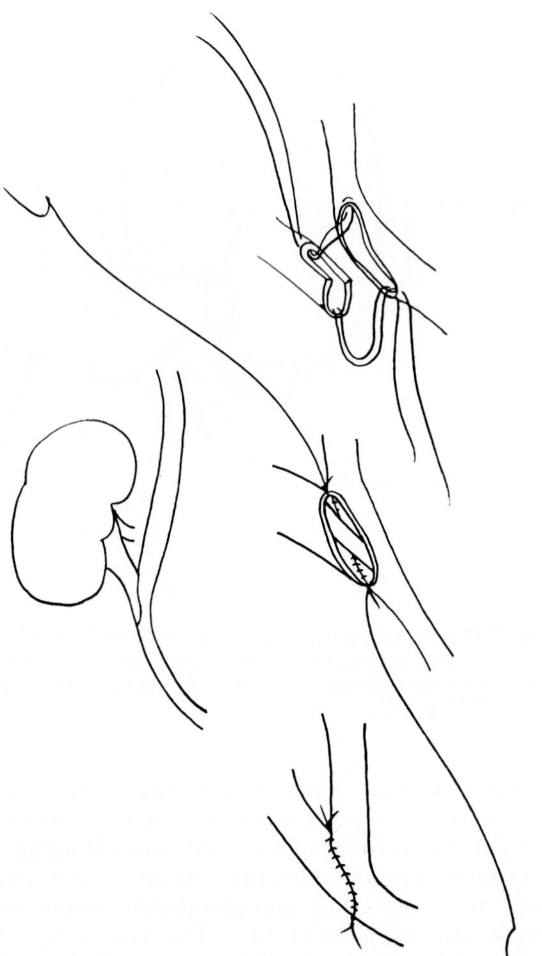

FIGURE 11-12 ■ Ureteropyelostomy and ureteroureterostomy. A double-pigtail stent is placed after the back wall suture line has been completed.

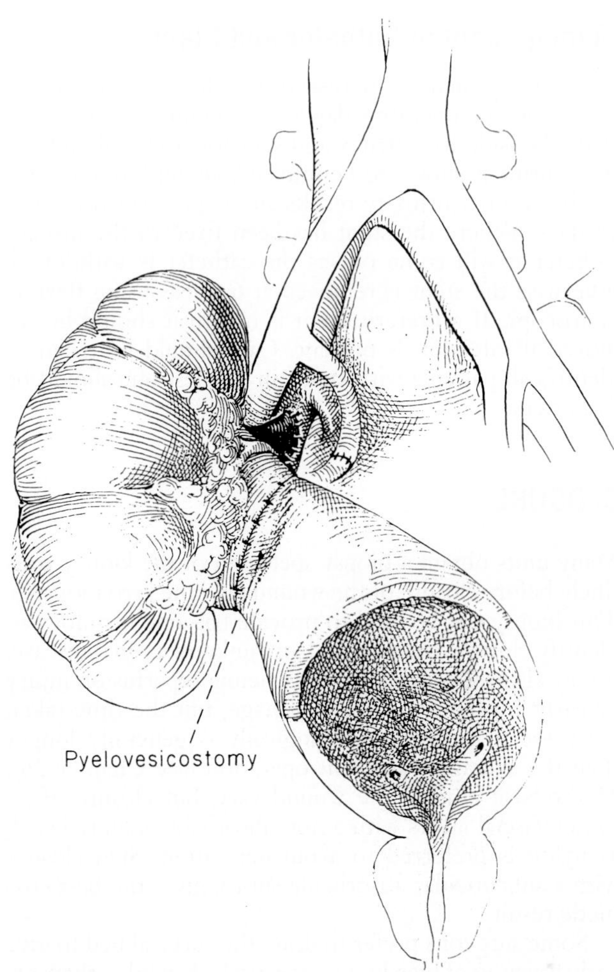

FIGURE 11-13 ■ Pyelovesicostomy. (From Firlit CF. Unique urinary diversions in transplantation. J Urol 1977;118:1043.)

ureteric reimplantation to treat reflux disease – in the latter case the blood supply to the ureter is severely compromised. By leaving the native ureter in continuity with its kidney, and anastomosing the pelvis or ureter of the renal transplant to the side of the native ureter, a good blood supply to the native ureter is guaranteed without the risk of an obstructed, hydronephrotic native kidney.

Pyelovesicostomy

Pyelovesicostomy has been described for urinary tract reconstruction when the native ureter and the renal transplant ureter are unsuitable or become so (Figure 11-13).[6,22,28] The bladder must reach the renal pelvis without tension. To achieve this the bladder may be mobilized and hitched to the psoas muscle or a bladder extension with a Boari flap may be needed.

Ureteroenterostomy

Ureteroenterostomy into an intestinal conduit or an intestinal pouch is indicated where the bladder has been removed or is unusable.[26,32] It is performed by slight distension of the conduit or pouch with antibiotic-containing irrigant and then using one of the extravesical ureteroneocystostomy techniques. Successful anastomosis of the transplant ureter to the afferent limb of an intestinal pouch has also been described.[27] If it is difficult to identify the intestinal conduit or pouch because of surrounding intestines, the addition of methylene blue dye to the irrigant stains the conduit or pouch and may make it easier to find.[69] This topic is discussed more completely in Chapter 12.

Ureteric Stents

Some surgeons use ureteric stents routinely to reduce the incidence of urological complications,[7,50] others only when there is concern about the potential for urinary leakage or temporary obstruction. Examples of the latter would include edema; periureteral bleeding; a thickened bladder; when a pyelopyelostomy, pyeloureterostomy, or ureteroureterostomy has been performed; or when the ureter has been anastomosed to an intestinal conduit or pouch. The ideal length of the stent is determined by the estimated distance between the renal pelvis of the kidney graft and the bladder (or its substitute). A double-pigtail 5F stent of 12-cm length is generally suitable for an adult transplant kidney located in the iliac fossa and anastomosed to the native bladder.

Management of Catheter and Stent

The urinary bladder or reservoir catheter usually is removed on postoperative day 5. Some units test the urine at the bedside for nitrites and sent for bacterial culture. If the urine is shown to be infected, an antibiotic is chosen based on sensitivity results and is prescribed for 10–14 days. Where the stent has been fixed to the urinary catheter it will come out as the catheter is withdrawn; otherwise the stent is removed at 6 weeks using flexible cystoscopy. If a ureteric stent is in situ it should be removed if infection is present. Care should be taken to identify all patients with stents in situ lest one should be forgotten.

CLOSURE

Many units obtain a biopsy specimen of the kidney routinely before closure of the wound (a "time zero biopsy"). This biopsy can be used to provide baseline histology to identify chronic changes and any unknown renal disease; it may also show evidence of ischemia reperfusion injury or early antibody-mediated damage, but the time taken for these to manifest histologically is generally longer than the average transplant operation (see Chapter 26). Methods of closing the wound vary, but closure of all musclofascial layers with a non-absorbable material such as nylon is preferred to avoid herniation. Skin closure with a subcuticular absorbable suture gives the best cosmetic result.

Some surgeons prefer to drain the surgical bed to give early warning of bleeding or urinary leak, while others argue that the drain is a portal for entry of microorganisms. If drainage is performed it should be a closed system and drains should be removed at the earliest opportunity. The exit site of the drain should be cleaned and dressed daily until the drain is removed.

The historical practice of capsulotomy of the transplanted kidney, where the renal capsule is carefully split along its convex border from pole to pole to minimize damage to the kidney as the parenchyma swelled in response to reperfusion injury, is no longer performed.[29,61]

PEDIATRIC RECIPIENT

For older children, the transplant procedure is the same as for adults if their weight is more than 20 kg.[5,20,49] The renal vessels are anastomosed end-to-side to the iliac vessels or to the aorta and vena cava.[9]

In smaller children (weight <20 kg), the right extraperitoneal space can be developed by extending the incision to the right costal margin,[48] or a transperitoneal approach can be used.[62] In the case of the latter, the abdomen is opened through the midline incision from the xyphoid to the pubis, and the retroperitoneum opened by incising the peritoneum lateral to the ascending colon, which is reflected medially. The terminal portion of the vena cava is dissected over 3–4 cm, ligating and dividing two to three lumbar veins posteriorly. The terminal aorta also is dissected free at its bifurcation, as is the right

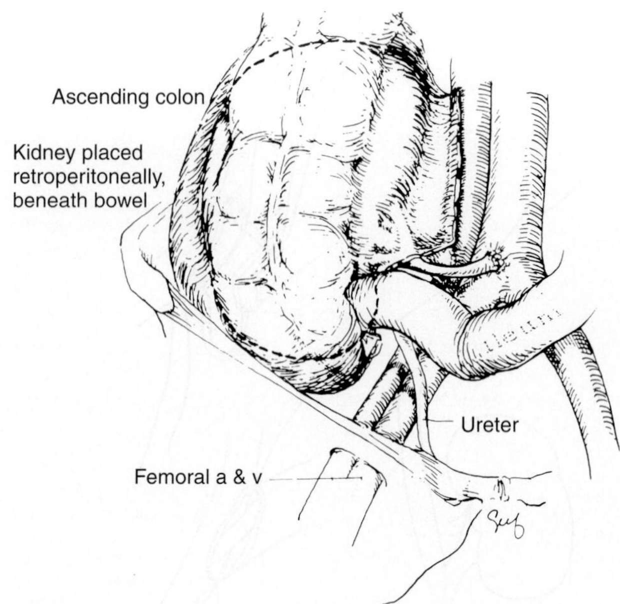

FIGURE 11-14 ■ Renal transplant in small children (<20 kg). (From Lee HM. Surgical techniques of renal transplantation. In: Morris PJ, editor. Kidney transplantation. London: Academic Press/Grune & Stratton; 1979. p. 159.)

common iliac artery. A partial occluding clamp is used to isolate the vena cava and aorta, in preference to full mobilization of vena cava and aorta and cross-clamping. The renal vein is anastomosed to the vena cava first in an end-to-side technique with non-absorbable monofilament vascular sutures (Figure 11-14).[40] The renal artery is then anastomosed to either the right common iliac artery or terminal aorta in an end-to-side fashion using fine non-absorbable monofilament vascular sutures. Occasionally a small aortic punch may be used to create a hole in the aorta to which the renal artery is anastomosed. This latter technique is said to reduce the chance of the renal artery lumen occluding if hypotension occurs. When the renal artery is anastomosed to the aorta it is usually brought in front of the vena cava, although on occasion it may lie best if passed behind the vena cava. Careful liaison with the anesthetist is required when clamping and declamping the vena cava and aorta, since the perfused kidney may remove a large part of the child's circulating volume, resulting in dramatic hemodynamic changes.

The ascending colon is placed back over the anterior surface of the kidney. No fixation is necessary. The ureter is brought down retroperitoneally crossing the common iliac artery at its midpoint and is implanted into the bladder as a ureteroneocystostomy.

End-to-end arterial anastomoses in growing children should be done wholly or partially interrupted; for end-to-side anastomoses, where there is a significant Carrel patch of donor vessel, continuous anastomoses may suffice.

PEDIATRIC DONOR

When a child's kidney is used as a donor kidney for an adult or child recipient, the surgical technique is essentially the same as has been described. Because of the small size of the renal vessels, use of aortic and vena caval patches generally is necessary. Interrupted sutures may be necessary for at least half the circumference of the anastomosis since the kidney will increase in size.

When pediatric kidneys are very small, double kidneys may be transplanted en bloc into adults and bigger children.[2,16,33,42,59]

For en bloc transplantation, both kidneys are removed with a segment of aorta and vena cava. The aorta and vena cava caudal to the renal vessels are removed and anastomosed to the aorta and vena cava cranial to the renal vessels, closing off the caudal aorta and cava of the donor. This technique allows the kidneys to be placed quite low over the iliac vessels and provides a short distance for the ureters to traverse to the bladder. Other techniques include simply oversewing the cranial ends of the aorta and vena cava, with anastomoses of the caudal ends of the aorta and vena cava end-to-side to the iliac vessels. Some surgeons advocate suturing the superior poles of the kidneys to the sides of the aorta to prevent torsion or kinking of renal vascular pedicles. Ureters are implanted to the bladder separately using the extravesical approach or are joined together to form a common funnel, as described earlier. Another technique is to remove segments of the recipient's external iliac artery and vein and anastomose the tubular aorta and inferior vena cava into the defects. A fourth technique is to incise longitudinally the posterior aorta and inferior vena cava and anastomose these vascular patches to the iliac vessels.

DOUBLE KIDNEY TRANSPLANT

Less than optimal kidneys are increasingly being used for transplantation, accepting less than perfect function in the knowledge that this is, nonetheless, superior to life on dialysis[1,54,65] Some centers routinely biopsy older donor kidneys,[53] and if the biopsy shows significant chronic changes then both donor kidneys are transplanted into one recipient, rather than transplanting one each into two separate recipients.

Double kidney transplantation can be performed in two ways.[17] Both kidneys can be transplanted on to the same side through an extended pararectal incision. The first kidney chosen should have the longest ureter, and is transplanted on to the common iliac artery and either the common iliac vein or vena cava; the second kidney is then implanted caudally on to the external iliac vessels. The ureters may be managed as described previously. It is important to transplant the cranial kidney first, since clamping the common iliac artery will remove the inflow to a kidney that has been transplanted to the external vessels below. The alternative method of transplantation is to implant kidneys bilaterally through separate incisions, one in each iliac fossa.

TRANSPLANT NEPHRECTOMY

Removal of a graft that has undergone chronic rejection and has been in place for many months or years can be extremely difficult and should be performed by an experienced transplant surgeon. The usual approach for the transplant nephrectomy is through the original transplant incision. An abdominal incision may be preferred in small children, particularly if the implantation was performed intra-abdominally. One also may use the abdominal approach to control the iliac vessels in case of a mycotic aneurysm or a perinephric abscess, where there is a risk of catastrophic hemorrhage. Prophylactic antibiotics should be given to cover skin and urinary pathogens, together with coverage of any other organism known to be prevalent.

In the early postoperative period, removal of the transplant in toto is simple with easy identification of the renal pedicle structures. The donor vessels may be simply ligated, with the ligated stumps of donor vessels either left in situ in the recipient or removed. Leaving stumps runs the risk of thrombosis or hemorrhage as the immune system attacks the donor endothelium, although this is less likely the more time that has elapsed since transplantation. Alternatively removal of the donor vessel stumps may necessitate vascular repair using an autologous saphenous vein patch to prevent narrowing of the native vessels.

The long-standing transplanted kidney is most easily removed subcapsularly. After deepening the original incision the false capsule is identified and incised. The kidney parenchyma is freed with blunt dissection all around the kidney in the plane within the capsule but outside the parenchyma. The vessels and ureter enter the capsule deep to the kidney, and it is usually necessary to incise the capsule around the hilum so as to isolate the vascular pedicle. Care should be taken to ensure that the native vessels, typically the external iliac artery and vein, are separate from the vascular pedicle. The pedicle is then mass-clamped with a Satinsky clamp and divided to remove the kidney. The vascular pedicle is oversewn with a monofilament vascular suture. The artery and the vein may be dissected and transfixed separately at this time, but this can be difficult and is usually unnecessary. Sometimes the segmental renal arteries and venous branches are ligated and divided as they appear during dissection within the renal hilar scar, obviating the need to control the pedicle. Transplant nephrectomy, therefore, leaves a small amount of donor material in the patient – the site of the anastomosis. Although theoretically at risk of rejection, this does not, in reality, appear to cause a problem.

If the wound is grossly contaminated or infected, it should be left open with packing, with secondary closure in mind.[34,60] Closed suction drainage may be used, according to surgeon's preference.

REFERENCES

1. Alfrey EJ, Lee CM, Scandling JD, et al. When should expanded criteria donor kidneys be used for single versus dual kidney transplants? Transplantation 1997;64:1142–6.
2. Amante AJ, Kahan BD. En bloc transplantation of kidneys from pediatric donors. J Urol 1996;155:852–6, discussion 856-7.
3. Barry JM, Lemmers MJ, Meyer MM, et al. Cadaver kidney transplantation in patients more than 65 years old. World J Urol 1996;14:243–8.
4. Barry JM, Pearse HD, Lawson RK, et al. Ureteroneocystostomy in kidney transplant with ureteral duplication. Arch Surg 1973;106:345–6.
5. Belzer FO, Schweitzer RT, Holliday M, et al. Renal homotransplantation in children. Am J Surg 1972;124:270–8.

6. Bennett AH. Pyelocystostomy in a renal allograft. Am J Surg 1973;125:633–5.
7. Benoit G, Blanchet P, Eschwege P, et al. Insertion of a double pigtail ureteral stent for the prevention of urological complications in renal transplantation: a prospective randomized study. J Urol 1996;156:881–4.
8. Bradic I, Pasini M, Vlatkovic G. Antireflux ureterocystostomy at the vertex of the bladder. Br J Urol 1975;47:525–30.
9. Broyer M, Gagnadoux MF, Beurton D, et al. Transplantation in children: technical aspects, drug therapy and problems related to primary renal disease. Proc Eur Dial Transplant Assoc 1981;18:313–21.
10. Carrel A. Le technique opératoire des anastomoses vasculaires et la transplantation des viscères. Lyon Med 1902;98:859.
11. Cohen J, Rees AJ, Williams G. A prospective randomized controlled trial of perioperative antibiotic prophylaxis in renal transplantation. J Hosp Infect 1988;11:357–63.
12. Cole BR. The psychosocial implications of pre-emptive transplantation. Pediatr Nephrol 1991;5:158–61.
13. Conlin MJ, Lemmers MJ, Barry JM. Extravesical ureteroneocystostomy for duplicated allograft ureters. J Urol 1994;152:1201–2.
14. Darouiche RO, Wall Jr MJ, Itani KM, et al. Chlorhexidine-alcohol versus povidone-iodine for surgical-site antisepsis. N Engl J Med 2010;362:18–26.
15. de Campos Freire Jr G, de Goes GM, de Campos Freire JG. Extravesical ureteral implantation in kidney transplantation. Urology 1974;3:304–8.
16. Dreikorn K, Rohl L, Horsch R. The use of double renal transplants from paediatric cadaver donors. Br J Urol 1977;49:361–4.
17. Ekser B, Baldan N, Margani G, et al. Monolateral placement of both kidneys in dual kidney transplantation: low surgical complication rate and short operating time. Transpl Int 2006;19:485–91.
18. Evans CM, Purohit S, Colbert JW, et al. Amoxycillin-clavulanic acid (Augmentin) antibiotic prophylaxis against wound infections in renal failure patients. J Antimicrob Chemother 1988;22:363–9.
19. Farouk K, Afridi Z, Bano U, et al. Electrocoagulation versus suture-ligation of lymphatics in kidney transplant recipient surgery. J Postgrad Med Inst 2006;4:398–403.
20. Fine RN, Korsch BM, Stiles Q, et al. Renal homotransplantation in children. J Pediatr 1970;76:347–57.
21. Fine RN, Tejani A, Sullivan EK. Pre-emptive renal transplantation in children: report of the North American Pediatric Renal Transplant Cooperative Study (NAPRTCS). Clin Transplant 1994;8:474–8.
22. Firlit C. Unique urinary diversions in transplantation. J Urol 1977;118:1043.
23. Fjeldborg O, Kim CH. Double ureters in renal transplantation. J Urol 1972;108:377–9.
24. Gil-Vernet JM, Gil-Vernet A, Caralps A, et al. Orthotopic renal transplant and results in 139 consecutive cases. J Urol 1989;142:248–52.
25. Hamburger J, Crosnier J, Dormont J. Experience with 45 renal homotransplantations in man. Lancet 1965;1:985–92.
26. Hatch DA, Belitsky P, Barry JM, et al. Fate of renal allografts transplanted in patients with urinary diversion. Transplantation 1993;56:838–42.
27. Heritier P, Perraud Y, Relave M, et al. Renal transplantation and Kock pouch: a case report. J Urol 1989;141:595–6.
28. Herwig KR, Konnak JW. Vesicopyelostomy: a method for urinary drainage of the transplanted kidney. J Urol 1973;109:955–7.
29. Hume DM. Kidney transplantation. In: Rapaport F, Dausset J, editors. Human transplantation. London: Grune & Stratton; 1968. p. 110.
30. Hume DM, Magee JH, Kauffman Jr. HM, et al. Renal homotransplantation in man in modified recipients. Ann Surg 1963;158:608–44.
31. Jaffers GJ, Cosimi AB, Delmonico FL, et al. Experience with pyeloureterostomy in renal transplantation. Ann Surg 1982;196:588–93.
32. Kelly WD, Merkel FK, Markland C. Ileal urinary diversion in conjunction with renal homotransplantation. Lancet 1966;1:222–6.
33. Kinne DW, Spanos PK, DeShazo MM, et al. Double renal transplants from pediatric donors to adult recipients. Am J Surg 1974;127:292–5.
34. Kohlberg WI, Tellis VA, Bhat DJ, et al. Wound infections after transplant nephrectomy. Arch Surg 1980;115:645–6.
35. Konnak JW, Herwig KR, Turcotte JG. External ureteroneocystostomy in renal transplantation. J Urol 1972;108:380–1.
36. Kootstra G. Kidney transplantation. In: Kremer B, Broelsch C, Henne-Bruns D, editors. Atlas of liver, pancreas, and kidney transplantation. Stuttgart: Georg Thieme Verlag; 1994. p. 128.
37. Kuss R, Tsenturier J, Milliez P. Quelques essais de greffes du rein chez l'homme. Mem Acad Chir 1951;77:755.
38. Lawler RH, West JW, Mc Nulty P, et al. Homotransplantation of the kidney in the human. JAMA 1950;144:844–5.
39. Leadbetter Jr GW, Monaco AP, Russell PS. A technique for reconstruction of the urinary tract in renal transplantation. Surg Gynecol Obstet 1966;123:839–41.
40. Lee HM. Surgical techniques of renal transplantation. In: Morris PJ, editor. Kidney transplantation. London: Academic Press/Grune & Stratton; 1979. p. 145.
41. Lich Jr. R. Obstructive diseases of the urinary tract in children. J Ark Med Soc 1961;58:127–30.
42. Lindstrom BL, Ahonen J. The use of both kidneys obtained from pediatric donors as en bloc transplants into adult recipients. Scand J Urol Nephrol 1975;71–2.
43. Lord RH, Pepera T, Williams G. Ureteroureterostomy and pyeloureterostomy without native nephrectomy in renal transplantation. Br J Urol 1991;67:349–51.
44. Masson D, Hefty T. A technique for the transplantation of 2 adult cadaver kidney grafts into 1 recipient. J Urol 1998;160:1779–80.
45. McDonald JC, Landreneau MD, Hargroder DE, et al. External ureteroneocystostomy and ureteroureterostomy in renal transplantation. Ann Surg 1987;205:428–31.
46. Merrill JP, Murray JE, Harrison JH, et al. Successful homotransplantation of the human kidney between identical twins. JAMA 1956;160:277–82.
47. Michon L, Hamburger J, Oeconomos N, et al. Une tentative de transplantation rénale chez l'homme: aspects medicaux et abiologiques. Presse Med 1953;61:1419–23.
48. Nahas WC, Mazzucchi E, Scafuri AG, et al. Extraperitoneal access for kidney transplantation in children weighing 20 kg or less. J Urol 2000;164:475–8.
49. Najarian JS, Simmons RL, Tallent MB, et al. Renal transplantation in infants and children. Ann Surg 1971;174:583–601.
50. Pleass HC, Clark KR, Rigg KM, et al. Urologic complications after renal transplantation: a prospective randomized trial comparing different techniques of ureteric anastomosis and the use of prophylactic ureteric stents. Transplant Proc 1995;27:1091–2.
51. Politano VA, Leadbetter WF. An operative technique for the correction of vesicoureteral reflux. J Urol 1958;79:932–41.
52. Prout Jr. GR, Hume DM, Williams GM, et al. Some urological aspects of 93 consecutive renal homotransplants in modified recipients. J Urol 1967;97:409–25.
53. Remuzzi G, Cravedi P, Perna A, et al. Long-term outcome of renal transplantation from older donors. N Engl J Med 2006;354:343–52.
54. Remuzzi G, Grinyo J, Ruggenenti P, et al. Early experience with dual kidney transplantation in adults using expanded donor criteria. Double Kidney Transplant Group (DKG). J Am Soc Nephrol 1999;10:2591–8.
55. Roake JA, Toogood GJ, Cahill AP, et al. Reducing renal ischaemia during transplantation. Br J Surg 1991;78:121.
56. Salehipour M, Salahi H, Fathikalajahi A, et al. Is perioperative intravesically applied antibiotic solution effective in the prophylaxis of urinary tract infections after renal transplantation? Urol Int 2010;85:66–9.
57. Salmela K, Eklund B, Kyllonen L, et al. The effect of intravesically applied antibiotic solution in the prophylaxis of infectious complications of renal transplantation. Transpl Int 1990;3:12–4.
58. Schiff Jr. M, Lytton B. Secondary ureteropyelostomy in renal transplant recipients. J Urol 1981;126:723–5.
59. Schneider JR, Sutherland DE, Simmons RL, et al. Long-term success with double pediatric cadaver donor renal transplants. Ann Surg 1983;197:439–42.
60. Schweizer RT, Kountz SL, Belzer FO. Wound complications in recipients of renal transplants. Ann Surg 1973;177:58–62.
61. Shackman R, Dempster WJ, Wrong OM. Kidney homotransplantation in the human. Br J Urol 1963;35:222–55.
62. Starzl T. Experience in renal transplantation. Philadelphia: WB Saunders; 1964.

63. Starzl TE, Marchioro TL, Dickinson TC, et al. Technique of renal homotransplantation. Experience with 42 cases. Arch Surg 1964;89:87–104.
64. Stevens A, Marshall V. Reimplantation of the ureter into the bladder. Surg Gynecol Obstet 1943;77:585.
65. Stratta RJ, Bennett L. Preliminary experience with double kidney transplants from adult cadaveric donors: analysis of United Network for Organ Sharing data. Transplant Proc 1997;29:3375–6.
66. Szmidt J, Karolak M, Sablinski T, et al. Transplantation of kidneys with nonvascular anatomical abnormalities. Transplant Proc 1988;20:767.
67. West MS, Stevens RB, Metrakos P, et al. Renal pedicle torsion after simultaneous kidney-pancreas transplantation. J Am Coll Surg 1998;187:80–7.
68. Wheatley TJ, Doughman TM, Veitch PS, et al. Subrectus pouch for renal transplantation. Br J Surg 1996;83:419.
69. Whitehead ED, Narins DJ, Morales PA. The use of methylene blue in the identification of the ileal conduit during re-operation. J Urol 1972;107:960–2.
70. Woodruff MF, Nolan B, Robson JS, et al. Renal transplantation in man. Experience in 35 cases. Lancet 1969;1:6–12.

CHAPTER 12

TRANSPLANTATION AND THE ABNORMAL BLADDER

Ricardo González • Julie Franc-Guimond • Barbara Ludwikowski

CHAPTER OUTLINE

The ability of the urinary bladder to store urine at low pressure and to empty completely at intervals with simultaneous relaxation of the sphincter complex is essential to preserve the integrity of the kidneys and to achieve continence. Although an abnormal urinary tract is not a contraindication to renal transplantation, bladder/sphincter dysfunction needs to be addressed before and after transplantation. In this chapter we shall discuss the causes, evaluation, and methods of treatment of bladder dysfunction.

Abnormal bladder function can be present in both adults and children with end-stage renal disease (ESRD) who are transplant candidates but the problem is more prevalent in the pediatric age group. About 20–30% of children who develop renal failure have potential bladder dysfunction.[14,29] Patients at risk for bladder dysfunction include those with a history of posterior urethral valve (PUV), prune-belly syndrome (PBS), neuropathic voiding dysfunction (NVD), bladder exstrophy, Ochoa and Hinman syndromes, patients with anorectal malformations, and persistence of the cloaca. In some of these conditions, the development of ESRD is frequently a consequence of the congenital anomaly associated with renal dysplasia (PUV, PBS, persistence of the cloaca)[57,82,100]; however in others, such as NVD, whether congenital or acquired, renal damage results from bladder dysfunction and is preventable with good management.[37]

When renal failure results from underlying urological anomalies (e.g., PUV, PBS, NVD), it can be assumed that the abnormal bladder that contributed to the damage of the native kidneys might adversely influence the outcome of the transplant. Many reports have shown that bladder dysfunction can negatively affect graft function if left untreated. Reinberg and colleagues[79] first pointed this out in 1988 for children with PUV. Other authors have reported similar findings.[13,59] Correction of structural anomalies and optimization of storage and emptying functions of the bladder are often recommended before transplantation.[48] In fact, improvement of bladder function can slow down the progression of renal insufficiency and allow the transplantation to be postponed.[68] Although in general all anticipated reconstructive procedures on the lower urinary tract are best performed before transplantation, this is not always possible for several reasons. For example, in children before toilet training it may be difficult to predict future continence. When polyuria is present, it may be difficult to predict how the bladder will behave once normal diuresis is restored. Likewise it is difficult to predict future bladder function after a prolonged period of oligo- or anuria.

It should also be kept in mind that bladders that seem to have normal function initially may become abnormal over time, such as is seen in cases of valve bladders or in children with tethered spinal cord. The opposite is also true. For example, a bladder that has inadequate capacity or compliance in the face of polyuria may function adequately after transplantation when normal urine output is restored.[58]

ASSESSMENT OF BLADDER FUNCTION

All patients in ESRD with known or suspected genitourinary abnormalities require evaluation of bladder function. A complete evaluation of the urinary tract before renal transplantation is necessary in all pediatric patients.

Errando et al. found it necessary to evaluate urodynamically 6.9% of 475 transplant recipients based on the following indications: (1) lower urinary tract symptoms; (2) defunctionalized bladder; and (3) complex urological history. These investigators found that 45% of the evaluated patients had abnormal urodynamic studies.[27] However, defunctionalized bladders which were normal before the onset of anuria as a rule recover function after diuresis is restored without specific management.[44] The same is not true of bladders with pre-existing abnormalities.

The evaluation starts with a complete history, including a log kept over several days recording voided volumes and frequency, incontinent episodes, and presence of nocturia or nocturnal enuresis. In anuric patients, the history before the onset of anuria is very valuable. In most cases of lower urinary tract anomalies, a voiding cystourethrogram is useful to estimate bladder capacity and to outline its contour. It is also essential to evaluate urethral anatomy and to determine the presence of vesicoureteral reflux when that information is necessary. Non-invasive urodynamics, including the pattern of the uroflow examination, the maximal and average flow rate, and the residual urine measured by bladder scanning are also important. In most patients without symptoms, a normal uroflow study and the absence of residual urine on ultrasonography are sufficient to rule out significant bladder dysfunction. Abnormal uroflow patterns or incomplete bladder emptying may be situational and should be repeated.[44,71]

Invasive urodynamic studies, including cystomanometry (with or without simultaneous intrarectal pressure measurements), and electromyography of the pelvic floor are needed when the bladder capacity and compliance are questionable, the uroflow pattern is abnormal, or there is a history of bladder dysfunction. The simultaneous performance of a voiding cystourethrogram and cystomanometry (videourodynamics) is most useful in such cases.

The pretransplant urological evaluation aims to diagnose, treat, and optimize any pre-existing bladder dysfunction.[29,50,78] Ramirez et al. retrospectively looked at 271 pediatric renal transplantations and found voiding cystourethrography (VCUG) useful in children less than 8 years of age and those with a history of urologic disease,[78] whereas in adults without a history of urologic disease or symptoms VCUG is not necessary.[36] Cystoscopy is indicated in cases in which the urinary flow is abnormal, residual urine volumes are elevated, or the urethra is difficult to catheterize. In these cases, if obstruction is ruled out, neurological investigation, including magnetic resonance imaging of the spinal cord, is necessary to rule out NVD.

After the evaluation is completed, one can make a judgment as to the adequacy of the lower urinary tract. Criteria for a usable bladder relate to bladder capacity, bladder compliance, the bladder's ability to empty completely, and urinary continence. The presence of vesicoureteral reflux also should be taken into consideration.

Bladder capacity varies with age. Known formulas exist to determine if the bladder capacity for age is satisfactory for a given patient. With the capacity of the newborn bladder at about 30 mL, and bladder capacity increasing by about 30 mL each year almost until puberty,[71] the formula (age in years $+1) \times 30 =$ bladder capacity in mL is useful. For infants we prefer the estimation of 7 mL/kg.[30] Although most calculations use the patient's age, assuming that the body habitus is within normal limits, this is often not the case in patients with spina bifida and ESRD. In this population we prefer the formula mentioned above, which assumes 7 mL of capacity for every kg of body weight.

Bladder compliance is defined as the change in bladder pressure for a given change in volume. It is calculated by dividing the volume change (ΔV) by the change in detrusor pressure (ΔP_{det}) — compliance $\Delta V/\Delta P$ detrusor — and is expressed in mL/cmH_2O. Decreased bladder compliance implies a poorly distensible bladder in which the pressure/volume curve is steep, and the pressure rise is rapid for low-volume increases. Although numerical values are often used to express compliance, interpretation of these numbers must take into consideration age and expected bladder capacity. The lowest full resting pressure is preferable regardless of the maximal bladder capacity.

McGuire and associates[63] stated that sustained detrusor pressures greater than 40 cmH_2O can cause upper tract damage.

GENERAL CONCEPTS OF MANAGEMENT OF BLADDER DYSFUNCTION

The general principles of making the bladder useful to receive a renal graft include: (1) providing a method for emptying when spontaneous voiding is not possible; (2) restoring bladder capacity and compliance; and (3) increasing outlet resistance when sphincter failure causes urinary incontinence. Although urinary incontinence may not affect the functional result of transplantation, restoring continence greatly enhances quality of life.[96]

A functional bladder may need to be re-evaluated over time if the waiting time for renal transplantation is prolonged or if new lower urinary tract symptoms occur. It also is known that bladder dysfunction in children and adolescents occurs after transplantation, even when the bladder was normal before renal transplantation, warranting careful follow-up.[42,98]

Methods to Enhance Bladder Emptying

Periodic, complete emptying of the bladder is important to prevent infections, keep the intravesical pressure low and allow for urinary continence. Chronic urinary retention leads to overflow incontinence, and urinary tract infection. When intravesical pressures are high, hydronephrosis with or without vesicoureteral reflux and renal damage develop. Medications that relax the bladder neck musculature such as alpha blockers may be used but are of unproven effectiveness in patients with NVD or PUV.[2,6] Symptomatic improvement of lower urinary tract symptoms in adults has been documented.[19,49] Botulinum A toxin injection to the sphincter mechanisms may be effective to improve bladder emptying in high spinal cord lesions but the effect is short-lived.[25] Therefore, in most cases of incomplete bladder emptying clean intermittent

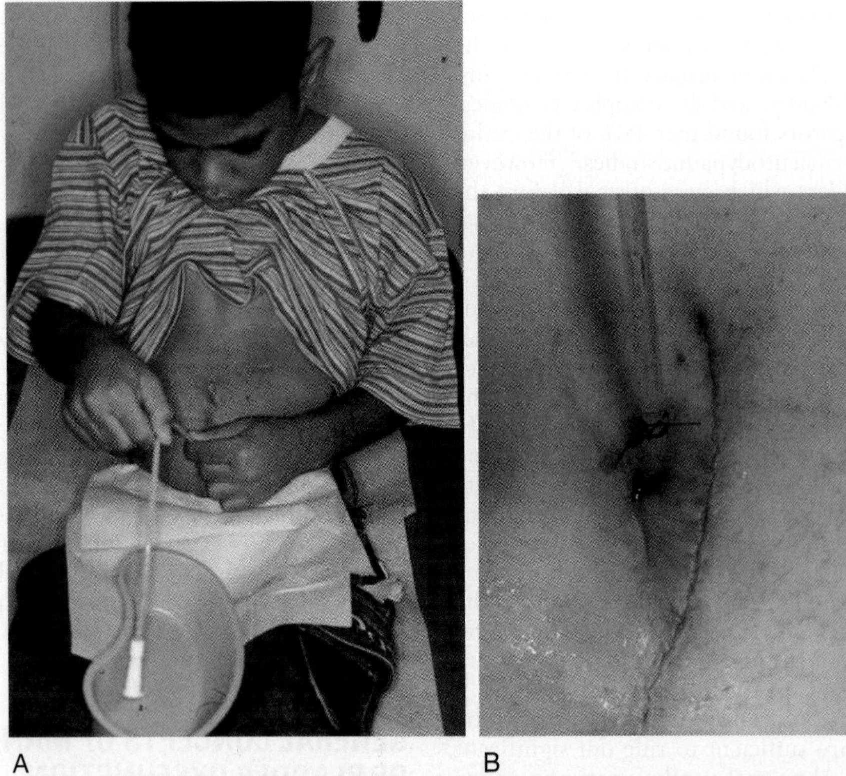

FIGURE 12-1 ■ (A) Catheterization through an umbilical stoma in a patient who had a continent catheterizable channel accomplished using the Mitrofanoff principle. (B) Creation of two stomas, on the right, umbilical stoma for appendicovesicostomy and on the left, V-rectangle stoma for appendicocecostomy for antegrade colon irrigations in patient with spina bifida and urine and stool incontinence.

catheterization is necessary. Forty years of experience leave no doubts about the effectiveness and safety of clean intermittent catheterization.[55] This is also true for renal transplant patients.[31]

When urethral catheterization is not possible because of anatomical reasons or lack of patient acceptance, the creation of a catheterizable channel with an abdominal stoma is necessary. First described by Mitrofanoff in 1980,[67] the popularization of continent appendicovesicostomy has permitted innumerable patients worldwide to live without incontinent urinary diversions. When the appendix is not available a reconfigured ileal or colonic conduit can be used.[75] The appendicular or intestinal channel should be implanted with a submucosal tunnel either in the native bladder or intestinal segment, used to augment the bladder with equally good results.[34] For cosmetic and anatomic reasons, we prefer placing the stoma at the umbilicus whenever possible (Figures 12-1 to 12-3).

Methods to Improve Capacity and Compliance

The causes of a small or poorly compliant bladder are multiple. A previously normal defunctionalized bladder because of anuria or supravesical diversion may be small but usually returns to normal capacity and compliance after refunctionalization by undiversion or transplantation. Cycling such bladders prior to transplantation is uncomfortable for the patient and unnecessary.[26]

A bladder may be anatomically small, as is often the case in patients with a history of bladder exstrophy or incontinent epispadias. A small bladder per se is not a threat to the upper tracts as long as the patient is incontinent. However, when bladder outlet resistance is surgically increased in an attempt to achieve dryness, high intravesical pressure and hydronephrosis will ensue. Such bladders require bladder augmentation by addition of a reconfigured segment of ileum or sigmoid colon.

Patients with NVD may have anatomically normal but functionally small bladders, that is small capacity at safe pressure (under 30 cmH_2O). When the cause of decreased capacity or compliance is hypertrophy of the detrusor muscle it may improve with antimuscarinic medications or botulin A toxin injected in the detrusor. Antimuscarinic drugs, although not without potential side effects, can be effective and well tolerated for long periods of time and thus must always be tried prior to surgical augmentation. Botulinum toxin injections on the other hand have a limited and temporary effect and are impractical for long-term management.[46] Both of these methods can only be effective when the cause of the decreased compliance lies in the detrusor. When increased collagen deposition is the cause, only bladder augmentation is effective.

Surgical augmentation of bladder capacity with its consequent improvement in compliance is normally accomplished by adding a reconfigured intestinal segment to the existing bladder. The majority of patients, particularly those with NVD, will require intermittent

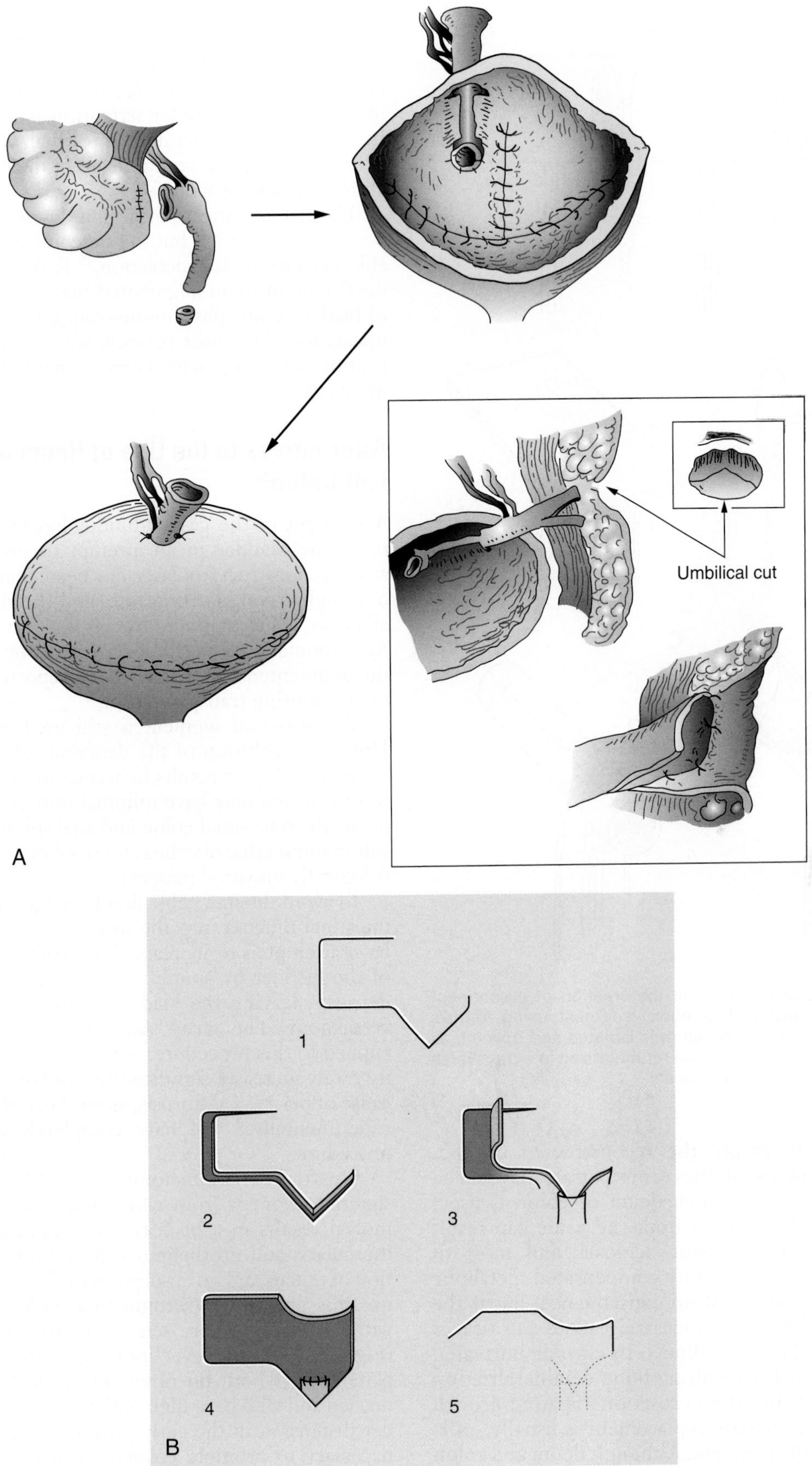

FIGURE 12-2 ■ (A) Illustration showing the creation of an appendicovesicostomy using the Mitrofanoff principle. (B) Creation of V-rectangle flaps for extraumbilical continent stoma.

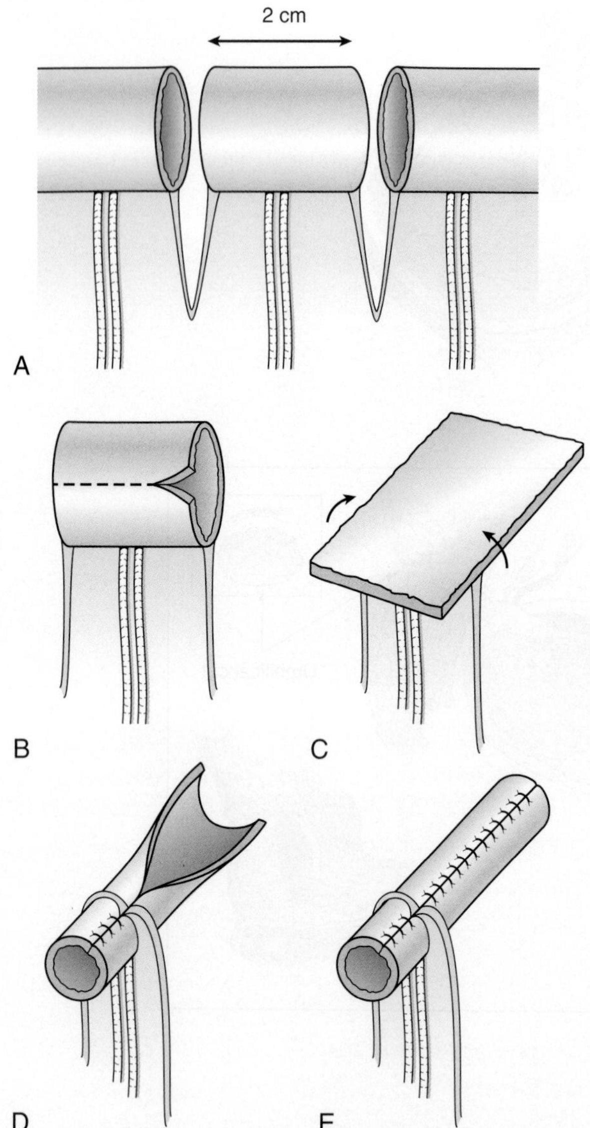

FIGURE 12-3 ■ Illustration showing the creation of a continent catheterizable channel with a bowel segment using Monti's principle. A 3-cm segment of ileum is isolated and opened, as shown in the illustration. It is then retubularized in a transverse fashion to create a 7-cm-long channel.

catheterization to empty the reconstructed bladder. Almost all segments of the urinary tract have been used for this purpose. When ileum or colon is used, the absorption of ammonia from the urine can result in hyperchloremic metabolic acidosis, and most of these patients have respiratory compensated metabolic acidosis.[73] This may be of no consequence, but if the kidneys are unable to compensate, carries the risk of serious acute and chronic illness. In chronic untreated cases a concern is the resulting bone demineralization which may result in osteoporosis or impaired growth in children.[69] Bicarbonate replacement is usually sufficient to correct the problem. Although ileum and colon are generally considered equal options, the exclusion of 30–40 cm of ileum from the gastrointestinal tract will invariably lead to vitamin B_{12} deficiency, needing replacement.[94] For this reason we prefer the use of the sigmoid colon. Its larger lumen, anatomical proximity, and thicker wall allow easy tunneled implantation of catheterizable channels or ureters (Figures 12-4 and 12-5). Mucus production and bladder stone formation occur equally often with ileum or colon and can be minimized by daily bladder irrigation with normal saline. In addition, postoperative intestinal obstruction from adhesions is more common after ileocystoplasty than after sigmoidcystoplasty.[88]

The risk of cancer developing in an augmented bladder is less than 5%[43] but the outcome is usually unfavorable because of late detection.[92] Risk factors for cancer development in an augmented bladder include a history of bladder exstrophy, immunosuppression, and *Bilharzia* infestation. For most patients with augmented bladder, routine screening with current methods is considered ineffective.[52]

Alternatives to the Use of Ileum or Left Colon[24]

A segment of the gastric fundus has been used to augment the bladder in an attempt to prevent metabolic acidosis. Gastrocystoplasty has been abandoned because of a higher complication rate, and the risk of metabolic alkalosis, which is more difficult to control than acidosis. Also spontaneous perforation caused by peptic ulcer in the augmented bladder has been reported in anuric patients awaiting transplantation.[80]

The ileocecal segment is still used in some centers. However, exclusion of the ileocecal valve from the gastrointestinal tract results in acceleration of the intestinal transit, which may have minimal impact in patients with normally innervated colon and anal sphincter but can result in intractable diarrhea and stool incontinence in neurologically impaired patients.[91]

To avoid the inevitable disadvantages of incorporating intestinal mucosa into the urinary tract, several authors have attempted to increase the capacity and compliance of the bladder by simply removing part or most of the detrusor, leaving the bladder urothelium as a large diverticulum. The term "autoaugmentation," sometimes applied to this procedure, is a misnomer since the capacity rarely increases significantly[56] and often decreases because of perivesical fibrosis, as has been shown to happen experimentally.[95] We have completely abandoned this procedure.

A partial detrusorectomy covered by a reconfigured sigmoid segment from which the mucosa has been removed results in a bladder wall composed of intestinal muscularis and urothelium with minimal or no production of mucus and no absorption of urine metabolites. We use this procedure (seromuscular colocystoplasty lined with urothelium) very selectively, with excellent results (Figure 12-6). However its indications are restricted to patients in whom no other intravesical procedures are needed and who have high outlet resistance to allow bladder distension in the early postoperative period. This is necessary to promote coaptation of the intestinal seromuscular segment with the urothelium.[38]

A dilated ureter has been used as material to enlarge the bladder.[10] Although appealing because of the urothelial lining, in practice ureterocystoplasty has very limited applications. Properly managed patients with

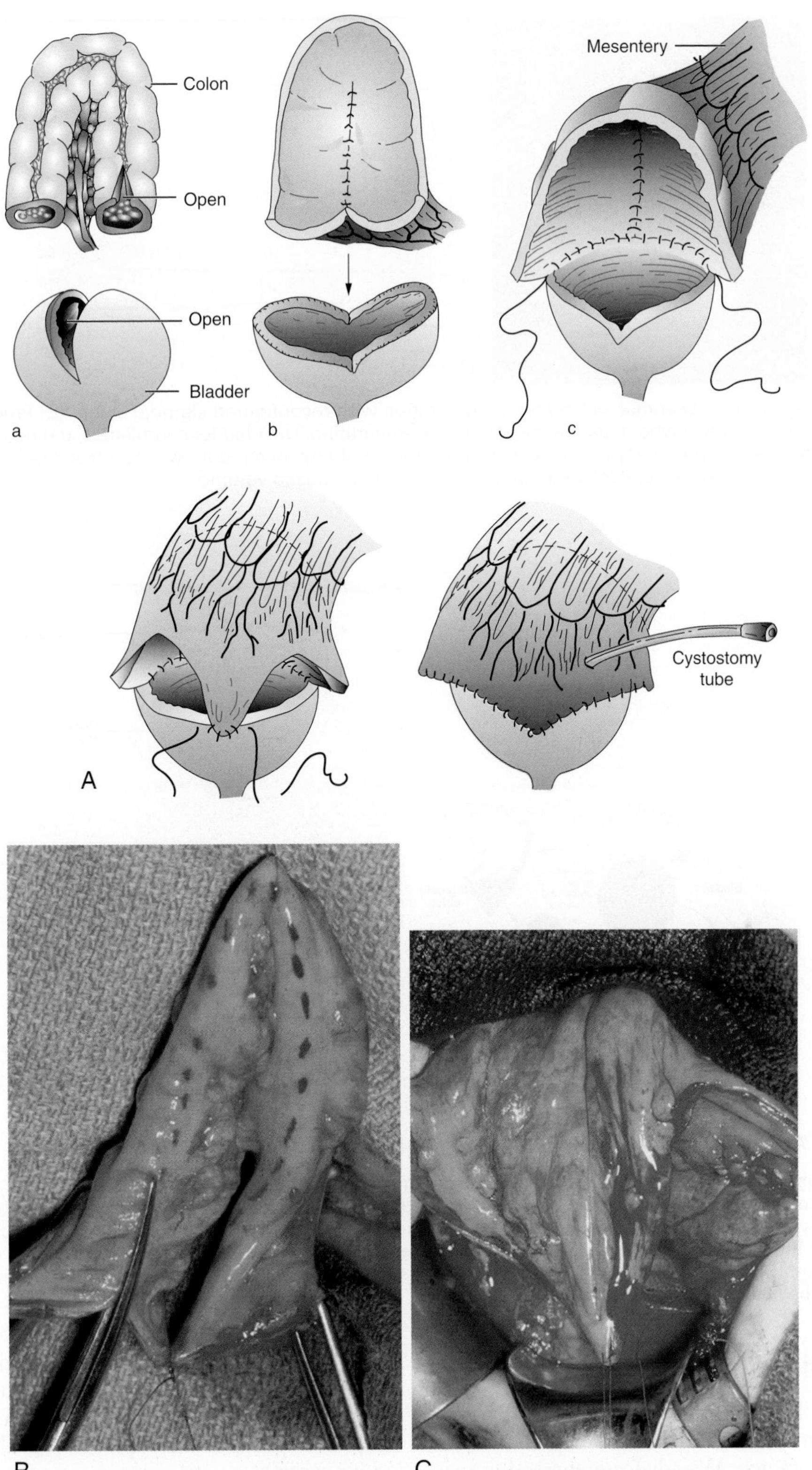

FIGURE 12-4 ■ (A) Bladder augmentation using reconfigured bowel segment. (B) Bowel segment used for bladder augmentation is detubularized on its antimesenteric border and folded in half to form a U shape. (C) The U-shaped flap is anastomosed to the opened bladder beginning in the midline posteriorly.

NVD should never develop ureteral dilatation of such magnitude as to be useful for augmentation.[37] Children with PUV may have massively dilated ureters but they are usually polyuric and, when augmentation is indicated, ureterocystoplasty rarely achieves the desired capacity.[76]

The futuristic idea of a bioengineered bladder constructed in vitro from cells harvested from the patient remains an elusive alternative to augmentation. If one considers that the majority of cases requiring bladder augmentation have an abnormal bladder innervation, the idea of replacing the bladder without correcting the neurological deficit loses appeal.[45]

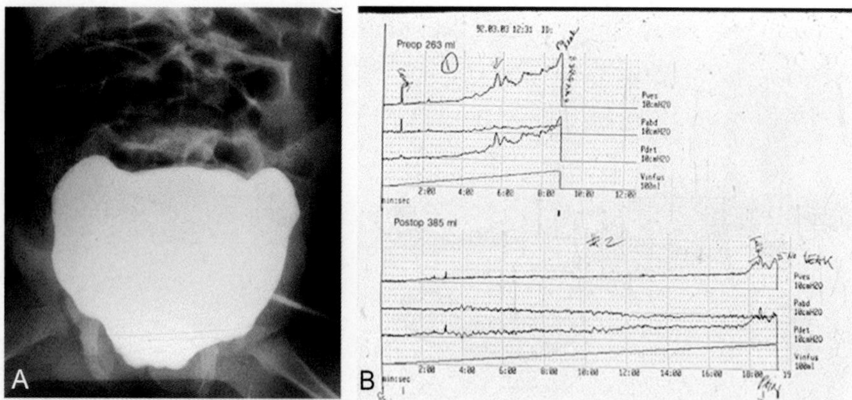

FIGURE 12-5 ■ (A) Radiographic appearance of bladder augmentation with reconfigured sigmoid colon. (B) Preoperative and postoperative cystometrogram in a patient who underwent a bladder augmentation. The bladder compliance, defined as the measure of the bladder's storage capability or Δvolume/Δpressure calculated for any volume increment, was decreased before surgery. Pves, bladder pressure; Pabd, abdominal pressure; Pdet, detrusor pressure; Vinfus, infused volume.

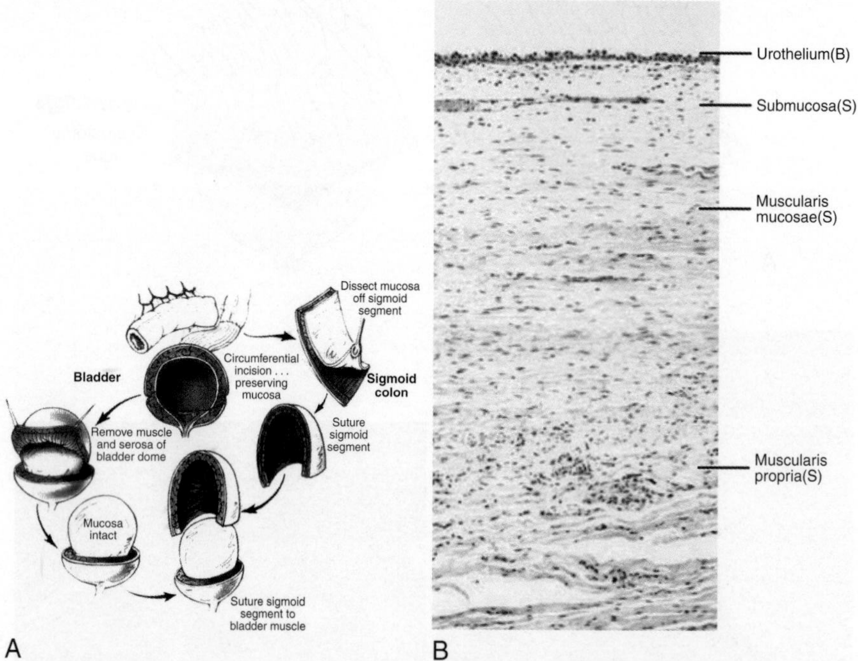

FIGURE 12-6 ■ (A) Seromuscular colocystoplasty lined with urothelium. Seventy-five percent of the detrusor is removed, leaving the urothelium intact. A colonic segment is isolated and reconfigured as for a conventional sigmoidcystoplasty after the mucosa has been removed, preserving the submucosa. The segment is then used to cover the denuded urothelium and thus prevent fibrosis. (B) Pathological aspect of the bladder wall after a seromuscular colocystoplasty lined with urothelium showing a new organ consisting of multilayer urothelium(B) (upper layer in picture) covering the submucosa and muscularis muscularis propria(S) of the colonic segment. Notice the absence of fibrosis.

Methods to Achieve Continence

Some patients with bladder abnormalities such as NVD and PUV when associated with ESRD may also suffer from urinary incontinence. We advocate correcting urinary incontinence prior to renal transplantation whenever possible. In general urinary incontinence can be caused by: (1) failure of the bladder to empty (overflow incontinence); (2) failure to store urine at low pressure; (3) incompetence of the sphincter mechanisms; or (4) bypass of the sphincter (ectopic ureters; fistulas). Frequently more than one factor is present. The anamnesis, imaging studies, and urodynamic evaluation are essential to establish the pathophysiology of incontinence in a given patient.

Overflow incontinence is managed by removal of the obstruction or, when the cause is failure of detrusor contractility, intermittent catheterization. The management of poor capacity and compliance was discussed in the previous section.

The management of sphincter failure requires simultaneous attention to the storage capacity of the bladder. In the authors' experience, injection of bulking agents in the bladder neck or proximal urethra has only a secondary role in enhancing continence and seldom achieves satisfactory results in cases of neuropathic sphincter failure.

Numerous procedures have been described in an attempt to "reconstruct" the bladder neck. With the possible exception of occasional success in cases of bladder exstrophy, we have been disappointed with the results of such procedures for neuropathic incontinence and have abandoned their use.

Implantation of an artificial urinary sphincter (AUS) is effective as an initial option to manage sphincter incompetence (Figure 12-7). The sphincter can be implanted at the bladder neck or, in postpubertal males, at the bulbous urethra. The failure rate is significantly increased when the device is implanted on a previously operated bladder neck or urethra. Therefore, it should be considered as an initial option and not as a rescue operation. Eighty percent continence rates have been reported from numerous centers.[54] Although in patients with normally innervated bladder spontaneous voiding is the rule, most patients with NVD required intermittent catheterization to empty. In about half of these cases bladder storage capacity needs to be enhanced by augmentation. The compatibility of the AUS with renal transplantation is well established.

Aponeurotic slings created with the patient's rectus fascia or other off-the-shelf biological materials (cadaveric fascia lata, porcine intestinal submucosa) are effective for females dependent on intermittent catheterization who have excellent bladder capacity and compliance, generally achieved by simultaneous bladder augmentation (Figure 12-8). Despite reports of favorable results, our experience with slings in males has been disappointing.[77]

Bladder neck closure with creation of a catheterizable channel should be contemplated when other methods have failed, although some authors use it as a first line of treatment in neurogenic incontinence.[11]

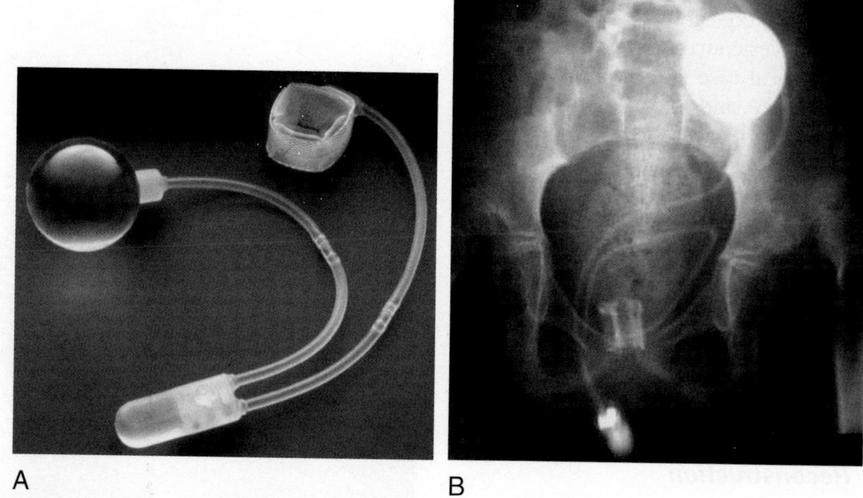

FIGURE 12-7 ■ (A) AMS-800 artificial urinary sphincter. It consists of a cuff implanted around the bladder neck or bulbous urethra (in adult males), a pressure-regulating balloon, and a pump which is implanted in the scrotum or labium major. (B) Plain radiograph of the abdomen showing the presence of the components of an artificial urinary sphincter that contains contrast media within the system, allowing good visualization of the device.

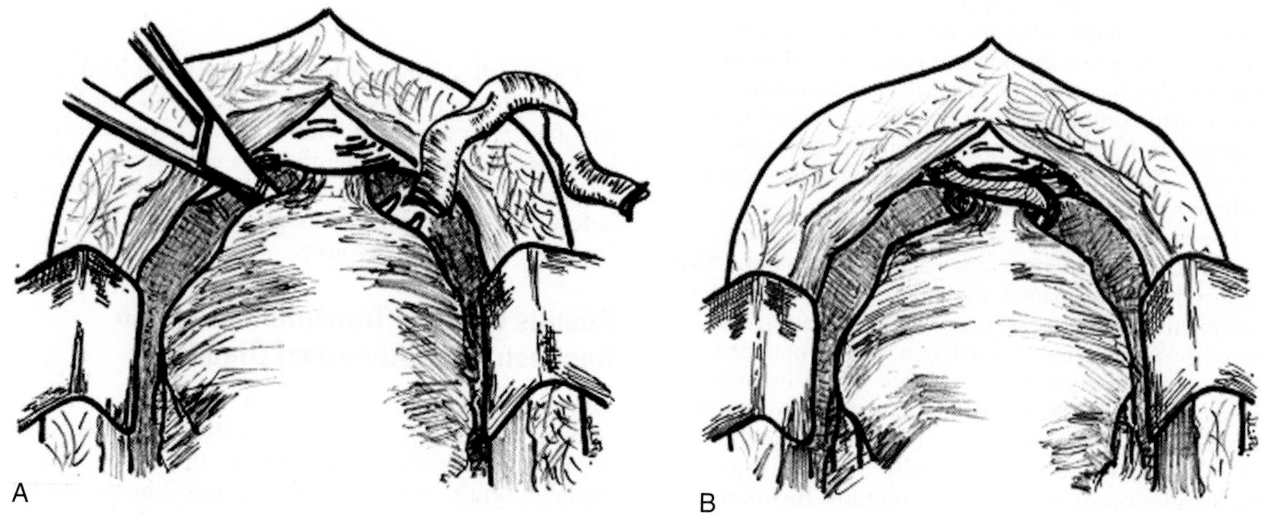

FIGURE 12-8 ■ Illustration showing the installation of a sling which can also can be done in pediatric patients. The sling (allograft fascial sling or autologous rectus fascia) is transferred around the bladder neck and crossed anteriorly. The ends are secured with permanent sutures and anchored suprapubically to Cooper's ligaments.

Urinary Diversion (Continent and Incontinent)

For patients without a bladder, an incontinent diversion such as an ileal or colonic conduit can be constructed. Success of transplantation into such conduits is well documented.[17,72] A continent urinary reservoir can also be used to avoid an incontinent stoma.[51]

Other Considerations in Patients with Abnormal Bladder

Reflux

High-grade vesicoureteral reflux that is left untreated after transplantation is accompanied by a higher risk of urinary tract infections, even if it was not a problem before transplantation.[12] Surgical options for treatment – ureteral reimplantation or nephrectomy – have been associated with a reduced risk of infection after transplantation.[28] Endoscopic injections of bulking agents also have been used to treat children with vesicoureteral reflux awaiting renal transplantation. A typical case is that of a boy with PUV with renal insufficiency and bilateral high-grade reflux (Figure 12-9). If there are no febrile urinary tract infections, the best course of action is to wait until the time for transplantation is near. An elective left laparoscopic nephroureterectomy about 6 weeks prior to transplantation followed by a right nephrectomy at the time of transplantation is the least invasive approach. Alternatively, bilateral native nephrectomy at the time of transplantation via midline incision is feasible. Earlier ureteral reimplantation in a valve bladder may lead to obstruction and acceleration of the course of renal insufficiency.[66]

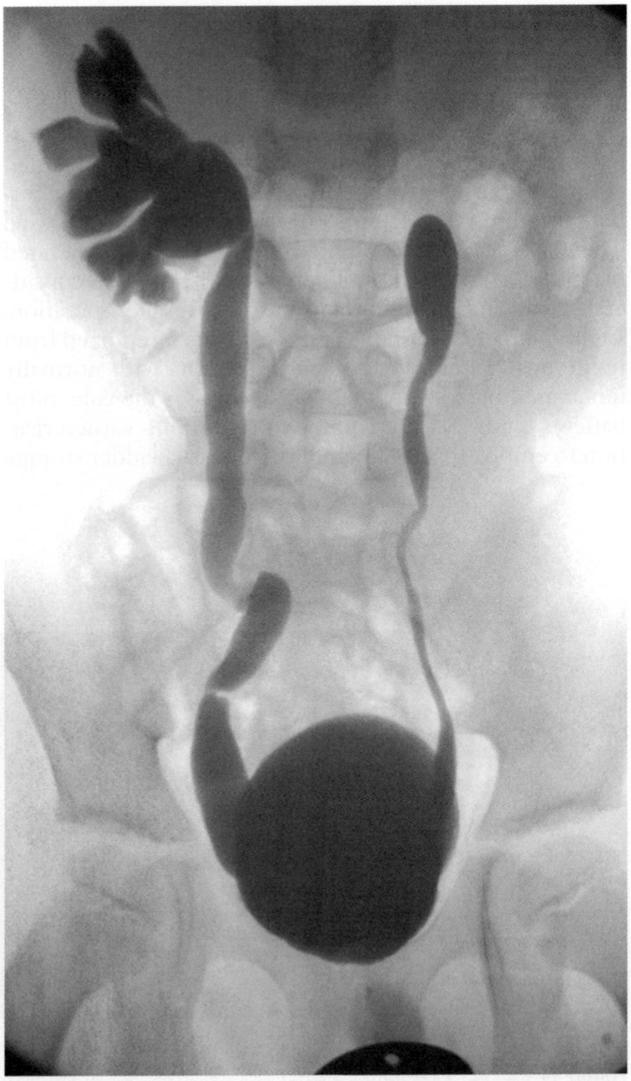

FIGURE 12-9 ■ Cystogram showing bilateral reflux in a child with end-stage renal disease awaiting transplantation. A laparoscopic left nephroureterectomy will be done 6 weeks before the transplantation. The right kidney will be removed at the time of transplantation though the same incision. (Courtesy of Dr. A Lignau, Berlin.)

Timing of Bladder Reconstruction

A challenge for pediatric urologists is the question of whether and when to augment the bladder in children with advanced renal insufficiency and reduced capacity and compliance. In children with a history of PUV, decreased storage capacity and incontinence may be related to polyuria from renal tubular dysfunction. The bladder that seems inadequate before the renal transplant may behave normally when the polyuria resolves.[16] Nevertheless, a bladder that has inadequate capacity and compliance for a given urine output may contribute to or accelerate the progression of renal failure[59] and improving capacity and emptying may delay the onset of ESRD. The same may apply to patients with NVD.[47]

The timing and type of bladder augmentation relative to the transplantation warrant comment. Most authors have performed the augmentation before the transplantation. This seems to be a safe approach but presents a management problem when the patient is anuric and expecting a cadaver donor organ because the bladder or neobladder must be kept sterile so as not to miss possible opportunities to use a well-matched organ. We usually recommend daily bladder irrigations and instillation of an antibiotic solution. Instillation of aminoglycosides, which is usually safe in patients with normal renal function, may lead to complications in patients with ESRD.[20]

The small number of cases in which the bladder was augmented after transplantation attests to the feasibility of such an approach when needed.[9] Nevertheless, it is generally recommended that if a conduit or a bladder augmentation is needed, it should be done several weeks before transplantation, although ureterocystoplasty may be performed simultaneously.

Results of Renal Transplantation into Reconstructed Abnormal Bladders

Our experience and the reviewed literature suggest that transplantation can be performed safely in patients with reconstructed bladders and urinary diversions with acceptable graft survival and function. Some authors reported an increased incidence of urological complications, such as urinary leak, ureteral stenosis, symptomatic urinary tract infections, metabolic acidosis, and calculi.

There are few controlled studies that permit meaningful comparisons between results of transplantation in native versus reconstructed bladders. Comparison among reported series is difficult because some fail to define the source of the graft, which is one of the best-known determinants of graft survival. Some series combine patients with bladder augmentation with patients with diversions; this is problematic because it is well recognized that nonrefluxing ureteroenterostomies, in contrast to ureteroneocystostomies, carry a risk of stenosis of greater than 10%.[93] Nevertheless, one retrospective controlled study that included mostly adult patients with urinary diversion failed to show any differences with control patients with normal bladders.[99] There is little question that, in patients who must have bladder augmentation to attain continence or prolong life of the native kidneys, such as patients with neurogenic bladder or after cystectomy, renal transplantation can be accomplished with satisfactory results.

Most authors agree that, although more complicated, it is feasible to proceed with renal transplantation in patients who are known to have an abnormal bladder with good results. Nahas and colleagues[70] reported on 24 patients (mean age 27.6 years), 21 of whom had the enterocystoplasty performed before transplantation. Seventeen transplants were from living donors. This is the largest series from a single center. In their series, the graft survival at a mean of 5 years was 78%, and the mean serum creatinine level was 141 μmol/L. Four patients died with functioning grafts. One patient died of bladder cancer 25 years after the augmentation, which was done because of tuberculosis of the bladder. The surgical complications mentioned included ureteral stenosis in 2 patients and a lymphocele in another. Urinary tract infections occurred at least once in 56% of patients and 32% required hospitalization.

The largest pediatric series reported is by Hatch and coworkers,[41] which consists of a retrospective review of children operated on in 16 North American centers over 28 years. The series includes patients with bladder augmentation ($n=17$) and patients with urinary diversion ($n=13$). Of the transplants, 45% were from living related donors. A surgical complication rate of 19% was reported. Surgical complications consisted of renal artery stenosis ($n=1$), urinary leak and fistula ($n=2$), bladder calculus ($n=1$), and wound dehiscence ($n=1$), or were related to the cutaneous stoma ($n=2$). Five patients developed metabolic acidosis (4 augmented). The incidence of postoperative urinary tract infections was not reported. Graft survival by donor type was not reported. The mean serum creatinine level for all patients was 133 μmol/L at 5 years and 221 μmol/L at 9 years. The graft survival was not significantly different for augmentation and diversion groups (78% versus 46%), but the trend suggests better results in the augmented group. More recently, Martín and associates[61] and DeFoor and coworkers[21] published good results using both enterocystoplasties and diversions.

Another multi-institutional review from 15 centers in France[85] included 20 patients with bladder augmentation, 8 with continent diversion, and 23 with incontinent diversion who received deceased donor renal transplants. The graft survival was 76% at 5 years, and there were no statistical differences between patients with augmentation or diversion. Data on renal function were not reported. Thirteen of 51 patients required repeat operations, including 3 for ureteral complications, 3 for lithiasis, and 1 for adenocarcinoma of the pouch. The incidence of urinary tract infections was 18%.

Another report from France[32] included 14 children (10 PUV), all with bladder augmentation (10 performed before transplantation). The graft survival was 84% and 73% at 5 years and 10 years, respectively. The serum creatinine level was less than 124 μmol/L in 9 of 14 patients after a mean follow-up of 80 months. Complications included symptomatic urinary tract infections in 4 patients, metabolic acidosis in 2, lithiasis in 2, and hematuria-dysuria syndrome in the only patient who underwent augmentation with stomach.

Koo and associates[53] reported on 18 children (mean age 8.4 years): 4 had an enterocystoplasty, 2 had a ureterocystoplasty, and 7 had a diversion (5 continent, 2 incontinent). The remaining 5 patients were transplanted into their native bladders. Eight had a history of PUV. Fifteen patients received kidneys from living related donors. Graft survival at a median follow-up of 4.4 years was 81%, and the mean serum creatinine level was 124 μmol/L. Complications included ureteral stenosis in 2 patients, incontinence in 1, lithiasis in 2, and stomal stenosis in 1. Allograft thrombosis occurred in 2 patients. Metabolic acidosis was observed in 12 patients, and urinary tract infections were seen in 10.

Power and colleagues[77] published results of 17 cadaver donor renal transplantations in 16 patients with spina bifida (mean age 20 years). Eight patients had enterocystoplasty, 5 had ileal conduits, and 3 had native bladders that emptied by clean intermittent self-catheterization. Graft survival was 65% at 53 months, and the mean creatinine level was 113 μmol/L. There were two deaths after failed transplantation.

A report of 9 children (7 augmentations, 2 continent diversions) from three centers included patients with PUV ($n=3$), urogenital sinus anomalies ($n=2$), and miscellaneous conditions ($n=4$).[89] Five augmentations were accomplished with stomach. Two patients had AUS. Graft survival (initial transplantation) was 56% at 29 months. At last follow-up, 8 of 9 patients were dialysis-free, and the mean creatinine level was 106 μmol/L. Complications occurred in 5 patients, including small-bowel obstruction ($n=1$), hematuria-dysuria syndrome ($n=1$), stomal stenosis ($n=1$), and ureteral obstruction ($n=2$).

Nguyen and colleagues[72] reported 17 patients with a mean age of 20 years who underwent 20 transplantations (14 living related donors). This was a retrospective controlled study, which included 7 patients with previously defunctionalized bladders, and 10 with either augmentation or diversion. There were no statistical differences in graft survival (70%) and patient survival (88%) among augmented/diverted bladders, previously defunctionalized bladders, and control patients. Mean serum creatinine level was 80 μmol/L for the previously defunctionalized bladders at 5 years and 106 μmol/L in the diversion/augmentation group at more than 5 years. There were no surgical complications in the previously defunctionalized bladders. In contrast, in patients with bowel incorporated into the urinary tract, there were 4 ureteral complications, 1 wound dehiscence, and 1 lithiasis. One patient developed metabolic acidosis, and 4 had urinary tract infections. Other authors looked at graft survival among augmented/diverted cases; although they reported better results in the diverted groups, the differences are not significant.[60,64,65,84,97]

A report on 13 patients transplanted into small bladders that had been defunctionalized for 3–20 years but not augmented (3 PUVs) indicated a graft survival of 62% at 4 years.[60] There were no surgical complications. Another 7 patients considered to have unusable bladders underwent transplantation into an existing urinary conduit. Their graft survival was 57% at 4 years.

Rigamonti and colleagues[84] published a distinctive study that looked at long-term results. From September 1987 to January 2005, 255 patients (161 males and 94 females) with a median age of 14 years (range 7 months to 39 years old) received 271 kidney transplants. The cause of ESRD was lower urinary tract disease in 83 cases. Among them, 23 had undergone bladder augmentation (n=16) or incontinent urinary diversion (n=7). Cumulative graft survival rates of all cases transplanted was 69.4% after 15 years; in the two investigated groups, augmented group and diverted group, graft survival was 80.7% (augmented group) and 55.5% (diverted group) (*P*-value not significant). The Italian authors concluded that bladder augmentation or urinary diversion is an appropriate management strategy when the native bladder is unsuitable and yields similar results to those obtained in the general population with normal lower urinary tracts.

Additional publications warrant comment. In a retrospective controlled study from Sweden[99] involving four institutions during a 15-year period, the outcomes of transplantation in patients with continent and incontinent diversion were compared with patients with normal bladders. The only difference among the groups was the surgical time, which was longer in the diverted group. Graft survival (70% versus 74%) and patient survival at greater than 5 years were similar. Likewise, there was no statistical difference in the 5-year serum creatinine level, but the data presented suggest a tendency toward a higher serum creatinine in the continent diversion group. Another controlled study published in 1994 by Griffin and coworkers[39] stated that graft survival and patient survival were comparable in patients with normal bladders and those with bladder dysfunction. Graft survival was 70% at 5 years for both groups and patient survival was 82% in dysfunctional bladders and 90% in normal bladders.

Riedmiller and associates[83] reported 12 patients (7 children) with renal transplantation (all cadaver donors) into continent diversion (4 with PUVs). Technical difficulties led to the need for reoperations in 6 of 12 patients, including 1 child requiring a second transplantation. At 32 months of follow-up, the mean creatinine level was 115 µmol/L, and 11 of 12 initial grafts were functioning. Bacteriuria was present in all cases, but no episodes of pyelonephritis were recorded. All of the aforementioned studies are summarized in Table 12-1.

Posterior Urethral Valves

Renal transplantation in patients with a history of PUV presents unique challenges. Some of these children have bladder dysfunction with poor compliance[15,74] and the proportion may be higher in children who have renal failure. Although many uncontrolled studies suggest that renal transplantation into the valve bladder is associated with good results,[18,86] close examination of every controlled study reported to date indicates that patients with renal transplantation into non-reconstructed valve bladders exhibit higher creatinine levels at the end of 5 years compared with controls. This higher creatinine level has been observed in virtually all studies reported and has been attributed to bladder dysfunction.[3,13,40,79] In 2000, Salomon and colleagues[87] reported worse results of transplantation in children with PUVs and symptomatic bladder dysfunction[86] than with children without such symptoms. The graft survival may be normal or marginally decreased in these cases.[23] Therefore it has been tempting to pursue an aggressive approach to the valve bladder in hopes of improving the life span of the native kidneys and the results of renal transplantation. However, others[8] have shown that patients with PUVs managed by a limited intervention approach had better outcomes than patients who underwent extensive urological procedures. Nonetheless, transplantation into a non-reconstructed valve bladder and into an augmented bladder can yield acceptable graft survival rates.[2] With the lack of controlled studies of patients with PUVs to define the possible advantages and risks of lower urinary tract reconstruction, no recommendations can be made based on the available evidence as to the indications of bladder augmentation in this condition.

In addition, one study indicates that the rate of post-transplantation urinary tract infections is greater in patients with a history of PUV, regardless of the presence of reflux.[80] This information is important, not to discourage renal transplantation in young patients with a history of PUV, but rather to pay particular attention to bladder care in these cases. It would seem rational to do everything feasible to optimize bladder function before transplantation by improving emptying, decreasing storage pressures, and providing adequate capacity. When evaluating these bladders, it must be remembered that what is considered adequate bladder capacity and compliance varies with the obligatory diuresis of a given patient. Inadequate capacity in a polyuric child with ESRD may become acceptable after the transplant when the urine output normalizes.

Prune-Belly Syndrome

Renal failure develops in a significant number of patients born with the PBS. The causes are renal dysplasia, obstruction, and pyelonephritis.[82] The first renal transplant in a patient with PBS was reported in 1976 by Shenasky and Whelchel,[90] followed by other single case reports. In 1989 Reinberg and colleagues reported on a series of children with PBS that were transplanted, with results similar to those of a control group.[81] These results were confirmed by Fontaine and colleagues[33] in 1997. This is

TABLE 12-1 **Significant Series Reporting on Graft and Patient Survival in Transplant Recipients with Reconstructed Bladders or Urinary Diversions**

		No. of Transplants			***Patient Survival***	***Cystoplasties***							
Reference	**No. of Graft Survival Patients**	**Total**	**Mean Serum LRD**	**DD**	**Mean Age (Years)**	**EC**	**GC**	**UDB**	**UC**	**CP**	**CD**	**ID**	**Rate**
Nahas et al.[70]	24	25	17	8	27.6	24							78% at 5 years
Hatch et al.[41]	30	31	14	17	12.1	11	1		5		1	12	78% at 5 years (cystoplasties); 46% at 5 years (urinary diversions); 60% at 10 years (overall survival)
Rischmann et al.[85]	51	51		51	NA	19	1				8	23	76% at 5 years
Fontaine et al.[33]	14	14		14	12.1	13	1						84% at 5 years; 73% at 10 years
Koo et al.[53]	18	21	15	6	8.4	4			2		5	2	81% at 4.4 years
Power et al.[77]	16	17		17	20.2	8						5	65% at 53 months
Sheldon et al.[89]	9	12	8	4	9.8	1	5		1		2		56% at 29 months
Nguyen et al.[72]	17	20	14	6	20	2		7				8	70% at >5 years
MacGregor et al.[60]	20	24	14	10	23			13				7	62% at 4 years (UDB); 57% at 4 years (ID)
Alfrey et al.[5]	10	8	NA	NA	12.8	3		7					NA
Warholm et al.[99]	22	22	NA	NA	32						5	17	93% (cases and controls) at 1 year* 70% (cases) versus 74% (controls) at 5 years*
Riedmiller et al.[83]	12	13		13	21.8						12		92% at 3 months
Martín et al.[61]	7	7		7	38.4	7							100% at 48 months
McInerney et al.[64]	21	21			NA	8						13	100% at 4.6 years and 3.2 years for conduits (8) and cutaneous ureterostomies (5); 75% of EC
Rigamonti et al.[84]	23	23			19 (EC) and 17 (ID)	16						7	55.5% (EC) and 80.7% (ID) at 15 years
Thomalla et al.[97]	8	8				8							50% (follow-up 6 months to 7 years)
DeFoor et al.[22]	20	20	15	5	4.5 (when reconstructed)	14				6			82% (7.3 years follow-up)
Griffin et al.[39]	23	23				20					3		70% at 5 years (similar to controls)
Mendizábal et al.[65]	15	18	1	17	13	4			3		1	6	77% and 62% at 1 year and 5 years

*Not statistically significant.

CD, continent diversion; CP, continent procedure; DD, deceased donor; EC, enterocystoplasty; GC, gastrocystoplasty; ID, incontinent diversion; LRD, living related donor; NA, not available; UC, ureterocystoplasty; UDB, undiverted bladder.

not surprising because bladder storage pressures are low in most cases of this syndrome. Later, an Italian group published their experience with a series of 5 boys and reported good results as well, but they stressed the need to address the lack of abdominal wall musculature by performing abdominal wall reconstruction in selected patients.[35] A unique complication specific to renal transplantation performed in patients with PBS is torsion of the graft. Whether this complication occurred because of the lax abdominal musculature or the fact that the kidney was grafted intraperitoneally is not clear.[1,62]

Neurogenic Bladder Dysfunction

Although the development of ESRD in patients with NVD is preventable with good management, transplantation in properly managed patients with NVD can be successful.[65]

CONCLUSION

ESRD caused by congenital genitourinary anomalies is common, especially in pediatric patients. Integrity of the lower urinary tract is mandatory, and proper investigation should be done in a given population. Graft implantation into the native bladder is always preferred. Surgical correction may be required, however, if the bladder is unsuitable. Planning ahead is crucial, and a multidisciplinary approach is advocated if possible. Bladder reconstruction and procedures to correct incontinence should be done before transplantation when clinically indicated.

Bladder reconstruction, although not exempt from complications, is an acceptable method for patients with abnormal lower urinary tract who are candidates for renal transplantation. Finally, even if the reported series of renal transplantation into abnormal bladders are small, and there are few controlled studies, the graft and patient survival rates in most series seem to be comparable to the rates for transplants into non-reconstructed bladders.

REFERENCES

1. Abbitt P, Chevalier R, Rodgers B, et al. Acute torsion of a renal transplant: cause of organ loss. Pediatr Nephrol 1990;4:174–5.
2. Abraham M, Nasir A, Sudarsanan B, et al. Role of alpha adrenergic blocker in the management of posterior urethral valves. Pediatr Surg Int 2009;25:1113–5.
3. Adams J, Mehls O, Wiesel M. Pediatric renal transplantation and the dysfunctional bladder. Transpl Int 2004;17:596–602.
4. Alexopoulos S, Lightner A, Concepcion W, et al. Pediatric kidney recipients with small capacity, defunctionalized urinary bladders receiving adult-sized kidney without prior bladder augmentation. Transplantation 2011;91:452–6.
5. Alfrey EJ, Conley SB, Tanney DC, et al. Use of an augmented urinary bladder can be catastrophic in renal transplantation. Transplant Proc 1997;29:154–5.
6. Austin P. The role of alpha blockers in children with dysfunctional voiding. Scientific World Journal 2009;1:880–3.
7. Barthold J, Rodríguez E, Freedman A, et al. Results of the rectus fascia sling or wrap procedures for treatment of neurogenic sphincteric incontinence. J Urol 1999;161:272–4.
8. Bartsch L, Sarwal M, Orlandi P, et al. Limited surgical interventions in children with posterior urethral valves can lead to better outcomes following renal transplantation. Pediatr Transplant 2002;6:400–5.
9. Basiri A, Otookesh H, Hosseini R, et al. Kidney transplantation before or after augmentation cystoplasty in children with high-pressure neurogenic bladder. BJU Int 2009;103:86–8.
10. Bellinger M. Ureterocystoplasty: a unique method for vesical augmentation in children. Urology 1993;149:811–3.
11. Bergman J, Lerman S, Kristo B, et al. Outcomes of bladder neck closure for intractable urinary incontinence in patients with neurogenic bladders. J Pediatr Urol 2006;2:528–33.
12. Bouchot O, Guillonneau B, Cantarovich D, et al. Vesicoureteral reflux in the renal transplantation candidate. Eur Urol 1991;20:26–8.
13. Bryant J, Joseph D, Kohaut E, et al. Renal transplantation in children with posterior urethral valves. J Urol 1991;146:1585–7.
14. Burns M, Watkins S, Mitchell M, et al. Treatment of bladder dysfunction in children with end-stage renal disease. J Pediatr Surg 1992;27:170–4.
15. Campaiola J, Perlmutter A, Steinhardt G. Noncompliant bladder resulting from posterior urethral valves. J Urol 1985;134:708–10.
16. Capozza N, Torino G, Collura G, et al. Renal transplantation in patients with "valve bladder": is bladder augmentation necessary? Transplant Proc 2010;42:1069–73.
17. Chaykovska L, Deger S, Wille A, et al. Kidney transplantation into urinary conduits with ureteroureterostomy between transplant and native ureter: single-center experience. Urology 2009;73:380–5.
18. Connolly J, Miller B, Bretan P. Renal transplantation in patients with posterior urethral valves: favorable long-term outcome. J Urol 1995;154:1153–5.
19. Costantini E, Lazzeri M, Bini V, et al. Open-label, longitudinal study of Tamsulosin for functional bladder outlet obstruction in women. Urol Int 2009;83:311–5.
20. de Jong T, Donckerwolcke R, Boemers T. Neomycin toxicity in bladder irrigation. J Urol 1993;150:1199.
21. DeFoor W, Minevich E, McEnery P, et al. Lower urinary tract reconstruction is safe and effective in children with end stage renal disease. J Urol 2003;170:1497–500.
22. DeFoor W, Tackett L, Minevich E, et al. Successful renal transplantation in children with posterior urethral valves. J Urol 2003;170:2402–4.
23. Dewan P, McMullin N, Barker A. Renal allograft survival in patients with congenital obstruction of the posterior urethra. Aust N Z J Surg 1995;65:27–30.
24. Duel B, González R, Barthold J. Alternative techniques for augmentation cystoplasty. J Urol 1998;159:998–1005.
25. Dykstra D, Sidi A. Treatment of detrusor-sphincter dyssynergia with Botulinum a toxin: a double-blind study. Arch Phys Med Rehabil 1990;71:24–6.
26. Errando C, Batista J, Caparros J, et al. Is bladder cycling useful in the urodynamic evaluation previous to renal transplantation? Urol Int 2005;74:341–5.
27. Errando C, Batista J, Caparros J, et al. Urodynamic evaluation and management prior to renal transplantation. Eur Urol 2000;38:415–8.
28. Erturk E, Burzon D, Orloff M, et al. Outcome of patients with vesicoureteral reflux after renal transplantation: the effect of pretransplantation surgery on posttransplant urinary tract infections. Urology 1998;51:27–30.
29. Ewalt D, Allen T. Urinary tract reconstruction in children undergoing renal transplantation. Adv Ren Replace Ther 1996;3:69–76.
30. Fairhurst J, Rubin C, Hyde I, et al. Bladder capacity in infants. J Pediatr Surg 1991;26:55–7.
31. Flechner S, Conley S, Brewer E, et al. Intermittent clean catheterization: an alternative to diversion in continent transplant recipients with lower urinary tract dysfunction. J Urol 1983;130:878–81.
32. Fontaine E, Gagnadoux M, Niaudet P, et al. Renal transplantation in children with augmentation cystoplasty: long-term results. J Urol 1998;159:2110–3.
33. Fontaine E, Salomon L, Gagnadoux M, et al. Long-term results of renal transplantation in children with the prune-belly syndrome. J Urol 1997;158:892–4.
34. Franc-Guimond J, González R. Effectiveness of implanting catheterizable channels into intestinal segments. J Pediatr Urol 2006;2:31–3.

35. Fusaro F, Zanon G, Ferreli A, et al. Renal transplantation in prune-belly syndrome. Transpl Int 2004;17:549–52.
36. Glazier D, Whang M, Geffner S, et al. Evaluation of voiding cystourethrography prior to renal transplantation. Transplantation 1996;62:1762–5.
37. González R. Editorial comment re: teapot ureterocystoplasty and ureteral mitrofanoff in bilateral megaureters: technical points and long-term results in neuropathic bladder by Kajbafzadeh AM et al. J Urol 2010;183:1175.
38. González R, Ludwikowski B, Horst M. Determinants of success and failure of seromuscular colocystoplasty lined with urothelium. J Urol 2009;182:1781–4.
39. Griffin P, Stephenson T, Brough S, et al. Transplanting patients with abnormal lower urinary tracts. Transpl Int 1994;7:288–91.
40. Groenewegen A, Sukhai R, Nauta J, et al. Results of renal transplantation in boys treated for posterior urethral valves. J Urol 1993;149:1517–20.
41. Hatch D, Koyle M, Baskin L, et al. Kidney transplantation in children with urinary diversion or bladder augmentation. J Urol 2001;165:2265–8.
42. Herthelius M, Oborn H. Bladder dysfunction in children and adolescents after renal transplantation. Pediatr Nephrol 2006;21:725–8.
43. Higuchi T, Granberg C, Fox J, et al. Augmentation cystoplasty and risk of neoplasia: fact, fiction and controversy. J Urol 2010;184:2492–6.
44. Hjälmås K. Urodynamics in normal infants and children. Scand J Urol Nephrol 1988;114:20–7.
45. Horst M, Madduri S, Gobet R, et al. Engineering functional bladder tissues. J Tissue Eng Regen Med (Epub ahead of print).
46. Horst M, Weber D, Bodmer C, et al. Repeated Botulinum-A toxin injection in the treatment of neuropathic bladder dysfunction and poor bladder compliance in children with myelomeningocele. Neurourol Urodyn 2011;30:1546–9.
47. Ivancić V, Defoor W, Jackson E, et al. Progression of renal insufficiency in children and adolescents with neuropathic bladder is not accelerated by lower urinary tract reconstruction. J Urol 2010;184:1768–74.
48. Kamal M, El-Hefnawy A, Soliman S, et al. Impact of posterior urethral valves on pediatric renal transplantation: a single-center comparative study of 297 cases. Pediatr Transplant 2011;15:482–7.
49. Kaplan S, Roehrborn C, Chancellor M, et al. Extended-release Tolterodine with or without Tamsulosin in men with lower urinary tract symptoms and overactive bladder: effects on urinary symptoms assessed by the international prostate symptom score. BJU Int 2008;102:1133–9.
50. Kashi S, Wynne K, Sadek S, et al. An evaluation of vesical urodynamics before renal transplantation and its effect on renal allograft function and survival. Transplantation 1994;57:1455–7.
51. Kocot A, Spahn M, Loeser A, et al. Long-term results of a staged approach: continent urinary diversion in preparation for renal transplantation. J Urol 2010;184:2038–42.
52. Kokorowski P, Routh J, Borer J, et al. Screening for malignancy after augmentation cystoplasty in children with spina bifida: a decision analysis. J Urol 2011;186:1437–43.
53. Koo H, Bunchman T, Flynn J, et al. Renal transplantation in children with severe lower urinary tract dysfunction. J Urol 1999;161:240–5.
54. Kryger J, González R, Barthold J. Surgical management of urinary incontinence in children with neurogenic sphincteric incompetence. J Urol 2000;163:256–63.
55. Lapides J, Diokno A, Silber S, et al. Clean, intermittent self-catheterization in the treatment of urinary tract disease. J Urol 1972;107:458–61.
56. Lindley R, Mackinnon A, Shipstone D, et al. Long-term outcome in bladder detrusorectomy augmentation. Eur J Pediatr Surg 2003;13:S7–12.
57. Lopez Pereira P, Espinosa L, Martinez Urrutina M, et al. Posterior urethral valves: prognostic factors. BJU Int 2003;91:687–90.
58. Lopez Pereira P, Jaureguizar E, Martinez Urrutia M, et al. Does treatment of bladder dysfunction prior to renal transplant improve outcome in patients with posterior urethral valves? Pediatr Transplant 2000;4:118–22.
59. Lopez Pereira P, Martinez Urrutia M, Espinosa L, et al. Bladder dysfunction as a prognostic factor in patients with posterior urethral valves. BJU Int 2002;90:308–11.
60. MacGregor P, Novick A, Cunningham R, et al. Renal transplantation in end stage renal disease patients with existing urinary diversion. J Urol 1986;135:686–8.
61. Martín M, Castro S, Castelo L, et al. Enterocystoplasty and renal transplantation. J Urol 2001;165:393–6.
62. Marvin R, Halff G, Elshihabi I. Renal allograft torsion associated with prune-belly syndrome. Pediatr Nephrol 1995;9:81–2.
63. McGuire E, Woodside J, Borden T, et al. Prognostic value of urodynamic testing in myelodysplastic patients. J Urol 1981;126:205–9.
64. McInerney P, Picramenos D, Koffman C, et al. Is cystoplasty a safe alternative to urinary diversion in patients requiring renal transplantation? Eur Urol 1995;27:117–20.
65. Mendizábal S, Estornell F, Zamora I, et al. Renal transplantation in children with severe bladder dysfunction. J Urol 2005;173:226–9.
66. Mildenberger H, Habenicht R, Zimmermann H. Infants with posterior urethral valves: a retrospective study and consequences for therapy. Prog Pediatr Surg 1989;23:104–12.
67. Mitrofanoff P. Trans-appendicular continent cystostomy in the management of the neurogenic bladder. Chir Pediatr 1980;21:297–305.
68. Montané B, Abitbol C, Seeherunvong W, et al. Beneficial effects of continuous overnight catheter drainage in children with polyuric renal failure. BJU Int 2003;92:447–51.
69. Mundy A, Nurse D. Calcium balance, growth and skeletal mineralisation in patients with cystoplasties. Br J Urol 1992;69:257–9.
70. Nahas W, Mazzucchi E, Arap M, et al. Augmentation cystoplasty in renal transplantation: a good and safe option – experience with 25 cases. Urology 2002;60:770–4.
71. Nevéus T, von Gontard A, Hoebeke P, et al. The standardization of terminology of lower urinary tract function in children and adolescents: report from the Standardisation Committee of the International Children's Continence Society. J Urol 2006;176:314–24.
72. Nguyen D, Reinberg Y, Gonzalez R, et al. Outcome of renal transplantation after urinary diversion and enterocystoplasty: a retrospective, controlled study. J Urol 1990;144:1349–51.
73. Nurse D, Mundy A. Metabolic complications of cystoplasty. Br J Urol 1989;63:165–70.
74. Peters C, Bauer S. Evaluation and management of urinary incontinence after surgery for posterior urethral valves. Urol Clin North Am 1990;17:379–87.
75. Piaggio L, Myers S, Figueroa T, et al. Influence of type of conduit and site of implantation on the outcome of continent catheterizable channels. J Pediatr Urol 2007;3:230–4.
76. Podestá M, Barros D, Herrera M, et al. Ureterocystoplasty: videourodynamic assessment. J Urol 2006;176:1721–5.
77. Power R, O'Malley K, Little D, et al. Long-term followup of cadaveric renal transplantation in patients with spina bifida. J Urol 2002;167:477–9.
78. Ramirez S, Lebowitz R, Harmon W, et al. Predictors for abnormal voiding cystourethrography in pediatric patients undergoing renal transplant evaluation. Pediatr Transplant 2001;5:99–104.
79. Reinberg Y, Gonzalez R, Fryd D, et al. The outcome of renal transplantation in children with posterior urethral valves. J Urol 1988;140:1491–3.
80. Reinberg Y, Manivel J, Froemming C, et al. Perforation of the gastric segment of an augmented bladder secondary to peptic ulcer disease. J Urol 1992;148:369–71.
81. Reinberg Y, Manivel J, Fryd D, et al. The outcome of renal transplantation in children with the prune belly syndrome. J Urol 1989;142:1541–2.
82. Reinberg Y, Manivel J, Pettinato G, et al. Development of renal failure in children with the prune belly syndrome. J Urol 1991;145:1017–9.
83. Riedmiller H, Gerharz E, Köhl U, et al. Continent urinary diversion in preparation for renal transplantation: a staged approach. Transplantation 2000;70:1713–7.
84. Rigamonti W, Capizzi A, Zacchello G, et al. Kidney transplantation into bladder augmentation or urinary diversion: long-term results. Transplantation 2005;80:1435–40.
85. Rischmann P, Malavaud B, Bitker M, et al. Results of 51 renal transplants with the use of bowel conduits in patients with impaired bladder function: a retrospective multicenter study. Transplant Proc 1995;27:2427–9.

86. Ross J, Kay R, Novick A, et al. Long-term results of renal transplantation into the valve bladder. J Urol 1994;151:1500–4.
87. Salomon L, Fontaine E, Guest G, et al. Role of the bladder in delayed failure of kidney transplants in boys with posterior urethral valves. J Urol 2000;163:1282–5.
88. Shekarriz B, Upadhyay J, Demirbilek S, et al. Surgical complications of bladder augmentation: comparison between various enterocystoplasties in 133 patients. Urology 2000;55:123–8.
89. Sheldon C, Gonzalez R, Burns M, et al. Renal transplantation into the dysfunctional bladder: the role of adjunctive bladder reconstruction. J Urol 1994;152:972–5.
90. Shenasky JH, Whelchel J. Renal transplantation in prune belly syndrome. J Urol 1976;115:112–3.
91. Sidi A, Aliabadi H, Gonzalez R. Enterocystoplasty in the management and reconstruction of the pediatric neurogenic bladder. J Pediatr Surg 1987;22:153–7.
92. Soergel T, Cain M, Misseri R, et al. Transitional cell carcinoma of the bladder following augmentation cystoplasty for the neuropathic bladder. J Urol 2004;172:1649–51.
93. Stein R, Fisch M, Ermert A, et al. Urinary diversion and orthotopic bladder substitution in children and young adults with neurogenic bladder: a safe option for treatment? J Urol 2000;163:568–73.
94. Stein R, Schröder A, Thüroff J. Bladder augmentation and urinary diversion in patients with neurogenic bladder: non-surgical considerations. J Pediatr Urol 2012;8:145–52.
95. Tapia Garibay J, Manivel J, González R. Effect of seromuscular colocystoplasty (SCLU) and partial detrusorectomy on a canine model of reduced bladder capacity. J Urol 1995; 154:903–6.
96. Thibodeau B, Metcalfe P, Koop P, et al. Urinary incontinence and quality of life in children. J Pediatr Urol 2013;9(1):78–83.
97. Thomalla J, Mitchell M, Leapman S, et al. Renal transplantation into the reconstructed bladder. J Urol 1989;141:265–8.
98. Van der Weide M, Cornelissen E, Van Achterberg T, et al. Lower urinary tract symptoms after renal transplantation in children. J Urol 2006;175:297–302.
99. Warholm C, Berglund J, Andersson J, et al. Renal transplantation in patients with urinary diversion: a case-control study. Nephrol Dial Transplant 1999;14:2937–40.
100. Warne S, Hiorns M, Curry J, et al. Understanding cloacal anomalies. Arch Dis Child 2011;96:1072–6.

CHAPTER 13

PERIOPERATIVE CARE OF PATIENTS UNDERGOING KIDNEY TRANSPLANTATION

Claus U. Niemann • C. Spencer Yost

CHAPTER OUTLINE

The first description of anesthesia for kidney transplantation (KTx) appeared in the early 1960s. It detailed the pioneering efforts in Boston with living related KTx between identical twins.[116]

The only monitors used in the 17 recipient cases described were a blood pressure cuff and an electrocardiogram (ECG). All recipients received neuraxial anesthesia. Within a few years, general anesthesia had become the norm and the first generation of immunosuppressants emerged, providing better deceased donor graft survival. As a result, the number of kidney transplants performed increased significantly.[62] Despite much progress, kidney transplant patients continue to be a challenge during the perioperative period because end-stage renal disease (ESRD) frequently results in the dysfunction of other major organ systems. Taken together, this often leads to less predictable responses to anesthetic drugs and techniques. In addition, their underlying disease puts these patients at high risk for cardiac and other perioperative complications.[25]

Today, KTx is performed in most countries in the world, with the most active ones being the United States, Canada, Australia, and most European countries, where the rate is greater than 35 per million citizens (http://www.transplant-observatory.org/Pages/home.aspx). Worldwide over 73 000 KTx were performed in 2010 with an average 5-year survival of 84%.

COMORBIDITIES IN END-STAGE RENAL DISEASE

The kidneys are essential for adjusting body fluid volume, electrolyte composition, acid–base balance, and hemoglobin levels. When kidney function declines, chronic renal insufficiency manifests as decreased glomerular filtration rate (GFR) and urine production. When GFR falls below 30 mL/min/1.72 m^2 (normal 120 mL/min/1.72 m^2) blood nitrogen waste accumulates and fluid and electrolytes are retained. When urine output falls below 400 mL/day, the patient is considered oliguric and will begin to develop abnormalities in Na^+, K^+, Ca^{2+}, Mg^{2+}, and phosphate levels.

Cardiovascular Complications

The two main cardiovascular complications of chronic renal failure are arterial hypertension and atherosclerosis, predisposing the patient to ischemic heart disease. The prevalence of preoperative hypertension in patients undergoing renal transplantation is about 80%.[114] Hypertension develops as a consequence of volume expansion secondary to salt and water retention.[10] If untreated, elevated systemic pressure within the kidney can cause sclerotic changes in the renal vasculature that further contribute to a vicious cycle of increasing hypertension and accelerated kidney injury. Additionally, alterations in levels of vasoactive humoral substances result in systemic and local changes in arterial tone.[41] Furthermore, when present, elevated renin levels cause increased systemic vascular resistance and blood pressure.

Hypertension in ESRD is mainly a result of fluid overload and increased systemic vascular resistance. This combination leads to increased myocardial afterload and wall stress. The balance of myocardial oxygen supply and demand may become disturbed since chronically elevated systemic pressure will cause left ventricular (LV) hypertrophy and increased myocardial oxygen requirements. At the same time a rise in LV end-diastolic pressure reduces subendocardial coronary perfusion. The elevated myocardial stress, in conjunction with uremia, can induce cardiomyopathic changes in the heart, which are in part reversible after successful KTx.

Indeed, even with the initiation of dialysis and the appropriate antihypertensive therapy, intrinsic cardiac dysfunction may improve. In patients in whom the hypertension cannot be controlled by dialysis alone, it has been suggested that an abnormal relationship may exist among plasma renin activity, intravascular fluid volume, blood pressure, and inappropriate levels of sympathetic activity.[18] Patients needing antihypertensive therapy in addition to dialysis are often refractory to single antihypertensive drug regimens and require a combination of antihypertensive drugs. This has implications for the perioperative period as significant drug interactions with volatile and intravenous anesthetic agents may be seen, especially during induction of general anesthesia in patients taking angiotensin-converting enzyme (ACE) inhibitors.[103,107]

Chronic kidney disease can accelerate the progression of atherosclerosis, and advanced renal disease modulates lipid metabolism, leading to increased concentrations of serum triglycerides and reduced levels of high-density lipoproteins.[44,93]

Cardiac disease is particularly prominent in ESRD patients with diabetes mellitus (DM). DM type 2 is the cause of ESRD in nearly 40% of patients and this comorbidity is present in a large percentage of patients awaiting kidney transplant.[120] Not surprisingly, nephropathy develops in nearly 60% of insulin-dependent diabetic patients. Patients with ESRD and DM have higher cardiovascular risk than do patients with uremia alone because of the acceleration of small-vessel atherosclerosis associated with DM and the frequently concomitant metabolic syndrome.[48] Diabetic patients have a higher incidence of autonomic neuropathy, which can have cardiovascular manifestations such as higher heart rate and blood pressure than in non-diabetic ESRD patients.[83] Diabetic patients also have higher rates of gastroparesis and overall hemodynamic instability.

Not surprisingly, cardiovascular disease is the predominant cause of death in patients with ESRD.[39] It remains one of the most important causes of death even after these patients have undergone renal transplantation.

The prevalence of coronary artery disease (CAD) in patients with ESRD has been reported in the range of 42–80%.[72] Acute myocardial infarction (MI), cardiac arrest of unknown etiology, cardiac arrhythmia, and cardiomyopathy account for over 50% of deaths in patients maintained on dialysis.[96] The death rate from cardiac causes in dialysis patients increases with age. It is approximately twofold higher for 45–64-year-olds and four times higher in patients older than 65 when compared with younger patients in the 20–44-year age range.[96] When echocardiography is performed on dialysis patients as a screening tool, a high incidence of abnormalities is found.[35] In one study, LV or right ventricular hypertrophy or pericarditis was detected in 60% of autopsies performed on dialysis patients.[3] Both dilated cardiomyopathy and concentric hypertrophy can develop in response to increases in intravascular volume and afterload. The accumulation of uremic toxins and metabolic acids also contributes to poor myocardial performance. Fluid overload and congestive heart failure occur when the kidneys cannot excrete the daily fluid intake, and hypervolemia ensues.

Humar and colleagues reported a 6.1% overall perioperative cardiac complication rate among 2694 renal transplant recipients.[58] Another large study by Gill and Pereira reported a 4.6% first-year all-cause mortality rate in 23 546 adult first-kidney transplant patients, with greater than 25% of these being secondary to cardiac causes.[42] The main predictors of adverse outcome were a past history of pretransplant cardiac disease or MI within the previous 6 months and age older than 40 years.

While still at elevated cardiovascular risk after receiving a KTx, the overall risk in KTx recipients is reduced when compared to the pretransplant cardiovascular morbidity of pretransplant ESRD patients.[6] Cho and colleagues documented that some patients with low ejection fractions secondary to uremic cardiomyopathy completely normalized their cardiac function after successful renal transplantation.[16] This beneficial effect is in part reflected in Figure 13-1, which shows that patients who remain on the transplant list without receiving a renal transplant have a persistent 3% per year incidence of MI, whereas patients who are transplanted have an initial rise in MI rate – probably due to perioperative stress – followed by a slower increase in the rate of MI compared to patients who do not receive a transplant.[61] Significantly depressed ventricular function is not necessarily a contraindication to renal transplantation; however, it may complicate the anesthetic management. Furthermore, the leading causes of posttransplant mortality are MI, infection, stroke, and malignancy. As also seen in Figure 13-1, patients go through a period of enhanced cardiovascular mortality in the first 4 months after KTx, with the incidence rising more slowly over the next 5–8 years.[61]

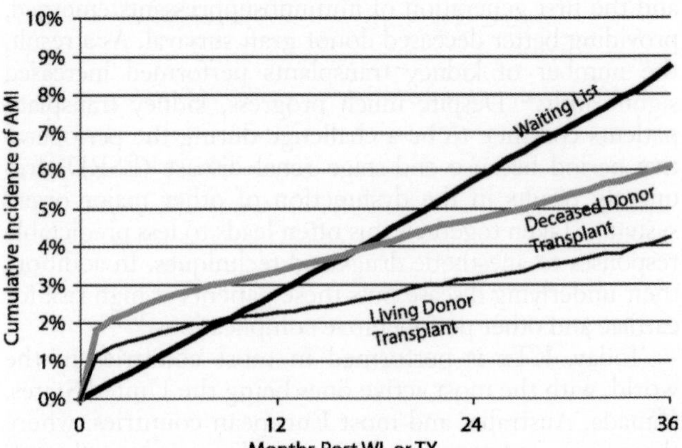

FIGURE 13-1 ■ Cumulative (Kaplan–Meier) incidence of acute myocardial infarction (AMI) on the waiting list (WL) and after kidney transplantation (TX). Most transplant recipients also spent time on the waiting list, but time was reset to "0" at transplantation. Most of the difference in AMI incidence in recipients of deceased versus living donor kidney transplants occurred very early after transplantation. Thereafter, the incidence of AMI was similar in deceased and living donor transplant recipients, with both eventually having a lower incidence than patients on the waiting list (From Kasiske BL, Maclean JR, Snyder JJ. Acute myocardial infarction and kidney transplantation. J Am Soc Nephrol 2006;17:900–7.)

Other cardiac conditions, such as pericardial disease and arrhythmia, may be encountered in patients with ESRD. Pericarditis, which may coexist with hemorrhagic pericardial effusion, may reverse with dialysis. The occurrence of arrhythmias may either be the consequence of electrolyte abnormalities or represent episodes of myocardial ischemia.

Hematologic Abnormalities

Patients in renal failure generally have normochromic, normocytic anemia that is usually due to impaired erythropoiesis secondary to decreased erythropoietin synthesis and release. Other factors contributing to anemia in renal failure include a decreased red blood cell lifespan, increased hemolysis and bleeding, repeated blood loss during hemodialysis, aluminum toxicity, uremia-induced bone marrow suppression, and iron, folate, and vitamin B_6 and B_{12} deficiencies. Treatment with recombinant erythropoietin can frequently raise hemoglobin levels to 10–13 g/dL,[33] which reduces symptoms of fatigue and improves cerebral and cardiac function.[74,76] In some patients, pre-existing hypertension can worsen with erythropoietin therapy,[33] raising questions about erythropoietin treatment and management goals.

An association between renal failure and bleeding tendency has long been recognized. The main abnormality of coagulation that has been described is a qualitative defect in platelet function produced by uremia. Platelet dysfunction – possibly related to decreased levels of platelet factor III resulting in poor platelet adhesion – appears to be central. However, no alteration in prothrombin or partial thromboplastin time can be measured. This product is removed by adequate dialysis to allow a return of normal platelet function. Other methods of treatment for uremic coagulopathy include platelet transfusion, cryoprecipitate, and infusions of DDAVP (desmopressin, 0.3 μg/kg).

Although a qualitative platelet defect can be identified in uremic patients, recent studies have pointed out that a prothrombotic state may also exist with uremia. A thromboelastographic study of whole blood clotting found increased coagulability and decreased fibrinolysis in uremic patients versus controls.[90] Platelet-derived microparticles (small vesicles with procoagulant activity released from activated platelets) may be involved in clinical thrombogenesis.[1] Despite these potential coagulation problems, blood loss during renal transplantation is normally less than 250 mL in experienced centers.

Uremia

Uremia may introduce central nervous system disturbances ranging from drowsiness, memory loss, and decreased concentration to myoclonus, seizures, stupor, and coma. However, severe uremic central nervous system disturbances are rarely seen in patients when appropriately dialyzed.

Chronic uremia may cause delayed gastric emptying. The mechanism for this malfunction is not completely known but gastric dysrhythmia with discoordinated myoelectrical activity has been found in uremic patients on maintenance hemodilysis.[66] In addition to delayed gastric emptying, renal failure patients have an increase in acidity and gastric volume[111] but this does not appear to be related to *Helicobacter pylori* infection.[102] There appears to be no difference in delayed gastric emptying whether patients are undergoing peritoneal dialysis or hemodialysis.

PREOPERATIVE CONSIDERATIONS

Preoperative assessment of a patient with ESRD should lead to correction or optimization of any persistent serious cardiorespiratory complications, such as congestive heart failure, treatable myocardial ischemia, and autonomic dysfunction in patients with DM. With increasing numbers of elderly and diabetic patients being accepted for renal transplantation, careful assessment of cardiorespiratory function is of paramount importance prior to listing a patient for transplantation. Although transplants involving deceased donor organs are often scheduled as urgent or emergency cases, prolonged cold preservation of the kidney is tolerated well (albeit cold ischemia times greater than approximately 20 hours increase the risk of delayed graft function, even in standard criteria donors) and should provide enough time for transplant candidates to be reasonably well prepared for surgery. Almost all patients receiving an organ from a deceased organ donor receive some form of dialysis prior to transplantation. Patients maintained on hemodialysis usually undergo a dialysis session at some point during the 24–36-hour period before transplantation to correct electrolyte imbalances and optimize volume status prior to surgery. Occasionally, patients are maintained on continuous ambulatory peritoneal dialysis as an alternative to hemodialysis, in which case volume status is more stable.

Patients not maintained on dialysis generally produce sufficient urine volume to prevent fluid overload. These patients are generally recipients of organs from living kidney donors. However, volume overload may still be present and electrolyte concentrations, particularly K^+ and HCO_3^-, may be abnormal and need to be monitored as clinically indicated. In patients on hemodialysis, calculation of the dry weight helps to estimate volume status. Patients undergoing hemodialysis may have fluid removed just before surgery to facilitate perioperative fluid management. Occasionally, removal of fluid may make patients hypovolemic and put them at risk for significant hypotension during surgery and especially during induction of anesthesia.

Potassium levels should be reviewed immediately before surgery, especially in patients who are dialysis-dependent and may have missed a regular dialysis appointment. Though unlikely after immediate preoperative dialysis, potassium levels greater than 6.0 mEq/L may require a delay in surgery and correction of potassium levels.

Cardiac risk assessment is an important component of the preoperative evaluation and is dictated by the underlying renal disease, its duration, and attendant comorbidities. A preoperative ECG and stress test may be sufficient for a patient who is young with newly diagnosed ESRD unrelated to diabetes, whereas a stress echocardiogram or a cardiac catheterization may be indicated for symptomatic patients or those with longstanding ESRD associated with diabetes. Many older and diabetic patients who are not able to undergo exercise ECG testing may have "silent" cardiac ischemia.[101] There is currently no absolute consensus on the optimal cardiac workup for ESRD patients being evaluated for KTx.

Several non-invasive screening tests have been studied for their ability to identify CAD in this patient population. In a prospective study, Herzog and colleagues performed dobutamine stress echocardiography (DSE) before quantitative coronary angiography in a mixed population of ESRD patients who were candidates for transplantation.[55] More than 50% of patients had some degree of CAD (defined as narrowing >50% in at least one coronary artery or main branch). However, the DSE displayed a sensitivity of only 52–75% and a specificity of 74–76% for identifying patients with CAD. These patients were monitored for up to 2 years. During this time, 20% of those with a negative DSE suffered cardiac death or MI or underwent coronary revascularization. The authors concluded that DSE was a useful, but imperfect tool for identifying patients needing further cardiac workup. However, while DSE detects functionally significant stenosis, most sudden cardiac deaths occur in functionally insignificant lesions (e.g., acute thrombosis in patients with coronary stenosis between 20% and 30%). Other non-invasive tests have limited use in identifying ESRD patients with CAD. In one study, dipyridamole thallium scintigraphy showed adequate sensitivity (80%) but poor specificity (37%) for CAD.[79] Molecular biomarkers such as troponin T have correlated with increased mortality in patients on the KTx waiting list and in post-KTx patients.[5,56]

A Cochrane Review meta-analysis studied the effectiveness of DSE and myocardial perfusion scanning (MPS) as screening tools for CAD in pretransplant patients.[118] This study identified 13 studies in which DSE was the screening test and nine studies in which MPS was the screening test. DSE was found to have aggregate sensitivity and specificity of 0.79 and 0.89 whereas MPS showed aggregate sensitivity and specificity of 0.67 and 0.70.

Other studies suggest that determination of cardiac risk should begin with the analysis of easily obtainable clinical variables rather than widely pursuing expensive tests with limited sensitivity and specificity.[46] For example, a history of chest pain is a helpful starting point in detecting CAD in these patients because it has a sensitivity and specificity of 65% for CAD.[101] A more comprehensive system, the revised cardiac risk index was originally derived from retrospective data and shown in a prospective population to be a good predictor of the cardiac risk for non-renal failure patients undergoing non-cardiac surgery.[70] It focuses on the presence or absence of six variables: (1) high-risk surgical procedure; (2) history of ischemic heart disease (excluding previous coronary revascularization); (3) history of heart failure; (4) history of stroke or transient ischemic attacks; (5) preoperative insulin therapy; and (6) preoperative creatinine levels higher than 2 mg/dL (152.5 µmol/L). These risk factors appear with high frequency in patients presenting for KTx. With zero or one risk factor, the rate of a major perioperative cardiac event is quite low; however, the rates rise rapidly to 6.6% and 11.0% when two or three or more of these risk factors are present. In addition, it is now widely understood that patients awaiting KTx require repeated cardiovascular surveillance. In the case of an initial negative cardiovascular evaluation, patients are risk-stratified (e.g., diabetic ESRD, non-diabetic risk factors) and assessed annually, biannually, or even less frequently. Patients with a positive initial cardiovascular workup (with or without a previous medical intervention) are mostly evaluated annually.[40]

Figure 13-2 displays one approach to preoperative cardiac evaluation. Patients can be initially stratified into

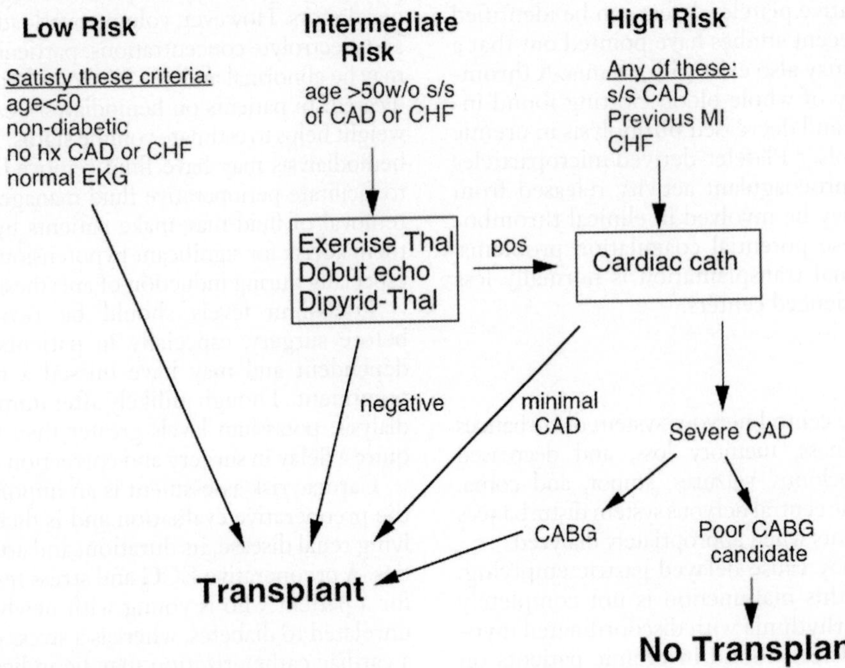

FIGURE 13-2 ■ Suggested guide for pretransplant cardiac evaluation. CAD, coronary artery disease; CHF, congestive heart failure; EKG, electrocardiogram; CABG, coronary artery bypass graft.

basic risk groups (low, medium, or high) based on history, symptoms, and basic exam. Low-risk patients may proceed to transplantation without additional workup while intermediate-risk patients should undergo a screening stress test such as DSE or radionuclide scintigraphy to help identify those transplant candidates with significant CAD. Coronary angiography is considered the gold standard for workup of CAD in high-risk patients but the transplant nephrologist must weigh the risk of contrast nephropathy in the patient who retains marginal renal function as well as the cost of the study and whether an intervention (e.g., coronary artery bypass graft or percutaneous coronary intervention (PCI)) is possible.

Depending on a patient's risk factors and the results of screening tests, pretransplant management may take the course of optimizing medical management or of having the patient undergo a revascularization procedure. The benefit of revascularization is controversial. Data from the CARP trial, where revascularization was performed prior to vascular surgery, showed no benefit of revascularization compared to medical management. In the COURAGE trial, an examination of the subgroup of patients with chronic kidney disease found no benefit of PCI versus medical management.[7,77,108] The high cardiac risk of these patients suggests that perioperative beta-blockade may be used as a means of decreasing perioperative risk during KTx. Several studies throughout the late 1990s established that perioperative beta-blockade provides significant protection from major cardiac events in high-risk, non-transplant patients. However, no prospective randomized trials have been conducted with perioperative beta-blockade in the kidney transplant population. Currently it is unknown whether such treatment can be applied safely to these patients, especially those with DM. Furthermore, patients needing antihypertensive treatment in addition to dialysis often require combinations of antihypertensive drugs (e.g., beta-blockers, ACE inhibiters, angiotensin receptor blockers) in large doses. Significant drug interactions between these antihypertensive drugs and volatile and intravenous anesthetic agents can be expected, especially during induction of general anesthesia.[103,107]

The time at which antiglycemic agents were last taken should also be determined. Oral agents should not be taken on the day of surgery because of the potential for unrecognized hypoglycemia under anesthesia. Insulin-dependent patients who are extremely brittle and have declining insulin levels are at risk for the development of ketosis and intraoperative acidemia.

Coagulation status, as reflected by the prothrombin time, international normalized ratio, partial thromboplastin time, fibrinogen, and platelet count, is routinely assessed before surgery. Although ESRD patients may be consuming protein-restricted diets, it is rare for such diets to cause a significant clotting factor deficiency. A helpful preoperative screen to predict bleeding is a carefully conducted history that includes family, dental, obstetric, surgical, transfusion, and drug histories. The bleeding time is not a useful screening test to predict intraoperative bleeding.[89] Patients who may be on anticoagulants or antiplatelet agents as maintenance medications to prevent thrombosis of their dialysis access or due to cardiovascular pathology should have their anticoagulation state reversed and should stop taking antiplatelet agents as soon as they are notified of a transplant. One center's review of 100 patients on a variety of anticoagulants and antiplatelet medications prior to KTx found no difference in reoperation rates and transfusion utilization compared to a control group of transplant patients not on these medications.[32] Because many patients are anxious at the time of transplantation, premedication is important. This anxiety may be suitably attenuated with an orally administered benzodiazepine (e.g., Valium, 5–10 mg). Intramuscular premedication is avoided because uremic patients tend to have bleeding disorders secondary to poor platelet function.

All patients presenting for KTx should be considered to have full stomachs, regardless of the period of preoperative fasting. Rapid-sequence induction should be considered, especially in patients with diabetes. The finding that gastric volumes greater than 0.4 mL/kg were seen in 50% of diabetic uremic patients but in only 4 of 24 (17%) non-diabetic uremics supports this recommendation.[95] The routine prophylactic administration of antacids may be advocated for patients with symptoms of esophageal reflux; a single dose of sodium citrate (30 mL) in the anesthetic room is appropriate. Histamine H_2-receptor antagonists (e.g., ranitidine 150 mg orally) or proton pump inhibitors (e.g., omeprazole) are given with the premedication to reduce gastric hyperacidity. Phenothiazine antiemetics and metoclopramide should be administered with care because they may cause prolonged sedation and extrapyramidal side effects in patients with renal failure.

INTRAOPERATIVE CONSIDERATIONS

Spinal anesthesia was used exclusively in the first reports of anesthesia for KTx performed in Boston.[116] Other centers have recently reported the successful use of regional anesthesia for these cases,[73] yet the vast majority of transplant centers now use general endotracheal anesthesia. Intraoperative management should focus on individualizing the anesthetic to the patient's medical status rather than on the type of general anesthesia used.[65] As previously mentioned, the spectrum of kidney transplant recipients ranges from young, relatively healthy patients suffering from IgA nephropathy to the elderly with severe hypertension and diabetes. Anesthetic depth and pharmacologic interventions need to be tailored to two different biological systems (the transplant recipient and the allograft) that require individual attention and may not always align when it comes to treatment options. For example, maintainance of adequate anesthetic depth to avoid intraoperative awareness may also reduce blood pressure and perfusion pressure to the newly reperfused graft. Aggressive fluid loading in order to optimize graft perfusion may be problematic in patients with a low ejection fraction and a history of congestive heart failure.

Standard ASA monitors may be all that are needed for these cases in patients with IgA nephropathy; however, patients with very advanced stages of comorbid medical conditions may require more extensive monitoring such as continuous arterial pressure or central venous pressure (CVP) monitoring, or both. Use of pulmonary artery catheter or transesophageal echocardiography is very rarely indicated. Nevertheless, there is no consensus on appropriate intraoperative monitoring, and most protocols are based on institutional preference and experience.

Significant acute changes in blood pressure may occur throughout the surgical procedure, with hypotension (49.6%) being more likely than hypertension (26.8%) in one series.[53] Both hypotension and hypertension have been associated with inferior patient and graft outcomes.

Hypertension is particularly seen during the induction phase, endotracheal intubation, emergence, and in the postoperative care unit. Patients with longstanding pre-existing hypertension that is not well controlled are at increased risk for large fluctuations in arterial blood pressure and heart rate. Several methods have been used to achieve adequate heart rate and blood pressure control during the critical periods of induction and endotracheal intubation. These include the use of moderate to large doses of opioids, such as fentanyl, that may blunt (but not reliably) the response to laryngoscopy. However, using moderate to large doses of opioids frequently results in difficulty maintaining adequate blood pressure without the use of vasoconstrictors after induction, especially since there is little surgical stimulation once the fascia is dissected. The short-acting opioid remifentanil, which is metabolized in the plasma, has been an effective drug for good heart rate control. Furthermore, the rate of remifentanil administration can be titrated to adjust anesthetic depth rapidly (Table 13-1). Alternatively, the short-acting beta-adrenergic blocker esmolol (0.5–1.0 mg/kg) is an excellent choice for blunting the hemodynamic response to endotracheal intubation and is well suited for kidney transplant patients with reasonable ventricular function. In patients with longstanding severe hypertension, esmolol often needs be administered at doses larger than 1 mg/kg and is best given in increments.

The single most common induction agent used during KTx is propofol. Other hypnotics such as thiopenthal and etomidate have also been succesfully used (Table 13-1). Several studies have demonstrated that the induction dose of propofol needed to achieve clinical hypnosis and reduction of the bispectral index to 50 was 40–60% higher in patients with end-stage kidney disease compared to normal patients.[45,64] However, caution is advised when considering these studies. In the study by Goyal and colleagues,[45] 0.2 mg/kg of propofol was titrated every 15 seconds to predefined end-points. The authors found a negative correlation between intraoperative propofol dose and preoperative hemoglobin levels. Study limitations and failure to identify an exact mechanism for this correlation do not support the use of a larger bolus induction dose in patients with end-stage kidney disease. Indeed, a larger induction dose is strongly discouraged in these patients, particularly when considering that they are dialyzed immediately prior to surgery and are possibly centrally volume-depleted.

Atracurium/cisatracurium or rocuronium/vecuronium is used most commonly[97] to achieve muscle relaxation for endotracheal intubation and surgical relaxation. Atracurium and cisatracurium are metabolized by spontaneous Hofmann degradation and plasma cholinesterase. Therefore, their duration of action is independent of either liver or kidney function.

Patients with ESRD have increased sensitivity to vecuronium, and this muscle relaxant has a prolonged duration of action in ESRD patients.[98] Rocuronium at a bolus dose of 0.6 mg/kg also has a prolonged duration of action (25% T1 recovery: 49 minutes versus 32 minutes with normal renal function).[97] Rocuronium and vecuronium can be safely used in patients with ESRD, but require appropriate clinical monitoring (Tables 13-2 and 13-3).

The use of succinylcholine is not absolutely contraindicated in patients with ESRD.[113] The increase in serum potassium after an intubating dose of succinylcholine was found to be the same, approximately 0.6 mEq/L, for patients with and without ESRD.[92] This increase can be tolerated without significant cardiac risk even by patients with an initial serum K^+ concentration greater than 5 mEq/L.

Overall, there is no evidence that the type of volatile anesthesic used during KTx is associated with patient and graft outcomes.

Most commonly, an inhaled technique is used with desflurane, isoflurane, or sevoflurane. All three of these volatile

TABLE 13-1 **Influence of End-Stage Renal Disease on Disposition Kinetics of Commonly Used Intravenous Induction Agents**

	Patients with Normal Renal Function				Patients with Impaired Renal Function			
	$T_{1/2}el$	Cl_p	V_{ss}	FF	$T_{1/2}el$	Cl_p	V_{ss}	FF
Propofol: Kirvela et al.[65]	1714	11.8	19.8	–	1638	12.9*	22.6	–
Ickx et al.[59]	420†	33.5†	5.8†	–	513†	32†	11.3†	–
Midazolam: Vinik et al.[117]	296	6.7	2.2	3.9	275	11.4*	3.8*	5.5*
Etomidate: Carlos et al.[12]	–	–	–	24.9	–	–	–	43.4*
Thiopental: Burch and Stanski[11]	611	3.2	1.9	15.7	583	4.5*	3*	28*
Christensen et al.[17]	588	2.7	1.4	11	1069	3.9*	3.2*	17.8*

*$P < 0.05$ versus healthy subjects.
†Median values.
$T_{1/2}el$, elimination half-life (min); Cl_p, systemic clearance (mL/kg/min); V_{ss}, apparent volume of distribution at steady state (L/kg); FF, free or unbound fraction of drug (%).
Note: Mean values are given except where indicated.

TABLE 13-2 Disposition of Neuromuscular Blocking Drugs in Patients with Chronic Renal Failure

	Patients with Normal Renal Function			***Patients with Impaired Renal Function***		
	$T_{1/2}el$	Cl_p	V_{ss}	$T_{1/2}el$	Cl_p	V_{ss}
Pancuronium: McLeod et al.[78]	104	1.8	0.34	489*	0.3*	0.24
Atracurium: Fahey et al.[34]	21	6.1	0.19	24	6.7	0.26
De Bros et al.[24]	17	5.9	0.14	21	6.9	0.21
Vecuronium: Lynam et al.[75]	53	5.3	0.20	83*	3.2*	0.24
Cisatracurium: Eastwood et al.[27]	30	4.2	–	34	3.8	–
Mivacurium: Head-Rapson et al.[51]	68	3.8	0.23	80	2.4*	0.24
Cis-cis						
Cis-trans	2	106	0.28	4.3	80	0.48
Trans-trans	2.3	57	0.21	4.2	47	0.27
Rocuronium: Szenohradszky et al.[112]	71	2.9	0.26	97	2.9	0.21
Cooper et al.[21]	104	3.7	0.21	97	2.5*	0.21

*$P < 0.05$.
$T_{1/2}el$, elimination half-life (min); Cl_p, systemic clearance (mL/kg/min); V_{ss}, apparent volume of distribution at steady state (L/kg).
Note: Mean values are given.

TABLE 13-3 Influence of Chronic Renal Failure on Disposition of Opioids in Anesthetized Patients

	Patients with Normal Renal Function				***Patients with Impaired Renal Function***			
	$T_{1/2}el$	Cl_p	V_{ss}	FF	$T_{1/2}el$	Cl_p	V_{ss}	FF
Morphine: Chauvin et al.[15]	186†	21.3	3.7	–	185†	17.1	2.8*	–
Sear et al.[106]	307†	11.4	3.8	–	302†	9.6	2.4*	–
Osborne et al.[87]	102†	27.3	3.2	–	120†	25.1	2.8*	–
Fentanyl: Duthie[26]	405†	14.8	7.7	–	594*	11.8	9.5	–
Sear and Hand[105]	175†	17.1	2.7	–	229†	18.5	3.6	–
Bower[8]	–	–	–	20.8	–	–	–	22.4
Koehntop and Rodman[67]	–	–	–	–	382†	7.5	3.1	–
Alfentanil: Chauvin et al.[14]	90†	3.1	0.3	11	107†	3.1	0.4*	19*
Bower and Sear[9]	120†	3.2	0.4	10.3	142†	5.3*	0.6	12.4*
Sufentanil: Davis et al.[23]	76†	12.8	1.3	–	90†	16.4	1.7	–
Sear[104]	195†	18.2	3.6	7.8	188†	19.2	3.8	8.6
Remifentanil: Hoke et al.[57]	4.0	33.2	0.19	–	4.9	35.4	0.25	–
Dahaba et al.[22]	16.4	46.3	0.57	–	18.9	28.0	0.36	–
Oxycodone: Kirvela et al.[63]	138†	16.7	2.39	–	234†	12.7	3.99	–

*$P < 0.05$ versus healthy subjects.
†Mean residence time (rather than elimination half-life).
$T_{1/2}el$, elimination half-life (min); Cl_p, systemic clearance (mL/kg/min); V_{ss}, apparent volume of distribution at steady state (L/kg); FF, free or unbound fraction of drug (%).
Note: Mean values are given throughout except for oxycodone, for which medians are given.

anesthetics have been reported to be safe during KTx. The metabolism of sevoflurane has been implicated in renal toxicity, but no controlled studies are available to identify clearly either safety concerns or harm associated with using sevoflurane in the setting of a newly transplanted kidney. There are two elements of concern with regard to renal toxicity: (1) production of fluoride ion from the metabolism of sevoflurane; and (2) generation of "compound A" from the breakdown of sevoflurane by sodium or barium hydroxide lime. Sevoflurane appears to have a very good safety record. It has been administered to millions of patients worldwide without conclusive evidence of renal toxicity. Two volunteer studies have found biochemical evidence of renal injury during sevoflurane anesthesia, whereas five other volunteer studies have not.[28–31,36,37,81] However, KTx may represent a situation of increased risk for renal injury, as defined by Artru.[4] Two studies have shown that sevoflurane, at fresh gas flow rates greater than 4L/min, did not change renal function indices or biochemical markers in patients with mildly impaired renal function (baseline creatinine >1.5 mg/dL).[20,82,115] In addition, one of the studies found that exposure to low-flow sevoflurane or low-flow isoflurane had no significant effect on renal function parameters such as serum creatinine or creatinine clearance in patients with baseline renal insufficiency (creatinine >1.5 mg/dL).[19]

Likewise, use of a balanced technique combining volatile anesthetics with opioids or use of total intravenous anesthesia with opioids and propofol had no significant effect on patient and graft outcomes.[65]

KTx is a moderately stimulating surgery with prolonged episodes of minimal stimulation. Blood loss rarely exceeds 300 mL and significant fluid shifts are not common. As a result, hypotension is frequently encountered, especially after the fascia is dissected, and may be further aggravated after unclamping of the iliac vessels and reperfusion of the graft.

Intraoperative managament during KTx should primarily focus on hemodynamic stability with preservation of good perfusion pressures to the graft. Individualized fluid management is the cornerstone of intraoperative management while pharmacologic support using vasoconstrictors with strong alpha-adrenergic effects, such as phenylephrine, is discouraged for reasons that will be subsequently discussed.

Maintenance of intravascular fluid status can be accomplished using natural colloids (albumin), synthetic colloids (hydroxyethyl starches, dextrans, gelatins), and crystalloids (normal saline, lactated Ringer's, plasmalyte). Given the minimal blood loss and few anticipated perioperative fluid shifts during KTx, crystalloids are sufficient for volume replacement and should be the preferred choice of fluid. Data for natural and synthetic colloids in KTx are sparse. Therefore, the use of these fluids in KTx cannot be generally recommended.

Indeed, a national survey of fluid choice at 49 hospitals in the United States found that >90% of patients receive normal saline or normal saline-based solutions during their kidney tranplants.[84] Concerns with administering crystalloid infusions are mainly centered around the impact on electrolytes and acid–base balance. In particular, hyperchloremic acidosis can occur with large infusions of normal saline and there is a perceived risk of hyperkalemia with Ringer's lactate in patients with end-stage kidney disease.

To address this concern, a prospective, randomized, double-blinded study compared normal saline to Ringer's lactate for intraoperative intravenous fluid therapy during KTx. Interestingly, the study demonstrated higher rates of severe hyperkalemia and metabolic acidosis in the normal saline group,[85] albeit the fluid administration in this study would have been considered excessive by most centers.

A different prospective, randomized, double-blinded study compared normal saline, Ringer's lactate, and plasmalyte for intra-operative intravenous fluid therapy during KTx. Primary end-points were changes in acid–base balance and electrolytes. Observed changes were predictable but none of them were clinically relevant. Plasmalyte was not associated with any changes in acid–base balance and electrolyes. The authors concluded that all three crystalloids can be safely used during KTx using a volume replacement algorithm of 20–30 mL/kg/h.[49] We also recommend a similar volume replacement algorithm of 30–40 mL/kg/h.

Whether CVP monitoring is truly required for adequate volume replacement during KTx continues to be debated. When CVP monitoring is in place, most centers recommend keeping the CVP in the range of 10–15 mmHg. The impact of timing and duration of volume replacement during KTx have been recently examined in a prospective randomized trial.[88] Patients were randomized to a continuous crystalloid infusion or a CVP-targeted crystalloid infusion with a low CVP target of 5 mmHg throughout most of the case and a CVP target of 15 mmHg at the end of renal vascular anastomoses (achieved by rapid infusion). Primary end-points were markers of allograft function within 5 postoperative days. Better early allograft function was observed in the CVP targeted-infusion group. However, several confounding factors in the study design warrant larger and better-controlled prospective studies.

Pharmacologic blood pressure support using alpha-agonist vasoconstrictors is usually discouraged based on some limited experimental animal data. Taken together, studies indicate that there is a substantial loss of renal hemodynamic responsiveness following ischemic injury when renal blood flow is attempted to be preserved using alpha-agonists. Furthermore, the studies suggest that the transplanted, denervated kidney loses its capacity for autoregulation and that the renal response to sympathomimetics is altered with a shift towards time-dependent flow reduction to the kidney. In one rat study, the hemodynamic autoregulation in the kidney graft declined following transplantation or denervation. Furthermore, the response to sympathomimetics in the transplanted kidney was shifted towards flow reduction. The authors postulated enhanced vasoconstriction via stimulation of alpha-adrenoceptors and blunted vasodilatation via stimulation of beta-adrenoceptors as a possible mechanism.[38,80]

Allograft function, as determined by intraoperative urine production, is typically optimized by maintaining adequate intraoperative perfusion pressure.[52] However, it is also frequently enhanced intraoperatively using mannitol and loop diuretics. Mannitol is freely filtered and not reabsorbed by the nephron, causing osmotic expansion of urine volume. It may also have a protective effect on the cells lining the renal tubule. It is usually administered during the warm ischemia phase; thus mannitol may protect against ischemic injury, as well as induce osmotic diuresis in the newly transplanted kidney. In most centers, relatively low doses of mannitol are administered, ranging between 0.25 and 0.5 mg/kg. Some data have shown that delayed graft function of the deceased donor renal allograft can be prevented by intraoperative administration of mannitol.[69]

Loop diuretics work by blocking the action of Na^+/K^+ pumps present in the thin ascending limb of Henle, thereby preventing reabsorption of electrolytes in this segment of the nephron. The high-osmolarity fluid that is carried along to the distal tubule prevents the reabsorption of water, resulting in the excretion of large volumes of urine with high electrolyte content (Tables 13-3 and 13-4).

TABLE 13-4 **Renal Excretion of Neuromuscular Blocking Drugs**

Quaternary Amines	
Suxamethonium	<10%
Benzylisoquinolinium Compounds	
Atracurium	10%
Doxacurium	25–30%
Mivacurium	<10%
Cisatracurium	?
Aminosteroid Compounds	
Pancuronium	35–50%
Vecuronium	15–20%
Pipercuronium	38%
Rocuronium	9%

Note: Expressed as a mean percentage (or range) of total drug elimination.

Low-dose dopamine (2–3 μg/kg/min) is commonly used to stimulate DA_1 dopaminergic receptors in the kidney vasculature and therefore induce vasodilation and increased urine output. Some small trials have shown improved urine output[47] and creatinine clearance[13] with low-dose dopamine during KTx, whereas other larger studies have shown no significant improvement in either parameter.[60,99] The utility of this approach has been questioned on the basis that a newly transplanted, denervated kidney may not respond to low-dose dopamine like normal kidneys do. Doppler ultrasound examination of newly transplanted kidneys found no significant change in blood flow with dopamine infusion rates of 1–5 μg/kg/min.[110]

Pain associated with surgery is moderate and is typically managed in the immediate postoperative phase with intravenous administration of opioids, often using patient-controlled analgesia. Opioids such as morphine, meperidine, and oxycodone should be used cautiously in patients with ESRD because they (or their active metabolites) are renally excreted and thus may accumulate in such patients.[2,63,104] This risk of opioid accumulation persists in the period after transplantation when the allograft may suffer from delayed graft function. In contrast, opioids such as fentanyl, sufentanil, alfentanil, and remifentanil have been shown to be safe alternatives, with fentanyl being the most commonly used opioid (Table 13-3).

POSTOPERATIVE CARE

All renal transplant patients should be considered for postoperative extubation using standard criteria. Postoperatively, most kidney transplant recipients are admitted to the postanesthesia care unit (PACU), with only a small percentage of these patients requiring admission to the intensive care unit (ICU).[68] However, there is institutional variability and some centers elect to admit all kidney transplant patients to the ICU.

In the PACU, these patients should be managed according to institutional protocols and PACU pain management guidelines should be tailored to ESRD patients, as previously discussed. Particular attention should be paid to graft function, which is mainly evaluated by urine output over time. Over 90% of living donor kidney transplant recipients have immediate graft function, as confirmed by urine production. However the rate of immediate graft function can drop off significantly in recipients of kidney grafts from standard criteria deceased donors and especially extended criteria donors. Poor graft function may be attributable to the graft itself, the vessels, the ureter, or clotting of the Foley catheter, all of which should be considered in the differential diagnosis. The Foley catheter should be irrigated to ensure that clot or tissue has not affected its patency. Flow in the arterial and venous anastomoses can be examined with ultrasound. Lastly, re-exploration of the wound should not be delayed if kinking of the vascular attachments or obstruction of the ureter along its course or at the site of bladder reimplantation is suspected.

ANESTHESIA FOR PATIENTS AFTER KIDNEY TRANSPLANTATION

Patients with good graft function as determined by laboratory values (blood urea nitrogen, creatinine) and with sufficient urine volume should be considered to have adequate renal function. The average GFR 6 months after deceased renal transplantation is almost 50 mL/min.[43] About 50% of patients will manifest a slow decline in GFR over the course of several years, but 30% will have a stable GFR. Given the improvement in patient survival following renal transplantation, it is likely that the rapid progression of cardiovascular disease seen in patients with ESRD is slowed, but not halted. These patients are still at higher cardiac risk than those who never had ESRD. Congestive heart failure (e.g., cardiomyopathy), LV hypertrophy, and ischemic heart disease remain important complications in renal transplant recipients. This is mainly due to persistent risk factors such as hypertension, diabetes, and dyslipidemia as well as new onset of metabolic syndrome and secondary hyperparathyroidism. Indeed, one study found considerable progression of coronary artery calcification in renal transplant patients at least 1 year after surgery. Findings were related to ethnicity of patients, blood pressure, body mass index, renal function, and baseline coronary artery calcification.[100] Aside from the residual traditional cardiac risk factors, graft rejection, viral infection, anemia,[91,96] and treatment with immunosuppressive drugs such as cyclosporine may also cause significant cardiovascular morbidity (e.g., hypertension). However, newer immunosuppressants are better tolerated.[71]

KIDNEY–PANCREAS TRANSPLANTATION

Patients with ESRD superimposed on DM will be subject to the same hemodynamic, fluid, volume, and electrolyte problems as those with ESRD alone. They will probably be maintained on some form of dialysis to manage fluid overload and accumulation of electrolytes. They may well have significant systemic hypertension for the reasons discussed in the section on cardiovascular complications, above. Accelerated atherosclerosis and autonomic nervous system dysfunction are also major cardiovascular changes present in diabetic patients. If ESRD is also present, the cardiovascular risk in these patients rises dramatically. Diabetic patients with severe CAD may not recognize anginal symptoms due to failure of the autonomic nervous system. Finally, they may also have the same problems of chronic anemia and uremic coagulopathy as those with renal failure alone.

After successful simultaneous pancreas–kidney (SPK) transplantation, cardiac pathology such as diastolic dysfunction and LV hypertrophy can improve or stabilize.[86] It has not been proved whether other manifestations of DM, such as accelerated atherosclerosis, neuropathy, or vascular insufficiency, will improve or stabilize following SPK.

Preoperative Considerations

Diabetic patients have a greater incidence of autonomic neuropathy, which can manifest as both higher heart rate and higher blood pressure compared to non-diabetic ESRD patients.[83] Type 2 diabetics often have metabolic syndrome, a combination of visceral obesity, atherogenic dyslipidemia (low levels of high-density lipoprotein and elevated levels of triglycerides), hypertension, and insulin resistance, which increases the risk for CAD and cardiovascular disease. The time at which antiglycemic agents were last taken should be determined. Orally administered antiglycemic agents should not be taken on the day of surgery to avoid unrecognized hypoglycemia under anesthesia. Insulin-dependent patients who are extremely brittle and have declining insulin levels are at risk for ketosis and intraoperative acidemia.

As noted earlier, diabetic patients, even those without renal dysfunction, have significant risk factors for cardiovascular complications during major surgery. Historically, the principal candidates for pancreas transplantation have been younger than those receiving kidney transplants, with up to 45% being in the 18–35-year age range. These patients tended to have fewer of the long-term manifestations of DM, such as atherosclerotic vascular disease and severe autonomic dysfunction. More recently, however, increasing numbers of older diabetic patients are being considered for pancreas transplantation. These patients will be at higher risk for major cardiovascular events perioperatively. An extensive cardiac workup is indicated in these older diabetic patients before surgery to rule out severe CAD. Preoperative evaluation by history and physical examination, ECG, treadmill testing, echocardiography with or without dobutamine stress, radionuclide scintigraphy, and cardiac angiography represent the full spectrum of workup that may be applicable.

It was suggested in the early 1990s that diabetic patients should be considered more difficult to intubate tracheally because of changes in their upper-airway tissues from exposure to high serum glucose levels. In fact, one study found a 31% incidence of difficult intubation conditions in this patient population.[94] Subsequently, a large study by the Mayo Clinic reviewed the anesthetic records of 150 patients with diabetes who underwent general anesthesia with tracheal intubation and found only a slightly increased incidence of "more difficulty visualizing" airway structures.[119] Halpern et al. reported only one difficult intubation in a series of 130 patients who underwent pancreas transplantation.[50] Thus, it appears that longstanding DM alone does not strongly predispose to airway difficulties but may be considered a contributing factor in patients with other potentially problematic airway features.

Intraoperative Considerations

Kidney–pancreas transplantations are long and surgically tedious operations involving extensive abdominal exposure. Therefore, general endotracheal anesthesia with muscle relaxation is the best anesthetic approach for these cases. Patients may have significant postoperative pain from the extensive abdominal dissection, so placement of an epidural catheter for postoperative pain control may be warranted. However, splanchnic perfusion to the transplanted organs is a major concern, and therefore some centers defer placement of an epidural catheter.

Because the pancreas seems to be a highly immunogenic organ, intensive immunosuppression is needed to prevent graft loss. The anesthesia team will need to deliver the initial dose of immunosuppressant so it is essential that the desired drugs be present and administered correctly in the operating room. Likewise, correct administration of the preoperative and intraoperative antibiotics requested by the surgical team is very important. Prophylaxis against enteric organisms introduced with transplanted bowel segments is crucial given the use of intense immunosuppression.

Standard monitors (five-lead ECG, non-invasive blood pressure measurement, pulse oximetry, end-tidal gas concentrations) plus arterial and central venous lines are required. The arterial line allows the anesthesia team to track blood pressure carefully and to draw samples for blood gas, glucose, and electrolyte determinations during these lengthy cases. The central venous catheter permits monitoring of cardiac filling pressure and central administration of drugs.

Due to their high incidence of autonomic dysfunction, diabetic patients are likely to have gastroparesis and large residual gastric volumes. This risk is even greater if the patient has ESRD and uremia. Administration of a nonparticulate antacid along with maintenance of cricoid pressure during rapid-sequence induction are mandatory in these patients.

Patients with autonomic neuropathy are often considered to be at greater risk for severe cardiovascular depression during induction of anesthesia. However, a study of uremic patients undergoing KTx found that diabetic patients with known pre-existing autonomic neuropathy had hemodynamic responses to induction that were similar to those of non-diabetic uremic patients.[50] Hemodynamic stability over long periods is probably best achieved using a balanced anesthetic technique. As with KTx alone, adequate blood pressure is desired to provide good perfusion pressure for a newly anastomosed pancreas.

One of the most challenging aspects of these cases is determining the amount and type of fluid to administer. On the one hand, a lengthy intra-abdominal procedure would indicate the need for significant amounts of fluid to compensate for large insensible and third-space losses. However, patients with ESRD may be significantly hypervolemic or hypertensive and may display hemodynamic pathology such as diastolic dysfunction, which can limit their ability to receive fluids. Therefore, fluid administration must be guided by cardiac preload, as indicated by chamber filling pressures, or by volume status, as determined by transesophageal echocardiography, for example. If fluid is necessary, it is probably best from a surgical standpoint to use colloid-based fluid rather than large volumes of crystalloid solution alone. Although no controlled studies have been conducted, swelling of the pancreas graft appears to be less with colloids than with crystalloids. Administration of blood products is indicated to provide adequate oxygen-carrying capacity and sufficient platelets or clotting factors if coagulation appears to be clinically impaired and is confirmed by laboratory analysis.

Abdominal muscle relaxation is essential for these extensive intra-abdominal procedures. The same issues outlined previously for patients undergoing KTx apply to choosing muscle relaxants for patients undergoing SPK. Because of the long duration of these cases, a continuous infusion of cisatracurium can be used to allow for titration of the level of block with reliable reversibility. Alternatively, intermittent administration of vecuronium, if titrated by train-of-four monitoring,[98] can produce excellent relaxation conditions. For patients who are undergoing pancreas transplant alone or pancreas after kidney and have adequate renal function, any intermediate-acting non-depolarizing muscle relaxant may be used without problems.

Intraoperative blood glucose control is important to prevent ketoacidosis in patients with unopposed counter-regulatory hormone secretion and to assess the function of the transplanted pancreas. Before the pancreas is unclamped, glucose should be checked hourly. Hyperglycemia may cause depressed immune function and impaired wound healing and may put patients at risk for more severe neurologic injury should brain ischemia occur.[109] After the pancreas is unclamped, glucose should be monitored every 30 minutes. Typically, glucose concentrations decrease by approximately 50 mg/dL/h after the pancreas is unclamped.

A randomized trial of insulin administration to insulin-dependent type 2 diabetics compared a continuous glucose-insulin infusion with intermittent intravenous insulin injections during both major and minor surgery. Very little difference was found in the ability to control intraoperative and postoperative glucose levels and metabolism.[54] Therefore, the manner of lowering glucose does not appear to be as critical as the glucose level itself.

Postoperative Care

Successful transplantation usually results in rapidly declining insulin requirements. Blood glucose levels should be monitored closely in the recovery room or the ICU to avoid hypoglycemia. If simultaneous KTx is also performed, urine output should also be closely monitored to detect reversible graft impingement. Postoperative pain control can be managed with epidural or patient-controlled analgesia.

REFERENCES

1. Ando M, Iwata A, Ozeki Y, et al. Circulating platelet-derived microparticles with procoagulant activity may be a potential cause of thrombosis in uremic patients. Kidney Int 2002;62(5):1757–63.
2. Angst MS, Buhrer M, Lotsch J. Insidious intoxication after morphine treatment in renal failure: delayed onset of morphine-6-glucuronide action. Anesthesiology 2000;92(5):1473–6.
3. Ansari A, Kaupke CJ, Vaziri ND, et al. Cardiac pathology in patients with end-stage renal disease maintained on hemodialysis. Int J Artif Organs 1993;16(1):31–6.
4. Artru AA. Renal effects of sevoflurane during conditions of possible increased risk. J Clin Anesth 1998;10(7):531–8.
5. Bagheri N, Taziki O, Falaknazi K. C-reactive protein, cardiac troponin T and low albumin are predictors of mortality in hemodialysis patients. Saudi J Kidney Dis Transpl 2009;20(5):789–93.
6. Bittar J, Arenas P, Chiurchiu C, et al. Renal transplantation in high cardiovascular risk patients. Transplant Rev (Orlando) 2009;23(4):224–34.
7. Boden WE, O'Rourke RA, Teo KK, et al. Optimal medical therapy with or without PCI for stable coronary disease. N Engl J Med 2007;356(15):1503–16.
8. Bower S. Plasma protein binding of fentanyl: the effect of hyperlipidaemia and chronic renal failure. J Pharm Pharmacol 1982;34:102.
9. Bower S, Sear JW. Disposition of alfentanil in patients receiving a renal transplant. J Pharm Pharmacol 1989;41:654.
10. Brown JJ, Dusredieck G, Fraser R, et al. Hypertension and chronic renal failure. Br Med Bull 1971;27(2):128–35.
11. Burch PG, Stanski DR. Decreased protein binding and thiopental kinetics. Clin Pharmacol Ther 1982;32:212.
12. Carlos R, Calvo R, Erill S. Plasma protein binding of etomidate in patients with renal failure or hepatic cirrhosis. Clin Pharmacokinet 1979;4:144.
13. Carmellini M, Romagnoli J, Giulianotti PC, et al. Dopamine lowers the incidence of delayed graft function in transplanted kidney patients treated with cyclosporine A. Transplant Proc 1994;26(5):2626–9.
14. Chauvin M, Lebrault C, Levron JC, et al. Pharmacokinetics of alfentanil in chronic renal failure. Anesth Analg 1987;66:53.
15. Chauvin M, Sandouk P, Scherrmann JM, et al. Morphine pharmacokinetics in renal failure. Anesthesiology 1987;66:327.
16. Cho WH, Kim HT, Park CH, et al. Renal transplantation in advanced cardiac failure patients. Transplant Proc 1997;29(1–2):236–8.
17. Christensen JH, Andreasen F, Jansen J. Pharmacokinetics and pharmacodynamics of thiopental in patients undergoing renal transplantation. Acta Anaesthesiol Scand 1983;27:513.
18. Converse Jr. RL, Jacobsen RN, Toto RD, et al. Sympathetic overactivity in patients with chronic renal failure. N Engl J Med 1992;327(27):1912–8.
19. Conzen PF, Kharash ED, Czerner SF, et al. Low-flow sevoflurane compared with low-flow isoflurane anesthesia in patients with stable renal insufficiency. Anesthesiology 2002;97(3):578–84.
20. Conzen PF, Nuscheler M, Melotte A, et al. Renal function and serum fluoride concentrations in patients with stable renal insufficiency after anesthesia with sevoflurane or enflurane. Anesth Analg 1995;81(3):569–75.
21. Cooper RA, Maddineni VR, Mirakhur RK, et al. Time course of neuromuscular effects and pharmacokinetics of rocuronium bromide (Org 9426) during isoflurane anaesthesia in patients with and without renal failure. Br J Anaesth 1993;71:222.
22. Dahaba AA, Oettl K, von Kobucar F, et al. End-stage renal failure reduces central clearance and prolongs the elimination of half-life of remifentanil. Can J Anaesth 2002;49:369.
23. Davis PJ, Stiller RL, Cook DR, et al. Pharmacokinetics of sufentanil in adolescent patients with chronic renal failure. Anesth Analg 1988;67:268.
24. De Bros FM, Lai A, Scott R, et al. Pharmacokinetics and pharmacodynamics of atracurium during isoflurane anesthesia in normal and anephric patients. Anesth Analg 1986;65:743.
25. de Lemos JA, Hillis LD. Diagnosis and management of coronary artery disease in patients with end-stage renal disease on hemodialysis. J Am Soc Nephrol 1996;7(10):2044–54.
26. Duthie DJR. Renal failure, surgery and fentanyl pharmacokinetics. Proceedings of VII European Congress of Anaesthesiology, volume II (main topics 7-12). Beitr Anaesthesiol Intensivmed 1987;20:374.
27. Eastwood NB, Boyd AH, Parker CJH, et al. Pharmacokinetics of 1R-cis 1R-cis atracurium besylate (51W89) and plasma laudanosine concentrations in health and chronic renal failure. Br J Anaesth 1995;75:431.
28. Ebert TJ, Frink Jr. EJ, Kharasch ED. Absence of biochemical evidence for renal and hepatic dysfunction after 8 hours of 1.25 minimum alveolar concentration sevoflurane anesthesia in volunteers. Anesthesiology 1998;88(3):601–10.
29. Ebert TJ, Messana LD, Uhrich TD, et al. Absence of renal and hepatic toxicity after four hours of 1.25 minimum alveolar anesthetic concentration sevoflurane anesthesia in volunteers. Anesth Analg 1998;86(3):662–7.
30. Eger 2nd EI, Gong D, Koblin DD, et al. Dose-related biochemical markers of renal injury after sevoflurane versus desflurane anesthesia in volunteers. Anesth Analg 1997;85(5):1154–63.
31. Eger 2nd EI, Koblin DD, Bowland T, et al. Nephrotoxicity of sevoflurane versus desflurane anesthesia in volunteers. Anesth Analg 1997;84(1):160–8.

32. Eng M, Brock G, Li X, et al. Perioperative anticoagulation and antiplatelet therapy in renal transplant: is there an increase in bleeding complication? Clin Transplant 2011;25(2):292–6.
33. Eschbach JW, Kelly MR, Haley NR, et al. Treatment of the anemia of progressive renal failure with recombinant human erythropoietin. N Engl J Med 1989;321(3):158–63.
34. Fahey MR, Rupp SM, Fisher DM, et al. The pharmacokinetics and pharmacodynamics of atracurium in patients with and without renal failure. Anesthesiology 1984;61:699.
35. Foley RN, Parfrey PS, Harnett JD, et al. Clinical and echocardiographic disease in patients starting end-stage renal disease therapy. Kidney Int 1995;47(1):186–92.
36. Frink Jr EJ, Malan P, Morgan S, et al. Renal concentrating function with prolonged sevoflurane or enflurane anesthesia in volunteers. Anesthesiology 1994;80(5):1019–25.
37. Frink Jr. EJ, Malan TP, Morgan SE, et al. Sevoflurane degradation product concentrations with soda lime during prolonged anesthesia. J Clin Anesth 1994;6(3):239–42.
38. Gabriels G, August C, Grisk O, et al. Impact of renal transplantation on small vessel reactivity. Transplantation 2003;75(5):689–97.
39. Gallon LG, Leventhal JR, Kaufman DB. Pretransplant evaluation of renal transplant candidates. Semin Nephrol 2002;22(6):515–25.
40. Gaston RS, Danovitch GM, Adams PL, et al. The report of a national conference on the wait list for kidney transplantation. Am J Transplant 2003;3(7):775–85.
41. Gavras H, Oliver JA, Cannon PJ. Interrelations of renin, angiotensin II, and sodium in hypertension and renal failure. Annu Rev Med 1976;27:485–521.
42. Gill JS, Pereira BJ. Death in the first year after kidney transplantation: implications for patients on the transplant waiting list. Transplantation 2003;75(1):113–7.
43. Gill JS, Tonelli M, Mix CH, et al. The change in allograft function among long-term kidney transplant recipients. J Am Soc Nephrol 2003;14(6):1636–42.
44. Goldberg IJ. Lipoprotein metabolism in normal and uremic patients. Am J Kidney Dis 1993;21(1):87–90.
45. Goyal P, Puri GD, Pandey CK, et al. Evaluation of induction doses of propofol: comparison between endstage renal disease and normal renal function patients. Anaesth Intensive Care 2002;30(5):584–7.
46. Grayburn PA, Hillis LD. Cardiac events in patients undergoing noncardiac surgery: shifting the paradigm from noninvasive risk stratification to therapy. Ann Intern Med 2003;138(6):506–11.
47. Grundmann R, Kindler J, Meider G, et al. Dopamine treatment of human cadaver kidney graft recipients: a prospectively randomized trial. Klin Wochenschr 1982;60(4):193–7.
48. Grundy SM. Hypertriglyceridemia, insulin resistance, and the metabolic syndrome. Am J Cardiol 1999;83(9B):25F–9F.
49. Hadimioglu N, Saadawy I, Saglam T, et al. The effect of different crystalloid solutions on acid–base balance and early kidney function after kidney transplantation. Anesth Analg 2008;107(1):264–9.
50. Halpern H, Miyoshi E, Kataoka LM, et al. Anesthesia for pancreas transplantation alone or simultaneous with kidney. Transplant Proc 2004;36(10):3105–6.
51. Head-Rapson AG, Devlin JC, Parker CJ, et al. Pharmacokinetics and pharmacodynamics of the three isomers of mivacurium in health, in end-stage renal failure and in patients with impaired renal function. Br J Anaesth 1995;75:31.
52. Heffron TG, Gadowski G, Buckingham F, et al. Laser Doppler blood flow measurement as a predictor of viability of renal allografts. Curr Surg 1990;47(6):431–2.
53. Heino A, Orko R, Rosenberg PH. Anaesthesiological complications in renal transplantation: a retrospective study of 500 transplantations. Acta Anaesthesiol Scand 1986;30(7):574–80.
54. Hemmerling TM, Schmid MC, Schmidt J, et al. Comparison of a continuous glucose-insulin-potassium infusion versus intermittent bolus application of insulin on perioperative glucose control and hormone status in insulin-treated type 2 diabetics. J Clin Anesth 2001;13(4):293–300.
55. Herzog CA, Marwick TH, Pheley AM, et al. Dobutamine stress echocardiography for the detection of significant coronary artery disease in renal transplant candidates. Am J Kidney Dis 1999;33(6):1080–90.
56. Hickson LT, El-Zoghby ZM, Lorenz EC, et al. Patient survival after kidney transplantation: relationship to pretransplant cardiac troponin T levels. Am J Transplant 2009;9(6):1354–61.
57. Hoke FJ, Shlugman D, Dershwitz M, et al. Pharmacokinetics and pharmacodynamics of remifentanil in persons with renal failure compared with healthy volunteers. Anesthesiology 1997;87:533.
58. Humar A, Kerr SR, Ramcharan T, et al. Peri-operative cardiac morbidity in kidney transplant recipients: incidence and risk factors. Clin Transplant 2001;15(3):154–8.
59. Ickx B, Cockshott ID, Barvais L, et al. Propofol infusion for induction and maintenance of anaesthesia in patients with end-stage renal disease. Br J Anaesth 1998;81:854.
60. Kadieva VS, Friedman L, Margolius LP, et al. The effect of dopamine on graft function in patients undergoing renal transplantation. Anesth Analg 1993;76(2):362–5.
61. Kasiske BL, Maclean JR, Snyder JJ. Acute myocardial infarction and kidney transplantation. J Am Soc Nephrol 2006;17(3):900–7.
62. Katz J, Kountz SL, Cohn R. Anesthetic considerations for renal transplant. Anesth Analg 1967;46(5):609–13.
63. Kirvela M, Lindgren L, Seppala T, et al. The pharmacokinetics of oxycodone in uremic patients undergoing renal transplantation. J Clin Anesth 1996;8(1):13–8.
64. Kirvela M, Olkkola KT, Rosenberg PH, et al. Pharmacokinetics of propofol and haemodynamic changes during induction of anaesthesia in uraemic patients. Br J Anaesth 1992;68(2):178–82.
65. Kirvela M, Yli-Hankala A, Lindgren L. Comparison of propofol/alfentanil anaesthesia with isoflurane/N_2O/fentanyl anaesthesia for renal transplantation. Acta Anaesthesiol Scand 1994;38(7):662–6.
66. Ko CW, Chang CS, Wu MJ, et al. Gastric dysrhythmia in uremic patients on maintenance hemodialysis. Scand J Gastroenterol 1998;33(10):1047–51.
67. Koehntop DE, Rodman JH. Fentanyl pharmacokinetics in patients undergoing renal transplantation. Pharmacotherapy 1997;17:746.
68. Kogan A, Singer P, Cohen J, et al. Readmission to an intensive care unit following liver and kidney transplantation: a 50-month study. Transplant Proc 1999;31(4):1892–3.
69. Koning OH, Ploeg RJ, van Bockel JH, et al. Risk factors for delayed graft function in cadaveric kidney transplantation: a prospective study of renal function and graft survival after preservation with University of Wisconsin solution in multi-organ donors. European Multicenter Study Group. Transplantation 1997;63(11):1620–8.
70. Lee TH, Marcantonio ER, Mangione CM, et al. Derivation and prospective validation of a simple index for prediction of cardiac risk of major noncardiac surgery. Circulation 1999;100(10):1043–9.
71. Legendre C, Campistol JM, Squifflet J-P, et al. Cardiovascular risk factors of sirolimus compared with cyclosporine: early experience from two randomized trials in renal transplantation. Transplant Proc 2003;35(3 Suppl.):151S–3S.
72. Lentine KL, Hurst FP, Jindal RM, et al. Cardiovascular risk assessment among potential kidney transplant candidates: approaches and controversies. Am J Kidney Dis 2010;55(1):152–67.
73. Linke CL, Merin RG. A regional anesthetic approach for renal transplantation. Anesth Analg 1976;55(1):69–73.
74. Lundin AP, Akerman MJ, Chester RM, et al. Exercise in hemodialysis patients after treatment with recombinant human erythropoietin. Nephron 1991;58(3):315–9.
75. Lynam DP, Cronnelly R, Castagnoli KP, et al. The pharmacodynamics and pharmacokinetics of vecuronium in patients anesthetized with isoflurane with normal renal function or with renal failure. Anesthesiology 1988;69:227.
76. Marsh JT, Brown WS, Wolcott D, et al. rHuEPO treatment improves brain and cognitive function of anemic dialysis patients. Kidney Int 1991;39(1):155–63.
77. McFalls EO, Ward HB, Moritz TE, et al. Coronary-artery revascularization before elective major vascular surgery. N Engl J Med 2004;351(27):2795–804.
78. McLeod K, Watson MJ, Rawlins MD. Pharmacokinetics of pancuronium in patients with normal and impaired renal function. Br J Anaesth 1976;48:341.
79. Mistry BM, Bastani B, Solomon H, et al. Prognostic value of dipyridamole thallium-201 screening to minimize perioperative cardiac complications in diabetics undergoing kidney or kidney-pancreas transplantation. Clin Transplant 1998;12(2):130–5.

80. Morita K, Seki T, Nonomura K, et al. Changes in renal blood flow in response to sympathomimetics in the rat transplanted and denervated kidney. Int J Urol 1999;6(1):24–32.
81. Munday IT, Stoddart PA, Jones RM, et al. Serum fluoride concentration and urine osmolality after enflurane and sevoflurane anesthesia in male volunteers. Anesth Analg 1995;81(2):353–9.
82. Nishimori A, Tanaka K, Ueno K, et al. Effects of sevoflurane anaesthesia on renal function. J Int Med Res 1997;25(2):87–91.
83. Norio K, Makisalo H, Isoniemi H, et al. Are diabetic patients in danger at renal transplantation? An invasive perioperative study. Eur J Anaesthesiol 2000;17(12):729–36.
84. O'Malley CM, Frumento RJ, Bennett-Guerrero E. Intravenous fluid therapy in renal transplant recipients: results of a US survey. Transplant Proc 2002;34(8):3142–5.
85. O'Malley CM, Frumento RJ, Hardy MA, et al. A randomized, double-blind comparison of lactated Ringer's solution and 0.9% NaCl during renal transplantation. Anesth Analg 2005;100(5):1518–24, table of contents.
86. Oppert M, Schneider U, Boksch W, et al. Improvement of left ventricular function and arterial blood pressure 1 year after simultaneous pancreas kidney transplantation. Transplant Proc 2002;34(6):2251–2.
87. Osborne R, Joel S, Grebenik K, et al. The pharmacokinetics of morphine and morphine glucuronides in kidney failure. Clin Pharmacol Ther 1993;54:158.
88. Othman MM, Ismael AZ, Hammouda GE. The impact of timing of maximal crystalloid hydration on early graft function during kidney transplantation. Anesth Analg 2010;110(5):1440–6.
89. Peterson P, Hayes TE, Arkin CF, et al. The preoperative bleeding time test lacks clinical benefit: College of American Pathologists' and American Society of Clinical Pathologists' position article. Arch Surg 1998;133(2):134–9.
90. Pivalizza EG, Abramson DC, Harvey A. Perioperative hypercoagulability in uremic patients: a viscoelastic study. J Clin Anesth 1997;9(6):442–5.
91. Ponticelli C, Villa M. Role of anaemia in cardiovascular mortality and morbidity in transplant patients. Nephrol Dial Transplant 2002;17(Suppl. 1):41–6.
92. Powell DR, Miller R. The effect of repeated doses of succinylcholine on serum potassium in patients with renal failure. Anesth Analg 1975;54(6):746–8.
93. Rapoport J, Aviram M, Chaimovitz C, et al. Defective high-density lipoprotein composition in patients on chronic hemodialysis. A possible mechanism for accelerated atherosclerosis. N Engl J Med 1978;299(24):1326–9.
94. Reissell E, Orko R, Maunuksela EL, et al. Predictability of difficult laryngoscopy in patients with long-term diabetes mellitus. Anaesthesia 1990;45(12):1024–7.
95. Reissell E, Taskinen MR, Orko R, et al. Increased volume of gastric contents in diabetic patients undergoing renal transplantation: lack of effect with cisapride. Acta Anaesthesiol Scand 1992;36(7):736–40.
96. Rigatto C. Clinical epidemiology of cardiac disease in renal transplant recipients. Semin Dial 2003;16(2):106–10.
97. Robertson EN, Driessen JJ, Booij LH. Pharmacokinetics and pharmacodynamics of rocuronium in patients with and without renal failure. Eur J Anaesthesiol 2005;22(1):4–10.
98. Sakamoto H, Takita K, Kemmotsu O, et al. Increased sensitivity to vecuronium and prolonged duration of its action in patients with end-stage renal failure. J Clin Anesth 2001;13(3):193–7.
99. Sandberg J, Tyden G, Groth CG. Low-dose dopamine infusion following cadaveric renal transplantation: no effect on the incidence of ATN. Transplant Proc 1992;24(1):357.
100. Schankel K, Robinson J, Bloom R, et al. Determinants of coronary artery calcification progression in renal transplant recipients. Am J Transplant 2007;7(9):2158–64.
101. Schmidt A, Stefenelli T, Schuster E, et al. Informational contribution of noninvasive screening tests for coronary artery disease in patients on chronic renal replacement therapy. Am J Kidney Dis 2001;37(1):56–63.
102. Schoonjans R, Van B, Vandamme W, et al. Dyspepsia and gastroparesis in chronic renal failure: the role of *Helicobacter pylori*. Clin Nephrol 2002;57(3):201–7.
103. Sear JW. Kidney transplants: induction and analgesic agents. Int Anesthesiol Clin 1995;33(2):45–68.
104. Sear JW. Sufentanil disposition in patients undergoing renal transplantation: influence of choice of kinetic model. Br J Anaesth 1989;63(1):60–7.
105. Sear JW, Hand CW. Fentanyl disposition in anaesthetized patient with renal failure using an iodine-labelled RIA. Br J Anaesth 2000;84:285.
106. Sear JW, Hand CW, Moore RA, et al. Studies on morphine disposition: influence of renal failure on the kinetics of morphine and its metabolites. Br J Anaesth 1989;62:28.
107. Sear JW, Jewkes C, Tellez JC, et al. Does the choice of antihypertensive therapy influence haemodynamic responses to induction, laryngoscopy and intubation? Br J Anaesth 1994;73(3):303–8.
108. Sedlis SP, Jurkovitz CT, Hartigan PM, et al. Optimal medical therapy with or without percutaneous coronary intervention for patients with stable coronary artery disease and chronic kidney disease. Am J Cardiol 2009;104(12):1647–53.
109. Sieber FE. The neurologic implications of diabetic hyperglycemia during surgical procedures at increased risk for brain ischemia. J Clin Anesth 1997;9(4):334–40.
110. Spicer ST, Gruenewald S, O'Connell PJ, et al. Low-dose dopamine after kidney transplantation: assessment by Doppler ultrasound. Clin Transplant 1999;13(6):479–83.
111. Strid H, Simren M, Stotzer PO, et al. Delay in gastric emptying in patients with chronic renal failure. Scand J Gastroenterol 2004;39(6):516–20.
112. Szenohradszky J, Fisher DM, Segredo V, et al. Pharmacokinetics of rocuronium bromide (ORG 9426) in patients with normal renal function or patients undergoing cadaver renal transplantation. Anesthesiology 1992;77:899.
113. Thapa S, Brull SJ. Succinylcholine-induced hyperkalemia in patients with renal failure: an old question revisited. Anesth Analg 2000;91(1):237–41.
114. Toto RD. Treatment of hypertension in chronic kidney disease. Semin Nephrol 2005;25(6):435–9.
115. Tsukamoto N, Hirabayashi Y, Shimizu R, et al. The effects of sevoflurane and isoflurane anesthesia on renal tubular function in patients with moderately impaired renal function. Anesth Analg 1996;82(5):909–13.
116. Vandam LD, Harrison JH, Murray JE, et al. Anesthetic aspects of renal homotransplantation in man. With notes on the anesthetic care of the uremic patient. Anesthesiology 1962;23:783–92.
117. Vinik HR, Reves JG, Greenblatt DJ, et al. The pharmacokinetics of midazolam in chronic renal failure patients. Anesthesiology 1983;59:390.
118. Wang LW, Fahirn MA, Hayen A, et al. Cardiac testing for coronary artery disease in potential kidney transplant recipients. Cochrane Database Syst Rev 2011;12:CD008691.
119. Warner ME, Contreras MG, Warner MA, et al. Diabetes mellitus and difficult laryngoscopy in renal and pancreatic transplant patients. Anesth Analg 1998;86(3):516–9.
120. Wolfe RA, Ashby VB, Milford EL, et al. Comparison of mortality in all patients on dialysis, patients on dialysis awaiting transplantation, and recipients of a first cadaveric transplant. N Engl J Med 1999;341(23):1725–30.

CHAPTER 14

EARLY COURSE OF THE PATIENT WITH A KIDNEY TRANSPLANT

Stuart J. Knechtle • Stephen Pastan

CHAPTER OUTLINE

A successful long-term outcome for a new kidney transplant recipient depends on the early perioperative management and course after surgery. Important factors affecting long-term outcome include the occurrence of delayed graft function (DGF)[10,73]; episodes of acute rejection[10]; early surgical complications,[5] such as obstruction, urine leak, or vascular complications; and sepsis.[10] Toxicity from calcineurin inhibitors (CNIs) can lead to chronic transplant damage later in the posttransplantation course.[47] Donor and recipient factors affect long-term outcome, particularly the use of expanded criteria donors[42] or highly sensitized recipients. The early management and amelioration of risk factors in the immediate postoperative period may lessen their long-term negative impact and improve outcome.

OVERVIEW

Perioperative Management

Management of the transplant recipient begins in the immediate preoperative period. An initial assessment of the recipient includes a careful assessment of pretransplant fluid status to determine the need for dialysis and a careful physical examination to exclude potential contraindications to transplantation, such as significant cardiac disease or vascular insufficiency, which could preclude successful surgery. Knowledge of the donor status also is helpful in the early postoperative management of the transplant recipient. With an ideal donor or a living related donor, the expected outcome is an immediately functioning transplant that may preclude posttransplant dialysis. Expanded criteria donors (donor age >60 years or age 50–59 years with death due to cerebrovascular accident, history of hypertension, or creatinine level >1.5 mg/dL) have a higher likelihood of DGF, which can lead to volume overload and the need for urgent dialysis.[13] Technical considerations include the need for vascular reconstruction, which may prolong surgery and contribute to postoperative DGF. Recipient factors also affect the early postoperative course. Significant risk factors for early posttransplant dysfunction include pretransplant sensitization, obesity, younger or older age, and anatomical considerations that complicate the surgery.

In the early perioperative period, attention to fluid and electrolyte balance is crucial. Careful monitoring of urine output is essential, and any decrease in urine flow must be evaluated carefully. The Kidney Disease: Improving Global Outcomes (KDIGO) guidelines recommend measuring urine volume every 1–2 hours for at least 24 hours after transplantation and daily until graft function is stable.[33] In addition, serum creatinine should be measured at least daily for 7 days or until hospital discharge, whichever occurs sooner. Creatinine should then be measured two to three times per week for a month, and a tapering frequency of measurements in ensuing weeks.[33] A decrease in urine volume may be due to acute tubular necrosis, hypovolemia, urinary leak, ureteric obstruction or, most significantly, vascular thrombosis or acute rejection. Assessment of the patient's volume status may help eliminate hypovolemia as a cause of decreasing urine output. DGF can be ascertained further with a nuclear scan or duplex ultrasonography to assess perfusion of the graft and to exclude renal artery or vein thrombosis. Duplex ultrasonography also allows the diagnosis of a urinary complication.

Measures to decrease the likelihood of DGF often are used during the operative procedure and in the perioperative period. Maintenance of adequate blood pressure and fluid status may be accomplished with intravenous albumin[18] or crystalloid, the latter being preferable. Shorter cold ischemia or pulsatile perfusion of the donor organ also may decrease the likelihood of postoperative DGF. Some centers have used intra-arterial calcium channel blockers, such as verapamil, to improve renal blood flow.[17] It is common practice to administer mannitol (12.5 g) about 10 minutes before the kidney is reperfused, which helps to trigger an osmotic diuresis and might be protective. Oral calcium channel blockers have been used to decrease the incidence of DGF.[16] There is controversy about the early initiation of CNIs because of the potential for nephrotoxicity. Some centers delay the use of CNIs until there is established diuresis. If additional immunosuppression is desired, polyclonal or monoclonal anti-T-cell antibodies may be used.

Graft Dysfunction

Early complications of renal transplantation may be mechanical/surgical or medical. Early medical problems are more common than posttransplant surgical problems (Table 14-1). The most common early posttransplant medical problem is DGF, which occurs in 20% of patients who received kidneys from ideal deceased donors and in nearly 40% of patients in whom the donors were older than age 55 years.[11] After or concomitant with DGF, acute rejection may become a significant clinical problem.[67,73,78]

TABLE 14-1 Early Surgical and Medical Complications after Transplantation

Surgical/Mechanical	Medical
Ureteral obstruction	Acute rejection
Hematuria	Delayed graft function
Urine leak	Acute calcineurin inhibitor nephrotoxicity
Arterial thrombosis/ stenosis	Prerenal/volume contraction
Renal vein thrombosis	Drug toxicity
Postoperative hemorrhage	Infection
Lymphocele	Recurrent disease

Other reasons for early medical complications include acute cyclosporine or tacrolimus nephrotoxicity, prerenal azotemia, other drug toxicity, infection, and early recurrent disease. An uncommon but serious posttransplantation medical problem is thrombotic microangiopathy (see below). Thrombotic microangiopathy may be induced by rejection or as a secondary event from cyclosporine, tacrolimus, or sirolimus therapy.[52] CNI blood levels should be measured regularly during the immediate postoperative period until target levels are reached,[33] as this measurement may indicate the likelihood of CNI toxicity versus rejection in the diagnosis of graft dysfunction. The level of mTORi (mammalian target of rapamycin inhibitor) should also be measured regularly if this class of drugs is used.

Mechanical problems usually are the result of complications of surgery or specific donor factors, such as multiple arteries, that lead to posttransplantation dysfunction. Mechanical/surgical factors include obstruction of the transplant, hematuria, urine leak or urinoma, and vascular problems such as renal artery or vein stenosis or thrombosis. Postoperative bleeding is another potential complication that may cause compression of the transplant because the transplant usually is placed in the retroperitoneal space. Posttransplant lymphoceles are another common cause of early transplant dysfunction. Lymph drainage from transected lymphatic channels accumulates in the perivascular and periureteral space and can cause ureteral obstruction or lower-extremity swelling from iliac vein compression.

SURGICAL COMPLICATIONS

Urinary Problems

Urinary Obstruction

After implantation of a living donor kidney transplant, urine output begins immediately or within minutes. (See Chapter 29 for a more complete discussion of urinary problems.) The same is not generally true of deceased donor kidneys, in which urine output may not be apparent for 1 hour or more after implantation and may be sluggish or non-existent for days if the kidney has been injured (DGF) by donor factors or preservation. If a kidney that was formerly making urine slows down or stops and does not respond to fluid administration, urinary obstruction has to be considered in the differential diagnosis. The initial evaluation is to check the patient's vital signs and physical exam to ensure adequate hydration and to check that the Foley catheter is functioning correctly. Obstruction of the Foley catheter by blood clots may occur easily and can be cleared by gentle irrigation. If these problems are not present, renal transplant ultrasound is the fastest, most accurate, and least expensive method to assess the renal pelvis for obstruction. Pelvicaliceal dilation seen by ultrasound implies distal obstruction. If the bladder is collapsed rather than full, the problem is likely to be ureteral obstruction. Treatment should be immediate decompression of the renal transplant pelvis by percutaneous insertion of a nephrostomy tube.

Subsequently (usually 1 or 2 days later to allow blood and edema to clear after nephrostomy tube placement), a nephrogram can be obtained to evaluate the ureter for stenosis or obstruction. The diagnosis is confirmed by a decline in the serum creatinine level after decompression of the renal pelvis.

After the Foley catheter is removed, the most common cause of urinary obstruction is not ureteral stenosis, but rather bladder dysfunction. This cause is particularly common in diabetic patients with neurogenic bladders. Initial management is replacement of the Foley catheter and a trial of an alpha-blocker, such as tamsulosin, doxazosin, or terazosin. If bladder dysfunction persists after one or two such trials, it may be necessary to start intermittent self-catheterization. In rare instances in which bladder dysmotility is severe and urinary tract infections are common, it may be preferable to drain the transplant ureter into an ileal conduit to the anterior abdominal wall. Ideally, a patient with a neurogenic bladder should have been evaluated before transplantation with urodynamic studies, and a decision should have been made about management at that time (see Chapters 4 and 12).

During the first 1 or 2 weeks after transplantation, obstruction usually is due to a technical problem related to surgery (see Chapter 29). If a ureteral stent was placed at the time of surgery, it is highly unusual to have obstruction. Possible explanations for obstruction are a twisted ureter or anastomotic narrowing. Generally, obstructions appear several weeks postoperatively, after the stent has been removed, and occur most frequently at the anastomosis between ureter and bladder.[27] Usually, these obstructions can be crossed by a guidewire and dilated percutaneously by an interventional radiologist (Figure 14-1). If the nephrostogram shows a long (>2 cm) stricture, especially a proximal or midureteral stricture, it is likely that the problem is not amenable to balloon dilation and that surgical repair is necessary (Figure 14-2). The operation of choice for a long stricture or one that has failed balloon dilation is ureteroureterostomy or ureteropyelostomy using the ipsilateral native ureter. The spatulated ends of the transplant and native ureters are anastomosed using running 5-0 absorbable suture. This anastomosis can be done over a 7 F double-J stent, which is left in place for 4–6 weeks. If no ipsilateral ureter is available, it may be necessary to use the contralateral ureter. If neither the ipsilateral ureter nor the contralateral ureter is available, alternatives include bringing the bladder closer to the kidney using a psoas hitch or fashioning a Boari flap,[19] but these measures are seldom necessary. Another method is endoureterotomy[23]; experience with this method is growing.[36] Even if urinary obstruction is clinically silent (i.e., the patient is asymptomatic with a normal creatinine value), urinary obstruction manifested by dilation of the pelvis and calices on ultrasound should be treated because it ultimately leads to thinning of the renal cortex and loss of renal function. Urinary obstruction should be treated immediately to minimize damage to the transplanted kidney.

Bleeding into the Urinary System

Gross hematuria is common immediately postoperatively because of surgical manipulation of the bladder. The Leadbetter–Politano procedure for ureteroneocystostomy is associated with more hematuria compared with the extravesical approach typified by the Lich technique or the technique described by us (see Chapter 11).[35] The advantage of this technique is that it effectively prevents reflux and can be done with excellent long-term results. Occasionally, continuous bladder irrigation is necessary if gross hematuria is associated with clots, although intermittent manual irrigation usually is adequate. Obstruction of the bladder outlet by a blood clot is an emergency; vigilant nursing care is required to ensure that it does not occur. It is preferable not to distend the bladder in the immediate postoperative period to avoid disrupting the bladder sutures or causing a leak, and continuous bladder irrigation and cystoscopy ideally are avoided. Minor hematuria without clots is common in the first 1 or 2 days regardless of the surgical method of ureteroneocystostomy and does not require treatment; it resolves over time without specific treatment.

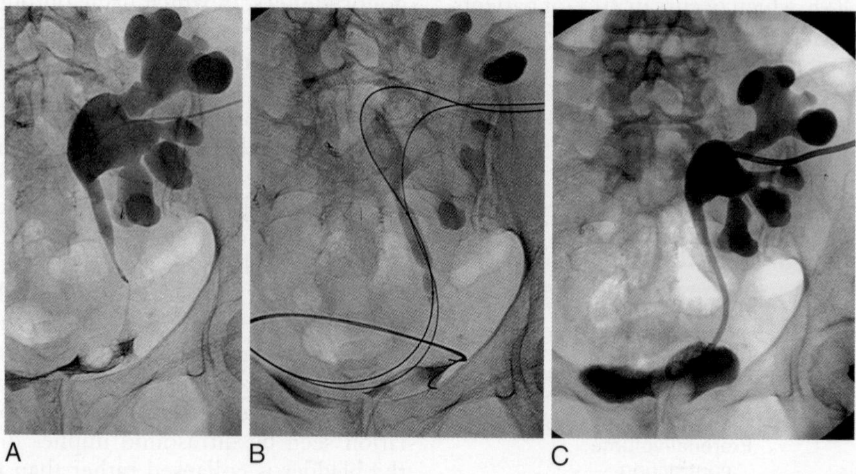

FIGURE 14-1 ■ This patient presented with an elevated creatinine level. Ultrasound showed pelvicaliceal dilation. (A) A percutaneous nephrostomy tube was placed, and the following day a nephrostogram was obtained. (B) The midureteral stenosis was crossed successfully with a guidewire, and the ureter was dilated with a balloon (the waist of the dilated balloon corresponds to the stricture). (C) Subsequently, a double-J stent was placed from the renal pelvis into the bladder across the dilated stricture.

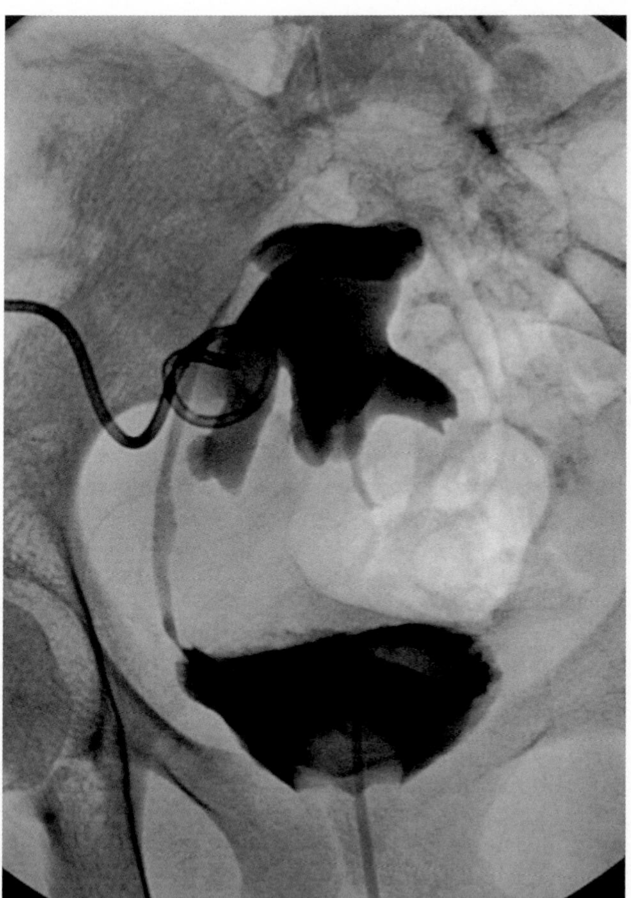

FIGURE 14-2 ■ This intra-abdominal kidney transplant was found by ultrasound to be obstructed. A nephrostomy tube was placed, and a nephrostogram was obtained the following day. The kidney had rotated medially and twisted the ureter proximally. The patient was managed operatively by placing the kidney laterally in a retroperitoneal pocket and performing ureteroureterostomy using the ipsilateral native ureter.

Urine Leak

A leak of urine from the transplanted kidney in the early postoperative period may be clinically obvious if the patient presents with abdominal pain, an increasing creatinine level, and a decrease in urine output. Urine in the peritoneal cavity causes peritonitis and pain. More commonly, assuming that the kidney was placed in the retroperitoneal position, a urinoma collects around the kidney and bladder and causes a bulge in the wound and pain with direct displacement of adjacent viscera, including the bladder. The diagnosis should be suspected if the serum creatinine level is increasing (or not decreasing appropriately). Adjunctive tests to help make the diagnosis of urine leak, if it is not obvious clinically, include a renal scan, which would show urine in the retroperitoneal space surrounding the bladder or around loops of bowel, or an ultrasound, which would show a fluid collection outside the bladder and which when aspirated has a high creatinine level. Urine leak generally is due to a surgical problem with the ureteroneocystostomy or ischemic necrosis of the distal ureter. Such a leak should be immediately repaired surgically because the risk of wound infection increases with delay in treatment.

Vascular Problems

Arterial Stenosis

Transplant renal artery stenosis may manifest in the early postoperative period by: (1) fluid retention; (2) elevated creatinine levels; and (3) hypertension.[24,77] (See Chapters 28 and 30 for a more complete discussion of vascular problems.) Commonly, the patient does not tolerate cyclosporine or tacrolimus because these drugs exacerbate the already existing ischemia at the glomerular arteriolar level. The aforementioned triad of clinical findings need not all be present, and the diagnosis should be suspected for any one of the three clinical signs. Cytomegalovirus (CMV) infection and DGF have been described as risk factors for transplant renal artery stenosis.[4] If the creatinine level is greater than 2 mg/dL, renal arteriography is best avoided because of the nephrotoxicity of the contrast dye. Magnetic resonance imaging angiography usually can give an accurate delineation of the arterial anatomy. Ultrasound also is safe, but not as discriminating, and may be helpful if jetting of flow beyond a stricture is seen.

As the population of renal transplant recipients has become older and includes more diabetic patients and patients with vascular disease, transplant renal artery pseudostenosis has become increasingly common. Pseudostenosis refers to arterial stenosis in the iliac artery proximal to the implantation of the transplant renal artery. Although the anastomosis and renal artery may be completely normal, a more proximal iliac artery stenosis can lead to hypoperfusion and resulting high renin output by the transplanted kidney.

Treatment of transplant renal artery stenosis and pseudostenosis includes balloon dilation and surgery. Generally, ostial stenosis, long areas of stenosis, and stenosis in tortuous arteries difficult to access radiographically are not treated as successfully with balloon dilation as with surgery. Stenoses within smaller branches of the renal artery may be treatable only by angioplasty. Iliac artery disease causing pseudostenosis may be treated by angioplasty, but risks embolization or dissection, leading to thrombosis or further ischemia. Surgical options include bypass of the stenosis using autologous saphenous vein, a prosthetic graft, or an allogeneic arterial graft procured from a deceased donor. The risk of the procedure has to be weighed against the potential benefit of improving renal transplant blood flow. In addition to the serum creatinine determination, a biopsy may be useful to assess the quality of the renal parenchyma. In advanced chronic rejection with a creatinine value greater than 2.5 mg/dL for more than 1 month, it may not be prudent to repair such arteries. Figure 14-3 shows a renal artery stenosis in the lower pole artery that was managed successfully by balloon angioplasty.

Arterial Thrombosis

Renal transplant arterial thrombosis usually occurs early (within 30 days) in the posttransplant period,[56] but should be a rare event because it is generally due to a technical error at the time of surgery. It usually is related to an intimal injury to the donor kidney during procurement or to anastomotic

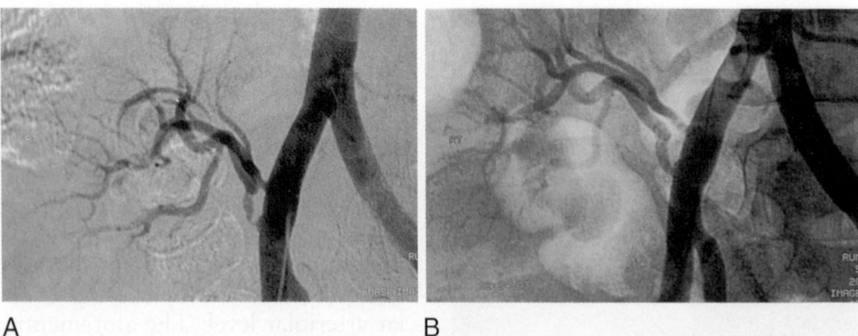

FIGURE 14-3 ■ This patient presented with fluid retention, hypertension, and an elevated creatinine level. (A) An arteriogram showed that the artery to the lower pole arising from a common aortic patch was stenotic proximally. (B) This stenosis was successfully treated with balloon angioplasty with resolution of the patient's symptoms.

narrowing or iliac artery injury during implantation. Kidneys from donors younger than 5 years old have been associated with a higher risk of thrombosis.[70] The kidney tolerates only 30–60 minutes of warm ischemia before it is irreversibly injured, making it difficult to diagnose and correct this problem before it is too late to salvage the kidney. The diagnosis should be suspected in a patient who has had a transplant hours to days before and has had a good urine output but who suddenly has a decrease in urine output. A high degree of suspicion has to be present, and the patient should be returned to the operating room promptly. If the patient had urine output preoperatively from the native kidneys, the diagnosis is difficult to make in a timely manner because urine output may continue after the renal transplant has thrombosed. The advantage of diagnostic ultrasound has to be weighed against the disadvantage of delaying a return to the operating room. Almost all kidney transplants with arterial thrombosis are lost because of ischemic injury.

In cases of more than one renal transplant artery in which arterial reconstruction is performed at implantation, there may be increased risk of thrombosis of one or more arteries. This increased risk particularly is a concern if there is a small accessory renal artery supplying the lower pole of the kidney and providing the ureteral blood supply. Thrombosis of a branch artery may manifest as an increase in serum creatinine levels associated with increased hypertension. Angiography shows partial thrombosis and loss of perfusion of a wedge-shaped section of renal parenchyma. The risk of this situation, in addition to potential long-term hypertension, is caliceal infarction and urine leak in the early postoperative period. Such kidneys, with partial infarction, generally can be salvaged. Urine leaks occurring through the outer cortex of the kidney after partial infarction may be managed by nephrostomy tube placement for urinary drainage and placement of another drain adjacent to the kidney to prevent urinoma. When the transplant ureter necroses as a result of arterial ischemia, alternative urinary drainage needs to be provided surgically; this would be managed most often by ureteropyelostomy using the ipsilateral native ureter.

Renal Vein Thrombosis

Renal vein thrombosis may occur when the donor renal vein was narrowed by repair of an injury or when the vein was twisted or compressed externally, but it may occur in the absence of a technical complication. The diagnosis is indicated by sudden onset of gross hematuria and decrease in urine output, associated with pain and swelling over the graft. Ultrasound shows absence of flow in the renal vein, diastolic reversal of flow in the renal artery (Figure 14-4), and an enlarged kidney, often with surrounding blood. Ultrasound can point to this diagnosis definitively. Only if it is immediately recognized and repaired can this problem be reversed. Immediate surgical repair of the vein and control of bleeding are required, and it is generally necessary to remove the kidney and revise the venous anastomosis. Bleeding from the swollen and cracked kidney surface usually can be controlled with hemostatic agents.

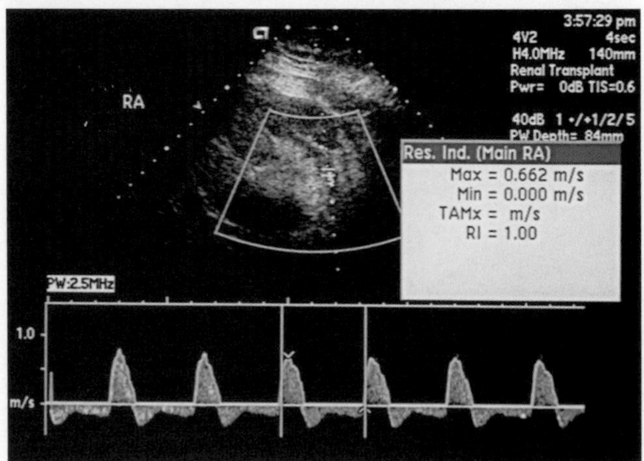

FIGURE 14-4 ■ Ultrasound shows absence of flow in the renal vein and reversal of diastolic flow in the renal artery. This kidney was enlarged to 14 cm in length with a surrounding fluid collection that represented blood. These ultrasound findings were pathognomonic of transplant renal vein thrombosis. The condition was treated surgically with excision of the kidney, placement of a venous extension graft using donor iliac vein obtained from a third-party donor, and reimplantation of the kidney. Three weeks later, the patient had a normally functioning kidney transplant.

Postoperative Bleeding

As with all surgery, postoperative bleeding may complicate renal transplant outcomes. Bleeding generally occurs during the first 24–48 hours after transplantation and is diagnosed by a decreasing hematocrit, swelling over the graft with a bulging incision, or significant blood seepage from the incision. Most often, bleeding occurs in patients taking anticoagulation agents for other medical problems. Patients treated with clopidogrel for underlying cardiac disease are at significant risk for postoperative bleeding; this class of medications should be avoided or discontinued 1 week before renal transplantation if acceptable from a cardiac perspective.[21] If the hematoma is not clinically obvious, an ultrasound or computed tomographic scan can define its size and help determine whether or not surgical evacuation is appropriate. Treatment includes immediate surgery and blood transfusions as necessary.

Graft Loss and Transplant Nephrectomy

During the early posttransplant period, if a renal transplant loses perfusion because of thrombosis or because of hyperacute, acute, or accelerated vascular rejection, it must be removed. Otherwise, the systemic toxicity of a necrotic kidney may cause fever, graft swelling or tenderness, and generalized malaise. Loss of perfusion can be assessed by nuclear scan or Doppler ultrasound. The technically easiest way to perform a transplant nephrectomy depends on how long the kidney has been in place. If nephrectomy is performed within 4 weeks, there are minimal adhesions, and the vessels are exposed easily for ligation and transplant nephrectomy. At later times, it is usually easiest to reopen the transplant incision and enter the subcapsular plane around the kidney. The kidney is dissected free in the subcapsular space, and a large vascular clamp is placed across the hilum. The kidney is amputated above the clamp, and 3-0 polypropylene (Prolene) is used to oversew the hilar vessels. The ureter also is oversewn (see Chapter 11).

REJECTION DURING THE EARLY POSTOPERATIVE PERIOD

Hyperacute Rejection

If a renal transplant is performed in the setting of ABO mismatch or a positive lymphocytotoxic crossmatch, the risk of hyperacute rejection or of antibody-mediated rejection (AMR) is increased (see Chapter 22). The incidence of hyperacute rejection is not 100%, presumably because some antibodies have lower affinity, lower density, do not bind complement, or cause accommodation.[60] It may be possible to prevent AMR by plasmapheresis to remove preformed antibodies and lower the total amount of alloantibody.[69] Cases of blood type A2 donors being transplanted to type O recipients have been reported because type A2 expresses less of the putative antigen, but this strategy also has increased risk of graft loss.[29] A crossmatch-negative, ABO-compatible recipient should be identified, or the kidney can be shipped to a center that has such a patient awaiting a kidney, potentially in exchange for a kidney to which the intended recipient has a negative crossmatch. A hyperacutely rejected kidney has no perfusion on renal scan because of microvascular thrombosis and needs to be removed.

Antibody-Mediated Rejection

Despite a negative T-cell crossmatch test preoperatively, some patients may develop an early aggressive form of rejection, termed AMR.[60] The criteria for AMR are: C4d staining of peritubular capillaries to document complement involvement; presence of donor-specific antibody in blood; histologic changes consistent with AMR, including polymorphonuclear leukocytes in peritubular capillaries, endotheliitis, and fibrin deposition.

This rejection is seen most often in sensitized patients with a high level of a panel-reactive antibody and in patients with a previous transplant. The time course of this type of rejection is typically within days to weeks of the transplant, although it may occur at any later time; it tends to be poorly responsive to steroids and occasionally resistant to all forms of antirejection therapy. Although successful prophylaxis of rejection has been described using intravenous immunoglobulin, rituximab, plasmapheresis, or thymoglobulin in highly sensitized patients,[30] when this form of rejection has started there is no standard treatment. The KDIGO guidelines recommend that such rejection be treated with one or more of the following with or without steroids: plasmapheresis, intravenous immunoglobulin, anti-CD20 antibody, or other lymphocyte-depleting antibody.[33] Randomized controlled trials are needed to determine which of these therapies (or combination of therapies) is most effective in treating AMR, and new agents are being investigated to identify more successful strategies of preventing or reversing AMR.[75]

Acute Rejection

The most common form of immunological rejection in the early posttransplant period is acute cellular rejection, mediated predominantly by host T lymphocytes responding to the allogeneic major histocompatibility complex (MHC) antigens on donor kidney. Acute rejection typically occurs 5–7 days after transplantation, but it can occur at virtually any time after this. The highest incidence of acute rejection is within the first 3 months, and overall rates of rejection vary from 5% to 40% within the first 6 months, depending on HLA matching and the immunosuppressive protocol. The clinical harbingers of acute rejection include an increasing creatinine level, weight gain, fever, and graft tenderness. With the use of cyclosporine and tacrolimus, fever and graft tenderness are seldom present. The diagnostic "gold standard" is kidney biopsy, which can be performed safely under local anesthesia. A biopsy needle is introduced under ultrasound guidance and removes a core of tissue that can be evaluated immediately for histological criteria of rejection (see Chapter 26). These criteria include tubulitis (invasion of tubules by lymphocytes), glomerulitis, and arteritis.[61] The importance of biopsy confirmation of rejection relates to the risk of increasing immunosuppression in patients whose graft dysfunction is not due to rejection but perhaps infection or other causes that might be exacerbated by increased immunosuppression.

First-line treatment of acute cellular rejection is bolus steroid therapy with methylprednisolone sodium succinate (Solu-Medrol). Many regimens are used successfully, but typical dose and duration are 10 mg/kg intravenously daily for 3 days (up to a maximum single dose of 1000 mg/day). About 85–90% of acute cellular rejection episodes are steroid-responsive. If the patient's serum creatinine level has not begun to decrease by day 4 of therapy, alternative treatment must be considered, such as antilymphocytic globulin, alemtuzumab (Campath-1H), or rituximab (anti-CD20) as lymphocytotoxic therapy. Many centers use antibody-depleting therapy first line for all severe vascular rejections (Banff 2A and 3), particularly if anti-IL-2 induction was used. Antibody-depleting therapies may be associated, however, with an increase in infectious complications when used to treat rejection compared with when used for induction.[43] Rejection that does not respond to treatment with steroids or antibody therapy occurs in less than 5% of patients, although more frequently in sensitized patients or repeat transplants with significant donor-specific antibody present.

The impact of acute cellular rejection on graft survival depends on the response to treatment, with minimal impact if treatment results in return to baseline function but negative impact with incomplete response or repeated rejection episodes.[46] Whether or not an early rejection episode predisposes the kidney to chronic rejection is controversial.

Borderline Rejection

If a protocol for kidney biopsy is interpreted as "borderline" by Banff criteria, we suggest treatment, as oral steroids may improve the outcome of subclinical rejection, but this matter awaits better evidence to substantiate.

MEDICAL COMPLICATIONS

Delayed Graft Function

DGF is defined as the need for dialysis during the first week after transplantation, and is the most frequent early posttransplant complication.[68] In the United States, the incidence of DGF has remained stable at about 25% since 1990.[8] DGF remains one of the main predictors of poor graft survival after deceased donor transplantation.[38] DGF has been estimated to decrease long-term renal allograft survival by 40%.[68]

Both donor and recipient factors contribute to the risk for DGF. The incidence of DGF is significantly higher in deceased versus living donor transplants. An analysis of 107 787 deceased donor kidney transplants reported to the United Network for Organ Sharing Scientific Renal Transplant Registry between October 1987 and 2001 showed an incidence of approximately 23% for standard criteria donors versus 34% for expanded criteria donors.[9] An increase in DGF has been noted with advancing donor age; young donors have a lower incidence of DGF (approximately 20%) compared with donors older than age 55 years (38%).[67] Prolonged cold ischemia time is a risk factor for developing DGF, but unlike other factors does not seem to have a significant effect on reducing graft survival.[32] DGF is less common in recipients receiving first deceased donor grafts than in patients undergoing repeat transplantation. Other recipient factors that increase the risk of DGF include male gender, African American race,[65] diabetes, obesity, longer waiting time on dialysis, and a mismatch in body size between the donor and the recipient.[22] It appears that the incidence of DGF can be reduced by the use of pulsatile perfusion of the procured renal allograft; however the effect of this technology on long-term graft outcomes is unclear.[41]

The diagnosis of DGF is apparent during the first 24 hours after transplantation; the most common clinical scenario is a decline in urine output unresponsive to a fluid challenge. The major differential diagnostic consideration in a patient with decreasing or absent urine output is volume depletion or an acute vascular or urological complication. Other conditions that can mimic DGF are rejection and recurrent focal segmental glomerulosclerosis (FSGS). This differential diagnosis can be evaluated with urgent ultrasound or radionuclide renal scanning. Typically, a transplant with DGF shows good renal perfusion and good parenchymal uptake of orthoiodohippurate (^{123}I-OIH) or mercaptoacetyltriglycine (^{99m}Tc-MAG3) with poor or no renal excretion. Kidney transplant biopsy is the "gold standard" for diagnosis. When the diagnosis of DGF is established, careful attention to fluid status is paramount to decrease the frequency and necessity for dialysis. The usual time course of DGF is 10–14 days.

A major concern for transplant recipients with DGF is the potential for early acute rejection. DGF may lead to activation of the immune system with release of cytokines and adhesion molecules (see Chapter 28).[26,38] This situation may result in an anti-MHC-directed alloimmune response, leading to an increased frequency of acute rejection. A recent study of pooled data reported 49% of DGF patients experienced an episode of acute rejection, compared with 35% of those without DGF.[79] This increase in rejection rate may contribute to the reported decrease in allograft survival in DGF patients.[51] The diagnosis of rejection in patients with DGF may be hindered because the primary clinical monitoring tool is a decrease in serum creatinine levels. Some centers use antilymphocyte therapy, such as thymoglobulin or alemtuzumab, to prevent early acute rejection, including acute rejection, which may occur in patients with DGF; alternatively, frequent biopsies in patients with DGF have been proposed as a way to detect early acute rejection episodes. Prevention of DGF and early recognition of rejection are important goals to help improve early and long-term graft survival.

Nephrotoxicity from Calcineurin Inhibitors

Early institution of the CNIs cyclosporine and tacrolimus at the time of transplantation is important to prevent acute rejection episodes. Because of the potential for additive nephrotoxicity, however, some centers avoid instituting CNIs until there is adequate function of the transplanted kidney. Centers that delay the onset of CNIs usually use antibody induction therapy to lower the incidence of early acute rejection.[51] Other centers, including ours, begin administering CNIs early in the posttransplant course, whether or not the allograft is functioning well or in DGF. Both of the CNIs cyclosporine and tacrolimus are effective in preventing acute rejection episodes, but they can lead to nephrotoxicity, primarily by decreasing renal blood flow in the afferent arteriole, leading to tubular injury.[40,57] Because of the variability of intestinal absorption in the early transplant period, underdosing and overdosing of these agents are common, which can lead to rejection episodes, or CNI nephrotoxicity. Although there are many clinical parameters that have been advocated to differentiate CNI nephrotoxicity from rejection, most clinical parameters are of insufficient sensitivity to predict confidently the cause of the transplant dysfunction. In patients with DGF, it may be more difficult to diagnose acute rejection or calcineurin nephrotoxicity reliably. Monitoring cyclosporine and tacrolimus levels is valuable in preventing significant increases in blood levels, which may lead to nephrotoxicity. Some centers routinely use a high-dose CNI protocol to prevent rejection and accept a certain level of nephrotoxicity as a consequence.

The most reliable way of differentiating calcineurin nephrotoxicity from rejection is percutaneous renal allograft biopsy. Generally, biopsies can be performed safely soon after transplantation, using real-time ultrasound imaging and automated biopsy needle devices. The histological hallmarks of calcineurin nephrotoxicity vary. Early functional nephrotoxicity is manifested most often by evidence of tubular injury. In patients with established calcineurin nephrotoxicity, reducing the dose or temporary discontinuation of cyclosporine or tacrolimus can lead to reversal of the renal injury. The avoidance of clinical or subclinical episodes of nephrotoxicity may be important in terms of long-term allograft histology and function.[71]

Prerenal Azotemia and Volume Depletion

Prerenal azotemia from volume depletion often may lead to deterioration of allograft function during the immediate postoperative period. Excessive use of diuretics and uncontrolled blood glucose are two common causes of prerenal azotemia from volume depletion. Because most patients are already receiving CNIs, which decrease renal blood flow, the concomitant insult of volume depletion may lead to elevated blood urea nitrogen and serum creatinine levels. It may be difficult to distinguish prerenal azotemia from an episode of acute rejection. Antihypertensive medications should be used carefully in the posttransplant period to avoid hypotension, which may further worsen renal blood flow. Meticulous attention to daily weights, intake and output, and assessment of orthostatic blood pressure changes can diagnose volume depletion as a contributing factor to renal allograft dysfunction. Volume repletion with intravenous or oral fluids is indicated.

Other Drug Toxicity

Transplant patients often have complex pharmacological regimens at the time of transplantation, which may include nephrotoxic medications or medications that may cause concomitant nephrotoxicity with CNIs.[37,74] Examples of the former include non-steroidal anti-inflammatory drugs and nephrotoxic antibiotics such as amphotericin and aminoglycosides. Tacrolimus and cyclosporine are metabolized by the cytochrome P-450-3A4 system (CYA P-450-3A4), and medications that are also metabolized by CYA P-450-3A4 may increase their blood levels. Examples of drugs that may interact with the metabolism of CNIs include non-dihydropyridine calcium channel blockers such as diltiazem and verapamil, erythromycin, ketoconazole, and fluconazole. Grapefruit juice also has been shown to increase the gastrointestinal absorption of cyclosporine (see Chapters 16 and 17).

Routine drug level monitoring is important when drugs that are metabolized by CYA P-450-3A4 are used. Adjustment of the daily dose of cyclosporine and tacrolimus to attain therapeutic blood levels helps prevent episodes of nephrotoxicity from the concomitant use of these agents. Avoidance of medications that interfere with drug metabolism is desirable. Selective serotonin reuptake inhibitor antidepressants are another class of pharmacological agents that need to be used with care. In particular, nefazodone and fluvoxamine are metabolized by CYA P-450-3A4 and may increase CNI blood levels.

Recurrent Disease

Most causes of renal failure do not recur in the transplanted kidney; when they do, it is usually later in the posttransplant course. (See Chapters 4 and 32 for further discussion of recurrent disease.) Two diseases may occur in the immediate posttransplant period and lead to significant graft dysfunction or graft loss if not treated aggressively. FSGS is the most common glomerular disease that can recur in the immediate postoperative period.[2,3] The overall recurrence rate is approximately 30–40%, with most cases recurring in the first posttransplant year[63,64]; presumably, a serum factor is present that causes glomerular injury and massive proteinuria.[63] Occasionally, FSGS may occur immediately after transplantation. The diagnosis is established by the development of nephrotic range proteinuria in a patient with a pretransplant diagnosis of FSGS, and is confirmed on biopsy. Electron microscopy shows diffuse foot process effacement, which is diagnostic in this setting. Various strategies have been used to treat recurrent FSGS, including high-dose CNIs, prednisone, and plasmapheresis. Currently, plasmapheresis seems to be the most effective treatment; however, some patients may have only a partial remission or may not respond to this modality.[3] In some cases, a course of plasmapheresis may need to be repeated if there is an initial response and subsequent relapse.

The other recurrent disease of concern in the immediate postoperative period is thrombotic microangiopathy, which can result from recurrent disease, endothelial injury from CNIs, hypercoagulable disorders, or AMR.[12] Thrombotic microangiopathy is multifactorial in origin. It is characterized clinically by a decrease in hematocrit or platelet count, or both, with evidence of a microangiopathic process on peripheral blood smear, increased lactate dehydrogenase levels, and transplant allograft dysfunction. Kidney biopsy specimens show fibrin deposition in the small arterioles of the kidney. Thrombotic microangiopathy has been noted to be induced by tacrolimus or cyclosporine. Discontinuation of the CNI and plasmapheresis have been beneficial in some series.[31] The use of anticoagulants and aspirin is of uncertain benefit. Eculizumab, an anti-C5 monoclonal antibody, has proven effective in treating renal transplant recipients with recurrent atypical hemolytic uremic syndrome related to genetic defects in complement regulatory proteins, and with thrombotic microangiopathy related to antiphospholipid antibodies.[48,82]

Infection

In the immediate postoperative period most infections are related to the surgical procedure and usually involve wound infection, bacteremia from a central line, urinary tract infection, or pneumonia.[62] (See Chapter 31 for a complete discussion of infection.) Prevention of these infections involves meticulous surgical technique, careful line care and use, removal of central lines and the Foley catheter as soon as possible, and early mobilization of the patient to prevent atelectasis or pneumonia. Most opportunistic infections do not occur until after the first 30 days. Of the opportunistic infections, CMV is still common after transplantation, particularly in recipients who are seronegative for CMV and who receive seropositive organs. Use of prophylactic oral antiviral drugs, such as valganciclovir, in patients receiving kidneys from CMV-positive patients has diminished the incidence and severity of clinical CMV infection[54]; however, after stopping valganciclovir CMV may still occur. Epstein–Barr virus infection may occur early after transplantation and usually is related to heightened immunosuppression in a previously seronegative patient. In the past, *Pneumocystis carinii* pneumonia was a frequent complication of transplantation; however, most centers now use routine prophylaxis with trimethoprim/sulfamethoxazole, which has nearly eliminated the occurrence of this infection in transplant patients. Other prophylactic agents include antifungal agents, such as fluconazole or clotrimazole troches, which can reduce the risk of mucosal *Candida* superinfection.

Highly resistant organisms have been detected with increasing frequency in transplant patients. Vancomycin-resistant *Enterococcus*[49,50,53] and *Candida* infections[45,55,59] are becoming significant causes of morbidity in hospitalized transplant patients. Risk factors for vancomycin-resistant *Enterococcus* include prolonged hospitalization in the intensive care unit, extensive surgical procedures, and intra-abdominal infection. Treatment options for this infection are limited. Quinupristin/dalfopristin (Synercid), linezolid (Zyvox), and daptomycin (Cubicin) may be useful for the control of serious vancomycin-resistant *Enterococcus* infections. The increase in *Candida* infection seems to be due to the routine use of clotrimazole or fluconazole to prevent *Candida* infection. Intravenous antibiotic use predisposes patients to fungal infection after transplantation. Infection with extended-spectrum beta-lactam-producing Gram-negative bacteria is becoming more common, particularly in the urinary tract.[39] Many of these patients require combination therapy which includes aminoglycoside antibiotics; the resulting nephrotoxicity can contribute to graft loss.

Clostridium difficile colitis is becoming an increasing problem in solid-organ transplant patients; one study found the peak incidence occurred 6–10 days posttransplant.[7] Early testing of stool for toxin, and institution of treatment with oral Flagyl should be carried out. In persistent or recurrent cases, oral vancomycin or rifaximin may be required.[72] Hands should be washed with soap and water, as alcohol-based hand scrubs may not kill the spores and prevent nosocomial transmission.

When an infection has occurred, aggressive management is indicated. This management may include removal of central venous catheters or Foley catheters. Any intra-abdominal fluid collections should be aspirated and drained if found to be infected. Urinary tract infections should be treated promptly, and the Foley catheter and ureteral stent should be removed as soon as possible.

Hypertension

Hypertension develops in nearly 80% of renal transplant recipients[14,15,25,58,81] (see Chapter 30). After kidney transplant, hypertension may be related to allograft dysfunction due to DGF or rejection, or to immunosuppressive medications. Cyclosporine, tacrolimus, and corticosteroids all may contribute to the development of hypertension. CNIs primarily cause hypertension through widespread arterial vasoconstriction, which increases systemic vascular resistance.[76] Vasoconstriction in the kidney activates the renin–angiotensin system, promotes sodium reabsorption and volume expansion, and increases endothelin release. CNIs also result in adverse changes in arachidonic acid metabolites, nitrous oxide production,[44] and sympathetic nerve activity.[34] Hypertension occurs more frequently with cyclosporine use than with tacrolimus. Corticosteroids also cause peripheral vasoconstriction, resulting in an acute rise in blood pressure[28]; further, they activate the mineralocorticoid receptor, resulting in volume expansion. Of note, up to 90% of patients are hypertensive prior to transplant[80]; pre-existing vascular calcification and arterial stiffness may persist and contribute to ongoing blood pressure elevation.[20] Transplant renal artery stenosis is a treatable cause of hypertension and should be ruled out in patients who have new-onset hypertension, or do not respond readily to antihypertensive therapy (see section above).[6,66] Because multiple causes may be present in the same patient, it often is difficult to ascertain the specific cause of hypertension after transplantation.

Patients with significant hypertension should be treated aggressively. Most centers prefer the use of calcium channel blockers and beta-blockers as first-line agents, although angiotensin-converting enzyme inhibitors or angiotensin II receptor blockers are being used more frequently. The major issues with the use of angiotensin-converting enzyme inhibitors or angiotensin II receptor blockers are anemia and hyperkalemia, which can be a particular problem in patients with decreased renal function. Table 14-2 presents the advantages and potential side effects of antihypertensive agents in transplant recipients.

TABLE 14-2 **Advantages and Potential Side Effects of Antihypertensive Agents in Transplant Recipients**

Class	Advantages/Indications	Side Effects
Diuretics	Salt-sensitive hypertension, volume expansion	Hyperuricemia Volume depletion
Beta-blockers	Large selection Selective agents preferred	Adverse effect on lipids Relative contraindication with asthma, diabetes, or peripheral vascular disease
Alpha-blockers	Useful with prostatic hypertrophy	Postural hypotension (first dose)
Central alpha-agonists	Clonidine useful in diabetic patients Clonidine available as transdermal patch	Dry mouth Rebound hypertension Fatigue
Calcium channel blockers	Improve renal blood flow May ameliorate cyclosporine nephrotoxicity (verapamil and diltiazem)	Drug interaction with CNI
ACE inhibitors and ARBs	Proteinuria	May cause renal insufficiency Hyperkalemia Anemia

ACE, angiotensin-converting enzyme; ARB, angiotensin II receptor blocker; CNI, calcineurin inhibitor.

Management of Graft Dysfunction

The diagnosis and treatment of graft dysfunction are integral components of the successful long-term management of the renal transplant recipient. Early diagnosis and directed therapy are crucial in the early posttransplant period to initiate appropriate therapy and avoid potential overimmunosuppression. Evaluation of graft dysfunction should start with a careful history to see if there is a potential for nephrotoxicity from drugs or if there is any likelihood of volume contraction contributing to the elevation of serum creatinine levels. A vigorous search for potential infection should follow, and if there is no obvious cause for deterioration in graft function, an ultrasound followed by a renal biopsy should be performed. If there is any clinical suspicion of renal artery or iliac artery stenosis, a magnetic resonance angiogram or arteriogram should be performed. We agree with the KDIGO indications for a kidney transplant biopsy, which are a persistently unexplained elevation in the serum creatinine, new-onset or unexplained proteinuria, and the failure of the serum creatinine to return to baseline values following treatment of acute rejection.[33] The KDIGO guidelines also recommend a kidney allograft biopsy every 7–10 days during DGF to evaluate for evidence of acute rejection. A percutaneous biopsy is often required to differentiate between CNI toxicity and rejection. Nephrotic-range proteinuria in a patient whose original disease was FSGS or thrombotic microangiopathy should prompt an immediate biopsy for diagnosis and potential treatment with plasmapheresis.

SUMMARY

Optimization of outcomes after renal transplantation depends on the rapid diagnosis and treatment of surgical and medical complications. In view of the invasiveness of the transplant procedure itself, the complexity of medical problems in this patient population, and the side effects of non-specific immunosuppressive therapy, close attention to the problems outlined in this chapter is crucial to avoid graft loss and patient death. Because the frequency of complications is greatest during the early posttransplant period, this is the time when vigilance should be highest.

REFERENCES

1. Almond PS, Matas A, Gillingham K, et al. Risk factors for chronic rejection in renal allograft recipients. Transplantation 1993;55(4):752–6, discussion 6–7.
2. Artero M, Biava C, Amend W, et al. Recurrent focal glomerulosclerosis: natural history and response to therapy. Am J Med 1992;92(4):375–83.
3. Artero ML, Sharma R, Savin VJ, et al. Plasmapheresis reduces proteinuria and serum capacity to injure glomeruli in patients with recurrent focal glomerulosclerosis. Am J Kidney Dis 1994;23(4):574–81.
4. Audard V, Matignon M, Hemery F, et al. Risk factors and long-term outcome of transplant renal artery stenosis in adult recipients after treatment by percutaneous transluminal angioplasty. Am J Transplant 2006;6(1):95–9.
5. Aultman DF, Sawaya DE, Zibari GB, et al. Are all successful renal transplants really successful? Am J Kidney Dis 1999;34(1):61–4.
6. Becker BN, Odorico JS, Becker YT, et al. Peripheral vascular disease and renal transplant artery stenosis: a reappraisal of transplant renovascular disease. Clin Transplant 1999;13(4):349–55.
7. Boutros M, Al-Shaibi M, Chan G, et al. *Clostridium difficile* colitis: increasing incidence, risk factors, and outcomes in solid organ transplant recipients. Transplantation 2012;93(10):1051–7.
8. Cecka JM. Kidney transplantation in the United States. Clin Transpl 2008;1–18.
9. Cecka JM. The UNOS renal transplant registry. In: Cecka JM, Terasaki PI, editors. Clinical transplants 2002. Los Angeles: UCLA Immunogenetics Center; 2003. p. 1–20.
10. Cecka JM. The UNOS scientific renal transplant registry – ten years of kidney transplants. Clin Transpl 1997;1–14.
11. Cecka JM. The UNOS scientific renal transplant registry. In: Cecka JM, Terasaki PI, editors. Clinical transplants 1998. Los Angeles: UCLA Tissue Typing Laboratory; 1999. p. 1–16.
12. Chiurchiu C, Ruggenenti P, Remuzzi G. Thrombotic microangiopathy in renal transplantation. Ann Transplant 2002;7(1):28–33.
13. Cho YW. Expanded criteria donors. In: Cecka JM, Terasaki PI, editors. Clinical transplants 1998. Los Angeles: Los Angeles Tissue Typing Lab; 1999. p. 421–36.
14. Curtis JJ. Hypertension following kidney transplantation. Am J Kidney Dis 1994;23(3):471–5.
15. Curtis JJ. Management of hypertension after transplantation. Kidney Int Suppl 1993;43:S45–9.

16. Dawidson I, Rooth P, Alway C, et al. Verapamil prevents posttransplant delayed function and cyclosporine A nephrotoxicity. Transplant Proc 1990;22(4):1379–80.
17. Dawidson I, Rooth P, Fry WR, et al. Prevention of acute cyclosporine-induced renal blood flow inhibition and improved immunosuppression with verapamil. Transplantation 1989;48(4):575–80.
18. Dawidson IJ, Sandor ZF, Coorpender L, et al. Intraoperative albumin administration affects the outcome of cadaver renal transplantation. Transplantation 1992;53(4):774–82.
19. del Pizzo JJ, Jacobs SC, Bartlett ST, et al. The use of bladder for total transplant ureteral reconstruction. J Urol 1998;159(3):750–2, discussion 2–3.
20. Delahousse M, Chaignon M, Mesnard L, et al. Aortic stiffness of kidney transplant recipients correlates with donor age. J Am Soc Nephrol 2008;19(4):798–805.
21. Dempsey CM, Lim MS, Stacey SG. A prospective audit of blood loss and blood transfusion in patients undergoing coronary artery bypass grafting after clopidogrel and aspirin therapy. Crit Care Resus 2004;6(4):248–52.
22. Doshi MD, Garg N, Reese PP, et al. Recipient risk factors associated with delayed graft function: a paired kidney analysis. Transplantation 2011;91(6):666–71.
23. Erturk E, Burzon DT, Waldman D. Treatment of transplant ureteral stenosis with endoureterotomy. J Urol 1999;161(2):412–4.
24. Fervenza FC, Lafayette RA, Alfrey EJ, et al. Renal artery stenosis in kidney transplants. Am J Kidney Dis 1998;31(1):142–8.
25. First MR, Neylan JF, Rocher LL, et al. Hypertension after renal transplantation. J Am Soc Nephrol 1994;4(Suppl. 8):S30–6.
26. Fuggle SV, Koo DD. Cell adhesion molecules in clinical renal transplantation. Transplantation 1998;65(6):763–9.
27. Ghasemian SM, Guleria AS, Khawand NY, et al. Diagnosis and management of the urologic complications of renal transplantation. Clin Transplant 1996;10(2):218–23.
28. Goodwin JE, Zhang J, Geller DS. A critical role for vascular smooth muscle in acute glucocorticoid-induced hypertension. J Am Soc Nephrol 2008;19(7):1291–9.
29. Hanto DW, Brunt EM, Goss JA, et al. Accelerated acute rejection of an A2 renal allograft in an O recipient: association with an increase in anti-A2 antibodies. Transplantation 1993;56(6):1580–3.
30. Jordan SC, Vo AA, Tyan D, et al. Current approaches to treatment of antibody-mediated rejection. Pediatr Transplant 2005;9(3):408–15.
31. Kaplan AA. Therapeutic apheresis for renal disorders. Ther Apher 1999;3(1):25–30.
32. Kayler LK, Srinivas TR, Schold JD. Influence of CIT-induced DGF on kidney transplant outcomes. Am J Transplant 2011;11(12):2657–64.
33. KDIGO clinical practice guideline for the care of kidney transplant recipients. Am J Transplant 2009;9(Suppl. 3):S1–155.
34. Klein IH, Abrahams AC, van Ede T, et al. Differential effects of acute and sustained cyclosporine and tacrolimus on sympathetic nerve activity. J Hypertens 2010;28(9):1928–34.
35. Knechtle SJ. Ureteroneocystostomy for renal transplantation. J Am Coll Surg 1999;188(6):707–9.
36. Kristo B, Phelan MW, Gritsch HA, et al. Treatment of renal transplant ureterovesical anastomotic strictures using antegrade balloon dilation with or without holmium:YAG laser endoureterotomy. Urology 2003;62(5):831–4.
37. Lake KD, Canafax DM. Important interactions of drugs with immunosuppressive agents used in transplant recipients. J Antimicrob Chemother 1995;36(Suppl. B):11–22.
38. Land W. Postischemic reperfusion injury and kidney transplantation. Prologue. Transplant Proc 1998;30(8):4210–3.
39. Linares L, Cervera C, Cofan F, et al. Risk factors for infection with extended-spectrum and AmpC beta-lactamase-producing Gram-negative rods in renal transplantation. Am J Transplant 2008;8(5):1000–5.
40. Mason J. Renal side-effects of cyclosporine. Transplant Proc 1990;22(3):1280–3.
41. Matsuoka L, Almeda JL, Mateo R. Pulsatile perfusion of kidney allografts. Curr Opin Organ Transplant 2009;14(4):365–9.
42. Metzger RA, Delmonico FL, Feng S, et al. Expanded criteria donors for kidney transplantation. Am J Transplant 2003;3(Suppl. 4): 114–25.
43. Morris PJ, Russell NK. Alemtuzumab (Campath-1H): a systematic review in organ transplantation. Transplantation 2006;81(10):1361–7.
44. Naesens M, Kuypers DR, Sarwal M. Calcineurin inhibitor nephrotoxicity. Clin J Am Soc Nephrol 2009;4(2):481–508.
45. Nampoory MR, Khan ZU, Johny KV, et al. Invasive fungal infections in renal transplant recipients. J Infect 1996;33(2):95–101.
46. Nankivell BJ, Alexander SI. Rejection of the kidney allograft. N Engl J Med 2010;363(15):1451–62.
47. Nankivell BJ, Borrows RJ, Fung CL, et al. The natural history of chronic allograft nephropathy. N Engl J Med 2003;349(24):2326–33.
48. Nester C, Stewart Z, Myers D, et al. Pre-emptive eculizumab and plasmapheresis for renal transplant in atypical hemolytic uremic syndrome. Clin J Am Soc Nephrol 2011;6(6):1488–94.
49. Newell KA, Millis JM, Arnow PM, et al. Incidence and outcome of infection by vancomycin-resistant *Enterococcus* following orthotopic liver transplantation. Transplantation 1998;65(3):439–42.
50. Orloff SL, Busch AM, Olyaei AJ, et al. Vancomycin-resistant *Enterococcus* in liver transplant patients. Am J Surg 1999;177(5):418–22.
51. Ortiz J, Parsikia A, Mumtaz K, et al. Early allograft biopsies performed during delayed graft function may not be necessary under thymoglobulin induction. Exp Clin Transplant 2012;10(3):232–8.
52. Oyen O, Strom EH, Midtvedt K, et al. Calcineurin inhibitor-free immunosuppression in renal allograft recipients with thrombotic microangiopathy/hemolytic uremic syndrome. Am J Transplant 2006;6(2):412–8.
53. Papanicolaou GA, Meyers BR, Meyers J, et al. Nosocomial infections with vancomycin-resistant *Enterococcus faecium* in liver transplant recipients: risk factors for acquisition and mortality. Clin Infect Dis 1996;23(4):760–6.
54. Paya C, Humar A, Dominguez E, et al. Efficacy and safety of valganciclovir vs. oral ganciclovir for prevention of cytomegalovirus disease in solid organ transplant recipients. Am J Transplant 2004;4(4):611–20.
55. Paya CV. Fungal infections in solid-organ transplantation. Clin Infect Dis 1993;16(5):677–88.
56. Penny MJ, Nankivell BJ, Disney AP, et al. Renal graft thrombosis. A survey of 134 consecutive cases. Transplantation 1994;58(5):565–9.
57. Perico N, Ruggenenti P, Gaspari F, et al. Daily renal hypoperfusion induced by cyclosporine in patients with renal transplantation. Transplantation 1992;54(1):56–60.
58. Pirsch JD, Friedman R. Primary care of the renal transplant patient. J Gen Intern Med 1994;9(1):29–37.
59. Pirsch JD, Odorico JS, D'Alessandro AM, et al. Posttransplant infection in enteric versus bladder-drained simultaneous pancreas-kidney transplant recipients. Transplantation 1998; 66(12):1746–50.
60. Racusen LC, Haas M. Antibody-mediated rejection in renal allografts: lessons from pathology. Clin J Am Soc Nephrol 2006;1(3):415–20.
61. Racusen LC, Solez K, Colvin RB, et al. The Banff 97 working classification of renal allograft pathology. Kidney Int 1999;55(2):713–23.
62. Rubin RH. Infectious diseases in transplantation/pre- and post-transplantation. In: Norman DJ, Suki WN, editors. Primer on transplantation. Thorofare, NJ: American Society of Transplant Physicians; 1998. p. 141–52.
63. Savin VJ, Sharma R, Sharma M, et al. Circulating factor associated with increased glomerular permeability to albumin in recurrent focal segmental glomerulosclerosis. N Engl J Med 1996;334(14):878–83.
64. Schachter ME, Monahan M, Radhakrishnan J, et al. Recurrent focal segmental glomerulosclerosis in the renal allograft: single center experience in the era of modern immunosuppression. Clin Nephrol 2010;74(3):173–81.
65. Schold JD, Srinivas TR, Braun WE, et al. The relative risk of overall graft loss and acute rejection among African American renal transplant recipients is attenuated with advancing age. Clin Transplant 2011;25(5):721–30.
66. Shames BD, Odorico JS, D'Alessandro AM, et al. Surgical repair of transplant renal artery stenosis with preserved cadaveric iliac artery grafts. Ann Surg 2003;237(1):116–22.

67. Shoskes DA, Cecka JM. Effect of delayed graft function on short- and long-term kidney graft survival. In: Cecka JM, Terasaki PI, editors. Clinical transplants 1997. Los Angeles: UCLA Tissue Typing Lab; 1998. p. 297.
68. Siedlecki A, Irish W, Brennan DC. Delayed graft function in the kidney transplant. Am J Transplant 2011;11(11):2279–96.
69. Singh N, Pirsch J, Samaniego M. Antibody-mediated rejection: treatment alternatives and outcomes. Transplant Rev (Orlando) 2009;23(1):34–46.
70. Singh A, Stablein D, Tejani A. Risk factors for vascular thrombosis in pediatric renal transplantation: a special report of the North American Pediatric Renal Transplant Cooperative Study. Transplantation 1997;63(9):1263–7.
71. Solez K, Vincenti F, Filo RS. Histopathologic findings from 2-year protocol biopsies from a U.S. multicenter kidney transplant trial comparing tacrolimus versus cyclosporine: a report of the FK506 Kidney Transplant Study Group. Transplantation 1998;66(12):1736–40.
72. Surawicz CM, Alexander J. Treatment of refractory and recurrent *Clostridium difficile* infection. Nat Rev Gastroenterol Hepatol 2011;8(6):330–9.
73. Troppmann C, Gillingham KJ, Benedetti E, et al. Delayed graft function, acute rejection, and outcome after cadaver renal transplantation. The multivariate analysis. Transplantation 1995;59(7):962–8.
74. Trotter JF. Drugs that interact with immunosuppressive agents. Semin Gastrointest Dis 1998;9(3):147–53.
75. Turgeon NA, Kirk AD, Iwakoshi NN. Differential effects of donor-specific alloantibody. Transplant Rev (Orlando) 2009;23(1):25–33.
76. Wadei HM, Textor SC. Hypertension in the kidney transplant recipient. Transplant Rev (Orlando) 2010;24(3):105–20.
77. Wong W, Fynn SP, Higgins RM, et al. Transplant renal artery stenosis in 77 patients – does it have an immunological cause? Transplantation 1996;61(2):215–9.
78. Woo YM, Jardine AG, Clark AF, et al. Early graft function and patient survival following cadaveric renal transplantation. Kidney Int 1999;55(2):692–9.
79. Yarlagadda SG, Coca SG, Formica Jr RN, et al. Association between delayed graft function and allograft and patient survival: a systematic review and meta-analysis. Nephrol Dial Transplant 2009;24(3):1039–47.
80. Young JB, Neumayer HH, Gordon RD. Pretransplant cardiovascular evaluation and posttransplant cardiovascular risk. Kidney Int Suppl 2010;118:S1–7.
81. Zeier M, Mandelbaum A, Ritz E. Hypertension in the transplanted patient. Nephron 1998;80(3):257–68.
82. Zuber J, Le Quintrec M, Sberro-Soussan R, et al. New insights into postrenal transplant hemolytic uremic syndrome. Nat Rev Nephrol 2011;7(1):23–35.

CHAPTER 15

AZATHIOPRINE

Sir Peter J. Morris

CHAPTER OUTLINE

INTRODUCTION

Azathioprine and steroids were the backbone of immunosuppression in renal transplantation for many years and the only form of immunosuppression from the early 1960s to the early 1980s, when cyclosporine first became available. After the introduction of cyclosporine, azathioprine and steroids were used in combination with cyclosporine or often after cessation of cyclosporine in so-called conversion protocols (see Chapter 17). One might wonder whether in the seventh edition of this book there still needs to be chapters on azathioprine and steroids, bearing in mind the introduction of mycophenolate mofetil (MMF) and sirolimus, both of which are antiproliferative agents but with different mechanisms of action. Certainly mycophenolate has largely replaced azathioprine in developed countries as a standard therapy with a calcineurin inhibitor and steroids (see Chapters 17–19). Nevertheless, the superiority of MMF compared with azathioprine is modest, to say the least. Azathioprine is an inexpensive agent, and it will continue to have a role in transplantation not only in the western world in combination with calcineurin inhibitors but also, in particular, in developing countries where the cost of immunosuppression is a major factor in determining immunosuppressive protocols.

Although steroids will continue to have a place in the prevention and treatment of rejection, the introduction of more powerful immunosuppressive agents is allowing steroid-sparing protocols to be developed. As outlined in the following chapter, the complications of steroids are considerable, and a major aim of current immunosuppressive protocols and trials is to diminish the use of steroids or indeed to avoid their use altogether.

6-Mercaptopurine was developed by Elion and Hitchings at Burroughs Wellcome as an anticancer agent in the 1950s.[6,7] Subsequently, 6-mercaptopurine was shown to be an immunosuppressive agent by Schwartz and Dameshek[29,30]; it suppressed the humoral response to a foreign protein and prolonged the survival of skin allografts in rabbits. The key paper by Schwartz and Dameshek on drug-induced immunological tolerance was noted by Calne in the United Kingdom and Hume in the United States, and independently these investigators showed that 6-mercaptopurine could delay or prevent rejection of renal allografts in dogs. In the original paper of Calne,[3] only two dogs survived the renal transplant operation for a short time, but when the dogs died from pneumonia at a little more than a month post transplantation, there was no histological evidence of rejection whatsoever, which was a unique finding at that time. Similar results in a much larger series of dog renal transplants in Hume's unit in Richmond, Virginia, were published at the same time.[36] Soon after that, Elion et al.[8,9] produced azathioprine, an imidazolyl derivative of 6-mercaptopurine, and this drug appeared to be somewhat less toxic than 6-mercaptopurine.[4] Azathioprine was first used in the clinic at the Peter Bent Brigham Hospital, Boston, in 1961.[21,22] Soon thereafter, azathioprine was introduced into renal transplantation in a rapidly increasing number of renal transplant units throughout the world.

Steroids first were used to treat rejection in patients on azathioprine[13] but then were added to azathioprine by Starzl to prevent rejection from the time of transplantation because rejection seemed inevitable.[33] From the beginning of this so-called azathioprine era, arbitrarily large doses of steroids were given from the time of transplantation, with a gradual reduction over 6–12 months to maintenance levels. The high doses of steroids used with azathioprine were responsible for most of the morbidity of transplantation (discussed in the next chapter). It was not until the 1970s that a series of randomized trials as well as observational studies led slowly to the realization that low-dose steroids were as effective as high-dose steroids in preventing rejection and that there was a major reduction in steroid complications of transplantation with low-dose regimens (see Chapter 16). By the late 1970s, azathioprine and low-dose steroids, sometimes used together with an antilymphocyte serum or globulin for induction (particularly in North America), were the standard immunosuppressive therapy until the introduction of cyclosporine in the early 1980s.

MECHANISM OF ACTION

Azathioprine and 6-mercaptopurine are thiopurines, and azathioprine is an imidazolyl derivative of 6-mercaptopurine. Azathioprine is metabolized in the liver before becoming active. One metabolic pathway is through its conversion to 6-mercaptopurine, the active metabolite of 6-mercaptopurine being 6-thioinosinic acid. Azathioprine also is metabolized by other pathways independently of 6-mercaptopurine. Azathioprine inhibits DNA and RNA synthesis by preventing interconversion among the precursors of purine synthesis and suppressing de novo purine synthesis. Azathioprine and 6-mercaptopurine block lymphocyte proliferation in vitro and the production of interleukin-2 (IL-2), which is probably an important aspect of its antiproliferative activity.[2] Xanthine oxidase has an important role in the catabolism of 6-mercaptopurine, and if allopurinol is used with azathioprine, it is mandatory to reduce the dosage of azathioprine significantly because the allopurinol inhibits the xanthine oxidase pathway.[9] This inhibition increases not only the immunosuppressive potency, but also the major side effect of azathioprine – marrow depression. Although the metabolites are excreted in the urine, these are inactive, and no reduction in dosage is required in the presence of a non-functioning kidney.[1] However, polymorphisms in the thiopurine *S*-methyltranferase enzyme which catalyses the *S*-methylation of 6-mercaptopurine and azathioprine may be associated with an increased likelihood of myelotoxicity and leukopenia.[10,16]

DOSAGE

Azathioprine is given as a single daily dose; if used with steroids alone, a suitable dose is 2.5 mg/kg/day. Careful monitoring of the leukocyte count is required, particularly in the early weeks post transplantation, when the dosage is reduced only in the presence of leukopenia. Although the dose of azathioprine may be reduced somewhat with time, a maintenance dose of azathioprine, particularly in the presence of low-dose steroids, should not be lower than 2 mg/kg/day. An important multicenter randomized trial was carried out in Australia to test low-dose versus high-dose steroids used with azathioprine after transplantation. The trial failed to show that low-dose steroids were as effective as high-dose steroids (in contrast to earlier but smaller trials), until it was realized that the poorer outcome with low-dose steroids was confined to units using low-dose azathioprine (i.e., <2 mg/kg/day).[5] A more recent analysis of data from the Collaborative Transplant Study also suggested that long-term graft survival was related to the dose of azathioprine that patients were receiving for maintenance. Patients on azathioprine and steroids only, who were receiving greater than 1.5 mg/kg, had better graft survival than those receiving a lower maintenance dose of azathioprine.[23]

When azathioprine is used with cyclosporine and steroids (triple therapy), lower doses are given. A fairly standard dose of azathioprine in a triple-therapy protocol is 1.5 mg/kg, or 100 mg/day. At this level, hematological toxicity is uncommon except in the presence of cytomegalovirus infection. There is some evidence in experimental models that azathioprine and cyclosporine are synergistic in terms of immunosuppression,[32] but there is no evidence of this in clinical studies.

Of interest is a 12-year follow-up report of a randomized trial where low-risk patients received either azathioprine and steroids or cyclosporine, azathioprine, and steroids. All patients received antilymphocyte globulin induction. Patient and graft survival were the same at 12 years, as was the incidence of rejection, but renal function was better in the arm not given cyclosporine.[14]

SIDE EFFECTS

The major complication of azathioprine therapy is bone marrow aplasia, most commonly evident as leukopenia, although in cases of more severe marrow depression, anemia and thrombocytopenia may be present. Regular monitoring of the leukocyte count is an important aspect of azathioprine therapy, and if the leukocyte count decreases to less than 3×10^9/L, the azathioprine dose should be reduced. Megaloblastic anemia has been described in association with the use of azathioprine.[17] As already mentioned, if allopurinol is required for the prevention of gout, the azathioprine dose should be reduced to 25% of the previous dose.

Hepatotoxicity has been attributed to azathioprine for many years, and although undoubtedly azathioprine is associated with hepatic dysfunction, this is probably rare (see Chapter 32). Other causes of hepatic dysfunction in the presence of azathioprine need to be sought energetically before attributing this to azathioprine. Hair loss is a common side effect of azathioprine when used in therapeutic doses. Early observations of an increased incidence of squamous cell cancer in transplant patients were attributed to azathioprine. There does not seem to be any evidence, however, that squamous cell cancers have a greater incidence in patients treated with azathioprine and steroids compared with patients treated with other immunosuppressive protocols such as cyclosporine and steroids. The major factor in the increased incidence of squamous cell cancer in immunosuppressed patients is due to the overall immunosuppressive load rather than any specific drug activity (see Chapters 34 and 36).

MONITORING OF AZATHIOPRINE THERAPY

Blood levels of azathioprine or its metabolites are not routinely monitored in clinical practice. As already suggested, the leukocyte count is monitored and the dose adjusted should leukopenia arise. It has been noted, however, that the development of leukopenia can also result from viral infection, leading to the suggestion that erythrocyte 6-thioguanine nucleotide levels may be a better indicator of azathioprine activity in transplant patients.[28]

A number of genetic variations in the thiopurine methyltransferase (TMPT) gene have been identified, which have been related to azathioprine-induced myelotoxicity.[10,16] Genotyping for this polymorphism prior to commencing azathioprine might allow the appropriate azathioprine dose for an individual to be determined.[27]

AZATHIOPRINE AND MYCOPHENOLATE MOFETIL

Three classical randomized controlled trials comparing azathioprine or placebo with two doses of MMF in a triple-therapy protocol with cyclosporine (Sandimmune) and steroids were carried out in the early 1990s (see Chapter 28). These three trials showed a significant reduction in the incidence of acute rejection, although patient and graft survival were not different at 1 year. Gradually this led to the replacement of azathioprine with MMF in most modern immunosuppressive protocols. However in recent years there has been some doubt cast on the superior efficacy of MMF over azathioprine, especially in the era of microemulsion formulations of cyclosporine and the newer calcineurin inhibitor, tacrolimus. For example, Remuzzi and colleagues carried out a trial comparing azathioprine with MMF but in which Neoral was used instead of Sandimmune, together with steroids.[26] They found no difference in rejection rates or in graft survival. This was attributed to the superior absorption of the Neoral formulation in comparison to Sandimmune. They also pointed out that the cost of MMF was some 15 times more than azathioprine. Another cohort study from UK Transplant compared the long-term outcome of deceased donor kidneys where one kidney went to a recipient who received azathioprine while the paired kidney went to a patient given MMF.[31] In this paired-kidney analysis there was no difference in patient or graft survival but increased rejection rates were noted in the MMF group. Another small trial compared MMF with azathioprine in combination with tacrolimus and steroids, and again found no difference in outcome.[20]

On the other hand a large randomized trial comparing tacrolimus, MMF, and steroids with tacrolimus, azathioprine, and steroids or cyclosporine (Neoral), MMF, and steroids showed that at 3 years all three regimens were safe and efficacious but the best overall results were with the tacrolimus–MMF–steroid combination.[12] An analysis of 49666 primary renal allograft recipients reported to the US Renal Data System suggested that continued therapy with MMF was associated with a protective effect against declining renal function at 1 year in comparison to azathioprine.[19] In contrast, data from the Collaborative Transplant Study registry show no improvement in graft survival at 5 years when mycophenolic acid is used with tacrolimus or cyclosporine.[24]

More recently, Knight and colleagues have carried out a systematic study of MMF versus azathioprine.[15] They identified 19 relevant randomized controlled trials which included a total of over 3000 patients. The significant results were, firstly, that MMF significantly reduced the risk of acute rejection when used in combination with any of the calcineurin inhibitors (Figure 15-1). However, there was a barely significant reduction in graft loss and no difference in patient survival or renal transplant function (Figure 15-2). Adverse events did not occur more commonly with either agent, other than diarrhea, which was far more common in patients receiving MMF. Thus there was a clinical benefit in terms of reduction of acute rejection whichever calcineurin inhibitor was used and there was a possible reduction in graft loss. When the cost of mycophenolate compared to azathioprine is taken into account, the benefits of MMF over azathioprine are relatively modest, if indeed they exist at all.

Study/subcategory	MMF (n/N)	AZA (n/N)	RR [95% CI]
1. CsA SIM			
Sollinger 1995	70/333	67/166	0.52 [0.39,0.69]
Keown 1996	66/337	60/166	0.54 [0.40,0.73]
Subgroup total	**670**	**332**	**0.53 [0.43,0.65]**
2. CsA ME			
Egfjord 1999	8/25	11/25	0.73 [0.353,1.50]
Suhail 2000	2/20	7/20	0.29 [0.067,1.21]
Miladipour 2002	4/40	10/40	0.40 [0.137,1.17]
Sadek 2002	27/162	43/157	0.61 [0.397,0.93]
Tuncer 2002	7/38	13/38	0.54 [0.242,1.20]
Remuzzi 2004	57/124	65/124	0.88 [0.680,1.13]
Merville 2004	5/37	7/34	0.66 [0.230,1.87]
Joh 2005	10/34	9/34	1.11 [0.517,2.39]
Weimer 2006	5/31	9/25	0.45 [0.172,1.17]
Subgroup total	**511**	**497**	**0.7 [0.58,0.85]**
3. Tacrolimus			
Mendez 1998	24/117	19/59	0.64 [0.38,1.07]
Johnson 2000	12/72	16/76	0.79 [0.40,1.56]
Wlodarczyk 2002	46/243	70/246	0.67 [0.48,0.92]
Subgroup total	**432**	**381**	**0.68 [0.52,0.87]**
4. CsA (unknown)			
Army Hospital Dehli 2002	1/17	3/16	0.31 [0.036,2.7]
Baltar 2002	1/14	5/12	0.17 [0.023,1.3]
Sun 2002	2/40	6/46	0.38 [0.082,1.8]
Subgroup total	**71**	**74**	**0.29 [0.1,0.82]**
Overall total	**1684**	**1284**	**0.62 [0.55,0.7]**

0.01 0.10 1.00 10.00
Relative Risk

FIGURE 15-1 ■ Forest plot shows the relative risk of acute rejection. Boxes represent relative risk (RR) in individual studies; diamonds represent summary effects. Relative risk less than 1 favors mycophenolate mofetil (MMF). Horizontal bars represent 95% confidence intervals (CI). CsA, cyclosporine; ME, microemulsion; SIM, Sandimmune; n, number of patients with acute rejection; N, total number of patients in study arm. (From Knight SR, Russell NK, Barcena L, et al. Mycophenolate mofetil decreases acute rejection and may improve graft survival in renal transplant recipients when compared with azathioprine: a systematic review. Transplantation 2009;87:785–94.)

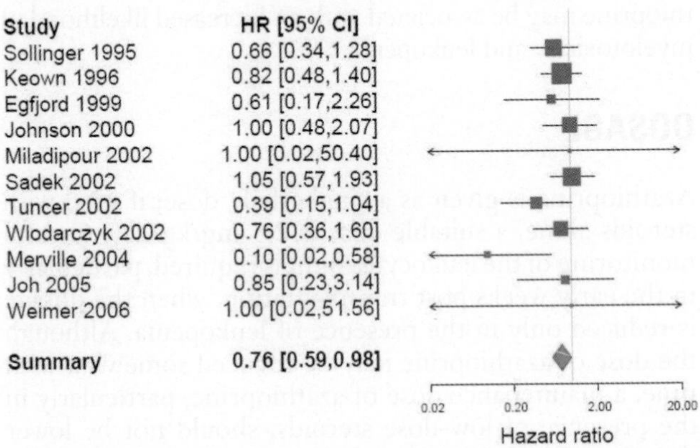

FIGURE 15-2 ■ Forest plot shows the hazard ratio (HR) for graft loss, including death with a functioning graft. Boxes represent hazard ratio in individual studies; diamond represents summary effect. Hazard ratio less than 1 favors mycophenolate mofetil. Horizontal lines represent 95% confidence intervals. (From Knight SR, Russell NK, Barcena L, et al. Mycophenolate mofetil decreases acute rejection and may improve graft survival in renal transplant recipients when compared with azathioprine: a systematic review. Transplantation 2009;87:785–94.)

An interesting recent study of immune responses in a selected group of patients in the Symphony study had suggested that tacrolimus/MMF had an effective impact on graft-protective Th2 responses and suppression of B-cell responses in comparison with tacrolimus/azathioprine, which was associated with normal IL-2 and IL-4 responses and a stronger humoral response.[35]

CYCLOSPORINE CONVERSION TO AZATHIOPRINE

Conversion of cyclosporine to azathioprine can be successfully achieved at 3–12 months after transplantation, with a resulting improvement in renal function, albeit with an increased risk of acute rejection. This has been well documented in Chapter 17 and will not be reiterated here.

AZATHIOPRINE CONVERSION TO MYCOPHENOLATE MOFETIL

There have been a number of studies in patients with chronic allograft nephropathy receiving a calcineurin inhibitor with azathioprine and steroids in whom azathioprine has been switched to MMF and the calcineurin inhibitor dosage either reduced or even eliminated. In general most of these studies, but not all, showed either stabilization or an improvement in renal function.[11,18,34]

TACROLIMUS AND AZATHIOPRINE

Several studies of tacrolimus with or without azathioprine suggest that azathioprine does not add anything to the immunosuppressive potency provided by tacrolimus. Indeed, one large randomized trial in Europe involving nearly 500 patients showed no difference in outcome at 3 years in respect of patient and graft survival, acute or chronic rejection.[25] This is discussed in more detail in Chapter 17.

CONCLUSION

Azathioprine was the cornerstone of immunosuppression from the early 1960s until cyclosporine was introduced in the early 1980s and continued to have a role when used with cyclosporine in so-called triple therapy. However, after the original trials comparing MMF and azathioprine in conjunction with Sandimmune found there was a very significant difference in the incidence of acute rejection, mycophenolate slowly replaced azathioprine. Today what is considered conventional therapy is tacrolimus, MMF, and steroids with or without induction. There is no question that MMF is more effective in terms of preventing acute rejection than azathioprine but the improvement in graft survival is modest. It is possible that azathioprine might have been discarded rather too early and does still have a place in renal transplantation, particularly where the cost of immunosuppressive drugs is a major factor.

REFERENCES

1. Bach JF, Dardenne M. The metabolism of azathioprine in renal failure. Transplantation 1971;12(4):253–9.
2. Bach JF. The mode of action of immunosuppressive agents. Oxford: North-Holland Publishing Company; 1975.
3. Calne RY. The rejection of renal homografts. Inhibition in dogs by 6-mercaptopurine. Lancet 1960;1:417–8.
4. Calne RY, Alexandre GP, Murray JE. A study of the effects of drugs in prolonging survival of homologous renal transplants in dogs. Ann N Y Acad Sci 1962;99:743–61.
5. d'Apice AJ, Becker GJ, Kincaid-Smith P, et al. A prospective randomized trial of low-dose versus high-dose steroids in cadaveric renal transplantation. Transplantation 1984;37(4):373–7.
6. Elion GB, Burgi E, Hitchings GH. Studies on condensed pyrimidine systems. IX. The synthesis of some 6-substituted purines. J Am Chem Soc 1952;74:411–4.
7. Elion GB, Bieber S, Hitchings GH. The fate of 6-mercaptopurine in mice. Ann N Y Acad Sci 1954;60(2):297–303.
8. Elion GB, Bieber S, Hitchings GH. A summary of investigations with 2-amino-6-[(1-methyl-4-nitro-5-imidazolyl)thio]purine (B.W. 57-323) in animals. Cancer Chemother Rep 1960;8:36–43.
9. Elion GB, Callahan S, Nathan H, et al. Potentiation by inhibition of drug degredation : 6-substituted purines and xanthine oxidase. Biochem Pharmacol 1963;12(1):85–93.
10. Fabre MA, Jones DC, Bunce M, et al. The impact of thiopurine *S*-methyltransferase polymorphisms on azathioprine dose 1 year after renal transplantation. Transpl Int 2004;17(9):531–9.
11. Garcia R, Pinheiro-Machado PG, Felipe CR, et al. Conversion from azathioprine to mycophenolate mofetil followed by calcineurin inhibitor minimization or elimination in patients with chronic allograft dysfunction. Transplant Proc 2006;38(9):2872–8.
12. Gonwa T, Johnson C, Ahsan N, et al. Randomized trial of tacrolimus+mycophenolate mofetil or azathioprine versus cyclosporine+mycophenolate mofetil after cadaveric kidney transplantation: results at three years. Transplantation 2003;75(12):2048–53.
13. Goodwin WE, Mims MM, Kaufman JJ. Human renal transplantation III. Technical problems encountered in six cases of kidney homotransplantation. Trans Am Assoc Genitourin Surg 1962;54:116–25.
14. Grimbert P, Baron C, Fruchaud G, et al. Long-term results of a prospective randomized study comparing two immunosuppressive regimens, one with and one without CsA, in low-risk renal transplant recipients. Transpl Int 2002;15(11):550–5.
15. Knight SR, Russell NK, Barcena L, et al. Mycophenolate mofetil decreases acute rejection and may improve graft survival in renal transplant recipients when compared with azathioprine: a systematic review. Transplantation 2009;87(6):785–94.
16. Kurzawski M, Dziewanowski K, Gawroska-Szklarz B, et al. The impact of thiopurine *S*-methyltransferase polymorphism on azathioprine-induced myelotoxicity in renal transplant recipients. Ther Drug Monit 2005;27(4):435–41.
17. Lennard L, Murphy MF, Maddocks JL. Severe megaloblastic anaemia associated with abnormal azathioprine metabolism. Br J Clin Pharmacol 1984;17(2):171–2.
18. Lezaic VD, Marinkovic J, Ristic S, et al. Conversion of azathioprine to mycophenolate mofetil and chronic graft failure progression. Transplant Proc 2005;37(2):734–6.
19. Meier-Kriesche HU, Steffen BJ, Hochberg AM, et al. Mycophenolate mofetil versus azathioprine therapy is associated with a significant protection against long-term renal allograft function deterioration. Transplantation 2003;75(8):1341–6.
20. Mucha K, Foroncewicz B, Paczek L, et al. 36-month follow-up of 75 renal allograft recipients treated with steroids, tacrolimus, and azathioprine or mycophenolate mofetil. Transplant Proc 2003;35(6):2176–8.
21. Murray JE, Merrill JP, Dammin GJ, et al. Kidney transplantation in modified recipients. Ann Surg 1962;156:337–55.
22. Murray JE, Merrill JP, Harrison JH, et al. Prolonged survival of human-kidney homografts by immunosuppressive drug therapy. N Engl J Med 1963;268:1315–23.
23. Opelz G, Dohler B. Critical threshold of azathioprine dosage for maintenance immunosuppression in kidney graft recipients. Collaborative Transplant Study. Transplantation 2000;69(5):818–21.

24. Opelz G, Dohler B, Collaborative Transplant Study. Influence of immunosuppressive regimens on graft survival and secondary outcomes after kidney transplantation. Transplantation 2009;87(6):795–802.
25. Pascual J, Segoloni G, Gonzalez Molina M, et al. Comparison between a two-drug regimen with tacrolimus and steroids and a triple one with azathioprine in kidney transplantation: results of a European trial with 3-year follow up. Transplant Proc 2003;35(5):1701–3.
26. Remuzzi G, Lesti M, Gotti E, et al. Mycophenolate mofetil versus azathioprine for prevention of acute rejection in renal transplantation (MYSS): a randomised trial. Lancet 2004;364(9433):503–12.
27. Sanderson J, Ansari A, Marinaki T, et al. Thiopurine methyltransferase: should it be measured before commencing thiopurine drug therapy? Ann Clin Biochem 2004;41(Pt 4):294–302.
28. Schutz E, Gummert J, Mohr FW, et al. Should 6-thioguanine nucleotides be monitored in heart transplant recipients given azathioprine? Ther Drug Monit 1996;18(3):228–33.
29. Schwartz R, Dameshek W. Drug-induced immunological tolerance. Nature 1959;183(4676):1682–3.
30. Schwartz R, Dameshek W. The effects of 6-mercaptopurine on homograft reactions. J Clin Invest 1960;39:952–8.
31. Shah S, Collett D, Johnson R, et al. Long-term graft outcome with mycophenolate mofetil and azathioprine: a paired kidney analysis. Transplantation 2006;82(12):1634–9.
32. Squifflet JP, Sutherland DE, Rynasiewicz JJ, et al. Combined immunosuppressive therapy with cyclosporin A and azathioprine. A synergistic effect in three of four experimental models. Transplantation 1982;34(6):315–8.
33. Starzl TE, Marchioro TL, Waddell WR. The reversal of rejection in human renal homografts with subsequent development of homograft tolerance. Surg Gynecol Obstet 1963;117:385–95.
34. Stoves J, Newstead CG, Baczkowski AJ, et al. A randomized controlled trial of immunosuppression conversion for the treatment of chronic allograft nephropathy. Nephrol Dial Transplant 2004;19(8):2113–20.
35. Weimer R, Deisz S, Dietrich H, et al. Impact of maintenance immunosuppressive regimens – balance between graft protective suppression of immune functions and a near physiological immune response. Transpl Int 2011;24(6):596–609.
36. Zukoski CF, Lee HM, Hume DM. The prolongation of functional survival of canine renal homografts by 6-mercaptopurine. Surg Forum 1960;11:470–2.

CHAPTER 16

STEROIDS

Simon R. Knight

CHAPTER OUTLINE

INTRODUCTION

When the first renal transplants were being performed in the early 1960s, the immunosuppressive properties of corticosteroids were already noted, and steroids were used successfully to reverse episodes of acute rejection.[24] In his 1964 book, Starzl described the use of steroids as a "pre-treatment" alongside azathioprine as prophylaxis against rejection, based on the premise that rejection was almost inevitable with azathioprine alone.[84] This work was soon followed by groups from Virginia, London, and Cleveland, with the use of steroids in combination with azathioprine from the time of transplantation and increased doses during episodes of acute rejection.[37,62,86] This combination of azathioprine and steroids became the mainstay of transplant immunosuppression for almost 20 years.

From the beginning of this so-called azathioprine era, arbitrarily large doses of steroids were given from the time of transplantation, with a gradual reduction over 6–12 months to maintenance levels. The high doses of steroids used with azathioprine were responsible for most of the morbidity of transplantation (discussed later). It was not until the 1970s that a series of randomized trials as well as observational studies led slowly to the realization that low-dose steroids were as effective as high-dose steroids in preventing rejection and that there was a major reduction in steroid complications of transplantation with low-dose regimens.

With the introduction of newer, more potent induction and maintenance agents there has been a great deal of interest over recent years in futher reducing steroid doses and either withdrawing them from maintenance immunosuppresive regimens or avoiding them altogether.

MECHANISM OF ACTION

Steroids are administered as prednisone or prednisolone. These agents are absorbed rapidly from the gut, and peak plasma concentrations occur 1–3 hours after administration. The mechanism of action of steroids is extremely complex and is still not understood fully.[14,20,76] Steroids are anti-inflammatory as well as being immunosuppressive. It was first noted by Billingham et al.[5] that cortisone would produce a modest prolongation of the life of skin allografts in the rabbit. In the treatment of acute rejection, it is probably the anti-inflammatory activity that produces the immediate response, whereas when used prophylactically it is the immunosuppressive activity that is predominant. A small randomized trial comparing prednisolone with a non-steroidal anti-inflammatory agent (ibuprofen) showed a higher rate of rejection in patients receiving the non-steroidal agent, confirming that the anti-inflammatory effect of steroids is not its major role in renal transplantation.[51]

Steroids are metabolized in the liver, where prednisone is converted to prednisolone. Although it has been estimated that the bioavailability of prednisone is approximately 80% of that achieved by prednisolone, no evidence exists in practice that there is a difference in outcome between prednisone (used most commonly in the United States) or prednisolone (used most commonly in Europe).[8,21] The half-life of steroids is short – about 60 minutes for prednisone and 200 minutes for prednisolone. These half-lives are increased substantially in the presence of hepatic dysfunction and are shorter in the presence of drugs such as phenytoin and rifampicin that induce hepatic enzymes. There is no evidence that these interactions have produced significant problems in clinical practice. It has also been shown that the clearance of prednisolone is slower in patients on cyclosporine compared with patients on azathioprine.[70] A later study suggested, however, that cyclosporine did not influence the metabolism of methylprednisolone, but the authors noted a considerable variation of the metabolism of methylprednisolone among patients.[90] The time- and dose-dependent induction of UDP-glucuronosyltransferase activity by steroids may increase the clearance of mycophenolic acid, reducing exposure to mycophenolate. Cattaneo et al. have demonstrated that, as steroids are tapered over the postoperative period, the mycophenolic acid area under the curve increases.[9] The pharmacokinetics of prednisolone during sirolimus therapy have also been studied, with some evidence for a minor interaction between sirolimus and prednisolone in some patients.[42]

Steroids do have a significant effect in vitro on T-cell proliferation, blocking interleukin-2 production.[65] A variety of other actions may augment their immunosuppressive activity (e.g., preventing the induction of interleukin-1 and interleukin-6 genes in macrophages).[50,95] Its anti-inflammatory activity perhaps is mediated by the inhibition of migration of monocytes to areas of inflammation,[20] and this same anti-inflammatory activity has a marked deleterious effect on wound healing.

STEROID RESISTANCE

The sensitivity of individuals to steroid therapy is highly variable. A study in healthy volunteers demonstrated a wide interindividual variation in the inhibition of lymphocyte proliferation by steroids.[31] Steroid resistance is frequently seen in patients with inflammatory conditions, and has been shown to correlate well with in vitro measurements of lymphocyte steroid sensitivity in patients suffering with rheumatoid arthritis,[47] ulcerative colitis,[30] asthma,[13] and systemic lupus erythematosus.[79]

In vitro studies of lymphocyte steroid sensitivity have demonstrated a higher incidence of resistance in patients with chronic renal failure than in healthy volunteers (52.9% versus 3.8%).[44] In renal transplant recipients, Langhoff and colleagues have demonstrated that pretransplant in vitro measurements of lymphocyte sensitivity are predictive of graft survival at 1 year in patients co-administered azathioprine, but less so in those receiving cyclosporine.[53] These results have been confirmed in vivo, with significantly higher sensitivity to methylprednisolone seen in those patients with graft function at 6 months when compared to patients with graft failure.[54] This difference in sensitivity is smaller in cyclosporine-treated patients than in those receiving azathioprine, suggesting that this effect may in part be offset by the use of newer, more potent immunosuppressant agents. Dialysis patients demonstrating steroid resistance have an increased risk of acute rejection and chronic allograft nephropathy posttransplant.[16] Interestingly, reduced lymphocyte prednisolone sensitivity correlates with impaired sensitivity to cyclosporine and tacrolimus, which may play a role in the high risk of allograft rejection in these patients.[44]

A number of potential mechanisms for this resistance to steroids have been suggested, including receptor downregulation by glucocorticoid exposure, negative inhibition by the beta isoform of the glucocorticoid receptor, or inhibition of the alpha isoform of the receptor by the proinflammatory transcription factor NK-κB in inflammatory conditions.[78]

DOSAGE

When used prophylactically with azathioprine, steroids were used initially in high doses (e.g., 100 mg/day), reducing to a maintenance dose of 20 mg/day over 6–9 months. McGeown and coworkers were the first to report consistently excellent graft survival with a low incidence of steroid-related complications using a lower prednisolone dose of 20 mg/day given orally as a single morning dose, with a further reduction occurring at 6 months to a baseline maintenance dose of 10 mg/day.[60] Because most of the Belfast patients had had bilateral nephrectomies and all had had more than 100 blood transfusions before transplantation, it was not clear whether the excellent results were related to the low dosage of steroids or to a transfusion effect, which was recognized widely as an important factor in improving graft outcome in the azathioprine era.

Trials of low-dose steroids versus high-dose steroids were carried out in Oxford, then in many other centers, all of which showed not only that low-dose steroids were as effective as high-dose steroids in preventing rejection but also that there was a significant reduction in steroid-related complications in patients receiving low-dose steroids.[7,10,11,17,36,38,61,71,83] The results of these trials led quickly to the wide adoption of low-dose steroid regimens with azathioprine. The results of a large multicenter trial reported by D'Apice et al.[15] demonstrated that low-dose steroids were only equally effective as high-dose steroids in preventing rejection if therapeutic doses of azathioprine were used (i.e., >2 mg/kg/day).

With the introduction of cyclosporine, steroids remained in use with or without azathioprine. In general, low-dose steroid protocols were continued, although there was a tendency, particularly in North America, to go back toward higher steroid dosage regimens in the first few weeks posttransplantation. This was a relatively transient practice and now with modern immunosuppressive protocols not only are low-dose steroids the norm but, indeed, discontinuation of steroids is becoming increasingly possible (see below).

Whether steroids should be given as a single daily dose in the morning or in divided doses has not been resolved. Because of the short half-life of prednisone and prednisolone, divided doses may be more rational, but it could be argued that a single morning daily dose would be more appropriate taking into account the diurnal rhythm of glucocorticoid metabolism.[25,64] There is no clinical evidence that one or the other protocol is more effective or less likely to produce side effects.

For many years, maintenance doses of prednisone or prednisolone of 10 mg/day were standard therapy in association with azathioprine. In patients with long-surviving grafts with good function, steroid dosages have been reduced to 5 or 6 mg/day. It is unlikely, however, that many patients who are on long-term azathioprine and steroids would be able to have their steroid dosage reduced to much less than 5 mg/day. Attempts in the past to withdraw steroids have often led to the onset of rejection when doses of less than 5 mg/day are reached. This is important to note as there are many long-surviving patients still on azathioprine and steroids. It should also be remembered that when patients have been on steroids for many years, their adrenocortical function may not recover from the long-standing suppression as the steroid dose is reduced, and this may produce clinical features of adrenocortical insufficiency.[63]

Alternate-day steroid therapy for maintenance has also been used widely, especially in children, in an attempt to reduce side effects, particularly growth retardation.[6,18,19,55,59,74] In children, alternate-day therapy may be associated with a greater incidence of rejection, but this is probably not the case in adults. A small randomized trial of alternate-day therapy failed to show any benefit over daily steroids, however.[59] Alternate-day therapy may lead to greater problems with respect to compliance, in contrast to a daily regimen of steroids.

It has been and still is common practice to administer a bolus of methylprednisolone prophylactically during the transplant operation with the aim of increasing immunosuppression and perhaps preventing delayed graft function, but a randomized prospective trial of bolus methylprednisolone versus placebo at the time of surgery did not show any benefit of the high perioperative intravenous dose of methylprednisolone.[45] Nevertheless it remains standard practice whatever the immunosuppressive regimen is to be.

TREATMENT OF ACUTE REJECTION

Steroids in high doses are the first approach to the treatment of an acute rejection episode. Early experience involved either increasing the oral dosage of steroids to high levels (e.g., 200 mg/day for 3 days), with a rapid reduction over 10 days to the dosage levels of steroids being given before the acute rejection episode, or boluses of intravenous methylprednisolone (e.g., 0.5–1 g/day for 3–5 days). Probably both approaches are equally effective. In an early randomized prospective trial in Oxford, however, high intravenous doses were as effective as high oral doses in reversing rejection, but there was a definite suggestion that steroid-related complications were lower in those who received intravenous therapy.[26] In a randomized study in children, a high intravenous dose of methylprednisolone (600 mg/m^2 daily for 3 days) was no more effective than low oral doses of prednisolone, reversing rejection in 70% as opposed to 72% of episodes.[69]

The commonest form of high-dose intravenous therapy to treat acute rejection has been 1 g of methylprednisolone given intravenously as a single bolus daily for 3 days. The intravenous bolus should be administered slowly over 5 minutes because the sudden injection of the bolus can lead to cardiac arrhythmias.[89] It is probable that 1 g of methylprednisolone is a much greater dose than required; in Oxford for many years now we have used 0.5 g of methylprednisolone daily intravenously for 3 days, whereas the Stockholm unit has used 0.25 g daily intravenously for 3 days. The lower intravenous doses do not appear to be associated with any greater incidence of steroid-resistant rejection, as originally suggested by a prospective trial of high-dose versus low-dose intravenous steroids to treat rejection.[46] Similarly, in a small double-blind, randomized trial, Stromstrad et al.[87] failed to show any therapeutic benefit of a 30 mg/kg bolus over a 3 mg/kg bolus, and similarly Lui et al.[56] failed to show any benefit of a bolus of 15 mg/kg of body weight over a bolus of 3 mg/kg.

SIDE EFFECTS

The side effects of continuous steroid therapy are numerous (Table 16-1). High-dose steroids were responsible for most complications of renal transplantation in the azathioprine era, and such complications have reduced markedly with the more recent widespread use of low-dose steroids. In a study of the cost of steroid side effects over 10 years in a cohort of 50 patients, the additional cost per patient attributable to a steroid complication was assessed at $5300 (US dollars).[91] Cost analysis in a recent randomized controlled trial of early steroid withdrawal from Egypt has shown a 2.9-fold increase in management costs for steroid-related morbidities in the steroid maintenance arm.[23]

Cushingoid Facies

Cushingoid facies used to be the hallmark of a renal transplant patient – a moon face, buffalo hump, acne, obese torso, and thin, easily bruised skin, all representing the cumulative effect of high-dose steroids. With lower-dose steroids, cushingoid facies is seen much less often, although most patients show modest changes in their facies in the early months posttransplantation. Most patients on low-dose steroids, which is the normal practice now with cyclosporine or tacrolimus, have relatively minimal facial changes related to steroids.

Wound Healing

The anti-inflammatory activity of steroids leads to poor wound healing. In the days of high-dose steroids, this was a major problem, influencing the healing not only of the incision, but also of the ureterovesical reconstruction. With low-dose steroids, poor wound healing is no longer a major problem.

TABLE 16-1 **Side Effects of Steroids After Renal Transplantation**

Cushingoid facies	Hypertension
Wound healing	Psychiatric disturbance
Growth retardation	Cataracts
Diabetes	Pancreatitis
Hyperlipidemia	Skin changes
Bone disease	Peptic ulceration
Obesity	

Growth Retardation

Growth retardation is of particular concern in children after renal transplantation. With modern lower doses of steroids, growth retardation is less of a problem.[77] As already discussed, the use of alternate-day steroids may reduce growth retardation, and further steroid reduction and withdrawal have also been successful in allowing catch-up growth in some studies (see below).

Diabetes

Glycosuria and insulin-dependent and non-insulin-dependent diabetes are common after transplantation. The occurrence of diabetes is related, in part, to steroid usage[39] but it has become commoner with the concomitant use of cyclosporine and tacrolimus, both of which can induce diabetes independently of steroids. In the presence of these two agents, the use of steroids augments the potential for diabetes, and often patients who become diabetic on cyclosporine or tacrolimus have a regression of the diabetes when steroid therapy is discontinued.

Hyperlipidemia

Hypercholesterolemia and hypertriglyceridemia are associated with steroid use. Hyperlipidemia has become a greater problem in the calcineurin inhibitor era as cyclosporine and tacrolimus both lead to an increased incidence, although this may be less of a problem with tacrolimus.[40] Withdrawal of steroids leads to improvements in the lipid profile (see below).

Bone Disease

Bone disease is a common and major problem posttransplantation, especially in the postmenopausal woman.[1,28,29,34,41,93] In the days of high-dose steroid therapy posttransplantation, avascular necrosis of bones, particularly of the head of the femur, was common, occurring with an incidence of approximately 10–15% within 2 years of transplantation (Figure 16-1). All the evidence suggests that this incidence was due to a cumulative effect of steroid dosage. As low-dose steroid protocols were introduced, the incidence of avascular necrosis decreased dramatically. However, the cumulative dose of steroids received by a patient on a high-dose steroid regimen, as opposed to a low-dose regimen, is not that much higher after 6 months.

Osteoporosis is associated with steroid therapy. In a randomized study, Hollander and colleagues showed that vertebral bone density was increased significantly in patients discontinuing steroids.[33] Similar evidence was reported by Aroldi et al.[3] in a randomized study of three different immunosuppressive protocols and vertebral bone density. These investigators showed that lumbar bone density decreased significantly in patients receiving cyclosporine and steroids but increased significantly in patients receiving cyclosporine alone without steroids. A recent meta-analysis of studies in transplant recipients has demonstrated a significant reduction in the risk of fractures and increase in bone mineral density with the use of bisphosphonates or vitamin D analogs, suggesting that the use of these agents should be considered particularly in recipients on long-term steroids.[85]

Many patients coming to renal transplantation have a degree of secondary hyperparathyroidism, and bone changes related to the hyperparathyroidism are enhanced by steroid therapy. Much more aggressive approaches to parathyroidectomy in patients with renal failure are being taken by most units now before transplantation. In patients after transplantation with raised parahormone levels, early parathyroidectomy also should be considered.

Obesity

Steroid therapy leads to a marked increase in appetite, and without any dietary restrictions after transplantation, all patients tend to gain weight, which is in addition to a weight increase resulting from salt and water retention. Many patients become obese (body mass index >30), and this adds to the risks of poor survival. Every attempt should be made to advise patients from the time of transplantation to restrict calorie intake carefully because once patients have gained weight in the presence of steroid therapy, it is extremely difficult for them to reduce their weight.

Hypertension

Hypertension after transplantation is common and is related in part to steroids as well as calcineurin inhibitor use. In steroid withdrawal protocols, hypertension improves once steroids are discontinued (see below).

Psychiatric Disturbance

Psychiatric disturbance is evident in patients on steroids in two ways. In the early days posttransplantation, particularly with the need for high-dose steroids to treat rejection, significant psychiatric mood changes may be observed. Later, when steroids are being withdrawn or reduced to low doses, psychiatric mood changes, especially depression, may also occur.

Cataracts

Steroid-related cataracts are common after renal transplantation, occurring in approximately 25% of patients.[80]

Pancreatitis

Acute pancreatitis occurs with a much greater incidence after renal transplantation than would be expected. Azathioprine and steroids have been associated with acute pancreatitis. The pancreatitis is probably related to overall immunosuppression and is often severe.[82] The clinical features of acute pancreatitis can be masked to some extent by steroids.

Skin Changes

Long-term steroids produced typical skin changes in renal transplant patients, the skin being thin, atrophic, easily bruised, and susceptible to knocks. A syndrome known

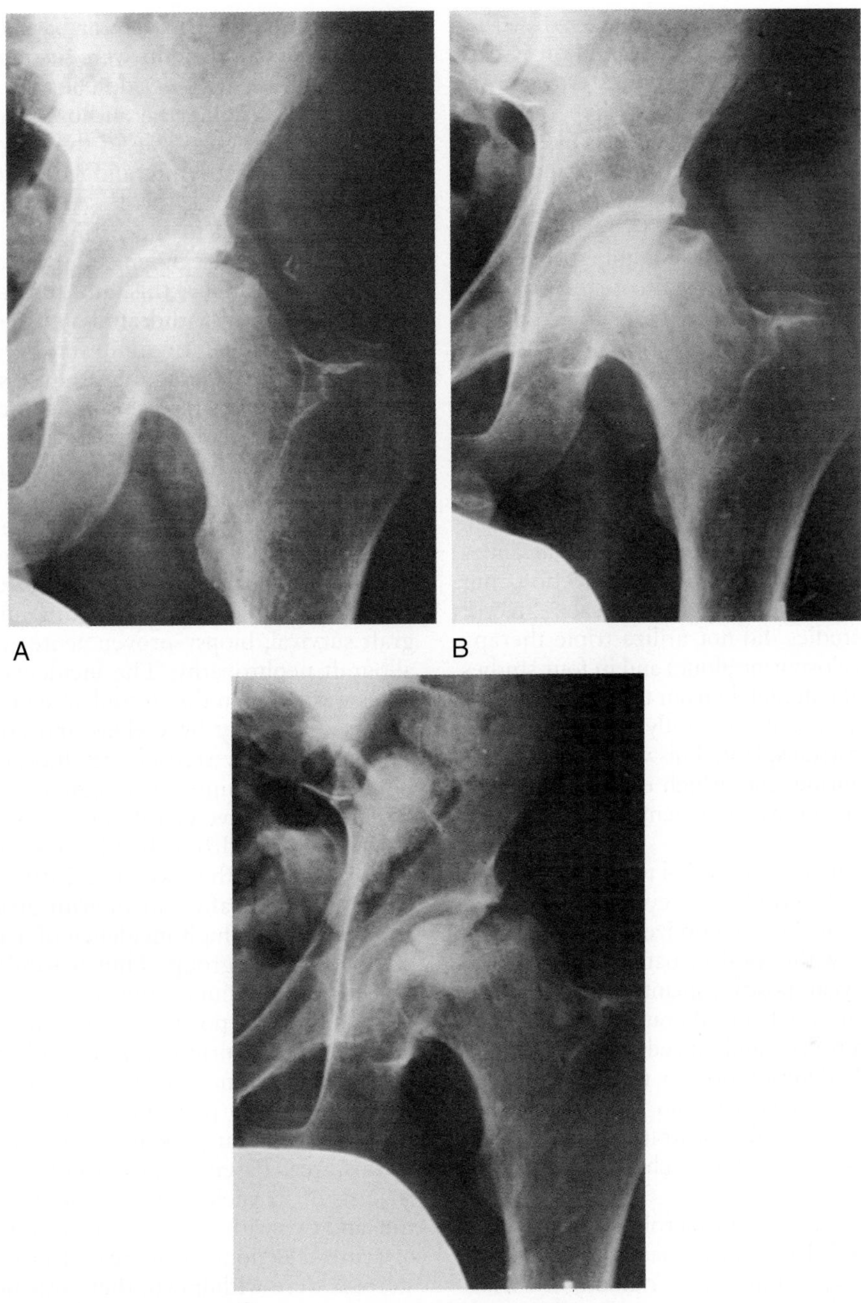

FIGURE 16-1 ■ The progression of avascular necrosis of the head of the femur. (A) Normal radiograph on first complaint of pain 1 year posttransplantation, (B) 5 months later, and (C) 20 months later. At this time, a hip replacement was performed.

as transplant leg is associated with long-term steroid usage; this occurs, for example, when a patient bumps into a chair or a table (a trivial injury), and a flap of skin is stripped or elevated from the lower leg.

Peptic Ulceration

Although it is debatable whether steroids do lead to the development of peptic ulceration, most units use prophylactic H_2 antagonists or proton pump inhibitors in the early months posttransplantation, when steroid doses are at their highest. The advent of low-dose steroid therapy has been associated with a dramatic diminution in the incidence of peptic ulceration after transplantation.

Acute Abdomen

In all renal transplant patients who present with an acute abdomen, steroids may mask the symptoms noted by the patient. If this fact is not remembered, diagnosis of diverticulitis or a perforated peptic ulcer may be delayed, with disastrous results.

STEROID WITHDRAWAL AND AVOIDANCE

The side effects of steroids, as outlined above, have generated a great deal of interest in withdrawal, or even complete avoidance, of these agents following renal transplantation. One of the major causes of death with a functioning graft following renal transplantation is cardiovascular disease, so the impact of long-term steroid use on cardiovascular risk factors such as hypertension, hyperlipidemia, and posttransplant diabetes is likely to be important.[66] Any advantage seen in terms of cardiovascular risk must be balanced against the reduction in immunosuppression and potential detriment to graft function, and such concerns have led to a large number of clinical trials investigating the risk and benefit of steroid withdrawal protocols.

In early patients treated with steroids and azathioprine, attempts to withdraw steroids resulted in almost inevitable acute rejection when the dose fell below 5–6 mg/day.[2,63] The introduction of cyclosporine led to renewed interest in such protocols, and spawned a number of clinical trials investigating steroid withdrawal at varying times posttransplant. An early meta-analysis of seven studies in cyclosporine-treated patients by Hricik and colleagues demonstrated an increased risk of acute rejection, but with no detriment to patient or graft survival.[35] Five of the seven included studies did not utilize triple therapy with azathioprine (cyclosporine alone) and in four studies steroids were avoided completely from the time of transplantation. Furthermore, only one study reported follow-up beyond 2 years posttransplant. This was the Canadian Multicentre Cyclosporine trial, which demonstrated superior long-term graft survival in patients who continued taking steroids.[81]

The results of this meta-analysis led to concerns about the early withdrawal of steroids from cyclosporine-based regimens, leading to further randomized controlled trials investigating late withdrawal in patients with stable renal function at 1 year posttransplant.[33,75] In the trial from Oxford, patients on triple therapy (cyclosporine, azathioprine, and steroids) randomized to stop steroids demonstrated a 10% deterioration in renal function at 1 year, which then stabilized with no increase in graft loss.[75] Both of these studies demonstrated beneficial effects in cardiovascular risk factors such as hypertension and blood lipids.

Following the introduction of tacrolimus and mycophenolate mofetil (MMF) to maintenance immunosuppressive regimens a large number of randomized trials with various combinations of induction and maintenance agents, as well as varying times of steroid withdrawal, have been published in the literature. In general the trend has been back towards earlier tapering and withdrawal of steroids, with withdrawal as early as 1 week posttransplant in a number of studies. One of the major concerns given the excess acute rejection seen in the early steroid withdrawal trials with cyclosporine is the impact of the reduction of immunosuppression on long-term graft and patient outcomes. Perhaps the most impressive study to date addressing this issue is the Astellas Steroid Withdrawal Study from Woodle and colleagues, in which patients receiving tacrolimus, MMF, and steroids were randomized at day 7 to withdraw steroids or continue a long-term maintenance dose of 5 mg/day from month 6.[94] Randomization and blinding were maintained for the duration of the 5-year follow-up. Whilst the study demonstrated an excess of mild, steroid-sensitive acute rejection in the withdrawal arm, 5-year patient and graft survival were unaffected. Benefits were seen in cardiovascular risk factors such as triglycerides, insulin requirements, and weight gain, leading the authors to conclude that early steroid withdrawal is safe in the longer term in patients treated with a tacrolimus and MMF regimen.

It was first noted by Pescovitz and colleagues that sirolimus may aid in the withdrawal of steroids from a calcineurin-based regimen.[73] Further observational studies appear to support this, and the use of sirolimus may also allow steroid withdrawal alongside reduction in the exposure to calcineurin inhibitors.[12,43,57,58]

The use of newer immunosuppressive agents such as MMF or sirolimus may also allow the safe withdrawal of steroids earlier than previously seen with cyclosporine-based regimens. Kumar and colleagues have reported a 3-year analysis of a large trial of 300 patients receiving basiliximab induction, a calcineurin inhibitor, and MMF or sirolimus in which patients were randomized to have steroids withdrawn on day 2 or to continue steroids.[52] There was no difference in graft function, patient and graft survival, biopsy-proven acute rejection, or chronic allograft nephropathy. The incidence of new-onset diabetes was lower in the steroid-free group.

A recent study by Gelens and colleagues attempted to combine early steroid withdrawal with a calcineurin inhibitor-free maintenance regimen.[22] Patients were randomized to receive tacrolimus and sirolimus, tacrolimus and MMF or daclizumab induction, sirolimus and MMF. Steroids were withdrawn after 2 days in all patients. The trial was halted after an interim analysis demonstrated an unacceptably high incidence of acute rejection in the calcineurin-free group. Thus it would appear that, even with modern immunosuppressant agents and antibody induction, it is not possible to combine the complete withdrawal of calcineurin inhibitors with steroid withdrawal.

More recent meta-analyses of steroid withdrawal protocols have been published to attempt to draw conclusions from the large body of randomized trial evidence in this area. Pascual and colleagues performed a meta-analysis of six such trials, four with MMF and cyclosporine and two with MMF and tacrolimus.[72] Whilst the risk of acute rejection was increased just over twofold when steroids were withdrawn, there was no significant difference in the incidence of graft failure. Unfortunately, this meta-analysis did not differentiate between the relative steroid-sparing potential of cyclosporine and tacrolimus. A similar meta-analysis from Tan and colleagues also demonstrated an increase in the risk of acute rejection, balanced by a reduction in the risk of opportunistic and urinary tract infections in a small subset of the included trials.[88]

A comprehensive meta-analysis from our own group included all steroid withdrawal and avoidance studies over a 27-year period, incorporating 34 studies and 5637 patients.[48] Overall analysis confirmed an increase in acute rejection with steroid avoidance or withdrawal (Figure 16-2; relative risk (RR) 1.56, $P<0.0001$), although no difference in steroid-resistant acute rejection was found, suggesting that these are mainly steroid-sensitive mild rejection episodes. Despite the increased rate of rejection and a small (clinically insignificant) increase in

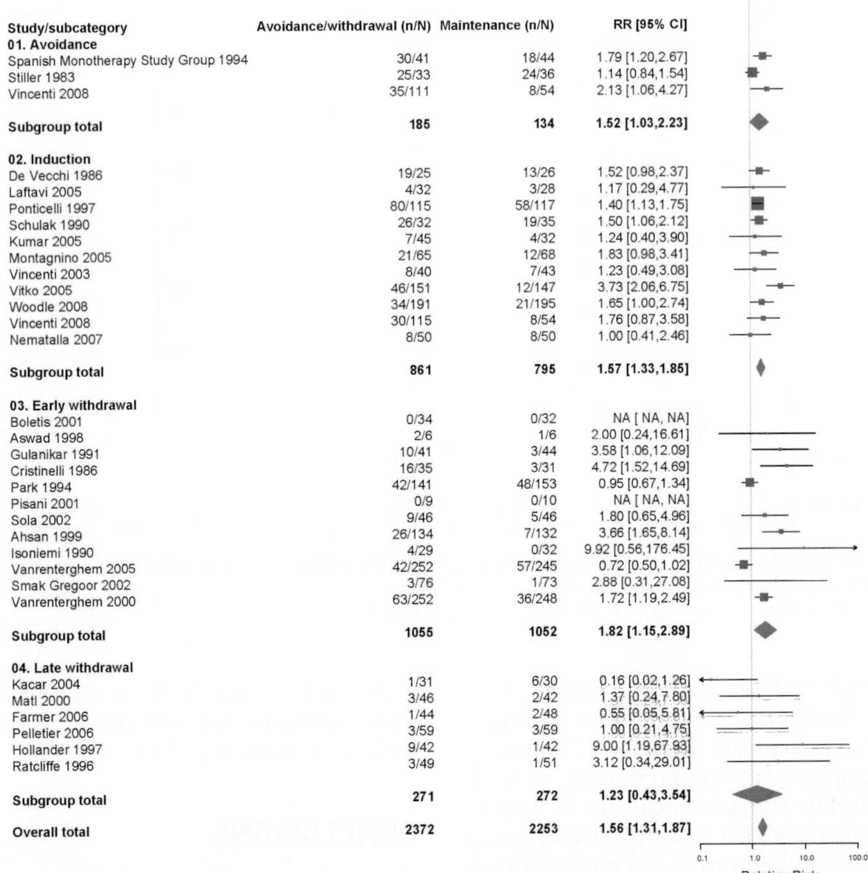

FIGURE 16-2 ■ Forest plot to show the relative risk of acute rejection with steroid avoidance or withdrawal at various times after transplantation. Blue boxes show treatment effect for individual studies. Red diamonds show summary treatment effect for each subgroup and overall analysis derived by random effects analysis. Horizontal lines show 95% confidence intervals. RR, relative risk; n, number of patients with acute rejection; N, total number of patients in study arm; CI, confidence interval. Subgroups are: (1) complete steroid avoidance; (2) induction steroids (≤7 days); (3) early steroid withdrawal (8 days to 12 months); and (4) late steroid withdrawal (>12 months). (From Knight SR, Morris PJ. Steroid avoidance or withdrawal after renal transplantation increases the risk of acute rejection but decreases cardiovascular risk. A meta-analysis. Transplantation 2010;89:1–14.)

serum creatinine, there was no difference in graft or patient survival. Significant benefits in cardiovascular risk factors were identified with steroid avoidance or withdrawal, with the incidence of hypertension (RR 0.90, $P<0.0001$), new-onset diabetes (RR 0.64, $P=0.0006$), and hypercholesterolemia (RR 0.76, $P<0.0001$) all reduced. Interestingly, no interaction was found between the use of induction immunosuppression, maintenance immunosuppression, and the time of steroid withdrawal on the ability to withdraw steroids. Post hoc analysis has however demonstrated a dose effect, with the cardiovascular benefit seen to be reduced when withdrawing lower doses of steroids.[49]

Whilst none of this randomized controlled trial data supports an effect on graft or patient survival with steroid withdrawal, registry data from the Collaborative Transplant Study[67] has suggested that patients with a functioning graft at 1 year who had steroids withdrawn had better graft and patient survival thereafter than patients remaining on steroids. The increased risk of acute rejection with steroid withdrawal was not seen in the registry data. The initial criticism of this study was that patients still on steroids at 1 year represented patients with poorer function as a result of rejection episodes or delayed graft function, but a subsequent analysis examining outcome only in patients with satisfactory renal function at 1 year found the same results. A more recent prospective study from the same group has confirmed a benefit in both graft and patient survival in renal and cardiac transplant patients in whom steroids are withdrawn greater than 6 months following transplantation, with no increase in incidence of acute rejection (Figure 16-3).[68] Benefits were also seen in cardiovascular parameters in the withdrawal group, with significantly fewer patients demonstrating elevated cholesterol levels. Whilst the number of patients and length of follow-up in this study are impressive (7 years), a major criticism is a lack of a randomized design, with the control cohort being retrospectively matched patients from the Collaborative Transplant Study registry.

A number of the studies described above include data from patients in whom steroids are avoided completely from the time of transplantation. Meta-analysis has shown no clear difference between subgroups of patients avoiding steroids compared to those continuing for a period following transplantation, although the number of studies is small and so the statistical power is limited. Individual studies have attempted to address the

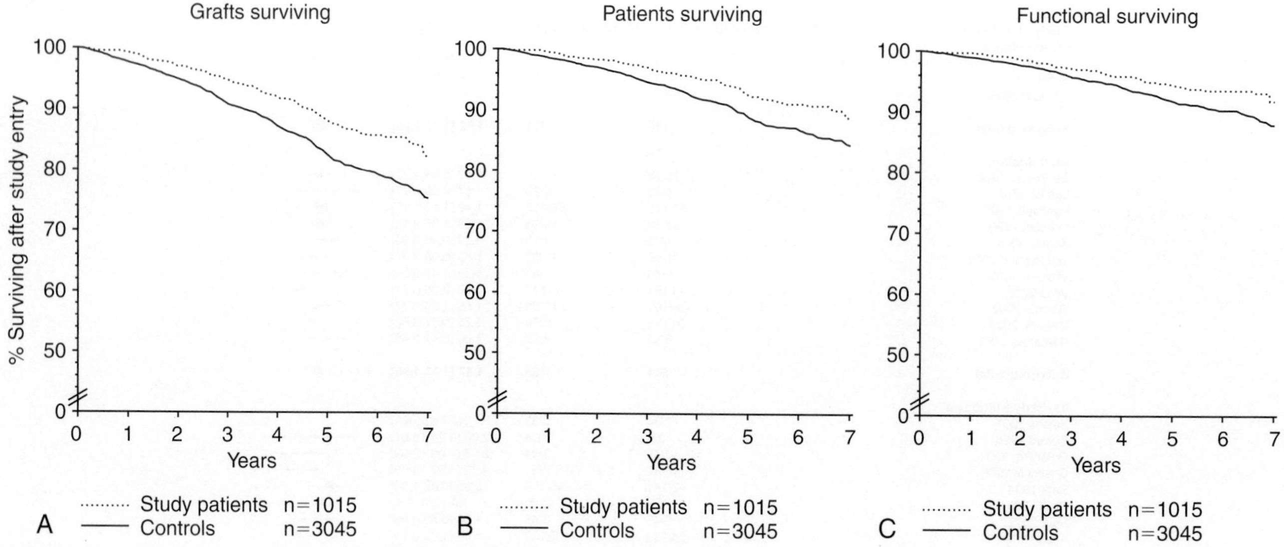

FIGURE 16-3 ■ Seven-year graft (A), patient (B), and functional graft (C) survival in renal transplant recipients after steroid withdrawal (study patients) or steroid continuation (matched controls). (From Opelz G, Dohler B, Laux G. Long-term prospective study of steroid withdrawal in kidney and heart transplant recipients. Am J Transplant 2005;5:720–8.)

timing of steroid withdrawal, most notably the three-arm FREEDOM study.[92] In this study, patients received basiliximab induction, mycophenolate sodium, and cyclosporine and were randomized to receive no steroids, steroids for 7 days, or to continue steroids. Incidence of biopsy-proven acute rejection was higher in the avoidance group compared to the withdrawal group (31.5% versus 26.1%), but no differences in graft survival or renal function were seen. The composite end-point at 12 months of biopsy-proven acute rejection, graft loss, or death was 36.0% in the steroid-free group, 29.6% with steroid withdrawal, and 19.3% with standard steroids, leading the authors to conclude that early withdrawal may be preferable to complete avoidance.

Steroid Withdrawal in Children

Given the detrimental effects of long-term corticosteroids on growth, there has been some interest in steroid withdrawal in pediatric transplant recipients. Benfield and colleagues performed a double-blind, randomized trial in children 6 months posttransplant either to continue maintenance steroids or withdraw gradually by 12 months.[4] Baseline immunosuppression was basiliximab induction, calcineurin inhibitor, and sirolimus. The study was stopped by the Drug Safety Monitoring Board after enrolment of 274 patients due to a very high incidence of posttransplant lymphoproliferative disorder (6.9%), probably relating to the very heavy baseline immunosuppression. The authors concluded that, whilst the immunosuppressive regimen used allowed for the safe withdrawal of steroids, it could not be recommended on safety grounds.

A more recent study reporting withdrawal of steroids beyond 1 year posttransplant from a more conventional regimen has demonstrated no excess in acute rejection at 2 years.[32] There was an improvement in growth and reduction in cardiovascular risk factors, with no detriment to graft survival or function. Similar benefits have also been demonstrated in the multicenter TWIST study, in which steroids were withdrawn at 4 days and replaced with daclizumab at induction.[27]

CONCLUSIONS

Corticosteroids remain an important part of the transplant immunosuppressive armory for the induction, maintenance, and treatment of acute rejection. Particularly in high doses, they are associated with a plethora of adverse effects and the overall trend is now towards reduction in steroid exposure with withdrawal or avoidance.

Steroid withdrawal is associated with an increased risk of acute rejection, but the evidence seems to suggest that this excess rejection is mild and treatable, and does not appear to be detrimental to longer-term graft survival and function. Withdrawal has significant benefits in terms of cardiovascular risk, bone complications, and growth.

Whilst the role of complete steroid avoidance is uncertain, early withdrawal in low-risk renal transplant recipients on a modern immunosuppressive regimen appears to be safe with significant benefits to the patient.

REFERENCES

1. Almond MK, Kwan JT, Evans K, et al. Loss of regional bone mineral density in the first 12 months following renal transplantation. Nephron 1994;66(1):52–7.
2. Anderton JL, Fananapazir L, Eccleston M. Minimum steroid requirements in renal transplant patients monitored by urinary fibrin degradation products and complement. Proc Eur Dial Transplant Assoc 1977;14:342–50.
3. Aroldi A, Tarantino A, Montagnino G, et al. Effects of three immunosuppressive regimens on vertebral bone density in renal transplant recipients: a prospective study. Transplantation 1997;63(3):380–6.
4. Benfield MR, Bartosh S, Ikle D, et al. A randomized double-blind, placebo controlled trial of steroid withdrawal after pediatric renal transplantation. Am J Transplant 2010;10(1):81–8.
5. Billingham RE, Krohn PL, Medawar PB. Effect of cortisone on survival of skin homografts in rabbits. Br Med J 1951;1(4716):1157–63.

6. Breitenfield RV, Hebert LA, Lemann Jr J, et al. Stability of renal transplant function with alternate-day corticosteroid therapy. JAMA 1980;244(2):151–6.
7. Buckels JA, Mackintosh P, Barnes AD. Controlled trial of low versus high dose oral steroid therapy in 100 cadaveric renal transplants. Proc Eur Dial Transplant Assoc 1981;18:394–9.
8. Burleson RL, Marbarger PD, Jermanovich N, et al. A prospective study of methylprednisolone and prednisone as immunosuppressive agents in clinical renal transplantation. Transplant Proc 1981;13(1 Pt 1):339–43.
9. Cattaneo D, Perico N, Gaspari F, et al. Glucocorticoids interfere with mycophenolate mofetil bioavailability in kidney transplantation. Kidney Int 2002;62(3):1060–7.
10. Chan L, French ME, Beare J, et al. Prospective trial of high-dose versus low-dose prednisolone in renal transplant patients. Transplant Proc 1980;12(2):323–6.
11. Chan L, French ME, Oliver DO, et al. High- and low-dose prednisolone. Transplant Proc 1981;13(1 Pt 1):336–8.
12. Citterio F, Sparacino V, Altieri P, et al. Addition of sirolimus to cyclosporine in long-term kidney transplant recipients to withdraw steroid. Transplant Proc 2005;37(2):827–9.
13. Corrigan CJ, Brown PH, Barnes NC, et al. Glucocorticoid resistance in chronic asthma. Peripheral blood T lymphocyte activation and comparison of the T lymphocyte inhibitory effects of glucocorticoids and cyclosporin A. Am Rev Respir Dis 1991;144(5):1026–32.
14. Cupps TR, Fauci AS. Corticosteroid-mediated immunoregulation in man. Immunol Rev 1982;65:133–55.
15. d'Apice AJ, Becker GJ, Kincaid-Smith P, et al. A prospective randomized trial of low-dose versus high-dose steroids in cadaveric renal transplantation. Transplantation 1984;37(4):373–7.
16. De Antonio SR, Saber LT, Chriguer RS, et al. Glucocorticoid resistance in dialysis patients may impair the kidney allograft outcome. Nephrol Dial Transplant 2008;23(4):1422–8.
17. De Vecchi A, Rivolta E, Tarantino A, et al. Controlled trial of two different methylprednisolone doses in cadaveric renal transplantation. Nephron 1985;41(3):262–6.
18. Diethelm AG, Sterling WA, Hartley MW, et al. Alternate-day prednisone therapy in recipients of renal allografts. Risk and benefits. Arch Surg 1976;111(8):867–70.
19. Dumler F, Levin NW, Szego G, et al. Long-term alternate day steroid therapy in renal transplantation. A controlled study. Transplantation 1982;34(2):78–82.
20. Fauci AS. Mechanisms of the immunosuppressive and anti-inflammatory effects of glucocorticosteroids. J Immunopharmacol 1978;1(1):1–25.
21. Gambertoglio JG, Frey FJ, Holford NH, et al. Prednisone and prednisolone bioavailability in renal transplant patients. Kidney Int 1982;21(4):621–6.
22. Gelens MA, Christiaans MH, van Heurn EL, et al. High rejection rate during calcineurin inhibitor-free and early steroid withdrawal immunosuppression in renal transplantation. Transplantation 2006;82(9):1221–3.
23. Gheith OA, Nematalla AH, Bakr MA, et al. Steroid avoidance reduces the cost of morbidities after live-donor renal allotransplants: a prospective, randomized, controlled study. Exp Clin Transplant 2011;9(2):121–7.
24. Goodwin WE, Mims MM, Kaufman JJ. Human renal transplantation III. Technical problems encountered in six cases of kidney homotransplantation. Trans Am Assoc Genitourin Surg 1962;54:116–25.
25. Grant SD, Forsham PH, DiRaimondo VC. Suppression of 17-hydroxycorticosteroids in plasma and urine by single and divided doses of triamcinolone. N Engl J Med 1965;273(21):1115–8.
26. Gray D, Shepherd H, Daar A, et al. Oral versus intravenous high-dose steroid treatment of renal allograft rejection. The big shot or not? Lancet 1978;1(8056):117–8.
27. Grenda R, Watson A, Trompeter R, et al. A randomized trial to assess the impact of early steroid withdrawal on growth in pediatric renal transplantation: the TWIST study. Am J Transplant 2010;10(4):828–36.
28. Grotz WH, Mundinger FA, Gugel B, et al. Bone fracture and osteodensitometry with dual energy X-ray absorptiometry in kidney transplant recipients. Transplantation 1994;58(8):912–5.
29. Grotz WH, Mundinger FA, Gugel B, et al. Bone mineral density after kidney transplantation. A cross-sectional study in 190 graft recipients up to 20 years after transplantation. Transplantation 1995;59(7):982–6.
30. Hearing SD, Norman M, Probert CS, et al. Predicting therapeutic outcome in severe ulcerative colitis by measuring in vitro steroid sensitivity of proliferating peripheral blood lymphocytes. Gut 1999;45(3):382–8.
31. Hearing SD, Norman M, Smyth C, et al. Wide variation in lymphocyte steroid sensitivity among healthy human volunteers. J Clin Endocrinol Metab 1999;84(11):4149–54.
32. Hocker B, Weber LT, Feneberg R, et al. Improved growth and cardiovascular risk after late steroid withdrawal: 2-year results of a prospective, randomised trial in paediatric renal transplantation. Nephrol Dial Transplant 2009;25(2):617–24.
33. Hollander AA, Hene RJ, Hermans J, et al. Late prednisone withdrawal in cyclosporine-treated kidney transplant patients: a randomized study. J Am Soc Nephrol 1997;8(2):294–301.
34. Horber FF, Casez JP, Steiger U, et al. Changes in bone mass early after kidney transplantation. J Bone Miner Res 1994;9(1):1–9.
35. Hricik DE, O'Toole MA, Schulak JA, et al. Steroid-free immunosuppression in cyclosporine-treated renal transplant recipients: a meta-analysis. J Am Soc Nephrol 1993;4(6):1300–5.
36. Hricik DE, Almawi WY, Strom TB. Trends in the use of glucocorticoids in renal transplantation. Transplantation 1994;57(7):979–89.
37. Hume DM, Lee HM, Williams GM, et al. Comparative results of cadaver and related donor renal homografts in man, and immunologic implications of the outcome of second and paired transplants. Ann Surg 1966;164(3):352–97.
38. Isoniemi H, Ahonen J, Eklund B, et al. Renal allograft immunosuppression. II. A randomized trial of withdrawal of one drug in triple drug immunosuppression. Transpl Int 1990;3(3):121–7.
39. Isoniemi H. Renal allograft immunosuppression V: glucose intolerance occurring in different immunosuppressive treatments. Clin Transplant 1991;5(3):268–72.
40. Jensik SC. Tacrolimus (FK 506) in kidney transplantation: three-year survival results of the US multicenter, randomized, comparative trial. FK 506 Kidney Transplant Study Group. Transplant Proc 1998;30(4):1216–8.
41. Julian BA, Laskow DA, Dubovsky J, et al. Rapid loss of vertebral mineral density after renal transplantation. N Engl J Med 1991;325(8):544–50.
42. Jusko WJ, Ferron GM, Mis SM, et al. Pharmacokinetics of prednisolone during administration of sirolimus in patients with renal transplants. J Clin Pharmacol 1996;36(12):1100–6.
43. Kahan BD, Podbielski J, Schoenberg L. Use of sirolimus to facilitate steroid withdrawal from a cyclosporine regimen. Transplant Proc 2006;38(9):2842–6.
44. Kang XX, Hirano T, Oka K, et al. Role of altered prednisolone-specific lymphocyte sensitivity in chronic renal failure as a pharmacodynamic marker of acute allograft rejection after kidney transplantation. Eur J Clin Pharmacol 1991;41(5):417–23.
45. Kauffman HM, Sampson D, Fox PS, et al. High dose (bolus) intravenous methylprednisolone at the time of kidney homotransplantation. Ann Surg 1977;186(5):631–4.
46. Kauffman Jr. HM, Stromstad SA, Sampson D, et al. Randomized steroid therapy of human kidney transplant rejection. Transplant Proc 1979;11(1):36–8.
47. Kirkham BW, Corkill MM, Davison SC, et al. Response to glucocorticoid treatment in rheumatoid arthritis: in vitro cell mediated immune assay predicts in vivo responses. J Rheumatol 1991;18(6):821–5.
48. Knight SR, Morris PJ. Steroid avoidance or withdrawal after renal transplantation increases the risk of acute rejection but decreases cardiovascular risk. A meta-analysis. Transplantation 2010;89(1):1–14.
49. Knight SR, Morris PJ. Interaction between maintenance steroid dose and the risk/benefit of steroid avoidance and withdrawal regimens following renal transplantation. Transplantation 2011;92(11):e63–4.
50. Knudsen PJ, Dinarello CA, Strom TB. Glucocorticoids inhibit transcriptional and post-transcriptional expression of interleukin 1 in U937 cells. J Immunol 1987;139(12):4129–34.
51. Kreis H, Chkoff N, Droz D, et al. Nonsteroid antiinflammatory agents as a substitute treatment for steroids in ATGAM-treated cadaver kidney recipients. Transplantation 1984;37(2):139–45.

52. Kumar MS, Heifets M, Moritz MJ, et al. Safety and efficacy of steroid withdrawal two days after kidney transplantation: analysis of results at three years. Transplantation 2006;81(6):832–9.
53. Langhoff E, Ladefoged J, Jakobsen BK, et al. Recipient lymphocyte sensitivity to methylprednisolone affects cadaver kidney graft survival. Lancet 1986;1(8493):1296–7.
54. Langhoff E, Ladefoged J. The impact of high lymphocyte sensitivity to glucocorticoids on kidney graft survival in patients treated with azathioprine and cyclosporine. Transplantation 1987;43(3):380–4.
55. Leb DE. Alternate day prednisone treatment may increase kidney transplant rejection. Proc Clin Dial Transplant Forum 1979;9:136–9.
56. Lui SF, Sweny P, Scoble JE, et al. Low-dose vs high-dose intravenous methylprednisolone therapy for acute renal allograft rejection in patients receiving cyclosporin therapy. Nephrol Dial Transplant 1989;4(5):387–9.
57. Mahalati K, Kahan BD. Sirolimus permits steroid withdrawal from a cyclosporine regimen. Transplant Proc 2001;33(1–2):1270.
58. Mahalati K, Kahan BD. A pilot study of steroid withdrawal from kidney transplant recipients on sirolimus-cyclosporine–a combination therapy. Transplant Proc 2001;33(7–8):3232–3.
59. McDonald FD, Horensten ML, Mayor GB, et al. Effect of alternate-day steroids on renal transplant function. A controlled study. Nephron 1976;17(6):415–29.
60. McGeown MG, Kennedy JA, Loughridge WG, et al. One hundred kidney transplants in the Belfast city hospital. Lancet 1977;2(8039):648–51.
61. Morris PJ, Chan L, French ME, et al. Low dose oral prednisolone in renal transplantation. Lancet 1982;1(8271):525–7.
62. Mowbray JF, Cohen SL, Doak PB, et al. Human cadaveric renal transplantation. Report of twenty cases. Br Med J 1965;2(5475):1387–94.
63. Naik RB, Chakraborty J, English J, et al. Serious renal transplant rejection and adrenal hypofunction after gradual withdrawal of prednisolone two years after transplantation. Br Med J 1980;280(6228):1337–40.
64. Nichols T, Nugent CA, Tyler FH. Diurnal variation in supression of adrenal function by glucocorticoids. J Clin Endocrinol Metab 1965;25:343–9.
65. Northrop JP, Crabtree GR, Mattila PS. Negative regulation of interleukin 2 transcription by the glucocorticoid receptor. J Exp Med 1992;175(5):1235–45.
66. Ojo AO, Hanson JA, Wolfe RA, et al. Long-term survival in renal transplant recipients with graft function. Kidney Int 2000;57(1):307–13.
67. Opelz G. Influence of treatment with cyclosporine, azathioprine and steroids on chronic allograft failure. The Collaborative Transplant Study. Kidney Int Suppl 1995;52:S89–92.
68. Opelz G, Dohler B, Laux G. Long-term prospective study of steroid withdrawal in kidney and heart transplant recipients. Am J Transplant 2005;5(4 Pt 1):720–8.
69. Orta-Sibu N, Chantler C, Bewick M, et al. Comparison of high-dose intravenous methylprednisolone with low-dose oral prednisolone in acute renal allograft rejection in children. Br Med J (Clin Res Ed) 1982;285(6337):258–60.
70. Ost L. Impairment of prednisolone metabolism by cyclosporine treatment in renal graft recipients. Transplantation 1987;44(4):533–5.
71. Papadakis J, Brown CB, Cameron JS, et al. High versus "low" dose corticosteroids in recipients of cadaveric kidneys: prospective controlled trial. Br Med J (Clin Res Ed) 1983;286(6371):1097–100.
72. Pascual J, Quereda C, Zamora J, et al. Steroid withdrawal in renal transplant patients on triple therapy with a calcineurin inhibitor and mycophenolate mofetil: a meta-analysis of randomized, controlled trials. Transplantation 2004;78(10):1548–56.
73. Pescovitz MD, Kahan BD, Julian BA, et al. Sirolimus (SRL) permits early steroid withdrawal from a triple therapy renal prophylaxis regimen. ASTP Abstracts 1997;62:261.
74. Potter DE, Holliday MA, Wilson CJ, et al. Alternate-day steroids in children after renal transplantation. Transplant Proc 1975;7(1):79–82.
75. Ratcliffe PJ, Dudley CR, Higgins RM, et al. Randomised controlled trial of steroid withdrawal in renal transplant recipients receiving triple immunosuppression. Lancet 1996;348(9028):643–8.
76. Rhen T, Cidlowski JA. Antiinflammatory action of glucocorticoids – new mechanisms for old drugs. N Engl J Med 2005;353(16):1711–23.
77. Rizzoni G, Broyer M, Guest G, et al. Growth retardation in children with chronic renal disease: scope of the problem. Am J Kidney Dis 1986;7(4):256–61.
78. Schaaf MJM, Cidlowski JA. Molecular mechanisms of glucocorticoid action and resistance. J Steroid Biochem Mol Biol 2002;83(1–5):37–48.
79. Seki M, Ushiyama C, Seta N, et al. Apoptosis of lymphocytes induced by glucocorticoids and relationship to therapeutic efficacy in patients with systemic lupus erythematosus. Arthritis Rheum 1998;41(5):823–30.
80. Shun-Shin GA, Ratcliffe P, Bron AJ, et al. The lens after renal transplantation. Br J Ophthalmol 1990;74(5):267–71.
81. Sinclair NR. Low-dose steroid therapy in cyclosporine-treated renal transplant recipients with well-functioning grafts. The Canadian Multicentre Transplant Study Group. CMAJ 1992;147(5):645–57.
82. Slakey DP, Johnson CP, Cziperle DJ, et al. Management of severe pancreatitis in renal transplant recipients. Ann Surg 1997;225(2):217–22.
83. Stabile C, Vincenti F, Garovoy M, et al. Is a "low" dose of prednisone better than a "high" dose at the time of renal transplantation? Braz J Med Biol Res 1986;19(3):355–66.
84. Starzl TE. Pretreatment with prednisolone. In: Starzl TE, editor. Experience in renal transplantation. Philadelphia: WB Saunders; 1964.
85. Stein EM, Ortiz D, Jin Z, et al. Prevention of fractures after solid organ transplantation: a meta-analysis. J Clin Endocrinol Metab 2011;96(11):3457–65.
86. Straffon RA, Hewitt CKW, Stewart BH, et al. Clinical experience with the use of 79 kidneys from cadavers for transplantation. Surg Gynecol Obstet 1966;123(3):483–92.
87. Stromstad SA, Kauffman HM, Sampson D, et al. Randomized steroid therapy of human kidney transplant rejection. Surg Forum 1978;29:376–7.
88. Tan JY, Zhao N, Wu TX, et al. Steroid withdrawal increases risk of acute rejection but reduces infection: a meta-analysis of 1681 cases in renal transplantation. Transplant Proc 2006;38(7):2054–6.
89. Thompson JF, Chalmers DH, Wood RF, et al. Sudden death following high-dose intravenous methylprednisolone. Transplantation 1983;36(5):594–6.
90. Tornatore KM, Walshe JJ, Reed KA, et al. Comparative methylprednisolone pharmacokinetics in renal transplant patients receiving double- or triple-drug immunosuppression. Ann Pharmacother 1993;27(5):545–9.
91. Veenstra DL, Best JH, Hornberger J, et al. Incidence and long-term cost of steroid-related side effects after renal transplantation. Am J Kidney Dis 1999;33(5):829–39.
92. Vincenti F, Schena FP, Paraskevas S, et al. A randomized, multicenter study of steroid avoidance, early steroid withdrawal or standard steroid therapy in kidney transplant recipients. Am J Transplant 2008;8(2):307–16.
93. Wolpaw T, Deal CL, Fleming-Brooks S, et al. Factors influencing vertebral bone density after renal transplantation. Transplantation 1994;58(11):1186–9.
94. Woodle ES, First MR, Pirsch J, et al. A prospective, randomized, double-blind, placebo-controlled multicenter trial comparing early (7 day) corticosteroid cessation versus long-term, low-dose corticosteroid therapy. Ann Surg 2008;248(4):564–77.
95. Zanker B, Walz G, Wieder KJ, et al. Evidence that glucocorticosteroids block expression of the human interleukin-6 gene by accessory cells. Transplantation 1990;49(1):183–5.

CHAPTER 17

Calcineurin Inhibitors

Juan C. Mejia • Amit Basu • Ron Shapiro

CHAPTER OUTLINE

Cyclosporine, introduced into clinical practice in the 1980s, and tacrolimus, introduced in the 1990s, are the current mainstream maintenance immunosuppressive medications used, with a shift toward a progressively higher utilization of tacrolimus-based regimens over the last 10 years. Both are immunosuppressive agents that improved clinical outcomes in liver and kidney transplant recipients.[46] The phase III trials leading to Food and Drug Administration (FDA) approval of tacrolimus (in 1994) were conducted first in liver rather than in kidney transplant recipients, in contrast to other immunosuppressive agents. Subsequent clinical trials in kidney transplantation led to FDA approval for kidney transplantation in 1997. By 2009, 84% of all new kidney transplant recipients and 90% of all new liver transplant recipients were receiving tacrolimus as maintenance immunosuppressive therapy before discharge[126]; these percentages have continued to increase over time.

Cyclosporine was first isolated from two strains of imperfect fungi (*Cylindrocarpon lucidum* Booth and *Trichoderma polysporum* Rifai) from soil samples by the Department of Microbiology at Sandoz (Basel, Switzerland) as an antifungal agent of limited activity.[34] Borel and colleagues demonstrated its potent immunosuppressive activity in a variety of in vitro and in vivo experiments.[11,12,43] It was first used clinically in England in the late 1970s by Calne and his associates in Cambridge. Initially, it was used with other drugs, such as prednisolone or Asta 036.5122 (cytimum, an analog of cyclophosphamide).[20,21] Cyclosporine revolutionized the field of transplantation, improving outcomes in renal transplantation, making it possible for routine liver and heart transplantation to be performed, and allowing the first clinical trials of pancreas and lung transplants. Tacrolimus (FK506, Prograf) was isolated in 1984 from the fermentation broth of *Streptomyces tsukubaensis*, a soil organism found at the foot of Mount Tsukuba near Tokyo. This compound was developed by researchers at the Chiba University of Japan. In the first clinical (rescue) trial, tacrolimus was administered to patients who were taking standard immunosuppressive therapy but who faced retransplantation because of ongoing organ rejection, or who had undesirable drug toxicities.[46] The initial clinical trial of tacrolimus as a primary immunosuppressive agent for the prophylaxis of rejection in liver transplant recipients began in the spring of 1990 at the University of Pittsburgh.[135] This work led eventually to multicenter randomized trials in liver and kidney transplantation.[97,111] Patients treated with tacrolimus had significantly fewer and less severe episodes of acute rejection than did patients given cyclosporine therapy. Tacrolimus also has shown efficacy as a rescue agent and as a primary maintenance immunosuppressive agent in heart, lung, pancreas, and small-bowel transplantation,[68,88,101,116,134] and was approved for heart transplantation in 2006.

MECHANISM OF ACTION

Calcineurin inhibitors exert their immunosuppressive effects by reducing interleukin-2 (IL-2) production and IL-2 receptor expression, leading to a reduction in T-cell activation. Tacrolimus inhibits T-lymphocyte activation by binding to FKBP-12, an intracellular protein. A complex is then formed of tacrolimus–FKBP-12, calcium, calmodulin, and calcineurin, which inhibits the phosphatase activity of calcineurin. This complex prevents the dephosphorylation and subsequent translocation of the nuclear factor of activated T cells (NF-AT), a nuclear component that initiates gene transcription for the formation of IL-2 (Figure 17-1). As a result, T-lymphocyte activation is inhibited.[46] The mechanism of action of cyclosporine is similar, except that the binding protein is cyclophilin. Tacrolimus is 10–100 times more potent than cyclosporine in its immunosuppressive effects.[112]

PHARMACOKINETIC PROPERTIES

The pharmacokinetic characteristics of calcineurin inhibitors show high interindividual and intraindividual variability, and the drugs have a narrow therapeutic index; therapeutic drug monitoring is necessary to optimize treatment. Because 90% of the agents is partitioned in the cellular components of blood, whole-blood concentrations correlate better with drug exposure (area under the curve) than do plasma concentrations.[27]

PHARMACOGENETICS

The absorption, bioavailability, and elimination of these drugs are primarily controlled by efflux pumps and enzymes of the cytochrome P (CYP) 450 family. DNA

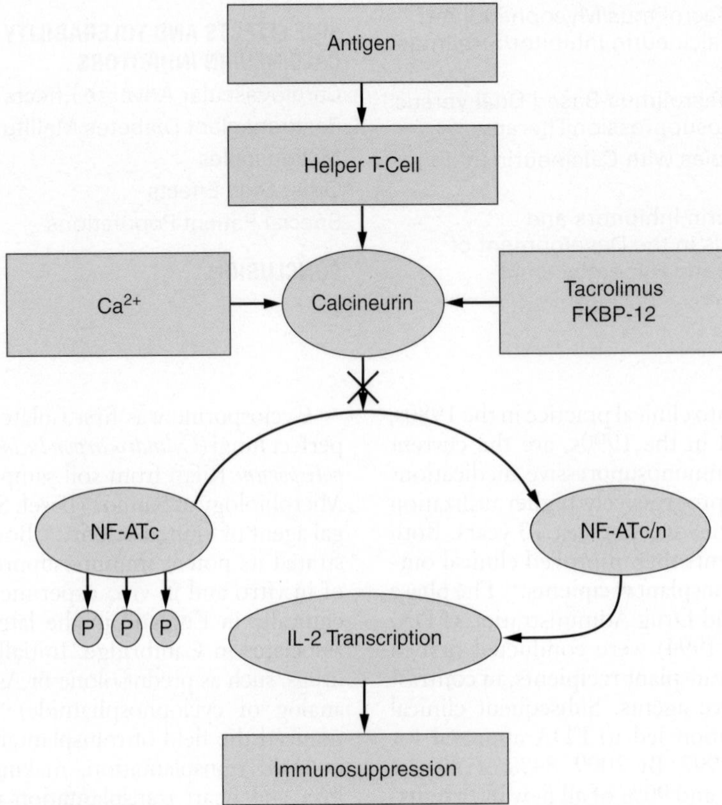

FIGURE 17–1 ■ Mechanism of action of tacrolimus. A complex is formed of tacrolimus–FKBP-12, calcium, calmodulin, and calcineurin, which inhibits the phosphatase activity of calcineurin. This prevents the dephosphorylation and subsequent translocation of nuclear factor of activated T cells (NF-AT), a nuclear component that initiates gene transcription for the formation of interleukin-2 (IL-2). C, cytoplasm; n, nucleus, P, phosphate. (From Fung JJ. Tacrolimus and transplantation: a decade in review. Transplantation 2004;77:S41.)

variants of the genes encoding these proteins contribute to the interindividual heterogeneity of the metabolism of calcineurin inhibitors. Cyclosporine and tacrolimus are metabolized by CYP3A4 and CYP3A5, and several single nucleotide polymorhphisms in the two genes have been associated with differences in drug clearance. Homozygotes for a common DNA variant that affects gene splicing (CYP3A5*3) may require a lower dose to remain within the target blood concentration. To date, this CYP3A5 variant is the only reported genetic factor to predict the appropriate starting dosage of tacrolimus.[30]

ABSORPTION AND DISTRIBUTION

The gastrointestinal absorption of calcineurin inhibitors is highly dependent on the presence of food, bile acids, and motility. They are rapidly but incompletely absorbed in the gastrointestinal tract, and peak concentrations in whole blood are attained 1–2 hours after oral administration.[142] Tacrolimus has low oral bioavailability (average 25%; range 4–93%).[142] The mean oral bioavailability of tacrolimus is comparable in adult (25%) and pediatric (31%) transplant recipients. The rate and extent of absorption of tacrolimus are reduced in the presence of food, with the peak concentration in whole blood compared with the fasting state decreased by approximately 50–75%, and the area under the curve decreased by 25–40% when the drug is taken after a meal.[112] Tacrolimus is highly bound to erythrocytes, in a concentration-dependent manner, with reduced ratios at higher drug concentrations related to binding saturation. Plasma protein binding may be 99%, with most of the drug bound to α_1-acid glycoprotein and albumin. Tacrolimus is widely distributed in most tissues, including the lungs, spleen, heart, kidney, pancreas, brain, muscle, and liver; tacrolimus crosses the placenta, with umbilical cord plasma concentrations one-third of those in maternal plasma.[112,142] Tacrolimus also is present in breast milk, but at extremely low levels (<2.5 ng/mL).

METABOLISM AND ELIMINATION

Cyclosporine is metabolized almost entirely in the liver, mostly through the CYP-450 system. Most of the drug is excreted in the bile, with only trace amounts being excreted in the urine. Tacrolimus is metabolized extensively in the liver as well and, to a much lesser extent, in the intestinal mucosa, with metabolism mediated at both sites by CYP3A4 isoenzymes.[112,142] Tacrolimus is converted by hydroxylation and demethylation to at least 15 metabolites, with the main metabolite being 13-*O*-dimethyltacrolimus. The mean clearance after intravenous administration of tacrolimus is as follows: 0.040 L/h/kg in healthy volunteers, 0.083 L/h/kg in adult kidney transplant patients, 0.053 L/h/kg in adult liver transplant patients, and 0.051 L/h/kg in adult heart transplant patients. When administered orally, fecal elimination accounts for 92.6±3.07% and urinary elimination accounts for 2.3 ±1.1% of the administered dose in healthy volunteers.[5]

TABLE 17-1 Drug Interactions Associated with Calcineurin Inhibitors

Drugs Increasing Tacrolimus Concentration (Cytochrome P-450 3A4 Inhibitors)
Calcium channel blockers: diltiazem, nicardipine, nifedipine, verapamil
Imidazole antifungal agents: clotrimazole, fluconazole, itraconazole, ketoconazole
Macrolide antibiotics: clarithromycin, erythromycin
Prokinetic agents: cisapride, metoclopramide
Other drugs: bromocriptine, cimetidine, corticosteroids, danazol, protease inhibitors
Grapefruit juice
Drugs Decreasing Tacrolimus Concentration (Cytochrome P-450 3A4 Inducers)
Anticonvulsants: carbamazepine, phenobarbital, phenytoin
Rifabutin/rifampicin, isoniazid
St. John's wort

The main drugs that interact with calcineurin inhibitors when administered simultaneously are either inducers or inhibitors of CYP3A4. CYP3A4 inhibitors potentially increase whole-blood concentrations, while CYP3A4 inducers decrease calcineurin inhibitor concentrations (Table 17-1).

SPECIAL PATIENT POPULATIONS

Three percent of patients require higher dosages (>0.4 mg/kg/day) to reach therapeutic tacrolimus concentrations. This is a reflection of the low bioavailability and, to a lesser extent, the high clearance of the drug.[142] In a non-blinded, parallel-group study, the bioavailability of tacrolimus was significantly ($P = 0.01$) lower in African American (11.9%) and Latin American (14.4%) patients than in white patients (18.8%).[94] A retrospective study in renal transplant recipients showed that African American recipients required higher dosages of tacrolimus on a milligram-per-kilogram basis.[142]

Children typically require higher tacrolimus dosages on a milligram-per-kilogram basis than adult patients, most likely reflecting the higher mean total body clearance and volume of distribution in children. Clinically relevant differences do not exist between adults and children, however, in terms of the time taken to reach maximal blood concentrations (2.1 hours in children versus 2 hours in adults), bioavailability (31% versus 25%), and mean terminal elimination half-life (11.5 hours versus 12 hours).[121] The mean clearance of tacrolimus in patients with renal dysfunction was similar to that in normal volunteers; tacrolimus pharmacokinetics after a single intravenous administration was similar in seven patients not receiving dialysis and five receiving dialysis.[5]

The mean clearance of tacrolimus in patients with mild hepatic dysfunction (mean Pugh score of 6.2) was not substantially different from that in normal volunteers after a single intravenous and oral dose. The mean clearance was substantially lower in patients with severe hepatic dysfunction (mean Pugh score >10), regardless of the route of administration.[5]

CLINICAL STUDIES IN KIDNEY TRANSPLANTATION

Rescue Therapy in Adults

The efficacy of tacrolimus in kidney transplantation was first shown in recipients with refractory rejection. Refractory rejection episodes in cyclosporine-treated patients were reversed by replacing cyclosporine with tacrolimus as the maintenance immunosuppressive agent. In contrast to antilymphocyte antibody preparations (e.g., OKT3 and polyclonal antibody preparations) that induce long-term suppression of T-cell responses, the immunosuppressive effects of tacrolimus could be titrated on a daily basis by following drug levels.[85]

An early large experience with tacrolimus in treating refractory acute renal allograft rejection in 77 patients receiving cyclosporine-based immunosuppressive therapy was reported from Pittsburgh.[74] Several conclusions were drawn from this study, as follows: (1) tacrolimus provided effective therapy for acute renal allograft rejection; (2) tacrolimus often provided effective therapy for vascular rejection in kidney transplants; and (3) the success of tacrolimus therapy for refractory acute renal allograft rejection was related to the severity and duration of rejection.

The 5-year follow-up of the Pittsburgh experience showed good long-term renal allograft function in patients undergoing tacrolimus rescue therapy.[72,73] A total of 169 patients were converted from cyclosporine to tacrolimus for refractory rejection, with a 74% success rate and a mean serum creatinine value of 2.3 ± 1.1 mg/dL (202 µmol/L). Of the patients receiving dialysis at the time of tacrolimus initiation, 46% were salvaged, with a mean serum creatinine level of 2.2 ± 0.4 mg/dL (189 µmol/L). Corticosteroid withdrawal was achieved in 22% of patients after conversion to tacrolimus, and the mean prednisone dose was reduced from 28 ± 1.1 to 8.5 ± 4.1 mg/day.

A prospective, randomized, multicenter comparative trial confirmed the efficacy of tacrolimus-based rescue therapy in patients with acute renal transplant rejection.[35] Rescue therapy with tacrolimus-based regimens reduced the incidence of recurrent acute rejection to 8.8% versus 34.1% (P = 0.002) in patients who remained on cyclosporine-based immunosuppression. Three-month Kaplan–Meier estimates for freedom from a second biopsy-proven acute rejection (BPAR) were 89.1% versus 61.4% (P = 0.002) in the tacrolimus-rescue and the cyclosporine continuation groups, respectively. Freedom from treatment failure was 72.6% versus 43% (P = 0.005), with treatment failure being defined as graft loss, second acute rejection, or withdrawal from treatment.

In a large European study on tacrolimus conversion for cyclosporine-induced toxicities, 73% of patients with cyclosporine-induced gingival hyperplasia (n = 32) showed significant resolution of hyperplasia, and recipients with cyclosporine-induced hypertrichosis (n = 116) showed marked improvement. The mean serum low-density lipoprotein (LDL) level decreased from 138 to 120 mg/dL, and the high-density lipoprotein levels remained unchanged in patients with cyclosporine-induced hyperlipidemia (n = 78). Finally, hypertension had markedly or completely resolved in 25% of patients (n = 75).[113]

Antibody-Mediated Rejection

Antibody-mediated rejection often occurs within the first 2 weeks after transplantation and is associated with oliguria, graft tenderness, fever, leukocytosis, and circulating antidonor antibodies. Before the introduction of tacrolimus, combinations of bolus corticosteroids, plasmapheresis, and antilymphocyte antibody preparations were used to treat acute humoral rejection, with inconsistent and unsatisfactory response rates. Tacrolimus-based regimens were developed for acute humoral rejection in renal transplant recipients, based on clinical experiences with tacrolimus in treating liver and heart transplants with acute humoral rejection.[110,154,155] Experimental evidence also supported the potential of tacrolimus in limiting antibody responses.[149,150]

Tacrolimus-based regimens for treating acute humoral rejection are based on the removal of circulating antibody at the time of the rejection episode (by plasmapheresis), suppressing the formation of new antidonor antibody with high-dose tacrolimus, and monitoring kidney allograft histology with protocol biopsies. Tacrolimus-based regimens were shown to reverse antibody-mediated rejection in renal allograft recipients.[153,156] In one series, all four patients had aggressive rejection episodes confirmed by immunohistopathology. These rejections were treated successfully with daily plasmapheresis for 5 days and high-dose tacrolimus (initial target levels 20–25 ng/mL) that resulted in reversal of rejection and allowed long-term graft survival. This regimen was not associated with life-threatening opportunistic infections or posttransplant diabetes mellitus (PTDM), despite high tacrolimus trough levels. The efficacy of tacrolimus in acute humoral rejection preceded the use of plasmapheresis and intravenous immunoglobulin regimens in the management of humoral rejection and highly sensitized patients (see Chapter 24),[153,156,159] and more recent work with bortezomib and eculizumab.

Maintenance Immunosuppression

The outcomes of kidney transplantation have improved with the advent of calcineurin inhibitors as part of highly effective immunosuppressive regimens. Several studies have addressed short-term outcomes of immunosuppression, including rates of acute rejection and patient and graft survival. Studies also have addressed medium- and long-term outcomes with calcineurin inhibitor-based immunosuppression, including 5-year patient and graft survival, renal function, cardiovascular events, and PTDM.

Comparison of Tacrolimus-Based and Cyclosporine-Based Regimens

The phase III US multicenter clinical trial compared the efficacy and safety of tacrolimus with that of the original formulation of cyclosporine.[111] At 1 year posttransplantation, 30.7% of tacrolimus-treated patients had experienced acute rejection compared with 46.4% of cyclosporine-treated patients (P = 0.001). The incidence of moderate to severe rejection was 10.8% in the tacrolimus-treated group compared with 26.5% in the cyclosporine-treated group. Intent-to-treat analysis revealed that the 1-year patient survival was 95.6% and 96.6% for the tacrolimus-treated and cyclosporine-treated patients, respectively (P = non-significant (NS)). The 1-year graft survival rate was 91.2% and 87.9% for the tacrolimus-treated and cyclosporine-treated patients, respectively (P = NS). The intent-to-treat analysis showed no significant differences in 5-year patient or graft survival between the tacrolimus-treated and the cyclosporine-treated patients. When crossover because of rejection was counted as graft failure, a statistically significant increase in graft survival was found in the tacrolimus group at 5 years (63.8% versus 53.8%; $P = 0.014$).[146] There also was a significant difference in the serum creatinine level between the tacrolimus-treated and cyclosporine-treated patients and in the number of patients who had a serum creatinine value greater than 1.5 mg/dL (tacrolimus 40.4% versus cyclosporine 62%; $P = 0.0017$). The patients treated with tacrolimus had a lower incidence of hirsutism and gingival hyperplasia, but a higher incidence of alopecia than patients treated with cyclosporine.

Racial differences also were evaluated for acute rejection in the US phase III multicenter clinical trial.[108] Among African Americans, 23.2% of patients in the tacrolimus-treated group developed acute rejection compared with 47.9% of patients in the cyclosporine-treated group ($P = 0.012$). When crossover because of rejection was counted as graft failure, there was a significant increase in the 5-year graft survival in African American patients in the tacrolimus-treated group (65.4% versus 42.6%; $P = 0.013$) compared with the cyclosporine-treated group.[145]

The US multicenter study that compared the efficacy and tolerability of tacrolimus versus cyclosporine also revealed that significantly fewer kidney transplant recipients required antihypertensive treatment in the tacrolimus-treated group compared with the cyclosporine-treated group.[69] In this 3-year multicenter comparative study, tacrolimus was associated with a significantly lower incidence of hypercholesterolemia than was cyclosporine (24% versus 38%; $P = 0.007$), and the need for lipid-lowering agents was significantly lower in the tacrolimus-treated patients (14% versus 38%; $P < 0.001$).[69] The projected graft half-life evaluated by the European Multicenter Renal Transplant Study also favored tacrolimus over cyclosporine (15.8 versus 10.8 years).[98]

All adult kidney transplants from 1995 to 2000 reported to United Network for Organ Sharing/Organ Procurement and Transplantation Network were analyzed by discharge immunosuppression.[14] The 1-, 3-, and 5-year adjusted actuarial graft survival rates with the tacrolimus-based regimens were 91.8%, 81.1%, and 69.8%, and for the cyclosporine-based regimens, these rates were 90.3%, 79.9%, and 67.5% ($P < 0.0001$).

Deceased donors reported to the Scientific Registry of Transplant Recipients Database between 1995 and 2002 were included in a study analyzing paired kidneys in which one kidney was allocated to a patient who was treated with cyclosporine microemulsion and the other kidney was allocated to a patient receiving tacrolimus therapy.[76] There was no difference in 5-year patient or graft survival. Renal function was superior in the tacrolimus-treated group at all time points. The 6-month inverse creatinine levels were significantly worse in the microemulsion cyclosporine arm compared with the tacrolimus arm ($P < 0.0001$). A study done on immunophenotyping of infiltrating cells of renal allograft biopsies from tacrolimus- or cyclosporine-treated patients showed reduced T-lymphocyte and macrophage interstitial infiltration at 4 and 6 months in the tacrolimus group compared to the cyclosporine-treated patients.[105]

In normal, healthy subjects, treatment with cyclosporine increased baseline creatinine level and blood pressure and reduced renal plasma flow and glomerular filtration rate (GFR) in otherwise normal kidneys. In contrast, treating normal human subjects with tacrolimus did not influence renal hemodynamic parameters, and the mean arterial blood pressure remained unchanged.[81]

A multicenter trial evaluated the effect of tacrolimus as secondary intervention in patients being treated with cyclosporine for 3 or more months after transplantation who had one of the following risk factors for chronic renal allograft failure: serum creatinine 2 mg/dL or greater for men and 1.7 mg/dL or greater for women, or a greater than 30% increase in the nadir posttransplant serum creatinine level. The trial randomly assigned 197 patients to convert to tacrolimus or remain on cyclosporine.[148] At 24 months, 56.8% of the patients in the tacrolimus-treated group and 87.5% in the cyclosporine-treated group had a serum creatinine level 2 mg/dL or greater ($P = 0.002$). Significantly fewer patients who were converted from cyclosporine to tacrolimus experienced a cardiovascular event compared with patients who continued treatment with cyclosporine (5.6% versus 24.3%; $P = 0.002$). Median serum cholesterol and LDL cholesterol levels were significantly lower in the tacrolimus-treated group compared with the cyclosporine-treated group. Therapeutic intervention with tacrolimus resulted in improved renal function, better lipid profiles, and fewer cardiovascular events in patients who were at risk for developing chronic renal allograft failure.[148]

Patients who have an acute rejection episode and hypercholesterolemia have a more than twofold greater risk of graft loss.[145] These combined risk factors were significantly different between treatment arms (tacrolimus 4.7% versus cyclosporine 17.4%; $P = 0.0008$). A randomized prospective study was done to compare the clinical and economic outcomes of tacrolimus versus cyclosporine in a regimen consisting of antithymocyte globulin (ATG) (Thymoglobulin) induction, and prednisone.[61] At 1 year, acute rejection, patient survival, graft survival, and the incidence of cytomegalovirus infection were similar. Creatinine levels were lower in the tacrolimus-treated group compared with the cyclosporine-treated group. The requirement for dyslipidemia treatment was statistically similar at 12 months after transplant (30% tacrolimus versus 35% cyclosporine). Total 12-month medication costs were similar ($17 723 ± $11 647 tacrolimus versus $16 515 ± $10 189 cyclosporine).[61]

A clinical study conducted in the early 1990s that compared treatment with cyclosporine versus tacrolimus found that significantly more patients who received tacrolimus-based immunosuppression developed PTDM.[146] A more recent study that compared treatment with tacrolimus versus cyclosporine found a similar incidence of PTDM for both regimens.[140] The decrease in insulin secretion caused by treatment with tacrolimus was dose-dependent and reversible. PTDM was reversible when tacrolimus blood levels were reduced. PTDM, however, did not seem to inhibit the widespread conversion from cyclosporine-to tacrolimus-based therapy in the pancreas transplant community (see below).

Comparison of Calcineurin Inhibitor/Azathioprine and Tacrolimus/Mycophenolate Mofetil Regimens

A randomized, prospective three-arm study compared the impact of immunosuppressive protocols using tacrolimus/azathioprine (n=76), tacrolimus/mycophenolate mofetil (MMF) (n=72), and cyclosporine microemulsion/MMF (n=75).[70] At 1 year, although there were no significant differences in overall rejection rates, there were significant differences in the total number of patients who required antilymphocyte antibody treatment (4.2% in the tacrolimus/MMF arm compared with 10.7% in the cyclosporine/MMF arm and 11.8% in the tacrolimus/azathioprine arm; P=0.05). There were no significant differences among the three groups in patient or graft survival at 1, 2, and 3 years.[2,49,70] In patients with delayed graft function, there was a trend toward improved graft survival in the tacrolimus-based treatment group at 1 year. This trend became significant when the tacrolimus/MMF arm was compared with the cyclosporine/MMF arm at 2 and 3 years. At 3 years, the serum creatinine level was significantly lower in the tacrolimus-treated patients than in the cyclosporine-treated patients.[49] A recent single-institution, prospective, open-labeled, randomized controlled trial comparing cyclosporine/azathioprine (n=146) versus tacrolimus/MMF (n=143) in 289 kidney transplant recipients treated with ATG and prednisone showed equal patient and graft survivals at 1 year; however, the tacrolimus/MMF group had better estimated GFR (cyclosporine/azathioprine 48±1 versus tacrolimus/MMF 53±1 mL/min/1.73 m^2, P=0.007), and a trend toward lower rates of BPAR, cyclosporine/azathioprine (14.4%) versus 11 (7.7%) with tacrolimus/MMF (P=0.07).[139]

Comparison of Tacrolimus/Mycophenolate Mofetil and Calcineurin Inhibitor/Sirolimus Regimens

Long-term posttransplant renal function is influenced by the incidence of acute rejection episodes, chronic allograft nephropathy, age of the kidney donor, and the use of calcineurin inhibitors.[146] Analysis of registry data examining the rate of change of creatinine clearance for patients who received kidney transplants between 1990 and 2000 showed that renal function improved in transplants performed after 1997. A more stable creatinine clearance was associated with tacrolimus versus cyclosporine therapy and with MMF versus azathioprine therapy.[51]

A randomized study comparing the combination of sirolimus or MMF with tacrolimus-based immunosuppression showed no significant differences in the incidence of biopsy-confirmed acute rejection (BCAR: 13% tacrolimus/sirolimus (n = 185) versus 11.4% tacrolimus/MMF (n = 176; P = 0.64).[50] Graft survival and patient survival were not significantly different between the groups at 6 months after transplantation. Significantly more recipients discontinued treatment with sirolimus (21.1% versus 10.8%; P = 0.0008). Renal function was significantly better in the tacrolimus/MMF group (serum creatinine 1.44 ± 0.45 mg/dL versus 1.77 ± 1.42 mg/dL; P = 0.018). The combination of tacrolimus and MMF was superior to tacrolimus and sirolimus in terms of improved renal function and a lower risk of hypertension and hyperlipidemia.[50]

The incidence of acute rejection was significantly higher in the tacrolimus/sirolimus arm (30% versus 2% for cyclosporine/sirolimus and 12% for tacrolimus/MMF) at 36 months in a randomized trial comparing these three regimens in renal transplantation.[57] Mean estimated GFR was consistently higher in the tacrolimus/MMF arm, epecially after controlling for donor age in a multivariate model during the first 30 months. There was not, however, a significant difference in actuarial graft survival at 8 years posttransplant among the groups. In another publication comparing the efficacy of tacrolimus and MMF with that of tacrolimus and sirolimus, the course of 97 kidney transplant patients treated with sirolimus and reduced-dose tacrolimus was reviewed. The outcomes of 19 patients who were converted to a tacrolimus/MMF protocol for various non-renal side effects were compared with 78 patients who remained on a tacrolimus/sirolimus protocol. Tacrolimus levels were increased in patients who were converted. Conversions from tacrolimus/sirolimus to tacrolimus/MMF led to improved renal function, however, despite increased tacrolimus levels after conversion.[6]

A prospective study compared the safety and efficacy of steroid avoidance in tacrolimus/MMF (n = 75) and tacrolimus/sirolimus (n = 75) in kidney transplantation. The primary end-point was acute rejection. Surveillance biopsies were done to analyze subclinical acute rejection and chronic allograft nephropathy. Clinical acute rejection and subclinical acute rejection were treated with methylprednisolone.[87] Two-year patient and graft survival, renal function, and adverse effects were monitored. Steroid avoidance under tacrolimus-based immunosuppression with MMF or sirolimus provided equivalent 2-year patient and graft survival, with a low incidence of acute rejection and new-onset diabetes mellitus. Subclinical acute rejection and chronic allograft nephropathy were lower in the tacrolimus/sirolimus group than in the tacrolimus/MMF group.

These optimistic findings were countered by an analysis of 44 915 adult renal transplants in the Scientific Renal Transplant Registry from 2000 to 2004. A total of 3524 (7.8%) patients received a baseline immunosuppressive regimen of tacrolimus/sirolimus, with an inferior overall survival (P < 0.001) and death-censored graft survival (P < 0.001) compared with tacrolimus/MMF (n = 27 007). In multivariate Cox models, the adjusted hazard ratio for overall graft loss with tacrolimus/sirolimus was 1.47 and with cyclosporine/sirolimus was 1.38 relative to tacrolimus/MMF. These effects were most apparent in high-risk transplants. Six-month acute rejection rates were low and did not differ among groups.[100] These data have to be interpreted in the context of the limitations of any retrospective database analysis.

A steroid-free randomized trial comparing sirolimus/tacrolimus, sirolimus/mycophenolate, and tacrolimus/mycophenolate showed higher than expected BCAR in the sirolimus/mycophenolate arm. The BCAR and graft survivial at 2 years for the sirolimus/tacrolimus group was 17.4% and 88.5% respectively, and for the tacrolimus/mycophenolate group 12.3% and 95.4%. Among the side effects, the sirolimus group had a higher incidence of delayed wound healing and hyperlipidemia.[44]

Comparison of Tacrolimus-Based Dual versus Triple Immunosuppression Therapy

Dual immunosuppression therapy refers to the use of tacrolimus with a second agent, such as a corticosteroid. Triple immunosuppression therapy refers to the use of tacrolimus and a corticosteroid with a third agent, such as azathioprine or MMF.

Dual therapy with tacrolimus-based immunosuppression provided similar efficacy to tacrolimus-based triple therapy for 36 months.[19,25,48,109,122,129] At 12 months, patient survival rates in the dual-therapy groups were ≥96% compared with ≥94% with triple therapy, with graft survival rates of ≥90% (dual-therapy groups) and ≥91% (triple-therapy groups). Three-year follow-up data are available from the Italian and Spanish trials, and graft survival was 87% in dual-therapy and triple-therapy groups. A similar percentage of patients experienced an acute rejection episode with dual-therapy or triple-therapy tacrolimus-based immunosuppressive regimens. Most of these episodes occurred in the first year after transplantation, with a 10–15-fold reduction in the incidence of rejection over the next 2 years.[39,109] In one study, the addition of MMF to tacrolimus plus corticosteroid therapy significantly ($P = 0.007$) reduced the incidence of rejection at 9 months.[117]

A prospective, randomized trial was performed to compare tacrolimus/prednisone with tacrolimus/azathioprine/prednisone from August 1, 1991, to October 11, 1992. With a mean follow-up of 9±4 months, the 1-year actuarial patient survival in the two-drug group was 95%, and for the three-drug group it was 91% (P=NS). One-year actuarial graft survival in the two-drug group was 90%, whereas in the three-drug group it was 82% (P=NS).[123] In another prospective, randomized trial reported from the same center, the combination of tacrolimus and prednisone was compared with tacrolimus, MMF, and prednisone in renal transplant recipients without induction therapy.[124] The combination of tacrolimus, steroids, and MMF was associated with excellent patient and graft survival and a lower incidence of rejection than the combination of tacrolimus and steroids.

Induction Therapies with Calcineurin Inhibitor Regimens

Margreiter et al.[96] studied the efficacy of alemtuzumab induction followed by tacrolimus monotherapy (n=65) compared to a control group of tacrolimus, MMF, and steroids (n=66). At 12 months the biopsy-proven rejection rate was 20% in the study group and 32% in the control group (P=0.09). Patient survival at 1 year was 98% for both groups. Graft survival was 96% for the study group versus 90% for the control group (P=0.18). A similar study compared alemtuzumab induction with tacrolimus monotherapy against daclizumab, tacrolimus, and mycophenolate therapy. The alemtuzumab and tacrolimus arm showed a survival with a functioning graft at 1 year of 97.6% versus 95.1% in the daclizumab arm and at 2 years of 92.6% versus 95.1% in the daclizumab group.[24] These results suggest that alemtuzumab induction together with tacrolimus monotherapy is at least as efficient as the daclizumab, tacrolimus, and mycophenolate or a tacrolimus, mycophenolate, and steroids regimen. The use of alemtuzumab induction with tacrolimus monotherapy was evaluated in 200 living donor kidney transplant recipients. The actuarial 3-year patient and graft survival in this study was 96.4% and 86.3%, respectively. The cumulative incidence of acute cellular rejection (ACR) at 3 years was 24%, about 88.7% of the ACR episodes were Banff 1, and of those, 82% were steroid-sensitive. The mean serum creatinine (mg/dL) and GFR (mL/min/1.73 m^2) at 3 years were 1.5±0.7 and 54.9±20.9, respectively.[132] The alemtuzumab/tacrolimus treatment was also evaluated in high immunological risk patients, as defined by a prior failed renal transplant, prior history of sensitization, or panel-reactive antibodies >20%. Patients were randomized to receive single-dose alemtuzumab prior to graft reperfusion, with tacrolimus monotherapy, or four doses of thymoglobulin with tacrolimus, mycophenolate, and steroids. One-year cumulative graft survival was 85.7% for the alemtuzumab group and 87.5% for the thymoglobulin group.[133] A similar study was done comparing the efficacy of alemtuzumab versus conventional induction therapy (basiliximab or rabbit ATG). In this trial patients were stratified according to acute rejection risk, with a high risk defined by a repeat transplant, a peak or current value of panel-reactive antibodies of 20% or more, or African American ethnicity. There were 139 high-risk patients, of whom 70 received alemtuzumab and 69 received rabbit ATG (rATG). The 335 low-risk patients were randomized to alemtuzumab (164 patients) or basiliximab (171 patients). All patients received tacrolimus and MMF and underwent a 5-day glucocorticoid taper in a regimen of early steroid withdrawal. By the first year after transplantation, BCAR was less frequent with alemtuzumab than with conventional therapy. The apparent superiority of alemtuzumab with respect to early BCAR was restricted to patients at low risk for transplant rejection; among high-risk patients, alemtuzumab and rabbit ATG had similar efficacy.[60]

In another study, alemtuzumab (n=113) or rATG (n=109) induction were compared in 180 (81%) kidney alone, 38 (17%) simultaneous pancreas–kidney (SPK), and four (2%) pancreas after kidney (PAK) transplants. Survival, initial length of stay, and maintenance immunosuppression (including early steroid elimination) were similar between alemtuzumab and rATG groups, but BPAR episodes occurred in 16 (14%) alemtuzumab patients compared with 28 (26%) rATG patients (P=0.02). Late BPAR (>12 months after transplant) occurred in one (8%) alemtuzumab patient and three (11%) rATG patients (P=NS). Infections and malignancy were similar between the two induction arms. The results of this study showed that alemtuzumab and rATG induction therapies were equally safe, but alemtuzumab was associated with less BPAR.[38]

Role of Calcineurin Inhibitors and Corticosteroids in the Development of Hypertension and Hyperglycemia

Although both calcineurin inhibitors and steroids have been associated with posttransplant hypertension and hyperglycemia, steroid dosing may have a major part in the development of these complications after transplantation (see Chapter 16). In one study, patients were evaluated 4 months after kidney transplantation; twice as many patients treated with tacrolimus and high-dose prednisone developed hypertension compared with patients treated with tacrolimus and low-dose prednisone (63% versus 32%; $P < 0.05$).[33]

Corticosteroids may promote the development of PTDM by inducing insulin resistance, decreasing insulin receptor number and affinity, impairing endogenous glucose production, and impairing glucose uptake by muscle.[120]

A study was done to assess the relative role of tacrolimus and corticosteroids in the development of glucose metabolic disorders.[10] Corticosteroid withdrawal in patients receiving tacrolimus-based immunosuppression led to a 22% decrease in fasting C-peptide levels ($P = 0.0009$). Fasting insulin levels and the insulin-to-glucose ratio also decreased but not significantly (P = NS). Steroid withdrawal also led to a reduction in lipid levels. Tacrolimus trough level reduction from 9.5 ng/mL to 6.4 ng/mL resulted in a 36% increase in pancreatic beta-cell secretion ($P = 0.04$), and insulin secretion increased by a similar rate. Hemoglobin A_{1c} improved from 5.9% to 5.3% ($P = 0.002$), although lipid levels did not change after trough level reduction.[10] Corticosteroid withdrawal resulted in a decrease in insulin resistance and a reduction in lipid levels; reduction of tacrolimus trough levels also improved glucose metabolism.

Early Corticosteroid Withdrawal Regimens

The safety of early corticosteroid withdrawal (see Chapter 14) was evaluated by a prospective, randomized, multicenter, double-blind study of early (7 days posttransplantation) corticosteroid cessation versus long-term maintenance with corticosteroids along with tacrolimus, MMF, and antibody induction in primary renal transplant patients.[158] Patient and graft survivals at 1 year were 98% and 96%, respectively. BPAR occurred in 9.8% of patients, and 4% were treated empirically for rejection. One-year analysis suggested that early withdrawal of corticosteroids was safe, resulting in excellent patient and graft survival, low acute rejection rates, and no graft loss to rejection.[152,158] Five-year results confirmed that early corticosteroid withdrawal provides a similar long-term renal allograft survival and function; however, early corticosteroid withdrawal is associated with a higher incidence of mild, Banff 1A, steroid-sensitive episodes of rejection. Steroid withdrawal provided improvements in cardiovascular risk factors (triglyceride, diabetes, weight gain).[152] A randomized trial comparing cyclosporine versus tacrolimus as long-term immunosuppression regimens following early steroid withdrawal 5 days after renal transplantation showed that tacrolimus was more effective in enabling patients to remain on a steroid-free regimen at 3 years (88% versus 65%; $P<0.001$).[117]

In another study, 101 patients underwent renal transplantation with tacrolimus, MMF, and 7 days of corticosteroids.[13] Anti-CD25 monoclonal antibody was administered to 25 patients at higher immunological risk. After a median follow-up of 51 months (range 36–62 months), patient survival was 97%, and graft survival was 91%. The incidence of acute rejection at 12 months was 19%. Only three further episodes of rejection occurred beyond 12 months. Graft function was stable during the study, with a mean estimated creatinine clearance of 57 mL/min at the end of follow-up. This steroid avoidance regimen was associated with excellent medium-term patient and graft outcomes and a low incidence of side effects. Most 10-year outcomes were described in a protocol incorporating discontinuation of steroids at postoperative day 7. The 10-year graft survival was 61% for living donor transplant and 51% for deceased donor transplants, comparable to 10-year Scientific Registry of Transplant Recipients national data.[115] The efficacy of early steroid withdrawal compared to chronic steroid maintenance has also been shown to be a reasonable approach in repeat kidney transplant recipients, with results showing similar graft and patient survivals at 1 and 5 years.[106]

Corticosteroid-Free Immunosuppression Regimens

A 6-month, open-label, multicenter, parallel-group study included 538 renal patients randomly assigned (1:1) to a daclizumab/tacrolimus/MMF regimen ($n = 260$) or a tacrolimus/MMF/corticosteroid regimen ($n = 278$).[116] The incidence of BPAR was 16.5% in both treatment groups; the incidence of biopsy-proven corticosteroid-resistant acute rejection was 4.3% and 5% in the tacrolimus/MMF/corticosteroids and daclizumab/tacrolimus/ MMF groups (P = NS). The median serum creatinine level at 6 months and overall safety profile were similar with both regimens.

A single-center, non-randomized, retrospective sequential study was used to evaluate outcomes in kidney transplant recipients given either alemtuzumab (Campath) ($n = 123$) or basiliximab ($n = 155$) in combination with a prednisone-free maintenance protocol using tacrolimus and MMF.[78] There was no significant difference in the 3-year graft and patient survival rates between the two groups. A lower rate of early (<3 months) rejection was observed in the alemtuzumab (4.1%) versus the basiliximab (11.6%) group, but rejection rates for both groups were equivalent at 1 year. Patient and graft survival and rejection rates were nearly identical between whites and

African Americans receiving alemtuzumab. The quality of renal function and the incidence of infectious complications were similar between the alemtuzumab and basiliximab groups.

Two corticosteroid-free, tacrolimus-based regimens were compared with standard triple therapy in a 6-month, phase III, open-label, parallel-group multicenter study.[147] A total of 451 patients were randomly assigned (1:1:1) to receive tacrolimus/MMF/corticosteroids, tacrolimus/MMF without induction, or tacrolimus monotherapy with basiliximab induction. The incidences of BPAR were 8.2% (triple therapy), 30.5% (tacrolimus/MMF), and 26.1% (basiliximab/tacrolimus) (P=0.001). The incidences of corticosteroid-resistant acute rejection were similar among the groups (P=NS). Graft and patient survival rates were similar among the groups. Overall safety profiles were similar. Differences were noted for anemia (24.5% versus 12.6% versus 14.5%), diarrhea (12.9% versus 17.9% versus 5.9%), and leukopenia (7.5% versus 18.5% versus 5.9%) for the triple-therapy, tacrolimus/MMF, and basiliximab/tacrolimus groups. Both corticosteroid-free regimens were equally effective in preventing acute rejection, with the basiliximab/tacrolimus regimen offering some safety benefits.[147] A prospective randomized trial was done comparing tacrolimus/sirolimus with tacrolimus/mycophenolate in renal transplant recipients using a prednisone-free regimen with over 8.5 years of follow-up. All patients received anti-IL-2 receptor antagonist (basiliximab). The tacrolimus/MMF group had overall better renal allograft survival (91% versus 70%, P=0.02); 13 patients (35.1%) in the tacrolimus/sirolimus group and 8 patients (17.8%) in the tacrolimus/MMF group experienced biopsy-proven ACR (P=0.07). By 3 months posttransplant, estimated GFR was significantly lower in the tacrolimus/sirolimus group compared with the tacrolimus/MMF group (47.7 versus 59.6 mL/min/1.73 m^2; P=0.0002), and this trend persisted throughout the follow-up period.[26]

Comparison of Corticosteroid-Sparing Regimens Using Tacrolimus-Based and Cyclosporine-Based Immunosuppression

Studies of corticosteroid-sparing protocols in patients treated with cyclosporine and MMF showed acute rejection rates to be unacceptably high among African American recipients.[1] A study examining corticosteroid withdrawal in 52 stable renal transplant recipients treated with tacrolimus and MMF showed a 98% patient survival and 92.3% graft survival.[15] The tacrolimus-based regimen was thought to promote compliance by facilitating steroid withdrawal and reducing cosmetic complications (see Chapter 16). A prospective randomized study comparing 5-year outcomes in kidney recipients maintained on four different calcineurin inhibitors based immunosuppression protocols (cyclosporine/MMF, cyclosporine/SRL, tacrolimus/MMF, tacrolimus/SRL) with basiliximab induction without long-term steroid therapy showed acceptable patient and graft survival at 5 years in all four groups.[86]

Calcineurin Inhibitor Avoidance and Low-Dose Tacrolimus Regimens

A prospective, randomized trial was performed in which 132 live donor renal allotransplant recipients were divided into two groups. Steroids and basiliximab induction were given to every patient.[59] Group A patients received low-dose tacrolimus/sirolimus as maintenance immunosuppression, whereas group B patients received MMF and sirolimus. No difference was noted in 1-year patient or graft survival between the two groups. The incidence of BPAR was slightly less in group B (P = NS). In addition, significantly better renal function was noted in group B patients 2 years after transplantation. One-year protocol biopsy specimens showed no significant differences in the chronic allograft damage index between groups. A prospective, randomized trial in renal transplantation compared sirolimus/MMF/prednisone (n = 81) with tacrolimus/MMF/prednisone (n = 84). The mean follow-up was 33 months. There was no difference in patient survival, graft survival, or the incidence of clinical acute rejection between the two groups. There also was no difference in the mean GFR measured by iothalamate clearance between the tacrolimus and sirolimus groups at 1 or 2 years.[91] At 1 year, chronicity using the Banff schema showed no difference in interstitial, tubular, or glomerular changes, but fewer chronic vascular changes in the sirolimus group. This study suggests that many of the promises of calcineurin inhibitor-free immunosuppression have perhaps not been achieved with short-term follow-up. The question of improved safety and efficacy in the longer term with calcineurin inhibitor-free immunosuppression has to be subjected to longer-term follow-up of the aforementioned study and similar studies.[99] Many previous studies of complete calcineurin inhibitor avoidance have used cyclosporine as the comparator drug. In one study, the GFR caculated by the abbreviated Modified Diet in Renal Disease in a group of patients receiving basiliximab induction and then randomized to sirolimus/MMF/steroids or cyclosporine/MMF/steroids was 66.6 mL/min and 50 mL/min at 5 years (P=0.0075) respectively.[42] In a similar study comparing sirolimus/MMF/steroid versus tacrolimus/MMF/steroid, the tacrolimus group had a iothalamate calculated GFR of 61 ± 17 mL/min at 2 years.[91] A meta-analysis of 19 randomized controlled trials with analysis of 3312 renal transplant recipients with median follow-up of 12 months showed that calcineurin inhibitor-sparing strategies with adjunctive mycophenolate can achieve comparable short-term graft function.[104]

A lower tacrolimus exposure regimen was evaluated by Ekberg et al.[37] In this trial, 1645 renal transplant recipients were randomly assigned to receive standard-dose cyclosporine, MMF, and corticosteroids, or daclizumab induction, MMF, and corticosteroids in combination with low-dose cyclosporine (target trough 50–100 ng/mL), low-dose tacrolimus (target trough 3–7 ng/mL), or low-dose sirolimus (target trough 3–7 ng/mL). At 12 months the mean calculated GFR was higher in patients receiving low-dose tacrolimus (65.4 mL/min) than in the other three groups. The rate of BPAR was lower in patients receiving low-dose tacrolimus (12.3%) than in those receiving standard-dose cyclosporine (25.8%), low-dose cyclosporine (24.0%), or low-dose sirolimus (37.2%). One-year allograft survival differed significantly among the four groups ($P=0.02$) and was highest in the low-dose tacrolimus group (94.2%), followed by the low-dose cyclosporine group (93.1%), the standard-dose cycloosporine group (89.3%), and the low-dose sirolimus group (89.3%).[37] An observational 2-year follow-up to this study showed that the mycophenolate and low-dose tacrolimus (GFR 68.6±23.8 mL/min) arm continued to have the highest GFR compared to standard-dose cyclosporine, low-dose cyclosporine, and low-dose sirolimus (65.9±26.2, 64.0±23.1, and 65.3±26.2 mL/min respectively), but the difference was not significant ($P=0.17$). The mycophenolate and low-dose tacrolimus arm also had the highest graft survival rate, but with reduced differences between groups over time, and the least acute rejection rate.[36]

Belatacept, a selective costimulation blocker, was designed to provide effective immunosuppression and avoid the renal and non-renal side effects associated with calcineurin inhibitors.[90] The BENEFIT study was a randomized 3-year, phase III study in adults receiving a kidney transplant from a living or standard criteria deceased donor. Patients were randomized to a more or less intensive regimen of belatacept, or cyclosporine. In all, 471/666 patients completed ≥3 years of therapy. A total of 92% (more intensive), 92% (less intensive), and 89% (cyclosporine) of patients survived with a functioning graft. The mean calculated GFR was ~21 mL/min/1.73 m^2 higher in the belatacept groups versus cyclosporine at year 3. From month 3 to month 36, the mean calculated GFR increased in the belatacept groups by +1.0 mL/min/1.73 m^2/year (more intensive) and +1.2 mL/min/1.73 m^2/year (less intensive) versus a decline of −2.0 mL/min/1.73 m^2/year (cyclosporine). One cyclosporine-treated patient experienced acute rejection between year 2 and year 3. Belatacept-treated patients at 3 years maintained a high rate of patient and graft survival that was comparable to cyclosporine-treated patients, despite an early increased occurrence of acute rejection and posttransplant lymphoproliferative disorder (PTLD).[144]

Other Calcineurin Inhibitors and Formulations

One of the major risk factors for graft failure is noncompliance with medication regimens. Advagraf (Tac-OD), a once-daily formulation, was introduced by Astellas in 2008 to contribute potentially to improve medication compliance. In phase I and II trials, Advagraf showed equivalent pharmacokinetic parameters (C_0 and area under the curve (AUC_{0-24})) of Tac-OD compared to the twice-daily Prograf formulation (Tac-BID) in healthy controls, de novo kidney transplant recipients, and stable kidney transplant recipients after conversion. However, several follow-up reports indicate that the use of Tac-OD in de novo or stable transplant recipients was associated with a considerably lower tacrolimus exposure, with studies reporting a systematic 10–20% lower AUC_{0-24} in comparison to Tac-BID.[31,64] Advagraf was not approved by the FDA in the United States.

Voclosporin (VCS, ISA247) is a novel calcineurin inhibitor in development for organ transplantation. PROMISE was a phase IIb, 6-month multicenter, randomized, open-label study of three ascending concentration-controlled groups of VCS (low, medium, and high) versus tacrolimus in 334 de novo kidney transplant recipients. This 6-month study showed VCS to be as efficacious as tacrolimus in preventing acute rejection (VCS low 10.7%, medium 9.1%, and high 2.3% versus tacrolimus 5.8%) with similar renal function in the low- and medium-exposure groups.[18]

Sandimmune, the original, oil-based formulation of cyclosporine (Sandimmune; Novartis, Basel, Switzerland) was introduced in 1983. Although a significant advance in immunosuppressive therapy, this formulation had numerous problems. Absorption was slow and showed a great deal of intrapatient and interpatient variability, making dosing difficult and increasing the risk of chronic rejection.[75,84]

In 1995, Neoral (Sandimmune Neoral; Novartis, Basel, Switzerland), a microemulsion formulation of cyclosporine, was approved for use by the FDA. This new formulation improved bioavailability with more rapid absorption and less variability in de novo and stable transplant patients.[83,84] Since its introduction, numerous randomized and non-randomized studies have showed lower acute rejection rates, although similar long-term patient and graft survival when compared to the Sandimmune formulation.[76,92,]

Pediatric Renal Transplantation (see Chapter 37)

The efficacy of tacrolimus as an immunosuppressive agent in pediatric renal transplantation has been shown in single-center experiences and in multicenter trials. A retrospective cohort study of 986 pediatric renal transplant recipients in the North American Pediatric Renal Transplant Cooperative Study (NAPRTCS) database (index renal transplant 1997 through 2000), who were treated with either cyclosporine/MMF/steroids ($n=766$) or tacrolimus/MMF/steroids ($n=220$), was performed to examine differences in outcome between these two groups.[107] In this analysis, tacrolimus and cyclosporine, in combination with MMF and steroids, were associated with similar rejection rates and graft survival in pediatric renal transplant recipients. Tacrolimus was associated with improved graft function at 1 and 2 years after transplantation. A 6-month, randomized, prospective, open, parallel-group study with an open extension phase was conducted in 18 centers from nine European countries to compare the efficacy and safety of tacrolimus with cyclosporine in pediatric renal transplant recipients.[40] The study randomly assigned (1:1) 196 pediatric patients (<18 years old) to receive either tacrolimus ($n=103$) or cyclosporine microemulsion ($n=93$), administered concomitantly with azathioprine and corticosteroids. The primary end-point was incidence and time to first acute rejection. At 1 year, tacrolimus therapy was associated with a significantly lower incidence of acute rejection (36.9%) compared with cyclosporine (59.1%; $P=0.003$). At 4 years, patient survival was similar, but graft survival significantly favored tacrolimus over cyclosporine (86% versus 69%; $P=0.025$). At 1, 2, 3, and 4 years, the mean

GFR was significantly better in the tacrolimus group than in the cyclosporine group. Three patients in each arm developed posttransplant lymphoproliferative disorder, and the incidence of diabetes mellitus was similar in the two groups. Tacrolimus was significantly more effective than cyclosporine in preventing acute rejection in pediatric renal transplant recipients. Renal function and graft survival also were superior with tacrolimus.[40] The addition of basiliximab to a tacrolimus-based regimen (tacrolimus/azathioprine/steroids) did not show any improved clinical efficacy at 6 months in a pediatric patient population with similar BPAR rates (20.4% without basiliximab versus 19.2% with basiliximab) and GFR (79.4 without basiliximab versus 77.6 mL/min/1.73 m^2 with basiliximab).[52]

The effect of corticosteroids on the epiphyseal growth plates is well recognized and results in irreversible growth stunting. Experience with corticosteroid withdrawal under tacrolimus therapy in pediatric patients has been associated with favorable outcomes. Two-thirds of the pediatric kidney transplant recipients were withdrawn successfully from corticosteroids, with a low incidence of graft dysfunction or acute rejection (23%).[125] Many of these patients had remarkable catch-up growth. Changes in kidney function, mixed lymphocyte culture, cell-mediated lympholysis, cytotoxic antibodies, lymphocyte populations, and cytokine response were studied in 14 pediatric renal transplant recipients with chronic rejection who were converted to tacrolimus. Serum creatinine levels decreased, creatinine clearance increased, and urinary protein excretion decreased after 6 months, and these values were maintained after 2 years under tacrolimus treatment.[39]

In one study eight pediatric renal transplant recipients (median age at transplant 2 years; range 1.2–12.9 years) were converted to tacrolimus and sirolimus-based immunosuppression as rescue therapy. All patients had biopsy-proven chronic allograft nephropathy. After the addition of sirolimus, the median dose required to keep tacrolimus blood trough concentrations within the target range increased by 71.2% (range 21.9–245.4%), and the dose-normalized tacrolimus exposure (area under the curve) decreased to 67.1%. Adding sirolimus to tacrolimus-based immunosuppression in young pediatric renal transplant recipients resulted in a significant decrease in tacrolimus exposure.[41]

CLINICAL STUDIES IN KIDNEY–PANCREAS TRANSPLANTATION (SEE CHAPTER 36)

The increase in the number of pancreas transplants has been made possible by technical improvements and improved immunosuppressive regimens. Treatment with tacrolimus-based immunosuppression has been associated with lower rejection rates, higher graft survival rates, and less nephrotoxicity compared to treatment with cyclosporine.[20,55]

Simultaneous Pancreas–Kidney Transplantation

In an analysis of 1194 pancreas transplantations performed at the University of Minnesota, the results were divided into five time periods ("eras") based on the technique and immunosuppressive regimen used.[130] In era II, the immunosuppressive regimen consisted of Minnesota antilymphocytic globulin (MALG) or muromonab-CD3 (OKT3) for induction and a combination of cyclosporine, azathioprine, and prednisone for maintenance. Duct management in eras II and III was by bladder drainage. In era III, tacrolimus was used for pancreas transplantation as soon as it was approved by the FDA in 1994. Induction was with equine ATG (Atgam), and OKT3 was used for treatment of rejection episodes. When MMF was approved a year later, it was added to the maintenance immunosuppressive regimen. In era IV, which began in March 1998, daclizumab, alone or in combination with the polyclonal anti-T-cell antibody (Atgam or ATG), was added to the induction regimen. Enteric drainage was the principal exocrine drainage technique. In patients with primary SPK transplantation, pancreas and kidney graft survival rates were significantly higher in eras III and IV than in era II. In eras III and IV combined, 1-year patient, pancreas, and kidney survival rates were 92%, 79%, and 88%, respectively; at 5 years, the corresponding figures were 88%, 73%, and 81%, respectively.[130]

In a prospective, randomized trial, 42 SPK recipients received ATG and daclizumab induction, with tacrolimus and steroids as baseline immunosuppression. Twenty-two patients were randomly assigned to receive MMF, and 20 patients received sirolimus in addition to tacrolimus and steroids. Actuarial patient, kidney, and pancreas allograft survivals were 100%, 100%, and 95%, respectively, at 6 months in the sirolimus group and 100%, 100%, and 100%, respectively, in the MMF group. The incidence of acute rejection was less than 10% and was limited to instances in which recipient immunosuppression was reduced.[16]

A prospective study of combined tacrolimus, MMF, and steroids without antibody induction was done in 17 SPK transplant patients. Low-dose intravenous tacrolimus was used as induction therapy. Clinical and biopsy-proven rejection occurred in four (23%) patients. Patients who developed rejection had low tacrolimus levels or had had discontinuation of MMF because of leukopenia, gastroparesis, or gastrointestinal side effects.[28] All rejection episodes responded to steroids.

Immunosuppression for SPK transplantation at Northwestern University was divided into four eras over an 8.5-year period.[79] In era I (March 1993 to February 1997), three immunosuppression combinations were used: cyclosporine/azathioprine/steroids (n = 28), cyclosporine/MMF/steroids (n = 8), or tacrolimus/MMF/steroids (n = 10); bladder drainage was used. In era II (July 1995 to February 1998), the combination of tacrolimus, MMF, and corticosteroids was used, with bladder drainage. In era III, combinations of tacrolimus (12-hour trough concentrations 10–12 ng/mL) and MMF (3 g/day) were used along with corticosteroids for maintenance immunosuppression; enteric drainage was used. In era IV, steroids were eliminated within 6 days of transplantation, and tacrolimus was combined with either MMF (n = 20) or sirolimus (n = 38); enteric drainage was used.

In eras I and II, all recipients received induction therapy with Atgam for 7–14 days after transplantation. In era III, for induction therapy, 17 patients were randomly assigned to a non-induction therapy arm, and 37 patients were randomly assigned to an anti-IL-2 receptor monoclonal antibody (daclizumab, $n = 35$; basiliximab, $n = 2$). Induction therapy in era IV consisted of rabbit ATG, 1 mg/kg intraoperatively and on postoperative days 1, 2, 4, 6, 8, 10, 12, and 14. One-year actuarial patient survival rates in eras III and IV were 96.3% and 100%, respectively; 1-year actuarial kidney survival rates in eras III and IV were 94.4% and 97.7%, respectively, and the 1-year actuarial pancreas survival rates were 88.9% and 100%, respectively. The 1-year rejection-free rate was 87.1% for era III and 96.6% for era IV. Compared with era I, kidney function significantly improved over the three eras. Rapid elimination of corticosteroids was successful in all recipients in era IV, with higher patient and graft survival rates than in the previous three eras. Rejection rates decreased further in era IV. The Northwestern group concluded that corticosteroids could be rapidly eliminated prospectively in all recipients without a decrease in graft survival rates or an increase in the rate of rejection.[79]

The incidence of cytomegalovirus and malignancies was not higher using tacrolimus/MMF compared with the cyclosporine/azathioprine regimen, with 5 years' follow-up.

A multicenter trial was done to assess the effect of antibody induction in SPK transplant recipients receiving tacrolimus, MMF, and corticosteroids.[17] The trial randomly assigned 174 SPK transplant recipients to induction ($n = 87$) or non-induction ($n = 87$), and the recipients were followed for 3 years. Induction agents included T-cell-depleting or IL-2 receptor antibodies. At 3 years, actual patient (94.3% and 89.7%) and pancreas (75.9% and 75.9%) survival rates were similar in the induction and non-induction groups. Actual kidney survival was significantly better in the induction group compared with the non-induction group at 3 years (92% versus 82%; $P = 0.04$).[17]

The EuroSPK Study Group, which compared tacrolimus and cyclosporine in primary SPK transplantation, enrolled 205 patients.[89] After antilymphocyte globulin induction, patients were randomly assigned to receive either tacrolimus or cyclosporine microemulsion together with MMF and steroids. At 1 year after transplantation, patient and kidney survival rates were excellent in both treatment groups. There was a significant difference in pancreas graft survival: 94.2% for tacrolimus and 73.9% for cyclosporine ($P = 0.00048$). There were significantly fewer grade 2 and grade 3 rejections with tacrolimus-based therapy. The EuroSPK group also presented data showing that 34 patients were switched from cyclosporine to tacrolimus, but only 6 patients receiving tacrolimus required conversion to alternative therapy during the course of the study.[9] The mean doses of MMF at 1 year also were lower in the tacrolimus group (1.36 g/day versus 1.67 g/day; $P = 0.007$). Good results have been shown in smaller studies as well (17 SPK transplantation, 5 PAK transplantation, and 6 pancreas transplant alone) with the use of alemtuzumab 30 mg induction, Prograf and mycophenolate immunosuppression, with patient and graft survival of 100% and 100% at 3 years.[138]

Steroid Withdrawal and Steroid-Free Protocols

Reduction of steroid use is extremely desirable in pancreas transplantation because long-term steroid use is associated with hypertension, hyperlipidemia, and glucose intolerance.[44] Complete steroid withdrawal was achieved in 58 (47%) of 124 patients transplanted at the University of Pittsburgh, with a mean time to steroid withdrawal of 15.2 ± 8 months.[71] Patient, pancreas, and kidney survival rates at 1 year were 100%, 100%, and 98%, respectively (off steroids) versus 97%, 91%, and 96%, respectively (on steroids; all P = NS). The cumulative risk of rejection was 74% for patients off steroids versus 76% for patients on steroids (these patients had not received antibody induction). The mean glycosylated hemoglobin levels were 5.2 ± 0.9% (off steroids) and 6.2 ± 2.1% (on steroids; $P = 0.02$). The Pittsburgh group concluded that steroid withdrawal could be achieved in pancreas transplant patients under tacrolimus-based immunosuppression and was associated with excellent patient and graft survival.[71]

A single-center, retrospective, sequential study from Northwestern University of 59 SPK patients demonstrated the efficacy of a steroid-free immunosuppresion regimen at 5 years with a kidney allograft survival of 90.7% and a pancreas allograft survival of 100% in the setting of thymoglobulin induction, tacrolimus/MMF regimen.[47]

The Minnesota Group reported a prospective trial of steroid withdrawal in pancreas transplantation.[56] Recipients with functioning grafts ≥6 and 36 months after SPK transplantation or PAK transplantation were enrolled. All patients received triple therapy for maintenance immunosuppression using tacrolimus and MMF, with the following inclusion criteria: (1) low maintenance steroid dose 0.075 mg/kg/day; (2) MMF dose ≥750 mg orally twice a day; and (3) tacrolimus levels ≥8 ng/mL. Fifty-five patients (29 SPK, 26 PAK) were randomly assigned to remain on steroids or to steroid withdrawal after 4–8 weeks. The median follow-up was 27 months in the SPK category and 26 months in the PAK category, and from randomization, 10 months in both categories. Steroid withdrawal 6 months after a successful pancreas transplant was not associated with a decrease in patient or graft survival, and it was not associated with an increase in the incidence of rejection or in the rate of graft loss from rejection. There was a better quality of life and a reduction in serum cholesterol levels in the steroid withdrawal group.[56]

Rapid corticosteroid elimination was carried out in 40 SPK recipients from Northwestern University in Chicago.[80] ATG was used for induction; maintenance immunosuppression was with tacrolimus/MMF in 20 patients and tacrolimus/sirolimus in 20 patients. Patient and graft survival rates and rejection rates were compared with historical controls ($n = 86$). One-year actuarial patient, kidney, and pancreas survival rates in the rapid corticosteroid elimination group were 100%, 100%, and 100%, respectively, and in the historical control group rates were 97%, 93%, and 97%, respectively. The 1-year rejection-free survival rate was 97% in the rapid corticosteroid elimination recipients versus 80% in the historical controls. Serum creatinine levels remained stable in all groups at 6 and 12 months after transplantation.[80]

Steroid-free immunosuppression has been used with excellent short-term results in low-risk pancreas–kidney transplantation recipients at the University of California at San Francisco.[45] Forty patients underwent pancreas–kidney transplantation from November 2000 to July 2002. ATG induction was combined with MMF, tacrolimus, and sirolimus for maintenance immunosuppression. Steroids were used as pretreatment only, given with ATG and discontinued by the end of the first postoperative week. Patient, kidney, and pancreas survival rates were 95%, 92.5%, and 87.5%, respectively. Biopsy-proven pancreas rejection rates at 1 and 3 months after transplantation were 2.5%, and kidney rejection rates at 1 and 3 months were 2.5%.[45]

Pancreas after Kidney Transplantation

According to data from the International Pancreas Transplant Registry, the current, nearly uniform use of tacrolimus/MMF in PAK transplantation makes a comparison with other regimens difficult, although graft survival rates have been significantly better than in the preceding era, when cyclosporine/azathioprine was used.[54]

In the overall analysis of tacrolimus/MMF-treated primary PAK transplant recipients, graft survival rates did not differ significantly whether or not antibody induction was given, although they tended to be numerically higher in PAK recipients given depleting or non-depleting antibody than in recipients not given antibody induction. In the PAK category, the relative risk of pancreas graft failure was reduced by the use of tacrolimus/MMF for immunosuppression.[54]

Between July 1, 1978, and April 30, 2002, 406 PAK transplants were performed at the University of Minnesota.[53] Immunosuppression was divided into eras. In era III, tacrolimus was used in combination with prednisone and initially azathioprine. MMF replaced azathioprine when it was approved by the FDA. Polyclonal antibody induction therapy with Atgam was used in 99%, and monoclonal antibody (OKT3) was used in 1% of patients; the median duration of antibody therapy was 5 days. In era IV, tacrolimus, MMF, and prednisone were the principal maintenance immunosuppressive agents. Daclizumab was used for induction either alone (21%) or in combination (79%) with a polyclonal antibody (Atgam or ATG). The median duration of antibody therapy was 3 days. Overall patient survival rates (deceased and living donor) at 1 and 3 years were 97% and 90%, respectively, and at 1 year in era IV overall survival was 96%. Overall pancreas graft survival rates (deceased and living donor) at 1 and 3 years in era III were 78% and 60%, respectively, and in era IV, at 1 year overall graft survival was 77%. Of technically successful transplants, pancreas graft loss rates to rejection in era III at 1 and 3 years were 10% and 19%, respectively; in era IV, at 1 year, it was 9%. PAK transplants now can be performed almost as successfully as SPK transplants; the introduction of tacrolimus and MMF in the mid-1990s contributed to this development.

Using tacrolimus-based and MMF-based immunosuppression, only 20% of recipients experiencing rejection episodes ultimately lost their pancreas graft to irreversible rejection. In eras III and IV, when tacrolimus was being used, there no longer existed a difference in outcome between primary transplants and second transplants.

SIDE EFFECTS AND TOLERABILITY OF CALCINEURIN INHIBITORS

The side-effect profile of tacrolimus is somewhat similar to that of cyclosporine (Table 17-2). The physiological effects, including reduction in renal blood flow and glomerular filtration, are also similar between tacrolimus and cyclosporine. The pathological manifestations of tacrolimus and cyclosporine toxicity are similar in that they include tubular vacuolization and arteriolar nodular hyalinosis that are indistinguishable. Microvascular changes involving arterioles or glomerular capillaries sometimes predominate, displaying a wide spectrum of severity from apoptosis and vacuolization of smooth-muscle cells to thrombotic microangiopathy.

A review of 21 patients with tacrolimus-associated thrombotic microangiopathy was published[136]; 17 of these occurred in kidney transplant recipients, whereas two cases occurred in liver transplant recipients and one each in heart and bone marrow transplant recipients. The mean time from transplantation to the onset of thrombotic microangiopathy was 9.3 ± 7.9 months. Clinical presentation varied from an absence of signs and symptoms of hemolysis to florid hemolytic anemia, thrombocytopenia, and azotemia. Renal biopsy specimens were obtained from the patients with a kidney transplant and showed acute thrombi within the glomerular capillaries, arterioles, or both. There are large circulating polymers of von Willebrand's factor in thrombotic microangiopathy, which increases the tendency for platelets to adhere to and aggregate on the subendothelium, resulting in thrombi and fibrin deposition. Treatment consists of reducing the dose of tacrolimus and substitution with cyclosporine or sirolimus. Other treatment modalities have included plasmapheresis, fresh frozen plasma exchange, and anticoagulation.[136]

TABLE 17-2 Adverse Effects Associated with Tacrolimus Therapy

Nephrotoxicity
Reduced renal blood flow, glomerular perfusion
Tubular and vascular toxicity
Neurotoxicity
Headaches, tremors, seizures, peripheral neuropathy, paresthesias
Metabolic disturbances
Hyperkalemic, hyperchloremic acidosis
Hypomagnesemia
Diabetes mellitus
Hyperuricemia
Hypercholesterolemia
Hypertension
Gastrointestinal disturbances
Diarrhea
Anorexia, nausea, and vomiting
Epigastric cramping
Cosmetic
Alopecia

Adverse events dictate the optimal dosage regimen of the drug. Decreasing the dosage of tacrolimus generally reduces its toxic effects, although some adverse effects are idiosyncratic and do not respond to such measures.[121] Tacrolimus treatment is associated with a higher incidence of diarrhea, disturbances in glucose metabolism, and some types of neurotoxicity, but a lower incidence of hypertension and hypercholesterolemia than with cyclosporine. Tacrolimus is only rarely associated with the cyclosporine-specific adverse effects of hirsutism, gum hyperplasia, and gingivitis, but it may cause alopecia and pruritus.

In a trial in renal transplant recipients, significantly fewer (all $P < 0.05$) tacrolimus recipients (compared with cyclosporine microemulsion recipients) experienced new-onset or worsening hypertension (15.7% versus 23.2%), urinary tract disorders (4.9% versus 9.2%), hypercholesterolemia (4.2% versus 8.9%), hyperbilirubinemia (0.3% versus 3.3%), gastrointestinal hemorrhage (0.3% versus 2.6%), cholestatic jaundice (0.3% versus 2.6%), hirsutism (0% versus 4.4%), and gum hyperplasia (0% versus 4.1%).[82] Tremor (12.2% versus 4.1% of patients), hypomagnesemia (6.6% versus 1.5%), thrombosis (4.5% versus 1.5%, mainly affecting the dialysis access vessels), and gastritis (3.1% versus 0.4%) were significantly (all $P < 0.05$) more common in the tacrolimus group. Another less common but serious side effect includes posterior reversible encephalopathy syndrome with an incidence of 0.49% in a recent report.[8]

Because tacrolimus and cyclosporine cause acute and chronic nephrotoxicity, concomitant use of these two agents is contraindicated. Nephrotoxicity related to tacrolimus treatment is dose-related and responds to dosage reduction.[127] Mean or median serum creatinine levels in renal transplant recipients were lower in tacrolimus-treated patients, with 5 years' follow-up, than in patients treated with cyclosporine microemulsion (or standard formulation).[58,145] Administration of other nephrotoxic agents simultaneously can exacerbate the adverse effects of tacrolimus. Examples of such agents include aminoglycosides, angiotensin-converting enzyme inhibitors, angiotensin receptor antagonists, amphotericin, and non-steroidal anti-inflammatory drugs.

Cardiovascular Adverse Effects

Hyperlipidemia occurs commonly after transplantation and is a risk factor for cardiovascular disease. Immunosuppression with tacrolimus-based regimens is associated with better lipid profiles than is immunosuppression with cyclosporine-based regimens.[4,95]

Analysis of the United States Renal Data System database showed that fewer tacrolimus (than cyclosporine) recipients had at least one new-onset hyperlipidemia code during the first year of treatment (11% versus 16%; $P = 0.0001$); a multivariate analysis showed that the risk of new-onset hypertension after transplantation was reduced by 35% under tacrolimus-based immunosuppression.[119] The 5-year follow-up results from a US randomized trial indicated that significantly fewer tacrolimus than cyclosporine recipients were receiving antihypertensive treatment (80.9% versus 91.3%; $P < 0.05$).[145]

Concentric increases in left ventricular posterior wall and interventricular septum thickness can occur with tacrolimus immunosuppression in 0.1% of patients.[29] This condition is reversible after dosage reduction or discontinuation of the drug.

Posttransplant Diabetes Mellitus

PTDM is a serious adverse effect of tacrolimus treatment; the complications of diabetes mellitus can result in decreased patient and graft survival.[103] PTDM is defined as insulin use for more than 30 consecutive days in the absence of pre-existing diabetes. The incidence of PTDM was significantly higher in tacrolimus-treated patients than cyclosporine-treated patients (9.8% versus 2.7%), according to a meta-analysis by Heisel et al.[63]

Disturbance in glucose metabolism, with rates as high as 26% for a cyclosporine-treated group compared to 33.6% in a tacrolimus group at 6 months, were reported in a recent study using a strict American Diabetes Association definition for new-onset diabetes after transplant and impaired fasting glucose.[143] In corticosteroid minimization trials, the 6-month incidence of PTDM (use of insulin >30 days) in the corticosteroid-free arm ranged from 0.4% to 1.4%.[23,71] Tacrolimus target trough levels have tended to be lower and more rapidly tapered in recent years; this also has led to a decrease in the incidence of PTDM.[102] The introduction of MMF and sirolimus and the use of combinations of these agents with tacrolimus has led to a reduction in acute rejection rates and a reduction in corticosteroid treatment for acute rejection episodes in the first year after transplantation; this also has resulted in a reduced incidence of PTDM in recent years.

A study from Cleveland compared the outcomes of 56 African American adult primary kidney transplant recipients treated with corticosteroids, sirolimus, and tacrolimus, targeted to low trough blood levels, with 65 white patients treated with steroids, MMF, and tacrolimus, targeted to higher blood levels. There were no significant differences in the actuarial 2-year patient, graft, and rejection-free graft survival rates between the two groups. PTDM occurred in 36% of the African American patients, however, despite similar doses of corticosteroids and lower trough levels of tacrolimus, compared with 15% of white patients ($P = 0.024$).[65]

Recipient-related risk factors for PTDM include an underlying glucose metabolic disorder (e.g., family history of diabetes mellitus, older recipient age, non-white ethnicity, sedentary lifestyle, higher body mass index) and hepatitis C virus positivity. Transplantation-related risk factors include acute rejection during first posttransplant year, high doses of corticosteroids, and high tacrolimus trough levels.

The risk of developing PTDM is highest in the first few months after transplantation, after which the incidence increases more slowly. The European multicenter trial found a 6-month PTDM incidence of 4.5% and an additional incidence of 0.4% from months 7 through 12.[82]

Many patients with PTDM can have reversal of diabetes mellitus, with eventual discontinuation of insulin. In the European trial, the 1-year cumulative incidence of

PTDM with tacrolimus was 8.3%, whereas the prevalence at 1 year was 5.5%.[97] In a US trial combining tacrolimus with MMF and corticosteroids, the 1-year incidence was 6.5%, and the 1-year prevalence was 2.2%.[70]

High levels of FKBP-12 are present in pancreatic beta cells, and this is associated with a decrease in insulin mRNA transcription and reduced insulin production in rats.[131] In the clinical setting, tacrolimus affects insulin secretion but does not affect insulin resistance. In addition, PTDM is probably not a separate entity but a consequence of an underlying glucose metabolic disorder that is uncovered by immunosuppression.[118] The effects of tacrolimus on insulin release are reversible, and after the early posttransplant period, tacrolimus and cyclosporine are equivalent in terms of their effect on glucose metabolism.[141]

Compared with cyclosporine-treated patients, the relative risk for developing PTDM in tacrolimus-treated patients was 1.53 ($P < 0.001$).[77] Compared with cyclosporine-treated patients, tacrolimus therapy was associated with a reduced risk of death (relative risk 0.65; $P < 0.001$) and graft failure (relative risk 0.70; $P < 0.001$). Under tacrolimus-based immunosuppression, the positive effects of lower blood pressure, less hypercholesterolemia, better renal function, and lower fibrinogen[7] offset the negative effect of PTDM.

Evidence from a meta-analysis suggests that targeting tacrolimus concentrations to less than 10 ng/mL minimizes graft loss and reduces the risk of diabetes mellitus without increasing the risk of acute rejection.[151] A recent trial by Hecking et al. suggests that treatment with basal insulin in the immediate postoperative period may reduce the incidence of new-onset diabetes mellitus after renal transplantation, presumably via insulin-mediated protection of B cells.[62]

Malignancies (see Chapters 34 and 35)

The use of immunosuppressive agents increases the risk of malignancy, the most common being malignancies of the skin and lymphoma. All agents increase these risks, and the risk is related to the intensity and duration of treatment. Epstein–Barr virus-related posttransplant lymphoproliferative disorder is associated with immunosuppressive treatment, with a lower risk in adults than in children. In the European Multicenter Renal Study, the incidence of posttransplant lymphoproliferative disorder at 1-year follow-up was 1% in the tacrolimus group and 0.7% in the cyclosporine microemulsion group.[97] The incidence of posttransplant lymphoproliferative disorder in pediatric renal transplant patients with tacrolimus immunosuppression was 0.96% based on an analysis of the NAPRTCS database.[32]

Other Side Effects

Tacrolimus-treated patients are more likely to have alopecia, tremor, headache, insomnia, dyspepsia, vomiting, diarrhea, and hypomagnesemia than cyclosporine-treated patients.[151] Cyclosporine-treated patients are more likely to have constipation, hirsutism, and gingival hyperplasia.

Special Patient Populations

In a large, randomized multicenter trial involving pediatric renal transplant recipients (children and adolescents), the most common (3% of patients) adverse events associated with tacrolimus-based primary immunosuppression were hypertension, infections, hypomagnesemia, increased mean serum creatinine, diarrhea, PTDM, and tremor.[137] Significantly more tacrolimus recipients experienced hypomagnesemia ($P = 0.001$) and diarrhea ($P < 0.05$) than cyclosporine recipients, and significantly fewer tacrolimus recipients experienced hypertrichosis ($P = 0.005$), flu syndrome ($P < 0.05$), and gum hyperplasia ($P < 0.05$).

The risks of tacrolimus during pregnancy are similar to the risks associated with cyclosporine. Data from the US National Transplantation Pregnancy Registry were used to compare outcomes in 19 tacrolimus recipients (24 pregnancies) with outcomes in 56 cyclosporine microemulsion recipients (71 pregnancies). Seventy-one percent of pregnancies resulted in live births in the tacrolimus group versus 80% of pregnancies in the cyclosporine microemulsion group; the mean gestational age was lower in the tacrolimus group than in the cyclosporine group (32.9 versus 35.8 weeks; $P = 0.0035$).[3] There were no other statistically significant differences in outcomes.

A single-center analysis was performed on 13 kidney transplant recipients and two SPK recipients who became pregnant under tacrolimus-based immunosuppression.[67] The 13 mothers after kidney transplantation delivered 19 infants, whereas the two mothers after SPK transplantation delivered three infants. All mothers survived the pregnancy. One infant was stillborn. Forty-one percent of the infants were either preterm or premature, and 27% of the infants were delivered by cesarean section. Toxemia of pregnancy or pre-eclampsia was seen in 23% of these pregnancies. None of the mothers experienced rejection during their pregnancy.

CONCLUSION

The studies discussed in this chapter have confirmed the primary place of calcineurin inhibitors, particularly tacrolimus for primary immunosuppression in adult and pediatric kidney and in adult kidney–pancreas transplantation. The key comparator for tacrolimus is cyclosporine microemulsion. Treating kidney transplant recipients with tacrolimus results in a 44% reduction in graft loss (censored for death) compared with cyclosporine-treated patients in the first 6 months after kidney transplantation.[151] On the basis of meta-analyses of data from randomized trials, treating 100 recipients at low risk (e.g., adult, well-matched, first transplants) with tacrolimus instead of cyclosporine would avoid 6 cases of acute rejection; this number increases to 17 cases if high-risk recipients are considered (e.g., sensitized recipients, second or third transplants, children). In contrast, treating with tacrolimus would lead to excess harm in an extra five recipients by causing them to develop insulin-dependent diabetes.[151] Both of the calcineurin inhibitors are nephrotoxic, and this can contribute to chronic allograft nephropathy directly via drug toxicity or indirectly via hypertension and dyslipidemia.[22,92,93,128]

Tacrolimus is associated with less hypertension and less hypercholesterolemia than cyclosporine. Tacrolimus use has steadily increased, and it is now used in more than 80% of kidney recipients. Despite its side effects, the superior immunosuppressive efficacy of tacrolimus has led to its preferential use in kidney and kidney–pancreas recipients.

REFERENCES

1. Ahsan N, Hricik D, Matas A, et al. Prednisone withdrawal in kidney transplant recipients on cyclosporine and mycophenolate mofetil: a prospective randomized study. Transplantation 1999;68:1865.
2. Ahsan N, Johnson C, Gonwa T, et al. Randomized trial of tacrolimus plus mycophenolate mofetil or azathioprine versus cyclosporine oral solution (modified) plus mycophenolate mofetil after cadaveric kidney transplantation: results at two years. Transplantation 2001;72:245.
3. Armenti VT, Corscia LA, McGrory CH, et al. National Transplantation Pregnancy Registry looks at outcomes with Neoral and tacrolimus. Nephrol News Issues 2000;14:S11.
4. Artz MA, Boots JMM, Ligtenberg G, et al. Randomized conversion from cyclosporine to tacrolimus in renal transplant patients: improved lipid profile and unchanged plasma homocysteine levels. Transplant Proc 2002;34:1793.
5. Astellas, Inc. Prograf prescribing information (US), Available online at: http://www.prograf.com/pdf/prograf_full_prescribing_information.pdf [accessed 22.01.07].
6. Augustine JJ, Chang PC, Knauss TC, et al. Improved renal function after conversion from tacrolimus/sirolimus to tacrolimus/mycophenolate mofetil in kidney transplant recipients. Transplantation 2006;81:1004.
7. Baid-Agrawal S, Delmonico FL, Tolkoff-Rubin NL, et al. Cardiovascular risk profile after conversion from cyclosporine A to tacrolimus in stable renal transplant recipients. Transplantation 2004;77:1199.
8. Barynski WS, Tan HP, Boardman JF, et al. Posterior reversible encephalopathy syndrome after solid organ transplantation. AJNR Am J Neuroradiol 2008;29:924.
9. Bechstein WO, Malaise J, Saudek F, et al. Efficacy and safety of tacrolimus compared with cyclosporine microemulsion in primary simultaneous pancreas-kidney transplantation: one year results of a large multicenter trial. Transplantation 2004;77:1221.
10. Boots J, Van Duijnhoven EM, Christiaans MH, et al. Glucose metabolism in renal transplant recipients on tacrolimus: the effect of steroid withdrawal and tacrolimus trough level reduction. J Am Soc Nephrol 2002;13:221.
11. Borel JF, Feurer C, Gubler HU, et al. Biological effects of cyclosporin A: a new antilymphocytic agent. Agents Actions 1976;6:468–75.
12. Borel JF, Feurer C, Magnee C, et al. Effects of the new anti-lymphocytic peptide cyclosporin A in animals. Immunology 1977;32:1017–25.
13. Borrows R, Chan K, Loucaidou M, et al. Five years of steroid sparing in renal transplantation with tacrolimus and mycophenolate mofetil. Transplantation 2005;80:125.
14. Bresnahan BA, Cherikh WS, Cheng Y, et al. Short-term benefit of tacrolimus versus cyclosporine therapy after renal transplantation: an analysis of UNOS/OPTN database. Am J Transplant 2003;3(Suppl. 5):462 (abstract 1213).
15. Buell JF, Kulkarni S, Grewal HP, et al. Early corticosteroid cessation at one week following kidney transplant under tacrolimus and mycophenolate mofetil (MMF) immunosuppression, three-year follow up. Transplantation 2000;69:S134 (abstract).
16. Burke GW, Ciancio G, Figueiro J, et al. Can acute rejection be prevented in SPK transplantation? Transplant Proc 2002;34:1913.
17. Burke GW, Kaufman DB, Millis JM, et al. Prospective randomized trial of the effect of antibody induction in simultaneous pancreas and kidney transplantation: three-year results. Transplantation 2004;77:1269.
18. Busque S, Cantarovich M, Mulgaonkar S. The PROMISE study: a phase 2b multicenter study of voclosporin (ISA247) versus tacrolimus in de novo kidney transplantation. Am J Transplant 2011;11:2675–84.
19. Calconi G, Vianello A. One-year follow up of a large European trial comparing dual versus triple tacrolimus-based immunosuppressive regimens following renal transplantation: Italian and Spanish Tacrolimus Study Group. Transplant Proc 2001;33:1021.
20. Calne RY, Rolles K, White DJ, et al. Cyclosporin A initially as the only immunosuppressant in 34 recipients of cadaveric organs: 32 kidneys, 2 pancreases, and 2 livers. Lancet 1979;1033–6.
21. Calne RY, Rolles K, White DJ, et al. Cyclosporin-A in clinical organ grafting. Transplant Proc 1981;13(1 Pt 1):349–58.
22. Campistol JM, Grinyo JM. Exploring treatment options in renal transplantation: the problems of chronic allograft dysfunction and drug-related nephrotoxicity. Transplantation 2001;71:S542.
23. Cantarovich D, Rostaing L, Mourad G. The combination of daclizumab, tacrolimus and MMF is an effective and safe steroid-free immunosuppressive regimen after renal transplantation: results of a large multicenter trial. Nephrol Dial Transplant 2003;18(Suppl 4):788.
24. Chan K, Taube D, Roufosse C, et al. Kidney transplantation with minimized maintenance: alemtuzumab induction with tacrolimus monotherapy – an open label, randomized trial. Transplantation 2011;92:774–80.
25. Chang R-WS, Snowden S, Palmer A, et al. European randomized trial of dual versus triple tacrolimus-based regimens for control of acute rejection in renal allograft recipients. Transpl Int 2001;14:384.
26. Chhabra D, Skaro AI, Leventhal JR, et al. Long-term kidney allograft function and survival in prednisone-free reigmens: tacrolimus/mycophenolate mofetil versus tacrolimus/sirolimus. Clin J Am Soc Nephrol 2012;7:504.
27. Christians U, Jacobsen W, Benet LZ, et al. Mechanisms of clinically-relevant drug interactions associated with tacrolimus. Clin Pharmacokinet 2002;41:813.
28. Ciancio G, LoMonte A, Buscemi G, et al. Use of tacrolimus and mycophenolate mofetil as induction and maintenance in simultaneous pancreas-kidney transplantation. Transpl Int 2000;13:S191.
29. Coley KC, Verrico MM, McNamara DM, et al. Lack of tacrolimus-induced cardiomyopathy. Ann Pharmacother 2001;35:985.
30. Coto E, Tavira B. Pharmacogenetics of calcineurin inhibitors in renal transplantation. Transplantation 2009;88:3S.
31. De Jonge H, Kuypers DR, Verbeke K, et al. Reduced CO concentrations and increased dose requirements in renal allograft recipients converted to the novel once-daily tacrolimus formulation. Transplantation 2010;90:523.
32. Dharnidharka VR, Ho P-L, Stablein DM, et al. Mycophenolate, tacrolimus and posttransplant lymphoproliferative disorder: a report of the North American Pediatric Renal Transplant Cooperative Study. Pediatr Transplant 2002;6:396.
33. Donahoo WT, Kosmiski LA, Eckel RH. Drugs causing dyslipoproteinemia. Endocrinol Metab Clin North Am 1998;27:677.
34. Dreyfuss M, Harri E, Hoftmann H, et al. Cyclosporin A and C: new metabolites from *Trichoderma polysporum*. Eur J Appl Microbiol 1976;3:125.
35. Dudley CRK. Conversion at first rejection: a prospective trial comparing cyclosporine microemulsion to tacrolimus in renal transplant recipients. Transplant Proc 2001;33:1034.
36. Ekberg H, Bernasconi C, Tedesco-Silva H, et al. Calcineurin inhibitor minimization in the symphony study: observational results 3 years after transplantation. Am J Transplant 2009;9:1876.
37. Ekberg H, Tedesco-Silva H, Demirbas A. Reduced exposure to tacrolimus inhibitors in renal transplantation. N Engl J Med 2007;357:25.
38. Farney AC, Doares W, Rogers J, et al. A randomized trial of alemtuzumab versus antithymocyte globulin induction in renal and pancreas transplantation. Transplantation 2009;88:810–9.
39. Ferrarris JR, Tambutti ML, Cardori RL, et al. Conversion from cyclosporine A to tacrolimus in pediatric kidney transplant recipients with chronic rejection. Transplantation 2004;77:532.
40. Filler G, Webb NJA, Milford DV, et al. Four-year data after pediatric renal transplantation: a randomized trial of tacrolimus vs. cyclosporine microemulsion. Pediatr Transplant 2005;9:498.
41. Filler G, Womiloju T, Feber J, et al. Adding sirolimus to tacrolimus-based immunosuppression in pediatric renal transplant recipients reduces tacrolimus exposure. Am J Transplant 2005;5:2005.

42. Flechner SM, Goldfarb D, Solez K, et al. Kidney transplantation with sirolimus and mycophenolate mofetil-based immunosupression: 5-year results of a randomized prospective trial compared to calcineurin inhibitor drugs. Transplantation 2007;83:7.
43. Flechner SM, Kurian SM, Solez K, et al. De novo kidney transplantation without use of calcineurin inhibitors preserves renal structure and function at two years. Am J Transplant 2004;4:1776.
44. Flenchner SM, Glyda M, Cockfield S, et al. The ORION study: comparison of two sirolimus-based regimens versus tacrolimus and mycophenolate mofetil in renal allograft recipients. Am J Transplant 2011;11:1633–44.
45. Friese CE, Sang-Mo K, Feng S, et al. Excellent short-term results with steroid-free maintenance immunosuppression in low-risk pancreas-kidney transplantation. Arch Surg 2003;138:1121.
46. Fung JJ. Tacrolimus and transplantation: a decade in review. Transplantation 2004;77:S41.
47. Gallon LG, Winoto J, Chhabra D, et al. Long-term renal transplant function in recipient of simultaneous kidney and pancreas transplant maintained with two prednisone free maintenance immunosuppressive combinations: tacrolimus/mycophenolate mofetil versus tacrolimus/sirolimus. Transplantation 2007;83:10.
48. Garcia I. Efficacy and safety of dual versus triple tacrolimus-based therapy in kidney transplantation: two year follow up. Transplant Proc 2002;34:1638.
49. Gonwa T, Johnson C, Ahsan N, et al. Randomized trial of tacrolimus and mycophenolate mofetil or azathioprine versus cyclosporine and mycophenolate mofetil after cadaveric kidney transplantation: results at three years. Transplantation 2003;75:2045.
50. Gonwa T, Mendez R, Yang HC, et al. Randomized trial of tacrolimus in combination with sirolimus or mycophenolate mofetil in kidney transplantation: results at six months. Transplantation 2003;75:1213.
51. Gourishankar S, Hunsicker LG, Jhangri GS, et al. The stability of the glomerular filtration rate after renal transplantation is improving. J Am Soc Nephrol 2003;14:2387.
52. Grenda R, Watson A, Vondrak K, et al. A prospective, randomized, multicenter trial of tacrolimus-based therapy with or without basiliximab in pediatric renal transplantation. Am J Transplant 2006;6:1666–72.
53. Gruessner AC, Sutherland DER, Dunn DL, et al. Pancreas after kidney transplants in post-uremic patients with type I diabetes mellitus. J Am Soc Nephrol 2001;12:2490.
54. Gruessner AC, Sutherland DER. Pancreas transplant outcomes for United States (US) and non-US cases as reported to the United Network for Organ Sharing (UNOS) and International Pancreas Transplant Registry as of October 2002. In: Cecka JM, Terasaki PI, editors. Clinical transplants 2002. Los Angeles: UCLA Tissue Typing Laboratory; 2003. p. 41.
55. Gruessner RW, Sutherland DE, Najarian JS, et al. Solitary pancreas transplantation for non-uremic patients with labile insulin-dependent diabetes mellitus. Transplantation 1997;64:1572.
56. Gruessner RWG, Sutherland DER, Parr E, et al. A prospective, randomized open-label study of steroid withdrawal in pancreas transplantation – a preliminary report with six months' follow up. Transplant Proc 2001;33:1663.
57. Guerra G, Ciancio G, Gaynor JJ, et al. Randomized trial of immunosuppression regimens in renal transplantation. J Am Soc Nephrol 2011;22:1758–68.
58. Halloran P, Ahsan N, Johnson C, et al. Three-year follow up of randomized multicenter kidney transplant study comparing tacrolimus (TAC)+azathioprine (AZA) versus cyclosporine modified (CsA)+mycophenolate mofetil (MMF) versus TAC+MMF. Am J Transplant 2001;1(Suppl 1):405.
59. Hamdy AF, El-Agroudy AE, Bakr MA, et al. Comparison of sirolimus with low-dose tacrolimus versus sirolimus-based calcineurin inhibitor-free regimen in live donor renal transplantation. Am J Transplant 2005;5:2531.
60. Hananay MJ, Woodle ES, Mulgaonkar S. Alemtuzumab induction in renal transplantation. N Engl J Med 2011;364:1909.
61. Hardinger KL, Bolul DL, Schnitzer MA, et al. A randomized, prospective, pharmacoeconomic trial of tacrolimus versus cyclosporine in combination with thymoglobulin in renal transplant recipients. Transplantation 2005;80:41.
62. Hecking M, Haidinger M, Doller D, et al. Early basal insulin therapy decreases new-onset diabetes after renal transplantation. J Am Soc Nephrol 2012;23:739.
63. Heisel O, Heisel R, Batshaw R, et al. New onset diabetes mellitus in patients receiving calcineurin inhibitors: a systematic review and meta-analysis. Am J Transplant 2004;4:583.
64. Hougardy JM, Broderers N, Kianda M, et al. Conversion from Prograf to Advagraf among kidney transplant recipients results in sustained decrease in tacrolimus exposure. Transplantation 2011;91:566.
65. Hricik DE, Anton HA, Knauss TC, et al. Outcomes of African-American kidney transplant recipients treated with sirolimus, tacrolimus and corticosteroids. Transplantation 2002;74:189.
66. Humar A, Parr E, Drangstveit MG, et al. Steroid withdrawal in pancreas transplant recipients. Clin Transplant 2000;14:75.
67. Jain AB, Shapiro R, Scantlebury VP, et al. Pregnancy after kidney and kidney-pancreas transplantation under tacrolimus: a single center's experience. Transplantation 2004;77:897.
68. Jamieson NV. Adult small intestinal transplantation in Europe. Acta Gastroenterol Belg 1999;62:239.
69. Jensik SCfor the FK506 Kidney Transplant Study Group. Tacrolimus (FK506) in kidney transplantation: three-year survival results of the U.S. multicenter, randomized, comparative trial. Transplant Proc 1998;30:1216.
70. Johnson C, Ahsan N, Gonwa T, et al. Randomized trial of tacrolimus (Prograf) in combination with azathioprine or mycophenolate mofetil versus cyclosporine (Neoral) with mycophenolate mofetil after cadaveric kidney transplantation. Transplantation 2000;69:834.
71. Jordan ML, Chakrabarti P, Luke P, et al. Results of pancreas transplantation after steroid withdrawal under tacrolimus immunosuppression. Transplantation 2000;69:265.
72. Jordan ML, Naraghi R, Shapiro R, et al. Tacrolimus rescue therapy for renal allograft rejection – five years' experience. Transplantation 1997;63:223.
73. Jordan ML, Naraghi RL, Shapiro R, et al. Five-year experience with tacrolimus rescue for renal allograft rejection. Transplant Proc 1997;29:306.
74. Jordan ML, Shapiro R, Jensen CWB, et al. FK506 conversion of renal allografts failing cyclosporine immunosuppression. Transplant Proc 1991;23:3078.
75. Kahan BD, Welsh M, Schoenberg L, et al. Variable oral absorption of cyclosporine: a biopharmaceutical risk factor for chronic renal allograft rejection. Transplantation 1996;62:599–606.
76. Kaplan B, Schold JD, Meier-Kriesche H-U. Long-term graft survival with neoral and tacrolimus: a paired kidney analysis. J Am Soc Nephrol 2003;14:2980.
77. Kasiske BL, Snyder JJ, Gilbertson D, et al. Diabetes mellitus after kidney transplantation in the United States. Am J Transplant 2003;3:178.
78. Kaufman DB, Leventhal JR, Axelrod D, et al. Alemtuzumab induction and prednisone-free maintenance immunotherapy in kidney transplantation: comparison with basiliximab induction – long-term results. Am J Transplant 2005;5:2539.
79. Kaufman DB, Leventhal JR, Gallon LG, et al. Technical and immunologic progress in simultaneous pancreas-kidney transplantation. Surgery 2002;132:545.
80. Kaufman DB, Leventhal JR, Koffron AJ, et al. A prospective study of rapid corticosteroid elimination in simultaneous pancreas-kidney transplantation. Transplantation 2002;73:169.
81. Klein IH, Abrahams A, van Ede T, et al. Different effects of tacrolimus and cyclosporine on renal hemodynamics and blood pressure in healthy subjects. Transplantation 2002;73:732.
82. Klinger M, Vitko S, Karja S, et al. Large prospective study evaluating steroid-free immunosuppression with tacrolimus/basiliximab and tacrolimus/MMF compared with tacrolimus/MMF/steroids in renal transplantation. Nephrol Dial Transplant 2003;18(Suppl 4):788.
83. Kovarik JM, Mueller EA, Richard F, et al. Evidence for earlier stabilization of cyclosporine pharmacokinetics in de novo renal transplant patients receiving a microemulsion formulation. Transplantation 1996;62:759–63.
84. Kovarik JM, Mueller EA, van Bree JB, et al. Cyclosporine pharmacokinetics and variability from a microemulsion formulation – a multicenter investigation in kidney transplant patients. Transplantation 1994;58:658–63.

85. Kulkarni S, Kopelan A, Woodle ES. Tacrolimus therapy in renal transplantation. In: Morris PJ, editor. Kidney transplantation: principles and practice. Philadelphia: Saunders; 2001. p. 251–62.
86. Kumar M, Saeed MI, Ranganna K, et al. Comparison of four different immunosuppression protocols without long-term steroid therapy in kidney recipients monitored by surveillance biopsy: five-year outcomes. Transpl Immunol 2008;20:32.
87. Kumar MSA, Heifets M, Fyfe B, et al. Comparison of steroid avoidance in tacrolimus/mycophenolate mofetil and tacrolimus/sirolimus combination in kidney transplantation monitored by surveillance biopsy. Transplantation 2005;80:807.
88. Kur F, Reichenspurner H, Meiser BM, et al. Tacrolimus (FK506) as primary immunosuppressant after lung transplantation. Thorac Cardiovasc Surg 1999;47:174.
89. Land W, Malaise J, Sandberg J, et al. Tacrolimus versus cyclosporine in primary simultaneous pancreas-kidney transplantation: preliminary results at one year of a large multicenter trial. Transplant Proc 2002;34:1911.
90. Larsen CP, Pearson TC, Adams AB, et al. Rational development of LEA29Y (belatacept), a high-affinity variant of CTLA4-Ig with potent immunosuppressive properties. Am J Transplant 2005;5:443–53.
91. Larson TS, Dean PG, Stegall MD, et al. Complete avoidance of calcineurin inhibitors in renal transplantation: a randomized trial comparing sirolimus and tacrolimus. Am J Transplant 2006;6:514.
92. Legendre C, Thervet E, Skhiri H, et al. Histological features of chronic allograft nephropathy revealed by protocol biopsies in kidney transplant recipients. Transplantation 1998;65:1506.
93. Ligtenberg G, Hené RJ, Blankestijn PJ, et al. Cardiovascular risk factors in renal transplant patients: cyclosporine A versus tacrolimus. J Am Soc Nephrol 2001;12:368.
94. Mancinelli LM, Frassetto L, Floren LC, et al. The pharmacokinetics and metabolic disposition of tacrolimus: a comparison across ethnic groups. Clin Pharmacol Ther 2001;69:24.
95. Mann M, Tanabe K, Tokumoto T, et al. Impact of tacrolimus on hyperlipidemia after renal transplantation: a Japanese single center experience. Transplant Proc 2000;32:1736.
96. Margreiter R, Klempnauer J, Neuhaus P, et al. Alemtuzumab (Campath-1H) and tacrolimus monotherapy after renal transplantation: results of a prospective randomized trial. Am J Transplant 2008;8:1480.
97. Mayer AD, Dmitrewski J, Squifflet JP, et al. Multicenter randomized trial comparing tacrolimus (FK506) and cyclosporine in the prevention of renal allograft rejection: a report of the European Tacrolimus Multicenter Renal Study Group. Transplantation 1997;64:436.
98. Mayer AD. Chronic rejection and graft half-life: five-year follow up of the European tacrolimus multicenter renal study. Transplant Proc 1998;34:1491.
99. Meier-Kriesche H-U, Hricik DE. Are we ready to give up on calcineurin inhibitors? Am J Transplant 2006;6:445.
100. Meier-Kriesche H-U, Schold JD, Srinivas TR, et al. Sirolimus in combination with tacrolimus is associated with worse renal allograft survival compared to mycophenolate mofetil combined with tacrolimus. Am J Transplant 2005;5:2273.
101. Meiser BM, Pfeiffer M, Schmidt D, et al. Combination therapy with tacrolimus and mycophenolate mofetil following cardiac transplantation; importance of mycophenolic acid therapeutic drug monitoring. J Heart Lung Transplant 1999;18:143.
102. Miller J, Mendez R, Pirsch JD, et al. Safety and efficacy of tacrolimus in combination with mycophenolate mofetil (MMF) in cadaveric renal transplant recipients. FK506/MMF Dose-Ranging Kidney Transplant Study Group. Transplantation 2000;63:977.
103. Montori VM, Basu A, Erwin PJ, et al. Post-transplantation diabetes: a systematic review of the literature. Diabetes Care 2002;25:583, 94.
104. Moore J, Middleton L, Cockwell, et al. Calcineurin inhibitor sparing with mycophenolate in kidney transplantation: a systematic review and meta-analysis. Transplantation 2009;87:4.
105. Moreso F, O'Valle F, Serón D, et al. Immunophenotype of infiltrating cells in protocol renal allograft biopsies from tacrolimus-versus cyclosporine treated patients. Transplantation 2007;83:649.
106. Mujtaba MA, Taber TE, Goggins WC, et al. Early steroid withdrawal in repeat kidney transplantation. Clin J Am Soc Nephrol 2011;6:404.
107. Neu AM, Ho PL, Fine RN, et al. Tacrolimus vs. cyclosporine A as primary immunosuppression in pediatric renal transplantation: a NAPRTCS study. Pediatr Transplant 2003;7:217.
108. Neylan JF for the FK506 Kidney Transplant Study Group. Racial differences in renal transplantation after immunosuppression with tacrolimus versus cyclosporine. Transplantation 1998;65:515.
109. Pascual J, Ortuno J. Simple tacrolimus-based immunosuppressive regimens following renal transplantation: a large multicenter comparison between double and triple therapy. Spanish and Italian Tacrolimus Study Group. Transplant Proc 2002;34:89.
110. Phelan DL, Thompson C, Henschell J, et al. Heart transplantation across preformed class I antibody using FK506. Hum Immunol 1992;34:70.
111. Pirsch JD, Miller J, Deiorhoi MH, et al. A comparison of tacrolimus (FK506) and cyclosporine for immunosuppression after cadaveric renal transplantation. Transplantation 1997;63:977.
112. Plosker GL, Foster RH. Tacrolimus: a further update of its pharmacology and therapeutic use in organ transplantation. Drugs 2000;59:323.
113. Pohanka E, Margreiter R, Sparacino V, et al. Switch to tacrolimus-based therapy for cyclosporine-related side effects: a large, prospective European study. Transplantation 2002;74(S):425 (abstract 2100).
114. Reddy KS, Stratta RJ, Shokouh-Amiri H, et al. Simultaneous kidney-pancreas transplantation without antilymphocyte induction. Transplantation 2000;69:49.
115. Rizzari MD, Suszynski TM, Gillingham KJ, et al. Ten-year outcome after rapid discontinuation of prednisone in adult primary kidney transplantation. Clin J Am Soc Nephrol 2012;7:494.
116. Rostaing L, Cantarovich G, Mourad G, et al. Corticosteroid-free immunosuppression with tacrolimus, mycophenolate mofetil and daclizumab induction in renal transplantation. Transplantation 2005;79:807.
117. Sandrini S, Aslam N, Tardanico R, et al. Tacrolimus versus cyclosporine for early steroid withdrawal after renal transplantation. J Nephrol 2012;25:1.
118. Sato T, Inagaki A, Uchida K, et al. Diabetes mellitus after transplant: relationship to pretransplant glucose metabolism and tacrolimus or cyclosporine A-based therapy. Transplantation 2003;76:1320.
119. Schnitzler MA, Lowell JA, Brennan DC. New-onset post-renal transplant hyperlipidemia with cyclosporine compared to tacrolimus. In: 2nd International Congress on Immunosuppression, San Diego; 2001 (abstract).
120. Schwimmer J, Zand MS. Management of diabetes mellitus after solid organ transplantation. Graft 2001;4:256.
121. Scott LJ, McKeage K, Kearn SJ, et al. Tacrolimus: a further update of its use in the management of organ transplantation. Drugs 2003;63:1247.
122. Segoloni G, Bonomini V, Maresca MC, et al. Tacrolimus is highly effective in both dual and triple therapy regimens following renal transplantation. Spanish and Italian Tacrolimus Study Group. Transpl Int 2000;13:S336.
123. Shapiro R, Jordan M, Scantlebury V, et al. A prospective, randomized trial of FK 506 in renal transplantation – a comparison between double and triple drug therapy. Clin Transplant 1994;8:508.
124. Shapiro R, Jordan ML, Scantlebury VP, et al. A prospective randomized trial of tacrolimus/prednisone versus tacrolimus/prednisone/ mycophenolate mofetil in renal transplant recipients. Transplantation 1999;67:411.
125. Shapiro R, Scantlebury VP, Jordan ML, et al. Pediatric renal transplantation under tacrolimus-based immunosuppression. Transplantation 1999;67:299.
126. Shapiro R, Young JB, Milford EL, et al. Immunosuppression: evolution in practice and trends, 1993–2003. Am J Transplant 2005;5:874.
127. Shimizu T, Tanabe K, Tokumoto T, et al. Clinical and histological analysis of acute tacrolimus (TAC) nephrotoxicity in renal allografts. Clin Transplant 1999;13(Suppl 1):48.
128. Solez K, Vincenti F, Filo RS. Histopathologic findings from 2-year protocol biopsies from a U.S. multicenter trial comparing tacrolimus versus cyclosporine: a report of the FK506 Kidney Transplant Study Group. Transplantation 1998;66:1736.
129. Squifflet JP, Bachman L, Claesson K, et al. Dose optimization of mycophenolate mofetil when administered with a low dose of tacrolimus in cadaveric renal transplant recipients. Transplantation 2001;72:63.

130. Sutherland DR, Gruessner RWG, Dunn DL, et al. Lessons learned from more than 1000 pancreas transplants at a single institution. Ann Surg 2001;233:463.
131. Tamura K, Fujimura T, Tsutsumi T, et al. Transcriptional inhibition of insulin by FK506 and possible involvement of FK506-binding protein-12 in pancreatic beta cell. Transplantation 1995;59:1606.
132. Tan HP, Donaldson J, Basu A, et al. Two hundred living donor kidney transplantations under alemtuzumab induction and tacrolimus monotherapy: 3-year follow-up. Am J Transplant 2009;9:355.
133. Thomas P, Woodside K, Lappin J, et al. Alemtuzumab (Campath 1H) induction with tacrolimus monotherapy is safe for high immunological risk renal transplantation. Transplantation 2007;83:11.
134. Thompson JS. Intestinal transplantation: experience in the United States. Eur J Pediatr Surg 1999;9:271.
135. Todo S, Fung JJ, Starzl TE, et al. Liver, kidney and thoracic organ transplantation under FK506. Ann Surg 1990;212:295.
136. Trimarchi HM, Truong LD, Brennan S, et al. FK-506 associated thrombotic microangiopathy: report of two cases and review of the literature. Transplantation 1999;67:539.
137. Trompeter R, Filler G, Webb NJ, et al. Randomized trial of tacrolimus versus ciclosporin microemulsion in renal transplantation. Pediatr Nephrol 2002;17:141.
138. Uemura T, Ramprasad V, Ramprasad V. Single dose of alemtuzumab induction with steroid-free maintenance immunosuppression in pancreas transplantation. Transplantation 2011;92:6.
139. Vacher-Coponat H, Moal V, Indreies M, et al. A randomized trial with steroids and anthithymocytes globulins comparing cyclosporine/azathioprine versus tacrolimus/mycophenolate mofetil (CATM2) in renal transplantation. Transplantation 2012;93:4.
140. Van Duijnhoven EM, Boots JM, Christiaans MH, et al. Metabolic aspects of tacrolimus in renal transplantation. Minerva Urol Nefrol 2003;55:1.
141. van Duijnhoven EM, Christiaans MH, Boots JM, et al. Glucose metabolism in the first 3 years after renal transplantation in patients receiving tacrolimus versus cyclosporine-based immunosuppression. J Am Soc Nephrol 2002;13:213.
142. Venkataramanan R, Swaminathan A, Prasad T, et al. Clinical pharmacokinetics of tacrolimus. Clin Pharmacokinet 1995;29:404.
143. Vicenti F, Friman S, Scheuermann E, et al. Results of an international randomized trial comparing glucose metabolism disorders and outcomes with cyclosporine versus tacrolimus. Am J Transplant 2007;7:1506.
144. Vicenti F, Larsen C, Alberu J, et al. Three-year outcomes from BENEFIT, a randomized, active-controlled, parallel-group study in adult kidney transplant recipients. Am J Transplant 2012;210:217.
145. Vincenti F, Jensik SC, Filo RS, et al. A long-term comparison of tacrolimus (FK506) and cyclosporine in kidney transplantation: evidence for improved allograft survival at 5 years. Transplantation 2002;73:775.
146. Vincenti F. A decade of progress in kidney transplantation. Transplantation 2004;77:S52.
147. Vitko S, Klinger M, Salmela K, et al. Two corticosteroid-free regimens – tacrolimus monotherapy after basiliximab administration and tacrolimus/mycophenolate mofetil – in comparison with a standard triple regimen in renal transplantation: results of the Atlas Study. Transplantation 2005;80:1734.
148. Waid TH. Prograf as secondary intervention versus continuation of cyclosporine in patients at risk for chronic renal allograft failure (CRAF) results in improved renal function, decreased CV risk, and no increased risk for diabetes. Am J Transplant 2003;3(Suppl 5):436 (abstract 1111).
149. Walliser P, Berizie CR, Kay JE. Inhibition of murine B lymphocyte proliferation by the novel immunosuppressant drug FK506. Immunology 1989;68:434.
150. Wasik M, Stepien-Sopniewska B, Lagodzinski Z, et al. Effect of FK506 and cyclosporine on human T and B lymphoproliferative responses. Immunopharmacology 1990;20:57.
151. Webster AC, Woodroffe RC, Taylor RS, et al. Tacrolimus versus ciclosporin as primary immunosuppression for kidney transplant recipients: meta-analysis and meta-regression of randomized trial data. BMJ 2005;331:810.
152. Woodle ES, First MR. A prospective, randomized, double-blind, placebo-controlled multicenter trial comparing early (7 day) corticosteroid cessation versus long-term, low-dose corticosteroid therapy. Ann Surg 2008;248:565.
153. Woodle ES, Newell KA, Haas M, et al. Reversal of accelerated renal allograft rejection with FK506. Clin Transplant 1997;11:2251.
154. Woodle ES, Pedrizet G, Brunt EM, et al. FK506: inhibition of humoral mechanisms of hepatic allograft rejection. Transplantation 1992;54:377.
155. Woodle ES, Pedrizet G, Brunt EM, et al. FK506: reversal of humorally-mediated rejection following ABO-incompatible liver transplantation. Transplant Proc 1991;23:2992.
156. Woodle ES, Spargo B, Ruebe M, et al. Treatment of acute glomerular rejection with FK506. Clin Transplant 1996;10:266.
157. Woodle ES, Thistlewaite JR, Gordon JH for the Tacrolimus Kidney Transplant Rescue Study Group. A multicenter trial of FK 506 (tacrolimus) therapy in acute refractory renal allograft rejection. Transplantation 1996;62:594.
158. Woodle ES. Fujisawa Corticosteroid Withdrawal Study Group. A prospective, randomized, multi-center, double-blind study of early corticosteroid cessation versus long-term maintenance of corticosteroid therapy with tacrolimus and mycophenolate mofetil in primary renal transplant recipients: one year report. Transplant Proc 2005;37:804.
159. Zachary AA, Montgomery RA, Ratner LE, et al. Specific and durable elimination of antibody to donor HLA antigens in renal transplant patients. Transplantation 2003;76:1519.

CHAPTER 18

MYCOPHENOLATES

Robert S. Gaston

CHAPTER OUTLINE

INTRODUCTION

While immunology has always been at the core of solid-organ transplantation, advances in clinical immunosuppression have typically preceded understanding of the mechanisms that beget their efficacy. Furthermore, utilization of immunosuppressants in the clinical arena often evolves away from the protocols documented to be safe and effective in clinical trials. There is, however, one clear exception: mycophenolic acid (MPA). Its immunosuppressive properties had been known for years; development of a readily absorbable oral preparation enabled initial clinical trials, with rapid government agency approval for use in routine practice. Despite numerous subsequent trials testing novel approaches to its administration, worldwide use of MPA in the majority of solid-organ transplant recipients is in keeping with basic tenets developed and tested over two decades ago. MPA preparations are now the most widely prescribed immunosuppressants in the world; their efficacy and basic tolerability have made them indispensable in solid-organ transplantation.

HISTORY OF MYCOPHENOLATES

MPA is a fermentation product of *Penicillium brevicompactum* and related fungi. It was first isolated by Gosio in 1896, named in 1913 by Alsberg and Black, and subsequently found to have weak antibacterial and antifungal activity.[43] Raistrick and colleagues published the structure of MPA in 1952. In the 1960s, it was found to have a strong antimitotic effect in mammalian cells, and was regarded as a potential antitumor agent. Subsequent work by Franklin and Cook documented its major mechanism of action (inhibition of the de novo pathway of purine synthesis).[43] At about the same time, a Japanese group documented MPA's immunosuppressive properties,[102] which were initially viewed as an impediment to clinical utility.

Discovery and development of cyclosporine (CsA) in the late 1970s and early 1980s changed the landscape for transplant immunosuppression. In a search for new agents targeting other pathways, Allison and Eugui, among others working first in the United Kingdom and subsequently at Syntex Pharmaceuticals, began examining in vitro the effect of MPA on lymphocyte function, documenting inhibition of cytotoxic T-cell generation, antibody formation, lymphocyte adhesion, and the mixed lymphocyte reaction.[3,4,38] Scientists at Syntex, via morpholinoethyl esterification of MPA, produced a prodrug (RS61443, mycophenolate mofetil, MMF) with substantially improved oral bioavailability in mammals and humans.[89]

Initial animal studies demonstrated the agent to be difficult to administer to dogs and primates with substantial gastrointestinal toxicity, especially at higher doses (>20 mg/kg).[106,119] Optimal kidney graft outcomes in dogs occurred when RS61443 was combined with low-dose CsA and prednisone. MMF monotherapy, even at substantially higher doses, demonstrated only limited efficacy. Initial human experience was in rheumatoid arthritis, where a dose of 2 g/day was associated with "significant clinical improvement" among refractory patients.[51] Side effects were minimal, and primarily of gastrointestinal origin (nausea, vomiting, abdominal pain, diarrhea). No other significant toxicities (including bone marrow suppression) were noted.

In 1988, it was elected to proceed with clinical trials in kidney transplantation. The initial study was a phase I/II trial involving 48 kidney recipients at two centers.[142] All patients received polyclonal antibody induction, CsA, and prednisone. Eight dosing groups of six subjects each received MMF in daily doses ranging from 100 to 3500 mg. The greatest efficacy in preventing acute rejection with an acceptable adverse event profile was seen in the 2000 and 3000 mg dosing groups, providing a basis for the design of three large registration trials.

The phase III MMF trials, commencing in 1992 and conducted across three continents, represented the first rigorously controlled studies involving large numbers of patients in solid-organ transplantation. Each enrolled approximately 500 subjects assigned to one of three treatment arms. Two of the groups in each study received MMF either 2 or 3 g/day in combination with CsA and corticosteroids. In the US trial, all patients underwent polyclonal antibody induction, with a comparator group receiving azathioprine instead of MMF.[140] In the tricontinental trial, treatment arms were identical, with an azathioprine control group, but without antibody induction.[151] In the European trial, there was no antibody induction and comparator patients received placebo instead of azathioprine.[39] Findings of all three trials were remarkably similar: a 50% reduction in rates of acute rejection (to less than 20% overall) within the first 6 months after transplantation, with identical graft and patient survival among treatment arms at 1 and 3 years (Figure 18-1). For most patients, the 2-g dose appeared to offer optimal efficacy with few adverse effects. Based on these findings, on May 3, 1995, the Food and Drug Administration (FDA) approved MMF (CellCept) 2–3 g/day for use in combination with CsA and corticosteroids, with global availability soon to follow.[24] A starting dose of 2 g/day became widely accepted in adults, and, by 2002, MMF was the most widely prescribed immunosuppressant in the United States.[76]

Over the last decade, there have been at least three other landmark developments impacting use of mycophenolates in transplantation. First, to address the gastrointestinal adverse events that plague some patients, Novartis developed an enteric-coated formulation, mycophenolate sodium (EC-MPS, Myfortic).[107] Designed to delay MPA release and absorption in the gut (with the assumption that gastric and early small-bowel exposure were major determinants of gastrointestinal toxicity), clinical trials documented EC-MPS efficacy equivalent to MMF, with a trend to fewer adverse gastrointestinal events. [15,126] EC-MPS became available in 2004. Second, in 2008, patent protection for the innovator formulation of MMF (CellCept) began expiring in the United States and globally.[37] The clinical impact of availability of multiple MMF preparations on patients and the marketplace is still to be determined. Finally, in 2009, the FDA approved the tacrolimus/MMF combination for use in kidney transplantation. Previously, use of MMF or EC-MPS with tacrolimus, the most common immunosuppressant combination in the world, had been "off-label," limiting its use as a comparator protocol in drug development.[160] This label change altered the landscape for new drug development, as well as providing guidance for MPA dosing in tacrolimus-based protocols.

MECHANISM OF ACTION

Among immunosuppressants, MPA is considered an antiproliferative agent (Figure 18-2). While calcineurin inhibitors (CsA and tacrolimus) block early signaling events and cytokine production, MPA exerts an effect downstream in the cell cycle, interfering with cytokine-dependent signals and lymphocyte proliferation.[2,38]

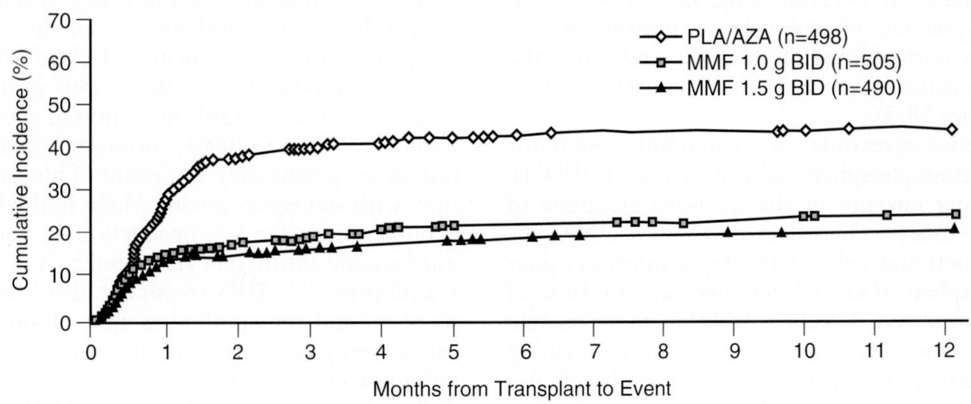

FIGURE 18-1 ■ Cumulative incidence of first biopsy-proven rejection in first year (excludes 1-year protocol biopsies; Kaplan–Meier estimates). Data from the pooled efficacy analysis of the three double-blind clinical studies in prevention of rejection.[60] The separation between the curves occurs in the first 2 months and is sustained to the end of the observation period. PLA, placebo; AZA, azathioprine; MMF, mycophenolate mofetil.

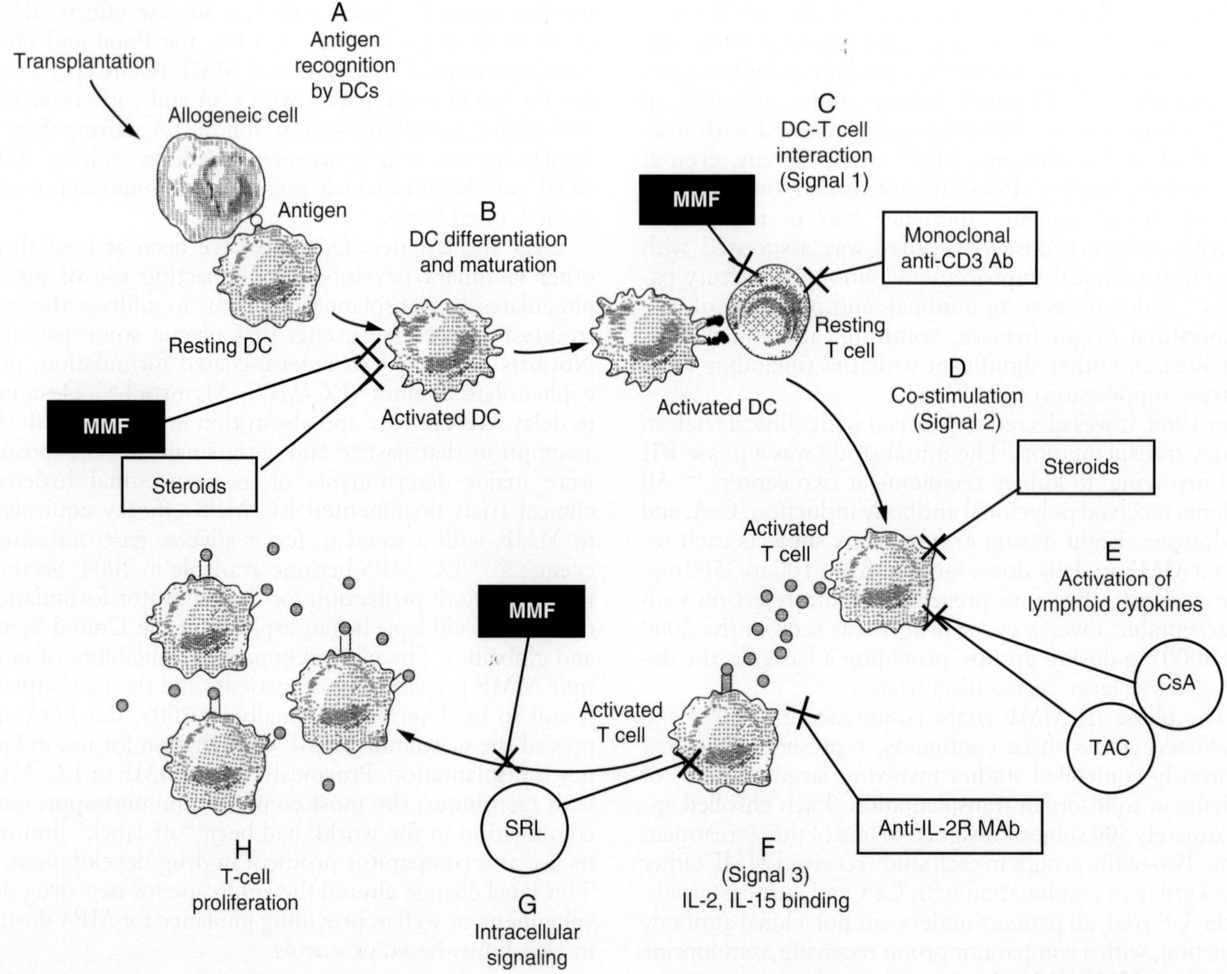

FIGURE 18-2 ■ **Steps in the activation of T cells, showing potential inhibition by mycophenolate mofetil (MMF) at sites B, C, and H. Ab, antibody; CsA, cyclosporine; DC, dendritic cell; IL-2R, interleukin-2 receptor; SRL, sirolimus; TAC, tacrolimus.** (Adapted from Shaw LM, Korecka M, Venkataramanan R, et al. Mycophenolic acid pharmacodynamics and pharmacokinetics provide a basis for rational monitoring strategies. Am J Transplant 2003;3:534.)

Given the documented immunosuppressive effect of a relatively non-specific inhibitor of nucleotide synthesis (azathioprine), MPA development in transplantation was based on the observation that inherited deletions in nucleic acid synthesis resulted in immunodeficiencies: children lacking adenosine deaminase show combined T-cell and B-cell deficits.[48] In contrast, subjects with absence of hypoxanthine-guanine phosphoribosyl transferase display essentially normal immune function,[3] indicating the purine salvage pathway as relatively unimportant in lymphocytes (Figure 18-3).

MPA acts as a reversible, non-competitive inhibitor of inosine 5'-monophosphate dehydrogenase (IMPDH), the rate-limiting enzyme in the de novo synthesis of guanine nucleotides.[38] This effect arrests new DNA synthesis in proliferating cells at the G_1/S interface; guanosine triphosphate (GTP) levels decrease to 10% of those in unstimulated T cells.[2] Addition of guanosine or deoxyguanosine reverses the inhibition, confirming the IMPDH target. T and B lymphocytes are highly dependent on this pathway for proliferation in response to stimulation. There are two isoforms of IMPDH, with type I expressed in most cell lines but type II the predominant isoform in activated T and B lymphocytes; IMPDH type II is four times more sensitive to MPA.[22] These two factors impart some degree of lymphocyte-specific selectivity to the impact of MPA on growth and proliferation. While monocyte and dendritic cell replication may also be affected by MPA, there is relatively little impact on neutrophils.[2,27]

The action at the G_1/S interface is selective. Neither the production of interleukin-2 nor the expression of its receptor is affected, showing a lack of influence on signal 1 of lymphocyte activation. This primary antiproliferative effect also retards induction of cytotoxic T cells.[38] Similarly, MPA mitigates primary and ongoing B-cell responses, presumably as a result of blockade of cell division, with subjects receiving MMF in the US pivotal trial demonstrating far less production of xenoantibody toward equine antithymocyte globulin (ATG) than those on azathioprine.[53,78] MPA treatment also blunts the synthesis of natural xenoantibodies after plasma exchange and splenectomy in rats, and inhibits the humoral response to influenza vaccine in humans.[41,139]

Another distinct mechanism of MPA activity may relate to the requirement for GTP to activate fucose and mannose transfer in glycoprotein synthesis, thus diminishing expression of adhesion molecules.[2,4] When

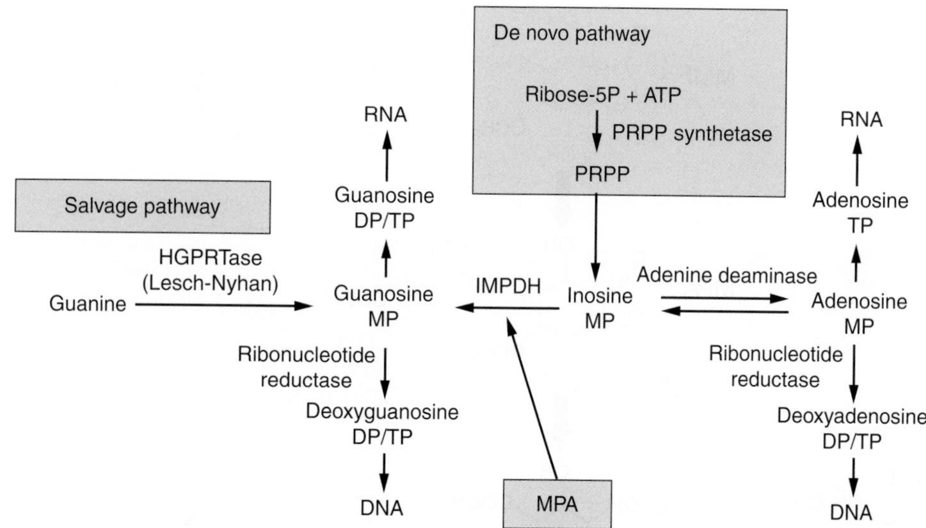

FIGURE 18-3 ■ Purine synthetic pathways showing site of inhibition by mycophenolic acid (MPA). ATP, adenosine triphosphate; DP, diphosphate; HGPRTase, hypoxanthine-guanine phosphoribosyl transferase; IMPDH, inosine monophosphate dehydrogenase; MP, monophosphate; PRPP, phosphoribosyl pyrophosphate;TP, triphosphate. (Adapted from Budde K, Glander P, Bauer S. Pharmacokinetics and pharmacodynamics of mycophenolic acid. A CME monograph. Berlin: Walter de Gruyter; 2004. p. 2–13.)

GTP is depleted as a consequence of MPA, adhesion of lymphocytes and monocytes to activated endothelial cells is decreased in a dose-dependent fashion.

Cell types other than lymphocytes may also be sensitive to MPA inhibition, with some models indicating vascular smooth-muscle cells,[104] mesangial cells,[63] and myofibroblasts[9] to display dampened proliferation. In a subhuman primate model of orthotopic allograft vasculopathy, intravascular ultrasound documented dose-dependent inhibition of the progression of intimal volume changes.[106] The efficacy of MMF was confirmed using aortic allografts in another subhuman primate model[79] and in a rodent chronic rejection system.[8] The effects were potentiated when MMF was administered with sirolimus, a combination that also reduced transforming growth factor-β_1 and its effects on extracellular matrix synthesis and degradation.[73,135]

CLINICAL PHARMACOLOGY AND BLOOD MONITORING

Dosing

In adults with kidney transplants, MMF is most commonly administered orally at a dose of 1 g twice daily.[24] In pediatric patients, the recommended dose of MMF oral suspension is 600 mg/m^2 at 12-hour intervals up to a maximum of 2 g daily. Intravenous MMF is administered at the same dose and frequency as the oral preparation, infused over 2 hours. EC-MPS is administered orally at a dose of 720 mg twice daily in adults.[107] The suggested dose of EC-MPS in stable pediatric patients is 400 mg/m^2 twice daily, but its use is not recommended in patients less than 5 years old.

Absorption

Orally delivered MMF is rapidly and almost completely absorbed in the stomach and upper intestine, then efficiently hydrolyzed to MPA (Figure 18-4). Drug absorption, as assessed by area under the curve (AUC), is not significantly altered by co-administered food, although the maximal concentration (C_{max}) is 40% lower in simultaneously fed renal transplant recipients.[24] The time to maximal concentration (T_{max}) of less than 1 hour is independent of hepatic or renal function. The T_{max} is slightly delayed, however, in the period immediately after transplantation (1.31 ± 0.76 hours) and in diabetic patients (1.59 ± 0.67 hours). In contrast, by 3 months it is 0.90 ± 0.24 hours. Metabolism of MMF to MPA yields 94% bioavailability. Over a range of 100–3000 mg/day, the MPA area under the concentration–time curve for 24 hours (AUC_{0-24}) is proportionate to dose in healthy subjects,[17] although a recent study of MMF kinetics in kidney transplant recipients revealed a non-linear relationship, with reduced bioavailability as doses increase from 250 to 2000 mg.[28] The magnitude of the non-linearity was greater (176% to 76%) in association with tacrolimus rather than CsA (123% to 90%). A recent multicenter crossover study comparing pharmacokinetics of two MMF preparations (Teva and Roche) in 43 stable kidney recipients found them to be comparable in all parameters studied.[146]

EC-MPS does not release MPA under acidic conditions (pH<5) as in the stomach but is highly soluble in a neutral-pH environment like the intestine.[5] Consistent with this property is a T_{max} of 1.5–2.75 hours, substantially delayed compared to MMF.[107] Gastrointestinal absorption is 93% and absolute bioavailability of MPA after administration of EC-MPS is 72%. There is substantial impact of food on MPA absorption with EC-MPS, although overall AUC is not affected; to avoid variability, it should always be taken on an empty stomach. Like MMF, EC-MPS pharmacokinetics are dose-proportional over its administration range, and its profile regarding metabolism and clearance (see below) is very similar as well. An EC-MPS dose of 720 mg most closely approximates the MPA exposure of 1000 mg of MMF.

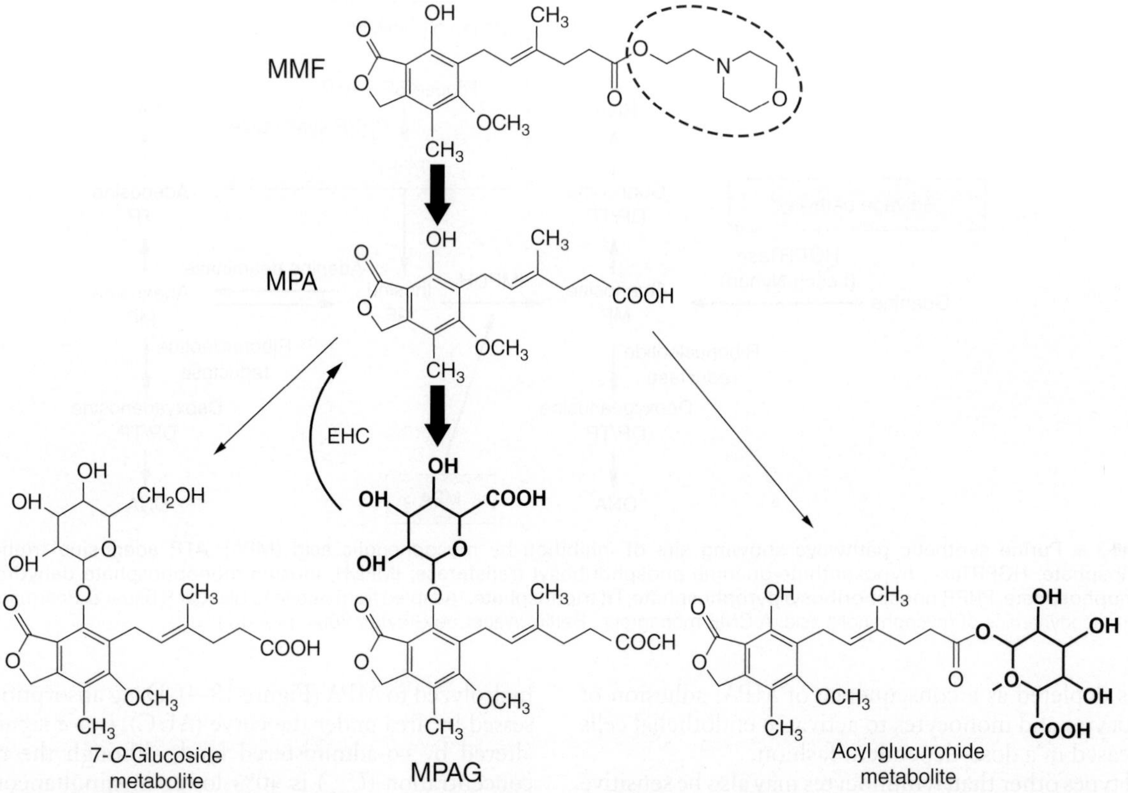

FIGURE 18-4 ■ **Metabolism of parent component mycophenolate mofetil (MMF) to mycophenolic acid (MPA) by cleavage of mofetil group (encircled) with primary metabolism to its glucuronide (MPAG), which may undergo enterohepatic recycling (EHC), and secondary acyl glucuronide and 7-*O*-glucoside metabolites.** (Adapted from Shaw LM, Korecka M, Venkataramanan R, et al. Mycophenolic acid pharmacodynamics and pharmacokinetics provide a basis for rational monitoring strategies. Am J Transplant 2003;3:534.)

Metabolism and Clearance

MPA is rapidly metabolized to an inactive glucuronide (MPAG) via one or more isoforms of the UGT1 gene family of uridine diphosphate–glucuronosyl transferases in the gastrointestinal tract, liver, and possibly kidney. Two minor metabolites also are formed: the acyl glucuronide and the phenolic glucoside[134] (Figure 18-4).

The apparent elimination half-life of MPA in healthy volunteers is 17.9 hours – a clearance of 11.6 L/h.[6] At 8–12 hours after oral drug administration, 37% of patients (range 10–61%) display a secondary peak in plasma MPA concentrations representing enterohepatic recirculation. The additional peak results from excreted MPAG in bile undergoing deglucuronidation by intestinal bacteria with subsequent reabsorption of MPA, and may account for up to 40–60% of the total dose interval MPA AUC.[17,18]

MPAG is the major urinary excretion product (93% of the radioactive parent compound); urinary excretion of MPA is negligible (1%). Fecal excretion accounts for 6%. Neither hemodialysis nor peritoneal dialysis significantly affects MPA plasma concentrations, although in multiple-dose studies either dialysis method may remove some MPAG. With renal dysfunction, there is a moderate increase in plasma MPA and a marked accumulation of MPAG. MPA binds tightly and extensively (97%), but reversibly, to serum albumin, decreasing its ability to inhibit IMPDH.[113] The free fraction, constituting 1–3% of the total amount in the blood of stable patients, is cleared by biliary and renal routes.

Hypoalbuminemia is associated with increased free MPA and greater MPA clearance. The impact of renal allograft dysfunction also increases the MPA free fraction because it decreases the binding of acidic drugs; in contrast, hepatic oxidative impairment produces no effect. Estimates of free MPA in ultrafiltrate samples have not been shown to offer any advantage over measurements of total MPA to predict therapeutic versus adverse reactions,[6,85] except in the presence of impaired early renal function, wherein there are increased concentrations of MPAG and other metabolites.[134]

Assays and Blood Monitoring

The MPA parent compound is readily measured in plasma by high-performance liquid chromatography.[65] In contrast, the widely available automated enzyme multiplier immunoassay technique (EMIT)[105] yields 15–20% higher results because its antibody reagent cross-reacts with the acyl-MPAG metabolite (Figure 18-4), which may contribute to both immunosuppressive and toxic effects.[90] Because of these properties, some have suggested that the EMIT assay may be preferable, and is the most widely utilized.

The gold-standard pharmacokinetic measure of MPA exposure is frequent sampling of blood over a 12-hour period, with calculation of the AUC concentration–time exposure. MPA AUC can be calculated from either full (8 or more samples over 12 hours) or limited (2–5 samples over 4 hours) sampling strategies.[77,158] Although the evidence is conflicting regarding utility, 12-hour predose (C_0) MPA levels are convenient to obtain and have been utilized effectively in some studies.[12,47] Correlation (r^2) of predose level with AUC for MMF ranges from 0.32 to 0.68, and may differ by concomitant calcineurin inhibitor usage[29,47] (Figure 18-5). For EC-MPS, variability in absorption means significantly poorer correlation between predose MPA level and AUC (r^2=0.02). Long-term, intrapatient variability of both AUC and trough levels is relatively low.[158]

After the first few weeks following transplantation, dose-normalized MPA exposure increases by 30–50%, reflecting perhaps decline in drug clearance, MPA saturation of tissues, or other factors.[59,153] MPA exposure/dose relationships may also differ in settings other than kidney transplantation (e.g., liver and small-bowel transplantation, bone marrow transplantation).[70,71] Typically, younger children require higher MMF doses per body mass index than older children or adults to achieve comparable MPA exposure.[166]

Considerable interpatient pharmacokinetic variability of MMF has been documented to be due to differences in hepatic/renal function, concurrent drug administration, and the presence of diarrhea, but not to ethnicity or gender.[118,133]

Pharmacodynamic monitoring of patients receiving MPA therapy has been studied. Peripheral blood lymphocytes (PBL) from patients on MMF demonstrate reduced response to stimulation assays, and diminished antibody production.[78,114] However, so many other factors affect the proliferative activity of PBL in this setting that the clinical utility of these assays is modest. IMPDH assays are technically demanding and difficult to reproduce; in addition, the whole-blood matrix may not reflect the impact in activated lymphocytes, which are the cells of interest. Estimates of IMPDH activity in isolated peripheral blood mononuclear cells display considerable interindividual variability. The time course of IMPDH inhibition, as measured by the production of xanthine monophosphate by isolated mononuclear cells, parallels the MPA plasma concentration.[14] Patients with lower IMPDH levels before transplantation, suggesting a genetically determined susceptibility to the drug, more frequently underwent dosage reductions within 6 months; pretransplant IMPDH activity has been suggested as a guide to MPA dosing in pediatric patients.[44,120] It is unclear, however, whether levels or fluctuations in IMPDH activity can be of utility in predicting either efficacy or toxicity of MMF in clinical transplantation.

Drug–Drug Interactions

In general, important drug–drug interactions with mycophenolates are rare. Cholestyramine may reduce MPA absorption.[24] Antibiotic therapy disrupting the gastrointestinal flora may interfere with deglucuronidation and enterohepatic recirculation, decreasing drug levels. Because acyclovir and ganciclovir compete with MPAG for tubular secretion, they may increase drug concentrations slightly, particularly among patients experiencing renal impairment. Co-administration of proton pump inhibitors has been reported to reduce exposure to MPA by 25–35%, but the clinical impact of this interaction is uncertain.[24]

Clearly, however, the most significant drug–drug interaction is with CsA: its importance is magnified since most dosing regimens of MMF and EC-MPS were established utilizing this combination. When either mycophenolate preparation is administered with CsA, subjects display lower MPA concentrations than those not receiving CsA or in whom the drug was discontinued.[54,56] This effect is the result of reduced enterohepatic

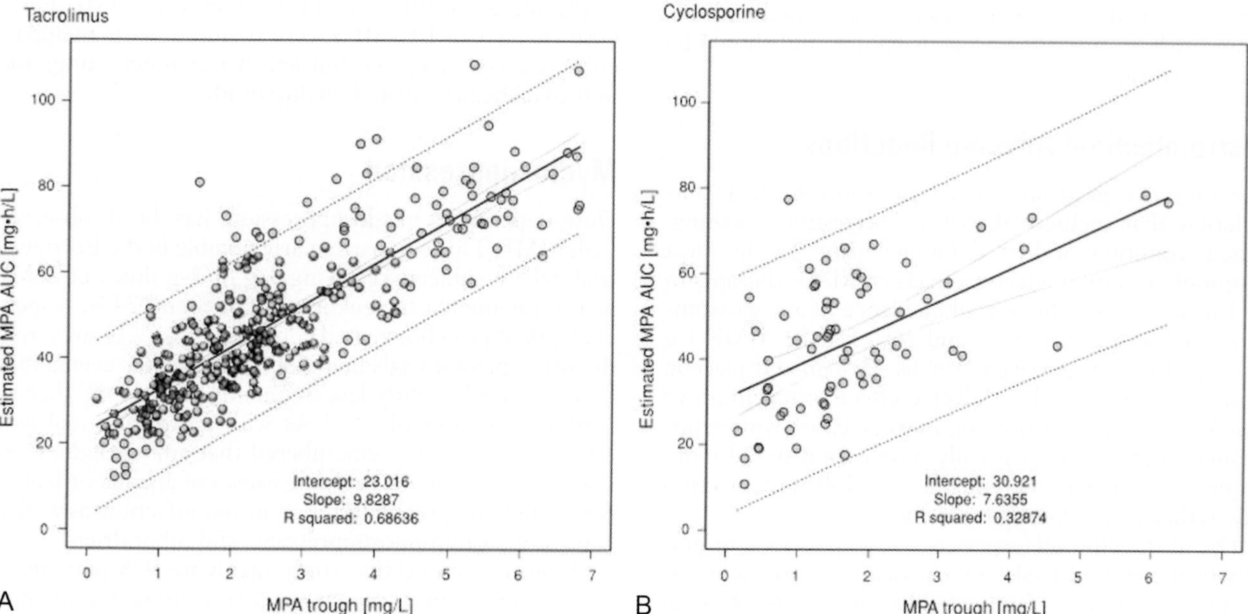

FIGURE 18-5 ■ **Linear regression analysis of the estimated mycophenolic acid (MPA) area under the concentration–time curve (AUC) versus trough in patients in the Opticept study receiving (A) tacrolimus and (B) cyclosporine.** (From Gaston RS, Kaplan B, Shah T, et al. Fixed- or controlled-dose MMF with standard- or reduced-dose calcineurin inhibitors: the Opticept trial. Am J Transplant 2009;9:1607.)

recirculation.[80] In contrast, co-administration with tacrolimus does not alter MPA exposure compared to placebo, and MPA exposure in combination with sirolimus is likewise higher than observed with CsA.[42,56,154] Similarly, the experimental Janus kinase inhibitor tofacitinib does not impact MPA pharmacokinetics.[86] This property resulted in 37% greater MPA exposure in tofacitinib- versus CsA-treated subjects in a recent phase IIb trial, with profound influence on the outcomes in kidney transplant recipients.[165] Finally, the corticosteroid component of most regimens increases MPAG slightly by inducing hepatic glucuronosyl transferase.[23]

CLINICAL TOXICITIES

The initial clinical trials of MMF suggested a lack of nephrotoxicity, neurotoxicity, or hepatotoxicity. The myelotoxicity and gastrointestinal side effects were reportedly "modest."[142] In general, adverse events, including invasive cytomegalovirus (CMV) infections, were more common in patients receiving 3 g (versus 2 g) of MMF daily, suggesting a dose-dependent relationship. In the pivotal trials, adverse events accounted for withdrawal of 15% of subjects in the MMF 3 g/day dose, 9% from MMF 2 g/day dose, and 5% from the comparator cohorts.[60] Early on, the occurrence of these side effects was thought to be linked to the MMF dose rather than to the plasma concentration of parent compound or its metabolites,[153] and indeed adverse events often respond to MMF dose reduction. However, while findings have been somewhat inconsistent, more recent evidence has correlated gastrointestinal and hematologic adverse events to MPA exposure as well as dose.[12,84] The frequency and severity of MMF-related adverse events are also influenced by the other immunosuppressants with which it is combined. Common clinical practice has been to reduce MMF dosing in response to adverse events; there is some evidence, however, that dose reduction can be associated with increased risk of rejection and graft failure, and should be approached cautiously.[20]

Gastrointestinal Adverse Reactions

One or more gastrointestinal symptoms from a constellation that includes diarrhea, indigestion, bloating, nausea, vomiting, and/or abdominal pain are the most commonly reported adverse effects of MMF therapy. In the European trial, the overall incidence of any gastrointestinal complaint was 53% and 46% for the MMF 3-g and 2-g doses, respectively, versus 42% in the placebo comparator arm.[40] These adverse effects often improve with MMF dose reduction, or, in some cases, with maintenance of the same total daily dose administered more frequently in smaller increments (e.g., 500 mg four times daily rather than 1000 mg twice daily).

The most common (experienced by up to 35% of subjects in the pivotal trials, almost twice the frequency as in comparator arms) and troublesome gastrointestinal adverse event is diarrhea.[60] Diarrhea occurs even more often, and with greater severity, when MMF is used in combination with tacrolimus rather than CsA (45% versus 25% in one study).[138] Since it also dramatically increases tacrolimus absorption and blood levels, clinical consequences of diarrhea may be greater with this combination as well.[94] In a registry analysis, Bunnapradist and colleagues found significantly increased risk of diarrhea (hazard ratio 1.37) associated with the tacrolimus/MMF combination, which, in turn, was linked to increased risk of graft failure (hazard ratio 2.13) and patient death (hazard ratio 2.04).[21] It must be remembered that, after renal transplantation, diarrhea can be due to a variety of causes other than immunosuppressant therapy, including pre-existing diabetic or uremic conditions, intercurrent infectious diseases, and concurrent antibiotic treatment.[93] Maes and colleagues reported 60% of 26 cases of diarrhea were due to an infectious origin – CMV, *Campylobacter*, or bacterial overgrowth, or, in another report, microsporidiosis.[58,93] In the other 40%, erosive enterocolitis was attributed to MMF, characterized by faster colonic transit, crypt distortion, and focal inflammation, thought to represent a toxic action of the acyl-MPAG metabolite on absorptive cells, leading to a predominance of goblet cells.[136] In the presence of persistent diarrhea, colonic biopsy specimens have shown apoptosis of intestinal gland epithelial cells[116] and atrophy of the intestinal villi, which in one patient was documented to disappear a few months after MMF withdrawal.[32]

EC-MPS was developed specifically to mitigate the gastrointestinal toxicities associated with MMF by delaying absorption in the gastrointestinal tract with a goal of reducing peak levels and delivering active drug to more distal portions of the bowel. Compared with MMF, EC-MPS showed equivalent efficacy and overall equivalent MPA drug exposure in kidney transplant patients, but very similar gastrointestinal adverse events when administered in randomized fashion (with CsA and corticosteroids) to either de novo or stable recipients.[15,126] Some conversion patients, however, showed marked improvement with EC-MPS, and, in another study of patients displaying gastrointestinal intolerance with MMF, fewer dose changes of EC-MPS were required, with an apparently reduced symptom burden, better functioning, and improved health-related quality of life.[25]

Myelosuppression

Dose-dependent myelosuppression has been observed with MMF. This was particularly notable in the European trial, where subjects receiving 3-g or 2-g doses of MMF had more anemia or leukopenia (26% and 24%, respectively) than placebo-treated controls (13%).[39] However, in the other pivotal trials hematopoietic adverse events may have occurred slightly less frequently with MMF than in azathioprine controls.[140,151] As with gastrointestinal side effects, it should be remembered that among kidney recipients there may be multiple causes of anemia or leukopenia, including renal dysfunction and infection, as well as concomitant immunosuppressants and other drugs.

A recent prospective study involving 978 patients at seven North American transplant centers found anemia (hemoglobin $\leq$10 g/dL) in 10%, and an association with recipient age, use of antiviral prophylaxis, and post-transplant dialysis.[69] In the recently completed Fixed

Dose–Concentration Controlled (FDCC) trial in Europe, anemia was reported in 38% of subjects.[13] Greater MMF dose and MPA predose (C_0) plasma concentrations have been correlated with decreased hemoglobin values among stable renal transplant recipients.[152] Another study suggested an even better correlation of anemia with MPA metabolites – MPAG and acyl-MPAG – than with MPA itself.[85] Conversely, others have found no association.[91,155] In a single nucleotide polymorphism analysis of kidney recipients with MMF-related anemia, one study found a protective effect of the HUS1 allele, with interleukin-12A and CYP2C8A genes associated with increased risk for anemia.[69] Other investigators, however, while confirming an association with CYP2C8A (but not the other genotypes) noted that expression of the "at-risk" phenotype is so rare (0.5% of population) as not to explain the observed frequency of anemia (or leukopenia).[13]

In the current era, leukopenia (fewer than 3000 leukocytes/mm^3) is reported in 14–23% of kidney transplant recipients.[13,69] A recent multivariable analysis (Cox regression) of Medicare-covered kidney recipients found a significant association between mycophenolate use and leukopenia (adjusted hazard ratio 1.21).[67] Other documented risk factors for leukopenia included corticosteroid-free regimens, weight, previous kidney transplant, deceased donor, and CMV seronegativity with a CMV-positive donor (and lengthier antiviral prophylaxis).[69] MMF-related leukopenia may be associated with markedly abnormal neutrophil morphology.[10] As with anemia, some, but not all, studies have shown MPA plasma concentrations and particularly free MPA AUC_{0-12h} to be significantly related to severe infections and leukopenia.[66,167] The leukopenia has been associated with stomatitis, particularly when combined with a sirolimus-based regimen.[157]

Infections

In the pivotal trials that utilized CsA with MMF, while viral infections (herpes simplex and zoster, and tissue-invasive CMV) were more common in MMF-treated recipients than controls, other opportunistic infections were not.[39,140,151] More recently, several studies have indicated significantly fewer herpes viral infections (especially CMV) with mTOR inhibitors than with mycophenolates.[110] However, widespread use of antiviral prophylaxis is now the norm, and most centers view CMV as a manageable problem.[81]

Recognition of BK virus infection and nephropathy coincided with the rapid assimilation of mycophenolates and tacrolimus into clinical practice, and most attribute its rise to more potent immunosuppression associated with these combinations.[64] Aggressive screening for BK viruria or viremia, with immunosuppressant dose reduction (focused on mycophenolates), has diminished the impact of BK nephropathy on risk of allograft failure.[62] Progressive multifocal leukoencephalopathy (PML) is a rare but debilitating central nervous system manifestation of polyomavirus infection, and has been associated with mycophenolate use. Registry analysis of PML in the United States found all reported cases in kidney recipients to be taking MMF, though MMF use was so ubiquitous that no statistical association could be documented.[111] Very recent analysis of reported cases of PML in the United States found a strong association with not only mycophenolates, but also azathioprine, CsA, cyclophosphamide, efalizumab, rituximab, and tacrolimus, among others, indicating a potential role for interactions among components of combination therapy.[128]

Introduction of MMF therapy has been reported to produce a significant increase in hepatitis C virus viremia in some, but not all, patients receiving concomitant CsA.[125] In contrast, MMF seems to show no significant effect on hepatitis B virus viremia despite in vitro studies that suggested that it inhibited viral replication.[95] Recent analysis of outcomes in kidney recipients with hepatitis C indicated no adverse impact of mycophenolate therapy on long-term graft or patient survival.[92]

Neoplastic Diseases

Early experience with MMF was associated with a numerical increase in subjects with lymphoma compared with placebo or azathioprine control groups.[60] Two large case-control studies, however, have indicated little or no additional adverse impact of mycophenolates on the risk of lymphoma or other malignancy in patients receiving pharmacologic immunosuppression.[45,123] Registry data also indicate malignancy risk associated with MMF use to be similar to other immunosuppressants.[74] Despite an emerging consensus that mTOR inhibitors may be associated with reduced malignancy risk, much of the anecdotal benefit is in comparison to calcineurin inhibitors rather than mycophenolates.[75,145]

Pregnancy and Reproduction

MMF demonstrated teratogenic effects at subclinical doses in animal studies,[31] which resulted in caution regarding its use in both males and females of reproductive age. Avoidance of mycophenolates in males fathering children is no longer recommended. However, fetal malformations have been reported in births to female kidney recipients taking MMF.[137] Mycophenolates are now categorized by the US FDA as category D agents in pregnancy (positive evidence of human fetal risk, but the benefits from use in pregnant women may be acceptable despite risk).[96] In a female recipient with stable kidney allograft function at least 1 year posttransplant who desires pregnancy, common practice is to convert from mycophenolate to azathioprine at least 6 weeks prior to discontinuing contraception.[96]

EARLY CLINICAL TRIALS OF MYCOPHENOLATES IN KIDNEY TRANSPLANTATION

A phase I/II dose-finding study of MMF in combination with polyclonal antibody induction, CsA, and corticosteroids in de novo kidney recipients indicated therapeutic benefit of MMF at doses of 2–3 g/day.[142] There was also suggested efficacy at these doses, demonstrated in the treatment settings of an ongoing or steroid-resistant acute renal rejection episode.[30,141] Three blinded, randomized phase III trials were initiated in 1992. Patients in each trial were assigned to one of three treatment arms: a control group or one of two groups receiving MMF 2 g or 3 g daily, respectively. All patients also received CsA and prednisone. The primary end-point of each study was prevention of acute rejection episodes during the first 6 months after transplantation, thought to be indicative of poorer 1-year and possibly long-term graft survival.

The European Mycophenolate Mofetil Study compared MMF to placebo with no antibody induction therapy.[39] At 6 months, 46% of those receiving placebo had experienced biopsy-proven acute rejection (BPAR), versus only 17% (2 g) and 14% (3 g) of those randomized to MMF. The US Renal Transplant Study, which required polyclonal antibody induction for all patients and included an azathioprine control arm, yielded corresponding acute rejection rates of 38%, 20%, and 18%, respectively.[140] The tricontinental study, which included an azathioprine comparator but without antibody induction, demonstrated BPAR in 36%, 20%, and 15% of subjects, respectively.[151] Each study also found significantly fewer histologically and clinically severe rejections among the MMF-treated cohorts. Thus, each trial documented similar benefit of MMF compared with azathioprine (or placebo) in prevention of early rejection episodes. Likewise, fewer patients in each trial withdrew from MMF than control for treatment failure, and there tended to be more adverse effects in the 3-g than the 2-g MMF groups.

Though none of the studies individually was sufficiently powered to test efficacy in terms of graft survival, a planned pooled analysis of 12-month data from the three studies, with a total of 1493 randomized subjects, confirmed the benefit of MMF on acute rejection episodes – 20% and 17% in the two MMF arms versus 41% in the control arms, yielding a relative risk ratio of 0.46.[60] There was significantly less steroid-resistant rejection in the MMF arms, and renal function at 1 year was substantially better (despite identical CsA exposure) in the MMF-treated patients. Despite a trend indicating fewer graft losses over time with MMF, the combined incidence of graft loss and death was 10%, 11%, and 12%, respectively, at 1 year (*P*=not significant). Longer-term follow-up failed to suggest a benefit of MMF versus azathioprine or placebo in the US Renal Transplant Study or tricontinental study, although data from the European trial revealed that the 2-g, but not the 3-g, dose of MMF reduced death-censored graft loss compared with placebo – 9%, 13%, and 16%, respectively (*P*=0.03).[40]

After FDA approval in 1995, MMF was rapidly incorporated into clinical practice in the United States. From the beginning, pharmacoeconomic analyses documented benefit: the cost of adding MMF to a regimen was more than offset by reduced costs associated with diagnosing and treating acute rejection and its consequences.[163,170] Subsequent analyses of clinical outcomes of almost 50 000 kidney recipients in the US Renal Data System (USRDS) suggested that prescription of MMF yielded significantly better early and late patient and graft survivals. The risk of late acute rejection episodes was reduced by 65%,[98] with the risk of long-term deterioration of graft function reduced by 20–34%.[99,115] By 1999, over 80% of US kidney recipients were on MMF, usually in combination with CsA.[76]

COMBINATION THERAPY UTILIZING MMF IN KIDNEY TRANSPLANTATION

The ascendancy of MMF in clinical practice was based on documented efficacy in reducing rejection (the pivotal trials), registry data indicating improved overall outcomes relative to azathioprine, and single-center experiences reporting better results with fewer complications in patients on the drug.[30,60,98,99] However, acceptance was not uniform, particularly as concomitant immunosuppression moved beyond corticosteroids and the original oil-based CsA formulation (Sandimmune) with which MMF was combined in its early trials.

Cyclosporines (see Chapter 16)

Shortly after the introduction of mycophenolates, CsA microemulsion (Neoral and generics, CsA-ME) began replacing Sandimmune. Data reported with the new CsA-ME/MMF combinations generally confirmed the initial experience cited above: rejection rates around 20%.[33,68,130] The ELITE-Symphony trial, enrolling over 1600 subjects, included two CsA-ME cohorts, normal- and reduced-dose (with MMF) after daclizumab induction.[36] Rejection rates after 1 year approximated 25%, similar to those observed previously. Alternatively, a multicenter European study using CsA-ME demonstrated only modest insignificant reductions in acute rejection episodes with MMF compared with azathioprine (34% and 35%, respectively, at 1 year), and questioned the value of a 10–15-fold cost differential.[121] Five-year follow-up likewise documented no evidence of a long-term benefit of MMF versus azathioprine with CsA-ME.[122]

Studies comparing MMF to sirolimus or everolimus in combination with CsA have typically shown comparable outcomes, with a differing side effect profile.[148] With a significant percentage of CsA-treated recipients on standard doses of MMF or EC-MPS not achieving adequate exposure to MPA early after transplantation (see section on therapeutic drug monitoring below), a European trial examined the effect of a "loading dose" approach. Investigators found more adverse events but substantially less early rejection (3% versus 17% of subjects) using higher than standard doses of EC-MPS (2880 then 2160 mg/day) for 6 weeks.[143]

African Americans are generally considered to be at greater immunologic risk than others, and a subgroup analysis of the US pivotal trial documented benefit of MMF for black recipients only in the 3-g dose group, with an acute rejection rate of 12% compared to 32% in the 2-g group and 48% in the azathioprine cohort.[112] These findings were seemingly confirmed in a single-center study: the standard 2-g dose of MMF produced no benefit in rejection risk among African Americans (relative risk 0.88) while white recipients fared much better (relative risk 0.35).[130] Registry data, however, supported overall benefit for African American recipients.[97] Review of data from the pivotal trial and other studies found that the excess acute rejections among African Americans, and others, occurred quite early after transplantation, a time when MPA pharmacokinetics are not stable and MPA exposure at standard doses is low in a substantial number of recipients on CsA-based protocols.[47,101,112,155] A subsequent study, conducted in stable renal allograft recipients, indicated no difference in MPA pharmacokinetics based on race or gender.[118] In current practice, there is no evidence supporting long-term use of a 3-g MMF dose in African Americans, nor for a 3-g dose in non-CsA-based regimens.

A 2003 paper regarding late kidney allograft failure identified chronic CsA-induced nephrotoxicity as its principal etiology.[108] The study was based on serial surveillance biopsies in recipients treated with CsA, azathioprine, and corticosteroids. A subsequent study from the same group, though, substituted MMF for azathioprine, and found substantially fewer changes suggestive of chronic allograft nephropathy, and interpreted the data as indicating that MMF must attenuate CsA nephrotoxicity.[109] Indeed, data from the earliest days of MMF use have suggested it might mitigate chronic allograft nephropathy.[115] Patients in the USRDS registry who were maintained on MMF for at least 2 years were reported to show a 34% reduced risk of worsening renal function, with significantly less late rejection.[98,115] A Spanish study indicated that MMF demonstrated benefit for patients with chronic allograft nephropathy even when introduced late after transplantation, though contradictory data exist.[49,52] It now appears that most late allograft failure is the result of immunologic mechanisms, with antibody-mediated injury playing a major role.[46,131] The putative benefit of MMF in preserving renal function and preventing late graft failure may actually reside in its efficacy as an immunosuppressant with both anti-T-cell and anti-B-cell effects.

Tacrolimus (see Chapter 17)

Studies evaluating the tacrolimus/MMF combination began appearing in the mid-1990s. A single-center, randomized study evaluated adding MMF to a tacrolimus/steroid regimen and documented reduction of acute rejection rates at 1 year from 44% to 27%.[132] A subsequent multicenter trial[101] reported 2 g/day of MMF reduced the incidence of acute rejection episodes compared with 1 g/day or azathioprine 9%, 32%, and 32%, respectively. The low acute rejection rate with the higher MMF dose, without overt evidence indicating greater risk of infection or malignancy, was thought to support the 2-g dose as optimal with tacrolimus; however, the mean time to rejection was 79 days, there were almost no rejections beyond 180 days in the 1-g MMF group, and, by 1 year, patients in the 2-g group had had doses reduced to a mean of 1.6 g/day (see section on therapeutic drug monitoring, below). In contrast, despite a 1-year rejection rate of 15% with the tacrolimus/MMF combination, another study failed to show a significant benefit of tacrolimus versus CsA-ME in combination with MMF on the incidence of acute rejection episodes, graft survival, or patient survival at 2 years among 223 subjects.[72] A subsequent analysis of Scientific Registry of Transplant Recipients data regarding living donor kidney transplants even showed, at 2 years, a significantly greater risk of graft failure with the tacrolimus/MMF than with the CsA-ME/MMF combination.[19] Eventually, efficacy and safety data obtained in two studies that compared tacrolimus to CsA-ME in combination with MMF led to the FDA's approval of the tacrolimus/MPA regimen in 2009. While the Symphony trial documented fewer rejection episodes (12%) and better graft survival with tacrolimus/MMF than two CsA-ME-based control groups,[36] a trial of modified-release tacrolimus documented efficacy and safety only similar to a CsA-ME/MMF control group.[138]

With tacrolimus/MMF established as a new standard, several reports document similar efficacy of tacrolimus-based protocols with sirolimus.[26,100] In a randomized, multicenter clinical trial comparing patients treated with MMF (n=176) versus sirolimus (n=185) (along with tacrolimus and steroids), there was no difference in rejection, graft survival, or patient survival. However, the MMF cohort displayed better renal function, less hypertension, and reduced hyperlipidemia.[100] Among patients on a tacrolimus-based regimen, improvements in renal function were observed in 19 patients converted from sirolimus to MMF compared with 78 recipients remaining on sirolimus.[7]

mTOR Inhibitors

Mycophenolates have been utilized with sirolimus in an attempt to avoid calcineurin inhibitors altogether. Patients receiving sirolimus (and presumably everolimus) in combination with mycophenolate have substantially greater MPA exposure than patients on CsA, and many of the side effects of the two drugs are similar (e.g., diarrhea, myelosuppression), making the combination difficult for some patients to tolerate.[42] However, an initial clinical study suggested that MMF plus sirolimus was at least as effective as MMF/CsA to prevent acute rejection.[82] In the Symphony study, one of four treatment groups received sirolimus after daclizumab induction in combination with MMF and corticosteroids.[36] Almost 40% of patients experienced acute rejection, with a high rate of study discontinuation, compromised graft survival, and relatively impaired glomerular filtration rate (GFR) at 1 year. In a conversion trial involving 830 patients switched between 6 and 120 months posttransplant from calcineurin inhibitors to sirolimus (in combination with MMF and corticosteroids), only subjects with a baseline estimated GFR$\geq$40 mL/min demonstrated improved GFR 2 years later.[127] Again, adverse effects were problematic, with converted patients experiencing more hyperlipidemia, anemia, diarrhea, stomatitis, and discontinuation from the study than those remaining on calcineurin inhibitor-based therapy. A very recent study of conversion from CsA-ME to everolimus demonstrated similar results: more acute rejection, with disappointing benefit in terms of GFR, adverse effects, and study discontinuations.[103] Nonetheless, some studies have demonstrated in patients able to tolerate the mTOR/mycophenolate combination stability of kidney function over time and a trend to fewer malignancies.[16,168]

Belatacept

Belatacept (Nulogix) is a monoclonal antibody that blocks costimulation of lymphocytes by inhibiting the interaction between CD80/86 and CD28. Approved for use in kidney recipients by US and European authorities in 2011, it is the first biologic agent to be utilized as maintenance therapy. It is administered intravenously at varying intervals after transplantation, and, from its earliest trials, has been combined with mycophenolate and corticosteroids.[162] Two treatment regimens (moderate and low intensity) of belatacept have now been studied in three large multicenter trials involving almost 1500 patients. Efficacy in preventing acute rejection and promoting graft and patient survival is comparable to CsA, with better preservation of renal function.[87,161,162] There may also be a benefit of the belatacept/MMF combination in reducing formation of de novo anti-HLA antibodies.[161] Adverse effects were more common in a "moderate-intensity" belatacept cohort that received more of the agent early after transplantation; the "low-intensity" regimen is now approved for clinical use. The belatacept/MMF combination was associated with more posttransplant lymphoproliferative disease than in comparator patients, particularly in those naïve for Epstein–Barr virus before transplantation; the combination is contraindicated in such patients. A single case of PML has also been reported.[55] At the time of writing, there appears to be no drug–drug interaction between belatacept and MMF.

USE OF MYCOPHENOLATES TO MINIMIZE OR AVOID OTHER IMMUNOSUPPRESSANTS

Minimization of Calcineurin Inhibitors

While calcineurin inhibitors have played a major beneficial role in the evolution of modern transplantation, their use is associated with significant toxicities, including glucose intolerance and renal impairment. The efficacy and relative tolerability of mycophenolate have enabled downward recalibration of what is considered therapeutic levels or doses of both CsA and tacrolimus, potentially reducing these toxic effects. Early on, dose reduction was typically performed late (beyond 6–12 months) in response to declining renal function.[117] More recently, the CAESAR trial tested full-dose versus low-dose CsA-ME (target C_0 150–300 ng/mL versus 50–100 ng/mL) in combination with MMF and corticosteroids from the time of transplantation, with half the low-dose patients randomized to withdraw CsA-ME after 6 months.[35] The withdrawal patients experienced significantly more acute rejection episodes, but only after CsA-ME was tapered and discontinued. The best outcomes were in the patients who remained on long-term, low-dose CsA-ME treatment, although glomerular filtration rate did not differ significantly from the full-dose patients. Likewise, in the Symphony trial, patients on low-dose CsA-ME fared comparably to those on full-dose CsA-ME.[36] However, patients on low-dose tacrolimus (target C_0 3–7 ng/mL) demonstrated fewer rejections, better renal function, and better graft survival than patients in any of three comparator groups. This effect remained evident with 3 years of follow-up.[34]

Withdrawal of Calcineurin Inhibitors

Mycophenolates have also been used in attempts to eliminate calcineurin inhibitors completely from a maintenance regimen, again with a goal of averting chronic nephrotoxicity.[108] One multicenter study of patients with deteriorating renal function at a mean of 6 years after transplantation documented significantly improved renal function at 6 and 12 months after stepwise withdrawal of CsA.[147] A multicenter study compared the 1-year outcomes of withdrawal at 3 months of either CsA (n=44) or MMF (n=40) from a three-drug regimen, including steroid therapy.[129] Withdrawal of CsA was associated with better renal function, decreased blood pressure, and more favorable lipid profiles despite a twofold increase in acute rejection episodes. Several studies have substituted sirolimus for calcineurin inhibitors in otherwise stable patients, with generally good results. In a trial designated "Spare-the-Nephron," stable patients 1–6 months posttransplant (on either tacrolimus or CsA-ME, as well as MMF and steroids) were randomized to remain on their calcineurin inhibitor (mostly tacrolimus) or switch to sirolimus.[168] Results at 2 years documented similar renal function between groups and a trend to less rejection and graft loss in the converted patients, with a different adverse event profile. The ZEUS trial randomized CsA-treated patients on EC-MPS to remain on calcineurin inhibitors or switch to everolimus at 4.5 months after transplantation.[16] Despite more rejections in the converted patients (13% versus 5%, P=0.01), patient and graft survival were similar at 3 years with better renal function in those on everolimus.

Avoidance of Calcineurin Inhibitors

Experience with an MMF/steroid maintenance regimen from the time of transplantation has typically not been good. In 98 low-risk kidney recipients, acute rejection episodes were observed in 53% within 12 months, requiring institution of calcineurin inhibitors.[163] A smaller study confined to recipients of living donor kidneys also observed more rejection and little or no overall benefit.[150] In contrast, a single-center report described 12 patients older than 50 years who received grafts from elderly donors and were successfully treated de novo with MMF, steroids, and an induction regimen of rabbit ATG.[149] Durability of benefit may also be an issue; in a Spanish study, 65% of MMF-treated patients remained on an avoidance regimen at 12 months, but only 36% were calcineurin inhibitor-free at 60 months.[57]

A more successful approach, though not uniformly so, has been substitution of another agent for calcineurin inhibitor at the time of transplantation. This was the basis of the belatacept experience (see above), and has also provided the underpinnings for development of tofacitinib.[165] Experience with mTOR inhibitors from the time of transplantation has been mixed, with Kreis in France and Flechner at the Cleveland Clinic reporting good results,[42,82] and Larson from the Mayo Clinic reporting neither advantage nor disadvantage from substituating sirolimus for tacrolimus.[88] However, multicenter studies, including Symphony, documented more rejection, a more problematic adverse event profile, and little or no benefit in renal function utilizing a MMF/sirolimus combination in de novo patients.[36,50]

Steroid Avoidance or Withdrawal

Availability of a potent agent like MMF was anticipated, in combination with CsA, to allow elimination of long-term corticosteroid therapy and its attendant complications. Again, however, results were mixed. A large National Institutes of Health-sponsored multicenter trial of steroid withdrawal at 3 months after transplantation using a CsA-ME/MMF regimen documented an increased risk of rejection episodes (particularly in minority patients), and resulted in early termination of the study.[1] More recently, the FREEDOM study examined steroid avoidance and withdrawal in patients on CsA and EC-MPS after basiliximab induction; a control group that remained on maintenance steroids clearly fared best.[164] In contrast, steroid withdrawal beginning at 3 months after transplantation showed no significant difference in rejection rates versus continued steroid therapy among European patients prescribed MMF/tacrolimus[144] or MMF/CsA-ME with antibody induction.[159] Although the superior results of the latter trials might be attributed to more potent baseline therapy, it might also represent a difference in patient populations.

After completion of these trials, philosophy regarding timing of steroid withdrawal changed: rather than in chronic, stable patients, the most advantageous time point might be early after transplantation, either avoiding steroids altogether or withdrawing under cover of heavier immunosuppression with closer monitoring. A European study showed success with only a single methylprednisolone dose at transplant along with daclizumab induction and tacrolimus/MMF maintenance therapy: 89% of patients were steroid-free at 6 months, with less posttransplant diabetes and stable kidney function.[124] In a large, randomized, blinded study where corticosteroids were withdrawn within 7 days of transplantation after lymphocyte depletion with rabbit ATG, a tacrolimus/MMF combination was equally effective with or without maintenance steroids over 5 years posttransplant.[169] In another large multicenter trial, depletional induction with alemtuzumab or rabbit ATG facilitated excellent outcomes over 3 years with a tacrolimus/MMF corticosteroid-free combination.[61] It should be remembered that, beyond the early avoidance philosophy, use of MMF at standard doses (as mandated in these trials) with tacrolimus is associated with substantially greater MPA exposure than the CsA-based trials noted in the previous paragraph, with the enhanced exposure perhaps influencing outcomes.

THERAPEUTIC DRUG MONITORING

Although fixed doses of MMF and EC-MPS have been the norm in most clinical trials and in practice, the marked interindividual variability in pharmacokinetics provides a rationale to implement therapeutic drug monitoring.[11] Despite some interest in pharmacodynamic monitoring, only pharmacokinetic monitoring has been widely tested or implemented. In an early study designed to provide a dataset of MPA exposure (AUC) in a cohort of kidney transplant recipients, 150 recipients were randomized to one of three dose groups of MMF (in combination with CsA and steroids).[153] The study documented poor bioavailability early after transplantation that seemed to stabilize by week 12, when AUCs were almost double those seen in the first 2 weeks posttransplant. There was substantially less acute rejection in patients with AUC >30 mg/h/L. Patients in the highest MPA target group experienced more adverse events, which in this trial resulted in study discontinuation, but no upper limit to define toxicity risk could be determined. While full 12-hour AUC measurement is unwieldy for clinical monitoring, limited sampling strategies correlate well with overall MPA exposure. Trough level monitoring correlates less well with AUC, but recent studies documented an r^2 of 0.68 for patients also receiving tacrolimus (less so for CsA-ME), and low intraindividual variability[47,158] (Figure 18-5). It should be reiterated that trough levels and AUC do not correlate (r^2=0.02) for EC-MPS. Finally, concomitant drug therapy matters. Kuypers and colleagues documented lowest risk for biopsy-proven acute rejection when both tacrolimus and MPA exposure were therapeutic, intermediate risk when one or the other (but not both) was therapeutic, and greatest risk when both drugs were subtherapeutic.[83]

Three large multicenter studies have prospectively tested the impact of therapeutic drug monitoring-based MMF dosing on clinical outcomes in kidney transplantation. In a French study (APOMYGRE), all subjects received CsA and steroids, and were randomized to receive fixed-dose or concentration-controlled (CC) MMF.[91] MMF exposure was measured via limited sampling AUC, and dose adjustments were made by study nurses according to Bayesian algorithm. There was significant benefit for the CC group at 12 months with less acute rejection and fewer treatment failures. The MMF dose was higher in the CC group at day 14 (P<0.0001), month 1 (P<0.0001), and month 3 (P<0.01), as were median AUCs on day 14 (34 versus 27 mg/h/L; P=0.0001) and at month 1 (45 versus 31 mg/h/L; P<0.0001). Adverse events did not differ between groups.

In contrast were two larger trials in Europe and the United States. The FDCC study enrolled 901 European kidney recipients, randomizing to either CC MMF dosing (target AUC 45 mg/h/L) or standard fixed dosing, in combination with calcineurin inhibitors (predominantly tacrolimus) and corticosteroids.[155] Dose changes in the FDCC trial (as well as Opticept[47]) were made by investigators without specific guidance as to frequency or scope. The two treatment groups were largely indistinguishable, with similar MPA exposure in both at all time points, and similar frequency of acute rejection episodes and treatment failure. Again, however, there was a strong relationship between MPA exposure and risk of acute rejection; 37% of subjects had AUC <30 mg/h/L at day 3, more commonly in those taking CsA-ME than tacrolimus. In the Opticept trial, conducted in the United States, 720

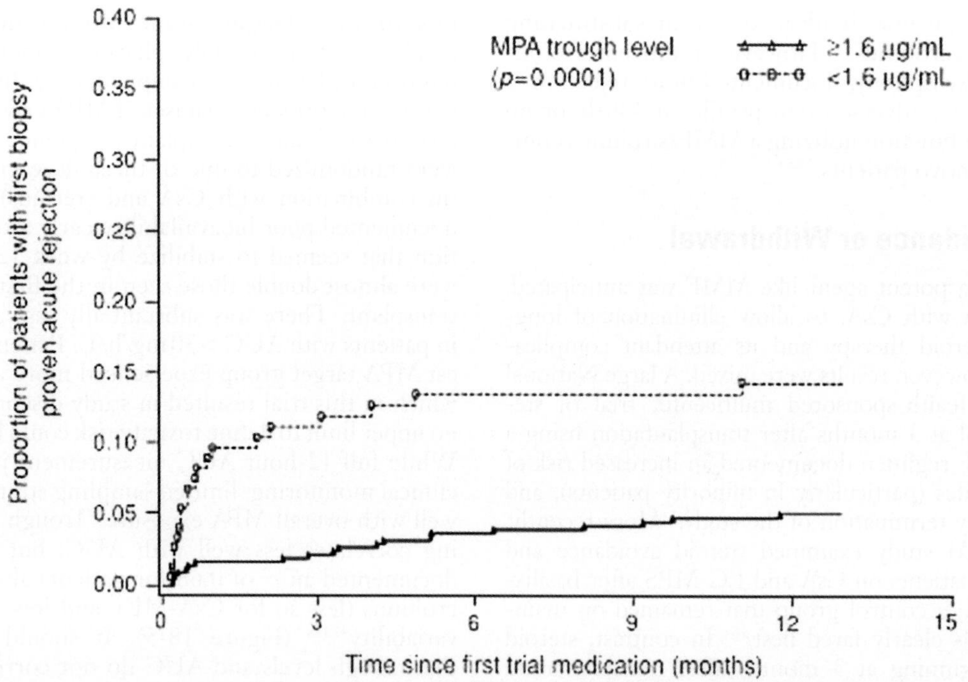

FIGURE 18-6 ■ Mycophenolic acid (MPA) exposure and time to first biopsy-proven acute rejection episode. Cox proportional hazards model estimate with the abbreviated MPA area under the concentration–time curve, baseline hypertension/diabetes, and treatment effect (controls versus concentration-controlled dosing) as covariates. Cutoff point of ≥1.6 µg/mL was based on receiver operating characteristic analysis of the study data. (From Gaston RS, Kaplan B, Shah T, et al. Fixed- or controlled-dose MMF with standard- or reduced-dose calcineurin inhibitors: the Opticept trial. Am J Transplant 2009;9:1607.)

patients were randomized to one of three groups: a control group on fixed-dose MMF and standard-dose calcineurin inhibitor (roughly 80% tacrolimus, 20% CsA) or one of two groups with CC MMF administration, and either standard dose or reduced-dose calcineurin inhibitor.[47] CC dosing of MMF was guided by trough MPA levels, with a target of 1.3 µL/mL for CsA patients, and 1.9 µL/mL for those on tacrolimus. Antibody induction was allowed, with approximately a third of patients receiving rabbit ATG, a third basiliximab, and a third no induction. Again, the groups were largely indistinguishable, with similar outcomes, though almost all tacrolimus patients (with a starting MMF dose of 2 g daily) quickly displayed therapeutic MPA exposure: there was a strong relationship in these patients between adequate exposure (trough MPA level ≥1.6 µg/mL) and reduced risk of acute rejection (Figure 18-6).

A recent consensus conference attempted to put these data into perspective, with recommendations for clinical practice.[90] AUC targets are 30–60 mg/h/L, with the upper limit established primarily as an indicator of no additional efficacy rather than association with toxicity. Recommended trough concentrations are C_0≥1.3 mg/L with CsA and C_0≥1.9 mg/L in patients on tacrolimus. In both the FDCC and Opticept trials, a standard 2-g daily dose of MMF produced adequate early MPA exposure in almost all tacrolimus-treated patients, while in a significant percentage of patients on CsA/MMF combinations, it did not.[47,155] In standard patients, there was no indication that therapeutic drug monitoring improved clinical outcomes. The greatest clinical benefit of therapeutic drug monitoring might be expected in patients on dual immunosuppression, patients undergoing calcineurin inhibitor- or steroid-sparing regimens, those at high immunologic risk, those with delayed graft function, or those with altered gastrointestinal, hepatic, or renal function.[90,156]

REFERENCES

1. Ahsan N, Hricik D, Matas A, et al. Prednisone withdrawal in kidney transplant recipients on cyclosporine and MMF – a prospective randomized study. Steroid Withdrawal Study Group. Transplantation 1999;68:1865.
2. Allison AC, Eugui EM. Mechanisms of action of mycophenolate mofetil in preventing acute and chronic allograft rejection. Transplantation 2005;80:S181.
3. Allison AC, Hovi T, Watts RW, et al. Immunological observations on patients with Lesch–Nyhan syndrome, and on the role of de-novo purine synthesis in lymphocyte transformation. Lancet 1975;2:1179.
4. Allison AC, Kowalski WJ, Muller CJ, et al. Mycophenolic acid and brequinar, inhibitors of purine and pyrimidine synthesis, block glycosylation of adhesion molecules. Transplant Proc 1993;25:67.
5. Arns W, Breuer S, Choudhury S, et al. Enteric-coated mycophenolate sodium delivers bioequivalent MPA exposure compared with MMF. Clin Transplant 2005;19:199–206.
6. Atcheson BA, Taylor PJ, Mudge DW, et al. Mycophenolic acid pharmacokinetics and related outcomes early after renal transplant. Br J Clin Pharmacol 2005;59:271.
7. Augustine JJ, Chang PC, Knauss TC, et al. Improved renal function after conversion from tacrolimus/sirolimus to tacrolimus/mycophenolate mofetil in kidney transplant recipients. Transplantation 2006;81:1004.
8. Azuma H, Binder J, Heemann U, et al. Effects of RS61443 on functional and morphological changes in chronically rejecting rat kidney allografts. Transplantation 1995;59:460.
9. Badid C, Vincent M, McGregor B, et al. Mycophenolate mofetil reduces myofibroblast infiltration and collagen III deposition in rat remnant kidney. Kidney Int 2000;58:51.
10. Banerjee R, Halil O, Bain BJ, et al. Neutrophil dysplasia caused by mycophenolate mofetil. Transplantation 2000;70:1608.

11. Bennett WM. Immunosuppression with mycophenolic acid: one size does not fit all. J Am Soc Nephrol 2003;14:2414.
12. Borrows R, Chusney G, Loucaidou M, et al. Mycophenolic acid 12-h trough level monitoring in renal transplantation: association with acute rejection and toxicity. Am J Transplant 2006;6:121.
13. Bouamar R, Elens L, Shuker N, et al. MPA-related anemia and leucopenia in renal transplant recipients are related to genetic polymorphisms in CYP2C8. Transplantation 2012;93:e39.
14. Budde K, Braun KP, Glander P, et al. Pharmacodynamic monitoring of mycophenolate mofetil in stable renal allograft recipients. Transplant Proc 2002;34:1748.
15. Budde K, Curtis J, Knoll G, et al. Enteric-coated mycophenolate sodium can be safely administered in maintenance renal transplant patients: results of a 1-year study. Am J Transplant 2004;4:237.
16. Budde K, Lehner F, Sommerer C, et al. Conversion from cyclosporine to everolimus at 4.5 months posttransplant: 3-year results from the randomized ZEUS study. Am J Transplant 2012;12:1528.
17. Bullingham R, Monroe S, Nicholls A, et al. Pharmacokinetics and bioavailability of mycophenolate mofetil in healthy subjects after single-dose oral and intravenous administration. J Clin Pharmacol 1996;36:315.
18. Bullingham R, Nicholls AJ, Kamm BR. Clinical pharmacokinetics of mycophenolate mofetil. Clin Pharmacokinet 1999;64:429.
19. Bunnapradist S, Daswani A, Takemoto SK. Graft survival following living-donor renal transplantation: a comparison of tacrolimus and cyclosporine microemulsion with mycophenolate mofetil and steroids. Transplantation 2003;76:10.
20. Bunnapradist S, Lentine KL, Burroughs TE, et al. MMF dose reductions and discontinuations after gastrointestinal complications are associated with renal transplant graft failure. Transplantation 2006;82:102.
21. Bunnapradist S, Neri L, Wong W, et al. Incidence and risk factors for diarrhea following kidney transplantation and association with graft loss and mortality. Am J Kidney Dis 2008;51:478.
22. Carr SF, Papp E, Wu JC, et al. Characterization of human type I and type II IMP dehydrogenases. J Biol Chem 1993;268:27286.
23. Cattaneo D, Perico N, Gaspari F, et al. Glucocorticoids interfere with mycophenolate mofetil bioavailability in kidney transplantation. Kidney Int 2002;62:1060.
24. Cell Cept® (mycophenolate mofetil) full prescribing information. Available online at: www.cellcept.com/cellcept/resources.htm [accessed 24.08.12].
25. Chan L, Mulgaonkar S, Walker R, et al. Patient-reported gastrointestinal symptom burden and health-related quality of life following conversion from mycophenolate mofetil to enteric-coated mycophenolate sodium. Transplantation 2006;81:1290.
26. Ciancio G, Burke GW, Gaynor JJ, et al. A randomized long-term trial of tacrolimus and sirolimus versus tacrolimus and mycophenolate mofetil versus cyclosporine (NEORAL) and sirolimus in renal transplantation, I: drug interactions and rejection at one year. Transplantation 2004;77:244.
27. Colic M, Stojic-Vukanic Z, Pavlovic B, et al. Mycophenolate mofetil inhibits differentiation, maturation and allostimulatory function of human monocyte-derived dendritic cells. Clin Exp Immunol 2003;134:63.
28. de Winter BC, Mathot RA, Sombogaard F, et al. Nonlinear relationship between MMF dose and mycophenolic acid exposure: implications for therapeutic drug monitoring. Clin J Am Soc Nephrol 2011;6:656.
29. de Winter BC, van Gelder T, Glander P, et al. Population pharmacokinetics of mycophenolic acid: a comparison between enteric-coated MPS and MMF in kidney transplant recipients. Clin Pharmacokinet 2008;47:827.
30. Deierhoi MH, Kauffman RS, Hudson SL, et al. Experience with mycophenolate mofetil (RS61443) in renal transplantation at a single center. Ann Surg 1993;217:476.
31. Downs SM. Induction of meiotic maturation in vivo in the mouse by IMP dehydrogenase inhibitors: effects on the developmental capacity of ova. Mol Reprod Dev 1994;38:293.
32. Ducloux D, Ottignon Y, Semhoun-Ducloux S, et al. Mycophenolate mofetil-induced villous atrophy. Transplantation 1998;66:1115.
33. Eckhoff DE, Young CJ, Gaston RS, et al. Racial disparities in renal allograft survival: a public health issue? J Am Coll Surg 2007;204:894.
34. Ekberg H, Bernasconi C, Tedesco-Silva H, et al. Calcineurin inhibitor minimization in the symphony study: observational results 3 years after transplantation. Am J Transplant 2009;9:1876.
35. Ekberg H, Grinyo J, Nashan B, et al. Cyclosporine sparing with MMF, daclizumab, and corticosteroids in renal allograft recipients: the CAESAR study. Am J Transplant 2007;7:560.
36. Ekberg H, Tedesco-Silva H, Demirbas A, et al. Reduced exposure to calcineurin inhibitors in renal transplantation. N Engl J Med 2007;357:2562.
37. Ensor CR, Trofe-Clark J, Gabardi S, et al. Generic maintenance immunosuppression in solid organ transplant recipients. Pharmacotherapy 2011;31:1111.
38. Eugui EM, Almquist SJ, Muller CD, et al. Lymphocyte-selective cytostatic and immunosuppressive effects of mycophenolic acid in vitro: role of deoxyguanosine nucleotide depletion. Scand J Immunol 1991;33:161.
39. European MMF Cooperative Study Group. Placebo-controlled study of mycophenolate mofetil combined with cyclosporine and corticosteroids for prevention of acute rejection. Lancet 1995;345:1321.
40. European MMF Cooperative Study Group. MMF in renal transplantation: 3-year results from the placebo-controlled trial. Transplantation 1999;68:391.
41. Figueroa J, Fuad SA, Kunjummen BD, et al. Suppression of synthesis of natural antibodies by mycophenolate mofetil (RS-61443): its potential use in discordant xenografting. Transplantation 1993;55:1371.
42. Flechner SM, Goldfarb D, Modlin C, et al. Kidney transplantation without calcineurin inhibitor drugs: a prospective, randomized trial of sirolimus versus cyclosporine. Transplantation 2002;74:1070.
43. Franklin TJ, Cook JM. The inhibition of nucleic acid synthesis by mycophenolic acid. Biochem J 1969;113:515.
44. Fukuda T, Goebel J, Thogersen H, et al. IMPDH activity as a pharmacodynamics biomarker of mycophenolic acid effects in pediatric kidney transplant recipients. J Clin Pharmacol 2011;51:309.
45. Funch DP, Ko HH, Travasso J, et al. Posttransplant lymphoproliferative disorder among renal transplant patients in relation to use of MMF. Transplantation 2005;80:1174.
46. Gaston RS, Cecka JM, Kasiske BL, et al. Evidence for antibody-mediated injury as a major determinant of late kidney allograft failure. Transplantation 2010;90:68.
47. Gaston RS, Kaplan B, Shah T, et al. Fixed- or controlled-dose MMF with standard- or reduced-dose calcineurin inhibitors: the Opticept trial. Am J Transplant 2009;9:1607.
48. Giblett ER, Anderson JE, Cohen F, et al. Adenosine-deaminase deficiency in two patients with severely impaired cellular immunity. Lancet 1972;2:1067.
49. Glicklich D, Gupta B, Schurter-Frey G, et al. Chronic renal allograft rejection: no response to mycophenolate mofetil. Transplantation 1998;66:398.
50. Glotz D, Charpentier B, Abramovicz D, et al. Thymoglobulin induction and sirolimus versus tacrolimus in kidney transplant recipients receiving MMF and steroids. Transplantation 2010;89:1511.
51. Goldblum R. Therapy of rheumatoid arthritis with mycophenolate mofetil. Clin Exp Rheumatol 1993;11(Suppl. 8):S117–9.
52. Gonzalez Molina M, Seron D, Garcia del Moral R, et al. Mycophenolate mofetil reduces deterioration of renal function in patients with chronic allograft nephropathy: a follow-up study by the Spanish Cooperative Study Group of Chronic Allograft Nephropathy. Transplantation 2004;77:215.
53. Grailer A, Nichols J, Hullett D, et al. Inhibition of human B cell responses in vitro by RS-61443, cyclosporine A and DAB486 IL-2. Transplant Proc 1991;23:314.
54. Gregoor PJ, de Sevaux RG, Hene RJ, et al. Effect of cyclosporine on mycophenolic acid trough levels in kidney transplant recipients. Transplantation 1999;68:1603.
55. Grinyo JM, Charpentier B, Pestana JM, et al. An integrated safety profile analysis of belatacept in kidney transplant recipients. Transplantation 2010;90:1521.
56. Grinyo JM, Ekberg H, Mamelok RD, et al. The pharmacokinetics of MMF in renal transplant recipients receiving standard-dose or low-dose cyclosporine, low-dose tacrolimus or low-dose sirolimus: the symphony pharmacokinetic substudy. Nephrol Dial Transplant 2009;24:2269.

57. Grinyo JM, Gil-Vernet S, Cruzado JM, et al. Calcineurin inhibitor-free immunosuppression based on antithymocyte globulin and mycophenolate mofetil in cadaveric kidney transplantation: results after 5 years. Transpl Int 2003;16:820.
58. Guerard A, Rabodonirina M, Cotte L, et al. Intestinal microsporidiosis occurring in two renal transplant recipients treated with mycophenolate mofetil. Transplantation 1999;68:699.
59. Hale MD, Nicholls AJ, Bullingham RE, et al. The pharmacokinetic–pharmacodynamic relationship for mycophenolate mofetil in renal transplantation. Clin Pharmacol Ther 1998;64:672.
60. Halloran P, Mathew T, Tomlanovich S, et al. Mycophenolate mofetil in renal allograft recipients: a pooled efficacy analysis of three randomized, double-blind, clinical studies in prevention of rejection. The International Mycophenolate Mofetil Renal Transplant Study Groups. Transplantation 1997;63:39.
61. Hanaway MJ, Woodle ES, Mulgaonkar S, et al. Alemtuzumab induction in renal transplantation. N Engl J Med 2011;364:1909.
62. Hardinger KL, Koch MJ, Bohl DJ, et al. BK-virus and the impact of pre-emptive immunosuppression reduction: 5 year results. Am J Transplant 2010;10:407.
63. Hauser IA, Renders L, Radeke HH, et al. Mycophenolate mofetil inhibits rat and human mesangial cell proliferation by guanosine depletion. Nephrol Dial Transplant 1999;14:58.
64. Hirsch HH, Brennan DC, Drachenberg CB, et al. Polyomavirus-associated nephropathy in renal transplantation: interdisciplinary analyses and recommendations. Transplantation 2005;79:1277.
65. Holt DW. Monitoring mycophenolic acid. Ann Clin Biochem 2002;39:173.
66. Hubner GI, Eismann R, Sziegoleit W. Relationship between mycophenolate mofetil side effects and mycophenolic acid plasma trough levels in renal transplant patients. Arzneimittelforschung 2000;50:936.
67. Hurst FP, Belur P, Nee R, et al. Poor outcomes associated with neutropenia after kidney transplantation: analysis of United States Renal Data System. Transplantation 2011;92:36.
68. Irish WD, Sherrill B, Brennan DC, et al. Three-year posttransplant graft survival in renal-transplant patients with graft function at 6 months receiving tacrolimus or cyclosporine microemulsion within a triple-drug regimen. Transplantation 2003;76:1686.
69. Jacobson PA, Schladt D, Oetting WS, et al. Genetic determinants of mycophenolate-related anemia and leukopenia after transplantation. Transplantation 2011;91:309.
70. Jacobson P, Huang J, Rydholm N, et al. Higher mycophenolate dose requirements in children undergoing hematopoietic cell transplant. J Clin Pharmacol 2008;48:485.
71. Jain A, Venkataramanan R, Kwong T, et al. Pharmacokinetics of mycophenolic acid in liver transplant patients after intravenous and oral administration of mycophenolate mofetil. Liver Transpl 2007;13:291.
72. Johnson C, Ahsan N, Gonwa T, et al. Randomized trial of tacrolimus (Prograf) in combination with azathioprine or mycophenolate mofetil versus cyclosporine (Neoral) with mycophenolate mofetil after cadaveric kidney transplantation. Transplantation 2000;69:834.
73. Jolicoeur EM, Qi S, Xu D, et al. Combination therapy of mycophenolate mofetil and rapamycin in prevention of chronic renal allograft rejection in the rat. Transplantation 2003;75:54.
74. Kasiske BL, Snyder JJ, Gilbertson DT, et al. Cancer after kidney transplantation in the United States. Am J Transplant 2004;4:905.
75. Kauffman HM, Cherikh WS, Cheng Y, et al. Maintenance immunosuppression with target-of-rapamycin inhibitors is associated with a reduced incidence of de novo malignancies. Transplantation 2005;80:883.
76. Kaufman DB, Shapiro R, Lucey MR, et al. Immunosuppression: practice and trends. Am J Transplant 2004;4(Suppl. 9):39.
77. Kiberd BA, Lawen J, Fraser AD, et al. Early adequate mycophenolic acid exposure is associated with less rejection in kidney transplantation. Am J Transplant 2004;4:1079.
78. Kimball JA, Pescovitz MD, Book BK, et al. Reduced human IgG anti-ATGAM antibody formation in renal transplant recipients receiving mycophenolate mofetil. Transplantation 1995;60:1379.
79. Klupp J, Dambrin C, Hibi K, et al. Treatment by mycophenolate mofetil of advanced graft vascular disease in non-human primate recipients of orthotopic aortic allografts. Am J Transplant 2003;3:817.
80. Kobayashi M, Saitoh H, Kobayashi M, et al. Cyclosporin A, but not tacrolimus, inhibits the biliary excretion of mycophenolic acid glucuronide possibly mediated by multidrug resistance-associated protein 2 in rats. J Pharmacol Exp Ther 2004;309:1029.
81. Kotton C, Kumar D, Caliendo AM, et al. International consensus guidelines on the management of cytomegalovirus in solid organ transplantation. Transplantation 2010;89:779.
82. Kreis H, Cisterne JM, Land W, et al. Sirolimus in association with mycophenolate mofetil induction for the prevention of acute graft rejection in renal allograft recipients. Transplantation 2000;69:1252.
83. Kuypers DRJ, Claes K, Evenepoel P, et al. Clinical efficacy and toxicity profile of tacrolimus and mycophenolic acid in relation to combined long-term pharmacokinetics in de novo renal allograft recipients. Clin Pharmacol Ther 2004;75:434.
84. Kuypers DRJ, de Jonge H, Naesens M, et al. Current target ranges of mycophenolic acid exposure and drug-related adverse events: a 5-year, open label, prospective clinical follow-up study in renal allograft recipients. Clin Ther 2008;30:673.
85. Kuypers DR, Vanrenterghem Y, Squifflet JP, et al. Twelve-month evaluation of the clinical pharmacokinetics of total and free mycophenolic acid and its glucuronide metabolites in renal allograft recipients on low dose tacrolimus in combination with mycophenolate mofetil. Ther Drug Monit 2003;25:609.
86. Lambda M, Tafti B, Melcher M, et al. Population pharmacokinetic analysis of mycophenolic acid coadministered with either tasocitinib (CP-690,550) or tacrolimus in adult renal allograft recipients. Ther Drug Monit 2010;32:778.
87. Larsen CP, Grinyo J, Medina-Pestana J, et al. Belatacept-based regimens versus a cyclosporine A-based regimen in kidney transplant recipients: 2-year results from the BENEFIT and BENEFIT-EXT studies. Transplantation 2010;90:1528.
88. Larson TS, Dean PG, Stegall MD, et al. Complete avoidance of calcineurin inhibitors in renal transplantation: a randomized trial comparing sirolimus and tacrolimus. Am J Transplant 2006;6:514.
89. Lee WA, Gu L, Miksztal AR, et al. Bioavailability improvement of mycophenolic acid through amino ester derivatization. Pharm Res 1990;7:161.
90. LeMeur Y, Borrows R, Pescovitz MD, et al. Therapeutic drug monitoring of mycophenolates in kidney transplantation: report of the Transplantation Society consensus meeting. Transplant Rev (Orlando) 2011;25:58.
91. LeMeur Y, Buchler M, Thierry A, et al. Individualized MMF dosing based on drug exposure significantly improves patient outcomes after renal transplantation. Am J Transplant 2007;7:2496.
92. Luan FC, Schaubel DE, Zhang H, et al. Impact of immunosuppressive regimen on survival of kidney transplant recipients with hepatitis C. Transplantation 2008;85:1601.
93. Maes BD, Dalle I, Geboes K, et al. Erosive enterocolitis in mycophenolate mofetil-treated renal-transplant recipients with persistent afebrile diarrhea. Transplantation 2003;75:665.
94. Maes BD, Lemahieu W, Kuypers D, et al. Differential effect of diarrhea on FK506 versus cyclosporine A trough levels and resultant prevention of allograft rejection in renal transplant recipients. Am J Transplant 2002;2:989.
95. Maes BD, van Pelt JF, Peeters JC, et al. The effect of mycophenolate mofetil on hepatitis B viral load in stable renal transplant recipients with chronic hepatitis B. Transplantation 2001;72:1165.
96. McKay DB, Josephson MA. Pregnancy after kidney transplantation. Clin J Am Soc Nephrol 2008;3(Suppl. 2):S117.
97. Meier-Kriesche HU, Ojo AO, Leichtman AB, et al. Effect of mycophenolate mofetil on long-term outcomes in African American renal transplant recipients. J Am Soc Nephrol 2000;11:2366.
98. Meier-Kriesche HU, Steffen BJ, Hochberg AM, et al. Long-term use of mycophenolate mofetil is associated with a reduction in the incidence and risk of late rejection. Am J Transplant 2003;3:68.
99. Meier-Kriesche HU, Steffen BJ, Hochberg AM, et al. Mycophenolate mofetil versus azathioprine therapy is associated with a significant protection against long-term renal allograft function deterioration. Transplantation 2003;75:1341.
100. Mendez R, Gonwa T, Yang HC, et al. A prospective, randomized trial of tacrolimus in combination with sirolimus or mycophenolate mofetil in kidney transplantation: results at 1 year. Transplantation 2005;80:303.

101. Miller J, Mendez R, Pirsch JD, et al. Safety and efficacy of tacrolimus in combination with mycophenolate mofetil (MMF) in cadaveric renal transplant recipients. FK506/MMF Dose-Ranging Kidney Transplant Study Group. Transplantation 2000;69:875.
102. Mitsui A, Suzuki S. Immunosuppressive effect of mycophenolic acid. J Antibiot (Tokyo) 1969;22:358.
103. Mjornstedt L, Sorensen SS, von Zur Muhlen B, et al. Improved renal function after early conversion from a calcineurin inhibitor to everolimus: a randomized trial in kidney transplantation. Am J Transplant 2012;12:2744–53.
104. Moon JI, Kim YS, Kim MS, et al. Effect of cyclosporine, mycophenolic acid, and rapamycin on the proliferation of rat aortic vascular smooth muscle cells: in vitro study. Transplant Proc 2000;32:2026.
105. Morris RG. Immunosuppressant drug monitoring: is the laboratory meeting clinical expectations? Ann Pharmacother 2005;39:119.
106. Morris RE, Wang J, Blum JR, et al. Immunosuppressive effects of the morpholinoethyl ester of mycophenolic acid (RS-61443) in rat and nonhuman primate recipients of heart allografts. Transplant Proc 1991;23:19.
107. Myfortic® (mycophenolic acid) delayed release tablets. Prescribing information. Available online at: www.pharma.us.novartis.com/product/pi/pdf/myfortic.pdf [accessed 24.08.12].
108. Nankivell BJ, Borrows RJ, Fung CL, et al. The natural history of chronic allograft nephropathy. N Engl J Med 2003;349:2326.
109. Nankivell BJ, Wavamunno MD, Borrows RJ, et al. MMF is associated with altered expression of chronic renal transplant histology. Am J Transplant 2007;7:366.
110. Nashan B, Gaston R, Emery V, et al. Review of cytomegalovirus infection findings with mammalian target of rapamycin inhibitor-based immunosuppressive therapy in de novo renal transplant recipients. Transplantation 2012;93:1075.
111. Neff RT, Hurst FP, Falta EM, et al. Progressive multifocal leukoencephalopathy and use of MMF after kidney transplantation. Transplantation 2008;86:1474.
112. Neylan JF for the U.S. Renal Transplant Mycophenolate Mofetil Study Group. Immunosuppressive therapy in high-risk transplant patients: dose dependent efficacy of mycophenolate mofetil in African-American renal allograft recipients. Transplantation 1997;64:1277.
113. Nowak I, Shaw LM. Mycophenolic acid binding to human serum albumin: characterization and relation to pharmacodynamics. Clin Chem 1995;41:1011.
114. Ogawa N, Nagashima N, Nakamura M, et al. Measurement of mycophenolate mofetil effect in transplant recipients. Transplantation 2001;72:422.
115. Ojo AO, Meier-Kriesche HU, Hanson JA, et al. Mycophenolate mofetil reduces late renal allograft loss independent of acute rejection. Transplantation 2000;69:2405.
116. Papadimitriou JC, Drachenberg CB, Beskow CO, et al. Graft-versus-host disease-like features in mycophenolate mofetil-related colitis. Transplant Proc 2001;33:2237.
117. Pascual M, Curtis J, Delmonico FL, et al. A prospective, randomized clinical trial of cyclosporine reduction in stable patients greater than 12 months after renal transplantation. Transplantation 2003;75:1501.
118. Pescovitz MD, Guasch A, Gaston R, et al. Equivalent pharmacokinetics of mycophenolate mofetil in African-American and Caucasian male and female stable renal allograft recipients. Am J Transplant 2003;3:1581.
119. Platz P, Sollinger HW, Hullett DA, et al. RS-61443: a new, potent immunosuppressant agent. Transplantation 1991;51:27.
120. Quemeneur L, Flacher M, Gerland LM, et al. Mycophenolic acid inhibits IL-2-dependent T cell proliferation, but not IL-2-dependent survival and sensitization to apoptosis. J Immunol 2002;169:2747.
121. Remuzzi G, Lesti M, Gotti E, et al. Mycophenolate mofetil versus azathioprine for prevention of acute rejection in renal transplantation (MYSS): a randomised trial. Lancet 2004;364:503.
122. Remuzzi G, Cravedi P, Costantini M, et al. MMF versus azathioprine for prevention of chronic allograft dysfunction in renal transplantation: the MYSS follow-up randomized, controlled clinical trial. J Am Soc Nephrol 2007;18:1973.
123. Robson R, Cecka JM, Opelz G, et al. Prospective registry-based observational cohort study of the long-term risk of malignancies in renal transplant patients treated with mycophenolate mofetil. Am J Transplant 2005;5:2954.
124. Rostaing L, Cantarovich D, Mourad G, et al. Corticosteroid-free immunosuppression with tacrolimus, mycophenolate mofetil, and daclizumab induction in renal transplantation. Transplantation 2005;79:807.
125. Rostaing L, Izopet J, Sandres K, et al. Changes in hepatitis C virus RNA viremia concentrations in long-term renal transplant patients after introduction of mycophenolate mofetil. Transplantation 2000;69:991.
126. Salvadori M, Holzer H, de Mattos A, et al. Enteric-coated mycophenolate sodium is therapeutically equivalent to mycophenolate mofetil in de novo renal transplant patients. Am J Transplant 2004;4:231.
127. Schena FP, Pascoe MD, Alberu J, et al. Conversion from calcineurin inhibitors to sirolimus maintenance therapy in renal allograft recipients: 24-month efficacy and safety results from the CONVERT trial. Transplantation 2009;87:233.
128. Schmedt N, Andersohn F, Garbe E. Signals of progressive multifocal leukoencephalopathy for immunosuppressants: a disproportionality analysis of spontaneous reports within the US adverse event reporting system. Pharmacoepidemiol Drug Saf 2012;21:1216–20.
129. Schnuelle P, van der Heide JH, Tegzess A, et al. Open randomized trial comparing early withdrawal of either cyclosporine or mycophenolate mofetil in stable renal transplant recipients initially treated with a triple drug regimen. J Am Soc Nephrol 2002;13:536.
130. Schweitzer EJ, Yoon S, Fink J, et al. Mycophenolate mofetil reduces the risk of acute rejection less in African-American than in Caucasian kidney recipients. Transplantation 1998;65:242.
131. Sellares J, de Freitas DG, Mengel M, et al. Understanding the causes of kidney transplant failure: the dominant role of antibody-mediated rejection and nonadherence. Am J Transplant 2012;12:388.
132. Shapiro R, Jordan ML, Scantlebury VP, et al. A prospective, randomized trial of tacrolimus/prednisone versus tacrolimus/prednisone/MMF in renal transplant recipients. Transplantation 1999;67:411.
133. Shaw LM, Korecka M, Aradhye S, et al. Mycophenolic acid area under the curve values in African American and Caucasian renal transplant patients are comparable. J Clin Pharmacol 2000;40:624.
134. Shaw LM, Korecka M, Venkataramanan R, et al. Mycophenolic acid pharmacodynamics and pharmacokinetics provide a basis for rational monitoring strategies. Am J Transplant 2003;3:534.
135. Shihab FS, Bennett WM, Yi H, et al. Combination therapy with sirolimus and mycophenolate mofetil: effects on the kidney and on transforming growth factor-beta1. Transplantation 2004;77:683.
136. Shipkova M, Armstrong VW, Oellerich M, et al. Acyl glucuronide drug metabolites: toxicological and analytical implications. Ther Drug Monit 2003;25:1.
137. Sifontis NM, Coscia LA, Constantinescu S, et al. Pregnancy outcomes in solid organ transplant recipients with exposure to MMF or sirolimus. Transplantation 2006;82:1698.
138. Silva HT, Yang HC, Abouljoud M, et al. One-year results with extended-release tacrolimus/MMF, tacrolimus/MMF, and cyclosporine/MMF in de novo kidney transplant recipients. Am J Transplant 2007;7:595.
139. Smith KG, Isbel NM, Catton MG, et al. Suppression of the humoral immune response by mycophenolate mofetil. Nephrol Dial Transplant 1998;13:160.
140. Sollinger HW. Mycophenolate mofetil for the prevention of acute rejection in primary cadaveric renal allograft recipients. U.S. Renal Transplant Mycophenolate Mofetil Study Group. Transplantation 1995;60:225.
141. Sollinger HW, Belzer FO, Deierhoi MH, et al. RS-61443 (mycophenolate mofetil): a multicenter study for refractory kidney transplant rejection. Ann Surg 1992;216:513.
142. Sollinger HW, Deierhoi MH, Belzer FO, et al. RS-61443 – a phase I clinical trial and pilot rescue study. Transplantation 1992;53:428.
143. Sommerer G, Glander P, Arns W, et al. Safety and efficacy of intensified versus standard dosing regimens of EC-MPS in de novo renal transplant patients. Transplantation 2011;91:779.
144. Squifflet JP, Vanrenterghem Y, van Hooff JP, et al. Safe withdrawal of corticosteroids or mycophenolate mofetil: results of a large, prospective, multicenter, randomized study. Transplant Proc 2002;34:1584.

145. Stallone G, Schena A, Infante B, et al. Sirolimus for Kaposi's sarcoma in renal-transplant recipients. N Engl J Med 2005;352:1317.
146. Sunder-Plassmann G, Reinke P, Rath T, et al. Comparative pharmacokinetic study of two mycophenolate mofetil formulations in stable kidney transplant patients. Transpl Int 2012;25:680–6.
147. Suwelack B, Gerhardt U, Hohage H. Withdrawal of cyclosporine or tacrolimus after addition of mycophenolate mofetil in patients with chronic allograft nephropathy. Am J Transplant 2004;4:655.
148. Tedesco Silva H, Cibrik D, Johnston T, et al. Everolimus plus reduced-exposure CsA versus mycophenolic acid plus standard-exposure CsA in renal transplant recipients. Am J Transplant 2010;10:1401.
149. Theodorakis J, Schneeberger H, Illner W-D, et al. Nephrotoxicity-free, MMF-based induction/maintenance immunosuppression in elderly recipients of renal allografts from elderly cadaveric donors. Transplant Proc 2000;32:9S.
150. Tran HT, Acharya MK, McKay DB, et al. Avoidance of cyclosporine in renal transplantation: effects of daclizumab, mycophenolate mofetil, and steroids. J Am Soc Nephrol 2000;11:1903.
151. Tricontinental Mycophenolate Mofetil Renal Transplantation Study Group. A blinded, randomized clinical trial of mycophenolate mofetil for the prevention of acute rejection in cadaveric renal transplantation. Transplantation 1996;61:1029.
152. van Besouw NM, van der Mast BJ, Smak Gregoor PJ, et al. Effect of mycophenolate mofetil on erythropoiesis in stable renal transplant patients is correlated with mycophenolic acid trough levels. Nephrol Dial Transplant 1999;14:2710.
153. van Gelder T, Hilbrands LB, Vanrenterghem Y, et al. A randomized double-blind, multicenter plasma concentration controlled study of the safety and efficacy of oral mycophenolate mofetil for the prevention of acute rejection after kidney transplantation. Transplantation 1999;68:261.
154. van Gelder T, Klupp J, Barten MJ, et al. Comparison of the effects of tacrolimus and cyclosporine on the pharmacokinetics of mycophenolic acid. Ther Drug Monit 2001;23:119.
155. van Gelder T, Silva HT, de Fijter JW, et al. Comparing mycophenolate mofetil regimens for de novo renal transplant recipients: the Fixed-Dose Concentration-Controlled Trial. Transplantation 2008;86:1043.
156. van Gelder T, Silva HT, de Fijter JW, et al. Renal transplant patients at high risk of acute rejection benefit from adequate exposure to mycophenolic acid. Transplantation 2010;89:595.
157. van Gelder T, ter Meulen CG, Hene R, et al. Oral ulcers in kidney transplant recipients treated with sirolimus and mycophenolate mofetil. Transplantation 2003;75:788.
158. van Hest RM, Mathot RA, Vulto AG, et al. Within-patient variability of mycophenolic acid exposure: therapeutic drug monitoring from a clinical point of view. Ther Drug Monit 2006;28:31.
159. Vanrenterghem Y, Lebranchu Y, Hene R, et al. Double-blind comparison of two corticosteroid regimens plus mycophenolate mofetil and cyclosporine for prevention of acute renal allograft rejection. Transplantation 2000;70:1352.
160. Vincenti F, Klintmalm G, Halloran PF. Open letter to the FDA: new drug trials must be relevant. Am J Transplant 2008;8:733–4.
161. Vincenti F, Larsen CP, Alberu J, et al. Three-year outcomes from BENEFIT, a randomized, active-controlled, parallel group study in adult kidney transplant recipients. Am J Transplant 2012;12:210.
162. Vincenti F, Larsen C, Durrbach A, et al. Costimulation blockade with belatacept in renal transplantation. N Engl J Med 2005;353:770.
163. Vincenti F, Monaco A, Grinyo J, et al. Multicenter randomized prospective trial of steroid withdrawal in renal transplant recipients receiving basiliximab, cyclosporine microemulsion and mycophenolate mofetil. Am J Transplant 2003;3:306.
164. Vincenti F, Schena FP, Paraskevas S, et al. A randomized, multicenter study of steroid avoidance, early steroid withdrawal or standard steroid therapy in kidney transplant recipients. Am J Transplant 2008;8:307.
165. Vincenti F, Tedesco Silva H, Busque S, et al. Randomized phase 2b trial of tofacitinib (CP-690,550) in de novo kidney transplant patients: efficacy, renal function, and safety at 1 year. Am J Transplant 2012;12:2446–56.
166. Weber LT, Hoecker B, Armstrong VW, et al. Long-term pharmacokinetics of mycophenolic acid in pediatric renal transplant recipients over 3 years posttransplant. Ther Drug Monit 2008;30:570.
167. Weber LT, Shipkova M, Armstrong VW, et al. The pharmacokinetic–pharmacodynamic relationship for total and free mycophenolic acid in pediatric renal transplant recipients: a report of the German study group on mycophenolate mofetil therapy. J Am Soc Nephrol 2002;13:759.
168. Weir MR, Mulgaonkar S, Chan L, et al. MMF-based immunosuppression with sirolimus in renal transplantation: a randomized, controlled spare-the-nephrons trial. Kidney Int 2011;79:897.
169. Woodle ES, First MR, Pirsch J, et al. A prospective, randomized, double-blind, placebo-controlled multicenter trial comparing early (7 day) corticosteroid cessation versus long-term, low-dose corticosteroid therapy. Ann Surg 2008;248:564.
170. Young M, Plosker GL. Mycophenolate mofetil: a pharmacoeconomic review of its use in solid organ transplantation. Pharmacoeconomics 2002;20:675.

CHAPTER 19

MTOR INHIBITORS: SIROLIMUS AND EVEROLIMUS

J. Andrew Bradley • Christopher J.E. Watson

CHAPTER OUTLINE

Sirolimus and its closely related analogue everolimus are potent immunosuppressive agents that impair lymphocyte activation and proliferation by inhibiting the mammalian target of rapamycin (mTOR). The mTOR inhibitors emerged in the 1990s as a completely new class of immunosuppressive agent and a promising alternative to calcineurin inhibitor (CNI)-based therapy in organ transplantation, particularly since mTOR inhibitors were not believed to cause nephrotoxicity, hitherto the Achilles heel of CNIs. Their appeal was further enhanced by the suggestion that they may have anti-tumor effects and also inhibitory effects on vascular smooth-muscle proliferation that might help prevent chronic rejection.

The early promise that mTOR inhibitors would replace CNI as the mainstay of immunosuppression after organ transplantation has not been fulfilled. Their side effects and limitations became increasingly apparent, and as a result their use in organ transplantation has been more limited than initially anticipated. As new information from clinical trials of the mTOR inhibitors emerges it is clear they still have an important role and are an effective alternative to CNI-based immunosuppressive therapy in a number of clinical situations.

DISCOVERY

Sirolimus (AY-22989, rapamycin, Rapamune) is a fermentation product of the bacterium *Streptomyces hygroscopicus*, first isolated from soil samples taken in 1965 from Easter Island, which is known locally as *Rapa Nui*, hence the subsequent decision to name the drug rapamycin. It was first investigated as an antifungal agent in the mid-1970s[8,136] and in 1977 it was also reported to have immunosuppressive effects in the rat, where it prevented the development of experimental allergic encephalomyelitis and adjuvant arthritis.[102] Twelve years later it was reported that administration of rapamycin prolonged the survival of heart allografts in rats and kidney allografts in pigs and dogs, although it was noted that some pigs developed interstitial pneumonitis,[20] an observation that was later to be noted in the clinic. More worryingly, rapamycin resulted in lethal vasculitis of the gastrointestinal tract in dogs[20] and this finding delayed further clinical evaluation of sirolimus. Tacrolimus, which shares structural similarity with sirolimus (Figure 19-1), also causes vasculitis in the dog,[26] but when used in humans in 1989 there was no sign of such toxicity,[144] which helped lead to a resumption in the clinical evaluation of sirolimus.

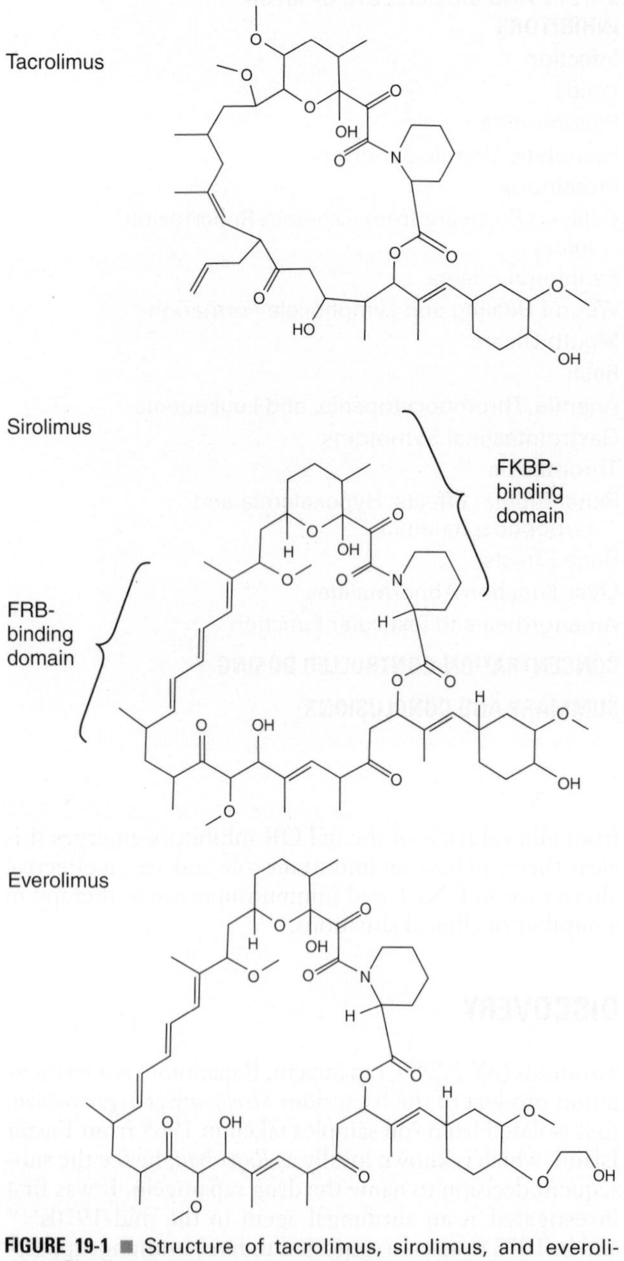

FIGURE 19-1 ■ Structure of tacrolimus, sirolimus, and everolimus. Sirolimus and everolimus are macrocyclic lactones with structural similarity to tacrolimus (FK506, Prograf). Everolimus has a 2-hydroxyethyl chain substitution at position 40 of the sirolimus structure. All three molecules have a common area that binds to a family of intracellular carrier proteins, the FK506 binding proteins (FKBPs), in particular the 12-kD protein FKBP12.

As the potential of sirolimus as a clinical immunosuppressive agent became apparent, chemists at Novartis synthesized everolimus (RAD001, SDZRAD, Certican, Zortress, Affinitor) by making a 2-hydroxyethyl chain substitution at position 40 of the sirolimus molecule (Figure 19-1), a drug which retained potent immunosuppressive activity with improved oral bioavailability.[134]

MECHANISM OF ACTION

The mTOR inhibitors sirolimus and everolimus exert their principal immunosuppressive effects by inhibiting the ability of the intracytoplasmic mTOR multiprotein enzyme complex to regulate the growth, proliferation, and survival of lymphocytes and other immunocompetent cells. mTOR (a 289-kD serine/threonine protein kinase) is a central component of two functionally distinct mTOR complexes called mTOR complex 1 and 2 (mTORC1 and mTORC2).[157] Both mTOR complexes exert their effects on other intracellular signaling molecules including Akt and S6 kinase. Sirolimus and everolimus are potent inhibitors of mTORC1, while the mTORC2 complex is relatively resistant to mTOR inhibition.

After entering into cells, the mTOR inhibitors bind to one of a family of immunophilins called FK506-binding proteins (FKBPs), particularly the 12-kD FKBP12 (Figure 19-2). Immunophilins are highly conserved and abundantly expressed cytosolic proteins whose natural function in the cell is the cis/trans isomerization of peptidyl–prolyl bonds and is completely distinct from their ability to act as receptors for certain immunosuppressant molecules and mediate immunosuppressive effects.[92] The sirolimus–FKBP12 or everolimus–FKBP12 molecular complex binds to the FKBP12-binding domain of mTOR and blocks association of Raptor with mTOR and the adaptor protein mLST8 that collectively comprise the functional mTORC1 complex within the cell.[55,157] This interferes with mTORC1-dependent intracellular signaling pathways, particularly those regulating cell growth and proliferation in response to signals from cytokines, growth factors, nutrients (especially amino acids), stress (e.g., hypoxia), and Toll-like receptor ligand engagement. In lymphoid cells, the important signals originate from the cell surface and are generated by cytokine receptor binding, such as binding of interleukin-2 to the interleukin-2 receptor complex, and ligand binding to coreceptors such as CD28.

The mTORC2 complex comprises mTOR, Rictor (rapamycin-insensitive companion of mTOR), mitogen-activated protein kinase-associated protein (mSIN1), protein observed with Rictor (Protor/PRR5), DEPTOR, and mLST8. While mTORC2 is resistant to acute inhibition by sirolimus (and everolimus), increasing evidence suggests that chronic exposure to sirolimus may block mTORC2 function. mTORC2 is involved in regulating cell morphology and maintaining the integrity of the cytoskeleton. It is also an important regulator of intracellular signaling pathways in both B and T cells, and mTORC2 inhibition may contribute to the immunosuppressive effects of sirolimus and everolimus.[83]

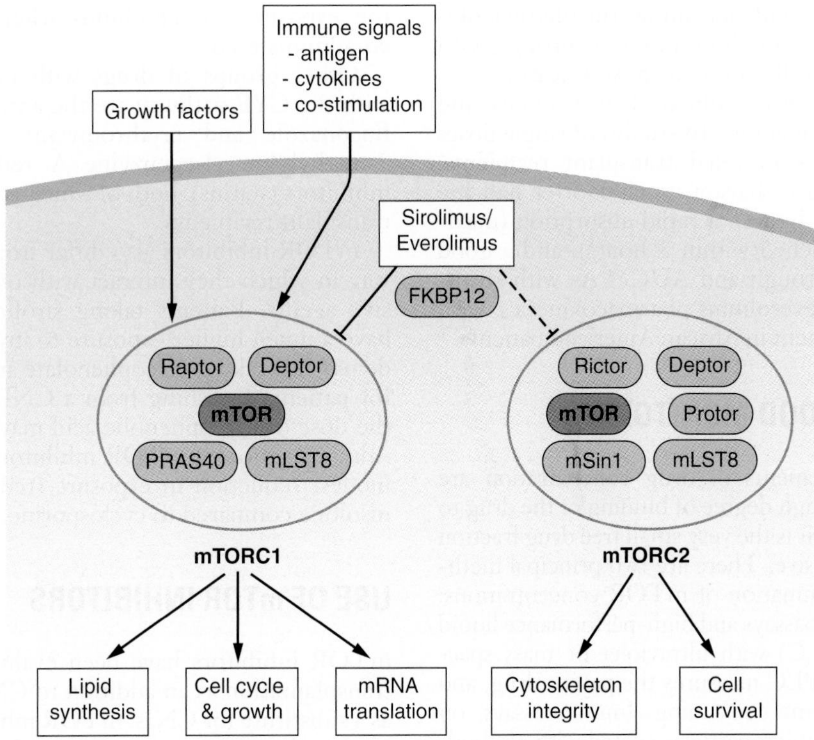

FIGURE 19-2 ■ Highly simplified schematic representation of the mechanism of action of mammalian target of rapamycin (mTOR) inhibitors. The mTOR inhibitors sirolimus and everolimus form an intracellular complex with FK506 binding protein 12 (FKBP12), and this complex inhibits the function of the TORC1 complex, possibly by preventing association of Raptor. TORC1 is important for cell proliferation in response to growth factor stimulation and regulates the S6K1 response to stimulation via the CD28 ligand in T cells. mTOR also forms the TORC2 complex, which is resistant to sirolimus and everolimus and is involved in cytoskeleton control.

Functionally distinct T-cell subsets exhibit differential susceptibility to mTOR inhibition[159] and, interestingly, mTOR inhibitors appear to promote preferentially the expansion of T-regulatory cells in humans,[13,129] which makes them attractive agents to include in experimental protocols aimed at promoting transplant tolerance.[56] The extent to which this property of mTOR inhibitors contributes to their clinical effectiveness as immunosuppressive agents remains to be defined.

While the principal immunosuppressive effect of mTOR inhibitors has been attributed to their inhibitory effect on T-cell proliferation, with activated lymphocytes showing cell cycle arrest in the late G1 phase, it is now clear that mTOR functions as a master regulator controlling many aspects of both innate and adaptive immunity.[131] The mechanisms of immunosuppression through mTOR inhibition are diverse, complex, and still not fully understood. For example, mTOR regulates T-cell trafficking through altered expression of cell surface molecules such as CCR7, and inhibition of mTOR alters lymphocyte migration patterns. mTOR plays an important role in regulating the differentiation of functionally distinct CD4+ T-cell subsets and mTOR blockade appears, as noted above, to promote preferentially the development of T-regulatory cells. mTOR also influences B-cell development and maturation, and inhibiting mTOR may interfere with B-cell responses. Inhibition of mTOR has been shown to have both immunosuppressive and immunostimulatory effects on dendritic cells, reducing and increasing their ability to stimulate T cells according to the type of dendritic cell. Paradoxically, inhibiting mTOR signaling may also have immunostimulatory effects on T cells and sirolimus may, for example, promote the generation of long-lived memory T cells.[5]

PHARMACOKINETICS

Sirolimus and everolimus are only available as oral formulations and both are marketed in tablet form; sirolimus is also available as an oral solution. They are rapidly absorbed from the intestine, although both have a relatively low and variable bioavailability (around 25%). Both sirolimus and everolimus have a narrow therapeutic index and therapeutic monitoring of blood levels is necessary to ensure effective and safe immunosuppression.

After absorption, sirolimus is extensively bound to erythrocytes, and less than 5% of the drug remains free in the plasma, where it is associated with the non-lipoprotein fraction.[158] It has a long half-life of about 60 hours in renal transplant patients, with rapid absorption time to maximal concentration at 1–2 hours and exposure that is proportional to dose, but with a large intersubject coefficient of variance (CV) of 52% and significant intrasubject variability (CV=26%).[45,94] The pharmacokinetic profiles of the tablet formulation and liquid formulation of sirolimus are similar apart from a lower maximal concentration with tablets.[71] With both formulations, the total drug exposure (area under the concentration–time curve (AUC) correlates well with maximal concentration and trough concentration.

Similar to cyclosporine and tacrolimus, the pharmacokinetics of sirolimus differ in different ethnic groups, with reduced oral bioavailability in African Americans.[33]

Everolimus is more water-soluble than sirolimus, and this increases its bioavailability. In studies of single doses of everolimus capsules in renal transplant recipients, everolimus was shown to have a much shorter half-life than sirolimus (16–19 hours), a rapid absorption (maximal concentration reached within 3 hours), and a good correlation between trough and AUC.[68] As with sirolimus, ethnicity affects everolimus pharmacokinetics, with a higher dose requirement in African American patients.[76]

THERAPEUTIC BLOOD MONITORING

Whole-blood measurements of drug concentration are performed due to the high degree of binding of the drug to erythrocytes, although it is the very small free drug fraction that is immunosuppressive. There are two principal methods used in the determination of mTOR concentrations: enzyme-linked immunoassays and high-performance liquid chromatography (HPLC) with ultraviolet or mass spectrometry detection. HPLC measures the parent drug, and is very accurate but time-consuming. Immunoassays, on the other hand, utilize microparticles coated with antibodies to the mTORs and provide a rapid assay, but one which overestimates the drug concentration due to crossreaction with drug metabolites in addition to the parent drug.[62,161]

PHARMACOGENETICS

Sirolimus and everolimus are metabolized in the liver and intestinal wall by the cytochrome P-450 (CYP) 3A enzyme subfamily (CYP3A4 and CYP3A5) and, to a minor extent, by CYP2C8. Polymorphisms of these enzymes are common and because of linkage disequilibrium (the genes lie adjacent on chromosome 7q21) may occur together. Polymorphisms of CYP3A enzymes are associated with lower drug concentration-to-dose ratios in patients expressing the least common genotypes.[4,84] An association between CYP3A5* genotype and dose requirement for sirolimus has been noted in some, but not all, studies, and a recent study in renal transplant patients found no association between CYP3A5 genotype and everolimus pharmacokinetics.[124]

DRUG INTERACTIONS

Since sirolimus and everolimus are metabolized primarily by CYP3A4, and to a lesser extent by CYP3A5 and CYP 2C8, drugs that affect these enzyme pathways alter the metabolism of the mTORs. Important among these are the CNIs, particularly cyclosporine, which can increase the concentration of mTOR inhibitors with a reciprocal increase in cyclosporine concentrations.[160] This drug interaction is particularly noticeable when the time interval between mTOR inhibitors and cyclosporine ingestion varies. It is thus important that patients receiving mTOR inhibitors and cyclosporine adhere to a regular pattern of medication and do not vary the interval between taking the two agents. Conversely, mTOR inhibitors reduce the exposure to tacrolimus when the two drugs are co-administered.[9,122]

Other groups of drugs with important interactions with the CYP pathway are the antimicrobials (especially fluconazole and erythromycin) and the 3-hydroxy-3-methylglutaryl-coenzyme A reductase (HMG-CoA) inhibitors (statins), both of which are widely used in renal transplant recipients.

mTOR inhibitors also differ from cyclosporine in the way in which they interact with other immunosuppressive agents. Patients taking sirolimus, like tacrolimus, have a much higher exposure to mycophenolic acid than do patients taking mycophenolate and cyclosporine,[15] and for patients switching from a CNI to mTOR inhibitor, the dose of mycophenolic acid may need to be adjusted. Administration of mTOR inhibitors may also result in a modest reduction in exposure (reduced AUC) to prednisolone compared to cyclosporine.[63]

USE OF mTOR INHIBITORS

mTOR inhibitors have been evaluated for use in renal transplantation as an addition to CNI-based therapy and as a substitute for CNIs. mTOR inhibitors have also been used as de novo treatment from the time of renal transplantation, as a later addition to CNIs to enhance immunosuppression in response to acute rejection, and as a substitute for CNIs to avoid CNI toxicity in the maintenance phase of immunosuppression.

Early in vitro and in vivo studies suggested that mTOR inhibitors and CNIs when used together had a synergistic immunosuppressive effect.[65,73] This might be anticipated given that CNIs and mTOR inhibitors each block different signals during T-cell activation and affect different stages of the cell cycle. Initially, it was envisaged that mTOR inhibitors might be best used along with CNIs to exploit this synergistic immunosuppressive effect, optimizing immunosuppression and minimizing agent-specific side effects. Evidence from rodent studies suggested, however, that sirolimus may exacerbate cyclosporine nephrotoxicity,[3] a finding that was subsequently confirmed in clinical studies.[67] Most of the initial work with sirolimus was done in conjunction with cyclosporine rather than tacrolimus because it was believed that competition for binding to the immunophilin FKBP12 would preclude co-administration of tacrolimus and sirolimus. It later became evident that there is an abundance of FKBP12 in the cytoplasm, and in vitro studies suggest that less than 5% of the available FKBP needs to be bound to cause half-maximal immunosuppression.[35] Tacrolimus and sirolimus can be administered simultaneously at therapeutic doses in humans without significant competition for FKBP12.[151]

De Novo Therapy with mTOR Inhibitors in the Absence of Calcineurin Inhibitors

Sirolimus has been investigated in numerous studies where it was the principal immunosuppressant. The first such studies were phase II trials conducted in Europe that examined concentration-controlled sirolimus dose regimens, rather than fixed-dose regimens. When sirolimus was administered as a component of triple therapy with azathioprine and prednisolone, it was associated with a similar incidence of acute rejection to that observed in patients on the old Sandimmune preparation of cyclosporine (41% versus 38% at 12 months).[52] A follow-up study substituted azathioprine with mycophenolate mofetil (MMF) and showed no significant difference in the incidence of acute rejection between sirolimus and cyclosporine, although there were numerically more acute rejection episodes in the sirolimus arm (27.5% versus 18.5%).[77] Patient and graft survivals were similar in the two study groups, although the studies were insufficiently powered to detect small differences. Pooled data from both studies showed significantly better renal function in patients receiving sirolimus.[110] These two early studies provided the first detailed insight into the toxicity profile of sirolimus in humans and suggested a side-effect profile that was different from that associated with CNIs (Table 19-1).

Subsequent studies further explored the use of sirolimus with MMF, together with anti-CD25 monoclonal antibody induction therapy. Early data suggested that the combination of sirolimus and MMF was superior to a cyclosporine-based regimen.[48] A subsequent randomized trial comparing sirolimus and tacrolimus (each given along with MMF and prednisolone) showed the two regimens to be comparable in terms of acute rejection rate and graft function.[82] A registry analysis suggested that renal allograft recipients treated with a combination of sirolimus and MMF had a higher rate of acute rejection and reduced allograft survival compared with recipients receiving alternative immunosuppressive regimens.[140]

A systematic review of randomized trials in which mTOR inhibitors were used in place of CNIs as initial therapy after kidney transplantation in studies published up to 2005 (eight different trials with a total of 750 participants) revealed that there was no difference in the incidence of acute rejection at 1 year, but the level of serum creatinine (a possible surrogate end-point for long-term graft survival) was lower in patients receiving mTOR inhibitors.[156]

Recent reports from two large-scale trials (ORION and Symphony) suggested that the combination of sirolimus and MMF is inferior to a low-dose tacrolimus and MMF-based triple therapy.

TABLE 19-1 Adverse Effects of Sirolimus Identified in Phase II Studies of Sirolimus Compared with Cyclosporine

	Sirolimus (*n* = 41+40)	Cyclosporine + Azathioprine (*n* = 42)	Cyclosporine + MMF (*n* = 38)
Metabolic			
Hypertriglyceridemia	21 + 29 = 50 (63%)	5 (12%)	19 (50%)
Hypercholesterolemia	18 + 26 = 44 (54%)	6 (14%)	17 (45)
Hyperglycemia	8 + 6 = 14 (17%)	3 (7%)	6 (16%)
IDDM	1 + 1 = 2 (2%)	1 (2%)	1 (3%)
ALT increase	8 + 8 = 16 (20%)	1 (2%)	3 (8%)
Hypokalemia	14 +8 = 22 (27%)	0	6 (16%)
Hypophosphatemia	6 + 6 = 12 (15%)	0	1 (3%)
Hyperuricemia	1 (3%)	–	7 (18%)
Hematological			
Thrombocytopenia	15 + 18 = 33 (41%)	0	3 (8%)
Leukopenia	16 + 11 = 27 (33%)	6 (14%)	7 (18%)
Anemia	15 + 17 = 32 (40%)	10 (24%)	11 (29%)
Infections			
CMV viremia	6 + 2 = 8 (10%)	5 (12%)	8 (21%)
Herpes simplex	10 + 6 = 16 (20%)	4 (10%)	6 (16%)
Herpes zoster	0 + 1 = 1 (1%)	1 (2%)	1 (3%)
Oral *Candida*	3 + 5 = 8 (10%)	0	3 (8%)
PCP	0 + 0	1 (2%)	0
Pyelonephritis/UTI	17 + 17 = 34 (42%)	12 (29%)	15 (39%)
Septicemia	6 + 2 = 8 (10%)	1 (2%)	1 (3%)
Pneumonia	7 + 6 = 13 (16%)	1 (2%)	2 (5%)
Wound infection	4 + 2 = 6 (7%)	2 (5%)	3 (8%)
Other			
Hypertension	7 + 16 = 23 (16%)	14 (33%)	18 (47%)
Arthralgia	8 (20%)	0	–
Tremor	1 + 2 = 3 (4%)	7 (14%)	8 (21%)
Gingival hyperplasia	0 + 0	4 (10%)	3 (8%)
Hirsutism	1 (3%)	–	4 (11%)
Diarrhea	15 (38%)	–	4 (11%)
Malignancies	0	2 (5%)	0

ALT, alanine aminotransferase; CMV, cytomegalovirus; IDDM, insulin-dependent diabetes mellitus; MMF, mycophenolate mofetil; PCP, *Pneumocystis jirovecii* pneumonia; UTI, urinary tract infection.

Data from Groth CG, Backman L, Morales JM, et al. Sirolimus (rapamycin)-based therapy in human renal transplantation: similar efficacy and different toxicity compared with cyclosporine. Sirolimus European Renal Transplant Study Group. Transplantation 1999;67:1036; and Kreis H, Cisterne JM, Land W, et al. Sirolimus in association with mycophenolate mofetil induction for the prevention of acute graft rejection in renal allograft recipients. Transplantation 2000;69:1252.

The ORION study was an open-label randomized multicenter international comparison of two sirolimus-based regimens with tacrolimus and MMF in adult first- or second-time recipients of living or deceased donor kidneys.[47] A total of 469 patients were recruited in 65 centers in North America, Europe, and Australia and randomly assigned to one of three groups. Group 1 received sirolimus (initial target trough levels 8–15 ng/mL) plus tacrolimus (target trough level 6–15 ng/mL), with stepwise withdrawal of tacrolimus after week 13 and continuation on sirolimus (maintenance trough levels of 12–20 ng/mL). Group 2 received sirolimus (initial target trough levels of 10–15 ng/mL reducing after 13 weeks to 8–15 ng/mL and after 26 weeks to 5–15 ng/mL) plus MMF (up to 2 g/day). Group 3 received tacrolimus (target trough levels of 8–15 ng/mL to week 26 and 5–15 ng/mL thereafter) and MMF (up to 2 g/day). The primary end-point of the study was Nankivell glomerular filtration rate (GFR) at 12 months,[112] and secondary end-points included GFR at 2 years, patient and graft survival, and biopsy-confirmed acute rejection. Study group 2 (sirolimus+MMF) was prematurely discontinued because of a higher-than-expected rate of acute rejection. No significant differences in the primary end-point were found. Patient survival was similar in all three groups (2-year patient survival 94.4% in group 1, 94.5% in group 2, and 97 % in group 3). Graft loss was numerically higher in the groups receiving sirolimus but not significantly so (2-year graft survival 88.5% in group 1, 89.9% in group 2, and 95.4% in group 3). The incidence of biopsy-proven acute rejection in the first 2 years was significantly higher in the CNI-free groups (group 1 17.4%, group 2 32.8%, and group 3 12.3%). Adverse events were the primary reason for patients not continuing in the study and this occurred in 34.2% of patients in group 1, 33.6% of patients in group 2, and 22.3% of patients in group 3. The authors concluded that sirolimus-based regimens were not associated with improved outcomes after kidney transplantation.

The Efficacy Limiting Toxicity Elimination (ELiTE)-Symphony study[40] was an open-label multicenter international randomized four-arm trial that examined the efficacy of reduced-dose sirolimus, tacrolimus, or cyclosporine when combined with daclizumab induction, MMF, and corticosteroids in adult renal transplant recipients. Both living donor and deceased donor transplants were included. The outcomes were also compared to those in recipients given standard-dose cyclosporine, MMF, and corticosteroids. The primary end-point was estimated GFR 12 months after transplantation. A total of 1645 patients were recruited from 15 participating countries. The study group given low-dose tacrolimus, MMF, and steroids had a significantly better 12-month GFR compared to the other three study groups. Acute rejection (biopsy-proven) in the first 6 months was three times higher in the low-dose sirolimus group (35.3%) compared to the low-dose tacrolimus group (11.3%). Allograft survival at 12 months (censored for death with a functioning transplant) was also significantly lower in the low-dose sirolimus and standard-dose cyclosporine groups (91.7% and 91.9% respectively) compared to the low-dose tacrolimus group (96.4%). Withdrawal from the study, mainly because of treatment failure (use of additional immunosuppressive agents and discontinuation of study drug), was highest in recipients randomized to low-dose sirolimus (48.9%). Serious adverse events occurred in 53.2% of patients in the low-dose sirolimus group compared with around 44% for the other study groups. In this study, therefore, low-dose sirolimus resulted in higher rates of biopsy-proven rejection and no improvement in renal function compared to the cyclosporine-based regimens.

In a subsequent report on this study, with an additional 2 years of follow-up based on around half of the patients originally recruited to the ELiTE-Symphony study,[39] renal function remained relatively stable overall and the incidence of graft rejection and graft loss remained low. The low-dose tacrolimus group continued to have the highest GFR but the difference with the other groups was no longer significant. However, the study was not powered to detect differences in the key end-points at 3 years. The number of patients in the low-dose sirolimus group who remained on sirolimus for the entire 3-year study period was low, although their average renal function at 3 years was numerically, but not significantly, slightly higher than that of patients remaining on the original agents in the other three groups.

De Novo Combination Therapy with mTOR Inhibitors and Calcineurin Inhibitors

One of the first studies of sirolimus in renal transplantation to be performed was a dose-ranging study that combined different doses of sirolimus (given as a fixed dose) in conjunction with a high-dose or low-dose Sandimmune cyclosporine (concentration-controlled).[66] All groups received steroids but no azathioprine or MMF. Small numbers of patients in the study and an unequal distribution of African Americans between the six study groups meant that the results were difficult to interpret. Nevertheless, the study showed that the combination of sirolimus and cyclosporine was more potent than cyclosporine alone in the prevention of acute rejection and that half-dose cyclosporine and sirolimus were as efficacious as full-dose cyclosporine and sirolimus. The higher incidence of acute rejection seen in African Americans in this study was also observed in subsequent studies.[64] The other important finding to emerge from this study was a high incidence of pneumocystis pneumonia in sirolimus-treated patients, mostly in patients from one center, where routine prophylaxis against *Pneumocystis jirovecii* was not given. Two large phase III studies of sirolimus followed shortly afterwards, one conducted in the United States[64] and the second worldwide (Table 19-2).[95] Similar to earlier studies, these studies used a fixed dose of sirolimus (2 or 5 mg/day) in combination with concentration-controlled cyclosporine. In the US study, the two different doses of sirolimus were compared with azathioprine, and all groups received steroids but no induction therapy.[64] Only patients with functioning renal allografts were recruited, in contrast to the global study in which function of the graft was not a prerequisite for enrollment.[95] The other major difference between the US and the global study was that the comparator in the global study was placebo rather than

TABLE 19-2 **Outcome of Two Phase III Sirolimus Adjuvant Therapy Studies**

	US Study (n = 719)			Global Study (n = 576)		
	Aza (n = 161)	SRL 2 mg (n = 284)	SRL 5 mg (n = 274)	Placebo (n = 130)	SRL 2 mg (n = 227)	SRL 5 mg (n = 219)
Acute rejection (%)	29.8	16.9*	12†	41.5	24.7‡	19.2§
Creatinine clearance (mL/min)	68.8	62.3	59.2	62.6		56.4
Graft survival (%)	94.4	94.3	92.7	87.7	89.9	90.9
Patient survival (%)	98.1	97.2	96	94.6	96.5	95

*$P = 0.002$ relative to the azathioprine arm.
†$P<0.001$ relative to the azathioprine arm.
‡$P=0.003$ relative to the placebo arm.
§$P<0.001$ relative to the placebo arm.
Aza, azathioprine; SRL, sirolimus.
Note: Acute rejection incidence and creatinine clearance (Nankivell formula) are 6-month values; graft and patient survivals are 12-month values.
From MacDonald A, for the Rapamune Global. Study Group. A worldwide, phase III, randomized, controlled, safety and efficacy study of a sirolimus/cyclosporine regimen for prevention of acute rejection in recipients of primary mismatched renal allografts. Transplantation 2001; 71:271.

azathioprine. Both studies showed a clear benefit in terms of reduction in the rate of acute rejection for patients receiving sirolimus, an effect that was more marked in patients receiving a higher dose of sirolimus. There was a difference in acute rejection rates, patient survival, and graft survival in the US study compared with the global study in all treatment arms, which likely reflects the different enrollment requirements, with only recipients with functioning grafts being entered into the US study.

These two pivotal studies in the development of sirolimus reveal much about how best to use sirolimus and its drawbacks. There was a high incidence of lymphocele formation (12–15% versus 3% in the azathioprine control group in the US study) and wound infection compared with the control arm. Of particular importance was the observation that the renal function of patients on a combination of sirolimus and cyclosporine was worse than that of patients on cyclosporine alone, with a 12-month calculated creatinine clearance of 67.5 mL/min in the azathioprine control group compared with 62 mL/min and 55.5 mL/min in the 2-mg and 5-mg sirolimus groups. A similar effect was seen in the global study.

The immunosuppressive synergy between cyclosporine and sirolimus in these studies was analyzed by median effect analysis of the pooled data.[67] This analysis showed that administration of sirolimus permitted a 2.2-fold reduction in cyclosporine exposure, and reciprocally cyclosporine permits a fivefold reduction in sirolimus dose to achieve the same immunosuppressive efficacy. Experimental data also suggest that synergism accounts for the increased nephrotoxicity.[125]

The combination of everolimus and cyclosporine has been evaluated in several multicenter clinical trials. An early multicenter clinical trial conducted predominantly in Europe compared two fixed doses of everolimus (1.5 and 3 mg/day) against MMF, with all three arms receiving corticosteroids and full-dose cyclosporine with target trough levels of 150–400 ng/mL until week 4 and then 100–300 ng/mL.[149,150] There was no significant difference between the three groups in the primary composite end-point at 6 months (biopsy-proven acute rejection, graft loss, death, and loss to follow-up). However, significantly worse renal function in both everolimus groups led to a protocol revision at 12 months with reduction in the target trough cyclosporine levels to 50–75 ng/mL. At 3 years renal function was similar in the low-dose everolimus and MMF groups, but significantly worse in the higher-dose everolimus group. A similar trial conducted predominantly in North America with the same composite end-point at 36 months and the same protocol amendment showed that all three groups were similarly efficacious but creatinine clearance was lower at 12 and 36 months in the everolimus groups.[90] Another multicenter randomized phase II study undertaken in the United States and Europe evaluated the efficacy and safety of everolimus 3 mg/day together with basiliximab induction, prednisolone, and either full-dose or reduced-dose cyclosporine (trough levels 125–250 ng/mL respectively), although a protocol amendment at 12 months reduced the cyclosporine trough target to 50–75 ng/mL in all patients.[114] The primary end-point was efficacy (composite of biopsy-proven acute rejection, graft loss, death, or loss to follow-up) and efficacy failure was significantly higher in the full-dose cyclosporine arm at 36 months (35.8% versus 17.2%). Creatinine clearance was similar in the two groups at 36 months.

Sirolimus has also been evaluated in combination with tacrolimus after an initial report suggesting that the theoretical misgivings about the combination are not seen in clinical practice.[103] As already noted above, the ORION study[47] included a group that received sirolimus plus tacrolimus but with stepwise withdrawal of tacrolimus after week 13 and continuation on sirolimus.

Sirolimus in combination with tacrolimus was compared with tacrolimus and MMF as primary immunosuppression after kidney transplantation in a randomized multicenter trial in the United States.[107] A total of 361 patients were recruited. Both arms of the study received corticosteroids and sirolimus was dosed to achieve blood levels of 4–12 ng/mL. At 1 year renal function was superior in the tacrolimus arm and patients receiving sirolimus had a higher incidence of study drug discontinuation (26.5%

versus 14.8%). The inferiority of sirolimus/tacrolimus in terms of renal function observed in this study was not found in a more recent European multicenter randomized phase II clinical trial involving 734 patients.[148] In this study primary immunosuppression using sirolimus plus tacrolimus was compared with tacrolimus plus MMF. Sirolimus was given according to a fixed-dose regimen of 2 mg for 28 days and 1 mg thereafter. Both study groups received steroids initially but these were tapered and discontinued after day 90. Renal function at 6 months, the primary end-point, was similarly good in the two study groups. Acute rejection and graft survival were similar in both groups, but premature withdrawal due to adverse events was twice as high in the sirolimus/tacrolimus arm (15.1% versus 6.3%).

Everolimus plus tacrolimus has also been evaluated for use as primary immunosuppression after renal transplantation. The first prospective study to evaluate this combination was a 6-month multicenter study performed in the United States. Ninety-two de novo renal transplant recipients were randomized to receive everolimus, steroids, and basiliximab together with either standard or low-exposure tacrolimus.[24] The differences in tacrolimus exposure achieved in the two study arms were relatively small but the study suggested that everolimus/tacrolimus-based immunosuppression was safe and effective and gave good renal function at 6 months.

In a global study performed in 13 countries (ASSET),[79] everolimus was given along with tacrolimus (target levels of 4–7 ng/mL) for the first 3 months in all patients and thereafter the two study arms comprised one maintained at the same target level of tacrolimus and a tacrolimus minimization group with target tacrolimus levels of 1.5–3.0 ng/mL. The study failed to demonstrate any benefit in the tacrolimus minimization group, possibly due to overlapping of achieved tacrolimus exposure in the two groups, but suggested that everolimus in combination with early tacrolimus minimization was associated with a low rejection rate, good graft survival and renal function, and an acceptable safety profile.

In conclusion, there is no convincing evidence that use of mTOR inhibitors as de novo therapy offers any advantage over CNI-based therapy. The 2009 Kidney Disease: Improving Global Outcomes (KIDIGO) clinical practice guidelines for the care of kidney transplant recipients recommend that the combined use of mTOR inhibitors and CNIs should be avoided, because they potentiate nephrotoxicity, particularly if used in the early period following transplantation.[72]

Maintenance Therapy with mTOR Inhibitors

Although available data suggest that mTOR inhibitors are as efficacious in terms of immunosuppressive potency as CNIs when used as the principal immunosuppressive agent, their use immediately after renal transplantation is undesirable because of their effects on wound healing and lymphocele formation. Because mTOR inhibitors used in the absence of CNIs do not have the same nephrotoxicity concerns as CNIs they are potentially attractive agents for use in the maintenance phase of the posttransplant course, especially in patients with CNI-associated problems, including chronic allograft nephropathy. The first major study to examine the efficacy of mTOR inhibitors in this context used sirolimus combined with cyclosporine and steroids as initial therapy, with the cyclosporine being stopped at 3 months in half the patients. Sirolimus was shown to provide sufficient immunosuppression during the maintenance phase, with superior calculated creatinine clearance compared with patients remaining on sirolimus and cyclosporine. Although the acute rejection rate was slightly higher in the no-cyclosporine group, this did not translate into poorer renal function.[61] Longer follow-up confirmed the sustained benefit of sirolimus maintenance therapy.[78,118] This study had no standard control group, and the subsequent finding of enhanced nephrotoxicity when CNIs are combined with sirolimus casts a shadow over the results.[64,95]

Smaller studies also suggest a benefit of sirolimus over CNIs as maintenance therapy after renal transplantation. A dual-center randomized controlled trial suggested that conversion to sirolimus in patients with impaired graft function results in a rapid improvement in measured GFR at 3 months, which was sustained to 2 years, whereas patients who remained on CNIs experienced deteriorating graft function.[155] Because of concerns about triggering acute rejection during the conversion from CNIs to sirolimus, some investigators have used a period of overlap of immunosuppression,[32] or covered the transition period with additional agents such as basiliximab,[146] but in patients who are greater than 6 months posttransplantation, it is unlikely that this is necessary.

Late conversion to sirolimus is associated with three dominant side effects that might limit its usefulness as a maintenance agent, in addition to the other side effects that are well recognized with sirolimus (see later). First, more than half of patients in some studies experience a rash, either an acneiform rash or a dermatitis-like rash affecting the hands and, in particular, the fingers. Second, the period of conversion to sirolimus is associated with the development of mouth ulcers that, in most patients, resolve within 4 weeks. If such ulcers fail to resolve, herpes simplex should be considered. Finally, patients with suboptimal renal function, particularly patients with proteinuria, are prone to develop marked proteinuria after conversion (see later).[30,87]

Despite the potential drawbacks in terms of side effects, evidence is accumulating that conversion from CNIs to mTOR inhibitors may be worthwhile in patients with chronic allograft nephropathy and, at least in the short term, may lead to improved graft function.[31] The optimal time for conversion in such patients is unclear, but early rather than late conversion may be best, before renal structural changes associated with chronic allograft nephropathy become extensive. Switching to mTOR inhibitors in patients who are experiencing other side effects from CNIs, such as neurotoxicity and diabetes, may also be a reasonable option. Conversion from CNIs to mTOR inhibitors for patients who develop hemolytic uremic syndrome should also be considered, although sirolimus itself has been identified as a cause of this condition.[10,133] Because mTOR inhibitors lead to an increased urinary excretion of uric acid, this is a further possible indication for the use of mTOR inhibitors in the management of severe gout in patients taking CNIs.

The ZEUS study, a multicenter, open-label, randomized controlled trial of everolimus-based, CNI-free immunosuppression, suggested that early replacement of CNIs with everolimus-based immunosuppression is advantageous for renal function.[16] A total of 503 adult recipients of renal transplants in 17 German and Swiss centers were recruited to the study and received initial therapy with basiliximab induction together with cyclosporine, mycophenolate, and prednisolone. At 4.5 months after transplantation recipients were randomized (n=300 or 60% of the total recruited) to continue on cyclosporine (n=145) or switch to an everolimus-based regimen (n=155) with everolimus trough concentrations of 6–10 ng/mL. Those recipients switched to everolimus showed a significant improvement in 12-month GFR (the primary end-point) compared to those who remained on cyclosporine (71.8 mL/min/1.73 m^2 versus 61.9 mL/min/1.73 m^2). Conversion to everolimus was associated with a 6% higher rate of postrandomization acute rejection than remaining on cyclosporine (10% versus 3%), but over the entire study period acute rejection rates were similar (15%). The overall efficacy and safety were similar in the two study groups.

mTOR INHIBITORS AND MALIGNANCY

mTOR Inhibitors as Antitumor Agents

The p13K/Akt/mTOR signaling pathway is often constitutively activated in malignant cells and stimulates cell proliferation and tumor growth as well as production of growth factors, such as vascular endothelial growth factor (VEGF), that stimulate angiogenesis, a key component of many tumors. Because of the central role of mTOR in regulating cellular processes in malignant cells, it is an attractive therapeutic target.[89] The ability of sirolimus to inhibit the growth of tumor cell lines in vitro and to prevent growth of transplanted tumors in rodent models has been long known and mTOR inhibitors represent a novel and important class of anticancer agents.[37] Although intuitively the immunosuppressive effects of mTOR might be expected to outweigh any beneficial effect on limiting tumor cell growth in patients with malignancy, this seems not to be the case and a number of new sirolimus derivatives have been developed specifically for use as antitumor agents, including temsirolimus (CC1-779), a sirolimus derivative formulated for intravenous administration. mTOR inhibitors have been evaluated for their efficacy and safety in a large number of phase I and phase II clinical trials for different types of malignancy and in some cases have progressed to evaluation in phase III trials. On the basis of available clinical evidence, everolimus has now been given approval in the United States and Europe for an increasing number of cancers that now include advanced renal cell carcinoma, subependymal giant cell astrocytoma, progressive neuroendocrine tumors, and advanced hormone receptor-positive HER-2-negative breast cancer. Food and Drug Administration approval for the latter was given in 2012, based on the results of a recently reported large randomized double-blind multicenter study (BOLERO-2) showing in an interim analysis a progression-free survival of 7.8 months for those receiving everolimus and 3.2 months for those given placebo.[11] The use of mTOR inhibitors is currently being tested in many of the other common types of cancer, including colorectal, ovarian, prostatic, gastric, and pancreatic cancer.

mTOR Inhibitors and Posttransplant Malignancy

Because patients after renal transplantation are at increased risk of developing most types of malignancy, particularly squamous cell cancer of the skin and lymphoma, the anticancer effects of mTOR inhibitors are of great relevance. Several reports suggest that maintenance immunosuppression with mTOR inhibitors after renal transplantation may be associated with a reduced risk of posttransplant malignancy. It is, however, important to bear in mind that this could, at least in part, reflect the ability of CNIs to increase the risk of malignancy rather than any direct protective effect of mTOR inhibitors. A multivariate analysis of posttransplant malignancy in 33 249 renal allograft recipients in the United States revealed that the incidence rates of any type of posttransplant malignancy were 0.6% in patients taking mTOR inhibitors, 0.6% for patients taking mTOR inhibitors plus CNIs, and 1.8% for patients taking CNIs alone.[70] Similarly, the incidence of posttransplant malignancy in adults randomly assigned to remain on sirolimus and CNIs was found to be greater than in subjects randomly assigned to early CNI withdrawal and an increased dose of sirolimus.[21]

mTOR Inhibitors and Non-Melanoma Skin Cancer

The most frequent type of cancer after renal transplantation is non-melanoma skin cancer which affects over half of all transplant recipients and is an important consideration when considering the optimal immunosuppressive regimen, especially for those patients considered at particularly high risk because of previous skin cancers or premalignant skin lesions.[43] A recently reported single-center randomized controlled trial showed that renal transplant recipients with premalignant skin lesions who were switched to sirolimus-based immunosuppression had less progression and in some cases even regression of premalignant skin lesions.[132] There were 25 patients assigned to the sirolimus arm and 19 to the control arm and, of the nine patients who developed histologically confirmed non-melanoma skin cancer during the 12-month follow-up period, only one was in the sirolimus arm. Another recently reported multicenter study (the TUMORAPA study) randomly assigned renal transplant recipients who were receiving calcineurin-based immunosuppression and had at least one invasive posttransplant cutaneous squamous cell carcinoma to switch to sirolimus or remain on CNIs.[44] New squamous cell cancers developed in 14 (22%) of those switched to sirolimus and 22 (39%) of those randomized to stay on calcineurin blockers, with a median term to onset of 16 versus 7 months respectively (*P*=0.02). Switching to sirolimus appears an effective strategy for reducing the risk of recurrent skin cancer and is a reasonable treatment option, although not without potential side effects. It was notable, however, that in the TUMORAPA study, twice as many serious adverse events occurred in those switched to sirolimus and 23% of patients discontinued sirolimus because of adverse events.

mTOR Inhibitors and Posttransplant Lymphoproliferative Disorder

Everolimus and sirolimus have been shown to inhibit markedly the growth of human posttransplant lymphoproliferative disorder-derived cell lines and Epstein–Barr virus-transformed B lymphocytes in vitro and in vivo.[99,100,116] Nevertheless there is relatively limited evidence to support the use of mTOR inhibitors in the management of posttransplant lymphoproliferative disorder, although a renal transplant recipient in whom disseminated posttransplant lymphoproliferative disorder resolved completely after conversion of immunosuppression to sirolimus has been reported.[27] In a pooled analysis from nine European centers, 19 renal transplant recipients with posttransplant lymphoproliferative disease were studied after conversion to mTOR inhibitors and subsequent withdrawal or minimization of CNIs.[121] Remission of disease was observed in 15 of the recipients, although since 12 of the recipients also received rituximab or chemotherapy with CHOP, it is difficult to know how much of the benefit was directly attributable to the use of mTOR inhibitors. Sirolimus did not appear to modify the risk of developing posttransplant lymphoproliferative disorder in an analysis of 25 127 patients who underwent renal transplantation in the United States, of whom 34 developed posttransplant lymphoproliferative disorder.[19]

mTOR Inhibitors and Kaposi's Sarcoma

mTOR inhibitors may have a useful role in the treatment of renal transplant recipients who develop Kaposi's sarcoma associated with herpesvirus-8, especially if the disease is confined to the skin. In a study of 15 patients who developed cutaneous Kaposi's sarcoma after renal transplantation while taking cyclosporine, switching them to sirolimus led to complete, histologically confirmed remission in all patients for the duration of the study (6 months) with preservation of graft function.[143] However response varies and may depend on the severity of disease. A retrospective analysis in which 14 renal transplant recipients with Kaposi's sarcoma (including several with visceral or advanced disease) were switched from CNIs to sirolimus showed that the switch was generally well tolerated. Complete remission was seen in two patients, and a partial response was seen in a further eight, although three of the partial responders with advanced disease relapsed after several months.[85] In patients who do not respond to mTOR inhibitors or show significant side effects it has been suggested that a combination of mTOR inhibitor and leflunomide (which inhibits Akt signaling upstream from mTOR) may act synergistically in the treatment of Kaposi's sarcoma.[12] The use of mTOR-based immunosuppression, however, does not necessarily prevent the development of posttransplant Kaposi's sarcoma.[6] Further studies are needed to evaluate the role of mTOR inhibitors in the treatment of Kaposi's sarcoma and to determine the optimal treatment strategy for patients with more advanced disease.

mTOR Inhibitors and BK Virus

Polyoma virus nephropathy due to BK virus is an increasingly recognized cause of kidney graft dysfunction. The incidence in patients with sirolimus-based immunosuppression has been reported to be relatively low, compared to other immunosuppressive regimens.[14] Moreover there are some reports that a sirolimus-based regimen may be associated with early resolution of nephropathy.[154] This observation is supported by some in vitro evidence suggesting that sirolimus may be working by blocking intracellular protein kinase pathways utilized by the virus, an effect that is complemented by the addition of leflunomide.[88]

SAFETY AND SIDE EFFECTS OF mTOR INHIBITORS

It was not until the phase II studies of sirolimus by Groth and Kreis and their colleagues[52,77] that the sirolimus-specific side effects became clear because until then the agent had been used in conjunction with CNIs. Table 19-1 shows the principal side effects found in these studies. In contrast to CNIs, it is notable that, although mTOR inhibitors may cause a range of agent-specific side effects, these do not include nephrotoxicity, neurotoxicity, hypertension, or gingival hyperplasia.

Infection

The incidence and pattern of infections reported in patients receiving mTOR inhibitors are broadly similar to those in patients receiving CNI-based immunosuppression. Neither the US study nor the global studies of de novo sirolimus use (Table 19-2) identified any particular problem with infection over and above that observed in the comparator groups, although the global study noted an increase in the incidence of mucosal lesions attributed (but without virological confirmation) to herpes simplex virus.[64,95] A meta-analysis of mTOR inhibitor use as primary immunosuppression after kidney transplantation confirmed the overall safety of mTOR inhibitors in terms of infection and noted that, when mTOR inhibitors were substituted for antimetabolites, there was a reduction in the incidence of cytomegalovirus infection.[156] Some studies have suggested that the incidence of pneumonia may be greater in patients receiving mTOR inhibitors, but the evidence for this remains inconclusive and confounded by the occurrence of drug-induced pneumonitis.

Lipids

One of the most concerning long-term problems associated with mTOR inhibitors is their metabolic effect on lipid metabolism. Two-thirds of patients may develop increased triglyceride levels, and half develop increased serum cholesterol levels. Fifty-three percent of sirolimus-treated patients required lipid-lowering agents compared with 24% in the cyclosporine groups combined. The full significance of the increased lipids associated with mTOR inhibitors is unclear, but it is a long-term concern. Lipids are implicated in the development of cardiovascular disease and in the genesis of chronic rejection.[104] What is unclear is whether these risks pertain in the presence of sirolimus. There is evidence in animal models that sirolimus inhibits graft vasculopathy,[58] an observation confirmed with everolimus in heart transplant recipients.[38] Sirolimus also seems able to prevent the accelerated vascular disease seen in cholesterol-fed, apolipoprotein E-deficient mice despite a high cholesterol diet.[42] The occurrence of lipid abnormalities seems to be, at least in part, genetically determined with polymorphisms in apolipoprotein A implicated.[101]

Pneumonitis

Pneumonitis is one of the most feared complications of mTOR inhibitors and may progress to pulmonary failure. It may occur at any time during treatment and presents as progressive dyspnea, dry cough, fatigue, and fever.[23,54] Imaging reveals bilateral pulmonary infiltrates (Figure 19-3), and pulmonary function tests may show a restrictive pattern. Open-lung biopsies have revealed granulomata in some cases. The effect is reversible with discontinuation of mTOR inhibitor. The true incidence of mTOR-associated pneumonitis is unclear, and it is probably under-recognized and under-reported. The first reports of sirolimus-associated pneumonitis were in 2000,[111] and these were followed by a disclosure from the US Food and Drug Administration of 31 other cases of interstitial pneumonitis associated with sirolimus use.[139] Earlier studies had reported an increased incidence of pneumonia (Table 19-1)[52], however, and one of the first studies reported an excess of pneumocystis pneumonia[66]; it is possible that some of these were in fact sirolimus-induced pneumonitis. Ten years previously, the complication had been noted as the principal cause of death in pigs undergoing renal transplantation with sirolimus.[20]

The etiology of sirolimus-associated pneumonitis is unclear. Reports suggest that it is more common in patients switching from a CNI to sirolimus, or having a CNI withdrawn from sirolimus/CNI combination, and having a high drug concentration.[23,51,139] A mortality of 12% was noted in the Food and Drug Administration report, although early recognition of the problem, with immediate discontinuation of sirolimus, should reduce the mortality from this complication.

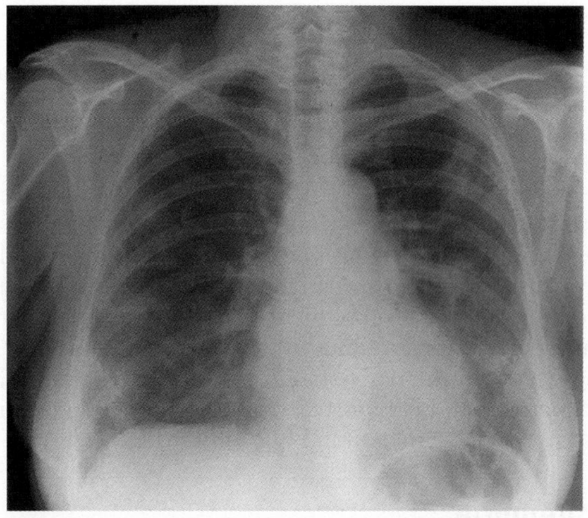

A

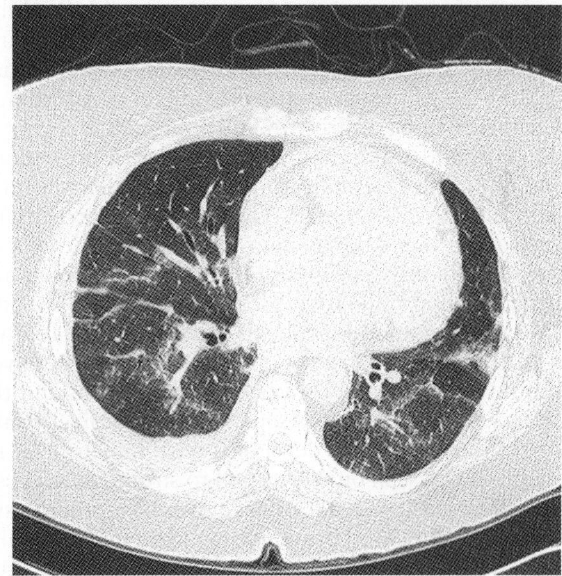

B

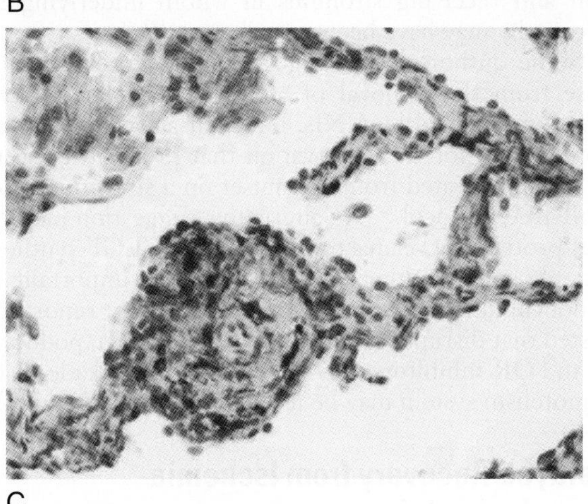

C

FIGURE 19-3 ■ Sirolimus-induced pneumonitis. (A) Plain chest radiograph shows bilateral interstitial infiltration. (B) High-resolution computed tomography scan shows patchy ground-glass opacification and interstitial reticular change. (C) Immunohistologic analysis of transbronchial lung biopsy specimen in sirolimus-induced pneumonitis shows heavy interstitial CD4T-cell infiltrate (immunoperoxidase, ×400). (A and B, courtesy of Dr. A. Tasker; C, courtesy of Dr. M. Griffiths.)

Hemolytic Uremic Syndrome

One of the main attractions of mTOR inhibitor therapy is its perceived lack of nephrotoxicity. Although sirolimus does not cause typical changes associated with CNI therapy, it is not entirely devoid of adverse effects on the kidney. The most serious of these is its association with hemolytic uremic syndrome (thrombotic microangiopathy). Hemolytic uremic syndrome was identified as a potential problem in patients taking cyclosporine and sirolimus,[81,127] but subsequent reports indicated that it could occur with sirolimus in the absence of CNIs.[10,133] It also occurs in the native kidneys of non-renal transplant recipients,[53] and is reported with everolimus, suggesting that it is a class effect of mTOR inhibitors.[90]

Proteinuria

Proteinuria is a common manifestation of mTOR inhibitor toxicity in patients converted to mTOR for renal impairment.[90] It is most common in patients who already have a degree of proteinuria at the time of conversion,[130] and it seems to be a direct mTOR effect that occurs in both adults and children.[18,87] The absence of proteinuria seems to be the best indicator of improvement in renal function after conversion.[17,30] The cause of the proteinuria is unclear. In one study of four patients who developed proteinuria, biopsy specimens revealed glomerulonephritis (membranoproliferative glomerulonephritis in one, membranous glomerulonephritis in another, and IgA nephropathy in the other two).[34] The proteinuria resolved when the patients were converted back to CNIs and the sirolimus was stopped. In a separate study of liver transplant recipients who had developed renal impairment, no proteinuria was seen on conversion to sirolimus, suggesting that pre-existing renal damage may be a prerequisite for the development of proteinuria.[29] Proteinuria has also been observed in patients undergoing islet transplantation and receiving sirolimus in whom underlying nephropathy may have been contributory.[137]

Some authors have suggested that proteinuria may arise from the removal of afferent arteriolar vasoconstriction afforded by CNIs, but such a mechanism cannot account for the observation that proteinuria occurs in patients treated from the outset on a sirolimus-based, CNI-free protocol.[145] An alternative suggestion has been that proteinuria relates to inhibition of VEGF synthesis, Akt phosphorylation, or other pathways important for podocyte function and integrity.[86,152] A recent report suggested that disruption of the autophagic flux in podocytes by mTOR inhibitors may play a role.[25] Blockade of the angiotensin system may be useful to limit proteinuria.[119]

Delayed Recovery from Ischemia-Reperfusion Injury

Delayed recovery of normal kidney function (delayed graft function) is a common manifestation of ischemia-reperfusion injury, more common in recipients of kidneys donated after circulatory death where both warm ischemia and cold ischemia contribute to renal injury. Reduced exposure to CNIs in the early posttransplant period is practiced in many transplant centers, so "non-nephrotoxic agents" such as mTOR inhibitors were an attractive alternative. However early experimental work in rats showed delayed recovery from ischemia-reperfusion injury,[50] and this has subsequently been observed in the clinic in small retrospective studies[105] and registry analyses.[138] The mechanism underlying this observation presumably relates to the inhibition of cell proliferation affecting tubular repair.[91] Although sirolimus is associated with a higher incidence of delayed graft function and prolonged recovery of function, renal function in the long term does not seem to suffer.[106,141]

Peripheral Edema

The occurrence of edema in patients taking mTOR inhibitors is well described. Most edema affects the lower limb[1] and may be unilateral (Figure 19-4) or bilateral; it is not necessarily ipsilateral to the kidney transplant. Angioedema affecting the eyelids and tongue has also been described.[49,108,142,153] The cause of this complication is unknown but typically resolves on discontinuation of mTOR inhibition.

Wound Healing and Lymphocele Formation

One of the most concerning complications of mTOR inhibitors is the potentially detrimental effect they have on the operative site. mTOR inhibitors not only impair wound healing but are also associated with a high incidence of lymphoceles after renal transplantation. The latter problem may be, in part, center-specific, suggesting a role for technical factors relating to the intraoperative management of lymphatics (whether divided, ligated, or left undisturbed). Wound problems

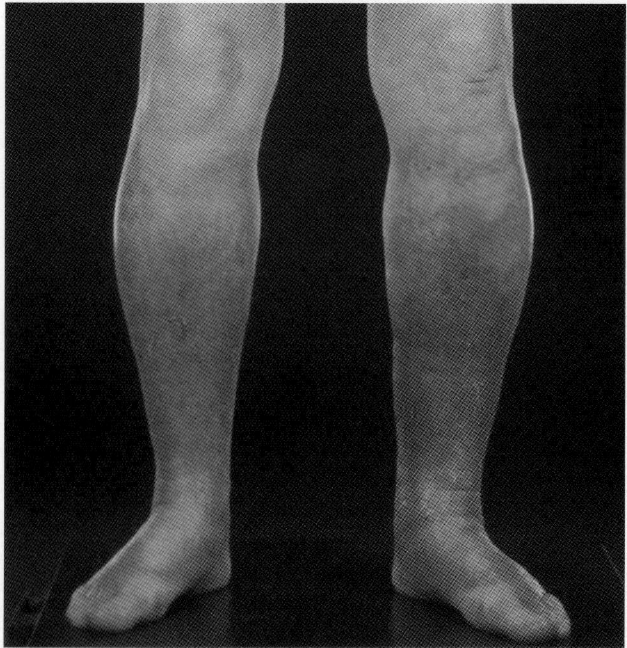

FIGURE 19-4 ■ Sirolimus-induced erythema and limb edema. Acute erythema and swelling in the limbs associated with sirolimus. The symptoms resolved after administration of steroids.

include fluid collections around the graft and beneath the skin, superficial infections, and late incisional hernia.[28] Anastomotic healing has not been reported as a problem after renal transplantation, but poor healing of the airway anastomosis has been cited after lung transplantation,[36,74] and there is evidence in the pig that ureteric anastomoses are less strong when performed in the presence of mTOR inhibitors.[69] The problems observed with wound healing may result from mTOR inhibition reducing the fibroblast response to fibroblast growth factor and to a lack of neovascularization of wounds due to decreased production of VEGF. A recently reported systematic review of randomized controlled trials of wound complications and lymphoceles after solid-organ transplantation supported the view that mTOR inhibitors are best avoided during the first few months after transplantation.[123] Pooled analysis showed a higher incidence of wound complications (odds ratio (OR) 1.77, confidence interval (CI) 1.31–2.37) and lymphoceles (OR 2.07, CI 1.62–2.65) for kidney transplant recipients receiving mTOR inhibitors along with calcineurin blockers. Wound complications (OR 3.00, CI 1.61–5.59) and lymphoceles (OR 2.13, CI 1.57–2.90) were also more common in recipients receiving mTOR inhibitors along with antimetabolites. Another recent but non-systematic review of wound-healing complications in relation to use of mTOR inhibitors suggested that wound complications may be less of a problem with the lower-exposure regimens of mTOR inhibitors that have now largely superseded the historical high-exposure regimens.[113] It has, however, been suggested that obesity may adversely influence wound healing in patients receiving mTOR inhibitors[147] and that it would be prudent to avoid their use in patients undergoing surgery, including transplantation, whose body mass index is greater than 32 kg/m^2 until more data are available.[113]

Mouth Ulcers

Oral ulceration (mucositis) manifesting as painful gingival or buccal mucosa leading to pain on eating is a well-documented and troublesome side effect of mTOR inhibition (Figure 19-5). The ulcers are usually small but multiple, and in some cases may be related to herpes simplex virus infection. In the global phase III study of de novo treatment with sirolimus, ulceration of the oral mucosa was observed in 19% of patients randomly assigned to 5 mg/day of sirolimus, 10% of patients assigned to 2 mg/day of sirolimus, and 9% of patients in the placebo group.[95] The lesions were all mild and resolved spontaneously without discontinuing sirolimus.[95]

Mouth ulcers are also common in patients converted to mTOR inhibitors. Again, such ulcers usually resolve spontaneously, but they can be problematic. In one prospective randomized study in which renal transplant recipients were converted at 1 year from a steroid-free regimen of tacrolimus and MMF to sirolimus and MMF, oral ulceration occurred in 9 of 15 converted patients. The mucosal lesions healed within 2 weeks of discontinuing sirolimus, but the problem led to premature cessation of the study.[139] The authors

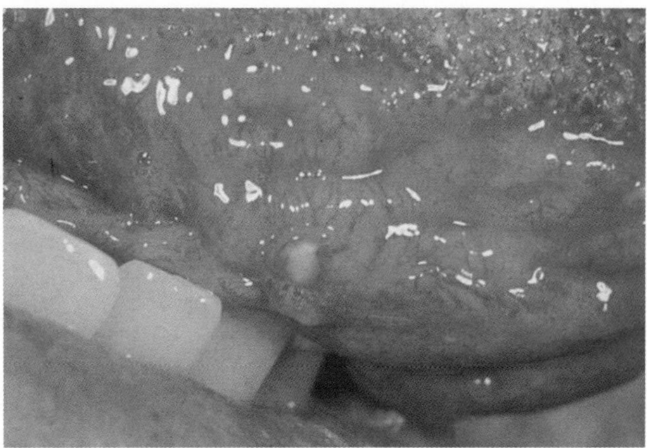

FIGURE 19-5 ■ Sirolimus-induced oral ulceration. Solitary aphthous-type ulcer on the undersurface of the tongue occurring several days after late (>6 months) conversion from calcineurin inhibitor to sirolimus. Such lesions are often multiple and painful and can be distressing for the patient. They usually resolve rapidly after adjustment of sirolimus to the lower end of the target range of 5–10 ng/mL.

postulated that the high incidence of oral ulceration may have been attributable to overimmunosuppression during conversion, the use of oral emulsion of sirolimus rather than tablets, and the lack of corticosteroids.[139] In a randomized study of conversion from CNIs to sirolimus after renal transplantation, aphthous-type mouth ulcers occurred in one-third of patients during the first 2 weeks after conversion, although all resolved with adjustment of sirolimus to the lower end of the target range of 5–15 ng/mL.[155] The association between mTOR inhibitors and mucosal ulceration may be attributable predominantly to their detrimental effect on wound healing, rather than any direct effect on initiating ulcer formation.

Rash

As already noted, rash is a common complication of mTOR inhibitor therapy and most commonly takes the form of an inflammatory acneiform eruption[96] or a dermatitis-like rash affecting the hands and, in particular, the fingers (Figure 19-6). This rash was apparent in both the early multicenter randomized trials of de novo sirolimus treatment after renal transplantation. In the US study, an acneiform rash was observed in 25% of recipients on 2 mg/day, 19% of recipients on 5 mg/day, and 11% in the azathioprine control group.[64] In the global phase III study, rash was observed in 14% of patients randomly assigned to 5 mg/day of sirolimus, 4% of patients assigned to 2 mg/day of sirolimus, and 5% of patients in the placebo group.[95]

In studies in which an indepth dermatological analysis has been undertaken, the incidence of dermatological side effects is considerably higher. A cross-sectional study of cutaneous adverse events in renal transplant recipients receiving long-term sirolimus-based immunosuppression reported the presence of an acne-like eruption in 46%, scalp folliculitis in 26%, and hidradenitis suppurativa in 12% of patients.[97] In the absence of a control group, it is difficult to attribute such findings exclusively to mTOR

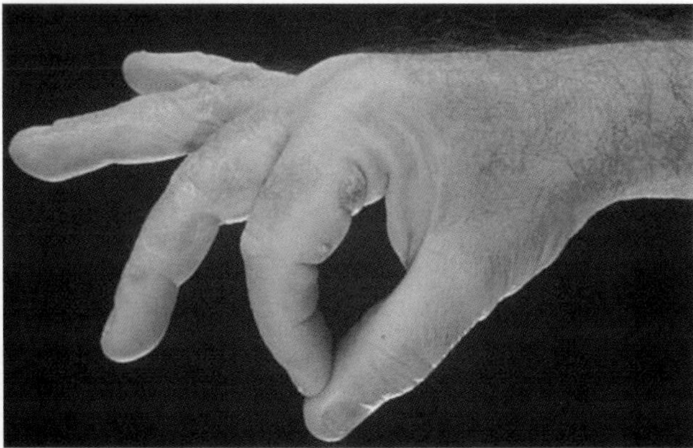

FIGURE 19-6 ■ Sirolimus-induced rash. After conversion from calcineurin inhibitor to sirolimus, patients commonly develop skin problems that may take the form of a dermatitis-like rash affecting the hands and, in particular, the fingers.

inhibitors, but both studies indicate the high frequency of dermatological complications associated with mTOR inhibitors. Although rashes are usually mild, they may be a reason for discontinuing mTOR inhibitors. In the randomized trial of late conversion to sirolimus in the authors' center, 68% of converted patients developed a rash, particularly acne, and 2 of the 19 converted patients discontinued sirolimus because of this.[155] The pathophysiology of rash in patients taking mTOR inhibitors is unclear, but may be attributable to their effect on the epidermal growth factor receptor, which is important in the differentiation and development of the hair follicle.[96]

Anemia, Thrombocytopenia, and Leukopenia

Anemia, thrombocytopenia, and leukopenia are all well-recognized side effects of mTOR inhibitor use. Although thrombocytopenia attracted the most attention in early studies, anemia has emerged as the most significant clinical problem. Anemia is a common complication during the first 6 months after renal transplantation regardless of the immunosuppressive regimen,[2] but the incidence is increased with use of mTOR inhibitors. In the global study of de novo sirolimus in renal transplantation, anemia was observed in 16% of recipients taking 2 mg/day and 27% of recipients taking 5 mg/day sirolimus. The incidence of anemia in the 5 mg/day group was significantly higher than in the placebo group (13%) receiving cyclosporine and steroids.[95] mTOR inhibitor dose adjustment may be required, and in some patients administration of erythropoietin may be necessary.

Anemia after renal transplantation most often results from iron deficiency and defective erythropoietin production, but the mechanisms responsible for mTOR inhibitor-induced anemia are unclear. Sirolimus blocks the in vitro response of bone marrow cells to several hematopoietic cytokines, including granulocyte colony-stimulating factor, interleukin-3, and kit ligand.[126] Although mTOR inhibitor-induced suppression of non-erythroid bone marrow cells contributes to leukopenia and thrombocytopenia, the extent to which they cause anemia by suppression of erythrocyte production is uncertain. Sirolimus has been observed to reduce hemoglobin levels without reducing the erythrocyte count in renal transplant recipients, arguing against a direct antiproliferative effect on erythroid bone marrow.[98] It was suggested instead that sirolimus may have a direct effect on iron homeostasis.[98]

Thrombocytopenia was identified as a side effect of sirolimus in the global and the US phase III randomized trials of de novo sirolimus and seemed to be dose-related.[64,95] In both studies, a few patients randomly assigned to the higher dose (5 mg/day) of sirolimus had to have sirolimus discontinued because of thrombocytopenia (6 of 208 (2.8%) in the global study and 3 of 274 (1.1%) in the US study), although none of the patients experienced severe thrombocytopenia or were reported to have had related hemorrhage. mTOR inhibitors may reduce circulating platelets as part of their inhibitory effect on hematopoietic cytokines. In addition, sirolimus has been shown to promote agonist-induced platelet aggregation in vitro,[7] and conceivably, if increased platelet aggregation occurs in vivo, it may promote increased removal of platelets by the spleen.

Although it is well recognized that mTOR inhibitors may reduce the platelet count, this is not usually of clinical significance and rarely requires cessation of therapy. Thrombocytopenia most often occurs within the first month of starting sirolimus, and its occurrence correlates with whole-blood trough levels of sirolimus that exceed 16 ng/mL. If the platelet count falls significantly, it usually responds well to dose reduction without the need to withdraw mTOR inhibitors.[57]

Finally, mTOR inhibitors may produce mild leukopenia, which is usually transient and dose-related.

Gastrointestinal Symptoms

Gastrointestinal side effects include abdominal pain, nausea, and vomiting, but the most common symptom is diarrhea, which is usually mild, dose-related, and does not require mTOR withdrawal. In the pivotal phase III studies of de novo sirolimus, mild diarrhea was observed in 27–32% of patients receiving 5 mg/day of sirolimus, 16–20% of those receiving 2 mg/day of sirolimus, and 11–13% of patients in the control groups.[64,95] Mild diarrhea is particularly common in patients receiving a combination of mTOR inhibitors and MMF[77] and may be related to pharmacokinetic interaction between the two agents[46]; concentration-controlled administration of MMF markedly reduces gastrointestinal symptoms.[46]

Thrombosis

Sirolimus, like CNIs, may increase platelet aggregation in vitro,[7] and it has been suggested that sirolimus, when used in combination with CNIs, may increase the risk of hepatic artery thrombosis after liver transplantation. There is no published evidence that mTOR inhibitors are associated with an increased risk of thromboembolic events after renal transplantation: mTOR-coated coronary stents are believed to have an increased incidence of thrombosis, although the evidence for this is poor.[120] In a retrospective single-center analysis of deep vein thrombosis, graft thrombosis, and pulmonary embolism in renal transplant recipients, the addition of sirolimus in recipients taking cyclosporine did not increase the risk of postoperative thrombotic events.[80] A strong correlation between the development of deep vein thrombosis and lymphocele was observed, however, in patients receiving sirolimus,[80] and the increased risk of deep vein thrombosis in patients developing lymphocele should be kept in mind.

In vitro sirolimus has been shown to reduce the expression of tissue plasminogen activator and induced the expression of plasminogen activator inhibitor by human umbilical vein endothelial cells, providing a possible underlying mechanism for the increased thromboembolic disease seen with mTOR inhibitors.[93]

Renal Tubular Effects: Hypokalemia and Hypophosphatemia

mTOR inhibitors may contribute to hypokalemia after renal transplantation, and in the phase II and III trials of primary treatment with sirolimus, values of serum potassium less than the normal range were recorded during the first 3 months in about half of patients.[110] Hypokalemia is usually mild and only about 10% of patients required a period of potassium supplementation, which readily corrected the problem.[110] Hypokalemia may be partially related to the dose of mTOR inhibitors given and seems to be due to mTOR inhibitor-induced alterations in tubular function leading to increased tubular secretion of potassium.[109]

Hypophosphatemia is also common in the first few weeks after renal transplantation and is multifactorial in etiology. Although reduced serum phosphate levels may be observed more often during the first 3 months in patients receiving mTOR inhibitors, this is rarely a clinically significant problem, and values return to normal with time and dose adjustment.[110] The mechanisms underlying mTOR inhibitor-associated hypophosphatemia are not completely understood, but mTOR inhibitors may impair renal tubular phosphate reabsorption, prolonging the phosphate leak.[135]

Bone Effects

Arthralgia was identified as a side effect of mTOR inhibitors in the global phase III study of sirolimus. It was observed in 27% of recipients on the higher dose (5 mg/day) of sirolimus compared with 16% and 13% of recipients on low-dose sirolimus or placebo.[95] Similar to the CNI-induced pain syndrome, bone pain associated with sirolimus affects weight-bearing areas, particularly the feet, ankles, and knees, although the pain may be unrelated to weight bearing. It is generally bilateral and symmetrical. The problem is much less common when lower doses of mTOR inhibitors are used, and symptoms may improve after dosage reduction or respond to treatment with bisphosphonates or alfacalcidol. mTOR inhibitor-induced bone pain and CNI-induced pain syndrome are likely due to a combination of increased adipocyte volume, reduced intraosseous perfusion, and marrow edema, giving rise to a "bone compartment syndrome."[41] The diagnosis usually can be confirmed by radionuclide bone scan (Figure 19-7) or magnetic resonance imaging that reveals hyperemia and marrow edema.

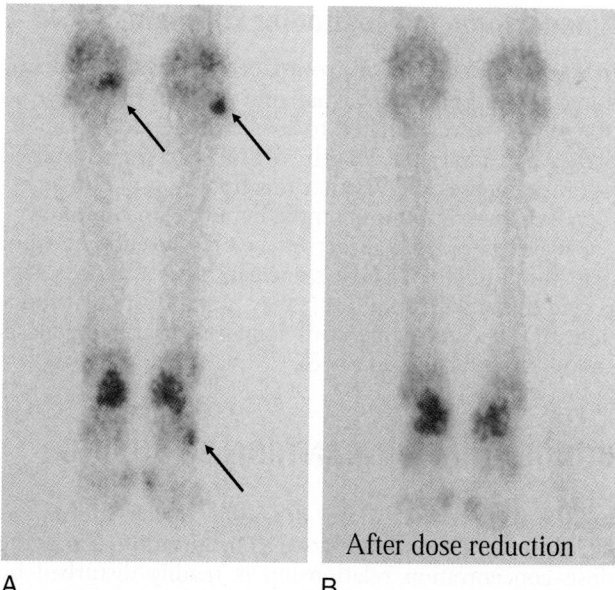

FIGURE 19-7 ■ Radionuclide bone scan in a patient with sirolimus-induced bone pain. The patient complained of pain affecting the feet, ankles, and knees. The diagnosis was confirmed by radioisotope scanning that revealed areas of increased uptake in the knees and at the ankles (arrows, A). After sirolimus dosage reduction, the symptoms resolved, and the bone scan returned to normal (B).

Osteoporosis and bone loss are common after renal transplantation, and there is evidence from preclinical and early clinical studies that mTOR inhibitors may have bone-sparing properties compared with CNIs. Although sirolimus is associated with bone remodeling, it does not result in a loss of trabecular bone volume in rat studies, in contrast to CNIs.[128] Similarly, everolimus inhibits osteoclast activity in vitro and reduces bone loss in an oophorectomized rat model.[75] Markers of bone turnover (serum osteocalcin and urinary *N*-telopeptides) also are significantly lower in renal transplant recipients taking de novo sirolimus compared with recipients taking cyclosporine.[22] Such studies suggest a possible advantage of mTOR inhibitors over CNIs, but more extensive clinical studies with extended follow-up are needed to confirm these early indications.

Liver Function Abnormalities

Sirolimus tends to cause increased levels of transaminases (alanine aminotransferase and aspartate aminotransferase) and lactate dehydrogenase. Whether this is clinically significant is unclear. There are two reports of hepatotoxicity in a renal transplant recipient[60,117] and a series of 10 liver transplant recipients in whom sirolimus was thought to be responsible for abnormal liver function tests, with two of the patients having liver biopsy specimens with eosinophilia and sinusoidal congestion.[115] This latter group of 10 patients underwent transplantation for hepatitis C, which had reinfected their grafts, making a clear association with sirolimus difficult.

Amenorrhea and Testicular Function

In a study of conversion from CNIs to sirolimus, it was noted that all three female patients younger than 40 years of age who were switched to sirolimus developed amenorrhea for a variable length of time and then resumed irregular menses.[155] Whether this finding is due to an effect of mTOR inhibitors on the hypothalamic–pituitary–gonadal axis or to a direct effect on the endometrium (e.g., inhibition of VEGF) is unclear. It has also been suggested that mTOR inhibitors may impair testicular function and are associated with impaired spermatogenesis and reduced fertility in males.[162]

CONCENTRATION-CONTROLLED DOSING

mTORs are critical-dose drugs in which efficacy is closely related to whole-blood concentration. Since the dose–concentration relationship is readily disturbed by interactions with other drugs commonly administered to transplant recipients, and adverse events are typically dose-related, mTOR dosage should be concentration-controlled; fixed-dose regimens run the risk of underimmunosuppression or toxicity and overimmunosuppression.

SUMMARY AND CONCLUSIONS

The mTOR inhibitors sirolimus and everolimus represent a distinct class of immunosuppressive agents and have been shown to be effective in preventing acute renal allograft rejection and preserving glomerular filtration. Their safety profile in terms of posttransplant infection is satisfactory and broadly comparable with that of patients receiving standard CNI-based therapy. The agent-specific side-effect profile of the mTOR inhibitors is also now well established and has relatively little overlap with that of CNIs.

Overall, the clinical impact of mTOR inhibitors for immunosuppression after renal transplantation has been less than anticipated when they were first introduced. They do not share the same nephrotoxicity as CNIs (although can cause proteinuria) and there is some evidence that they may limit chronic allograft nephropathy. However, the problems of impaired wound healing and lymphocele formation argue against the immediate use of mTOR inhibitors after renal transplantation, and the adverse effects of mTOR inhibitors on the lipid profile and the low but significant risk of life-threatening pneumonitis are concerns with long-term use.

What then is their role? They are an attractive alternative for patients who cannot tolerate CNIs. They are also an appealing option for recipients whose graft function is declining because of chronic nephropathy. They have a role for recipients who have a high risk of malignant disease, particularly those with previous skin cancer, and they may be a useful option in recipients with troublesome BK nephropathy.

The optimal timing for the introduction of mTOR inhibitors after renal transplantation is still unclear and better ways to manage the troublesome mucosal and dermatological complications that are commonly encountered need to be found. Most importantly, long-term studies are needed to determine whether the early benefits observed with mTOR inhibitors in terms of preservation of renal function translate into improved long-term graft survival and protection from chronic allograft nephropathy, particularly in light of adverse registry data on graft and patient survival.[59] There is also still a need to determine the extent to which any such benefits outweigh the long-term side effects of mTOR inhibitors, particularly their adverse effects on the lipid profile.

REFERENCES

1. Aboujaoude W, Milgrom ML, Govani MV. Lymphedema associated with sirolimus in renal transplant recipients. Transplantation 2004;77:1094–6.
2. Afzali B, Al-Khoury S, Shah N, et al. Anemia after renal transplantation. Am J Kidney Dis 2006;48:519–36.
3. Andoh TF, Lindsley J, Franceschini N, et al. Synergistic effects of cyclosporine and rapamycin in a chronic nephrotoxicity model. Transplantation 1996;62:311–6.
4. Anglicheau D, Le Corre D, Lechaton S, et al. Consequences of genetic polymorphisms for sirolimus requirements after renal transplant in patients on primary sirolimus therapy. Am J Transplant 2005;5:595–603.
5. Araki K, Ellebedy AH, Ahmed R. TOR in the immune system. Curr Opin Cell Biol 2011;23:707–15.
6. Babel N, Eibl N, Ulrich C, et al. Development of Kaposi's sarcoma under sirolimus-based immunosuppression and successful treatment with imiquimod. Transpl Infect Dis 2008;10:59–62.
7. Babinska A, Markell MS, Salifu MO, et al. Enhancement of human platelet aggregation and secretion induced by rapamycin. Nephrol Dial Transplant 1998;13:3153–9.
8. Baker H, Sidorowicz A, Sehgal SN, et al. Rapamycin (AY-22,989), a new antifungal antibiotic. III. In vitro and in vivo evaluation. J Antibiot (Tokyo) 1978;31:539–45.
9. Baldan N, Rigotti P, Furian L, et al. Co-administration of sirolimus alters tacrolimus pharmacokinetics in a dose-dependent manner in adult renal transplant recipients. Pharmacol Res 2006;54:181–5.
10. Barone GW, Gurley BJ, Abul-Ezz SR, et al. Sirolimus-induced thrombotic microangiopathy in a renal transplant recipient. Am J Kidney Dis 2003;42:202–6.
11. Baselga J, Campone M, Piccart M, et al. Everolimus in postmenopausal hormone-receptor-positive advanced breast cancer. N Engl J Med 2012;366:520–9.
12. Basu G, Mohapatra A, Manipadam MT, et al. Leflunomide with low-dose everolimus for treatment of Kaposi's sarcoma in a renal allograft recipient. Nephrol Dial Transplant 2011;26:3412–5.
13. Battaglia M, Stabilini A, Migliavacca B, et al. Rapamycin promotes expansion of functional CD4+CD25+FOXP3+ regulatory T cells of both healthy subjects and type 1 diabetic patients. J Immunol 2006;177:8338–47.
14. Benavides CA, Pollard VB, Mauiyyedi S, et al. BK virus-associated nephropathy in sirolimus-treated renal transplant patients: incidence, course, and clinical outcomes. Transplantation 2007;84:83–8.
15. Buchler M, Lebranchu Y, Beneton M, et al. Higher exposure to mycophenolic acid with sirolimus than with cyclosporine cotreatment. Clin Pharmacol Ther 2005;78:34–42.
16. Budde K, Becker T, Arns W, et al. Everolimus-based, calcineurin-inhibitor-free regimen in recipients of de-novo kidney transplants: an open-label, randomised, controlled trial. Lancet 2011;377:837–47.
17. Bumbea V, Kamar N, Ribes D, et al. Long-term results in renal transplant patients with allograft dysfunction after switching from calcineurin inhibitors to sirolimus. Nephrol Dial Transplant 2005;20:2517–23.
18. Butani L. Investigation of pediatric renal transplant recipients with heavy proteinuria after sirolimus rescue. Transplantation 2004;78:1362–6.
19. Caillard S, Dharnidharka V, Agodoa L, et al. Posttransplant lymphoproliferative disorders after renal transplantation in the United States in era of modern immunosuppression. Transplantation 2005;80:1233–43.

20. Calne RY, Collier DS, Lim S, et al. Rapamycin for immunosuppression in organ allografting. Lancet 1989;2:227.
21. Campistol JM, Eris J, Oberbauer R, et al. Sirolimus therapy after early cyclosporine withdrawal reduces the risk for cancer in adult renal transplantation. J Am Soc Nephrol 2006;17:581–9.
22. Campistol JM, Holt DW, Epstein S, et al. Bone metabolism in renal transplant patients treated with cyclosporine or sirolimus. Transpl Int 2005;18:1028–35.
23. Champion L, Stern M, Israel-Biet D, et al. Brief communication: sirolimus-associated pneumonitis: 24 cases in renal transplant recipients. Ann Intern Med 2006;144:505–9.
24. Chan L, Greenstein S, Hardy MA, et al. Multicenter, randomized study of the use of everolimus with tacrolimus after renal transplantation demonstrates its effectiveness. Transplantation 2008;85:821–6.
25. Cina DP, Onay T, Paltoo A, et al. Inhibition of MTOR disrupts autophagic flux in podocytes. J Am Soc Nephrol 2012;23:412–20.
26. Collier DS, Calne R, Thiru S, et al. FK-506 in experimental renal allografts. Transplant Proc 1987;19:3975–7.
27. Cullis B, D'Souza R, McCullagh P, et al. Sirolimus-induced remission of posttransplantation lymphoproliferative disorder. Am J Kidney Dis 2006;47:e67–72.
28. Dean PG, Lund WJ, Larson TS, et al. Wound-healing complications after kidney transplantation: a prospective, randomized comparison of sirolimus and tacrolimus. Transplantation 2004;77:1555–61.
29. Dervaux T, Caillard S, Meyer C, et al. Is sirolimus responsible for proteinuria? Transplant Proc 2005;37:2828–9.
30. Diekmann F, Budde K, Oppenheimer F, et al. Predictors of success in conversion from calcineurin inhibitor to sirolimus in chronic allograft dysfunction. Am J Transplant 2004;4:1869–75.
31. Diekmann F, Campistol JM. Conversion from calcineurin inhibitors to sirolimus in chronic allograft nephropathy: benefits and risks. Nephrol Dial Transplant 2006;21:562–8.
32. Diekmann F, Fritsche L, Neumayer HH, et al. Sirolimus dosage during and after conversion from calcineurin inhibitor therapy to sirolimus in chronic kidney transplant patients. Kidney Blood Press Res 2004;27:186–90.
33. Dirks NL, Huth B, Yates CR, et al. Pharmacokinetics of immunosuppressants: a perspective on ethnic differences. Int J Clin Pharmacol Ther 2004;42:701–18.
34. Dittrich E, Schmaldienst S, Soleiman A, et al. Rapamycin-associated post-transplantation glomerulonephritis and its remission after reintroduction of calcineurin-inhibitor therapy. Transpl Int 2004;17:215–20.
35. Dumont FJ, Kastner C, Iacovone Jr F, et al. Quantitative and temporal analysis of the cellular interaction of FK-506 and rapamycin in T-lymphocytes. J Pharmacol Exp Ther 1994;268:32–41.
36. Dutly AE, Gaspert A, Inci I, et al. The influence of the rapamycin-derivate SDZ RAD on the healing of airway anastomoses. Eur J Cardiothorac Surg 2003;24:154–8, discussion 8.
37. Easton JB, Houghton PJ. mTOR and cancer therapy. Oncogene 2006;25:6436–46.
38. Eisen HJ, Tuzcu EM, Dorent R, et al. Everolimus for the prevention of allograft rejection and vasculopathy in cardiac-transplant recipients. N Engl J Med 2003;349:847–58.
39. Ekberg H, Bernasconi C, Tedesco-Silva H, et al. Calcineurin inhibitor minimization in the Symphony study: observational results 3 years after transplantation. Am J Transplant 2009;9:1876–85.
40. Ekberg H, Tedesco-Silva H, Demirbas A, et al. Reduced exposure to calcineurin inhibitors in renal transplantation. N Engl J Med 2007;357:2562–75.
41. Elder GJ. From marrow oedema to osteonecrosis: common paths in the development of post-transplant bone pain. Nephrology (Carlton) 2006;11:560–7.
42. Elloso MM, Azrolan N, Sehgal SN, et al. Protective effect of the immunosuppressant sirolimus against aortic atherosclerosis in apo E-deficient mice. Am J Transplant 2003;3:562–9.
43. Euvrard S, Kanitakis J, Claudy A. Skin cancers after organ transplantation. N Engl J Med 2003;348:1681–91.
44. Euvrard S, Morelon E, Rostaing L, et al. Sirolimus and secondary skin-cancer prevention in kidney transplantation. N Engl J Med 2012;367:329–39.
45. Ferron GM, Mishina EV, Zimmerman JJ, et al. Population pharmacokinetics of sirolimus in kidney transplant patients. Clin Pharmacol Ther 1997;61:416–28.
46. Flechner SM, Feng J, Mastroianni B, et al. The effect of 2-gram versus 1-gram concentration controlled mycophenolate mofetil on renal transplant outcomes using sirolimus-based calcineurin inhibitor drug-free immunosuppression. Transplantation 2005;79:926–34.
47. Flechner SM, Glyda M, Cockfield S, et al. The ORION study: comparison of two sirolimus-based regimens versus tacrolimus and mycophenolate mofetil in renal allograft recipients. Am J Transplant 2011;11:1633–44.
48. Flechner SM, Goldfarb D, Modlin C, et al. Kidney transplantation without calcineurin inhibitor drugs: a prospective, randomized trial of sirolimus versus cyclosporine. Transplantation 2002;74:1070–6.
49. Fuchs U, Zittermann A, Berthold HK, et al. Immunosuppressive therapy with everolimus can be associated with potentially life-threatening lingual angioedema. Transplantation 2005;79:981–3.
50. Fuller TF, Freise CE, Serkova N, et al. Sirolimus delays recovery of rat kidney transplants after ischemia-reperfusion injury. Transplantation 2003;76:1594–9.
51. Garrean S, Massad MG, Tshibaka M, et al. Sirolimus-associated interstitial pneumonitis in solid organ transplant recipients. Clin Transplant 2005;19:698–703.
52. Groth CG, Backman L, Morales JM, et al. Sirolimus (rapamycin)-based therapy in human renal transplantation: similar efficacy and different toxicity compared with cyclosporine. Sirolimus European Renal Transplant Study Group. Transplantation 1999;67:1036–42.
53. Hachem RR, Yusen RD, Chakinala MM, et al. Thrombotic microangiopathy after lung transplantation. Transplantation 2006;81:57–63.
54. Haydar AA, Denton M, West A, et al. Sirolimus-induced pneumonitis: three cases and a review of the literature. Am J Transplant 2004;4:137–9.
55. Heitman J, Movva NR, Hall MN. Targets for cell cycle arrest by the immunosuppressant rapamycin in yeast. Science 1991;253:905–9.
56. Hester J, Schiopu A, Nadig SN, et al. Low-dose rapamycin treatment increases the ability of human regulatory T cells to inhibit transplant arteriosclerosis in vivo. Am J Transplant 2012;12:2008–16.
57. Hong JC, Kahan BD. Sirolimus-induced thrombocytopenia and leukopenia in renal transplant recipients: risk factors, incidence, progression, and management. Transplantation 2000;69:2085–90.
58. Ikonen TS, Gummert JF, Hayase M, et al. Sirolimus (rapamycin) halts and reverses progression of allograft vascular disease in non-human primates. Transplantation 2000;70:969–75.
59. Isakova T, Xie H, Messinger S, et al. Inhibitors of mTOR and risks of allograft failure and mortality in kidney transplantation. Am J Transplant 2012;12:379–87.
60. Jacques J, Dickson Z, Carrier P, et al. Severe sirolimus-induced acute hepatitis in a renal transplant recipient. Transpl Int 2010;23:967–70.
61. Johnson RW, Kreis H, Oberbauer R, et al. Sirolimus allows early cyclosporine withdrawal in renal transplantation resulting in improved renal function and lower blood pressure. Transplantation 2001;72:777–86.
62. Johnson-Davis KL, De S, Jimenez E, et al. Evaluation of the Abbott ARCHITECT i2000 sirolimus assay and comparison with the Abbott IMx sirolimus assay and an established liquid chromatography-tandem mass spectrometry method. Ther Drug Monit 2011;33:453–9.
63. Jusko WJ, Ferron GM, Mis SM, et al. Pharmacokinetics of prednisolone during administration of sirolimus in patients with renal transplants. J Clin Pharmacol 1996;36:1100–6.
64. Kahan BD. Efficacy of sirolimus compared with azathioprine for reduction of acute renal allograft rejection: a randomised multicentre study. The Rapamune US Study Group. Lancet 2000;356:194–202.
65. Kahan BD, Gibbons S, Tejpal N, et al. Synergistic effect of the rapamycin-cyclosporine combination: median effect analysis of in vitro immune performances by human T lymphocytes in PHA, CD3, and MLR proliferative and cytotoxicity assays. Transplant Proc 1991;23:1090–1.
66. Kahan BD, Julian BA, Pescovitz MD, et al. Sirolimus reduces the incidence of acute rejection episodes despite lower cyclosporine doses in caucasian recipients of mismatched primary renal allografts: a phase II trial. Rapamune Study Group. Transplantation 1999;68:1526–32.

67. Kahan BD, Kramer WG. Median effect analysis of efficacy versus adverse effects of immunosuppressants. Clin Pharmacol Ther 2001;70:74–81.
68. Kahan BD, Wong RL, Carter C, et al. A phase I study of a 4-week course of SDZ-RAD (RAD) quiescent cyclosporine-prednisone-treated renal transplant recipients. Transplantation 1999;68:1100–6.
69. Kahn D, Spearman CW, Mall A, et al. The effect of rapamycin on the healing of the ureteric anastomosis and wound healing. Transplant Proc 2005;37:830–1.
70. Kauffman HM, Cherikh WS, Cheng Y, et al. Maintenance immunosuppression with target-of-rapamycin inhibitors is associated with a reduced incidence of de novo malignancies. Transplantation 2005;80:883–9.
71. Kelly PA, Napoli K, Kahan BD. Conversion from liquid to solid rapamycin formulations in stable renal allograft transplant recipients. Biopharm Drug Dispos 1999;20:249–53.
72. Kidney Disease: Improving Global Outcomes (KDIGO) Transplant Work Group. KDIGO clinical practice guideline for the care of kidney transplant recipients. Am J Transplant 2009;9(Suppl. 3):S1–157.
73. Kimball PM, Kerman RH, Kahan BD. Production of synergistic but nonidentical mechanisms of immunosuppression by rapamycin and cyclosporine. Transplantation 1991;51:486–90.
74. King-Biggs MB, Dunitz JM, Park SJ, et al. Airway anastomotic dehiscence associated with use of sirolimus immediately after lung transplantation. Transplantation 2003;75:1437–43.
75. Kneissel M, Luong-Nguyen NH, Baptist M, et al. Everolimus suppresses cancellous bone loss, bone resorption, and cathepsin K expression by osteoclasts. Bone 2004;35:1144–56.
76. Kovarik JM, Kahan BD, Rajagopalan PR, et al. Population pharmacokinetics and exposure-response relationships for basiliximab in kidney transplantation. The U.S. Simulect Renal Transplant Study Group. Transplantation 1999;68:1288–94.
77. Kreis H, Cisterne JM, Land W, et al. Sirolimus in association with mycophenolate mofetil induction for the prevention of acute graft rejection in renal allograft recipients. Transplantation 2000;69:1252–60.
78. Kreis H, Oberbauer R, Campistol JM, et al. Long-term benefits with sirolimus-based therapy after early cyclosporine withdrawal. J Am Soc Nephrol 2004;15:809–17.
79. Langer RM, Hene R, Vitko S, et al. Everolimus plus early tacrolimus minimization: a phase III, randomized, open-label, multicentre trial in renal transplantation. Transpl Int 2012;25:592–602.
80. Langer RM, Kahan BD. Sirolimus does not increase the risk for postoperative thromboembolic events among renal transplant recipients. Transplantation 2003;76:318–23.
81. Langer RM, Van Buren CT, Katz SM, et al. De novo hemolytic uremic syndrome after kidney transplantation in patients treated with cyclosporine-sirolimus combination. Transplantation 2002;73:756–60.
82. Larson TS, Dean PG, Stegall MD, et al. Complete avoidance of calcineurin inhibitors in renal transplantation: a randomized trial comparing sirolimus and tacrolimus. Am J Transplant 2006;6:514–22.
83. Lazorchak AS, Su B. Perspectives on the role of mTORC2 in B lymphocyte development, immunity and tumorigenesis. Protein Cell 2011;2:523–30.
84. Le Meur Y, Djebli N, Szelag JC, et al. CYP3A5*3 influences sirolimus oral clearance in de novo and stable renal transplant recipients. Clin Pharmacol Ther 2006;80:51–60.
85. Lebbe C, Euvrard S, Barrou B, et al. Sirolimus conversion for patients with posttransplant Kaposi's sarcoma. Am J Transplant 2006;6:2164–8.
86. Letavernier E, Bruneval P, Vandermeersch S, et al. Sirolimus interacts with pathways essential for podocyte integrity. Nephrol Dial Transplant 2009;24:630–8.
87. Letavernier E, Pe'raldi MN, Pariente A, et al. Proteinuria following a switch from calcineurin inhibitors to sirolimus. Transplantation 2005;80:1198–203.
88. Liacini A, Seamone ME, Muruve DA, et al. Anti-BK virus mechanisms of sirolimus and leflunomide alone and in combination: toward a new therapy for BK virus infection. Transplantation 2010;90:1450–7.
89. LoPiccolo J, Blumenthal GM, Bernstein WB, et al. Targeting the PI3K/Akt/mTOR pathway: effective combinations and clinical considerations. Drug Resist Updat 2008;11:32–50.
90. Lorber MI, Mulgaonkar S, Butt KM, et al. Everolimus versus mycophenolate mofetil in the prevention of rejection in de novo renal transplant recipients: a 3-year randomized, multicenter, phase III study. Transplantation 2005;80:244–52.
91. Loverre A, Ditonno P, Crovace A, et al. Ischemia-reperfusion induces glomerular and tubular activation of proinflammatory and antiapoptotic pathways: differential modulation by rapamycin. J Am Soc Nephrol 2004;15:2675–86.
92. Lucke C, Weiwad M. Insights into immunophilin structure and function. Curr Med Chem 2011;18:5333–54.
93. Ma Q, Zhou Y, Nie X, et al. Rapamycin affects tissue plasminogen activator and plasminogen activator inhibitor I expression: a potential prothrombotic mechanism of drug-eluting stents. Angiology 2012;63:330–5.
94. MacDonald A, Scarola J, Burke JT, et al. Clinical pharmacokinetics and therapeutic drug monitoring of sirolimus. Clin Ther 2000;22(Suppl. B):B101–21.
95. MacDonald AS. A worldwide, phase III, randomized, controlled, safety and efficacy study of a sirolimus/cyclosporine regimen for prevention of acute rejection in recipients of primary mismatched renal allografts. Transplantation 2001;71:271–80.
96. Mahe E, Morelon E, Lechaton S, et al. Acne in recipients of renal transplantation treated with sirolimus: clinical, microbiologic, histologic, therapeutic, and pathogenic aspects. J Am Acad Dermatol 2006;55:139–42.
97. Mahe E, Morelon E, Lechaton S, et al. Cutaneous adverse events in renal transplant recipients receiving sirolimus-based therapy. Transplantation 2005;79:476–82.
98. Maiorano A, Stallone G, Schena A, et al. Sirolimus interferes with iron homeostasis in renal transplant recipients. Transplantation 2006;82:908–12.
99. Majewski M, Korecka M, Joergensen J, et al. Immunosuppressive TOR kinase inhibitor everolimus (RAD) suppresses growth of cells derived from posttransplant lymphoproliferative disorder at allograft-protecting doses. Transplantation 2003;75:1710–7.
100. Majewski M, Korecka M, Kossev P, et al. The immunosuppressive macrolide RAD inhibits growth of human Epstein–Barr virus-transformed B lymphocytes in vitro and in vivo: a potential approach to prevention and treatment of posttransplant lymphoproliferative disorders. Proc Natl Acad Sci U S A 2000;97:4285–90.
101. Maluf DG, Mas VR, Archer KJ, et al. Apolipoprotein E genotypes as predictors of high-risk groups for developing hyperlipidemia in kidney transplant recipients undergoing sirolimus treatment. Transplantation 2005;80:1705–11.
102. Martel RR, Klicius J, Galet S. Inhibition of the immune response by rapamycin, a new antifungal antibiotic. Can J Physiol Pharmacol 1977;55:48–51.
103. McAlister VC, Gao Z, Peltekian K, et al. Sirolimus-tacrolimus combination immunosuppression. Lancet 2000;355:376–7.
104. McLaren AJ, Fuggle SV, Welsh KI, et al. Chronic allograft failure in human renal transplantation: a multivariate risk factor analysis. Ann Surg 2000;232:98–103.
105. McTaggart RA, Gottlieb D, Brooks J, et al. Sirolimus prolongs recovery from delayed graft function after cadaveric renal transplantation. Am J Transplant 2003;3:416–23.
106. McTaggart RA, Tomlanovich S, Bostrom A, et al. Comparison of outcomes after delayed graft function: sirolimus-based versus other calcineurin-inhibitor sparing induction immunosuppression regimens. Transplantation 2004;78:475–80.
107. Mendez R, Gonwa T, Yang HC, et al. A prospective, randomized trial of tacrolimus in combination with sirolimus or mycophenolate mofetil in kidney transplantation: results at 1 year. Transplantation 2005;80:303–9.
108. Mohaupt MG, Vogt B, Frey FJ. Sirolimus-associated eyelid edema in kidney transplant recipients. Transplantation 2001;72:162–4.
109. Morales JM, Andres A, Dominguez-Gil B, et al. Tubular function in patients with hypokalemia induced by sirolimus after renal transplantation. Transplant Proc 2003;35:154S–6S.
110. Morales JM, Wramner L, Kreis H, et al. Sirolimus does not exhibit nephrotoxicity compared to cyclosporine in renal transplant recipients. Am J Transplant 2002;2:436–42.
111. Morelon E, Stern M, Kreis H. Interstitial pneumonitis associated with sirolimus therapy in renal-transplant recipients. N Engl J Med 2000;343:225–6.

112. Nankivell BJ, Gruenewald SM, Allen RD, et al. Predicting glomerular filtration rate after kidney transplantation. Transplantation 1995;59:1683–9.
113. Nashan B, Citterio F. Wound healing complications and the use of mammalian target of rapamycin inhibitors in kidney transplantation: a critical review of the literature. Transplantation 2012;94:547–61.
114. Nashan B, Curtis J, Ponticelli C, et al. Everolimus and reduced-exposure cyclosporine in de novo renal-transplant recipients: a three-year phase II, randomized, multicenter, open-label study. Transplantation 2004;78:1332–40.
115. Neff GW, Ruiz P, Madariaga JR, et al. Sirolimus-associated hepatotoxicity in liver transplantation. Ann Pharmacother 2004;38:1593–6.
116. Nepomuceno RR, Balatoni CE, Natkunam Y, et al. Rapamycin inhibits the interleukin 10 signal transduction pathway and the growth of Epstein-Barr virus B-cell lymphomas. Cancer Res 2003;63:4472–80.
117. Niemczyk M, Wyzgal J, Perkowska A, et al. Sirolimus-associated hepatotoxicity in the kidney graft recipient. Transpl Int 2005;18:1302–3.
118. Oberbauer R, Segoloni G, Campistol JM, et al. Early cyclosporine withdrawal from a sirolimus-based regimen results in better renal allograft survival and renal function at 48 months after transplantation. Transpl Int 2005;18:22–8.
119. Oroszlan M, Bieri M, Ligeti N, et al. Sirolimus and everolimus reduce albumin endocytosis in proximal tubule cells via an angiotensin II-dependent pathway. Transpl Immunol 2010;23:125–32.
120. Palmerini T, Biondi-Zoccai G, Della Riva D, et al. Stent thrombosis with drug-eluting and bare-metal stents: evidence from a comprehensive network meta-analysis. Lancet 2012;379:1393–402.
121. Pascual J. Post-transplant lymphoproliferative disorder – the potential of proliferation signal inhibitors. Nephrol Dial Transplant 2007;22(Suppl. 1):i27–35.
122. Pascual J, del Castillo D, Cabello M, et al. Interaction between everolimus and tacrolimus in renal transplant recipients: a pharmacokinetic controlled trial. Transplantation 2010;89:994–1000.
123. Pengel LH, Liu LQ, Morris PJ. Do wound complications or lymphoceles occur more often in solid organ transplant recipients on mTOR inhibitors? A systematic review of randomized controlled trials. Transpl Int 2011;24:1216–30.
124. Picard N, Rouguieg-Malki K, Kamar N, et al. CYP3A5 genotype does not influence everolimus in vitro metabolism and clinical pharmacokinetics in renal transplant recipients. Transplantation 2011;91:652–6.
125. Podder H, Stepkowski SM, Napoli KL, et al. Pharmacokinetic interactions augment toxicities of sirolimus/cyclosporine combinations. J Am Soc Nephrol 2001;12:1059–71.
126. Quesniaux VF, Wehrli S, Steiner C, et al. The immunosuppressant rapamycin blocks in vitro responses to hematopoietic cytokines and inhibits recovering but not steady-state hematopoiesis in vivo. Blood 1994;84:1543–52.
127. Robson M, Cote I, Abbs I, et al. Thrombotic micro-angiopathy with sirolimus-based immunosuppression: potentiation of calcineurin-inhibitor-induced endothelial damage? Am J Transplant 2003;3:324–7.
128. Romero DF, Buchinsky FJ, Rucinski B, et al. Rapamycin: a bone sparing immunosuppressant? J Bone Miner Res 1995;10:760–8.
129. Ruggenenti P, Perico N, Gotti E, et al. Sirolimus versus cyclosporine therapy increases circulating regulatory T cells, but does not protect renal transplant patients given alemtuzumab induction from chronic allograft injury. Transplantation 2007;84:956–64.
130. Ruiz JC, Diekmann F, Campistol JM, et al. Evolution of proteinuria after conversion from calcineurin inhibitors (CNI) to sirolimus (SRL) in renal transplant patients: a multicenter study. Transplant Proc 2005;37:3833–5.
131. Saemann MD, Haidinger M, Hecking M, et al. The multifunctional role of mTOR in innate immunity: implications for transplant immunity. Am J Transplant 2009;9:2655–61.
132. Salgo R, Gossmann J, Schofer H, et al. Switch to a sirolimus-based immunosuppression in long-term renal transplant recipients: reduced rate of (pre-)malignancies and nonmelanoma skin cancer in a prospective, randomized, assessor-blinded, controlled clinical trial. Am J Transplant 2010;10:1385–93.
133. Sartelet H, Toupance O, Lorenzato M, et al. Sirolimus-induced thrombotic microangiopathy is associated with decreased expression of vascular endothelial growth factor in kidneys. Am J Transplant 2005;5:2441–7.
134. Schuler W, Sedrani R, Cottens S, et al. SDZ RAD, a new rapamycin derivative: pharmacological properties in vitro and in vivo. Transplantation 1997;64:36–42.
135. Schwarz C, Bohmig GA, Steininger R, et al. Impaired phosphate handling of renal allografts is aggravated under rapamycin-based immunosuppression. Nephrol Dial Transplant 2001;16:378–82.
136. Sehgal SN, Baker H, Vezina C. Rapamycin (AY-22,989), a new antifungal antibiotic. II. Fermentation, isolation and characterization. J Antibiot (Tokyo) 1975;28:727–32.
137. Senior PA, Paty BW, Cockfield SM, et al. Proteinuria developing after clinical islet transplantation resolves with sirolimus withdrawal and increased tacrolimus dosing. Am J Transplant 2005;5:2318–23.
138. Simon JF, Swanson SJ, Agodoa LY, et al. Induction sirolimus and delayed graft function after deceased donor kidney transplantation in the United States. Am J Nephrol 2004;24:393–401.
139. Singer SJ, Tiernan R, Sullivan EJ. Interstitial pneumonitis associated with sirolimus therapy in renal-transplant recipients. N Engl J Med 2000;343:1815–6.
140. Srinivas TR, Schold JD, Guerra G, et al. Mycophenolate mofetil/sirolimus compared to other common immunosuppressive regimens in kidney transplantation. Am J Transplant 2007;7:586–94.
141. Stallone G, Di Paolo S, Schena A, et al. Addition of sirolimus to cyclosporine delays the recovery from delayed graft function but does not affect 1-year graft function. J Am Soc Nephrol 2004;15:228–33.
142. Stallone G, Infante B, Di Paolo S, et al. Sirolimus and angiotensin-converting enzyme inhibitors together induce tongue oedema in renal transplant recipients. Nephrol Dial Transplant 2004;19:2906–8.
143. Stallone G, Schena A, Infante B, et al. Sirolimus for Kaposi's sarcoma in renal-transplant recipients. N Engl J Med 2005;352:1317–23.
144. Starzl TE, Todo S, Fung J, et al. FK 506 for liver, kidney, and pancreas transplantation. Lancet 1989;2:1000–4.
145. Stephany BR, Augustine JJ, Krishnamurthi V, et al. Differences in proteinuria and graft function in de novo sirolimus-based vs. calcineurin inhibitor-based immunosuppression in live donor kidney transplantation. Transplantation 2006;82:368–74.
146. Sundberg AK, Rohr MS, Hartmann EL, et al. Conversion to sirolimus-based maintenance immunosuppression using daclizumab bridge therapy in renal transplant recipients. Clin Transplant 2004;18(Suppl. 12):61–6.
147. Tiong HY, Flechner SM, Zhou L, et al. A systematic approach to minimizing wound problems for de novo sirolimus-treated kidney transplant recipients. Transplantation 2009;87:296–302.
148. Van Gurp E, Bustamante J, Franco A, et al. Comparable renal function at 6 months with tacrolimus combined with fixed-dose sirolimus or MMF: results of a randomized multicenter trial in renal transplantation. J Transplant 2010;2010:731426.
149. Vitko S, Margreiter R, Weimar W, et al. Three-year efficacy and safety results from a study of everolimus versus mycophenolate mofetil in de novo renal transplant patients. Am J Transplant 2005;5:2521–30.
150. Vitko S, Margreiter R, Weimar W, et al. Everolimus (Certican) 12-month safety and efficacy versus mycophenolate mofetil in de novo renal transplant recipients. Transplantation 2004;78:1532–40.
151. Vu MD, Qi S, Xu D, et al. Tacrolimus (FK506) and sirolimus (rapamycin) in combination are not antagonistic but produce extended graft survival in cardiac transplantation in the rat. Transplantation 1997;64:1853–6.
152. Vuiblet V, Birembaut P, Francois A, et al. Sirolimus-based regimen is associated with decreased expression of glomerular vascular endothelial growth factor. Nephrol Dial Transplant 2012;27:411–6.
153. Wadei H, Gruber SA, El-Amm JM, et al. Sirolimus-induced angioedema. Am J Transplant 2004;4:1002–5.
154. Wali RK, Drachenberg C, Hirsch HH, et al. BK virus-associated nephropathy in renal allograft recipients: rescue therapy by sirolimus-based immunosuppression. Transplantation 2004;78:1069–73.
155. Watson CJ, Firth J, Williams PF, et al. A randomized controlled trial of late conversion from CNI-based to sirolimus-based immunosuppression following renal transplantation. Am J Transplant 2005;5:2496–503.

156. Webster AC, Lee VW, Chapman JR, et al. Target of rapamycin inhibitors (sirolimus and everolimus) for primary immunosuppression of kidney transplant recipients: a systematic review and meta-analysis of randomized trials. Transplantation 2006;81:1234–48.
157. Wullschleger S, Loewith R, Hall MN. TOR signaling in growth and metabolism. Cell 2006;124:471–84.
158. Yatscoff R, LeGatt D, Keenan R, et al. Blood distribution of rapamycin. Transplantation 1993;56:1202–6.
159. Zeiser R, Leveson-Gower DB, Zambricki EA, et al. Differential impact of mammalian target of rapamycin inhibition on CD4+CD25+Foxp3+ regulatory T cells compared with conventional CD4+ T cells. Blood 2008;111:453–62.
160. Zimmerman JJ, Harper D, Getsy J, et al. Pharmacokinetic interactions between sirolimus and microemulsion cyclosporine when orally administered jointly and 4 hours apart in healthy volunteers. J Clin Pharmacol 2003;43:1168–76.
161. Zochowska D, Bartlomiejczyk I, Kaminska A, et al. High-performance liquid chromatography versus immunoassay for the measurement of sirolimus: comparison of two methods. Transplant Proc 2006;38:78–80.
162. Zuber J, Anglicheau D, Elie C, et al. Sirolimus may reduce fertility in male renal transplant recipients. Am J Transplant 2008;8:1471–9.

CHAPTER 20

ANTILYMPHOCYTE GLOBULIN, MONOCLONAL ANTIBODIES, AND FUSION PROTEINS

Allan D. Kirk

CHAPTER OUTLINE

Renal transplantation is the preferred treatment for most end-stage renal diseases. The success of transplantation has been counterbalanced, however, by its dependence on immunosuppressive drugs with their related infectious, metabolic, and malignant complications. Consequently, a common goal throughout the history of clinical transplantation has been the minimization and individualization of immunosuppressive therapy. Typically, drugs with highly specific mechanisms of action have been preferred over drugs with broad effects, and the search for increasingly specific drugs has provided a major impetus for the development of immunosuppressive therapies in general, and of antibodies and fusion proteins in particular.

Antibodies and other glycoprotein cell surface receptors are defined by their ability to bind to a particular ligand with unambiguous specificity. Although they may mediate diverse effects through associated downstream signaling pathways, their function is characterized by fidelity to distinct binding motifs. This trait has been long recognized as having great potential for targeted therapeutic use with minimal unintended effects, and organ transplantation historically has been a preferred testing ground for receptor-based therapeutics, such as monoclonal antibodies (MAbs), polyclonal antibody preparations, and engineered glycoprotein receptor–antibody hybrids known as fusion proteins, collectively known as biologics.

The initial success of biologics in transplantation has more recently led to an explosion in the number developed for clinical use.[252] In addition to transplant-related indications, biologics have been developed for the treatment of many oncologic and autoimmune conditions, and there are now at least 200 preparations in some level of clinical or preclinical development.[63,251] Importantly, although renal allograft rejection was the original indication for MAb therapy,[69] most modern development has been spurred by indications serving larger population bases. In addition to using agents developed for transplantation, clinicians are increasingly adopting therapies from other immunologically relevant indications. This so-called off-label use is now increasingly common and is becoming a primary means of biologics development for transplantation.

This chapter provides an overview of antibody-based and receptor-based therapies for kidney transplantation. Drugs developed and approved for use in transplantation are described; drugs with relevant actions that have been developed for other indications but evaluated in transplantation also are described. Investigational agents that have been tested clinically are reviewed.

HISTORICAL PERSPECTIVE

The early experiences in renal transplantation were marked by very high rates of rejection and complications related to the effects of the two available immunosuppressants of the day, glucocorticosteroids and azathioprine; this, combined with the recognition that lymphocytes were the predominant effectors in rejection, stimulated interest in alternative lymphocyte-directed strategies. By the mid-1960s, several investigators had shown that animals injected with lymphocytes would produce sera containing lymphocyte-specific antibodies, which could be used to reduce the lymphocyte counts when injected into other experimental animals. This technology gave rise to the initial lymphocyte depletion trials using antilymphocyte antibody preparations – antilymphocyte serum, antilymphocyte globulin, and antithymocyte globulin.[28,72,78,294] These agents were collectively called polyclonal preparations because they were composed of antibodies with many, largely undefined specificities. Their ability to prevent and reverse rejection, particularly in patients refractory to the drugs of the day, led to their increasing use over the ensuing decade.[68]

The increased use of polyclonals made many of their limitations apparent. The imprecise in vivo methods for producing polyclonal antibodies resulted in preparations with promiscuous binding to many non-lymphocyte cell types. Although each antibody in the preparation bound to a single target, collectively the preparation bound to a broad array of cell surface molecules. Cross-reactivity with many hematopoietic cells made anemia, neutropenia, and thrombocytopenia dose limiting. The method of production also led to wide batch-to-batch variability. The clinical effect of the agent varied considerably, making it difficult to establish prospectively proper dosages and to estimate the magnitude of anticipatable side effects. In addition, because the preparations were made in animals, usually rabbits or horses, they contained proteins that were antigenic to humans.[212,306] They had the potential to induce a neutralizing antibody response and evoke adverse effects, such as serum sickness or anaphylaxis.[240] Finally, some lymphocyte cell surface receptors, when bound by antibody, would induce cell activation, leading to a release of anaphylatoxins and cytokines, producing a syndrome of flu-like and, in extreme cases, septic-like symptoms, subsequently termed cytokine release syndrome.

In the 1970s, Kohler and Milstein[169] presented a landmark development in the field of protein therapeutics – a means of producing antibody preparations with a single, genetically defined monoclonal specificity. The development of MAbs addressed many of the shortcomings associated with polyclonal preparations, particularly specificity and variability. The first such preparation approved for clinical use was muromonab (OKT3), a MAb of mouse origin specific for human cluster of differentiation (CD) 3 (described later).[69] OKT3 rapidly and specifically cleared T cells from the peripheral circulation and was shown to be a very effective treatment for allograft rejection.[69,91,221,234,265] Although many of the problems associated with the diffuse nature of polyclonal antibodies were addressed, some were not. The immune response against heterologous animal proteins and the cytokine release syndrome remained. OKT3's heightened specificity for the T-cell receptor (TCR) not only produced more reliable T-cell clearance but also more reliable T-cell activation and cytokine release. The antimouse antibody response also limited prolonged dosing in a subset of patients.[140]

With the genetic engineering advances of the 1980s, the production of MAbs became much more efficient, theoretically allowing any surface molecules to be targeted. Effort was redirected from pan-T-cell depletion toward fine targeting of relevant T-cell subsets and blockade of functions unique to effector T-cell activation. An example was the high-affinity interleukin (IL)-2 receptor, CD25 (described later), expressed predominantly on activated T cells. Additionally, methods of genetic engineering were developed to allow DNA encoding for binding sites from heterologous proteins to be grafted on to genetic sequences encoding the monomorphic scaffold of human antibodies to create chimeric or humanized MAbs.[33,141,202] These techniques also allowed for unique fusion proteins to be created, combining the Fc portions of antibodies with non-antibody receptors and ligands, and allowing for cell surface molecules to be created in a soluble form with prolonged half-lives.

The humanization of antibodies and the use of human-derived receptors has practically eliminated the problem of antibody clearance and opened the possibility for prolonged treatment regimens. More recently, the production of fully human antihuman antibodies has become a practical reality.[346] Techniques including phage display mutagenesis and the transgenic production of mice containing human immunoglobulin genes that respond to immunization with human antibody now offer the promise of highly specific, non-immunogenic, well-tolerated protein reagents. Human and humanized biologics are now making possible prolonged therapy with highly specific therapeutic agents.

Multiple surface molecules have been targeted by biologics investigationally, and several are now accepted as clinical therapies in transplantation and other indications. Biologic therapy is being increasingly adopted into standard practice, with 83% of kidney transplants performed in the United States now using prophylactic antibody therapy of some sort.[268] Despite this general trend, however, it has not been established whether this strategy is necessary in all cases. Although antibody induction reduces acute rejection rates in the first year after transplantation, the lasting effects of induction remain incompletely defined.[303,304] The modern era is now characterized by the availability of many promising agents and the challenge of understanding their most appropriate clinical use.

ANTIBODY STRUCTURE AND FUNCTION

The clinical effects of MAbs in transplantation relate closely to the physiological effects and structural characteristics of antibodies in general. Antibodies are one of two common glycoprotein antigen receptors that result from somatic gene rearrangements in specialized lymphocytes, the other being TCRs.[104,135] Five different heavy-chain loci (μ, γ, α, ε, and δ) and two light-chain loci (κ and λ), each with variable, diversity, or junctional (V, D, or J) and constant (C) regions, are brought together randomly by the recombination associated gene (RAG)-1 and RAG-2 apparatus to form a functional antigen receptor with highly variable binding ability. Antibodies have a basic structure of two identical heavy chains and two identical light chains (Figure 20-1). The heavy-chain usage defines the immunoglobulin type as being IgM, IgG, IgA, IgE, or IgD. This structure forms two identical antigen-binding sites brought together on a common region known as the Fc portion of the antibody. Although all of these subtypes have therapeutic potential, IgG antibodies have been the most commonly used clinically. IgG molecules are the most common result of peripheral immunization and are structurally easier to produce and manipulate.

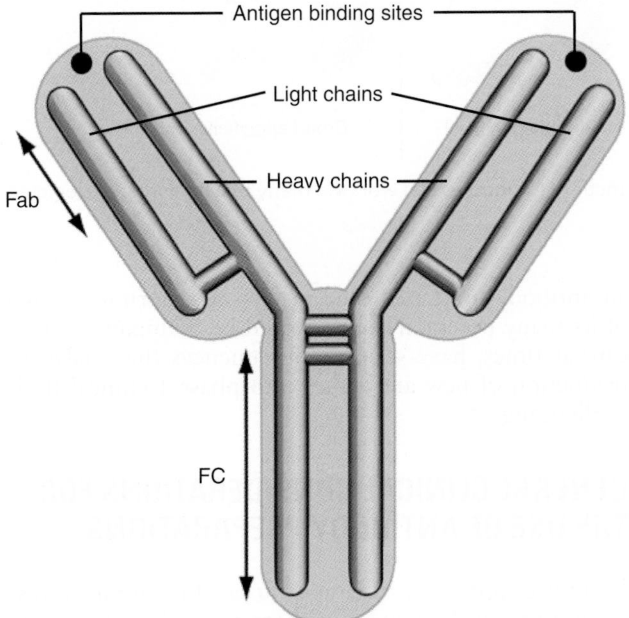

FIGURE 20-1 ■ General antibody structure. The prototypic structure of an IgG molecule is shown.

Physiologically, antibodies exist as surface molecules on B cells, facilitating their antigen-specific activation and, importantly, are secreted into the serum to bind to and neutralize circulating antigens. Heterologous nonhuman antibodies are sufficiently similar to their human counterparts to facilitate most physiological effector functions when used in humans. Antibodies produced by mice, rabbits, and horses can be used in humans and still evoke biologically important effects. There is no animal that is a priori superior, however, and all heterologous antibodies have the potential to induce a neutralizing antibody response.

Antibodies can have a broad range of effects when they bind (Figure 20-2). They can mimic the native ligand of a molecule and lead to signal transduction, or they can bind to the molecule in such a way as to prevent it from binding to its intended ligand.[314,348] Antibodies can be either activating or inhibiting, and the predominant effect can be determined only through empirical in vivo analysis. Antibodies can bind to cells in such a way as to have no appreciable effect.[142] Thus, antibody binding cannot be equated with functional significance. In some cases, a combined effect occurs whereby the antibody activates the targeted molecule but induces surface molecule internalization, effectively clearing the molecule from the cell surface and inhibiting its subsequent function.[151] This transient activation effect can lead to a burst of target cell activity (e.g., cytokine release), resulting in undesirable side effects, or can simply lead to surface modulation of the targeted molecule. Antibodies cannot target molecules that are not present on the cell surface. Although they can influence intracellular pathways, they cannot bind intracellular molecules directly in vivo.

Antibodies also activate the classical complement cascade and in doing so can induce complement-mediated lysis of a targeted cell. In addition, many phagocytic cells have receptors for the constant Fc region of antibodies and preferentially engulf cells coated with antibody through a process known as antibody-dependent cellular cytotoxicity (ADCC). Both of these activities facilitate the most noticeable effect of antibody therapies – target cell depletion. Depletion is only the most obvious effect of antibody therapy, however, and should not be assumed to be the most relevant or desired. Additionally, these effects depend on their antigen-binding region and their non-variable Fc region for effectiveness.[93] The importance of Fc segment effects is shown by non-specific antibody infusion, which can mediate important effects, presumably by neutralizing complement or saturating Fc receptors.[49,245]

It has become apparent that the maturation state of the targeted cells also can influence the response to antibody treatments. Specifically, cells that have matured into a memory phenotype have some degree of resistance to antibody-mediated depletion.[228] The mechanisms involved in depletion resistance remain to be defined, but memory

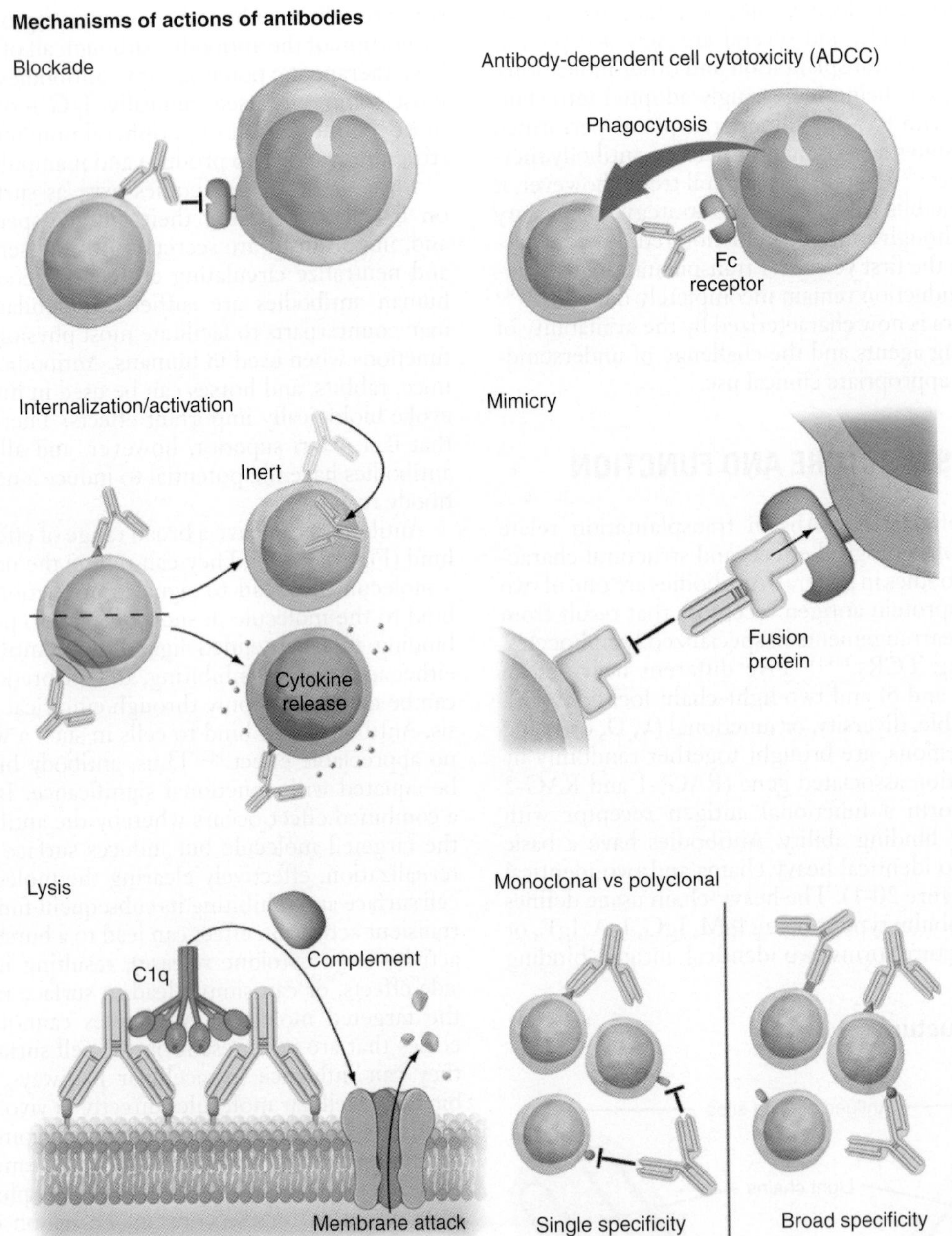

FIGURE 20-2 ■ Mechanisms of action for antibody and fusion protein function. Antibodies can work via many mechanisms, as depicted here and described in more detail in the text.

cells differ from naïve cells in many potentially relevant ways, including enhanced antiapoptotic and complement regulatory gene expression. The ultimate effect of antibody therapy may vary not only with the antibody preparation but also with the phenotype of the targeted cell and even the immune history of the recipient.

All of these effects can alter the function of molecules and cells, giving antibodies broad therapeutic potential. This array of effects makes antibody development difficult, however. Minor changes in antibody structure can radically alter their effects, and at present it is impossible to predict an antibody's properties on a structural basis alone. Certain IgG isotypes support complement and ADCC functions better than others, but generally an antibody must be tested in vivo to determine which of its many potential effects would be dominant.[109] This can, at times, have serious consequences that make introduction of new antibodies into phase I clinical trials challenging.[299]

GENERAL CLINICAL CONSIDERATIONS FOR THE USE OF ANTIBODY PREPARATIONS

Immunosuppressive regimens used for organ transplantation can be generally characterized as induction, maintenance, or rescue therapies. Induction immunosuppression is intense treatment designed to inhibit immune responsiveness prophylactically at the time of transplantation. It is usually potent to the point that its prolonged use is prohibitively toxic. Maintenance immunosuppression is of lesser potency, but is tolerable for long-term use and forms the basis of most immunosuppressive regimens. Rescue therapy is similar to induction in that it is intense, effective, and chronically intolerable, but differs in that it is used to reverse established rejection. Immunosuppressive medications can conceivably fall into any or all of these categorizations based on the dose and route used. Biologics currently are primarily indicated as rescue agents and are used in approximately 20% of all acute rejection episodes.[341] Their use as induction agents is growing: 83% of patients undergoing kidney transplantation now receive biologic induction.[268]

Antibody preparations also have been generally classified as depleting or non-depleting based on whether or not they deplete cells expressing the targeted antigen. Generally, T-cell-depleting antibody preparations are primarily indicated for the treatment of refractory (e.g., steroid-resistant) acute cellular rejections, acute rejections occurring in high-risk settings (e.g., marginal kidneys), and particularly aggressive vascular (e.g., Banff grade 2 or 3) rejections. Depleting antibodies also are being increasingly used as induction agents, although this is often an off-label use. Non-depleting antibody preparations and fusion proteins have been most commonly studied as induction agents and typically have less efficacy in rescue indications. Maintenance applications of biologics have been made possible by the ability to produce human biologics, and as such are just beginning to be explored. The first biologic maintenance agent, belatacept, was approved for use as a calcineurin inhibitor replacement for kidney transplantation in June 2011.[176,326,329] It is a fusion protein with specificity for the B7 costimulatory molecules and will be considered fully in Chapter 21.

Many depleting and non-depleting antibody preparations have been studied in randomized trials and have been proven efficacious in reducing the rate of acute rejection when used as an induction agent combined with standard maintenance regimens and compared with bolus methylprednisolone induction. Few prospective studies compare the prominent agents, however, and no agent has distinguished itself as clearly superior in all clinical circumstances. Most trials have used the surrogate endpoint of acute rejection, rather than more definitive outcome measures, such as patient or graft survival.

When considered as a whole, biologics have been convincingly shown to be more effective than steroids in reversing acute rejection.[341] When used as induction agents, they reduce the incidence of acute rejection in the first 6 months of transplantation in kidney recipients, particularly recipients who are sensitized or experiencing delayed graft function, compared with the historical standard of bolus methylprednisolone induction and maintenance with cyclosporine, azathioprine, and prednisone.[303,304] Despite these benefits, there is no evidence that biologics alter long-term patient or graft survival in the era of modern immunosuppression.[303,304,341] Long-term analysis suggests that a measurable effect in kidney transplantation disappears after 5 years. This analysis may indicate that the side effects of maintenance therapy or patient comorbidities supersede early graft outcome and are the dominant determinants of outcome over time.

Antibody preparation use does not generally influence the rate of technical complications[136] but seems to reduce the risk of graft thrombosis in children.[282] Several induction strategies, in particular polyclonal antibodies and OKT3, have been shown, however, to increase measurably the risk of posttransplantation lymphoproliferative disease (PTLD) and death from malignancy when combined with conventional maintenance immunosuppression.[59,191,197,229,230] PTLD is a product of the intensity of the overall immunosuppressive therapy in combination with the recipient's preexisting immunity to the causative agent, Epstein–Barr virus. Specifically, the expected PTLD rate is 0.5% in patients who do not receive antibody induction or who receive CD25-specific therapy. OKT3 induction carries a significantly higher rate of 0.85%, as does polyclonal depletion at 0.81%, particularly in recipients newly exposed to Epstein–Barr virus at transplantation.[59] Interestingly, the use of alemtuzumb, a CD52-specific MAb with potent depletional properties similar in magnitude but differing in spectrum to polyclonal preparations or OKT3, has been shown to have a low PTLD incidence that approximates that of the non-depletional CD25-specific MAbs.[155] This likely relates to alemtuzumab's B-cell-depleting properties, with B cells being the dominant reservoir of Epstein–Barr virus, although practice patterns associated with alemtuzumab also may account for the difference.

Other early complications, including cardiovascular and infectious deaths, correlate with antibody use, but the interpretation of this relationship is confounded by the preferential use of antibodies in high-risk patients.[42,197] Viral infection is a substantial concern, however, when using potent antibody therapy, particularly agents associated with T-cell depletion. When used for induction or rescue, antibody preparations should be accompanied by broad prophylaxis against opportunistic infection. Antiviral therapy, such as ganciclovir or acyclovir,[16,125,317] should be initiated and continued for at least 3 months. The choice of agent is based on the pretransplant status of the donor and recipient. Oral candidiasis prophylaxis with nystatin or clotrimazole and *Pneumocystis* therapy with trimethoprim/sulfamethoxazole also should be considered for several months. Individual clinical risks often dictate substantially longer periods of prophylaxis. Each antibody preparation has a unique side-effect profile and indication, which are discussed subsequently.

The use of antibody preparations for maintenance therapy had been limited until more recently by the immune response formed against the antibody itself. Recombinant humanized or chimeric antibodies and fusion proteins have essentially eliminated this as a concern, however. One agent, belatacept, is now available as a maintenance agent (discussed in Chapter 21), and it is likely that future development of other molecules will explore the role of antibodies in sustained preventive therapy.

POLYCLONAL ANTIBODY PREPARATIONS

Heterologous antibody preparations can be derived from many animals immunized with human tissues, cells (e.g., human lymphocytes), or cell lines (e.g., Jurkatt cells). When reinfused into humans, these antibodies bind to antigens expressed on the original immunogen, where they mediate the effects discussed earlier. Given that these preparations are produced through whole-cell immunization, the resulting preparations contain a vast array of antibodies binding many epitopes expressed on the immunogen cells – some intended, and some not. Because each animal produces a unique immune response to an antigen, clinical-grade preparations are generally the result of pooled responses from many animals. For practical reasons, most polyclonal preparations are derived from rabbit or horse immunizations.

Ideally, a single renewable cell type equivalent to the effector cell in rejection could be used as a reproducible immunogen free from elements such as stromal tissue and neutrophils. No such cell has been identified or developed, however. Commercially available polyclonal preparations continue to be made using heterogeneous cell populations or tissues such as thymus obtained from deceased donors or surgical specimens, or from a T-cell line, the Jurkatt cell line, that is thought to approximate the antigenic spectrum of allospecific T cells. After immunization, the immunized animals are bled to obtain hyperimmune serum. The serum is typically absorbed against platelets, erythrocytes, and selected proteins to remove antibodies that could result in undesirable effects such as thrombocytopenia. Historically, hyperimmune serum was administered without additional purification, but now all commercially available products are purified to obtain only IgG isotypes. Even so, polyclonal antibody preparations are not fractionated to separate relevant from irrelevant antibodies pre-existent from the environmental immune responses of the immunized animals. Greater than 90% of antibodies found in polyclonal preparations are likely not involved in therapeutically relevant antigen binding.[32,34,248,281]

Many groups have prepared polyclonal antibody preparations for their own institutional use, and this practice gave rise to a highly variable literature with little standardization or objective comparisons between products.[132,297,298,311] More recently, three dominant commercial polyclonal preparations have emerged: two rabbit-derived antibody preparations, antithymocyte globulin–rabbit (ATG-R, Thymoglobulin, Genzyme-Sanofi) and antithymocyte globulin–Fresenius (ATG-F, Fresenius), and one horse-derived product (ATGAM, Pfizer). Of these, Thymoglobulin is used most commonly in North America,[268] with both rabbit preparations used in Europe. ATGAM is primarily used for the treatment of aplastic anemia, but can be used for patients who have a hypersensitivity to rabbits.

As discussed earlier, antibodies can mediate many effects when they bind to their target antigen, and a significant factor determining their effect is the antigenic specificity of the preparation. By their very nature, polyclonal preparations are composed of a wide variety of antibodies, and complete characterization has remained elusive.[32,34,248] Detected specificities include many T-cell molecules involved in antigen recognition (CD3, CD4, CD8, and TCR), adhesion (CD2, lymphocyte function antigen (LFA)-1, and intracellular adhesion molecule (ICAM)-1), and costimulation (CD28, CD40, CD80, CD86, and CD154), and non-T-cell molecules (CD16 and CD20) and class I and class II major histocompatibility complex (MHC) molecules (Figure 20-3). Although all of these targets hypothetically can influence

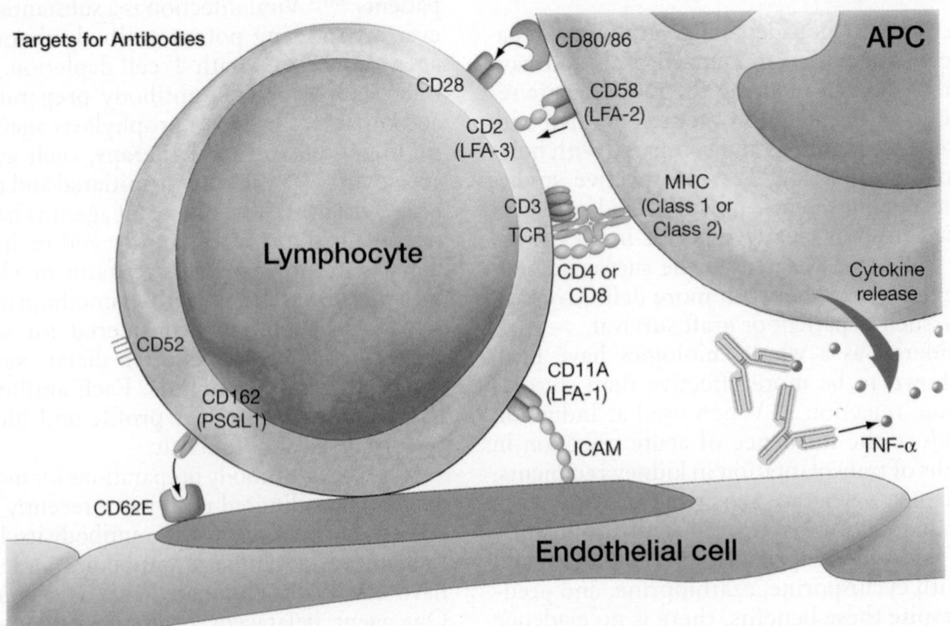

FIGURE 20-3 ■ Sites of action for antibody and fusion proteins in clinical use. Shown are the surface molecules that have been targeted in clinical transplant trials and their respective ligands when known. APC, antigen-presenting cell; ICAM, intracellular adhesion molecule; LFA, lymphocyte function antigen; MHC, major histocompatibility complex; TCR, T-cell receptor; TNF-α, tumor necrosis factor-α.

an immune response, and when studied individually they do, it is unclear which of these specificities are crucial to the ultimate therapeutic effect. This broad reactivity with adhesion molecules and other receptors upregulated on activated endothelium has led many authors to advocate the preferential use of polyclonal antibody preparations in situations, such as prolonged ischemic times, where endothelial activation and ischemia-reperfusion injury is anticipated.[20,53]

Most polyclonal antibodies have prolonged serum half-lives of several weeks.[41,249] Non-depleted cells have been shown to be coated with heterologous antibody for months, suggesting that these preparations could influence the function of lymphocytes long after treatment has stopped. Lymphocyte subsets are abnormal for years after therapy, with particularly low $CD4^+$ T-cell counts.[206] It also is reasonable to assume that antibodies targeting differing specificities would have variable effective half-lives based on the rates of surface molecule recycling, the affinity of the binding interaction, and the mechanism of action. Stimulating antibodies may have effects whenever they are bound, whereas inhibitory compounds could mediate an effect only when the natural ligand being antagonized is present. Polyclonal preparations likely have mechanisms of action that vary by batch, circumstance of use, and degradation state. It is unlikely that any single generalized mechanism exists. For the purposes of following the clinical effect, bulk T-cell depletion is used as a general estimate of antibody potency, and polyclonal antibody preparations are considered depletional agents.

SPECIFIC CLINICAL APPLICATIONS OF POLYCLONAL ANTIBODY PREPARATIONS

Polyclonal antibody preparations have been used in transplantation to achieve immunosuppression since the 1960s.[294] They are used as induction and rescue therapies, but the immune response to the proteins has precluded attempts to use them as maintenance drugs. As discussed previously, no single mechanism of action has been established, and they likely mediate their antirejection properties through depletion and other effects, including costimulation blockade, adhesion molecule modulation, and, to a lesser extent, B-cell depletion.[32,34,239,248]

Induction

Historically, polyclonal antibody preparations were used to bolster the effect of steroids and azathioprine in an attempt to reduce the unacceptably high rejection rates typical of the 1960s and 1970s. Generally, a 2–3-week course of a polyclonal antibody delayed the onset of acute rejection and reduced the requirement for high-dose steroids in the early postoperative period without significantly altering long-term survival.[69,72,134,298,342] After the introduction of cyclosporine, the use of polyclonal antibody induction fell from favor with the realization that this potent combination was associated with increased infectious and malignant morbidity.[199,224] With improved viral prophylaxis, a better understanding of the infectious etiology of PTLD, and more standardized commercial polyclonal products, there has been a marked resurgence of interest in polyclonal antibody induction.[268]

Most modern trials have evaluated polyclonal antibodies added to an otherwise rigorous maintenance regimen (typically triple immunosuppressive therapy). This intense regimen has statistically reduced acute rejection rates, but has reciprocated with increased infectious morbidity without changing long-term outcome.[55,204] This increased infectious risk may be acceptable in selected higher-risk patient populations, such as recipients of donation after cardiac death donors, recipients of extended criteria donation, and patients with a high risk of rejection, such as retransplant recipients and recipients with delayed graft function,[20,50,51,53,105,277,297] particularly when avoidance of prolonged calcineurin inhibitors is desired.[84,270,285] A recent randomized trial between ATG-R and CD25-specific (basiliximab) induction showed that ATG-R reduced the incidence and severity of acute rejection but not the incidence of delayed graft function.[35] Early patient and graft survival were not influenced by the choice of induction regimen, but a follow-up study suggested a graft survival benefit with ATG-R.[37]

Other recent trials have attempted to address the increased infectious risk by pairing aggressive polyclonal induction with substantially reduced maintenance therapy. Two pilot studies have shown that ATG-R induction facilitates reduced maintenance immunosuppression in highly selected, closely followed patients, leading to graft and patient survivals comparable to the current standard.[293,302] These studies have emphasized administration before reperfusion, theoretically to take maximal advantage of antiadhesion molecule effects, and relatively high-dose therapy, to limit the proinflammatory effects of reperfusion and to achieve rapid and lasting T-cell depletion. Although these studies indicate that such an approach is possible, it remains to be seen if it can be generalized to non-investigational settings.

Rescue

Although induction therapy remains an off-label indication for polyclonal antibodies, their use for the treatment of steroid-refractory rejection is an established indication. Many polyclonal preparations have shown their utility in this setting, spanning several decades of associated maintenance regimens. The first randomized trial showing that antilymphocyte serum was superior to high-dose steroids for the treatment of established rejection was reported in 1979.[276] In the context of azathioprine and prednisone maintenance immunosuppression, antilymphocyte serum reversed rejection faster than bolus glucocorticosteroids, reduced the rate of recurrent rejection, and led to improved survival at 1 year.[210] Most rejection episodes occurring in the cyclosporine era and beyond respond to bolus steroids. Polyclonal agents have been indicated as a second-line therapy for steroid-resistant acute cellular rejection.[25,101,195,254] Recurrent rejection can be treated with repeated courses of polyclonal antibodies in situations where antirabbit (or antihorse) antibodies have not been formed.[30,192]

Of the currently available polyclonal preparations, ATG-R is used most commonly for rescue. It has been shown to be superior to ATGAM in terms of reversal of steroid-resistant rejection and persistence of a rejection-free state.[101] This difference has not been shown, however, to influence patient or graft survival.

Non-T-cell-specific polyclonal antibody preparations also reverse established cellular acute rejection. Although not typically considered alongside T-cell-depleting polyclonal antibody preparations, high-dose human IgG fractions (intravenous immunoglobulin) are polyclonal antibodies of random specificity pooled from human donors. Because they are not derived from animals, are not the products of heterologous immunization, and do not target a specific cell type, most of the adverse effects associated with polyclonal antibodies are not applicable. Nevertheless, high-dose human IgG fractions have been shown to reverse rejection despite the absence of any T-cell-depleting abilities. Although a course of polyclonal anti-T-cell antibody typically consists of 5–20 mg/kg given over several days, intravenous immunoglobulin is infused at much higher doses, 500–1000 mg/kg over 1–3 days, and at this dose has been shown to reverse established rejection with the same overall reversal rate as OKT3.[49] At least at high dose, non-specific antibody infusion can modulate immune responses, perhaps through complement sequestration and Fc receptor binding with resultant downregulatory effects of Fc receptor-expressing antigen-presenting cells (APCs).[150]

Administration and Adverse Effects

The polyclonal preparations used in modern clinical practice are generally given through a large-caliber central vein to avoid thrombophlebitis. In experienced hands, a dialysis fistula can be accessed for this purpose. More recent reports have suggested that polyclonal antibodies can be administered peripherally when diluted and formulated with heparin, hydrocortisone, or bicarbonate solutions.[246,347] An in-line filter is recommended to prevent infusion of precipitates that may develop during storage. The protein content should not exceed 4 mg/mL, and dextrose-containing solutions should be avoided because they induce protein precipitation.

Given the weeks-long half-lives of polyclonal antibodies, divided doses are not required for steady-state levels. The tolerability of these compounds is markedly improved, however, by spaced dosing. The rate of infusion is associated with the severity of side effects, and the course of therapy is generally over several days, with individual doses given over 4–6 hours. This time course depends on the dose used and is most applicable to the standard doses of ATG-R and ATG-F (1.5 mg/kg/dose for a total of 7.5–10 mg/kg) or ATGAM (15 mg/kg/dose for a total of 75–100 mg/kg). More recent investigational induction studies have employed substantially higher doses given over 12–24 hours or, alternatively, while the patient is anesthetized.[105,293,302] With a growing emphasis being placed on reduced length of stay after transplantation, larger infusions over fewer days are being employed.

Generally, rabbit-derived polyclonal preparations seem to be significantly better tolerated and more efficacious than ATGAM when used in a quadruple regimen for renal transplantation.[36,117] The most common acute symptoms associated with polyclonal antibody use are the result of transient cytokine release. Chills and fevers occur in at least 20% of patients and are generally treatable by premedication with methylprednisolone, antipyretics, and antihistamines. The use of polyclonal antibodies, particularly in the treatment of rejection, has been associated with an increase in the reactivation and development of primary viral disease caused by cytomegalovirus, herpes simplex virus, Epstein–Barr virus, and varicella.[1,107] It is likely, however, that this is not a class-specific association, but rather an indication of more intensive immunosuppression in general.

Dosage adjustment is warranted to counter leukopenia and thrombocytopenia. Peripheral cell counts drawn immediately after infusion tend to exaggerate cytopenic effects, and most side effects are promptly remedied by time. T-cell counts or, more easily, absolute lymphocyte counts can be monitored to ensure that the preparation is achieving its desired effect. Absolute lymphocyte counts less than 100 cells/μL are typical. Attempts to tailor therapy to a specific peripheral cell count have been made to limit the use of these costly preparations. Rejection can occur and persist with very low T-cell counts, however, and there is little evidence that dose variation by cell count alters efficacy.

As discussed earlier, polyclonal antibody preparations evoke a humoral immune response to themselves.[212,240,306] This response can be detected by enzyme-linked immunosorbent assay-based assays for antirabbit or antihorse antibody, but these tests typically are unavailable in most clinical settings. Failure to achieve significant T-cell depletion suggests the presence of these antibodies. Serum sickness and anaphylaxis also can occur.[240] Pre-emptive skin testing is not practiced often because these tests have not correlated well with clinical outcome.[27,38] Rather, slow infusion rates should be employed during the initial exposure. Antianimal antibodies are most likely to occur in individuals with prior exposure to the preparation involved, but also can exist in individuals with significant prior exposure to the animals themselves.

The most common adverse symptoms related to polyclonal antibodies are fever, urticaria, rash, and headache. These are most likely related to the release of pyrogenic cytokines, such as tumor necrosis factor (TNF)-α, IL-1, and IL-6, which results from activating antibody binding to targeted cell surface receptors and subsequent cell lysis.[56,81,321] Infrequently, pulmonary edema and severe hypertension or hypotension can result in death. As the number of target cells decreases with repeated dosing, this response typically abates. The most concerning response is within the first 24 hours of the first dose, and patients should be monitored closely during this period. The response is limited considerably by methylprednisolone premedication. The rash associated with polyclonal antibody administration conversely tends to occur late in the treatment or at times after the last dose. It is generally self-limiting and requires only symptomatic treatment for urticaria. Antiendothelial antibodies in polyclonal antibodies have been suggested to bind to donor endothelia and activate complement, inducing humoral rejection in some patients.[65]

MONOCLONAL ANTIBODY PREPARATIONS

MAb preparations differ from polyclonal preparations in that all antibody molecules are derived from a single genetic template and are identical. Batch-to-batch variation is eliminated, allowing the mechanism of action and half-life to be extrapolated based on a single ligand receptor interaction (although this still can be influenced by many individualized circumstances). This preparation narrows the scope of effect, however, making the use of these drugs more dependent on precise knowledge of the pathology involved.

Historically, MAbs are the product of clonally immortalized B-cell hybridomas. More recently, genetically engineered mammalian cells have been the source. Use of other production methods, including viral and prokaryotic, or even plant cells, is being investigated.[8] As the production cell becomes increasingly distant from human, the resultant antibodies have increasingly aberrant glycosylation, which can radically alter their efficacy.[93] Regardless of the production cell, the resultant antibody can be purified of any extraneous proteins or other antibodies and used as an infused drug.

The most common method for deriving an MAb typically has been to immunize a mouse with a cell or cell fraction containing the antigen desired. Splenocytes are isolated from the immunized animal, and fused with an immortalized cell, producing many diverse antibody-producing cells. These cells are cloned (grown from single cell suspensions), and the supernatant from each clone is tested for reactivity against the desired antigen. A single robust clone with the desired antibody production characteristics is chosen and grown either in vitro or in a carrier animal. The supernatant from the clone is purified for therapeutic use. Because many MAbs are made by mouse B cells, they are mouse antibodies. Similar to animal-derived polyclonal antibodies, they can be cleared from the circulation by an antibody-directed immune response.[57] This immune response can cause anaphylaxis and neutralize the effect of the MAb in subsequent administrations.[267]

To improve the efficiency of antibody production and eliminate animal-derived protein epitopes, the gene fragment encoding the binding site of murine antibodies can be isolated and engineered on to the gene that encodes for non-polymorphic regions of a human antibody, such as IgG1.[33,120,202] The resultant hybrid antibody gene can be transfected into a high-expressing eukaryotic cell line and grown in vitro to produce antibodies that are predominantly human antibody, yet still bind to a specific human epitope (Figure 20-4). These hybrid antibodies can be considered chimeric, if the entirety of the murine antibody-binding site is used in the construct, or humanized, if the only murine portion is the specific complementary determining regions of the parent antibody.[141] Generally, chimeric antibodies preserve the specificity of the original antibody better, whereas humanized antibodies have less chance of evoking a neutralizing response.[87] Practically speaking, both are effective strategies that help avoid the problem of antibody clearance.

The entire IgG gene has been transgenically expressed in a mouse.[346] This animal, when immunized, makes human, not mouse, antibody, which can be prepared for monoclonal production. This method is likely to be more efficient for producing truly human antihuman antibodies without the need to engineer each antibody individually.

When approved for clinical use, MAbs must be named based on their structural characteristics (Table 20-1). The generic name of a MAb gives the practitioner a reasonable understanding of the origins and specificity of the MAb.

MONOCLONAL ANTIBODIES IN CURRENT CLINICAL TRANSPLANTATION PRACTICE

Because each MAb has a singular specificity, each agent available for general clinical use is considered individually (Figure 20-3). Most MAbs are defined based on their targeted cell surface protein, and these generally are classified based on the CD nomenclature. A numerical CD designation does not define an antigen, but rather defines a molecule or group of molecules. MAbs that bind to the same CD molecule can bind to the same or different epitopes and have similar or different effects.

Muromonab (OKT3; Murine Anti-CD3)

OKT3 (muromonab) is no longer available for clinical use. However, it is considered here given its unique place in the historical continuum of MAb therapy. OKT3 is CD3-specific; CD3 is a transmembrane complex of

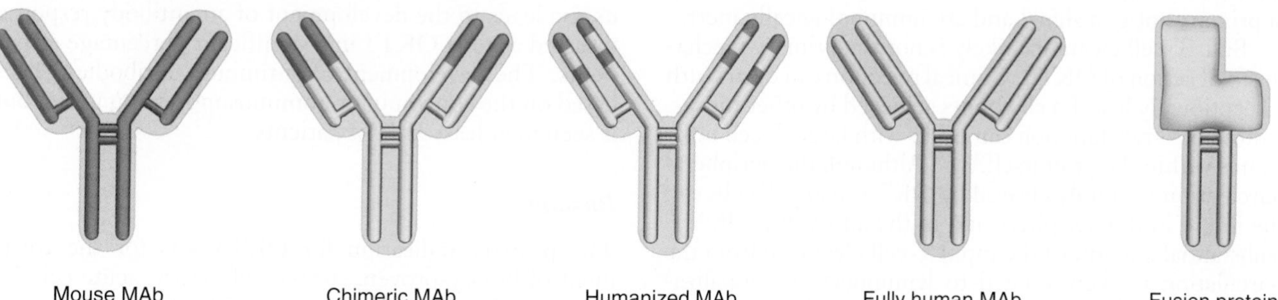

FIGURE 20-4 ■ Types of monoclonal antibodies (MAb) and fusion proteins. Dark areas represent portions of the molecule of non-human origin, and light areas represent human proteins.

TABLE 20-1 **Nomenclature for Monoclonal Antibodies**

	Target		Source		Suffix
Varies based on preference of developer	-vi(r)-	Viral	-u-	Human	-mab
	-ba(c)-	Bacterial	-o-	Mouse	
	-li(m)-	Immune	-a-	Rat	
	-le(s)-	Infectious lesions	-e-	Hamster	
	-ci(r)-	Cardiovascular	-i-	Primate	
	-co(l)-	Colonic tumor	-xi-	Chimeric	
	-me(l)-	Melanoma	-zu-	Humanized	
	-ma(r)-	Mammary tumor			
	-go(t)-	Testicular tumor			
	-go(v)-	Ovarian tumor			
	-pr(o)-	Prostate tumor			
	-tu(m)-	Miscellaneous tumor			

proteins that links to the TCR and conveys its activating signal to the nucleus via a calcineurin-dependent pathway, thus serving as the fundamental signal in antigen-specific T-cell activation. CD3 is present on essentially all T cells, defining the cell type. The TCR signal is generally known as signal 1 because it is primarily required for T-cell activation and defines the antigen specificity of the T cell. Given that T cells are a crucial mediator of acute cellular rejection, CD3 was one of the first molecules to be targeted with MAbs, and OKT3 (muromonab) was the first MAb to gain clinical approval for therapeutic use in humans.[221]

Although the molecular target of OKT3 is singular and precise, its effects are many. The mechanism by which OKT3 mediates its immunosuppressive effect remains ill defined. OKT3 is an IgG2a mouse antibody that binds to the ε component of human CD3. On binding, the antibody mediates complement-dependent cell lysis and ADCC and in doing so rapidly clears T cells from the peripheral circulation.[321] This binding event also leads to pan-T-cell activation before their elimination, resulting in systemic cytokine release. The result is a marked cytokine release syndrome that is responsible for most of the adverse effects associated with the drug (see later).

When antigen binds to the TCR, TCR-CD3 internalization occurs; physiologically, this ensures that antigen binding is reflective of antigen burden and avoids activation mediated by continuous binding of a low-prevalence antigen. Similarly, OKT3 binding to CD3 leads to TCR-CD3 internalization.[56] T cells that are not cleared are often rendered void of surface TCR. These T cells that fail to express the TCR are incapable of receiving a primary antigen signal and are immunologically inert.

Bulk T-cell clearance likely is not the primary mechanism of action of OKT3. Clinical rejection can occur with exceptionally low T-cell counts achieved by other means, and stable graft function can occur with large T-cell infiltrates within the graft itself.[131,156] Although the peripheral circulation is rapidly cleared by OKT3, many T cells can be found in the periphery and in the allograft itself.[151] A substantial amount of the rapid T-cell clearance from the circulation is likely related to lymphocyte marginalization, perhaps induced by the cytokines released and by the methylprednisolone that is given with OKT3. The overall effect of OKT3 is likely an aggregate effect of interrupted TCR binding, TCR internalization, cytokine-mediated regulatory changes, disrupted trafficking, and cell depletion. OKT3 has proven efficacy as an induction and rescue agent. Its immunogenicity has prevented its use as a maintenance agent, and the drug is effective only in combination with other immunosuppressive compounds.[324]

Induction

Initial trials with OKT3 have shown that this MAb is an efficacious induction agent in kidney transplantation,[2,82,200,217] but only when combined with otherwise effective maintenance immunosuppression.[324] OKT3 cannot prevent rejection beyond the period of its actual infusion without additional maintenance therapy. Its usefulness as an induction agent is most pronounced in sensitized patients[220] and patients with delayed graft function, in whom it facilitates the delay of calcineurin inhibitor administration and the resultant nephrotoxicity.[24,145] It reduces the number of acute rejection episodes and the time to first rejection episode. In more recent literature, OKT3 has been shown to reduce acute rejection episodes compared with cyclosporine, azathioprine, or mycophenolate mofetil and steroids without changing patient or graft survival,[3,122,216] but to be equivalent to intravenous cyclosporine induction in children.[22] Despite its early prominence, use of OKT3 as an induction agent dramatically declined in recent years, primarily as a result of its side-effect profile, and this led to its voluntary withdrawal from the market in 2009.

Because OKT3 is an entirely mouse-derived antibody, its use leads to the development of an antibody response directed against OKT3 in a significant percentage of patients. The development of antimouse antibodies varies based on the concomitant immunosuppression given, but is seen in at least 30% of patients.

Rescue

The primary indication for OKT3 was for the treatment of biopsy-proven, steroid-refractory, acute cellular rejection. In this indication, the side-effect profile was deemed justifiable, and the efficacy of OKT3 was undeniable.[69,86,221,308–310] OKT3 was successful in providing sustained reversal of approximately 80% of these vigorous rejections. It was effective even in the presence of prior aggressive lymphocyte depletion, suggesting that its mechanism of action was not primarily a result of bulk T-cell depletion.[75,156,234] The incidence of steroid-refractory rejection, defined as failure to respond to 3 consecutive days of bolus methylprednisolone (e.g., 500 mg daily), declined considerably with improved maintenance immunosuppressive agents, as did the incidence of rejection in general. Thus, the need for OKT3 was reduced considerably. That, combined with its unfavorable side-effect profile relative to newer agents, led to its withdrawal from the US market in 2009. Sporadic use based on existing stocks of the drug continued into 2010.

Interleukin-2 Receptor (CD25)-Specific Monoclonal Antibodies

The receptor for IL-2 is composed of three chains (α, β, and γ), of which the α and γ chains are constitutively expressed, and the β chain is induced with activation. The presence of the β chain, now designated as CD25, indicates prior T-cell activation and identifies cells that have undergone some degree of effector maturation. CD25 has been targeted to suppress activated cells, while sparing resting cells.

Two commercially available anti-CD25 antibodies have been developed, both of which have been engineered to avoid antimurine antibody responses. Daclizumab is a humanized anti-CD25 IgG1, and basiliximab is a chimeric mouse–human anti-CD25 IgG1. Both agents avoid immune clearance and can be used for prolonged periods without inducing a neutralizing antibody.[7,170,264,328] CD25 was the first molecule to be targeted successfully with a humanized MAb in transplantation.[164] These agents also avoid the serum sickness associated with mouse-derived, rabbit-derived, or horse-derived proteins. Daclizumab is no longer available for commercial use. Its withdrawal in 2009 was voluntary and largely based on market rather than biological considerations. It is being considered for reintroduction in non-transplant settings. Basiliximab thus remains the only CD25-specific MAb available for use in transplantation. Studies for both of these agents are considered as the efficacy and mechanisms of action of these agents appear to be practically interchangeable.

Anti-CD25 antibodies are thought to work primarily through steric hindrance of IL-2 binding to CD25 and deprive T cells of this cytokine during early activation. There is little evidence for a depletional effect, or if there is one, it is limited to a few cells. More recently, it has become clear that CD25 induction is involved not only in the activation of cytotoxic T cells but also in the activation of cells with potentially salutary effects on the allograft, such as T-regulatory cells.[300] T cells that have been previously activated and are responding in an anamnestic response are less dependent on IL-2 for proliferation. Heterologous responses (cross-reactive responses between a previously encountered pathogen and an alloantigen) or memory alloimmune responses seem not to be affected significantly by CD25 interruption. Given this biology primarily focused on naïve T-cell early activation, CD25-directed antibodies have found a role in induction, but have no role in the treatment of established rejection. Although there has been anecdotal experience using these antibodies for maintenance immunosuppression in the setting of calcineurin inhibitor toxicity with recurrent rejection,[100] no study has formally evaluated this approach.

Induction

Many anti-CD25 antibodies, including anti-Tac,[164] 33B3.1,[287] LO-Tact-1,[126] and BT563,[322] have been tested in humans and been shown to delay modestly or reduce the onset of acute rejection when used with conventional maintenance immunosuppression. The experimental rodent antibodies have been generally abandoned in favor of the humanized/chimerized antibodies.

Daclizumab and basiliximab have been shown to reduce modestly the incidence of acute cellular rejection compared with methylprednisolone induction when used in triple or double immunosuppressive regimens, with exceptional patient tolerability in kidney and extrarenal transplantation.[23,124,144,208,209,211,271,327] Studies comparing basiliximab with polyclonal antibodies in regimens using cyclosporine, mycophenolate mofetil, and steroids have shown comparable outcomes.[178,205,284] The use of depletional agents appears to be preferable in high-risk situations.[35,37,116] The magnitude of the antirejection effect seen with anti-CD25 therapy depends to some extent on the intensity of the maintenance regimen, with earlier trials using cyclosporine-based and azathioprine-based regimens showing a 25% reduction and later trials in the tacrolimus/mycophenolate mofetil era showing a more modest 10% improvement. Anti-CD25 induction also has been used successfully in steroid-free regimens in kidney transplantation.[31,257,290] The use of anti-CD25 has not been shown, however, to facilitate more aggressive maintenance reduction regimens, such as monotherapy or calcineurin avoidance.[225,331]

Administration and Adverse Effects

Although the efficacy of anti-CD25 therapies is modest, the safety profile is highly favorable.[23,124,144,208,209,211,271,284,327] Binding of anti-CD25 antibodies does not mediate T-cell activation, and no perceptible cytokine release occurs. Clinical trials generally have shown no increase in infectious complications or delayed wound healing. The risk of PTLD with anti-CD25 induction is similar to that when no induction agent is employed.[59,155]

Alemtuzumab (Humanized Anti-CD52)

Given the reduction in rejection achieved with prolonged polyclonal antibody-mediated T-cell depletion, the ease of administration and consistency of MAbs, and the benefits of humanization, clinicians have sought agents with a combination of these traits. The CD52-specific humanized MAb alemtuzumab has emerged as a promising depletional MAb.[29,116,190,336,339]

Alemtuzumab (Campath-1H) is a humanized IgG1 derivative of a rat antihuman CD52.[336] CD52 is a non-modulating, glycosylphosphatidylinositol-anchored membrane protein of unknown function found in high density on most T cells, B cells, and monocytes.[113] CD52 is not found on hematopoietic precursor cells and does not seem to be an adhesion molecule; it is not necessary for T-cell activation. Several versions of the non-humanized anti-CD52 predecessors of alemtuzumab have been studied and been shown to be effective in mediating rapid T-cell depletion and reversing steroid-resistant rejection. The humanized form has been studied in several indications and is currently approved for the treatment of lymphogenous malignancies.

Although not approved for use in solid-organ transplantation, alemtuzumab has been used off-label as an induction agent.[272,273] Its mechanism of action seems to be predominantly related to bulk T-cell depletion, with lesser depletion of B cells and monocytes. It rapidly depletes CD52-expressing lymphocytes centrally and peripherally in renal transplant recipients.[156] The use of alemtuzumab as a rescue drug is burgeoning, and there has been anecdotal investigation in this drug as a maintenance therapy. Alemtuzumab is currently unavailable for commercial use in transplantation, but is being supplied for transplant use by its maker (Sanofi). The drug is being positioned in the market as Lemtrada, for use in patients with multiple sclerosis.

Induction

In preliminary, uncontrolled studies, alemtuzumab has been shown to facilitate reduced-maintenance immunosuppressive requirements without an apparent increase in infectious or malignant complications in kidney and extrarenal transplantation compared with historical controls.[14,45,46,112,147,148,156,161,166,167,196,272,305,319] Specifically, alemtuzumab has been used to achieve perioperative depletion in combination with triple immunosuppression and early steroid weaning; steroid-free regimens with calcineurin inhibitors and mycophenolate mofetil maintenance; and with monotherapy regimens of cyclosporine, tacrolimus, or sirolimus. Graft and patient survivals have been comparable to contemporaneously reported registry data, although the incidence of reversible rejection has predictably increased with decreases in concomitant maintenance therapy. Prospective comparison with other regimens is just beginning. Alemtuzumab has been shown to provide similar outcomes in low-risk patients compared to basiliximab induction, and similar outcomes in high-risk patients compared to ATG-R.[116]

Mechanistic studies investigating alemtuzumab induction have shown that, although it depletes all T-cell subsets to some degree, it has modest selectivity for naïve cell types.[228] Non-depleted T cells exhibit a memory phenotype and seem to be most susceptible to calcineurin inhibitors. Maintenance regimens including calcineurin inhibitors seem to do best in alemtuzumab-based maintenance reduction strategies. The rapid and profound depletion has allowed for a delay in the initiation of therapeutic calcineurin inhibitor levels, however, and has made this an attractive option for patients with delayed graft function.[166]

Although alemtuzumab depletes B cells, its effect on T cells is more profound and lasting. It does not clear plasma cells. Some investigators have associated alemtuzumab administration with an increase in antibody-mediated rejection or at least posttransplant development of donor-specific alloantibody.[44] Whether this association is related to the effects of the antibody, the reductionist maintenance regimens used with alemtuzumab, or specifics of patient selection and screening for HLA-specific antibodies remains to be determined. There appears to be a homeostatic response to the B-cell-depleting effect leading to high levels of BAFF and concomitant increases in activated B cells emerging after alemtuzumab administration that is a potential mechanistic explanation for a rise in alloantibody production.[29]

Rescue

The rodent antihuman CD52 predecessors of alemtuzumab, Campath-1M and Campath-1G, were originally tested as rescue agents.[95–97,114] In the original studies using anti-CD52 for steroid-resistant rejection, the antibodies were used with triple immunosuppression and steroid bolus therapy, leading to a prohibitively immunosuppressive regimen with excess infectious morbidity and mortality. With the success of alemtuzumab as an induction agent, there has been a resurgence of interest in its use as a rescue agent. Several anecdotal reports have recently emerged.[62,15,74,320] Additional study is required to define its role in this setting, although its predilection for naïve cells may limit its efficacy after sensitization.

Administration and Adverse Effects

Alemtuzumab can be administered through a peripheral intravenous catheter and can be dosed as a 30-mg flat dose or at 0.3 mg/kg dose over 3 hours. Almost total elimination of peripheral $CD3^+$ T cells can be expected within 1 hour of the first infusion, although secondary lymphoid depletion requires 48 hours and at least two doses.[156,228] Higher doses have not been shown to be of additional benefit in transplantation.

The rapid depletion characteristic of alemtuzumab is associated with a cytokine release phenomenon similar to, but typically less severe than, that seen with polyclonal antibodies or OKT3. Administration should be preceded by a bolus of methylprednisolone, diphenhydramine, and acetaminophen. The first dose should be given in a setting capable of dealing with hypotension, anaphylaxis, and other sequelae of cytokine release. Neutralizing antibodies have not been described for alemtuzumab.

Early trials investigating alemtuzumab as a therapy for multiple sclerosis suggested an association between its use and the development of autoimmune thyroiditis.[64] Specifically, patients with multiple sclerosis receiving high-dose investigational therapy with alemtuzumab had a significantly increased risk of hyperthyroidism developing 1–3 years after therapy. It has been hypothesized that T-cell depletion, particularly depletion that selectively spares activated cells, could disrupt T-cell regulation and unmask autoreactive clones. This effect could be most evident in individuals with low-level adjuvant maintenance immunosuppression, as was the case in the multiple sclerosis trials. There has been a case report of autoimmune thyroiditis in an alemtuzumab-treated renal transplant patient, leaving the potential for autoimmune disease as an unresolved matter of concern.[157]

Rituximab (Humanized Anti-CD20)

Rituximab is a chimeric MAb specific for CD20. CD20 is a cell surface glycoprotein involved in B-cell activation and maturation whose natural ligand is unknown.[79] Similar to alemtuzumab, it has been developed and approved for use in lymphogenous malignancies, particularly CD20+ B-cell lymphomas and PTLD.[111] Given its specificity for B cells (and despite its lack of specificity for antibody-producing plasma cells), rituximab has been suggested to be a therapy for antibody-mediated rejection and rejections involving vasculitis.[18,19] Rituximab also has been used in regimens designed to facilitate transplantation in sensitized individuals, such as ABO-incompatible donor-recipient pairs or transplants across a positive crossmatch following antibody removal.[99,102,250,286,318,332] At present, the role of rituximab in transplantation is largely investigational; however, similar to alemtuzumab, its off-label use is increasing considerably.

The mechanism of action of rituximab is presumed to be depletional, primarily through induced apoptosis.[80,307] Treatment with this antibody rapidly and specifically clears CD20+ cells from the circulation. The role of CD20+ cells in alloimmune responses is currently incompletely defined. Although these cells are precursors to antibody-producing plasma cells, they do not produce antibody without further maturation. Their role in acute antibody production is not well established, and it is unlikely that they have a direct effector cell role in rejection. Several authors have documented CD20+ infiltrates as a marker for particularly recalcitrant acute rejection.[128,263] These cells are known to have APC function and it has been postulated that they serve to facilitate intragraft antigen presentation. Currently, rituximab is being used in induction and rescue indications.

Induction

The use of rituximab as an induction agent has been limited to patients with known donor-specific sensitization. In particular, rituximab has been suggested to be a surrogate for recipient splenectomy in patients undergoing donor desensitization with plasmapheresis or intravenous immunoglobulin infusion, or both.[286,318] It has not been prospectively studied, but rituximab seems to have some effect in reducing the rebound of alloantibody in these complex patients.

Rescue

Several reports have emerged suggesting that rituximab has a role in the treatment of vascular rejection (Banff classification 2 and 3) and in reversing emerging alloantibody formation.[18,19,90] This would be presumed to be relevant for allograft infiltrates shown to contain CD20+ cells, although specific guidelines for the use of rituximab remain forthcoming. As with its use as an induction therapy, use of rituximab as a rescue agent remains investigational.

Rituximab's most important indication in organ transplantation is not as a rescue agent for rejection, but rather as a primary treatment for PTLD.[301] Although immunosuppression reduction is the primary therapeutic maneuver in PTLD, rituximab has emerged as an effective and well-tolerated maneuver to be interjected between immunosuppressive withdrawal and more aggressive chemotherapy.

Administration and Adverse Effects

Rituximab can be administered through a peripheral vein and is associated with few overt side effects. As with all proteins, anaphylaxis can occur, and initial doses should be given in a monitored environment. When used as a treatment for PTLD, it is typically given at a dose of 375 mg/m^2. Dosing as an immunosuppressant has empirically followed this regimen. Rituximab persists in the circulation for weeks to months, and a single dose effectively eliminates CD20+ cells for a similarly prolonged period. The presence of rituximab in the serum artificially produces a pan-positive B-cell crossmatch by complement-dependent cytotoxicity and flow techniques. Characterization of alloantibody after the use of rituximab requires alloantigen-specific methods, such as solid-phase bead array assays.

Numerous other humanized and fully human CD20-specific MAbs are under development for a host of immune and oncologic indications.[17,321] Their use in transplantation remains expectant.

FUSION PROTEINS

Fusion proteins are molecules that have been engineered from a single receptor targeting a ligand of interest fused to another protein that provides another salutary property. In transplantation, this secondary molecule is typically the Fc portion of an IgG molecule that gives the receptor an antibody-like half-life and/or opsonization properties.[146,176,183] Fusion proteins also can involve the fusion of a specific toxin to a MAb to facilitate epitope-directed drug delivery.[168] Fusion proteins are similar to MAbs because they have a single homogeneous specificity and can be composed of human or humanized components, limiting their immune clearance and opening their use for prolonged administration. One fusion protein, belatacept, is now approved for use in transplantation and will be considered specifically in Chapter 21. There are notable examples of other transplant-relevant fusion proteins in development that are discussed subsequently.

Monoclonal Antibodies and Fusion Proteins in Clinical Transplantation Investigation

The promise of MAb therapy has led to the development of a rapidly expanding number of antibodies and fusion proteins targeting a wide variety of surface molecules.[325] Several of these agents have shown efficacy in large-animal transplant models and in early clinical transplant trials. Even more have been developed for autoimmune indications, such as psoriasis and rheumatoid arthritis, but their immunomodulating effects have clear potential in transplant indications. The following agents have been studied in early-phase clinical transplant trials or have received approval for clinical use in non-transplant indications and have preclinical trials suggesting efficacy in transplantation. These agents are discussed based on their targeted ligand. All new antibodies under clinical development are now humanized or fully human.[252] Numerous agents have been tested and shown promise in preclinical studies, but will not be specifically addressed here.

CD2-Specific Approaches

CD2, also known as LFA-2, is an adhesion molecule expressed on T cells and natural killer cells that binds to CD58 (LFA-3) on APCs and facilitates TCR binding and signal transduction. It has been targeted by the rat IgG2b anti-CD2 MAb BTI-322, and more recently by siplizumab (also known as MEDI-507), a humanized IgG1 version of BTI-322. BTI-322 was investigated initially as an induction and rescue agent for deceased donor renal and hepatic allografts and for graft-versus-host disease, and was shown to have biological activity and to give results consistent with the standard therapies available at the time.[182,203,243,290]

Clinical trials in psoriasis using siplizumab began in 1999 and were met with an unexpected propensity toward agent immunogenicity.[170] This agent has been used in non-human primate transplant tolerance trials with success in mixed chimerism-directed approaches[149] and has been used clinically as part of a non-myeloablative conditioning regimen to achieve mixed hematopoietic chimerism.[288] Siplizumab has been investigated in phase I and II trials for T-lymphocytic malignancies, graft-versus-host disease and psoriasis.[63] There are no active trials with siplizumab registered in ClinicalTrials.gov.[63]

Alefacept is a human fusion protein of the CD2 ligand (CD58, LFA-3) with IgG1 that has been shown to inhibit T-cell proliferation. Its administration also has been shown to have a relative selective depleting effect on effector memory T cells, the same cells that have been relatively spared by other depleting MAbs and polyclonal preparations.[106,265] It gained increased attention more recently in experimental transplantation. Alefacept is currently approved for the treatment of plaque-like psoriasis. Preclinical trials in non-human primate transplantation have shown that alefacept has minimal effect on graft survival when used alone, but that it does extend graft survival when used with adjuvant therapies.[88,338] In particular, its pairing with belatacept was shown to eliminate belatacept-resistant memory T cells and facilitate belatacept-based maintenance therapy in non-human primates and in vitro in humans.[184,338]

Alefacept was recently studied in a phase II trial pairing it with tacrolimus-based maintenance immunosuppression. Although the results remain unpublished, the outcomes were not viewed as sufficient to continue the development of the drug in transplantation. Presently, there is one registered trial investigating alefacept in graft-versus-host disease.[63]

CD3-Specific Antibodies

Targeting CD3 is a proven strategy, as shown by the success of OKT3. Significant effort has been directed toward modernizing the anti-CD3 approach to avoid the many side effects associated with CD3 activation. Several CD3-specific antibodies, including huOKT3γ1 (MGA031, teplizumab), aglycosyl CD3 (otelixizumab), and visilizumab (HuM291), have been humanized and otherwise engineered to eliminate their undesirable activating properties and immunogenicity.[94,218,351,352] Phase I studies have indicated that modified versions of a CD3-specific antibody can achieve T-cell depletion without the confounding problems of cytokine release or an antibody neutralization. Phase II trials using visilizumab in marrow transplantation have shown initial efficacy against graft-versus-host disease,[48] and teplizumab has shown promise as a prophylactic agent in new-onset diabetes mellitus.[123,275] These studies have shown that the side effects related to OKT3 use are not inherent in CD3-directed therapies, opening the door for more refined targeting of this receptor complex. Currently, teplizumab has completed a single clinical study in islet transplantation, the results of which have yet to be reported.[63] Visilizumab has completed phase III trials for ulcerative colitis, but there are no ongoing registered trials for visilizumab.[63]

CD4-Specific Antibodies

CD4 is a cell surface glycoprotein that binds to a monomorphic region of MHC class II molecules and in doing so stabilizes the interaction between the TCR and MHC class II. It is expressed on approximately two-thirds of peripheral T cells and has partially defined several functional T-cell subsets, including helper T cells and T-regulatory cells. CD4 also is expressed by peripheral monocytes and other APCs, where its function is poorly characterized. It likely plays a crucial role in facilitating cell-to-cell communication among lymphoid cells, and it has lesser effects on physiological effector functions. Given its central role in cellular immune responses, CD4 has long been a target for immune manipulation, and several antibodies have been tested in transplantation. Generally, the efficacy has been exceptional in defined rodent models and modest in more clinically relevant settings; this may relate to the growing recognition that $CD4^+$ T cells have a potential role in tempering immune responses.[5,300,335]

Many studies have shown that anti-CD4 antibody induction dramatically inhibits the development of acute rejection in rodents, particularly when combined with supplementary donor antigen, such as donor-specific transfusion.[189,259,278,349] Given that the distribution of MHC class II molecules differs substantially between rodents and humans, however, these studies have not been predictive of the anticipated effect in humans. Depleting[85,236,260] and non-depleting[10,71,77,179,214,344] antibodies have shown an effect in experimental models, suggesting that cell elimination, disruption of cell-cell communication, or signal transduction through CD4 may be mechanistically relevant. Two humanized anti-CD4 preparations have shown significant prolongation of non-human primate renal allograft survival.[71,236]

Initial clinical transplantation trials using anti-CD4 MAbs employed murine-derived antibodies, including OKT4A, BL4, MT151, and B-F5.[76,85,175] Predictably, these agents were subject to immune clearance, but nevertheless were shown to lead to CD4⁺ T-cell clearance. Regardless, patients experienced rejection rates of 50%, and the agents were not sufficiently efficacious to warrant further development. Subsequent trials investigating the humanized OKT4A[67] and the chimeric cM-T412[198] have been evaluated in conjunction with cyclosporine-based maintenance therapy in kidney and heart transplant recipients.[255] In both cases, the antibody was well tolerated, and treated patients had low rates of rejection, suggesting that this approach is promising. Antibody responses toward the remnant murine portions of the MAb were surprisingly frequent, however. $CD4^+$ T-cell depletion was not achieved using OKT4A, but was common with cM-T412.

The mouse antihuman CD4 MAb, Max.16H5, has been tested in pilot fashion as a clinical rescue agent.[253] Max.16H5 depleted $CD4^+$ T cells and was associated with reversal of rejection in most treated patients. Neutralizing antibodies were not detected. No trials investigating humanized anti-CD4 MAbs have been reported for rescue therapy.

Many human or humanized CD4-specific MAbs, including HuMax-CD4 (zanolimumab), TNX355, MT412, and 4162W94,[60,174,283] have been evaluated in phase I, II, and III trials for non-transplant indications, such as psoriasis and rheumatoid arthritis, as well as oncological indications. These studies have shown that CD4-specific antibodies can influence immune responses and that their use is relatively safe in humans. Currently, there are no active anti-CD4 MAb trials registered in transplantation.[63]

Costimulation-Based Therapies

Interest in the costimulation pathways as targets for immune manipulation has exploded in recent years.[118] Generally, these agents interfere with pathways that act to influence the outcome of antigen binding to the TCR. Costimulatory molecules can exert positive or negative influences on the efficiency of antigen presentation and recognition and alter the threshold for activation of naive T lymphocytes without having a primary activating or inhibitory function. Costimulatory molecule manipulation influences only cells with ongoing TCR activation and should have effects only on cells actively undergoing antigen recognition; this has been thought to allow for antigen-specific immune manipulation.

The most studied costimulatory receptor on T cells is CD28. It has two known ligands, CD80 (B7-1) and CD86 (B7-2), both of which are expressed on APCs. CD28 is constitutively expressed on most T cells and on ligation reduces the threshold for TCR activation.[143] CD152 (cytotoxic T-lymphocyte-associated antigen 4 (CTLA-4)) is an induced molecule expressed on T-cell activation that is structurally similar to CD28 and competitively binds CD80 and CD86, transmitting an inhibitory signal that acts to terminate the immune response.[337] CD28 and CD152 serve reciprocal roles, both stimulated by the B7 molecules and facilitating (CD28) or quelling (CD152) a T-cell response.

An additional receptor-ligand pair that has gained considerable attention involves CD40 and CD154. CD154, also known as CD40 ligand, is expressed on activated T cells and other cells, including platelets.[11,108,121,153] CD40 is expressed on APCs. Although the specific effect of CD154 on T cells is incompletely defined, CD40 has a major influence on APC activation. CD40 ligation leads to marked APC activation, including increased expression of the B7 molecules and MHC, and stimulatory cytokine production, greatly facilitating antigen presentation.[52] CD154 is released from the alpha granules of activated platelets and acts locally to greatly augment alloimmune responses.[54] It can serve as the sole source of CD154 responsible for rejection.[354] CD154 exists as a large inducible reservoir that can be triggered by platelet activation and augment antigen presentation at the time of a traumatic injury, including a transplant procedure. Its release is local and governed by alpha degranulation.[54] Many other costimulatory molecules have been investigated, but none has yet been exploited as a target in the clinic.[61,63]

Costimulatory molecules can be targeted with blocking MAbs to inhibit their stimulatory effects. Because it is difficult to determine prospectively whether a MAb is stimulatory or inhibitory in vivo, and because costimulatory molecules have stimulatory and inhibitory effects, it has been challenging to find therapeutically reliable agents. Because CD152 and CD154 are upregulated on activated T cells, these costimulatory molecules also may serve as targets for selective elimination of activated effector cells.[201] Selective targeting of CD152 with the MAb ipilimumab has been used to augment immunity in the setting of metastatic melanoma, with salutary oncologic results balanced by considerable induction of autoimmune side effects.[129,130]

Although most experimental use of MAbs directed against costimulatory molecules in transplantation has focused on tolerance induction (elimination of a need for any maintenance therapy), the clinical focus has been on pairing costimulation-directed biologics with maintenance minimization strategies, particularly calcineurin-sparing approaches. Agents interfering with the CD28/B7 and the CD40/CD154 pathways have reached clinical trials, with one B7-specific fusion protein, belatacept, achieving approval for use in kidney transplantation (discussed in depth in Chapter 21). Two humanized MAbs specific for CD154, hu5c8 and IDEC-131, have been shown in non-human primates to prevent acute rejection for months to years without additional immunosuppression and have been paired with sirolimus monotherapy and donor-specific transfusion to lead to operational tolerance in some cases.[154,158,238,353] Early human trials with hu5c8 were hindered by unimpressive efficacy and concerns for thromboembolic risk.[160]

CD154-specific therapies have not been studied clinically in recent years, and most preclinical attention has turned toward intervention with CD40 as opposed to CD154.[4] Pursuant to CD40 blockade, one agent, ASKP1240 (also known as 4d11), has reached the clinic and completed phase I trials.[63] ASKP1240 is a fully human CD40-specific MAb that has been shown in numerous non-human primate studies to prevent kidney and liver allograft rejection, particularly when used in combination with tacrolimus.[9,137,152,223] Phase II trials are imminent. Investigational interest in CD154 manipulation also remains intense.

A cocktail of two humanized MAbs specific for the B7 molecules CD80 and CD86 has been shown to facilitate prolonged renal allograft survival in non-human primates.[162] These antibodies reached clinical trials in organ transplantation and were shown to have initial safety in humans. Their development has not been pursued. A similar approach has been exploited with the fusion protein belatacept (covered in Chapter 21).[176]

Although there are many costimulation molecules that have been targeted in rodents, with dramatic results, no MAbs have been successfully transitioned to the clinic. This situation likely relates to the fundamental role that costimulation molecules have in general immunity and immune homeostasis. In addition to the thromboembolic concerns, marked adverse reactions have been associated with costimulation-directed MAbs. Severe autoimmune enteritis and vasculitis have been triggered by the CD152-specific ipilimumab, showing that CTLA-4 signaling and its resultant negative T-cell regulation is vital to preserving a balance with the activating effects of CD28 signaling.[129,130] Similarly, severe septic-like responses have been reported after the administration of TGN1412, a CD28-specific MAb tested in phase I trials.[299] There seems to be a fundamental balance between the two B7-specific T-cell molecules CD28 and CD152 that is required to avoid dysregulated autoimmunity. Greater success has been achieved with agents that target the B7 molecules CD80 and CD86, providing inhibition of potential CD28 and CD152 signals; this has been achieved through the use of B7-specific fusion proteins. However, the conceptual promise of CD28-specific blockade has led to the development of numerous agents, including single-chain domain-specific antibodies that have proven themselves efficacious in non-human primate transplantation.[231,232] Their clinical translation is anticipated.

Tumor Necrosis Factor-α-Based Approaches

Sequestration of cytokines using MAbs has long been contemplated as a therapeutic strategy in many inflammatory diseases. Although many cytokine-specific agents have been developed, only TNF-α-specific agents have gained widespread clinical use. TNF-α is a cytokine produced by many immune cells that is ubiquitously present in most inflammatory responses and has numerous general proinflammatory effects, including increased chemotaxis, vascular permeability, and fever. It has been considered as an attractive target for many inflammatory aspects of transplantation, including depletion-associated cytokine release syndrome, ischemia-reperfusion injury, and rejection. Three TNF-α-specific agents are currently approved for non-transplant conditions, and their use in transplantation is emerging, particularly in islet transplantation.

Infliximab is a chimeric IgG1 MAb that binds to cell-bound and circulating TNF-α, sequestering it from the TNF receptor and inhibiting TNF-dependent proinflammatory effects. It has been developed for the treatment of numerous autoimmune disorders, including rheumatoid arthritis (its primary approved clinical use), psoriasis, Crohn's disease, and ulcerative colitis.[279,345] It has been used in pilot studies of many transplant indications, including renal, bone marrow, intestinal, and islet transplantation, with suggestive success. Its predominant therapeutic effect in transplantation seems to be to limit paracrine cytokine-mediated activation within the graft and to mute the clinical sequelae of rejection without altering the overall infiltrate of inciting allosensitization.[73,98,226] Similarly, adalimumab is a TNF-α-specific MAb that has been approved for the treatment of psoriatic arthritis.[345]

Etanercept is a soluble recombinant TNF receptor–IgG fusion protein that acts to absorb soluble TNF-α and limit its availability in the circulation. It is approved for the treatment of rheumatoid arthritis and has been increasingly evaluated for a role in the treatment of graft-versus-host disease.[139] Use of etanercept in islet transplantation has recently been reported.[21,232]

Golimumab is a fully human TNF-α-specific MAb that is in phase II trials for rheumatoid arthritis. No reports have been made of this agent in transplantation, although there are numerous trials in autoimmune indications.[63]

Several other cytokine-directed MAbs are now approved for immune indications outside of transplantation and are likely to have relevance to transplantation. Ustakinimab is a humanized MAb specific for the p40 subunit common to the receptors for both IL-12 and IL-23.[340] It is approved for clinical use in the treatment of psoriasis,[181] particularly in patients who have failed therapy with etanercept. The IL-12/23 axis is increasingly recognized as relevant in transplantation, particularly in the setting of costimulation blockade-resistant rejection, and it is likely that ustakinimab will be evaluated as an adjuvant therapy in combination with costimulation blockade-based strategies in the foreseeable future. Similarly, tocilizumab is an IL-6 receptor MAb approved for use in rheumatoid arthritis.[323] Given the role of IL-6 in alloantibody production, one trial has been initiated using tocilizumab in patients awaiting kidney transplantation with hopes that it will attenuate alloantibody production in sensitized individuals.[63]

Targeting Cell Adhesion

Given the fundamental requirement for adhesion molecules in most inflammatory responses, there has been long-standing interest in blocking adhesion interactions to prevent platelet and leukocyte adherence and infiltration. As discussed previously, polyclonal antibodies are thought to bind to and inhibit some adhesion molecules. Several MAbs have been developed to target adhesion pathways.[26]

Among the most prominent is the LFA-1/ICAM-1 pathway. LFA-1 (the heterodime integrin molecule CD11a/CD18) is expressed on mature T cells and binds to ICAM-1 (CD54) expressed on APCs and endothelial cells.[193,258,289] The pathway greatly facilitates initial lymphocyte recruitment at sites of injury and inflammation.[207] Adhesion pathways have been studied in several preclinical settings, including rodents[138,244] and non-human primates,[70,146,251] with survival being markedly prolonged in rodents and prolonged 30 days in primates. Recent data pairing the LFA-1-specific MAb TS1/22 with belatacept has led to exceptionally prolonged survival in non-human primate islet transplantation.[13]

Enlimomab, a murine anti-CD54 MAb, was successfully tested in a phase I trial involving high-risk deceased donor kidneys[119] and subsequently evaluated in a placebo-controlled phase II study combined with conventional triple-drug maintenance therapy.[261] No significant difference was detected between the treated and the placebo groups, and further development was not pursued. Similarly, odulimomab, a murine anti-LFA-1 MAb, was studied as an induction agent compared with R-ATG in renal transplantation, with no significant difference being found between the groups.[133] A single rescue trial using the anti-LFA-1 murine MAb 25-3 failed to show efficacy.[180]

The most promising and well-studied LFA-1-specific MAb is efalizumab. Efalizumab (Raptiva) is a recombinant humanized MAb that binds to human CD11a and inhibits the LFA-1/ICAM-1 interaction.[83,213] Efalizumab has been tested in phase I/II studies for renal transplantation where it was paired with conventional triple immunosuppression. In that setting, the combined regimen was overly immunosuppressive and its development waned.[330] It re-emerged recently in two clinical islet trials as the centerpiece maintenance immunosuppressant. In these trials, the efalizumab-based regimen was shown to facilitate initial engraftment and function, and to prevent islet rejection successfully.[235,316] Trials based on efalizumab as a calcineurin alternative were initiated in kidney transplantation but had to be halted when the maker of efalizumab withdrew the drug from the market.[63] It was used clinically and approved by the Food and Drug Administration (FDA) for treatment of mild-to-moderate psoriasis. However, its use was associated with a low incidence of progressive multifocal leukoencephalopathy (approximately 1/10 000 exposures), which was cited as an undue risk for patients with psoriasis. In general, this risk profile, while perhaps adverse for psoriasis, is acceptable in kidney transplantation, and there is genuine hope that this agent will resurface for use in transplant indications in the future.

Other integrin-based adhesion molecules have been shown to be clearly involved in peripheral immune responses, the most studied of which is VLA4 (α_4-integrin). The MAb natalizumab targets this molecule and has gained FDA approval for the treatment of multiple sclerosis.[233] It was subsequently withdrawn from the market due to an elevated risk of progressive multifocal encephalopathy, but returned with more robust warning relative to this side effect. VLA-4 specific MAbs have been shown to attenuate costimulation blockade-resistant rejection in mice,[165] and promising preliminary results in non-human primates have been observed. Its availability for off-label use in the clinic may facilitate clinical transplant trials in the foreseeable future.

PSGL1-Ig (YSPSL) is a fusion protein combining the extracellular domains of P-selectin glycoprotein ligand-1 (CD162) with the Fc portion of IgG1. CD162 is a ligand for P-selectin, E-selectin, and L-selectin, all of which have been shown to facilitate leukocyte and platelet adhesion. Because cell adhesion has been implicated as a primary event in reperfusion injury and in allorecognition, this drug has been contemplated as a therapy to limit the impact of events occurring during initial implantation. Treatment with PSGL1-Ig has been shown to attenuate ischemia-reperfusion injury, most prominently in rodent models of hepatic warm ischemia.[47,89,92] This agent has recently completed testing in a phase I/II evaluation in liver transplantation showing that it attenuates the clinical and biochemical syndrome of hepatic ischemia-reperfusion injury.[43] Testing in the setting of kidney transplantation has been performed to determine its efficacy in preventing reperfusion injury. These studies have completed enrollment and results are pending.[63]

Targeting the T-Cell Receptor

T cells bind their cognate antigen through their heterodimeric glycoprotein TCR. There are two general forms, an α/β form, expressed on 95% of peripheral T cells and responsible for specifying most alloimmune responses, and a γ/δ form, which is involved in innate immune responses and appears late in allograft rejection.[159] The TCR is a result of somatic gene rearrangement similar to that seen in antibody formation, and the specificity of each T cell can be defined by its individual TCR. Rejections based on specific TCR/MHC interactions select for specific TCR types, showing that each MHC mismatch is recognized by a few clones, rather than by the entire T-cell repertoire.[115] Although this finding fostered initial enthusiasm for targeting antigen-specific T cells through custom MAbs specific for a given TCR, this approach has been deemed impractical given the vast number of TCRs generated during T-cell maturation and their variable crossreactivity with variable MHC polymorphisms. Nevertheless, the success of targeting TCR-associated proteins such as CD3 has generated some interest in targeting monomorphic portions of the TCR directly. More recently, the realization that TCR signaling is required for T-cell apoptosis and regulation has made preservation of the TCR a competing strategy.

T10B9, also known as Medi-500, is a murine IgM specific for a monomorphic determinant on α/β and γ/δ TCRs. It is effective in mediating T-cell depletion in vitro and in vivo[40] and has been studied as a rescue and induction agent in renal and cardiac transplantation.[333,334] In both trials, the antibody-mediated T-cell depletion was well tolerated. Its efficacy as a rescue agent seemed to be similar to that of OKT3, and the cardiac trial suggested efficacy as an induction agent. Nevertheless, the agent has not been developed further in organ transplantation, likely as a result of comparably effective humanized MAbs. T10B9 has been studied as a conditioning agent of bone marrow transplantation,[313] and a phase III trial using T10B9 as an ex vivo depletional agent for bone marrow transplantation has been completed.[63]

TOL101 is an IgM MAb that is specific for the α/β TCR. It has been shown to have numerous depletional and non-depletional effects on human T cells.[103,280] The drug has entered phase I/II testing in kidney transplantation with a favorable initial safety interim analysis.[111]

Targeting Complement

Proteins of the complement cascade have long been known to be crucial in mediating antibody-associated cytotoxicity.[66] Many approaches have been contemplated to achieve complement elimination in the setting of antibody presensitization, including plasmapheresis and intravenous immunoglobulin administration. More recently, it has been shown that complement, specifically that produced locally within the kidney itself, is a contributing factor facilitating peripheral T-cell maturation and rejection.[237] Polymorphisms in complement expression have been shown to influence the incidence of rejection and renal allograft survival in ways not previously recognized.[39]

Two complement-specific agents have been used clinically and have been shown to be biologically active with promise for application in transplantation. Eculizumab is a humanized MAb specific for C5a, a key initiation factor in complement membrane attack complex formation. It has been shown to be a potentially effective therapy for paroxysmal nocturnal hemoglobinuria and is currently in phase III trials for this indication.[63,127,350] Numerous single-center studies and case reports have recently shown that eculizumab, when used as part of a multimodal treatment strategy, can facilitate the prevention or reversal of numerous complement-mediated maladies, including hemolytic uremic syndrome and antibody-mediated rejection.[173,185–187,295,355,356.] Accordingly, there are now numerous ongoing clinical trials investigating the systematic use of this agent in kidney transplantation,[63] and it is likely that this agent will become an established part of the transplant armamentarium in the future.

TP-10 (soluble complement receptor type 3) is a recombinant soluble protein that binds and inactivates the central activating component of the complement cascade, C3. It has been used in numerous preclinical settings and shown to be effective in preventing humoral xenograft rejection in a pig-to-non-human primate model.[241] It was investigated in a clinical trial for its role in preventing cardiopulmonary bypass-related complications, with disappointing results.[63] Despite its clear ability to arrest C3-mediated complement activation, it has not been systematically investigated in clinical transplantation.

Other Experimental Antibodies and Fusion Proteins

Almost all surface molecules expressed by leukocytes have been considered for therapeutic targeting. Many have been formally investigated in early clinical trials without sufficient promise to warrant additional clinical development. Others have significant promise in advanced preclinical settings but have yet to be tested in humans. This section will call out additional agents in which there is some clinical experience. Knowledge of these agents is useful for a complete understanding of the field.

Targeting CD5

CD5 is an adhesion molecule that is constitutively expressed on T cells and a subset of B cells.[247] It binds to CD72 and is thought to regulate the intensity of antigen receptor signal transduction. Its primary function may be costimulatory or inhibitory, but mounting evidence suggests that it has a role in self-tolerance. XomaZyme-CD5 Plus (XomaZyme H65) is a ricin-conjugated CD5-specific MAb that has been evaluated in clinical trials to prevent graft-versus-host disease after bone marrow transplantation, rheumatoid arthritis, and systemic lupus erythematosus, without apparent efficacy.[194,219,242,291] As the biology of this molecule is better understood, its re-evaluation as a therapeutic target may be warranted.

Targeting CD6

The human CD6 is a cell surface glycoprotein expressed by T cells and a subset of B cells. It has been shown to act as a costimulatory molecule and can stimulate T cells when crosslinked with CD28.[222] Anti-CD6 MAbs inhibit the interaction of CD6 with its ligand, activated leukocyte cell adhesion molecule.[292] Anti-T12, an anti-CD6 MAb, has been evaluated clinically, but has not shown consistent efficacy.[163] More recently, an anti-CD6 has been used ex vivo to T-cell-deplete bone marrow before its use in marrow transplantation, with promising short- and long-term results.[227,262]

Targeting CD7

CD7 is a cell surface costimulatory molecule expressed on human T and natural killer cells and on cells in the early stages of T-, B-, and myeloid cell differentiation.[269,296] Its expression is augmented on activated alloimmune-responsive T cells. CD7 has been thought to be an attractive target for MAbs, offering the possibility of alloimmune-activated T-cell-specific depletion.

SDZCHH380 is a chimeric mouse antihuman CD7 IgG1 that has been studied in initial clinical renal transplant trials.[177] SDZCHH380 induction was prospectively compared with OKT3 induction, with comparable results. At 4 years, SDZCHH380-treated patients had good allograft function and did not develop neutralizing antibodies.[274] Additional development has not been reported.

Targeting CD8

CD8 is a glycoprotein present on approximately one-third of T cells in lieu of CD4. Similar to CD4, it binds to a monomorphic region MHC, although it binds to class I rather than to class II antigens. CD8 defines cytotoxic effector cells and perhaps subsets of natural killer and regulatory cells. It facilitates binding between the TCR and class I molecules and is important in protective immune lysis of virally infected parenchymal cells. $CD8^+$ T cells are known to infiltrate allografts and to participate in allograft rejection.[256] Despite this demonstrated role in rejection, CD8 has not been successfully targeted in transplantation, perhaps because $CD8^+$ T cells are recruited late in an alloimmune response and have less regulatory control over immune responses than $CD4^+$ T cells. The CD8-specific MAb anti-Leu2a has been shown to deplete peripheral blood $CD8^+$ cells in humans; however, when tested as a rescue agent, it had limited effects in reversing renal allograft rejection.[343] More recently, 76-2-11, a mouse anti-swine CD8-specific MAb, has been shown to delay the onset of cardiac allograft vasculopathy in a miniature swine model of cardiac transplantation, suggesting that there may be a limited role for this approach.[6] Additionally, ex vivo depletion of $CD8^+$ T cells with anti-Leu2a has been investigated as a means of reducing graft-versus-host disease, with promising preliminary results.[215] Anti-CD8 induction has not been investigated clinically in solid-organ transplantation.

Targeting CD45

CD45 is a transmembrane protein tyrosine phosphatase expressed on T cells. It is physically associated with the TCR and facilitates the signal transduction function of CD3 through interactions with the zeta and zeta-associated protein-70 components of CD3.[188] CD45 exists in several isoforms (CD45RA, CD45RB, and CD45RO) that result from RNA spliced variants, and these are differentially expressed on T cells with varying degrees of maturity and activation. Of these, CD45RB has been most aggressively targeted as T cells expressing high amounts of this isoform skew toward an aggressive T helper type 1 phenotype. CD45RB-specific MAbs have been shown to induce transplant tolerance in some rodent models and to prolong the survival of non-human primate renal allografts significantly.[58,188] Several antibodies, including those linked to the yttrium isotope ^{90}Y, have entered phase I trials for oncologic indications,[63] and at least one humanized anti-CD45RB has been anticipated to enter early-phase clinical trials in renal transplantation.[340] ChA6, a chimeric MAb binding CD45RB and CD45RO (an isotype found on memory T cells), has been shown to prevent islet allograft rejection in mice by deleting memory T cells and being permissive for the persistence of protolerant regulatory T cells.[110]

Immunotoxins

Antibodies that have been joined either chemically or genetically with a specific cytotoxic agent (e.g., ricin or diphtheria toxin) have been termed immunotoxins.[171] These compounds have the specificity of MAbs but can exert a cytotoxic effect beyond that related to complement or ADCC. Many immunotoxins are now being investigated as tumor-specific cytotoxic agents for malignancies and have been shown to have potent antitumor effects. Two CD25-specific immunotoxins currently in clinical trials for lymphoblastic leukemia, LMB-2 and RFT5.dgA, have shown the ability to clear $CD25^+$ cells effectively from the circulation.[12,63,172] These agents could be envisioned to perform in a means analogous to the CD25-specific MAbs currently available, with a more potent depletional effect rather than acting predominantly through steric inhibition of CD25. Similarly, a CD22-specific immunotoxin is in trials for $CD22^+$ lymphoblastic leukemia and might be envisioned as an agent similar to other B-cell-specific MAbs such as rituximab.[63,266]

Although immunotoxins have not been clinically tested in transplantation, ample preclinical data suggest that they have great therapeutic potential. Specifically, a macaque CD3-specific diphtheria immunotoxin, FN18-CRM9, has been used in non-human primate renal transplantation, with remarkable success.[168,312] Treatment with FN18-CRM9 induces a rapid 3-log-fold depletion of T cells in the peripheral circulation and in the secondary lymphoid organs. Rhesus monkeys so treated before transplantation experience markedly prolonged allograft survival with no other maintenance immunosuppression, and a significant proportion survive for years after T-cell repopulation. Although most of these animals eventually develop chronic allograft nephropathy,[315] the induction effect is impressive, and it has served as the conceptual inspiration for many clinical trials using T-cell depletion.[45,156,167] Because most adults have antibodies against diphtheria toxin, this approach has not been successfully transferred to a human-specific MAb. Nevertheless, this is a promising approach for future development.

CONCLUSION

Antibodies are now established as valuable agents for the treatment and prevention of allograft rejection. Currently, several polyclonal and monoclonal anti-T-cell antibodies have proven roles in the treatment of steroid-resistant acute rejection. The last 15 years have seen increasing justification for the use of antibodies as induction agents. Antibody induction has been shown to be an effective means of achieving very low rates of acute rejection in renal transplantation. The trials performed to date have shown, however, that antibodies produce a modest benefit over regimens with calcineurin inhibitors, antiproliferative agents, and steroids, or that they are associated with increased morbidity. Nevertheless, it is appropriate to consider antibody induction as emerging from an adolescence of sorts, and less morbid target strategies and reduced maintenance regimens are expected to improve the side-effect profile of antibody induction schemes. The use of these agents to facilitate calcineurin inhibitor avoidance, particularly when paired with costimulation blockade-based therapies such as belatacept (Chapter 21), is likely to be a focus of the coming several years.

The optimal use of antibody induction is still being determined, but it is increasingly clear that the benefits derived from antibodies will be determined by their appropriate application. Modern immunosuppressive regimens should be individualized, specifically pairing induction agents based on their mechanism of action to a specific clinical need, and combining them with complementary maintenance therapies.

The future of transplantation continues to be cloaked by a need for more specific therapies with broader therapeutic indices. Antibodies are highly specific and have proved to be safe and effective drugs whose side effects are generally confined to the specific effects of the target antigen bound. Although the early hopes of clinicians have been slow to materialize, the technology associated with antibody design, construction, and production has consistently improved to yield a diverse array of agents to be tested and added to the transplant armamentarium. The future is likely to see almost exclusive use of humanized or human antibodies and fusion proteins as opposed to xenogeneic protein constructs. Past problems of antigenicity and severe cytokine release effects are surmountable, and as the targeted antigens become more rationally selected based on growing understanding of biology, antibodies and fusion proteins are expected to continue to establish themselves as crucial agents not only for induction and rescue but also, importantly, for maintenance therapy. Trials are beginning to explore this facet of antibody and fusion protein administration. Additionally, the use of antibody combinations may become an attractive way of manipulating the immune response. Transplant clinicians will need to become increasingly aware of immune therapies developed for autoimmune and malignant indications.

REFERENCES

1. Abbott KC, Hypolite IO, Viola R, et al. Hospitalizations for cytomegalovirus disease after renal transplantation in the United States. Ann Epidemiol 2002;12:402.
2. Abramowicz D, Goldman M, De Pauw L, et al. The long-term effects of prophylactic OKT3 monoclonal antibody in cadaver kidney transplantation – a single-center, prospective, randomized study. Transplantation 1992;54:433.
3. Abramowicz D, Pradier O, Marchant A, et al. Induction of thromboses within renal grafts by high-dose prophylactic OKT3. Lancet 1992;339:777.
4. Adams AB, Shirasugi N, Jones TR, et al. Development of a chimeric anti-CD40 monoclonal antibody that synergizes with LEA29Y to prolong islet allograft survival. J Immunol 2005;174:542.
5. Akl A, Luo S, Wood KJ. Induction of transplantation tolerance – the potential of regulatory T cells. Transpl Immunol 2005;14:225.
6. Allan JS, Choo JK, Vesga L, et al. Cardiac allograft vasculopathy is abrogated by anti-CD8 monoclonal antibody therapy. Ann Thorac Surg 1997;64:1019.
7. Amlot PL, Rawlings E, Fernando ON, et al. Prolonged action of a chimeric interleukin-2 receptor (CD25) monoclonal antibody used in cadaveric renal transplantation. Transplantation 1995;60:748.
8. Andersen DC, Reilly DE. Production technologies for monoclonal antibodies and their fragments. Curr Opin Biotechnol 2004;15:456.
9. Aoyagi T, Yamashita K, Suzuki T, et al. A human anti-CD40 monoclonal antibody, 4D11, for kidney transplantation in cynomolgus monkeys: induction and maintenance therapy. Am J Transplant 2009;9:1732–41.
10. Arima T, Lehmann M, Flye MW. Induction of donor specific transplantation tolerance to cardiac allografts following treatment with nondepleting (RIB 5/2) or depleting (OX-38) anti-CD4 mAb plus intrathymic or intravenous donor alloantigen. Transplantation 1997;63:284.
11. Armitage RJ, Fanslow WC, Strockbine L, et al. Molecular and biological characterization of a murine ligand for CD40. Nature 1992;357:80.
12. Arons E, Sorbara L, Raffeld M, et al. Characterization of T-cell repertoire in hairy cell leukemia patients before and after recombinant immunotoxin BL22 therapy. Cancer Immunol Immunother 2006;55:1100.
13. Badell IR, Russell MC, Thompson PW, et al. LFA-1-specific therapy prolongs allograft survival in rhesus macaques. J Clin Invest 2010;120:4520–31.
14. Bartosh SM, Knechtle SJ, Sollinger HW. Campath-1H use in pediatric renal transplantation. Am J Transplant 2005;5:1569.
15. Basu A, Ramkumar M, Tan HP, et al. Reversal of acute cellular rejection after renal transplantation with Campath-1H. Transplant Proc 2005;37:923.
16. Batiuk TD, Bodziak KA, Goldman M. Infectious disease prophylaxis in renal transplant patients: a survey of US transplant centers. Clin Transplant 2002;16:1.
17. Bayes M, Rabasseda X, Prous JR. Gateways to clinical trials. Methods Find Exp Clin Pharmacol 2005;27:49.
18. Becker YT, Becker BN, Pirsch JD, et al. Rituximab as treatment for refractory kidney transplant rejection. Am J Transplant 2004;4:996.
19. Becker YT, Samaniego-Picota M, Sollinger HW. The emerging role of rituximab in organ transplantation. Transpl Int 2006;19:621.
20. Beiras-Fernandez A, Chappell D, Hammer C, et al. Influence of polyclonal anti-thymocyte globulins upon ischemia-reperfusion injury in a non-human primate model. Transpl Immunol 2006;15:273.
21. Bellin MD, Kandaswamy R, Parkey J, et al. Prolonged insulin independence after islet allotransplants in recipients with type 1 diabetes. Am J Transplant 2008;8:2463–70.
22. Benfield MR, Tejani A, Harmon WE, et al. A randomized multicenter trial of OKT3 mAbs induction compared with intravenous cyclosporine in pediatric renal transplantation. Pediatr Transplant 2005;9:282.
23. Beniaminovitz A, Itescu S, Lietz K, et al. Prevention of rejection in cardiac transplantation by blockade of the interleukin-2 receptor with a monoclonal antibody. N Engl J Med 2000;342:613.
24. Benvenisty AI, Cohen D, Stegall MD, et al. Improved results using OKT3 as induction immunosuppression in renal allograft recipients with delayed graft function. Transplantation 1990;49:321.
25. Benvenisty AI, Tannenbaum GA, Cohen DI, et al. Use of antithymocyte globulin and cyclosporine to treat steroid-resistant episodes in renal transplant recipients. Transplant Proc 1987;19:1889.
26. Berlin PJ, Bacher JD, Sharrow SO, et al. Monoclonal antibodies against human T cell adhesion molecules – modulation of immune function in nonhuman primates. Transplantation 1992;53:840.
27. Bielory L, Wright R, Niehuis AW, et al. Antithymocyte globulin hypersensitivity in bone marrow failure patients. JAMA 1988;260:3164.
28. Bishop G, Cosimi AB, Voynow NK, et al. Effect of immunosuppressive therapy for renal allografts on the number of circulating sheep red blood cells rosetting cells. Transplantation 1975;20:123.
29. Bloom D, Chang Z, Pauly K, et al. BAFF is increased in renal transplant patients following treatment with alemtuzumab. Am J Transplant 2009;9:1835–45.
30. Bock HA, Gallati H, Zurcher RM, et al. A randomized prospective trial of prophylactic immunosuppression with ATG-Fresenius versus OKT3 after renal transplantation. Transplantation 1995;59:830.
31. Boillot O, Mayer DA, Boudjema K, et al. Corticosteroid-free immunosuppression with tacrolimus following induction with daclizumab: a large randomized clinical study. Liver Transpl 2005;11:61.
32. Bonnefoy-Berard N, Vincent C, Revillard J. Antibodies against functional leukocyte surface molecules in polyclonal antilymphocyte and antithymocyte globulins. Transplantation 1991;51:669.
33. Boulianne GL, Hozumi N, Shulman MJ. Production of functional chimaeric mouse/human antibody. Nature 1984;312:643.
34. Bourdage JS, Hamlin DM. Comparative polyclonal antithymocyte globulin and antilymphocyte/antilymphoblast globulin anti-CD antigen analysis by flow cytometry. Transplantation 1995;59:1194.
35. Brennan DC, Daller JA, Lake KD, et al. Rabbit antithymocyte globulin versus basiliximab in renal transplantation. N Engl J Med 2006;355:1967–77.
36. Brennan DC, Flavin K, Lowell JA, et al. A randomized, double-blinded comparison of thymoglobulin versus ATGAM for induction immunosuppressive therapy in adult renal transplant recipients. Transplantation 1999;67:1011.
37. Brennan DC, Schnitzler MA. Long-term results of rabbit antithymocyte globulin and basiliximab induction. N Engl J Med 2008;359:1736–8.
38. Brooks CD, Karl KJ, Francom SF. ATGAM skin test standardization: comparison of skin testing techniques in horse-sensitive and unselected human volunteers. Transplantation 1994;58:1135.
39. Brown KM, Kondeatis E, Vaughan RW, et al. Influence of donor C3 allotype on late renal-transplantation outcome. N Engl J Med 2006;354:2014.
40. Brown SA, Lucas BA, Waid TH, et al. T10B9 (MEDI-500) mediated immunosuppression: studies on the mechanism of action. Clin Transplant 1996;10:607.
41. Bunn D, Lea CK, Bevan DJ, et al. The pharmacokinetics of anti-thymocyte globulin (ATG) following intravenous infusion in man. Clin Nephrol 1996;45:29.

42. Bunnapradist S, Daswani A, Takemoto SK. Patterns of administration of antibody induction therapy and their associated outcomes. In: Cecka JM, Terasaki PI, editors. Clinical transplants 2002. Los Angeles: UCLA Immunogenetics Center; 2003. p. 351.
43. Busuttil RW, Lipshutz GS, Kupiec-Weglinski JW, et al. rPSGL-Ig for improvement of early liver allograft function: a double-blind, placebo-controlled, single-center phase II study. Am J Transplant 2011;11:786–97.
44. Cai J, Terasaki PI, Bloom DD, et al. Correlation between human leukocyte antigen antibody production and serum creatinine in patients receiving sirolimus monotherapy after Campath-1H induction. Transplantation 2004;78:919.
45. Calne R, Friend P, Moffatt S, et al. Preop tolerance, perioperative campath 1H, and low-dose cyclosporin monotherapy in renal allograft recipients. Lancet 1998;351:1701.
46. Calne R, Moffatt SD, Friend PJ, et al. Campath IH allows low-dose cyclosporine monotherapy in 31 cadaveric renal allograft recipients. Transplantation 1999;68:1613.
47. Carmody IC, Meng L, Shen XD, et al. P-selectin knockout mice have improved outcomes with both warm ischemia and small bowel transplantation. Transplant Proc 2004;36:263.
48. Carpenter PA, Lowder J, Johnston L, et al. A phase II multicenter study of visilizumab, humanized anti-CD3 antibody, to treat steroid-refractory acute graft-versus-host disease. Biol Blood Marrow Transplant 2005;11:465.
49. Casadei DH, del C Rial M, Opelz G, et al. A randomized and prospective study comparing treatment with high-dose intravenous immunoglobulin with monoclonal antibodies for rescue of kidney grafts with steroid-resistant rejection. Transplantation 2001;71:53.
50. Cecka JM, Gjertson D, Terasaki P. Do prophylactic antilymphocyte globulins (ALG and OKT3) improve renal transplant in recipient and donor high-risk groups? Transplant Proc 1993;25:548.
51. Cecka JM, Terasaki PI. The UNOS scientific renal transplant registry 1991. In: Terasaki P, editor. Clinical transplants 1991. Los Angeles: UCLA Tissue Typing Laboratory; 1991. p. 1.
52. Cella M, Scheidegger D, Palmer-Lehmann K, et al. Ligation of CD40 on dendritic cells triggers production of high levels of interleukin-12 and enhances T cell stimulatory capacity: T-T help via APC activation. J Exp Med 1996;184:747.
53. Chappell D, Beiras-Fernandez A, Hammer C, et al. In vivo visualization of the effect of polyclonal antithymocyte globulins on the microcirculation after ischemia/reperfusion in a primate model. Transplantation 2006;81:552.
54. Charafeddine AH, Kim EJ, Maynard DM, et al. Platelet-derived CD154: ultrastructural localization and clinical correlation in organ transplantation. Am J Transplant 2012;12:3143–51.
55. Charpentier B, Rostaing L, Berthoux F, et al. A three-arm study comparing immediate tacrolimus therapy with antithymocyte globulin induction therapy followed by tacrolimus or cyclosporine A in adult renal transplant recipients. Transplantation 2003;75:844.
56. Chatenoud L, Ferran C, Legendre C, et al. In vivo cell activation following OKT3 administration: systemic cytokine release and modulation by corticosteroids. Transplantation 1990;49:697.
57. Chatenoud L, Jonker M, Villemain F, et al. The human immune response to the OKT3 monoclonal antibody is oligoclonal. Science 1986;232:1406.
58. Chen G, Luke PP, Yang H, et al. Anti-CD45RB monoclonal antibody prolongs renal allograft survival in cynomolgus monkeys. Am J Transplant 2007;7:27–37.
59. Cherikh WS, Kauffman HM, McBride MA, et al. Association of the type of induction immunosuppression with posttransplant lymphoproliferative disorder, graft survival, and patient survival after primary kidney transplantation. Transplantation 2003;76:1289.
60. Choy EH, Panayi GS, Emery P, et al. Repeat-cycle study of high-dose intravenous 4162W94 anti-CD4 humanized monoclonal antibody in rheumatoid arthritis: a randomized placebo-controlled trial. Rheumatology 2002;41:1142.
61. Clarkson MR, Sayegh MH. T-cell costimulatory pathways in allograft rejection and tolerance. Transplantation 2005;80:555.
62. Clatworthy MR, Friend PJ, Calne RY, et al. Alemtuzumab (CAMPATH-1H) for the treatment of acute rejection in kidney transplant recipients: long-term follow-up. Transplantation 2009;87:1092–5.
63. Clinicaltrials.gov. Available online at: http://www.clinicaltrials.gov/ [accessed 19.09.12].
64. Coles AJ, Wing M, Smith S, et al. Pulsed monoclonal antibody treatment and autoimmune thyroid disease in multiple sclerosis. Lancet 1999;354:1691.
65. Colovai AI, Vasilescu ER, Foca-Rodi A, et al. Acute and hyperacute humoral rejection in kidney allograft recipients treated with anti-human thymocyte antibodies. Hum Immunol 2005;66:501.
66. Colvin RB, Smith RN. Antibody-mediated organ-allograft rejection. Nat Rev Immunol 2005;5:807.
67. Cooperative Clinical Trials in Transplantation Research Group. Murine OKT4A immunosuppression in cadaver donor renal allograft recipients: a Cooperative Clinical Trials in Transplantation pilot study. Transplantation 1997;63:1087.
68. Cosimi AB. The clinical value of antilymphocyte antibodies. Transplant Proc 1981;13:462.
69. Cosimi AB, Burton RC, Colvin RB, et al. Treatment of acute renal allograft rejection with OKT3 monoclonal antibody. Transplantation 1981;32:535.
70. Cosimi AB, Conti D, Delmonico FL, et al. In vivo effects of monoclonal antibody to ICAM-1 (CD54) in nonhuman primates with renal allografts. J Immunol 1990;144:4604.
71. Cosimi AB, Delmonico FL, Wright JK, et al. Prolonged survival of nonhuman primate renal allograft recipients treated only with anti-CD4 monoclonal antibody. Surgery 1990;108:406.
72. Cosimi AB, Wortis HH, Delmonico FL, et al. Randomized clinical trial of antithymocyte globulin in cadaver renal allograft recipients: importance of T cell monitoring. Surgery 1976;80:155.
73. Couriel D, Saliba R, Hicks K, et al. Tumor necrosis factor alpha blockade for the treatment of steroid-refractory acute GVHD. Blood 2004;104:649.
74. Csapo Z, Benavides-Viveros C, Podder H, et al. Campath-1H as rescue therapy for the treatment of acute rejection in kidney transplant patients. Transplant Proc 2005;37:2032.
75. D'Alessandro AM, Pirsch JD, Stratta RJ, et al. OKT3 salvage therapy in a quadruple immunosuppressive protocol in cadaveric renal transplantation. Transplantation 1989;47:297.
76. Dantal J, Ninin E, Hourmant M, et al. Anti-CD4 MoAb therapy in kidney transplantation – a pilot study in early prophylaxis of rejection. Transplantation 1996;62:1502.
77. Darby CR, Bushell A, Morris PJ, et al. Nondepleting anti-CD4 antibodies in transplantation: evidence that modulation is far less effective than prolonged CD4 blockade. Transplantation 1994;57:1419.
78. Davis RC, Nabseth DC, Olsson CA, et al. Effect of rabbit ALG on cadaver kidney transplant survival. Ann Surg 1972;176:521.
79. Deans JP, Kalt L, Ledbetter JA, et al. Association of 75/80-kDa phosphoproteins and the tyrosine kinases Lyn, Fyn, and Lck with the B cell molecule CD20: evidence against involvement of the cytoplasmic regions of CD20. J Biol Chem 1995;270:22632.
80. Deans JP, Li H, Polyak MJ. CD20-mediated apoptosis: signalling through lipid rafts. Immunology 2002;107:176.
81. Debets JMH, Leunissen KML, van Hooff HJ, et al. Evidence of involvement of tumor necrosis factor in adverse reactions during treatment of kidney allograft rejection with antithymocyte globulin. Transplantation 1989;47:487.
82. Debure A, Chekoff N, Chatenoud L, et al. One-month prophylactic use of OKT3 in cadaver kidney transplant recipients. Transplantation 1988;45:546.
83. Dedrick RL, Walicke P, Garovoy M. Anti-adhesion antibodies efalizumab, a humanized anti-CD11a monoclonal antibody. Transpl Immunol 2002;9:181.
84. Deierhoi MH, Sollinger HW, Kalayoglu M, et al. Quadruple therapy for cadaver renal transplantation. Transplant Proc 1987;19:1917.
85. Delmonico FL, Cosimi AB. Anti-CD4 monoclonal antibody therapy. Clin Transplant 1996;10:397.
86. Delmonico FL, Cosimi AB. Monoclonal antibody treatment of human allograft recipients. Surg Gynecol Obstet 1988;166:89.
87. Delmonico FL, Cosimi AB, Kawai T, et al. Non-human primate responses to murine and humanized OKT4A. Transplantation 1993;55:722.
88. Dhanireddy KK, Bruno DA, Zhang X, et al. Alefacept (LFA3-Ig), portal venous donor specific transfusion, and sirolimus prolong renal allograft survival in non-human primates. J Am Coll Surg 2006;203:S92.
89. Dulkanchainun TS, Goss JA, Imagawa DK, et al. Reduction of hepatic ischemia/reperfusion injury by a soluble P-selectin glycoprotein ligand-1. Ann Surg 1998;227:832.

90. Faguer S, Kamar N, Guilbeaud-Frugier C, et al. Rituximab therapy for acute humoral rejection after kidney transplantation. Transplantation 2007;83:1277–80.
91. Farges C, Samuel D, Bismuth H. Orthoclone OKT3 in liver transplantation. Transplant Sci 1992;2:16.
92. Farmer DG, Anselmo D, Da Shen X, et al. Disruption of P-selectin signaling modulates cell trafficking and results in improved outcomes after mouse warm intestinal ischemia and reperfusion injury. Transplantation 2005;80:828.
93. Ferrant JL, Benjamin CD, Cutler AH, et al. The contribution of Fc effector mechanisms in the efficacy of anti-CD154 immunotherapy depends on the nature of the immune challenge. Int Immunol 2004;16:1583.
94. Friend PJ, Hale G, Chatenoud L, et al. Phase I study of an engineered aglycosylated humanized CD3 antibody in renal transplant rejection. Transplantation 1999;68:1632.
95. Friend PJ, Hale G, Waldmann H, et al. Campath-1M-prophylactic use after kidney transplantation: a randomized controlled clinical trial. Transplantation 1989;48:248.
96. Friend PJ, Rebello P, Oliveira D, et al. Successful treatment of renal allograft rejection with a humanized antilymphocyte monoclonal antibody. Transplant Proc 1995;27:869.
97. Friend PJ, Waldmann H, Hale G, et al. Reversal of allograft rejection using the monoclonal antibody, Campath-1G. Transplant Proc 1991;23:2253.
98. Froud T, Ricordi C, Baidal DA, et al. Islet transplantation in type 1 diabetes mellitus using cultured islets and steroid-free immunosuppression: Miami experience. Am J Transplant 2005;5:2037.
99. Fuchinoue S, Ishii Y, Sawada T, et al. The 5-year outcome of ABO-incompatible kidney transplantation with rituximab induction. Transplantation 2011;91:853–7.
100. Gabardi S, Catella J, Martin ST, et al. Maintenance immunosuppression with intermittent intravenous IL-2 receptor antibody therapy in renal transplant recipients. Ann Pharmacother 2011;45:e48.
101. Gaber AO, First MR, Tesi RJ, et al. Results of the double-blind, randomized, multicenter, phase III clinical trial of Thymoglobulin versus Atgam in the treatment of acute graft rejection episodes after renal transplantation. Transplantation 1998;66:29.
102. Genberg H, Kumlien G, Wennberg L, et al. ABO-incompatible kidney transplantation using antigen-specific immunoadsorption and rituximab: a 3-year follow-up. Transplantation 2008;85:1745–54.
103. Getts DR, Wiseman AC, Mulgaonkar S, et al. Evaluating safety and efficacy of TOL101 induction to prevent kidney transplant rejection, part a interim analysis. Transpl Int 2011;24:93.
104. Gill JI, Gulley ML. Immunoglobulin and T cell receptor gene rearrangement. Hematol Oncol Clin North Am 1994;8:751.
105. Goggins WC, Pascual MA, Powelson JA, et al. A prospective, randomized, clinical trial of intraoperative versus postoperative Thymoglobulin in adult cadaveric renal transplant recipients. Transplantation 2003;76:798.
106. Gordon KB, Vaishnaw AK, O'Gorman J, et al. Treatment of psoriasis with alefacept: correlation of clinical improvement with reductions of memory T-cell counts. Arch Dermatol 2003;139:1563.
107. Gourishankar S, McDermid JC, Jhangri GS, et al. Herpes zoster infection following solid organ transplantation: incidence, risk factors and outcomes in the current immunosuppressive era. Am J Transplant 2004;4:108.
108. Graf D, Korthauer U, Mages HW, et al. Cloning of TRAP, a ligand for CD40 on human T cells. Eur J Immunol 1992;22:3191.
109. Greenwood J, Clark M, Waldmann H. Structural motifs involved in human IgG antibody effector functions. Eur J Immunol 1993;23:1098.
110. Gregori S, Mangia P, Bacchetta R, et al. An anti-CD45RO/RB monoclonal antibody modulates T cell responses via induction of apoptosis and generation of regulatory T cells. J Exp Med 2005;201:1293.
111. Grillo-Lopez AJ, White CA, Varns C, et al. Overview of the clinical development of rituximab: first monoclonal antibody approved for the treatment of lymphoma. Semin Oncol 1999;26 (5 Suppl. 14):66.
112. Gruessner RW, Kandaswamy R, Humar A, et al. Calcineurin inhibitor- and steroid-free immunosuppression in pancreas-kidney and solitary pancreas transplantation. Transplantation 2005; 79:1184.
113. Hale G. The CD52 antigen and development of the CAMPATH antibodies. Cytotherapy 2001;3:137.
114. Hale G, Waldmann H, Friend P, et al. Pilot study of CAMPATH-1, a rat monoclonal antibody that fixes human complement, as an immunosuppressant in organ transplantation. Transplantation 1986;42:308.
115. Hall BL, Hand SL, Alter MD, et al. Variables affecting the T cell receptor V-β repertoire heterogeneity of T cells infiltrating human renal allografts. Transpl Immunol 1993;1:217.
116. Hanaway MJ, Woodle ES, Mulgaonkar S, et al. Alemtuzumab induction in renal transplantation. N Engl J Med 2011;364:1909–19.
117. Hardinger KL, Schnitzler MA, Miller B, et al. Five-year follow up of thymoglobulin versus ATGAM induction in adult renal transplantation. Transplantation 2004;78:136.
118. Harlan DM, Kirk AD. The future of organ and tissue transplantation: can T-cell costimulatory pathway modifiers revolutionize the prevention of graft rejection? JAMA 1999;282:1076.
119. Haug CE, Colvin RB, Delmonico FL, et al. A phase I trial of immunosuppression with anti-ICAM-1 (CD54) mAb in renal allograft recipients. Transplantation 1993;55:766.
120. Heinrich G, Gram H, Kocher HP, et al. Characterization of a human T cell-specific chimeric antibody (CD7) with human constant and mouse variable regions. J Immunol 1989;143:3589.
121. Henn V, Slupsky JR, Grafe M, et al. CD40 ligand on activated platelets triggers an inflammatory reaction of endothelial cells. Nature 1998;391:591.
122. Henry ML, Pelletier RP, Elkhammas EA, et al. A randomized prospective trial of OKT3 induction in the current immunosuppression era. Clin Transplant 2001;15:410.
123. Herold KC, Hagopian W, Auger JA, et al. Anti-CD3 monoclonal antibody in new-onset type 1 diabetes mellitus. N Engl J Med 2002;346:1692.
124. Hershberger RE, Starling RC, Eisen HJ, et al. Daclizumab to prevent rejection after cardiac transplantation. N Engl J Med 2005;352:2705.
125. Hibberd PL, Tolkoff-Rubin NE, Cosimi AB, et al. Symptomatic cytomegalovirus disease in the cytomegalovirus antibody seropositive renal transplant recipient treated with OKT3. Transplantation 1992;53:68.
126. Hiesse C, Lantz O, Kriaa F, et al. Treatment with Lo-Tact-1, a monoclonal antibody to the interleukin-2 receptor, in kidney transplantation. Presse Med 1991;20:2036.
127. Hill A, Hillmen P, Richards SJ, et al. Sustained response and long-term safety of eculizumab in paroxysmal nocturnal hemoglobinuria. Blood 2005;106:2559.
128. Hippen BE, DeMattos A, Cook WJ, et al. Association of CD20 infiltrates with poorer clinical outcomes in acute cellular rejection of renal allografts. Am J Transplant 2005;5:2248.
129. Hodi FS, Mihm MC, Soiffer RJ, et al. Biologic activity of cytotoxic T lymphocyte-associated antigen 4 antibody blockade in previously vaccinated metastatic melanoma and ovarian carcinoma patients. Proc Natl Acad Sci U S A 2003;100:4712.
130. Hodi FS, O'Day SJ, McDermott DF, et al. Improved survival with ipilimumab in patients with metastatic melanoma. N Engl J Med 2010;363:711–23.
131. Hoffmann SC, Hale DA, Kleiner DE, et al. Functionally significant renal allograft rejection is defined by transcriptional criteria. Am J Transplant 2005;5:573.
132. Hoitsma AJ, van Lier LH, Reekers P, et al. Improved patient and graft survival after treatment of acute rejections of cadaveric renal allografts with rabbit antithymocyte globulin. Transplantation 1985;39:274.
133. Hourmant M, Bedrossian J, Durand D, et al. A randomized multicenter trial comparing leukocyte function-associated antigen-1 monoclonal antibody with rabbit antithymocyte globulin as induction treatment in first kidney transplantations. Transplantation 1996;62:1565.
134. Howard RJ, Condie RM, Sutherland DER, et al. The use of antilymphoblast globulin in the treatment of renal allograft rejection. Transplant Proc 1981;13:473.
135. Hozumi N, Tonegawa S. Evidence for somatic rearrangement of immunoglobulin genes coding for variable and constant regions. Proc Natl Acad Sci U S A 1976;73:3628.

136. Humar A, Ramcharan T, Denny R, et al. Are wound complications after a kidney transplant more common with modern immunosuppression? Transplantation 2001;72:1920.
137. Imai A, Suzuki T, Sugitani A, et al. A novel fully human anti-CD40 monoclonal antibody, 4D11, for kidney transplantation in cynomolgus monkeys. Transplantation 2007;84:1020–8.
138. Isobe M, Yagita H, Okumura K, et al. Specific acceptance of cardiac allograft after treatment with antibodies to ICAM-1 and LFA-1. Science 1992;255:1125.
139. Jacobsohn DA, Vogelsang GB. Anti-cytokine therapy for the treatment of graft-versus-host disease. Curr Pharm Des 2004;10:1195.
140. Jaffers GJ, Fuller TC, Cosimi AB, et al. Monoclonal antibody therapy: anti-idiotype and non-anti-idiotype antibodies to OKT3 arising despite intense immunosuppression. Transplantation 1986;41:572.
141. Jones PT, Dear PH, Foote J, et al. Replacing the complementarity-determining regions in a human antibody with those from a mouse. Nature 1986;321:522.
142. Jonker M, Malissen B, Mawas C. The effect of in vivo application of monoclonal antibodies specific for human cytotoxic T cells in rhesus monkeys. Transplantation 1983;35:374.
143. June CH, Ledbetter JA, Gillespie MM, et al. T-cell proliferation involving the CD28 pathway is associated with cyclosporine-resistant interleukin 2 gene expression. Mol Cell Biol 1987;7:4472.
144. Kahan BD, Rajagopalan PR, Hall M, et al. Reduction of the occurrence of acute cellular rejection among renal allograft recipients treated with basiliximab, a chimeric anti-interleukin-2-receptor monoclonal antibody. Transplantation 1999;67:276.
145. Kahana L, Ackermann J, Lefor W, et al. Uses of orthoclone OKT3 for prophylaxis of rejection and induction in initial nonfunction in kidney transplantation. Transplant Proc 1990;22:1755.
146. Kaplon RJ, Hochman PS, Michler RE, et al. Short course single agent therapy with an LFA-3-IgG fusion protein prolongs primate cardiac allograft survival. Transplantation 1996;61:356.
147. Kaufman DB, Leventhal JR, Axelrod D, et al. Alemtuzumab induction and prednisone-free maintenance immunotherapy in kidney transplantation: comparison with basiliximab induction – long-term results. Am J Transplant 2005;5:2539.
148. Kaufman DB, Leventhal JR, Gallon LG, et al. Alemtuzumab induction and prednisone-free maintenance immunotherapy in simultaneous pancreas-kidney transplantation comparison with rabbit antithymocyte globulin induction long-term results. Am J Transplant 2006;6:331.
149. Kawai T, Wee SL, Bazin H, et al. Association of natural killer cell depletion with induction of mixed chimerism and allograft tolerance in non-human primates. Transplantation 2000;70:368.
150. Kazatchkine MD, Kaveri SV. Immunomodulation of autoimmune and inflammatory diseases with intravenous immune globulin. N Engl J Med 2001;345:747.
151. Kerr PG, Atkins RC. The effects of OKT3 therapy on infiltrating lymphocytes in rejecting renal allografts. Transplantation 1989;48:33.
152. Kirk AD. 4D11: The second mouse? Am J Transplant 2009;9:1701–2.
153. Kirk AD, Blair PJ, Tadaki DK, et al. The role of CD154 in organ transplant rejection and acceptance. Philos Trans R Soc Lond B Biol Sci 2001;356:691.
154. Kirk AD, Burkly LC, Batty DS, et al. Treatment with humanized monoclonal antibody against CD154 prevents acute renal allograft rejection in nonhuman primates. Nat Med 1999;5:686.
155. Kirk AD, Cherikh WS, Ring M, et al. Dissociation of depletional induction and posttransplant lymphoproliferative disease in kidney recipients treated with alemtuzumab. Am J Transplant 2007;7:2619–25.
156. Kirk AD, Hale DA, Mannon RB, et al. Results from a human renal allograft tolerance trial evaluating the humanized CD52-specific monoclonal antibody alemtuzumab (CAMPATH-1H). Transplantation 2003;76:120.
157. Kirk AD, Hale DA, Swanson SJ, et al. Autoimmune thyroid disease after renal transplantation using depletional induction with alemtuzumab. Am J Transplant 2006;6:1084.
158. Kirk AD, Harlan DM, Armstrong NN, et al. CTLA4-Ig and anti-CD40 ligand prevent renal allograft rejection in primates. Proc Natl Acad Sci U S A 1997;94:8789.
159. Kirk AD, Ibrahim S, Dawson DV, et al. Characterization of T cells expressing the γδ antigen receptor in human renal allograft rejection. Hum Immunol 1993;36:11.
160. Kirk AD, Knechtle SJ, Sollinger H, et al. Preliminary results of the use of humanized anti-CD154 in human renal allotransplantation. Am J Transplant 2001;1:S191.
161. Kirk AD, Mannon RB, Kleiner DE, et al. Results from a human renal allograft tolerance trial evaluating T-cell depletion with alemtuzumab combined with deoxyspergualin. Transplantation 2005;80:1051.
162. Kirk AD, Tadaki DK, Celniker A, et al. Induction therapy with monoclonal antibodies specific for CD80 and CD86 delays the onset of acute renal allograft rejection in non-human primates. Transplantation 2001;72:377.
163. Kirkman RL, Araujo JL, Busch GJ, et al. Treatment of acute renal allograft rejection with monoclonal anti-T12 antibody. Transplantation 1983;36:620.
164. Kirkman RL, Shapiro ME, Carpenter CB, et al. A randomized prospective trial of anti-Tac monoclonal antibody in human renal transplantation. Transplantation 1991;51:107.
165. Kitchens WH, Haridas D, Wagener ME, et al. Integrin antagonists prevent costimulatory blockade-resistant transplant rejection by CD8(+) memory T cells. Am J Transplant 2012;12:69–80.
166. Knechtle SJ, Fernandez LA, Pirsch JD, et al. Campath-1H in renal transplantation: the University of Wisconsin experience. Surgery 2004;136:754.
167. Knechtle SJ, Pirsch JD, Fechner H, et al. Campath-1H induction plus rapamycin monotherapy for renal transplantation: results of a pilot study. Am J Transplant 2003;3:722.
168. Knechtle SJ, Vargo D, Fechner J, et al. FN18-CRM9 immunotoxin promotes tolerance in primate renal allografts. Transplantation 1997;63:1.
169. Kohler G, Milstein C. Continuous cultures of fused cells secreting antibody of predefined specificity. Nature 1975;256:495.
170. Kovarik JM, Burtin P. Immunosuppressants in advanced clinical development for organ transplantation and selected autoimmune diseases. Expert Opin Emerg Drugs 2003;8:47.
171. Kreitman RJ. Toxin-labeled monoclonal antibodies. Curr Pharm Biotechnol 2001;2:313.
172. Kreitman RJ, Wilson WH, White JD, et al. Phase I trial of recombinant immunotoxin anti-Tac(Fv)-PE38 (LMB-2) in patients with hematologic malignancies. J Clin Oncol 2000;18:1622.
173. Krid S, Roumenina LT, Beury D, et al. Renal transplantation under prophylactic eculizumab in atypical hemolytic uremic syndrome with CFH/CFHR1 hybrid protein. Am J Transplant 2012;12:1938–44.
174. Kuritzkes DR, Jacobson J, Powderly WG, et al. Antiretroviral activity of the anti-CD4 monoclonal antibody TNX-355 in patients infected with HIV type 1. J Infect Dis 2004;189:286.
175. Land W. Monoclonal antibodies in 1991: new potential options in clinical immunosuppressive therapy. Clin Transplant 1991;5:493.
176. Larsen CP, Pearson TC, Adams AB, et al. Rational development of LEA29Y (belatacept), a high-affinity variant of CTLA4-Ig with potent immunosuppressive properties. Am J Transplant 2005;5:443.
177. Lazarovits AI, Rochon J, Banks L, et al. Human mouse chimeric CD7 monoclonal antibody for the prophylaxis of kidney transplant rejection. J Clin Invest 1993;150:5163.
178. Lebranchu Y, Bridoux F, Buchler M, et al. Immunoprophylaxis with basiliximab compared with antithymocyte globulin in renal transplant patients receiving MMF-containing triple therapy. Am J Transplant 2002;2:48.
179. Lehmann M, Sternkopf F, Metz F, et al. Induction of long-term survival of rat skin allografts by a novel, highly effective anti-CD4 monoclonal antibody. Transplantation 1992;54:959.
180. Le Mauff B, Hourmant M, Rougier JP, et al. Effect of anti-LFA1 (CD11a) monoclonal antibodies in acute rejection in human kidney transplantation. Transplantation 1991;52:291.
181. Leonardi CL, Kimball AB, Papp KA, et al. Efficacy and safety of ustekinumab, a human interleukin-12/23 monoclonal antibody, in patients with psoriasis: 76-week results from a randomised, double-blind, placebo-controlled trial (PHOENIX 1). Lancet 2008;371:1665–74.
182. Lerut J, Van Thuyne V, Mathijs J, et al. Anti-CD2 monoclonal antibody and tacrolimus in adult liver transplantation. Transplantation 2005;80:1186.
183. Linsley PS, Wallace PM, Johnson J, et al. Immunosuppression in vivo by a soluble form of the CTLA-4 T cell activation molecule. Science 1992;257:792.

184. Lo DJ, Weaver TA, Stempora L, et al. Selective targeting of human alloresponsive CD8+ effector memory T cells based on CD2 expression. Am J Transplant 2011;11:22–33.
185. Locke JE, Magro CM, Singer AL, et al. The use of antibody to complement protein C5 for salvage treatment of severe antibody-mediated rejection. Am J Transplant 2009;9:231–5.
186. Lonze BE, Dagher NN, Simpkins CE, et al. Eculizumab, bortezomib and kidney paired donation facilitate transplantation of a highly sensitized patient without vascular access. Am J Transplant 2010;10:2154–60.
187. Lonze BE, Singer AL, Montgomery RA. Eculizumab and renal transplantation in a patient with CAPS. N Engl J Med 2010;362:1744–5.
188. Luke PP, O'Brien CA, Jevnikar AM, et al. Anti-CD45RB monoclonal antibody-mediated transplantation tolerance. Curr Mol Med 2001;5:533.
189. Madsen JC, Peugh WN, Wood KJ, et al. The effect of anti-L3T4 monoclonal antibody treatment on first set rejection of murine cardiac allografts. Transplantation 1987;44:849.
190. Magliocca JF, Knechtle SJ. The evolving role of alemtuzumab (Campath-1H) for immunosuppressive therapy in organ transplantation. Transpl Int 2006;19:705.
191. Malatack JF, Gartner JCJ, Urbach AH, et al. Orthotopic liver transplantation, Epstein–Barr virus, cyclosporine, and lymphoproliferative disease: a growing concern. J Pediatr 1991;118:667.
192. Malinow L, Walker J, Klassen DK, et al. Antilymphocyte induction immunosuppression in the post-Minnesota antilymphocyte globulin era: incidence of renal dysfunction and delayed graft function: a single center experience. Clin Transplant 1996;10:237.
193. Marlin SD, Springer TA. Purified intercellular adhesion molecule-1 (ICAM-1) is a ligand for lymphocyte function-associated antigen 1 (LFA-1). Cell 1987;51:813.
194. Martin PJ, Nelson BJ, Appelbaum FR, et al. Evaluation of a CD5-specific immunotoxin for treatment of acute graft-versus-host disease after allogeneic marrow transplantation. Blood 1996;88:824.
195. Matas AJ, Tellis VA, Quinn T, et al. ALG treatment of steroid-resistant rejection in patients receiving cyclosporine. Transplantation 1986;41:579.
196. McCurry KR, Iacono A, Zeevi A, et al. Early outcomes in human lung transplantation with Thymoglobulin or Campath-1H for recipient pretreatment followed by posttransplant tacrolimus near-monotherapy. J Thorac Cardiovasc Surg 2005;130:528.
197. Meier-Kriesche HU, Arndorfer JA, Kaplan B. Association of antibody induction with short- and long-term cause-specific mortality in renal transplant recipients. J Am Soc Nephrol 2002;13:769.
198. Meiser BM, Reiter C, Reichenspurner H, et al. Chimeric monoclonal CD4 antibody – a novel immunosuppressant for clinical heart transplantation. Transplantation 1994;58:419.
199. Merion M, White DJG, Thiru S, et al. Cyclosporine: five years experience in cadaveric renal transplantation. N Engl J Med 1984;310:148.
200. Millis JM, McDiarmid SV, Hiatt JR, et al. Randomized prospective trial of OKT3 for early prophylaxis of rejection after liver transplantation. Transplantation 1989;47:82.
201. Monk NJ, Hargreaves RE, Marsh JE, et al. Fc-dependent depletion of activated T cells occurs through CD40L-specific antibody rather than costimulation blockade. Nat Med 2003;9:1275.
202. Morrison SL, Johnson MJ, Herzenberg LA, et al. Chimeric human antibody molecules: mouse antigen-binding domains with human constant region domains. Proc Natl Acad Sci U S A 1984;81:6851.
203. Mourad M, Besse T, Malaise J, et al. BTI-322 for acute rejection after renal transplantation. Transplant Proc 1997;29:2353.
204. Mourad G, Garrigue V, Squifflet JP, et al. Induction versus noninduction in renal transplant recipients with tacrolimus-based immunosuppression. Transplantation 2001;72:1050.
205. Mourad G, Rostaing L, Legendre C, et al. Sequential protocols using basiliximab versus antithymocyte globulins in renal-transplant patients receiving mycophenolate mofetil and steroids. Transplantation 2004;78:584.
206. Muller TF, Grebe SO, Neumann MC, et al. Persistent long-term changes in lymphocyte subsets induced by polyclonal antibodies. Transplantation 1997;64:1432.
207. Nakajima H, Sano H, Nishimura T, et al. Role of vascular cell adhesion molecule 1/very late activation antigen 4 and intercellular adhesion molecule 1/lymphocyte function-associated antigen 1 interactions in antigen-induced eosinophil and T cell recruitment into the tissue. J Exp Med 1994;179:1145.
208. Nashan B, Light S, Hardie IR, et al. Reduction of acute renal allograft rejection by daclizumab. Transplantation 1999;67:110.
209. Nashan B, Moore R, Amlot P, et al. Randomized trial of basiliximab versus placebo for control of acute cellular rejection in renal allograft recipients. CHIB201 International Study Group. Lancet 1997;350:1193.
210. Nelson PW, Cosimi AB, Delmonico FL, et al. Antithymocyte globulin as the primary treatment for renal allograft rejection. Transplantation 1983;36:587.
211. Neuhaus P, Clavien PA, Kittur D, et al. Improved treatment response with basiliximab immunoprophylaxis after liver transplantation: results from a double-blind randomized placebo-controlled trial. Liver Transpl 2002;8:132.
212. Niblack G, Johnson K, Williams T, et al. Antibody formation following administration of antilymphocyte serum. Transplant Proc 1987;19:1896.
213. Nicolls MR, Gill RG. LFA-1 (CD11a) as a therapeutic target. Am J Transplant 2006;6:27.
214. Niimi M, Witzke O, Bushell A, et al. Nondepleting anti-CD4 monoclonal antibody enhances the ability of oral alloantigen delivery to induce indefinite survival of cardiac allografts: oral tolerance to alloantigen. Transplantation 2000;70:1524.
215. Nimer SD, Giorgi J, Gajewski JL, et al. Selective depletion of CD8 cells for prevention of graft-versus-host disease after bone marrow transplantation: a randomized controlled trial. Transplantation 1994;57:82.
216. Norman DJ, Kahana L, Stuart Jr FP, et al. A randomized clinical trial of induction therapy with OKT3 in kidney transplantation. Transplantation 1993;55:44.
217. Norman DJ, Shield III. CF, Barry J, et al. Early use of OKT3 monoclonal antibody in renal transplantation to prevent rejection. Am J Kidney Dis 1988;11:107.
218. Norman DJ, Vincenti F, de Mattos AM, et al. Phase I trial of HuM291, a humanized anti-CD3 antibody, in patients receiving renal allografts from living donors. Transplantation 2000;70:1707.
219. Olsen NJ, Brooks RH, Cush JJ, et al. A double-blind, placebo-controlled study of anti-CD5 immunoconjugate in patients with rheumatoid arthritis. The Xoma RA Investigator Group. Arthritis Rheum 1996;39:1102–8. Erratum in: Arthritis Rheum 1996;39:1575.
220. Opelz G. Efficacy of rejection prophylaxis with OKT3 in renal transplantation. Collaborative Transplant Study. Transplantation 1995;60:1220.
221. Ortho Multicenter Transplant Study Group. A randomized clinical trial of OKT3 monoclonal antibody for acute rejection of cadaveric renal transplants. N Engl J Med 1985;313:337.
222. Osorio LM, Rottenberg M, Jondal M, et al. Simultaneous cross-linking of CD6 and CD28 induces cell proliferation in resting T cells. Immunology 1998;93:358.
223. Oura T, Yamashita K, Suzuki T, et al. Long-term hepatic allograft acceptance based on CD40 blockade by ASKP1240 in nonhuman primates. Am J Transplant 2012;12:1740–54.
224. Oyer PE, Stinson EB, Jamieson SW, et al. Cyclosporin-A in cardiac allografting: a preliminary experience. Transplant Proc 1983;15:1247.
225. Parrott NR, Hammad AQ, Watson CJ, et al. Multicenter, randomized study of the effectiveness of basiliximab in avoiding addition of steroids to cyclosporine a monotherapy in renal transplant recipients. Transplantation 2005;79:344.
226. Pascher A, Radke C, Dignass A, et al. Successful infliximab treatment of steroid and OKT3 refractory acute cellular rejection in two patients after intestinal transplantation. Transplantation 2003;76:615.
227. Patel NC, Chinen J, Rosenblatt HM, et al. Long-term outcomes of nonconditioned patients with severe combined immunodeficiency transplanted with HLA-identical or haploidentical bone marrow depleted of T cells with anti-CD6 mAb. J Allergy Clin Immunol 2008;122:1185–93.
228. Pearl JP, Parris J, Hale DA, et al. Immunocompetent T-cells with a memory-like phenotype are the dominant cell type following antibody-mediated T-cell depletion. Am J Transplant 2005;5:465.
229. Penn I. Cancers complicating organ transplantation. N Engl J Med 1990;323:1767.

230. Penn I. The problem of cancer in organ transplant recipients: an overview. Transplant Sci 1994;4:23.
231. Poirier N, Blancho G, Vanhove B. CD28-specific immunomodulating antibodies: what can be learned from experimental models? Am J Transplant 2012;12:1682–90.
232. Poirier N, Mary C, Dilek N, et al. Preclinical efficacy and immunological safety of FR104, an antagonist anti-CD28 monovalent Fab′ antibody. Am J Transplant 2012;12:2630–40.
233. Polman CH, O'Connor PW, Havrdova E, et al. A randomized, placebo-controlled trial of natalizumab for relapsing forms of multiple sclerosis. N Engl J Med 2006;354:899–910.
234. Ponticelli C, Rivolta E, Tarantino A, et al. Treatment of severe rejection of kidney transplant with Orthoclone OKT3. Clin Transplant 1987;1:99.
235. Posselt AM, Bellin MD, Tavakol M, et al. Islet transplantation in type 1 diabetics using an immunosuppressive protocol based on the anti-LFA-1 antibody efalizumab. Am J Transplant 2010;10:1870–80.
236. Powelson JA, Knowles RW, Delmonico FL, et al. CDR-grafted OKT4A monoclonal antibody in cynomolgus renal allograft recipients. Transplantation 1994;57:788.
237. Pratt JR, Basheer SA, Sacks SH. Local synthesis of complement component C3 regulates acute renal transplant rejection. Nat Med 2002;8:582.
238. Preston EH, Xu H, Dhanireddy KK, et al. IDEC-131 (anti-CD154), sirolimus and donor-specific transfusion facilitate operational tolerance in non-human primates. Am J Transplant 2005;5:1032.
239. Preville X, Flacher M, LeMauff B, et al. Mechanisms involved in antithymocyte globulin immunosuppressive activity in a nonhuman primate model. Transplantation 2001;71:460.
240. Prin Mathieu C, Renoult E, Kennel De March A, et al. Serum anti-rabbit and anti-horse IgG, IgA, and IgM in kidney transplant recipients. Nephrol Dial Transplant 1997;12:2133.
241. Pruitt SK, Kirk AD, Bollinger RR, et al. The effect of soluble complement receptor type 1 on hyperacute rejection of porcine xenografts. Transplantation 1994;57:363.
242. Przepiorka D, LeMaistre CF, Huh YO, et al. Evaluation of anti-CD5 ricin A chain immunoconjugate for prevention of acute graft-vs.-host disease after HLA-identical marrow transplantation. Ther Immunol 1994;1:77–82.
243. Przepiorka D, Phillips GL, Ratanatharathorn V, et al. A phase II study of BTI-322, a monoclonal anti-CD2 antibody for treatment of steroid-resistant acute GVHD. Blood 1998;92:4066.
244. Qin L, Chavin KD, Lin J, et al. Anti-CD2 receptor and anti-CD2 ligand (CD48) antibodies synergize to prolong allograft survival. J Exp Med 1994;179:341.
245. Raghavan M, Bjorkman PJ. Fc receptors and their interactions with immunoglobulins. Annu Rev Cell Dev Biol 1996;12:181.
246. Rahman GF, Hardy MA, Cohen DJ. Administration of equine anti-thymocyte globulin via peripheral vein in renal transplant recipients. Transplantation 2000;69:1958.
247. Raman C. CD5, an important regulator of lymphocyte selection and immune tolerance. Immunol Res 2002;26:255.
248. Rebellato LM, Gross U, Verbanac KM, et al. A comprehensive definition of the major antibody specificities in polyclonal rabbit antithymocyte globulin. Transplantation 1994;57:685.
249. Regan JF, Lyonnais C, Campbell K, et alUS Thymoglobulin Multi-Center Study Group. Total and active thymoglobulin levels: effects of dose and sensitization on serum concentrations. Transpl Immunol 2001;9:29.
250. Rehman S, Meier-Kriesche HU, Scornik J. Use of intravenous immune globulin and rituximab for desensitization of highly human leukocyte antigen-sensitized patients awaiting kidney transplantation. Transplantation 2010;90:932.
251. Reichert JM. Therapeutic monoclonal antibodies: trends in development and approval in the US. Curr Opin Mol Ther 2002;4:110.
252. Reichert JM, Rosensweig CJ, Faden LB, et al. Monoclonal antibody successes in the clinic. Nat Biotechnol 2005;23:1073.
253. Reinke P, Kern F, Fietze W, et al. Anti-CD4 monoclonal antibody therapy of late acute rejection in renal allograft recipients – CD4 T cells play an essential role in the rejection process. Transplant Proc 1995;27:859.
254. Richardson AJ, Higgins RM, Liddington M, et al. Antithymocyte globulin for steroid resistant rejection in renal transplant recipients immunosuppressed with triple therapy. Transpl Int 1989;2:27.
255. Robbins RC, Oyer PE, Stinson EB, et al. The use of monoclonal antibodies after heart transplantation. Transplant Sci 1992;2:22.
256. Rocha PN, Plumb TJ, Crowley SD, et al. Effector mechanisms in transplant rejection. Immunol Rev 2003;196:51.
257. Rostaing L, Cantarovich D, Mourad G, et al. Corticosteroid-free immunosuppression with tacrolimus, mycophenolate mofetil, and daclizumab induction in renal transplantation. Transplantation 2005;79:807.
258. Rothlein R, Dustin ML, Marlin SD, et al. A human intercellular adhesion molecule (ICAM-1) distinct from LFA-1. J Immunol 1986;137:1270.
259. Sablinski T, Hancock WW, Tilney NL, et al. CD4 monoclonal antibodies in organ transplantation – a review of progress. Transplantation 1991;52:579.
260. Sablinski T, Sayegh MH, Kut JP, et al. The importance of targeting the CD4+ T cell subset at the time of antigenic challenge for induction of prolonged vascularized allograft survival. Transplantation 1992;53:219.
261. Salmela K, Wramner L, Ekberg H, et al. A randomized multicenter trial of the anti-ICAM-1 monoclonal antibody (Enlimomab), for the prevention of acute rejection and delayed onset of graft function in cadaveric renal transplantation. Transplantation 1999;67:729.
262. Sao H, Kitaori K, Kasai M, et al. A new marrow T cell depletion method using anti-CD6 monoclonal antibody-conjugated magnetic beads and its clinical application for prevention of acute graft-vs.-host disease in allogeneic bone marrow transplantation: results of a phase I–II trial. Int J Hematol 1999;69:27.
263. Sarwal M, Chua MS, Kambham M, et al. Molecular heterogeneity in acute renal allograft rejection identified by DNA microarray profiling. N Engl J Med 2003;349:125.
264. Sarwal MM, Ettenger R, Dharnidharka V, et al. Complete steroid avoidance is effective and safe in children with renal transplants: a multicenter randomized trial with three-year follow-up. Am J Transplant 2012;12:2719–29.
265. Scheinfeld N. Alefacept: a safety profile. Expert Opin Drug Saf 2005;4:975.
266. Schnell R, Vitetta E, Schindler J, et al. Treatment of refractory Hodgkin's lymphoma patients with an anti-CD25 ricin A-chain immunotoxin. Leukemia 2000;14:129.
267. Schroeder TJ, First MR, Mansour ME, et al. Antimurine antibody formation following OKT3 therapy. Transplantation 1990;49:48.
268. Scientific Registry of Transplant Recipients (SRTR) and Organ Procurement and Transplantation Network (OPTN). SRTR/OPTN 2010 annual data report. Am J Transplant 2012;12(Suppl. 1).
269. Sempowski GD, Lee DM, Kaufman RE, et al. Structure and function of the CD7 molecule. Crit Rev Immunol 1999;19:331.
270. Shaffer D, Langone A, Nylander WA, et al. A pilot protocol of a calcineurin-inhibitor free regimen for kidney transplant recipients of marginal donor kidneys or with delayed graft function. Clin Transplant 2003;17:31.
271. Shapiro AM, Lakey JR, Ryan EA, et al. Islet transplantation in seven patients with type 1 diabetes mellitus using a glucocorticoid-free immunosuppressive regimen. N Engl J Med 2000;343:230.
272. Shapiro R, Basu A, Tan H, et al. Kidney transplantation under minimal immunosuppression after pretransplant lymphoid depletion with Thymoglobulin or Campath. J Am Coll Surg 2005;200:505.
273. Shapiro R, Young JB, Milford EL, et al. Immunosuppression: evolution in practice and trends, 1993–2003. Am J Transplant 2005;5:874.
274. Sharma LC, Muirhead N, Lazarovits AI. Human mouse chimeric CD7 monoclonal antibody (SDZCHH380) for the prophylaxis of kidney transplant rejection: analysis beyond 4 years. Transplant Proc 1997;29:323.
275. Sherry N, Hagopian W, Ludvigsson J, et al. Teplizumab for treatment of type 1 diabetes (Protégé study): 1-year results from a randomised, placebo-controlled trial. Lancet 2011;378:487–97.
276. Shield CF, Cosimi AB, Tolkoff-Rubin NE, et al. Use of antithymocyte globulin for reversal of acute allograft rejection. Transplantation 1979;28:461.
277. Shield CF, Edwards EB, Davies DB, et al. Antilymphocyte induction therapy in cadaver renal transplantation. Transplantation 1997;63:1257.
278. Shizuru JA, Seydel KB, Flavin TF, et al. Induction of donor-specific unresponsiveness to cardiac allografts in rats by pretransplant anti-CD4 monoclonal antibody therapy. Transplantation 1990;50:366.

279. Siddiqui MA, Scott LJ. Infliximab: a review of its use in Crohn's disease and rheumatoid arthritis. Drugs 2005;65:2179.
280. Siemenow M, Brown SA, Thompson JS, et al. TOL101; a novel alphabeta TCR targeting monoclonal antibody. Am J Transplant 2010;10:36.
281. Simpson MA, Monaco AP. Clinical uses of polyclonal and monoclonal antilymphoid sera. In: Chatenoud L, editor. Monoclonal antibodies in transplantation. Austin, TX: RG Landes; 1995. p. 1.
282. Singh A, Stablein D, Tejani A. Risk factors for vascular thrombosis in pediatric renal transplantation: a special report of the North American Pediatric Renal Transplant Cooperative Study. Transplantation 1997;63:1263.
283. Skov L, Kragballe K, Zachariae C, et al. HuMax-CD4: a fully human monoclonal anti-CD4 antibody for the treatment of psoriasis vulgaris. Arch Dermatol 2003;139:1433.
284. Sollinger H, Kaplan B, Pescovitz MD, et al. Basiliximab versus antithymocyte globulin for prevention of acute renal allograft rejection. Transplantation 2001;72:1915.
285. Sommer BG, Henry ML, Ferguson RM. Sequential antilymphoblast globulin and cyclosporine for renal transplantation. Transplant Proc 1987;19:1879.
286. Sonnenday CJ, Warren DS, Cooper M, et al. Plasmapheresis, CMV hyperimmune globulin, and anti-CD20 allow ABO-incompatible renal transplantation without splenectomy. Am J Transplant 2004;4:1315.
287. Soulillou JP, Cantarovich D, Le MB, et al. Randomized controlled trial of a monoclonal antibody against the interleukin-2 receptor (33B3.1) as compared with rabbit antithymocyte globulin for prophylaxis against rejection of renal allografts. N Engl J Med 1990;322:1175.
288. Spitzer TR, McAfee SL, Dey BR, et al. Nonmyeloablative haploidentical stem-cell transplantation using anti-CD2 monoclonal antibody (MEDI-507)-based conditioning for refractory hematologic malignancies. Transplantation 2003;75:1748.
289. Springer TA, Dustin ML, Kishimoto TK, et al. The lymphocyte function associated LFA1, CD2 and LFA3 molecules: cell adhesion receptors of the immune system. Annu Rev Immunol 1987;5:223.
290. Squifflet JP, Besse T, Malaise J, et al. BTI-322 for induction therapy after renal transplantation: a randomized study. Transplant Proc 1997;29:317.
291. Stafford FJ, Fleisher TA, Lee G, et al. A pilot study of anti-CD5 ricin A chain immunoconjugate in systemic lupus erythematosus. J Rheumatol 1994;21:2068–70.
292. Starling GC, Whitney GS, Siadak AW, et al. Characterization of mouse CD6 with novel monoclonal antibodies which enhance the allogeneic mixed leukocyte reaction. Eur J Immunol 1996;26:738.
293. Starzl TE, Murase N, Abu-Elmagd K, et al. Tolerogenic immunosuppression for organ transplantation. Lancet 2003;361:1502.
294. Starzl TE, Porter KA, Iwasaki Y, et al. The use of heterologous antilymphocyte globulins in human homotransplantation. In: Wolstenholme GEW, O'Connor M, editors. Antilymphocyte serum. Boston: Little, Brown; 1967. p. 1.
295. Stegall MD, Diwan T, Raghavaiah S, et al. Terminal complement inhibition decreases antibody-mediated rejection in sensitized renal transplant recipients. Am J Transplant 2011;11:2405–13.
296. Stillwell R, Bierer BE. T cell signal transduction and the role of CD7 in costimulation. Immunol Res 2001;24:31.
297. Stratta RJ, D'Alessandro AM, Armbrust MJ, et al. Sequential antilymphocyte globulin/cyclosporine immunosuppression in cadaveric renal transplantation: effect of duration of ALG therapy. Transplantation 1989;47:96.
298. Streem SB, Novick AC, Braun WE, et al. Low-dose maintenance prednisone and antilymphoblast globulin for the treatment of acute rejection. Transplantation 1983;35:420.
299. Suntharalingam G, Perry MR, Ward S, et al. Cytokine storm in a phase 1 trial of the anti-CD28 monoclonal antibody TGN1412. N Engl J Med 2006;355:1018.
300. Suri-Payer E, Amar AZ, Thornton AM, et al. CD4 CD25 T cells inhibit both the induction and effector function of autoreactive T cells and represent a unique lineage of immunoregulatory cells. J Immunol 1998;160:1212.
301. Svoboda J, Kotloff R, Tsai DE. Management of patients with post-transplant lymphoproliferative disorder: the role of rituximab. Transpl Int 2006;19:259.
302. Swanson SJ, Hale DA, Mannon RB, et al. Kidney transplantation with rabbit antithymocyte globulin induction and sirolimus monotherapy. Lancet 2003;360:1662.
303. Szczech LA, Berlin JA, Aradhye S, et al. Effect of anti-lymphocyte induction therapy on renal allograft survival: a meta-analysis. J Am Soc Nephrol 1997;8:1771.
304. Szczech LA, Berlin JA, Feldman HI. The effect of antilymphocyte induction therapy on renal allograft survival: a meta-analysis of individual patient-level data. Anti-Lymphocyte Antibody Induction Therapy Study Group. Ann Intern Med 1998;128:817.
305. Tan HP, Kaczorowski DJ, Basu A, et al. Living donor renal transplantation using alemtuzumab induction and tacrolimus monotherapy. Am J Transplant 2006;6:2409.
306. Tatum AH, Bollinger RR, Sanfilippo F. Rapid serologic diagnosis of serum sickness from antilymphocyte globulin therapy using enzyme immunoassay. Transplantation 1984;38:582.
307. Taylor RP, Lindorfer MA. Immunotherapeutic mechanisms of anti-CD20 monoclonal antibodies. Curr Opin Immunol 2008;20:444–9.
308. Tesi RJ, Elkhammas EA, Henry ML, et al. OKT3 for primary therapy of the first rejection episode in kidney transplants. Transplantation 1993;55:1023.
309. Thistlethwaite Jr JR, Cosimi AB, Delmonico FL, et al. Evolving use of OKT3 monoclonal antibody for treatment of renal allograft rejection. Transplantation 1984;38:695.
310. Thistlethwaite Jr JR, Gaber AO, Haag BW, et al. OKT3 treatment of steroid-resistant renal allograft rejection. Transplantation 1987;43:176.
311. Thomas F, Cunningham P, Thomas J, et al. Superior renal allograft survival and decreased rejection with early high-dose and sequential multi-species antilymphocyte globulin therapy. Transplant Proc 1987;19:1874.
312. Thomas JM, Neville DM, Contreras JL, et al. Preclinical studies of allograft tolerance in rhesus monkeys. Transplantation 1997;64:124.
313. Thompson JS, Pomeroy C, Kryscio RJ, et al. Use of a T cell-specific monoclonal antibody, T10B9, in a novel allogeneic stem cell transplantation protocol for hematologic malignancy high-risk patients. Biol Blood Marrow Transplant 2004;10:858.
314. Tite JP, Sloan A, Janeway CJ. The role of L3T4 in T cell activation: L3T4 may be both an Ia-binding protein and a receptor that transduces a negative signal. J Mol Cell Immunol 1986;2:179.
315. Torrealba JR, Fernandez LA, Kanmaz T, et al. Immunotoxin-treated rhesus monkeys: a model for renal allograft chronic rejection. Transplantation 2003;76:524.
316. Turgeon NA, Avila JG, Cano JA, et al. Experience with a novel efalizumab-based immunosuppressive regimen to facilitate single donor islet cell transplantation. Am J Transplant 2010;10:2082–91.
317. Turgeon N, Fishman JA, Basgoz N, et al. Effect of oral acyclovir or ganciclovir therapy after preemptive intravenous ganciclovir therapy to prevent cytomegalovirus disease in cytomegalovirus seropositive renal and liver transplant recipients receiving antilymphocyte antibody therapy. Transplantation 1998;66:1780.
318. Tyden G, Kumlien G, Genberg H, et al. ABO incompatible kidney transplantations without splenectomy, using antigen-specific immunoadsorption and rituximab. Am J Transplant 2005;5:145.
319. Tzakis AG, Tryphonopoulos P, Kato T, et al. Preliminary experience with alemtuzumab (Campath-1H) and low-dose tacrolimus immunosuppression in adult liver transplantation. Transplantation 2004;77:1209.
320. Upadhyay K, Midgley L, Moudgil A. Safety and efficacy of alemtuzumab in the treatment of late acute renal allograft rejection. Pediatr Transplant 2012;16:286–93.
321. Vallhonrat H, Williams WW, Cosimi AB, et al. In vivo generation of C4b, Bb, iC3b, and SC5b-9 after OKT3 administration in kidney and lung transplant recipients. Transplantation 1999;67:253.
322. van Gelder T, Zietse R, Mulder AH, et al. A double-blind, placebo-controlled study of monoclonal anti-interleukin-2 receptor antibody (BT563) administration to prevent acute rejection after kidney transplantation. Transplantation 1995;60:248.
323. Venkiteshwaran A. Tocilizumab. MAbs 2009;1:432–8.
324. Vigeral P, Chkoff N, Chatenoud L, et al. Prophylactic use of OKT3 monoclonal antibody in cadaver kidney recipients: utilization of OKT3 as the sole immunosuppressive agent. Transplantation 1986;41:730.

325. Vincenti F. New monoclonal antibodies in renal transplantation. Minerva Urol Nefrol 2003;55:57.
326. Vincenti F, Charpentier B, Vanrenterghem Y, et al. A phase III study of belatacept-based immunosuppression regimens versus cyclosporine in renal transplant recipients (BENEFIT study). Am J Transplant 2010;10:535–46.
327. Vincenti F, Kirkman R, Light S, et al. Interleukin-2-receptor blockade with daclizumab to prevent acute rejection in renal transplantation. Daclizumab Triple Therapy Study Group. N Engl J Med 1998;338:161.
328. Vincenti F, Lantz M, Birnbaum J, et al. A phase I trial of humanized anti-interleukin-2 receptor antibody in renal transplantation. Transplantation 1997;63:33.
329. Vincenti F, Larsen CP, Durrbach A, et al. Belatacept (LEA29Y) for maintenance immunosuppression after renal transplantation. N Engl J Med 2005;353:770.
330. Vincenti F, Mendez R, Pescovitz M, et al. A phase I/II randomized open-label multicenter trial of efalizumab, a humanized anti-CD11a, anti-LFA-1 in renal transplantation. Am J Transplant 2007;7:1770–7.
331. Vincenti F, Ramos E, Brattstrom C, et al. Multicenter trial exploring calcineurin inhibitors avoidance in renal transplantation. Transplantation 2001;71:1282.
332. Vo AA, Peng A, Toyoda M, et al. Use of intravenous immune globulin and rituximab for desensitization of highly HLA-sensitized patients awaiting kidney transplantation. Transplantation 2010;89:1095–102.
333. Waid TH, Lucas BA, Thompson JS, et al. Treatment of renal allograft rejection with T10B9.1A31 or OKT3: final analysis of a phase II clinical trial. Transplantation 1997;64:274.
334. Waid TH, Thompson JS, McKeown JW, et al. Induction immunotherapy in heart transplantation with T10B9.1A-31: a phase I study. J Heart Lung Transplant 1997;16:913.
335. Waldmann H. Therapeutic approaches for transplantation. Curr Opin Immunol 2001;13:606.
336. Waldmann H, Hale G. CAMPATH: from concept to clinic. Philos Trans R Soc Lond B Biol Sci 2005;360:1707.
337. Walunas TL, Bakker CY, Bluestone JA. CTLA-4 ligation blocks CD28-dependent T cell activation. J Exp Med 1996;183:2541.
338. Weaver TA, Charafeddine AH, Agarwal A, et al. Alefacept promotes co-stimulation blockade based allograft survival in nonhuman primates. Nat Med 2009;15:746–9.
339. Weaver TA, Kirk AD. Alemtuzumab. Transplantation 2007;84:1545–7.
340. Weber J, Keam SJ. Ustekinumab. BioDrugs 2009;23:53–61.
341. Webster A, Pankhurst T, Rinaldi F, et al. Polyclonal and monoclonal antibodies for treating acute rejection episodes in kidney transplant recipients. Cochrane Database Syst Rev 2006; 19, CD004756.
342. Wechter WJ, Morrell RM, Bergan J, et al. Extended treatment with antilymphocyte globulin (ATGAM) in renal allograft recipients. Transplantation 1979;28:365.
343. Wee SL, Colvin RB, Phelan JM, et al. Fc-receptor for mouse IgG1 (Fc gamma RII) and antibody-mediated cell clearance in patients treated with Leu2a antibody. Transplantation 1989;48:1012.
344. Wee SL, Stroka DM, Preffer FL, et al. The effects of OKT4A monoclonal antibody on cellular immunity of nonhuman primate renal allograft recipients. Transplantation 1992;53:501.
345. Weinberg JM, Bottino CJ, Lindholm J, et al. Biologic therapy for psoriasis: an update on the tumor necrosis factor inhibitors infliximab, etanercept, and adalimumab, and the T-cell-targeted therapies efalizumab and alefacept. J Drugs Dermatol 2005; 4:544.
346. Weiner LM. Fully human therapeutic monoclonal antibodies. J Immunother 2006;29:1.
347. Wiland AM, Fink JC, Philosophe B, et al. Peripheral administration of thymoglobulin for induction therapy in pancreas transplantation. Transplant Proc 2001;33:1910.
348. Wong JT, Eylath AA, Ghobrial I, et al. The mechanism of anti-CD3 monoclonal antibodies: mediation of cytolysis by inter-T cell bridging. Transplantation 1990;50:683.
349. Wood KJ, Pearson TC, Darby C, et al. CD4: a potential target molecule for immunosuppressive therapy and tolerance induction. Transplant Rev 1991;5:150.
350. Woodle ES, Baldwin 3rd. WM. Of mice and men: terminal complement inhibition with anti-C5 monoclonal antibodies. Am J Transplant 2011;11:2277–8.
351. Woodle ES, Xu D, Zivin RA, et al. Phase I trial of a humanized, Fc receptor nonbinding OKT3 antibody, huOKT3gamma1(Ala-Ala) in the treatment of acute renal allograft rejection. Transplantation 1999;68:608.
352. Xu D, Alegre M-L, Varga SS, et al. In vitro characterization of five humanized OKT3 effector function variant antibodies. Cell Immunol 2000;200:16–26.
353. Xu H, Montgomery SP, Preston EH, et al. Studies investigating pretransplant donor-specific blood transfusion, rapamycin, and the CD154-specific antibody IDEC-131 in a nonhuman primate model of skin allotransplantation. J Immunol 2003;170:2776.
354. Xu H, Zhang X, Mannon RB, et al. Platelet-derived or soluble CD154 induces vascularized allograft rejection independent of cell-bound CD154. J Clin Invest 2006;116:769.
355. Zimmerhackl LB, Hofer J, Cortina G, et al. Prophylactic eculizumab after renal transplantation in atypical hemolytic-uremic syndrome. N Engl J Med 2010;362:1746–8.
356. Zuber J, Quintrec ML, Krid S, et al. Eculizumab for atypical hemolytic uremic syndrome recurrence in renal transplantation. Am J Transplant 2012;12:3337–54.

CHAPTER 21

BELATACEPT

Blayne A. Sayed • Allan D. Kirk • Thomas C. Pearson • Christian P. Larsen

CHAPTER OUTLINE

INTRODUCTION: TWO SIGNALS

As discussed in Chapter 20, the targeting of T-cell costimulatory pathways as adjuncts to, or even replacement for, current immunotherapy following renal transplantation has become a clinical reality.[9,18,39–41] As crucial mediators and controllers of the adaptive immune response, T cells require multiple signals for effective and appropriate activation.[42] This paradigm was first described by Bretscher and Cohn in the context of B-cell activation and later extended to T-cell activation by Lafferty and Cunningham (reviewed here[30]). As is well appreciated by most students of immunology, engagement of the T-cell receptor (TCR) with peptide antigen presented by major histocompatibility complex (MHC) expressed on antigen presenting cells (APCs) provides the primary activation signal and determines the antigen-specific nature of the response. However, it is important to distinguish that the specificity of a response does not dictate its character; a T cell can "respond" in many ways, including evoking antigen-specific cytotoxicity, anergy, or regulation. Thus, the character of a response is shaped largely through contemporaneous binding of additional molecules to include T-cell costimulatory receptors. Costimulatory molecules bind to their ligands, generally expressed by APCs, which provide a second signal that decreases intracellular activation thresholds and helps shape the nature of the T-cell response.

The paradigm of a two-signal requirement for T-cell activation is based on the necessity for immune self-discrimination. As compared to foreign antigen, self peptide is vastly more abundant in vivo. In this context simple engagement of the TCR with peptide-bearing MHC would generate an exceedingly high incidence of autoreactive T-cell clones. As such, secondary signals whose expression is regulated as part of the "danger" signal to pathogens, as termed by Matzinger,[28] is necessary for driving T-cell responses directed against foreign antigens. Conversely, costimulatory signals are not only required for effective T-cell activation but their absence of inhibitory signaling is also essential for curtailing an immune response and likely for generation of tolerance. TCR engagement in the absence of costimulatory signals leads to T-cell anergy or generation of tolerogenic T-cell clones, and, indeed, there are T-cell costimulatory molecules that have a primary mollifying effect.

The costimulatory signal is not a simple binary on/off switch but rather induces a network of signals that influences the quantitative and qualitative nature of the ensuing T-cell response.[4] TCR engagement in the presence of positive costimulatory signaling pathways induces cellular proliferation, cytokine production, upregulation of activation molecules, and T-helper cell differentiation.[44] Activation of negative costimulatory signaling pathways results in inhibition of cellular proliferation and cytokine production, and even apoptosis. Under certain conditions, these signals also lead to the development of regulatory T-cell subsets that actively suppress the immune response. The more we understand costimulatory pathways and their fine control over adaptive immune responses, the more attractive they have become as therapeutic targets. Posttransplant immunosuppression has been long dependent on drugs such as calcineurin inhibitors (CNI) that do little to eradicate or alter the function of alloresponsive T cells. They simply provide a "chemical blindfold" which, once removed, results in resumed graft rejection.[28] Harnessing the function of costimulatory molecules, inherent regulators of T-cell activation and tolerance, therefore provides a more logical means of immunomodulation.

COSTIMULATORY PATHWAYS

The most well known activating costimulatory pathway consists of the CD28 receptor, which is constitutively expressed on T cells, and its ligands CD80/CD86 (B7-1/B7-2), which are upregulated on activated APCs and cells with surrogate APC function. Engagement of CD28 in the context of TCR activation induces T-cell proliferation, survival, clonal expansion, and cytokine expression, including paracrine expression of the T-cell trophic factor

IL-2.[29,36] In contrast, cytotoxic T-lymphocyte-associated antigen 4 (CTLA-4, CD152) functions as an alternative receptor that is quickly upregulated on activated T cells, competitively binds CD80 and CD86 and functions to terminate ongoing immune responses.[43] Mice with a targeted deletion of CTLA-4 develop a fatal lymphoproliferative disorder and T cells derived from these animals show an exuberant proliferative and cytokine response to stimulation.[25] Thus the in vivo illustration of this pathway is as such: inflammation, for example after tissue injury, drives sustained APC activation and B7 expression and creates an excess of B7 that allows for saturation of CD28 mediated positive costimulation. As the injury and its related APC activation subsides, declining B7 expression becomes a rate limiting factor and costimulation becomes dominated by the higher-affinity inhibitory CD152 signaling. Thus, in an elegant display of efficiency, the costimulatory pathways that initiate an immune response reflexively curtail the response as well, and in doing so, minimize the risk of unregulated or pathological immune injury.

Another receptor ligand pair, best known for its role in B-cell isotype switching but also known to play an important role in T-cell activation, is CD40 and CD154. CD154, also known as CD40 ligand (CD40L), is widely expressed on a variety of cell types, including activated T cells. CD40, a member of the tumor necrosis factor (TNF) receptor superfamily, is constitutively expressed on most APCs and on activated endothelium.[19] Binding of CD40/CD40L enhances APC function and longevity by inducing expression of MHC and the B7 molecules, other activation molecules, cytokines, by enhancing nuclear factor (NF)-κB-responsive pathways and by inhibiting Fas-mediated apoptosis. Although not as well understood, the cross-linking of CD154 is known to induce T-cell production of cytokines essential for T helper cell differentiation, including interleukins IL-4 and IL-10.[3]

Numerous other costimulatory pathways have since been discovered with both positive and negative properties. While their description is beyond the scope of this chapter, their biology has been reviewed by Sayegh et al.[24] It is also important to note that a third signal is now generally accepted to establish the ultimate magnitude of an immune response. Cytokine and chemokine receptors form the basis for signal 3, and once specificity and character are established by signals 1 and 2, the magnitude and dispersion of their influence is defined by alterations in cytokine and chemokine receptors. In all, immune responses should be seen as nuanced controlled processes rather than binary responses used solely for cytotoxic effector functions.

COSTIMULATION BLOCKADE

Given their essential role in T-cell activation, costimulatory molecules have long been a target for blockade in the transplant setting. In the laboratory, the primary means of testing costimulatory blockers has been to measure their effectiveness in inhibiting T-cell function, preventing graft rejection and inducing durable graft tolerance. In the clinical setting, however, a more pragmatic approach has been employed to pair costimulation blockade with minimization and/or withdrawal of conventional immunotherapies, particularly CNIs.

One of the early high-impact studies that signaled the potentially groundbreaking role of costimulation blockade came from Larsen and Pearson, who demonstrated that simultaneous blockade of the CD28 and CD40 pathways with CTLA-4 Ig and anti-CD154 inhibited T-cell responses in vitro and that perioperative blockade provided durable protection for murine cardiac and skin allografts in vivo.[17] Kirk and Knechtle extended these findings to an outbred non-human primate (NHP) model, heralding their likely clinical applicability,[14] and subsequently broke new ground by documenting that monotherapy with a humanized mouse anti-CD154 antibody prevents MHC-mismatched renal allograft rejection and exerted a sustained antirejection effect in NHPs.[13] As discussed previously (Chapter 20), although murine and NHP studies demonstrated much promise by targeting the CD40/CD154 pathway, human trials were hindered by poor efficacy and concern for development of thromboembolism; further studies are still pending.[12–14] Early experiments that directly inhibited or disrupted the CD28 or B7 also yielded promising results but were highly context-dependent and did little to promote long-term tolerance. Finally, the use of CTLA-4 fusion proteins as indirect inhibition of the CD28 pathway proved to be highly efficacious and led to the development of belatacept, the first costimulatory targeted therapy added to the transplant armamentarium and the focus of this chapter.

Costimulation Blockade: CD28-B7

Direct targeting of the CD28-B7 pathway through the use of B7-1 and B7-2 blocking antibodies has a dose-dependent inhibitory effect on primary mixed leukocyte reactions (MLR), an in vitro model of direct alloreactivity. However, only modest effects in graft survival are evident when CD28-deficient mice are the recipients of cardiac allografts.[33] Other studies utilizing the heterotopic murine cardiac allograft model found no graft survival benefit when utilizing a CD28-deficient host background, but instead indicated that disrupting recipient, but not donor, B7 expression results in long-term cardiac allograft survival.[27,37] This effect appears to be tissue-specific as the B7-1/B7-2 knockout mice are able to reject allogeneic skin grafts in the absence of previous antigen exposure or even in the presence of functional cardiac allografts. More recent data demonstrate that use of an anti-CD28 antibody that causes CD28 internalization prevents chronic rejection and promotes long-term allograft survival in a rat renal transplantation model.[10,22] Thus, CD28 pathway blockade is not a definitive go/no go immune switch, but rather skews the likelihood of a response towards an aggressive phenotype.

In NHP, a brief induction course with either anti-B7-1 or anti-B7-2 monotherapy is sufficient to delay renal allograft rejection, although combination induction therapy with both anti-B7-1 and anti-B7-2 antibodies has a more notable effect.[16] The combination of anti-B7-1 and B7-2 antibodies with either cyclosporine A (CsA) or sirolimus (SRL) also proved to be effective for prolonging allograft function, although neither regimen was sufficient to induce long-term tolerance.[2,11,31] Paradoxically, Hausen et al.[11] noted that CsA alone was inferior to CsA in combination with anti-B7-1 and B7-2 antibodies, whereas Ossevoort et al.[31] noted no difference between the groups, although NHP treated with the latter combination therapy did appear to have reduced incidence of vascular rejection. Taken together, the majority of small-animal and NHP data suggested that direct disruption of the CD28/B7 pathway holds promise for induction and potentially maintenance therapy, but that it falls short of developing long-term host allograft tolerance.

Costimulation Blockade: CTLA-4 Ig

Linsley et al. developed abatacept, studied preclinically as CTLA-4 Ig, a chimeric molecule incorporating the extracellular domain of human CTLA-4 and the Fc portion of human immunoglobulin (Ig) that binds with high affinity to the B7 molecules.[25] The CTLA-4 portion of the molecule provides the specificity for binding, whereas the Fc portion of the IgG molecule provides opsonization properties and antibody-like half-life.[26] CTLA-4 Ig effectively blocks the T-cell component of the CD28/CD152 pathway by competing for B7 binding. In vitro CTLA-4 Ig inhibits T-cell proliferation and T-helper cell-induced B-cell antibody production.[25] Addition of CTLA-4 Ig to an MLR also inhibits dendritic cell-induced T-cell proliferation.[21]

In vivo, treatment with CTLA-4 Ig has a profound impact on short-term murine cardiac allograft survival, although the effects are limited to the treatment period and shortly afterwards, with a failure to induce long-term tolerance.[38] Using the rat renal allograft model, Sayegh et al. documented that close to 90% of rats receiving one dose of CTLA-4 Ig on day 2 posttransplant had prolonged survival with preserved renal function as well as long-term donor-specific tolerance, as compared to control animals that uniformly progressed to allograft rejection and death.[35] Further, early addition of CTLA-4 Ig to a cyclosporine regimen virtually prevents chronic rejection and late addition is sufficient to rescue graft function.[1,5] Presaging the complexity of clinical dosing, the timing of CTLA-4 Ig has an important effect on outcome, with CTLA-4 dosing on day 0 being only a third as effective as dosing on day 2 posttransplantation.

Interestingly, trials of CTLA-4 Ig in NHPs proved less promising. In combination CTLA-4 Ig and anti-CD154 prolonged the survival of MHC-mismatched renal allografts, but CTLA-4 Ig alone had more modest and transient effects.[14] In an NHP model of allogeneic pancreatic islet transplantation, 40% of animals treated with CTLA-4 Ig showed prolonged graft survival – again, a modest result – although all animals had suppressed humoral responses.[23]

Rational Development of Belatacept (LEA29Y)

The disappointing results in NHP set the stage for the development of belatacept, a second-generation form of CTLA-4 Ig/abatacept. Early work identified the regions of CTLA-4 Ig essential for binding to CD80, and site-directed mutagenesis confirmed the ability to abolish or augment binding affinity.[32] Although CTLA-4 Ig has a high affinity for CD80, it demonstrates low-avidity binding for monomeric CD86.[8] Blockade of both CD80 and CD86 is essential for durable inhibition of allograft rejection in murine and NHP transplant models.[16,33] Taken together, these results suggested that mutating CTLA-4 Ig to induce higher-avidity binding, especially for CD86, could generate a molecule with enhanced immunosuppressive function.

Belatacept (LEA29Y) is the result of this effort. It is a second-generation form of abatacept with two amino acid substitutions (L104E and A29Y), which increase the binding affinity to CD86 and CD80 approximately fourfold and twofold, respectively, as compared to its parent compound.[20] These changes resulted in an approximately 10-fold increase in T-cell inhibitory activity in vitro. Most importantly, however, in an NHP kidney transplant model belatacept provided apparently better allograft protection than prior experience with its parent compound as a monotherapy and also added significant benefit to a conventional immunosuppressive combination therapy regimen.

CLINICAL APPLICATION OF BELATACEPT

Given these results, a phase II study was designed to compare the efficacy of belatacept as a maintenance immunosuppressant to the standard CNI cyclosporine in combination with steroids, mycophenolate mofetil (MMF), and a basiliximab induction.[41] The study involved approximately 200 human recipients of de novo renal transplants and demonstrated that belatacept, given as an intravenous infusion every 4 or 8 weeks, did not increase rates of acute rejection at 6 months as compared to cyclosporine. Further, belatacept-based immunotherapy also resulted in improved renal function at 1 year and trends towards lower incidence of CNI-related toxicities, including hypertension and posttransplant diabetes.

The Belatacept Evaluation of Nephroprotection and Efficacy as First-line Immunosuppression Trial (BENEFIT) was as an international phase III trial designed to evaluate belatacept-versus cyclosporine-based regimens in approximately 650 adult patients receiving kidney transplants from living or standard criteria deceased donors.[39] Based on the results of the phase II study, the objectives of the phase III trial were to assess at 12 months whether less intensive (LI) and more intensive (MI) belatacept-based immunosuppression could maintain similar rates of acute rejection and patient and graft survival as well as superior renal function, as compared to cyclosporine-based therapy. By most measures the study was successful. Belatacept was well tolerated by patients and resulted in equivalent patient and graft survival, superior renal function (Figure 21-1), and a trend toward less chronic allograft nephropathy. Belatacept-based therapy also generated a trend towards improved cardiovascular and metabolic profiles. Interestingly, the rates and grades of acute allograft rejection were higher in the belatacept-based MI and LI

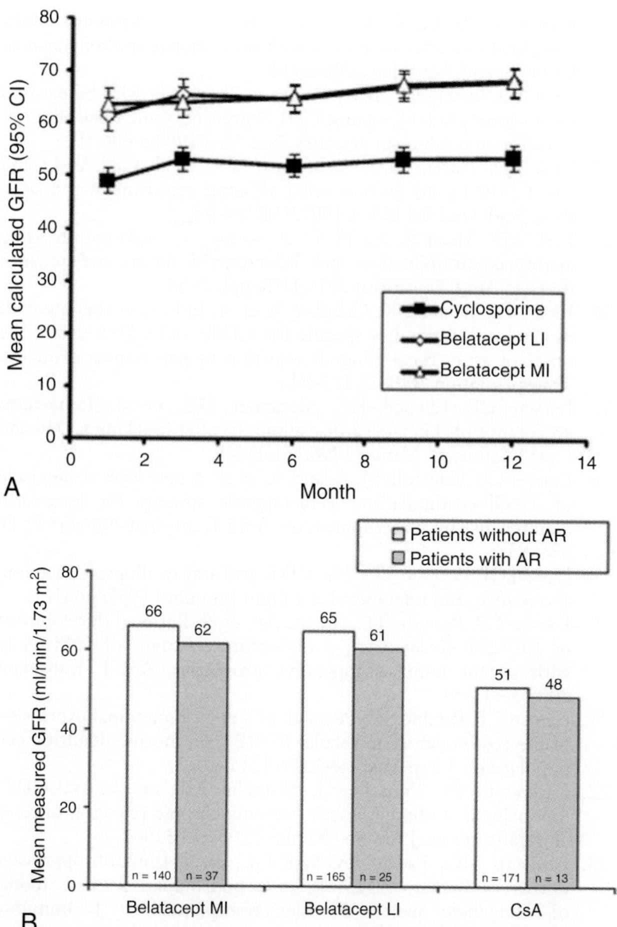

FIGURE 21-1 ■ Renal function from the Belatacept Evaluation of Nephroprotection and Efficacy as First-line Immunosuppression Trial (BENEFIT) trial. (A) Glomerular filtration rate (GFR) of patients treated with a more intensive (MI) or less intensive (LI) belatacept-based regimen compared to a cyclosporine (CsA)-based control group, indicating that belatacept-treated patients enjoy improved renal function throughout the first posttransplant year. (B) GFR is shown for the MI, LI, and CsA groups, indicating that, while rejection leads to lower GFR in all groups, the GFR in belatacept-treated patients who have experienced rejection still exceeds that in the non-rejecting CsA patients. AR, acute rejection. (From Vincenti F, Charpentier B, Vanrenterghem Y, et al. A phase III study of belatacept-based immunosuppression regimens versus cyclosporine in renal transplant recipients (BENEFIT study). Am J Transplant 2010;10:535–46.)

regimens (22% and 17%, respectively) versus the cyclosporine group (7%) (Figure 21-2). The majority of the acute rejection episodes occurred early (within the first 3 months), showed no sign of recurrence, and resolved with treatment.

The subsequent 3-year BENEFIT follow-up confirmed equivalent rates of patient and graft survival.[40] As expected, the belatacept-based regimens demonstrated advantages for long-term renal function which remained stable throughout follow-up, unlike the cyclosporine group, which declined over time. There were also no cases of acute rejection from year 2 to year 3 in the belatacept groups, confirming that those episodes tended to occur in the immediate time period after transplantation and were subsequently unlikely to recur. Posttransplant

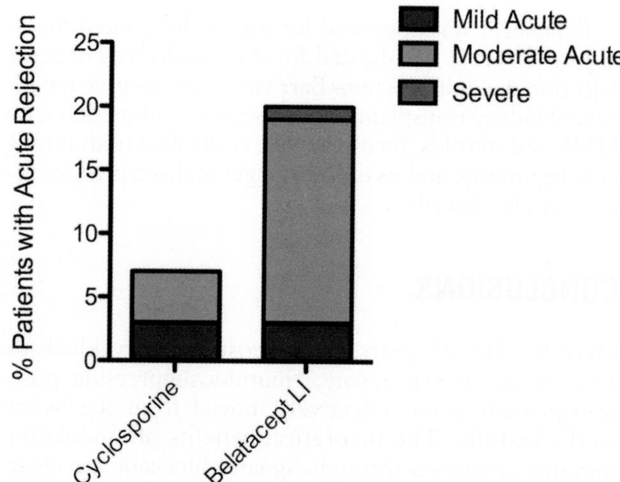

FIGURE 21-2 ■ Increased rate and grade of rejection in patients treated with belatacept from the BENEFIT trial. Shown are rejection rates and grades for belatacept (LI, less intensive – the regimen forming the basis for the Food and Drug Administration approval)-treated patients compared to cyclosporine-treated patients. Belatacept is associated with more rejection and with higher grades of rejection.

lympoproliferative disorder, although rare, was more common in the belatacept groups, particularly amongst patients in the MI cohort who were Epstein–Barr virus-negative recipients.

The BENEFIT-EXT study examined similar outcome measures in adults receiving allografts from extended criteria donors at 12 months and 3 years.[6,34] Extended criteria donors include donors older than 60 years, donors older than 50 with at least two other risk factors (cerebrovascular accident, hypertension, serum creatinine >1.5 mg/dL), cold ischemia time greater than 24 hours, or donation after cardiac death. At 12 months and 3 years belatacept-based immunosuppressive regimens resulted in comparable rates of acute rejection and patient and graft survival, as compared to the cyclosporine-based regimen. Additionally, belatacept use leads to better renal function and improved cardiovascular and metabolic profiles.

Other exploratory open-label phase II trials recently have examined whether the use of belatacept-based immunosuppression can entirely preclude CNIs and corticosteroids.[7,15] Ferguson et al. randomized recipients of living and standard criteria deceased donors to receive belatacept-MMF, belatacept-SRL, or tacrolimus (TAC)-MMF, a standard steroid avoidance regimen.[7] The belatacept-MMF group had a higher rate of acute rejection at 6 months (12%) versus the belatacept-SRL (4%) and TAC-MMF (3%) groups, although 12% is actually much lower than reported in other CNI- or steroid-avoiding regimens. Belatacept-based therapy also appeared to confer superior renal function, as compared to TAC. In an ongoing study, Kirk et al. have investigated a combined therapy with alemtuzumab, SRL, and belatacept, indicating that this base regimen facilitates a low rate of steroid-sensitive acute rejection (5%), and facilitates a long-term therapy of belatacept monotherapy in selected recipients of live donor kidneys.[15] These trials provide insight into the potential uses of belatacept.

Belatacept was approved for use in the United States in June 2011. It is indicated for the prophylaxis of acute rejection in adult, Epstein–Barr virus-seropositive recipients of kidney transplants when used in combination with MMF and steroids. Its use outside controlled trials is only now beginning, and its efficacy in generalized practice remains to be described.

CONCLUSIONS

Over the last 25 years, T-cell costimulatory blockade as a means of maintenance immunosuppression post-transplantation has effectively moved from the bench to the bedside. The theoretical benefits of modulating immune responses through signal 2 blockade are clear: preservation of antigen specificity, potential for sustained effect, and elimination of off-target side effects. However, the limited requirement for costimulation in established immune responses likely will conscribe the use of belatacept somewhat, placing a demand upon the clinician to find the ideal adjuvant therapies for use with belatacept and to identify the patient population most likely to benefit from this approach. The coming years will help shape the optimal use of belatacept in particular, and pave the way for costimulation-based approaches in general.

REFERENCES

1. Azuma H, Chandraker A, Nadeau K, et al. Blockade of T-cell costimulation prevents development of experimental chronic renal allograft rejection. Proc Natl Acad Sci U S A 1996;93:12439–44.
2. Birsan T, Hausen B, Higgins JP, et al. Treatment with humanized monoclonal antibodies against CD80 and CD86 combined with sirolimus prolongs renal allograft survival in cynomolgus monkeys. Transplantation 2003;75:2106–13.
3. Blotta MH, Marshall JD, DeKruyff RH, et al. Cross-linking of the CD40 ligand on human CD4+ T lymphocytes generates a costimulatory signal that up-regulates IL-4 synthesis. J Immunol 1996;156:3133–40.
4. Bour-Jordan H, Bluestone JA. Regulating the regulators: costimulatory signals control the homeostasis and function of regulatory T cells. Immunol Rev 2009;229:41–66.
5. Chandraker A, Azuma H, Nadeau K, et al. Late blockade of T cell costimulation interrupts progression of experimental chronic allograft rejection. J Clin Invest 1998;101:2309–18.
6. Durrbach A, Pestana JM, Pearson T, et al. A phase III study of belatacept versus cyclosporine in kidney transplants from extended criteria donors (BENEFIT-EXT study). Am J Transplant 2010;10:547–57.
7. Ferguson R, Grinyo J, Vincenti F, et al. Immunosuppression with belatacept-based, corticosteroid-avoiding regimens in de novo kidney transplant recipients. Am J Transplant 2011;11:66–76.
8. Greene JL, Leytze GM, Emswiler J, et al. Covalent dimerization of CD28/CTLA-4 and oligomerization of CD80/CD86 regulate T cell costimulatory interactions. J Biol Chem 1996;271:26762–71.
9. Harlan DM, Kirk AD. The future of organ and tissue transplantation: can T-cell costimulatory pathway modifiers revolutionize the prevention of graft rejection? JAMA 1999;282:1076–82.
10. Haspot F, Seveno C, Dugast AS, et al. Anti-CD28 antibody-induced kidney allograft tolerance related to tryptophan degradation and TCR class II B7 regulatory cells. Am J Transplant 2005;5:2339–48.
11. Hausen B, Klupp J, Christians U, et al. Coadministration of either cyclosporine or steroids with humanized monoclonal antibodies against CD80 and CD86 successfully prolong allograft survival after life supporting renal transplantation in cynomolgus monkeys. Transplantation 2001;72:1128–37.
12. Kawai T, Andrews D, Colvin RB, et al. Thromboembolic complications after treatment with monoclonal antibody against CD40 ligand. Nat Med 2000;6:114.
13. Kirk AD, Burkly LC, Batty DS, et al. Treatment with humanized monoclonal antibody against CD154 prevents acute renal allograft rejection in nonhuman primates. Nat Med 1999;5:686–93.
14. Kirk AD, Harlan DM, Armstrong NN, et al. CTLA4-Ig and anti-CD40 ligand prevent renal allograft rejection in primates. Proc Natl Acad Sci U S A 1997;94:8789–94.
15. Kirk AD, Mead S, Xu H, et al. Kidney transplantation using alemtuzumab induction and belatacept/sirolimus maintenance therapy. Am J Transplant 2011;11(Suppl. 2):S45.
16. Kirk AD, Tadaki DK, Celniker A, et al. Induction therapy with monoclonal antibodies specific for CD80 and CD86 delays the onset of acute renal allograft rejection in non-human primates. Transplantation 2001;72:377–84.
17. Larsen CP, Elwood ET, Alexander DZ, et al. Long-term acceptance of skin and cardiac allografts after blocking CD40 and CD28 pathways. Nature 1996;381:434–8.
18. Larsen CP, Knechtle SJ, Adams A, et al. A new look at blockade of T-cell costimulation: a therapeutic strategy for long-term maintenance immunosuppression. Am J Transplant 2006;6(5 Pt 1): 876–83.
19. Larsen CP, Pearson TC. The CD40 pathway in allograft rejection, acceptance, and tolerance. Curr Opin Immunol 1997;9:641–7.
20. Larsen CP, Pearson TC, Adams AB, et al. Rational development of LEA29Y (belatacept), a high-affinity variant of CTLA4-Ig with potent immunosuppressive properties. Am J Transplant 2005;5:443–53.
21. Larsen CP, Ritchie SC, Pearson TC, et al. Functional expression of the costimulatory molecule, B7/BB1, on murine dendritic cell populations. J Exp Med 1992;176:1215–20.
22. Laskowski IA, Pratschke J, Wilhelm MJ, et al. Anti-CD28 monoclonal antibody therapy prevents chronic rejection of renal allografts in rats. J Am Soc Nephrol 2002;13:519–27.
23. Levisetti MG, Padrid PA, Szot GL, et al. Immunosuppressive effects of human CTLA4Ig in a non-human primate model of allogeneic pancreatic islet transplantation. J Immunol 1997;159:5187–91.
24. Li XC, Rothstein DM, Sayegh MH. Costimulatory pathways in transplantation: challenges and new developments. Immunol Rev 2009;229:271–93.
25. Linsley PS, Brady W, Urnes M, et al. CTLA-4 is a second receptor for the B cell activation antigen B7. J Exp Med 1991;174:561–9.
26. Linsley PS, Wallace PM, Johnson J, et al. Immunosuppression in vivo by a soluble form of the CTLA-4 T cell activation molecule. Science 1992;257:792–5.
27. Mandelbrot DA, Furukawa Y, McAdam AJ, et al. Expression of B7 molecules in recipient, not donor, mice determines the survival of cardiac allografts. J Immunol 1999;163:3753–7.
28. Matzinger P. Graft tolerance: a duel of two signals. Nat Med 1999;5:616–7.
29. McAdam AJ, Schweitzer AN, Sharpe AH. The role of B7 co-stimulation in activation and differentiation of CD4+ and CD8+ T cells. Immunol Rev 1998;165:231–47.
30. Mueller DL, Jenkins MK, Schwartz RH. Clonal expansion versus functional clonal inactivation: a costimulatory signalling pathway determines the outcome of T cell antigen receptor occupancy. Annu Rev Immunol 1989;7:445–80.
31. Ossevoort MA, Ringers J, Kuhn EM, et al. Prevention of renal allograft rejection in primates by blocking the B7/CD28 pathway. Transplantation 1999;68:1010–8.
32. Peach RJ, Bajorath J, Brady W, et al. Complementarity determining region 1 (CDR1)- and CDR3-analogous regions in CTLA-4 and CD28 determine the binding to B7-1. J Exp Med 1994;180:2049–58.
33. Pearson TC, Alexander DZ, Corbascio M, et al. Analysis of the B7 costimulatory pathway in allograft rejection. Transplantation 1997;63:1463–9.
34. Pestana JO, Grinyo JM, Vanrenterghem Y, et al. Three-year outcomes from BENEFIT-EXT: a phase III study of belatacept versus cyclosporine in recipients of extended criteria donor kidneys. Am J Transplant 2012;12:630–9.
35. Sayegh MH, Akalin E, Hancock WW, et al. CD28-B7 blockade after alloantigenic challenge in vivo inhibits Th1 cytokines but spares Th2. J Exp Med 1995;181:1869–74.

36. Sayegh MH, Turka LA. The role of T-cell costimulatory activation pathways in transplant rejection. N Engl J Med 1998;338:1813–21.
37. Szot GL, Zhou P, Sharpe AH, et al. Absence of host B7 expression is sufficient for long-term murine vascularized heart allograft survival. Transplantation 2000;69:904–9.
38. Turka LA, Linsley PS, Lin H, et al. T-cell activation by the CD28 ligand B7 is required for cardiac allograft rejection in vivo. Proc Natl Acad Sci U S A 1992;89:11102–5.
39. Vincenti F, Charpentier B, Vanrenterghem Y, et al. A phase III study of belatacept-based immunosuppression regimens versus cyclosporine in renal transplant recipients (BENEFIT study). Am J Transplant 2010;10:535–46.
40. Vincenti F, Larsen CP, Alberu J, et al. Three-year outcomes from BENEFIT, a randomized, active-controlled, parallel-group study in adult kidney transplant recipients. Am J Transplant 2012;12:210–7.
41. Vincenti F, Larsen C, Durrbach A, et al. Costimulation blockade with belatacept in renal transplantation. N Engl J Med 2005;353:770–81.
42. Vincenti F, Luggen M. T cell costimulation: a rational target in the therapeutic armamentarium for autoimmune diseases and transplantation. Annu Rev Med 2007;58:347–58.
43. Walunas TL, Bakker CY, Bluestone JA. CTLA-4 ligation blocks CD28-dependent T cell activation. J Exp Med 1996;183:2541–50.
44. Yamada A, Salama AD, Sayegh MH. The role of novel T cell costimulatory pathways in autoimmunity and transplantation. J Am Soc Nephrol 2002;13:559–75.

CHAPTER 22

OTHER FORMS OF IMMUNOSUPPRESSION

Ben Sprangers • Jacques Pirenne • Chantal Mathieu • Mark Waer

CHAPTER OUTLINE

SMALL MOLECULES

Leflunomide and Malononitrilamides

Leflunomide, initially developed as an agriculture herbicide, was explored as an immunosuppressant because of its ability to inhibit the enzyme dihydroorotate dehydrogenase.[14] The potential of leflunomide as an immunosuppressant in the field of transplantation was extensively demonstrated in various experimental studies, but its long half-life (several days) poses the problem of potential overimmunosuppression in transplant patients. Analogues of the active metabolite of leflunomide have been developed and are called malononitrilamides (MNAs). FK778 (also known as MNA715 or HMR1715) is the best studied synthetic MNA, and as it has a much shorter half-life than leflunomide (6–45 hours versus 15–18 days) it was believed to represent an attractive alternative to leflunomide for application in organ transplantation.[112]

Chemical Structure and Pharmacology

Leflunomide (*N*-(4)) trifluoro-methylphenyl-5-methylisoxawol-4-carboximide) is a prodrug and is rapidly converted to its biologically active metabolite teriflunomide

(A771703). Serum levels of teriflunomide are referred to as leflunomide levels. The half-life of teriflunomide is long in humans (approximately 15 days). The drug enters the enterohepatic recirculation and is excreted by the intestinal and urinary systems in equal proportions. Leflunomide is insoluble in water and is suspended in 1% carboxymethylcellulose for oral administration.

The MNAs are designed to be structurally similar to A771726. Oral bioavailability of FK778 is not substantially affected by food, and no gender effect on pharmacokinetics was observed in phase I studies.

Mechanism of Action

Leflunomide and its analogues have strong antiproliferative effects on both T lymphocytes and B lymphocytes, thus limiting the formation of antibodies.[41,228] Inhibition of pyrimidine synthesis is the most important mechanism of action as leflunomide directly inhibits the enzyme dihydroorotate dehydrogenase.[289] Lymphocytes rely entirely on the de novo pathway of pyrimidine biosynthesis and cannot use another, the so-called "pyrimidine salvage pathway." Dihydroorotate dehydrogenase inhibition leads to depletion of the nucleotide precursors uridine triphosphate and cytidine triphosphate which are necessary for the synthesis of RNA and DNA, and hence strongly suppress DNA and RNA synthesis.

The in vivo mechanism of action of leflunomide may depend on factors such as drug levels, disposable uridine pools, and the immune activation pathway involved. Studies have indicated that, in addition to inhibition of dihydroorotate dehydrogenase, leflunomide and the MNAs may act through inhibition of tyrosine kinases. Phosphorylation of the epidermal growth factor receptor of human fibroblasts has been shown to be inhibited by leflunomide.[160] It was shown that leflunomide directly inhibited the interleukin (IL)-2-stimulated protein tyrosine kinase activity of p56lck and p59fyn,[160] which is associated with activation through the T-cell receptor/CD3 complex. At higher concentrations, A771726 also inhibited IL-2-induced tyrosine phosphorylation of Janus kinase (JAK)1 and JAK3 protein tyrosine kinases.[60] Leflunomide analogues have also been shown to possess strong inhibitory activity on the antiapoptotic tyrosine kinase Bruton's tyrosine kinase, a key factor for T-cell-independent antibody formation.[150] The hypothesis that leflunomide may exhibit more than one mechanism of action in vivo was further illustrated in mice where uridine restored proliferation and IgM production by lipopolysaccharide-stimulated B cells, whereas suppression of IgG production was not reversed. This phenomenon correlated in a dose-dependent manner with tyrosine phosphorylation of JAK3 and STAT6 proteins, known to be involved in IL-4-induced signal transduction pathways.[228] This double in vivo mechanism of action was confirmed in rats, in which xenoreactivity was counteracted by the administration of uridine, whereas alloreactivity was not.[42]

Also inhibition of various macrophage functions by leflunomide and MNAs has been described; in particular, inhibition of the production of oxygen radicals,[15,116,156] the inhibition of IgE-mediated hypersensitivity responses,[110] the expression of IL-8 receptor type A, as well as tumor necrosis factor (TNF)-mediated nuclear factor kappa B (NF-κB) activation.[155] Tacrolimus also inhibits maturation of dendritic cells by preventing upregulation of activation markers and IL-12 production, and this phenomenon was not reversible by exogenous uridine. FK778 has equivalent or stronger immunosuppressive activity than leflunomide, both in vitro and in vivo.[112] The immunosuppressive effect is synergistic with that of calcineurin inhibitors (CNI) and mycophenolate mofetil (MMF).[21,53]

Interestingly, FK778 and leflunomide have been shown to possess antiviral effects, although the precise mechanism is unclear: inhibition of viral replication of members of the herpesvirus family by preventing tegument acquisition by viral nucleocapsids during the late stage of virion assembly has been implicated.[65,121] Leflunomide is effective against multidrug-resistant cytomegalovirus (CMV) in vitro,[284] although this in vitro activity is modest and the selectivity index is low.[67] This anti-CMV effect of leflunomide and FK778 was confirmed in a rat model of heterotopic heart transplantation.[43,298] Another interesting feature is that both leflunomide and FK778 have vasculoprotective effects, independent of the inhibition of dihydroorotate dehydrogenase.[54,216]

Experimental Experience

In various rodent transplantation studies, leflunomide was shown to be at least equally potent as cyclosporine,[14] and able to synergize with cyclosporine to induce tolerance.[143] Specific characteristics of leflunomide-mediated immunosuppression in rats were its ability to interrupt ongoing acute rejections,[288] and its efficacy in preventing and treating chronic vascular rejection.[291]

One of the most attractive characteristics of leflunomide and the MNAs is their strong capacity to delay xenograft rejection and to induce partial xenograft tolerance.[142] This may be related to the strong suppressive effects of leflunomide on T-cell-independent xenoantibody formation, and on its capacity to induce natural killer cell nonresponsiveness and to modulate xenoantigen expression.[38]

Monotherapy with FK778 in rats,[183] and its combination with microemulsified cyclosporine in dogs[129] or tacrolimus in non-human primates,[197] reduced chronic allograft nephropathy[183] and significantly prolonged renal allograft survival.[129,183,197]

Clinical Experience

The main role of leflunomide in renal transplantation nowadays is the treatment of BK virus nephropathy (BKVN).[115,287] Based on the in vitro effective anti-BK concentration, an in vivo target level of 50–100 mg/mL has been proposed. In a prospective study, 26 renal transplant recipients with biopsy-proven BKVN were treated with leflunomide in combination with discontinuation of MMF and reduction of tacrolimus to a 4–6 ng/mL range.[287] Although the leflunomide levels were in the lower range (on average 50 mg/mL), a significant reduction in serum and urine BKV titers was obtained, allograft function stabilized, and the overall graft loss rates because of BKV were only 15%.[115] Less encouraging results were obtained in another prospective open-label study in which viral clearance was only obtained in 40% of patients with significant toxicity, resulting in discontinuation of the drug in 17% of patients.[66] The contribution of reduction of immunosuppressive agents and leflunomide to the efficacy of BKVN treatment is unclear at this moment.[59,114,265] Based on recent in vitro data, it has been suggested that the combination of sirolimus with leflunomide might be an effective treatment approach.[140] FK778 has also been studied in the context of BKVN, but although it was able to decrease BK viral load, FK778 treatment was associated with more acute rejections, decreased renal function, and more adverse events compared with reduction of immunosuppression.[94]

In animal studies, leflunomide was able to reverse acute and chronic rejection. Two clinical studies reported that leflunomide was capable of stabilizing allograft function in patients with worsening allograft function due to chronic allograft dysfunction.[135]

A phase II multicenter study was performed with FK778 involving 149 renal transplant patients,[276] where FK778 was combined with tacrolimus and corticosteroids. The patients receiving FK778 experienced a reduced number of acute rejections, but there was no effect on graft survival at week 16.[276] The reduction of acute rejection episodes was most pronounced in the subgroup in which target levels were obtained in the second week. Of note, mean total and low-density lipoprotein cholesterol levels were 20% lower in the FK778 group versus the placebo group.[276] The validity of these results was hampered by the design of the study, and, at this time, the development of FK778 in the field of organ transplantation has ceased.

Toxicity

Although rats tolerate leflunomide well, dogs readily develop anemia and gastrointestinal ulcerations. Reportedly, the most frequent side effects in arthritis patients receiving long-term leflunomide treatment were diarrhea (17%), nausea (10%), alopecia (8%), and rash (10%), leading to a dropout rate of ±5%.[230] Recently, thrombotic microangiopathy attributed to leflunomide was reported in patients treated for BKVN.[135] In the above-mentioned phase II study involving FK778, there was a dose-dependent increase in side effects, including anemia, hypokalemia, symptomatic myocardial ischemia, and esophagitis.[276] Other reported side effects are pneumonitis and peripheral neuropathy.[39,118] Leflunomide has teratogenic effects in both animals and humans, and a washout period with cholestyramine is advised for both women and men before considering conception.[177] Combining leflunomide with methotrexate might increase the risk for bone marrow suppression and liver toxicity.[47,241] Furthermore, rifampin accelerates the conversion of leflunomide to teriflunomide, and might increase the levels. Combination with warfarin potentially increases the international normalized ratio.

Conclusion

The role of leflunomide in renal transplantation is limited to the treatment of patients with BKVN and some promising results have been reported in this respect. The MNAs – because of their shorter half-life – were considered a promising class of immunosuppressants but results in randomized clinical trials have been disappointing, and the development of these agents in organ transplantation has been halted.

FTY720 or Fingolimod

Chemical Structure and Pharmacology

FTY720 or 2-amino-2-[2-(4-octylphenyl)ethyl]-1,3-propanediol hydrochloride is a synthetic structural analogue of myriocin, a metabolite of the ascomycete *Isaria sinclairii*, a type of vegetative wasp.[79,80,215] Maximal concentration and area under the curve are proportional to the dose, indicating that the pharmacokinetic profile of FTY720 is linear. The volume of distribution is largely superior to the blood volume, indicating a widespread tissue penetration. FTY720 undergoes hepatic metabolism and has a long half-life (around 100 hours).

Mechanism of Action

FTY720 has a unique mechanism of action as it mainly affects lymphocyte trafficking.[38,97,154,159] FTY720 acts as a high-affinity agonist of the sphingosine 1-phosphate receptor-1 (S1PR1 or Edg1). Binding of its receptor results in internalization of S1PR1, rendering lymphocytes unable to respond to the naturally occurring gradient of S1P (low concentrations in thymus and secondary lymphoid organs, high concentrations in lymph and plasma) retaining lymphocytes in the low-S1P environment of lymphoid organs.[159,186] Following FTY720 administration in mice, B and T cells immediately leave the peripheral blood and migrate to the peripheral lymph nodes, mesenteric lymph nodes. and Peyer's patches. The cells return to the peripheral blood after withdrawal of the drug without undergoing apoptotic death.[297] This altered cell trafficking is accompanied by a reduction of lymphocyte infiltration into grafted organs.[96,297,299] Interestingly, lymphocytes treated ex vivo with FTY720 and reintroduced in vivo similarly migrate to the peripheral lymphoid tissues, indicating that FTY720 acts directly on lymphocytes. This process of accelerated homing was completely blocked in vivo by co-administration of anti-CD62L, anti-CD49d, and anti-CD11a monoclonal antibody.[38] In vitro, FTY720 in the presence of TNF-α increases the expression of certain intercellular adhesion molecules on human endothelial cells.[139] Thus, alteration of cell trafficking by FTY720 may result not only from its direct action on lymphocytes, but also from an effect on endothelial cells.

Interestingly, it has been suggested that $CD4^+CD25^+$ regulatory T cells are differently affected by FTY720 compared to T-effector cells.[217] $CD4^+CD25^+$ regulatory T cells express lower levels of $S1P_1$ and $S1P_4$ receptors and, hence, show reduced response to FTY720. Furthermore, in vitro FTY720-treated $CD4^+CD25^+$ T-regulatory cells possess an increased suppressive activity in an antigen-specific proliferation assay.[217,300]

Unlike CNI, FTY720 is a poor inhibitor of T-cell function in vitro.[267] In particular, FTY720 does not influence antigen-induced IL-2 production. In vitro exposure to high FTY720 concentrations (4×10^{-6}) induces chromatin condensation, typical DNA fragmentation, and formation of apoptotic bodies. Whether administration of FTY720 in vivo is also associated with significant apoptosis is a matter of debate.[38,158]

S1PR are also present on murine dendritic cells. Upon administration of FTY720, dendritic cells in lymph nodes and spleen are reduced, the expression of CD11b, CD31/PECAM-1, CD54/ICAM-1, and CCR-7 is down-regulated, and transendothelial migration to CCL19 is diminished.[132] In a recent study it was demonstrated that FTY720 inhibited lymphangiogenesis and thus prolonged allogeneic islet survival in mice.[295]

Experimental Experience

FTY720 given daily by oral gavage has marked antirejection properties in mice, rats, dogs, and monkeys.[158,249,267,294] FTY720 (0.1–10 mg/kg) prolongs survival of skin allografts in highly allogeneic rodent models.[37] In a DA to LEW rat combination, a short course of peritransplant oral FTY720 (5 mg/kg; days –1 and 0) prolongs cardiac allograft survival and is as efficient as a 10-day posttransplant treatment with tacrolimus at 1 mg/kg.[292] Cardiac and liver allograft survival is prolonged in the ACI to Lew rat model by either induction or maintenance treatment with FTY720.[247] Even delayed administration of FTY720 interrupts an ongoing allograft rejection, suggesting a role for FTY720 as a rescue agent.[248,293] FTY720 blocks not only rejection but also graft-versus-host disease after rat intestinal transplantation.[163] FTY720 may also protect form ischemia-reperfusion injury, partially through its cytoprotective actions.[52,82,153,242]

Both small- and large-animal models provide evidence that FTY720 acts in synergy with CNI, and that this benefit does not result from pharmacokinetic interactions.[248] An induction course with FTY720 acts in synergy with posttransplant tacrolimus in prolongating cardiac allograft survival in rats.[293] A similar phenomenon has been observed when FTY720 is used posttransplant in combination with cyclosporine in rat skin and heart allografts.[102,248] FTY720 shows synergistic effect with CNI in heart and liver transplant in the ACI to Lew rat model.[294] FTY720 shows synergy with cyclosporine in dog kidney (0.1–5 mg/kg/day) and monkey kidney (0.1–1 mg/kg/day) transplantation.[267] Finally, FTY720 (0.1 mg/kg) synergizes with CNI in dog liver transplantation.[250] Synergy between FTY720 and rapamycin was also observed in rat cardiac transplantation.[286]

KRP-203 or 2-amino-2-(2-[4-3(-benzyloxyphenylthio)-2-cholorophenyl]ethyl)-1,3-propanediol hydrochloride has a similar molecular structure as FTY720. KRP-203 alone or in combination with low-dose cyclosporine or MMF prolonged skin, heart, and renal allograft survival.[78,224,246]

Clinical Experience

Stable renal transplant patients maintained on cyclosporine tolerate well one oral dose of FTY720 (0.25–3.5 mg). Similarly to its effect in animals, single doses of FTY720 cause a lymphopenia that is dose-dependent in intensity and duration, and that equally affects CD4 cells, CD8 cells, memory T cells, naïve T cells, and B cells.[29]

In phase II and III studies in de novo renal transplantation, it was shown that 2.5 mg FTY720 in combination with full-dose cyclosporine and steroids is as effective as MMF in combination with full-dose cyclosporine and steroids, although the FTY720-treated patients had lower creatinine clearance at 12 months.[260,261] FTY720 5 mg did not allow a 50% reduction in cyclosporine exposure.[214,260] FTY720 2.5 mg in combination with reduced-dose cyclosporine resulted in underimmunosuppression.[165] Also in combination with tacrolimus, FTY720 2.5 mg was not superior to MMF in a recent study in de novo renal transplant recipients.[100] Recently, it was reported that FTY720 in combination with everolimus was not beneficial with regard to prevention of acute rejection and preservation of allograft function in renal transplant recipients at high risk for delayed graft function.[259]

Toxicity

The side effects of FTY720 are in general similar to those of other immunosuppressants, with hypertension, anemia, constipation, and nausea most commonly reported. Side effects specific for FTY720 are bradycardia, macular/retinal edema, dyspnea, and a transient rise in liver function tests.[165,214] Although it is considered a main impediment of further clinical development, reduction of heart rate after the first dose of FTY720 is transient and does not persist in the maintenance phase.[61,176] Importantly, typical side effects of CNI – nephrotoxicity, neurotoxicity, and diabetogenicity – have not been observed with FTY720.

Conclusion

FTY720 has a unique mechanism of action. The available clinical studies show that FTY720 is not superior to standard care and therefore its future in organ transplantation is uncertain.

1,25-Dihydroxyvitamin D_3 and its Analogues

Chemical Structure and Pharmacology

1,25-Dihydroxyvitamin D_3 ($1,25(OH)_2D_3$) and some of its new synthetic structural analogues are promising immunomodulators with effects in autoimmunity and transplantation immunology. Besides its well-known role in mineral and bone homeostasis, non-classical effects of vitamin D have been increasingly recognized, such as modulation of growth, differentiation, and function of various cell types, regulation of immune responses, cardiovascular processes, and cancer prevention.[20,277] Local vitamin D metabolism allows immune cells to modulate immune response autonomously. Optimal immune functioning of this autocrine and/or paracrine circuit crucially depends on the availability of circulating $1,25(OH)_2D_3$. The exact levels of circulating $1,25(OH)_2D_3$ needed to meet the requirements of "vitamin D sufficiency" are still a matter of debate, especially in the light of the non-classical effects of vitamin D.

Mechanism of Action

A role for $1,25(OH)_2D_3$ in immune regulation is suggested by the presence of its receptor (vitamin D receptor or VDR) in almost all immune cells, including activated CD4 and CD8 cells, B cells, neutrophils, and antigen-presenting cells, hence modulating both innate and adaptive immune responses.[196,251] Moreover, the VDR expression in some immune cells is controlled by immune signals.[10] Furthermore, most immune cells express vitamin D metabolizing enzymes such as CYP27B1 in T and B lymphocytes, and CYP2R1 in dendritic cells.[178,236] This allows for the local conversion of 25(OH)D_3 into 1,25$(OH)_2D_3$, and represents an important mechanism by which immune cells can reach supraphysiological levels of 1,25$(OH)_2D_3$ needed to influence immune responses without affecting systemic levels of 1,25$(OH)_2D_3$. Furthermore, the expression of CYP27B1 in immune cells is controlled by immune signals. For example, CYP27B1 expression by monocytes/macrophages is upregulated by interferon-γ (IFN-γ), lipopolysaccharide, *Mycobacterium tuberculosis*-derived 19 kDa lipoprotein and viral infections. Moreover, CYP27B1 expression in macrophages and dendritic cells is not suppressed by 1,25$(OH)_2D_3$ itself, allowing for massive local production of 1,25$(OH)_2D_3$ by macrophages in patients with granulomatous diseases. As an alternative negative-feedback loop 1,25$(OH)_2D_3$ upregulates CYP24 in immune cells.[56]

Upon exposure to 1,25$(OH)_2D_3$ monocytes acquire phenotypical features of macrophages, and macrophages obtain increased chemotactic and phagocytic activities.[91] Moreover, Toll-like receptor activation of monocytes/macrophages results in upregulation of VDR and VDR target genes leading to the induction of cathelicidin antimicrobial peptide and killing of *Mycobacterium tuberculosis*.[144] 1,25$(OH)_2D_3$ inhibits dendritic cell maturation (decreased levels of major histocompatibility complex class II and costimulatory molecules), enhances endocytic capacity, inhibits the production of IL-12 and IL-23, and enhances the release of IL-10 and macrophage inflammatory protein-3α. Dendritic cells are thereby deviated towards a more immature or tolerogenic phenotype, having in vitro as well as in vivo the capacity to induce the development of regulatory T cells.[89,188,275]

Upon T-cell activation, VDR expression is dramatically increased. Furthermore, 1,25$(OH)_2D_3$ also directly alters the cytokine profile of T cells by inhibiting the production of inflammatory Th1-cytokines such as IL-2 and IFN-γ, as well as the Th17-derived cytokines IL-17 and IL-21.[111,257] $CD4^+CD25^{high}CD127^{low}$ regulatory T cells were induced after vitamin D exposure and IL-10 was selectively induced within CD4T cells. The molecular pathways by which 1,25$(OH)_2D_3$ modulates the expression of these and other genes in the immune system varies widely (reviewed in reference 11). Next to the classical interaction with VDR-specific binding sites in the promoter region of target genes (vitamin D-responsive elements), as in the inhibition of IFN-γ,[45] 1,25$(OH)_2D_3$ also interferes with other pathways of transcription regulation. For example, 1,25$(OH)_2D_3$-mediated inhibition of IL-2 is due to impairment of nuclear factor of activated T cells/activating protein-1 (AP-1) complex formation and subsequent association with its binding site within the IL-2 promoter.[5,253]

Exposing B cells to 1,25$(OH)_2D_3$ inhibits the proliferation, plasma cell differentiation, immunoglobulin secretion (IgG and IgM), and memory B-cell generation, and induces B-cell apoptosis.[36] Finally, 1,25$(OH)_2D_3$ was put forward as an important regulator of lymphocyte trafficking. Active 1,25$(OH)_2D_3$ imprints activated T cells and terminally differentiating B cells with skin-homing properties via induction of the skin-homing receptor CCR10.[225,229]

Experimental Experience

The fact that 1,25$(OH)_2D_3$ and its analogues influence the immune system by immunomodulation through the induction of immune shifts and regulator cells makes these products very appealing for clinical use, especially in the treatment and prevention of autoimmune diseases. In the NOD mouse, upregulation of regulator cells and a shift away from Th1 towards Th2 could be observed in 1,25$(OH)_2D_3$-treated mice, both locally in the pancreas as well as in the peripheral immune system.[90,179] Moreover, a restoration of the defective sensitivity to apoptosis characteristic for NOD T lymphocytes was observed, resulting in a better elimination of autoreactive effector cells.[33,51] This increased sensitivity to apoptosis has been described for different apoptosis-inducing signals. This mechanism may explain why an early and short-term 1,25$(OH)_2D_3$ treatment before the clinical onset of autoimmunity can lead to long-term protection and restoration of self-tolerance.

A clear additive and even synergistic effect was observed between 1,25$(OH)_2D_3$ or its analogues and other more classical immunosuppressants such as cyclosporine, sirolimus, or MMF, both in vitro and in several in vivo autoimmune disease models, such as autoimmune diabetes[34,95] and experimental autoimmune encephalomyelitis.[26,27,272]

Moreover, 1,25$(OH)_2D_3$ and its analogues were investigated in various transplantation models such as pancreatic islet allo- and xenotransplantation in mice,[89,95] allogeneic heart[113] and skin transplantation in mice,[18,278] allogeneic aorta,[199] bone marrow,[180] heart,[106,136] kidney,[201] and liver transplantation in rats.[202] The overall conclusion that can be drawn from these studies is that, as monotherapy, 1,25$(OH)_2D_3$ and its analogues provoke only a modest prolongation of graft function. This is not surprising in view of the rather weak intrinsic effects of 1,25$(OH)_2D_3$ and its analogues on T cells. However, in conjunction with other immunosuppressants, strong synergistic effects often can be observed. In addition, in view of its effect on antigen presentation and on directing the immune system in the Th2 direction, 1,25$(OH)_2D_3$ may help to induce tolerance.[89]

Clinical Experience

Multiple groups have reported a correlation between vitamin D deficiency and susceptibility to respiratory infections, especially in the context of infections by *Mycobacterium tuberculosis* and Gram-negative bacteria.[105] Autier and Gandini performed a meta-analysis including 18 independent randomized controlled trials, demonstrating that administration of vitamin D supplementation is associated with a decrease in overall mortality rates (relative risk 0.93, 95% confidence interval 0.87–0.99).[9] There is still a lack of non-biased large cohort studies that can sustain the proposed benefits of vitamin D supplementation for optimal immune function.

Mutations in the CYP2R1 gene, as well as in the CYP17B1 gene, impairing their enzymatic activity, have been described and polymorphisms in these genes have been proposed to be associated with type 1 diabetes mellitus susceptibility.[146,200] Analogues of vitamin D could successfully block progression of insulitis in prediabetic NOD mice, along with preventing recurrence of autoimmune diabetes in NOD mice after syngeneic islet transplantation, when combined with other immunomodulating agents.[34,89]

Toxicity

A major concern remains the side effects of $1,25(OH)_2D_3$ on calcium and bone metabolism. The use of $1,25(OH)_2D_3$ analogues which have maintained or amplified immunomodulatory effects in combination with reduced effects on calcium and bone partially conquer this problem.[273] The additional use of calcium-lowering conditions, such as limited nutrient calcium intake, and bone resorption inhibitors, such as bisphosphonates, aid in further bypassing the negative side effects of hypercalcemia and excessive bone resorption,[271] thereby facilitating the step towards the clinical applicability of $1,25(OH)_2D_3$ and its analogues for their potent immunomodulatory properties.

Conclusion

With the discovery of VDRs and vitamin D-metabolizing enzymes in immune cells, it is now evident that $1,25(OH)_2D_3$ exerts a plethora of effects targeting both the innate and adaptive immune compartment. The emerging data linking inadequate vitamin D levels to immune anomalies, such as increased infection rates and autoimmunity, are of interest in this context. VDR agonists, and especially hypocalcemic vitamin D analogues, are plausible candidates for the prevention and/or treatment of infections such as tuberculosis and several autoimmune disorders.

Bredinin or Mizoribine

Chemical Structure and Pharmacology

Bredinin, 4-carbamoyl-1-β-D-ribofurano-syhmidazolium-5-olate, is a nucleoside analogue that is structurally similar to ribavirin. It was first isolated from the culture media of the ascomycetes *Eupenicillium brefeldianum* harvested from the soil of Hachijo Island (Japan, 1971). It has weak antibiotic activity against *Candida albicans*.[164]

Mechanism of Action

Bredinin exerts its immunosuppressive function through selective inhibition of the enzymes inosine monophosphate dehydrogenase and guanosine monophosphate synthetase, both of which are required for the generation of guanosine monophosphate from inosine monophosphate in the de novo pathway. In contrast to azathioprine, bredinin is not incorporated into nucleic acids in the cells, resulting in fewer side effects, such as myelosuppression and hepatoxicity. Bredinin was found to inhibit both humoral and cellular immunity by selectively inhibiting lymphocyte proliferation.[108]

Experimental and Clinical Experience

In a canine model of renal transplantation, bredinin prolonged graft survival. In humans, as compared to azathioprine, bredinin showed equally potent immunosuppressive activity and fewer adverse effects.[8,122,254,256] As expected based on its similarity in structure to ribavirine, bredinin exhibits in vitro antiviral activity against CMV, respiratory syncytial virus, measles, hepatitis C, corona virus, parainfluenza, and influenza virus.[103,169,210,223] In a recent study, bredinin was substituted for MMF in patients with BKV in their urine. BKV DNA in the urine became negative in five out of seven patients.[83] In the remaining two patients, there was a significant decrease in urinary BKV DNA. No acute rejection or deterioration of graft function occurred during the study period.[83]

Toxicity

The principal adverse reactions associated with the use of bredinin were leukopenia, abnormal hepatic function, rash, increased levels of uric acid, and vomiting.

Conclusion

Bredinin has mainly been used in Japan and is infrequently used elsewhere. As a consequence, experience with bredinin is limited, but results show that it is a safe and effective immunosuppressant in human kidney transplantation. Because of its antiviral activity, bredinin might be yet another drug to be evaluated in the setting of BKVN.

JAK3 Inhibitors: CP-690,550, Tasocitinib, or Tofacitinib

Several JAK3 inhibitors have been developed, e.g., tyrphostin AG-490, PNU156804, dimethoxyquinazoline compounds (WHI-P131), CP-690,550 and Mannich base NC1153, and several of them have been shown to possess immunosuppressive properties.[17,119,126,235] Given the lymphocyte-restricted role of JAK3, JAK3 inhibitors are considered an interesting novel class of immunosuppressive drugs.

Chemical Structure and Pharmacology

Of the multiple potential candidate compounds, one has entered clinical trials – the ATP congener CP-690,550 (CP; tasocitinib or tofacitinib, Pfizer, NJ), which binds to the ATP catalytic site on JAK molecules. It has been proposed that analysis of P-STAT5 at the cellular level could be an adequate means to monitor the immunomodulatory effect of CP-690,550.[198]

Mechanism of Action

JAK3 is a tyrosine kinase essential for the signal transduction from the common gamma-chain of the cytokine receptors for IL-2, IL-4, IL-7, IL-9, IL-15, and IL-21 to the nucleus. As the expression of the receptors is restricted to immune cells, this makes them an attractive target for new immunosuppressants. Signal transduction mediated by JAK3 is obligatory for lymphocyte activation, differentiation, and homeostasis, as evidenced by the finding that deficiency in JAK3 results in severe combined deficiency syndrome.[148,204,206,207] A possible detrimental effect of interference with IL-2 signaling relates to the fact that tolerance induction is essentially dependent on the IL-2 pathway.[128,151,152] Thus, the challenge for immunosuppressive drug design has been to achieve selective inhibition of JAK3 versus JAK2 activities. Although Pfizer claimed a 20-fold selectivity for JAK3 using an in vitro assay, clinical data suggest that this ratio is far less than 20-fold. This narrow selectivity was confirmed by the work of Karaman et al.[117]

Experimental Experience

CP-690,550 is the most potent (inhibitory potency of 1 nM) and selective JAK3 inhibitor developed to date. In both rodents and non-human primates, CP-690,550 exerted strong suppression of immune reactions and prolonged the survival of cardiac and renal allografts. In monotherapy it significantly delayed the onset of rejection in kidney allografts.[24,25,35] In non-human primates, CP-690,550 significantly reduced IL-2-enhanced IFN-γ production and CD25 and CD71 expression by T cells. Furthermore, CP-690,550 inhibited cellular alloimmune responses in vitro.[35,184] Administration in vivo resulted in a reduction of NK cell and T-cell numbers, whereas CD8 effector memory T-cell levels were unaltered.[46,184] Recently, it was shown that CP-690,550 selectively inhibits T-cell effector function while preserving the suppressive activity of CD4$^+$CD25^{high} regulatory T cells.[222]

Clinical Experience

CP-690,550 was evaluated as induction and maintenance therapy in a phase IIA, multicenter, open-label, randomized controlled trial in kidney transplant recipients.[31] All patients received induction therapy, MMF, and steroids. Patients in group 1 received tacrolimus, while patients in groups 2 and 3 were administered CP-690,550 15 mg and 30 mg twice a day, respectively.[31] Because of the high incidence of BKVN in the CP-690,550 groups, the protocol was adjusted to stop MMF and decrease the steroid exposure. Compared to tacrolimus, both CP-690,550 groups showed similar rates of acute rejection episodes and allograft function, but experienced greater incidences of hyperlipidemia and infections (suggestive of additional JAK2 inhibition).[31] A phase IIB trial compared cyclosporine at standard dosage versus CP-690,550 15 mg twice a day for 6 months then 10 mg twice a day, or CP-690,550 15 mg twice a day for 3 months then 10 mg twice a day. All patients received in addition induction therapy, MMF, and steroids. Unexpectedly, the lower CP-690,550 dosage arm showed a trend toward the lowest rejection rate and a superior allograft function. However, in this study there were important adverse events, including increased CMV infection rates, and BKVN in both CP-690,550 arms (data presented at 2011 American Transplant Congress).

Toxicity

In a dose escalation study, the most frequent adverse events were infection and gastrointestinal side effects. CP-690,550 15 mg and 30 mg twice a day were associated with a mean decrease in hemoglobin from baseline of 11%.[274] There was in addition a decrease in natural killer cells and B cells. There were no changes in the number of neutrophils, total lymphocytes, platelets, or CD4 or CD8 T cells.[274]

Conclusion

In summary, combination of CP-690,550 with MMF resulted in acceptable rates of acute rejection with evidence of overimmunosuppression when CP-690,550 30 mg twice a day was combined with MMF. CP-690,550 15 mg twice a day co-administered with MMF resulted in similar outcomes while associated with modest lipid elevations and a higher rate of viral infections. In our opinion, considering the known side-effect profile of CNI, further evaluation of CP-690,550 is warranted. Given the side effects reported with the use of CP-690,550, the challenge remains to develop immunosuppressive drugs with truly selective inhibition of JAK3 versus JAK2 activities. The lack of success in developing a selective antagonist of JAK3 probably relates to the focus on chemical analogues of ATP while more success is to be expected from developing molecules displaying allosteric inhibition via binding of non-catalytic sites.

AEB071 or Sotrastaurin

Chemical Structure and Pharmacology

Sotrastaurin (AEB071) is a low-molecular-weight, synthetic compound that potently and reversibly inhibits all 10 isoforms of protein kinase C (PKC) – most importantly, PKC-θ, PKC-α, and PKC-β, with lesser activity on PKC-δ.[123] Sotrastaurin is primarily metabolized through hepatic CYP3A4 into inactive metabolites and *N*-desmethyl-sotrastaurin, which has similar potency as sotrastaurin and is present at low blood concentrations (less than 5% of the parent exposure). Renal excretion of sotrastaurin is negligible and only a small amount is excreted in the bile (1% of the dose). The elimination half-life of sotrastaurin averages 6 hours. In clinical trials, it is recommended that patients administer sotrastaurin consistently either with or without food to avoid food-related fluctuations in drug exposure over time.[123]

Clinical drug interaction studies to date have demonstrated that sotrastaurin increases the area under the concentration–time curve of everolimus (1.2-fold) and of tacrolimus (2-fold).[124] Sotrastaurin increased tacrolimus concentration inasmuch as the tacrolimus dose needed to achieve a given C_0 was up to 47% lower when combined with sotrastaurin versus MMF.[124] Conversely, sotrastaurin area under the concentration–time curve is increased up to 1.8-fold by cyclosporine and 4.6-fold by ketoconazole.[125]

Mechanism of Action

PKC is a family of serine/threonine-specific protein kinases involved in diverse signal transduction pathways that modulate a whole range of cellular processes, including activation, proliferation, differentiation, apoptosis, and autophagy.[231] PKC-θ has been shown to be essential in the T-cell receptor/CD3 signal transduction pathway. PKC-α modulates Th1 responses, including IFN-γ production. PKC-β controls B-cell receptor-induced NF-κB transactivation and T-independent B-cell responses. Finally, PKC-ε influences macrophage function.[161,255]

Experimental Experience

Of note, sotrastaurin was demonstrated to be non-toxic when added to human islet cultures.[162] These results suggest AEB071 to be an appropriate immunosuppressive candidate for clinical trials in islet transplantation. Recently, it was shown in non-human primates that sotrastaurin in combination with cyclosporine at subtherapeutic doses resulted in markedly prolonged renal allograft survival, indicating synergistic immunosuppressive effects.[19]

Clinical Experience

In a phase II randomized controlled trial, sotrastaurin with standard or reduced tacrolimus was compared with standard tacrolimus alone, in addition to induction therapy and steroids.[30] Three months posttransplant, stable patients on sotrastaurin were switched from tacrolimus to MMF. The three arms showed equal efficacy up to 3 months; at the end of the study there was no difference in allograft function, although the incidence of acute rejection was significantly higher in the standard tacrolimus with sotrastaurin arm.[30] Because of lack of efficacy, this study was prematurely discontinued. In another recent trial in de novo renal transplant recipients with immediate graft function, study subjects were randomized to sotrastaurin or tacrolimus.[73] All patients received basiliximab, MMF, and steroids. This study demonstrated a lower degree of efficacy but better renal function with the CNI-free regimen of sotrastaurin with MMF versus the tacrolimus-based control.[73] A study combining sotrastaurin with everolimus is currently ongoing.

Toxicity

In the above-mentioned clinical trial, there was a 12% incidence of tachycardia and 18% of serious infections.[30,73] A dose-dependent chronotropic effect has been observed in preclinical and phase I sotrastaurin studies; therefore the higher heart rate and tachycardia observed with the sotrastaurin in combination with MMF were not unexpected. All tachycardia adverse events were mild and the majority occurred soon after transplantation.

Conclusion

Sotrastaurin blocks PKC-mediated early T-cell activation,[20] providing a new approach for immunosuppression distinct from CNI. However, the efficacy results of this phase II study do not support the combination of sotrastaurin 300 mg twice a day with MMF as a CNI-free regimen. Based on the results recently reported by Bigaud et al. in non-human primates,[19] sotrastaurin as a CNI-sparing agents warrants further evaluation in future clinical trials.

Bortezomib

Chemical Structure and Pharmacology

Bortezomib is a proteasomal inhibitor approved by the Food and Drug Administration for the treatment of multiple myeloma. Bortezomib is increasingly used in the setting of solid-organ transplantation. Bortezomib was administered in four doses of 1.3 mg/m^2 intravenously in 3-5-minute infusions over an 11-day period in kidney transplant recipients. Prior to bortezomib administration, patients need to be premedicated with methylprednisolone. Peak serum concentration is reached at 30 minutes and the drug is cleared within 1 hour.[62]

Mechanism of Action

Bortezomib is a selective inhibitor of the 26S proteasome, preventing the activation of NF-κB.[244] It induces apoptosis of rapidly dividing, metabolically active cells with extensive protein synthesis. The ability of bortezomib to target plasma cells spurred interest as a new therapeutic approach in the treatment or prevention of alloantibody formation in organ transplantation.

Experimental Experience

In vitro, bortezomib was associated with a reduction in the number of bone marrow-derived plasma cells and attenuated alloantibody production.[193] Bortezomib primarily acts through plasma cell depletion, resulting in reduced antibody production to T-dependent antigens. As marginal zone B cells are resistant to bortezomib-mediated effects, T-independent type 2 responses are less affected.[133] In a mouse model of lupus, bortezomib depleted both short- and long-lived plasma cells, resulting in a reduction of anti-double-stranded DNA antibody production.[170] Vogelbacher et al. recently established that bortezomib alone or in combination with sirolimus can also prevent alloantibody formation in a rat model of kidney transplantation.[279]

Clinical Experience

Bortezomib therapy for antibody-mediated rejection has resulted in mixed results.[55,63,218] Everly et al. administered bortezomib to 6 patients with antibody-mediated rejection with concomitant acute cellular rejection refractory to currently available therapies.[63] Bortezomib administration resulted in resolution of antibody-mediated rejection in all 6 patients, a decrease of donor-specific antibody levels, and improvement of allograft function.[63]

In another study, Walsh et al. reported the results of bortezomib treatment in 28 patients with antibody-mediated rejection.[285] Bortezomib treatment was associated with variable results, with better responses in early (occurring in the first 6 months after transplantation) versus late (occurring 6 months or more after transplantation) antibody-mediated rejection.[285] In contrast, in the study of Sberro-Soussan et al., bortezomib treatment did not result in a decrease of donor-specific antibody mean fluorescence intensity when used as sole desensitization therapy in four renal transplant recipients with subacute antibody-mediated rejection with persistent donor-specific antibodies.[218] However, in this study bortezomib therapy was not initiated until weeks or months following the diagnosis of antibody-mediated rejection, and repeat biopsies were not performed following bortezomib treatment.[218]

Toxicity

The most common side effects associated with bortezomib treatment are gastrointestinal toxicity, thrombocytopenia, and neuropathy.[63] These can be potentially severe and disabling. To date, no increase in rate of opportunistic infections has been reported. Importantly, although bortezomib is associated with substantial reductions in donor-specific antibody levels, it does not result in a decrease in protective antibody levels.[64]

Conclusion

Proteasome inhibitor therapy has potential in the treatment of antibody-mediated rejection in kidney transplant recipients both as primary and rescue therapy. Optimal responses with bortezomib are obtained when antibody-mediated rejection occurs early posttransplant and bortezomib treatment is initiated promptly. Bortezomib has recently also been shown to provide effective therapy for antibody-mediated rejection in heart and lung transplant recipients.[57,171]

Others

Cladiribine is an adenosine deaminase-resistant analogue of deoxyadenosine and is used in the treatment of leukemia and lymphoma. A number of studies have explored the immunosuppressive capacity of cladiribine. In vitro, cladribine inhibits both B- and T-cell proliferation.[86] In vivo, cladiribine monotherapy was shown to prolong skin allograft survival in mice,[87] in combination with cyclosporine it prolonged liver and heart allograft survival in rats,[221] and was more effective than cyclosporine monotherapy in small-bowel allografts.[174] However, no clinical trials are published to date.

The farnesyltransferase inhibitor A 228839 was developed as an anticancer compound that inhibits Ras GTPases. A 228839 inhibited lectin-induced proliferation and antigen-presenting cell-induced T-cell proliferation. The compound also inhibited lymphocyte Th1 cytokine production and promoted apoptosis in lectin-activated lymphocytes.[227] Another farnesyltransferase inhibitor, ABT-100 was shown in vitro to block the secretion of IFN-γ and IL-4 by naïve T cells and suppressed alloreactivity. In a rat heterotopic cardiac transplant model, ABT-100 alone or in combination with subtherapeutic dose of cyclosporine delayed the development of acute rejection.[226] Given its combined antirejection and antioncogenic effects, farnesyltransferase inhibitors could represent an attractive new class of immunosuppressants in malignancy-prone organ transplant recipients if future clinical trials confirm their efficacy.

When a T-cell receptor recognizes its specific antigen the lymphoid cell-specific kinase lck is phosphorylated and, together with the receptor-associated CD3 complex, phosphorylates zinc-associated phosphorylase 70. These events trigger the downstream cascade that increases intracellular calcium, activating calcineurin. Inhibitors of lck have become available recently. A-770041 and structurally similar molecules have been shown to prolong the survival of heterotopic murine heart and renal subcapsular islet grafts as well as to blunt the production of immunoglobulin IgG2a. Emodin ($C_{15}H_{10}O_5$), the cyclic derivative from rhubarb root and rhizomes, has been shown to prolong murine skin graft survival and to dampen IL-2 production.[145] However, neither of these archetypal compounds shows sufficient specificity for lck versus other kinases to warrant clinical development.[227]

FR 252921, an immunosuppressive agent isolated from the culture of *Pseudomonas fluorescens*, inhibits AP-1 transcription activity, and acts predominantly against antigen-presenting cells. FR 252921 demonstrated synergy with tacrolimus in vitro and in vivo. In murine models of skin transplantation, compared with the optimal dose of tacrolimus alone, the combination of FR 252921 and tacrolimus prolonged graft survival.[75–77]

Brequinar sodium exerts its immunosuppressive effects through the inhibition of the enzyme dihydroorotate dehydrogenase, resulting in inhibition of both T and B lymphocytes. Although the characteristics of brequinar suggest that it would be an attractive immunosuppressant, the suboptimal pharmacologic profile jeopardizes its use in transplant patients. The future use of this drug in the field of transplantation will require the development of analogues exhibiting a shorter half-life and reduced toxicity.

Spergualin was originally isolated from the culture filtrate of *Bacillus laterosporus*, and explored as a new anticancer or antibiotic substance. Its analogue 15-deoxyspergualin subsequently became widely known as a promising new immunosuppressant. The precise mode of action of 15-deoxyspergualin is largely unknown and, because of its poor oral bioavailability, 15-deoxyspergualin must be delivered parenterally, which hampers its widespread clinical use.[263] Its efficacy has been demonstrated in the treatment of kidney allograft rejection, ABO-incompatible kidney transplantation, and transplantation in sensitized patients.[6,93,252] Until analogues are developed that allow oral administration,[134] the major clinical indication of 15-deoxyspergualin is limited to the treatment of rejection crises where 15-deoxyspergualin may be an interesting alternative to steroids or antilymphocyte agents. The fact that it remains effective after recurrent administration is promising.

Upon cellular uptake, cyclophosphamide is extensively metabolized into its active compounds phosphoramide mustard and acrolein.[22,49] The reaction of the phosphoramide mustard with DNA results in cell death.[50] Because of its limited efficacy and multiple side effects, the only standard indication for cyclophosphamide in transplantation today is the desensitization of highly sensitized recipients prior to kidney transplantation.[1] Most of these protocols involve repeated plasmapheresis, in combination with cyclophosphamide, either with or without continuation of steroids, until a kidney transplant becomes available.

TOTAL LYMPHOID IRRADIATION

For several decades, total lymphoid irradiation (TLI) has been used for the treatment of Hodgkin's disease. The possibility of applying TLI as an immunosuppressive regimen rather than an anticancer treatment was discovered by investigators at Stanford University.[81]

Procedure

TLI is delivered through two ports. A first so-called mantle port includes the lymph nodes of the neck, axilla, and mediastinum. The other port is called the "inverted Y" and encompasses aortic, iliac and pelvic lymph nodes, and spleen. Usually, a total dose of 40–50 Gy (1 Gy = 100 rad) is administered in daily fractions of 1.5–2.5 Gy.

Mechanisms of Action

Much of the currently available experimental evidence on the immunological mechanisms underlying TLI-induced tolerance points to the importance of suppressor cells. The group of Strober identified post-TLI suppressors cells as host-type natural killer T cells, as the protective effect of TLI against graft-versus-host disease was abrogated in mice with a CD1d inactivated gene.[130] These host-type natural killer T cells produced IL-4 and stimulated donor-type cells to produce IL-4 also.[130,131] Definitive evidence of the functional importance and activity of these suppressor cells was delivered by the demonstration that they could prevent graft-versus-host disease in vivo.[99] Post-TLI attenuation of effector T-lymphocyte reactivity was equally proposed to be responsible for the observed immunosuppressed state after TLI.[16,68,69] This intrinsic T-cell defect was dependent on the irradiation of both thymus and extrathymic tissues.[181] After TLI, anergized T cells were shown to be incapable of proliferating even in the presence of exogenous IL-2.[71] In other studies, TLI was shown to lead to thymic clonal deletion of donor- or host-reactive lymphocytes.[211] TLI-treated mice also exhibited decreased antidonor cytotoxic T-cell precursor frequencies.[72] Finally, Strober's group showed that Th2 lymphocytes recover soon after TLI, whereas Th1 lymphocytes remain deficient for several months,[15] and showed that this defect can also be prevented by thymic shielding during irradiation.[16] This Th2 dominance after TLI has been confirmed by other groups in rodents[70] and in large animals.[233] Recently, Nador et al. demonstrated that tolerance induction after conditioning with TLI and antithymocyte globulin (ATG) depends upon the ability of naturally occurring regulatory natural killer T cells and regulatory T cells to suppress the residual alloreactive T cells that are capable of rejecting the allograft.[167]

Experimental Experience

TLI-treated BALB/c mice receiving fully allogeneic C57BL6 bone marrow and skin graft on the first day after TLI became stable hematopoietic chimeras without signs of graft-versus-host disease, and developed permanent donor-specific tolerance with preserved anti-third-party reactivity.[239] Tolerance induction was critically dependent on the width of the irradiation field, the time of transplantation after TLI, the total dose of TLI, and the absence of presensitization.[239,280,281]

Although bone marrow chimerism could be easily induced, tolerance to either heart[88] or kidney allografts[104] was not obtained, suggesting that TLI-induced bone marrow chimerism does not necessarily create tolerance toward organ-specific antigens.

The combination of TLI and low-dose cyclosporine was found to be effective and clinically safe in rats,[208] and TLI with postoperative ATG induced permanent and specific transplantation tolerance toward heart allografts in about 40% of transplanted dogs.[238] These encouraging results led to a similar trial in clinical kidney transplantation. Myburgh et al. applied a modified TLI regimen in baboons, with low dosage and wide-field exposure, and showed that tolerance can be achieved in larger animals without concomitant bone marrow transplantation.[166]

Also, in heart or heart–lung transplantation experiments between xenogeneic non-human primate species, preoperative TLI, when administered in combination with cyclosporine and ATG,[209] cyclosporine and splenectomy[23] or cyclosporine and medrol,[185] was more efficient than any other treatment regimen. Pretransplant TLI, combined with cyclosporine and methotrexate in a pig heart-into-baboon model, resulted in a graft survival time of more than 2 weeks. This regimen was able to inhibit xenoreactive natural antibody production but not the xenoreactivity of macrophages. In a pig islet-into-rat xenograft model, TLI in combination with deoxyspergualin was extremely effective,[262] and even in a discordant lamb-into-pig model, TLI synergized with cyclosporine and azathioprine to provoke a 30-fold increase of the mean xenograft survival time.[264]

The principal disadvantage for the clinical application of TLI is that the complete regimen of fractionated daily irradiations needs to be administered and completed before, and sufficiently close to, the moment of transplantation, and finding a suitable donor organ within such a restricted timeframe is problematic. Investigators have therefore explored the possibility of using TLI after transplantation. In mouse and rat heart allograft models, posttransplant TLI significantly prolonged graft survival when combined with monoclonal anti-CD4 antibodies[266] or with infusion of donor-type dendritic cell precursors.[98]

Clinical Experience

The first clinical kidney transplants utilizing TLI were performed at the University of Minnesota in 20 patients who had previously rejected a renal allograft.[168] Because similar results (an increase of about 30% 1-year graft survival compared with historical control data) were achieved in this patient population using cyclosporine, and because of the ease of administration, the investigators concluded to prefer cyclosporine over TLI.

In the 1980s, a controlled trial was performed at the University of Leuven, in which end-stage diabetic nephropathy patients received cadaveric kidney allografts, investigating the effect of pretransplant TLI (20 daily fractions of 1 Gy, followed by 1 weekly TLI dose until a suitable donor was found) followed by low-dose posttransplant prednisone maintenance treatment.[283] Long-term (8-year) follow-up revealed that rejection episodes were more frequent, and patient and graft survival significantly inferior in the TLI-treated group.[282] The excess mortality in the TLI-treated patients was due to sepsis, resulting from high-dose steroid therapy needed to treat rejection crises. This clinical experience confirmed the animal data that also showed that TLI by itself is insufficient to provoke long-term graft survival or tolerance and that extra manipulations are needed.

In a study at Stanford University, 24 patients received a first, and one patient a second, cadaveric renal allograft using TLI and ATG.[138] The actuarial graft survival was 76% and 68% at 1 and 2 years, respectively. Ten of the 25 patients never had a rejection crisis despite an overall poor HLA-matching between donor and recipient. In follow-up studies, a specific antidonor mixed lymphocyte culture hypo- or non-responsiveness was demonstrated[44] and, in some patients, all immunosuppressive drugs could be withdrawn.[237] An evaluation in a larger group of 52 patients treated with the same protocol at the same center showed a 3-year graft survival of about 50%, which is less than in cyclosporine-treated patients (around 75%).[138]

Posttransplant TLI in combination with anti-CD3 monoclonal antibodies, or with ATG and donor-specific blood transfusions, seemed very effective in a rat heart allograft model. On the basis of these results, the efficacy of TLI was evaluated in heart transplant patients with therapy-resistant or early vascular rejection.[107,137,213] This resulted in a significant reduction of rejection recurrences, an effect which was maintained for at least 2 years. In the meantime, these favorable results have been confirmed by several other groups. Also, TLI-treated patients develop less coronary atherosclerosis than matched controls despite multiple rejection episodes.[7,40,149,187,270]

Scandling et al. have reported the use of TLI to induce tolerance in the setting of combined kidney/hematopoietic stem cell transplantation between HLA-matched donor/recipient pairs.[219,220] Patients received a conditioning regimen of 10 doses of TLI (80–120 cGy), five doses of rabbit ATG, MMF for 1 month, and cyclosporine for at least 6 months. Donor hematopoietic stem cells were injected intravenously on day 11 in the outpatient infusion center.[220] The majority of patients (8/12) were able to discontinue antirejection medications, and all patients had excellent graft function at the last observation point. The reason for continued immunosuppressive therapy was recurrence of focal segmental glomerulosclerosis in one of four patients and rejection episodes during the tapering of cyclosporine in the three other patients.[220]

Conclusion

TLI has been shown to be a safe immunosuppressive regimen. It has been abandoned in clinical practice for organizational reasons, except for the treatment of therapy-resistant rejection of heart or heart–lung transplant. However, its ability to induce tolerance – in combination with ATG and hematopoietic stem cell transplantation – might renew interest in this treatment modality. To date, no evidence of radiation-related late effects has been documented with TLI.[141]

PHOTOPHERESIS

Extracorporeal photopheresis is a technique in which leukocytes, removed from patients by leukopheresis, are exposed to 8-methoxypsoralen and ultraviolet A light. It was developed as an immunoregulatory treatment for erythrodermic cutaneous T-cell lymphoma.[58] Subsequently, the procedure was shown to be safe as an alternative treatment for various human immune and autoimmune diseases.[192] Furthermore, in rats[191] and monkeys,[189] the regimen was shown to result in extended skin allograft and cardiac allograft and xenograft survival.

Different mechanisms have been shown to contribute to the immunomodulatory effect of photopheresis: selective inhibition of effector cells,[190,191] induction of a high rate of apoptosis,[296] increased capacity to phagocytose apoptotic T cells, resulting in the induction of anticlonotypic immune responses,[205] shift towards Th2 immune activation,[12] and induction of regulatory CD4 and CD8 cells.[84,92]

In clinical transplantation, photopheresis has been applied as both a therapeutic and prophylactic option. It has been applied in the treatment of recurrent or resistant acute rejection in renal transplant patients,[12,48,85,101,127,243,290] but the number of patients included in these studies is limited, and prospective randomized trials are needed. The safety and efficacy of photopheresis in the prevention of acute rejection of cardiac allografts have been evaluated in primary cardiac allograft recipients, randomly assigned to standard triple-drug immunosuppressive therapy (cyclosporine, azathioprine, and prednisone) alone or in conjunction with 24 photopheresis sessions performed during the first 6 months after transplantation. After 6 months of follow-up, photopheresis-treated patients developed significantly fewer multiple rejections, and there were no significant differences in the rates or types of infection. Although there was no significant effect on graft survival rates at 6 or 12 months, this study indicated that photopheresis may be an effective new immunosuppressive regimen in transplant recipients.[13] In patients with refractory bronchiolitis obliterans after lung transplantation, photopheresis resulted in a stabilization of graft function and/or in some of these patients in histological reversal of rejection.[173,212]

SPLENECTOMY

Pretransplant splenectomy in the recipient before transplantation was first proposed by Starzl et al. in 1963 as a means of improving graft survival.[234] Although splenectomy is a standard procedure for patients who develop hypersplenism or azathioprine-associated leukopenia, evidence on the role of splenectomy in enhancing graft survival is controversial.[175,195,234,240] A large prospective randomized trial in Minneapolis showed splenectomy improved graft survival significantly,[74] but longer-term follow-up showed loss of beneficial effects because of an increased infection-related mortality.[245] Several other single-center studies have shown an alarming risk of sepsis and death, nullifying any early benefits of splenectomy on graft survival,[2,194] and a multicenter analysis from the South Eastern Organ Procurement Foundation confirmed a modest improvement in graft survival after splenectomy, but a relentless increase in patient mortality.[147]

Splenectomy has a place in the preparation of a recipient who is to receive an ABO-incompatible graft, a practice that is likely to become more widely employed in living related donor transplantation, where an ABO-incompatible but otherwise suitable donor is the only available donor. Alexandre et al. reported a series of 38 such ABO-incompatible living donor transplants in which the recipient was prepared by plasmapheresis, donor-specific platelet transfusion, and splenectomy.[3,203,232] Although the authors believe that the need for plasmapheresis and donor-specific platelet transfusion should be re-evaluated, splenectomy was thought to be important, since 3 of 38 recipients who did not have a splenectomy lost their grafts from acute vascular rejection, in contrast to only 5 of 33 who did undergo splenectomy. A small-scale but successful experience with postsplenectomy ABO-incompatible living donor kidney transplantation has also been reported by Ishikawa et al. in Japan.[109] In the setting of ABO-incompatible kidney transplantation, antigen-specific immunoadsorption, rituximab, and bortezomib treatment have been developed as alternatives to plasmapheresis and splenectomy. This will further reduce the indications for splenectomy in organ transplantation.[268,269]

PLASMAPHERESIS

Plasmapheresis has been applied in three settings related to organ transplantation. The first is in the treatment of steroid-resistant acute rejection that is morphologically predominantly vascular, and considered to be antibody-mediated rather than cell-mediated. Although some initial reports suggested a beneficial effect,[32] controlled trials were unconvincing.[4,120] Nojima et al. reported the successful treatment of antibody-mediated acute renal allograft rejection by combining plasmapheresis with 15-deoxyspergualin.[172] The second setting is in the preparation of recipients of ABO-incompatible living donor kidneys, referred to earlier,[3,203,232] although Bryngier et al. have reported some successful ABO-incompatible grafts without prior plasmapheresis of the recipient.[28] In a third setting, plasmapheresis is used in an attempt to reduce the titer and the broad reactivity of HLA antibodies in highly sensitized candidate transplant dialysis patients, where it is combined with cyclophosphamide/rituximab therapy to prevent reappearance of the antibodies.[157] Encouraging early results of this approach have been reported, although they were associated with considerable morbidity.[258] Immunoabsorption has been applied as an alternative to plasmapheresis, and was found to be an equally efficient method.[182,268] Studies of this approach in highly sensitized candidate transplant recipients are continuing.

REFERENCES

1. Alarabi A, Backman U, Wikstrom B, et al. Plasmapheresis in HLA-immunosensitized patients prior to kidney transplantation. Int J Artif Organs 1997;20:51.
2. Alexander JW, First MR, Majeski JA, et al. The late adverse effect of splenectomy on patient survival following cadaveric renal transplantation. Transplantation 1984;37:467.
3. Alexandre GP, Squifflet JP, De Bruyere M, et al. Present experiences in a series of 26 ABO-incompatible living donor renal allografts. Transplant Proc 1987;19:4538.
4. Allen NH, Dyer P, Geoghegan T, et al. Plasma exchange in acute renal allograft rejection. A controlled trial. Transplantation 1983;35:425.
5. Alroy I, Towers TL, Freedman LP. Transcriptional repression of the interleukin-2 gene by vitamin D3: direct inhibition of NFATp/AP-1 complex formation by a nuclear hormone receptor. Mol Cell Biol 1995;15:5789.
6. Amemiya H, Koyama I, Kyo M, et al. Outline and long-term prognosis in 15-deoxyspergualin-treated cases. Japan Collaborative Transplant Study Group of NKT-01. Transplant Proc 1996;28:1156.
7. Asano M, Gundry SR, Razzouk AJ, et al. Total lymphoid irradiation for refractory rejection in pediatric heart transplantation. Ann Thorac Surg 2002;74:1979.
8. Aso K, Uchida H, Sato K, et al. Immunosuppression with low-dose cyclosporine combined with bredinin and prednisolone. Transplant Proc 1987;19:1955.
9. Autier P, Gandini S. Vitamin D supplementation and total mortality: a meta-analysis of randomized controlled trials. Arch Intern Med 2007;167:1730.
10. Baeke F, Korf H, Overbergh L, et al. Human T lymphocytes are direct targets of 1,25-dihydroxyvitamin D3 in the immune system. J Steroid Biochem Mol Biol 2010;121:221.
11. Baeke F, Takiishi T, Korf H. Vitamin D: modulator of the immune system. Curr Opin Pharmacol 2010;10:482.
12. Baron ED, Heeger PS, Hricik DE, et al. Immunomodulatory effect of extracorporeal photopheresis after successful treatment of resistant renal allograft rejection. Photodermatol Photoimmunol Photomed 2001;17:79.
13. Barr ML, Meiser BM, Eisen HJ, et al. Photopheresis for the prevention of rejection in cardiac transplantation. Photopheresis Transplantation Study Group. N Engl J Med 1998;339:1744.
14. Bartlett RR, Dimitrijevic M, Mattar T, et al. Leflunomide (HWA 486), a novel immunomodulating compound for the treatment of autoimmune disorders and reactions leading to transplantation rejection. Agents Actions 1991;32:10.
15. Bass H, Mosmann T, Strober S. Evidence for mouse Th1- and Th2-like helper T cells in vivo. Selective reduction of Th1-like cells after total lymphoid irradiation. J Exp Med 1989;170:1495.
16. Bass H, Strober S. Deficits in T helper cells after total lymphoid irradiation (TLI): reduced IL-2 secretion and normal IL-2 receptor expression in the mixed leukocyte reaction (MLR). Cell Immunol 1990;126:129.
17. Behbod F, Erwin-Cohen RA, Wang ME, et al. Concomitant inhibition of Janus kinase 3 and calcineurin-dependent signaling pathways synergistically prolongs the survival of rat heart allografts. J Immunol 2001;166:3724.

18. Bertolini DL, Araujo PR, Silva RN, et al. Immunomodulatory effects of vitamin D analog KH1060 on an experimental skin transplantation model. Transplant Proc 1999;31:2998.
19. Bigaud M, Wieczorek G, Beerli C, et al. Sotrastaurin (AEB071) alone and in combination with cyclosporine A prolongs survival times of non-human primate recipients of life-supporting kidney allografts. Transplantation 2012;93:156.
20. Bikle D. Nonclassic actions of vitamin D. J Clin Endocrinol Metab 2009;94:26.
21. Bilolo KK, Ouyang J, Wang X, et al. Synergistic effects of malononitrilamides (FK778, FK779) with tacrolimus (FK506) in prevention of acute heart and kidney allograft rejection and reversal of ongoing heart allograft rejection in the rat. Transplantation 2003;75:1881.
22. Boddy AV, Yule SM. Metabolism and pharmacokinetics of oxazaphosphorines. Clin Pharmacokinet 2000;38:291.
23. Bollinger RR, Fabian MA, Harland RC, et al. Total lymphoid irradiation for cardiac xenotransplantation in nonhuman primates. Transplant Proc 1991;23:587.
24. Borie DC, Larson MJ, Flores MG, et al. Combined use of the JAK3 inhibitor CP-690,550 with mycophenolate mofetil to prevent kidney allograft rejection in nonhuman primates. Transplantation 2005;80:1756.
25. Borie DC, O'Shea JJ, Changelian PS. JAK3 inhibition, a viable new modality of immunosuppression for solid organ transplants. Trends Mol Med 2004;10:532.
26. Branisteanu DD, Mathieu C, Bouillon R. Synergism between sirolimus and 1,25-dihydroxyvitamin D3 in vitro and in vivo. J Neuroimmunol 1997;79:138.
27. Branisteanu DD, Waer M, Sobis H, et al. Prevention of murine experimental allergic encephalomyelitis: cooperative effects of cyclosporine and 1alpha,25-(OH)2D3. J Neuroimmunol 1995;61:151.
28. Brynger H, Rydberg L, Samuelsson B, et al. Renal transplantation across a blood group barrier – 'A2' kidneys to 'O' recipients. Proc Eur Dial Transplant Assoc 1983;19:427.
29. Budde K, Schmouder L, Nashan B, et al. Pharmacodynamics of single doses of the novel immunosuppressant FTY720 in stable renal transplant patients. Am J Transplant 2003;3:846.
30. Budde K, Sommerer C, Becker T, et al. Sotrastaurin, a novel small molecule inhibiting protein kinase C: first clinical results in renal-transplant recipients. Am J Transplant 2010;10:571.
31. Busque S, Leventhal J, Brennan DC, et al. Calcineurin-inhibitor-free immunosuppression based on the JAK inhibitor CP-690,550: a pilot study in de novo kidney allograft recipients. Am J Transplant 2009;9:1936.
32. Cardella CJ, Sutton DM, Falk JA, et al. Effect of intensive plasma exchange on renal transplant rejection and serum cytotoxic antibody. Transplant Proc 1978;10:617.
33. Casteels K, Waer M, Bouillon R, et al. 1,25-Dihydroxyvitamin D3 restores sensitivity to cyclophosphamide-induced apoptosis in non-obese diabetic (NOD) mice and protects against diabetes. Clin Exp Immunol 1998;112:181.
34. Casteels KM, Mathieu C, Waer M, et al. Prevention of type I diabetes in nonobese diabetic mice by late intervention with nonhypercalcemic analogs of 1,25-dihydroxyvitamin D3 in combination with a short induction course of cyclosporin A. Endocrinology 1998;139:95.
35. Changelian PS, Flanagan ME, Ball DJ, et al. Prevention of organ allograft rejection by a specific Janus kinase 3 inhibitor. Science 2003;302:875.
36. Chen S, Sims GP, Chen XX, et al. Modulatory effects of 1,25-dihydroxyvitamin D3 on human B cell differentiation. J Immunol 2007;179:1634.
37. Chiba K, Hoshino Y, Suzuki C, et al. FTY720, a novel immunosuppressant possessing unique mechanisms. I. Prolongation of skin allograft survival and synergistic effect in combination with cyclosporine in rats. Transplant Proc 1996;28:1056.
38. Chiba K, Yanagawa Y, Masubuchi Y, et al. FTY720, a novel immunosuppressant, induces sequestration of circulating mature lymphocytes by acceleration of lymphocyte homing in rats. I. FTY720 selectively decreases the number of circulating mature lymphocytes by acceleration of lymphocyte homing. J Immunol 1998;160:5037.
39. Chikura B, Lane S, Dawson JK. Clinical expression of leflunomide-induced pneumonitis. Rheumatology (Oxford) 2009;48:1065.
40. Chin C, Hunt S, Robbins R, et al. Long-term follow-up after total lymphoid irradiation in pediatric heart transplant recipients. J Heart Lung Transplant 2002;21:667.
41. Chong AS, Gebel H, Finnegan A, et al. Leflunomide, a novel immunomodulatory agent: in vitro analyses of the mechanism of immunosuppression. Transplant Proc 1993;25:747.
42. Chong AS, Huang W, Liu W, et al. In vivo activity of leflunomide: pharmacokinetic analyses and mechanism of immunosuppression. Transplantation 1999;68:100.
43. Chong AS, Zeng H, Knight DA, et al. Concurrent antiviral and immunosuppressive activities of leflunomide in vivo. Am J Transplant 2006;6:69.
44. Chow D, Saper V, Strober S. Renal transplant patients treated with total lymphoid irradiation show specific unresponsiveness to donor antigens the mixed leukocyte reaction (MLR). J Immunol 1987;138:3746.
45. Cippitelli M, Santoni A. Vitamin D3: a transcriptional modulator of the interferon-gamma gene. Eur J Immunol 1998;28:3017.
46. Conklyn M, Andresen C, Changelian P, et al. The JAK3 inhibitor CP-690550 selectively reduces NK and CD8+ cell numbers in cynomolgus monkey blood following chronic oral dosing. J Leukoc Biol 2004;76:1248.
47. Curtis JR, Beukelman T, Onofrei A, et al. Elevated liver enzyme tests among patients with rheumatoid arthritis or psoriatic arthritis treated with methotrexate and/or leflunomide. Ann Rheum Dis 2010;69:43.
48. Dall'Amico R, Murer L, Montini G, et al. Successful treatment of recurrent rejection in renal transplant patients with photopheresis. J Am Soc Nephrol 1998;9:121.
49. de Jonge ME, Huitema AD, Rodenhuis S, et al. Clinical pharmacokinetics of cyclophosphamide. Clin Pharmacokinet 2005;44:1135.
50. de Jonge ME, Huitema AD, van Dam SM, et al. Population pharmacokinetics of cyclophosphamide and its metabolites 4-hydroxycyclophosphamide, 2-dechloroethylcyclophosphamide, and phosphoramide mustard in a high-dose combination with Thiotepa and Carboplatin. Ther Drug Monit 2005;27:756.
51. Decallonne B, van Etten E, Giulietti A, et al. Defect in activation-induced cell death in non-obese diabetic (NOD) T lymphocytes. J Autoimmun 2003;20:219.
52. Delbridge MS, Shrestha BM, Raftery AT, et al. Reduction of ischemia-reperfusion injury in the rat kidney by FTY720, a synthetic derivative of sphingosine. Transplantation 2007;84:187.
53. Deuse T, Schrepfer S, Reichenspurner H. Immunosuppression with FK778 and mycophenolate mofetil in a rat cardiac transplantation model. Transplantation 2003;76:1627.
54. Deuse T, Schrepfer S, Schafer H, et al. FK778 attenuates lymphocyte-endothelium interaction after cardiac transplantation: in vivo and in vitro studies. Transplantation 2004;78:71.
55. Diwan TS, Raghavaiah S, Burns JM, et al. The impact of proteasome inhibition on alloantibody-producing plasma cells in vivo. Transplantation 2011;91:536.
56. Dusso AS, Kamimura S, Gallieni M, et al. gamma-Interferon-induced resistance to 1,25-(OH)2 D3 in human monocytes and macrophages: a mechanism for the hypercalcemia of various granulomatoses. J Clin Endocrinol Metab 1997;82:2222.
57. Eckman PM, Thorsgard M, Maurer D, et al. Bortezomib for refractory antibody-mediated cardiac allograft rejection. Clin Transpl 2009;475.
58. Edelson R, Berger C, Gasparro F, et al. Treatment of cutaneous T-cell lymphoma by extracorporeal photochemotherapy. Preliminary results. N Engl J Med 1987;316:297.
59. Egli A, Kohli S, Dickenmann M, et al. Inhibition of polyomavirus BK-specific T-cell responses by immunosuppressive drugs. Transplantation 2009;88:1161.
60. Elder RT, Xu X, Williams JW, et al. The immunosuppressive metabolite of leflunomide, A77 1726, affects murine T cells through two biochemical mechanisms. J Immunol 1997;159:22.
61. Ettenger R, Schmouder R, Kovarik JM, et al. Pharmacokinetics, pharmacodynamics, safety, and tolerability of single-dose fingolimod (FTY720) in adolescents with stable renal transplants. Pediatr Transplant 2011;15:406.
62. Everly JJ, Walsh RC, Alloway RR, et al. Proteasome inhibition for antibody-mediated rejection. Curr Opin Organ Transplant 2009;14:662.

63. Everly MJ, Everly JJ, Susskind B, et al. Bortezomib provides effective therapy for antibody- and cell-mediated acute rejection. Transplantation 2008;86:1754.
64. Everly MJ, Terasaki PI, Hopfield J, et al. Protective immunity remains intact after antibody removal by means of proteasome inhibition. Transplantation 2010;90:1493.
65. Evers DL, Wang X, Huong SM, et al. 3,4′,5-Trihydroxy-trans-stilbene (resveratrol) inhibits human cytomegalovirus replication and virus-induced cellular signaling. Antiviral Res 2004;63:85.
66. Faguer S, Hirsch HH, Kamar N, et al. Leflunomide treatment for polyomavirus BK-associated nephropathy after kidney transplantation. Transpl Int 2007;20:962.
67. Farasati NA, Shapiro R, Vats A, et al. Effect of leflunomide and cidofovir on replication of BK virus in an in vitro culture system. Transplantation 2005;79:116.
68. Field EH, Becker GC. The immunosuppressive mechanism of total lymphoid irradiation. I. The effect on IL-2 production and IL-2 receptor expression. Transplantation 1989;48:499.
69. Field EH, Becker GC. Blocking of mixed lymphocyte reaction by spleen cells from total lymphoid-irradiated mice involves interruption of the IL-2 pathway. J Immunol 1992;148:354.
70. Field EH, Rouse TM. Alloantigen priming after total lymphoid irradiation alters alloimmune cytokine responses. Transplantation 1995;60:695.
71. Field EH, Steinmuller D. Nondeletional mechanisms of tolerance in total-lymphoid irradiation-induced bone marrow chimeras. Transplantation 1993;56:250.
72. Florence LS, Jiang GL, Ang KK, et al. In vitro analysis of T cell-mediated cytotoxicity displayed by rat heart allograft recipients rendered unresponsive by total-lymphoid irradiation and extracted donor antigen. Transplantation 1990;49:436.
73. Friman S, Arns W, Nashan B, et al. Sotrastaurin, a novel small molecule inhibiting protein-kinase C: randomized phase II study in renal transplant recipients. Am J Transplant 2011;11:1444.
74. Fryd DS, Sutherland DE, Simmons RL, et al. Results of a prospective randomized study on the effect of splenectomy versus no splenectomy in renal transplant patients. Transplant Proc 1981;13:48.
75. Fujine K, Abe F, Seki N, et al. FR252921, a novel immunosuppressive agent isolated from *Pseudomonas fluorescens* no. 408813. II. In vitro property and mode of action. J Antibiot (Tokyo) 2003;56:62.
76. Fujine K, Tanaka M, Ohsumi K, et al. FR252921, a novel immunosuppressive agent isolated from *Pseudomonas fluorescens* no. 408813. I. Taxonomy, fermentation, isolation, physico-chemical properties and biological activities of FR252921, FR252922 and FR256523. J Antibiot (Tokyo) 2003;56:55.
77. Fujine K, Ueda H, Hino M, et al. FR252921, a novel immunosuppressive agent isolated from *Pseudomonas fluorescens* no. 408813. III. In vivo activities. J Antibiot (Tokyo) 2003;56:68.
78. Fujishiro J, Kudou S, Iwai S, et al. Use of sphingosine-1-phosphate 1 receptor agonist, KRP-203, in combination with a subtherapeutic dose of cyclosporine A for rat renal transplantation. Transplantation 2006;82:804.
79. Fujita T, Inoue K, Yamamoto S, et al. Fungal metabolites. Part 11. A potent immunosuppressive activity found in *Isaria sinclairii* metabolite. J Antibiot (Tokyo) 1994;47:208.
80. Fujita T, Inoue K, Yamamoto S, et al. Fungal metabolites. Part 12. Potent immunosuppressant, 14-deoxomyriocin, (2S,3R,4R)-(E)-2-amino-3,4-dihydroxy-2-hydroxymethyleicos-6-enoic acid and structure-activity relationships of myriocin derivatives. J Antibiot (Tokyo) 1994;47:216.
81. Fuks Z, Strober S, Bobrove AM, et al. Long term effects of radiation of T and B lymphocytes in peripheral blood of patients with Hodgkin's disease. J Clin Invest 1976;58:803.
82. Fuller TF, Hoff U, Kong L, et al. Cytoprotective actions of FTY720 modulate severe preservation reperfusion injury in rat renal transplants. Transplantation 2010;89:402.
83. Funahashi Y, Hattori R, Kinukawa T, et al. Conversion from mycophenolate mofetil to mizoribine for patients with positive polyomavirus type BK in urine. Transplant Proc 2008;40:2268.
84. Gatza E, Rogers CE, Clouthier SG, et al. Extracorporeal photopheresis reverses experimental graft-versus-host disease through regulatory T cells. Blood 2008;112:1515.
85. Genberg H, Kumlien G, Shanwell A, et al. Refractory acute renal allograft rejection successfully treated with photopheresis. Transplant Proc 2005;37:3288.
86. Gorski A, Grieb P, Korczak-Kowalska G, et al. Cladribine (2-chloro-deoxyadenosine, CDA): an inhibitor of human B and T cell activation in vitro. Immunopharmacology 1993;26:197.
87. Gorski A, Grieb P, Makula J, et al. 2-Chloro-2-deoxyadenosine – a novel immunosuppressive agent. Transplantation 1993;56:1253.
88. Gottlieb M, Strober S, Hoppe RT, et al. Engraftment of allogeneic bone marrow without graft-versus-host disease in mongrel dogs using total lymphoid irradiation. Transplantation 1980;29:487.
89. Gregori S, Casorati M, Amuchastegui S, et al. Regulatory T cells induced by 1 alpha,25-dihydroxyvitamin D3 and mycophenolate mofetil treatment mediate transplantation tolerance. J Immunol 2001;167:1945.
90. Gregori S, Giarratana N, Smiroldo S, et al. A 1alpha,25-dihydroxyvitamin D(3) analog enhances regulatory T-cells and arrests autoimmune diabetes in NOD mice. Diabetes 2002;51:1367.
91. Griffin MD, Xing N, Kumar R. Vitamin D and its analogs as regulators of immune activation and antigen presentation. Annu Rev Nutr 2003;23:117.
92. Griffith TS, Kazama H, VanOosten RL, et al. Apoptotic cells induce tolerance by generating helpless CD8+ T cells that produce TRAIL. J Immunol 2007;178:2679.
93. Groth CG. Deoxyspergualin in allogeneic kidney and xenogeneic islet transplantation: early clinical trials. Ann N Y Acad Sci 1993;685:193.
94. Guasch A, Roy-Chaudhury P, Woodle ES, et al. Assessment of efficacy and safety of FK778 in comparison with standard care in renal transplant recipients with untreated BK nephropathy. Transplantation 2010;90:891.
95. Gysemans C, Waer M, Laureys J, et al. A combination of KH1060, a vitamin D(3) analogue, and cyclosporin prevents early graft failure and prolongs graft survival of xenogeneic islets in nonobese diabetic mice. Transplant Proc 2001;33:2365.
96. Habicht A, Clarkson MR, Yang J, et al. Novel insights into the mechanism of action of FTY720 in a transgenic model of allograft rejection: implications for therapy of chronic rejection. J Immunol 2006;176:36.
97. Halin C, Scimone ML, Bonasio R, et al. The S1P-analog FTY720 differentially modulates T-cell homing via HEV: T-cell-expressed S1P1 amplifies integrin activation in peripheral lymph nodes but not in Peyer patches. Blood 2005;106:1314.
98. Hayamizu K, Huie P, Sibley RK, et al. Monocyte-derived dendritic cell precursors facilitate tolerance to heart allografts after total lymphoid irradiation. Transplantation 1998;66:1285.
99. Hertel-Wulff B, Palathumpat V, Schwadron R, et al. Prevention of graft-versus-host disease by natural suppressor cells. Transplant Proc 1987;19:536.
100. Hoitsma AJ, Woodle ES, Abramowicz D, et al. FTY720 combined with tacrolimus in de novo renal transplantation: 1-year, multicenter, open-label randomized study. Nephrol Dial Transplant 2011;26:3802.
101. Horina JH, Mullegger RR, Horn S, et al. Photopheresis for renal allograft rejection. Lancet 1995;346:61.
102. Hoshino Y, Suzuki C, Ohtsuki M, et al. FTY720, a novel immunosuppressant possessing unique mechanisms. II. Long-term graft survival induction in rat heterotopic cardiac allografts and synergistic effect in combination with cyclosporine A. Transplant Proc 1996;28:1060.
103. Hosoya M, Shigeta S, Ishii T, et al. Comparative inhibitory effects of various nucleoside and nonnucleoside analogues on replication of influenza virus types A and B in vitro and in ovo. J Infect Dis 1993;168:641.
104. Howard RJ, Sutherland DE, Lum CT, et al. Kidney allograft survival in dogs treated with total lymphoid irradiation. Ann Surg 1981;193:196.
105. Hughes DA, Norton R. Vitamin D and respiratory health. Clin Exp Immunol 2009;158:20.
106. Hullett DA, Cantorna MT, Redaelli C, et al. Prolongation of allograft survival by 1,25-dihydroxyvitamin D3. Transplantation 1998;66:824.
107. Hunt SA, Strober S, Hoppe RT, et al. Total lymphoid irradiation for treatment of intractable cardiac allograft rejection. J Heart Lung Transplant 1991;10:211.
108. Ichikawa Y, Ihara H, Takahara S, et al. The immunosuppressive mode of action of mizoribine. Transplantation 1984;38:262.

109. Ishikawa A, Itoh M, Ushlyama T, et al. Experience of ABO-incompatible living kidney transplantation after double filtration plasmapheresis. Clin Transplant 1998;12:80.
110. Jarman ER, Kuba A, Montermann E, et al. Inhibition of murine IgE and immediate cutaneous hypersensitivity responses to ovalbumin by the immunomodulatory agent leflunomide. Clin Exp Immunol 1999;115:221.
111. Jeffery LE, Burke F, Mura M, et al. 1,25-Dihydroxyvitamin D3 and IL-2 combine to inhibit T cell production of inflammatory cytokines and promote development of regulatory T cells expressing CTLA-4 and FoxP3. J Immunol 2009;183:5458.
112. Jin MB, Nakayama M, Ogata T, et al. A novel leflunomide derivative, FK778, for immunosuppression after kidney transplantation in dogs. Surgery 2002;132:72.
113. Johnsson C, Tufveson G. MC 1288–a vitamin D analogue with immunosuppressive effects on heart and small bowel grafts. Transpl Int 1994;7:392.
114. Johnston O, Jaswal D, Gill JS, et al. Treatment of polyomavirus infection in kidney transplant recipients: a systematic review. Transplantation 2010;89:1057.
115. Josephson MA, Gillen D, Javaid B, et al. Treatment of renal allograft polyoma BK virus infection with leflunomide. Transplantation 2006;81:704.
116. Karaman A, Fadillioglu E, Turkmen E, et al. Protective effects of leflunomide against ischemia-reperfusion injury of the rat liver. Pediatr Surg Int 2006;22:428.
117. Karaman MW, Herrgard S, Treiber DK, et al. A quantitative analysis of kinase inhibitor selectivity. Nat Biotechnol 2008;26:127.
118. Kho LK, Kermode AG. Leflunomide-induced peripheral neuropathy. J Clin Neurosci 2007;14:179.
119. Kirken RA, Erwin RA, Taub D, et al. Tyrphostin AG-490 inhibits cytokine-mediated JAK3/STAT5a/b signal transduction and cellular proliferation of antigen-activated human T cells. J Leukoc Biol 1999;65:891.
120. Kirubakaran MG, Disney AP, Norman J, et al. A controlled trial of plasmapheresis in the treatment of renal allograft rejection. Transplantation 1981;32:164.
121. Knight DA, Hejmanowski AQ, Dierksheide JE, et al. Inhibition of herpes simplex virus type 1 by the experimental immunosuppressive agent leflunomide. Transplantation 2001;71:170.
122. Kokado Y, Ishibashi M, Jiang H, et al. A new triple-drug induction therapy with low dose cyclosporine, mizoribine and prednisolone in renal transplantation. Transplant Proc 1989;21:1575.
123. Kovarik JM, Slade A. Overview of sotrastaurin clinical pharmacokinetics. Ther Drug Monit 2010;32:540.
124. Kovarik JM, Steiger JU, Grinyo JM, et al. Pharmacokinetics of sotrastaurin combined with tacrolimus or mycophenolic acid in de novo kidney transplant recipients. Transplantation 2011;91:317.
125. Kovarik JM, Stitah S, Slade A, et al. Sotrastaurin and cyclosporine drug interaction study in healthy subjects. Biopharm Drug Dispos 2010;31:331.
126. Kudlacz E, Perry B, Sawyer P, et al. The novel JAK-3 inhibitor CP-690550 is a potent immunosuppressive agent in various murine models. Am J Transplant 2004;4:51.
127. Kumlien G, Genberg H, Shanwell A, et al. Photopheresis for the treatment of refractory renal graft rejection. Transplantation 2005;79:123.
128. Kundig TM, Schorle H, Bachmann MF, et al. Immune responses in interleukin-2-deficient mice. Science 1993;262:1059.
129. Kyles AE, Gregory CR, Griffey SM, et al. Immunosuppression with a combination of the leflunomide analog, FK778, and microemulsified cyclosporine for renal transplantation in mongrel dogs. Transplantation 2003;75:1128.
130. Lan F, Zeng D, Higuchi M, et al. Host conditioning with total lymphoid irradiation and antithymocyte globulin prevents graft-versus-host disease: the role of CD1-reactive natural killer T cells. Biol Blood Marrow Transplant 2003;9:355.
131. Lan F, Zeng D, Higuchi M, et al. Predominance of NK1.1+TCR alpha beta+ or DX5+TCR alpha beta+T cells in mice conditioned with fractionated lymphoid irradiation protects against graft-versus-host disease: "natural suppressor" cells. J Immunol 2001;167:2087.
132. Lan YY, De Creus A, Colvin BL, et al. The sphingosine-1-phosphate receptor agonist FTY720 modulates dendritic cell trafficking in vivo. Am J Transplant 2005;5:2649.
133. Lang VR, Mielenz D, Neubert K, et al. The early marginal zone B cell-initiated T-independent type 2 response resists the proteasome inhibitor bortezomib. J Immunol 2010;185:5637.
134. Lebreton L, Annat J, Derrepas P, et al. Structure-immunosuppressive activity relationships of new analogues of 15-deoxyspergualin. 1. Structural modifications of the hydroxyglycine moiety. J Med Chem 1999;42:277.
135. Leca N. Leflunomide use in renal transplantation. Curr Opin Organ Transplant 2009;14:370.
136. Lemire JM, Archer DC, Khulkarni A, et al. Prolongation of the survival of murine cardiac allografts by the vitamin D3 analogue 1,25-dihydroxy-delta 16-cholecalciferol. Transplantation 1992;54:762.
137. Levin B, Bohannon L, Warvariv V, et al. Total lymphoid irradiation (TLI) in the cyclosporine era – use of TLI in resistant cardiac allograft rejection. Transplant Proc 1989;21:1793.
138. Levin B, Hoppe RT, Collins G, et al. Treatment of cadaveric renal transplant recipients with total lymphoid irradiation, antithymocyte globulin, and low-dose prednisone. Lancet 1985;2:1321.
139. Li XK, Enosawa S, Kakefuda T, et al. FTY720, a novel immunosuppressive agent, enhances upregulation of the cell adhesion molecular ICAM-1 in TNF-alpha treated human umbilical vein endothelial cells. Transplant Proc 1997;29:1265.
140. Liacini A, Seamone ME, Muruve DA, et al. Anti-BK virus mechanisms of sirolimus and leflunomide alone and in combination: toward a new therapy for BK virus infection. Transplantation 2010;90:1450.
141. Lim TS, O'Driscoll G, Freund J, et al. Short-course total lymphoid irradiation for refractory cardiac transplantation rejection. J Heart Lung Transplant 2007;26:1249.
142. Lin Y, Goebels J, Xia G, et al. Induction of specific transplantation tolerance across xenogeneic barriers in the T-independent immune compartment. Nat Med 1998;4:173.
143. Lin Y, Vandeputte M, Waer MA. short-term combination therapy with cyclosporine and rapamycin or leflunomide induces long-term heart allograft survival in a strongly immunogenic strain combination in rats. Transpl Int 1996;9(Suppl 1):S328.
144. Liu PT, Stenger S, Li H, et al. Toll-like receptor triggering of a vitamin D-mediated human antimicrobial response. Science 2006;311:1770.
145. Liu YX, Shen NY, Liu C, et al. Immunosuppressive effects of emodin: an in vivo and in vitro study. Transplant Proc 2009;41:1837.
146. Lopez ER, Regulla K, Pani MA, et al. CYP27B1 polymorphisms variants are associated with type 1 diabetes mellitus in Germans. J Steroid Biochem Mol Biol 2004;89–90:155.
147. Lucas BA, Vaughn WK, Sanfilippo F, et al. Effects of pretransplant splenectomy: univariate and multivariate analyses. Transplant Proc 1987;19:1993.
148. Macchi P, Villa A, Giliani S, et al. Mutations of Jak-3 gene in patients with autosomal severe combined immune deficiency (SCID). Nature 1995;377:65.
149. Madden BP, Barros J, Backhouse L, et al. Intermediate term results of total lymphoid irradiation for the treatment of non-specific graft dysfunction after heart transplantation. Eur J Cardiothorac Surg 1999;15:663.
150. Mahajan S, Ghosh S, Sudbeck EA, et al. Rational design and synthesis of a novel anti-leukemic agent targeting Bruton's tyrosine kinase (BTK), LFM-A13 [alpha-cyano-beta-hydroxy-beta-methyl-N-(2, 5-dibromophenyl) propenamide]. J Biol Chem 1999;274:9587.
151. Malek TR, Bayer AL. Tolerance, not immunity, crucially depends on IL-2. Nat Rev Immunol 2004;4:665.
152. Malek TR, Yu A, Vincek V, et al. CD4 regulatory T cells prevent lethal autoimmunity in IL-2Rbeta-deficient mice. Implications for the nonredundant function of IL-2. Immunity 2002;17:167.
153. Man K, Ng KT, Lee TK, et al. FTY720 attenuates hepatic ischemia-reperfusion injury in normal and cirrhotic livers. Am J Transplant 2005;5:40.
154. Mandala S, Hajdu R, Bergstrom J, et al. Alteration of lymphocyte trafficking by sphingosine-1-phosphate receptor agonists. Science 2002;296:346.
155. Manna SK, Aggarwal BB. Immunosuppressive leflunomide metabolite (A77 1726) blocks TNF-dependent nuclear factor-kappa B activation and gene expression. J Immunol 1999;162:2095.

156. Manna SK, Mukhopadhyay A, Aggarwal BB. Leflunomide suppresses TNF-induced cellular responses: effects on NF-kappa B, activator protein-1, c-Jun N-terminal protein kinase, and apoptosis. J Immunol 2000;165:5962.
157. Marfo K, Lu A, Ling M, et al. Desensitization protocols and their outcome. Clin J Am Soc Nephrol 2011;6:922.
158. Masubuchi Y, Kawaguchi T, Ohtsuki M, et al. FTY720, a novel immunosuppressant, possessing unique mechanisms. IV. Prevention of graft versus host reactions in rats. Transplant Proc 1996;28:1064.
159. Matloubian M, Lo CG, Cinamon G, et al. Lymphocyte egress from thymus and peripheral lymphoid organs is dependent on S1P receptor 1. Nature 2004;427:355.
160. Mattar T, Kochhar K, Bartlett R, et al. Inhibition of the epidermal growth factor receptor tyrosine kinase activity by leflunomide. FEBS Lett 1993;334:161.
161. Mecklenbrauker I, Saijo K, Zheng NY, et al. Protein kinase Cdelta controls self-antigen-induced B-cell tolerance. Nature 2002;416:860.
162. Merani S, McCall M, Pawlick RL, et al. AEB071 (sotrastaurin) does not exhibit toxic effects on human islets in vitro, nor after transplantation into immunodeficient mice. Islets 2011;3:338.
163. Mitsusada M, Suzuki S, Kobayashi E, et al. Prevention of graft rejection and graft-versus-host reaction by a novel immunosuppressant, FTY720, in rat small bowel transplantation. Transpl Int 1997;10:343.
164. Mizuno K, Tsujino M, Takada M, et al. Studies on bredinin. I. Isolation, characterization and biological properties. J Antibiot (Tokyo) 1974;27:775.
165. Mulgaonkar S, Tedesco H, Oppenheimer F, et al. FTY720/cyclosporine regimens in de novo renal transplantation: a 1-year dose-finding study. Am J Transplant 2006;6:1848.
166. Myburgh JA, Smit JA, Stark JH, et al. Total lymphoid irradiation in kidney and liver transplantation in the baboon: prolonged graft survival and alterations in T cell subsets with low cumulative dose regimens. J Immunol 1984;132:1019.
167. Nador RG, Hongo D, Baker J, et al. The changed balance of regulatory and naive T cells promotes tolerance after TLI and anti-T-cell antibody conditioning. Am J Transplant 2010;10:262.
168. Najarian JS, Ferguson RM, Sutherland DE, et al. Fractionated total lymphoid irradiation as preparative immunosuppression in high risk renal transplantation: clinical and immunological studies. Ann Surg 1982;196:442.
169. Naka K, Ikeda M, Abe K, et al. Mizoribine inhibits hepatitis C virus RNA replication: effect of combination with interferon-alpha. Biochem Biophys Res Commun 2005;330:871.
170. Neubert K, Meister S, Moser K, et al. The proteasome inhibitor bortezomib depletes plasma cells and protects mice with lupus-like disease from nephritis. Nat Med 2008;14:748.
171. Neumann J, Schio S, Tarrasconi H, et al. Bortezomib in lung transplantation: a promising start. Clin Transpl 2009;421.
172. Nojima M, Yoshimoto T, Nakao A, et al. Combined therapy of deoxyspergualin and plasmapheresis: a useful treatment for antibody-mediated acute rejection after kidney transplantation. Transplant Proc 2005;37:930.
173. O'Hagan AR, Stillwell PC, Arroliga A, et al. Photopheresis in the treatment of refractory bronchiolitis obliterans complicating lung transplantation. Chest 1999;115:1459.
174. Oberhuber G, Schmid T, Thaler W, et al. Evidence that 2-chlorodeoxyadenosine in combination with cyclosporine prevents rejection after allogeneic small bowel transplantation. Transplantation 1994;58:743.
175. Opelz G, Terasaki PI. Effect of splenectomy on human renal transplants. Transplantation 1973;15:605.
176. Oppenheimer F, Mulgaonkar S, Ferguson R, et al. Impact of long-term therapy with FTY720 or mycophenolate mofetil on cardiac conduction and rhythm in stable adult renal transplant patients. Transplantation 2007;83:645.
177. Ostensen M. Disease specific problems related to drug therapy in pregnancy. Lupus 2004;13:746.
178. Overbergh L, Decallonne B, Valckx D, et al. Identification and immune regulation of 25-hydroxyvitamin D-1-alpha-hydroxylase in murine macrophages. Clin Exp Immunol 2000;120:139.
179. Overbergh L, Decallonne B, Waer M, et al. 1alpha,25-dihydroxyvitamin D3 induces an autoantigen-specific T-helper 1/T-helper 2 immune shift in NOD mice immunized with GAD65 (p524-543). Diabetes 2000;49:1301.
180. Pakkala I, Taskinen E, Pakkala S, et al. MC1288, a vitamin D analog, prevents acute graft-versus-host disease in rat bone marrow transplantation. Bone Marrow Transplant 2001;27:863.
181. Palathumpat VC, Vandeputte MM, Waer M. Effects of thymus irradiation on the immune competence of T cells after total-lymphoid irradiation. Transplantation 1990;50:95.
182. Palmer A, Taube D, Welsh K, et al. Removal of anti-HLA antibodies by extracorporeal immunoadsorption to enable renal transplantation. Lancet 1989;1:10.
183. Pan F, Ebbs A, Wynn C, et al. FK778, a powerful new immunosuppressant, effectively reduces functional and histologic changes of chronic rejection in rat renal allografts. Transplantation 2003;75:1110.
184. Paniagua R, Si MS, Flores MG, et al. Effects of JAK3 inhibition with CP-690,550 on immune cell populations and their functions in nonhuman primate recipients of kidney allografts. Transplantation 2005;80:1283.
185. Panza A, Roslin MS, Coons M, et al. One-year survival of heterotopic heart primate xenografts treated with total lymphoid irradiation and cyclosporine. Transplant Proc 1991;23:483.
186. Pappu R, Schwab SR, Cornelissen I, et al. Promotion of lymphocyte egress into blood and lymph by distinct sources of sphingosine-1-phosphate. Science 2007;316:295.
187. Pelletier MP, Coady M, Macha M, et al. Coronary atherosclerosis in cardiac transplant patients treated with total lymphoid irradiation. J Heart Lung Transplant 2003;22:124.
188. Penna G, Adorini L. 1Alpha,25-dihydroxyvitamin D3 inhibits differentiation, maturation, activation, and survival of dendritic cells leading to impaired alloreactive T cell activation. J Immunol 2000;164:2405.
189. Pepino P, Berger CL, Fuzesi L, et al. Primate cardiac allo-and xenotransplantation: modulation of the immune response with photochemotherapy. Eur Surg Res 1989;21:105.
190. Perez M, Edelson R, Laroche L, et al. Inhibition of antiskin allograft immunity by infusions with syngeneic photoinactivated effector lymphocytes. J Invest Dermatol 1989;92:669.
191. Perez MI, Edelson RL, John L, et al. Inhibition of antiskin allograft immunity induced by infusions with photoinactivated effector T lymphocytes (PET cells). Yale J Biol Med 1989;62:595.
192. Perotti C, Torretta L, Viarengo G, et al. Feasibility and safety of a new technique of extracorporeal photochemotherapy: experience of 240 procedures. Haematologica 1999;84:237.
193. Perry DK, Burns JM, Pollinger HS, et al. Proteasome inhibition causes apoptosis of normal human plasma cells preventing alloantibody production. Am J Transplant 2009;9:201.
194. Peters TG, Williams JW, Harmon HC, et al. Splenectomy and death in renal transplant patients. Arch Surg 1983;118:795.
195. Pierce JC, Hume DM. The effect of splenectomy on the survival of first and second renal homotransplants in man. Surg Gynecol Obstet 1968;127:1300.
196. Provvedini DM, Tsoukas CD, Deftos LJ, et al. 1,25-dihydroxyvitamin D3 receptors in human leukocytes. Science 1983;221:1181.
197. Qi S, Zhu S, Xu D, et al. Significant prolongation of renal allograft survival by delayed combination therapy of FK778 with tacrolimus in nonhuman primates. Transplantation 2003;75:1124.
198. Quaedackers ME, Mol W, Korevaar SS, et al. Monitoring of the immunomodulatory effect of CP-690,550 by analysis of the JAK/STAT pathway in kidney transplant patients. Transplantation 2009;88:1002.
199. Raisanen-Sokolowski AK, Pakkala IS, Samila SP, et al. A vitamin D analog, MC1288, inhibits adventitial inflammation and suppresses intimal lesions in rat aortic allografts. Transplantation 1997;63:936.
200. Ramos-Lopez E, Kahles H, Weber S, et al. Gestational diabetes mellitus and vitamin D deficiency: genetic contribution of CYP27B1 and CYP2R1 polymorphisms. Diabetes Obes Metab 2008;10:683.
201. Redaelli CA, Wagner M, Gunter-Duwe D, et al. 1alpha,25-dihydroxyvitamin D3 shows strong and additive immunomodulatory effects with cyclosporine A in rat renal allotransplants. Kidney Int 2002;61:288.

202. Redaelli CA, Wagner M, Tien YH, et al. 1alpha,25-Dihydroxycholecalciferol reduces rejection and improves survival in rat liver allografts. Hepatology 2001;34:926.
203. Reding R, Squifflet JP, Pirson Y, et al. Living-related and unrelated donor kidney transplantation: comparison between ABO-compatible and incompatible grafts. Transplant Proc 1987;19:1511.
204. Roberts JL, Lengi A, Brown SM, et al. Janus kinase 3 (JAK3) deficiency: clinical, immunologic, and molecular analyses of 10 patients and outcomes of stem cell transplantation. Blood 2004;103:2009.
205. Rook AH, Suchin KR, Kao DM, et al. Photopheresis: clinical applications and mechanism of action. J Investig Dermatol Symp Proc 1999;4:85.
206. Russell SM, Johnston JA, Noguchi M, et al. Interaction of IL-2R beta and gamma c chains with Jak1 and Jak3: implications for XSCID and XCID. Science 1994;266:1042.
207. Russell SM, Tayebi N, Nakajima H, et al. Mutation of Jak3 in a patient with SCID: essential role of Jak3 in lymphoid development. Science 1995;270:797.
208. Rynasiewicz JJ, Sutherland DE, Kawahara K, et al. Total lymphoid irradiation: critical timing and combination with cyclosporin A for immunosuppression in a rat heart allograft model. J Surg Res 1981;30:365.
209. Sadeghi AM, Laks H, Drinkwater DC, et al. Heart-lung xenotransplantation in primates. J Heart Lung Transplant 1991;10:442.
210. Saijo M, Morikawa S, Fukushi S, et al. Inhibitory effect of mizoribine and ribavirin on the replication of severe acute respiratory syndrome (SARS)-associated coronavirus. Antiviral Res 2005;66:159.
211. Salam A, Vandeputte M, Waer M. Clonal deletion and clonal anergy in allogeneic bone marrow chimeras prepared with TBI or TLI. Transpl Int 1994;7(Suppl. 1):S457.
212. Salerno CT, Park SJ, Kreykes NS, et al. Adjuvant treatment of refractory lung transplant rejection with extracorporeal photopheresis. J Thorac Cardiovasc Surg 1999;117:1063.
213. Salter SP, Salter MM, Kirklin JK, et al. Total lymphoid irradiation in the treatment of early or recurrent heart transplant rejection. Int J Radiat Oncol Biol Phys 1995;33:83.
214. Salvadori M, Budde K, Charpentier B, et al. FTY720 versus MMF with cyclosporine in de novo renal transplantation: a 1-year, randomized controlled trial in Europe and Australasia. Am J Transplant 2006;6:2912.
215. Sasaki S, Hashimoto R, Kiuchi M, et al. Fungal metabolites. Part 14. Novel potent immunosuppressants, mycestericins, produced by *Mycelia sterilia*. J Antibiot (Tokyo) 1994;47:420.
216. Savikko J, Von Willebrand E, Hayry P. Leflunomide analogue FK778 is vasculoprotective independent of its immunosuppressive effect: potential applications for restenosis and chronic rejection. Transplantation 2003;76:455.
217. Sawicka E, Dubois G, Jarai G, et al. The sphingosine 1-phosphate receptor agonist FTY720 differentially affects the sequestration of CD4+/CD25+ T-regulatory cells and enhances their functional activity. J Immunol 2005;175:7973.
218. Sberro-Soussan R, Zuber J, Suberbielle-Boissel C, et al. Bortezomib as the sole post-renal transplantation desensitization agent does not decrease donor-specific anti-HLA antibodies. Am J Transplant 2010;10:681.
219. Scandling JD, Busque S, Dejbakhsh-Jones S, et al. Tolerance and chimerism after renal and hematopoietic-cell transplantation. N Engl J Med 2008;358:362.
220. Scandling JD, Busque S, Shizuru JA, et al. Induced immune tolerance for kidney transplantation. N Engl J Med 2011;365:1359.
221. Schmid T, Hechenleitner P, Mark W, et al. 2-Chlorodeoxyadenosine (cladribine) in combination with low-dose cyclosporin prevents rejection after allogeneic heart and liver transplantation in the rat. Eur Surg Res 1998;30:61.
222. Sewgobind VD, Quaedackers ME, van der Laan LJ, et al. The Jak inhibitor CP-690,550 preserves the function of CD4CD25FoxP3 regulatory T cells and inhibits effector T cells. Am J Transplant 2010;10:1785.
223. Shigeta S. Recent progress in antiviral chemotherapy for respiratory syncytial virus infections. Expert Opin Investig Drugs 2000;9:221.
224. Shimizu H, Takahashi M, Kaneko T, et al. KRP-203, a novel synthetic immunosuppressant, prolongs graft survival and attenuates chronic rejection in rat skin and heart allografts. Circulation 2005;111:222.
225. Shirakawa AK, Nagakubo D, Hieshima K, et al. 1,25-Dihydroxyvitamin D3 induces CCR10 expression in terminally differentiating human B cells. J Immunol 2008;180:2786.
226. Si MS, Ji P, Lee M, et al. Potent farnesyltransferase inhibitor ABT-100 abrogates acute allograft rejection. J Heart Lung Transplant 2005;24:1403.
227. Si MS, Ji P, Tromberg BJ, et al. Farnesyltransferase inhibition: a novel method of immunomodulation. Int Immunopharmacol 2003;3:475.
228. Siemasko K, Chong AS, Jack HM, et al. Inhibition of JAK3 and STAT6 tyrosine phosphorylation by the immunosuppressive drug leflunomide leads to a block in IgG1 production. J Immunol 1998;160:1581.
229. Sigmundsdottir H, Pan J, Debes GF, et al. DCs metabolize sunlight-induced vitamin D3 to 'program' T cell attraction to the epidermal chemokine CCL27. Nat Immunol 2007;8:285.
230. Smolen JS, Kalden JR, Scott DL, et al. Efficacy and safety of leflunomide compared with placebo and sulphasalazine in active rheumatoid arthritis: a double-blind, randomised, multicentre trial. European Leflunomide Study Group. Lancet 1999;353:259.
231. Spitaler M, Cantrell DA. Protein kinase C and beyond. Nat Immunol 2004;5:785.
232. Squifflet JP, De Meyer M, Malaise J, et al. Lessons learned from ABO-incompatible living donor kidney transplantation: 20 years later. Exp Clin Transplant 2004;2:208.
233. Stark JH, Smit JA, Myburgh JA. Nonspecific mixed lymphocyte culture inhibitory antibodies in sera of tolerant transplanted baboons conditioned with total lymphoid irradiation. Transplantation 1994;57:1103.
234. Starzl TE, Marchioro TL, Waddell WR. Human renal homotransplantation in the presence of blood group incompatibilities. Proc Soc Exp Biol Med 1963;113:471.
235. Stepkowski SM, Kao J, Wang ME, et al. The Mannich base NC1153 promotes long-term allograft survival and spares the recipient from multiple toxicities. J Immunol 2005;175:4236.
236. Stoffels K, Overbergh L, Bouillon R, et al. Immune regulation of 1alpha-hydroxylase in murine peritoneal macrophages: unravelling the IFNgamma pathway. J Steroid Biochem Mol Biol 2007;103:567.
237. Strober S, Dhillon M, Schubert M, et al. Acquired immune tolerance to cadaveric renal allografts. A study of three patients treated with total lymphoid irradiation. N Engl J Med 1989;321:28.
238. Strober S, Modry DL, Hoppe RT, et al. Induction of specific unresponsiveness to heart allografts in mongrel dogs treated with total lymphoid irradiation and antithymocyte globulin. J Immunol 1984;132:1013.
239. Strober S, Slavin S, Gottlieb M, et al. Allograft tolerance after total lymphoid irradiation (TLI). Immunol Rev 1979;46:87.
240. Stuart FP, Reckard CR, Ketel BL, et al. Effect of splenectomy on first cadaver kidney transplants. Ann Surg 1980;192:553.
241. Suissa S, Ernst P, Hudson M, et al. Newer disease-modifying antirheumatic drugs and the risk of serious hepatic adverse events in patients with rheumatoid arthritis. Am J Med 2004;117:87.
242. Suleiman M, Cury PM, Pestana JO, et al. FTY720 prevents renal T-cell infiltration after ischemia/reperfusion injury. Transplant Proc 2005;37:373.
243. Sunder-Plassman G, Druml W, Steininger R, et al. Renal allograft rejection controlled by photopheresis. Lancet 1995;346:506.
244. Sunwoo JB, Chen Z, Dong G, et al. Novel proteasome inhibitor PS-341 inhibits activation of nuclear factor-kappa B, cell survival, tumor growth, and angiogenesis in squamous cell carcinoma. Clin Cancer Res 2001;7:1419.
245. Sutherland DE, Fryd DS, Strand MH, et al. Results of the Minnesota randomized prospective trial of cyclosporine versus azathioprine-antilymphocyte globulin for immunosuppression in renal allograft recipients. Am J Kidney Dis 1985;5:318.
246. Suzuki C, Takahashi M, Morimoto H, et al. Efficacy of mycophenolic acid combined with KRP-203, a novel immunomodulator, in a rat heart transplantation model. J Heart Lung Transplant 2006;25:302.

247. Suzuki S, Enosawa S, Kakefuda T, et al. Long-term graft acceptance in allografted rats and dogs by treatment with a novel immunosuppressant, FTY720. Transplant Proc 1996;28:1375.
248. Suzuki S, Enosawa S, Kakefuda T, et al. A novel immunosuppressant, FTY720, with a unique mechanism of action, induces long-term graft acceptance in rat and dog allotransplantation. Transplantation 1996;61:200.
249. Suzuki S, Kakefuda T, Amemiya H, et al. An immunosuppressive regimen using FTY720 combined with cyclosporin in canine kidney transplantation. Transpl Int 1998;11:95.
250. Suzuki T, Jin MB, Shimamura T, et al. A new immunosuppressant, FTY720, in canine kidney transplantation: effect of single-drug, induction and combination treatments. Transpl Int 2004;17:574.
251. Takahashi K, Nakayama Y, Horiuchi H, et al. Human neutrophils express messenger RNA of vitamin D receptor and respond to 1alpha,25-dihydroxyvitamin D3. Immunopharmacol Immunotoxicol 2002;24:335.
252. Takahashi K, Tanabe K, Ooba S, et al. Prophylactic use of a new immunosuppressive agent, deoxyspergualin, in patients with kidney transplantation from ABO-incompatible or preformed antibody-positive donors. Transplant Proc 1991;23:1078.
253. Takeuchi A, Reddy GS, Kobayashi T, et al. Nuclear factor of activated T cells (NFAT) as a molecular target for 1alpha,25-dihydroxyvitamin D3-mediated effects. J Immunol 1998;160:209.
254. Takeuchi N, Ohshima S, Matsuura O, et al. Immunosuppression with low-dose cyclosporine, mizoribine, and steroids in living-related kidney transplantation. Transplant Proc 1994;26:1907.
255. Tan SL, Parker PJ. Emerging and diverse roles of protein kinase C in immune cell signalling. Biochem J 2003;376:545.
256. Tanabe K, Tokumoto T, Ishikawa N, et al. Long-term results in mizoribine-treated renal transplant recipients: a prospective, randomized trial of mizoribine and azathioprine under cyclosporine-based immunosuppression. Transplant Proc 1999;31:2877.
257. Tang J, Zhou R, Luger D, et al. Calcitriol suppresses antiretinal autoimmunity through inhibitory effects on the Th17 effector response. J Immunol 2009;182:4624.
258. Taube DH, Williams DG, Cameron JS, et al. Renal transplantation after removal and prevention of resynthesis of HLA antibodies. Lancet 1984;1:824.
259. Tedesco-Silva H, Lorber MI, Foster CE, et al. FTY720 and everolimus in de novo renal transplant patients at risk for delayed graft function: results of an exploratory one-yr multicenter study. Clin Transplant 2009;23:589.
260. Tedesco-Silva H, Pescovitz MD, Cibrik D, et al. Randomized controlled trial of FTY720 versus MMF in de novo renal transplantation. Transplantation 2006;82:1689.
261. Tedesco-Silva H, Szakaly P, Shoker A, et al. FTY720 versus mycophenolate mofetil in de novo renal transplantation: six-month results of a double-blind study. Transplantation 2007;84:885.
262. Thomas F, Pittman K, Ljung T, et al. Deoxyspergualin is a unique immunosuppressive agent with selective utility in inducing tolerance to pancreas islet xenografts. Transplant Proc 1995;27:417.
263. Thomas FT, Tepper MA, Thomas JM, et al. 15-Deoxyspergualin: a novel immunosuppressive drug with clinical potential. Ann N Y Acad Sci 1993;685:175.
264. Tixier D, Levy C, Le Bourgeois JP, et al. Discordant heart xenografts. Experimental study in pigs conditioned by total lymphoid irradiation and cyclosporine A. Presse Med 1992;21:1941.
265. Topalis D, Lebeau I, Krecmerova M, et al. Activities of different classes of acyclic nucleoside phosphonates against BK virus in primary human renal cells. Antimicrob Agents Chemother 2011;55:1961.
266. Trager DK, Banks BA, Rosenbaum GE, et al. Cardiac allograft prolongation in mice treated with combined posttransplantation total-lymphoid irradiation and anti-L3T4 antibody therapy. Transplantation 1989;47:587.
267. Troncoso P, Stepkowski SM, Wang ME, et al. Prophylaxis of acute renal allograft rejection using FTY720 in combination with subtherapeutic doses of cyclosporine. Transplantation 1999;67:145.
268. Tyden G, Kumlien G, Genberg H, et al. ABO incompatible kidney transplantations without splenectomy, using antigen-specific immunoadsorption and rituximab. Am J Transplant 2005;5:145.
269. Tyden G, Kumlien G, Genberg H, et al. ABO-incompatible kidney transplantation and rituximab. Transplant Proc 2005;37:3286.
270. Valentine VG, Robbins RC, Wehner JH, et al. Total lymphoid irradiation for refractory acute rejection in heart-lung and lung allografts. Chest 1996;109:1184.
271. van Etten E, Branisteanu DD, Overbergh L, et al. Combination of a 1,25-dihydroxyvitamin D3 analog and a bisphosphonate prevents experimental autoimmune encephalomyelitis and preserves bone. Bone 2003;32:397.
272. van Etten E, Branisteanu DD, Verstuyf A, et al. Analogs of 1,25-dihydroxyvitamin D3 as dose-reducing agents for classical immunosuppressants. Transplantation 2000;69:1932.
273. van Etten E, Decallonne B, Verlinden L, et al. Analogs of 1alpha,25-dihydroxyvitamin D3 as pluripotent immunomodulators. J Cell Biochem 2003;88:223.
274. van Gurp E, Weimar W, Gaston R, et al. Phase 1 dose-escalation study of CP-690 550 in stable renal allograft recipients: preliminary findings of safety, tolerability, effects on lymphocyte subsets and pharmacokinetics. Am J Transplant 2008;8:1711.
275. van Halteren AG, van Etten E, de Jong EC, et al. Redirection of human autoreactive T-cells upon interaction with dendritic cells modulated by TX527, an analog of 1,25 dihydroxyvitamin D(3). Diabetes 2002;51:2119.
276. Vanrenterghem Y, van Hooff JP, Klinger M, et al. The effects of FK778 in combination with tacrolimus and steroids: a phase II multicenter study in renal transplant patients. Transplantation 2004;78:9.
277. Verstuyf A, Carmeliet G, Bouillon R, et al. Vitamin D: a pleiotropic hormone. Kidney Int 2010;78:140.
278. Veyron P, Pamphile R, Binderup L, et al. New 20-epi-vitamin D3 analogs: immunosuppressive effects on skin allograft survival. Transplant Proc 1995;27:450.
279. Vogelbacher R, Meister S, Guckel E, et al. Bortezomib and sirolimus inhibit the chronic active antibody-mediated rejection in experimental renal transplantation in the rat. Nephrol Dial Transplant 2010;25:3764.
280. Waer M, Ang KK, van der Schueren E, et al. Allogeneic bone marrow transplantation in mice after total lymphoid irradiation: influence of breeding conditions and strain of recipient mice. J Immunol 1984;132:991.
281. Waer M, Ang KK, van der Schueren E, et al. Influence of radiation field and fractionation schedule of total lymphoid irradiation (TLI) on the induction of suppressor cells and stable chimerism after bone marrow transplantation in mice. J Immunol 1984;132:985.
282. Waer M, Leenaerts P, Vanrenterghem Y, et al. Factors determining the success rate of total lymphoid irradiation in clinical kidney transplantation. Transplant Proc 1989;21:1796.
283. Waer M, Vanrenterghem Y, Roels L, et al. Total lymphoid irradiation in renal cadaveric transplantation in diabetics. Lancet 1985;2:1354.
284. Waldman WJ, Knight DA, Lurain NS, et al. Novel mechanism of inhibition of cytomegalovirus by the experimental immunosuppressive agent leflunomide. Transplantation 1999;68:814.
285. Walsh RC, Everly JJ, Brailey P, et al. Proteasome inhibitor-based primary therapy for antibody-mediated renal allograft rejection. Transplantation 2010;89:277.
286. Wang ME, Tejpal N, Qu X, et al. Immunosuppressive effects of FTY720 alone or in combination with cyclosporine and/or sirolimus. Transplantation 1998;65:899.
287. Williams JW, Javaid B, Kadambi PV, et al. Leflunomide for polyomavirus type BK nephropathy. N Engl J Med 2005;352:1157.
288. Williams JW, Xiao F, Foster P, et al. Leflunomide in experimental transplantation. Control of rejection and alloantibody production, reversal of acute rejection, and interaction with cyclosporine. Transplantation 1994;57:1223.
289. Williamson RA, Yea CM, Robson PA, et al. Dihydroorotate dehydrogenase is a high affinity binding protein for A77 1726 and mediator of a range of biological effects of the immunomodulatory compound. J Biol Chem 1995;270:22467.
290. Wolfe JT, Tomaszewski JE, Grossman RA, et al. Reversal of acute renal allograft rejection by extracorporeal photopheresis: a case presentation and review of the literature. J Clin Apher 1996;11:36.

291. Xiao F, Shen J, Chong A, et al. Control and reversal of chronic xenograft rejection in hamster-to-rat cardiac transplantation. Transplant Proc 1996;28:691.
292. Xu M, Pirenne J, Antoniou EA, et al. Effect of peritransplant FTY720 alone or in combination with post-transplant tacrolimus in a rat model of cardiac allotransplantation. Transpl Int 1998;11:288.
293. Xu M, Pirenne J, Antoniou S, et al. FTY720 compares with FK 506 as rescue therapy in rat heterotopic cardiac transplantation. Transplant Proc 1998;30:2221.
294. Yamashita K, Nomura M, Omura T, et al. Effect of a novel immunosuppressant, FTY720, on heart and liver transplantations in rats. Transplant Proc 1999;31:1178.
295. Yin N, Zhang N, Xu J, et al. Targeting lymphangiogenesis after islet transplantation prolongs islet allograft survival. Transplantation 2011;92:25.
296. Yoo EK, Rook AH, Elenitsas R, et al. Apoptosis induction of ultraviolet light A and photochemotherapy in cutaneous T-cell lymphoma: relevance to mechanism of therapeutic action. J Invest Dermatol 1996;107:235.
297. Yuzawa K, Stephkowski SM, Wang M, et al. FTY720 blocks allograft rejection by homing of lymphocytes in vivo. Transplant Proc 2000;32:269.
298. Zeng H, Waldman WJ, Yin DP, et al. Mechanistic study of malononitrileamide FK778 in cardiac transplantation and CMV infection in rats. Transplantation 2005;79:17.
299. Zhang Q, Chen Y, Fairchild RL, et al. Lymphoid sequestration of alloreactive memory CD4 T cells promotes cardiac allograft survival. J Immunol 2006;176:770.
300. Zhou PJ, Wang H, Shi GH, et al. Immunomodulatory drug FTY720 induces regulatory CD4(+)CD25(+) T cells in vitro. Clin Exp Immunol 2009;157:40.

CHAPTER 23

Approaches to the Induction of Tolerance

Kathryn J. Wood

CHAPTER OUTLINE

INTRODUCTION

Historical Perspective

In 1951, Billingham and Medawar published a landmark article entitled "Technique of free skin grafting in mammals."[14] These classic experiments provided the foundation for what would become the field of transplantation immunology and laid the groundwork for many concepts in immunology, including immunologic memory.[14] Further work, based upon the early writings of Ray D. Owen,[141] involved skin grafting dizygotic mammalian twin calves. The observations that these grafts are accepted by both hosts led to the hypothesis that a phenomenon of immunological tolerance to the skin grafts was achieved secondary to "foreign" blood cells persistent in each twin, as a consequence of placental fusion.[13]

These breakthroughs in research translated to the clinic in 1954, when Joseph Murray and colleagues performed the first successful kidney transplant between monozygotic twins at the Peter Bent Brigham Hospital in Boston, Massachusetts. The success of this feat was in part due to the lack of immunosuppression needed in the transplant of monozygotic twins. Allografts that were attempted subsequently failed because of uncontrolled acute rejection responses mounted by the immune system. The quest to identify methods of both immunosuppression and tolerance induction in transplantation began.[218]

Definition of "Tolerance"

Generally, the concept of tolerance (operational) refers to the persistent survival of a transplanted allograft in the absence of continuing immunosuppressive therapy and an ongoing destructive immune response targeting the graft. This functional definition is appropriate as multiple immunological mechanisms and donor–recipient factors are involved in both inducing and maintaining tolerance to a defined set of donor antigens *in vivo*. Achieving functional tolerance in transplant recipients will mandate that specific allograft-destructive responses are "switched off" while the global immune response to pathogens and carcinogens remains intact. The most robust form of transplantation tolerance therefore has to be donor-specific, as opposed to mere immuno-incompetence, a requirement that can be tested experimentally by grafting third-party transplants and by challenging tolerant recipients to respond to virus infections and tumor loads. The concept of graft-specific tolerance is essential, both to maintain long-term survival of graft and host and to eliminate the adverse events associated with lifelong non-specific immunosuppression.

Need for Tolerance in Clinical Transplantation

The immune response to an allograft is an ongoing dialogue between the innate and adaptive immune system that, if left unchecked, will lead to the rejection of transplanted cells, tissues, or organs (see Chapter 2[216]). Elements of the innate immune system, including macrophages, neutrophils, and complement, are activated as a consequence of tissue injury sustained during cell isolation or organ retrieval, as well as ischemia-reperfusion. Activation of the innate immune system inevitably leads to the initiation and amplification of the adaptive response that involves T cells, B cells, and antibodies. T cells require a minimum of two signals for activation – antigen recognition (often referred to as signal 1) and costimulation (referred to as signal 2). The majority of B cells require help from T cells to initiate antibody production. Antibodies reactive to donor antigens, including major and minor histocompatibility antigens and blood group antigens, can trigger or contribute to rejection, early as well as late, after transplantation.

Multiple factors are taken into account in making this decision, including where the antigen is "seen" and the conditions that are present at the time, in particular the presence or absence of inflammation associated with activation of the innate response. The innate response is neither specific nor is it altered significantly with multiple antigenic challenges. In contrast, the adaptive response is specific for a particular antigen or combination of antigens and "remembers" when it encounters the same antigen again, augmenting its activity and the rapidity of the response at each encounter. When the immune system encounters an antigen, it has to decide which type of response to make. In most cases, even though one component of the immune system may dominate and lead to rejection, the process is usually multifactorial, resulting from the integration of multiple mechanisms.

Understanding the molecular and cellular mechanisms that lead to allograft rejection has provided insights leading to the development of therapeutics that suppress this unwanted immune response. A diverse collection of small-molecule and biological immunosuppressive agents are available for clinical use that have the potential to control or inhibit allograft rejection. In the context of solid-organ transplantation, the drugs that are currently available for clinical use include azathioprine, cyclosporine, tacrolimus, mycophenolate mofetil, rapamycin, antithymocyte globulin, anti-CD25 monoclonal antibodies, belatacept, and steroids (Table 23-1). Each immunosuppressive agent acts on a different aspect of the immune response to an allograft and can therefore be used effectively in combination. Unfortunately, all of these agents are globally non-specific in their suppressive activity and each has some deleterious side effects.

These immunosuppressive drugs can be used successfully to prevent or control acute allograft rejection; however, they are less effective at controlling the long-term

TABLE 23-1 **Immunosuppressive Agents Used in Solid-Organ Transplantation**

Class of Agent	Agent
Corticosteroid	Prednisone Methyl prednisolone
Antiproliferative	Azathioprine Mycophenolate mofetil Mycophenolate sodium
Calcineurin inhibitor	Cyclosporine Tacrolimus
mTOR inhibitor	Sirolimus Everolimus
Polyclonal antilymphocyte antibodies	ALG ATG
Monoclonal antibodies (with target)	Muromonab (CD3) Basiliximab (IL-2α receptor CD25) Alemtuzumab (CD52) Rituximab (CD20)
Costimulation blockade	Belatacept (LEA29Y – CTLA-4-Ig)

ALG, antilymphocyte globulin; ATG, antithymocyte globulin; CTLA-4, cytotoxic T lymphocyte antigen-4; IL, interleukin; mTOR, mammalian target of rapamycin.

response to injury and activation of the immune system. They also appear to be unable to promote the development of unresponsiveness or tolerance to the donor alloantigens consistently, at least in the way they are used clinically at present. For nearly all transplant recipients, the continued survival of the allograft depends on lifelong administration of several immunosuppressive drugs. The exception to this statement is liver transplantation where, in a proportion of pediatric and adult recipients, it is possible to wean patients treated with immunosuppressive drugs off their immunosuppression in the longer term.[45,120,189]

The inability of current immunosuppressive drug regimens to induce tolerance to donor antigens in the majority of patients may be due, in part, to the non-specific nature of the immunosuppression resulting from their inability to distinguish between the potentially harmful immune response mounted against the organ graft and immune responses that could be beneficial, protecting the recipient from infectious pathogens as well as providing mechanisms to control the development of malignant cells. In general, the drugs act by interfering with lymphocyte activation and/or proliferation irrespective of the antigen specificity of the responding cells (Figure 23-1). This lack of immunological specificity means that the immune system of a patient treated with one or more of these therapeutic agents is compromised not only in its ability to respond to the transplant, but also in its ability to respond to any other antigenic stimuli that may be encountered after transplantation. Therefore patients are more susceptible to infections (see Chapter 31[61]) and are at a higher risk for developing cancer (see Chapters 34 and 35[210]).

The development of immunological tolerance or specific unresponsiveness to donor alloantigens in the short term or the long term after transplantation appears to offer the best possibility of achieving effectiveness and

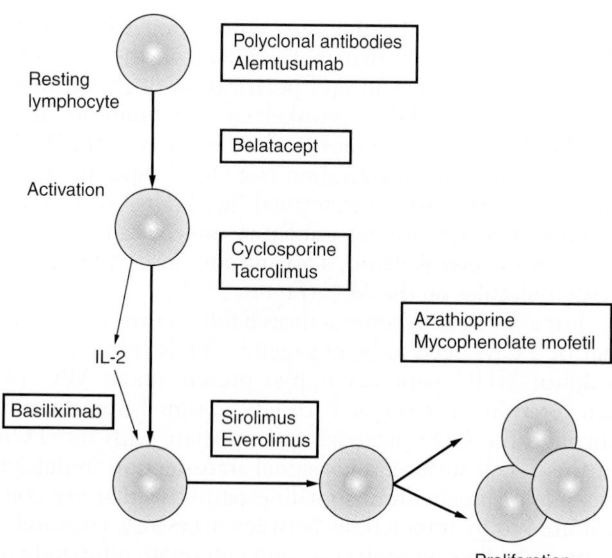

FIGURE 23-1 ■ Schematic indicating the sites of action of common immunosuppressive agents during an immune response. Each immunosuppressive agent targets a specific step in the activation and proliferation of T lymphocytes. IL-2, interleukin-2.

specificity in the control of the immune system after transplantation in either the absence, or at least reduced loads of, non-specific immunosuppressive agents. If tolerance to donor alloantigens could be achieved reliably, it would ensure that only lymphocytes in the patient's immune repertoire responding to donor antigens were suppressed or controlled, leaving the majority of lymphocytes immune competent and able to perform their normal functions after transplantation, including protecting the body from infection and cancer after transplantation. This chapter is, therefore, dedicated to the discussion of the mechanisms underlying tolerance induction and strategies utilized to induce unresponsiveness in transplanted allografts.

UNDERSTANDING THE IMMUNOLOGIC MECHANISMS BEHIND TOLERANCE INDUCTION

Overview of T-Cell Activation

An understanding of the cellular and molecular mechanisms of activation and regulation of the immune system is important for the development of novel approaches for tolerance induction in the context of transplantation as well as autoimmunity. The following section sets the scene by discussing the different approaches to tolerance induction being explored most actively at present.

Hematopoietic stem cells (HSCs) present in the bone marrow give rise to all of the leukocyte populations that participate in innate and adaptive immune responses. The thymus is the key organ that shapes the T-cell repertoire. T-cell precursors leave the bone marrow and migrate to the thymus, where they rearrange the genes that encode the antigen recognition structure, the T-cell receptor (TCR). Thymocytes that express TCRs with low affinity for self antigen presented by self major histocompatibility complex (MHC) molecules are "neglected" and die, as they will be of no use to the host. In contrast, thymocytes expressing TCRs with a high affinity for self antigen undergo programmed cell death and are "deleted" from the repertoire as they could create a response to self antigens in the periphery and be harmful to the host. This leaves the T cells with receptors that have an intermediate affinity to enter the bloodstream where they recirculate between blood and peripheral lymphoid tissue. A third population of T cells, which will be discussed later, so-called thymus-derived or naturally occurring regulatory T cells (Treg), are also selected in the thymus and migrate to the periphery. Through thymic selection a mature T-cell repertoire is developed that is not only diverse, but can also react to foreign antigen while still remaining tolerant to self antigens.

Naïve T cells encounter antigen in the form of a peptide–MHC complex on the surface of antigen presenting cells (APCs). Antigen presentation to T cells can be performed by a variety of APCs, including dendritic cells (DCs), macrophages, and B cells, although DCs are the most immunostimulatory of all the APCs and the most potent at stimulating naïve T cells to respond.[181]

As a direct consequence of organ retrieval and implantation the tissue within the transplant is injured and stressed.[43,131,143] Cells of the innate immune system express invariant pathogen-associated pattern recognition receptors (PRRs) that enable them to detect not only repeating structural units expressed by pathogens, referred to as pathogen-associated molecular patterns (PAMPs),[190] but also markers of tissue injury or damage-associated molecular patterns (DAMPs). Local tissue damage and ischemia-reperfusion injury generate many potential DAMPs, including reactive oxygen species, heat shock proteins, heparin sulfate and high-mobility group box (HMBG)-1, following capture by the receptor for advanced glycation end-products (RAGE) complex and fibrinogen, that can bind to PRRs. There are several families of PRRs, including transmembrane proteins present at the cell surface, such as Toll-like receptors (TLRs). The sensing of DAMPs by PRRs results in the potent activation of the inflammasome,[139] upregulating the transcription of genes and production of microRNAs[3] involved in inflammatory responses, setting up amplification and feedback loops that augment the response and trigger adaptive immunity. The end result is the production of inflammatory mediators, including the proinflammatory cytokines, interleukin (IL)-1, IL-6, and tumor necrosis factor (TNF), type I interferons (IFNs), chemokines (chemoattractant cytokines),[24,109] and the rapid expression of P-selectin (CD62P) by endothelial cells. These events identify the transplant as a site of injury and inflammation, modifying the activation status, permeability, and viability of endothelial cells lining the vessels, triggering the release of soluble molecules, including antigens from the graft, inducing the production of acute-phase proteins, including complement factors systemically, as well as in some cases by the organ itself, stimulating the maturation and migration of donor-derived APCs and DCs from the transplant to recipient lymphoid tissue.[95,203] This process results in upregulation of donor MHC, costimulatory and adhesion molecules by the donor-derived APCs, enabling them to become potent stimulators of naïve T cells. The presentation of donor alloantigens to recipient T cells by donor-derived APCs results in T-cell activation via the direct pathway of allorecognition.[1]

Activation of the innate immune system within the allograft also triggers the recruitment of inflammatory leukocytes of recipient origin into the graft. These recipient APCs have the capacity to acquire donor histocompatibility antigens from the graft tissue and process them into peptides that can be presented to T cells via the indirect pathway of allorecognition. A third pathway of presentation of alloantigen to T cells has also been described, the so-called semidirect pathway of allorecognition whereby, as a result of close contact between recipient APCs and donor cells, sections of membrane containing histocompatibility molecules are transferred from one cell to the other for presentation to T cells.[1]

The interaction between APCs of donor or recipient origin and T lymphocytes is pivotal to the adaptive arm of the immune response. Immunostimulatory APCs are brought into close proximity with naïve T cells that may have TCRs capable of recognizing either intact donor alloantigens via the direct or semidirect pathways of allorecognition or donor peptides presented by recipient MHC molecules via the indirect pathway. An immunologic synapse is formed by the close interaction between the APC and the T cell that is dependent on the successful dynamic rearrangement and polarization of the filamentous actin in the DCs' cytoskeletal membrane to bring the MHC–peptide complex in close relation to the TCR, thereby initiating an activation response.[47] Specific T-cell membrane compartments, termed "lipid rafts," serve as recruitment centers for costimulatory molecules to concentrate on the cytoskeleton, allowing for closer interactions with molecules on the APC (Figure 23-2).

For a T cell to become activated fully, a threshold number of TCRs need to be engaged.[113] TCR recognition of a donor MHC–peptide complex present on an APC, often referred to as signal 1, results in signal transduction through the CD3 proteins that associate with the TCR at the T-cell surface. This signal transduction initiates a cascade of biochemical signaling pathways that are contributed to by interactions between accessory, costimulatory, and adhesion molecules and culminate ultimately in cytokine production and proliferation of the triggered T cell and its differentiation into an effector cell.

Accessory and costimulatory molecules that have been shown to be important in triggering T-cell activation on the T-cell side include CD4, CD11b/CD18 (leukocyte function associated antigen-1 (LFA-1)), CD28, and CD154 (CD40 ligand).[88] These molecules

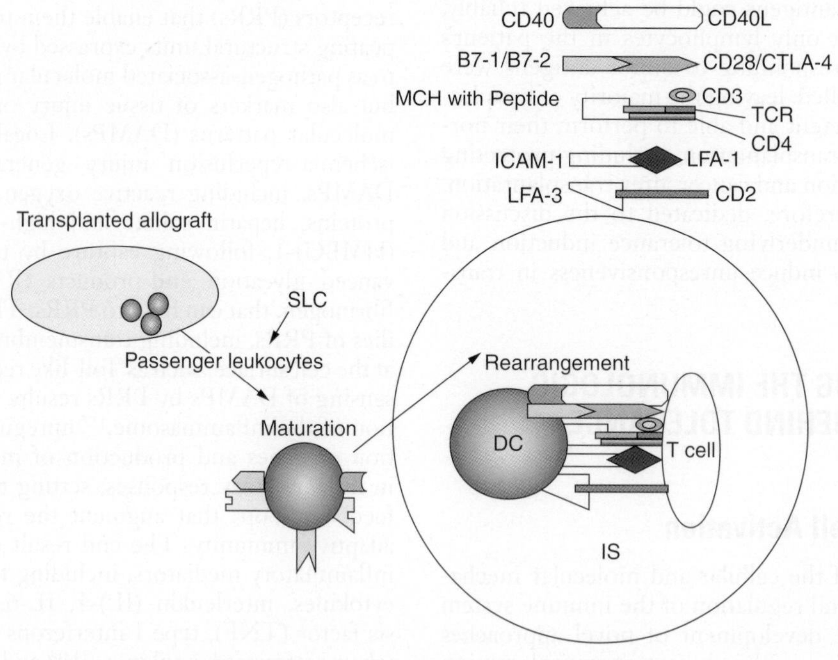

FIGURE 23-2 ■ Formation of the immunologic synapse. Passenger leukocytes from a transplanted allograft emigrate from the organ and, under the influence of secondary lymphoid tissue chemokine (SLC), migrate to the lymph nodes and spleen. En route these dendritic cells (DC) undergo maturation and upregulation/rearrangement of their cell surface markers using mechanisms linked to lipid rafting. Once in the lymph node T-cell activation ensues upon the formation of the immunologic synapse (IS). T-cell activation requires at least two signals. Signal 1 is delivered to the T cell when major histocompatibility complex (MHC) class II–peptide complexes on the antigen presenting cell (APC) are recognized specifically by the T-cell receptor (TCR)–CD3 complex, expressed by the T cell. CD4 (T cell) interacts with the MHC class II molecule, fulfilling an adhesion and a signaling function. Second signals or costimulation is provided by additional cell surface interactions. CD28 (T cell) can bind to B7-2 (CD86) and B7-1 (CD80), expressed by the APC. This interaction delivers a signal to the T cell that lowers the threshold for T-cell activation. C40 on the APC can bind to its ligand, CD40L (CD154) (T cell). This interaction provides additional signals to the T cell but, in contrast to the CD28 pathway, also delivers signals to the APC, resulting in an increase in expression of B7-1 and B7-2. To ensure that the T cell engages the APC for sufficient time for the signaling events to occur, adhesion molecules, including intracellular adhesion molecule 1 (ICAM-1) and lymphocyte function antigen 1 (LFA-1), also engage each other.

must engage their ligands on APCs, MHC class II, intercellular cell adhesion molecule (ICAM), CD86/80 (B7-1/B7-2), and CD40 respectively to ensure that once antigen recognition by TCR signal 1, has occurred, the threshold for activation of a naïve T cell is overcome by delivering signal 2.

The two-signal model of T-cell activation is well accepted, but it is important to note that this is a simplification. The cytokine and chemokine milieu present at the time these molecular engagements occur affects the differentiation pathway a T cell takes and the course of the response. Cytokines and chemokines can modulate the expression of the cell surface molecules mentioned previously, as well as the expression of cytokine and chemokine receptors themselves. This modulation can result in differential signaling in the T cell and APC, tipping the balance of the response from full to partial activation or, in some circumstances, inactivation of the cells involved, modifying dramatically the downstream events (i.e., cell migration patterns and the generation of effector cells). Activation signals in the form of cytokines propagate the responses initiated by signals 1 and 2 and are often referred to as the third signal in T-cell activation.

Mechanisms of Tolerance to Donor Antigens

The human immune system has evolved naturally to respond to challenges in a precise and controlled way. A constant balance exists to ensure an effective, but not excessive, response to any unwanted stimuli. Therefore, it may be possible to take advantage of these mechanisms to induce or maintain tolerance to donor antigens. Many mechanisms of tolerance are, in fact, continuously utilized by the body to prevent reactions against self antigens which would ultimately lead to autoimmune pathologies.[138] Many of these mechanisms and regulatory cell populations can be harnessed to induce and maintain tolerance to alloantigens.[213,217]

The mechanisms identified as responsible for inducing or maintaining tolerance to donor antigens include the following:

- Deletion of donor-reactive cells centrally in the thymus as well as in the periphery
- T-cell ignorance, or a state of T-cell unresponsiveness that is relevant to grafts placed at "immunologically privileged" sites such as the cornea or brain
- Exhaustion, in which the ability of donor-reactive cells is eliminated as a result of overstimulation and cell death
- Anergy, defined as a state of unresponsiveness that is refractory to further stimulation
- Immunoregulation – an active process whereby the immune response to an allograft is controlled by populations of regulatory immune cells.

To exploit regulation of the immune response to an organ graft for therapeutic purposes, a clearer understanding of the mechanisms by which this phenomenon operates is required. Although, theoretically, regulation could be operating exclusively through a single mechanism, such as deletion that could result in the elimination of donor-reactive T cells and B cells from the repertoire, as will be discussed below, at present there is little evidence to support this as the only, or even the dominant, mechanism for inducing and maintaining unresponsiveness to cell and organ transplants. The more likely scenario is that different mechanisms work in concert and that distinct combinations of mechanisms are brought into play depending on donor and recipient characteristics, immunosuppression, infection, and so on.

Mechanisms of Tolerance Induction and Maintenance

Persistence of Donor Antigen

An overriding feature in all of the mechanisms of tolerance mentioned above is the persistent presence of donor antigen throughout the period of tolerance *in vivo*. Many experimental models have established that donor antigen must be present continuously to maintain a tolerant state, before or after transplantation, irrespective of the precise mechanisms involved.[21,67,170] The source of the antigen can be donor-derived cells introduced before transplantation, as is the case in models of mixed chimerism,[86] or the graft itself after transplantation.[67] In the absence of antigen, tolerance is lost gradually because the mechanisms responsible for maintaining tolerance are no longer stimulated. During the induction phase and the maintenance phase of tolerance, the presence of alloantigen is the key factor driving the outcome. As is often the case with the immune system, the same element can influence the response both positively and negatively. In the case of donor antigen, presentation in the wrong context, as in a proinflammatory environment, as outlined above, could lead to activation with the potential of destroying the tolerant state and triggering graft rejection, but once tolerance is established it is critical for maintaining the tolerant state.

Deletion of Donor-Reactive Leukocytes

T cells. The death or deletion of lymphocytes that can recognize and respond to self antigens or, after transplantation, donor alloantigens is a very effective mechanism for eliminating lymphocytes from the immune repertoire that have the potential to damage the host or the graft, thereby creating unresponsiveness or tolerance to self or donor alloantigens. Both T cells and B cells can be deleted from the repertoire in this manner and, if this is the only mechanism in operation, deletion needs to be sustained to maintain tolerance in the long term.

Central tolerance by clonal deletion of T cells in the thymus is the major mechanism by which tolerance to self antigens is induced and can be exploited as a mechanism for inducing tolerance to donor antigens.

Central deletion of donor alloantigen-reactive T cells has been particularly successful in the context of therapeutic strategies using donor bone marrow in combination with non-myeloablative therapy, such as T-cell depletion or costimulation blockade, for the induction of tolerance.[187] The clinical applicability of this strategy can be demonstrated by kidney transplant recipients who have previously undergone bone marrow transplantation from the same donor due to hematologic indications.[178] Macrochimerism in these patients leads to long-term graft acceptance without immunosuppression. In mixed allogeneic chimeras in the mouse, donor-derived DCs have been shown to reside and persist in the recipient thymus.[116,197] As a result, there is continuous deletion of donor-reactive thymocytes, leading to the absence of donor-reactive T cells in the periphery and tolerance to donor alloantigens.

The challenge of these approaches is to achieve a sufficient level of chimerism reliably without using a treatment regimen that is excessively toxic. Moreover, data regarding the necessity for durable chimerism are conflicting. Data from clinical studies suggest that transient, rather than persistent, chimerism may be sufficient in the presence of other immunosuppressive agents to achieve tolerance in some individuals.[81] In contrast, primate studies have shown that even in the presence of persistent chimerism rejection can occur.[157]

Intrathymic injection of donor antigen or allopeptides directly into the thymus results in the deletion of donor-reactive cells.[76,152] If this injection of antigen is combined with leukocyte or T-cell depletion in the periphery, it can lead to the successful induction of operational donor-specific tolerance (DST) in rodents.[76]

Antigen-reactive T cells may also be deleted from the T-cell repertoire in the periphery.[209] The introduction of high doses of defined antigens intravenously or orally has been shown to result in deletion of mature T cells in the peripheral lymphoid organs.[8,82] Both $CD4^+$ and $CD8^+$ T cells can be eliminated by peripheral deletion, but in many cases deletion is incomplete, even when high doses of antigen are used. However, this approach might also enable another mechanism of control to be developed, the generation or expansion of regulatory T cells.[145]

The mechanisms by which T cells are deleted in the thymus and the periphery have been an area of active investigation. Two distinct modes of apoptosis have been implicated as the mechanism essential for T-cell death in these settings. Activation-induced cell death (AICD) is a process through which T cells undergo cell death in the periphery.[93] Following restimulation through TCR, a number of different molecules, including CD95 (Fas), TNF receptor 1 (TNFR1), and TNF-related apoptosis-inducing ligand receptor (TRAILR), can play a role in AICD depending on the circumstances, triggering a complex series of signaling events which ultimately lead to caspase activation, DNA fragmentation, cytoskeletal degradation, and cell death. Either high doses of antigen or repetitive stimulation is necessary for AICD in the periphery.[211]

The Fas pathway may also play a role, in combination with other mechanisms, in the deletion of T cells at particular sites in the periphery, so-called immune-privileged sites that include the testis and the eye.[7] At these sites, transplantation of allogeneic tissues results in the prolonged survival of the transplanted tissue relative to the survival obtained after transplantation of the same tissue at other sites. Fas ligand expression has been shown to be an important contributor enabling these sites to maintain their immune-privileged status. The Fas pathway also has been implicated in deletional tolerance after administration of allogeneic bone marrow.[55] However, attempts that have been made to harness the immunologic potential of these immune-privileged sites have been met with varying degrees of success,[202] suggesting that multiple mechanisms are involved.

In addition to the Fas pathway, other peripheral mechanisms have been implicated in clonal downsizing after the elimination of antigen, including upregulation of expression of CD152 (CTLA-4), a negative regulator of T-cell activation on T cells.[207] Another immunoinhibitory costimulatory molecule, programmed cell death 1 receptors (PD-1), can inhibit lymphocyte activation when it binds to its ligands, PD-L1 and PD-L2.[49]

The reappearance of donor-reactive cells at a functional level can be controlled or prevented by the continuing presence of donor antigen in the form of the organ graft (discussed above) and/or active immunoregulation. This process results in the long-term survival of the graft, provided that the rate of deletion is maintained or that additional mechanisms that can promote tolerance to the graft are induced.

B cells. The elimination of B cells from the repertoire is also a mechanism that has evolved to ensure that B cells that are polyreactive and capable of binding self antigens are eliminated in the bone marrow before they enter the periphery. As rearrangement of immunoglobulin genes occurs at random to enable as many foreign protein and carbohydrate antigens to be recognized as possible, it inevitably leads to the generation of B cells that express B-cell receptors (BCR) that can recognize self antigens. Estimates vary, but suggest that up to 70% of the immature B cells produced are self-reactive. Of the order of one-third of these immature B cells are eliminated by receptor editing, whereby new gene rearrangements result in the production of an alternate light chain that can pair with the existing heavy chain, altering the antigen recognition properties of the expressed BCR. When an immature B cell recognizes self antigen with high avidity, it rapidly internalizes the antigen and undergoes a period of developmental arrest. Lymph node homing receptors, such as CD62 ligand (CD62L), are not expressed, and the receptors for B-cell-activating factor (BAFF), a cytokine required for B-cell survival, are not induced. In addition, recombinase activating genes remain switched on, which allows the BCR to be replaced by editing the light chain. Any B cell undergoing this process will die after 1–2 days if it fails to express a non-autoreactive receptor. Death through this pathway does not require Fas and is, in part, due to antigen-induced expression of the Bcl-2 interacting mediator of cell death (Bim), which inhibits B-cell survival proteins from the Bcl-2 family.

Receptor editing is a mechanism that could be used to delete immature B cells capable of recognizing donor alloantigens from the repertoire, particularly in situations where the repertoire is reshaped following leukocyte depletion or the induction of mixed chimerism, as well as when organs are transplanted into young infants.

If receptor editing fails to eliminate all of the self-reactive B cells generated, residual immature B cells expressing highly self-reactive receptors are triggered to die by interaction with self antigen. This mechanism of control or regulation has been studied using immunoglobulin transgenic mice and the data obtained suggest that B cells are deleted efficiently when the antigen they recognize is membrane-bound. The efficiency of this process was found to be dependent on the probability that the immature B cells encountered the relevant self antigen and therefore its efficiency is clearly related to antigen density/frequency.

Deletion of B cells capable of recognizing donor alloantigens from the repertoire of a transplant recipient is a mechanism that can be harnessed in transplantation. This mechanism of regulation is most efficient when the antigens recognized are present at high doses. Infant recipients of ABO-incompatible heart allografts have been shown to delete B cells capable of making antibodies to blood group antigens presented on the heart transplant.[44] Mixed chimerism strategies that result in the coexistence of donor and recipient bone marrow should also enable donor-reactive B cells to be deleted if the level of chimerism achieved is sufficient to ensure that B cells encounter donor cells.[188]

Regulation of Immune Responses

Although the concept of antigen-specific suppression is not new, over the past 10 years there has been a resurgence of interest in the characterization and functional dissection of T-cell-mediated suppression, now more often called immunoregulation.

Suppression was described first in the 1970s after the demonstration that antigen-specific unresponsiveness could be transferred from one recipient to another.[56] Importantly, transplantation provided some of the earliest evidence for suppression or immune regulation by T cells *in vivo*. Data from neonatal tolerance studies suggested that additional mechanisms beyond deletion of donor-reactive cells were involved.[12,215]

Different populations of immune regulatory cells can play a role in controlling the immune response after transplantation, including Treg, regulatory B cells (Breg), myeloid-derived suppressor cells (MDSCs), DCs, and regulatory macrophages.[213]

Regulatory T Cells

Many different types of T cells with regulatory activity have been described, including $CD4^+$ T cells,[166,217] $CD8^+$ T cells,[107,160,205] $CD4^-CD8^-$ double-negative T cells,[194] natural killer (NK) T cells,[128] and γδT cells.[71] As $CD4^+$ T cells with regulatory functions have been studied in greater depth to date, this section will focus on this population of regulatory cells.

$CD25^+FOXP3^+$ Treg can arise via two distinct developmental pathways. First, as mentioned above, thymus-derived or naturally occurring regulatory cells (nTreg) differentiate in the thymus and are thought to function primarily to suppress responses to self antigen and hence prevent autoimmune disease. Evidence for this comes from studies in patients with rare genetic defects and in mice with either naturally occurring or genetically engineered defects. For example, profound immune dysregulation leading to autoimmunity is observed in patients with the immune dysregulation polyendocrinopathy enteropathy X-linked (IPEX) syndrome. IPEX patients have been found to have a point mutation in the gene encoding factor forkhead box P3 (FOXP3),[11,92] the master gene for T-cell regulation, resulting in functional impairment of Treg activity *in vitro*.[5] Scurfy mice also have mutations in FOXP3 and a related immune profile.[158] Second, when $CD4^+$ T cells encounter antigen in a tolerogenic microenvironment in the periphery, such as when antigen is presented by immature DCs or in the presence of immunosuppressive cytokines, the $CD4^+$ T cells differentiate into "adaptive" or antigen-induced Treg (iTreg).[77] In the context of transplantation, it can be argued that this pathway may be the more important route to generating donor alloantigen-reactive Treg after transplantation.[214] Moreover, this pathway may be used to sustain the unresponsive state through a process often referred to as infectious tolerance. Immunoregulatory cells have been shown to be able to transfer unresponsiveness from a transplant recipient with a long-term surviving graft to a fresh naïve recipient through many generations of cells, suggesting that, in the presence of donor antigen, Treg can generate further cohorts by influencing the differentiation patterns of naïve cells *in vivo*.[84,154] These cells appear to function not by eliminating donor-reactive aggressive leukocytes, but by silencing their functional activity *in vivo*. Interestingly, despite their distinct developmental origins, both nTreg and iTreg rely on sustained expression of high levels of the transcription of FOXP3 for their suppressive function.

A clear indication that long-term allograft survival in the absence of long-term immunosuppression, a status referred to as operational transplantation tolerance, involved the presence of T cells with the ability to regulate the function of naïve alloreactive T cells, thereby preventing the rejection of a fresh graft, was reported.[64,65] Subsequently, this form of cellular regulation was found to be associated with $CD4^+$ T cells and Hall and colleagues were the first to suggest that CD25 might be a useful marker for identifying $CD4^+$ T cells with regulatory activity.[66] Similar data were obtained in a rat renal allograft model where operational tolerance was induced by donor-specific blood transfusion.[155,156] As a direct demonstration that $CD4^+$ T cells expressing high levels of CD25 could regulate rejection, Hara and colleagues showed that cotransfer of $CD4^+CD25^+$ T cells from tolerant animals led to indefinite skin graft survival in 80% of immunodeficient mice reconstituted with naïve CBA effector T cells.[69]

In the absence of any previous exposure to alloantigen there are usually insufficient numbers of nTreg to prevent rejection of a fully allogeneic (MHC + minor histocompatibility antigen mismatched) graft, as the frequency of T cells present in the repertoire capable of making a destructive response to the graft far outnumbers the relatively small numbers of nTreg present and rejection occurs.[69] The fact that nTreg cannot prevent destruction of an allograft in the absence of immunosuppression does not mean that the cells do not function. However, under these circumstances, the balance between rejection and regulation is against regulation, as the suppressive activity of any Treg present is overwhelmed by the destructive response mediated by effector T cells. The presence of pre-existing donor alloantigen-reactive memory T cells in the recipient can also overwhelm immune regulation as the kinetics of activation of the memory cells is very rapid and, unless very high numbers of Tregs are present at the outset of the response, the balance between rejection and regulation is pushed markedly in favor of rejection.[221] Importantly, this critical balance between graft destruction and acceptance can be shifted in a number of ways, notably by employing strategies that increase the relative frequency and/or the activation status and consequently the functional activity of a Treg that can then respond to donor alloantigens before or in the early period after transplantation,[48,59] or by inhibiting or reducing the activity of the effector cells.

Whilst the observation that mice with long-term surviving allografts contain populations of alloantigen-reactive CD25$^+$ Treg was important, these experiments were unable to distinguish between Treg that were generated by the induction strategy itself and those that arose simply by the presence of the accepted allograft. In terms of developing potential clinical approaches, it is important to clarify whether induction strategies that ultimately lead to long-term operational tolerance can drive Treg development independently of the graft itself. Data demonstrating that exposure to alloantigen in the absence of a transplant can lead to the induction of CD4$^+$CD25$^+$ Treg were obtained in a number of studies. For example, when CD4$^+$CD25$^+$ were isolated from mice 28 days after pretreatment with donor alloantigen in combination with non-depleting anti-CD4 therapy, these cells prevented rejection of a test skin graft in a sensitive adoptive transfer model.[87] Critically, protection of the test graft was not observed with similar populations isolated from naïve mice, or mice treated with anti-CD4 only or DST only, demonstrating that tolerance mediated by CD25$^+$ Treg can indeed be induced *in vivo* before transplantation if recipients are exposed to donor alloantigen under permissive conditions. Moreover, data have been reported demonstrating that the presence of the allograft alone can lead to the development of T cells with regulatory properties that can protect a challenged graft from rejection,[67] even when the allograft itself has been rejected.[201] Both of these examples demonstrate that T cells with regulatory activity can be induced in the presence of alloantigen in the form of the allograft or an infusion of alloantigen, or indeed both, and that these cells can contribute to controlling subsequent responses to alloantigen *in vivo*.

Another important issue that has been under investigation is where Treg that can control allograft rejection function most effectively and where they can be found or detected *in vivo*. There is evidence that the location in which Treg function may change with time after transplantation. Early in the response after transplantation, Treg have been shown to be present and functionally active in the draining lymph nodes, while later in the posttransplant course Treg have been shown to function within the allograft itself.[25] Indeed, there is increasing evidence that an important site of immune regulation is within the allograft itself, where Treg function to create an environment that is permissive of control.[58,83,84] Moreover, re-exposing Treg to antigen in a tissue may enable them to become more potent suppressors and therefore more effective at controlling rejection.[162]

Although a significant body of work has demonstrated that Treg can control responses to alloantigen, most studies have used either *in vitro* assays or experimental models whereby cells are adoptively transferred into immunodeficient recipients, where allograft rejection is driven by relatively small numbers of effector T cells compared to the number that would be found in a full immune repertoire *in vivo*. Arguably, a much more relevant question for clinical application of this approach is: What role do Treg play in an intact immune system? In transplantation Treg-specific inactivation was used to show that, in the anti-CD4/DST tolerance induction model described above, the survival of primary heart allografts in normal, lymphoreplete recipients is also unequivocally dependent on iTreg driven by the tolerance induction protocol.[22] These data suggest that it should indeed be possible to boost the function of Tregs in non-lymphopenic transplant patients.

The mechanisms used by Treg to control the activity of other cell populations include cell–cell contact. CD152 has been shown to play a critical role in this respect,[87] as well as the creation of a microenvironment through molecules such as IL-10[69] and transforming growth factor-β (TGF-β).[78]

The microenvironment created by the presence of Treg in the lymphoid tissues and the allograft contributes to the phenomenon of linked unresponsiveness, a powerful mechanism that allows tolerance to "spread" from the initiating antigen to those present on cells in the immediate vicinity (Figure 23-3). For example, if a recipient's immune system is exposed to a defined alloantigen before transplantation either alone or in combination with immunomodulating agents, the immune response to that antigen will be modulated and subsequently the unresponsiveness achieved will be linked to other molecules present on the transplanted tissue.[33,115]

Regulatory B Cells

B cells with the capacity to suppress the development of autoimmune diseases in mice were first described in the 1980s. Breg express high levels of CD1d, CD21, CD24, and IgM and moderate levels of CD19, although some heterogeneity has been described, suggesting that different subsets of Breg may exist.[122] One of the characteristics of B cells with regulatory activity is their ability to secrete IL-10. CD40 stimulation appears to be required to stimulate IL-10 production and has been reported to be necessary for activation of Breg, enabling them to manifest their functional activity and suppress Th1 differentiation. It has been suggested that there is a link between regulatory B cells and T cells, with Breg acting as potent generators of Treg. Breg have been described in both mouse and human. Mouse Breg express T-cell Ig domain and mucin domain protein 1 (Tim-1).[37] Human regulatory B cells share some properties with their mouse counterparts, including an immature phenotype, and comprise a small subset of the total B-cell pool.

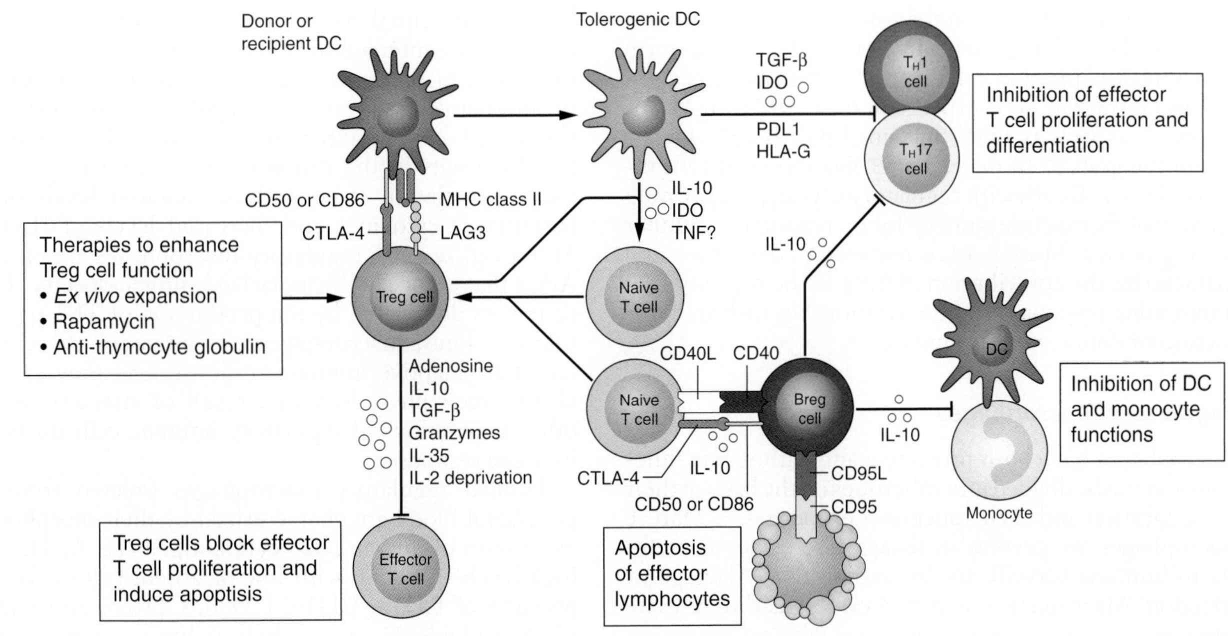

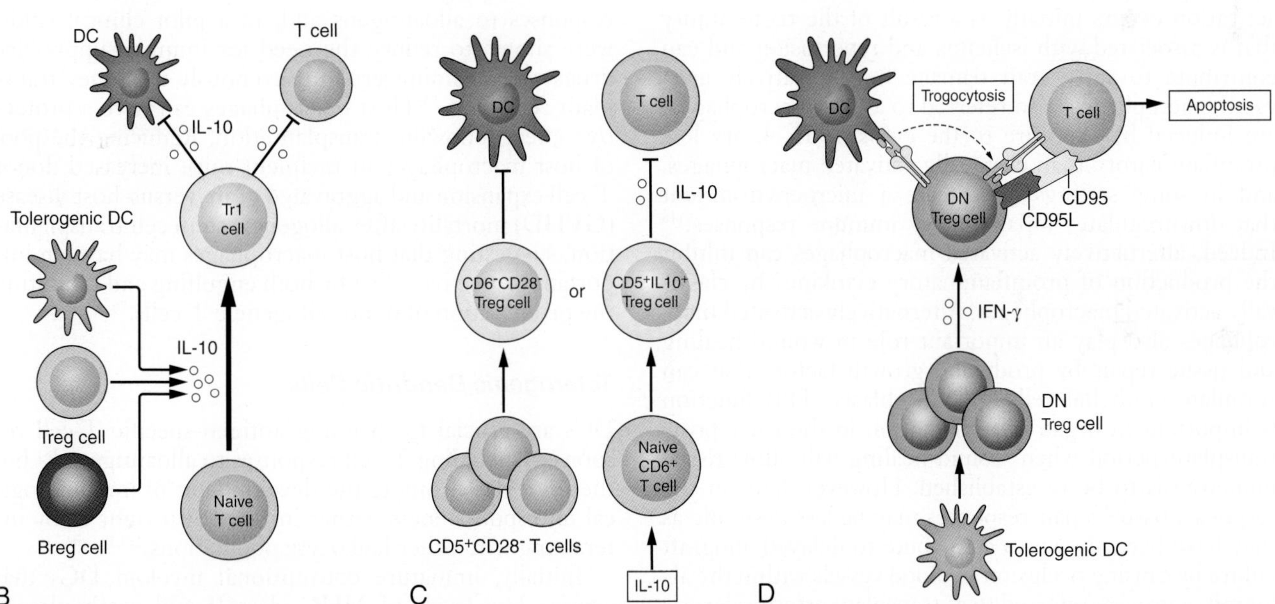

FIGURE 23-3 ■ Mechanisms used by adaptive regulatory immune cells in transplantation. (A) nTreg cells that can respond to donor alloantigens through crossreactivity will be present in the recipient at the time of transplantation. These will be recruited to the allograft where they can suppress ischemia-reperfusion injury. In the draining lymphoid tissue nTreg cells will inhibit T-cell proliferation. Breg and tolerogeneic dendritic cells (DC) will engage naïve T cells, inducing iTreg cells that will contribute to Treg cell-mediated suppression of allograft rejection within the allograft through a variety of mechanisms, including production of interleukin-10 (IL-10) and transforming growth factor-β (TGF-β), inhibition of antigen presenting cell (APC) function as well as through alteration of amino acid and energy metabolism. (B) Tr1 cells are FOXP3-regulatory T cells induced in the presence of IL-10 produced by Treg cells, tolerogenic DC, or Breg, either in the draining lymphoid tissue or within the allograft. They can suppress both APC and T-cell function. (C) $CD8^+$ Treg cells contribute to immune regulation. $CD8^+CD28^-$ cells can inhibit APC function, while in the presence of IL-10 naïve $CD8^+$ T cells can be converted to $CD8^+$Tr cells that function in a similar manner to Tr1 cells. (D) $CD4^-CD8^-$ (DN) T cells function by downregulating the expression of costimulatory molecules, thereby inhibiting the ability of APC to stimulate an immune response and inducing apoptosis of DC. In addition, DN T cells can acquire alloantigen through trogocytosis, enabling them to present antigen to T cells, resulting in T-cell apoptosis. (Reproduced with permission from Wood KJ, Bushell A, Hester J. Regulatory immune cells in transplantation. Nat Rev Immunol 2012;12:417–30.)

In transplantation, there is only indirect evidence that Breg may play a role in controlling immune responses to alloantigens. Interestingly, in renal transplant recipients who have a functioning graft in the absence of immunosuppression, a B-cell signature was found to be associated with this state of operational tolerance to donor alloantigens.[135,165] A distinct, but also B-cell-dominated, signature of tolerance was identified in a separate cohort of long-term immunosuppression-free renal transplant recipients.[144]

Experimental studies on the role of Breg in transplantation are limited at present. In a rat model of long-term kidney transplantation tolerance, a shift in both peripheral and intragraft gene expression from IgG to IgM was observed, as well as IgM$^+$, but not IgG$^+$, B-cell clusters within the graft.[101] In mice, Tim-1 ligation on B cells induced Tim-1$^+$ B cells with regulatory activity,[37] suggesting a potential therapeutic strategy for increasing the number of Breg *in vivo*. More work is required to determine and characterize the contribution of Breg in the regulation of alloimmune responses and the relationship with the production of donor-specific antibody.[28]

Regulatory Macrophages

Macrophages have both protective and pathogenic functions and can be divided into subgroups on the basis of their tissue location and their functional properties.[132] Mature macrophages are present in tissues where they contribute to immune surveillance by sensing tissue damage or infection. Macrophages activated via TLRs differentiate into classically activated macrophages (also referred to as M1 macrophages) and produce inflammatory cytokines, including TNF and IL-1. In transplantation, macrophage activation occurs initially as a result of the tissue injury that is associated with ischemia and reperfusion and can contribute to early graft damage.[106] Alternatively activated macrophages (also referred to as M2 macrophages) are induced by exposure to the cytokine IL-4, are less proinflammatory than classically activated macrophages, and in some settings can create a microenvironment that downregulates inflammatory immune responses.[118] Indeed, alternatively activated macrophages can inhibit the production of proinflammatory cytokines by classically activated macrophages. Alternatively activated macrophages also play an important role in wound healing and tissue repair by producing growth factors that can stimulate epithelial cells and fibroblasts. This function is important in organ transplantation in the early post-transplant period when wound healing will allow tissue homeostasis to be re-established. However, later in the response, tissue repair responses may be less desirable as they have been shown to contribute to delayed allograft failure by causing occlusion of blood vessels within the allograft, a process referred to as transplant arteriosclerosis or transplant-associated vasculopathy.

It has been proposed that regulatory macrophages may represent an additional distinct macrophage population whose main physiological role is to dampen inflammatory immune responses and prevent the immunopathology associated with prolonged classical macrophage activation.[46] However, to date, no stable, convenient surface markers specific for regulatory macrophages have been identified. Regulatory macrophages produce high amounts of IL-10, a common feature of leukocytes with immunoregulatory properties, usually following costimulation with two ligands, for example, TLR and immune complexes. Unlike alternatively activated macrophages, regulatory macrophages do not express arginase and are not dependent on STAT6 signaling.

Macrophages are positioned within the lymphoid architecture to interact with lymphocytes, and therefore have the potential to influence each other's functional activity. The interaction of Treg cells with macrophages can result in the macrophages acquiring the properties of alternatively activated or regulatory macrophages[195] (Figure 23-2). The interaction of macrophages with B1 B cells results in the formation of a regulatory macrophage population that produces reduced levels of inflammatory cytokines and increased levels of IL-10.[212] Moreover, *in vitro*, regulatory macrophages are efficient APCs that induce highly polarized antigen-specific T-cell responses dominated by the production of Th2-type cytokines. Thus, macrophages can influence the character of an adaptive immune response, and they can also change their physiology as a result of interactions with other populations of regulatory immune cells during an immune response.

Human regulatory macrophages isolated from the peripheral blood are characterized by their morphology, expression of human leukocyte antigen (HLA)-DR, and high levels of CD86 with low or absent cell surface expression of CD14, CD16, CD80, CD163, and CD282 (TLR2) (Table 23-1) and their ability to suppress mitogen-driven T-cell proliferation *in vitro*. Human regulatory macrophages have the capacity to regulate immune responses to alloantigens and, in a pilot clinical study, were shown to reduce the need for immunosuppressive drugs when administered intravenously to kidney transplant recipients.[73] Host macrophages can have a protective effect following transplantation. Reducing the pool of host macrophages in recipient mice increased donor T-cell expansion and aggravated graft-versus-host disease (GVHD) mortality after allogeneic stem cell transplantation, suggesting that host macrophages may have an important protective effect by both engulfing and inhibiting the proliferation of donor allogeneic T cells.[70]

Tolerogenic Dendritic Cells

DCs are crucial for priming antigen-specific T-cell responses, including T-cell responses to alloantigens,[181] but they can also promote the development of immunological unresponsiveness, either in their own right or by interacting with other leukocyte populations.[129,182,203,215]

Initially, immature conventional myeloid DCs that express low levels of MHC class II and costimulatory molecules at the cell surface were identified as the dominant form of DC that had the capacity to induce T-cell tolerance.[112] Indeed, immature DCs can promote tolerance to solid-organ allografts and bone marrow grafts[129] and their tolerogenic effects can be enhanced by other immunomodulatory agents, such as drugs that block the CD40–CD40L costimulatory axis.[111] However, as the characterization of DCs has progressed, it is clear that the state of maturity of the DCs is not the only factor that enables them to induce unresponsiveness.

Plasmacytoid DCs (pDCs) produce type I IFNs in response to single-stranded nucleic acids, which activate pDCs via both TLR-dependent and TLR-independent pathways, thus promoting antiviral innate and adaptive immune responses. Compared with conventional DCs, pDCs express lower levels of the costimulatory molecules CD80 and CD86 and higher levels of the inhibitory molecule PD-L1, and consequently exhibit poor immunostimulatory activity. Indeed, pDC interaction with naïve T cells has been shown to promote the generation of Treg cells in the thymus and in the periphery. The molecular mechanisms used by pDCs to promote tolerance are complex.[186] In experimental models, pDCs can acquire alloantigen in the allograft and then migrate to the draining lymphoid tissue where they interact with T cells and induce the generation of $CCR4^+CD4^+CD25^+Foxp3^+$ Treg cells.[137] In mice, pre-pDC appear to be the principal cell type that facilitates HSC engraftment and induction of donor-specific skin graft tolerance in allogeneic recipients.[57]

In humans, pDCs produce significant amounts of IL-10, low levels of IFN-γ, and no detectable IL-4, IL-5, or TGF-β, creating a microenvironment that promotes immune regulation.[57] Tolerogenic human DCs that secrete high levels of IL-10 in the absence of IL-12 induce adaptive IL-10-producing regulatory type-1 (Tr1) T cells.[103] Data demonstrating that DCs regulate the suppressive ability, expansion, and/or differentiation of Treg cells, with the loss of DCs resulting in reduced numbers of Treg cells, have been reported in mice.[32] Thus tolerogenic DCs and T cells with regulatory activity may be linked and act in concert with one another in some situations.

The tolerogenic phenotype of human DCs has been characterized by high cell surface expression of the inhibitory receptor ILT3.[27] In DCs, ILT3 signaling on binding cognate ligands such as MHC class I, HLA-G, and CD1d inhibits tyrosine phosphorylation, NF-κB and MAPK p38 activity, transcription of certain costimulatory molecules, and the secretion of proinflammatory cytokines and chemokines. In addition, ILT3 can interact with its ligands on T cells to promote inhibitory signaling in T cells. Stimulation through ILT3 appears to be a prerequisite for DC tolerization. Both $ILT3^{high}$ tolerogenic DCs and soluble ILT3 have been shown to induce $CD4^+$ T-cell anergy and differentiation of antigen-specific $CD8^+$ suppressor T cells.[206]

Higher numbers of pDCs than myeloid DCs have been found in the peripheral blood of pediatric liver transplant recipients who were operationally tolerant to their allograft as well as those receiving low-dose immunosuppressive therapy during prospective immunosuppressive drug weaning, compared with patients on maintenance immunosuppression.[123] In addition, higher levels of expression of PD-L1 and CD86 by pDC were found to correlate with elevated numbers of $CD4^+CD25^{high}FOXP3^+$ Treg cells in liver transplant recipients who were free from immunosuppressive drug regimens.[196] These data suggest that pDCs and Treg cells may contribute to immune regulation in liver transplant recipients.

The ability of different populations of DCs to induce tolerance, combined with clinical observations, suggests that both myeloid DCs and pDCs can promote tolerance to alloantigens, and that DC maturation in itself is not the distinguishing feature that separates immunogenic DC functions from tolerogenic ones.[121] Indeed, maturation is more of a continuum than an "on-off" switch, and a "semimature" state, in which DCs are phenotypically mature but remain poor producers of proinflammatory cytokines, appears to be better linked with tolerogenic function. The use of DCs to facilitate the induction of operational tolerance is not without risk. DCs are arguably better known for the ability to prime the immune system. Indeed, DCs pulsed with antigen are being used clinically as vaccines to stimulate immune responses to tumor antigens. Using DCs as a cellular therapy in transplantation may carry the risk of sensitizing the recipient. One possible approach to reducing this risk is to combine DC administration with costimulatory blockade with the objective of presenting donor alloantigens to induce T-cell unresponsiveness.

Myeloid-Derived Suppressor Cells

MDSCs have been associated with many antigen specific and non-specific suppressive functions, including regulation of innate immunity, T-cell activation, and tumor immunity. MDSCs are a heterogeneous population of progenitor cells that can accumulate in tissues during an inflammatory immune response, where they differentiate into macrophages, DCs, and granulocytes. The expansion and activation of MDSCs are regulated by factors produced by other cells that are present in the same microenvironment, including stromal cells, activated T cells and, in tumors, the tumor cells themselves.

Several MDSC subsets have been described in both mice and humans.[16] Despite their heterogeneity, common phenotypical markers are expressed by most MDSCs, including Gr1 and CD11b in mice, and CD33, CD11b, CD34 and low levels of MHC class II in humans. Activated MDSCs suppress proliferation and cytokine production by effector T cells, B cells, and NK cells *in vitro* through mechanisms that include their expression of inducible nitric oxide synthase 1, which induces nitric oxide production, and expression of arginase 1, which depletes arginine. MDSCs also appear to be able to inhibit T-cell proliferation and modify T-cell differentiation pathways. For example, they can promote Treg cell differentiation in a process requiring IFN-γ and IL-10.[63] Interestingly, interactions between MDSCs and macrophages result in a shift of macrophages towards an alternatively activated phenotype and the increased production of IL-10 by MDSCs.[51]

In experimental transplant models, MDSCs have been shown to promote tolerance to alloantigens. Direct evidence of a tolerogenic role for MDSCs has been obtained for heart and islet allografts in mice[29,52] and by iNOS-expressing MDSCs in a rat kidney allograft model.[40] In bone marrow transplantation, indirect evidence for a role of MDSCs has come from the observation that transplantation tolerance could not be induced in mice that did not express MHC class II on circulating leukocytes, despite the fact that many other leukocyte populations may also be altered in this setting.[220] The mechanisms used by MDSCs to promote tolerance to alloantigens require further clarification. Some evidence suggests that they may act partly through the induction or sparing of Treg.[40] Alternatively, MDSCs have been found to upregulate heme oxygenase 1, an enzyme that has immunoregulatory activity through the inhibition of DC maturation and preservation of IL-10 function as well as cytoprotective properties.[35]

Mesenchymal Stromal Cells

Mesenchymal stromal cells (MSCs) are a subpopulation of multipotent cells within the bone marrow that support hematopoiesis and possess immunomodulatory and reparative properties.[41] Bone marrow-derived MSCs have the ability to migrate to sites of inflammation, including to an allograft.[39] When MSCs are exposed to an inflammatory microenvironment they have been found capable of regulating many immune effector functions through specific interactions with leukocytes that participate in both innate and adaptive responses. The proinflammatory cytokines IFN-γ, TNF-α, and/or IL-1β have been shown to activate bone marrow-derived MSCs.[161] *In vivo*, activation by IFN-γ has been shown to be essential for preventing GVHD by MSCs.[151] Once activated, MSCs can control the activity of T cells,[172] B cells,[4] DCs,[176] NKs,[177] and macrophages,[4,134] either through direct cell–cell contact or indirectly through the release of soluble factors into the local microenvironment. The cocktail of factors secreted by MSCs includes matrix metalloproteinases (MMPs),[38,39,110] with the production of MMP2 being linked directly to a decrease in CD25 expression on $CD4^+$ T cells and the inhibition of alloantigen-driven proliferation resulting in long-term survival of allogeneic islets of Langerhans.[39]

MSCs have been shown to promote the generation of Treg cells *in vitro* and *in vivo* through mechanisms involving prostaglandin E_2, TGF-β, and cell–cell contact.[26,42] The impact of MSCs on the generation of Treg cells may also be indirect as MSCs can influence the maturation of DCs. DCs repeatedly exposed to MSCs are maintained in an immature-like state, indicated by the downregulation of CD11c, CD80, CD86, and CD40 and upregulation of CD11b.[222] In transplantation, retrieval and transplantation of the allograft inevitably result in ischemia and reperfusion injury creating an inflammatory microenvironment within the graft. The recruitment of MSCs to the graft in the early posttransplant period could potentially lead to the conversion of T cells, also recruited into the allograft, into Treg cells. The immunomodulatory properties of MSCs on B-cell function could also contribute to suppressing graft rejection by inhibiting alloantibody production.[54]

Information from Analyzing Tolerant Recipients

Operational tolerance, whereby an allograft remains functional and rejection-free for over 1 year without immunosuppression, is often described as the holy grail of transplantation. Clearly, to be able to achieve operational tolerance would have a major benefit for the patient, reducing the morbidity and mortality associated with lifelong immunosuppression. However, operational tolerance remains a relatively rare event in the clinical setting.

A small number of bone marrow transplant recipients who subsequently required a renal transplant were transplanted with a kidney from their bone marrow donor.[75,167,175] In these cases, long-term immunosuppression was unnecessary because the recipient was already unresponsive to the donor alloantigens as a result of the allogeneic chimerism that developed after the successful bone marrow transplant. Clinical reports of patients exhibiting spontaneous tolerance to an allograft, after withdrawal of immunosuppression in the absence of a bone marrow transplant, are still infrequent but are increasing in number.[17,4,142,163,189] Based on these case reports, a number of groups proposed that, by studying these patients in depth, it would be possible to define a molecular signature of tolerance in immunosuppression-free kidney and liver transplant recipients (see below).[104,120,135,165]

The majority of patients who are able to stop immunosuppression without rejection of their allograft arrive at that point as a result of either discontinuation of immunosuppression by the clinical team as a consequence of the side effects of immunosuppression or non-adherence/compliance or as a result of weaning of immunosuppression based on a clinical protocol (particularly in liver transplant recipients) designed to minimize immunosuppressive drugs without compromising the function of the allograft. There is also a smaller group of patients who have been treated with protocols designed with the deliberate aim of inducing tolerance to a kidney transplant; this will be discussed in detail below.[81,102,168,178,184]

It is generally accepted that there is a hierarchy with respect to the ease of inhibition or suppression of immune response directed against different organs. Liver allografts and skin grafts are at the two opposite ends of this spectrum. In experimental transplantation liver allografts are sometimes accepted spontaneously in the absence of any immunosuppression or immunomodulation.[23] Furthermore, in clinical transplantation it is often noted that the liver "protects" other organs that are transplanted alongside it from the full force of the rejection response – the so-called liver effect. Based upon these observations it has been suggested that liver allografts have the capacity to promote the development of immunological unresponsiveness. A number of mechanisms have been proposed to account for the liver effect, including many of those discussed above; for example, the large antigen load delivered by the liver itself, the presence of a large number of passenger leukocytes that could result in the deletion of donor-reactive cells, and the establishment of long-lasting microchimerism in some recipients as well as the production of soluble MHC class I by the liver.[180] As a result, liver transplant recipients have proved to be an interesting population of immunosuppression-free patients for investigations designed to determine if a molecular signature of tolerance exists.

Estimates vary, but in the order of 25–60% of liver transplant recipients appear to have the potential to be weaned from immunosuppression without the risk of rejection.[45,189] Early investigations focused on phenotyping the populations of leukocytes that were present in immunosuppression-free liver transplant recipients; the majority were weaned from immunosuppression as a result of participation in well-controlled clinical weaning protocols.[189] Analysis of the peripheral blood from immunosuppression-free liver transplant recipients revealed an increase in $CD25^+CD4^+$ T cells with regulatory activity *in vitro* as well as a skewing of other T-cell subsets, notably γδ T cells, compared to the profiles found in age-matched controls.[104,120] Interestingly, FOXP3+ cells were also found to be a prominent component of lymphocytes infiltrating the liver allografts.[108] Further analysis using transcriptional profiling demonstrated that there was a molecular signature of tolerance associated with tolerance in immunosuppression-free liver transplant recipients[15,119] and that this signature can be used to guide weaning off immunosuppression. In other words, the molecular signature can be used to provide a risk assessment of which patients are more likely to wean from immunosuppression without the risk of rejection – an exciting development for the future of clinical liver transplantation.[15]

In kidney transplantation, there are far fewer patients able to continue to have a functioning allograft in the absence of immunosuppression. Nevertheless, a small number of patients who are immunosuppression-free can be identified and have been studied to determine if there is a molecular signature of tolerance after kidney transplantation. Two independent studies, one in Europe and the other in the United States, found that there was a signature of tolerance in immunosuppression-free kidney transplant recipients that could be cross-validated between the two cohorts of patients studied. Interestingly, the signature of tolerance in kidney transplant recipients was distinct from that identified in immunosuppression-free liver transplant recipients. In immunosuppression-free kidney transplant recipients a predominance of B cells in the peripheral blood in the absence of donor-specific antibody was found in the signature. At first sight this finding was somewhat surprising, but may suggest that B cells with regulatory properties are present (see above). Gene expression analysis demonstrated that there was a pattern of gene expression associated with immunosuppression-free graft survival, nine of which were found to be most significant.[165] Further work is required to determine if the molecular signature of tolerance identified in kidney transplant recipients can be used to identify patients currently on immunosuppression who would benefit from withdrawal or minimization of immunosuppression if it could be withdrawn safely, i.e., without risk to the graft.

STRATEGIES WITH THE POTENTIAL TO INDUCE IMMUNOLOGIC TOLERANCE TO AN ALLOGRAFT

The strategies for tolerance induction being explored most actively at present invoke one or more of the mechanisms of tolerance outlined above, including the continuous deletion of donor-reactive leukocytes by establishing the presence of high levels of donor cells in the recipient (mixed chimerism), short-term depletion, and/or deletion of donor-reactive leukocytes combined with the establishment of immunoregulation and suppression of responses to donor alloantigens in the longer term after transplantation and costimulation blockade, leading to the induction of T-cell unresponsiveness in the presence of an organ graft.[74] Data emerging from the analysis of samples from patients enrolled in tolerance induction protocols again suggest that no single mechanism can account for or dominate the tolerance induction or maintenance process in transplant recipients.[135,165]

Most of the approaches being explored, with the exception of some protocols for inducing mixed chimerism, do not aim to induce tolerance to donor antigens before transplantation. Instead they attempt to use novel strategies that are relatively non-specific in their mode of action at the time of transplantation to create an environment that promotes the development of operational tolerance to the graft in the long term in the presence of the allograft. This often means that patients are treated with immunosuppressive drugs in the short term after transplantation with weaning of immunosuppression later in the transplant course. Although in an ideal world it could be argued that it would be preferable to switch off the immune response to donor antigens before the graft is transplanted, in the short term this may not be realistic with the therapeutic agents currently available. Moreover, the safety of the patient is a prime concern and therefore the development of tolerance to the graft in the long term still has major benefits for patients because it enables the total amount of immunosuppressive drug therapy to be reduced and, in some patients, eliminated over the transplant course, resulting in significant benefits for patients by reducing the side effects of lifelong immunosuppression.

Mixed Chimerism

The coexistence of stable mixtures of donor and recipient cells resulting in a state of allospecific tolerance is an idea that was initially restricted to the field of bone marrow and HSC transplantation. As mentioned above, a small number of bone marrow transplant recipients who subsequently required a renal transplant, and were transplanted with a kidney from their bone marrow donor, exhibited tolerance to donor alloantigens.[75,167,175] Obviously, bone marrow or HSC transplantation is not an appropriate approach to consider for most recipients on transplant waiting lists as achieving fully allogeneic chimerism requires a conditioning regimen that is relatively toxic and has the drawback of reducing the immunocompetence of the recipient's immune system in some situations. Nevertheless, these cases provided a foundation for the development of non-myeloablative conditioning protocols wherein donor bone marrow cells are introduced into recipients under conditions allowing for the development and maintenance of macrochimerism and long-term allograft survival.

Many different approaches have been used to achieve macrochimerism. Total lymphoid irradiation alone or in combination with bone marrow infusion has been shown to be effective at inducing tolerance in some recipients in rodents, primates, and human patients.[133,168,174,183] Despite the requirement for irradiation that has arguably inhibited the development and clinical application of these protocols to their fullest extent, strategies using total lymphoid irradiation have continued to be refined, leading to more recent reports that this approach can be used safely and effectively to induce tolerance to a kidney transplant. For example, Scandling and colleagues reported that a conditioning regimen of total lymphoid irradiation and antithymocyte globulin after transplantation resulted in the engraftment of donor HSC. The persistent mixed chimerism achieved enabled immunosuppression to be discontinued without rejection episodes or clinical manifestations of GVHD.[168]

The limitations of myeloablative therapy prompted the development and refinement of alternative approaches in animal models to enable high-dose bone marrow infusions in combination with non-myeloablative conditioning regimens that promote deletion of donor-reactive cells in the thymus. Interestingly, both costimulation blockade and T-cell depletion (see below) have been shown to be potentially useful in this context.[164] The demonstration that transient macrochimerism, via non-myeloablative conditioning, could achieve tolerance to renal allografts transplanted along with donor bone marrow in non-human primate models was the impetus for the translation of this approach to clinical transplantation.[80,126,164]

Mixed chimerism was first used successfully to treat a patient with multiple myeloma who had end-stage renal failure and received a kidney from an HLA-identical living donor.[178] The pretransplant workup included thymic irradiation, whole-body irradiation, splenectomy, and donor marrow infusion, and then relied on the administration of a short course of cyclosporine posttransplantation. As in the primate studies, macrochimerism was only detectable in the early period after transplantation, and after the first 2 months the percentage of donor cells declined. Nevertheless, withdrawal of immunosuppressive therapy (cyclosporine) at 10 weeks posttransplantation did not trigger rejection and immunosuppression-free survival, i.e., operational tolerance, persisted. To date, nine patients with end-stage renal failure who had an HLA-identical donor have been treated with this protocol,[19] with only one recipient developing evidence of renal allograft rejection after stopping immunosuppression that could be treated successfully by temporary reintroduction of immunosuppression. Although chimerism was lost in all of these patients, data suggesting that there was enrichment for $CD25^+$ CD4 T cells with regulatory activity after transplant were obtained,[50] suggesting that the maintenance of the macrochimeric state up to the time of transplantation may be sufficient to enable other mechanisms to be induced, enabling the graft to function in the absence of long-term immunosuppressive drug therapy.

As a result of these encouraging data and further refinement of the protocols in experimental models, the mixed chimerism approach for tolerance induction was extended to HLA-mismatched kidney transplants.[81] The first two patients enrolled in this trial were treated successfully and immunosuppression was withdrawn. However, the third patient developed irreversible humoral rejection 10 days after transplantation. Careful review of this case showed that this patient had high levels of pre-existing alloantibody activity, but no detectable donor-specific antibody before transplantation. The protocol was therefore modified to include rituximab (anti-CD20). Stable renal allograft function has been maintained in seven of the eight subjects in whom immunosuppression was discontinued, although long-term monitoring of all of these patients continues.

The analysis of samples from patients enrolled in this trial showed that the chimeric state was achieved but persisted only transiently. Evidence for unresponsiveness to donor alloantigens was obtained through *in vitro* assays and data supporting the idea that regulatory mechanisms were operating were obtained by analyzing FOXP3 expression by polymerase chain reaction.[81]

Costimulation Blockade

As discussed previously, the activation of a T cell is dependent upon multiple signals.[88] When antigen recognition occurs in the absence of costimulation, T cells become anergic or undergo apoptosis.[169] Monoclonal antibodies and recombinant fusion proteins targeting costimulatory molecules are capable of inducing unresponsiveness to donor antigens *in vivo* by allowing antigen recognition to take place in the absence of costimulation. The molecules that participate in costimulation pathways have attracted interest as targets for the development of novel therapeutics not only because they have immunosuppressive properties and the ability to prevent rejection but also to facilitate the induction of immunological unresponsiveness to donor alloantigens.

Members of the immunoglobulin and TNF:TNF receptor superfamilies make up many of the costimulatory molecules that are integral to positive and negative costimulation of T-cell responses. Research and development has been focused on two pairs of ligand–receptor interactions that seem to play key roles in positive costimulation: CD80/CD86 interacting with CD28 expressed by T cells and CD40 interacting with CD154, which are members of the Ig and TNF:TNFR superfamilies respectively. CD28 blockade by a mutated version of CTLA-4-Ig (belatacept) for transplantation has been licensed for clinical use (by the US Food and Drug Administration (FDA) in June 2011 and the European Medicines Agency (EMA) in April 2011).[204]

The B7:CD28/CTLA-4 Pathway

CD80 (B7-1) and CD86 (B7-2) are expressed as cell surface molecules by APCs and are responsible for delivering additional or second signals to T cells when they interact with their ligands CD28 and CD152 (CTLA-4). CD28 is expressed constitutively by T cells, while CD152 is only expressed later in the activation response. CD86 appears to interact preferentially with CD28 and may be the most important ligand for T-cell activation. CD80 may bind preferentially to CD152.[179,193] In contrast to CD28, CD152 negatively regulates T-cell activation when it engages its ligand on the APC. Thus targeting CD28 will inhibit T-cell activation, whereas targeting CD152 will potentiate T-cell activation. Both approaches are of interest in different contexts, as demonstrated by the development of CTLA-4-Ig for preventing allograft rejection and the development of anti-CD152 as a cancer therapy.[171] Interestingly, CD152 is constitutively expressed and plays a key role in the functional activity of regulatory T cells.[87,159]

When CTLA-4-Ig, an immunoglobulin fusion protein of CTLA-4, was produced, it was shown to inhibit graft rejection in xenogeneic and allogeneic systems.[99,100]

In rodent models, CTLA-4-Ig therapy alone was found capable of inducing tolerance to the graft,[100] an effect that was enhanced when donor antigen was included in the treatment protocol.[147] However, this effect did not translate to primate models where CTLA-4-Ig monotherapy was not found to induce long-term graft survival.[90] Indeed, a mutated form of CTLA-4-Fc, LEA29Y or belatacept, was found to be a more potent inhibitor of allograft rejection than the native molecule, in primate renal transplant models.[98] Belatacept differs from CTLA-4-Ig by two amino acid sequences, which confers an approximately twofold greater binding capacity to CD80 and CD86. Belatacept has been approved for clinical use for the indication of prophylaxis of organ rejection in adult kidney transplant recipients (by the FDA in June, 2011 and EMA in April, 2011) when used in conjunction with basiliximab induction, mycophenolate mofetil, and corticosteroids as maintenance immunosuppression.

Other reagents which target CD28 have also been developed. A CD28 superagonist, TGN1412, showed enhanced expansion of regulatory T cells in preclinical studies and was taken into a phase I clinical trial. However, six healthy volunteers treated with TGN1412 experienced a massive expansion of inflammatory T cells that resulted in a cytokine storm. The trial was terminated as all volunteers experienced multiorgan failure.[185] Despite this, the development of antibody-mediated selective costimulatory blockade remains an attractive therapeutic strategy as specifically blocking CD28, for example, would still allow CTLA-4 signaling, potentially enhancing T-cell suppression. Monovalent Fab fragments (Fv) which selectively block CD28 have been developed to prevent signals through CD28 whilst allowing negative signals via CTLA-4 to remain intact. CD28 single-chain Fv (scFv) fragments have been shown to prolong allograft survival significantly in primates, increasing the number of Treg in the periphery as well as in the graft,[150] and is in clinical development.

CD40-CD154 Pathway

The CD40-CD154 pathway has been targeted using monoclonal antibody therapy to inhibit graft rejection.[94] CD154, or CD40 ligand, is a type 2 membrane protein of the TNF family and is expressed predominantly by activated $CD4^+$ T cells and by a small proportion of $CD8^+$ T cells, NK cells, and eosinophils,[30] and, more recently, CD154 has also been found on platelets.[2,96] Structural models predict that CD154 forms a homotrimer that binds to its ligand, CD40, on the surface of APCs. CD40 is expressed by B cells, macrophages, DCs, and thymic epithelium, and is inducible on the surface of endothelial cells and fibroblasts.[97]

The CD40-CD154 pathway interaction is pivotal for the induction of humoral and cellular responses, with the importance of CD154 for B-cell activation first being demonstrated in *in vitro* studies. A CD40-Ig fusion protein and a blocking monoclonal antibody to CD154 were shown to inhibit B-cell cycling, proliferation, and differentiation into plasma cells in response to T-cell-dependent antigens.[136] *In vivo* studies using the anti-CD154 monoclonal antibody, CD40 or CD154 knockout mice[79,219] all demonstrated a crucial role for this interaction in the generation of primary and secondary humoral responses to T-cell-dependent antigens, class switching to antigen switching RGG1 responses and development of germinal centers. The lack of humoral response in the absence of CD40–CD40L interaction is due not only to a lack of signaling through CD40 on the B-cell surface, but also the inhibition of priming of $CD4^+$ T cells through CD40L[60] as a result of the bidirectional nature of the CD40-CD154 pathway. Signals through CD40 have been shown to upregulate expression of CD80 and CD86 as well as induce IL-12.[62] Activation of DCs through CD40 promotes their ability to present antigen to T cells; this may explain why targeting CD154 and blocking its ability to interact with CD40 have profound effects on T-cell-dependent immune responses *in vivo*. Thus targeting CD40-CD154 could act to prevent both cell-mediated and antibody-mediated rejection.

Anti-CD154 was found capable of inducing long-term acceptance of cardiac, renal, and islet allografts in several murine and non-human primate models either when used as monotherapy or in conjunction with anti-CD28.[89,90,94,117,146] Disappointingly, anti-CD154 therapy was found to have the unexpected complication of thrombogenesis when it was translated to the clinic.[91] Indeed, it was found subsequently that CD154 plays a key role in coagulation implicated in platelet activation and the stabilization of thrombi.[2]

Targeting CD3 and Accessory Molecules

Initially, administration of depleting anti-CD4 and anti-CD8 monoclonal antibodies was shown to result in prolonged graft survival.[31,114,173] That this treatment strategy resulted in antigen-specific tolerance was first shown most clearly when a protein antigen was administered in conjunction with a depleting anti-CD4 monoclonal antibody.[9,10] Refinements of these types of protocols have resulted in the ability to achieve long-term T-cell unresponsiveness to protein and alloantigens in the absence of T-cell depletion in experimental models. In fact, many other accessory molecules, other than anti-CD4 and anti-CD8, have been targeted and shown capable of inducing tolerance to alloantigens.

OKT3, a mouse anti-human CD3 monoclonal antibody, received approval for human use in 1986 in kidney transplant patients undergoing rejection and later in liver and cardiac transplant recipients.[140] Although widely used, OKT3 brought with it the undesired complications of the human antimouse antibody response as well as a first dose reaction characterized by fevers, chills, gastrointestinal, respiratory, and cardiac complications,[53,192] as a result of T-cell activation and subsequent cytokine release. As a result, many investigators have invested time in the construction of pharmacotherapeutics that mimic the efficacy of OKT3 with less immunogenicity. In preliminary studies a few of these OKT3-derived molecules, such as hu12F6, hOKT3γ1(Ala-Ala), and ChAglyCD3, have proven to be more effective in T-cell suppression and less immunogenic when compared to OKT3.[72,85,105]

Along with anti-CD3, antibodies to CD11a (LFA-1) and its ligands, ICAM-1, -2, and -3, have been investigated and have suggested prolonged graft survival.[6,153] However, an adverse side effect profile in clinical trials has resulted in withdrawal of efalizumab (anti-LFA-1) from clinical development.

Operational tolerance induced by these strategies has been shown to develop over several weeks after the initial antigen encounter[148,170] and is dependent on the amount of antigen infused.[149] With high doses of donor bone marrow, deletion may also be used as one of the mechanisms of tolerance initially,[8,20] while with lower doses of antigen, immunoregulation is the mechanism in operation. In mice and rats, this type of tolerance has been shown to be infectious[83,154]; in other words, it can be transferred from one generation of cells to another. The maintenance of tolerance in these systems requires the persistent presence of antigen in the form of the organ when the thymus is still functional.[67]

LEUKOCYTE DEPLETION AT THE TIME OF TRANSPLANTATION

Many tolerance induction strategies that have been investigated in small- and large-animal studies result in the depletion of leukocytes (antithymocyte globulin, anti-CD52) or T cells (anti-CD3 with or without immunotoxin, CD2, CD4, and CD8). In small animals, the short-term depletion of T cells appears to be sufficient in some situations for tolerance to develop and be maintained in the long term. The success rate can be enhanced by removing the thymus before transplantation to prevent repopulation of the periphery with T cells after transplantation.[127] However, in humans, leukocyte depletion with the anti-CD52 monoclonal antibody alemtuzemab in combination with immunosuppressive drugs is not sufficient to induce operational tolerance, but can enable minimization of immunosuppression to control residual donor-reactive cells.[68,130,199,200,208]

CELL THERAPY

Cellular therapies using Treg, regulatory macrophages, and MSCs to suppress rejection or GVHD are being developed for use in clinical transplantation as a strategy to promote the development of specific unresponsiveness.[124]

Treg Cell Therapy

Tregs have been infused into bone marrow transplant recipients with the objective of limiting GVHD. Expanded Tregs were used to treat two patients who developed GVHD following bone marrow transplantation, with clinical improvement demonstrated in both patients.[198] No safety concerns were reported from two dose escalation studies when *ex vivo* expanded cord blood or donor-derived Tregs were infused into adult patients receiving hematopoietic stem cell transplantation.[18,36] Moreover, in the second study GVHD was prevented in the absence of any immunosuppressive treatment regimen, and lymphoid reconstitution occurred with improved immunity to opportunistic pathogens, and no loss of the graft-versus-leukemia effect.[36] In organ transplantation, the ONE study, a multicenter phase I/II study funded by the European Union FP7 program, will investigate the safety of infusion of *ex vivo* expanded nTreg and Tr1 cells into kidney transplant recipients (www.onestudy.org).

Regulatory Macrophage Cell Therapy

Regulatory macrophages isolated from the organ donor have been administered intravenously to two living donor kidney transplant recipients with no deleterious impact on graft function, enabling tacrolimus immunosuppressive therapy to be reduced within the first 24 weeks after transplantation.[73] A follow-up study using regulatory macrophages in kidney transplant recipients will be performed as part of the ONE study.

Mesenchymal Stromal Cell Therapy

Although over 100 clinical trials investigating the immunomodulatory and proreparative effects of MSCs are in progress (www.clinicaltrials.gov), this form of cell therapy is still at an early stage of development.

Not all clinical studies using MSCs to modulate immune reactivity have reported positive data. The activation status of the MSCs at the time of infusion may explain these inconsistencies. A significant placebo effect was observed in phase III clinical trials that used third-party MSCs to treat GVHD.[125] In contrast, treatment with MSCs was found to correlate with a significant improvement in patients with steroid-resistant liver or gastrointestinal GVHD.[125] In kidney transplantation, infusion of autologous MSCs resulted in a lower incidence of acute rejection, a decreased risk of opportunistic infection, and better estimated renal function at 1 year posttransplantation.[191]

Acknowledgments

The work from the authors' own laboratory described in this review was supported by grants from The Wellcome Trust, Medical Research Council, British Heart Foundation, and the European Union ONE Study, Optistem, TRIAD and BioDRIM networks.

REFERENCES

1. Afzali B, Lombardi G, Lechler RI. Pathways of major histocompatibility complex allorecognition. Curr Opin Organ Transplant 2008;13:438–44.
2. Andre P, Prasad KSS, Denis CV, et al. CD40L stabilizes arterial thrombi by a β3 integrin-dependent mechanism. Nat Med 2002;8:247–52.
3. Anglicheau D, Muthukumar T, Suthanthiran M. MicroRNAs: small RNAs with big effects. Transplantation 2010;90:105–12.
4. Asari S, Itakura S, Ferreri K, et al. Mesenchymal stem cells suppress B-cell terminal differentiation. Exp Hematol 2009;37:604–15.
5. Bacchetta R, Passerini L, Gambineri E, et al. Defective regulatory and effector T cell functions in patients with FOXP3 mutations. J Clin Invest 2006;116:1713–22.
6. Badell IR, Russell MC, Thompson PW, et al. LFA-1-specific therapy prolongs allograft survival in rhesus macaques. J Clin Invest 2010;120:4520–31.
7. Bellgrau D, Duke R. Apoptosis and CD95 ligand in immune privileged sites. Int Rev Immunol 1999;18:547–62.
8. Bemelman F, Honey K, Adams E, et al. Bone marrow transplantation induces either clonal deletion or infectious tolerance depending on the dose. J Immunol 1998;160:2645–8.

9. Benjamin RJ, Cobbold SP, Clark MR. Tolerance to rat monoclonal antibodies: implications for serotherapy. J Exp Med 1986;163:1539–52.
10. Benjamin RJ, Qin S, Wise MP, et al. Mechanisms of monoclonal antibody-facilitated tolerance induction: a possible role for the CD4 (L3T4) and CD11a (LFA-1) molecules in self-non-self discrimination. Eur J Immunol 1988;18:1079–88.
11. Bennett CL, Christie F, Ramsdell F, et al. The immune dysregulation, polyendocrinopathy, enteropathy, X-linked syndrome (IPEX) is caused by mutations of FOXP3. Nat Genet 2001;27:20–1.
12. Billingham RE, Brent L, Medawar PB. Actively acquired tolerance of foreign cells. Nature 1953;172:603–6.
13. Billingham RE, Lampkin GH, Medawar PB, et al. Tolerance to homografts, twin diagnosis, and the freemarting condition in cattle. Heredity 1952;6:201–12.
14. Billingham RE, Medawar PB. Technique of free skin grafting in mammals. J Exp Biol 1951;28:385–91.
15. Bohne F, Martínez-Llordella M, Lozano J-J, et al. Intra-graft expression of genes involved in iron homeostasis predicts the development of operational tolerance in human liver transplantation. J Clin Invest 2012;122:368–82.
16. Boros P, Ochando JC, Chen S-H, et al. Myeloid-derived suppressor cells: natural regulators for transplant tolerance. Hum Immunol 2010;71:1061–6.
17. Brouard S, Dupont A, Giral M, et al. Operationally tolerant and minimally immunosuppressed kidney recipients display strongly altered blood T-cell clonal regulation. Am J Transplant 2005;5:330–40.
18. Brunstein CG, Miller JS, Cao Q, et al. Infusion of ex vivo expanded T regulatory cells in adults transplanted with umbilical cord blood: safety profile and detection kinetics. Blood 2011;117:1061–70.
19. Buhler L, Spitzer T, Sykes M, et al. Induction of kidney allograft tolerance after transient lymphohematopoietic chimerism in patients with multiple myeloma and end-stage renal disease. Transplantation 2002;74:1405–9.
20. Bushell A, Jones E, Gallimore A, et al. The generation of CD25+CD4+ regulatory cells that prevent allograft rejection does not compromise immunity to a viral protein. J Immunol 2005;174:3290–7.
21. Bushell A, Morris P, Wood K. Anti-CD4 antibody combined with random blood transfusion leads to authentic transplantation tolerance in the mouse: a protocol with significant clinical potential. Transplantation 1994;58:133–40.
22. Bushell A, Wood K. GITR ligation blocks allograft protection by induced CD25+CD4+ regulatory T cells without enhancing effector T-cell function. Am J Transplant 2007;7:759–68.
23. Calne RY, Sells RA, Pena JR, et al. Induction of immunological tolerance by porcine liver allografts. Nature 1969;223:472–6.
24. Carvalho-Gaspar M, Billing JS, Spriewald BM, et al. Chemokine gene expression during allograft rejection: comparison of two quantitative PCR techniques. J Immunol Methods 2005;301:41–52.
25. Carvalho-Gaspar M, Jones ND, Luo S, et al. Location and time-dependent control of rejection by regulatory T cells culminates in a failure to generate memory T cells. J Immunol 2008;180:6640–8.
26. Casiraghi F, Azzollini N, Cassis P, et al. Pretransplant infusion of mesenchymal stem cells prolongs the survival of a semiallogeneic heart transplant through the generation of regulatory T cells. J Immunol 2008;181:3933–46.
27. Chang C, Ciubotariu R, Manavalan J, et al. Tolerization of dendritic cells by T(S) cells: the crucial role of inhibitory receptors ILT3 and ILT4. Nat Immunol 2002;3:237–43.
28. Chong AS, Sciammas R. Matchmaking the B-cell signature of tolerance to regulatory B cells. Am J Transplant 2011;11:2555–60.
29. Chou H-S, Hsieh C-C, Charles R, et al. Myeloid-derived suppressor cells protect islet transplants by B7-H1 mediated enhancement of T regulatory cells. Transplantation 2012;93:272–82.
30. Clarkson MR, Sayegh MH. T-cell costimulatory pathways in allograft rejection and tolerance. Transplantation 2005;80:555–63.
31. Cobbold S, Waldmann H. Skin allograft rejection by L3T4[+] and LYT-2[+] T cell subsets. Transplantation 1986;41:634–9.
32. Darrasse-Jèze G, Deroubaix S, Mouquet H, et al. Feedback control of regulatory T cell homeostasis by dendritic cells in vivo. J Exp Med 2009;206:1853–62.
33. Davies JD, Leong LY, Mellor A, et al. T cell suppression in transplantation tolerance through linked recognition. J Immunol 1996;156:3602–7.
34. Devlin J, Doherty D, Thomson L, et al. Defining the outcome of immunosuppression withdrawal after liver transplantation. Hepatology 1998;27:926–33.
35. De Wilde V, Van Rompaey N, Hill M, et al. Endotoxin-induced myeloid-derived suppressor cells inhibit alloimmune responses via heme oxygenase-1. Am J Transplant 2009;9:2034–47.
36. Di Ianni M, Falzetti F, Carotti A, et al. Tregs prevent GVHD and promote immune reconstitution in HLA-haploidentical transplantation. Blood 2011;117:3921–8.
37. Ding Q, Yeung M, Camirand G, et al. Regulatory B cells are identified by expression of TIM-1 and can be induced through TIM-1 ligation to promote tolerance in mice. J Clin Invest 2011;121:3645–56.
38. Ding Y, Bushell A, Wood KJ. Mesenchymal stem-cell immunosuppressive capabilities: therapeutic implications in islet transplantation. Transplantation 2010;89:270–3.
39. Ding Y, Xu D, Feng G, et al. Mesenchymal stem cells prevent the rejection of fully allogenic islet grafts by the immunosuppressive activity of matrix metalloproteinase-2 and -9. Diabetes 2009;58:1797–806.
40. Dugast A-S, Haudebourg T, Coulon F, et al. Myeloid-derived suppressor cells accumulate in kidney allograft tolerance and specifically suppress effector T cell expansion. J Immunol 2008;180:7898–906.
41. English K, French A, Wood KJ. Mesenchymal stromal cells: facilitators of successful transplantation? Cell Stem Cell 2010;7:431–42.
42. English K, Ryan JM, Tobin L, et al. Cell contact, prostaglandin E-2 and transforming growth factor beta 1 play non-redundant roles in human mesenchymal stem cell induction of CD4(+) CD25(High)forkhead box P3(+) regulatory T cells. Clin Exp Immunol 2009;156:149–60.
43. Famulski KS, Broderick G, Einecke G, et al. Transcriptome analysis reveals heterogeneity in the injury response of kidney transplants. Am J Transplant 2007;7:2483–95.
44. Fan X, Ang A, Pollock-Barziv S, et al. Donor-specific B-cell tolerance after ABO-incompatible infant heart transplantation. Nat Med 2004;10:1227–33.
45. Feng S, Lobritto SJ, Demetris AJ, et al. Complete immunosuppression withdrawal and subsequent allograft function among pediatric recipients of parental living donor liver transplants. JAMA 2012;307:283–93.
46. Fleming BD, Mosser DM. Regulatory macrophages: setting the threshold for therapy. Eur J Immunol 2011;41:2498–502.
47. Fooksman DR, Vardhana S, Vasiliver-Shamis G, et al. Functional anatomy of T cell activation and synapse formation. Annu Rev Immunol 2010;28:79–105.
48. Francis RS, Feng G, Tha-In T, et al. Induction of transplantation tolerance converts potential effector T cells into graft protective regulatory T cells. Eur J Immunol 2011;41:726–38.
49. Francisco LM, Sage PT, Sharpe AH. The PD-1 pathway in tolerance and autoimmunity. Immunol Rev 2010;236:219–42.
50. Fudaba Y, Spitzer TR, Shaffer J, et al. Myeloma responses and tolerance following combined kidney and nonmyeloablative marrow transplantation: in vivo and in vitro analyses. Am J Transplant 2006;6:2121–33.
51. Gallina G, Dolcetti L, Serafini P, et al. Tumors induce a subset of inflammatory monocytes with immunosuppressive activity on CD8+ T cells. J Clin Invest 2006;116:2777–90.
52. Garcia MR, Ledgerwood L, Yang Y, et al. Monocytic suppressive cells mediate cardiovascular transplantation tolerance in mice. J Clin Invest 2010;120:2486–96.
53. Gaston RS, Deierhoi MH, Patterson T, et al. OKT3 first-dose reaction: association with T cell subsets and cytokine release. Kidney Int 1991;39:141–8.
54. Ge W, Jiang J, Baroja ML, et al. Infusion of mesenchymal stem cells and rapamycin synergize to attenuate alloimmune responses and promote cardiac allograft tolerance. Am J Transplant 2009;9:1760–72.
55. George J, Sweeney S, Kirklin J, et al. An essential role for Fas ligand in transplantation tolerance induced by donor bone marrow. Nat Med 1998;4:333–5.
56. Gershon R, Kondo K. Infectious immunlogical tolerance. Immunology 1971;21:903–14.
57. Gilliet M, Liu Y-J. Generation of human CD8 T regulatory cells by CD40 ligand-activated plasmacytoid dendritic cells. J Exp Med 2002;195:695–704.

58. Graca L, Cobbold SP, Waldmann H. Identification of regulatory T cells in tolerated allografts. J Exp Med 2002;195:1641–6.
59. Graca L, Thompson S, Lin C-Y, et al. Both CD4+CD25+ and CD4+CD25- regulatory cells mediate dominant transplantation tolerance. J Immunol 2002;168:5558–65.
60. Grewal I, Foellmer H, Grewal K, et al. Requirement for CD40 ligand in costimulation induction, T cell activation, and experimental allergic encephalomyelitis. Science 1996;274:1864–7.
61. Grossi PA, Costa AN, Fehily D, et al. Infections and organ transplantation: new challenges for prevention and treatment – a colloquium. Transplantation 2012;93:S4–39.
62. Gurunathan S, Irvine K, Wu C, et al. CD40 ligand/trimer DNA enhances both humoral and cellular immune responses and induces protective immunity to infectious and tumor challenge. J Immunol 1998;161:4563–71.
63. Haile LA, von Wasielewski R, Gamrekelashvili J, et al. Myeloid-derived suppressor cells in inflammatory bowel disease: a new immunoregulatory pathway. Gastroenterology 2008;135:871–81.
64. Hall BM, Jelbart ME, Dorsch SE. Suppressor T cells in rats with prolonged cardiac allograft survival after treatment with cyclosporine. Transplantation 1984;37:595–600.
65. Hall B, Jelbart M, Gurley K, et al. Specific unresponsiveness in rats with prolonged cardiac allograft survival after treatment with cyclosporine. Mediation of specific suppression by T helper/inducer cells. J Exp Med 1985;162:1683–94.
66. Hall B, Pearce N, Gurley K, et al. Specific unresponsiveness in rats with prolonged cardiac allograft survival after treatment with cyclosporine. III. Further characterisation of the CD4+ suppressor cell and its mechanisms of action. J Exp Med 1990;171:141–57.
67. Hamano K, Rawsthorne M, Bushell A, et al. Evidence that the continued presence of the organ graft and not peripheral donor microchimerism is essential for the maintenance of tolerance to alloantigen in anti-CD4 treated recipients. Transplantation 1996;62:856–60.
68. Hanaway MJ, Woodle ES, Mulgaonkar S, et al. Alemtuzumab induction in renal transplantation. N Engl J Med 2011;364:1909–19.
69. Hara M, Kingsley C, Niimi M, et al. IL-10 is required for regulatory T cells to mediate tolerance to alloantigens in vivo. J Immunol 2001;166:3789–96.
70. Hashimoto D, Chow A, Greter M, et al. Pretransplant CSF-1 therapy expands recipient macrophages and ameliorates GVHD after allogeneic hematopoietic cell transplantation. J Exp Med 2011;208:1069–82.
71. Hayday A, Tigelaar R. Immunoregulation in the tissues by γδ T cells. Nat Rev Immunol 2003;3:233–42.
72. Herold KC, Gitelman SE, Masharani U, et al. A single course of anti-CD3 monoclonal antibody hOKT3γ1(Ala-Ala) results in improvement in C-peptide responses and clinical parameters for at least 2 years after onset of type 1 diabetes. Diabetes 2005;54:1763–9.
73. Hutchinson JA, Riquelme P, Sawitzki B, et al. Cutting edge: immunological consequences and trafficking of human regulatory macrophages administered to renal transplant recipients. J Immunol 2011;187:2072–8.
74. Issa F, Wood KJ. Translating tolerogenic therapies to the clinic – where do we stand? Frontiers Immunol 2012;3:.
75. Jacobsen N, Taaning E, Ladefoged J, et al. Tolerance to an HLA-B. DR disparate kidney allograft after bone marrow transplantation from the same donor. Lancet 1994;343:800.
76. Jones N, Fluck N, Mellor A, et al. Deletion of alloantigen-reactive thymocytes as a mechanism of adult transplantation tolerance induction following intrathymic antigen administration. Eur J Immunol 1997;27:1591–600.
77. Josefowicz SZ, Rudensky A. Control of regulatory T cell lineage commitment and maintenance. Immunity 2009;30:616–25.
78. Josien R, Douillard P, Guillot C, et al. A critical role for transforming growth factor beta in donor transfusion induced allograft tolerance. J Clin Invest 1998;102:1920–6.
79. Kawabe T, Naka T, Yoshida K, et al. The immune responses in CD40-deficient mice: impaired immunoglobulin class switching and germinal centre formation. Immunity 1994;1:167–78.
80. Kawai T, Cosimi A, Colvin R, et al. Mixed allogeneic chimerism and renal allograft tolerance in cynomolgus monkeys. Transplantation 1995;59:256–62.
81. Kawai T, Cosimi AB, Spitzer TR, et al. HLA-mismatched renal transplantation without maintenance immunosuppression. N Engl J Med 2008;358:353–61.
82. Kearney E, Pape K, Loh D, et al. Visualisation of peptide-specific T cell immunity and peripheral tolerance induction in vivo. Immunity 1994;1:327–39.
83. Kendal AR, Chen Y, Regateiro FS, et al. Sustained suppression by Foxp3+ regulatory T cells is vital for infectious transplantation tolerance. J Exp Med 2011;208:2043–53.
84. Kendal AR, Waldmann H. Infectious tolerance: therapeutic potential. Curr Opin Immunol 2010;22:560–5.
85. Keymeulen B, Vandemeulebroucke E, Ziegler AG, et al. Insulin needs after CD3-antibody therapy in new-onset type 1 diabetes. N Engl J Med 2005;352:2598–608.
86. Khan A, Tomita Y, Sykes M. Thymic dependence of loss of tolerance in mixed allogeneic bone marrow chimeras after depletion of donor antigen. Transplantation 1996;62:380–7.
87. Kingsley CI, Karim M, Bushell AR, et al. CD25+CD4+ regulatory T cells prevent graft rejection: CTLA-4- and IL-10-dependent immunoregulation of alloresponses. J Immunol 2002;168:1080–6.
88. Kinnear G, Jones ND, Wood KJ. Costimulation blockade: current perspectives and implications for therapy. Tranplantation 2013; [in press].
89. Kirk A, Burkly L, Batty D, et al. Treatment with humanised monolconal antibody against CD154 prevents acute renal allograft rejection in nonhuman primates. Nat Med 1999;5:686–93.
90. Kirk A, Harlan D, Armstrong N, et al. CTLA4-Ig and anti-CD40 ligand prevent renal allograft rejection in primates. Proc Natl Acad Sci U S A 1997;94:8789–94.
91. Kirk AD, Knechtle SJ, Sollinger HW, et al. Preliminary results of the use of humanized anti-CD154 in human renal allotransplantation. Am J Transplant 2001;1:S191.
92. Kobayashi I, Shiari R, Yamada M, et al. Novel mutations of FOXP3 in two Japanese patients with immune dysregulation, polyendocrinopathy, enteropathy, X linked syndrome (IPEX). J Med Genet 2001;38:874–6.
93. Krammer PH, Arnold R, Lavrik IN. Life and death in peripheral T cells. Nat Rev Immunol 2007;7:532–42.
94. Larsen C, Alexander D, Hollenbaugh D, et al. CD40-gp39 interactions play a critical role during allograft rejection. Transplantation 1996;61:4–9.
95. Larsen C, Morris P, Austyn J. Migration of dendritic leukocytes form cardiac allografts into host spleens: a novel pathway for initiation of rejection. J Exp Med 1990;171:307–14.
96. Larsen CP, Knechtle SJ, Adams A, et al. A new look at blockade of T-cell costimulation: a therapeutic strategy for long-term maintenance immunosuppression. Am J Transplant 2006;6:876–83.
97. Larsen CP, Pearson TC. The CD40 pathway in allograft rejection, acceptance, and tolerance. Curr Opin Immunol 1997;9:641–7.
98. Larsen CP, Pearson TC, Adams AB, et al. Rational development of LEA29Y (belatacept), a high-affinity variant of CTLA4-Ig with potent immunosuppressive properties. Am J Transplant 2005;5:443–53.
99. Larsen P, Elwood E, Alexander D, et al. Long-term acceptance of skin and cardiac allografts after blocking CD40 and CD28 pathways. Nature 1996;381:434–8.
100. Lenschow DJ, Zeng Y, Thistlethwaite JR, et al. Long-term survival of xenogeneic pancreatic islet grafts induced by CTLA4Ig. [see comments]. Science 1992;257:789–92.
101. Le Texier L, Thebault P, Lavault A, et al. Long-term allograft tolerance is characterized by the accumulation of B cells exhibiting an inhibited profile. Am J Transplant 2010;11:429–38.
102. Leventhal J, Abecassis M, Miller J, et al. Chimerism and tolerance without GVHD or engraftment syndrome in HLA-mismatched combined kidney and hematopoietic stem cell transplantation. Sci Transl Med 2012;4:124ra28.
103. Levings MK, Gregori S, Tresoldi E, et al. Differentiation of Tr1 cells by immature dendritic cells requires IL-10 but not CD25+CD4+ Tr cells. Blood 2005;105:1162–9.
104. Li Y, Koshiba T, Yoshizawa A, et al. Analyses of peripheral blood mononuclear cells in operational tolerance after pediatric living donor liver transplantation. Am J Transplant 2004;4:2118–25.
105. Li B, Wang H, Dai J, et al. Construction and characterization of a humanized anti-human CD3 monoclonal antibody 12F6 with effective immunoregulation functions. Immunology 2005;116:487–98.
106. Li XC. The significance of non-T-cell pathways in graft rejection: implications for transplant tolerance. Transplantation 2010;90:1043–7.

107. Li XL, Ménoret S, Bezie S, et al. Mechanism and localization of CD8 regulatory T cells in a heart transplant model of tolerance. J Immunol 2010;185:823–33.
108. Li Y, Zhao X, Cheng D, et al. The presence of Foxp3 expressing T cells within grafts of tolerant human liver transplant recipients. Transplantation 2008;86:1837–43.
109. Lo DJ, Weaver TA, Kleiner DE, et al. Chemokines and their receptors in human renal allotransplantation. Transplantation 2011;91:70–7.
110. Lu C, Li XY, Hu Y, et al. MT1-MMP controls human mesenchymal stem cell trafficking and differentiation. Blood 2010;115:221–9.
111. Lu L, Li W, Fu F, et al. Blockade of the CD40-CD40 ligand pathway potentiates the capacity of donor-derived dendritic cell progenitors to induce long-term cardiac allograft survival. Transplantation 1997;64:1808–15.
112. Lu L, McCaslin D, Starzl TE, et al. Bone marrow-derived dendritic cell progenitors (NLDC 145+, MHC class II+, B7-1dim, B7-2-) induce alloantigen-specific hyporesponsiveness in murine T lymphocytes. Transplantation 1995;60:1539–45.
113. Macagno A, Napolitani G, Lanzavecchia A, et al. Duration, combination and timing: the signal integration model of dendritic cell activation. Trends Immunol 2007;28:227–33.
114. Madsen JC, Peugh WN, Wood KJ, et al. The effect of anti-L3T4 monoclonal antibody on first-set rejection of murine cardiac allografts. Transplantation 1987;44:849–52.
115. Madsen JC, Superina RA, Wood KJ, et al. Immunological unresponsiveness induced by recipient cells transfected with donor MHC genes. Nature 1988;332:161–4.
116. Manilay J, Pearson D, Sergio J, et al. Intrathymic deletion of alloreactive T cells in mixed bone marrow chimeras prepared with a nonmyeloablative conditioning regime. Transplantation 1998;66:96–102.
117. Markees T, Phillips N, Noelle R, et al. Prolonged survival of mouse skin allografts in recipients treated with donor splenocytes and antibody to CD40 ligand. Transplantation 1997;64:329–35.
118. Martinez FO, Helming L, Gordon S. Alternative activation of macrophages: an immunologic functional perspective. Annu Rev Immunol 2009;27:451–83.
119. Martínez-Llordella M, Lozano JJ, Puig-Pey I, et al. Using transcriptional profiling to develop a diagnostic test of operational tolerance in liver transplant recipients. J Clin Invest 2008;118:2845–57.
120. Martinez-Llordella M, Puig-Pey I, Orlando G, et al. Multiparameter immune profiling of operational tolerance in liver transplantation. Am J Transplant 2007;7:309–19.
121. Matta BM, Castellaneta A, Thomson AW. Tolerogenic plasmacytoid DC. Eur J Immunol 2010;40:2667–76.
122. Mauri C, Blair PA. Regulatory B cells in autoimmunity: developments and controversies. Nat Rev Rheumatol 2010;6:636–43.
123. Mazariegos GV, Zahorchak AF, Reyes J, et al. Dendritic cell subset ratio in tolerant, weaning and non-tolerant liver recipients is not affected by extent of immunosuppression. Am J Transplant 2005;5:314–22.
124. McMurchy AN, Bushell A, Levings MK, et al. Moving to tolerance: clinical application of T regulatory cells. Semin Immunol 2011;23:304–13.
125. Mills CR. Osiris therapeutics announces preliminary results for prochymal phase III GvHD trials. Cited 1 November 2009. Available online at: http://investor.osiris.com/releasedetail.cfm?ReleaseID=407404.
126. Monaco AP, Medawar P. Chimerism in organ transplantation: conflicting experiments and clinical observations. Transplantation 2003;75:13S–6S.
127. Monaco AP, Wood ML, Russel PS. Studies on heterologous anti-lymphocyte serum in mice: III. Immunologic tolerance and chimerism produced across the H-2 locus with adult thymectomy and anti-lymphocyte serum. Ann N Y Acad Sci 1966;129:190–206.
128. Monteiro M, Almeida CF, Caridade M, et al. Identification of regulatory Foxp3+ invariant NKT cells induced by TGF-β. J Immunol 2010;185:2157–63.
129. Morelli AE, Thomson AW. Tolerogenic dendritic cells and the quest for transplant tolerance. Nat Rev Immunol 2007;7:610–21.
130. Morgan RD, O'Callaghan JM, Knight SR, et al. Alemtuzumab induction therapy in kidney transplantation: a systematic review and meta-analysis. Transplantation 2012;93:1179–88.
131. Mühlberger I, Perco P, Fechete R, et al. Biomarkers in renal transplantation ischemia reperfusion injury. Transplantation 2009;88:S14–9.
132. Murray PJ, Wynn TA. Protective and pathogenic functions of macrophage subsets. Nat Rev Immunol 2011;11:723–37.
133. Myburgh JA, Smit JA, Stark JH, et al. Total lymphoid irradiation in kidney and liver transplantation in the baboon: Prolonged graft survival and alteration in cell subsets with low cumulative dose regimens. J Immunol 1984;132:1019–25.
134. Nemeth K, Leelahavanichkul A, Yuen PST, et al. Bone marrow stromal cells attenuate sepsis via prostaglandin E-2-dependent reprogramming of host macrophages to increase their interleukin-10 production. Nat Med 2009;15:42–9.
135. Newell KA, Asare A, Kirk AD, et al. Identification of a B cell signature associated with renal transplant tolerance in humans. J Clin Invest 2010;120:1836–47.
136. Noelle R, Roy M, Shepherd D, et al. A 39-kDa protein on activated helper T cells binds CD40 and transduces the signal for cognant activation of B cells. Proc Natl Acad Sci U S A 1992;89:6550–4.
137. Ochando JC, Homma C, Yang Y, et al. Alloantigen-presenting plasmacytoid dendritic cells mediate tolerance to vascularized grafts. Nat Immunol 2006;7:652–62.
138. O'Garra A, Vieira P. Regulatory T cells and mechanisms of immune system control. Nat Med 2004;10:801–5.
139. Ogura Y, Sutterwala FS, Flavell RA. The inflammasome: first line of the immune response to cell stress. Cell 2006;126:659–62.
140. Ortho Multicenter Transplant Study Group. A randomized clinical trial of OKT3 monoclonal antibody for acute rejection of cadaveric renal transplants. N Engl J Med 1985;313:337–42.
141. Owen R. Erythrocyte antigens and tolerance phenomena. Proc R Soc Lond B Biol Sci 1956;146:8–18.
142. Owens MI, Maxwell J, Goodnight J, et al. Discontinuance of immunosuppression in renal transplant patients. Arch Surg 1975;110:1450–1.
143. Pallet N, Fougeray S, Beaune P, et al. Endoplasmic reticulum stress: an unrecognized actor in solid organ transplantation. Transplantation 2009;88:605–13.
144. Pallier A, Hillion S, Danger R, et al. Patients with drug-free long-term graft function display increased numbers of peripheral B cells with a memory and inhibitory phenotype. Kidney Int 2010;78:503–13.
145. Pape K, Merica R, Mondino A, et al. Direct evidence that functionally impaired CD4+ T cells persist in vivo following the induction of peripheral tolerance. J Immunol 1998;160:4719–29.
146. Parker D, Greiner D, Phillips N, et al. Survival of mouse pancreatic islet allografts in recipients treated with allogeneic small lymphocytes and antibody to CD40 ligand. Proc Natl Acad Sci U S A 1995;92:9560–4.
147. Pearson T, Alexander D, Hendrix R, et al. CTLA4-Ig plus bone marrow induces long-term allograft survival and donor-specific unresponsiveness in the murine model. Transplantation 1996;61:997–1004.
148. Pearson TC, Darby C, Bushell AR, et al. The assessment of transplantation tolerance induced by anti-CD4 monoclonal antibody in the murine model. Transplantation 1993;55:361–7.
149. Pearson TC, Madsen JC, Larsen C, et al. Induction of transplantation tolerance in the adult using donor antigen and anti-CD4 monoclonal antibody. Transplantation 1992;54:475–83.
150. Poirier N, Azimzadeh AM, Zhang T, et al. Inducing CTLA-4-dependent immune regulation by selective CD28 blockade promotes regulatory T cells in organ transplantation. Sci Transl Med 2010;2:17ra10.
151. Polchert D, Sobinsky J, Douglas GW, et al. IFN-gamma activation of mesenchymal stem cells for treatment and prevention of graft versus host disease. Eur J Immunol 2008;38:1745–55.
152. Posselt AM, Barker CF, Tomaszewski JE, et al. Induction of donor-specific unresponsiveness by intrathymic islet transplantation. Science 1990;249:1293–5.
153. Posselt AM, Szot GL, Frassetto LA, et al. Islet transplantation in type 1 diabetic patients using calcineurin inhibitor-free immunosuppressive protocols based on T-cell adhesion or costimulation blockade. Transplantation 2010;90:1595–601.
154. Qin S, Cobbold SP, Pope H, et al. "Infectious" transplantation tolerance. Science 1993;259:974–7.
155. Quigley RL, Wood KJ, Morris J. Mediation of antigen-induced suppression of renal allograft rejection by a CD4 ($W3/25^{+}$) T cell. Transplantation 1989;47:684–8.

156. Quigley RL, Wood KJ, Morris PJ. Transfusion induces blood donor-specific suppressor cells. J Immunol 1989;142:463.
157. Ramakrishnan SK, Page A, Farris AB, et al. Evidence for kidney rejection after combined bone marrow and renal transplantation despite ongoing whole-blood chimerism in rhesus macaques. Am J Transplant 2012;12:1755–64.
158. Ramsdell F. Foxp3 and natural regulatory T cells: key to a cell lineage? Immunity 2003;19:165–8.
159. Read S, Malmstrom V, Powrie F. Cytotoxic T lymphocyte associated antigen 4 plays an essential role in the function of CD25+CD4+ regulatory cells that control intestinal inflammation. J Exp Med 2000;192:295–302.
160. Reibke R, Garbi N, Ganss R, et al. CD8+ regulatory T cells generated by neonatal recognition of peripheral self-antigen. Proc Natl Acad Sci 2006;103:15142–7.
161. Ren GW, Zhang LY, Zhao X, et al. Mesenchymal stem cell-mediated immunosuppression occurs via concerted action of chemokines and nitric oxide. Cell Stem Cell 2008;2:141–50.
162. Rosenblum MD, Gratz IK, Paw JS, et al. Response to self antigen imprints regulatory memory in tissues. Nature 2011;480:538–42.
163. Roussey-Kesler G, Giral M, Moreau A, et al. Clinical operational tolerance after kidney transplantation. Am J Transplant 2006;6:736–46.
164. Sachs DH, Sykes M, Kawai T, et al. Immuno-intervention for the induction of transplantation tolerance through mixed chimerism. Semin Immunol 2011;23:165–73.
165. Sagoo P, Perucha E, Sawitzki B, et al. Development of a cross-platform biomarker signature to detect renal transplant tolerance in humans. J Clin Invest 2010;120:1848–61.
166. Sakaguchi S, Miyara M, Costantino CM, et al. FOXP3+ regulatory T cells in the human immune system. Nat Rev Immunol 2010;10:490–500.
167. Sayegh M, Fine N, Smith J, et al. Immunologic tolerance to renal allografts after bone marrow transplants from the same donors. Ann Intern Med 1991;114:954.
168. Scandling JD, Busque S, Dejbakhsh-Jones S, et al. Tolerance and chimerism after renal and hematopoietic-cell transplantation. N Engl J Med 2008;358:362–8.
169. Schwartz RH. A cell culture model for T lymphocyte clonal anergy. Science 1990;248:1349–56.
170. Scully R, Qin S, Cobbold S, et al. Mechanisms in CD4 antibody-mediated transplantation tolerance: kinetics of induction, antigen dependency and role of regulatory T cells. Eur J Immunol 1994;24:2383–92.
171. Sharma P, Wagner K, Wolchok JD, et al. Novel cancer immunotherapy agents with survival benefit: recent successes and next steps. Nat Rev Cancer 2011;11:805–12.
172. Sheng HM, Wang Y, Jin YQ, et al. A critical role of IFN gamma in priming MSC-mediated suppression of T cell proliferation through up-regulation of B7-H1. Cell Res 2008;18:846–57.
173. Shizuru JA, Gregory AK, Chao CT-B, et al. Islet allograft survival after a single course of treatment of recipient with antibody to L3T4. Science 1987;237:278–80.
174. Slavin S, Strober S, Fuks Z, et al. Induction of specific tissue transplantation tolerance using fractionated total lymphoid irradiation in adult mice: long-term survival of allogeneic bone marrow and skin grafts. J Exp Med 1977;146:34–48.
175. Sorof J, Koerper M, Portale A, et al. Renal transplantation without chronic immunosuppression after T cell depleted HLA-mismatched bone marrow transplantation. Transplantation 1995;59:1633–5.
176. Spaggiari GM, Abdelrazik H, Becchetti F, et al. MSCs inhibit monocyte-derived DC maturation and function by selectively interfering with the generation of immature DCs: central role of MSC-derived prostaglandin E-2. Blood 2009;113:6576–83.
177. Spaggiari GM, Capobianco A, Abdelrazik H, et al. Mesenchymal stem cells inhibit natural killer-cell proliferation, cytotoxicity, and cytokine production: role of indoleamine 2,3-dioxygenase and prostaglandin E2. Blood 2008;111:1327–33.
178. Spitzer T, Delmonico F, Tolkoff-Rubin N, et al. Combined histocompatibility leukocyte antigen-matched donor bone marrow and renal transplantation for multiple myeloma with end stage renal disease: the induction of allograft tolerance through mixed lymphohematopoietic chimersim. Transplantation 1999;68:480–4.
179. Stamper CC, Zhang Y, Tobin JF, et al. Crystal structure of the B7-1/CTLA-4 complex that inhibits human immune responses. Nature 2001;410:608–11.
180. Starzl T, Murase N, Thomson A, et al. Liver transplants contribute to their own success. Nat Med 1996;2:163–5.
181. Steiman R, Witmer M. Lymphoid dendritic cells are potent stimulators of the primary mixed leukocyte reaction in mice. Proc Natl Acad Sci 1978;75:5132–6.
182. Steinman RM, Hawiger D, Nussenzweig MC. Tolerogenic dendritic cells. Annu Rev Immunol 2003;21:685–711.
183. Strober S, Dhillon M, Schubert M, et al. Acquired immune tolerance to cadaveric renal allografts: a study of three patients treated with total lymphoid irradiation. N Engl J Med 1989;321:28–33.
184. Strober S, Slavin S, Gottlieb M, et al. Allograft tolerance after total lymphoid irradiation (TLI). Immunol Rev 1979;46:87–112.
185. Suntharalingam G, Perry MR, Ward S, et al. Cytokine storm in a phase 1 trial of the anti-CD28 monoclonal antibody TGN1412. N Engl J Med 2006;355:1018–28.
186. Swiecki M, Colonna M. Unraveling the functions of plasmacytoid dendritic cells during viral infections, autoimmunity, and tolerance. Immunol Rev 2010;234:142–62.
187. Sykes M. Hematopoietic cell transplantation for tolerance induction: animal models to clinical trials. Transplantation 2009;87:309–16.
188. Sykes M, Sachs D. Mixed chimerism. Philos Trans R Soc Lond B Biol Sci 2001;356:707–26.
189. Takatsuki M, Uemoto S, Inomata Y, et al. Weaning of immunosuppression in living donor liver transplant recipients. Transplantation 2001;72:449–54.
190. Takeuchi O, Akira S. Pattern recognition receptors and inflammation. Cell 2010;140:805–20.
191. Tan J, Wu W, Xu X, et al. Induction therapy with autologous mesenchymal stem cells in living-related kidney transplants. JAMA 2012;307:1169–77.
192. Thistlethwaite Jr JR, Stuart JK, Mayes JT, et al. Complications and monitoring of OKT3 therapy. Am J Kidney Dis 1988;11:112–9.
193. Thompson C. Distinct roles for the costimulatory ligands B7-1 and B7-2 in T helper cell differentiation? Cell 1995;81:879–982.
194. Thomson C, Lee B, Zhang L. Double-negative regulatory T cells. Immunol Res 2006;35:163–77.
195. Tiemessen MM, Jagger AL, Evans HG, et al. CD4+CD25+Foxp3+ regulatory T cells induce alternative activation of human monocytes/macrophages. Proc Natl Acad Sci 2007;104:19446–51.
196. Tokita D, Mazariegos GV, Zahorchak AF, et al. High PD-L1/CD86 ratio on plasmacytoid dendritic cells correlates with elevated T-regulatory cells in liver transplant tolerance. Transplantation 2008;85:369–77.
197. Tomita Y, Khan A, Sykes M. Role of intrathymic clonal deletion and peripheral anergy in transplantation tolerance induced by bone marrow transplantation in mice conditioned with a non-myeloablative regimen. J Immunol 1994;153:1087–98.
198. Trzonkowski P, Bieniaszewska M, Juscinska J, et al. First-in-man clinical results of the treatment of patients with graft versus host disease with human ex vivo expanded CD4+CD25+CD127- T regulatory cells. Clin Immunol 2009;133:22–6.
199. Trzonkowski P, Zilvetti M, Chapman S, et al. Homeostatic repopulation by CD28-CD8+ T cells in alemtuzumab-depleted kidney transplant recipients treated with reduced immunosuppression. Am J Transplant 2008;8(2):338–47.
200. Trzonkowski P, Zilvetti M, Friend P, et al. Recipient memory-like lymphocytes remain unresponsive to graft antigens after CAMPATH-1H induction with reduced maintenance immunosuppression. Transplantation 2006;82:1342–51.
201. Tullius S, Nieminen M, Bechstein W, et al. Chronically rejected rat kidney allografts induce donor-specific tolerance. Transplantation 1997;64:158–61.
202. Turvey S, Gonzalez-Nicolini V, Kingsley C, et al. Fas ligand transfected myoblasts and islet cell transplantation. Transplantation 2000;70:1641–9.
203. van Kooten C, Lombardi G, Gelderman KA, et al. Dendritic cells as a tool to induce transplantation tolerance: obstacles and opportunities. Transplantation 2011;91:2–7.
204. Vincenti F, Larsen C, Durrbach A, et al. Costimulation blockade with belatacept in renal transplantation. N Engl J Med 2005;353:770–81.
205. Vlad G, Cortesini R, Suciu-Foca N. CD8+ T suppressor cells and the ILT3 master switch. Hum Immunol 2008;69:681–6.
206. Vlad G, D'Agati VD, Zhang Q-Y, et al. Immunoglobulin-like transcript 3-Fc suppresses T-cell responses to allogeneic human islet transplants in hu-NOD/SCID mice. Diabetes 2008;57:1878–86.

207. Walunas T, Lenschow D, Bakker C, et al. CTLA-4 can function as a negative regulator of T cell activation. Immunity 1994;1: 405–13.
208. Watson C, Bradley J, Friend P, et al. Alemtuzumab (CAMPATH 1H) induction therapy in cadaveric kidney transplantation – efficacy and safety after five years. Am J Transplant 2005;5:1347–53.
209. Webb SR, Sprent J. Induction of neonatal tolerance to Mlsa antigens by CD8+ T cells. Science 1990;248:1643–6.
210. Webster AC, Craig JC, Simpson JM, et al. Identifying high risk groups and quantifying absolute risk of cancer after kidney transplantation: a cohort study of 15 183 recipients. Am J Transplant 2007;7:2140–51.
211. Wells A, Li X, Li Y, et al. Requirement for T cell apoptosis in the induction of peripheral transplantation tolerance. Nat Med 1999;5:1303–7.
212. Wong S-C, Puaux A-L, Chittezhath M, et al. Macrophage polarization to a unique phenotype driven by B cells. Eur J Immunol 2010;40:2296–307.
213. Wood KJ, Bushell A, Hester J. Regulatory immune cells in transplantation. Nat Rev Immunol 2012;12:417–30.
214. Wood KJ, Bushell A, Jones ND. Immunologic unresponsiveness to alloantigen in vivo: a role for regulatory T cells. Immunol Rev 2011;241:119–32.
215. Wood KJ, Bushell AR, Jones ND. The discovery of immunological tolerance: now more than just a laboratory solution. J Immunol 2010;184:3–4.
216. Wood KJ, Goto R. Mechanisms of rejection: current perspectives. Transplantation 2012;93:1–10.
217. Wood KJ, Sakaguchi S. Regulatory T cells in transplantation tolerance. Nat Immunol Rev 2003;3:199–210.
218. Woodruff M, Anderson N. Effect of lymphocyte depletion by thoracic duct fistula and administration of antilymphocyte serum on the survival of skin homografts in rats. Nature 1963;200:702.
219. Xu J, Foy T, Laman J, et al. Mice deficient for the CD40 ligand. Immunity 1994;1:423–31.
220. Yamada A, Chandraker A, Laufer TM, et al. Cutting edge: recipient MHC class II expression is required to achieve long-term survival of murine cardiac allografts after costimulatory blockade. J Immunol 2001;167:5522–6.
221. Yang J, Brook M, Carvalho-Gaspar M, et al. Allograft rejection mediated by memory T cells is resistant to regulation. Proc Natl Acad Sci U S A 2007;104:19954–9.
222. Zhang B, Liu R, Shi D, et al. Mesenchymal stem cells induce mature dendritic cells into a novel Jagged-2-dependent regulatory dendritic cell population. Blood 2009;113:46–57.

CHAPTER 24

Transplantation in the Sensitized Recipient and Across ABO Blood Groups

Mark D. Stegall

CHAPTER OUTLINE

Naturally occurring antibodies against blood group antigens and acquired alloantibodies against donor human leukocyte antigens (HLAs) may pose major barriers to a successful renal transplantation. Since approximately 20% of renal allograft candidates may be blood group-incompatible with their living donor and more than one-third will demonstrate some level of anti-HLA antibody pretransplant, understanding the unique issues pertaining to antidonor antibody is important for the proper management of these patients.

Over the past decade, "desensitization" protocols involving either multiple plasma exchange treatments or high-dose intravenous immune globulin (IVIG) have been developed to achieve a transplant with good short-term success despite the presence of antibodies. In addition, programs involving either paired living donation or acceptable mismatches for deceased donor allocation have provided additional options for patients with antidonor antibodies. This chapter discusses the rationale for transplanting kidneys in the setting of anti-HLA antibodies and/or antibodies against blood group and the currently observed outcomes. Specific emphasis is placed on what is known regarding the mechanisms and treatment of both early and late antibody-mediated injury, including the results of some recent therapeutic trials. Finally, what is known regarding the mechanism of antibody production in the setting of renal transplantation is outlined, highlighting important gaps in current knowledge in this emerging field.

SENSITIZED PATIENTS

Historically, some of the first evidence for alloantibody was the retrospective study of Patel and Terasaki in 1969.[45] This study showed that the ability of a recipient's serum to lyse donor cells in vitro was associated with allograft loss within hours of transplantation in a high percentage of cases. Since that time, the presence of a "positive crossmatch" due to donor-specific alloantibody (DSA) generally has been considered an absolute contraindication to kidney transplantation. Thus, the presence of DSA in a potential renal allograft recipient severely limits the options for successful kidney transplantation. Recently, however, new technologies have greatly increased the chances of transplantation in sensitized patients.

ALLOANTIBODY DETECTION

To understand the therapeutic options for sensitized patients, one first must understand the various assays used to determine the presence of alloantibody (Table 24-1). A more detailed description of these assays is presented elsewhere in this book (see Chapter 10).

The sensitivity of the assay is important in determining the presence and amount of antibody. For example, complement-dependent cytotoxicity (CDC) assays in which the recipient serum is tested for its ability to lyse target lymphocytes is of low sensitivity. For class I detection, the

TABLE 24-1 **Alloantibody Detection Assays**

Screening Assays	
Panel-reactive antibody (T-cell only)	
Solid phase bead or ELISA assays	
Donor-specific alloantibody detection assays	
Anti–Class I	
T cell cytotoxicity (NIH-CDC) assay	Very low sensitivity
T cell AHG-CDC assay	Low sensitivity
T cell FXM assay	High sensitivity
Solid phase bead or ELISA assay	Highest sensitivity
Anti–Class I or Anti–Class II (or Both)	
B cell cytotoxicity (NIH-CDC) assay	Low sensitivity
B cell FXM assay	High sensitivity
Solid phase bead or ELISA assay	Highest sensitivity

AHG-CDC, antihuman globulin–Centers for Disease Control and Prevention; ELISA, enzyme-linked immunosorbent assay; FXM, flow cytometric crossmatch; NIH-CDC, National Institutes of Health–Centers for Disease Control and Prevention.

sensitivity of the CDC assays can be enhanced by adding antihuman globulin (T-cell AHG). Flow cytometry is a more sensitive method of detecting DSA than with CDC techniques. Finally, solid-phase assays in which single HLAs are bound to microspheres or enzyme-linked immunosorbent assay (ELISA) plates are even more sensitive and have the added ability of determining the specificity of almost all of the alloantibodies that might be present in a patient's serum. For solid-phase assays such as the commonly used LABscreen, the level of alloantibody usually is expressed as the mean fluorescence intensity (MFI).[47] Levels that laboratories and transplant programs consider to be positive tend to vary, but an MFI level of >1000 generally is accepted as positive.

A solid-phase assay commonly is used as the initial screening tool to determine the presence of alloantibody. It also can be used to determine the breadth of sensitization against HLA, termed the panel-reactive antibody (PRA).[16] The PRA seeks to identify the different anti-HLA specificities in a sensitized patient's serum and then uses a formula to calculate the chances that the recipient will have DSA against kidneys from the deceased donor pool. The PRA was originally determined from a panel of cells that represented the donor pool (hence the name "panel-reactive antibody").

The PRA per se does not give information regarding the level of alloantibody, but does provide information regarding the probability of finding a donor against whom the recipient has no DSA. Thus, the PRA is commonly used as a factor in deceased donor kidney allocation. Candidates with high PRAs commonly are given extra allocation priority "points" in deceased donor kidney allocation.

If a specific donor is being considered for kidney transplant, a crossmatch assay usually is performed to verify the presence or absence of DSA against donor cells.[16] The first crossmatches were cell-based cytotoxicity assays in which recipient serum was mixed with donor lymphocytes – either T cells or B cells. The T-cell cytotoxicity crossmatch assay is now routinely performed with AHG enhancement and is termed the T-cell AHG crossmatch. This assay was the most commonly performed assay for DSA detection for many years. Because the primary goal of the crossmatch assays at that time was to avoid hyperacute rejection, a positive T-cell AHG crossmatch was (and usually still is) considered an absolute contraindication to kidney transplantation.

Subsequently, the use of flow cytometric crossmatch (FXM) techniques allowed for the detection of lower levels of alloantibody and non-cytotoxic alloantibody. The ability to detect low levels of DSA stimulated a new discussion. Were these alloantibody levels too low to cause hyperacute rejection? Before the development of FXM techniques, some patients had been transplanted unknowingly with low levels of DSA and apparently had done well. The significance of a positive FXM remained unclear for many years, with some experts considering it an absolute contraindication to kidney transplantation and others considering it an unimportant finding that merely represented yet another barrier for sensitized patients. Most experiences, including our own, have suggested that patients with a negative T-cell AHG crossmatch and a positive T-cell FXM are at very low risk for hyperacute rejection, but are at increased risk early after transplantation for humoral or cellular rejection, or both.

Another historically controversial area surrounds the significance of a positive B-cell crossmatch. Because B cells express class I and class II, a positive B-cell crossmatch may be due to the presence of anti-class I antibody or anti-class II antibody, or a combination of both. In addition, some B-cell crossmatches may be positive secondary to non-HLA antibodies or innocuous autoantibodies. Finally, because most sensitized patients have a combination of anti-class I and anti-class II antibodies, a positive B-cell crossmatch in the absence of a positive T-cell crossmatch is rare, limiting further the ability to study the importance of alloantibody against class II. Our own data, described in detail subsequently, suggest that a B-cell crossmatch secondary to anti-donor class II alloantibody can lead to hyperacute rejection in rare cases, but is a risk factor for early antibody-mediated rejection (AMR). A positive B-cell crossmatch due to high levels of class II DSA may be a particularly bad risk for the development of chronic antibody-mediated injury (see below).

A major source of confusion regarding the significance of the various cell-based assays is a general lack of standardization in the manner in which crossmatches are done in different laboratories. Registry data of sensitized patients contain heterogeneous information, and most published reports are based on small numbers of patients from single centers. The introduction of so-called solid-phase assays has brought significant changes to alloantibody characterization, but laboratories continue to perform significant modifications of these assays.

IMMUNOLOGICAL RISK

Clinicians now have the ability to estimate DSA levels across a spectrum ranging from very high to very low. In clinical practice today, DSA detected as a positive crossmatch or in solid-phase assays is no longer considered an absolute contraindication to kidney transplantation, but rather it represents the immunological risk of antibody-mediated injury.[18] This concept of immunological risk has emerged as one of the core principles in the transplantation of sensitized patients. The increased immunological risk ranges from an increased risk of hyperacute rejection, such as that seen in sensitized patients with high levels of DSA, to an increased risk of early humoral rejection, such as that seen in sensitized patients with low levels of DSA. Very low levels may represent little increased risk at all compared to unsensitized recipients. Quantifying this risk is an important aspect of designing protocols to enable successful kidney transplantation in sensitized patients. As described later, a combination of the various previously described assays allows clinicians to better determine the risk of antibody-mediated graft damage in sensitized patients. Current assays cannot completely determine the entire immunological risk of all patients. In addition, sensitized patients are at increased risk for T-cell-mediated rejection, and patients may possess antibodies against antigens not detected by current assays.

CLINICAL APPROACHES TO SENSITIZED PATIENTS

Deceased Donor Transplantation

If sensitized patients have no prospective living donors, their only transplant option is to be placed on the deceased donor waiting list. Since, by definition, a candidate with a 90% calculated PRA (cPRA) has alloantibody that reacts with 90% of the deceased donors, the rate of transplantation via this approach is low. In the United States, the assay used to determine cPRA varies among transplant programs; however, most use sensitive solid-phase assays. Approximately 30 000 patients on the Organ Procurement and Transplantation Network/United Network for Organ Sharing (UNOS) cadaver donor kidney waiting list are "sensitized"[72] and approximately 9000 are sensitized broadly with a cPRA greater than 90%. In the United States, candidates with high cPRAs are given extra allocation point so that they are given priority for kidneys against which they have no antibody. In addition, kidneys that are O-ABDR HLA-mismatched are allocated preferentially to highly sensitized patients. Despite this, fewer than 500 of these patients are transplanted each year.[61] Most sensitized patients never receive a transplant. In addition, the graft survival of patients who do receive a transplant is decreased, with the risk of graft loss at 1 year 1.8 times that of unsensitized patients. Another 7000 or so waitlisted candidates have a PRA of 20–80%. Currently, these patients receive no points for being sensitized and have approximately half the transplantation rate of unsensitized patients.

A more aggressive approach to transplanting sensitized patients with deceased donor kidneys is the Acceptable Mismatch Program of Eurotransplant.[11] In this program, anti-HLA antibodies are identified using a CDC assay. Highly sensitized patients (PRA >85%) are placed at the top of the kidney match run and organs are allocated based on the absence of DSA against the donor HLA (i.e., "acceptable mismatch" for HLA). In this program, approximately 60% of the highly sensitized patients are transplanted within 2 years after inclusion in the acceptable mismatch program and the short-term graft survival appears similar to that of unsensitized patients. Low levels of DSA that are present at the time of transplant are not considered at the time of allocation, and it is unclear what the long-term outcomes will be in this program.

A similar approach using an apparently more sensitive assay for anti-HLA antibody detection has been used at Emory University.[3] In a report of this approach from 1999 to 2003, 25% of sensitized patients were transplanted, representing a 47% increase in the transplant rate. Five-year outcomes appeared similar in sensitized and unsensitized recipients.

Desensitization protocols have been tried sparingly in deceased donor candidates. The major goal of desensitization protocols has been to achieve a negative CDC crossmatch at the time of transplant. In a multicenter, double-blinded study, 101 sensitized renal allograft candidates received high-dose IVIG (2 g/kg monthly × 4) or equivalent volume placebo.[33] Baseline PRA levels as determined by a T-cell cytotoxicity assay were similar in both groups (80% in both). IVIG treatment decreased the PRA by approximately 10% by 4 months, but the PRA returned to baseline at 6 months (2 months after the last IVIG infusion) and was equal to that of placebo-treated patients at that time point. Among dose-adherent patients, 35% (n=16) IVIG and 17% (n=8) placebo patients were able to be transplanted. Nine of 17 patients transplanted after IVIG infusion had a rejection episode, however, compared with only 1 of 10 placebo-treated patients.

The fact that desensitization protocols involving multiple plasmapheresis treatments require coordination of the timing of transplantation severely limits their applicability to cadaver donor kidney transplantation.

Paired Donation

If a sensitized candidate has potential living donors, these donors should be HLA-typed in order to find a crossmatch-negative donor. If no such donor can be found, sensitized candidates may opt to enter into one of the growing number of paired living donor programs.[9,20,39,51,55] These "exchange" schemas have been shown to increase the transplantation rate of ABO-incompatible and sensitized patients. Paired schemas employ the same "unacceptable antigen" schema described earlier to find a crossmatch-negative donor for sensitized patients. Although these programs increase the number of potential donors for sensitized patients, patients with antibodies against a wide variety of HLA types may still not be able to find a crossmatch-negative donor, even if the donor pool is very large. One of the central questions in paired donation is: How long should a sensitized patient wait for a crossmatch-negative donor versus proceeding to a transplant using a donor against whom the recipient has DSA? Since many sensitized patients may not find a DSA-negative donor, most paired donor programs employ "optimization" protocols that seek to identify donors for sensitized patients with lower levels of DSA than their original donor, with hopes of improving their outcome. Thus, transplantation of a sensitized patient in this setting might employ both paired donation and desensitization. Paired donation is discussed in more detail in the next chapter (Chapter 25).

Living Donor Kidney Transplantation with DSA: Desensitization Protocols

A viable option for sensitized candidates is to perform the living donor kidney transplant despite the presence of a DSA.[4,22,27,40,62,64,68] Overall, recent data suggest that patient survival is improved in patients undergoing a DSA-positive transplant compared to remaining on dialysis, but that many problems remain, including a decrease in long-term graft survival compared to DSA-negative transplants (Figure 24-1).[41] Montgomery et al.[41] compared 211 sensitized patients who underwent HLA-incompatible living donor kidney transplantation at Johns Hopkins Hospital to control groups from the UNOS kidney transplant waiting list matched for factors such as PRA, age, blood type, and number of years of renal replacement therapy. Five-year Kaplan–Meier estimates of patient survival were 80% in patients receiving an HLA-incompatible transplant compared to 51.5% in patients who remained on dialysis and 65.6% who waited on dialysis to receive a HLA-compatible deceased donor graft.

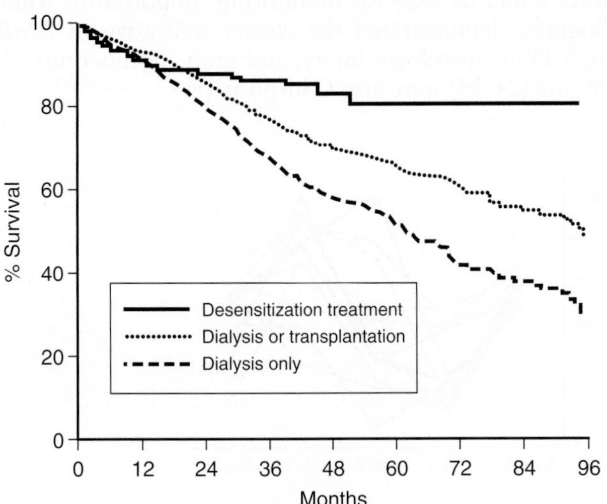

No. at Risk

Desensitization treatment	210	170	143	110	75	58	42	28	14
Dual therapy	1027	854	688	497	321	230	157	96	41
Dialysis only	1012	822	626	419	250	159	93	54	17

FIGURE 24-1 ■ Survival benefit of desensitization in human leukocyte antigen (HLA)-incompatible kidney recipients. Kaplan–Meier estimate showing improved patient survival for patients who underwent desensitization treatment compared to matched patients who either remained on dialysis (dialysis only) or underwent HLA-compatible transplantation (dialysis or transplantation). (From Montgomery RA, Lonze BE, King KE, et al. Desensitization in HLA-incompatible kidney recipients and survival. N Engl J Med 2011;365:318, with permission.)

One-year graft survival rates of nearly 100% are being reported in recent studies involving sensitized patients transplanted using desensitization protocols.[64,68] Long-term allograft outcome data are sparse, but most studies suggest that long-term renal allograft survival in the setting of DSA appears to be lower than that of transplants without DSA. The 5-year graft survival was 70.7% in 19 patients transplanted with a positive crossmatch against their living donor at the University of Maryland.[30] Recently, we found that the actual 5-year death-censored graft survival in 102 sensitized patients with DSA also was 70.7% compared to 88.0% in non-sensitized recipients matched for age and sex ($P<0.01$).[37] Thus, an increased chance of chronic injury is emerging as one of the important problems facing sensitized patients.

Specific Issues Related to DSA

The major problems encountered in DSA-positive transplants pertain to the risk of antibody-mediated injury. These can be categorized broadly as hyperacute rejection, early acute antibody-mediated rejection and chronic antibody-mediated injury. These will be discussed individually, but can be summarized here. The incidence of hyperacute rejection is related to the level of DSA at the time of transplantation. The incidence of early acute AMR depends primarily on the development of high levels of DSA and the activation of terminal complement in the first few weeks after transplantation. The mechanisms of chronic antibody-mediated injury are less dependent on DSA levels. Transplant glomerulopathy is the hallmark of chronic antibody-mediated damage and is more closely associated with the presence of anticlass II DSA and the development of cellular infiltrates in the glomeruli and peritubular capillaries.

Hyperacute Rejection and Very High Levels of DSA

The primary goal of "desensitization" is the avoidance of the catastrophic occurrence of hyperacute rejection. The exact level of DSA that leads to this complication is unclear, but most programs consider a positive T-cell AHG crossmatch a high risk for hyperacute rejection. Indeed, early in our experience, we transplanted 10 patients who, despite multiple plasmapheresis treatments (mean 10 treatments), were unable to achieve a negative T-cell AHG crossmatch.[62] Given that these highly sensitized patients had almost no other option at that time, we performed the transplant despite the persistence of low titers in the T-cell AHG crossmatch (undiluted to 1:8) on the day of transplantation. Of these 10 patients, two developed hyperacute rejection. The incidence of early AMR in this group was 70% and the 1-year graft survival was only 50%. From these data, we conclude that the inability to achieve a negative T-cell AHG crossmatch by the day of transplantation resulted in such poor outcomes that we now consider it a contraindication to transplantation. In our program, this correlated with a baseline B-flow cytometric crossmatch (BFXM) of 450. New therapy will be needed in order to achieve a better outcome in these patients. Recently, we have demonstrated that pretransplant treatment with bortezomib depletes alloantibody secreting cells and improves the response to PE in these patients with very high levels of DSA, allowing some to undergo a successful transplant (see below).[10]

Although no randomized trial has directly compared the ability of IVIG and PE to achieve a negative CDC crossmatch pretransplant in patients with high levels of DSA, in one published study both therapies were equally effective in patients with a T-cell AHG of 1:8 at baseline.[62]

Early Acute Antibody-Mediated Rejection

Even if hyperacute rejection is avoided, patients with DSA still have a high incidence of acute AMR in the first few weeks after transplantation. Indeed, early AMR has emerged as one of the major complications of transplantation of highly sensitized renal transplant recipients.

While many cases of AMR in conventional kidney transplant recipients occur in combination with acute cellular rejection (ACR), recipients with DSA at the time of transplant tend to have a "pure" form of acute AMR that commonly occurs in the first month after transplantation and is relatively straightforward to diagnose. The Banff classification for acute AMR includes the presence of DSA in the serum, evidence of C4d deposition in the peritubular capillaries, and histologic evidence of tissue injury (including vascular microthrombi, peritubular capillaritis, and/or acute tubular injury).[50] The presence or absence of graft dysfunction differentiates clinical from subclinical acute AMR. In particular, the development of C4d staining, an inert byproduct of complement activation that binds covalently to endothelium, has been an important breakthrough in providing histologic correlations with AMR.[14,31,43]

In single-center reports involving +XMKTx, the incidence of acute AMR ranges from 30% to 40%, with higher levels of baseline DSA correlating with higher rates of early acute AMR.[4,40,68] In a series from Hôpital St. Louis in Paris, the incidence of AMR was 36.4% with a baseline DSA MFI of 3001–6000 and 51.3% with a baseline DSA MFI of >6000.[37]

The incidence of early acute AMR appears to correlate with the development of high levels of DSA after transplantation. Our group examined the natural history of DSA early after transplantation and its relationship with AMR in 70 positive crossmatch kidney transplant recipients.[4] The overall incidence of AMR was 36%, with the mean time to diagnosis of approximately 10 days and all episodes occurring within 1 month of transplantation. All but one AMR episode was associated with graft dysfunction (increase in serum creatinine over nadir >0.3 mg/dL in the first month), but in many instances, evidence of histologic injury preceded the increase in serum creatinine.

The time course changes in DSA posttransplant correlated well with the development of AMR (Figure 24-2). Overall, mean DSA levels decreased by day 4 and remained low in patients who did not develop AMR. By day 10, however, DSA levels increased in patients developing AMR, with 92% (23/25) of patients with a FXM >359 (molecules of equivalent soluble fluorochrome units of approximately 34000) developing AMR. The BFXM and the total DSA measured by LABscreen beads correlated well across a wide spectrum, suggesting that either could be used for monitoring. Importantly, when allografts demonstrated the cluster indicative of AMR (high DSA, histologic injury, and graft dysfunction), all but one (24/25) were also C4d-positive.

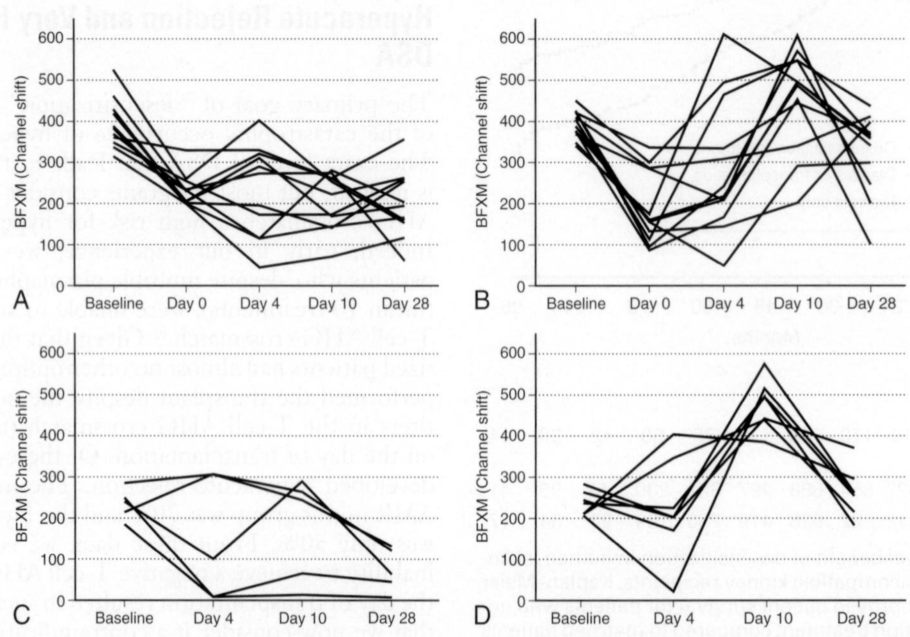

FIGURE 24-2 ■ Correlation between donor-specific alloantibody (DSA) levels and early acute antibody-mediated rejection (AMR). (A) DSA levels from baseline to 28 days posttransplant for the high DSA patients without AHR; (B) high DSA patients with resulting AHR; (C) low DSA patients without AHR; and (D) low DSA patients with resulting AHR. BFXM, B-cell flow crossmatch. (From Burns JM, Cornell LD, Perry DK, et al. Alloantibody levels and antibody mediated rejection early after positive crossmatch kidney transplantation. Am J Transplant 2008;8:2684, with permission.)

Treatment of AMR

Treatment of AMR in this clinical setting usually involves the immediate institution of PE therapy to reduce DSA levels.

Vo et al. described high-dose IVIG (e.g., 2 g/kg) for the treatment of AMR in their protocols that employed high-dose IVIG for desensitization.[68] However, they also employ PE in AMR that does not respond to IVIG. Since most PE-based protocols also employ lower doses of IVIG (usually 10 mg/kg) after each PE to replace serum immunoglobulin levels, it is unclear what role IVIG might also play in PE-based treatments of AMR. However, one recent study has suggested that PE was more effective than IVIG in reversing AMR.[36]

The role of splenectomy in the treatment of AMR also remains unclear and overall its use seems to be declining. In our series, splenectomy was performed for severe AMR in the setting of a rising serum creatinine (usually >2.0) and rising serum DSA levels despite daily PE treatments. Splenectomy was performed in 43% of the patients that developed AMR, all but one of whom regained normal renal function.[64]

Several reports have described the use of bortezomib for the treatment of AMR.[13,49,66,69] In most of these reports, the AMR episode occurred in conjunction with ACR and developed months to years after transplantation. AMR in this setting may be different from the pure AMR described in sensitized recipients in that the DSA production may be due to a de novo immune response that might involve shortlived plasmablasts and coordination between antigen-presenting cells, T helper cells and naïve B cells. While it is difficult to demonstrate the efficacy of bortezomib in these studies without controls, it is remarkable that, in the judgment of the various authors, bortezomib appeared to generally decrease DSA and reverse either pure AMR or AMR in combination with ACR.

Prevention of AMR

We performed a single-center, open-label study to determine if treatment with eculizumab could reduce the incidence of AMR in the first 3 months after +XMKTx.[64] The incidence of biopsy-proven AMR in 26 highly sensitized renal transplant recipients was compared to a historical control group of 51 sensitized patients treated with a similar PE-based desensitization protocol without eculizumab. The treatment regimen is outlined in Figure 24-3. The incidence of AMR was 7.7% (2/26) in the eculizumab group compared to 41.2% (21/51) in the control group (P=0.0031). Eculizumab-treated patients did not routinely receive posttransplant PE and the same percentage developed high levels of DSA after transplant (BFXM >350 or MFI >10 000) compared to the control group (50% versus 43%). Thus, eculizumab did not appear to affect DSA levels. However, in the control group, 100% of patients who developed high DSA after transplant developed AMR. In contrast, in the eculizumab group only 15% (2/13) developed AMR. Importantly, all biopsies in both groups of patients with high DSA were positive for C4d. Thus, eculizumab prevented AMR despite high levels of DSA and proximal complement deposition in the allograft.

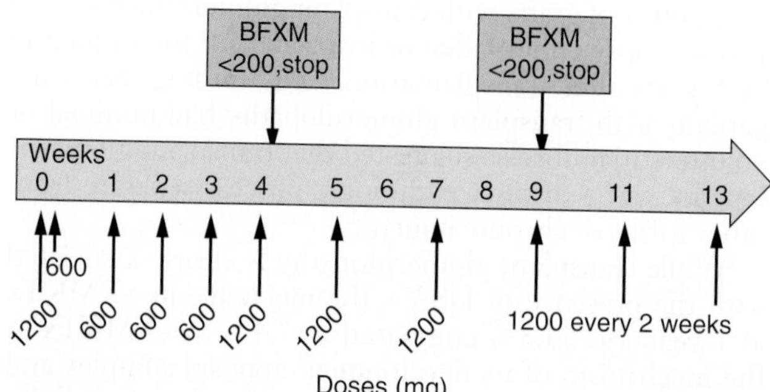

FIGURE 24-3 ■ Eculizumab treatment protocol for the prevention of antibody-mediated rejection (AMR). The dosing regimen consisted of 1200 mg immediately prior to transplantation, 600 mg on postoperative day 1, and then 600 mg weekly for 4 weeks thereafter. At week 4, assessment of donor-specific alloantibody (DSA) levels was performed. Eculizumab was discontinued in patients whose DSA had a significantly decreased B-flow cytometric crossmatch (BFXM: channel shift <200). In patients with persistently high DSA and thus believed to be at continued risk for AMR, eculizumab was continued (1200 mg week 5 and then every 2 weeks). Another DSA assessment was performed at week 9 and eculizumab was discontinued if the BFXM channel shift was <200. (From Stegall MD, Diwan T, Raghavaih S, et al. Terminal complement inhibition decreases antibody mediated rejection in sensitized renal transplant recipients. Am J Transplant 2011; 11: 2405, with permission.)

The two cases of AMR in the eculizumab group occurred on posttransplant days 7 and 14, in the setting of an increasing serum creatinine, increased DSA, and a biopsy that showed C4d staining with glomerular microthrombi. Compared to AMR in the control group, these two episodes were relatively mild and easy to reverse with PE. Both grafts recovered completely and were functioning at 1 year after transplantation. The cause of AMR in these two patients remains unclear, but in both cases anti-C5 levels were therapeutic and the hemolytic assay was completely blocked, suggesting that terminal complement was inhibited. Thus, a C5-independent mechanism is likely the cause of AMR in eculizumab-treated patients.

Since high levels of DSA and C4d-positive staining are common in eculizumab-treated patients, the diagnosis of AMR relies heavily on "evidence of graft injury" and graft dysfunction. Currently, a randomized, open-label, multicenter study is being conducted to validate the findings of our single-center study.

CHRONIC ANTIBODY-MEDIATED INJURY

Chronic antibody-mediated injury has become increasingly implicated as a major cause of late renal allograft loss.[5,12,24,35,38,71] This is especially common in patients with DSA at the time of transplantation.

The major histologic lesion that is associated with chronic antibody-mediated injury is transplant glomerulopathy.[2,24,32] This lesion is characterized by duplication of the glomerular basement membrane. Transplant glomerulopathy generally carries one of the worst prognoses for any histologic lesion found on surveillance biopsy. In one study, 60% of grafts with transplant glomerulopathy on a 1-year biopsy either failed or lost >50% of their function by 5 years after transplantation.[5] The finding that some patients with transplant glomerulopathy had minimal or no interstitial fibrosis suggested that transplant glomerulopathy was a distinct pathologic process separate from other forms of chronic injury.[24]

While transplant glomerulopathy is clearly associated with the presence of DSA – the incidence in +XMKTx at 1 year was 54.5% compared to 7.4% in –XMKTx[2] – the mechanism of its development appears complex and may depend more on the presence of a chronic cellular infiltrate than on the continued deposition of DSA and complement activation.

Several recent studies suggest that subclinical cellular infiltration distinct from ACR portends poor graft outcome.[2,21,25,26,29,38] These studies showed that the presence of macrophages, neutrophils, and lymphocytes in the peritubular capillaries (termed peritubular capillaritis) was common in patients with DSA and was associated with the development of transplant glomerulopathy and graft loss. Loupy et al. showed that, while the persistence of C4d-positive staining in the peritubular capillaries carried a higher risk from chronic injury, many grafts in patients with DSA developed chronic injury despite low DSA levels and being C4d-negative.[38] Indeed, the presence of peritubular capillaritis has emerged as the major risk factor for subsequent transplant glomerulopathy.

Taken together, these data suggest that the initiation of chronic injury might be due to the deposition of DSA and complement activation. This leads to chemotaxis of inflammatory cells. The subsequent development of chronic glomerulopathy (CG) might be due to the persistence of peritubular capillaritis, which could be independent of DSA and complement. Another possibility is that chronic injury might be dependent on either very low levels of DSA and complement that are not detected by our current methods or by intermittent activation that is missed by infrequent surveillance biopsies. Yet another possible mechanism of the development of transplant glomerulopathy might involve direct activation of endothelium by DSA. Data showing that DSA alone can activate endothelial cells in vitro suggest that complement-independent mechanisms of damage also might exist.[67]

However, there are several reasons to continue to interpret these early histologic studies with caution. First, light microscopy has been shown to underestimate the amount of inflammation and damage. For example, electron microscopy can identify endothelial cell activation in patients with DSA early after transplantation and months prior to the development of CG. Similarly, we recently demonstrated that almost all patients with a positive crossmatch at the time of transplant show gene expression evidence of inflammation and cellular infiltration, even when peritubular capillaritis and CG are absent by light microscopy.[8] Second, the variable progression of chronic inflammation and transplant glomerulopathy as seen by light microscopy suggests that there are factors that we are not identifying that are important in its pathogenesis.[73] Finally, the finding that DSA against donor class II is more likely to cause chronic injury needs to be incorporated into the overall model of chronic antibody-mediated injury.[2]

The role of complement in either the development of peritubular capillaritis or transplant glomerulopathy could be tested using prolonged eculizuamb therapy. Unfortunately, the current studies using eculizumab for the treatment of early AMR were designed to discontinue C5 inhibition early after transplantation if DSA levels fell below a predetermined low level (BFXM channel shift <200 in our single-center study). Thus, in the first 10 patients followed to 1 year, eight stopped drug at 1 month, while two were treated for an entire year.[64] While the overall incidence of peritubular capillaritis did appear to be lower at 3 months in the eculizumab group, two patients treated with drug for 1 year for high levels of DSA did develop peritubular capillaritis while on treatment. Several others have developed transplant glomerulopathy in the months to years after stopping the drug and two patients lost their graft due to chronic antibody-mediated injury at 2 years after transplantation. Thus, a relatively short peritransplant course of eculizuamb that prevents early AMR has not prevented the development of chronic antibody-mediated injury. A study design involving prolonged treatment with eculizumab for months to years after transplantation is needed to answer the question of whether or not C5 plays a role in chronic injury.

Prevention of chronic AMR might best be managed by pre-emptive treatment of increased DSA levels early after transplantation. One study by Trivedi et al.[66] described their experience with 11 patients treated with bortezomib for the de novo development of anti-HLA antibodies. Within 22 days, 9 of 11 patients had a decrease in antibody levels. The authors suggest that this pre-emptive use of bortezomib may avoid chronic antibody-mediated damage, but long-term results are not yet available.

ABO-INCOMPATIBLE KIDNEY TRANSPLANTATION

Historically, the presence of antibody against donor blood group also has been considered a contraindication to kidney transplantation, with high antibody levels associated with hyperacute and early humoral rejection. However, similar to sensitized patients, several options now exist for patients who are ABO-incompatible with their living donors. These include[60]: (1) being placed on the deceased donor waiting list; (2) entering into a paired living donor program; or (3) undergoing a desensitization protocol and receiving the ABO-incompatible living donor kidney despite the presence of antidonor antibody.

Being placed on the deceased donor waiting list is the most commonly used option. Because most ABO-incompatible candidates are blood group O (78% in our series),[23] their current mean waiting time for a deceased donor kidney is approximately 5 years in the United States. This long waiting time translates into increased morbidity and mortality pre- and posttransplantation, especially in older patients and diabetics.

In countries with fewer deceased donor kidney transplants, ABO-incompatible kidney transplantation may be the only option.[16,58] Numerous studies have shown that ABO-incompatible living donor kidney transplantation has higher early graft loss rates than ABO-compatible grafts, but long-term survival is comparable, ranging from 79% to 98% at 5 years.[1,16,17,19,23,42,63,65] The reason for the improved long-term survival of ABO-incompatible compared to DSA-positive transplants is unclear. The development of accommodation or even tolerance to blood group antibody may occur despite the continued presence of antiblood group antibody.[46,52,70] A recent histologic study suggests that ABO-incompatible renal allografts have less peritubular capillaritis and less transplant glomerulopathy compared to DSA-positive grafts at 5 years.[1]

The level of antiblood group antibody that causes hyperacute rejection has not been determined exactly and may vary. Several groups have shown that antiblood group isohemagglutination titers of less than 1:8 or 1:16 seems to be "safe" at the time of transplantation in that evidence of antibody deposition is not seen on 30-minute postreperfusion surveillance biopsy specimens. Achieving these "safe" levels of antibody can be difficult in some patients, however. Patients who at baseline (before any therapy) have high levels of antiblood group antibody (e.g., >1:512) rarely can be "desensitized" (have antidonor antibody reduced to safe levels) using our current protocols. Performing splenectomy either before or at the time of transplantation might allow successful ABO-incompatible transplantation even in patients with very high antiblood group antibody levels.

Protocols have evolved to include pre-emptive plasmapheresis treatments, and antibody monitoring aimed at maintaining low levels of antidonor antibody in the first 2 weeks after transplantation. Most protocols aim to maintain the isoagglutination antiblood group antibody titer less than 1:16 for 2 weeks.[16,17,19,23,42,65] Due to the lack of prospective, randomized trials, many important questions regarding ABO-incompatible kidney transplantation remain unanswered, including: (1) What is the maximum blood group titer that is acceptable at the time of transplant?[63] (2) Do immunoabsorption columns that specifically remove antiblood group antibody really have less morbidity and better outcomes than standard PE?[19] (3) What is the role of rituximab in these protocols? (4) Is steroid-free immunosuppression possible in ABO-incompatible transplantation?[17] (5) How does one generate and measure accommodation and tolerance to ABO-incompatible transplantation in both adults and children?[46,70]

A major barrier to the widespread application of ABO-incompatible kidney transplantation is the increased cost compared with conventional transplants. We performed a retrospective study comparing 40 ABO-incompatible with 77 matching ABO-compatible living donor renal allografts with respect to complications, resource use, and cost from day 14 to 90 days posttransplantation.[54] Overall, surgery-related complications and resource use were increased in the ABO-incompatible group, primarily because of the desensitization protocol and AMR. In the absence of rejection, the mean number of complications was similar for both groups. ABO-incompatible kidney transplantation cost approximately $38 000 more than ABO-compatible transplants, but was cost-effective compared with maintaining the patient on dialysis while waiting for a blood group-compatible deceased donor kidney.

While paired donation has significantly decreased the need for ABO-incompatible living donor kidney transplantation, it remains a viable option for some patients, albeit with greater morbidity, but shorter waiting times compared to ABO-compatible transplants.

MECHANISTIC VIEW OF ANTIBODY PRODUCTION AND INJURY

Over the past decade, the pathway to antibody production has been clearly delineated in numerous animal and human studies.[48,59,63] The phenotypes of the various B-cell subsets are shown in Table 24-2. The bone marrow continuously generates a large variety of naïve B cells expressing cell surface immunoglobulin. Although each naïve B cell's immunoglobulin is unique, as a population these naïve B cells are capable of interacting with an enormous variety of antigens, including all types of class I and class II HLA molecules. These mature, but naïve, B cells remain in a quiescent state until they encounter antigen in secondary lymphoid tissue, such as the spleen. Activation of B cells, which requires T-cell help, may lead to the development of plasma cells (either short-lived or long-lived) and to the development of memory B cells. Naïve B cells express cell surface immunoglobulin, yet only plasma cells are capable of antibody secretion. Memory B cells also express cell surface immunoglobulin and are capable of rapid conversion to plasma cells within hours of reexposure to antigen. Memory B cells do not secrete immunoglobulin, however.

Long-lived plasma cells can persist for years in special microenvironments of the marrow and spleen, continuously producing antibody even in the absence of antigenic stimulation. They are terminally differentiated and are resistant to most pharmacologic agents. Most of the anti-HLA antibody detected in sensitized recipients is likely produced by long-lived plasma cells.

Plasma cells seem to be resistant to most immunomodulatory agents commonly in use in clinical transplantation.[48,49] They do not use interleukin-2 for their function and are not significantly inhibited by either

TABLE 24-2 **Cell Surface Phenotypes of B-Cell Subsets**

Naïve B Cell	Memory B Cell	Plasma Cell
$CD20^+/CD27^-$	$CD27^+/CD20^{+/-}$	$CD27^-/CD20^-$
$CD38^-/CD138^-$	$CD38^-/CD138^-$	$CD38^+/CD138^+$
Intracytoplasmic Immunoglobulin Negative	Intracytoplasmic Immunoglobulin Negative	Intracytoplasmic Immunoglobulin Positive

calcineurin inhibitors or antibodies against the interleukin-2 receptors. They do not express CD52, the target for alemtuzumab. They also do not express CD20 and would seem to be resistant to treatment with the anti-CD20 antibody, rituximab. Indeed, recent studies by our group have demonstrated that plasma cells are resistant to desensitization with IVIG, rituximab, and Thymoglobulin.[48,49]

The presence of DSA is only the first step in the development of humoral rejection. The next step is the binding of antibody to allograft. Using immunohistological techniques, donor-specific IgG and IgM are not detectable on renal allograft vascular endothelium, even in the setting of clear-cut AMR.[15,50] Indirect evidence of antibody binding to an allograft has been the demonstration of C4d in the peritubular capillaries, but C4d is inactive and does not damage renal allografts.[14,43] More distal terminal complement activation is associated with kidney damage, however.[44] The presence of membrane attack complex of C5b-9 has been shown to mediate neutrophil influx and synthesis of proinflammatory cytokines and may cause direct cell injury, apoptosis, and necrosis.[34,56] Similarly, the anaphylatoxin C5a is a chemoattractant for neutrophils and macrophages. The C5a receptor on endothelial cells, neutrophils, and macrophages activates these and other cells to produce cytokines, chemokines, and adhesion molecules,[6,7] and may regulate apoptosis.[28,57] Antibody also has been shown to cause endothelial cell damage by complement-independent mechanisms.[67]

It has been suggested in clinical and experimental studies that organ allografts seem to develop resistance to antigraft antibody. This was first described and is well established in ABO-incompatible allografts. Other investigators have shown evidence for this process in allosensitized recipients of renal allografts.[52] The mechanisms of accommodation are unknown; however, data suggest that the stimulation of antiapoptotic molecules, such as hemoxygenase 1, Bcl-xl, and Bcl-2, may be important early.[52] Our group showed that normally functioning ABO-incompatible renal allografts 1 year after transplantation develop a unique intragraft gene expression profile different from ABO-compatible grafts.[46] There is molecular evidence of accommodation in human ABO-incompatible grafts. In our opinion, the evidence for accommodation is much stronger for ABO-incompatible grafts than for positive-crossmatch renal allograft recipients.

Combining what is known about antibody production with existing clinical studies, a mechanistic model of alloantibody production and antibody-mediated damage in sensitized renal allograft recipients can be constructed. In this model, baseline DSA is the product of long-lived plasma cells that generally are resistant to current therapy. Desensitization therapy primarily removes or blocks DSA without significantly affecting ongoing antibody production. After transplantation, alloantibody is the product of persistent production by pre-existing plasma cells and the recruitment of memory B cells to become plasma cells. This conversion of memory B cells to plasma cells is the major mechanism by which patients with low levels of DSA at baseline develop humoral rejection after transplant.

Humoral rejection in patients with high levels of DSA at baseline involves a memory B-cell response and ongoing DSA production by pre-existing plasma cells. We hypothesize that the recruitment of naïve B cells is not a mechanism of antibody production either at baseline or during a humoral rejection episode. The basis for this assumption is our clinical observation that humoral rejection occurs despite treatment with either rabbit antithymocyte globulin (Thymoglobulin) (which would decrease T-cell help) or rituximab (which removes naïve T cells).

Since DSA at baseline is primarily produced by long-lived plasma cells, we and others have attempted to find agents that might deplete plasma cells in sensitized recipients. In vitro, bortezomib caused apoptosis of plasma cells, but this was not observed with rituximab, IVIG, or Thymoglobulin.[48,49] We then performed a dose escalation study of the impact of bortezomib monotherapy in highly sensitized patients.[10] Bortezomib caused significant depletion of bone marrow-derived plasma cells in some patients (Figure 24-4). This potentiated the ability of PE to lower DSA levels and allowed for the transplantation of some patients who were not able to be transplanted using PE alone. However, the impact of bortezomib may be limited by its poor bioavailability and another recent report of two patients failed to show an impact of bortezomib alone when PE was not used.[53]

Taken together, existing evidence suggests that bortezomib therapy has a modest impact on plasma cells. Developed for the treatment of multiple myeloma, clinicians in that area have moved to more prolonged treatment schedules. However, prolonged treatment increases the incidence of toxicity and it is unclear if more prolonged treatment will lead to improved depletion of plasma cells and greater reduction of DSA levels in the serum in sensitized patients.

The development of therapy to control antibody production and its impact on renal allografts is in its infancy. It is likely that the next few years will see important advances in this area.

CONCLUSION

The treatment options for renal transplant candidates who have DSA or who are blood group-incompatible with their living donor continue to evolve. In many instances, paired donation or acceptable mismatch programs are able to avoid these antibody barriers. However, for some patients, a DSA-positive or ABO-incompatible kidney transplant may be the best treatment option. The immunological risk of patients varies from very low to prohibitively high, and protocols can be tailored to the risk of antibody-mediated damage. Novel new therapies such as the use of eculizumab to prevent early AMR in DSA-positive transplants suggest that this major complication is becoming more manageable. However, chronic injury remains a major unsolved problem in these patients. Future research efforts focusing on the mechanisms of antibody production and its impact on the graft should provide for continued progress in this new and challenging field.

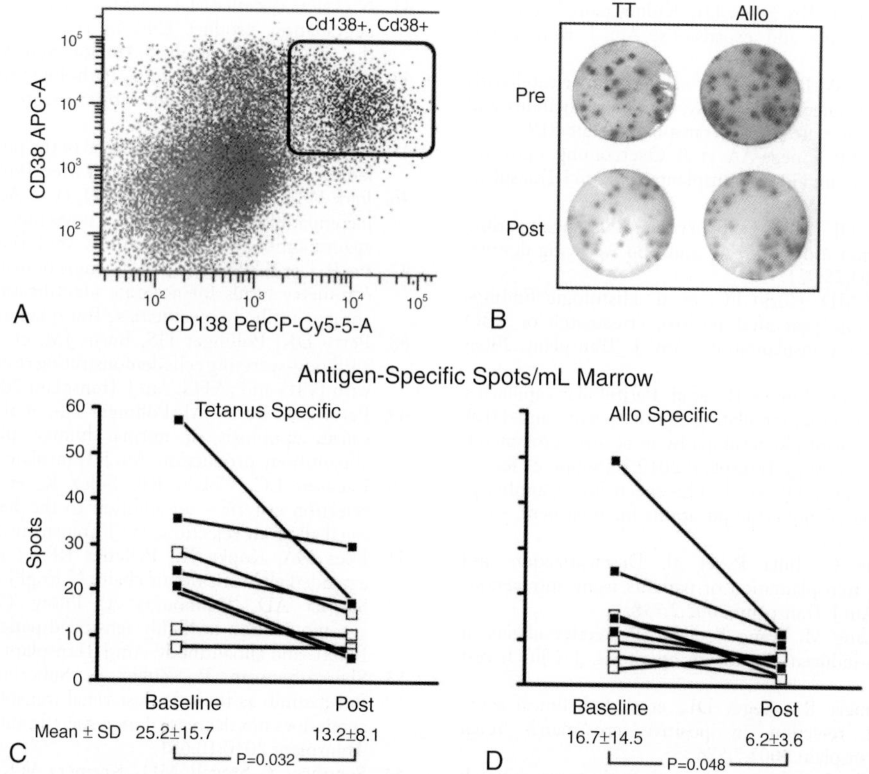

FIGURE 24-4 ■ Proteasome inhibition depletes antigen-specific marrow-derived plasma cells. (A) Representative flow cytometry of the bone marrow population enriched for plasma cells (CD138+, CD38+). (B) Representative ELISPOT showing numerous individual plasma cells (spots) specific for tetanus toxoid (TT) and HLA (Allo) pretreatment and a reduction in number of antigen-specific plasma cells with proteasome inhibition (*P*=0.032 for tetanus-specific plasma cells and *P*=0.048 for HLA-specific plasma cells). Four patients received one four-dose cycle (open squares) and four received four four-dose cycles (closed squares). (From Diwan T, Raghavaiah S, Burns J, et al. Proteasome inhibition depletes normal human plasma cells and enhances anti-donor antibody reduction in sensitized renal allograft candidates. Transplantation 2011;91:536, with permission.)

REFERENCES

1. Bentall A, Herrera LP, Dean PG, et al. ABO incompatible vs positive crossmatch kidney transplants: do differences in capillaritis correlate with outcome? Am J Transplant 2012;12(s3):151.
2. Bentall A, Cornell LD, Gloor JM, et al. Five year outcomes in living donor kidney transplants with a positive crossmatch. Am J Transplant 2013;13(1):76-85. Epub 2012 Oct 16. doi: 10.1111/j.1600-6143.2012.04291.x.
3. Bray RA, Nolen JDL, Larsen C, et al. Transplanting the highly sensitized patient: the Emory Algorithm. Am J Transplant 2006;6:2307.
4. Burns JM, Cornell LD, Perry DK, et al. Alloantibody levels and antibody mediated rejection early after positive crossmatch kidney transplantation. Am J Transplant 2008;8:2684.
5. Cosio FG, Grande JP, Wadei H, et al. Predicting subsequent decline in kidney allograft function from early surveillance biopsies. Am J Transplant 2005;5:2464.
6. Cragg MS, Howat WJ, Bloodworth L, et al. Complement mediated cell death is associated with DNA fragmentation. Cell Death Differ 2000;7:48.
7. Czermak BJ, Sarma V, Bless M, et al. In vitro and in vivo dependency of chemokine generation on C5a and TNF-α. J Immunol 1999;162:2321.
8. Dean PG, Park WD, Cornell LD, et al. Intragraft gene expression in positive crossmatch kidney allografts: ongoing inflammation mediated chronic antibody-mediated damage. Am J Transplant 2012;12:1551–63.
9. de Klerk M, Witvliet MD, Haase-Kromwijk BJ, et al. A highly-efficient living donor kidney exchange program for both blood type and crossmatch incompatible recipient combinations. Transplantation 2006;82:1616.
10. Diwan T, Raghavaiah S, Burns J, et al. Proteasome inhibition depletes normal human plasma cells and enhances anti-donor antibody reduction in sensitized renal allograft candidates. Transplantation 2011;91:536.
11. Doxiadis IIN, Class FHJ. Transplantation of highly sensitized patients via the acceptable mismatch program or desensitization? We need both. Curr Opin Organ Transplant 2009;14:410.
12. El-Zoghby ZM, Stegall MD, Lager DJ, et al. Identifying specific causes of kidney allograft loss. Am J Transplant 2009;9:527.
13. Everly MJ, Everly JJ, Arend LJ, et al. Bortezomib provides effective therapy for antibody and cell-mediated rejection. Transplantation 2008;86:1754.
14. Feucht HE, Schneeberger H, Hillebrand G, et al. Capillary deposition of C4d complement fragment and early renal graft loss. Kidney Int 1993;43:1333.
15. Fidler ME, Gloor JM, Lager DJ, et al. Histologic findings of antibody-mediated rejection in ABO blood-group-incompatible living-donor kidney transplantation. Am J Transplant 2004;4:101.
16. Fuchinoue S, Ishii Y, Sawada T, et al. The 5-year outcome of ABO-incompatible kidney transplantation with rituximab induction. Transplantation 2011;91:853.
17. Galliford J, Charif R, Chan KK, et al. ABO incompatible living renal transplantation with a steroid sparing protocol. Transplantation 2008;86:901.
18. Gebel HM, Bray RA, Nickerson P. Pre-transplant assessment of donor-reactive HLA-specific antibodies in renal transplantation: contraindication vs. risk. Am J Transplant 2003;3:1488.
19. Genberg H, Kumlien G, Wennberg L, et al. ABO-incompatible kidney transplantation using antigen-specific immunoadsorption and rituximab: a 3 year follow-up. Transplantation 2008;85:1745.

20. Gentry SE, Montgomery RA, Segev DL. Kidney paired donation: fundamentals, limitations and expansions. Am J Kidney Dis 2011;57:144.
21. Gibson IW, Gwinner W, Brocker V, et al. Peritubular capillaritis in renal allografts: prevalence, scoring system, reproducibility and clinicopathological correlates. Am J Transplant 2008;8:819.
22. Gloor JM, DeGoey SR, Pineda AA, et al. Overcoming a positive crossmatch in living donor kidney transplantation. Am J Transplant 2003;3:1017.
23. Gloor JM, Lager DJ, Moore SB, et al. ABO-incompatible kidney transplantation using both A2 and non-A2 living donors. Transplantation 2003;75:971.
24. Gloor JM, Stegall MD, Cosio FC, et al. Histologic findings in renal allografts one year after positive crossmatch or ABO incompatible kidney transplantation. Am J Transplant 2006; 6:1841.
25. Gloor JM, Cornell LD, Winters JL, et al. Peritubular capillaritis and C4D immunostaining, circulating donor specific anti-HLA antibodies, and transplant glomerulopathy in positive crossmatch kidney transplantation. Am J Transplant 2010;10(Suppl. 4):46.
26. Gloor J, Cosio F, Lager DJ, et al. The spectrum of antibody-mediated renal allograft injury: implications for treatment. Am J Transplant 2008;8:1367.
27. Glotz D, Antoine C, Julia P, et al. Desensitization and subsequent kidney transplantation of patients using intravenous immunoglobulin. Am J Transplant 2002;2:758.
28. Guo RF, Huber-Lang M, Wang X, et al. Protective effects of anti-C5a in sepsis-induced thymocyte apoptosis. J Clin Invest 2000;106:1271.
29. Haas M, Montgomery RA, Segev DL, et al. Subclinical acute antibody-mediated rejection in positive crossmatch renal allografts. Am J Transplant 2007;7:576.
30. Haririan A, Nogueira J, Kukuruga D, et al. Positive cross-match living donor kidney transplantation: longer-term outcomes. Am J Transplant 2009;9:536.
31. Herzenberg AM, Gill JS, Djurdev O, et al. C4d deposition in acute rejection: an independent long-term prognostic factor. J Am Soc Nephrol 2002;13:234.
32. Isssa N, Cosio FG, Gloor JM, et al. Transplant glomerulopathy: risk and prognosis related to anti-human leukocyte antigen class II antibody levels. Transplantation 2008;15:681.
33. Jordan SC, Tyan D, Stablein DM, et al. Evaluation of intravenous immunoglobulin as an agent to lower allosensitization and improve transplantation in highly sensitized adult patients with end-stage renal disease: report of the NIH IG02 trial. J Am Soc Nephrol 2004;15:3256.
34. Kilgore KS, Ward PA, Warren JS. Neutrophil adhesion to human endothelial cells is induced by the membrane attack complex: the roles of P-selectin and platelet activating factor. Inflammation 1998;22:583.
35. Lee P-C, Terasaki PI, Takemoto SK, et al. All chronic rejection failures of kidney transplants were preceded by the development of HLA antibodies. Transplantation 2003;74:1192.
36. Lefaucheur C, Nochy D, Andrade J, et al. Comparison of combination plasmapheresis IVIg/anti-CD20 versus high-dose IVIg in the treatment of antibody mediated rejection. Am J Transplant 2009;9:1099.
37. Lefaucher C, Loupy A, Hill GS, et al. Preexisting donor-specific HLA antibodies predict outcome in kidney transplantation. J Am Soc Nephrol 2010;21:1398.
38. Loupy A, Suberbielle-Boissel C, Hill GS, et al. Outcome of subclinical antibody-mediated rejection in kidney transplant recipients with preformed donor-specific alloantibody. Am J Transplant 2009;9:2561.
39. Montgomery RA, Zachary AA, Ratner LE, et al. Clinical results from transplanting incompatible live donor kidney donor/recipient pairs using kidney paired donation. JAMA 2005;294:1655.
40. Montgomery RA, Zachary AA. Transplanting patients with a positive donor-specific crossmatch: a single center's perspective. Pediatr Transplant 2004;8:535.
41. Montgomery RA, Lonze BE, King KE, et al. Desensitization in HLA-incompatible kidney recipients and survival. N Engl J Med 2011;365:318.
42. Montgomery JR, Berger JC, Warren DS, et al. Outcomes of ABO-incompatible kidney transplantation in the United States. Transplantation 2012;93:603.
43. Nickeleit V, Zeiler M, Gudat F, et al. Detection of the complement degradation product C4d in renal allografts: diagnostic and therapeutic implications. J Am Soc Nephrol 2002;13:242.
44. Nishi S, Imai N, Ito Y, et al. Pathologic study on the relationship between C4d, CD59 and C5b-9 in acute renal allograft rejection. Clin Transplant 2004;11:18.
45. Patel R, Terasaki PI. Significance of the positive crossmatch test in kidney transplantation. N Engl J Med 1969;280:735.
46. Park WD, Grande JP, Ninova D, et al. Accommodation in ABO-incompatible kidney allografts, a novel mechanism of self-protection against antibody-mediated injury. Am J Transplant 2003;3:952.
47. Pei R, Lee JH, Shih N-J, et al. Single human leukocyte antigen flow cytometry beads for accurate identification of human leukocyte antigen antibody specificities. Transplantation 2003;75:43.
48. Perry DK, Pollinger HS, Burns JM, et al. Two novel essays of antibody-secreting cells demonstrating resistance to desensitization with IVIG and rATG. Am J Transplant 2008;8:133.
49. Perry DK, Burns JM, Pollinger HS, et al. Proteasome inhibition causes apoptosis of normal human plasma cells preventing alloantibody production. Am J Transplant 2009;9:201.
50. Racusen LC, Colvin RB, Solez K, et al. Antibody-mediated rejection criteria – an addition to the Banff '97 classification of renal allograft rejection. Am J Transplant 2003;3:708.
51. Rees MA, Kopke JE, Pelletier RP, et al. A non-simultaneous extended altruistic donor chain. N Engl J Med 2009;360:1096.
52. Salama AD, Delikouras A, Pusey CD, et al. Transplant accommodation in highly sensitized patients: a potential role for Bcl-xL and alloantibody. Am J Transplant 2001;1:260.
53. Sberro-Soussan R, Zuber J, Suberbielle-Boissel C, et al. Boretzomib as the sole post-renal transplantation desensitization agent does not decrease donor-specific anti-HLA antibodies. Am J Transplant 2010;10:681.
54. Schwartz J, Stegall MD, Kremers WK, et al. Complications, resource utilization, and cost of ABO incompatible living donor kidney transplantation. Transplantation 2006;82:155.
55. Segev DL, Gentry SE, Warren DS, et al. Kidney paired donation and optimizing the use of live donor organs. JAMA 2005;293:1883.
56. Shibata T, Cosio FG, Birmingham DJ. Complement activation induces the expression of decay-accelerating factor on human mesangial cells. J Immunol 1991;147:3901.
57. Shieferdecker HL, Schlaf G, Jungermann K, et al. Functions of anaphylatoxin C5a in rat liver: direct and indirect actions on nonparenchymal and parenchymal cells. Int Immunopharmacol 2001;1:469.
58. Shimmura H, Tanabe K, Ishida H, et al. Lack of correlation between results of ABO-incompatible living kidney transplantation and anti-ABO blood type antibody titers under our current immunosuppression. Transplantation 2005;80:985.
59. Slifka MK, Antia R, Whitmire JK, et al. Humoral immunity due to long-lived plasma cells. Immunity 1998;8:363.
60. Stegall MD, Dean PG, Gloor JM. ABO-incompatible kidney transplantation. Transplantation 2004;78:635.
61. Stegall MD, Dean PG, McBride MA, et al. Organ Procurement and Transplantation Network/United Network for Organ Sharing Kidney/Pancreas Transplantation Committee: Survival of mandatorily shared cadaveric kidneys and their paybacks in the zero mismatch era. Transplantation 2002;74:670.
62. Stegall MD, Gloor JM, Winters J, et al. A comparison of plasmapheresis vs high-dose IVIG desensitization in renal allograft recipients with high levels of donor specific alloantibody. Am J Transplant 2006;6:346.
63. Stegall MD, Dean PG, Gloor JM. Mechanisms of alloantibody production in sensitized renal allograft recipients. Am J Transplant 2009;9:998.
64. Stegall MD, Diwan T, Raghavaih S, et al. Terminal complement inhibition decreases antibody mediated rejection in sensitized renal transplant recipients. Am J Transplant 2011;11:2405.
65. Tanabe K, Takahashi K, Sonda K, et al. Long-term results of ABO-incompatible living kidney transplantation. Transplantation 1998;65:224.
66. Trivedi HL, Terasaki PI, Feroz A, et al. Abrogation of anti-HLA antibodies via proteasome inhibition. Transplantation 2009;87:1555.
67. Valenzuela NM, Reed EF. The link between major histocompatibility complex antibodies and cell proliferation. Transplant Rev 2011;25:154.

68. Vo AA, Lukovsky M, Toyoda M, et al. Rituximab and intravenous immune globulin for desensitization during renal transplantation. N Engl J Med 2008;359:242.
69. Walsh RC, Everly JJ, Brailey P, et al. Proteasome inhibitor-based primary therapy for antibody-mediated renal allograft rejection. Transplantation 2010;89:277.
70. West LJ. ABO-incompatible hearts for infant transplantation. Curr Opin Organ Transplant 2011;16:548.
71. Worthington JE, Martin S, Al-Husseini DM, et al. Post-transplant production of donor HLA-specific antibodies as a predictor of renal transplant outcome. Transplantation 2003;75:1034.
72. United Network for Organ Sharing. Available online at: www.unos.org [accessed 18.05.12].
73. Wavamunno MD, O'Connell PJ, Vitalone M, et al. Transplant glomerulopathy: ultrastructural abnormalities occur early in longitudinal analyses of protocol biopsies. Am J Transplant 2007;7:2757.

CHAPTER 25

KIDNEY PAIRED DONATION PROGRAMS FOR LIVING DONORS

Sommer E. Gentry • Dorry L. Segev

CHAPTER OUTLINE

There are far more eligible transplant candidates worldwide than there are organs available. One emerging modality, kidney paired donation (KPD), otherwise referred to as kidney exchange or paired exchange, increases living kidney donation by enabling would-be donors who are not compatible with their intended recipients to participate in a mutually beneficial exchange of organs. This requires a coordinated effort to collect data about incompatible pairs and about other types of participants such as non-directed (altruistic) donors and compatible pairs, and to select appropriate matches[28] by a manual or algorithmic process.

In this chapter, we examine the common features and the idiosyncrasies of several successful KPD efforts around the world,[6] including Korea, the Netherlands, Canada, the United Kingdom, and the United States. In doing so, the main elements of modern KPD are reviewed. Furthermore, reviewing these differences may be reassuring for groups working to implement this exciting new modality; for each potential snag that might have delayed or limited one program's efforts, there are counterexamples in which that aspect of KPD was not an impediment.

BEGINNINGS OF KIDNEY PAIRED DONATION

In a traditional two-way or three-way KPD (Figure 25-1), two or more incompatible pairs exchange kidneys so that two or more compatible matches result. This requires reciprocal matches, so that every individual who donates a kidney is assured that the intended recipient will be matched with another donor and will undergo transplantation. This also requires that all donors who are part of the arrangement donate simultaneously, to avoid a situation where an individual donates but the intended recipient does not receive a transplant because another donor decides against donation.

THE ROLE OF HLA MATCHING

KPD may have the longest history in Korea, which established a program in 1991. By 2003, paired donations comprised more than 10% of living kidney donations at one Korean center.[23] Korea's approach to living donor kidney transplantation emphasizes close human leukocyte antigen (HLA) matching between donors and recipients. Living donors are only accepted as compatible if they share more than one DR antigen or two of four A/B antigens with their recipients. Of pairs deemed incompatible, 30% had HLA mismatching beyond these criteria, 65% were blood type-incompatible, and only 5% had a positive crossmatch test.[12] In the Netherlands, by comparison, about half of incompatible pairs have positive crossmatch and half are blood type-incompatible.[26] The Korean restriction requiring close HLA matches for living donation may have directed more candidate/donor pairs into the KPD group, but may have ruled out more potential exchanges. In most other programs, only pairs with donor-specific anti-HLA (or anti-ABO) antibody are considered incompatible, rather than pairs simply with HLA mismatch. Also, degree of HLA matching is not usually considered important in KPD matching priorities, except for favoring the rare zero-HLA-mismatch opportunities.

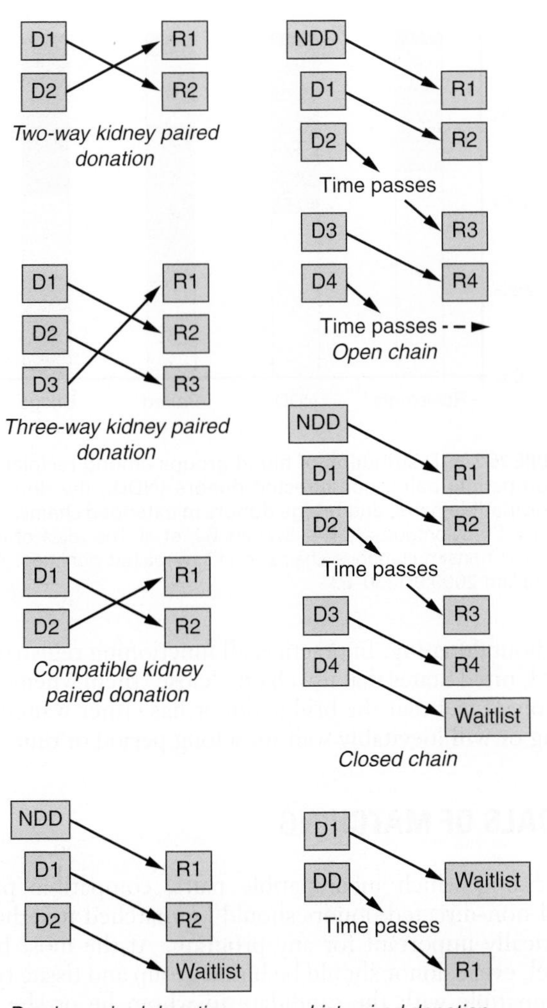

FIGURE 25-1 ■ Terminology for various forms of paired donation. Pictured are non-directed or altruistic donors (NDD), recipients (R) who are paired with their incompatible donors (D), and waitlist recipients, in a variety of paired donation arrangements. (Reprinted with permission from Gentry SE, Montgomery RA, Segev DL. Kidney paired donation: fundamentals, limitations, and expansion. Am J Kidney Dis 2011;57:144–51.)

LEGAL RESTRICTIONS

Legal restrictions on living organ donation have played a significant role in the evolution of KPD in many countries. In 2005, in the United States, the term "kidney paired donation" rather than "kidney exchange" was adopted to emphasize that these arrangements should not be seen as violating the National Organ Transplantation Act's (NOTA's) prohibition on selling living donor organs (phrased as "exchanging for valuable consideration"). In December 2007, the United States enacted a new law – HR 710, the Charlie W. Norwood Living Donation Act – clarifying that KPD was not illegal under NOTA. This law made possible the efforts of the United Network for Organ Sharing in building a national KPD registry funded and overseen by the US government. In the United Kingdom, only relatives and those with strong emotional ties to the candidate were permitted to be living organ donors, until legislation allowing kidney exchange was enacted in 2006.[14] In India, every paired exchange performed must be individually approved by the Authorization Committee of the particular state,[22] effectively discouraging intrastate arrangements.

ANONYMITY

The conventional practice in the United States is to maintain strict anonymity among the KPD participants before surgery, with meetings possible after surgery if desired by all parties.[21] In the Netherlands, patients in a pilot study expressed a strong preference for anonymity, and so that country's exchange program maintains anonymity throughout the process.[17] In Germany, anonymous KPD is prohibited, so exchanges can only proceed after incompatible pairs meet and socialize.[11] In Romania, a single-center program transplanted 56 pairs between 2001 and 2005,[18] and this group felt that maintaining anonymity among pairs involved in KPD was unnecessary and would be too logistically difficult, so they encouraged open interaction before and after the transplants.

DONOR TRAVEL AND ORGAN TRANSPORT

In the Netherlands, a compact country which is densely populated, donors travel to the transplant center where their paired recipients are being transplanted and cared for.[6] In the United States, which has a much larger geographic footprint, donor organs are now routinely transported to the recipient center.[29] US physicians became more comfortable with transporting living donor kidneys for this purpose after a large-scale registry study showed that up to 8 hours of cold ischemia time did not have negative repercussions for a live donor kidney[30] and a case report demonstrated the feasibility of this practice.[20] In Canada, the standard is for donors to travel.[7]

FINANCIAL ISSUES

In the United States, financial arrangements are frequently a complicating factor in KPD. There is no obvious party responsible for paying the expenses incurred in donor evaluations for incompatible donors, some of whom never donate, nor for the tissue typing and administrative costs of maintaining a paired donation registry to locate suitable matches. Some have called for extending the concept of the standard acquisition charge, used in the United States to recoup expenses related to acquiring deceased donor organs, to KPD[25]; this seems to be an approach favored by the insurance payer community as well.[13]

EXPANSIONS BEYOND INCOMPATIBLE PAIRS

In every KPD program, many incompatible pairs will fail to find a match opportunity. Because blood group O donors are most likely to be compatible with their recipients, there will be a blood group imbalance, with too few

O donors for too many O recipients, in any population of incompatible pairs.[9] Some populations are also enriched for highly sensitized candidates, who are difficult to match in an exchange that seeks a compatible pairing. This imbalance limits exchange opportunities and leads to innovations (Figure 25-1) such as extending match arrangements to three or more pairs,[27] desensitization as part of the exchange program,[19] and the inclusion of compatible pairs[10] and non-directed donors,[24] all of which can enhance the proportion of incompatible pairs successfully transplanted. One less common variant shown in Figure 25-1 was implemented in the New England region of the United States: in a list paired donation (also known as list exchange), a candidate whose incompatible living donor donates to a stranger on the deceased donor waitlist is given preferential placement on the waitlist for a future, compatible deceased donor.

THE ROLE OF NON-DIRECTED DONORS

In the arrangements referred to as chains or as domino paired donations, a non-directed or altruistic donor starts a sequence of paired donations by donating to a paired recipient whose donor then becomes available for the next recipient (Figure 25-1). At the end of the sequence, one incompatible pair's donor is left unmatched. This donor might donate immediately to a candidate on the deceased donor waiting list, creating a closed chain (domino paired donation). Alternatively, the last donor might wait (for a few months or longer) as a bridge donor, subsequently donating to another incompatible pair to begin another sequence of donations (open chain, or non-simultaneous extended altruistic donor chain).

Non-directed donors are particularly valuable in paired donation because non-directed donors are not paired with one particular candidate who must receive a kidney, easing the reciprocal compatibility requirement. Furthermore, a renege will not directly harm a pair (because no individual donates without his or her paired recipient receiving a transplant), even though a renege will cause the chain to break and, therefore, the final patient on the deceased donor waiting list (the one who would have closed the chain) does not receive a transplant. Finally, blood group O donors are more prevalent among non-directed donors than paired donors (Figure 25-2).

In programs where non-directed donors have been incorporated into KPD, non-directed donor chains often comprise a majority of the transplants arranged. In the Netherlands, non-directed donors are only matched to incompatible pairs after the pairs have tried to find a traditional kidney exchange with other pairs. Also, non-directed donors in the Netherlands are allocated on a center basis rather than by the national program.[26]

There has been some debate about whether open chains or closed chains will facilitate more transplants. Open chains hold a promise of indefinite continuation that is intuitively appealing, but, in practice, bridge donors have a blood group distribution (Figure 25-2) that makes them hard to match.[8] Long delays between the recipient's transplant and the donor's operation might cause an unknown number of bridge donors to withdraw without donating. In practice, all functioning registries in the United States that use chains "close" them when those involved feel that the bridge donor has either waited too long or will inevitably wait for a long period of time.

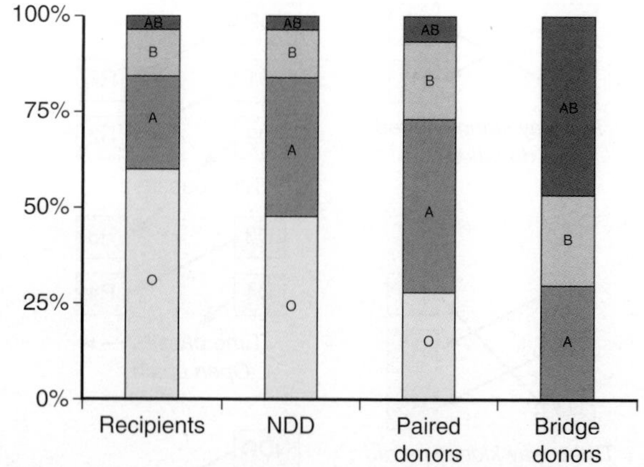

FIGURE 25-2 ■ **Distribution of blood groups among recipients of incompatible pairs, non-directed donors (NDD), the donors of incompatible pairs, and bridge donors in extended chains.** (From Gentry SE, Montgomery RA, Swihart BJ, et al. The roles of dominos and nonsimultaneous chains in kidney paired donation. Am J Transplant 2009;9:1330–6.)

GOALS OF MATCHING

Deciding which incompatible pairs, compatible pairs, and non-directed donors should be matched together is critically important for any program. At the most basic level, every donor should be blood group and tissue type-compatible with the candidate to whom he or she will donate. There are exceptions to this rule: some transplant centers have experience with desensitization protocols for ABO-incompatible or HLA-incompatible transplants, or both. These centers may wish to combine desensitization with kidney exchange in order to obtain transplants for their hardest-to-match patients.[19]

MATCHING ALGORITHMS

Beyond simply understanding which donors could successfully donate to which candidates in a KPD registry, matching participants together so that the largest number of people can achieve the greatest benefit requires sophisticated mathematics and specialized optimization algorithms.[28] This holds true for any of the variations or expansions of KPD described herein. We refer to a "match" as a single two-way, three-way, or chain of transplants, as in Figure 25-1. For a fixed pool of participants in a paired donation registry, "matching" means selecting a non-overlapping set of matches to proceed to transplant.

Matching decisions in a KPD registry are necessarily interconnected, because choosing one match means that other potentially useful matches involving any of those same participants will not be possible. Some seemingly effective matching heuristics neglect the interconnectedness of these decisions. For instance, it is not optimal to rank all possible matches and then choose the highest-ranked match first, the next highest-ranked available match second, and so on. This match rank heuristic, which has been used in some operational registries,[15] might transplant fewer people than would be possible with better matching algorithms.

There are only two correct approaches to find the best set of matches among a specific list of participants: exhaustive search or integer programming (optimization). In exhaustive search, a computer generates every possible set of matches and then compares them to select the best set of matches, as in the Korean registry.[16] Exhaustive search is only possible for small registries, because the number of different sets of matches possible grows incredibly quickly. Integer programming models, including some algorithms specialized for the paired donation problem,[1] use mathematical techniques to locate and verify the best set of matches without having to describe all possible sets of matches explicitly.

REGISTRY SIZE

Although the matching algorithm is important, the most significant factor in increasing the fraction of incompatible pairs matched is increasing the number of participants in a registry. All candidates benefit from increasing pool size, but the benefit is particularly pronounced for sensitized candidates. For instance, a nationwide registry in the United States would create a sixfold increase in kidney exchange opportunities for sensitized candidates.[28]

The advantage of large over small programs has implications for the organization of registries around the world. Canada, the United Kingdom, and the Netherlands, each with a population in the tens of millions, have established national KPD registries.[6] In South Korea, KPD is generally conducted within large single-center programs.[6] One single-center program in the United States, by relying on compatible pairs, has grown its program to be more than one-third of its live donor kidney volume.[3] In the United States, there are many models competing: there are single-center programs, several multicenter consortia, and an effort by the United Network for Organ Sharing to establish a national registry integrated with the national deceased donor allocation system.[2] The various registries in the United States serve different but overlapping populations, because many incompatible pairs are registered for more than one of these. Because fewer incompatible pairs and many fewer sensitized candidates will find matches if participants are divided into smaller pools than if the participants were in one larger pool, the proliferation of multiple registries is of concern, as discussed in a recent national consensus conference.[5]

BEYOND NATIONAL LINES

In North America, at least one KPD has occurred between the United States and Canada.[29] In June 2012, a couple in Greece became part of a KPD chain in the United States, after Greek law was amended to allow unrelated organ donors and permit KPD for the first time. There have been calls for establishing international KPD systems to facilitate the flow of organs around the world,[4] although the logistics of doing so will no doubt remain challenging.

FUTURE OF KIDNEY PAIRED DONATION

KPD is proving to be a viable strategy to circumvent living donor incompatibility. In 2001 there were only 12 US transplants from paired donation, but there were 574 a decade later in 2011 (representing 10% of living donor kidney transplants that year), making KPD by far the most rapidly growing category of living donor transplants. Media attention to this modality, and greater physician familiarity with its variations, will be positive forces in expanding access to paired donation. We believe innovations in this field will allow more candidates with incompatible donors to benefit from kidney transplantation.

REFERENCES

1. Abraham DJ, Blum A, Sandholm T. Clearing algorithms for barter exchange markets: enabling nationwide kidney exchanges. In: Proceedings of the 8th ACM conference on Electronic commerce. San Diego, California, USA: ACM; 2007. p. 295–304.
2. Akkina SK, Muster H, Steffens E, et al. Donor exchange programs in kidney transplantation: rationale and operational details from the north central donor exchange cooperative. Am J Kidney Dis 2011;57:152–8.
3. Bingaman AW, Wright Jr FH, Kapturczak M, et al. Single-center kidney paired donation: the Methodist San Antonio experience. Am J Transplant 2012;12:2125–32.
4. Connolly JS, Terasaki PI, Veale JL. Kidney paired donation – the next step. N Engl J Med 2011;365:868–9.
5. Feng S, Melcher ML, Blosser C, et al. Dynamic challenges inhibiting optimal adoption of kidney paired donation: findings of a consensus conference. Am J Transplant 2013; (in press).
6. Ferrari P, de Klerk M. Paired kidney donations to expand the living donor pool. J Nephrol 2009;22:699–707.
7. Fortin MC, Williams-Jones B. Who should travel in kidney exchange programs: the donor, or the organ? Open Med 2011;e23–5.
8. Gentry SE, Montgomery RA, Swihart BJ, et al. The roles of dominos and nonsimultaneous chains in kidney paired donation. Am J Transplant 2009;9:1330–6.
9. Gentry SE, Segev DL, Montgomery RA. A comparison of populations served by kidney paired donation and list paired donation. Am J Transplant 2005;5:1914–21.
10. Gentry SE, Segev DL, Simmerling M, et al. Expanding kidney paired donation through participation by compatible pairs. Am J Transplant 2007;7:2361–70.
11. Giessing M, Deger S, Roigas J, et al. Cross-over kidney transplantation with simultaneous laparoscopic living donor nephrectomy: initial experience. Eur Urol 2008;53:1074–8.
12. Huh KH, Kim MS, Ju MK, et al. Exchange living-donor kidney transplantation: merits and limitations. Transplantation 2008;86:430–5.
13. Irwin FD, Bonagura AF, Crawford SW, et al. Kidney paired donation: a payer perspective. Am J Transplant 2012;12:1388–91.
14. Johnson RJ, Allen JE, Fuggle SV, et al. Early experience of paired living kidney donation in the United Kingdom. Transplantation 2008;86:1672–7.
15. Keizer KM, de Klerk M, Haase-Kromwijk BJ, et al. The Dutch algorithm for allocation in living donor kidney exchange. Transplant Proc 2005;37:589–91.
16. Kim BS, Kim YS, Kim SI, et al. Outcome of multipair donor kidney exchange by a web-based algorithm. J Am Soc Nephrol 2007;18:1000–6.
17. Kranenburg LW, Visak T, Weimar W, et al. Starting a crossover kidney transplantation program in the Netherlands: ethical and psychological considerations. Transplantation 2004;78:194–7.
18. Lucan M. Five years of single-center experience with paired kidney exchange transplantation. Transplant Proc 2007;39:1371–5.

19. Montgomery RA. Living donor exchange programs: theory and practice. Br Med Bull 2011;98:21–30.
20. Montgomery RA, Katznelson S, Bry WI, et al. Successful three-way kidney paired donation with cross-country live donor allograft transport. Am J Transplant 2008;8:2163–8.
21. Montgomery RA, Zachary AA, Ratner LE, et al. Clinical results from transplanting incompatible live kidney donor/recipient pairs using kidney paired donation. JAMA 2005;294:1655–63.
22. Pahwa M, Saifee Y, Tyagi V, et al. Paired exchange kidney donation in India: a five-year single-center experience. Int Urol Nephrol 2012;44:1101–5.
23. Park K, Lee JH, Huh KH, et al. Exchange living-donor kidney transplantation: diminution of donor organ shortage. Transplant Proc 2004;36:2949–51.
24. Rees MA, Kopke JE, Pelletier RP, et al. A nonsimultaneous, extended, altruistic-donor chain. N Engl J Med 2009;360:1096–101.
25. Rees MA, Schnitzler MA, Zavala EY, et al. Call to develop a standard acquisition charge model for kidney paired donation. Am J Transplant 2012;12:1392–7.
26. Roodnat JI, Zuidema W, van de Wetering J, et al. Altruistic donor triggered domino-paired kidney donation for unsuccessful couples from the kidney-exchange program. Am J Transplant 2010;10:821–7.
27. Saidman SL, Roth AE, Sonmez T, et al. Increasing the opportunity of live kidney donation by matching for two and three way exchanges. Transplantation 2006;81:773–82.
28. Segev DL, Gentry SE, Warren DS, et al. Kidney paired donation and optimizing the use of live donor organs. JAMA 2005;293:1883–90.
29. Segev DL, Veale JL, Berger JC, et al. Transporting live donor kidneys for kidney paired donation: initial national results. Am J Transplant 2011;11:356–60.
30. Simpkins CE, Montgomery RA, Hawxby AM, et al. Cold ischemia time and allograft outcomes in live donor renal transplantation: is live donor organ transport feasible? Am J Transplant 2007;7:99–107.

CHAPTER 26

PATHOLOGY OF KIDNEY TRANSPLANTATION

Alton B. Farris, III • Lynn D. Cornell • Robert B. Colvin

CHAPTER OUTLINE

RENAL ALLOGRAFT BIOPSY

Renal biopsy remains the "gold standard" for the diagnosis of episodes of graft dysfunction that occur commonly in patients after transplantation.[410] Studies have indicated that the results of a renal allograft biopsy change the clinical diagnosis in 30–42% and therapy in 38–83% of patients, even after the first year.[183,185,295,410] Most importantly, unnecessary immunosuppression was avoided in 19% of patients.[295] The biopsy is also a gold mine of information on pathogenetic mechanisms, a generator of hypotheses that can be tested in experimental animal studies and in clinical trials. Finally, the biopsy serves, in turn, to validate the hypothesis tested in such trials. Renal biopsy interpretation currently relies primarily on histopathology complemented by immunological molecular probes, and perhaps in the future, with quantitative gene expression.

This chapter describes the relevant light, immunofluorescence, and electron microscopy (EM) findings of the most common lesions affecting the renal allograft and their differential diagnosis, citing references largely limited to human pathological studies after 1990. The discussion is broadly divided into allograft rejection and non-rejection pathology, with an emphasis on differential diagnosis of acute and chronic allograft dysfunction. Grading systems of acute and chronic rejection are discussed further in those sections.

Optimal Tissue

At least seven non-sclerotic glomeruli and two arteries (bigger than arterioles) are recommended for adequate evaluation.[59,366] Using these criteria, the sensitivity of a single core is approximately 90%, and the predicted sensitivity of two cores is about 99%.[59] However, adequacy depends entirely on the lesions seen in the biopsy: one artery with endarteritis is sufficient for the diagnosis of acute cellular rejection (ACR), even if no glomerulus is present; similarly, immunofluorescence or EM of one glomerulus is adequate to diagnose membranous glomerulonephritis (MGN). In contrast, a large portion of cortex with a minimal infiltrate does not exclude rejection. Subcapsular cortex often shows inflammation and fibrosis and is not representative. Diagnosis of certain diseases is even possible with only medulla (acute humoral rejection (AHR), polyomavirus tubulointerstitial nephritis (PTN)). However, a normal medulla does not rule out rejection.[403] Frozen sections for light microscopy are of limited value; the diagnostic accuracy of frozen sections was 89% when compared with paraffin sections.[50] Rapid processing in formalin/paraffin processing is preferred.

Microscopy

The biopsy is examined for glomerular, tubular, vascular, and interstitial pathology, including: (1) transplant glomerulitis, glomerulopathy, and de novo or recurrent glomerulonephritis; (2) tubular injury, isometric vacuolization, tubulitis, atrophy, or intranuclear viral inclusions; (3) endarteritis, fibrinoid necrosis, thrombi, myocyte necrosis, nodular medial hyalinosis, or chronic allograft arteriopathy; (4) interstitial infiltrates of activated mononuclear cells, edema, or neutrophils, fibrosis, and scarring. Arteries and arterioles are particularly scrutinized, as well as peritubular capillaries (PTCs), since the diagnostic lesions often lie in the vessels.

Our standard immunofluorescence panel detects IgG, IgA, IgM, C3, C4d, albumin, and fibrin in cryostat sections. C4d, a complement fragment, is used to identify antibody-mediated rejection (AMR); the other stains are primarily for recurrent or de novo glomerulonephritis.[53] Immunohistochemistry in paraffin sections may be used for C4d. EM is valuable when de novo or recurrent glomerular disease is suspected and to evaluate PTC basement membranes.[164]

Classification of Pathologic Diagnoses in the Renal Allograft

The ideal diagnostic classification of renal allograft pathology should be based on pathogenesis, have therapeutic relevance, and be reproducible. The current classification, based on Banff and other systems (Table 26-1), meets these criteria.[61,237]

TABLE 26-1 Pathological Classification of Renal Allograft Disease

I. Immunological rejection
  A. Hyperacute rejection
  B. Acute rejection
    1. Acute T-cell-mediated rejection (acute cellular rejection, C4d⁻)
      a. Tubulointerstitial (Banff type I)
      b. Endarteritis (Banff type II)
      c. Arterial fibrinoid necrosis/transmural inflammation (Banff type III)
      d. Glomerular (transplant glomerulitis; no Banff type)
    2. Acute antibody-mediated rejection (acute humoral rejection, C4d⁺)
      a. Tubular injury
      b. Capillaritis/thrombotic microangiopathy
      c. Arterial fibrinoid necrosis
  C. Chronic rejection
    1. Chronic T-cell-mediated rejection (with T-cell activity)
    2. Chronic antibody-mediated rejection (with antibody activity, C4d⁺)
II. Alloantibody/autoantibody-mediated diseases of allografts
  A. Anti-GBM disease in Alport's syndrome
  B. Nephrotic syndrome in nephrin-deficient recipients
  C. Anti-TBM disease in TBM antigen-deficient recipients
  D. De novo membranous glomerulonephritis
  E. Anti-angiotensin II receptor autoantibody syndrome
III. Non-rejection injury
  A. Acute ischemic injury (acute tubular necrosis)
  B. Drug toxicity
    1. Calcineurin inhibitor (cyclosporine, tacrolimus)
    2. mTOR inhibitors (sirolimus, everolimus, rapamycin)
  C. Acute tubulointerstitial nephritis (drug allergy)
  D. Infection (viral, bacterial, fungal)
  E. Major artery/vein thrombosis
  F. Mechanical
    1. Obstruction
    2. Urine leak
  G. Renal artery stenosis
  H. Arteriosclerosis
  I. De novo glomerular disease
  J. Posttransplant lymphoproliferative disease
  K. Chronic allograft nephropathy, not otherwise classified (interstitial fibrosis and tubular atrophy)
IV. Recurrent primary disease
  A. Immunological (e.g., IgA nephropathy, lupus nephritis, anti-GBM disease)
  B. Metabolic (e.g., amyloidosis, diabetes, oxalosis)
  C. Unknown (e.g., dense deposit disease, focal segmental glomerulosclerosis)

mTOR, mammalian target of rapamycin; GBM, glomerular basement membrane; TBM, tubular basement membrane.
From Colvin RB, Nickeleit V. Renal transplant pathology. In: Jennette JC, Olson JL, Schwartz MM, et al., editors. Heptinstall's pathology of the kidney. Philadelphia: Lippincott-Raven, 2006. p. 1347.

DONOR KIDNEY BIOPSY

Biopsy of the deceased donor kidney is sometimes used to determine the suitability of the kidney for transplantation. Objective pathologic criteria based on outcome that could be applied to the renal biopsy as a screening test have not been established, as donor biopsies are not routinely performed and controlled trials have not been done. One of the major problems in assessing the donor kidney is that this is usually done with cryostat sections, often by non-renal pathologists in the middle of the night. Even though many other studies try to correlate fibrosis or vascular disease, reproducibility of scoring these lesions, even on permanent sections by expert renal pathologists in broad daylight, is notoriously poor.[105] Arbitrary criteria risk that kidneys will be discarded needlessly. In two large studies, the outcome at 1–5 years was not measurably correlated with pathological lesions.[44,284] However, as rejection and patient death from complications diminish, the influence of the quality of the graft is likely to increase.

Glomerulosclerosis can be readily assessed in frozen section, by the most casual observers, and has been a popular parameter for judging the quality of the donor kidney. Glomerulosclerosis >20% correlates with poor graft outcome in some, but not all, studies.[89,109,310] The odds ratio remained significant after adjustment for donor age, rejection episodes, or panel-reactive antibody.[310] However, other large studies have failed to detect a major effect of glomerulosclerosis >20%, if adjusted for the age of the donor[301] or renal function.[84] At least 25 glomeruli are needed to correlate with outcome.[402] A wedge biopsy may not be representative, since it includes mostly outer cortex, the zone where glomerulosclerosis and fibrosis due to vascular disease are most severe; therefore a needle biopsy is recommended.

Other lesions may cause the transplant surgeon or pathologist to argue against use of the graft. Arterial intimal fibrosis increases the risk of delayed graft function (DGF)[172] and has a slight effect on 2-year graft survival (6% decrease).[383] Thrombotic microangiopathy (TMA), with widespread but less than 50% glomerular thrombi, increases the likelihood of DGF and primary non-function,[301] but is compatible with unaltered 2-year graft survival.[225] Reversal of diabetic glomerulosclerosis[1] and IgA nephropathy have been reported,[169] as well as MGN,[261] lupus nephritis,[204] membranoproliferative glomerulonephritis (MPGN),[39] and endothelialosis due to pre-eclampsia (personal observation). Mathematically combined scores of pathological lesions have been proposed as a guide,[314] including, most recently, the Maryland Aggregate Pathology Index.[254] In addition to glomerulosclerosis, the score includes interstitial fibrosis, glomerular size, periglomerular fibrosis, arterial wall-to-lumen ratio, and arteriolar hyalinosis. Further, whether this will provide an efficient separation of beneficial organs will depend on prospective validation studies.

At this time histological evaluation is recommended in donors with any evidence of renal dysfunction, a family history of renal disease, or those whose age is >60 years. Histological selection of kidneys from donors over 60 years can result in a graft survival rate similar to that of grafts from younger patients.[314]

HYPERACUTE REJECTION

Hyperacute rejection refers to immediate rejection (typically within 10 minutes to an hour) of the kidney upon perfusion with recipient blood, where the recipient is presensitized to alloantigens on the surface of the graft endothelium. During surgery, the graft kidney becomes soft, flabby and livid, mottled, purple or cyanotic in color; urine output ceases. The kidney subsequently swells and widespread hemorrhagic cortical necrosis and medullary congestion appear. The large vessels are sometimes thrombosed.

Early lesions show marked accumulation of platelets in glomerular capillary lumens that appear as amorphous pale pink, finely granular masses in hematoxylin and eosin-stained slides (negative on periodic acid–Schiff (PAS) stains). Neutrophil and platelet margination then occurs over the next hour or so along damaged endothelium of small arteries, arterioles, glomeruli, and PTCs and the capillaries fill with sludged (compacted) red cells and fibrin.[409] The larger arteries are usually spared. The neutrophils do not infiltrate initially but form "chain-like" figures in the PTCs without obvious thrombi.[409] The endothelium is stripped off the underlying basal lamina, and the interstitium becomes edematous and hemorrhagic. Intravascular coagulation occurs and cortical necrosis ensues over 12–24 hours. The medulla is relatively spared, but is ultimately affected as the whole kidney becomes necrotic.[184] Widespread microthrombi are usually found in the arterioles and glomeruli and can be detected even in totally necrotic samples. The small arteries may show fibrinoid necrosis. Mononuclear infiltrates are typically sparse. A T-cell component may be present, as judged by $CD3^+$ cells in the adventitia of small arteries.[108] By EM, neutrophils attach to injured glomerular endothelial cells.[409] The endothelium is swollen, separated from the glomerular basement membrane (GBM) by a lucent space. Capillary loops and PTCs are often bare of endothelium. Platelet, fibrin thrombi, and trapped erythrocytes occlude capillaries.[61]

The site of antibody and complement deposition is determined by the site of the target endothelial alloantigens. Hyperacute rejection due to pre-existing anti-human leukocyte antigen (HLA) class I antibodies may show C3, C4d, and fibrin throughout the microvasculature.[138] ABO antibodies (primarily IgM) also deposit in all vascular endothelium. Cases with anticlass II antibodies may have IgG/IgM primarily in glomerular and PTCs, where class II is normally conspicuous.[3] In the antiendothelial monocyte antigen cases, IgG is primarily in PTCs, rather than glomeruli or arteries.[297] Often antibodies cannot be detected in the vessels,[352] even though they can be eluted from the kidney.[211,241] In these cases C4d should be positive in PTCs[53] and more useful than immunoglobulin stains. Occasional cases, particularly intraoperative biopsies, may be negative for C4d, perhaps related to focally decreased perfusion or insufficient time to generate substantial C4d amounts.

The differential diagnosis of hyperacute rejection includes ischemia and major vascular thrombosis. The major diagnostic feature of hyperacute rejection is C4d deposition in PTCs and the prominence of neutrophils in capillaries. While the finding of antibody and C4d deposition in PTCs is diagnostic when present, negative immunofluorescence stains do not exclude hyperacute rejection. Exogenous antibody (rabbit or horse antilymphocyte serum) can cause severe endothelial injury, sometimes with C4d deposition mimicking hyperacute rejection.[54] Hyperacute rejection typically has more hemorrhage, necrosis, and neutrophil accumulation in glomeruli and PTCs than acute tubular necrosis (ATN), although glomerular neutrophils alone are associated with ischemia.[107] Major arterial thrombosis has predominant necrosis with little hemorrhage or microthrombi and PTC neutrophils are not that prominent. Renal vein thrombosis shows marked congestion and relatively little neutrophil response.

ACUTE RENAL ALLOGRAFT REJECTION

Acute rejection typically develops in the first 2–6 weeks after transplantation, but can arise in a normally functioning kidney from 3 days to 10 years or more, or in a graft affected by other conditions, such as ATN, calcineurin inhibitor toxicity (CNIT), or chronic rejection. Acute rejection may be caused by T cell or antibody injuring the graft, acting separately or together (Table 26-1). Only since 1999 has the distinction between the two pathogenetic pathways been clearly made in the literature and the criteria continue to be refined. Since these respond to different immunosuppressive therapies, the distinction is of considerable clinical importance.

Acute T-Cell-Mediated Rejection

Acute T-cell-mediated rejection, also known as ACR, is caused by T cells reacting to donor histocompatibility antigens expressed in the tubules, interstitium, vessels, and glomeruli, separately or in combination (Table 26-2). The donor ureter is also affected, but rarely sampled.[106]

TABLE 26-2 Banff/Types of Acute T-Cell-Mediated Rejection*

Borderline/Suspicious	Any tubulitis (1 cell/tubule or more (t1, t2, or t3))+infiltrate 0–25% (i0 or i1) or mild tubulitis (1–4 cells/tubule) (t1) and infiltrate >25% (i2 or i3)
Type I	Tubulitis >4 cells/tubule + infiltrate >25%
A	With 5–10 cells/tubule (t2)
B	With >10 cells/tubule (t3)
Type II	Mononuclear cells under arterial endothelium
A	<25% luminal area (v1)
B	≥25% luminal area (v2)
Type III	Transmural arterial inflammation, *or* fibrinoid arterial necrosis with accompanying lymphocytic inflammation (v3)†

*All cases should be analyzed for C4d deposition. If C4d is present, an additional diagnosis of concurrent antibody-mediated rejection is made.

†Cases with these features are often due to alloantibody. To use as a category of T-cell-mediated rejection requires C4d in peritubular capillaries to be negative.

From Colvin RB, Nickeleit V. Renal transplant pathology. In: Jennette JC, Olson JL, Schwartz MM, et al., editors. Heptinstall's pathology of the kidney. Philadelphia: Lippincott-Raven, 2006. p. 1347.

Tubulointerstitial Rejection (Type I)

The prominent microscopic feature of ACR is a pleiomorphic interstitial infiltrate of mononuclear cells, accompanied by interstitial edema and sometimes hemorrhage (Figure 26-1). The infiltrate is typically patchy, both in the cortex and medulla. The infiltrating cells are primarily T cells and macrophages. Activated T cells (lymphoblasts) with increased basophilic cytoplasm, nucleoli, and occasional mitotic figures indicate increased synthetic and proliferative activity.[182] Granulocytes are not uncommonly present but rarely prominent. When neutrophils are conspicuous, the possibility of AMR or pyelonephritis should be considered. Eosinophils are present in about 30% of biopsies with rejection and can be abundant, but are rarely more than 2–3% of the infiltrate.[8,274] Abundant eosinophils (10% of infiltrate) are associated with endarteritis (Banff type II).[233] Mast cells increase, as judged by tryptase content, and correlate with edema.[72] Acute rejection with abundant plasma cells has been described as early as the first month, associated with poor graft survival.[4,48,228] Infiltrating T cells express cytotoxic molecules, namely perforin,[175,294] FasL,[5,294] granzyme A and B,[191,236,294,324] TIA-1/GMP-17,[230,236] and tumor necrosis factor (TNF)-β (lymphotoxin).[281]

Mononuclear cells invade tubules and insinuate between tubular epithelial cells, a process termed "tubulitis" (Figure 26-1B), which is best appreciated in sections stained with PAS or a silver stain to delineate the tubular basement membrane (TBM). All cortical tubules (proximal and distal) as well as the medullary tubules and the collecting ducts may be affected. Tubular cell apoptosis occurs,[15,162,230,282] which correlates with the number of cytotoxic cells and macrophages in the infiltrate.[230,282] Tubular epithelial cells express HLA-DR, intercellular adhesion molecule (ICAM)-1, and vascular cell adhesion molecule (VCAM)-1 in increased amounts in ACR[21,29,35,93,101–103,269,289,401] and express the costimulatory molecules CD80 and CD86.[276] Tubules also synthesize TNF-α,[252] transforming growth factor-β_1, interleukin (IL)-15, osteopontin, and vascular endothelial growth factor.[7,290,411] Increased expression of S100A4 and smooth-muscle α-actin signals a differentiation toward mesenchymal cells, a process sometimes termed epithelial to mesenchymal transition.[190,319] This does not seem to be accompanied by migration of the cells out of the tubule.[91,237]

Not all events in the graft rejection are causing injury. Some tubular cell-derived molecules have the potential to inhibit acute rejection, such as protease inhibitor-9, the only known inhibitor of granzyme B[324] and IL-15, which inhibits expression of perforin.[411] T cells that downregulate the immune response are also present, as judged by their expressioin of the transcription factor Foxp3.[399] Foxp3 cells are also prominent in accepted grafts in humans[176] and mice[62,248] and may help distinguish harmful from beneficial infiltrates.[27,28,126]

CD8$^+$ and CD4$^+$ cells invade tubules.[392] Intratubular T cells with cytotoxic granules,[230] and CD4$^+$FOXP3$^+$ cells[398]

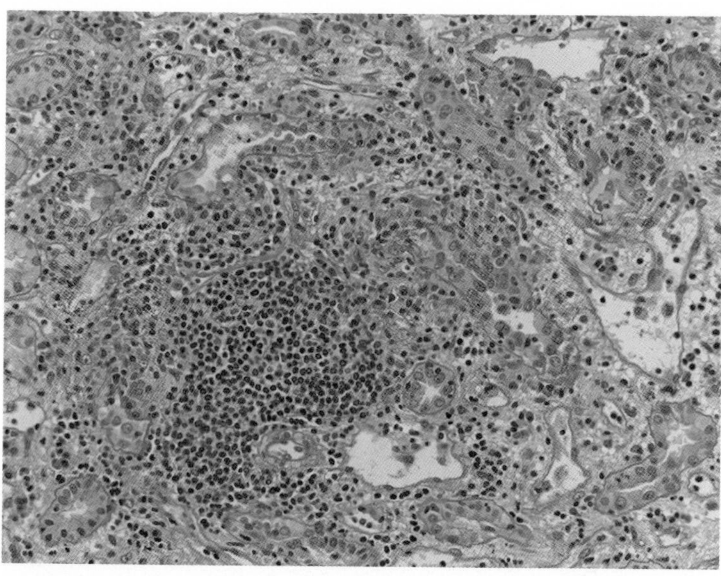

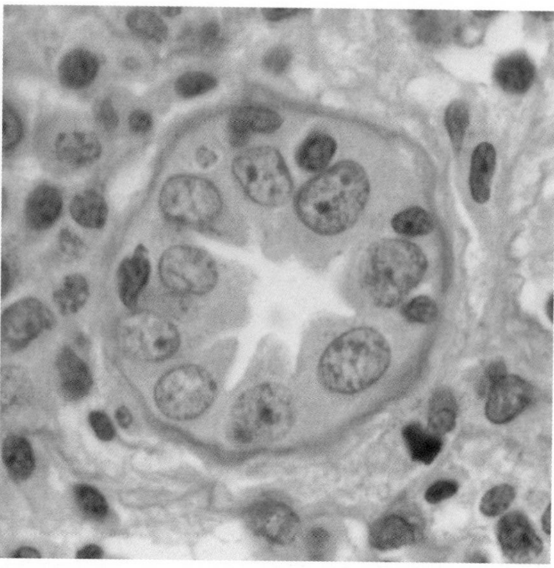

FIGURE 26-1 ■ Acute cellular rejection, type I. (A) Mononuclear cells, composed of activated lymphocytes and macrophages, infiltrate the edematous interstitium and invade tubules. Tubulitis affects proximal and other tubules, where mononuclear cells are interposed between the tubular epithelial cells (B). The invading mononuclear cells appear dark with scant cytoplasm, which distinguishes them from tubular epithelial cells. The tubular basement membranes are stained red by the periodic acid–Schiff stain, which is useful to delineate the boundary between the tubule and the interstitium.

accumulate selectively in the tubules, compared with the interstitial infiltrate. T cells proliferate once inside the tubule, as judged by the marker Ki67 (MIB-1), which contributes to their concentration within tubules, in addition to selective invasion.[230,320] Increased tubular HLA-DR,[29,102] TNF-α,[252] interferon-γ (IFN-γ) receptor,[281] IL-2 receptor,[187] and IL-8 are detectable by immunoperoxidase study in ACR. Several adhesion molecules are increased on tubular cells during rejection, including ICAM-1 (CD54) and VCAM-1, that correlate with the degree of T-cell infiltration.[35]

Signs of tubular cell injury can be detected by TdT-uridine-nick end label (TUNEL) apoptosis assay. Increased numbers of TUNEL$^+$ tubular cells are present in acute rejection, compared with normal kidneys.[162,230] The frequency was significantly lower in cyclosporine toxicity or ATN.[230] The degree of apoptosis correlates with the cytotoxic cells in the infiltrate, consistent with a pathogenetic relationship.[230] Prominent apoptosis of the infiltrating T cells has also been detected at a frequency comparable to that in the normal thymus (1.8% of cells).[230] Apoptosis probably occurs in infiltrating T cells as a result of activation-induced cell death and would thereby serve to limit the immune reaction.[230] Little, if any, immunoglobulin deposition is found by immunofluorescence in ACR, which is characterized primarily by extravascular fibrin accumulation in the interstitium and not uncommonly increased C3 along the TBM. The C3 is largely derived from tubular cells.[11] C3 may have a role in the pathogenesis of acute rejection, since C3-deficient mouse kidneys have prolonged survival.[305]

Gene expression studies of graft tissue have revealed that transcripts for proteins of cytotoxic T lymphocytes (CTLs), such as granzyme B, perforin, and Fas ligand[76,152,205,347,376,377,381] and the master transcription factor for CTLs, T-bet, are characteristic of ACR.[152] Graft CTL-associated transcripts (CATs) precede tubulitis in mouse kidney grafts.[86] Treatment of rejection is followed by a measurable decrease in CATs.[377] However, knockout of either granzyme or perforin does not prevent acute rejection, suggesting they are not essential.[85] Other genes associated with acute rejection are IFN-γ, TNF-β, TNF-α, RANTES, and macrophage inflammatory protein (MIP)-1α.[152]

Endarteritis (Type II Rejection)

Infiltration of mononuclear cells under arterial and arteriolar endothelium is the defining lesion of type II ACR (Figure 26-2). Many terms have been used for this process, including "endothelialitis," "endothelitis," "endovasculitis," "intimal arteritis," or "endarteritis." We prefer endarteritis, which emphasizes the type of vessel (artery versus vein) involved and the site of inflammation. Mononuclear cells, that are sometimes attached to the endothelial surface, are insufficient for the diagnosis of endarteritis; however, they probably represent the early phase of this lesion. Endarteritis in ACR must not be confused with fibrinoid necrosis of arteries. The latter is characteristic of acute AMR and can also be seen in thrombotic vasculopathy.

Endarteritis has been reported historically in 35–56% of renal biopsies with ACR[22,59,188,274,338] and it may be more common in patients on belatacept.[400] Many do not find the lesion as often; this may possibly be ascribed to inadequate sampling, overdiagnosis of rejection (increasing the denominator), patient population with respect to medication adherence (severity of rejection), or the timing of the biopsy with respect to antirejection therapy. Endarteritis lesions affect arteries of all sizes, including the arteriole, although the lesions affect larger vessels preferentially. For example, in a detailed analysis, 27% of the artery cross-sections were affected, versus 13% of the arterioles.[274] A sample of four arteries would have an estimated sensitivity of about 75% in the detection of

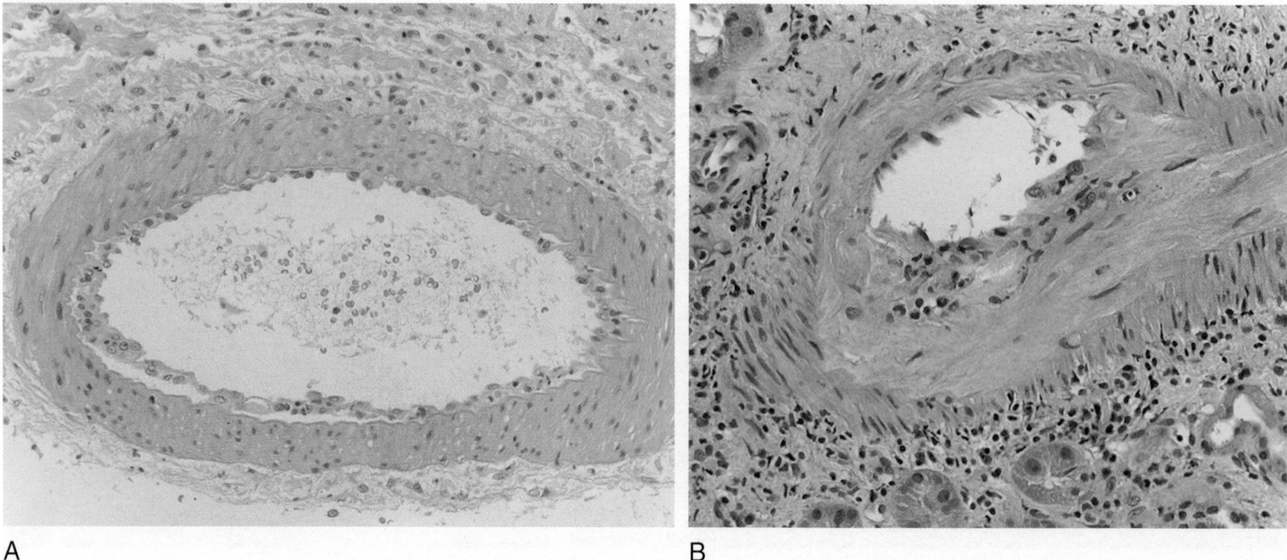

FIGURE 26-2 ■ Acute cellular rejection, type II. (A) Endarteritis in a medium-sized artery. The endothelium is lifted by undermining mononuclear cells, without involvement of the media. (B) Subendothelial infiltration in a small artery with underlying arteriosclerosis (donor disease). This acute process should be distinguished from chronic transplant arteriopathy.

type II rejection.[274] Thus a sample may not be considered adequate to rule out endarteritis unless several arteries are included. "Arteriolitis" has the same significance as endarteritis.[23] Endarteritis can occur in cases with little or no interstitial infiltrate or tubulitis, arguing that it has a distinct pathogenetic mechanism.[61] Recent studies have suggested that endarteritis may also be related to anti-donor antibodies,[197] and such lesions can be produced in mice by adoptive transfer of donor-specific antibodies.[149]

Endothelial cells are typically reactive with increased cytoplasmic volume and basophilia. The endothelium shows disruption and lifting from supporting stroma by infiltrating inflammatory cells.[10] Occasionally endothelial cells are necrotic or absent; however, thrombosis is rare. Endothelial apoptosis occurs[162,230] and increased numbers of endothelial cells appear in the circulation.[413] The medium usually shows little change. In severe cases a transmural mononuclear infiltrate may be seen (termed type III rejection). The cells infiltrating the endothelium and intima are T cells and monocytes, but not B cells.[10] Both $CD8^+$ and $CD4^+$ cells invade the intima in early grafts, but later $CD8^+$ cells predominate,[392] suggesting that class I antigens are the primary target.[230] Vascular endothelial cell apoptosis can be detected in sites of endarteritis.[162,230]

Normal arterial endothelial cells express class I antigens, weak ICAM-1, and little or no class II antigens, or VCAM-1. During acute rejection the endothelium of arteries expresses increased HLA-DR[101,392] and ICAM-1 and VCAM-1.[36,93] This adhesion molecule upregulation occurs in association with $CD3^+$[35] and $CD25^+$[103] infiltrating mononuclear cells. Endothelial cells also have decreased endothelin expression in rejection with endarteritis, but not in tubulointerstitial rejection.[404]

Glomerular Lesions

In most ACR cases, glomeruli are spared or show minor changes, typically a few scattered mononuclear cells (T cells and monocytes) and occasionally segmental endothelial damage (as in Figure 26-3A).[390] A severe form of this glomerular injury, termed "transplant glomerulitis" or "acute allograft glomerulopathy," develops in a minority of cases (<5%), manifested by hypercellularity, injury, and enlargement of endothelial cells, infiltration of glomeruli by mononuclear cells and by webs of PAS-positive material.[317] Crescents and thrombi are rare. The glomeruli contain numerous $CD3^+$ and $CD8^+$ T cells and monocytes.[145,392] Fibrin and scant immunoglobulin and complement deposits are found in glomeruli. Endarteritis often accompanies the transplant glomerulitis.[240] Glomerulitis is more often related to AMR, and evidence for this (C4d, donor-specific antibodies) should be sought in these cases.

Atypical Rejection Syndromes

Unique patterns of rejection have been observed under novel immunosuppression regimens. For example, pronounced lymphocyte depletion results from alemtuzumab (Campath-1H) and ACR in this setting has a prominent monocyte population (i.e., an acute monocytic rejection).[115,181,182] Much of the interstitial rejection infiltrate stains for CD68, correlating with renal dysfunction and tubular stress, shown by HLA-DR staining of the tubules. Under these conditions, T cells did not correlate with renal dysfunction or HLA-DR staining.[115]

Studies have recently included simultaneous bone marrow and kidney transplantation protocols in an attempt to induce tolerance to the transplanted organ. In these studies, HLA-mismatched renal transplants have been performed; withdrawal of maintenance immunosuppression has been accomplished in some of the patients with relatively preserved renal function.[176] In several of these patients, a capillary leak or engraftment syndrome has been observed around 10 days after a simultaneous kidney/bone marrow transplant preceded by a non-myeloablative conditioning regimen. In this "engraftment syndrome," acute tubular injury is accompanied by congested PTCs containing mononuclear cells

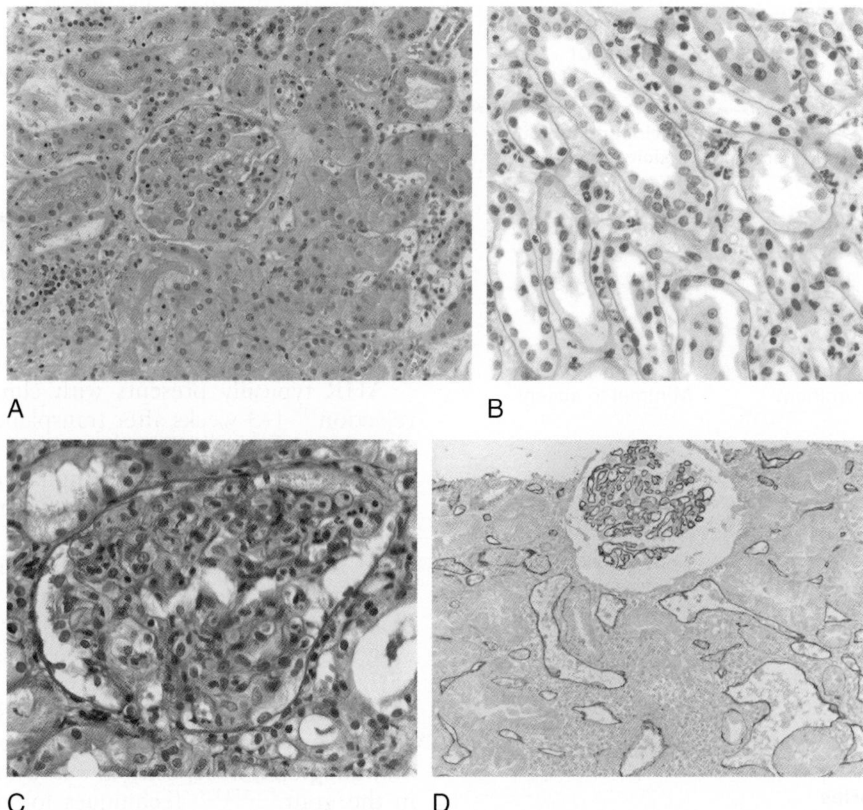

FIGURE 26-3 ■ Acute humoral rejection. (A) Low power shows mild interstitial inflammation, focal hemorrhage, neutrophils, and thrombi in glomerular capillaries and dilated peritubular capillaries with leukocytes. (B) At high power neutrophils can be seen in the peritubular capillaries with little tubulitis. Periodic acid–Schiff stain. (C) Acute transplant glomerulitis is prominent in this case of acute humoral rejection. Glomerular endothelial cells are swollen and the capillaries are filled with mononuclear cells, probably mostly macrophages. Periodic acid–Schiff stain. (D) C4d stain of a case of acute humoral rejection shows prominent, diffuse staining of dilated peritubular capillaries, sometimes containing inflammatory cells, and linear staining along the glomerular basement membrane. Immunohistochemistry with a polyclonal anti-C4d rabbit antibody.

and red blood cells. Immunohistochemistry shows that the cells are primarily $CD68^+MPO^+$ mononuclear cells and $CD3^+CD8^+$ T cells, the latter with a high proliferation index ($Ki67^+$). XY chromosome fluorescence in situ hybridization has been used to demonstrate that the PTC cells are recipient-derived, correlating with chimerism studies showing a simultaneous decline in circulating donor cells and recovery of recipient circulating cells. PTC endothelial injury can also be seen on EM in these cases.[92,176] Similar pathologic features have been observed in recipients of autologous mesenchymal stem cells (Remuzzi et al., personal communication). The etiology of the syndrome remains undefined, and others have performed combined kidney and bone marrow transplants without observing this phenomenon.[201]

Differential Diagnosis

Interstitial mononuclear inflammation and tubulitis occur in a variety of diseases other than acute rejection. Tubulitis has been documented in renal transplants with dysfunction due to lymphoceles (obstruction) and in urine leaks, possibilities that need to be considered and excluded by other techniques.[71] Acute obstruction typically has some dilation of the collecting tubules, especially in the outer cortex. Edema and a mild mononuclear infiltrate are also common.[59,71,216] When eosinophils are more abundant than usual for rejection and eosinophils invading tubules are identified, then drug allergy may be favored over rejection. The presence of endarteritis permits a definitive diagnosis of active rejection.[274] Lymphocytes commonly surround vessels (without medial involvement), a nonspecific feature, and must not be confused with endarteritis. Tubulitis is often present in atrophic tubules and does not indicate acute rejection. The diagnosis of acute pyelonephritis should be raised when active inflammation and abundant intratubular neutrophils are present. A note of caution, though: in AHR, neutrophilic tubulitis with neutrophil casts can be seen[222]; a C4d stain and urine culture will help in distinguishing between these.[61] Prominent tubulitis does favor acute rejection over ATN, particularly in the proximal tubules.[216]

The usual diagnostic feature of polyomavirus interstitial nephritis (BK virus) is the enlarged, hyperchromatic tubular nuclei with lavender viral nuclear inclusions, often in collecting ducts. However, these may be inconspicuous, and diligent study of multiple sections may be required. Other clues are prominent apoptosis of tubular cells, abundant plasma cells, which invade tubules. Immunohistochemistry for the polyoma SV40 large T antigen or in situ hybridization for BK polyomavirus and EM (even of paraffin) will confirm the diagnosis. Sometimes BK virus infection, with its exuberant plasmacytic infiltration and activated

TABLE 26-3 **Differentiation between Acute Rejection and Acute Calcineurin Inhibitor Toxicity**

	Acute Rejection	Calcineurin Inhibitor Toxicity
Interstitium		
Infiltrate	Moderate to marked	Absent to mild
Edema	Usual	Can be present
Tubules		
Tubular injury	Usual	Usual
Vacuoles	Occasional	Common
Tubulitis	Prominent	Minimal to absent
Arterioles		
Endotheliitis	Can be present	Absent
Smooth muscle	Absent	Sometimes degeneration present
Mucoid intimal	Absent	Sometimes thickening with present red blood cells (TMA)
Arteries		
Endotheliitis	Common	Absent (rare mononuclear TMA)
Peritubular Capillaries		
C4d	May be positive	Negative
Glomeruli		
Mononuclear cells	Often	Rare
Thrombi	Occasional	Occasionally prominent (TMA)

TMA, thrombotic microangiopathy.

immunoblasts, may be confused with the plasmacytic hyperplasia form of posttransplant lymphoproliferative disease (PTLD),[61] which also should be considered in the differential diagnosis of ACR. Rarer infections, including cytomegalovirus and microsporidia, should also be considered in biopsies with interstitial inflammation.

Patients with CNIT typically have a minimal mononuclear cell infiltrate (Table 26-3). Endarteritis or C4d+ is found extremely rarely, if ever, in CNIT and if either is present, is the most discriminating feature for acute rejection.[265,353,384]

Acute Antibody-Mediated Rejection

Acute AMR (also known as AHR) is due to damage by circulating antibodies that react to donor alloantigens on endothelium. These antigens include most commonly HLA class I and class II antigens[53,137,344] and in ABO-incompatible grafts the ABO blood group antigens.[96] Other proposed antigens on the endothelium (allo- or autoantigens) may also contribute. The clearest evidence of non-major histocompatibility complex (MHC) alloantigens comes from the rare observation of AHR in HLA-identical grafts.[52,125] AHR may occur in the absence of evidence for T-cell-mediated injury, particularly in positive-crossmatch transplants[42,199,346]; however, it is not uncommon for both to be present, particularly in the later posttransplant period (months to years).[53]

The main risk factors for the development of anti-HLA antibodies are blood transfusion, pregnancy, and prior transplant.[208] Donor-specific antibody (DSA), which typically refers to anti-HLA antibody, may arise de novo in the posttransplant period, or alloantibody may be present prior to transplantation in the case of positive-crossmatch or ABO blood group-incompatible transplants with preconditioning regimens to lower the alloantibody level prior to transplantation.

AHR typically presents with clinically severe acute rejection[137] 1–3 weeks after transplantation, but also can arise months to years later, associated with decreased immunosuppression or non-compliance.[382] With current therapy, approximately 5–7% of recipients develop an episode of AHR, and about 25% of biopsies taken for acute rejection have pathological evidence of an AHR component.[61] The main risk factor is presensitization by blood transfusion, pregnancy, or prior transplant[208]; however, the majority have a negative cross-match at the time of transplantation.[61]

Traditionally, identification of AHR in biopsies is difficult since none of the histologic features is diagnostic and immunoglobulin deposition was usually not detectable in the graft.[221,270,323] Techniques for demonstrating C4d in PTCs, pioneered by Feucht et al.,[95] substantially improved detection of this condition[53,69,222,306,323]; most studies since 1999 have employed it as a criterion for AHR. New evidence points to AHR with little or no C4d deposition (discussed below).

Serologic testing for DSA has become more sensitive in the past decade due to the widespread use of solid-phase assays over the older cell-based assays.[47,113] These assays can be used prior to transplantation and for posttransplant monitoring for DSA. These more sensitive methods of detecting DSA have brought to light the spectrum of alloantibody-mediated damage (e.g., capillaritis) that may not have been recognized in previous studies.[65]

Diagnostic Criteria

The three diagnostic criteria for AHR are: (1) histologic evidence of acute injury (neutrophils in capillaries, acute tubular injury, fibrinoid necrosis); (2) evidence of antibody interaction with tissue (typically C4d in PTCs); and (3) serologic evidence of circulating antibodies to antigens expressed by donor endothelium (typically HLA).[222,306] If only two of the three major criteria are established (for example, when antibody is negative or not done), the diagnosis is considered suspicious for AHR. Biopsies meeting criteria for both AHR and ACR type I or II are considered to have both forms of rejection. Some biopsies show prominent capillaritis and glomerulitis in association with DSA but little or no C4d. These C4d-negative cases also are "suspicious" for active AMR by the current definitions, but may be mediated by antibodies via cellular rather than complement mechanisms. This rarely occurs in the acute setting, and is discussed further in the chronic AMR section.

Pathologic Features

Histologic findings are typically scant to moderate mononuclear interstitial infiltrates, sometimes with prominent neutrophils[142,222,313,390] and increased numbers of macrophages[212] (Figure 26-3B). The extent of mononuclear infiltration often does not meet the criteria for ACR.[313] PTCs have neutrophils in about 50% of cases and are classically dilated (Figure 26-3B). Interstitial edema and hemorrhage can be prominent. Glomeruli have accumulations of macrophages (~50% of cases) and neutrophils (~25% of cases) (Figure 26-3C)[222,275,313,390] and occasionally fibrin thrombi or segmental necrosis.[137,222,390] Acute tubular injury, sometimes severe, can be identified in many cases and may be the only initial manifestation of AHR. Focal necrosis of whole tubular cross-sections, similar to cortical necrosis, has been reported; 38–70% of AHR cases may have patchy infarction.[206,390] Little mononuclear cell tubulitis is found, although a neutrophilic tubulitis with or without neutrophil casts may be prominent,[390] resembling acute pyelonephritis. Plasma cells can be abundant in AHR, either early[4] or late[75,300] after transplantation, sometimes associated with severe edema and increased IFN-γ production in the graft.[75] B cells can be also present, but have no apparent diagnostic value.[61]

In about 15% of cases small arteries show fibrinoid necrosis, with little mononuclear infiltrate in the intima or adventitia but with neutrophils and karyorrhexic debris (Figure 26-4).[206,390] Arterial thrombosis can be found in 10% and a pattern resembling TMA has also been reported.[206] Around 75% of cases with fibrinoid necrosis are C4d-positive.[142,222,275,390] Presumably the C4d-negative cases had T-cell-mediated rejection or TMA. Antibodies to the angiotensin II type 1 receptor have been detected in a few cases with arterial fibrinoid necrosis, in the absence of capillary C4d deposition.[83] The presence of mononuclear endarteritis in cases of AHR strongly suggests a component of T-cell-mediated rejection.[390]

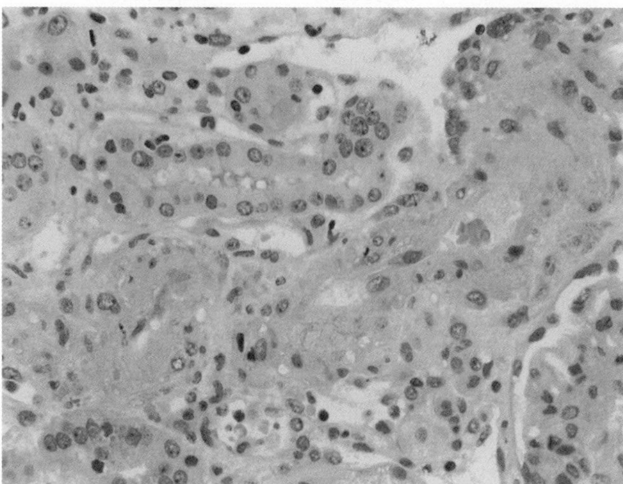

FIGURE 26-4 ■ Fibrinoid arterial necrosis: an arteriole with destruction of the medial wall smooth-muscle cells by fibrinoid necrosis. Some neutrophils are present underneath the reactive and swollen endothelium. This vascular change is distinctly different from endarteritis (compare with Figure 26-2) and can be seen in both acute humoral rejection and type III acute rejection. This case had positive C4d.

By EM the PTCs are dilated, containing neutrophils. The endothelium is reactive and shows loss of fenestrations. The glomerular endothelium is separated from the GBM by a widened lucent space with endothelial cell swelling[390] and loss of endothelial fenestrations, indicative of injury. Platelets, fibrin, and neutrophils are found in glomerular and PTCs. The small arteries with fibrinoid necrosis show marked endothelial injury and loss, smooth-muscle necrosis, and deposition of fibrin. [61]

C4d Interpretation

Feucht and colleagues first drew attention to C4d as a possible marker of an antibody-mediated component of severe rejection.[95] C4d, a fragment of complement component C4, is released during activation of the classical complement pathway by antigen–antibody interaction. C4d binds to tissue components via a thioester bond at the local site of activation. The covalent linkage explains why C4d remains for several days after alloantibody disappears, since antibody binds to cell surface antigens that can be lost by modulation, shedding, or cell death. C4d deposition can precede histological evidence of AHR by 5–34 days.[133] C4d in 1-week protocol biopsies was followed by clinical acute rejection in 82% of cases[380] and was associated with donor-reactive antibodies.[186]

Although immunoglobulin deposition is found in only a minority of cases, C4d is characteristically detected in a widespread, uniform ring-like distribution in the PTCs by immunofluorescence in cryostat sections[53,95]. Deposition occurs in both the cortex and medulla.

In a comparison of methods for C4d, the triple-layer immunofluorescence technique[53] proved the most sensitive, although the difference with immunohistochemistry in paraffin-embedded tissue was small.[259] Using immunohistochemistry in formalin-fixed, paraffin-embedded tissue, C4d has a similar pattern (Figure 26-3D), although the intensity is variable. With fixed tissue, plasma in the capillaries and interstitium may stain for C4d, which interferes with interpretation.[61] "Plasma staining" is a fixation artifact of C4d immunohistochemistry, and so PTCs must show clear circumferential staining to be called positive by this technique. Glomerular capillary staining also occurs, but is hard to distinguish from C4d normally found in the mesangium in frozen sections stained by immunofluorescence. Formalin fixation eliminates this background staining and demonstrates glomerular C4d in about 30% of AHR cases.[313]

PTC C4d deposition is associated with concurrent circulating antibodies to donor HLA class I or II antigens in 88–95% of recipients with acute rejection.[33,132,222] False-negative antibody assays are probably due most often to absorption by the graft, as shown by elution from rejected grafts in patients who had no detectable circulating antibody.[217] Alternatively, non-HLA antigens may be the target.[52,125]

Other components of the complement system have been sought. C3d, a degradation product of C3, was found in PTCs in 39–60% of biopsies from HLA-mismatched grafts with diffuse C4d.[132,142,193,380] C3d was usually,[132] but not always,[193] associated with C4d. C3d correlated with AHR in all studies, and was associated with increased risk of graft loss in two series, compared to C3d-negative cases, but C3d provided no convincing additional risk compared with C4d+. The interpretation of C3d stains is complicated by the common presence of C3d along the TBM.[132] Even though C3d should indicate more complete complement activation, it added no diagnostic value to C4d in grafts showing histologic features of AHR, except in the setting of ABO-incompatible grafts.[132] Other complement components, such as C1q, C5b-9, and C-reactive protein, are not conspicuous in PTCs in acute rejection.[166,277] Lectin pathway components, which activate C4 by binding to microbial carbohydrates, are sometimes detected.[159,380]

Natural killer (NK) cells have been the focus of recent research in antibody-mediated graft injury.[6,148] Microarray analysis has indicated that several DSA-specific gene transcripts show high expression in NK cells, and immunohistochemistry also shows prominent numbers of PTC NK cells in these cases.[144] Depletion of NK cells with anti-NK1.1 significantly reduced DSA-induced chronic allograft vasculopathy in a murine cardiac allograft model.[148]

The prognosis of AHR is uniformly worse than ACR,[53,137,188,206,390,417] but outcome has generally improved with early recognition and vigorous therapy. In one series, 75% of the 1-year graft losses from acute rejection were in the C4d+ AHR group.[222] However, some of those who recover from the acute episode of AHR have a similar long-term outcome,[390] suggesting that the pathogenetic humoral response can be transient if treated effectively.

While most approaches for treatment or prevention of AHR involve removing alloantibody from the circulation (by plasmapheresis) or decreasing production of alloantibody (e.g., by antiplasma cell drugs), another technique to prevent graft damage by antibody is by inhibiting complement. Eculizumab, a humanized monoclonal antibody directed against the terminal complement component C5, is now being applied in renal transplantation, particularly in sensitized (positive-crossmatch) patients at a high risk for early AHR. C5 is downstream of C4d in the complement cascade; thus, with DSA activation of complement, diffuse C4d deposition would be expected even with effective C5 inhibition. Early surveillance biopsies in eculizumab-treated patients have shown diffuse C4d deposition but absent morphological signs of AHR, including a lack of endothelial cell activation by EM. The absence of respective pathology suggests endothelial protection by eculizumab, and moreover supports the notion that most cases of early AHR are complement-mediated. However, AHR was observed in a few patients despite eculizumab therapy, and may be due to IgM DSA not detected by the usual DSA testing methods.[24] Notably, a subset of patients still developed features of chronic humoral rejection (CHR), including transplant glomerulopathy (TG), although the time of treatment with eculizumab varied between patients, from 1 month to 1 year.[370] While effective in preventing early AHR in positive-crossmatch transplants, it appears that complement inhibition alone does not entirely prevent chronic, antibody-mediated microcirculation injury. Furthermore, the limited diagnostic reliability for AHR of C4d and serum DSA is apparent in this setting, suggesting that diagnostic criteria refinements are needed.

Differential Diagnosis

For differential diagnosis, it is helpful that both ATN[323,389] and TMA in native kidneys are C4d-negative. Among 26 cases of TMA/hemolytic uremic syndrome in native kidneys, none had positive C4d, including cases with lupus anticoagulant and antiphospholipid antibodies.[323] In five cases of recurrent hemolytic uremic syndrome in transplant recipients, C4d was also negative.[14] Among native kidney diseases, only lupus nephritis[198,323] and endocarditis[198] have been reported to have PTC C4d. Glomerular C4d deposits, of course, are not specific, since they occur in many forms of immune complex glomerulonephritis in native kidneys. Arterial intimal fibrosis often stains for C4d, even in native kidneys, and should not be taken as evidence of AMR.[323]

The comparative features of "pure" humoral and ACR are given in Table 26-4. In AHR neutrophils are the predominant inflammatory cells in PTCs, glomeruli, tubules, and the interstitium, with or without accompanying fibrinoid necrosis. The vascular lesion of AHR, if present, is fibrinoid necrosis of the wall while in ACR endarteritis is the usual lesion. C4d deposition in PTCs (immunofluorescence microscopy) is typically only present in AHR, but not in ACR.[61]

Classification Systems

The most widely used system currently is the "Banff working schema" ("Banff" for short). Banff started as an international collaborative effort led by Kim Solez, Lorraine Racusen, and Philip Halloran to achieve a consensus that would be useful for drug trials and routine

TABLE 26-4 **Differentiation between Acute Humoral Rejection and Acute Cellular Rejection**

	Acute Humoral Rejection	Acute Cellular Rejection
Interstitium		
Infiltrate	Variable	Moderate to severe
Edema	Present	Present
Peritubular capillaries	Neutrophils	Mononuclear cells
C4d*	Positive	Negative
Tubules		
Acute tubular necrosis	Can be present	Usually absent
Tubulitis	Neutrophils	Mononuclear cells
Vessels		
Endarteritis	Can be present	Present in type II
Fibrinoid necrosis	Typically present	Present in type III
Glomeruli		
Inflammatory cells	Neutrophils	Mononuclear cells
Fibrinoid necrosis	Can be present	Typically absent

*C4d staining in peritubular capillaries indicates activation of the classical complement pathway by humoral antibody (monoclonal antibody, immunofluorescence microscopy).

diagnosis.[237,365,366] Banff is still growing and remodeling, undergoing revisions based on data presented and debated at the biennial Banff meeting. These included restructuring that separated the category of endarteritis, according to the National Institutes of Health Cooperative Clinical Trials in Transplantation criteria,[59,307] the addition of acute[306] and chronic AMR,[367] and the birth[366] and death[367] of "chronic allograft nephropathy (CAN)."[367]

Banff scores three elements to assess acute rejection: tubulitis (t); the extent of cortical mononuclear infiltrate (i); and vascular inflammation (intimal arteritis or transmural inflammation) (v). Mononuclear cell glomerulitis (g) is scored but not yet part of the classification of rejection. Banff recognizes three major categories of acute T-cell-mediated rejection (tubulointerstitial, endarteritis, and arterial fibrinoid necrosis) (Table 26-2). The threshold for type I (tubulointerstitial) ACR is >25% cortical mononuclear inflammation in the non-atrophic areas, provided tubulitis of at least 5–10 cells/tubule is present.[307] Cases with no tubulitis, regardless of the extent of infiltrate, are not considered ACR. Biopsies with C4d+ PTCs are considered to have an additional component of AMR, which occurs in 20–30% of cases.[143] Cases with tubulitis are termed "suspicious for rejection" or "borderline" in the current Banff system. Many, but not all, of these cases are early or mild acute rejection: 75–88% of patients with suspicious/borderline category and graft dysfunction improve renal function with increased immunosuppression,[332,342] comparable to the response rate in type I rejection (86%).[332] A minority (28%) of untreated suspicious/borderline cases progress to frank acute rejection in 40 days.[232] Almost all with suspicious/borderline findings do well, provided there is no element of concurrent AMR, which commonly has a suspicious/borderline pattern, although care must be taken not to misinterpret peritubular capillaritis as interstitial inflammation.[65,313] The suspicious category is not counted as acute rejection in most clinical trials – a major omission in our opinion.

The interobserver reproducibility of the present Banff classification is sufficient but needs improvement. In a Canadian study, the agreement rate for rejection was 74%, but there was only 43% agreement on the suspicious/borderline cases,[122] similar to a European series.[397] Among a group of 21 European pathologists, the agreement rate was poor for all of the acute Banff scores (t, i, v, g) in transplant biopsy slides (all kappa scores <0.4).[105] Agreement for t and v scores improved significantly when participants were asked to grade a lesion in a photograph (kappa scores of 0.61 and 0.69, respectively), arguing that the challenge is primarily finding the lesion in the glass slide. Lack of improvement in the other categories (g, i) argues that the definitions are faulty. Despite these considerations, Banff is fully accepted as a scoring system of drug trials and is used widely in clinical practice (although not necessarily with an individual score report).[61]

LATE GRAFT DISEASES

Although acute rejection has diminished in clinical importance in the last decade, allografts are still lost by slow, progressive diseases that cause a 3–5% annual attrition rate. The specific causes of this are many and sometimes difficult to ascertain, particularly if only an end-stage kidney is examined. Unfortunately two terms, "chronic rejection" and "CAN," have been used in past literature to lump together these myriad diseases. The role of the pathologist in interpreting the biopsy is to provide the most specific diagnosis possible and indicate the activity of the process. While some have argued that the renal biopsy is not useful in analyzing graft dysfunction after 1 year, the data show that in 8–39% of patients the biopsy led to a change in management that improved renal function.[185,295] Here we will discuss the criteria used to distinguish some of these diseases and those that remain idiopathic. The term "chronic rejection" is best defined as chronic injury primarily mediated by an immune reaction to donor alloantigens.

Chronic Antibody-Mediated Rejection

Circulating anti-HLA antibodies have long been associated with increased risk of late graft loss.[155,386] Chronic, active AMR (CHR) was first reported in 2001[223] and is now recognized as a separate category in the Banff schema.[367] CHR differs from AHR in the usual lack of evidence of acute inflammation (neutrophils, thrombi, necrosis) and the presence of matrix synthesis (basement membrane multilamination, fibrosis in arterial intima and the interstitium). CHR commonly arises late (>6 months after transplantation) and usually occurs in patients with or without a history of AHR, although C4d in early biopsies is a risk factor for later TG with C4d.[117,119,131,312] In the setting of de novo DSA, many patients have reduced levels of immunosuppression (absorption, iatrogenic, or non-compliance).[406] In these cases, a combination of CHR and AHR may be seen, along with a component of T-cell-mediated rejection.[199]

Patients with CHR typically present with late graft dysfunction (average of 4–5 years posttransplant), with proteinuria and circulating DSA. Most do not have a previous episode of AHR and, indeed, present with no obvious preceding clinical event. The major risk factor identified is reduced immunosuppression due to non-compliance.[406] Iatrogenic and physiologic causes also contribute.

The criteria of CHR are the triad of: (1) one of the following morphologic features: TG (duplication or "double contours" in GBMs), multilamination of the PTC basement membrane, PTC loss and interstitial fibrosis, or chronic arteriopathy with fibrous intimal thickening (without duplication of the internal elastica); (2) diffuse C4d deposition in PTCs; and (3) circulating DSA. If only two elements of the triad are present, the diagnosis is considered "suspicious." Although helpful when positive, C4d deposition and serum DSA are particularly problematic in the chronic setting: they are less sensitive markers due to serum DSA level variability with time posttransplant. Two features point to ongoing immunologic activity: the presence of C4d and mononuclear cells in glomerular and PTCs.

TG, defined by duplication of the GBM by light microscopy in the absence of specific de novo or recurrent glomerular disease, was one of the first lesions to be linked to DSA. TG has been associated with anti-HLA antibodies (especially anti-class II), with the risk increasing if the antibodies were donor-specific.[117] TG is best revealed in PAS or silver stains (Figure 26-5A, B). The glomeruli may show an increase in mesangial cells and matrix with various degrees of scarring and adhesions. In some cases mesangiolysis or webbing of the mesangium may be prominent as well as segmental or global sclerosis. EM reveals duplication or multilamination of the GBM (Figure 26-5C), often accompanied by cellular (mononuclear or mesangial cell) interposition, widening or lucency of the subendothelial space, and a moderate increase in mesangial matrix and cells.[135] Glomeruli may show focal and segmental glomerulosclerosis (FSGS), especially in more advanced TG, and some cases with collapsing

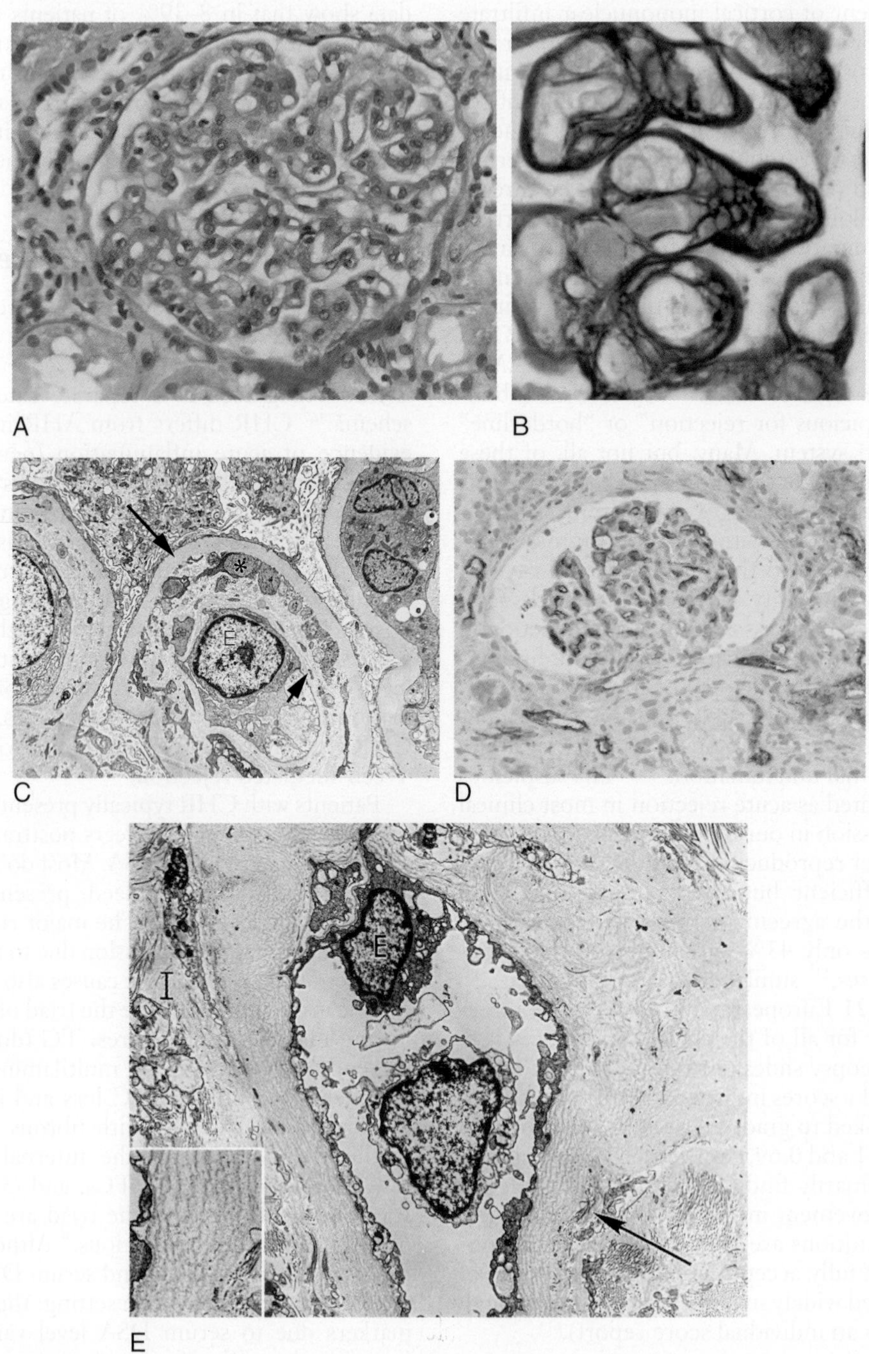

FIGURE 26-5 ■ Chronic allograft glomerulopathy. (A) Widespread duplication of the glomerular basement membrane (GBM) with mild mesangial hypercellularity and increased mononuclear cells in the glomerular capillaries. Periodic acid–Schiff stain. (B) GBM multilamination at high power in a silver stain. (C) Electron microscopy: high power of a glomerular capillary showing duplication of the GBM; the new or second layer of GBM (short arrow) forms underneath the endothelium (E) and is separated from the old GBM layer (long arrow) by the cellular (mononuclear or mesangial cell) interposition (*). (D) Immunohistochemistry stain for C4d in paraffin sections shows prominent C4d deposition in glomerular and peritubular capillaries. (E) Electron microscopy: high magnification of a peritubular capillary with multilamination (arrow) of the basement membrane. Inset: higher magnification of the area marked by arrow. E, endothelium; I, interstitium.

FSGS lesions have been observed. EM detects 40% more cases of TG than light microscopy.[163] The GBM typically has rarefactions, microfibrils, and cellular debris but few or no deposits.[43,158,304] Endothelial cells may appear reactive with loss of fenestrae, probably undergoing "dedifferentiation."[57,158,304] Podocyte foot process effacement ranges from minimal to quite extensive,[158] corresponding to the degree of proteinuria. The non-duplicated GBM may become slightly thickened, attributable to compensatory hypertrophy.

Peritubular Capillary and Tubulointerstitial Lesions

PTCs may be dilated and prominent, with thick basement membranes, or may altogether disappear, leaving only occasional traces of the original basement membrane behind.[30,160] In a subset of patients, PTCs have prominent C4d deposition (as in Figure 26-3D), which is associated with circulating antidonor HLA class I or II reactive antibodies.[223] Other allografts with CHR features may show focal or multifocal C4d staining of PTCs by immunofluorescence or immunohistochemistry, or dim C4d staining by immunofluorescence. EM reveals splitting and multilayering of the PTC basement membrane (Figure 26-5E), first described by Monga.[224,250] Each ring probably represents the residue of one previous episode of endothelial injury, going from oldest (outer) to most recent (inner). Quantitation is necessary to establish diagnostic specificity. Scoring of multilamination requires EM, not always available for transplant biopsies, and quantitative assessment of the number of layers, since to distinguish from other common causes of lamination, more than six layers have to be present.[163] Only in chronic rejection were three or more PTCs found with 5–6 circumferential layers or one PTC with seven or more circumferential layers.[163] PTC lamination correlates with TG,[163,224] C4d deposition,[312] and loss of PTCs.[160] Marked multilamination (5–6 layers in three capillaries or >6 in one) was found in 50% of cases with interstitial fibrosis that lacked arterial or glomerular changes, and may point to past episodes of rejection as the cause of the fibrosis.[224]

Transplant Arteriopathy

Alloantibodies to graft class I antigens are a specific risk factor for chronic transplant arteriopathy in human renal allografts.[73,168] Typically, transplant arteriopathy is recognized by thickening of the arterial intima with mononuclear inflammatory cells ($CD3^+$ T cells or $CD68^+$ monocytes/macrophages) within the thickened intima. In a recent study, patients with preformed DSA showed accelerated arteriosclerosis on serial biopsies.[146,147] While the transplant arteriopathy lesions were attributable to DSA on serial biopsies from the same allografts, transplant arteriopathy may not be distinguishable from the arterial intimal thickening seen in hypertension.[146] Careful study of the progression of arteriosclerosis in allografts has shown that DSA exacerbates the process, similar to accelerated aging of the kidney.[146] Experiments in animals show that transplant arteriopathy can be initiated by passive transfer of donor-reactive MHC antibodies in recipients with no functional T cells.[223,312] Transplant arteriopathy is also believed to be due to chronic T-cell-mediated injury and is further described in that section. The relative contribution of these two pathways is far from clear and no criteria exist to distinguish them at the level of the arteries.

Accommodation

Not all patients with circulating DSA have clinical or pathologic evidence of chronic graft injury. This paradox was observed in ABO grafts and termed "accommodation."[17] Accommodation is thought to represent a process of endothelial cell adaptation to antibody and complement over time. In accommodation, DSAs may be detectable; however, morphologic signs of tissue injury are absent. Subclinical interaction of antibody with graft endothelium (accommodation) has been revealed by the demonstration of diffuse C4d in PTCs, found in 2.0% of routine protocol biopsies,[234] and a higher frequency among presensitized patients (17%) or patients with ABO-incompatible grafts (51%).[96,132] The stability of such accommodation, referring to the presence of PTC C4d deposition in the absence of other evidence of antibody-mediated injury, has not been established.

In renal allografts PTC C4d deposition in the absence of other evidence of antibody-mediated injury is observed without signs of acute or chronic rejection; more specifically, there is no ATN-like minimal inflammation, no glomerulitis (g0), no chronic TG (cg0), no peritubular capillaritis (ptc0), and no PTC basement membrane multilamination (<5 layers by EM). Current Banff criteria refer to this situation as "C4d deposition without evidence of active rejection." If there are simultaneous borderline changes, the cases are considered to be indeterminate.[360] Accommodation is common in the setting of ABO-incompatible allografts, with at least 80% of normal surveillance biopsies showing C4d deposition in PTCs with no apparent long-term consequences.[132] However, evidence from patients[406] and non-human primates[362] suggests that DSA and C4d deposition (and/or capillaritis) lead to chronic graft pathology and loss and these patients should be closely monitored and efforts made to reduce DSA levels.

Longitudinal Studies. CHR is a process that evolves over several years, typically beginning entirely subclinically. In non-human primates with MHC-incompatible grafts and no immunosuppression, C4d deposition predicts chronic rejection with glomerulopathy and arteriopathy and ultimate graft loss with a high degree of certainty.[361] A sequence of four stages has been demonstrated in protocol biopsies. The process begins with antibody production, followed by C4d deposition, and later, morphologic and functional changes.[361] A similar sequence, with the addition of capillaritis and glomerulitis, has been reported in patients.[406]

C4d-Negative Antibody-Mediated Rejection

Attention has recently been drawn to so-called "C4d-negative" AMR. These cases have DSA and varying degrees of morphological evidence of antibody-mediated injury but lack detectable C4d deposition in PTC endothelium.[128–130] This has been described in two settings: late indication biopsies (with features of chronic AMR), and early protocol biopsies in stable patients who were presensitized.[130,210] In these cases other signs of endothelial injury were detected (capillaritis or increased endothelial gene expression). Negative C4d might be explained by time-dependent degradation of C4d deposits in the microcirculation, complement-independent antibody-mediated injury, or issues with the C4d stain itself (sensitivity, interpretation of a positive).[129] Molecular studies have uncovered a subset of cases with morphological features of antibody-mediated injury and DSA showing increased endothelial cell-associated transcript expression, indicative of endothelial cell activation and stress. These data suggest that 50–60% of late AMR may lack C4d positivity. It is probably much less common in AHR: we have only rarely seen such cases (as a consult). Cases are missed by current Banff criteria due to C4d negativity.[359] It would appear that there is another category of AMR that is between acute and chronic, in that neutrophils and rapid decline in graft dysfunction are absent, as well as no evidence of chronic matrix production (duplication of basement membranes, fibrosis of interstitium or intima). This is characterized by capillaritis and glomerulitis with mononuclear cells, with or without C4d, in association with DSA. This was described clearly in 3-month protocol biopsies in clinically stable presensitized patients and carried an increased risk of development of chronic lesions (TG) at 1 year.[209] Eventually, this will likely be added to the Banff diagnostic armamentarium as a distinct category of AMR; however, data are still being gathered by a respective Banff Working Group regarding the significance of this entity in an attempt to provide diagnostic criteria.[237] At present we suggest the term "smoldering" AMR for this condition.

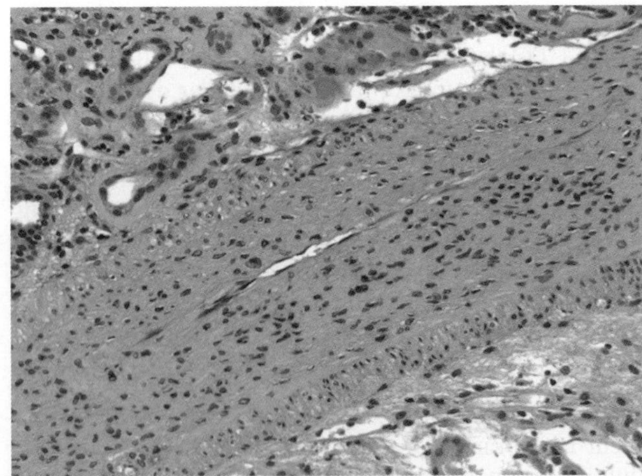

FIGURE 26-6 ■ Chronic allograft arteriopathy: an interlobular artery with prominent intimal fibroplasia. The presence of scattered mononuclear cells in the intima and the lack of duplication of the internal elastica are characteristic of chronic rejection. This biopsy was positive for C4d.

Chronic T-Cell-Mediated Rejection

There is no doubt that T cells can cause chronic graft injury, yet the specific criteria are not well developed and subject to refinement. Using the CHR model, the current Banff classification defines "chronic active T-cell-mediated rejection" as showing morphologic features of chronicity (arterial intimal fibrosis without elastosis) combined with features indicative of ongoing T-cell activity (mononuclear cells in the intima). Interstitial fibrosis with a mononuclear infiltrate and tubulitis is in some instances also probably part of this condition, as surveillance follow-up biopsies after an episode of ACR not uncommonly show continued inflammation.[110] However, at present the arterial lesions are the most definitive. It is anticipated that molecular gene expression studies will help in the future to document the activity of the infiltrate. Other non-specific features that are commonly present in association with transplant arteriopathy are loss of PTCs and interstitial fibrosis and tubular atrophy (IFTA).[160]

Chronic Allograft Arteriopathy

Small and large arteries, as early as 1 month after transplantation, can begin to develop severe intimal proliferation and luminal narrowing.[41,58,146] The intimal change is most prominent in the larger arteries, but can be seen at all levels, from interlobular arteries to the main renal artery. The intima shows pronounced concentric fibrous thickening with invasion and proliferation of spindle-shaped myofibroblasts (Figure 26-6). This vascular change has been termed chronic transplant arteriopathy and, when combined with an infiltrate of mononuclear cells in the intima, is characteristic of chronic T-cell-mediated rejection. Subendothelial mononuclear cells are one of the most distinctive features and argue that the endothelium itself is a target. T cells ($CD4^+$, $CD8^+$, $CD45RO^+$), macrophages, and dendritic cells infiltrate the intima.[124,285,335] T cells express cytotoxic markers, including perforin[99] and GMP-17,[230] and markers of proliferation (proliferating cell nuclear antigen).[124] No B cells (CD20) are detected.[124] It is imagined that this is a dampened version of the endarteritis of acute rejection.

The second distinctive feature is the lack of multilamination of the elastica interna (fibroelastosis), best appreciated in elastin stains. Fibroelastosis, typical of hypertensive, atrophic, and aging arterial changes provide useful differential diagnostic features from rejection. Foamy macrophages containing lipid droplets are sometimes seen along the internal elastica and can be found as early as 4 weeks after transplantation. The endothelium expresses increased adhesion molecules, notably ICAM-1 and VCAM-1. Antagonism of ICAM-1 binding/expression inhibits chronic rejection[329] and in humans certain ICAM-1 genetic polymorphisms (e.g., exon 4, the Mac-1 binding site) appear to confer a higher risk factor for chronic rejection.[226] The endothelium remains of donor origin[157,345]; however, some of the spindle-shaped cells that contribute to the intimal thickening are of recipient origin.[178,285] The myointimal cells stain prominently for smooth-muscle actin, sometimes so strikingly that a "double media" seems to be formed.[333] This phenomenon has also been described as the development of a new artery inside and concentric with the old,[156] with elastic laminae and a muscular media, separated from the old internal elastic lamina poorly by cellular tissue. By EM, the thickened intima consists of myofibroblasts, collagen fibrils, basement membrane material, and a loose amorphous electron-lucent ground substance.[302] The matrix consists of collagen, fibronectin, tenascin, proteoglycans (biglycan and decorin), and acid mucopolysaccarides.[56,123,227] Fibronectin has the extra domain of cellular fibronectin, typical of embryonic or wound-healing fibronectin.[123] Several growth factors/cytokines have been detected. Platelet-derived growth factor (PDGF) A chain protein is primarily in endothelial cells, while the B chain is in macrophages and smooth-muscle cells.[9] Enhanced PDGF B-type receptor protein was found on intimal cells and on smooth-muscle cells of the proliferating vessels.[94] Fibroblast growth factor-1 and its receptor are present in the thickened intima.[179] TNF-α is in the smooth muscle of vessels with chronic rejection in contrast to normal kidneys.[280]

Sequence of Arterial Lesions

T-cell-mediated arterial lesions can be divided into three stages, which probably differ in mechanism and reversibility.[57] The stage I lesion is endarteritis, characteristic of type II ACR. This lesion lacks matrix formation. This acute stage is believed to be T-cell-mediated endothelial injury. Stage II lesions have intimal matrix production and accumulation of myofibroblasts forming a “neointima.” This stage also contains mononuclear cells (T cells and macrophages), believed to be active in the intimal proliferation and accumulation of matrix. Intermediate stages between stage I and II lesions are sometimes found, with lymphocytes admixed with fibrin and fibromuscular proliferation, well documented in a non-human primate model of chronic rejection.[407] Secondary factors probably become increasingly important as the lesion progresses to stage III, where the intima is fibrous and inflammatory cells are scant. A fourth category, resembling natural atherosclerosis with cholesterol clefts and calcification, has also been proposed.[124]

A large body of experimental evidence supports the concept that the arterial lesions are immunologically mediated[57]: (1) the lesions do not routinely arise in isografts; (2) the target antigens can be either major or minor histocompatibility antigens[2,68,331]; (3) the specific initiator is probably T cells followed by antibody (antibody is necessary and sufficient for the fibrous lesion in mice); (4) the target cell is probably the endothelium, but the smooth muscle may also be affected; (5) secondary non-immunologic mechanisms analogous to those in atherosclerosis are important in the progression of the lesion; and ultimately (6) the process may be independent of specific antidonor immunological activity. T cells are sufficient to initiate cellular vascular lesions in B-cell-deficient mice, but these lesions do not readily progress to fibrosis in the absence of antibody.[328] Fibrous lesions are also markedly reduced in strain combinations that fail to elicit a humoral antibody response. The best evidence for T-cell mechanisms of chronic allograft injury in humans is that subclinical or late clinical cellular rejection is associated with progressive graft fibrosis and dysfunction[63,263,327] and endarteritis is associated with later transplant arteriopathy.[192] As mentioned previously, antibodies likely conspire to accelerate the process of allograft arteriopathy/arteriosclerosis.[146,147]

Differential Diagnosis of Late Biopsies

The diagnosis of the cause of late graft dysfunction remains a challenge for several reasons: the diagnostic features may have been lost or obscured over time (e.g., loss of viral antigens or C4d) and typically more than one pathological process is present, analogous to the layers of failed civilizations in an archeological dig. The most important questions for the pathologist and clinician, and the prime reason for the biopsy, are whether the disease is active and whether the graft is potentially salvageable, so that additional therapy can be proposed.

Transplant Glomerulopathy

Duplication of the GBM has many other causes, such as TMA and MPGN; however these do not have C4d in PTC unless there is more than one concurrent pathologic process. Also in CHR, GBMs may show multilamination extending completely around the capillary, even between the endothelium and the mesangium, less likely to be seen in other conditions.[49] With immunohistochemical techniques in paraffin sections, C4d is present along the glomerular capillary walls in about 10–30% of TG.[312,354] Although officially required for diagnosis by the Banff schema, it is now recognized that approximately 30% of TG due to CHR is C4d-negative.[180] Notably, while most cases of TG are due to CHR, this pattern is also seen in allografts with chronic TMA and in patients with hepatitis C virus (HCV) infection.[19] Crescents or diffuse immunoglobulin deposits suggest recurrent or de novo glomerulonephritis.[116,287,303]

Arteriosclerosis. Transplant arteriopathy is traditionally distinguished from chronic allograft arteriopathy by the presence of fibroelastosis (increased elastic fibers in the intima) in the former. To distinguish intimal fibrosis due to hypertension from that due to chronic rejection, an elastin stain is valuable, since in hypertension, but not necessarily in rejection, the elastica interna is multilayered (“elastosis”), and in chronic rejection the elastica is not duplicated, but may be fractured. Foam cells and mononuclear cells in the intima also favor rejection. A recent study, however, suggested that some lesions of vascular intimal thickening due to alloantibody are indistinguishable from those due to hypertension.[146]

Chronic CNIT has been traditionally diagnosed by the presence of nodular hyaline replacement of individual smooth-muscle cells, which may form distinctive deposits on the outer side of the arteriole, as described by Mihatsch as cyclosporine arteriolopathy.[243–247] Ordinary hyalinosis due to diabetes, hypertension, or aging typically is subendothelial. However, peripheral nodular hyalinosis, while more common in patients on CNI, can be seen in a substantial fraction (28%) of biopsies at 10 years in patients never exposed to CNI.[364]

CHR. The features that point to a component of CHR are discussed above and include most specifically the presence of C4d in PTC and/or glomeruli and capillaritis and glomerulitis. Multilamination of the GBM or PTC basement membranes is also typical. In the absence of C4d in PTC, other causes of lamination of the GBM must be excluded.

Polyomavirus. Demonstration of polyomavirus by immunohistochemistry in previous biopsies can point to a causal role in the late graft damage, even when the virus is no longer detectable.[61]

Obstruction, usually difficult to diagnose by histology, archetypically shows dilated collecting ducts, especially in the outer cortex, lymphatics filled with Tamm–Horsfall protein, occasionally ruptured tubules with granulomas, and sometimes acute tubular injury.[61]

Renal artery stenosis causes tubular atrophy (or even acute injury) accompanied by relatively little fibrosis or intraparenchymal arteriolar/arterial lesions.[61]

Recurrent and de novo glomerular diseases are generally identified by their light, immunofluorescence, and EM criteria in native kidneys.[61]

Interstitial Fibrosis. IFTA do not serve to distinguish rejection from other causes, such as CNI toxicity and previous BK polyomavirus infection. Some of these cases may be the end-stage of active processes in which the etiologic agent is no longer appreciable (e.g., late effects of polyomavirus or TMA). Others may represent burned-out or inactive rejection. This might be the case for TG or arteriopathy without C4d deposition.

The term "CAN" was created in Banff in 1993 to draw attention to the fact that not all late graft injury was due to rejection, and that, to make the diagnosis of rejection, certain more specific features than interstitial fibrosis and tubular atrophy needed to be present (notably chronic glomerular or arterial lesions). However, the unintended consequence was that "CAN" itself became a diagnosis that inhibited the search for specific, and perhaps treatable, causes. CAN has been replaced in Banff 2005 with category 5: "IF and TA, no evidence of any specific etiology." This now includes only those cases for which no specific etiologic features can be defined, and excludes those with pathologic features of CHR, chronic CNIT, hypertensive renal disease, PTN, obstruction, or other de novo or recurrent renal disease.[367]

ACUTE TUBULAR INJURY

The morphologic basis of DGF is usually acute ischemic injury (also known as ATN). The most common feature histologically is loss of the brush borders of proximal tubular cells, best shown on a PAS stain with focal interstitial edema and mononuclear cell accumulation (Figure 26-7). The tubular lumen appears larger than normal and lacks the usual artifactual sloughing of the apical cytoplasm in human renal biopsies (this sloughing has occurred in vivo and was washed downstream). The other features of ATN include flattening of the cytoplasm and loss of cell nuclei due to apoptosis/death of individual tubular epithelial cells and covering of the TBM by the remaining cells. The lumen contains individual apoptotic detached cells ("anoikis") and inflammatory cells. Reactive changes in the tubular epithelium are seen after 24–48 hours, including large basophilic nuclei with prominent nucleoli, increased cytoplasmic basophilia, and occasionally mitoses. Focal interstitial, PTC, and glomerular capillary neutrophils may be seen but are not as prominent as in AHR; and C4d is negative. Mechanical flushing of cadaveric kidneys with organ preservation fluid immediately before transplantation (as advocated by some) was associated with abnormal cellular debris within the tubules and eosinophilic proteinaceous material within Bowman's capsule and an increased frequency of DGF.[318] DGF has other causes; and if function has not recovered in 1–2 weeks, a diagnostic biopsy is recommended to ascertain the presence of occult acute rejection, found in 18% of patients with DGF at 7 days.[167]

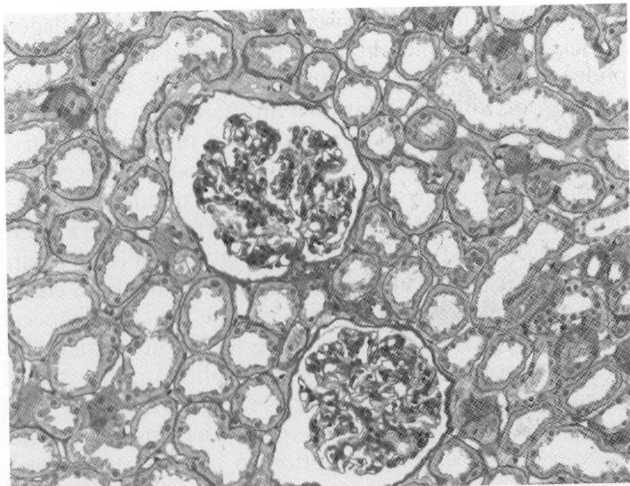

FIGURE 26-7 ■ Acute tubular necrosis. Dilated "rigid"-appearing tubular lumens with loss of brush borders, occasional loss of nuclei, and cytoplasmic thinning. Mild edema is present but there is little inflammation. Glomeruli are normal. Periodic acid–Schiff stain.

CALCINEURIN INHIBITOR NEPHROTOXICITY

The CNI class of drugs, including cyclosporine and tacrolimus, causes both acute and chronic nephrotoxicity that includes ischemic injury without morphologic features, vacuolar tubulopathy, acute endothelial injury (TMA), and arteriolar hyalinosis.[245,247] These cause secondary pathological effects, such as tubular atrophy, interstitial fibrosis and global or segmental glomerulosclerosis. As judged by protocol biopsies, chronic CNIT is universal in renal transplants after about 5 years.[263] Chronic CNIT can also damage native kidneys in patients with other organ transplants, and contributes to the 7–21% prevalence of end-stage renal disease in non-renal transplant recipients after 5 years.[286]

Acute CNI Toxicity

Toxic Tubulopathy

The biopsy features of acute toxicity are quite variable. A normal biopsy is found in "functional CNIT," which is due to reversible vasospasm.[315] In toxic tubulopathy,

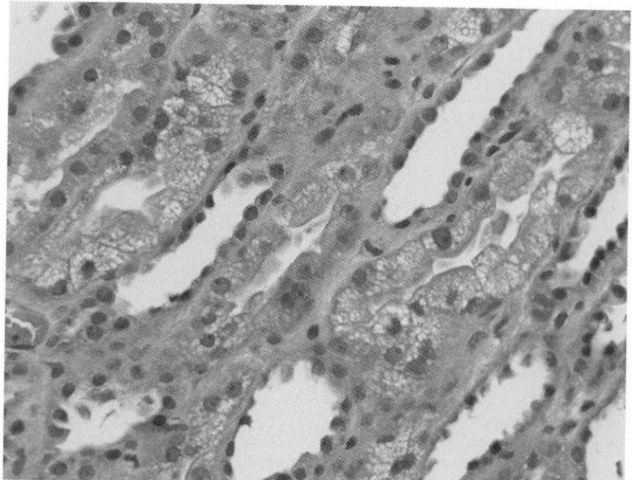

FIGURE 26-8 ■ Acute calcineurin inhibitor nephrotoxicity with isometric vacuolization of tubular epithelium. This change can also be seen in other causes of tubular injury, including ischemia, osmotic diuretics, and intravenous immunoglobulin.

proximal tubules show the most conspicuous morphologic changes with loss of brush borders and isometric (uniformly sized), clear, fine vacuolization (or microvacuoles) in the epithelial cells (Figure 26-8). The microvacuoles contain clear aqueous fluid rather than lipid, and are indistinguishable from those caused by osmotic diuretics or ischemia. EM shows that the vacuoles in cyclosporine toxicity are due to dilation of the endoplasmic reticulum and appear empty.[246] Isometric vacuolization may begin in the straight portion of the proximal tubule,[246] although it can extend to the convoluted portion. The degree of vacuolization does not correlate with drug levels; some patients with CNIT lack the vacuolar change,[218] and isometric vacuoles can be found in a minority of patients with stable renal function.[368] However, reduction of the CNI dosage causes disappearance of tubular vacuolization.[381]

Acute Arteriolar Toxicity and Thrombotic Microangiopathy

Arterioles are a significant target of CNIT. The most characteristic acute changes include individual medial smooth-muscle cell degeneration, necrosis/apoptosis, and loss.[246] The apoptotic smooth-muscle cells are later replaced by rounded, "lumpy" protein deposits or hyalinosis, which is the beginning of a more chronic arteriolopathy.[246] Accumulation of glycogen (PAS-positive, diastase-sensitive) in smooth-muscle cells has been described on high doses.[195] Endothelial cells can have prominent vacuolization and some swelling. Immunofluorescence microscopy of the vessels often shows deposits of IgM, C3 and sometimes fibrin/fibrinogen, but these changes are non-specific.[26]

TMA due to CNI was first reported in bone marrow transplant recipients treated with cyclosporine[351] and occurs in about 1–4% of renal allograft recipients, even with careful attention to drug levels, suggesting that it is dose-independent and probably idiosyncratic.[46,151] Most cases present with a delayed onset and a slow loss of function 1–5 months posttransplant.[369]

The pathologic changes are believed to be an exaggeration of CNI-induced endothelial and smooth-muscle damage. The small arteries and arterioles have mucoid intimal thickening with acid mucopolysaccarides and extravasated red cells and fragments; fibrinoid necrosis and thrombi may be prominent. Apoptosis of endothelial and smooth-muscle cells is seen. The medial smooth muscle can develop a mucoid appearance with loss of a clear definition of the cells.[265] The arterioles may show hypertrophy of the endothelial cells and have a "constricted" appearance.[265] The vascular lumens may be partially or completely obliterated by the intimal proliferation and endothelial swelling. The vascular lesions are most severe in the interlobular and arcuate-sized arteries, and can lead to cortical infarction.[369] By immunofluorescence microscopy, the vessels stain with IgM, C3, and fibrin.[61]

The glomeruli typically have swollen bloodless capillaries with scattered fibrin-platelet thrombi (Figure 26-9A), particularly in the hilum,[351] the so-called pouch lesion.[242] The endothelial cells are swollen and may completely obliterate the capillary lumens. The GBM is segmentally duplicated with cellular (mononuclear or mesangial cell) interposition best seen by EM, which also shows the loss of fenestrae and swelling of the endothelial cytoplasm. Variable mesangial expansion, sclerosis, and mesangiolysis[242] may be seen. Marked congestion and focal, global, or segmental necrosis can be present.[394]

Differential Diagnosis

Acute tubular toxicity of cyclosporine may be indistinguishable from ischemia or tubulopathy from intravenous immunoglobulin or mannitol, which all have vacuoles by light microscopy.[134] By EM a coarser and more varied vacuolization is typical of ATN and the periphery of infarcts[246] compared with the isometric (uniform) vacuoles of cyclosporine toxicity. The vacuoles of osmotic diuretic injury do not involve the endoplasmic reticulum, as do those of cyclosporine toxicity.[242] Necrosis of tubular cells is more common in ATN (0.5% of tubules), characteristically involving whole tubular cross-sections.[368] Acute medial apoptosis/degeneration in arterioles is the only definitive finding favoring CsA toxicity.

Morphology alone cannot distinguish the various etiologies of TMA,[207,279] which in renal transplants are most commonly CNI, AHR, HCV, and recurrent TMA. Recurrence should be the first choice when the recipient's original disease was TMA, unless associated with a diarrheal illness. C4d deposition in PTCs is present in AHR but absent in CNI-associated TMA (as in Figure 26-9B; see section on AHR). Serum should also be tested for anti-HLA class I and class II, and antiendothelial antibodies. HCV-positive renal allograft recipients may develop TMA with associated elevation of circulating anticardiolipin antibody[18]; thus hepatitis serology and anticardiolipin antibody determination could help distinguish between HCV versus CNI in the etiology of TMA. The healing phase of TMA may leave intimal fibrosis that resembles chronic rejection, even with a few intimal mononuclear cells.[61]

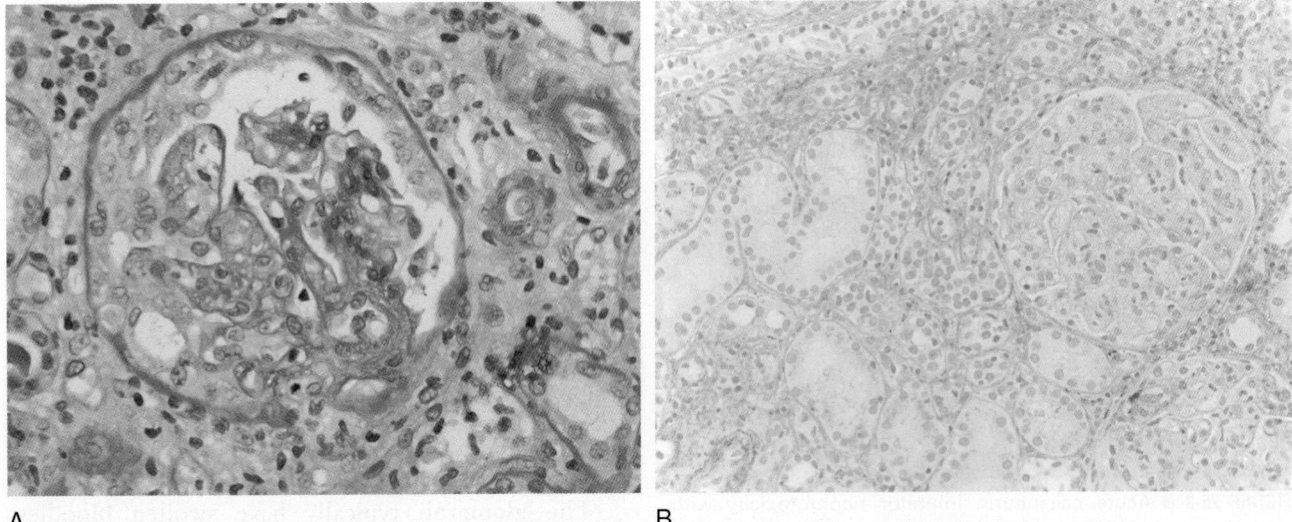

FIGURE 26-9 ■ Thrombotic microangiopathy associated with calcineurin inhibitors. (A) A glomerulus with widespread endothelial swelling, segmental glomerular basement membrane duplication, and focal collapse resembling a crescent. Arterioles show endothelial swelling and occasional peripheral hyaline nodules. Periodic acid–Schiff stain. (B) No glomerular or peritubular capillary C4d deposition is detected in this case. Immunohistochemistry for C4d in paraffin, using rabbit polyclonal anti-C4d.

Chronic CNI Toxicity

Irreversible chronic renal failure due to CNIT was first demonstrated in native kidneys of heart transplant patients who received cyclosporine for more than a year.[256] Similar lesions arise in patients on tacrolimus.[311] Biopsies showed IFTA, arteriolar hyalinosis, and sometimes focal glomerular scarring. These findings have been confirmed and extended in numerous other studies.[26] Since many features resemble chronic rejection in the kidney, the most convincing pathology data come from non-renal transplant patients on cyclosporine.[78,278]

CNI Arteriolopathy

The chronic phase of CNI arteriolopathy is characterized by replacement of the degenerated medial smooth-muscle cells with hyaline-like deposits, in a beaded pattern along the peripheral, outer media (Figure 26-10A). This has been referred to as "nodular protein (hyaline) deposits"[244] in a "pearl-like pattern"[26] and "peripheral medial nodular hyalinosis," and is now called "CNI arteriolopathy." The current evidence supports the view that this type of arteriolopathy is more common but not specific for CNI,[364] despite extensive historical evidence to the contrary.[278] Evidence of apoptosis is sometimes found in the form of

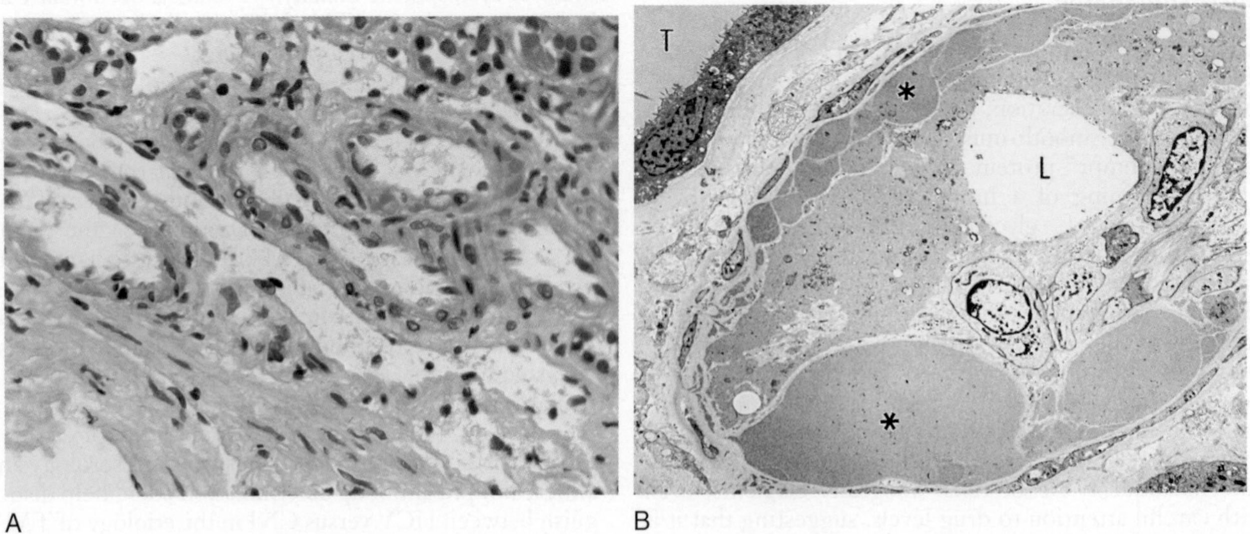

FIGURE 26-10 ■ Calcineurin inhibitor arteriolopathy. (A) Several arterioles with peripheral nodular hyalinosis, where hyalin deposits replace necrotic/apoptotic smooth-muscle cells in the outermost media. (B) Electron microscopy: an artery that has "beads" of hyalin (*) along the outer media. L, arteriolar lumen; T, tubule. (Periodic acid–Schiff 800×; electron microscopy 2700×)

karyorrhexic debris in the medium, but fibrinoid necrosis is not observed.[257] In severe cases the medium is nearly devoid of smooth-muscle cells.[257]

EM reveals a distinctive replacement of individual smooth-muscle cells of afferent arterioles with amorphous electron-dense material, which contains cell debris and protrudes into the adventia (Figure 26-10B). This gives rise to the beaded hyalinosis distribution in the outer medium noted by light microscopy. The myocyte nuclei are sometimes condensed (apoptotic), or have two nuclei or mitotic figures.[415] The cytoplasm is vacuolated, with dilated endoplasmic reticulum, and has degenerated mitochondria, lipofuscin granules, multivesicular bodies, and a disarray of microfibrils and reduced intercellular junctions. The endothelium sometimes appears "swollen," protruding into and narrowing the lumen, and having reduced cell junctions; aggregates of platelets are rare.[13,415] These findings support the view that the smooth-muscle myocyte of the afferent arteriole is a primary target of CNI injury. Immunofluorescence microscopy shows IgM and C3 in a relatively non-specific, but conspicuous, sheathing of the arterioles.[26]

CNI arteriolopathy begins and predominates in the afferent arterioles but may progress to the small arteries and efferent arterioles.[26,415] Decreased renin immunostaining in the juxtaglomerular apparatus suggests that the prime target of CNI is the renin-producing smooth-muscle cell in the afferent arteriole.[378] The frequency of arterioles affected with hyalinosis is typically small (<15%) and the lesions can easily be overlooked.[379] In renal transplant patients on cyclosporine, 15% of protocol biopsies at 6 months showed CNI arteriolopathy which increased to 45% in 18-month protocol biopsies[336]; "non-specific" hyalinosis showed no progressive increase. Ten-year protocol biopsies showed a 2.4-fold increased risk of peripheral nodular hyaline in patients treated with CNI compared to those never on CNI, but even 28% of the latter had the lesion.[364] The arteriolar lesions also develop in native kidneys of patients who receive even low doses of cyclosporine for 2 years.[299,418] Mihatsch has suggested a scoring system of CNI arteriolopathy with improved reproducibility (personal communication).[358]

Glomerular Lesions

After 1 year on cyclosporine, glomeruli show increased numbers with global or segmental sclerosis.[78,278] Focal, segmental sclerosis was more common in CNI-treated bone marrow (13%) and heart transplant (27%) recipients at autopsy than their respective CNI-free controls (0% and 14%).[278] Heart transplant recipients have an increase in the heterogeneity of glomerular volume and size, with more small and large glomeruli (compensatory hypertrophy) compared with controls (living kidney donors).[257] The shift to smaller glomeruli becomes more extreme with chronic renal failure and the hypertrophied glomeruli disappear.[255] Thus hyperfiltration injury probably causes the progressive glomerular proteinuria and sclerosis. Bone marrow and heart transplant patients at autopsy show glomerular collapse in 59% of patients on CNI versus 8% of those not on CNI.[278] This can develop into florid collapsing glomerulopathy, attributed to the severe CNI arteriolopathy.[120]

Immunofluorescence findings are non-specific (IgM and C3 in scarred areas). EM in cardiac and liver transplant recipients showed diffuse expansion of the mesangial matrix, with little hypercellularity, GBM, or podocyte lesions.[78,257] Those with frank collapsing glomerulopathy have podocyte foot process effacement and detachment of podocytes from the GBM.[120] The endothelium shows loss of its normal fenestrae, perhaps reflecting a component of TMA.[61]

Tubules and Interstitium

IFTA was recognized as a feature of CNIT in the early studies.[387] The interstitium had prominent patchy fibrosis, with a scanty infiltrate. Band-like narrow zones of IFTA ("striped fibrosis") were once regarded as characteristic of CNIT[90,322,353]; however, indistinguishable "stripes" occur in patients not maintained on CNI,[74] casting doubt on the specificity of that pattern. Interstitial fibrosis also develops in native kidneys in patients on CNI[243,291,418,419] and remains for at least a month after discontinuing the drug.[239] Thus even low doses of cyclosporine can cause significant and presumably permanent loss of renal function by inducing chronic tubulointerstitial nephritis.[61]

Differential Diagnosis

Distinction between chronic rejection and chronic CNIT is a challenge (Table 26-5). The nodular arteriolopathy is supportive of CNIT but not decisive. The arterioles are relatively spared in chronic rejection, compared with

TABLE 26-5 Differentiation between Chronic Rejection and Chronic Calcineurin Inhibitor Toxicity

	Chronic Rejection	Calcineurin Inhibitor Toxicity
Interstitium		
Infiltrate	Plasma cells	Mild
Fibrosis	Patchy	Patchy, "striped"
Peritubular Capillaries		
C4d	Often positive	Negative
Multilamination BM	Usual	Absent
Tubules		
Tubular atrophy	Usual	Usual
Vacuoles	Occasional	Occasional
Arterioles		
Smooth muscle	Absent	Usual degeneration
External nodular	Absent	Present hyalinosis
Arteries		
Intimal fibrosis	Usual	Can be present but unrelated
Mononuclear cells	Common	Absent intima
Glomeruli		
Duplication GBM	Usual	Absent
Mesangial expansion	Can be present	Can be present

BM, basement membrane; GBM, glomerular basement membrane.

chronic CNIT, and the arteries are more affected, with proliferative intimal fibrosis without elastosis.[245] PTC C4d deposits or mononuclear cells in the arterial intima are the most useful signs of an active rejection process. An inflammatory infiltrate, including plasma cells, is less common in CNIT than rejection.[260] Other features are not decisive. IFTA and glomerular sclerosis are found in either. GBM duplication and endothelial dedifferentiation can also be seen in either, although perhaps more commonly in chronic rejection.[61]

TARGET OF RAPAMYCIN INHIBITOR TOXICITY

Inhibitors of the mammalian target of rapamycin (TORi) (rapamycin, everolimus, sirolimus) can cause DGF due to tubular toxicity that resembles myeloma cast nephropathy. Pathologically, in addition to acute tubular injury, eosinophilic debris and macrophages were present in tubular lumina, that mimicked myeloma casts, but the casts stain for keratin, rather than immunoglobulin light chains.[363] TORi can also cause TMA, indistinguishable from that due to CNI.[316]

Increased proteinuria is common on patients switched from CNI to TORi because they had developed severe CNIT. In these patients, GFR improves but increased proteinuria develops in about 30%.[200] CNI exposure is not necessary for the proteinuric response to TORi. Conversion from azathioprine to TORi can also cause increased proteinuria.[393] Patients started on TORi without CNI had double the risk of proteinuria at 6–12 months compared with those on CNI.[372]

Few pathological studies have been published. One reported a variety of glomerular diseases typical of native kidneys, suggesting recurrent disease.[79] A recipient begun on TORi developed 12 g/day proteinuria in the first week after transplantation, which remitted after the drug was discontinued.[375] Biopsy showed no obvious glomerular disease was evident by light, immunofluorescence, or EM, suggesting the proteinuria was due to failure of tubular reabsorption. One notable case report described collapsing glomerulopathy in a patient with Kaposi's sarcoma converted to TORi from azathioprine.[165] We have seen two cases of FSGS in patients started on TORi: one had collapsing glomerulopathy (Cornell et al., unpublished). More pathology studies are clearly needed, particularly on those patients started on TORi.[61]

DRUG-INDUCED ACUTE TUBULOINTERSTITIAL NEPHRITIS

Drug induced interstitial nephritis in the allograft is similar to that in the native kidney, and resembles tubulointerstitial rejection. Both are characterized by an intense mononuclear interstitial infiltrate and tubulitis, and have variable numbers of eosinophils. Acute rejection occasionally has a prominent eosinophilic infiltrate[8,136,154,189,385,405]; conversely, drug-induced interstitial nephritis may have no eosinophils, especially that due to non-steroidal anti-inflammatory drugs.[60] Endarteritis, if present, is unequivocal evidence for rejection. Strong, but not absolute, evidence for a drug etiology is the invasion of multiple tubules by eosinophils, and eosinophils in tubular casts (Colvin, unpublished observation), usually attributed to prophylactic trimethaprim-sulfamethoxazole (Bactrim). We have also seen one case of severe acute interstitial nephritis and serum sickness-like syndrome secondary to the horse antithymocyte globulin.[61]

INFECTIONS

Many organisms can infect the transplanted kidney, ranging from mycobacteria and candida[229] to herpes simplex virus[355] and human herpesvirus-1.[355] In addition, viruses such as cytomegalovirus and HCV can have indirect effects on the transplant, promoting rejection or immune-mediated disease.[66,317,392] Here we will discuss the three most important types of infections: polyomavirus, adenovirus, and bacterial pyelonephritis.

Polyomavirus Tubulointerstitial Nephritis

PTN has emerged since 1996 as a significant cause of early and late graft damage.[80,81,219,268,272,292] Among various series of patients on tacrolimus/mycophenolate mofetil, PTN arises in about 5%, similar to the prevalence of acute rejection. The virus was originally isolated from BK, a Sudanese patient who had distal donor ureteral stenosis, 3 months after a living related transplant.[111] BK virus is related to JC virus (which also inhabits the human urinary tract) and to simian virus SV40. These viruses are members of the papovavirus group, which includes the papillomaviruses. The BK virus commonly infects urothelium but rarely causes morbidity in immunocompetent individuals. However, in renal transplant recipients three lesions have been attributed to BK virus: hemorrhagic cystitis, ureteral stenosis, and interstitial nephritis.[51,112,153]

PTN is characterized by a patchy mononuclear infiltrate associated with tubulitis and tubular cell injury (Figure 26-11B).[292] The infiltrate often contains plasma cells, which sometimes invade the tubules. Concurrent ACR may be present. Tubular cell apoptosis is prominent, as well as "dedifferentiation" of tubular epithelial cells, with loss of polarity and a spindly shape. PTN has three recognized stages: stage A has only minimal inflammation; stage B shows marked tubular injury, denudation of the TBMs and interstitial edema with a mixed, mild to marked inflammatory cell infiltrate; stage C has marked IFTA.[81,82,150,271,272]

The recognition of viral nuclear inclusions is the key step in diagnosis. The affected nuclei are usually enlarged with a smudgy, amorphous lavender inclusion (Figure 26-11B). Other nuclear changes found less commonly are eosinophilic, granular inclusions with or without a halo, and a vesicular variant with coarsely clumped, irregular basophilic material.[268,269,273] These nuclear inclusions tend to be grouped in tubules, particularly collecting ducts in the cortex and outer medulla, and can often be spotted at low power. Immunohistochemistry and EM confirm the diagnosis. Monoclonal antibodies are commercially available which react with BK-specific

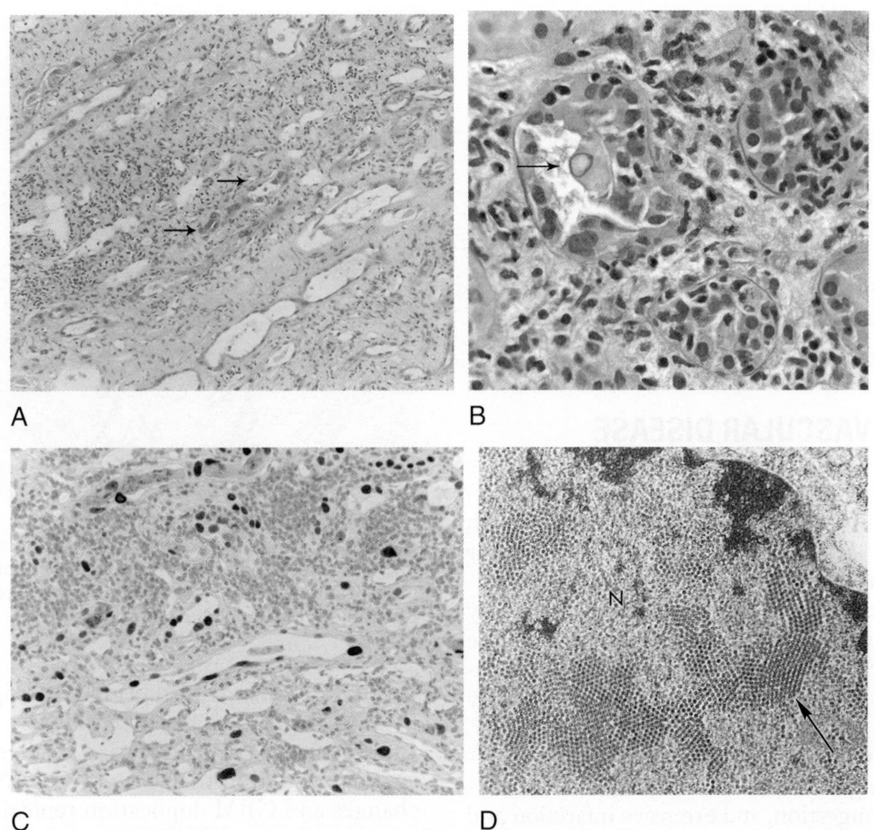

FIGURE 26-11 ■ Polyoma (BK) virus infection. (A) Low-power view showing patchy mononuclear inflammation in the medulla with groups of atypical nuclei in tubular epithelium (arrows). (B) Higher power shows polyomavirus inclusion (arrow), marked tubulitis, and tubular cell apoptosis. (C) Immunohistochemistry: monoclonal antibody to SV40 large T antigen (homologous to BK, JC, and other polyoma viruses), many tubular epithelial cell nuclei appear dark brown due to immunoreactivity for polyoma virus. (D) Electron microscopy: high magnification of a tubular cell nucleus (N) containing polyoma virions (arrow), that are rounded, 30–35 nm in diameter, and organized in arrays (from *Cynomolgus* monkey). (From van Gorder MA, Della Pelle P, Henson JW, et al. Cynomolgus polyoma virus infection: a new member of the polyoma virus family causes interstitial nephritis, ureteritis, and enteritis in immunosuppressed cynomolgus monkeys. Am J Pathol 1999;154:1273-84.)[396]

determinants and with the large T antigen of several polyoma species (Figure 26-11C). EM will reveal the characteristic intranuclear paracrystalline arrays of viral particles of about 40 nm diameter (Figure 26-11D). Other tests useful for monitoring patients at risk are urine cytology ("decoy cells") and polymerase chain reaction quantitation of virus in the blood, although these are not specific enough to make a PTN diagnosis.[61]

Polyomavirus infections may cause an immune complex deposition along the TBM, as described in 43% of cases in a series from Seattle, being the most common cause of IgG deposits in the TBM of transplants.[34] Granular IgG, C3, and C4d are focally present by immunofluorescence and amorphous electron-dense deposits by EM. The prognostic significance is not known.[61]

Late graft fibrosis and scarring/"CAN" may be caused by polyomavirus, even though the virus is no longer demonstrable. The virus is cytopathic for tubular cells and leads to characteristically destructive tubular lesions, with only TBM remaining. The diagnosis is sometimes only possible by review of prior biopsies. Suspicion of PTN is heightened if tubular destruction is severe. The process may be clinically silent: protocol biopsies have shown a subclinical incidence of PTN of 1.2%.[40] Furthermore, PTN can affect native kidneys of recipients of non-renal allografts; only a few cases have been reported, but this may be in part due to a presumption of CNIT and a lack of renal biopsies in this setting.[203]

Adenovirus

Adenovirus, most frequently serotype 11, causes hemorrhagic cystitis and also occasionally tubulointerstitial nephritis in renal allografts, which may resemble a space-occupying lesion by imaging studies.[202,414] Biopsy shows necrotizing inflammation with neutrophils and tubular destruction, interstitial hemorrhage and red cell casts, granulomatous inflammation,[38,161,267,357] or a zonal inflammation localized to the outer medulla.[220] Tubular cells have intranuclear ground-glass inclusions with a distinct halo surrounded by a ring of marginated chromatin and glassy smudged nuclei. The diagnosis is established by immunoperoxidase stains for viral antigen in tubular cells, and EM to reveal the intranuclear crystalline arrays of 75–80-nm viral particles. Immune complexes may also contribute to the injury. Decreased immunosuppression has been followed by recovery.[61]

Acute Pyelonephritis

Pyelonephritis is a potentially devastating complication of transplantation. Pyelonephritis can present as acute renal failure[114,416] and cause graft loss.[139,171] Pyelonephritis arises most often 1 year or more after transplantation (80% of episodes).[298] *Escherichia coli* was the most common organism (80%). Acute pyelonephritis is a not uncommon finding on renal biopsy, despite the expectation that the process is patchy.[416] Renal biopsies are not the usual method of diagnosis; however, if neutrophils are abundant, especially if they form destructive abscesses and casts in tubules, the diagnosis should be at the top of the list. Other variants are emphysematous pyelonephritis, due to gas-producing organisms,[171] xanthogranulomatous pyelonephritis,[87,170] and malakoplakia.[373]

MAJOR RENAL VASCULAR DISEASE

Most arterial thromboses develop in the early posttransplant period and produce acute infarction with microthrombi and scant inflammation.[20] Evidence for underlying rejection should be sought by careful examination of the larger arteries for endarteritis. Renal artery stenosis (typically at the anastomosis site), a cause of late graft dysfunction, can be deceptive clinically and pathologically.[37,356] Biopsies show tubular injury or atrophy with relatively little inflammation or fibrosis.

Renal vein thrombosis causes a swollen and purple kidney, sometimes with graft rupture.[334] The cortex shows severe hemorrhagic congestion, and extensive infarction and necrosis,[238] sometimes with diffuse microcapillary thrombi. Intracapillary leukocytes can be a clue as in native kidneys. Late renal vein thrombosis is associated with proteinuria due to MGN or TG, sometimes with graft loss.[340] Lupus anticoagulant has been detected in a few patients.[215]

DE NOVO GLOMERULAR DISEASE

Patients without previous glomerular disease occasionally develop lesions in the allograft that resemble a primary glomerular disease, rather than the usual chronic allograft glomerulopathy. While some are no doubt coincidental, at least three are related to an alloimmune response to the allograft: MGN, anti-GBM disease in Alport's syndrome, and recurrent nephrotic syndrome in congenital nephrosis. A fourth, relatively common de novo glomerular disease, FSGS, is believed to be related to hyperfiltration injury of the allograft or marked microvascular compromise due to CNIT.[61]

Membranous Glomerulonephritis

De novo MGN is typically a late complication, with a prevalence of about 1–2%.[70,141,251] In contrast, recurrent MGN can present early.[321] The risk factors for de novo MGN include time after transplant, de novo MGN in a first graft,[141] and HCV infection.[70,251] Light microscopy usually shows rather mild GBM changes. Mesangial hypercellularity is found in about 33%. Mononuclear cells can be abundant in glomerular capillaries, raising the possibility of transplant glomerulitis or renal vein thrombosis.[249] Immunofluorescence shows granular deposits along the GBM that stain for IgG, C3, C4d, and factor H[67]; about 35% are more irregular and segmental in distribution than typical primary (idiopathic) MGN.[249,391] By EM subepithelial electron-dense deposits are present (Figure 26-12), which are smaller and more irregular in distribution than primary MGN.[249,391] Endothelial changes and GBM duplication typical of TG are present in half of the cases.[249,391] Repeat biopsies have shown persistence or progression of the deposits in most cases and occasional resolution.[12,249] The pathogenesis of de novo MGN has not been established. The literature supports the hypothesis that de novo MGN may be a form of AMR or directed at minor histocompatibility antigen(s) in the glomerulus, presumably on the podocyte or a special type of chronic rejection.[57,389,391] The common presence of TG is consistent with this hypothesis.[249,391]

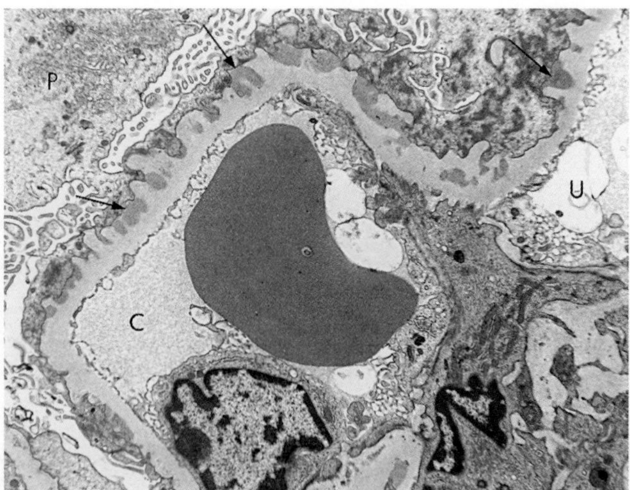

FIGURE 26-12 ■ De novo membranous glomerulonephritis: subepithelial electron-dense deposits (arrows) along the glomerular basement membrane with intervening basement membrane spikes. Podocyte (P) foot processes are effaced. C, capillary lumen; U, urinary space.

Anti-GBM Nephritis

Patients with Alport's syndrome or hereditary nephritis commonly develop anti-GBM alloantibodies, because they genetically lack self-tolerance to GBM collagen components. However this leads to glomerulonephritis in only a minority. Overall, de novo crescentic and necrotizing glomerulonephritis due to anti-GBM antibodies after transplantation is uncommon, seen in only 5% of male adult renal allograft recipients with typical Alport's syndrome.[173,174,16] The pathology is similar to that in native kidney with prominent crescents (not a feature of allograft rejection), segmental necrosis, and red cell casts. Second transplantation with and without recurrent anti-GBM nephritis have both been reported.[77,121,395] The 5-year graft survival may be equal to that of non-Alport's recipients.[119]

De Novo Podocytopathy in Congenital Nephrosis

Congenital nephrotic syndrome of the Finnish type, an autosomal recessive disease due to mutations in the nephrin gene NPHS1, paradoxically leads to posttransplant nephrotic syndrome.[213,283] The podocyte pathology resembles minimal-change disease and usually responds to cyclophosphamide.[98,194] De novo "minimal-change disease" is thought to be caused by the alloantibodies to nephrin in some cases.[296]

Focal Segmental Glomerulosclerosis

De novo FSGS has been described in adult recipients of pediatric kidneys,[266,412] in which the presumed pathogenesis is hyperfiltration injury, in long-standing grafts, in which parenchymal loss due to CNIT or chronic rejection leads to hyperfiltration injury of residual glomeruli, and as the collapsing variant of FSGS, probably related to CNI arteriolopathy.[231]

De novo collapsing glomerulopathy presents months to years after transplantation with proteinuria (2–12 g/day).[231,258,374] Diffuse or focal, global, or segmental collapse of glomeruli was evident with prominent hyperreactive podocytes (Figure 26-13). Arteriolar hyalinosis,

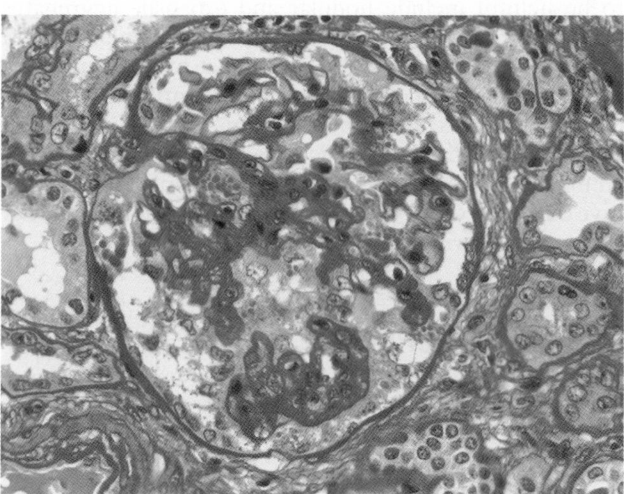

FIGURE 26-13 ■ De novo collapsing glomerulopathy: collapsed glomerular capillaries and prominent podocyte proliferation, hypertrophy, and abundant reabsorption droplets. Severe arteriolar hyalinosis with peripheral nodules typical of calcineurin inhibitor arteriolopathy was present. This is a native kidney in a patient with a heart–lung transplant. Periodic acid–Schiff stain. (From Goes N, Colvin RB. Renal failure nine years after a heart-lung transplant. N Engl J Med 2006;6:671–9.)[120]

arteriosclerosis, and interstitial fibrosis were also present. A rapid progression to renal failure occurred in 80% of the patients (2–12 months). The cause is unknown; all patients were human immunodeficiency virus-negative. Collapsing glomerulopathy can also develop in native kidneys in patients on CNI (Figure 26-13).[120]

RECURRENT RENAL DISEASE

Recurrent disease (e.g., dense deposit in Figure 26-14) is a significant cause of allograft failure.[45,97,308] The frequency and clinical significance of recurrence vary with the disease (Table 26-6). In one study, glomerular diseases, including recurrent and de novo glomerulonephritis and TG, were responsible for 37% of cases of graft loss; 14% of death-censored graft losses were due to recurrent glomerular disease.[88] Recurrence of immune-mediated disease may become a greater problem in the future with longer graft survival and development of tolerance protocols that require no immunosuppression. The reader is referred to a comprehensive review elsewhere for detailed information regarding specific diseases.[61]

Transplantation also can uniquely illuminate the early pathologic events that precede clinical signs and determine the reversibility of pre-existing lesions in the donor kidney (e.g., diabetes, IgA nephropathy). For example, early recurrent MGN – as early as 2 weeks posttransplant the glomeruli can show staining in a membranous pattern by immunofluorescence for IgG, C4d, and kappa and lambda light chains, but corresponding electron-dense deposits may not be present ultrastructurally; these features can be seen on biopsy without proteinuria clinically.[321] Later biopsies of the allografts show a more typical membranous pattern with subepithelial deposits by EM. Diabetic nephropathy begins with an increase in allograft glomerular volume at 6 months,[288] followed by increases in mesangial volume.[408] Thickening of the GBM is first evident after 2–3 years[32,408] and nodular diabetic glomerulosclerosis at 5–15 years posttransplant (Figure 26-15).[140] Tubulointerstitial diseases may also recur, such as with recurrent oxalate nephropathy in primary hyperoxaluria.[25]

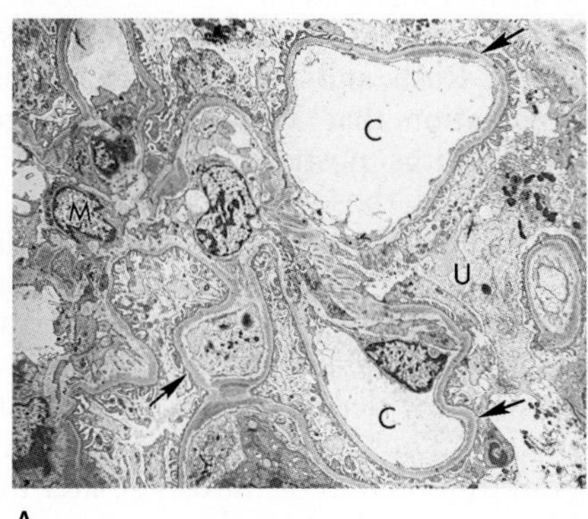

A

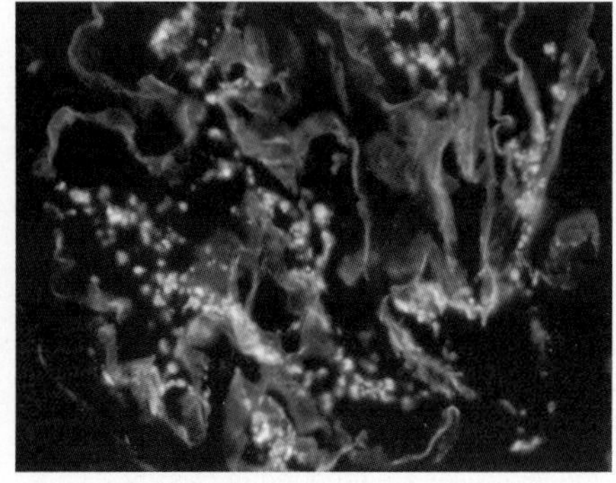

B

FIGURE 26-14 ■ Recurrent dense deposit disease. (A) Electron microscopy: widespread very electron-dense deposits that are continuous, linear, and embedded in the glomerular basement membrane proper, i.e., intramembranous (arrows). Similar deposits are also seen in the mesangium (M). C, capillary lumen; U, urinary space. (B) Immunofluorescence microscopy: staining for C3 shows broad linear ribbon-like deposits along the glomerular basement membrane and blob-like deposits in the mesangium (mesangial rings).

TABLE 26-6 **Classification of Recurrent Renal Disease**

Usually Recur (>50% of Patients)	
Adverse effect*	Primary hemolytic uremic syndrome
	Primary oxalosis
	Dense deposit disease
	Collapsing FSGS†
Little or no adverse effect	Immunotactoid/fibrillary glomerulopathy†
	Systemic light-chain disease†
	Diabetes mellitus‡
Commonly Recur (5–50%)	
Adverse effect	FSGS
	Membranoproliferative GN, type I
	Membranous GN
	ANCA-related diseases
	Wegener's granulomatosis
	Pauci-immune GN
	Microscopic polyarteritis
	Progressive systemic sclerosis
	Sickle cell nephropathy†
Little or no adverse effect	IgA nephropathy
	Henoch–Schönlein purpura
	Amyloidosis
Rarely Recur (<5%)	
Adverse effect	Anti-GBM disease
Little or no adverse effect	Systemic lupus erythematosus
	Fabry's disease
	Cystinosis
Recurrence reported§	Thrombotic thrombocytopenic purpura
	Adenosine phosphoribosyl transferase deficiency
	Familial fibronectin glomerulopathy
	Lipoprotein glomerulopathy
	Malacoplakia
Never Recur (0%)	
Unique complications	Hereditary nephritis/Alport's syndrome (anti-GBM disease)
	Congenital nephrosis (nephrotic syndrome; nephrin autoantibody)
No unique complications	Polycystic disease (all genetic types)
	Osteo-onychodysplasia (nail-patella)†
	Acquired cystic disease
	Secondary hemolytic uremic syndrome (infection)
	Secondary FSGS
	Familial FSGS†
	Postinfectious acute glomerulonephritis†

*Adverse effect defined as graft loss of >5% (when disease recurs).
†Limited experience: few cases reported (*n*<10).
‡Arteriolar and glomerular lesions recur to some degree in most, if not all, cases, but nodular glomerulosclerosis delayed until >5 years.
§Recurrence occurs, but too few cases are reported to classify frequency or consequences.
ANCA, antineutrophil cytoplasmic antibody; FSGS, focal segmental glomerulosclerosis; GBM, glomerular basement membrane; GN, glomerulonephritis.

Posttransplant Lymphoproliferative Disease

Immunosuppression leads to an increased risk of malignancy, particularly those neoplasms caused by viruses and ultraviolet radiation. These malignancies are presumptively suppressed by immune responses which recognize the viral or mutation-derived neoantigens. The major viral-related tumors are Kaposi's sarcoma (human herpesvirus-8), cervical cancer (human papillomavirus), and PTLD (Epstein–Barr virus). Of these, PTLD not uncommonly affects the kidney, sometimes presenting as graft dysfunction.

PTLD involving the kidney can resemble ACR, in having a widespread mononuclear infiltrate invading tubules and even vessels.[228,309,337] In our experience, a useful clue that favors PTLD is when the infiltrate forms a dense sheet of monomorphic lymphoblasts without edema or granulocytes (Figure 26-16A). Serpiginous necrosis of the lymphoid cells (irregular patches) is distinctive, but not always present.[309] The other features found to be helpful include nodular and expansile aggregates of immature lymphoid cells; the nuclei are enlarged and vesicular with prominent nucleoli that may be multiple. Immunohistochemistry is helpful in identifying the predominance of B cells in the infiltrate, which is never seen in rejection alone. If the cells have a monoclonal kappa or lambda phenotype the diagnosis is confirmed. The definitive diagnosis of PTLD is in situ hybridization for EBER (Epstein–Barr virus-encoded RNA) (Figure 26-16B).

PROTOCOL BIOPSIES

"Protocol" or "surveillance" biopsies taken at predetermined times for evaluation of the status of the renal allograft, independent of renal function, are currently the standard of care at several leading transplant centers[64,177,253,263,327,341,371] and widely used in clinical trials to evaluate efficacy.[55] Protocol biopsies have the potential ability to reveal mechanisms of late graft loss and to identify active processes that might be interrupted therapeutically before irreversible injury has occurred.[88] The risk of protocol biopsy is low. There were no deaths or graft losses in the Hannover series of over 1000 biopsies[339] and graft loss was 0.04%.[104]

The current interest in protocol biopsies started with David Rush and colleagues, who made the surprising observation that 30% of biopsies from stable patients 1–3 months posttransplant showed histological rejection[325] and those with these lesions show later loss of renal function.[326,327] Many other studies have confirmed this result.[64,177,253,263,327,341] Mononuclear inflammation that meets the Banff criteria for ACR or borderline acute rejection is found in 5–50% of protocol biopsies in the first 12 months, depending on therapy and patient populations.[264] Those with inflammation have a higher risk of graft dysfunction or fibrosis at later time points.[65,178,254,264] Grafts with both inflammation and fibrosis do the worst.[64,214,253,350] In one study, the best predictor of allograft function 1 year after transplantation was persistent inflammation, of any type, including those patterns considered in Banff to be irrelevant to the diagnosis of acute rejection

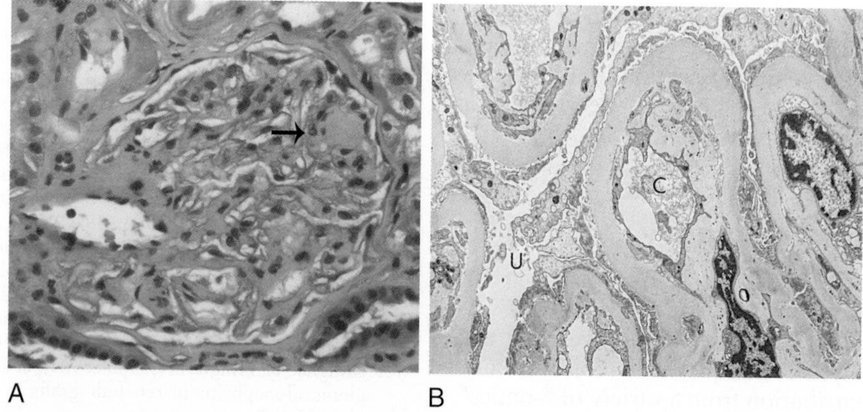

FIGURE 26-15 ■ Recurrent diabetic nephropathy 12 years after transplant. (A) Glomerulus with prominent Kimmelstiel–Wilson mesangial nodules (arrow) and arteriolar hyalinosis. Periodic acid–Schiff stain. (B) Electron microscopy of another case shows homogeneous thickening of the glomerular basement membrane up to 1100 nm. C, capillary lumen; U, urinary space.

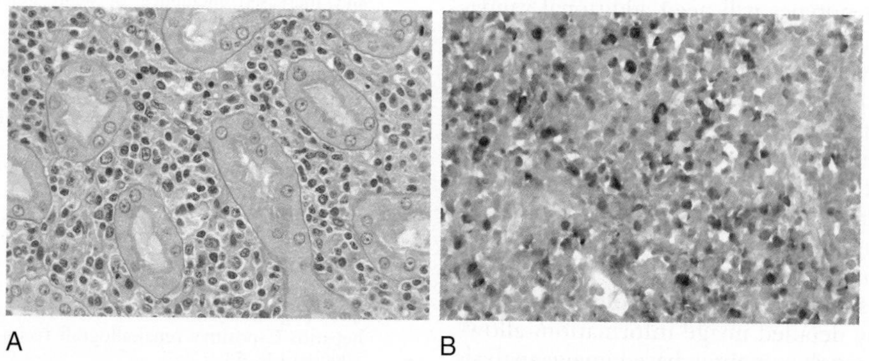

FIGURE 26-16 ■ Posttransplant lymphoproliferative disease. (A) Dense mononuclear cell infiltrate in the interstitium that permeates between the tubules without tubulitis (although tubulitis may occur in posttransplant lymphoproliferative disease (PTLD)). The monomorphic infiltrate and the lack of edema distinguish PTLD from the usual cellular rejection. (B) In situ hybridization: nuclei of mononuclear cells stain dark, brown-black for Epstein–Barr virus-encoded RNA (EBER), which is the definitive test for the diagnosis of PTLD.

(in areas of interstitial fibrosis, around large blood vessels, in nodules, or in subcapsular areas).[235] Infiltrates in areas of atrophy correlated with IFTA at 6 months and graft dysfunction at 2 years. In another study, protocol biopsies at 1 year posttransplant that showed fibrosis and inflammation predicted a worse GFR at 5 years compared to biopsies with fibrosis and no inflammation and compared to normal biopsies.[293] These results suggest that these infiltrates are part of the pathogenesis of slow, progressive renal injury.[55,214]

Grafts in recipients that are developing tolerance also typically have graft infiltrates, sometimes termed the "acceptance reaction,"[349] which spontaneously disappears and is followed by indefinite graft survival.[31,330] The acceptance reaction had less infiltration by CD3+ T cells and macrophages, less T-cell activation, long-lasting apoptosis of graft-infiltrating T cells, less IFN-γ and more IL-10 than rejecting grafts.

What differentiates infiltrates in patients with stable and unstable graft function? In stable grafts endarteritis is found rarely (0.3% in one series)[234] and can herald an impending acute episode.[325] Among the interstitial infiltrates, only the diffuse pattern (rich in macrophages and granzyme B CTLs) was more common in biopsies taken for acute dysfunction.[235] In contrast, nodular infiltrates (rich in B cells and activated T cells) were more common in protocol biopsies. Similarly, infiltrates rich in activated macrophages distinguished biopsies with clinical versus subclinical acute rejection.[127] Molecular studies have shown that increased levels of transcripts for T-bet (a Th1 master transcription factor), FasL (cytotoxic mediator) and CD152 (CTLA-4, an inhibitory costimulatory molecule) are associated with graft dysfunction.[152]

Foxp3 cells are on the list of suspects to distinguish non-aggressive infiltrates.[31,348] Recent evidence shows that regulatory T cells (Treg) that express the Foxp3 transcription factor infiltrate tolerated grafts in mice treated with costimulatory blockade.[196] Foxp3 cells can also be found in grafts with infiltrates interpreted as acute rejection.[398] Although the significance of Foxp3+ cells has yet to be determined, high numbers of such Treg cells are likely beneficial,[248] in view of the known suppressor functions of these cells. The hope of much ongoing research is the discovery of markers that predict graft acceptance in a clinical setting.[100,248]

The most important question is whether treatment of subclinical rejection is beneficial (and then what therapy is optimal). No study has dared to randomize treatment in patients with acute rejection on protocol biopsy. The closest to a controlled trial was that of Rush and colleagues, who found that patients with protocol biopsies, treated with steroid boluses if they had subclinical rejection, had a better outcome than a group of patients who declined a renal biopsy (and were presumed to have a similar frequency of subclinical rejection).[327] Other diseases revealed by the "eye of the needle" clearly benefit from altered therapy, including CNIT[262,263] and polyomavirus infection.[40]

FUTURE DIRECTIONS IN BIOPSY ASSESSMENT

Biopsy assessment will likely further improve from advances in image analysis techniques and molecular understanding. The contribution from a variety of "-omics" fields and technologies has led to improvements in allograft biopsy assessment.[235,343] Molecular phenotypes have been characterized for a variety of pathologic states in renal allograft biopsies; however, the clinical utility of these molecular phenotypes will need additional validation before it is understood in what circumstances molecular assessment can be superior to histopathology. In addition, before molecular biopsy assessment is clinically feasible as an adjunct to histopathology, additional improvements are needed in molecular method turnaround time, cost, and the reporting required for high-dimensional "-omics" data.

In addition, digital microscopic techniques (e.g., whole-slide scanning) are emerging which will likely improve biopsy assessment. Whole histology slide images contain highly detailed image information, allowing data mining through computer-based image analysis techniques. For example, interstitial fibrosis assessment can be automated; and automation can likely make interstitial fibrosis assessment more reproducible.[91] Multiparameter staining techniques can also be coupled with digital imaging and analysis algorithms to provide more objective and quantitative assessment of molecular derangements in the renal biopsies. The advancements in technology and pathologic understanding will likely provide a more complete picture and allow enhanced patient care.

Acknowledgments

Many thanks to Dr. Shamila Mauiyyedi, a coauthor of the prior version, and to Dr. Paul J. Kurtin, for his useful suggestions on the manuscript.

REFERENCES

1. Abouna GM, Al Adnani MS, Kremer GD, et al. Reversal of diabetic nephropathy in human cadaveric kidneys after transplantation into non-diabetic recipients. Lancet 1983;2:1274–6.
2. Adams DH, Tilney NL, Collins JJJ, et al. Experimental graft arteriosclerosis. I. The Lewis-to-F-344 allograft model. Transplantation 1992;53:1115–9.
3. Ahern AT, Artruc SB, DellaPelle P, et al. Hyperacute rejection of HLA-AB-identical renal allografts associated with B lymphocyte and endothelial reactive antibodies. Transplantation 1982;33:103–6.
4. Aiello FB, Calabrese F, Rigotti P, et al. Acute rejection and graft survival in renal transplanted patients with viral diseases. Mod Pathol 2004;17:189–96.
5. Akasaka Y, Ishikawa Y, Kato S, et al. Induction of Fas-mediated apoptosis in a human renal epithelial cell line by interferon-gamma: involvement of Fas-mediated apoptosis in acute renal rejection. Mod Pathol 1998;11:1107–14.
6. Akiyoshi T, Hirohashi T, Alessandrini A, et al. Role of complement and NK cells in antibody mediated rejection. Hum Immunol 2012;73:1226–32.
7. Alchi B, Nishi S, Kondo D, et al. Osteopontin expression in acute renal allograft rejection. Kidney Int 2005;67:886–96.
8. Almirall J, Campistol JM, Sole M, et al. Blood and graft eosinophilia as a rejection index in kidney transplant. Nephron 1993;65:304–9.
9. Alpers CE, Davis CL, Barr D, et al. Identification of platelet-derived growth factor A and B chains in human renal vascular rejection. Am J Pathol 1996;148:439–51.
10. Alpers CE, Gordon D, Gown AM. Immunophenotype of vascular rejection in renal transplants. Mod Pathol 1990;3:198–203.
11. Andrews PA, Finn JE, Lloyd CM, et al. Expression and tissue localization of donor-specific complement C3 synthesized in human renal allografts. Eur J Immunol 1995;25:1087–93.
12. Antignac C, Hinglais N, Gubler MC, et al. De novo membranous glomerulonephritis in renal allografts in children. Clin Nephrol 1988;30:1–7.
13. Antonovych TT, Sabnis SG, Austin HA, et al. Cyclosporine A-induced arteriolopathy. Transplant Proc 1988;20(Suppl. 3):951–8.
14. Artz MA, Steenbergen EJ, Hoitsma AJ, et al. Renal transplantation in patients with hemolytic uremic syndrome: high rate of recurrence and increased incidence of acute rejections. Transplantation 2003;76:821–6.
15. August C, Schmid KW, Dietl KH, et al. Prognostic value of lymphocyte apoptosis in acute rejection of renal allografts. Transplantation 1999;67:581–5.
16. Bach D, Peters A, Rowemeier H, et al. Anti-basal membrane glomerulonephritis after homologous kidney transplantation in hereditary Alport's nephropathy. Dtsch Med Wochenschr 1991;116:1752–6.
17. Bach FH, Turman MA, Vercellotti GM, et al. Accommodation: a working paradigm for progressing toward clinical discordant xenografting. Transplant Proc 1991;23:205–7.
18. Baid S, Pascual M, Williams Jr WW, et al. Renal thrombotic microangiopathy associated with anticardiolipin antibodies in hepatitis C-positive renal allograft recipients. J Am Soc Nephrol 1999;10:146–53.
19. Baid-Agrawal S, Farris 3rd AB, Pascual M, et al. Overlapping pathways to transplant glomerulopathy: chronic humoral rejection, hepatitis C infection, and thrombotic microangiopathy. Kidney Int 2011;80:879–85.
20. Bakir N, Sluiter WJ, Ploeg RJ, et al. Primary renal graft thrombosis. Nephrol Dial Transplant 1996;11:140–7.
21. Barrett M, Milton AD, Barrett J, et al. Needle biopsy evaluation of class II major histocompatibility complex antigen expression for the differential diagnosis of cyclosporine nephrotoxicity from kidney graft rejection. Transplantation 1987;44:223–7.
22. Bates WD, Davies DR, Welsh K, et al. An evaluation of the Banff classification of early renal allograft biopsies and correlation with outcome. Nephrol Dial Transplant 1999;14:2364–9.
23. Bellamy CO, Randhawa PS. Arteriolitis in renal transplant biopsies is associated with poor graft outcome. Histopathology 2000;36:488–92.
24. Bentall A, Cornell LD, Gloor JM, et al. Five-year outcomes in living donor kidney transplants with a positive crossmatch. Am J Transplant 2012;142:634–41.
25. Bergstralh EJ, Monico CG, Lieske JC, et al. Transplantation outcomes in primary hyperoxaluria. Am J Transplant 2010;10:2493–501.
26. Bergstrand A, Bohmann SO, Farnsworth A, et al. Renal histopathology in kidney transplant recipients immunosuppressed with cyclosporin A: results of an international workshop. Clin Nephrol 1985;24:107–19.
27. Bestard O, Cruzado JM, Mestre M, et al. Achieving donor-specific hyporesponsiveness is associated with FOXP3+ regulatory T cell recruitment in human renal allograft infiltrates. J Immunol 2007;179:4901–9.
28. Bestard O, Cruzado JM, Rama I, et al. Presence of FoxP3+ regulatory T cells predicts outcome of subclinical rejection of renal allografts. J Am Soc Nephrol 2008;19:2020–6.
29. Bishop GA, Hall BM, Duggin GG, et al. Immunopathology of renal allograft rejection analyzed with monoclonal antibodies to mononuclear cell markers. Kidney Int 1986;29:708–17.
30. Bishop GA, Waugh JA, Landers DV, et al. Microvascular destruction in renal transplant rejection. Transplantation 1989;48:408–14.

31. Blancho G, Gianello PR, Lorf T, et al. Molecular and cellular events implicated in local tolerance to kidney allografts in miniature swine. Transplantation 1997;63:26–33.
32. Bohman SO, Tyden G, Wilczek H, et al. Prevention of kidney graft diabetic nephropathy by pancreas transplantation in man. Diabetes 1985;34:306–8.
33. Bohmig GA, Exner M, Habicht A, et al. Capillary C4d deposition in kidney allografts: a specific marker of alloantibody-dependent graft injury. J Am Soc Nephrol 2002;13:1091–9.
34. Bracamonte ER, Furmanczyk PS, Smith KD, et al. Tubular basement membrane immune deposits associated with polyoma virus nephropathy in renal allografts. Mod Pathol 2006;19:259A.
35. Briscoe DM, Pober JSS, Harmon WE, et al. Expression of vascular cell adhesion molecule-1 in human renal allografts. J Am Soc Nephrol 1992;3:1180–5.
36. Brockmeyer C, Ulbrecht M, Schendel DJ, et al. Distribution of cell adhesion molecules (ICAM-1, VCAM-1, ELAM-1) in renal tissue during allograft rejection. Transplantation 1993;55:610–5.
37. Bruno S, Remuzzi G, Ruggenenti P. Transplant renal artery stenosis. J Am Soc Nephrol 2004;15:134–41.
38. Bruno B, Zager RA, Boeckh MJ, et al. Adenovirus nephritis in hematopoietic stem-cell transplantation. Transplantation 2004;77:1049–57.
39. Brunt EM, Kissane JM, Cole BR, et al. Transmission and resolution of type I membranoproliferative glomerulonephritis in recipients of cadaveric renal allografts. Transplantation 1988;46:595–8.
40. Buehrig CK, Lager DJ, Stegall MD, et al. Influence of surveillance renal allograft biopsy on diagnosis and prognosis of polyomavirus-associated nephropathy. Kidney Int 2003;64:665–73.
41. Burke BA, Chavers BM, Gillingham KJ, et al. Chronic renal allograft rejection in the first 6 months posttransplant. Transplantation 1995;60:1413–7.
42. Burns JM, Cornell LD, Perry DK, et al. Alloantibody levels and acute humoral rejection early after positive crossmatch kidney transplantation. Am J Transplant 2008;8:2684–94.
43. Busch GJ, Galvanek EG, Reynolds ES. Human renal allografts. Analysis of lesions in long-term survivors. Hum Pathol 1971;2:253–98.
44. Cahen R, Dijoud F, Couchoud C, et al. Evaluation of renal grafts by pretransplant biopsy. Transplant Proc 1995;27:2470.
45. Cameron JS. Recurrent primary disease and de novo nephritis following renal transplantation. Pediatr Nephrol 1991;5:412–21.
46. Candinas D, Keusch G, Schlumpf R, et al. Hemolytic-uremic syndrome following kidney transplantation: prognostic factors. Schweiz Med Wochenschr 1994;124:1789–99.
47. Cecka JM. Current methodologies for detecting sensitization to HLA antigens. Curr Opin Organ Transplant 2011;16:398–403.
48. Charney DA, Nadasdy T, Lo AW, et al. Plasma cell-rich acute renal allograft rejection. Transplantation 1999;68:791–7.
49. Chicano SL, Cornell LD, Selig MK, et al. Distinctive ultrastructural features of chronic allograft glomerulopaithy: new formation of circumferential glomerular basement membrane. Mod Pathol 2006;19(Suppl. 1):260A–1A, 1207.
50. Cohen AH, Gonzalez S, Nast CC, et al. Frozen-section analysis of allograft renal biopsy specimens. Reliable histopathologic data for rapid decision making. Arch Pathol Lab Med 1991;115:386–9.
51. Coleman DV, MacKenzie EFD, Gardner SD, et al. Human polyoma virus (BK) infection and ureteric stenosis in renal allograft recipients. J Clin Pathol 1978;31:338–47.
52. Collins AB, Chicano S, Cornell LD, et al. Putative antibody-mediated rejection with C4d deposition in HLA-identical, ABO compatible renal allografts. Transplant Proc 2006;38:3427–9.
53. Collins AB, Schneeberger EE, Pascual MA, et al. Complement activation in acute humoral renal allograft rejection: diagnostic significance of C4d deposits in peritubular capillaries. J Am Soc Nephrol 1999;10:2208–14.
54. Colovai AI, Vasilescu ER, Foca-Rodi A, et al. Acute and hyperacute humoral rejection in kidney allograft recipients treated with anti-human thymocyte antibodies. Hum Immunol 2005;66:501–12.
55. Colvin RB. Eye of the needle. Am J Transplant 2006;354:2803–13.
56. Colvin RB. Pathology of renal allografts. In: Colvin RB, Bhan AK, McCluskey RT, editors. Diagnostic immunopathology. 2nd ed. New York: Raven Press; 1995. p. 329–66.
57. Colvin RB. Renal transplant pathology. In: Jennette JC, Olson JL, Schwartz MM, et al., editors. Heptinstall's Pathology of the Kidney. 5th ed. Philadelphia: Lippincott-Raven; 1998. p. 1409–540.
58. Colvin R, Chase C, Winn H, et al. Chronic allograft arteriopathy: insights from experimental models. In: Orosz C, editor. Transplant vascular sclerosis. Austin, TX: R.G. Landes Biomedical Publishers; 1995. p. 7–34.
59. Colvin RB, Cohen AH, Saiontz C, et al. Evaluation of pathologic criteria for acute renal allograft rejection: reproducibility, sensitivity, and clinical correlation. J Am Soc Nephrol 1997;8:1930–41.
60. Colvin RB, Fang LS-T. Interstitial nephritis. In: Tisher CC, Brenner BM, editors. Renal pathology. 2nd ed. Philadelphia, PA: JB Lippincott; 1994. p. 723–68.
61. Colvin RB, Nickeleit V. Renal transplant pathology. In: Jennette JC, Olson JL, Schwartz MM, et al., editors. Heptinstall's pathology of the kidney. 6th ed. Philadelphia, PA: Lippincott Williams & Wilkins; 2006. p. 1347–490.
62. Cook CH, Bickerstaff AA, Wang JJ, et al. Spontaneous renal allograft acceptance associated with "regulatory" dendritic cells and IDO. J Immunol 2008;180:3103–12.
63. Cornell LD, Colvin RB. Chronic allograft nephropathy. Curr Opin Nephrol Hypertens 2005;14:229–34.
64. Cosio FG, Grande JP, Wadei H, et al. Predicting subsequent decline in kidney allograft function from early surveillance biopsies. Am J Transplant 2005;5:2464–72.
65. Cosio FG, Lager DJ, Lorenz EC, et al. Significance and implications of capillaritis during acute rejection of kidney allografts. Transplantation 2010;89:1088–94.
66. Cosio FG, Roche Z, Agarwal A, et al. Prevalence of hepatitis C in patients with idiopathic glomerulonephritis in native and transplant kidneys. Am J Kidney Dis 1996;28:752–8.
67. Cosyns JP, Kazatchkine MD, Bhakdi S, et al. Immunohistochemical analysis of C3 cleavage fragments, factor H, and the C5b-9 terminal complex of complement in de novo membranous glomerulonephritis occurring in patients with renal transplant. Clin Nephrol 1986;26:203–8.
68. Cramer DV, Qian SQ, Harnaha J, et al. Cardiac transplantation in the rat. I. The effect of histocompatibility differences on graft arteriosclerosis. Transplantation 1989;47:414–9.
69. Crespo M, Pascual M, Tolkoff-Rubin N, et al. Acute humoral rejection in renal allograft recipients: I. Incidence, serology and clinical characteristics. Transplantation 2001;71:652–8.
70. Cruzado JM, Carrera M, Torras J, et al. Hepatitis C virus infection and de novo glomerular lesions in renal allografts. Am J Transplant 2001;1:171–8.
71. Curtis JJ, Julian BA, Sanders CE, et al. Dilemmas in renal transplantation: when the clinical course and histological findings differ. Am J Kidney Dis 1996;27:435–40.
72. Danilewicz M, Wagrowska-Danilewicz M. Immunohistochemical analysis of the interstitial mast cells in acute rejection of human renal allografts. Med Sci Monit 2004;10:BR151–6.
73. Davenport A, Younie ME, Parsons JE, et al. Development of cytotoxic antibodies following renal allograft transplantation is associated with reduced graft survival due to chronic vascular rejection. Nephrol Dial Transplant 1994;9:1315–9.
74. Dell'Antonio G, Randhawa PS. "Striped" pattern of medullary ray fibrosis in allograft biopsies from kidney transplant recipients maintained on tacrolimus. Transplantation 1999;67:484–6.
75. Desvaux D, Le Gouvello S, Pastural M, et al. Acute renal allograft rejections with major interstitial oedema and plasma cell-rich infiltrates: high γ-interferon expression and poor clinical outcome. Nephrol Dial Transplant 2004;19:933–9.
76. Desvaux D, Schwarzinger M, Pastural M, et al. Molecular diagnosis of renal-allograft rejection: correlation with histopathologic evaluation and antirejection-therapy resistance. Transplantation 2004;78:647–53.
77. Diaz JI, Valenzuela R, Gephardt G, et al. Anti-glomerular and anti-tubular basement membrane nephritis in a renal allograft recipient with Alport's syndrome. Arch Pathol Lab Med 1994;118(7):728–31.
78. Dische FE, Neuberger J, Keating J, et al. Kidney pathology in liver allograft recipients after long-term treatment with cyclosporin A. Lab Invest 1988;58:395–402.
79. Dittrich E, Schmaldienst S, Soleiman A, et al. Rapamycin-associated post-transplantation glomerulonephritis and its remission after reintroduction of calcineurin-inhibitor therapy. Transpl Int 2004;17:215–20.
80. Drachenberg CB, Beskow CO, Cangro CB, et al. Human polyoma virus in renal allograft biopsies: morphological findings and correlation with urine cytology. Hum Pathol 1999;30:970–7.

81. Drachenberg CB, Hirsch HH, Ramos E, et al. Polyomavirus disease in renal transplantation: review of pathological findings and diagnostic methods. Hum Pathol 2005;36:1245–55.
82. Drachenberg CB, Papadimitriou JC, Hirsch HH, et al. Histological patterns of polyomavirus nephropathy: correlation with graft outcome and viral load. Am J Transplant 2004;4:2082–92.
83. Dragun D, Muller DN, Brasen JH, et al. Angiotensin II type 1-receptor activating antibodies in renal-allograft rejection. N Engl J Med 2005;352:558–69.
84. Edwards EB, Posner MP, Maluf DG, et al. Reasons for non-use of recovered kidneys: the effect of donor glomerulosclerosis and creatinine clearance on graft survival. Transplantation 2004;77:1411–5.
85. Einecke G, Fairhead T, Hidalgo LG, et al. Tubulitis and epithelial cell alterations in mouse kidney transplant rejection are independent of CD103, perforin or granzymes A/B. Am J Transplant 2006;6:2109–20.
86. Einecke G, Melk A, Ramassar V, et al. Expression of CTL associated transcripts precedes the development of tubulitis in T-cell mediated kidney graft rejection. Am J Transplant 2005;5:1827–36.
87. Elkhammas EA, Mutabagani KH, Sedmak DD, et al. Xanthogranulomatous pyelonephritis in renal allografts: report of 2 cases. J Urol 1994;151:127–8.
88. El-Zoghby ZM, Stegall MD, Lager DJ, et al. Identifying specific causes of kidney allograft loss. Am J Transplant 2009;9:527–35.
89. Escofet X, Osman H, Griffiths DF, et al. The presence of glomerular sclerosis at time zero has a significant impact on function after cadaveric renal transplantation. Transplantation 2003;75:344–6.
90. Farnsworth A, Hall BM, Ng A, et al. Renal biopsy morphology in renal transplantation. Am J Surg Pathol 1984;8:243–52.
91. Farris AB, Colvin RB. Renal interstitial fibrosis: mechanisms and evaluation. Curr Opin Nephrol Hypertens 2012;21:289–300.
92. Farris AB, Taheri D, Kawai T, et al. Acute renal endothelial injury during marrow recovery in a cohort of combined kidney and bone marrow allografts. Am J Transplant 2011;11:1464–77.
93. Faull RJ, Russ GR. Tubular expression of intercellular adhesion molecule-1 during renal allograft rejection. Transplantation 1989;48:226–30.
94. Fellström B, Klareskog L, Heldin CH, et al. Platelet-derived growth factor receptors in the kidney – upregulated expression in inflammation. Kidney Int 1989;36:1099–102.
95. Feucht HE, Felber E, Gokel MJ, et al. Vascular deposition of complement-split products in kidney allografts with cell-mediated rejection. Clin Exp Immunol 1991;86:464–70.
96. Fidler ME, Gloor JM, Lager DJ, et al. Histologic findings of antibody-mediated rejection in ABO blood-group-incompatible living-donor kidney transplantation. Am J Transplant 2004;4:101–7.
97. Floege J. Recurrent glomerulonephritis following renal transplantation: an update. Nephrol Dial Transplant 2003;18:1260–5.
98. Flynn JT, Schulman SL, deChadarevian JP, et al. Treatment of steroid-resistant post-transplant nephrotic syndrome with cyclophosphamide in a child with congenital nephrotic syndrome. Pediatr Nephrol 1992;6:553–5.
99. Fox WM, Hameed A, Hutchins GM, et al. Perforin expression localizing cytotoxic lymphocytes in the intimas of coronary arteries with transplant-related accelerated arteriosclerosis. Hum Pathol 1993;24:477–82.
100. Fudaba Y, Spitzer TR, Shaffer J, et al. Myeloma responses and tolerance following combined kidney and nonmyeloablative marrow transplantation: in vivo and in vitro analyses. Am J Transplant 2006;6:2121–33.
101. Fuggle SV, McWhinnie DL, Chapman JR, et al. Sequential analysis of HLA class II antigen expression in human renal allografts: induction of tubular class II antigens and correlation with clinical parameters. Transplantation 1985;42:144–50.
102. Fuggle SV, McWhinnie DL, Morris PJ. Precise specificity of induced tubular HLA-class II antigens in renal allografts. Transplantation 1987;44:214–20.
103. Fuggle SV, Sanderson JB, Gray DW, et al. Variation in expression of endothelial adhesion molecules in pretransplant and transplanted kidneys – correlation with intragraft events. Transplantation 1993;55:117–23.
104. Furness PN, Philpott CM, Chorbadjian MT, et al. Protocol biopsy of the stable renal transplant: a multicenter study of methods and complication rates. Transplantation 2003;76:969–73.
105. Furness PN, Taub N, Assmann KJ, et al. International variation in histologic grading is large, and persistent feedback does not improve reproducibility. Am J Surg Pathol 2003;27:805–10.
106. Fusaro F, Murer L, Busolo F, et al. CMV and BKV ureteritis: which prognosis for the renal graft? J Nephrol 2003;16:591–4.
107. Gaber LW, Gaber AO, Tolley EA, et al. Prediction by postrevascularization biopsies of cadaveric kidney allografts of rejection, graft loss, and preservation nephropathy. Transplantation 1992;53:1219–25.
108. Gaber LW, Gaber AO, Vera SR, et al. Successful reversal of hyperacute renal allograft rejection with the anti-CD3 monoclonal OKT3. Transplantation 1992;54:930–2.
109. Gaber LW, Moore LW, Alloway RR, et al. Glomerulosclerosis as a determinant of posttransplant function of older donor renal allografts. Transplantation 1995;60:334–9.
110. Gago M, Cornell LD, Kremers WK, et al. Kidney allograft inflammation and fibrosis, causes and consequences. Am J Transplant 2012;12:1199–207.
111. Gardner SD, Field AM, Coleman DV, et al. New human papovavirus (B.K.) isolated from urine after renal transplantation. Lancet 1971;1:1253–7.
112. Gardner SD, MacKenzie EF, Smith C, et al. Prospective study of the human polyomaviruses BK and JC and cytomegalovirus in renal transplant recipients. J Clin Pathol 1984;37:578–86.
113. Gebel HM, Bray RA. The evolution and clinical impact of human leukocyte antigen technology. Curr Opin Nephrol Hypertens 2010;19:598–602.
114. Gillum DM, Kelleher SP. Acute pyelonephritis as a cause of late transplant dysfunction. Am J Med 1985;78:156–8.
115. Girlanda R, Kleiner DE, Duan Z, et al. Monocyte infiltration and kidney allograft dysfunction during acute rejection. Am J Transplant 2008;8:600–7.
116. Glassock RJ, Feldman D, Reynolds ES, et al. Human renal isografts: a clinical and pathologic analysis. Medicine 1968;47:411–24.
117. Gloor JM, Sethi S, Stegall MD, et al. Transplant glomerulopathy: subclinical incidence and association with alloantibody. Am J Transplant 2007;7:2124–32.
118. Gloor JM, Winters JL, Cornell LD, et al. Baseline donor-specific antibody levels and outcomes in positive crossmatch kidney transplantation. Am J Transplant 2010;10:582–9.
119. Gobel J, Olbricht CJ, Offner G, et al. Kidney transplantation in Alport's syndrome: long-term outcome and allograft anti-GBM nephritis. Clin Nephrol 1992;38:299–304.
120. Goes N, Colvin RB. Renal failure nine years after a heart-lung transplant. N Engl J Med 2006;6:671–9.
121. Goldman M, Depierreux M, De Pauw L, et al. Failure of two subsequent renal grafts by anti-GBM glomerulonephritis in Alport's syndrome: case report and review of the literature. Transpl Int 1990;3:82–5.
122. Gough J, Rush D, Jeffery J, et al. Reproducibility of the Banff schema in reporting protocol biopsies of stable renal allografts. Nephrol Dial Transplant 2002;17:1081–4.
123. Gould VE, Martinez LV, Virtanen I, et al. Differential distribution of tenascin and cellular fibronectins in acute and chronic renal allograft rejection. Lab Invest 1992;67:71–9.
124. Gouldesbrough DR, Axelsen RA. Arterial endothelialitis in chronic renal allograft rejection: a histopathological and immunocytochemical study. Nephrol Dial Transplant 1994;9:35–40.
125. Grafft CA, Cornell LD, Gloor JM, et al. Antibody-mediated rejection following transplantation from an HLA-identical sibling. Nephrol Dial Transplant 2010;25:307–10.
126. Grimbert P, Mansour H, Desvaux D, et al. The regulatory/cytotoxic graft-infiltrating T cells differentiate renal allograft borderline change from acute rejection. Transplantation 2007;83:341–6.
127. Grimm PC, McKenna R, Nickerson P, et al. Clinical rejection is distinguished from subclinical rejection by increased infiltration by a population of activated macrophages. J Am Soc Nephrol 1999;10:1582–9.
128. Haas M. C4d-negative antibody-mediated rejection in renal allografts: evidence for its existence and effect on graft survival. Clin Nephrol 2011;75:271–8.
129. Haas M. Pathologic features of antibody-mediated rejection in renal allografts: an expanding spectrum. Curr Opin Nephrol Hypertens 2012;21:264–71.

130. Haas M, Mirocha J. Early ultrastructural changes in renal allografts: correlation with antibody-mediated rejection and transplant glomerulopathy. Am J Transplant 2011;11:2123–31.
131. Haas M, Montgomery RA, Segev DL, et al. Subclinical acute antibody-mediated rejection in positive crossmatch renal allografts. Am J Transplant 2007;7:576–85.
132. Haas M, Rahman MH, Racusen LC, et al. C4d and C3d staining in biopsies of ABO- and HLA-incompatible renal allografts: correlation with histologic findings. Am J Transplant 2006;6:1829–40.
133. Haas M, Ratner LE, Montgomery RA. C4d staining of perioperative renal transplant biopsies. Transplantation 2002;74:711–7.
134. Haas M, Sonnenday CJ, Cicone JS, et al. Isometric tubular epithelial vacuolization in renal allograft biopsy specimens of patients receiving low-dose intravenous immunoglobulin for a positive crossmatch. Transplantation 2004;78:549–56.
135. Habib R, Broyer M. Clinical significance of allograft glomerulopathy. Kidney Int Suppl 1993;43:S95–8.
136. Hallgren R, Bohman SO, Fredens K. Activated eosinophil infiltration and deposits of eosinophil cationic protein in renal allograft rejection. Nephron 1991;59:266–70.
137. Halloran PF, Schlaut J, Solez K, et al. The significance of the anti-class I antibody response. II. Clinical and pathologic features of renal transplants with anti-class I-like antibody. Transplantation 1992;53:550–5.
138. Halloran PF, Wadgymar A, Ritchie S, et al. The significance of the anti-class I antibody response. I. Clinical and pathologic features of anti-class I-mediated rejection. Transplantation 1990;49:85–91.
139. Hansen BL, Rohr N, Svendsen V, et al. Bacterial urinary tract infection in cyclosporine-A immunosuppressed renal transplant recipients. Scand J Infect Dis 1988;20:425–7.
140. Hariharan S, Smith RD, Viero R, et al. Diabetic nephropathy after renal transplantation. Clinical and pathologic features. Transplantation 1996;62:632–5.
141. Heidet L, Gagnadoux ME, Beziau A, et al. Recurrence of de novo membranous glomerulonephritis on renal grafts. Clin Nephrol 1994;41:314–8.
142. Herman J, Lerut E, Van Damme-Lombaerts R, et al. Capillary deposition of complement C4d and C3d in pediatric renal allograft biopsies. Transplantation 2005;79:1435–40.
143. Herzenberg AM, Gill JS, Djurdjev O, et al. C4d deposition in acute rejection: an independent long-term prognostic factor. J Am Soc Nephrol 2002;13:234–41.
144. Hidalgo LG, Sis B, Sellares J, et al. NK cell transcripts and NK cells in kidney biopsies from patients with donor-specific antibodies: evidence for NK cell involvement in antibody-mediated rejection. Am J Transplant 2010;10:1812–22.
145. Hiki Y, Leong AY, Mathew TH, et al. Typing of intraglomerular mononuclear cells associated with transplant glomerular rejection. Clin Nephrol 1986;26:244–9.
146. Hill GS, Nochy D, Bruneval P, et al. Donor-specific antibodies accelerate arteriosclerosis after kidney transplantation. J Am Soc Nephrol 2011;22:975–83.
147. Hill GS, Nochy D, Loupy A. Accelerated arteriosclerosis: a form of transplant arteriopathy. Curr Opin Organ Transplant 2010;15:11–5.
148. Hirohashi T, Chase CM, Della Pelle P, et al. A novel pathway of chronic allograft rejection mediated by NK cells and alloantibody. Am J Transplant 2012;12:313–21.
149. Hirohashi T, Uehara S, Chase CM, et al. Complement independent antibody-mediated endarteritis and transplant arteriopathy in mice. Am J Transplant 2010;9:1–8.
150. Hirsch HH, Brennan DC, Drachenberg CB, et al. Polyomavirus-associated nephropathy in renal transplantation: interdisciplinary analyses and recommendations. Transplantation 2005;79:1277–86.
151. Hochstetler LA, Flanigan MJ, Lager DJ. Transplant-associated thrombotic microangiopathy: the role of IgG administration as initial therapy. Am J Kidney Dis 1994;23:444–50.
152. Hoffmann SC, Hale DA, Kleiner DE, et al. Functionally significant renal allograft rejection is defined by transcriptional criteria. Am J Transplant 2005;5:573–81.
153. Hogan TF, Borden EC, McBain JA, et al. Human polyomavirus infections with JC virus and BK virus in renal transplant patients. Ann Intern Med 1980;92:373–8.
154. Hongwei W, Nanra RS, Stein A, et al. Eosinophils in acute renal allograft rejection. Transpl Immunol 1994;2:41–6.
155. Hourmant M, Cesbron-Gautier A, Terasaki PI, et al. Frequency and clinical implications of development of donor-specific and non-donor-specific HLA antibodies after kidney transplantation. J Am Soc Nephrol 2005;16:2804–12.
156. Howie AJ, Bryan RL, Gunson BK. Arteries and veins formed within renal vessels: a previously neglected observation. Virchows Arch 1992;420:301–4.
157. Hruban RH, Long PP, Perlman EJ, et al. Fluorescence in situ hybridization for the Y-chromosome can be used to detect cells of recipient origin in allografted hearts following cardiac transplantation. Am J Pathol 1993;142:975–80.
158. Hsu HC, Suzuki Y, Churg J, et al. Ultrastructure of transplant glomerulopathy. Histopathology 1980;4:351–67.
159. Imai N, Nishi S, Alchi B, et al. Immunohistochemical evidence of activated lectin pathway in kidney allografts with peritubular capillary C4d deposition. Nephrol Dial Transplant 2006;21:2589–95.
160. Ishii Y, Sawada T, Kubota K, et al. Injury and progressive loss of peritubular capillaries in the development of chronic allograft nephropathy. Kidney Int 2005;67:321–32.
161. Ito M, Hirabayashi N, Uno Y, et al. Necrotizing tubulointerstitial nephritis associated with adenovirus infection. Hum Pathol 1991;22:1225–31.
162. Ito H, Kasagi N, Shomori K, et al. Apoptosis in the human allografted kidney. Analysis by terminal deoxynucleotidyl transferase-mediated DUTP-botin nick end labeling. Transplantation 1995;60:794–8.
163. Ivanyi B, Fahmy H, Brown H, et al. Peritubular capillaries in chronic renal allograft rejection: a quantitative ultrastructural study. Hum Pathol 2000;31:1129–38.
164. Ivanyi B, Kemeny E, Szederkenyi E, et al. The value of electron microscopy in the diagnosis of chronic renal allograft rejection. Mod Pathol 2001;14:1200–8.
165. Izzedine H, Brocheriou I, Frances C. Post-transplantation proteinuria and sirolimus. N Engl J Med 2005;353:2088–9.
166. Jabs WJ, Logering BA, Gerke P, et al. The kidney as a second site of human C-reactive protein formation in vivo. Eur J Immunol 2003;33:152–61.
167. Jain S, Curwood V, White SA, et al. Sub-clinical acute rejection detected using protocol biopsies in patients with delayed graft function. Transpl Int 2000;13(Suppl. 1):S52–5.
168. Jeannet M, Pinn VW, Flax MH, et al. Humoral antibodies in renal allotransplantation in man. N Engl J Med 1970;282:111–7.
169. Ji S, Liu M, Chen J, et al. The fate of glomerular mesangial IgA deposition in the donated kidney after allograft transplantation. Clin Transplant 2004;18:536–40.
170. Jones BF, Nanra RS, Grant AB, et al. Xanthogranulomatous pyelonephritis in a renal allograft: a case report. J Urol 1989;141:926–7.
171. Kalra OP, Malik N, Minz M, et al. Emphysematous pyelonephritis and cystitis in a renal transplant recipient – computed tomographic appearance. Int J Artif Organs 1993;16:41–4.
172. Karpinski J, Lajoie G, Cattran D, et al. Outcome of kidney transplantation from high-risk donors is determined by both structure and function. Transplantation 1999;67:1162–7.
173. Kashtan CE. Alport syndrome and thin glomerular basement membrane disease. J Am Soc Nephrol 1998;9:1736–50.
174. Kashtan CE. Alport syndrome: renal transplantation and donor selection. Ren Fail 2000;22:765–8.
175. Kataoka K, Naomoto Y, Shiozaki S, et al. Infiltration of perforin-positive mononuclear cells into the rejected kidney allograft. Transplantation 1992;53:240–2.
176. Kawai T, Cosimi AB, Spitzer TR, et al. HLA-mismatched renal transplantation without maintenance immunosuppression. N Engl J Med 2008;358:353–61.
177. Kee TY, Chapman JR, O'Connell PJ, et al. Treatment of subclinical rejection diagnosed by protocol biopsy of kidney transplants. Transplantation 2006;82:36–42.
178. Kennedy LJ, Weissman IL. Dual origin of intimal cells in cardiac allograft arteriosclerosis. N Engl J Med 1971;285:884–8.
179. Kerby JD, Verran DJ, Luo KL, et al. Immunolocalization of FGF-1 and receptors in glomerular lesions associated with chronic human renal allograft rejection. Transplantation 1996;62:190–200.
180. Kieran N, Wang X, Perkins J, et al. Combination of peritubular c4d and transplant glomerulopathy predicts late renal allograft failure. J Am Soc Nephrol 2009;20:2260–8.
181. Kirk AD, Hale DA, Mannon RB, et al. Results from a human renal allograft tolerance trial evaluating the humanized CD52-specific monoclonal antibody alemtuzumab (CAMPATH-1H). Transplantation 2003;76:120–9.

182. Kirk AD, Mannon RB, Kleiner DE, et al. Results from a human renal allograft tolerance trial evaluating T-cell depletion with alemtuzumab combined with deoxyspergualin. Transplantation 2005;80:1051–9.
183. Kiss D, Landman J, Mihatsch M, et al. Risks and benefits of graft biopsy in renal transplantation under cyclosporin-A. Clin Nephrol 1992;38:132–4.
184. Kissmeyer-Nielsen F, Olsen S, Petersen VP, et al. Hyperacute rejection of kidney allografts, associated with pre-existing humoral antibodies against donor cells. Lancet 1966;2:662–5.
185. Kon SP, Templar J, Dodd SM, et al. Diagnostic contribution of renal allograft biopsies at various intervals after transplantation. Transplantation 1997;63:547–50.
186. Koo DD, Roberts IS, Quiroga I, et al. C4d deposition in early renal allograft protocol biopsies. Transplantation 2004;78:398–403.
187. Kooijmans-Coutinho MF, Bruijn JA, Hermans J, et al. Evaluation by histology, immunohistology and PCR of protocollized renal biopsies 1 week post-transplant in relation to subsequent rejection episodes. Nephrol Dial Transplant 1995;10:847–54.
188. Kooijmans-Coutinho MF, Hermans J, Schrama E, et al. Interstitial rejection, vascular rejection, and diffuse thrombosis of renal allografts. Predisposing factors, histology, immunohistochemistry, and relation to outcome. Transplantation 1996;61:1338–44.
189. Kormendi F, Amend W. The importance of eosinophil cells in kidney allograft rejection. Transplantation 1988;45:537–9.
190. Kriz W, Kaissling B, Le Hir M. Epithelial-mesenchymal transition (EMT) in kidney fibrosis: fact or fantasy? J Clin Invest 2011;121:468–74.
191. Kummer J, Wever P, Kamp A, et al. Expression of granzyme A and B proteins by cytotoxic lymphocytes involved in acute renal allograft rejection. Kidney Int 1995;47:70–7.
192. Kuypers DR, Chapman JR, O'Connell PJ, et al. Predictors of renal transplant histology at three months. Transplantation 1999;67:1222–30.
193. Kuypers DR, Lerut E, Evenepoel P, et al. C3d deposition in peritubular capillaries indicates a variant of acute renal allograft rejection characterized by a worse clinical outcome. Transplantation 2003;76:102–8.
194. Lane PH, Schnaper HW, Vernier RL, et al. Steroid-dependent nephrotic syndrome following renal transplantation for congenital nephrotic syndrome. Pediatr Nephrol 1991;5:300–3.
195. Larsen S, Brun C, Duun S, et al. Early arteriolopathy following "high-dose" cyclosporine in kidney transplantation. APMIS 1988;(Suppl. 4);66–73.
196. Lee I, Wang L, Wells AD, et al. Recruitment of Foxp3+ T regulatory cells mediating allograft tolerance depends on the CCR4 chemokine receptor. J Exp Med 2005;201:1037–44.
197. Lefaucheur C, Loupy A, Vernerey D, et al. Antibody-mediated vascular rejection of kidney allografts: a population-based study. Lancet 2013;381:313–9.
198. Lerut E, Kuypers D, Van Damme B. C4d deposition in the peritubular capillaries of native renal biopsies. Histopathology 2005;47:430–2.
199. Lerut E, Kuypers DR, Verbeken E, et al. Acute rejection in non-compliant renal allograft recipients: a distinct morphology. Clin Transplant 2007;21:344–51.
200. Letavernier E, Pe'raldi MN, Pariente A, et al. Proteinuria following a switch from calcineurin inhibitors to sirolimus. Transplantation 2005;80:1198–203.
201. Leventhal J, Abecassis M, Miller J, et al. Chimerism and tolerance without GVHD or engraftment syndrome in HLA-mismatched combined kidney and hematopoietic stem cell transplantation. Sci Transl Med 2012;4:124–8.
202. Lim AK, Parsons S, Ierino F. Adenovirus tubulointerstitial nephritis presenting as a renal allograft space occupying lesion. Am J Transplant 2005;5:2062–6.
203. Limaye AP, Smith KD, Cook L, et al. Polyomavirus nephropathy in native kidneys of non-renal transplant recipients. Am J Transplant 2005;5:614–20.
204. Lipkowitz GS, Madden RL, Kurbanov A, et al. Transplantation and 2-year follow-up of kidneys procured from a cadaver donor with a history of lupus nephritis. Transplantation 2000;69:1221–4.
205. Lipman ML, Stevens AC, Strom TB. Heightened intragraft CTL gene expression in acutely rejecting renal allografts. J Immunol 1994;152:5120–7.
206. Lobo PI, Spencer CE, Stevenson WC, et al. Evidence demonstrating poor kidney graft survival when acute rejections are associated with IgG donor-specific lymphocytotoxin. Transplantation 1995;59:357–60.
207. Loomis LJ, Aronson AJ, Rudinsky R, et al. Hemolytic uremic syndrome following bone marrow transplantation: a case report and review of the literature. Am J Kidney Dis 1989;14:324–8.
208. Lorenz M, Regele H, Schillinger M, et al. Risk factors for capillary C4d deposition in kidney allografts: evaluation of a large study cohort. Transplantation 2004;78:447–52.
209. Loupy A, Hill GS, Suberbielle C, et al. Significance of C4d Banff scores in early protocol biopsies of kidney transplant recipients with preformed donor-specific antibodies (DSA). Am J Transplant 2011;11:56–65.
210. Loupy A, Suberbielle-Boissel C, Hill GS, et al. Outcome of subclinical antibody-mediated rejection in kidney transplant recipients with preformed donor-specific antibodies. Am J Transplant 2009;9:2561–70.
211. Lucas ZJ, Coplon N, Kempson R, et al. Early renal transplant failure associated with subliminal sensitization. Transplantation 1970;10:522–8.
212. Magil AB, Tinckam K. Monocytes and peritubular capillary C4d deposition in acute renal allograft rejection. Kidney Int 2003;63:1888–93.
213. Mahan JD, Maver SM, Sibley RK, et al. Congenital nephrotic syndrome: evolution of medical management and results of transplantation. J Pediatr 1984;105:549–57.
214. Mannon RB, Matas AJ, Grande J, et al. Inflammation in areas of tubular atrophy in kidney allograft biopsies: a potent predictor of allograft failure. Am J Transplant 2010;10:2066–73.
215. Marcen R, Pascual J, Quereda C, et al. Lupus anticoagulant and thrombosis of kidney allograft vessels. Transplant Proc 1990;22:1396–8.
216. Marcussen N, Lai R, Olsen TS, et al. Morphometric and immunohistochemical investigation of renal biopsies from patients with transplant ATN, native ATN, or acute graft rejection. Transplant Proc 1996;28:470–6.
217. Martin L, Guignier F, Mousson C, et al. Detection of donor-specific anti-HLA antibodies with flow cytometry in eluates and sera from renal transplant recipients with chronic allograft nephropathy. Transplantation 2003;76:395–400.
218. Marucci G, Morandi L, Macchia S, et al. Fibrinogen storage disease without hypofibrinogenaemia associated with acute infection. Histopathology 2003;42:22–5.
219. Mathur VS, Olson JL, Darragh TM, et al. Polyomavirus-induced interstitial nephritis in two renal transplant recipients: case reports and review of the literature. Am J Kidney Dis 1997;29:754–8.
220. Mathur SC, Squiers EC, Tatum AH, et al. Adenovirus infection of the renal allograft with sparing of pancreas graft function in the recipient of a combined kidney-pancreas transplant. Transplantation 1998;65:138–41.
221. Mauiyyedi S, Colvin RB. Humoral rejection in kidney transplantation: new concepts in diagnosis and treatment. Curr Opin Nephrol Hypertens 2002;11:609–18.
222. Mauiyyedi S, Crespo M, Collins AB, et al. Acute humoral rejection in kidney transplantation: II. Morphology, immunopathology, and pathologic classification. J Am Soc Nephrol 2002;13:779–87.
223. Mauiyyedi S, Pelle PD, Saidman S, et al. Chronic humoral rejection: identification of antibody-mediated chronic renal allograft rejection by C4d deposits in peritubular capillaries. J Am Soc Nephrol 2001;12:574–82.
224. Mazzucco G, Motta M, Segoloni G, et al. Intertubular capillary changes in the cortex and medulla of transplanted kidneys and their relationship with transplant glomerulopathy: an ultrastructural study of 12 transplantectomies. Ultrastruct Pathol 1994;18:533–7.
225. McCall SJ, Tuttle-Newhall JE, Howell DN, et al. Prognostic significance of microvascular thrombosis in donor kidney allograft biopsies. Transplantation 2003;75:1847–52.
226. McLaren AJ, Marshall SE, Haldar NA, et al. Adhesion molecule polymorphisms in chronic renal allograft failure. Kidney Int 1999;55:1977–82.
227. McManus BM, Malcom G, Kendall TJ, et al. Prominence of coronary arterial wall lipids in human heart allografts. Implications for pathogenesis of allograft arteriopathy. Am J Pathol 1995;147:293–308.
228. Meehan SM, Domer P, Josephson M, et al. The clinical and pathologic implications of plasmacytic infiltrates in percutaneous renal allograft biopsies. Hum Pathol 2001;32:205–15.

229. Meehan SM, Josephson MA, Haas M. Granulomatous tubulointerstitial nephritis in the renal allograft. Am J Kidney Dis 2000;36:E27.
230. Meehan S, McCluskey R, Pascual M, et al. Cytotoxicity and apoptosis in human renal allografts: identification, distribution, and quantitation of cells with a cytotoxic granule protein GMP-17 (TIA-1) and cells with fragmented nuclear DNA. Lab Invest 1997;76:639–49.
231. Meehan SM, Pascual M, Williams WW, et al. De novo collapsing glomerulopathy in renal allografts. Transplantation 1998;65:1192–7.
232. Meehan SM, Siegel CT, Aronson AJ, et al. The relationship of untreated borderline infiltrates by the Banff criteria to acute rejection in renal allograft biopsies. J Am Soc Nephrol 1999;10:1806–14.
233. Meleg-Smith S, Gauthier PM. Abundance of interstitial eosinophils in renal allografts is associated with vascular rejection. Transplantation 2005;79:444–50.
234. Mengel M, Bogers J, Bosmans JL, et al. Incidence of C4d stain in protocol biopsies from renal allografts: results from a multicenter trial. Am J Transplant 2005;5:1050–6.
235. Mengel M, Gwinner W, Schwarz A, et al. Infiltrates in protocol biopsies from renal allografts. Am J Transplant 2006;6:747–52.
236. Mengel M, Mueller I, Behrend M, et al. Prognostic value of cytotoxic T-lymphocytes and CD40 in biopsies with early renal allograft rejection. Transpl Int 2004;17:293–300.
237. Mengel M, Sis B, Haas M, et al. Banff 2011 Meeting report: new concepts in antibody-mediated rejection. Am J Transplant 2012;12:563–70.
238. Merion RM, Calne RY. Allograft renal vein thrombosis. Transplant Proc 1985;17:1746–50.
239. Messana JM, Johnson KJ, Mihatsch MJ. Renal structure and function effects after low dose cyclosporine in psoriasis patients: a preliminary report. Clin Nephrol 1995;43:150–3.
240. Messias NC, Eustace JA, Zachary AA, et al. Cohort study of the prognostic significance of acute transplant glomerulitis in acutely rejecting renal allografts. Transplantation 2001;72:655–60.
241. Metzgar RS, Seigler HF, Ward FE, et al. Immunological studies on elutes from human renal allografts. Transplantation 1972;13:131–7.
242. Mihatsch MJ, Gudat F, Ryffel B, et al. Cyclosporine nephropathy. In: Tisher CC, Brenner BM, editors. Renal pathology: with clinical and functional correlations. 2nd ed. Philadelphia: JB Lippincott; 1994. p. 1641–81.
243. Mihatsch MJ, Helmchen U, Casanova P, et al. Kidney biopsy findings in cyclosporine-treated patients with insulin-dependent diabetes mellitus. Klin Wochenschr 1991;69:354–9.
244. Mihatsch MJ, Morozumi K, Strom EH, et al. Renal transplant morphology after long-term therapy with cyclosporine. Transplant Proc 1995;27:39–42.
245. Mihatsch MJ, Ryffel B, Gudat F. The differential diagnosis between rejection and cyclosporine toxicity. Kidney Int 1995;52(Suppl.):S63–9.
246. Mihatsch MJ, Thiel G, Ryffel B. Cyclosporine nephrotoxicity. Adv Nephrol Necker Hosp 1988;17:303–20.
247. Mihatsch MJ, Theil G, Spichtin HP, et al. Morphological findings in kidney transplants after treatment with cyclosporine. Transplant Proc 1983;15(Suppl. 1):2821–35.
248. Miyajima M, Chase CM, Alessandrini A, et al. Early acceptance of renal allografts in mice is dependent on foxp3(+) cells. Am J Pathol 2011;178(4):1635–45.
249. Monga G, Mazzucco G, Basolo B, et al. Membranous glomerulonephritis (MGN) in transplanted kidneys: investigation on 256 renal allografts. Mod Pathol 1993;6:249–58.
250. Monga G, Mazzucco G, Messina M, et al. Intertubular capillary changes in kidney allografts: a morphologic investigation on 61 renal specimens. Mod Pathol 1992;5:125–30.
251. Morales JM, Pascual-Capdevila J, Campistol JM, et al. Membranous glomerulonephritis associated with hepatitis C virus infection in renal transplant patients. Transplantation 1997;63:1634–9.
252. Morel D, Normand E, Lemoine C, et al. Tumor necrosis factor alpha in human kidney transplant rejection – analysis by in situ hybridization. Transplantation 1993;55:773–7.
253. Moreso F, Ibernon M, Goma M, et al. Subclinical rejection associated with chronic allograft nephropathy in protocol biopsies as a risk factor for late graft loss. Am J Transplant 2006;6:747–52.
254. Munivenkatappa RB, Schweitzer EJ, Papadimitriou JC, et al. The Maryland aggregate pathology index: a deceased donor kidney biopsy scoring system for predicting graft failure. Am J Transplant 2008;8:2316–24.
255. Myers BD, Newton L, Boshkos C, et al. Chronic injury of human renal microvessels with low-dose cyclosporine therapy. Transplantation 1988;46:694–703.
256. Myers BD, Ross J, Newton L, et al. Cyclosporine-associated chronic nephropathy. N Engl J Med 1984;311:699–705.
257. Myers BD, Sibley R, Newton L, et al. The long-term course of cyclosporine-associated chronic nephropathy. Kidney Int 1988;33:590–600.
258. Nadasdy T, Allen C, Zand MS. Zonal distribution of glomerular collapse in renal allografts: possible role of vascular changes. Hum Pathol 2002;33:437–41.
259. Nadasdy GM, Bott C, Cowden D, et al. Comparative study for the detection of peritubular capillary C4d deposition in human renal allografts using different methodologies. Hum Pathol 2005;36:1178–85.
260. Nadasdy T, Krenacs T, Kalmar KN, et al. Importance of plasma cells in the infiltrate of renal allografts. An immunohistochemical study. Pathol Res Pract 1991;187:178–83.
261. Nakazawa K, Shimojo H, Komiyama Y, et al. Preexisting membranous nephropathy in allograft kidney. Nephron 1999;81:76–80.
262. Nankivell BJ, Borrows RJ, Fung CL, et al. Calcineurin inhibitor nephrotoxicity: longitudinal assessment by protocol histology. Transplantation 2004;78:557–65.
263. Nankivell BJ, Borrows RJ, Fung CL, et al. The natural history of chronic allograft nephropathy. N Engl J Med 2003;349:2326–33.
264. Nankivell BJ, Chapman JR. The significance of subclinical rejection and the value of protocol biopsies. Am J Transplant 2006;6:2006–12.
265. Neild GH, Taube DH, Hartley RB, et al. Morphological differentiation between rejection and cyclosporin nephrotoxicity in renal allografts. J Clin Pathol 1986;39:152–9.
266. Neumayer HH, Huls S, Schreiber M, et al. Kidneys from pediatric donors: risk versus benefit. Clin Nephrol 1994;41:94–100.
267. Nickeleit V. Critical commentary to: acute adenoviral infection of a graft by serotype 35 following renal transplantation. Pathol Res Pract 2003;199:701–2.
268. Nickeleit V, Hirsch HH, Binet IF, et al. Polyomavirus infection of renal allograft recipients: from latent infection to manifest disease. J Am Soc Nephrol 1999;10:1080–9.
269. Nickeleit V, Hirsch HH, Zeiler M, et al. BK-virus nephropathy in renal transplants-tubular necrosis, MHC-class II expression and rejection in a puzzling game. Nephrol Dial Transplant 2000;15:324–32.
270. Nickeleit V, Mihatsch MJ. Kidney transplants, antibodies and rejection: is C4d a magic marker? Nephrol Dial Transplant 2003;18:2232–9.
271. Nickeleit V, Mihatsch MJ. Polyomavirus nephropathy: pathogenesis, morphological and clinical aspects. In: Kreipe HH, editor. Verh Dtsch Ges Pathol, vol. 88. Tagung. Munich: Urban & Fischer; 2004. p. 69–84.
272. Nickeleit V, Mihatsch MJ. Polyomavirus nephropathy in native kidneys and renal allografts: an update on an escalating threat. Transpl Int 2006;19:960–73.
273. Nickeleit V, Steiger J, Mihatsch MJ. BK virus infection after kidney transplantation. Graft 2002;5(Suppl.):S46–57.
274. Nickeleit V, Vamvakas EC, Pascual M, et al. The prognostic significance of specific arterial lesions in acute renal allograft rejection. J Am Soc Nephrol 1998;9:1301–8.
275. Nickeleit V, Zeiler M, Gudat F, et al. Detection of the complement degradation product C4d in renal allografts: diagnostic and therapeutic implications. J Am Soc Nephrol 2002;13:242–51.
276. Niemann-Masanek U, Mueller A, Yard BA, et al. B7-1 (CD80) and B7-2 (CD 86) expression in human tubular epithelial cells in vivo and in vitro. Nephron 2002;92:542–56.
277. Nishi S, Imai N, Ito Y, et al. Pathological study on the relationship between C4d, CD59 and C5b-9 in acute renal allograft rejection. Clin Transplant 2004;18(Suppl. 11):18–23.
278. Nizze H, Mihatsch MJ, Zollinger HU, et al. Cyclosporine-associated nephropathy in patients with heart and bone marrow transplants. Clin Nephrol 1988;30:248–60.
279. Noris M, Remuzzi G. Thrombotic microangiopathy after kidney transplantation. Am J Transplant 2010;10:1517–23.
280. Noronha IL, Eberlein-Gonska M, Hartley B, et al. In situ expression of tumor necrosis factor-alpha, interferon-gamma, and interleukin-2 receptors in renal allograft biopsies. Transplantation 1992;54:1017–24.

281. Noronha IL, Hartley B, Cameron JS, et al. Detection of IL-1 beta and TNF-alpha message and protein in renal allograft biopsies. Transplantation 1993;56:1026–9.
282. Noronha IL, Oliveira SG, Tavares TS, et al. Apoptosis in kidney and pancreas allograft biopsies. Transplantation 2005;79:1231–5.
283. Nyberg G, Friman S, Svalander C, et al. Spectrum of hereditary renal disease in a kidney transplant population. Nephrol Dial Transplant 1995;10:859–65.
284. Nyberg G, Hedman L, Blohme I, et al. Morphologic findings in baseline kidney biopsies from living related donors. Transplant Proc 1992;24:355–6.
285. Oguma S, Banner B, Zerbe T, et al. Participation of dendritic cells in vascular lesions of chronic rejection of human allografts. Lancet 1988;2:933–6.
286. Ojo AO, Held PJ, Port FK, et al. Chronic renal failure after transplantation of a nonrenal organ. N Engl J Med 2003;349:931–40.
287. Olsen S, Bohman SO, Petersen VP. Ultrastructure of the glomerular basement membrane in long term renal allografts with transplant glomerular disease. Lab Invest 1974;30:176–89.
288. Østerby R, Nyberg G, Karlberg I, et al. Glomerular volume in kidneys transplanted into diabetic and non-diabetic patients. Diabet Med 1992;9:144–9.
289. Ozdemir BH, Aksoy PK, Haberal AN, et al. Relationship of HLA-DR expression to rejection and mononuclear cell infiltration in renal allograft biopsies. Ren Fail 2004;26:247–51.
290. Ozdemir BH, Ozdemir FN, Haberal N, et al. Vascular endothelial growth factor expression and cyclosporine toxicity in renal allograft rejection. Am J Transplant 2005;5:766–74.
291. Palestine AG, Austin III HA, Balow JE, et al. Renal histopathologic alterations in patients treated with cyclosporine for uveitis. N Engl J Med 1986;314:1293–8.
292. Pappo O, Demetris AJ, Raikow RB, et al. Human polyoma virus infection of renal allografts: histopathologic diagnosis, clinical significance, and literature review. Mod Pathol 1996;9:105–9.
293. Park WD, Griffin MD, Cornell LD, et al. Fibrosis with inflammation at one year predicts transplant functional decline. J Am Soc Nephrol 2010;21:1987–97.
294. Pascoe MD, Marshall SE, Welsh KI, et al. Increased accuracy of renal allograft rejection diagnosis using combined perforin, granzyme B, and Fas ligand fine-needle aspiration immunocytology. Transplantation 2000;69:2547–53.
295. Pascual M, Vallhonrat H, Cosimi AB, et al. The clinical usefulness of the renal allograft biopsy in the cyclosporine era: a prospective study. Transplantation 1999;67:737–41.
296. Patrakka J, Ruotsalainen V, Reponen P, et al. Recurrence of nephrotic syndrome in kidney grafts of patients with congenital nephrotic syndrome of the Finnish type: role of nephrin. Transplantation 2002;73:394–403.
297. Paul L, Class F, van Es L, et al. Accelerated rejection of a renal allograft associated with pretransplantation antibodies directed against donor antigens on endothelium and monocytes. N Engl J Med 1979;300:1258–9.
298. Pearson JC, Amend Jr WJ, Vincenti FG, et al. Post-transplantation pyelonephritis: factors producing low patient and transplant morbidity. J Urol 1980;123:153–6.
299. Pei Y, Scholey JW, Katz A, et al. Chronic nephrotoxicity in psoriatic patients treated with low-dose cyclosporine. Am J Kidney Dis 1994;23:528–36.
300. Poduval RD, Kadambi PV, Josephson MA, et al. Implications of immunohistochemical detection of C4d along peritubular capillaries in late acute renal allograft rejection. Transplantation 2005;79:228–35.
301. Pokorna E, Vitko S, Chadimova M, et al. Proportion of glomerulosclerosis in procurement wedge renal biopsy cannot alone discriminate for acceptance of marginal donors. Transplantation 2000;69:36–43.
302. Porter KA. Renal transplantation. In: Heptinstall RH, editor. The pathology of the kidney. 4th ed. Boston: Little, Brown; 1990. p. 1799–933.
303. Porter KA, Andres GA, Calder MW, et al. Human renal transplants. II. Immunofluorescence and immunoferritin studies. Lab Invest 1968;18:159–75.
304. Porter KA, Dossetor JB, Marchioro TL, et al. Human renal transplants. I. Glomerular changes. Lab Invest 1967;16:153–81.
305. Pratt JR, Basheer SA, Sacks SH. Local synthesis of complement component C3 regulates acute renal transplant rejection. Nat Med 2002;8:582–7.
306. Racusen LC, Colvin RB, Solez K, et al. Antibody-mediated rejection criteria – an addition to the Banff 97 classification of renal allograft rejection. Am J Transplant 2003;3:708–14.
307. Racusen LC, Solez K, Colvin RB, et al. The Banff 97 working classification of renal allograft pathology. Kidney Int 1999;55:713–23.
308. Ramos EL, Tisher CC. Recurrent diseases in the kidney transplant. Am J Kidney Dis 1994;24:142–54.
309. Randhawa PS, Magnone M, Jordan M, et al. Renal allograft involvement by Epstein–Barr virus associated post-transplant lymphoproliferative disease. Am J Surg Pathol 1996;20:563–71.
310. Randhawa PS, Minervini MI, Lombardero M, et al. Biopsy of marginal donor kidneys: correlation of histologic findings with graft dysfunction. Transplantation 2000;69:1352–7.
311. Randhawa PS, Shapiro R, Jordan ML, et al. The histopathological changes associated with allograft rejection and drug toxicity in renal transplant recipients maintained on FK506. Clinical significance and comparison with cyclosporine. Am J Surg Pathol 1993;17:60–8.
312. Regele H, Bohmig GA, Habicht A, et al. Capillary deposition of complement split product C4d in renal allografts is associated with basement membrane injury in peritubular and glomerular capillaries: a contribution of humoral immunity to chronic allograft rejection. J Am Soc Nephrol 2002;13:2371–80.
313. Regele H, Exner M, Watschinger B, et al. Endothelial C4d deposition is associated with inferior kidney allograft outcome independently of cellular rejection. Nephrol Dial Transplant 2001;16:2058–66.
314. Remuzzi G, Cravedi P, Perna A, et al. Long-term outcome of renal transplantation from older donors. N Engl J Med 2006;354:343–52.
315. Remuzzi G, Perico N. Cyclosporine-induced renal dysfunction in experimental animals and humans. Kidney Int Suppl 1995;52:S70–4.
316. Reynolds JC, Agodoa LY, Yuan CM, et al. Thrombotic microangiopathy after renal transplantation in the United States. Am J Kidney Dis 2003;42:1058–68.
317. Richardson WP, Colvin RB, Cheeseman SH, et al. Glomerulopathy associated with cytomegalovirus viremia in renal allografts. N Engl J Med 1981;305:57–63.
318. Roake JA, Fawcett J, Koo DD, et al. Late reflush in clinical renal transplantation. Protection against delayed graft function not observed. Transplantation 1996;62:114–6.
319. Robertson H, Ali S, McDonnell BJ, et al. Chronic renal allograft dysfunction: the role of T cell-mediated tubular epithelial to mesenchymal cell transition. J Am Soc Nephrol 2004;15:390–7.
320. Robertson H, Wheeler J, Thompson V, et al. In situ lymphoproliferation in renal transplant biopsies. Histochem Cell Biol 1995;104:331–4.
321. Rodriguez EF, Cosio FG, Nasr SH, et al. The pathology and clinical features of early recurrent membranous glomerulonephritis. Am J Transplant 2012;12:1029–38.
322. Rosen S, Greenfeld Z, Brezis M. Chronic cyclosporine-induced nephropathy in the rat. Transplantation 1990;49:445–52.
323. Rotman S, Collins AB, Colvin RB. C4d deposition in allografts: current concepts and interpretation. Transplant Rev 2005;19:65–77.
324. Rowshani AT, Florquin S, Bemelman F, et al. Hyperexpression of the granzyme B inhibitor PI-9 in human renal allografts: a potential mechanism for stable renal function in patients with subclinical rejection. Kidney Int 2004;66:1417–22.
325. Rush DN, Henry SF, Jeffery JR, et al. Histological findings in early routine biopsies of stable renal allograft recipients. Transplantation 1994;57:208–11.
326. Rush DN, Jeffery JR, Gough J. Sequential protocol biopsies in renal transplant patients. Clinico-pathological correlations using the Banff schema. Transplantation 1995;59:511–4.
327. Rush D, Nickerson P, Gough J, et al. Beneficial effects of treatment of early subclinical rejection: a randomized study. J Am Soc Nephrol 1998;9:2129–34.
328. Russell PS, Chase CM, Colvin RB. Alloantibody- and T cell-mediated immunity in the pathogenesis of transplant arteriosclerosis: lack of progression to sclerotic lesions in B cell-deficient mice. Transplantation 1997;64:1531–6.

329. Russell PS, Chase CM, Colvin RB. Coronary atherosclerosis in transplanted mouse hearts. IV Effects of treatment with monoclonal antibodies to intercellular adhesion molecule-1 and leukocyte function-associated antigen-1. Transplantation 1995;60:724–9.
330. Russell PS, Chase CM, Colvin RB, et al. Kidney transplants in mice. An analysis of the immune status of mice bearing long-term, H-2 incompatible transplants. J Exp Med 1978;147:1449–68.
331. Russell PS, Chase CM, Winn HJ, et al. Coronary atherosclerosis in transplanted mouse hearts. I. Time course and immunogenetic and immunopathological considerations. Am J Pathol 1994;144:260–74.
332. Saad R, Gritsch HA, Shapiro R, et al. Clinical significance of renal allograft biopsies with "borderline changes," as defined in the Banff schema. Transplantation 1997;64:992–5.
333. Sacchi G, Bertalot G, Cancarini C, et al. Atheromatosis and double media: uncommon vascular lesions of renal allografts. Pathologica 1993;85:183–94.
334. Said R, Duarte R, Chaballout A, et al. Spontaneous rupture of renal allograft. Urology 1994;43:554–8.
335. Salomon RN, Hughes CC, Schoen FJ, et al. Human coronary transplantation-associated arteriosclerosis. Evidence for a chronic immune reaction to activated graft endothelial cells. Am J Pathol 1991;138:791–8.
336. Savoldi S, Scolari F, Sandrini S, et al. Cyclosporine chronic nephrotoxicity: histologic follow up at 6 and 18 months after renal transplant. Transplant Proc 1988;20(S3):777–84.
337. Schmidtko J, Wang R, Wu CL, et al. Posttransplant lymphoproliferative disorder associated with an Epstein–Barr-related virus in cynomolgus monkeys. Transplantation 2002;73:1431–9.
338. Schroeder TJ, Weiss MA, Smith RD, et al. The efficacy of OKT3 in vascular rejection. Transplantation 1991;51:312–5.
339. Schwarz A, Gwinner W, Hiss M, et al. Safety and adequacy of renal transplant protocol biopsies. Am J Transplant 2005;5:1992–6.
340. Schwarz A, Krause PH, Offermann G, et al. Impact of de novo membranous glomerulonephritis on the clinical course after kidney transplantation. Transplantation 1994;58:650–4.
341. Schwarz A, Mengel M, Gwinner W, et al. Risk factors for chronic allograft nephropathy after renal transplantation: a protocol biopsy study. Kidney Int 2005;67:341–8.
342. Schweitzer EJ, Drachenberg CB, Anderson L. Significance of the Banff borderline biopsy. Am J Kidney Dis 1996;28:585–91.
343. Schwimmer JA, Markowitz GS, Valeri AM, et al. Secondary focal segmental glomerulosclerosis in non-obese patients with increased muscle mass. Clin Nephrol 2003;60:233–41.
344. Scornik JC, LeFor WM, Cicciarelli JC, et al. Hyperacute and acute kidney graft rejection due to antibodies against B cells. Transplantation 1992;54:61–4.
345. Sedmak D, Sharma H, Czajka C, et al. Recipient endothelialization of renal allografts. An immunohistochemical study utilitizing blood group antigens. Transplantation 1988;46:907–10.
346. Sellares J, de Freitas DG, Mengel M, et al. Understanding the causes of kidney transplant failure: the dominant role of antibody-mediated rejection and nonadherence. Am J Transplant 2012;12:388–99.
347. Sharma VK, Bologa RM, Li B, et al. Molecular executors of cell death – differential intrarenal expression of Fas ligand, Fas, granzyme B, and perforin during acute and/or chronic rejection of human renal allografts. Transplantation 1996;62:1860–6.
348. Shimizu A, Yamada K, Meehan SM, et al. Acceptance reaction: intragraft events associated with tolerance to renal allografts in miniature swine. J Am Soc Nephrol 2000;11:2371–80.
349. Shimizu A, Yamada K, Meehan SM, et al. Intragraft cellular events associated with tolerance in pig allografts: the "acceptance reaction". Transplant Proc 1997;29:1155.
350. Shishido S, Asanuma H, Nakai H, et al. The impact of repeated subclinical acute rejection on the progression of chronic allograft nephropathy. J Am Soc Nephrol 2003;14:1046–52.
351. Shulman H, Striker G, Deeg HJ, et al. Nephrotoxicity of cyclosporin A after allogeneic marrow transplantation. Glomerular thromboses and tubular injury. N Engl J Med 1981;305:1392–5.
352. Sibley RK, Payne W. Morphologic findings in the renal allograft biopsy. Semin Nephrol 1985;5:294–306.
353. Sibley RK, Rynasiewicz J, Ferguson RM, et al. Morphology of cyclosporine nephrotoxicity and acute rejection in patients immunosuppressed with cyclosporine and prednisone. Surgery 1983;94:225–34.
354. Sijpkens YW, Joosten SA, Wong MC, et al. Immunologic risk factors and glomerular C4d deposits in chronic transplant glomerulopathy. Kidney Int 2004;65:2409–18.
355. Silbert PL, Matz LR, Christiansen K, et al. Herpes simplex virus interstitial nephritis in a renal allograft. Clin Nephrol 1990;33:264–8.
356. Simmons RL, Tallent MB, Kjellstrand CM, et al. Renal allograft rejection simulated by arterial stenosis. Surgery 1970;68:800–4.
357. Singh HK, Nickeleit V. Kidney disease caused by viral infections. Curr Diag Pathol 2004;10:11–21.
358. Sis B, Dadras F, Khoshjou F, et al. Reproducibility studies on arteriolar hyaline thickening scoring in calcineurin inhibitor-treated renal allograft recipients. Am J Transplant 2006;6:1444–50.
359. Sis B, Jhangri GS, Bunnag S, et al. Endothelial gene expression in kidney transplants with alloantibody indicates antibody-mediated damage despite lack of C4d staining. Am J Transplant 2009;9:2312–23.
360. Sis B, Mengel M, Haas M, et al. Banff '09 meeting report: antibody mediated graft deterioration and implementation of Banff working groups. Am J Transplant 2010;10:464–71.
361. Smith RN, Kawai T, Boskovic S, et al. Chronic antibody mediated rejection of renal allografts: pathological, serological and immunologic features in nonhuman primates. Am J Transplant 2006;6:1790–8.
362. Smith RN, Kawai T, Boskovic S, et al. Four stages and lack of stable accommodation in chronic alloantibody-mediated renal allograft rejection in *Cynomolgus* monkeys. Am J Transplant 2008;8:1662–72.
363. Smith KD, Wrenshall LE, Nicosia RF, et al. Delayed graft function and cast nephropathy associated with tacrolimus plus rapamycin use. J Am Soc Nephrol 2003;14:1037–45.
364. Snanoudj R, Royal V, Elie C, et al. Specificity of histological markers of long-term CNI nephrotoxicity in kidney-transplant recipients under low-dose cyclosporine therapy. Am J Transplant 2011;11:2635–46.
365. Solez K. History of the Banff classification of allograft pathology as it approaches its 20th year. Curr Opin Organ Transplant 2010;15:49–51.
366. Solez K, Axelsen RA, Benediktsson H, et al. International standardization of criteria for the histologic diagnosis of renal allograft rejection: the Banff working classification of kidney transplant pathology. Kidney Int 1993;44:411–22.
367. Solez K, Colvin RB, Racusen L, et al. Banff '05 meeting report: differential diagnosis of chronic injury and elimination of chronic allograft nephropathy ("CAN") in the Banff schema. Am J Transplant 2007;7:518–26.
368. Solez K, Racusen LC, Marcussen N, et al. Morphology of ischemic acute renal failure, normal function, and cyclosporine toxicity in cyclosporine-treated renal allograft recipients. Kidney Int 1993;43:1058–67.
369. Sommer BG, Innes JT, Whitehurst RM, et al. Cyclosporine-associated renal arteriopathy resulting in loss of allograft function. Am J Surg 1985;149:756–64.
370. Stegall MD, Diwan T, Raghavaiah S, et al. Terminal complement inhibition decreases antibody-mediated rejection in sensitized renal transplant recipients. Am J Transplant 2011;11:2405–13.
371. Stegall MD, Park WD, Larson TS, et al. The histology of solitary renal allografts at 1 and 5 years after transplantation. Am J Transplant 2011;11:698–707.
372. Stephany BR, Augustine JJ, Krishnamurthi V, et al. Differences in proteinuria and graft function in de novo sirolimus-based vs. calcineurin inhibitor-based immunosuppression in live donor kidney transplantation. Transplantation 2006;82:368–74.
373. Stern SC, Lakhani S, Morgan SH. Renal allograft dysfunction due to vesicoureteric obstruction by nodular malakoplakia. Nephrol Dial Transplant 1994;9:1188–90.
374. Stokes MB, Davis CL, Alpers CE. Collapsing glomerulopathy in renal allografts: a morphological pattern with diverse clinicopathologic associations. Am J Kidney Dis 1999;33:658–66.
375. Straathof-Galema L, Wetzels JF, Dijkman HB, et al. Sirolimus-associated heavy proteinuria in a renal transplant recipient: evidence for a tubular mechanism. Am J Transplant 2006;6:429–33.
376. Strehlau J, Pavlakis M, Lipman M, et al. Quantitative detection of immune activation transcripts as a diagnostic tool in kidney transplantation. Proc Natl Acad Sci 1997;94:695–700.

377. Strehlau J, Pavlakis M, Lipman M, et al. The intragraft gene activation of markers reflecting T-cell-activation and -cytotoxicity analyzed by quantitative RT-PCR in renal transplantation. Clin Nephrol 1996;46:30–3.
378. Strom EH, Epper R, Mihatsch MJ. Ciclosporin-associated arteriolopathy: the renin producing vascular smooth muscle cells are more sensitive to ciclosporin toxicity. Clin Nephrol 1995;43:226–31.
379. Strom EH, Thiel G, Mihatsch MJ. Prevalence of cyclosporine-associated arteriolopathy in renal transplant biopsies from 1981 to 1992. Transplant Proc 1994;26:2585–7.
380. Sund S, Hovig T, Reisaeter AV, et al. Complement activation in early protocol kidney graft biopsies after living-donor transplantation. Transplantation 2003;75:1204–13.
381. Suthanthiran M. Molecular analyses of human renal allografts: differential intragraft gene expression during rejection. Kidney Int 1997;58(Suppl.):S15–21.
382. Takemoto SK, Zeevi A, Feng S, et al. National conference to assess antibody-mediated rejection in solid organ transplantation. Am J Transplant 2004;4:1033–41.
383. Taub HC, Greenstein SM, Lerner SE, et al. Reassessment of the value of post-vascularization biopsy performed at renal transplantation: the effects of arteriosclerosis. J Urol 1994;151:575–7.
384. Taube DH, Neild GH, Williams DG, et al. Differentiation between allograft rejection and cyclosporin nephrotoxicity in renal transplant recipients. Lancet 1985;2:171–4.
385. Ten RM, Gleich GJ, Holley KE, et al. Eosinophil granule major basic protein in acute renal allograft rejection. Transplantation 1989;47:959–63.
386. Terasaki PI, Ozawa M. Predictive value of HLA antibodies and serum creatinine in chronic rejection: results of a 2-year prospective trial. Transplantation 2005;80:1194–7.
387. Thiru S, Maher ER, Hamilton DV, et al. Tubular changes in renal transplant recipients on cyclosporine. Transplant Proc 1983;15:2846–51.
388. Thoenes GH, Pielsticker K, Schubert G. Transplantation-induced immune complex kidney disease in rats with unilateral manifestations in the allografted kidney. Lab Invest 1979;41:321–9.
389. Thurman JM, Lucia MS, Ljubanovic D, et al. Acute tubular necrosis is characterized by activation of the alternative pathway of complement. Kidney Int 2005;67:524–30.
390. Trpkov K, Campbell P, Pazderka F, et al. Pathologic features of acute renal allograft rejection associated with donor-specific antibody. Analysis using the Banff grading schema. Transplantation 1996;61:1586–92.
391. Truong L, Gelfand J, D'Agati V, et al. De novo membranous glomerulonephropathy in renal allografts: a report of ten cases and review of the literature. Am J Kidney Dis 1989;14:131–44.
392. Tuazon TV, Schneeberger EE, Bhan AK, et al. Mononuclear cells in acute allograft glomerulopathy. Am J Pathol 1987;129:119–32.
393. van den Akker JM, Wetzels JF, Hoitsma AJ. Proteinuria following conversion from azathioprine to sirolimus in renal transplant recipients. Kidney Int 2006;70:1355–7.
394. Van den Berg-Wolf MG, Kootte AM, Weening JJ, et al. Recurrent hemolytic uremic syndrome in a renal transplant recipient and review of the Leiden experience. Transplantation 1988;45:248–51.
395. Vangelista A, Frasca GM, Martella D, et al. Glomerulonephritis in renal transplantation. Nephrol Dial Transplant 1990;1:42–6.
396. van Gorder MA, Della Pelle P, Henson JW, et al. Cynomolgus polyoma virus infection: a new member of the polyoma virus family causes interstitial nephritis, ureteritis, and enteritis in immunosuppressed cynomolgus monkeys. Am J Pathol 1999;154:1273–84.
397. Veronese FV, Manfro RC, Roman FR, et al. Reproducibility of the Banff classification in subclinical kidney transplant rejection. Clin Transplant 2005;19:518–21.
398. Veronese FJ, Rotman S, Smith RN, et al. FOXP3+ Cells infiltrate renal allografts during acute cellular rejection: pathological and clinical correlates of putative intragraft T regulatory cells. Am J Transplant 2006; WTC 2006 Abstract.
399. Veronese F, Rotman S, Smith RN, et al. Pathological and clinical correlates of FOXP3(+) cells in renal allografts during acute rejection. Am J Transplant 2007;7:914–22.
400. Vincenti F, Larsen C, Durrbach A, et al. Costimulation blockade with belatacept in renal transplantation. N Engl J Med 2005;353:770–81.
401. Waltzer WC, Miller F, Arnold A, et al. Immunohistologic analysis of human renal allograft dysfunction. Transplantation 1987;43:100–5.
402. Wang HJ, Kjellstrand CM, Cockfield SM, et al. On the influence of sample size on the prognostic accuracy and reproducibility of renal transplant biopsy. Nephrol Dial Transplant 1998;13:165–72.
403. Wang H, Nanra RS, Carney SL, et al. The renal medulla in acute renal allograft rejection: comparison with renal cortex. Nephrol Dial Transplant 1995;10:1428–31.
404. Watschinger B, Vychytil A, Attar M, et al. Pattern of endothelin immunostaining during rejection episodes after kidney transplantation. Clin Nephrol 1994;41:86–93.
405. Weir MR, Hall-Craggs M, Shen SY, et al. The prognostic value of the eosinophil in acute renal allograft rejection. Transplantation 1986;41:709–12.
406. Wiebe C, Gibson IW, Blydt-Hansen TD, et al. Evolution and clinical pathologic correlations of de novo donor-specific HLA antibody post kidney transplant. Am J Transplant 2012;12:1157–67.
407. Wieczorek G, Bigaud M, Menninger K, et al. Acute and chronic vascular rejection in non-human primate kidney tranplantation. Am J Transplant 2006;6:459–66.
408. Wilczek HE, Jaremko G, Tyden G, et al. Evolution of diabetic nephropathy in kidney grafts. Evidence that a simultaneously transplanted kidney exerts a protective effect. Transplantation 1995;59:51–7.
409. Williams GM, Hume DM, Huson Jr RP, et al. "Hyperacute" renal-homograft rejection in man. N Engl J Med 1968;279:611–5.
410. Williams WW, Taheri D, Tolkoff-Rubin N, et al. Clinical role of the renal transplant biopsy. Nat Rev Nephrol 2012;8:110–21.
411. Wong WK, Robertson H, Carroll HP, et al. Tubulitis in renal allograft rejection: role of transforming growth factor-beta and interleukin-15 in development and maintenance of CD103+ intraepithelial T cells. Transplantation 2003;75:505–14.
412. Woolley AC, Rosenberg ME, Burke BA, et al. De novo focal glomerulosclerosis after kidney transplantation. Am J Med 1988;84:310–4.
413. Woywodt A, Schroeder M, Gwinner W, et al. Elevated numbers of circulating endothelial cells in renal transplant recipients. Transplantation 2003;76:1–4.
414. Yagisawa T, Nakada T, Takahashi K, et al. Acute hemorrhagic cystitis caused by adenovirus after kidney transplantation. Urol Int 1995;54:142–6.
415. Yamaguchi Y, Teraoka S, Yagisawa T, et al. Ultrastructural study of cyclosporine-associated arteriolopathy in renal allografts. Transplant Proc 1989;21:1517–22.
416. Yang CW, Kim YS, Yang KH, et al. Acute focal bacterial nephritis presented as acute renal failure and hepatic dysfunction in a renal transplant recipient. Am J Nephrol 1994;14:72–5.
417. Yard B, Spruyt-Gerritse M, Claas F, et al. The clinical significance of allospecific antibodies against endothelial cells detected with an antibody-dependent cellular cytotoxicity assay for vascular rejection and graft loss after renal transplantation. Transplantation 1993;55:1287–93.
418. Young EW, Ellis CN, Messana JM, et al. A prospective study of renal structure and function in psoriasis patients treated with cyclosporin. Kidney Int 1994;46:1216–22.
419. Zachariae H, Hansen HE, Kragballe K, et al. Morphologic renal changes during cyclosporine treatment of psoriasis. Studies on pretreatment and posttreatment kidney biopsy specimens. J Am Acad Dermatol 1992;26:415–9.

CHAPTER 27

CHRONIC ALLOGRAFT FAILURE

Brian J. Nankivell

CHAPTER OUTLINE

INTRODUCTION: THE PROBLEM OF GRAFT LOSS

Despite the success of modern transplantation, which can produce early acute rejection rates below 15% and 1-year graft survival rates above 90%, long-term graft attrition rates have remained unchanged at 4% graft loss per year.[55,56] Progressive transplant renal dysfunction often leads to graft failure and return to dialysis, accompanied by substantial morbidity and mortality. This chapter will evaluate the causes of chronic transplant failure, its pathophysiology, and diagnostic pathology, and present a therapeutic approach.

Kidney allografts are damaged from both immune and non-immune mechanisms. The histopathology of a chronically failing allograft usually shows interstitial fibrosis, tubular atrophy, glomerulosclerosis, and vascular abnormalities (Figure 27-1) (see Chapter 26). These features represent the summated effects of tissue injury from multiple pathogenic insults combined with the kidney's fibrotic healing response, which is influenced by alloimmunity and recipient immunosuppression (Figure 27-2 and Table 27-1). These end-pathway phenotypes are expressed within local anatomical compartments (tubular, interstitial, microvascular, and glomerular) by tissues with a limited repertoire of response (Table 27-1). Different drivers of nephron damage have a differential incidence and rate of progression where the relative mix alters according to time after transplantation, but can operate simultaneously.

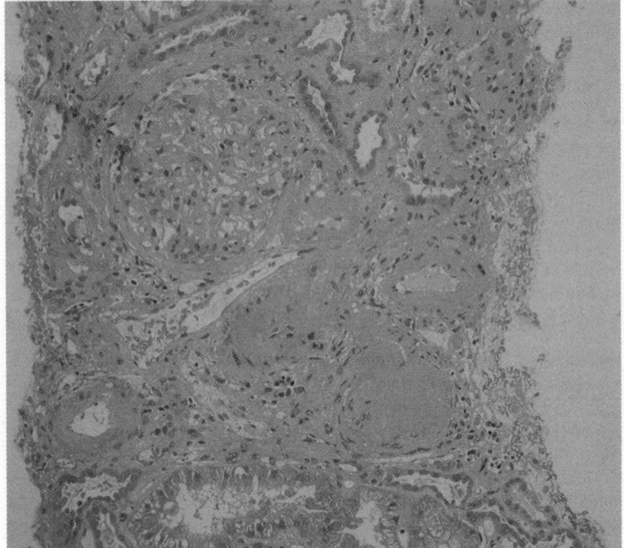

FIGURE 27-1 ■ Chronic allograft nephropathy showing chronic interstitial fibrosis and tubular atrophy, accompanied by glomerulosclerosis, increased mesangial matrix, and vascular changes.

PATHOPHYSIOLOGY OF CHRONIC ALLOGRAFT DAMAGE

Models of Chronic Kidney Transplant Injury

Risk factors for chronic allograft loss include donor organ quality, ischemia-reperfusion injury with delayed graft function (DGF) immune factors, including human leukocyte antigen (HLA) mismatch, donor-specific and MICA antibodies, and acute rejection, and recipient factors such as hypertension, proteinuria, smoking, and medication

TABLE 27-1 Causes of Allograft Damage (Events and Risks)

Non-immune
Deceased donor
Older donor age, donor vascular disease, and extended criteria donor
Donor brain death and autonomic storm, inotropic use, donor renal failure
Ischemia-reperfusion injury (warm and cold ischemia times, perfusion, and organ transport)
Delayed graft function (clinical) and acute tubular necrosis (biopsy)
Ascending urinary tract infection with allograft pyelonephritis
Transplant ureteric obstruction
Polyomavirus nephropathy
Calcineurin inhibitor nephrotoxicity
Recurrent or de novo glomerulonephritis
Hypertension
Proteinuria
Hyperlipidemia
Recipient smoking
Alloimmune
Young recipient age
Ethnicity
Altered handling of immunosuppressive agents (pharmacokinetics)
Variable trough levels (malabsorption or compliance)
Therapy non-compliance
Histoincompatibility, CREG mismatches
Recipient presensitization (panel-reactive antibodies)
Hyperacute rejection (rare)
Early antibody-mediated acute rejection
Acute rejection (severe or steroid-resistant, vascular, late, or undiagnosed/untreated)
Subclinical rejection
True chronic rejection with fibrointimal vascular hyperplasia
Late de novo anti-HLA antibody formation
Chronic antibody-mediated rejection with transplant glomerulopathy

CREG, cross-reactive groups.

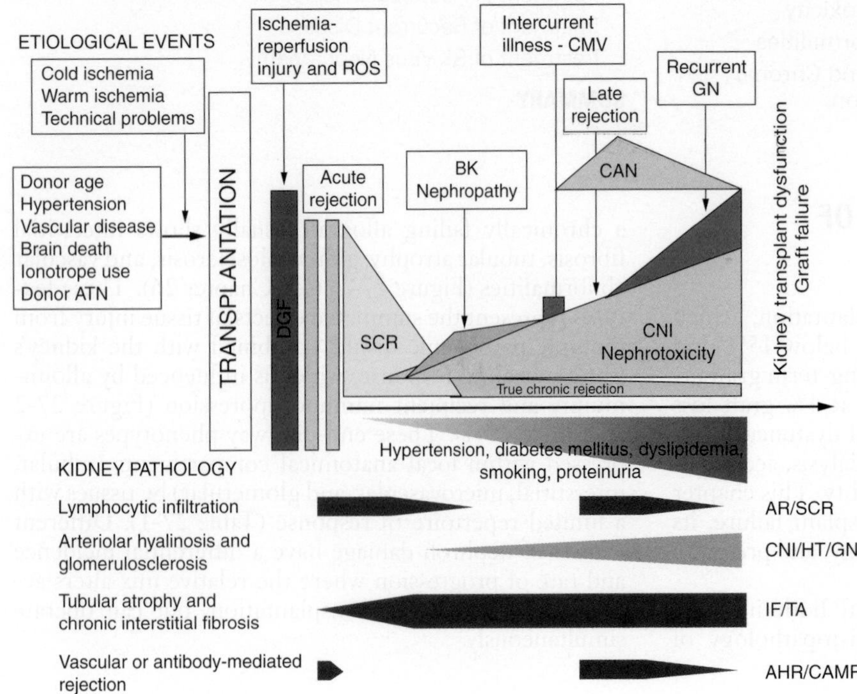

FIGURE 27-2 ■ Immune and non-immune events leading to allograft damage and transplant failure. ATN, acute tubular necrosis; CAN, chronic allograft nephropathy; CMV; cytomegalovirus; CNI, calcineurin inhibitors; DGF, delayed graft function; GN; glomerulonephritis; ROS, reactive oxygen species; SCR, subclinical rejection.

non-adherence[71] (Table 27-1). The pathophysiology of chronic allograft failure can be ascribed to one of several unified hypotheses. Specific additional pathophysiological mechanisms of graft injury have also been proposed, although these paradigms are not mutually exclusive.

Originally, kidney allograft damage and late graft failure were usually simply attributed to "chronic rejection," with pathology of chronic lymphocytic interstitial infiltration, sometimes accompanied by specific vascular or glomerular abnormalities. While commonly described in the prednisolone-azathioprine era,[38] this pattern became less common with more potent immunosuppression regimes incorporating calcineurin inhibitors (CNIs). Risk factor profiling showing alternative risk factors, and unchanged long-term graft survival despite lower acute rejection rates and stronger antirejection therapies suggest that other mechanisms of graft injury may also be important. However, acute and chronic rejection still remain clinically relevant in immunologically active patients, those with excessive prescribed reductions of immunosuppressive therapy or with treatment non-compliance, where chronic low-level alloimmune activity can be manifested by persistent cellular interstitial inflammation, fibrointimal hyperplasia, or with transplant glomerulopathy associated with circulating donor-specific antibody (DSA) and tissue C4d.

The input-stress model is a composite model that describes the interaction between the starting "input" of the transplanted kidney (the overall quality or condition of the organ and early events, including procurement, preservation, and reimplantation injury) with a series of subsequent immune and non-immune stresses, including cellular infiltration, antibody-mediated alloimmunity, and other non-immune ("load") mechanisms, including hypertension, hyperfiltration, proteinuria, dyslipidemia, nephrotoxic drugs, and infection. These stressors have been postulated to drive cells from a normal state into a senescent phenotype, exhaust repair processes, and deplete the finite nephron supply, leading to graft failure.[31]

The cumulative damage hypothesis is based on sequential observational pathology and assumes that chronic allograft damage is the end result of a series of time-dependent immune and non-immune insults inflicted on the transplanted kidney, resulting in permanent nephron damage. The number of nephrons within the transplanted kidney is finite, and nephrons, after destruction, cannot be replaced, although hypertrophy of remaining nephrons may occur to compensate partially for losses. The transplanted kidney gradually fails from the summated and incremental loss of individual nephrons, combined with additional internal structural damage leading to overall organ malfunction. Nephron damage is mediated by a multitude of alloimmune, ischemic, and inflammatory stimuli, yielding lethal or sublethal tubular injury with a profibrotic healing response. Multiple pathways and mediators result in cumulative structural damage to all compartments within the transplanted kidney (Figure 27-2).

Mechanisms of Chronic Allograft Progression

The cytokine excess theory postulates that chronic allograft damage is due to acute and repeated tissue injury inducing excessive cytokine production (e.g., interferon-γ), leading to interstitial and vascular fibrosis (by transforming growth factor (TGF)-β_1). Cytokines and chemokines play key roles in the recruitment, activation, and ingress of inflammatory T cells and monocyte/macrophages. A role for other mediators, such as vascular endothelial growth factor, endothelin-1, plasminogen-activating factor-1, monocyte chemoattractant protein-1, platelet-derived growth factor A and B, RANTES, bone morphogenetic protein 7, hepatocyte growth factor, connective tissue growth factor, and advanced glycation end products, is supported by their altered expression in experimental and human chronic rejection or graft fibrosis.[3,18,28,73,93] Similarly, uncontrolled or excessive reactive oxygen species (ROS) production from tubular cell mitochondria may cause cellular injury, apoptosis, and expression of a senescent phenotype. Studies have shown that interstitial inducible nitric oxide synthase protein expression, nitrotyrosine, and ex vivo ROS production are increased in chronic allograft nephropathy (CAN).[2] The nephrotoxic injury from CNI therapy also constitutes an important continuing non-immune stressor of the kidney allograft.[15,23,70,73,96]

The hyperfiltration theory implies that, when individual nephrons are progressively lost, the metabolic load and tubular protein reabsorption from the ultrafiltrate fall on to a diminishing number of remaining nephrons. Hyperfiltration with glomerular hypertension can result in further tubular and glomerular damage, although the human evidence is weak. Estimates of single nephron hyperfiltration in transplant recipients are only modestly increased after transplantation, being partially ameliorated by reduced overall transplant glomerular filtration rate (GFR) and single nephron load. Results of graft survival in donor–recipient size mismatch have been contradictory or non-supportive, with many studies showing no effect. Registry data show no effect on change in calculated GFR and lack of an expected inflexion point of progression of renal dysfunction at lower GFR.[26] The classic hyperfiltration lesions of focal segmental glomerulosclerosis (FSGS) are uncommon. Hyperfiltration may have a deleterious effect only when substantial glomerular loss has occurred, such as in advanced chronic allograft damage or when a small infant donor kidney is transplanted into a large adult, so its overall contribution seems minor.

Proteinuria is a powerful composite risk factor as a marker of kidney damage and has been implicated in tubular injury from ultrafiltration of toxic substances, cytokines, and other mediators. Urinary protein excretion greater than 0.5 g/day has been associated with progressive graft dysfunction and failure[19,99] and may be due to glomerular protein leak (glomerular proteinuria) or failed tubular reabsorption from atrophic tubules (tubular proteinuria), or both.

Hypertension is common before and after transplantation and has been associated with graft failure and death using registry analysis, although direct histological evidence linking it to chronic allograft damage is limited. It occurs in 70–90% of recipients, related to pretransplant hypertension and vascular disease, glucocorticoid and cyclosporine use, graft dysfunction, or transplant renal artery stenosis. Chronic hypertensive changes recognizable in a kidney transplant include fibrointimal thickening with duplication of the internal elastic lamina in small muscular arteries, arteriolar hyalinosis, and ischemic glomerulosclerosis.[71,74] Other adverse factors associated with graft progression include recipient smoking, dyslipidemia, and diabetes mellitus.

Failure to Resolve Chronic Inflammation

Normal wound healing after acute injury usually results in self-limited healing with complete resolution of the inflammatory and fibrogenic process. Fibrosis in the allograft differs from normal healing in that repeated episodes of acute injury occur, which may be followed sometimes by a partial or incomplete resolution of inflammation. An ongoing cycle of non-specific injury causing tubular inflammation, enhanced allorecognition, and additional immune-mediated injury may then be created, becoming self-perpetuating and failing to resolve. The total inflammation burden irrespective of its location is a better predictor of graft survival than the Banff i score alone.[60] In one study, patients with intragraft Foxp3$^+$ T (regulatory) cells within the subclinical rejection (SCR) infiltrate experienced better 5-year graft function, suggestive of a protective effect.[4] Persistent chronic inflammatory cells are commonly observed within areas of atrophic tubules and fibrosis in failing grafts and, along with SCR, have been associated with progressive functional impairment, increased tubular damage in sequential biopsy studies, and greater death-censored graft failure.[52,60,63,68]

Epithelial–Mesenchymal Transition-Induced Fibrosis

Epithelial–mesenchymal transition (EMT) describes a phenotypical change induced in tubular epithelial cells which lose their cell-to-cell basement membrane contacts and structural polarity, and transform into spindle-shaped cells that resemble mesenchymal or myofibroblast-type cells. With the exception of the distal collecting duct, the renal tubular cells originate from fetal mesenchyme, undergoing transition to cells of an epithelial phenotype during development of the embryonic kidney. These cells retain their ability to back-differentiate or "transition" into mesenchymal cells with the appropriate stimuli, providing a potential source of interstitial fibroblasts (so-called type II EMT). Sublethal tubular injury or exposure to stimuli such as TGF-β_1, hypoxic injury, or interleukin-1 can induce a series of genetically programmed steps initiated by impaired cell-to-cell adhesion and loss of the tubular cell's morphogenetic clues and signals. Transition from tubular epithelial cells into myofibroblasts begins with loss of tight junctions and adherent junctions, desmosomes, and E-cadherin (an epithelial marker). This is followed by reorganization of F-actin stress fibers and de novo expression of α-smooth-muscle actin (a mesenchymal marker), filopodia, and lamellipodia for movement controlled by molecular reprogramming of the cell (Figure 27-3). The final stages of EMT are cellular migration into the interstitial space and transition into fibroblasts, secreting interstial matrix proteins, collagen, and fibronectin. EMT may be potentially reversible; surviving cells can repopulate injured denuded tubules with new functional epithelia (so-called mesenchymal-to-epithelial transition).[10]

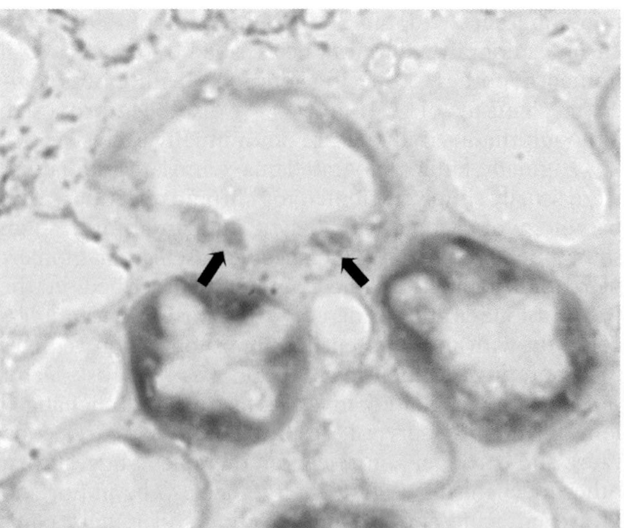

FIGURE 27-3 ■ Epithelial mesenchymal transition illustrated by dual staining of E-cadherin (blue) and α-smooth-muscle actin (brown) in a tubular epithelial cell.

Early experimental support for EMT came with genetically tagged epithelial cells which showed that 36% of all FSP1-positive matrix-producing fibroblasts originate from renal proximal tubules in a model of unilateral ureteral obstruction.[43] However, these early Cre/Lox results have not been supported by several recent cell lineage-tracing studies, casting doubt on the tubular EMT hypothesis as the source of interstitial myofibroblasts. Instead they suggest that some fibroblasts may originate from resident capillary endothelial cells, via endothelial-to-mesenchymal transition.[29] Profibrotic growth factors within the peritubular microenvironment, generated from injured tubular cells, infiltrating inflammatory cells or residential activated fibroblasts, can induce or promote EMT. TGF-β, basic fibroblast growth factor, connective tissue growth factor, angiotensin II, matrix metalloproteinase-2 and tissue-type plasminogen activator are balanced against inhibitors such as bone morphogenetic protein-7, as well as therapeutic agents, including sirolimus, vitamin D, stains, and angiotensin II type I receptor blockers. TGF-β/Smad, integrin-linked kinase, and Wnt/β-catenin signaling are important intracellular signal transduction pathways controlling the process of EMT.[10]

The main clinical drivers of EMT in kidney transplantation are immune infiltration, CNI immunosuppression, and oxidative stress. Epithelial phenotype changes suggestive of EMT, defined by pathology expressing both epithelial and mesenchymal markers (e.g., β-catenin and vimentin) or by EMT-associated gene expression, correlate with histological cyclosporine A nephrotoxicity with tubular dilatation and vacuolation,[22,100] allograft dysfunction, SCR, or lymphocytic cellular infiltration (Banff total i scores), prolonged ischemic times, and with interstitial fibrosis.[34,100]

Attributing a mechanistic role of EMT for progressive interstitial fibrosis and tubular atrophy in vivo versus that of resident or infiltrating fibroblasts is challenging, with sequential transplant biopsy studies reporting mixed results.[32,101] Changes of tubular cells to a mesenchymal phenotype are commonly reported from cross-sectional observational studies.[16,32,34,101,102] However, EMT may be incomplete, with transformed cells sloughing off into the tubular lumen instead of crossing the basement membrane. In human transplantation, interstitial fibroblasts were predominantly of recipient origin using Y chromosomal DNA analysis of sex-mismatched donor–recipient pairs.[30]

Donor Age and Replicative Senescence

Cellular replicative senescence is the normal aging process of cells that eventually leads to exhaustion and irreversible growth arrest and has been postulated as an explanation of the poorer actuarial graft survival from older donor kidneys.[31,57,59] Cultured somatic cells stop cycling and become senescent after a fixed number of doublings, known as the Hayflick limit. This "mitotic clock" is largely controlled in humans by telomeres, that shorten with each mitotic division until they ultimately arrest in the G1 phase of the cell cycle. Shortened telomeres have been observed in native and transplanted older kidneys (driven by oxidative stress and aging), but with little evidence of a role in human chronic allograft damage. Senescent cells have altered shape and cytoskeletal collagen, increased expression of tumor suppressor genes, senescence-associated β-galactosidase activity, deposition of lipofuscin, activation of p53 and p16 pathways, and additional markers – predominantly within the tubulointerstitial compartment.[58] The senescent phenotype in CAN is not mediated by accelerated telomere shortening, but rather by altered expression of cell cycling pathways.[66]

Alternative explanations for the poor outcomes from older donor kidneys include a differential response to injury with age, an impaired ability to withstand stress, limited ability to repair damage once incurred, and amplification of external insults by pre-existing structural abnormalities (such as donor vascular disease) commonly present in older kidneys.

Cortical Ischemia

Tubular epithelial cells are supplied by the peritubular capillary (PTC) network that is downstream from the efferent arterioles of the glomerular tuft. These cells are metabolically active cells, being rich in mitochondria that power the electrolyte pumps and endocytotic protein reabsorption machinary. Tubular cells are susceptible to ischemia from upstream vascular narrowing, caused by partial or total glomerulosclerosis, arteriolar hyalinosis, and vasoconstriction induced by CNIs and other factors, fibrointimal hyperplasia, hypertension, or donor changes in small muscular arteries, and capillary rarefaction associated with interstitial fibrosis, which reduces blood supply and oxygen diffusion. Hypoxic stress provokes an adaptive survival response of the cell which includes switching to anaerobic glycolysis and activation of antiapoptotic molecular programs. Hypoxia-inducible factors (e.g., HIF-1α) are central regulators of this response, activating a multitude of genes regulating glucose metabolism, cell proliferation and survival, as well as angiogenesis, chemotaxis of inflammatory cells, and formation and turnover of extracellular matrix via profibrotic cytokines such as TGF-α, platelet-derived growth factor, connective tissue growth factor, and vascular endothelial growth factor.[45]

Injury of the PTCs begins activation and nuclear swelling of endothelial cells, loss of fenestrae, and apoptosis and cellular detachment from the basement membrane, finally leading to collapse and occlusion of the capillary. Cross-sectional studies have associated chronic antibody-mediated rejection (CAMR) and CAN with progressive loss of the PTC network and small muscular arteries, endothelial cell apoptosis, and multilamination of the basement membrane. Attenuation of the microvasculature occurred regardless of the cause of chronic allograft damage and has been reported in chronic cellular rejection, C4d$^+$ chronic rejection, and sclerosing CAN. Greater allograft damage paralleled loss of PTC surface area, allograft dysfunction, and proteinuria.[39]

In experimental ischemic acute renal failure, early and permanent rarefaction of the PTC network occurred in the inner stripe of the outer medulla, followed by tubulointerstitial fibrosis and reduced urinary concentrating ability. Although current human evidence is consistent and reproducible in transplantation,[39,40,94] it cannot distinguish cause from effect – whether microvascular loss causes localized tubular ischemia and interstitial fibrosis, whether tubular loss reduces supportive angiogenic factors, or whether angioregression associated with the fibrotic healing response of chronic allograft damage is a paraphenomenon reflecting a common insult.

Internal Structural Failure

Function within the transplanted kidney may be impaired by structural damage at the level of the individual nephron or the intact whole organ. Major damage to any component along the length of the nephron causes functional failure of the whole unit. Glomerular damage may manifest as global or partial glomerulosclerosis, transplant glomerulopathy, or the formation of atubular glomeruli, which develop after severe irreversible damage and disconnection of downstream tubules.[6] Tubular malfunction may occur because of localized apoptosis to individual tubular cells, tubular atrophy involving the tubular cross-section, or luminal obstruction from cellular debris.

In addition, the transplant kidney may malfunction from internal architectural disruption, leading to loss of ability to modify the tubular ultrafiltrate to form concentrated and acidified urine. Segmentally injured glomeruli may form adhesions attached to Bowman's capsule (synechiae), which can misdirect the glomerular ultrafiltrate into paraglomerular or paratubular channels leading to the interstitial space. Inflammatory necrosis tends to progress to obliterative fibrosis during healing, with loss of tubular basement membrane integrity and reduced overall functional efficiency.[6] Functional failure of the transplanted kidney is a combination of the summated loss of individual nephrons with additional disturbance of its internal architecture.

TIME COURSE OF HISTOLOGICAL DAMAGE

The pathway of progression from donor kidney to end-stage transplant failure comprises a time-dependent series of pathological insults causing histological injury that is sequentially overlaid on earlier stages of damage (Figure 27-4). There are two broad overlapping phases of allograft damage observed by sequential biopsy studies, starting with early tubulointerstitial injury followed by the addition of later microvascular and glomerular abnormalities and further progressive interstitial fibrosis and tubular atrophy.[70]

Most tubular loss and chronic interstitial fibrosis begins soon after transplantation involving mechanisms of ischemia-reperfusion injury, severe acute rejection, and persistent SCR. Later, tubular injury is less intense and may be driven by residual alloimmune mechanisms or BK virus nephropathy, and may be accompanied by glomerular, microvascular, and capillary histological changes from CNI nephrotoxicity, chronic antibody-mediated rejeciton and recurrent glomerulonephritis, as well as the effects of hypertension, dyslipidemia, and diabetes mellitus. Further acute injury may occur with an episode of late acute rejection.

Donor Abnormalities and Procurement Injury

Inherited donor changes strongly influence subsequent allograft structure, graft function, graft response to injury and, ultimately, long-term graft survival. Implantation biopsy histology is needed to define accurately the contribution of donor disease and is recommended as a standard of care. Important donor pathological features include the extent of glomerulosclerosis (>20% is severe, and these kidneys are often discarded), glomerulomegaly (with implied nephron loss and hyperfiltration), and microvascular disease (a persistent histological abnormality associated with donor age, hypertension, and death from cerebrovascular disease).

Donor brain death influences graft outcome by nonspecific pathophysiological effects and by potentiation of graft immunogenicity and alloresponsiveness. Registry data

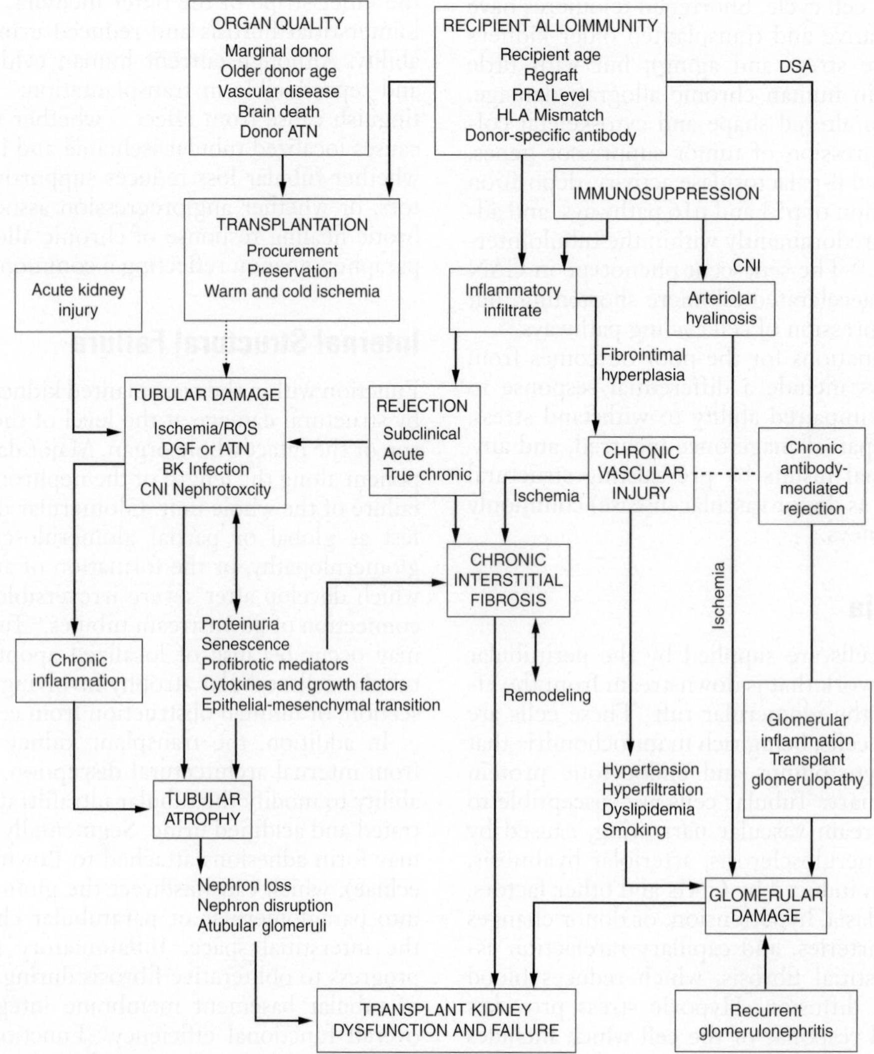

FIGURE 27-4 ■ Interaction between donor organ quality, transplantation events, and immunosuppression on differing histological compartments leading to allograft damage. ATN, acute tubular necrosis; CNI, calcineurin inhibitors; DGF, delayed graft function; DSA, donor-specific antibody; HLA, human leukocyte antigen; PRA, panel-reactive antibodies; ROS, reactive oxygen species.

demonstrate excellent and identical survival rates of living unrelated and one haplotype-matched living related donor kidneys, despite greater genetic and HLA differences, compared with cadaver donor transplants. The transplanted organ is not inert, but can be immunologically altered by proinflammatory mediators released by brain death, leading to cellular infiltration of the allograft with increased acute rejection episodes. Injured tissues express innate danger receptors or Toll receptor system ligands (normally protecting against infectious pathogens), which promote immune cell maturation, activation, and rejection. Experimental brain death provokes a cascade of chemokines, cytokines, proinflammatory lymphokines (tumor necrosis factor-α, interferon-γ), and adhesion molecules (intercellular adhesion molecule, vascular cell adhesion molecule, leukocyte function-associated antigen 1), and expression of major histocompatibility complex (MHC) class I and II antigens, which trigger a more rapid and intense host alloimmune response.

The "autonomic storm" generated by brain death is accompanied by chaotic blood pressure fluctuations, initially with a hypertensive phase from brainstem herniation and massive circulating catecholamine release, followed by hypotension from hypothalamic-pituitary dysfunction, diabetes insipidus, electrolyte abnormalities, reduced thyroid and cortisol levels, hypothermia, core temperature dysregulation, pulmonary changes, and coagulopathies. Systemic hypotension, cardiovascular instability, and adrenergic vasoconstriction may lead to donor ischemic acute kidney injury. Other histological abnormalities associated with brain death include early glomerular hyperemia, glomerulitis, periglomerulitis, endothelial cell proliferation, tubular vacuolation from osmotic agents (e.g., mannitol), and later tubular degeneration with intracellular biochemical disturbances, necrosis, and atrophy. Transplant dysfunction is greatest from hemodynamically unstable donors experiencing prolonged hypotension after brain death. The physiological effect is clinically manifested by DGF and acute tubular necrosis seen on implantation biopsy.

Delayed Graft Function and Ischemic Injury

DGF is defined by need for dialysis after transplantation, and has increased from 15% to about 22% over two decades[86] as kidneys from older deceased donors with vascular comorbidity (expanded criteria donors), or following cardiac death (non-heart-beating donors) are increasingly transplanted because of organ shortages. These marginal kidneys result in inferior initial function rates, patient and allograft survival relative to standard criteria donors, but still improve overall recipient survival compared with remaining on dialysis. The incidence of DGF correlates with donor age, organ size and quality (older donor, hypotension, diabetes, renal impairment, and hypertension), and prolonged ischemia times (from shipping or perioperative surgical reperfusion). DGF increases long-term graft loss by 41% by systematic meta-analysis.[104]

Renal tubular epithelial cells are metabolically active and consequently vulnerable to ischemia which depletes oxygen, and limits cellular metabolism and Na^+/K^+-ATPase exchanger function. Reperfusion injury from oxygenated blood generates ROS, leading to DNA breakdown, lipid peroxidation, apoptosis, and cellular necrosis of tubular cells and injury to vascular endothelial cells. Reducing the proinflammatory state and graft immunogenicity from procurement and perioperative ischemia may improve transplanted organ quality and function. Proposed therapies to ameliorate these effects include better organ preservation techniques and preservation solutions, ischemic preconditioning, and use of vasodilators or antiapoptotic molecules. Optimal intensive care unit management, pulsatile ex vivo machine perfusion, rapid transfer of organs, and prompt implantation all help reduce transplant organ stresses.

Ischemic tubular injury can recover if the basement membrane remains intact and sufficient residual tubular cells survive to replenish the nephron. Injury beyond this threshold results in permanent nephron loss. Repair of tubular injury is initiated by inflammatory and fibrogenic signaling followed by interstitial infiltration of mononuclear cells and macrophages and a variable proliferation of fibroblasts. Tissue remodeling occurs with deposition of extracellular matrix. The pattern of interstitial fibrosis and tubular atrophy is the sequela of prior tubular injury combined with the kidney's response. It is clinically accompanied by low-level proteinuria, hypertension, allograft dysfunction, and shortened graft survival.

Early Tubulointerstitial Damage

Injury to tubular cells soon after kidney transplantation occurs from many factors, including ischemia-reperfusion injury, acute tubular necrosis, acute rejection and SCR, polyomavirus infection, and CNI nephrotoxicity, which is superimposed on donor disease. CNI nephrotoxicity also may contribute to tubular injury with isometric vacuolization, patchy necrosis with microcalcification, and cytoplasmic inclusion bodies that represent giant mitochondria with abnormal cristae when high doses are used. Early interstitial fibrosis may be increased by CNI therapy compared with sirolimus-treated grafts. Tubular atrophy with loss of height of the tubular cross-section, loss of nuclei, and dilation of the tubular lumen are associated with the deposition of chronic interstitial fibrosis. Alloimmune mononuclear infiltration increases profibrotic factors, including TGF-β and the expression of the tissue inhibitor of metalloproteinases (TIMP) family of enzymes in kidney tissue. An activated cellular infiltrate within areas of tubular scarring may further aggravate later damage and fibrosis.[14,68]

The extracellular matrix is a dynamic network of proteins and proteoglycans, which accumulate from increased synthesis and decreased breakdown; this is partially mediated by TGF-β_1, angiotensin, and immunosuppressive therapy. Cyclosporine generates a profibrotic cytokine profile with increased TGF-β_1 and TIMP-1, leading to interstitial fibrosis in humans and experimental models. Abrogation by angiotensin II blockade suggests mediation by the renin–angiotensin system and a potential treatment target, although not proven in clinical practice. In contrast, cell cycle inhibitors, such as mycophenolic acid, reduce interstitial cellular proliferation, myofibroblast infiltration, and collagen deposition in vivo and in experimental chronic rejection. Some evidence shows that sirolimus also limits tubular atrophy, vascular hyperplasia, and possibly the extent of interstitial fibrosis, although these analyses are confounded by increased early alloimune injury, when compared against a more potent CNI.[21]

Acute Rejection and Alloimmune Mechanisms

Acute rejection episodes have been a consistant risk factor for reduced graft half-life and actuarial graft survival (especially for deceased donors). As the incidence of acute rejection decreases with newer immunosuppression, the individual impact of a rejection is enhanced, with severe rejection episodes remaining.

Other important alloimmune risk factors for graft loss include recipient sensitization and HLA matching (see Chapter 10). The MHC is the principal target of the alloimmune response, with reduced registry graft survival associated with HLA mismatching persisting even with modern immunosuppression. Cross-reactive groups share MHC class I antigen epitopes, and mismatch increases acute and chronic rejection rates and graft dysfunction. Cross-reactive group sharing improves long-term graft survival. Pretransplant antibodies to HLA antigens may be provoked by blood transfusions, pregnancy or miscarriage, or prior transplantation. More sensitive and specific cross-matching techniques such as antihuman globulin-augmented complement-dependent cytotoxicity crossmatch, flow cytometric or solid-phase serum screening better identify pretransplant DSA and have reduced early antibody-mediated rejection.

After renal transplantation, formation of de novo DSA has been correlated with subsequent allograft failure from chronic rejection in prospective studies. A role for antibody-mediated graft loss is supported by $C4d^+$ biopsy specimens in failing allografts with chronic rejection or transplant glomerulopathy. Rarely, antibodies against non-classic HLA antigens (e.g., endothelial cells, AT1 receptor, glomerular antigens such as heparin sulfate, and renal basement membrane) can also be pathogenic.

The influence of allograft rejection contributing to chronic injury depends on the type, timing, severity, and persistence of rejection episodes. When diagnosed and treated promptly, acute interstitial cellular rejection usually resolves without sequelae. In contrast, episodes of vascular or steroid-resistant rejection, recurrent rejection, untreated SCR, true chronic interstitial rejection, or late rejection (usually defined as >3 months after transplantation) can cause allograft damage.[55,70] Silent interstitial cellular rejection increases later interstitial fibrosis in biopsy series, and episodes of vascular rejection can be followed by later chronic vascular damage.

Subclinical Rejection

SCR is conventionally defined as histologically proven acute rejection with a tubulointerstitial mononuclear infiltration (Figure 27-5) but without concurrent functional deterioration, and is diagnosed only on biopsy specimens taken per protocol. It is clinically distinct from acute rejection, which is accompanied by rapid functional impairment and diagnosed by indication-driven pathology. There is substantial variation in the reported frequency of SCR among studies, likely related to differences in patient recipient immunological risk, HLA mismatch, prior acute rejection episodes, ethnicity, baseline immunosuppression protocol, transplant era, and timing of the biopsy after transplantation. The prevalence of acute SCR (Banff grade 1A) in 3-month protocol biopsy specimens ranges from 3% to 31%, with borderline SCR occurring in 11–41%.[70,85]

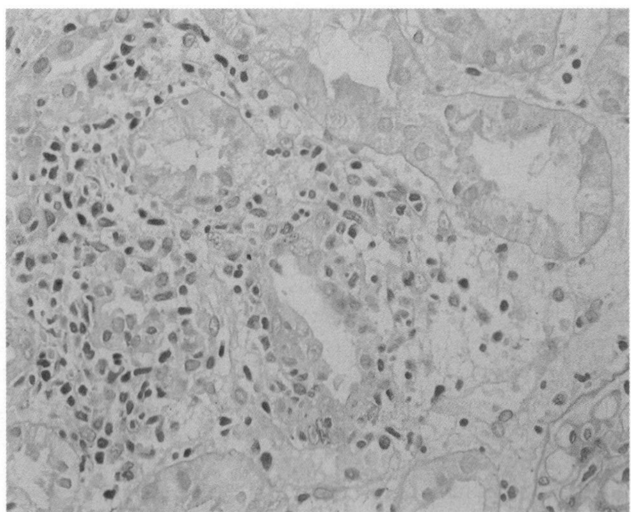

FIGURE 27-5 ■ Subclinical rejection with interstitial lymphocytic infiltration with low-level tubulitis, but unchanged renal transplant function.

Allografts with SCR result in greater subsequent histological damage, renal dysfunction, and impaired graft survival.[69,79,85] SCR is associated with chronic interstitial fibrosis and tubular atrophy, mediated by several pathways. Lymphocytes, activated macrophages, and inflammatory mediators all can generate interstitial fibrosis, controlled by profibrotic signals, including interleukin-1, interleukin-6, tumor necrosis factor-α, adhesion molecules, and TGF-β. Use of more powerful immunosuppression with control of SCR is followed by less tubulointerstitial damage in cohort studies.

The first randomized prospective study for SCR showed that corticosteroid therapy significantly decreased acute rejection episodes and chronic tubulointerstitial scores at 6 months and improved renal function by 2 years after transplantation, with a trend toward better survival by 4 years, using cyclosporine-based immunosuppression and a background SCR prevalence of 30%.[80] A second trial of SCR treatment in patients using both cyclosporine and tacrolimus (28% SCR prevalence) showed better estimated GFR (eGFR) at 6 and 12 months,[50] but no benefit could be demonstrated in a third trial using tacrolimus in low-immune risk patients, where the SCR prevalence was 4.7%.[78]

Evidence for a pathogenic role of SCR comes from the compartment-specific nature of histological injury occurring where previous or current subclinical lymphocytic infiltration is co-localized; the temporal sequence, in which SCR occurs before the onset of tubular damage; a dose-dependent relationship, in which the intensity of SCR correlates with the severity of later chronic damage; its biological plausibility; and its confirmation in several transplant populations. In sequential biopsy studies, the early interstitial mononuclear infiltration (coded by the Banff i score) usually resolves in a quasi-exponential fashion. In some individuals, however, SCR may persist at low levels on repeated biopsy specimens as chronic T-cell-mediated rejection. In compliant patients at intermediate or low immunological risk using CNI-based therapy, chronic rejection seems to be uncommon, but it may generate interstitial fibrosis and tubular atrophy in non-compliant or high-immunological-risk patients, or those using low-level immunosuppression or steroid withdrawal.

Subclinical antibody-mediated rejection can also be seen in protocol biopsies associated with a C4d-positive peritubular staining, leukocyte capillaritis with margination, and DSA. It is relatively common in positive-crossmatch or sensitized recipients, or following treatment of late antibody-associated rejection, but can also occur in 10% of standard risk recipients. Persistent sublethal microcirculation injury from circulating DSA can activate glomerular endothelial cells and widen the subendothelial space with glomerular basement membrane (GBM) reduplication, which sometimes evolves into chronic transplant glomerulopathy.[51,90]

Tubulointerstitial Injury from BK Virus Nephropathy (see Chapters 29 and 32)

BK virus is an endemic polyomavirus infection of high prevalence, low morbidity, and long latency that can asymptomatically reactivate in immunocompetent individuals.[36] After primary childhood infection, it can persist in the renal cortex and medulla, and be transmitted within a transplanted kidney. Asymptomatic reactivation can occur in 10–68% of recipients using CNI-based immunosuppression, with graft dysfunction in 1–10%. Severe BK virus nephropathy can develop with tubulointerstitial nephritis, leading to progressive renal dysfunction and graft loss (incidence 5% where 46% fail).[44] Polyomavirus allograft nephropathy is a term encompassing kidney transplant infection from BK virus or, rarely, with JC virus. Although incipient infection occurs soon after transplantation, asymptomatic BK viremia may occur within 3 months initially without graft dysfunction, and subsequently with the onset of clinical renal impairment between 3 and 12 months.

In the early phases of infection, focal virus replication in the medulla produces a mild cytopathic effect and minimal functional impairment. Viral replication within tubules forms intranuclear inclusions, which gradually enlarge with smudgy nuclear chromatin, cellular atypia, and anisocytosis (Figure 27-6). Tubular epithelial cells degenerate with rounding, detachment, and finally apoptosis or necrosis, which slough into the tubular lumen and can be seen as diagnostic urinary "decoy" cells. As multifocal viral activation advances, a cytopathic inflammatory response of monocytes, polymorphonuclear cells, and plasmacytoid cells is generated, which may resemble acute interstitial rejection (but lacks arteritis, C4d deposition, or HLA-DR expression).

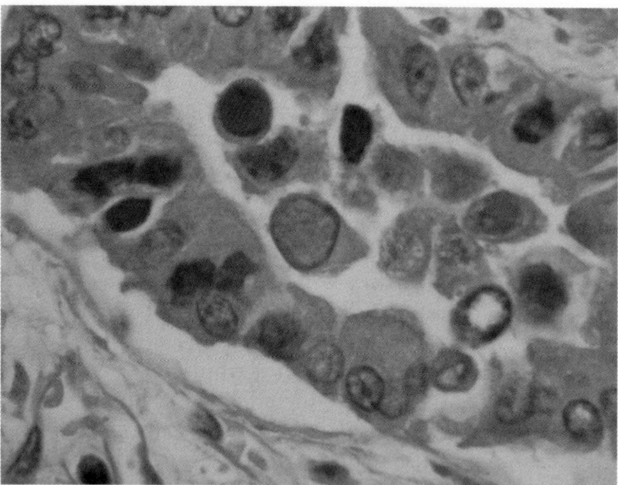

FIGURE 27-6 ■ BK virus nephropathy infecting a renal tubule. Tubular cells are abnormal with some "ground-glass" nuclear changes, smudging, tubular necrosis, and sloughing into the lumen, eventually forming urinary decoy cells.

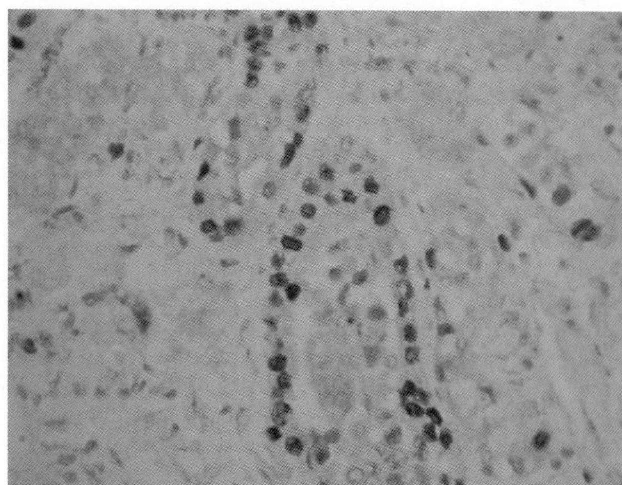

FIGURE 27-7 ■ Immunoperoxidase stain (SV40T) of BK-infected renal tubular cells (brown) – diagnostic of polyoma viral nephropathy.

When confronted by suspicious pathology, confirmation of BK viral infection should be undertaken by tissue SV40T immunochemistry (Figure 27-7) and quantification of viremia by polymerase chain reaction. Electron microscopy demonstrates the characteristic 35–38-nm intranuclear paracrystalline viral arrays which are distinguished by size and shape from adenovirus (at 70–90 nm), cytomegalovirus, and enveloped herpes simplex (at 120–160 nm). As viral infection progresses, chronic tubulointerstitial scarring with flattened and atrophic tubules can produce a non-specific pattern of fibrosis, and may be accompanied by dystrophic microcalcification and low-grade chronic inflammation, although BK virus nephropathy remains as a specific differential diagnostic entity.[36,72,76]

Progressive and Late-Stage Chronic Allograft Damage

As the transplanted kidney ages, phenotypical abnormalities may appear within the glomerular and microvascular compartments, accompanied by progressive tubulointerstitial damage.[70] Drivers for ongoing tubular injury (Figure 27-2) include residual SCR and inflammation (chronic T-cell rejection), late acute rejection (sometimes associated with antibody), CNI nephrotoxicity, BK viral infection, and late acute kidney injury secondary to an intercurrent illness. Acute late rejection from iatrogenic underimmunosuppression or non-compliance often results in severe tubular damage and the initiation of persistent subclinical or chronic rejection, leading to progressive renal dysfunction and graft failure (Figure 27-2). Microvascular attenuation and glomerulosclerosis are characteristic of late allograft pathology[39,70] and have multiple potential causes, including CNI nephrotoxicity, CAMR with transplant glomerulopathy, recurrent glomerulonephritis, diabetic microvascular disease, hypertensive glomerulosclerosis, and the effects of smoking and dyslipidemia (Figure 27-2).

Chronic T-Cell-Mediated Interstitial Rejection

The Banff schema mandates recognition of morphological features of chronic rejection, with arterial and capillary changes being emphasized as discriminating features. Chronic interstitial rejection mediated by T cells is less commonly reported in compliant patients with CNI-based therapy and involves T cells ($CD4^+$ or $CD8^+$) and macrophages. The vascular changes of chronic rejection observed in small muscular arteries include medial fibrointimal hyperplasia, focal destruction of the internal elastic lamina, and infiltration of smooth-muscle cells into the neointima, which are relatively uncommon, although some may progress to complete vascular occlusion (Figures 27-8 and 27-9). Although still classified within the T-cell-mediated umbrella, some may be accompanied by DSA. Donor disease, prior vascular rejection, hyperlipidemia, hypertension, and smoking also modulate small muscular arterial changes, expressed as chronic fibrointimal thickening (reported as the Banff cv score) (Figure 27-10), and should be considered in biopsy interpretation.

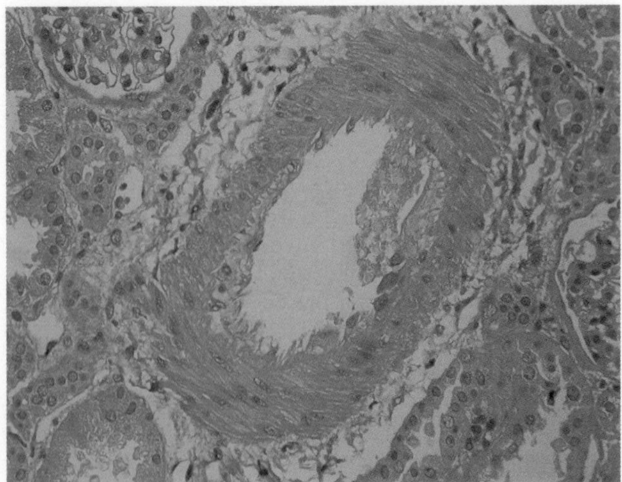

FIGURE 27-8 ■ Early vascular changes of chronic antibody-mediated rejection in a small muscular artery. Intimal and endothelial cells are abnormal with edema and early neointimal formation present. A small, partially adherent thrombus is seen in the lumen.

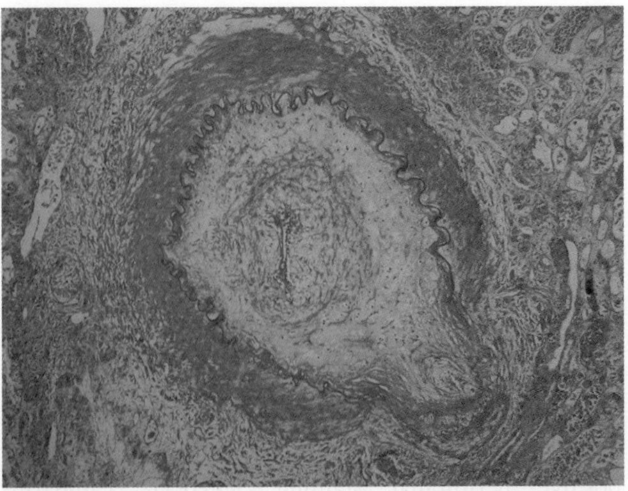

FIGURE 27-9 ■ More advanced subacute vascular changes with extensive neointimal formation (within the internal elastic lamina boundary), characterized by invading myofibroblasts, deposition of matrix proteins, collagen, and edema, resulting in near occlusion of the vascular lumen. Masson trichrome stain.

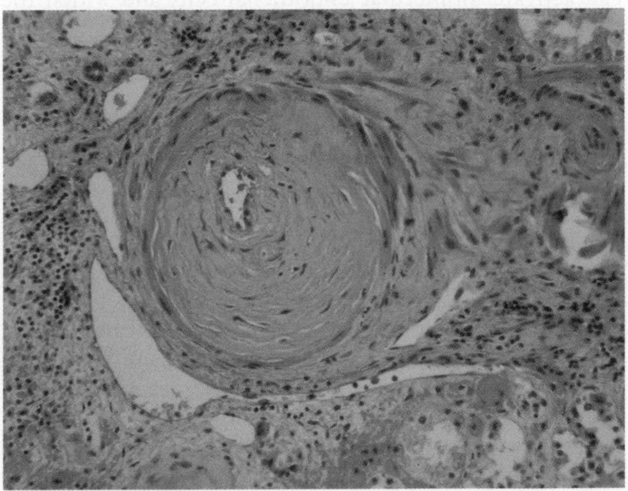

FIGURE 27-10 ■ Chronic fibrointimal hyperplasia in chronic rejection (severe), with concentric layers of smooth-muscle cells and collagen and near occlusion of the vessel.

Calcineurin Inhibitor Nephrotoxicity

The introduction of cyclosporine revolutionized kidney transplantation, sunstantially improving the 1-year graft survival and permitting transplantation of non-renal solid organs. CNIs are well tolerated and have become the backbone of modern immunosuppression (see Chapter 17), but are pleiomorphic nephrotoxins, causing histological abnormalities within all anatomical compartments of the transplanted kidney. This constitutes a significant diagnostic and management problem for their use in long-term therapy.

The classic histological features of CNI nephrotoxicity include de novo or increasing arteriolar

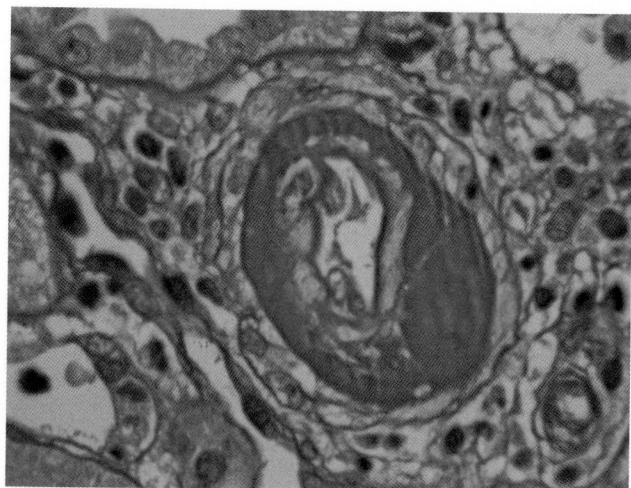

FIGURE 27-11 ■ Arteriolar hyalinosis, with a large, eccentrically located nodule within the media of the arteriole.

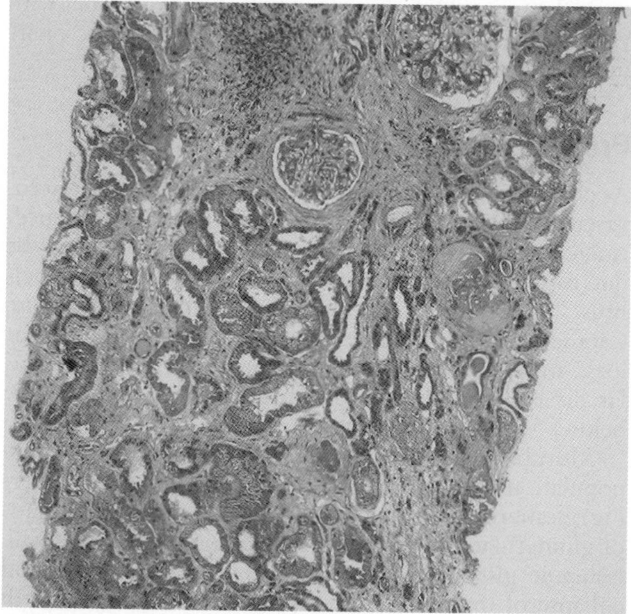

FIGURE 27-12 ■ Striped fibrosis. Demarcated areas of striped fibrosis near adjacent normal cortex, associated with interstitial fibrosis. Masson trichrome stain stains collagen green.

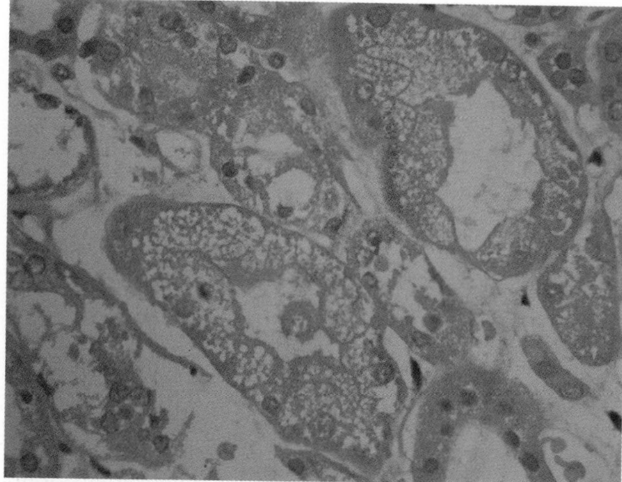

FIGURE 27-13 ■ Isometric vacuolation in the proximal tubular cells from cyclosporine tubulopathy.

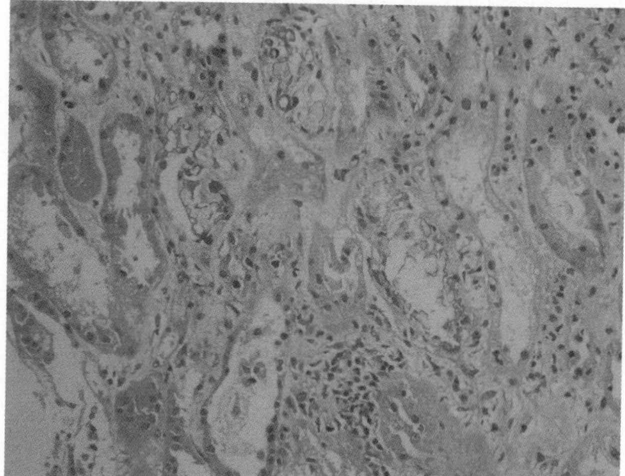

FIGURE 27-14 ■ Tubular microcalcification (blue staining) within tubular epithelial cells associated with cyclosporine nephrotoxicity.

hyalinosis (Figure 27-11) and striped cortical fibrosis (Figure 27-12), supported by isometric tubular vacuolization (Figure 27-13) and tubular microcalcification (unrelated to other causes, such as tubular necrosis and hyperparathyroidism) (Figure 27-14). Other reported diagnostic lesions include peritubular and glomerular capillary congestion (diagnostically unreliable), diffuse interstitial fibrosis (important but non-specific), toxic tubulopathy (seen predominantly with high-dose cyclosporine therapy), and juxtaglomerular hyperplasia (uncommonly seen and non-specific). Tacrolimus and cyclosporine are indistinguishable by pathology, and most data come from older studies using cyclosporine. The pathological diagnosis of CNI nephrotoxicity is hampered because of the paucity of reliable diagnostic markers and expression of an incomplete constellation of histological features in any one biopsy sample. The most reliable and specific abnormality is de novo or increasing arteriolar hyalinosis, classically described in a peripheral and nodular pattern (rather than a subendothelial and diffuse distribution) but with appropriate clinical exclusions and caveats (see later).

Striped fibrosis is a subjectively defined area of dense striped cortical fibrosis and atrophic tubules demarcated against areas of normal adjacent cortex, and probably represents watershed infarction of interlobular or arcuate arteries (Figure 27-12). Originally regarded as pathognomonic of CNI nephrotoxicity, it lacks sensitivity and specificity. Tubular microcalcification has been associated with chronic cyclosporine nephrotoxicity but can be due to localized cell necrosis from any cause (Figure 27-14), or residual hyperparathyroidism. Proximal tubular cells display isometric vacuolation in early studies using high-dose cyclosporine therapy (corresponding to dilated and stressed endoplasmic reticulum in the proximal straight tubules), cytoplasmic inclusion bodies as abnormal giant mitochondria with deranged cristae, EMT, and ultimately necrosis or apoptosis. Chronic diffuse tubulointerstitial damage has multiple causes and is diagnostically non-specific.

CNI-induced arteriolopathy has been attributed to vacuolation and necrosis of arteriolar smooth muscle and endothelial cells, followed by insudation of protein to form nodular hyaline deposits. The presence of arteriolar hyalinosis is associated with acute clinical nephrotoxicity and cyclosporine dose and trough levels.[67] Interpretative problems include variations of vascular cross-section appearance according to the plane of section, lack of accurate definition of "nodularity," early and mild CNI-related arteriolar hyalinosis initially manifesting as a circumferential lesion that later progresses to a nodular deposit, and substantial intrabiopsy variation, so evaluation of several sections is recommended. An attempt to grade circular versus non-circular involvement of arterioles and the number affected marginally improved pairwise agreement, but at the expense of useful clinical information.[8,89] Early hyalinosis may be mild and patchy, intermittently observed on sequential biopsy specimens, and is often reversible with CNI dosage reduction. These early arteriolar lesions are correlated with older donor age and inferior graft function.[8] Later arteriolar hyalinosis lesions have been associated with high-grade and progressive microvascular narrowing, increasing ischemic glomerulosclerosis, and further chronic tubulointerstitial damage; these lesions are less reversible.[67] Severe arteriolar hyalinosis gradually results in vascular narrowing and downstream ischemic glomerulosclerosis (Figure 27-15).

When arteriolar hyalinosis occurs in a failing allograft, the diagnosis of CNI nephrotoxicity is strengthened by the presence of nodularity, progression compared with baseline histology (Figure 27-11), and exclusion of alternative explanations, including donor disease (in implantation biopsy seen with older hypertensive donors), ischemic arteriolar injury, dyslipidemia, diabetes mellitus, and hypertensive nephrosclerosis (distinguished histologically by subendothelial hyalinosis, elastic lamina reduplication, and medial hyperplasia in small arteries and verified by clinical information).[8,37,67] Progressive arteriolar hyalinosis currently remains the best diagnostic marker of CNI nephrotoxicity.

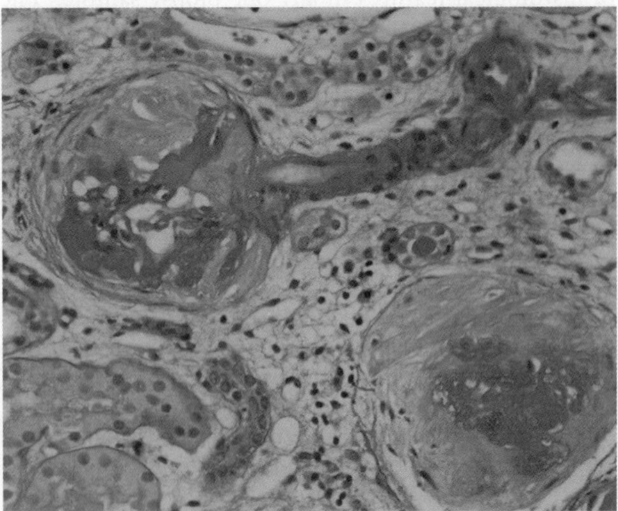

FIGURE 27-15 ■ Severe arteriolar hyalinosis of the feeding afferent arteriole leading to collapse of the glomeruli from calcineurin nephrotoxicity.

Evidence that CNI nephrotoxicity contributes to late graft injury is inferred from several lines of evidence, including the unchanged long-term graft attrition rates despite suppression of early acute rejection, the characteristic toxicity lesions in longitudinal histopathology studies,[67] shown by results of clinical trials of CNI avoidance, early withdrawal and dose reduction or late withdrawal demonstrating functional or structural improvement, and the finding of the classical histopathology lesions of CNI nephrotoxicity and renal failure occurring in either native kidneys of non-renal solid-organ transplant recipients or from patients treated with CNI for autoimmune diseases. Arteriolar hyalinosis is associated with downstream glomerulosclerosis and a common secondary diagnosis in 30% of "troubled transplants,"[27] and becomes increasingly prevalent from sustained chronic exposure and older transplant age. By one decade after transplantation it is present in the vast majority, but with variable individual severity that suggests intrinsic pharmacodynamic susceptibility.[67,70]

Progressive Glomerular Abnormalities

As chronic allograft damage progresses within the microvascular and glomerular compartments, increasing arteriolar hyalinosis and severe vascular narrowing may be due to CNI nephrotoxicity, but also from diabetes mellitus, hypertension, dyslipidemia, smoking, and aging. Glomerular abnormalities include ischemic glomerular loss, atubular glomeruli formation, recurrent glomerular disease, and chronic transplant glomerulopathy (see below).

Morphometric analysis of CAN has identified separate populations of smaller (ischemic) and larger (hyperfiltering) glomeruli, widening the base of frequency histograms of glomerular size. These separate populations of small, ischemic glomeruli are characterized by wrinkling and collapse of the glomerular capillary wall associated with extracapillary fibrotic material, and are contrasted with larger, hyperfiltering glomeruli. Ischemic glomerulosclerosis may occur secondary to early ischemic podocyte injury, associated with proteinuria and glomerulosclerosis, or later vascular or endothelial cell injury from CNIs, hypertension, or alloimmune injury. Vascular narrowing of small arteries or afferent arterioles irrespective of cause may result in downstream ischemic glomerulosclerosis.

Severe tubular injury can result in a perfused glomerulus that is functionally disconnected from its downstream proximal tubule. Atubular glomeruli are usually smaller than normal or contracted within an enlarged glomerular cyst and may be surrounded by periglomerular fibrosis. Bowman's capsule is lined by abnormal podocytes with intact interdigitating pedicles of uncertain origin. Bowman's space is filled by inspissated proteinaceous material from residual glomerular filtration and local reabsorption.[24] These atubular glomeruli are common in native tubulointerstitial kidney diseases, such as chronic pyelonephritis and lithium and cisplatin nephrotoxicity, and are diagnosed in research settings by serial sections with three-dimensional reconstruction or freeze fracture scanning electron microscopy. In normal living and cadaver donor kidneys, 1–2% of glomeruli are atubular, increasing to 17–18% with CAN and 29% with cyclosporine nephrotoxicity.[24] Although atubular glomeruli are a consequence of irreversible obliteration of the tubular lumen, many remain perfused but non-functional, whereas others progress to global glomerulosclerosis after a variable lag period of several years.

Transplant Glomerulopathy and Chronic Antibody-Mediated Rejection

Chronic transplant glomerulopathy comprises a spectrum of abnormalities, which include chronic glomerular changes of thickening or duplication of the glomerular capillary basement membrane, double contour formation, and mesangial interposition (Figures 27-16 and 27-17). Chronic glomerulopathy scores (designated as Banff cg) are determined by the extent of peripheral capillary loop involvement of the most affected of non-sclerotic glomeruli, preferably using periodic acid–Schiff stains.[70] Transplant glomerulopathy is the morphological expression of persistent CAMR, from chronic glomerular endothelial injury to the capillary loops.[13] It is reported in 5–15% of failing and failed grafts,[17,53,88,95] and associated with glomerular infiltration of activated T cells, natural killer cells, or monocytes/macrophages, endothelial C4d deposition in glomeruli or PTCs, or both, and circulating antidonor HLA antibodies.[77,87] The prevalence of C4d deposition ranges from 36% to 91% in biopsy specimens with transplant glomerulopathy,[88] 12–61% in biopsy specimens with chronic rejection and renal dysfunction,[54,77] to only 2% in well-functioning protocol biopsy specimens.[59] The prevalence varies by center, clinical scenario, methodology, and definition of C4d positivity (Figure 27-20).

Electron microscopy demonstrates glomerular endothelial swelling and activation, subendothelial widening with deposition of flocculent or fibrillary material (Figure 27-18), GBM duplication, and mesangial matrix expansion. Other associated histological features include multilamination, or multilayering, of the PTC basement membranes (Figure 27-19) and endothelial cell phenotype changes with loss of fenestrae. Moderate (five to six layers) or severe (seven or more layers) multilamination may be present in 38% of failed transplants ascribed to chronic rejection. Smaller amounts of multilamination (generally averaging two to three layers or less) may signify antibody effect in kidney transplantation, but have been reported in some native kidney diseases such as obstructive uropathy, analgesic nephropathy, radiation nephritis, reflux-dysplastic syndrome, and thrombotic microangiopathy.[42] Transplant glomerulopathy is clinically accompanied by proteinuria, reduced renal function, and graft survival.[14,88]

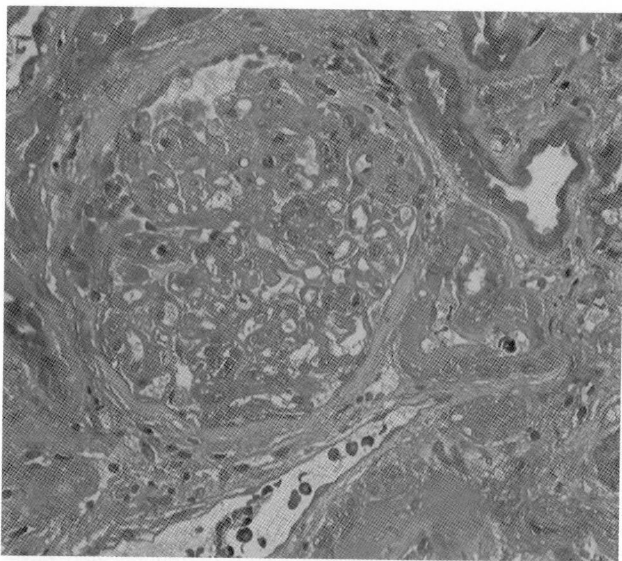

FIGURE 27-17 ■ Light microscopic appearance of transplant glomerulopathy showing increased mesangial matrix, thickened capillary loops, and partial closure of the capillary loops.

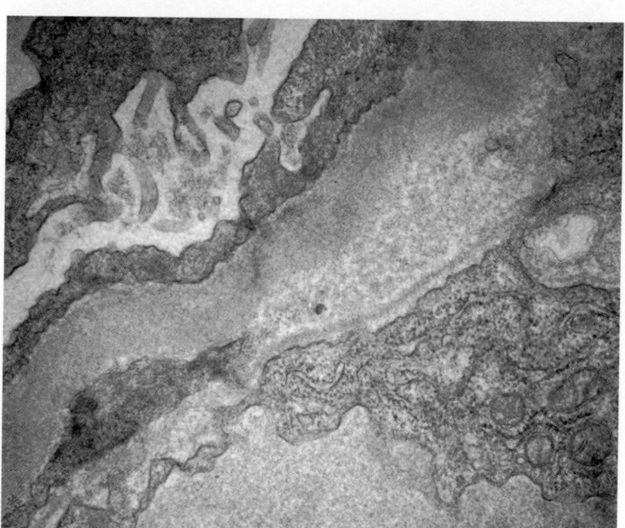

FIGURE 27-18 ■ Subendothelial fibrillary material in transplant glomerulopathy by electron microscopic examination.

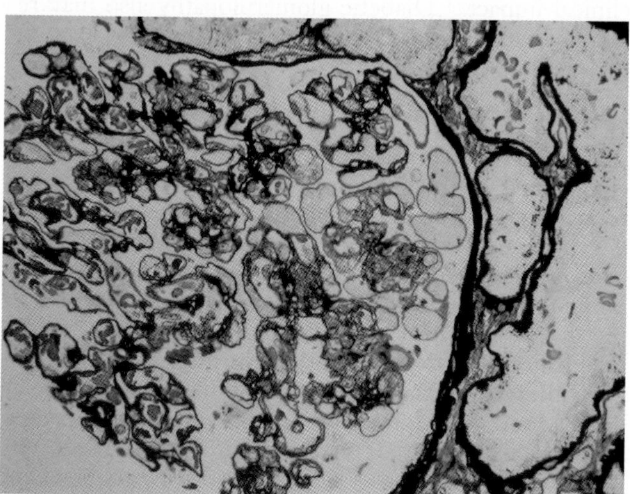

FIGURE 27-16 ■ Transplant glomerulopathy by methamine silver stain light microscopy, showing double contours of the glomerular capillary loops (seen as a parallel pair of lines).

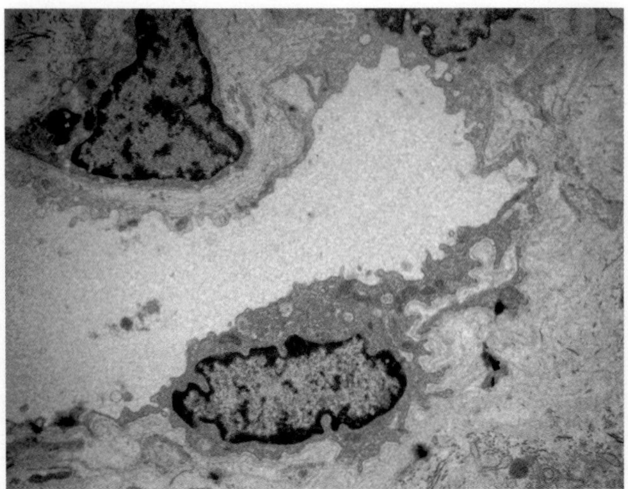

FIGURE 27-19 ■ Peritubular multilamination of the basement membrane in chronic antibody-mediated rejection (transplant glomerulopathy). Note multiple layers of reduplicated basement membrane.

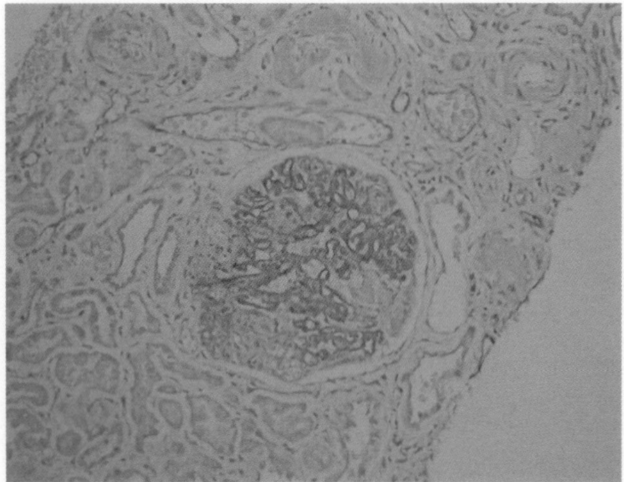

FIGURE 27-20 ■ Immunoperoxidase stain for C4d in glomerular capillary loops and peritubular capillaries in chronic antibody-mediated rejection.

The diagnostic triad of chronic (or late) antibody-mediated rejection in the context of organ dysfunction includes the following[12,61,88,90,91]:

1. Morphological features of transplant glomerulopathy (Banff score ≥cg1, with double contours on light microscopy), supported by activation of glomerular endothelial cells and widening of the subendothelial space with fibrillary material, and PTC basement membrane multilamination by electron microscopy.
2. C4d deposition in peritubular capillaries ("focal": 10% positive on immunohistochemistry) or in glomeruli (assessable only by paraffin sections), or in both – the "footprint" of classical complement activation by antibody (but relatively insensitive and may be negative).
3. The presence of circulating DSA to donor HLA or other endothelial antigens.

Mononuclear inflammatory cells adherent within the PTCs, such as glomerulitis, chronic arteriopathy with fibrous intimal thickening, and splintering of elastica, or a plasma cell interstitial infiltrate, are also supportive of CAMR. A Banff diagnosis "suggestive of chronic antibody-mediated rejection" is made when chronic capillary changes are present with one other feature of the triad. The differential diagnosis of transplant glomerulopathy includes thrombotic microangiopathy which may produce similar glomerular histology and requires clinical exclusion by blood film examination, haptoglobin levels, and lactate dehydrogenase levels (differential diagnosis includes infection, recurrent hemolytic uremic syndrome, and anticardiolipin antibody thrombotic microangiopathy), and hepatitis C mesangiocapillary glomerulonephritis (excluded by serology, viremia, and absence of GBM deposits).

Recurrent Glomerular Disease

Because glomerular disease (including diabetes) accounts for most end-stage renal failure, some recipients develop recurrence of their original disease in the allograft. Recurrent glomerulonephritis is diagnosed by exclusion of donor-transmitted disease and de novo glomerulonephritis. It has a negative impact on graft survival and causes 8.4% of allograft losses by 10 years in recipients with renal failure from glomerulonephritis.[7] The relative impact of recurrent glomerulonephritis increases as graft survival lengthens, or in some populations in whom primary glomerulonephritis is prevalent or severe. The clinical course and severity of recurrent glomerular disease often recapitulate that of the patient's original disease,[11] except for patients with vasculitis or lupus nephritis; these conditions are usually controlled by transplant immunosuppression.

FSGS (20–50% recurrence rates) and dense deposit disease (50–90% recurrence) have the worst prognosis and together constitute 55–60% of all recurrent glomerulonephritis. Membranous glomerulonephritis recurs in 29–50%; membranoproliferative glomerulonephritis type 1 recurs in 20–33%; and IgA nephropathy recurs in 58%, although with limited early (but increased later) clinical impact.[11] Diabetic glomerulopathy also may recur, but with variable clinical effect (Figure 27-21).

Late Acute Rejection and Intercurrent Illness

Acute rejection arising beyond 3 months from non-compliance or iatrogenic underimmunosuppression can present with subacute or acute renal dysfunction. While it can develop in sensitized patients, it usually occurs from medication non-compliance or iatrogenic under-immunosuppression (e.g., following severe infection or the diagnosis of cancer). Pathology usually shows well-established rejection with extensive interstitial lymphocytic infiltration, chronic interstitial fibrosis with tubular destruction, and glomerulosclerosis, often accompanied by antibody-mediated rejection (circulating DSA, endothelialitis, and tissue C4d) or vascular rejection. Late transplant acute kidney injury can accompany medical or surgical events, such as myocardial infarction, sepsis, or abdominal emergencies.

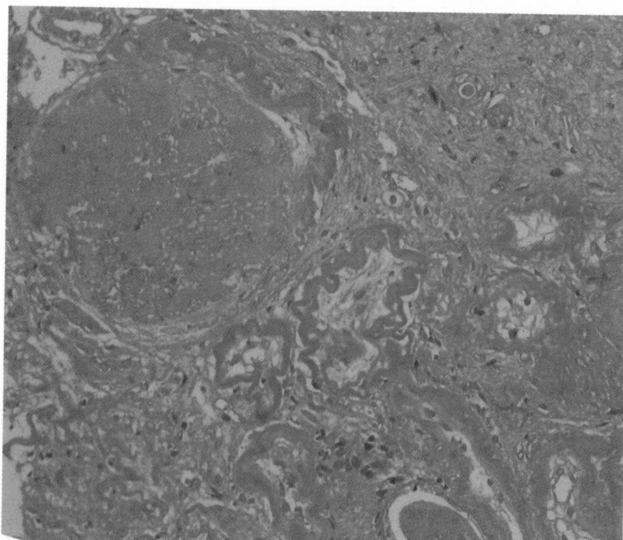

FIGURE 27-21 ■ Recurrence of diabetic nephropathy in a renal transplant showing thickened tubular basement membranes and diffuse diabetic glomerulopathy with massively increased mesangial matrix and thickened glomerular basement membrane (green).

APPROACH TO A FAILING ALLOGRAFT

Monitoring of Renal Function

Transplant renal function depends predominantly on the extent of tubulointerstitial damage, with a contribution from sclerosed glomeruli and glomerular abnormalities. Serum creatinine and calculated GFR formulas, although inexpensive and simple, are imperfect compared with the more expensive and accurate isotopic GFR methods. Errors are related to differential creatine generation (e.g., muscle loss from corticosteroids, malnutrition, and sepsis), the variable tubular secretion of creatinine, the non-linear relationship with GFR, and inaccuracies and laboratory differences in biochemical measurement. Serum creatinine underestimates the extent of tubulointerstitial damage, and early biopsy should be considered before the occurrence of severe renal dysfunction.

Proteinuria and Urinalysis

Proteinuria is a powerful and independent risk factor for graft and patient survival, and it represents a composite of several adverse diagnostic groupings such as transplant glomerulopathy, recurrent FSGS and glomerulonephritis causing glomerular proteinuria, and severe non-specific CAN with tubular proteinuria. Urine protein excretion may increase with hypertension, hyperfiltration, obesity, and mTOR inhibitor therapy, and be reduced by renin–angiotensin blockade, CNI therapy, ischemia, and poor transplant function. Residual proteinuria from native kidneys may obscure interpretation; however, this usually declines by 1–2 months after transplantation. Proteinuria that fails to decrease or increases (quantified by serial urine protein-to-creatinine ratios) occurs in 31–45% of recipients and portends a worse prognosis. Persistent, high-grade, increasing, or de novo proteinuria, or hematuria combined with proteinuria should prompt a diagnostic biopsy.

Renal Transplant Imaging

Diagnostic ultrasonography can measure transplant size, exclude ureteric obstruction as a cause of dysfunction, and evaluate vascular supply by Doppler to detect areas of cortical infarction (e.g., from a thrombosed polar artery) or renal artery stenosis. Ultrasound is excellent for the diagnosis of surgical complications, but suboptimal for either acute rejection (the features of which include increased renal volume, reduced cortical echogenicity, loss of corticomedullary differentiation, and splaying of the medullary pyramids) or chronic allograft damage. The chronic parenchymal changes of irregular cortical outline, reduced cortical width, increased echogenicity, and loss of corticomedullary junction differentiation are observed only after significant damage has occurred.

The resistance index (RI) of the kidney transplant is a non-invasive measure of intrarenal compliance calculated from early segmental renal transplant arteries as the index of peak systolic blood velocity (V_{max}) relative to the minimal diastolic velocity (V_{min}), expressed as $1-(V_{min}/V_{max})$. Higher RI values imply decreased diastolic blood flow and augmented downstream vascular resistance, and correlate with intra-abdominal pressure, older age, and pulse pressure profile and inversely with pulse rate. An RI exceeding 0.80 adversely correlates with renal impairment, graft failure, and fractional interstitial fibrosis.[75] Renal transplant angiography of chronic rejection demonstrates severely "pruned" vessels from vascular attenuation associated with chronic interstitial fibrosis. Doppler techniques can quantify intragraft blood flow where allograft perfusion decreases with parenchymal damage, and a phase-sensitive, two-dimensional speckle-tracking technique which reflects the altered elastic properties with renal allograft fibrosis. All techniques are relatively insensitive for detection of early damage.

Research techniques include magnetic resonance imaging (MRI), which can accurately quantify kidney transplant volume loss, detecting microstructural changes and blood flow alterations secondary to parenchymal damage. T1-weighted pulse sequences can distinguish acute rejection from CNI nephrotoxicity using intensity differences at the corticomedullary demarcation, and, while sensitive for parenchymal disease, is not specific and was poorly correlated with biopsy diagnosis.[98] Similary, gadolinium-enhanced dynamic turbo fast low-angle shot (FLASH) imaging, which enhances corticomedullary demarcation, also yields diagnostic overlap in severe renal dysfunction. Other techniques such as gadolinium MRI perfusion and blood oxygenation level-dependent (BOLD) MRI have been used to distinguish acute rejection from acute tubular necrosis, with medullary perfusion reduced with rejection.

Immune Surveillance Tests

Urinary Diagnostics

Urinary excretion of low-molecular-weight proteins, including β_2-microglobulin and the tubular enzymes (alanine aminopeptidase, γ-glutamyl transpeptidase, and alkaline phosphatase), α_1-microglobulinuria, *N*-acetyl-D-glucosaminidase and neutrophil gelatinase-associated lipocalin, are markers of proximal tubular injury, but are not routinely used for failing allografts. Urinary β_2-microglobulin is strongly associated with acute rejection. Urinary mRNA levels of FOXP3, a specific marker for regulatory T lymphocytes, were increased with acute rejection compared with CAN and normal biopsy specimens, and although low levels identified risk of graft failure, considerable overlap between groups limited clincial application.[65] Gene expression of other molecules from tubultar cells excreted into the urine, including cytotoxic T-lymphocyte markers, CD3 (a T-cell marker), CD103 (CD8 cytotoxic T-lymphocyte intraepithelial homing marker), perforin, granzyme A and CD25 (T-cell activation markers), interferon-inducible protein 10, and chemokine receptor CXCR3, has been correlated with acute rejection, but not with chronic rejection or normal biopsy specimens.[65] Urinary TGF-β, detected by coculture with luciferase-expressing cells or by TGF-β1 mRNA levels, increased with chronic renal allograft rejection or CAN.

Serum Immune Surveillance Markers

Non-invasive markers of immune activity are being developed as potential replacements for transplant biopsy. ELISPOT assays of activated lymphocytes secreting interferon-γ correlate with kidney transplant dysfunction,[5] and mitogen-stimulated CD4 T-cell reactivity[48] quantifies risks of infection and rejection, but diagnostic overlap, moderate specificity, and lack of independent validation and utility studies currently obscure their clinical value. Serum neopterin (an activated macrophage marker) is a sensitive marker for acute immunologic activity (increased in early or severe rejection), but is non-specific (being elevated in cytomegalovirus infection and renal dysfuction). Serum soluble CD30 levels (a T-cell helper type 2 immune response marker), while correlated with chronic rejection, are also increased by infection and influenced by CNI therapy, limiting their clinical specificity.

Kidney Transplant Biopsy

Principles Guiding Clinical Biopsy

Chronic allograft damage is best characterized by transplant histology (Tables 27-2 and 27-3; see Chapter 27). A diagnostic renal biopsy is recommended in patients with progressive chronic allograft dysfunction with the following caveats:

1. Transplant biopsy should be considered after clinical exclusion of obvious causes of acute dysfunction (see below).
2. An early biopsy should be undertaken before substantial deterioration in transplant function because late histology is often non-specific, hampering the definition of a specific diagnosis; established damage is less responsive to therapy.
3. Biopsy samples containing at least 10 glomeruli and two arteries are needed for adequacy – preferably two cores of cortex as some pathological features are patchy.

   Samples also should include arterioles (defined as two or less muscle layers and absent or incomplete internal elastic lamina) for assessment of CNI-induced hyalinosis, and small muscular arteries for assessment of immune-mediated fibrointimal hyperplasia (scored as Banff cv). Glomerular and microvascular changes provide an important etiological diagnosis. Tubulointerstitial damage can be appreciated easily on small histological samples and defines the severity of nephron loss. Older transplants may be surrounded by a dense fibrotic capsule that may need careful penetration.
4. Fibrosis may be difficult to appreciate, standardize, and quantify, especially if it is patchy, as with striped fibrosis, or variably diffuse between tubules. Objective assessment linked to a validated image analysis using trichrome or Sirius Red staining can detect collagen and early fibrosis, although other matrix proteins may not be stained. Biological

TABLE 27-2 Clinical Scenarios and Kidney Transplant Pathology

Clinical Scenarios	Key Defining Features	Associated Features
Extended or marginal donor	Arterial (cv) and arteriolar (ah) disease, glomerulosclerosis	Interstitial fibrosis
Early ischemia-reperfusion injury	Tubular necrosis or interstitial edema or both	Tubular atrophy and chronic interstitial fibrosis
Subclinical rejection	Interstitial infiltration of mononuclear cells and tubulitis	Tubulointerstitial damage
Chronic interstitial rejection	Interstitial cells and tubulitis, fibrointimal hyperplasia	Tubulointerstitial damage
Chronic antibody-mediated rejection	Transplant glomerulopathy, C4d⁺ (PTC) donor-specific antibody Mesangial matrix	Double contours, PTC-BM ML by EM mesangial matrix Proteinuria, decreased GFR
Calcineurin inhibitor nephrotoxicity	Progressive arteriolar hyalinosis, striped fibrosis	Microcalcification, diffuse fibrosis, tubulopathy
Polyomavirus nephropathy	Inflammatory tubular necrosis, viral nuclear changes, histochemistry (SV40T antigen) Blood BK virus PCR	Tubular cell virus by EM, urinary decoy cells, blood BK PCR Urinary decoy cells
Hypertensive nephrosclerosis	Arterial vascular changes, IEL reduplication	Glomerulosclerosis, arteriolar changes

ah, arteriolar hyalinosis; cv, chronic vascular changes; EM, electron microscopy; GFR, glomerular filtration rate; IEL, internal elastic lamina; PCR, polymerase chain reaction; PTC, peritubular capillary; PTC-BM ML, peritubular capillary basement membrane multilamination.

TABLE 27-3 **Kidney Transplant Diagnostic Pathology**

Banff Qualifier (Banff Code)	Interstitial Mononuclear Infiltration (i)	Tubulitis (t)	Chronic Interstitial Fibrosis (ci)	Tubular Atrophy (ct)	Fibrointimal Thickening or Glomerulopathy (cv or cg)	Arteriolar Hyalinosis (ah)	Glomerular Sclerosis	Comments
Acute tubular injury	0 to +			(+ some acute tubular loss)				Tubular injury with necrosis, nuclear changes, or tubular dilation; changes may be minimal
Acute cellular rejection	++ to +++	++ to +++						Acute renal dysfunction; i1 and t1 is borderline; occasionally arteritis with i0 and t0
Subclinical rejection	+ to +++	+ to +++						Normal renal function; acute or borderline; rarely arteritis
Sclerosing CAN "TA/IF tubulointerstitial not otherwise specified"				+ to +++	+ to +++		0 to +++	Non-specific damage; often cellular inflammation in areas of damage; very common
Chronic (interstitial or cellular) rejection	+ to +++	+ to +++	+ to +++	+ to +++	cv 0 to +++ (cg variable)		Variable	Fibrointimal hyperplasia, neointima and neomedia formation, internal elastic lamina disruption, and intimal inflammation as defining features; may be C4d+
Chronic antibody-mediated rejection with glomerulopathy	Variable	Variable	Variable	cg + to +++	(+)	+ to +++		Capillary loop double contours, capillary interposition, increased mesangial matrix, PTC multilamination by EM; usually C4d+ and donor antibody-positive
Hypertensive nephrosclerosis					cv + to +++	0 to ++	+ (wrinkled)	Internal elastic lamina reduplication, hyperplastic small arteries, small arterial hyaline may be present
Recurrent glomerulonephritis			Variable	Variable		common late	0 to +++	Proliferative glomerular changes; diagnostic IF and EM needed
Chronic CNI toxicity	(+)		+ to +++ (striped diffuse)	+ to +++ (vacuolation)	cv 0 to + (myxoid)	+ to +++ (±wrinkled)	±0 to +++	± Microcalcification and isometric vacuolation of tubules; rarely, acute thrombotic microangiopathy and juxtaglomerular hyperplasia

CAN, chronic allograft nephropathy; CNI, calcineurin inhibitor; EM, electron microscopy; IF, immunofluorescence; i1, Banff acute mild interstitial inflammation; PTC, peritubular capillary; T1, mild tubulitis; TA/IF, tubular atrophy/interstitial fibrosis.

variability, inadequate sample size, and subjective differences in the pathologist's scores can lower the diagnostic reliability of histology. Although reproducibility between pathologists is imperfect, with consistent undergrading or overgrading of scores, interobserver agreement for major chronic scores (e.g., ci and ct) is generally good compared with alloimmune markers and acute rejection parameters.

5. Implantation or postperfusion biopsy specimens are important to distinguish pre-existing donor pathology from newer changes and allow comparison of changes over time with other interval biopsy specimens. A temporal sequence of histology, interpreted in the context of interval clinical events and therapy, is important in the etiological assessment of graft dysfunction.
6. The biopsy specimen from a chronically failing graft should be processed similarly to a specimen from native kidney disease. Light microscopy assesses the presence, extent, and grade of chronic allograft damage and nephron loss, along with any accompanying specific diagnoses, such as rejection, CNI nephrotoxicity, hypertensive vascular disease, BK virus nephropathy, or transplant glomerulonephritis. Periodic acid–Schiff stain highlights basement membranes and arteriolar hyalinosis, silver stains allow identification of double contours in transplant glomerulopathy, and trichrome stains of collagen deposition define the extent of chronic fibrosis. Immunofluorescence or immunoperoxidase techniques are usually negative or non-specific in most biopsy specimens from failing allografts, but are helpful to diagnose recurrent or de novo glomerulonephritis, allograft viral infection (e.g., BK virus or cytomegalovirus stains), or CAMR (for peritubular C4d deposition). Electron microscopy can detect early transplant glomerulopathy or electron-dense deposits to confirm transplant glomerulonephritis.
7. Adequate clinical information should be provided to the interpreting pathologist, including current function; donor quality; relevant previous clinical events, such as delayed function or acute rejection; and the cause of recipient end-stage renal failure. Key diagnostic questions should be formulated. A collaborative clinicopathological diagnosis is the optimal way to interpret transplant histology (see Tables 27-2 and 27-3).

Risk and Safety of Transplant Biopsies

Needle core biopsy has an excellent safety profile with a low risk of graft loss and minimal risk of morbidity. The risk of major complications, such as substantial bleeding, macroscopic hematuria with ureteric obstruction, peritonitis, or graft loss, is approximately 1%. Minor complications reported are gross hematuria in 3.5%, perirenal hematomas in 2.5%, and asymptomatic arteriovenous fistulas in 7.3%.[82] The risk of graft loss from protocol biopsy is 0.03%, although this is increased with indication-driven procedures, when adult kidneys are placed in either an extraperitoneal or a transperitoneal position in infants, or when a needle exceeding 18-gauge is used. Safety should be maximized by using a skilled operator employing ultrasound guidance and an automated gun.

Diagnostic Algorithm for a Chronically Failing Graft

A serum creatinine that is gradually deteriorating or remains persistently elevated should be evaluated initially by exclusion of reversible causes, which include dehydration (by fluid state examination, diarrhea, diuretic use), acute CNI nephrotoxicity (by CNI blood levels), use of nephrotoxins (e.g., angiotensin-converting enzyme (ACE) inhibitors, and angiotensin receptor II blockers, non-steroidal anti-inflammatory drug or cyclooxygenase-2 inhibitors) which reduce GFR, early recurrent glomerular disease (by urinalysis for hematuria or proteinuria), and ureteric obstruction or vascular impairment (by ultrasound imaging).

Transplant biopsy can provide a specific etiologic diagnosis of a chronically failing graft, essential in the formulation of rational treatments directed towards underlying pathophysiological cause(s). Because tubulointerstitial damage is the final result of multiple previous insults, assigning a specific etiological diagnosis presents a practical difficulty for pathologists, especially if the allograft is approaching end stage, as severely damaged grafts lose their diagnostic specificity. Any kidney transplant pathology may have multiple and overlaid causes, which may be difficult to distinguish, especially in the absence of prior histology.

Broadly, the primary cause(s) of transplant deterioration should be classified as: (1) non-immune causes of tubular injury (e.g., early ischemia-reperfusion damage with DGF, donor disease); (2) alloimmune causes (acute, chronic antibody or T-cell-mediated rejection, or mixed patterns); (3) a specific diagnostic entity (e.g., recurrent glomerulonephritis, CNI nephrotoxicity, hypertensive nephrosclerosis). Rejection should be considered, as many late biopsies for cause are secondary to acute or chronic rejection, often from treatment non-compliance or iatrogenic underimmunosuppression. The dominant pathological cause of graft dysfunction should be listed, along with other secondary diagnoses. Pointers for primary treatment assignment (either increasing or decreasing immunosuppression) should include recent graft pathology (alloimmune histological clues include fibrointimal hyperplasia of small arteries, interstitial lymphocytic infiltration, lymphocytes in peritubular capillaries, transplant glomerulopathy, or positive C4d staining), the recipient's prior rejection and non-compliance history, and level of sensitization, which aids risk assesssment.

TREATMENT OF A FAILING ALLOGRAFT

Long-Term Immunosuppression

Induction and maintenance regimens currently used produce good early results; however validations of the optimal combination of immunosuppressive agents

TABLE 27-4 **Management of Chronic Allograft Nephropathy and Chronic Allograft Damage**

Prevention and Screening
Minimize ischemia-reperfusion damage (shortest ischemic times, optimal procurement and transport)
Minimize donor–recipient histoincompatibility
Rapid diagnosis and effective treatment of acute rejection
Early optimal immunosuppression (including early CNI and interleukin-2 receptor antibody in recipients with medium to high immune risk)

Control of Early Subclinical Rejection
Prophylaxis for CMV with valganciclovir or valaciclovir
Early BK virus screening (especially with high-dose immunosuppression)
Monitoring of renal function, urinalysis (for glomerulonephritis), and imaging (for ureteric obstruction)
Regular compliance review
Control of progression factors
Control hypertension (ACE inhibitor and ARB preferred to limit scarring, calcium channel blocker or beta-blocker may be added, diuretic may often may be needed)
No added salt, stop smoking, control lipids, limit weight gain
Control diabetes and urinary tract infections (if present)
Reduce (eliminate or substitute) long-term CNI in recipients with low to medium immune risk (if chronic allograft nephropathy or CNI nephrotoxicity develops)
Avoid late underimmunosuppression (risk of subclinical rejection)
Match immunosuppression to immunological risk and rejection history
Clinical management of acute interval recipient events (e.g., sepsis, acute tubular necrosis) with restitution of appropriate immunosuppression with stability of acute insult
Monitoring and preventive strategies for neoplasia and cardiovascular risk factors in patient

ACE, angiotensin-converting enzyme; ARB, angiotensin receptor blocker; CMV, cytomegalovirus; CNI, calcineurin inhibitor.

by long-term clinical studies are more limited in their follow-up (Table 27-4; see also Chapters 15–22). Most units use CNI-based triple therapy; some withdraw corticosteroids routinely, most intermittent undertake dosage adjustments, or switch therapies according to changing clinical scenarios. The ideal long-term immunosuppressive agents should be effective and well tolerated, and have minimal side effects. Desirable properties include:

1. Alloimmune effectiveness – to be able to provide adequate immunosuppression to suppress acute rejection, chronic T-cell-mediated rejection, or CAMR
2. Lack of nephrotoxicity or even renoprotective properties
3. Few or minimal cosmetic and subjective side effects to optimize compliance
4. Neutral or antineoplasic properties (e.g., mTOR inhibitors), as opposed to some properties of CNIs or antiproliferative agents that may promote cancer or metastases
5. Minimal or absent enhancement of comorbidity (e.g., lipids, posttransplant diabetes mellitus, cardiovascular disease)
6. Simple oral dosing regimes.

General Treatment Principles

Several ideas for the treatment of chronic kidney transplant damage are as follows:

1. Chronic allograft damage is the end result of multiple pathophysiological pathways of injury (Figure 27-2). Hence no single "magic bullet" is likely to be sufficient for its treatment, but rather several therapies and approaches would be needed to counteract the specific and varied etiological insults (Table 27-4). Optimal and adequate immunosuppression is of key importance. Other potentially useful treatments could include specific antagonists targeted at fibrogenic mechanisms, or indirect clinical approaches, such as the treatment of hypertension, lipids, infections, and smoking.
2. Drivers of injury are time-dependent, and therapy ideally should be initiated before or during periods of ongoing injury. Experimental and clinical data suggest that treatments have different windows of benefit. Some may only help early after transplantation, and others may be detrimental if used late. Therapeutic flexibility of immunosuppression should be maintained and adjusted to changing clinical circumstances. An example would be potent front-loaded CNI therapy to suppress early rejection, followed by minimal levels to limit nephrotoxicity or other complications.
3. Prevention is better than cure. Chronic allograft fibrosis and tubular atrophy reflect the later expression of prior pathogenic insults. Nephrons, once lost from the transplanted kidney, cannot be replaced. Early injury should be minimized by procuring an optimal donor organ, limiting ischemia-reperfusion injury, using adequate initial and maintenance immunosuppression, and implementing appropriate monitoring.
4. Therapy should be tailored according to individual requirements and immunological risk and adjusted for different and changing clinical scenarios. Examples would be CNI minimization strategies with DGF or late CNI nephrotoxicity, or conversely, strengthening of immunosuppression when subclinical, chronic, or late rejection has developed. Optimal immunosuppression appropriate to each individual patient's immunological risk category should be instituated, as well as implementing early (biopsy) diagnosis and adequate treatment for severe or resistant rejection. Severe rejection may result in persistent SCR, so follow-up biopsy may be considered.
5. Technical advances in tissue pathology, such as gene complementary DNA microarrays, microRNA, proteomics, and metabolomics, are expected to yield diagnostic advances and mechanistic information. Allograft transcriptome changes occur before histological fibrosis, and improved diagnostics may yield better disease classification, allowing optimization of treatment strategies.

Treatment Approach by Specific Diagnosis

A specific etiologic diagnosis of transplant dysfunction is essential for rational treatment directed towards the underlying pathophysiological cause(s).

Interstitial Fibrosis and Tubular Atrophy

The most common pathology of slowly progressive graft failure is chronic interstitial fibrosis and tubular atrophy, usually accompanied by vascular changes and glomerulosclerosis.[70] Formally designated as sclerosing chronic allograft nephropathy,[92] the interstitial fibrosis and tubular atrophy pattern occurs in 27–45% of late graft losses,[17,27] and most biopsies taken late after transplantation.[14,27,64,70,81] It represents the final common pathway of nephron injury with its fibrotic healing response, rather than a specific diagnostic entity. While several pathogenic pathways can lead to interstitial fibrosis and tubular atrophy, the alloimmune response remains an important cause.[68,70]

The clinical approach to a failing graft with interstitial fibrosis and tubular atrophy should consider potential immune and non-immune etiologies, by collating clinical, biological and histological information. Interstitial fibrosis and tubular atrophy should be classified by pathophysiology as primarily attributable to: (1) early non-immune causes, such as donor disease or ischemia-reperfusion damage; (2) immune injury, from acute, severe, persistent, or late rejection; (3) other specific diagnostic entities, such as recurrent disease, BK virus nephropathy, hypertension, and CNI toxicity. Several causes of injury may coexist at one time, or be differentially expressed over the graft's lifetime; hence several diagnoses may be present on a single biopsy (Table 27-2).

One treatment strategy for the interstitial fibrosis and tubular atrophy–CAN pattern is CNI minimization, on the assumption than CNI nephrotoxicity is its primary cause. CNI-sparing regimes supplemented by mycophenolate increase transplant GFR in meta-analyses of randomized controlled trials and tend to improve graft survival, with acute rejection only being increased in trials of mandated CNI elimination, but not for avoidance or dysfunction.[62] A large randomized study of transplant dysfunction (where CAN was proven in 91.3%) substituted sirolimus for CNI, but failed its primary eGFR difference end-point versus continued CNI, and was futile with severe transplant dysfunction (eGFR <40 mL/min) or when proteinuria exceeded 0.5 g/day.[81] In other controlled trials, CNI elimination with sirolimus substitution or initial avoidance reduced vascular and tubulointerstitial damage.[20,64]

Approach to Calcineurin Inhibitor Nephrotoxicity

Isolated CNI nephrotoxicity (either acute cyclosporine-mediated glomerular vasoconstriction or chronic structural nephrotoxicity without rejection), if recognized early, generally has a relatively good outcome when treated by CNI-sparing regimes.[27] CNI withdrawal reverses the functional decline and improves eGFR in failing transplants.[20] Randomized trials of reduction or withdrawal of CNI improved renal function in 90% of patients, with a small risk of rejection and graft loss.[1] Patients interconverted from cyclosporine to low-dose tacrolimus showed improved renal function, lipids, hypertension, and cardiovascular markers, but without a change in 5-year graft survival.[84]

When deteriorating function from CNI nephrotoxicity occurs in low immune-risk patients (and SCR is excluded by biopsy), then CNI withdrawal and maintenance with concentration-controlled mycophenolate mofetil and corticosteroids are recommended.[33] When CNI nephrotoxicity occurs in recipients of higher immune risk, retransplants or previous rejection(s), then CNI can be either minimized or substituted with sirolimus or everolimus, with serum creatinine monitoring (the rejection risk for withdrawal approximates 10%).[46] These mTOR inhibitors are weaker immunosuppressive agents which are poorly tolerated at higher doses with side effects, including mouth ulcers, peripheral edema, proteinuria, anemia, or thrombocytopenia, causing discontinuation in 30–45% of patients.

Newer, non-nephrotoxic immunosuppressive agents may also be considered, although long-term clinical data are incomplete. Belatacept (targeting the CD28-CD80/86 pathway and T-cell costimulation) and tofacitinib (a Janus kinase 1/3 inhibitor) when combined with mycophenolate decreased graft failure (odds ratio 0.61; 95% confidence interval 0.39–0.96) in a meta-analysis of CNI-sparing trials.[83] Voclosporine, a cyclosporine analogue which is immunologically non-inferior to tacrolimus, has claimed reduced nephrotoxicity. The CD2-specific fusion protein alefacept (targeting the LFA3-CD2 pathway and selectively eliminating memory T cells) and sotrastaurin (a protein kinase C inhibitor reducing T-lymphocyte activation and cytokine release) are currently in preclinical development.

Chronic Antibody-Mediated Rejection

CAMR may occur from unrecognized pre-existing DSA or the development of de novo antibodies after transplantation,[95,97] which are often anti-HLA class II and secondary to treatment non-compliance or underimmunosuppression.

Evidence for treatment of CAMR is limited to uncontrolled cohort studies, which have been adapted from acute antibody-mediated rejection. Strengthened baseline immunosuppression with increased tacrolimus and mycophenolate dosages (suppressing B- and T-cell expansion) and use of corticosteroids (which are re-added if patients are steroid-free) are suggested. ACE inhibitors or angiotensin II receptor blockers to limit proteinuria may be added. Aggressive treatments, such as plasmapheresis to remove circulating DSA with intravenous immunoglobulin, supplemented by rituximab (a monoclonal antibody against CD20-bearing B cells but not plasma cells), produce variable results. The roles of bortezomib, a proteasome inhibitor of plasma cells, and eculizumab, an anti-C5 antibody inhibitor, in the treatment of CAMR show some promise but require further evaluation.

Chronic Active T-Cell-Mediated Rejection

Chronic active T-cell-mediated rejection is characterized by the presence of persistent interstitial T-lymphocyte infiltration with associated tubulitis, B cells and macrophages, and represents a failure of maintenance immunosuppression to control residual alloimmune activity. Rarely, fibrointimal hyperplasia of small muscular arteries occurs, and can progress to vascular occlusion.

Suggested treatment involves strengthened immunosuppression, such as conversion from cyclosporine to tacrolimus,[103] azathioprine to mycophenolate mofetil,[47] and addition of corticosteroids to dual therapy. Compliance checks, review of appropriate target blood drug levels, and exclusion of interfering agents (e.g., St. John's wort or phenytoin inducing metabolizing enzymes and reducing CNI levels) are prudent.

Treatment of Acute Late Rejection

Acute rejection can develop late after transplantation in sensitized patients but more commonly occurs from medication non-compliance or medical underimmunosuppression. Clinically severe, frequently steroid-resistant and difficult to reverse, the histology displays widespread tubulointerstitial damage, interstitial infiltration with eosinophils, plasma cells, and macrophages, and is often associated with de novo DSA and vascular rejection.

Initial treatment by pulse corticosteroids and strengthening baseline immunosuppression has limited success, and use of antithymocyte globulin and/or plasma exchange with intravenous immunoglobulin or rituximab requires careful consideration of recipient risk and the potential graft salvageability. Uncontrolled chronic rejection leading to progressive graft failure is common.

Treatment of Recurrent Disease

Recurrent or de novo glomerulonephritis fails in up to 8.4% of grafts,[7,25,41] with clinical clues of hematuria or proteinuria. Generally, blood pressure control and renin–angiotensin system blockade, which appear beneficial in cohort studies, are suggested. Specific treatment of recurrent glomerulonephritis is summarized below according to disease.

Recurrent focal segmental glomerulosclerosis. FSGS has a most significant clinical impact because of its high recurrence rate, poor intermediate outcome, and the number of young patients with FSGS who undergo transplantation. FSGS affects glomerular visceral epithelial cells (podocytes) from either genetic mutations in critical podocyte proteins or from circulating protein "toxic permeability factors" which injure the podocyte and increase glomerular permeability. Idiopathic FSGS recurs in 20–50% and approximately half fail within 5 years. FSGS with an early childhood onset, rapid progression to dialysis, diffuse mesangial hypercellularity or glomerular collapse, or fulminant recurrence in previous allografts is an adverse risk factor. Graft loss from recurrent FSGS predicts recurrence in 70% of subsequent allografts, and most of these fail, potentially precluding that individual from future transplantation.

Proteinuria may recur within hours, but usually is seen by 1–2 weeks after transplantation. Recurrence of FSGS is suspected by increasing weekly spot urine protein/creatinine ratios and proven by biopsy where podocyte foot process effacement seen on electron microscopy is the earliest marker, occurring well before segmental glomerulosclerosis on light microscopy. Plasma exchange to remove circulating protein, high-dose cyclosporine, corticosteroids, and ACE inhibitors (or angiotensin II receptor blockers) can achieve complete or partial remission in 80–90%.[9] TOR inhibitors, which affect the podocyte and cause proteinuria, should be avoided.

Membranous Glomerulonephritis. Membranous glomerulonephritis recurs in 10–30% of patients and is the most common de novo glomerular disease. Recurrent disease occurs slightly sooner (1–2 years) than de novo membranous glomerulonephritis (2–3 years), and both usually manifest as nephrotic syndrome. The 10-year graft loss rate is approximately 50%, with increased risk in male recipients, recipients with aggressive original disease, and recipients of living related transplants. Subepithelial immune complexes, containing terminal complement, insert into podocyte membranes, causing sublytic cellular activation, oxidant and protease production, and damage to the underlying GBM. Immunosuppression with mycophenolate mofetil or azathioprine, corticosteroids to reduce antibody formation, or rituximab may have a role.

Other Recurrent Diseases. Immunosuppression usually controls most immune-mediated renal diseases, including antineutrophil cytoplasmic antibody vasculitis, lupus nephritis, and Goodpasture's disease. IgA nephropathy commonly recurs but generally with a mild clinical impact, and treatment using corticosteroids and mycophenolate is suggested. Rapid corticosteroid withdrawal approximately triples the risk of recurrent glomerulonephritis.[49] Light-chain deposition disease often recurs. Dense deposit disease recurs in 50–90% with graft failure but case reports suggest benefit with eculizumab. Fabry disease recurs late after transplantation, requiring specific agalsidase treatment. Transplant diabetic nephropathy also reappears late with proteinuria and graft dysfunction and characteristic tissue pathology.

Treatment of BK Virus Nephropathy

Current antiviral agents are ineffective against BK, and correspondingly, preventive strategies of avoidance of excessive immunosuppression and regular viral surveillance by blood nucleic acid (polymerase cahin reaction) testing are recommended. Early detection of viremia before graft dysfunction occurs is treated by cautious reduction of immunosuppresion, which often reduces or eliminates circulating virus before destructive parenchymal infection.

BK viral allograft nephropathy is difficult to eradicate once established, especially if accompanied by high-grade interstitial inflammation.[44,72] Ciprofloxacin, low-dose cidofovir, elimination or substitution of mycophenolate with either leflunonide (all weak antiviral agents) or azathioprine, conversion from tacrolimus to low-dose cyclosporine or 50% reduction in the CNI dose, or regular intravenous immunoglobulin therapy (for BK infection coexisting with "rejection") are all potential therapies demonstrating limited benefit in small uncontrolled studies.[35,46]

SUMMARY

Progressive late allograft failure and chronic allograft damage are best conceptualized as the consequence of cumulative transplant damage from time-dependent immune and non-immune insults resulting in a final common pathway of nephron loss and its fibrotic healing response. Allograft damage is common, progressive, time-dependent, and remains clinically important, despite improvements in immunosuppression and the control of early acute rejection episodes.

An early phase of tubulointerstitial damage occurs soon after transplantation, secondary to causes such as ischemia-reperfusion injury, acute tubular necrosis, acute rejection and SCR, polyomavirus nephropathy, and CNI tubular nephrotoxicity, which are superimposed on any pre-existing donor disease. Subsequently, cellular infiltration and alloimmune injury gradually lessen, although chronic T-cell-mediated rejection can persist in some. Microvascular and glomerular abnormalities are progressively added from causes including CNI nephrotoxicity, hypertension, chronic antibody-mediated rejection with transplant glomerulopathy, and recurrent or de novo glomerulonephritis.

These pathogenic insults are associated with disruption of the internal architecture of the transplanted kidney, cortical ischemia from microvascular attenuation, and the persistent chronic inflammation that fails to resolve, and cytokine, chemokine and growth factor-promoting genetic and phenotypical tubular changes with excessive fibrosis.

Progressive allograft dysfunction is detected by serial monitoring of serum creatinine concentration and investigated by evaluation of therapeutic drug levels, urinalysis, imaging, and a timely diagnostic biopsy. A careful collaborative etiological diagnosis should consider acute or chronic rejection against non-immune factors such as pre-existing donor quality or early ischemia-reperfusion injury, recurrent glomerular disease, allograft BK viral infection and CNI nephrotoxicity, and accelerating factors such as hypertension, proteinuria, dyslipidemia, and smoking. Treatment should be targeted towards the dominant pathophysiological diagnosis.

Acknowledgments

I am grateful for the excellent photomicrographs provided by Dr. Rajathurai Murugasa and Prof. Ranjit S. Nanra, of John Hunter Hospital, Newcastle, and by Dr. Moses D. Wavamunno and Mr. Matthew J. Vitalone of CTRR, Westmead Hospital.

REFERENCES

1. Abramowicz D, Del Carmen Rial M, Vitko S, et al. Cyclosporine withdrawal from a mycophenolate mofetil-containing immunosuppressive regimen: results of a five-year, prospective, randomized study. J Am Soc Nephrol 2005;16(7):2234–40.
2. Albrecht EW, van Goor H, Smit-van Oosten A, et al. Long-term dietary L-arginine supplementation attenuates proteinuria and focal glomerulosclerosis in experimental chronic renal transplant failure. Nitric Oxide 2003;8(1):53–8.
3. Benigni A, Bruzzi I, Mister M, et al. Nature and mediators of renal lesions in kidney transplant patients given cyclosporine for more than one year. Kidney Int 1999;55(2):674–85.
4. Bestard O, Cunetti L, Cruzado JM, et al. Intragraft regulatory T cells in protocol biopsies retain foxp3 demethylation and are protective biomarkers for kidney graft outcome. Am J Transplant 2011;11(10):2162–72.
5. Bestard O, Nickel P, Cruzado JM, et al. Circulating alloreactive T cells correlate with graft function in longstanding renal transplant recipients. J Am Soc Nephrol 2008;19(7):1419–29.
6. Bonsib SM, Abul-Ezz SR, Ahmad I, et al. Acute rejection-associated tubular basement membrane defects and chronic allograft nephropathy. Kidney Int 2000;58(5):2206–14.
7. Briganti EM, Russ GR, McNeil JJ, et al. Risk of renal allograft loss from recurrent glomerulonephritis. N Engl J Med 2002;347(2):103–9.
8. Brocker V, Schubert V, Scheffner I, et al. Arteriolar lesions in renal transplant biopsies: prevalence, progression, and clinical significance. Am J Pathol 2012;180(5):1852–62.
9. Canaud G, Zuber J, Sberro R, et al. Intensive and prolonged treatment of focal and segmental glomerulosclerosis recurrence in adult kidney transplant recipients: a pilot study. Am J Transplant 2009;9(5):1081–6.
10. Carew RM, Wang B, Kantharidis P. The role of EMT in renal fibrosis. Cell Tissue Res 2012;347(1):103–16.
11. Chadban S. Glomerulonephritis recurrence in the renal graft. J Am Soc Nephrol 2001;12(2):394–402.
12. Colvin RB. Antibody-mediated renal allograft rejection: diagnosis and pathogenesis. J Am Soc Nephrol 2007;18(4):1046–56.
13. Colvin RB, Smith RN. Antibody-mediated organ-allograft rejection. Nat Rev Immunol 2005;5(10):807–17.
14. Cosio FG, Grande JP, Wadei H, et al. Predicting subsequent decline in kidney allograft function from early surveillance biopsies. Am J Transplant 2005;5(10):2464–72.
15. Davies DR, Bittmann I, Pardo J. Histopathology of calcineurin inhibitor-induced nephrotoxicity. Transplantation 2000;69(12 Suppl.):SS11–3.
16. Djamali A, Reese S, Yracheta J, et al. Epithelial-to-mesenchymal transition and oxidative stress in chronic allograft nephropathy. Am J Transplant 2005;5(3):500–9.
17. El-Zoghby ZM, Stegall MD, Lager DJ, et al. Identifying specific causes of kidney allograft loss. Am J Transplant 2009;9(3):527–35.
18. Evans NJ, White SA, Bicknell GR, et al. The expression of endothelin and inducible nitric oxide synthase in human renal allografts and their role in chronic renal allograft nephropathy. Transplant Proc 2001;33(1–2):1181.
19. Fernandez-Fresnedo G, Plaza JJ, Sanchez-Plumed J, et al. Proteinuria: a new marker of long-term graft and patient survival in kidney transplantation. Nephrol Dial Transplant 2004;19(Suppl. 3): iii47–51.
20. Flechner SM, Kobashigawa J, Klintmalm G. Calcineurin inhibitor-sparing regimens in solid organ transplantation: focus on improving renal function and nephrotoxicity. Clin Transplant 2008;22(1):1–15.
21. Flechner SM, Kurian SM, Solez K, et al. De novo kidney transplantation without use of calcineurin inhibitors preserves renal structure and function at two years. Am J Transplant 2004;4(11):1776–85.
22. Galichon P, Vittoz N, Xu-Dubois YC, et al. Epithelial phenotypic changes detect cyclosporine in vivo nephrotoxicity at a reversible stage. Transplantation 2011;92(9):993–8.
23. Gallagher MP, Hall B, Craig J, et al. A randomized controlled trial of cyclosporine withdrawal in renal-transplant recipients: 15-year results. Transplantation 2004;78(11):1653–60.
24. Gibson IW, Downie TT, More IA, et al. Atubular glomeruli and glomerular cysts – a possible pathway for nephron loss in the human kidney? J Pathol 1996;179(4):421–6.
25. Golgert WA, Appel GB, Hariharan S. Recurrent glomerulonephritis after renal transplantation: an unsolved problem. Clin J Am Soc Nephrol 2008;3(3):800–7.
26. Gourishankar S, Hunsicker LG, Jhangri GS, et al. The stability of the glomerular filtration rate after renal transplantation is improving. J Am Soc Nephrol 2003;14(9):2387–94.
27. Gourishankar S, Leduc R, Connett J, et al. Pathological and clinical characterization of the 'troubled transplant': data from the DeKAF study. Am J Transplant 2010;10(2):324–30.
28. Grandaliano G, Di Paolo S, Monno R, et al. Protease-activated receptor 1 and plasminogen activator inhibitor 1 expression in chronic allograft nephropathy: the role of coagulation and fibrinolysis in renal graft fibrosis. Transplantation 2001;72(8):1437–43.
29. Grgic I, Duffield JS, Humphreys BD. The origin of interstitial myofibroblasts in chronic kidney disease. Pediatr Nephrol 2012;27(2):183–93.
30. Grimm PC, Nickerson P, Jeffery J, et al. Neointimal and tubulointerstitial infiltration by recipient mesenchymal cells in chronic renal-allograft rejection. N Engl J Med 2001;345(2):93–7.

31. Halloran PF, Melk A, Barth C. Rethinking chronic allograft nephropathy: the concept of accelerated senescence. J Am Soc Nephrol 1999;10(1):167–81.
32. Hazzan M, Hertig A, Buob D, et al. Epithelial-to-mesenchymal transition predicts cyclosporine nephrotoxicity in renal transplant recipients. J Am Soc Nephrol 2011;22(7):1375–81.
33. Hazzan M, Labalette M, Copin MC, et al. Predictive factors of acute rejection after early cyclosporine withdrawal in renal transplant recipients who receive mycophenolate mofetil: results from a prospective, randomized trial. J Am Soc Nephrol 2005;16(8):2509–16.
34. Hertig A, Verine J, Mougenot B, et al. Risk factors for early epithelial to mesenchymal transition in renal grafts. Am J Transplant 2006;6(12):2937–46.
35. Hilton R, Tong CY. Antiviral therapy for polyomavirus-associated nephropathy after renal transplantation. J Antimicrob Chemother 2008;62(5):855–9.
36. Hirsch HH, Steiger J. Polyomavirus BK. Lancet Infect Dis 2003;3(10):611–23.
37. Horike K, Takeda A, Yamaguchi Y, et al. Is arteriolar vacuolization a predictor of calcineurin inhibitor nephrotoxicity? Clin Transplant 2011;25(Suppl. 23):23–7.
38. Hume DM, Merrill JP, Miller BF, et al. Experiences with renal homotransplantation in the human: report of nine cases. J Clin Invest 1955;34(2):327–82.
39. Ishii Y, Sawada T, Kubota K, et al. Injury and progressive loss of peritubular capillaries in the development of chronic allograft nephropathy. Kidney Int 2005;67(1):321–32.
40. Ishii Y, Shimizu A, Sawada T, et al. Injury of peritubular capillaries correlates with graft function in chronic renal allograft nephropathy. Transplant Proc 2001;33(1–2):1213–4.
41. Ivanyi B. A primer on recurrent and de novo glomerulonephritis in renal allografts. Nat Clin Pract Nephrol 2008;4(8):446–57.
42. Ivanyi B, Fahmy H, Brown H, et al. Peritubular capillaries in chronic renal allograft rejection: a quantitative ultrastructural study. Hum Pathol 2000;31(9):1129–38.
43. Iwano M, Plieth D, Danoff TM, et al. Evidence that fibroblasts derive from epithelium during tissue fibrosis. J Clin Invest 2002;110(3):341–50.
44. Johnston O, Jaswal D, Gill JS, et al. Treatment of polyomavirus infection in kidney transplant recipients: a systematic review. Transplantation 2010;89(9):1057–70.
45. Kaelin Jr. WG, Ratcliffe PJ. Oxygen sensing by metazoans: the central role of the HIF hydroxylase pathway. Mol Cell 2008;30(4):393–402.
46. Kasiske BL, Zeier MG, Chapman JR, et al. KDIGO clinical practice guideline for the care of kidney transplant recipients: a summary. Kidney Int 2010;77(4):299–311.
47. Knight SR, Russell NK, Barcena L, et al. Mycophenolate mofetil decreases acute rejection and may improve graft survival in renal transplant recipients when compared with azathioprine: a systematic review. Transplantation 2009;87(6):785–94.
48. Kowalski RJ, Post DR, Mannon RB, et al. Assessing relative risks of infection and rejection: a meta-analysis using an immune function assay. Transplantation 2006;82(5):663–8.
49. Kukla A, Chen E, Spong R, et al. Recurrent glomerulonephritis under rapid discontinuation of steroids. Transplantation 2011;91(12):1386–91.
50. Kurtkoti J, Sakhuja V, Sud K, et al. The utility of 1- and 3-month protocol biopsies on renal allograft function: a randomized controlled study. Am J Transplant 2008;8(2):317–23.
51. Lerut E, Naesens M, Kuypers DR, et al. Subclinical peritubular capillaritis at 3 months is associated with chronic rejection at 1 year. Transplantation 2007;83(11):1416–22.
52. Mannon RB, Matas AJ, Grande J, et al. Inflammation in areas of tubular atrophy in kidney allograft biopsies: a potent predictor of allograft failure. Am J Transplant 2010;10(9):2066–73.
53. Matas AJ, Leduc R, Rush D, et al. Histopathologic clusters differentiate subgroups within the nonspecific diagnoses of CAN or CR: preliminary data from the DeKAF study. Am J Transplant 2010;10(2):315–23.
54. Mauiyyedi S, Pelle PD, Saidman S, et al. Chronic humoral rejection: identification of antibody-mediated chronic renal allograft rejection by C4d deposits in peritubular capillaries. J Am Soc Nephrol 2001;12(3):574–82.
55. McDonald S, Russ G, Campbell S, et al. Kidney transplant rejection in Australia and New Zealand: relationships between rejection and graft outcome. Am J Transplant 2007;7(5):1201–8.
56. Meier-Kriesche HU, Schold JD, Kaplan B. Long-term renal allograft survival: have we made significant progress or is it time to rethink our analytic and therapeutic strategies? Am J Transplant 2004;4(8):1289–95.
57. Melk A. Senescence of renal cells: molecular basis and clinical implications. Nephrol Dial Transplant 2003;18(12):2474–8.
58. Melk A, Schmidt BM, Takeuchi O, et al. Expression of p16INK4a and other cell cycle regulator and senescence associated genes in aging human kidney. Kidney Int 2004;65(2):510–20.
59. Mengel M, Bogers J, Bosmans JL, et al. Incidence of C4d stain in protocol biopsies from renal allografts: results from a multicenter trial. Am J Transplant 2005;5(5):1050–6.
60. Mengel M, Reeve J, Bunnag S, et al. Scoring total inflammation is superior to the current Banff inflammation score in predicting outcome and the degree of molecular disturbance in renal allografts. Am J Transplant 2009;9(8):1859–67.
61. Mengel M, Sis B, Haas M, et al. Banff 2011 meeting report: new concepts in antibody-mediated rejection. Am J Transplant 2012;12(3):563–70.
62. Moore J, Middleton L, Cockwell P, et al. Calcineurin inhibitor sparing with mycophenolate in kidney transplantation: a systematic review and meta-analysis. Transplantation 2009;87(4):591–605.
63. Moreso F, Ibernon M, Goma M, et al. Subclinical rejection associated with chronic allograft nephropathy in protocol biopsies as a risk factor for late graft loss. Am J Transplant 2006;6(4):747–52.
64. Mota A, Arias M, Taskinen EI, et al. Sirolimus-based therapy following early cyclosporine withdrawal provides significantly improved renal histology and function at 3 years. Am J Transplant 2004;4(6):953–61.
65. Muthukumar T, Dadhania D, Ding R, et al. Messenger RNA for FOXP3 in the urine of renal-allograft recipients. N Engl J Med 2005;353(22):2342–51.
66. Naesens M. Replicative senescence in kidney aging, renal disease, and renal transplantation. Discov Med 2011;11(56):65–75.
67. Nankivell BJ, Borrows RJ, Fung CL, et al. Calcineurin inhibitor nephrotoxicity: longitudinal assessment by protocol histology. Transplantation 2004;78(4):557–65.
68. Nankivell BJ, Borrows RJ, Fung CL, et al. Delta analysis of posttransplantation tubulointerstitial damage. Transplantation 2004;78(3):434–41.
69. Nankivell BJ, Borrows RJ, Fung CL, et al. Natural history, risk factors, and impact of subclinical rejection in kidney transplantation. Transplantation 2004;78(2):242–9.
70. Nankivell BJ, Borrows RJ, Fung CL, et al. The natural history of chronic allograft nephropathy. N Engl J Med 2003;349(24):2326–3433.
71. Nankivell BJ, Kuypers DR. Diagnosis and prevention of chronic kidney allograft loss. Lancet 2011;378(9800):1428–37.
72. Nickeleit V, Singh HK, Mihatsch MJ. Polyomavirus nephropathy: morphology, pathophysiology, and clinical management. Curr Opin Nephrol Hypertens 2003;12(6):599–605.
73. Pilmore HL, Dittmer ID. Calcineurin inhibitor nephrotoxicity: reduction in dose results in marked improvement in renal function in patients with coexisting chronic allograft nephropathy. Clin Transplant 2002;16(3):191–5.
74. Ponticelli C, Cucchiari D, Graziani G. Hypertension in kidney transplant recipients. Transpl Int 2011;24(6):523–33.
75. Radermacher J, Mengel M, Ellis S, et al. The renal arterial resistance index and renal allograft survival. N Engl J Med 2003;349(2):115–1124.
76. Randhawa PS, Finkelstein S, Scantlebury V, et al. Human polyoma virus-associated interstitial nephritis in the allograft kidney. Transplantation 1999;67(1):103–9.
77. Regele H, Bohmig GA, Habicht A, et al. Capillary deposition of complement split product C4d in renal allografts is associated with basement membrane injury in peritubular and glomerular capillaries: a contribution of humoral immunity to chronic allograft rejection. J Am Soc Nephrol 2002;13(9):2371–80.
78. Rush D, Arlen D, Boucher A, et al. Lack of benefit of early protocol biopsies in renal transplant patients receiving TAC and MMF: a randomized study. Am J Transplant 2007;7(11):2538–45.
79. Rush DN, Jeffery J, Nickerson P. Subclinical acute rejection: is it a cause of chronic rejction in renal transplantation? J Am Soc Nephrol 2000;14(3):131–7.
80. Rush D, Nickerson P, Gough J, et al. Beneficial effects of treatment of early subclinical rejection: a randomized study. J Am Soc Nephrol 1998;9(11):2129–34.

81. Schena FP, Pascoe MD, Alberu J, et al. Conversion from calcineurin inhibitors to sirolimus maintenance therapy in renal allograft recipients: 24-month efficacy and safety results from the CONVERT trial. Transplantation 2009;87(2):233–42.
82. Schwarz A, Gwinner W, Hiss M, et al. Safety and adequacy of renal transplant protocol biopsies. Am J Transplant 2005;5(8):1992–6.
83. Sharif A, Shabir S, Chand S, et al. Meta-analysis of calcineurin-inhibitor-sparing regimens in kidney transplantation. J Am Soc Nephrol 2011;22(11):2107–18.
84. Shihab FS, Waid TH, Conti DJ, et al. Conversion from cyclosporine to tacrolimus in patients at risk for chronic renal allograft failure: 60-month results of the CRAF Study. Transplantation 2008;85(9):1261–9.
85. Shishido S, Asanuma H, Nakai H, et al. The impact of repeated subclinical acute rejection on the progression of chronic allograft nephropathy. J Am Soc Nephrol 2003;14(4):1046–52.
86. Siedlecki A, Irish W, Brennan DC. Delayed graft function in the kidney transplant. Am J Transplant 2011;11(11):2279–96.
87. Sijpkens YW, Bruijn JA, Paul LC. Chronic allograft nephropathy categorised in chronic interstitial and vascular rejection. Transplant Proc 2001;33(1–2):1153.
88. Sis B, Campbell PM, Mueller T, et al. Transplant glomerulopathy, late antibody-mediated rejection and the ABCD tetrad in kidney allograft biopsies for cause. Am J Transplant 2007;7(7):1743–52.
89. Sis B, Dadras F, Khoshjou F, et al. Reproducibility studies on arteriolar hyaline thickening scoring in calcineurin inhibitor-treated renal allograft recipients. Am J Transplant 2006;6(6):1444–50.
90. Sis B, Jhangri GS, Bunnag S, et al. Endothelial gene expression in kidney transplants with alloantibody indicates antibody-mediated damage despite lack of C4d staining. Am J Transplant 2009;9(10):2312–23.
91. Sis B, Mengel M, Haas M, et al. Banff '09 meeting report: antibody mediated graft deterioration and implementation of Banff working groups. Am J Transplant 2010;10(3):464–71.
92. Solez K, Axelsen RA, Benediktsson H, et al. International standardization of criteria for the histologic diagnosis of renal allograft rejection: the Banff working classification of kidney transplant pathology. Kidney Int 1993;44(2):411–22.
93. Song E, Zou H, Yao Y, et al. Early application of Met-RANTES ameliorates chronic allograft nephropathy. Kidney Int 2002;61(2):676–85.
94. Steegh FM, Gelens MA, Nieman FH, et al. Early loss of peritubular capillaries after kidney transplantation. J Am Soc Nephrol 2011;22(6):1024–9.
95. Stegall MD, Gloor JM. Deciphering antibody-mediated rejection: new insights into mechanisms and treatment. Curr Opin Organ Transplant 2010;15(1):8–10.
96. Szolar DH, Preidler K, Ebner F, et al. Functional magnetic resonance imaging of human renal allografts during the post-transplant period: preliminary observations. Magn Reson Imaging 1997;15(7):727–35.
97. Terasaki PI, Cai J. Human leukocyte antigen antibodies and chronic rejection: from association to causation. Transplantation 2008;86(3):377–83.
98. te Strake L, Schultze Kool LJ, Paul LC, et al. Magnetic resonance imaging of renal transplants: its value in the differentiation of acute rejection and cyclosporin A nephrotoxicity. Clin Radiol 1988;39(3):220–8.
99. Veronese FV, Noronha IL, Manfro RC, et al. Prevalence and immunohistochemical findings of subclinical kidney allograft rejection and its association with graft outcome. Clin Transplant 2004;18(4):357–64.
100. Vitalone MJ, Naesens M, Sigdel T, et al. The dual role of epithelial-to-mesenchymal transition in chronic allograft injury in pediatric renal transplantation. Transplantation 2011;92(7):787–95.
101. Vitalone MJ, O'Connell PJ, Jimenez-Vera E, et al. Epithelial-to-mesenchymal transition in early transplant tubulointerstitial damage. J Am Soc Nephrol 2008;19(8):1571–83.
102. Vongwiwatana A, Tasanarong A, Rayner DC, et al. Epithelial to mesenchymal transition during late deterioration of human kidney transplants: the role of tubular cells in fibrogenesis. Am J Transplant 2005;5(6):1367–74.
103. Webster AC, Woodroffe RC, Taylor RS, et al. Tacrolimus versus ciclosporin as primary immunosuppression for kidney transplant recipients: meta-analysis and meta-regression of randomised trial data. BMJ 2005;331(7520):810.
104. Yarlagadda SG, Coca SG, Formica Jr RN, et al. Association between delayed graft function and allograft and patient survival: a systematic review and meta-analysis. Nephrol Dial Transplant 2009;24(3):1039–47.

CHAPTER 28

VASCULAR AND LYMPHATIC COMPLICATIONS AFTER KIDNEY TRANSPLANTATION

Richard D.M. Allen

CHAPTER OUTLINE

INTRODUCTION

The enduring techniques of vascular anastomoses described by Alexis Carrel more than a century ago have not changed significantly (see Chapter 1). His simple test of satisfactory vascular anastomosis was observation of a viable kidney transplant producing urine within minutes of completion. No matter how many times it has been witnessed before, this observation will always puts a smile on the face of everyone in the kidney transplant operating room. However, the progressive improvement in kidney graft survival has focused greater emphasis on surgeon-related causes of kidney graft loss. Surgical misadventure after kidney transplantation, once ranked low as a cause of graft loss in the first 6 months after transplantation, is now three times more likely to occur than graft loss as a result of rejection (Figure 28-1).

The transplanted kidney is a highly vascular organ. Ten to 15% of cardiac output at rest, accounting for between 500 and 750 mL/min, passes through the kidney. A graphic example of the magnitude of the renal blood flow is the simple temporary occlusion of the transplant renal vein with a pair of forceps at the time of surgery, described clinically as the Hume test, which results in rapid and pulsatile engorgement of a well-perfused kidney transplant. Equally, a breach in the continuity of the transplanted artery or vein can result in catastrophic blood loss and circulatory failure within minutes, particularly in the presence of a recipient left ventricle already compromised by coexisting coronary artery disease, long-term effects of systemic hypertension, or uremic cardiomyopathy.

The kidney is also unforgiving of interruption of blood flow, with the cortex more sensitive to hypoxia than

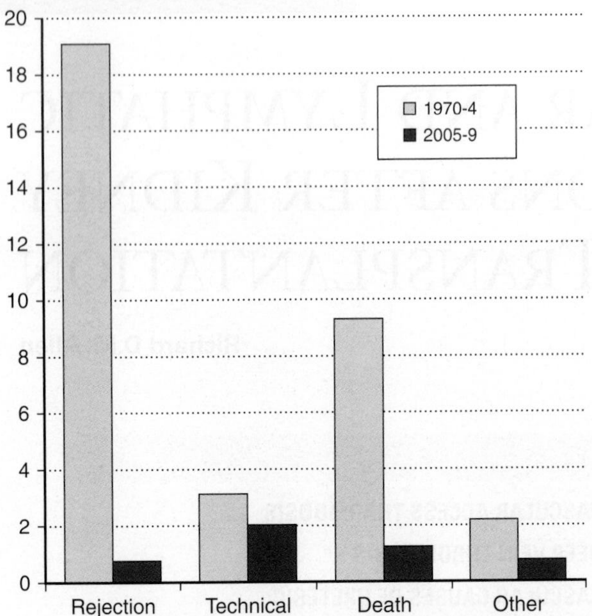

FIGURE 28-1 ■ Causes of graft loss in the first 6 months after kidney transplantation reported to ANZDATA Registry in Australia for recipients of living and deceased donors, comparing 5-year time periods 1970 through 1974 ($n = 1118$ transplants) and 2005 through 2009 ($n = 4014$ transplants).

the medulla. The magnitude of the effect of acute and complete interruption of blood flow during the transplantation procedure depends on the quality of the donor kidney, length of ischemia time, temperature of the kidney, and extent of intrarenal thrombosis that might occurr during a period of stasis or reduced renal blood flow. Irreversible cortical necrosis can occur within minutes, and even in the most favorable situations is inevitable by the 20-minute mark. Incomplete interruption of blood flow has a more subtle effect. Arterial pressure sensors within the kidney detect pressures capable of triggering a cascade of autoregulatory changes to increase systemic pressures to satisfy the requirements of the kidney, sometimes at the expense of the recipient's well-being. Impaired venous drainage is probably better tolerated, although sudden occlusion of a previously well-perfused kidney can lead to dramatic rupture of the cortex with uncontrolled bleeding from intrarenal veins.

TECHNICAL COMPLICATIONS AND THEIR PREVENTION

Informed Consent

A description of the possible complications of kidney transplantation to a patient when obtaining informed consent before surgery can cause alarm. The possibilities should be put into the context of the individual transplant center's own published results of patient and graft survival at 1 year. Ideally, the individual transplant surgeon's own results will be peer-reviewed on a regular basis both within and outside the surgeon's own transplant center.

Kidney transplantation involves placement of a kidney in a heterotopic position. By comparison, cardiothoracic and liver transplant surgeons have an easier task, placing size-matched donor organs into an orthotopic position after removal of the failed recipient organ. In deceased donor kidney transplantation, the surgeon must cope with the computer-allocated pairing of the donor kidney and recipient. Donor kidneys, particularly from an extended criteria deceased donor, are not new engine parts that can be taken off a spare parts shelf. They are preowned and have no regenerative capacity. The good kidney transplant surgeon is one who recognizes the small margin for surgical error, and avoids difficult situations by careful preparation and anticipation of the potential pitfalls. The incidence of vascular complications will vary according to the quality of the recipient evaluation, the donor kidney, and surgical technique of implantation. These are discussed in detail in Chapters 4, 8, and 11, but some of these points relating to prevention of vascular complications are worth reiterating here. When complications do occur, the surgeon attempts salvage of the situation, balancing risks to both the recipient and the donor kidney.

Preoperative Assessment

An accessible patent iliac artery and vein with unimpeded proximal blood flow that are able to be sutured are essential, and should be evaluated by a senior member of the transplant surgery team before the patient is placed on the transplant waiting list. Surgical access can be difficult because of a polycystic kidney, obesity, or a failed previous kidney transplant. Extensive mural arterial calcification can make clamping and suturing impossible without disruption of the artery. Placement of a patient on a kidney transplant waitlist without surgical assessment and resolution of identified problems, and lack of systems in place to ensure access to results of the assessment at all times, is considered medically negligent in the event of an avoidable vascular complication.

Right or Left Donor Kidney

Despite single-center reports claiming that results of transplantation of the right donor kidney are the same as those for the left,[22] transplant surgeons always prefer the left donor kidney because of its longer renal vein and shorter artery. When given the choice of a living left donor kidney with two arteries or a right kidney with one artery, most surgeons choose the former.[17] The longer left renal vein is less fragile and more easily sutured to the more deeply situated external iliac vein than the short right renal vein. Equally, the right renal artery anastomosis is more difficult to site because of its propensity to kink. Objective evidence to support the greater ease of transplantation of the left kidney is found in Australian registry data that compared outcomes of left and right deceased donor kidney pairs.[54] The data of paired kidneys from 2396 heart-beating brain-dead donors showed that recipients of right-sided kidneys were at significantly greater risk of developing delayed graft function and had inferior graft function because of greater risk of graft loss in the 3 months after transplantation, but principally because of surgical misadventure. The authors recommended that the more experienced surgeons within a transplant center be allocated the right donor kidneys to implant.

Anastomosis of the deceased donor right renal vein can be facilitated by vein elongation using the adjacent donor inferior vena cava (Figure 28-2) or a donor iliac vein extension graft. Alternatively, as is frequently the need in

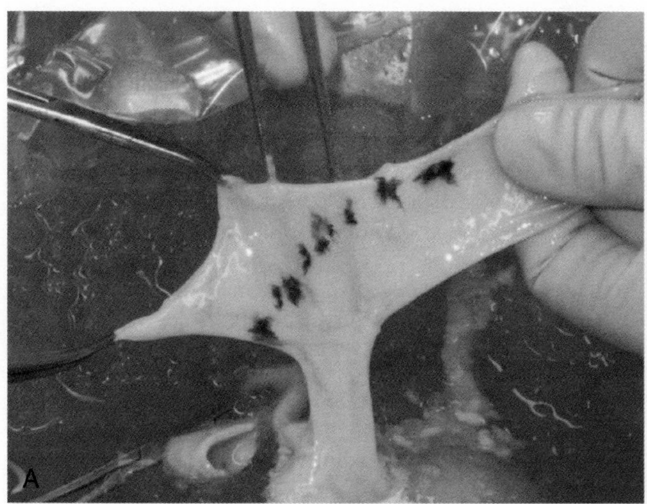

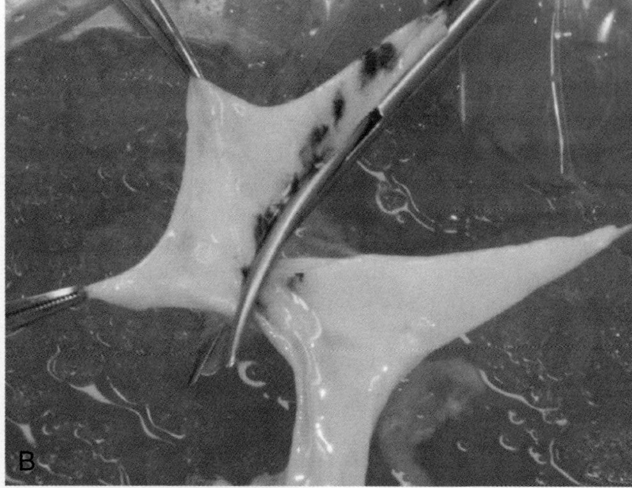

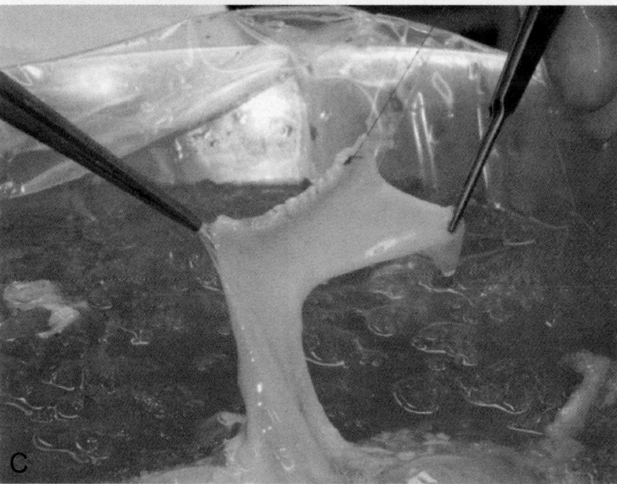

FIGURE 28-2 ■ Extension of the right renal vein using adjacent deceased donor inferior vena cava (IVC). (A) Marking the portion of IVC proposed for elongation. (B) Fashioning of the IVC. (C) Elongated renal vein ready for transplantation.

living donor right kidneys, the recipient external iliac vein can be mobilized by dividing the internal iliac veins.

Back Table Preparation

All donor kidneys require back table preparation, and failure of the surgeon to examine the deceased donor kidney before starting the recipient procedure can create problems if the kidney is not "as advertised" by the retrieval surgeon. Accessory arteries may have been missed or divided (Figure 28-3). Atheromatous plaque, clot, or an intimal flap may be impinging on the lumen of the renal artery. Inadvertent traction or a donor surgeon's wayward scissor may have torn or injured the donor renal vein. If problems are identified and corrected before surgery, operating and anastomosis times are kept to a minimum and surgical options are retained, such as preservation of the inferior epigastric artery for anastomosis to a lower-pole artery. For living donor kidneys, a missed accessory artery in the living donor kidney is apparent at the time of initial cool perfusion at the back table. This is not the case for the in-situ cool-perfused deceased donor kidney. Donor artery and vein are mobilized as necessary, with perirenal adipose tissue trimmed, the gonadal vein ligated and removed and, in the case of a deceased donor kidney, the adrenal gland is removed. Hemostasis after revascularization of the transplanted kidney is easier if vein tributaries and small hilar vessels associated with trimmed tissue are ligated.

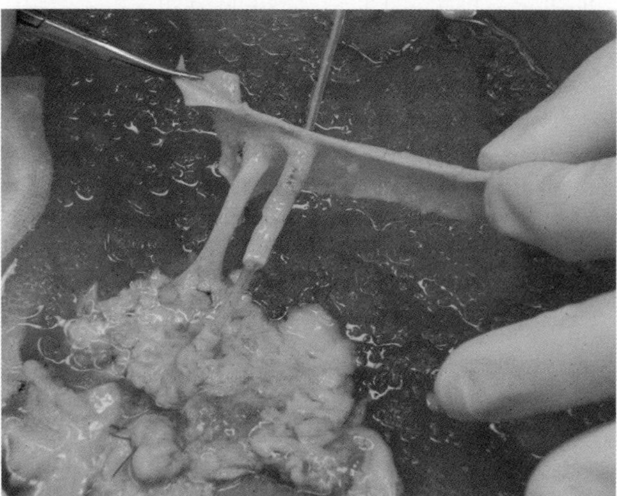

FIGURE 28-3 ■ Right-sided deceased donor kidney with two renal arteries. The lower artery was divided at the time of multiorgan donor retrieval surgery.

Repeat flushing of a deceased donor kidney with a small volume of preservation solution has several advantages.

Residual venous blood, if present, can be cleared. Leaking vessels can be identified and ligated before revascularization. There is also clinical evidence that the subsequently "freshened" deceased donor kidney is more likely to avoid graft dysfunction.[39] Finally, the kidney vasculature is accurately oriented. The superior and inferior margins of the artery and vein can be marked to reduce the risk of twisting the vessels at the time of anastomosis (Figure 28-4). To reduce handling of the donor kidney during the surgical procedure and for ease of surgery, the kidney can be placed in a temporary stocking, or a surgical glove surrounded by ice slush. The back table with ice slush and preservation fluid should be available until the vascular anastomoses are completed in the event that it is necessary to cool the kidney again.

Transplant Renal Vein Anastomosis

The technical details of the anastomosis have been described in Chapter 11 but one or two points are worth reiterating. Unless there is a recipient history of factors predisposing to venous thrombosis, systemic heparinization for the vascular anastomoses is unnecessary in a dialysis-dependent patient, even in the era of widespread use of synthetic erythropoietin agents. The site of the iliac vein anastomosis can be marked with a sterile surgical marking pen before applying the venous clamps to reduce the risk of vein rotation during clamp application. Accurate sizing of the venotomy length prevents stretching of the end of the transplant renal vein to accommodate a venotomy that is too long. Stretching leads to a long stenosed anastomosis. After opening the vein, the surgeon searches for pairs of valve cusps and disrupts them if they are adjacent to the anastomosis. A stay suture is applied to the midpoint of at least one of the sides of the venotomy to reduce the risk of catching the opposite wall of the anastomosis with the continuous running vein suture.

The external iliac veins in an obese recipient or a short muscular male patient with a deep pelvis and almost vertically disposed external iliac vein can be challenging, particularly for right-sided donor kidneys placed in the left iliac fossa. For ease of access, it is tempting to place the venous anastomosis close to the inguinal ligament but there is a risk of compression of the renal vein during wound closure. Options include lengthening of the donor renal vein or the sometimes difficult task of mobilization of the external iliac vein by dividing the internal iliac vein and its tributaries. The surgeon should ensure that there are long stumps on the ligated veins. Lost ligatures can result in massive blood loss within minutes from the large and thin-walled labyrinth of pelvic and presacral veins that are prone to retracting into the depths of the surgical wound. In such instances, bleeding is best managed by carefully packing the depths of the wound and applying pressure, a request for blood products, and systematic control of venous bleeding by application of metal clips or polypropylene (Prolene) sutures.

A thrombosed or stenosed external iliac vein is preferably identified by color Doppler ultrasound scanning (CDUS) before surgery and should be considered in patients with a history of deep vein thrombosis (DVT), previous transplant surgery, unilateral leg swelling, or emergency dialysis access via the femoral vein (Figure 28-5). When encountered at the time of surgery, the common

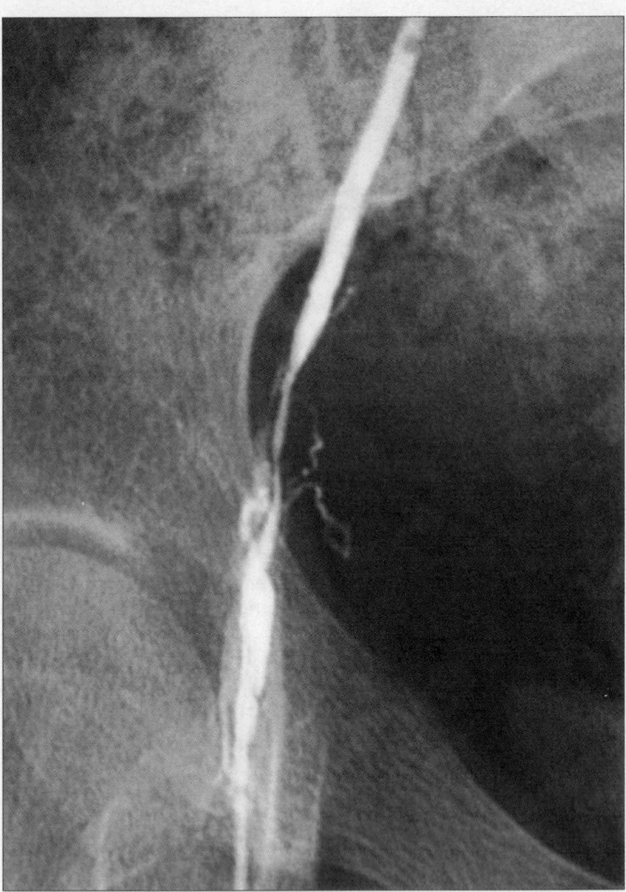

FIGURE 28-5 ■ Ascending venogram shows a long stenosis of the right iliac vein in a patient with a history of temporary hemodialysis cannulas and a previous thigh arteriovenous fistula.

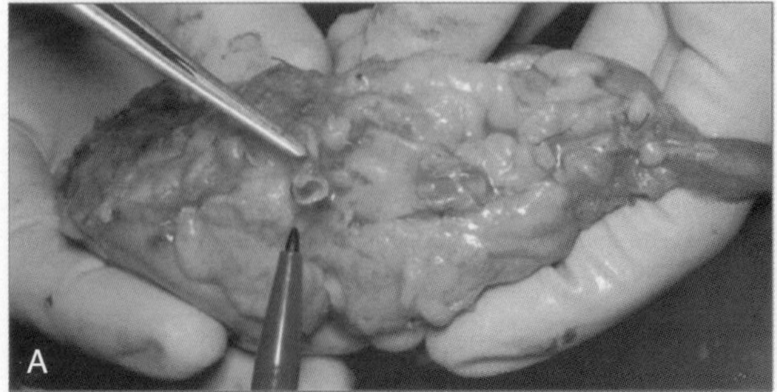

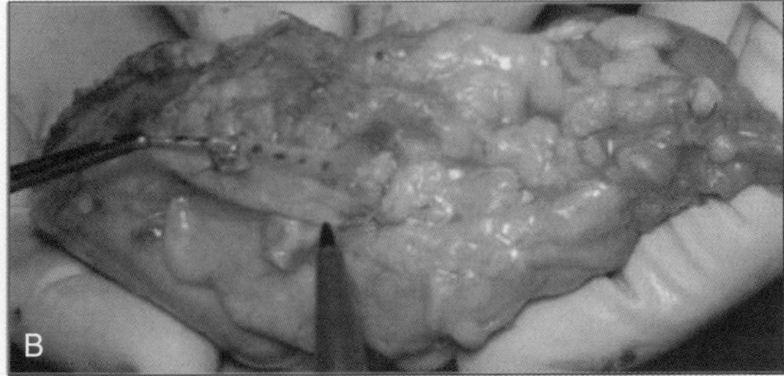

FIGURE 28-4 ■ Marking of the vessels of a left-sided living donor kidney transplant prior to transplantation for the purpose of assisting their orientation at the time of surgery. (A) Superior margin of the renal artery. (B) Inferior margin of the renal vein.

iliac vein often has a preserved lumen and can be used for the transplant renal vein anastomosis. Alternatively, the surgeon can close the wound and transplant the kidney into the opposite iliac fossa.

Transplant Renal Artery Anastomosis

The extent of the dissection of the iliac artery should be limited to diminish the risk of disruption of adjacent lymphatic channels. If the internal iliac artery is to be used, the surgeon fully mobilizes the bifurcation of the common iliac artery and carefully examines the origin for an atheromatous plaque. Use of the internal iliac artery is avoided if the opposite side artery has been involved in a previous transplant (Figure 28-6). The bifurcation or trifurcation of the internal iliac artery should be preserved to reduce the risk of buttock claudication. If both internal iliac arteries have been used for transplantation claudication is inevitable, as is impotence. An unusual Vietnamese study involving internal iliac artery anastomoses in male live donor kidney recipients should allay concerns that the erect penis will deviate to the side of the ligated internal iliac artery (Prof. Tran Ngoc Sinh, Cho Ray Hospital, Ho Chi Minh City, Vietnam, personal communication).

Arterial clamps are applied with care. Clamps with silicone inserts applied horizontally are less likely to disrupt calcified plaque commonly situated on the posterior aspect of the artery. Endarterectomy can often be avoided by carefully selecting a soft segment of artery. To avoid kinking during wound closure, the renal artery length can be adjusted by resecting the donor aortic patch. Equally, the shortened artery of the right kidney can be anastomosed to the end of the internal iliac artery. This has the added advantage of deeper placement of the transplant anastomoses, less tension on the short right renal vein, and easy positioning of the kidney after revascularization.

Multiple renal arteries are encountered more commonly with the increasing popularity of laparoscopic living kidney donation and the preference for the left kidney.[17] At least 20% of left kidneys have more than one artery after living donation. Small accessory renal arteries, particularly at the upper pole, can be ligated without problem, but not lower-pole arteries that often contribute blood supply to the donor ureter.[10] Anastomosis of two arteries close together on an aortic patch of a left-sided deceased donor kidney is comparatively straightforward but dual arteries to a right-sided kidney make positioning of the kidney difficult without kinking one or the other artery.

Individual transplant surgeons will have their own views about how best to manage multiple arteries of a living kidney donor. Despite longer anastomosis times, the author's preference is for two separate anastomoses, particularly if the arteries are of nearly equal size. This approach avoids the need for a complex anastomosis with a theoretical increased risk of thrombosis. The exception is a small upper-pole or lower-pole accessory artery that can be anastomosed, on the back table, to the side of a main renal artery and away from the end of the renal artery (see Chapter 11 for more technical details).

Reperfusion

Reperfusion is the high point of the transplant procedure – there is no turning back. Before completing the arterial anastomosis, air is excluded from the clamped vessels by injecting heparinized saline. Fixed retractors that might compress proximal iliac vessels are reviewed and individual anastomoses are tested before revascularization of the transplanted kidney. Imperfect anastomoses are managed more easily beforehand (Figure 28-7). The proximal arterial clamp and venous clamps are released first. The last clamp removed is the distal iliac artery clamp after systemic blood pressure has stabilized following reperfusion of the kidney. Observation of urine within a couple of minutes is a reassuring sight – a pink,

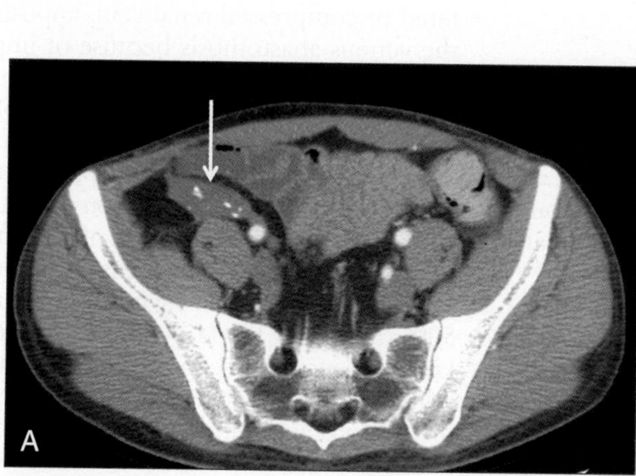

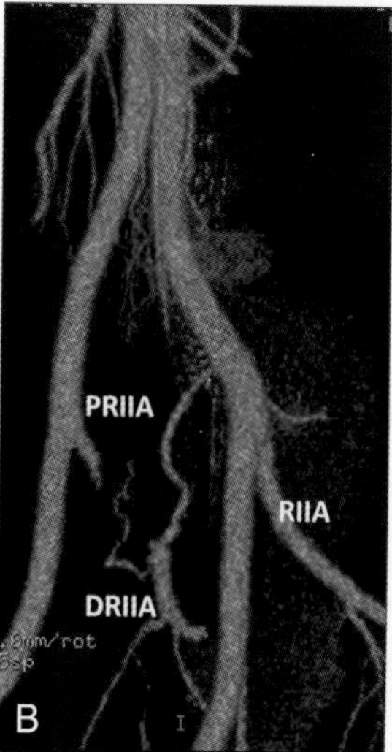

FIGURE 28-6 ■ Computed tomography scan of male patient with avascular right living donor kidney transplant that failed because of chronic rejection. The arterial anastomosis was to the right internal iliac artery. (A) Axial view of small avascular kidney transplant (arrow) adjacent to the common iliac artery. (B) Oblique perspective of vascular reconstruction of aortoiliac arteries demonstrating proximal stump of right internal iliac artery (PRIIA), retrograde filling of distal right iliac artery (DRIIA), and patent left internal iliac artery (LIIA).

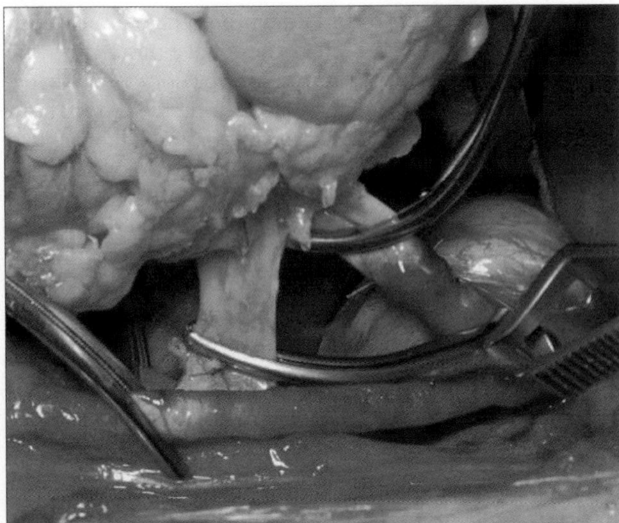

FIGURE 28-7 ■ Testing the integrity of the end-to-end right internal iliac artery to transplant renal artery anastomosis before revascularization of the kidney transplant.

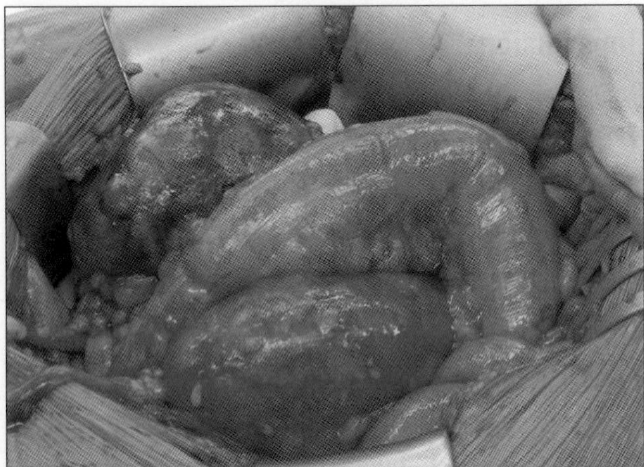

FIGURE 28-8 ■ Sigmoid colon separating the dual kidney transplants from a marginal cadaver donor. The left-sided kidney was transplanted first and is of uniform appearance. The right kidney is of mottled appearance 10 minutes after revascularization. Ten minutes later, it had the same appearance as the left kidney transplant.

firm, and well-perfused kidney is the next best thing. If neither is observed, the surgeon should actively look for problems. Kidneys from marginal donors or with long renal ischemia times may have a "blotchy" or mottled appearance with dark, less well-perfused areas. An encouraging sign is the gradual reduction in extent of the dark areas until the kidney is uniformly pink (Figure 28-8).

A flaccid, poorly perfused kidney is reason for concern. Modern tissue typing and crossmatching techniques have essentially excluded hyperacute rejection as a cause (see Chapter 10). The surgeon starts with inspection of the renal artery to exclude kinking or twisting and resolves it if possible by repositioning the kidney. Next is confirmation of pulsatility of the iliac artery proximal to the anastomosis and its continuity into the transplant renal artery to the hilum of the kidney. Interruption of flow can be due to an intimal flap, particularly in recipients with underlying arterial disease and kidney from older donors. Management is not easy. The most likely site of an intimal flap would be at the anastomosis or the proximal clamp site.

The decision to revise the arterial anastomosis or the "safety-first option" of removing the transplanted kidney and reperfusing with preservation solution can be difficult. If revision is undertaken, the recipient is heparinized, the transplant artery flushed with at least 50 mL of heparinized saline, and the renal vein clamped.

Extrarenal arterial spasm is a not uncommon finding and likely the result of undue traction on the renal artery during donor or implantation surgery. The spasm may be segmental. The kidney is soft but not necessarily discolored. Anecdotal reports suggest that placement of a swab generously soaked in papaverine around the artery and excision of affected artery adventitial tissue may help. Alternatively, and with permission of the anesthetist, the iliac artery distal to the arterial anstomosis is clamped and diluted glycerol trinitate injected into the proximal iliac artery. Spasm is usually self-limiting but can cause concern and warrant systemic heparinization. If no arterial inflow problem can be identified and systemic blood pressure is satisfactory, the surgeon should be patient, particularly if the kidney swells when the renal vein is temporarily occluded (Hume test). A small incision into the capsule of the kidney followed by evidence of bright arterial bleeding can also be reassuring, as can an on-table CDUS examination.

Catastrophic bleeding after removing all vascular clamps is unlikely to occur if the anastomoses have been assessed before revascularization. If present, however, it is usually venous in nature and either from a tributary vein, or worse, from a disrupted venous anastomosis because of traction on a thin-walled and right-sided living donor kidney renal vein. Because of the continuous nature of the suture, simple repair is usually impossible and, if attempted, results in excessive blood loss or anastomotic stenosis, or both. Removal of the kidney, reperfusion with preservation solution, and calmly starting all over is a sensible solution. The observation of a tense, engorged, and pulsatile kidney with marked capsular bleeding is indicative of venous outflow obstruction. Causes can be a rotated or compressed renal vein, apposition of the sides of the venous anastomosis because of imperfect suturing or inclusion of external iliac vein valve cusps in the anastomosis. Because of the relatively controlled situation, revision of the anastomosis usually can be undertaken within 10 minutes, after systemic heparinization, clamping the renal artery, and exsanguination of the transplant. An uncommon cause is compression of the left common iliac vein as it passes under the right common iliac artery, described as the May–Thurner syndrome.[3] Probably, the extra 500–750 mL of blood per minute from the transplanted kidney is enough to compromise the narrowed iliac vein at that point. If recognized at time of surgery, a more proximal venous anastomosis can be attempted or the internal iliac artery divided to allow mobilization of the right common iliac artery. If recognized after transplantation, endovascular stenting of the iliac vein may be an option.

A disappointing observation on completion of the vascular anastomoses is the finding of a well-perfused transplant but with the ureter pointing in the wrong direction, away from the bladder. The kidney has been transplanted upside down and this is more likely to occur with a living donor kidney in the absence of the full length of renal vein and the aortic patch to assist with orientation. One option is to remove the kidney, reperfuse, and start again. Alternatively, the kidney can be left in place and, provided there is an adequate length of ureter, it can be provided with a more circuitous route to the recipient bladder. Personal communications from several surgeons suggest that the latter option is reasonable.

Positioning the Kidney and Wound Closure

The ureteroneocystostomy should be the relaxing part of the kidney transplant operation. The kidney is positioned to avoid compression of the vascular pedicle and, all being well, urine is being produced. A suction drain is inserted with the transplanted kidney in view. Avulsion of a tenuous venous anastomosis with the forceful push of the surgeon's hand is not easy to cope with at this stage of the operation!

During apposition of the abdominal wall muscles, the potential for kinking of the kidney transplant vasculature increases, particularly in thin patients receiving large kidneys, male patients with a narrow deep pelvis, a venous anastomosis too close to the inguinal ligament, or an incision too close to the anterior superior iliac spine. Mobilizing the peritoneum in a medial direction off the undersurface of the anterior abdominal wall may help. Monitoring transplant arterial perfusion during wound closure with CDUS can be reassuring.

Failing this, a reliable "surgical escape" is to place the kidney into the peritoneal cavity by creating a longitudinal window in the peritoneum, adjacent to the kidney and more anterior to the vascular anastomoses. The kidney is positioned anterolateral to the cecum on the right side and the sigmoid colon on the left side. The greater omentum can be used to separate the bowel from the kidney. Percutaneous biopsy subsequently is still feasible after placement of local anesthetic agent at the level of the peritoneum.

Postoperative Recovery

An experienced member of the surgical team remains with the recipient in the early recovery phase and until there is conclusive evidence of satisfactory perfusion of the transplanted kidney. The careful positioning of kidney at time of surgery can be undone readily by a restless recipient flexing the hips because of pain, urinary catheter intolerance, and hypoxia, or an unhelpful radiographer determined that the recipient sits bolt upright for a mobile chest X-ray. Transplanted kidneys producing urine at the end of the surgical procedure are easier to manage, particularly if urine is being produced in volumes that could not be achieved by residual native kidney function. The better the urine volume, the less likely that clots will form in the bladder.

If no urine has been seen on the operating table or in recovery, and the recipient is hemodynamically stable with a central venous pressure of at least 5 cmH_2O, a CDUS examination is always indicated before the recipient leaves the operating suite complex, particularly if difficulty was encountered with kidney positioning during wound closure. Out of routine working hours, it helps if the transplant surgeon is adept with the use of an ultrasound machine dedicated to the transplant unit. An inadequate arterial signal and significant collections are indications for an immediate return to the operating room. A presurgery expectation of poor initial transplant function, on the basis of donor factors, is not sufficient reason to postpone CDUS examination of the anuric transplant recipient.

The need for an additional arterial anastomosis is also good reason for an early CDUS in the presence of the operating surgeon with knowledge of the surgical vascular anatomy. Patency of an accessory renal artery is difficult to determine in the early postoperative phase by observation of urine output alone. These smaller vessels are more prone to thrombosis or kinking, and longer-term consequences include poor graft function and hypertension. An avascular segment of kidney can occur, at least initially, without noticeable effect.

Because of the quality of modern CDUS, indications for formal angiography in the early phase after kidney transplantation are few. They are perhaps limited to the suspicion of proximal iliac artery disease or clamp injury and an obese recipient in whom visualization of the renal artery and iliac vessels is not technically feasible. Helical computed tomography (CT) angiography is usually easier and faster to obtain.

Drain Tube

Removal of a suction drain should be a straightforward task. Without suction it is withdrawn slowly with a twisting motion to dislodge fatty tissue trapped in the small side holes of the drain as a result of the suction. Small pediatric kidneys have been known to undergo torsion of the vascular pedicle on removal of the drain with resultant loss of graft function.

The timing of drain tube removal depends on the volume and nature of the drained fluid. It is not unusual to record 100–200 mL of heavily blood-stained drainage in the first few hours of transplantation. Drainage volume can be an unreliable gauge of active bleeding, particularly if brisk. Patient discomfort, tachycardia, hypotension, and abdominal findings of an enlarging mass around the transplant are indicators of a significant bleed requiring urgent surgical exploration. Large-volume drainage of less heavily blood-stained fluid generally indicates residual peritoneal dialysate (if the peritoneum was breached), lymph, or urine. Urine is excluded by biochemical analysis or absence of glucose on dipstick testing.

Compartment Syndrome

All can be well with a transplanted kidney while the recipient is in a supine or near-supine position. CDUS is also performed with the recipient in a supine position. However, when the patient is placed in a sitting or standing position, downward movement of abdominal contents can cause external compression of the transplanted

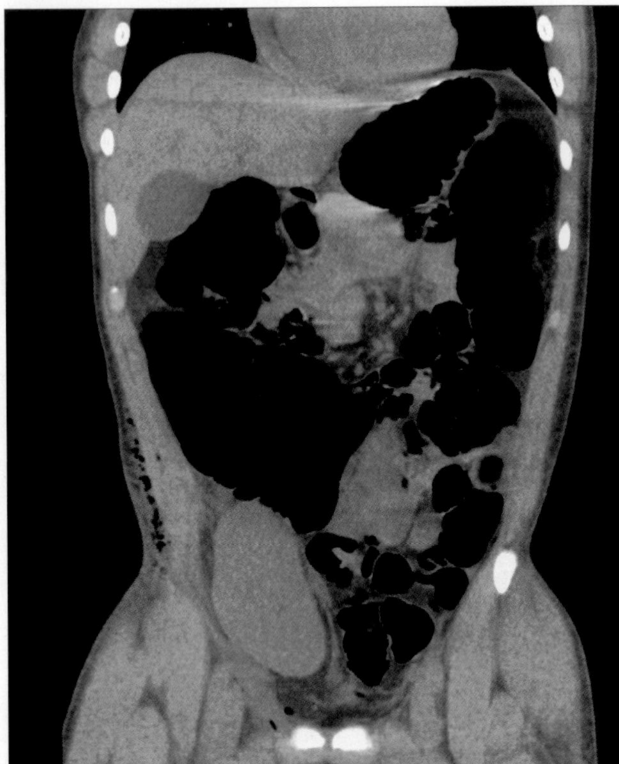

FIGURE 28-9 ■ Computed tomography scan with coronal view of abdomen 24 hours after kidney transplantation. The perfusion of the kidney transplant in the right iliac fossa was compromised by gross pseudo-obstruction of the large and small bowel.

kidney or change its position. Contributing factors include a large polycystic kidney, heavy fat-laden small-bowel mesentery, and greater omentum in a patient with truncal obesity. Hematoma, urinoma, lymphocele, or paralytic ileus can do likewise, even with the patient in a supine position. The contribution of the compartment syndrome to initial poor kidney transplant function should not be underestimated (Figure 28-9). Reversible factors should be resolved without delay. A paralytic ileus or pseudo-obstruction of the large bowel can be frustrating to manage in the first week after transplantation. The latter may require a rectal tube to deflate the large bowel under supervision of the colorectal surgery team.

HEMATOMA

Hematoma formation is a not uncommon finding after kidney transplantation during the initial inpatient period, particularly in anticoagulated recipients or those receiving antiplatelet agents, Thymoglobulin, or plasmapheresis. Most hematomas are small and insignificant ultrasound findings that resolve spontaneously. Those associated with discomfort, hypotension, transplant dysfunction, and falling hemoglobin are not. Extreme examples are surgical emergencies after rupture of the kidney cortex or arterial anastomosis disruption (Figure 28-10). Others expand progressively within the retroperitoneal space with inevitable external pressure on the transplant and adverse effect on arterial blood inflow or venous outflow. The extent of the hematoma by CT scanning is best

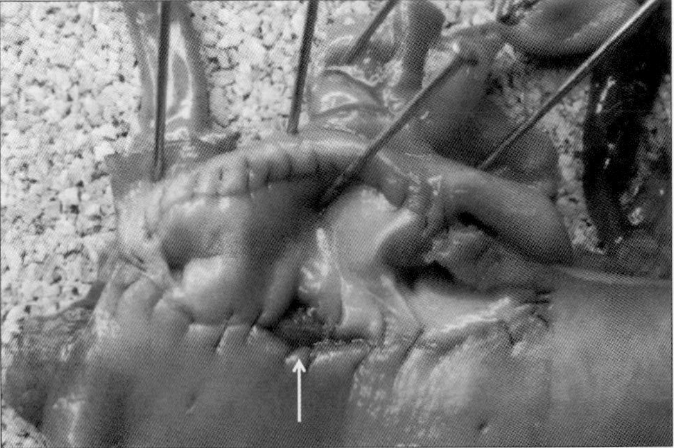

FIGURE 28-10 ■ Postmortem preparation of recipient external iliac artery and two donor renal arteries on an atheromatous donor aortic patch. It demonstrates a small disruption of the anastomosis (arrow) that led to catastrophic bleeding 10 days after transplant surgery.

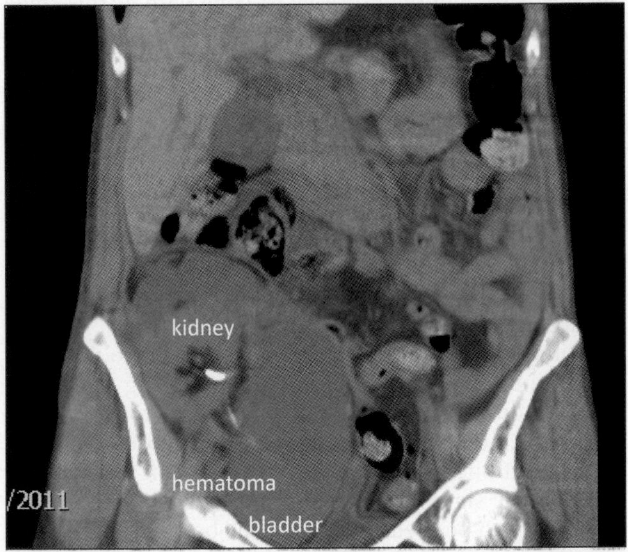

FIGURE 28-11 ■ Computed tomography scan (without vascular contrast material) with coronal view of abdomen showing compression of the kidney transplant by an anteriorly placed hematoma.

shown as a heterogeneous crescentic peritransplant collection (Figure 28-11). The CT findings change with time after the bleeding event, with evidence of recent bleeding of more concern. CDUS examination is appropriate to assess transplant perfusion but because of surrounding bowel gas is unreliable for assessment of hematoma size.

Percutaneous drainage of the hematoma is unlikely to be successful. Indications for surgical exploration of the transplanted kidney include symptoms, progression of size, ongoing blood loss, and transplant dysfunction. The original wound is reopened and care taken to remove the hematoma, always being alert to the possibility of dislodging clot that is providing tenuous hemostasis at the site of bleeding. Surgical exploration in the first day or so after transplantation for hematoma evacuation might locate active bleeding from a hilar vessel, a retroperitoneal vein, or divided abdominal wall muscle. Thereafter, a more common finding is a stable hematoma without obvious cause. Invariably, transplant perfusion and function improve after hematoma evacuation. Bruising in dependent subcutaneous areas lateral to and below the transplant, such as the labia or the scrotum, is often seen several days later. The risk of hematoma formation is increased by the use of anticoagulants, particularly in patients receiving heparin by infusion for prophylaxis against vascular thrombosis.[26] Careful titration of heparin infusion rate to maintain an activated partial thromboplastin time of 60 seconds is not easy. The reported risk of need for surgical intervention in patients heparinized after transplantation is 30–60%. Heparinized patients positive for lupus anticoagulant are especially difficult to manage with heparin.[35] Greater safety can be achieved with the use of thromboelastography to direct judicious use of heparin, during and after transplant surgery in patients at risk.[8] Anecdotally at least, hematoma formation is more common in the presence of antiplatelet agents such as aspirin and/or clopidogrel. They are prescribed increasingly on a long-term basis by cardiologists and nephrologists in patients with significant cardiovascular disease or in the belief – for which there is as yet no evidence – that fistula patency is improved. Their use is not a contraindication to transplantation. However, they do reduce the margin for surgical error and dictate the need for meticulous hemostasis at time of surgery.

VASCULAR THROMBOSIS AND THROMBOPHILIA

Early kidney transplant loss as a result of thrombosis of artery or vein is a devastating complication, with a 2% incidence (Figure 28-1). Compared with other forms of vascular surgery, the incidence of thrombosis is low, perhaps because of the highly vascular nature of the kidney. The low incidence may also support the traditional view that renal failure is associated with a bleeding tendency secondary to platelet and clotting factor dysfunction.[11] Arterial thrombosis or infarction of a denervated kidney is often painless and heralded only by loss of graft function. By the time the diagnosis is confirmed by imaging, kidney salvage is not a practical option (Figure 28-12). Interruption of the venous drainage can be spectacular with graft rupture and bleeding. It has an equally disappointing prospect for kidney salvage because of the rapidity of the process after occlusion of the renal vein has occurred. Thrombotic complications are minimized by identification and management of risk at the time of transplantation.

Thrombosis of the kidney vasculature is the end result of stasis, endothelial changes, and procoagulant factors and can be multifactorial. Causes of stasis are largely technical in nature and readily identifiable at the time of transplant exploration. They include poorly constructed anastomoses, malpositioning of the transplant, rotation of the kidney, or external compression. Recipient hypovolemia and inadequate cardiac output, for whatever reason, are contributory but not causal factors. The contribution of intrarenal causes, such as acute vascular rejection and acute tubular necrosis (ATN), is less quantifiable, but can be diagnosed by histological examination provided viable

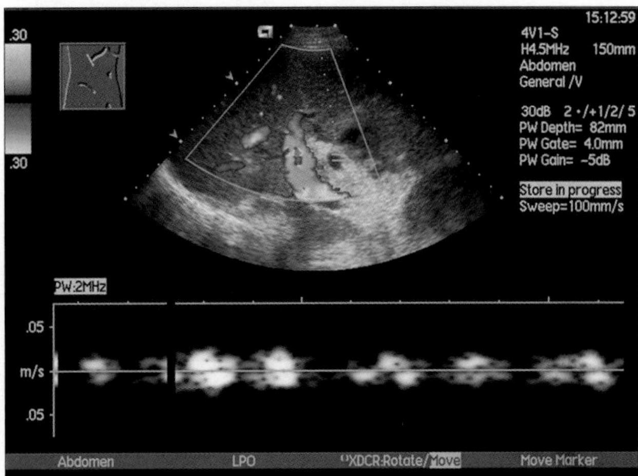

FIGURE 28-12 ■ Color duplex ultrasound shows minimal blood flow into kidney transplant as a result of almost complete occlusion by thrombus of the transplant renal artery 5 days after transplantation. The transplanted kidney was not viable when explored soon afterward.

cortical tissue can be obtained. Because this is often not the case, intrarenal causes are probably underestimated and underdiagnosed.

Epidemiological studies have attempted to identify other risk factors, particularly those amenable to preventive strategies.[11,21] Those that cannot be modified are recipient and donor age, recipient and donor vascular pathology, diabetes mellitus and, at least in the view of some recipients, morbid obesity. A large registry-based and case-matched study has shown that half of all cases of kidney transplant vascular thrombosis occur in repeat transplant recipients.[43] The implication is that transplanted kidneys in the setting of retransplantation are more likely to have endothelial inflammation and development of microthrombi after exposure to the recipient immune system. Strategies exist to minimize this risk in selected, highly sensitized recipients with a negative donor lymphocytotoxicity crossmatch (see Chapter 10). ATN attributable to the reperfusion injury is also associated with endothelial changes, and, together with hydronephrosis, is associated with increased intrarenal pressures, making perfusion of the transplanted kidney more difficult. Recipients dependent on peritoneal dialysis before transplantation are more likely to have thrombotic complications, likely due to intravascular hypovolemia.

The introduction of recombinant human erythropoietin (rEPO) has revolutionized the treatment of anemia associated with end-stage kidney disease, reducing the need for routine blood transfusion and improving quality of life and patient survival. rEPO dose is titrated to provide recipient hemoglobin in the range of 100–120 g/L. With higher hemoglobin values, there is an increased risk of adverse cardiac events. Nevertheless, the current widespread use of rEPO in patients presenting for kidney transplantation has not resulted in an increased risk of vascular thrombosis.[21]

Erythrocytosis, defined as hematocrit greater than 51% or hemoglobin greater than 160 g/L, occurs in 10–15% of recipients 6 months to 2 years after kidney transplantation.[47] About a quarter regress spontaneously, with the remainder persisting for several years and remitting as graft function diminishes. Thromboembolic events and symptoms of lethargy, malaise, and headache necessitate repeated venepuncture and may be necessary in up to 30% of these patients. The problem is more common in male patients, smokers, and patients with a rejection-free course. Erythropoietin levels are usually in the normal range. By chance, patients introduced to small doses of an angiotensin-converting enzyme inhibitor for the management of hypertension were noted to have progressive reduction of hematocrit to more normal levels. The suggestion is that angiotensin II is a growth factor for red blood cells.

Thrombophilic Factors

After exclusion of technical causes in a hemodynamically stable kidney transplant recipient, thrombosis may be explained by one of the numerous hypercoagulable or thrombophilic states. Many are inherited, but are more frequently acquired.[21,25] These include deficiencies of antithrombin III, protein C, and protein S, each occurring in less than 1% of the dialysis patients. When a thrombotic event of any kind occurs in a patient older than 45 years and in the absence of a family history, these deficiencies are unlikely.

Inheritance of factor V Leiden (FVL) or prothrombin G20210A mutations can increase the risk of thrombosis, usually venous, of the transplant vasculature by at least threefold. FVL mutation is present in 2–5% of the normal population and is not more common in patients with kidney disease. It is found, however, in 15–20% of patients with venous thromboembolism and 60% of patients with a family history of thromboembolism. When these mutations are present in kidney transplant recipients, the risk of major thrombotic events, particularly renal vein thrombosis (RVT), is 40%.[59] The presence of FVL or prothrombin G20210A mutations is also associated with shorter graft survival, probably as a result of greater microvascular thrombosis in renal vessels affected by rejection or intimal thickening. A case could therefore be made for routine genetic screening for these polymorphisms in patients awaiting a renal transplant. It should be mandatory if there is a history of thromboembolism.

The presence of acquired antiphospholipid antibodies (APAs), including anticardiolipin antibody and lupus anticoagulant, is common in patients awaiting transplantation. Although present in about 10% of patients, related clinical events are less common. When associated with a history of thrombotic events, these patients, often with systemic lupus erythematosus, are labeled as having APA syndrome. They have a universal incidence of graft loss to thrombosis when prophylaxis is not employed. Equally, anticoagulation after transplantation offers protection against graft loss.[1] The presence of APAs without a history of thrombosis is seemingly not a problem.

Contribution of Immunosuppressive Agents

The introduction of cyclosporine, usually at doses of 15 mg/kg or more, was associated with an increased incidence of graft thrombosis, particularly RVT, in the first week after transplantation.[47] Cyclosporine was subsequently shown to have procoagulant properties, increasing factor VIII, and release of tissue factors from monocytes and von Willebrand factor and P-selectin from endothelium. This is likely a dose–response effect, for in recent years meticulous cyclosporine drug dosing based on drug level monitoring has resulted in fewer reports of RVT. Mammalian target of rapamycin (mTOR) inhibitors are not thought to contribute to thromboembolic events after kidney transplantation.

Hemolytic uremic syndrome/thrombotic thrombocytopenic purpura is an infrequent but well-described complication of cyclosporine use. The diagnosis, seen soon after transplantation, is based on deteriorating renal function, decreasing platelet count, and characteristic glomerular thrombi seen in core biopsy specimens. Most resolve with discontinuation of cyclosporine and conversion to tacrolimus. Reports also describe the same presentation with tacrolimus, which responds with conversion to cyclosporine. The alternative would be to introduce an mTOR inhibitor.

Prolonged use of heparin can lead to the development of measurable antibodies against platelet factor 4 (PF4) in up to 20% of patients. Heparin-induced thrombocytopenic syndrome (HITS) is an immune-mediated thrombocytopenia together with thrombotic complications occurring within 24 hours of a patient's re-exposure to heparin during the transplant procedure. The subsequent immune complex activates platelets, predisposes the patient to clotting of veins and arteries, and causes the platelets to be consumed. The diagnosis of HITS for the first time in a transplant recipient is uncommon, but is likely underreported, particularly in pre-emptive live donor kidney recipients and patients treated by peritoneal dialysis. A proven past diagnosis of HITS (involving measurable PF4 antibody) mandates absolute avoidance of any form of heparin during the transplant procedure. Anticoagulation can be provided with direct thrombin inhibitors such as epirudin, argatroban, or bivalirudin.

Renal Vein Thrombosis

Occlusion of the renal vein by thrombus soon after transplantation is now an unusual event and invariably associated with a technical problem. However, in the era of high cyclosporine dosing, the incidence of the seemingly spontaneous RVT was as high as 6% and occurred classically towards the end of the first week of transplantation in an otherwise uncomplicated transplant kidney.[49] Witnessing the dramatic presentation over a couple of hours is an unforgettable experience. Rapid onset of oliguria and hematuria is accompanied by graft enlargement and rupture associated with extreme patient discomfort and life-threatening bleeding. RVT can happen during the course of a morning ward round. The Oxford Transplant Unit response almost two decades ago was to introduce daily aspirin from the time of surgery, the effect of which was to decrease the incidence of RVT from 5.6% to 1.2%.[49]

The CDUS findings are of a swollen graft with a crescent of clot along the convex margin of the kidney and covering a longitudinal rupture of the cortex. In this

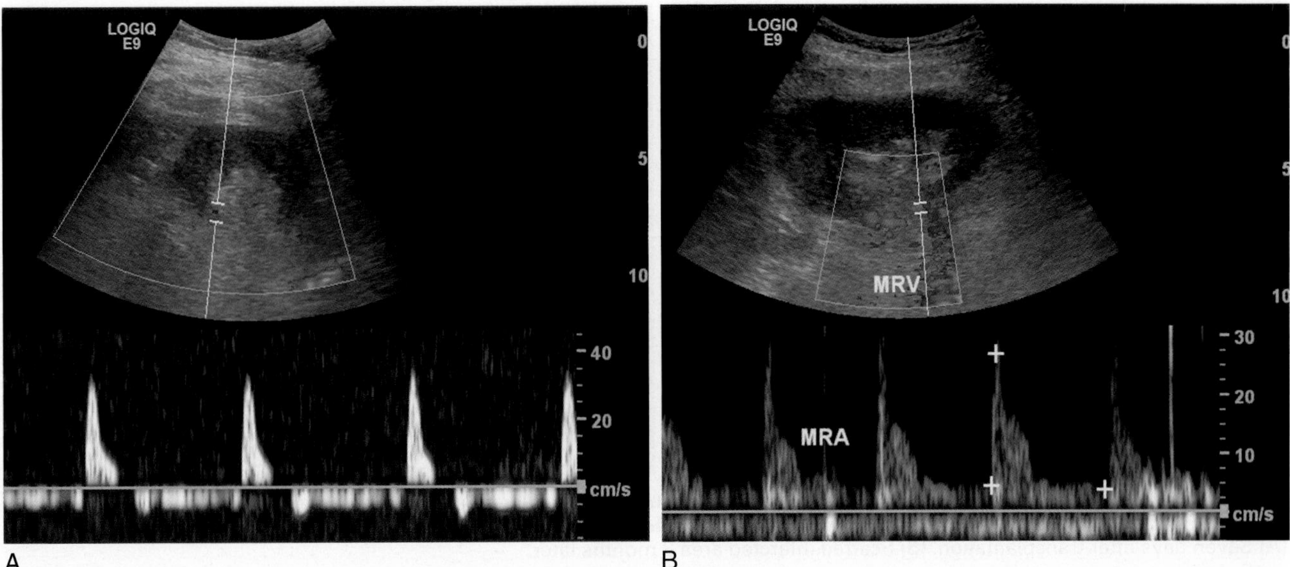

FIGURE 28-13 ■ Color Doppler ultrasound findings in a patient presenting with acute renal vein thrombosis 24 hours after kidney transplantation. (A) Immediately before renal vein thrombectomy and demonstrating reverse diastolic flow in the main transplant renal artery. (B) Restoration of normal flow pattern 2 hours after urgent graft exploration, thrombectomy, and disruption of a valve leaflet caught in the venous anastomosis to the external ilac vein. MRV, magnetic resonance venography; MRA, magnetic resonance angiography.

setting, reverse diastolic flow of the arterial waveform is diagnostic (Figure 28-13A). Potentially, the transplant can be saved following early diagnosis if the patient is taken directly to the operating room by the surgical team (Figure 28-13B). The operative findings will match the ultrasound description along with active arterial bleeding from the ruptured cortex. The presentation, apart from evidence of reverse diastolic flow, is similar to the description of graft rupture seen with severe ATN in the era before brain death legislation. Some surgeons of that era performed prophylactic division of the kidney capsule to allow the kidney to cope better with the inevitable parenchymal swelling associated with tubular necrosis.

The technical causes of RVT include an iliac vein valve cusp sutured into the anastomosis, kinking of the long left-sided donor kidney vein, and compression of the short right donor renal vein.

Surgical management of an acutely occluded renal vein is difficult. If identified in the early period after transplantation, simple reopening of the wound and making more space for the transplanted kidney may be associated with a rapid improvement in appearance of the kidney. Placement of the kidney in the peritoneal cavity may prevent the same from happening again. If thrombus is present in the renal vein of a right-sided donor kidney, removal of the kidney and reperfusion with preservation solution may be the only practical option. The donor kidney is retransplanted with consideration given to provision of greater mobilization of the iliac vein and more proximal siting of the venous anastomosis.

RVT is uncommon beyond the early period after transplantation, suggesting that transplant renal vein is comparatively resistant to anastomotic stenosis and perhaps protected by high renal vein blood flow. It can be seen in a subacute situation associated with secondary causes, such as iliofemoral vein thrombosis, de novo membranous nephropathy, glomerulonephritis, and thrombophilic states. Because of the time of presentation many months after surgery, percutaneous combined mechanical and chemical thrombolysis is feasible.[36]

Renal Artery Thrombosis

Spontaneous thrombosis of the renal artery is uncommon. It usually is due to technical reasons such as arterial kinking or torsion of the renal vascular pedicle. Contributing factors include poor cardiac output, hypotension, intravascular volume depletion, and thrombophilic states, or increased intrarenal pressure resulting from ATN, hydronephrosis, or cellular rejection. The renal arteries of kidneys that have failed because of chronic rejection often remain patent for many years.

Apart from loss of graft function, the signs and symptoms are negligible. Kidney graft loss is "silent." The diagnosis is made by CDUS or surgical exploration. Arterial thrombosis is a terminal event that can be averted only if arterial inflow is considered as a cause of poor graft function, and immediate intervention undertaken; hence, the importance of recognition of an arterial problem before thrombosis occurs. Routine CDUS assessment of the extrarenal transplant artery and the presence of worsening hypertension and poor graft function are good starting points.

Segmental Arterial Thrombosis

About 15% of deceased donor kidneys will have more than one renal atery and the number is likely greater for living donor kidneys in the era of laparoscopic donor nephrectomy. The arterial supply to the kidney parenchyma has no collateral circulation. Hence, failure to anastomose an accessory artery, or thrombosis of an accessory artery

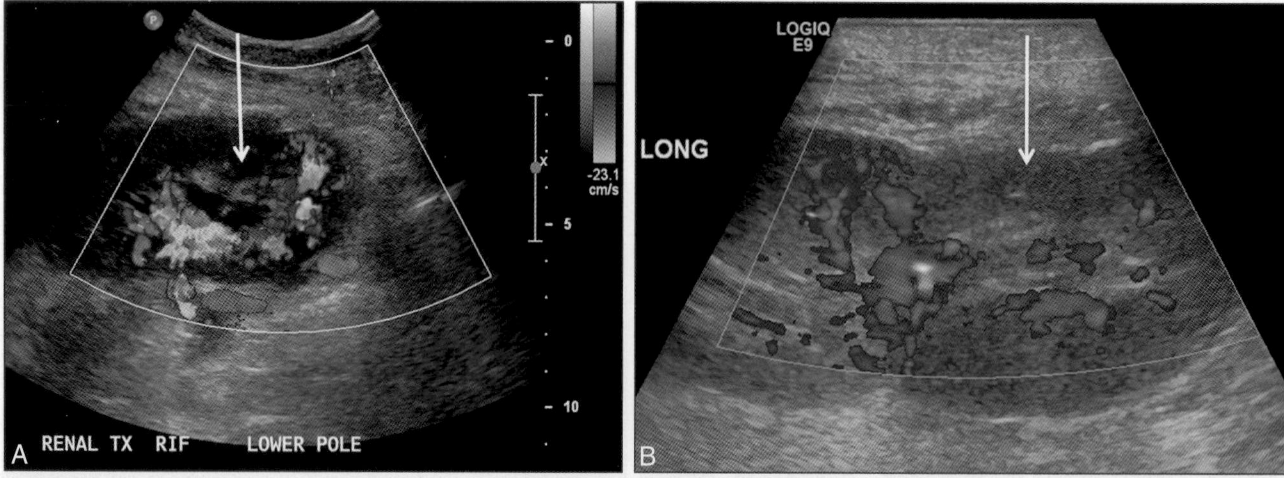

FIGURE 28-14 ■ Color Doppler ultrasound demonstrating wedge-shaped avascular area (arrow) of lower pole of a deceased donor kidney transplant with four renal arteries, one of which was shown to be thrombosed at the time of subsequent transplant exploration. (A) Seven days after transplantation. (B) Scarred infarcted area 3 months later.

or branch, will lead inevitably to a wedge-shaped infarct of the kidney. Inability to transplant a small upper-pole accessory artery or branch is a not uncommon event and is usually of little significance. It will be obvious at the time of transplantation as an ischemic area on the cortex of the kidney and a small perfusion defect may be apparent with CDUS examination. Larger accessory vessel or branch vessel occlusion will have a more significant impact on the transplanted kidney.

In the acute phase, evidence of segmental infarction is a lactate dehydrogenase level greater than 500 IU/L.[23] CDUS will demonstrate an obvious wedge-shaped area of absent renal perfusion (Figure 28-14A). A core biopsy will provide a histological diagnosis of necrotic kidney parenchyma. If the necrosis is full thickness, from capsule to calyceal system, urine leakage and formation of a urinoma may occur from about the fifth day after transplantation. It is not inevitable, and if not apparent by the end of the second week of transplantation, urine leakage is unlikely to occur (see Chapter 29 for management). Longer term, the infarcted segment of the kidney transplant will be replaced by scar tissue (Figure 28-14B).

Thrombosis Prevention Strategies

Acknowledging that vascular thrombosis is a multifactorial event, prevention necessitates the need for a combination of general and specific measures that make up Virchow's classic triad of contributing factors. Endothelial injury and inflammation will be reduced by minimizing factors leading to ATN at the multiorgan donor procedure, avoidance of prolonged cold and warm ischemia, and early core biopsy in a poorly functioning kidney to diagnose and aggressively manage vascular and antibody-mediated rejection. Stasis at the time of and after transplant surgery will be minimized by optimal surgical technique and fluid management – there is no margin for surgical error and beware of the transplant surgeon who blames the patient for his or her own surgical shortcomings!

The recognition of thrombophilic states as a major contributor to vascular thrombosis after kidney transplantation introduces the possible need for routine screening and, in turn, directed therapy to reduce the risk of thrombosis. Some centers do but there is no consensus for either strategy. Routine screening is expensive, and most thrombophilic states are rare. The most common are APAs, but, in the absence of a previous thrombotic event, the risk of allograft thrombosis is low. It would therefore be reasonable to limit investigation to potential recipients with previous or family history of thrombotic events, including deep and superficial vein thromboses, pulmonary emboli, thrombosed fistulas, multiple occlusions of central venous dialysis catheters, and problematic clotting of dialysis lines. To this list could be added patients undergoing pre-emptive transplantation with a living donor kidney.

Management of thrombophilic states is individualized to the patient's risk factors. For known thrombophilia and a history of clinical events, perioperative heparinization followed by long-term anticoagulation with warfarin has proven efficacy, including successful retransplantation.[12] The risk of bleeding seems acceptable in view of the incidence of thrombotic complications. Recommendations are less clear for patients with known risk factors but no history of thrombotic events. In a prospective study of 310 kidney transplant recipients in which all were given daily low-dose aspirin therapy, there was no difference in thrombotic events in patients with or without measurable thrombophilic factors.[42] Hence, known thrombophilia in the absence of a positive history might be appropriately managed by long-term low-dose aspirin alone. A role for other platelet inhibitors has yet to be defined.

TORSION

Rotation of the kidney about its own vascular pedicle only occurs when placed in an intraperitoneaal position (Figure 28-15). The need is usually prompted by difficulty closing the abdominal musculature without

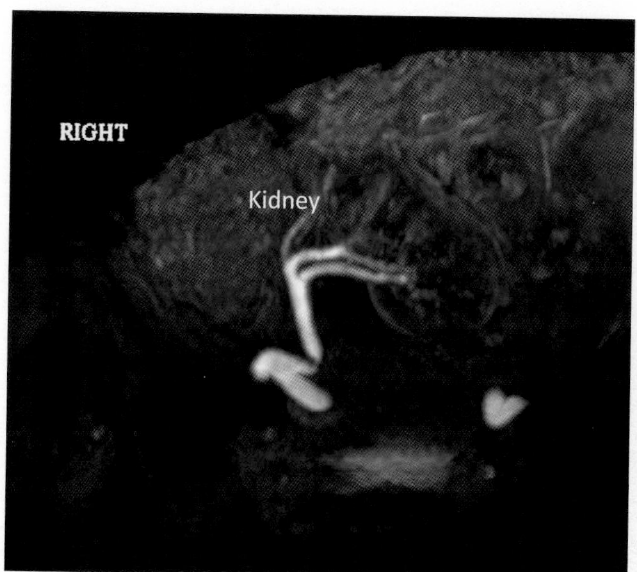

FIGURE 28-15 ■ Magnetic resonance imaging (MRI) angiogram demonstrating torsion of a transplant renal artery of a kidney transplant in the right iliac fossa. The kidney had been placed in an intraperitoneal position when transplanted 3 months earlier in a patient receiving mammalian target of rapamycin (mTOR) inhibitor immunosuppression. The kidney transplant was subsequently lost despite emergency exploration after MRI angiography.

compromising the transplant kidney vasculature. It is also performed routinely for diabetic patients receiving simultaneous pancreas and kidney transplants (SPK) through a midline incision. For these patients, the kidney is placed on the left side, lateral to the sigmoid colon, perhaps explaining why kidney transplant torsion is rarely reported after SPK.

Because of its very low incidence, the diagnosis of torsion is often overlooked and possible warning signs of pain, nausea, and oliguria are missed. Imaging is likely to show absence or very limited perfusion of the kidney transplant. A review of 16 cases described a successful outcome after graft exploration of 25%, and recommends prophylactic nephropexy to prevent torsion of kidneys placed in the peritoneal cavity, particularly if immunosuppression includes use of a TOR inhibitor.[29]

VASCULAR ACCESS THROMBOSIS

The arteriovenous fistula acts as a lifeline for dialysis-dependent patients, with effective vascular access surveillance being clinical examination and longitudinal assessment of pump speeds and pressure readings.[40] After transplantation, it provides reassurance for the recipient with delayed graft function, and even after succesful transplatation, recipients and clinicians are reluctant to ligate the fistula. However, with less surveillance, progressive intimal hyperplasia leads in the majority to eventual and "silent" loss of the fistula flow that is not worthy of resuscitation. In others, the size of the native vein fistula continues to grow, with the feeding artery and vein continuing to adapt to the low-resistance fistula circuit by becoming progressively more ectatic and tortuous. In turn, cardiac output increases progressively with 3, 4, and more liters of blood passing through the fistula anastomosis each minute. Tortuosity may lead to progressive kinking of the fistula vein and eventual stasis, and thrombosis which extends proximally. Painful thrombophlebitis intervenes and and anticoagulation may be necessary.

In the current era of good long-term transplant graft function, a case can now be made for a more proactive approach to ligation of native vein fistulae 6–12 months after transplantation, particularly in patients with ectatic feeding arteries or concerns about the effect of the fistula circuit on cardiac output. If left, the feeding artery will become progressively aneurysmal with tension in the artery wall proportional to the radius and arterial pressure. Intraluminal mural thombus forms, from which emboli head towards the distal arteries. Figure 28-16 represents an extreme example of this scenario.

DEEP VEIN THROMBOSIS

After any major surgery, a hypercoagulable state persists for 4 weeks. An early retrospective Oxford study based on clinical findings in a kidney transplant population in which specific DVT prophylaxis was not used, showed an incidence of 8.3% in 480 patients. However, the peak incidence was not early after transplantation but in the fourth month and usually associated with an event necessitating bed rest or pelvic pathology, such as a lymphocele.[2] Unpublished data from a 40-year Korean study of 1695 patients, presented at the International Congress of the Transplantation Society, Vancouver, 2010 (I.S. Moon – abstract 36) also demonstrated a low overall incidence of early symptomatic DVT and a mean presentation time of 6 years after kidney transplantation. By implication kidney transplant recipients are at low risk because of the protective bleeding tendency afforded by end-stage kidney disease and the preceding hemodialysis. The subsequent absence of reports of change of early DVT incidence in the rEPO era suggests the protective effect is not related to anemia. A prospective assessment of the incidence of DVT after transplant surgery has not been published.

Stable kidney transplant function, however, places recipients at the same risk as the general population with no unique risk factors, apart perhaps from the presence of a lymphocele (Figure 28-17). The physical presence of the kidney transplant itself, situated in the iliac fossa, does not seem to be a risk factor. Equally, proximal extension of an iliofemoral DVT is an uncommon event, probably because of the volume of blood entering the iliac vein from the transplanted kidney. Nevertheless, it can happen, presenting with dramatic ipsilateral leg swelling followed by loss of graft function. It is associated with a poor outcome if not recognized quickly.[46] Suggested management is anticoagulation with heparin, placement of a temporary caval filter via the contralateral femoral vein, followed by thrombolysis through a cannula placed in the ipsilateral popliteal vein with the patient lying prone on the interventional radiology table.

Adoption of universal measures for DVT prophylaxis has merit in a kidney transplant unit, despite the

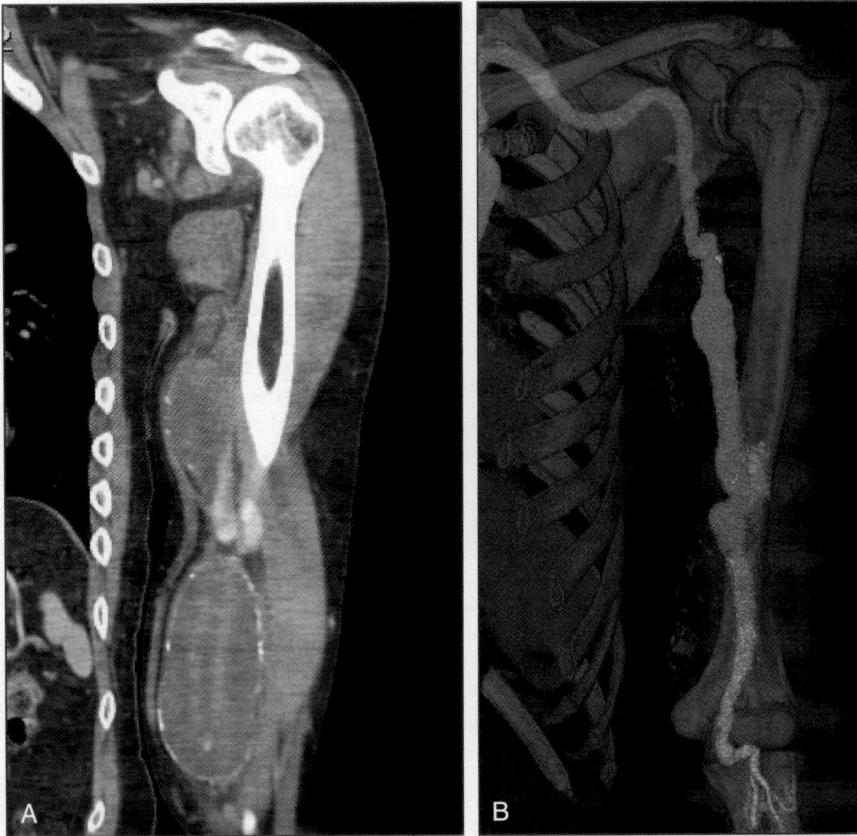

FIGURE 28-16 ■ Computed tomography angiogram of the left brachial artery in a transplant recipient presenting with clinical evidence of emboli in digital arteries 10 years after transplantation and 5 years after ligation of left brachiocephalic fistula. (A) Thrombus in two fusiform aneurysms of the brachial artery measuring 5 and 4 cm in diameter. (B) Arterial reconstruction of the lumen brachial artery.

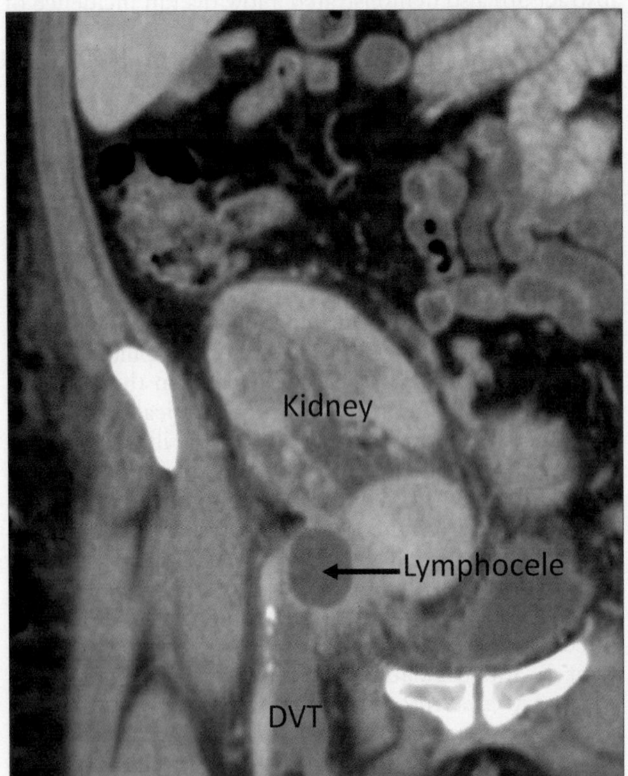

FIGURE 28-17 ■ Computed tomography scan (coronal view) with vascular contrast material demonstrates a small lymphocele compressing the distal right external iliac vein with resultant thrombosis of the more distal common femoral. DVT, deep vein thrombosis.

low incidence of DVT in the early period after kidney transplantation and the reassuring absence of reports showing an increase in incidence in the rEPO era. These prophylactic measures include the fitting of below-knee antithrombosis stockings before surgery and the use of intermittent calf compression during surgery. They are considered to be as effective as subcutaneous heparin, provided that the stockings are worn throughout the inpatient stay, and early ambulation and calf exercises are undertaken. If these low-risk measures become routine practice, they are less likely to be overlooked in the higher-risk patients with a history of pulmonary emboli or DVT and obese patients. In these patients, subcutaneous heparin can be added, with unfractionated preferred to long-acting fractionated heparin because of its ability to reverse in situations such as troublesome hematuria or the need for a kidney transplant biopsy.

VASCULAR CAUSES OF URETERIC COMPLICATIONS

The transplant ureter blood supply is totally dependent on the renal artery, and if present, an accessory lower-pole artery. The relationship between an accessory vessel and ureter is unpredictable and difficult to preserve, particularly for kidneys from obese donors (Figure 28-18). Failure to preserve increases the risk of necrosis or stenosis of the distal end of the ureter. Equally, preservation of the relationship between the lower-pole accessory artery and

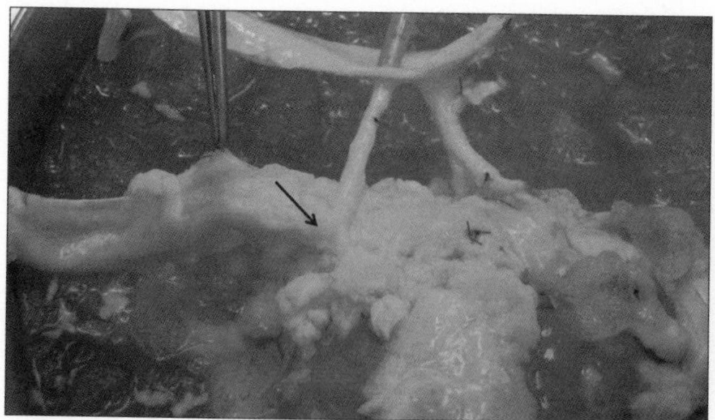

FIGURE 28-18 ■ Left-sided kidney from an obese deceased donor with an accessory lower-pole renal artery (cannulated) providing a branch (arrow) to supply the ureter (held by forceps).

the ureter can compromise the ureter by causing external compression after heterotopic positioning of the transplant, as demonstrated in Figure 28-19. The problem is usually diagnosed when the recipient presents with a hydronephrosis after removal of the ureteric stent placed at the time of transplantation. Surgical correction is challenging and involves either anastomosis of the native ureter to the transplant renal pelvis or a new transplant ureteroneocystostomy to be performed after mobilization of bladder and viable transplant ureter (see Chapter 29).

MYCOTIC ANEURYSM

An infected false aneurysm involving the anastomosis of the donor aortic patch to the iliac artery is an uncommon but potentially lethal vascular complication resulting from bacteremic shock or massive acute blood loss. It presents in the second or third week after transplantation as an acute febrile illness with possible evidence of distal thromboemboli in the ipsilateral lower limb. Alternatively, it can be a ligated transplant renal artery stump infected at the time of graft nephrectomy. A site of infection may be identified elsewhere, such as an infected venous cannula. The organism can be a bacterium or fungus that lodges in a defect in the intima of the aortic patch caused by suturing or ulceration of atheromatous plaque. Subsequent artery wall infection leads to anastomosis rupture. If contained locally, an infected false aneurysm is obvious on CDUS examination.

Management is individualized with life-saving measures undertaken first.[28,45] Nephrectomy is usually undertaken with repair of the arterial defect using a vein patch and followed by prolonged administration of appropriate antimicrobial agents. Reports also exist of successful local or endovascular repair of small unruptured mycotic aneurysms together with prolonged antimicrobial use.

BIOPSY-RELATED VASCULAR COMPLICATIONS

A needle core biopsy gun with a small spring-loaded 18G-caliber needle can be a dangerous weapon, even in experienced ultrasound-guided hands. Informed consent is taken beforehand. Cessation of antiplatelet agents is likely to reduce the incidence of minor, but not major, complications.[31] Hematoma formation is common, if not inevitable, in the first week or two after transplantation. Clot is seen outside of and adjacent to the kidney transplant and often extending upwards in the retroperitoneal plane. CT scanning without vascular contrast provides a better imaging than CDUS, which tends to underestimate the extent of the hematoma. Biopsy of an established kidney transplant can be associated with a subcapsular hematoma that can quickly compromise transplant function and viability (Figure 28-20). The author has vivid memories of performing an uneventful

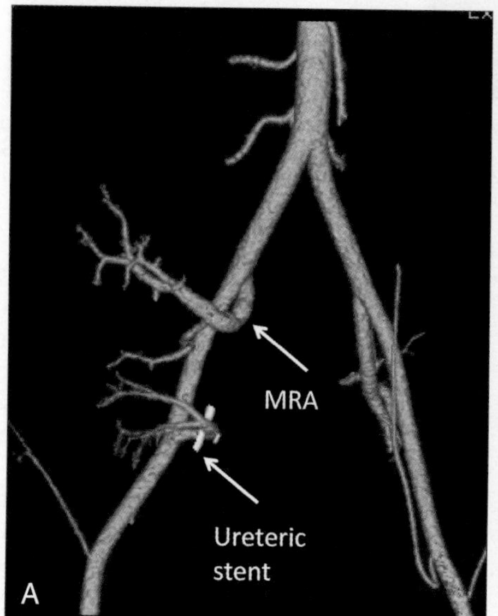

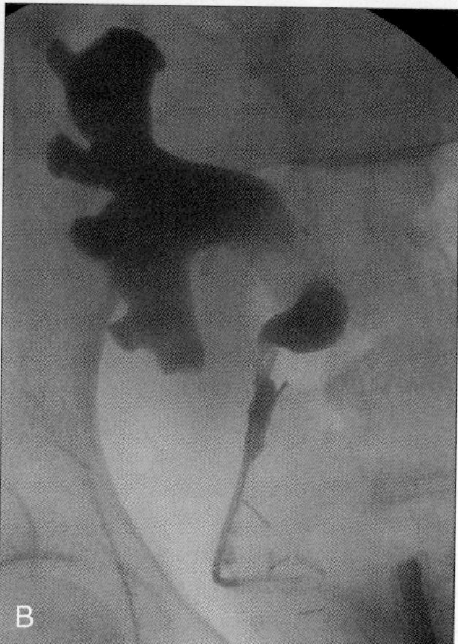

FIGURE 28-19 ■ External compression of the proximal transplant ureter in a patient receiving a left-sided living donor kidney with two renal arteries separtely transplanted into the right iliac fossa. (A) The relationship of the transplant ureteric stent (arrow) to the lower-pole accessory renal artery which is anastomosed to the distal right external iliac artery. The main renal artery is anastomosed end to end to the right internal iliac artery. (B) Retrograde pyelogram to investigate hydronephrosis 2 weeks after elective removal of the transplant ureteric stent.

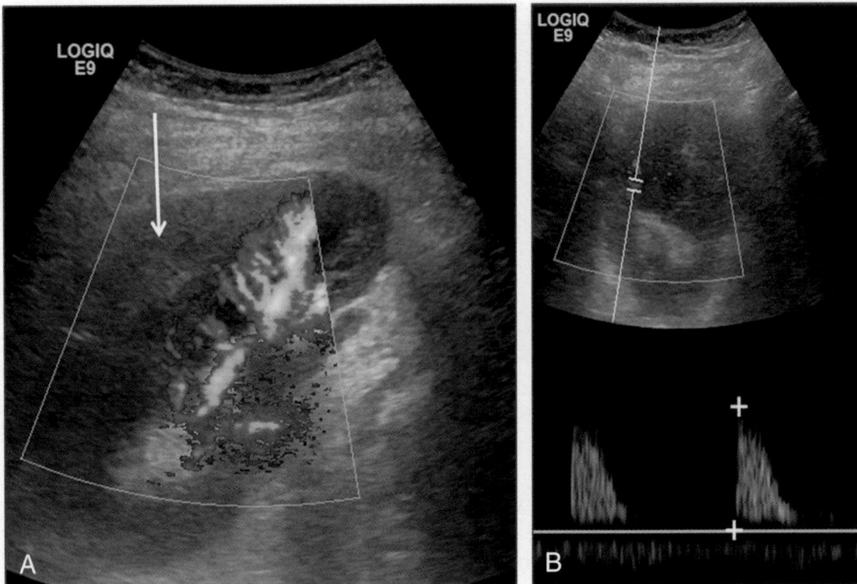

FIGURE 28-20 ■ Color Doppler ultrasound in a transplant recipient to investigate anuria following a protocol kidney core biopsy 3 months after transplantation. (A) Large subcapsular hematoma compressing kidney parenchyma. (B) Hilar artery waveforms demonstrating poor arterial blood flow into the transplant.

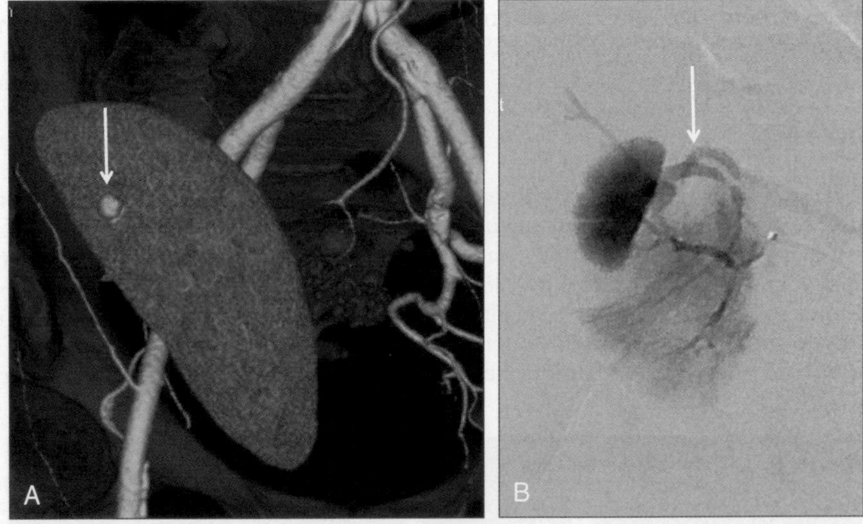

FIGURE 28-21 ■ Incidental finding of an upper-pole biopsy-related false aneurysm at time of computed tomography angiography. (A) Vascular reconstruction demonstrating 1-cm aneurysm (arrow) and draining arteriovenous fistula. (B) Selective angiography 3 months later to treat the then 2.5-cm partially thrombosed aneurysm and fistula (arrow). Both spontaneously thrombosed during selective angiography.

1-year protocol core biopsy without ultrasound guidance. Three mornings later, the patient returned anuric after a night of "rock and roll" dancing. CDUS demonstrated a large subcapsular hematoma compressing an avascular kidney transplant. The earlier biopsy demonstrated cortex and medulla separated by a segment of artery. The event prompted the purchase of a dedicated ultrasound machine for the transplant unit.

Microscopic hematuria is also an almost universal finding after core biopsy. Macroscopic hematuria is seen after about 10% of percutaneous biopsies. Problematic bleeding is usually self-limiting with bed rest, although retrograde ureteric stenting may be necessary. Small false aneurysms and arteriovenous fistulas within the transplant kidney are less common. They are shown by CDUS examination and CT angiography, usually as incidental findings (Figure 28-21). If an acute problem, a regimen of bed rest, intermittent ultrasound with local compression, and temporary cessation of antiplatelet agents and heparin is usually successful in managing a false aneurysm. Occasionally, CDUS will detect an arteriovenous fistula between bigger vessels within the kidney. They are usually asymptomatic, although an impressive bruit may be present on auscultation. In most cases, conservative management is successful, even for large fistulas, as shown in Figure 28-22. Interventional embolization is a more practical option than open surgery to control intrarenal bleeding into the urinary collecting system, or to treat significant vascular steal from the kidney transplant.

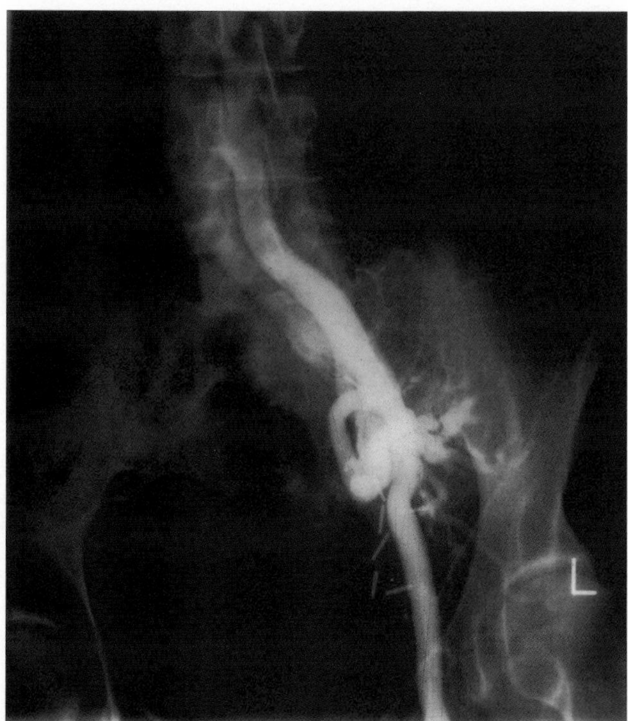

FIGURE 28-22 ■ Angiogram of a left-sided kidney transplant shows rapid passage of vascular contrast material into the common iliac vein, consistent with a large intrarenal arteriovenous fistula secondary to a percutaneous 14-gauge core biopsy of the kidney. The fistula was managed conservatively.

TRANSPLANT RENAL ARTERY STENOSIS

Transplant renal artery stenosis (TRAS) is the commonest vascular complication after kidney transplantation. Although the etiology is variable, it is a potentially treatable cause of hypertension and graft dysfunction. If severe and left untreated, it can lead to graft loss or may be fatal.

Definition and Incidence

There is no consensus definition of TRAS. At one end of the spectrum is the classic presentation of a bruit over the transplant, refractory hypertension, deteriorating renal function, life-threatening congestive cardiac failure secondary to fluid retention, and dramatic reversal by correction of the stenosis.[14] It presents most commonly 3 months to 2 years after transplantation[18] with symptoms and signs caused by activation of the renin–angiotensin system. At the other end of the spectrum is the incidental finding of a stenosis on CDUS examination of 50% or greater reduction in renal artery lumen diameter in a normotensive patient in the absence of graft dysfunction. In between is the common finding of hypertension which is multifactorial and an independent risk factor for long-term graft survival (see Chapter 30). Hence, any measure to improve blood pressure control may be valid provided the intervention has few inherent risks, and even if it may not provide measurable benefit for the kidney transplant recipient in the short to medium term, it may in the long term.

The reported incidence of TRAS varies widely from 1% to 23% depending on the definition used. The higher figure dates back to Hamburger's 14-year experience, published in 1973.[27] His transplant recipients underwent formal angiography on a routine basis. CDUS examination is the modern-day equivalent. Its safety and low cost make it an indispensable tool in the transplant clinic as the first-line screening tool to investigate graft dysfunction. It provides qualitative and quantitative assesment of the kidney and has made a major contribution to the continuing improvement in graft survival.[13] Protocol-driven CDUS examination of the transplant renal artery will also raise awareness of unappreciated arterial pathology contributing to the cause of hypertension.

The comparative ease and safety of interventional radiology techniques to correct the problem initially identified by CDUS examination have resulted in an increased reporting of TRAS managed by intervention. However, having identified flow disturbance in the transplant renal artery, there are key unresolved questions that will be answered only by standardized reporting and management of those findings.[9] Is the stenosis progressive in the long term? Is hypertension alone an indication for intervention? How do we determine a hemodynamically significant stenosis? When and how do we intervene? In the kidney transplant setting, only observational studies with varying reporting criteria and methodology exist to provide answers. Furthermore, the natural history of TRAS is uncertain, and the long-term benefit of intervention is unknown. Do TRAS behave, and should they be managed, in the same way as native renal artery stenoses?[57] Meaningful answers will not come from retrospective analysis of registry data[18] but rather from a longitudinal study of unselected patients undergoing surveillance CDUS at defined time points and intervention, as indicated by clinical parameters such as graft function and hypertension.

In the interim, the author's suggested definition of TRAS is one based on a diagnosis of hypertension requiring increasing antihypertensive therapy, with or without deterioration in graft function, in the presence of a renal artery stenosis which, when corrected, results in improvement of blood pressure control or renal function, or both. If such a definition were used, the incidence of TRAS would be closer to 1% than to 23%. Surveillance CDUS of the extrarenal transplant artery, 6 weeks after transplantation, has been routine at Royal Prince Alfred Hospital in Sydney since 2003. Using the suggested diagnostic criteria, the incidence of TRAS is 4.5%.

Pathogenesis

The stenosis is usually situated near the anastomosis of the renal artery to an iliac artery and can be short, diffuse, or at multiple sites, and occur at different times, in line with the multiple possisble causes for TRAS. In a large series of TRAS, Voiculescu et al.[56] reported that most stenoses are identified in the first 6 months. Fibrosis accounted for 40%, donor artery atherosclerosis for 27%, and renal artery kinking for 21%. Stenoses at the anastomosis site are more likely to be technical and apparent from time of transplantation and probably stable. End-to-side anastomoses may be more of a problem than end-to-end

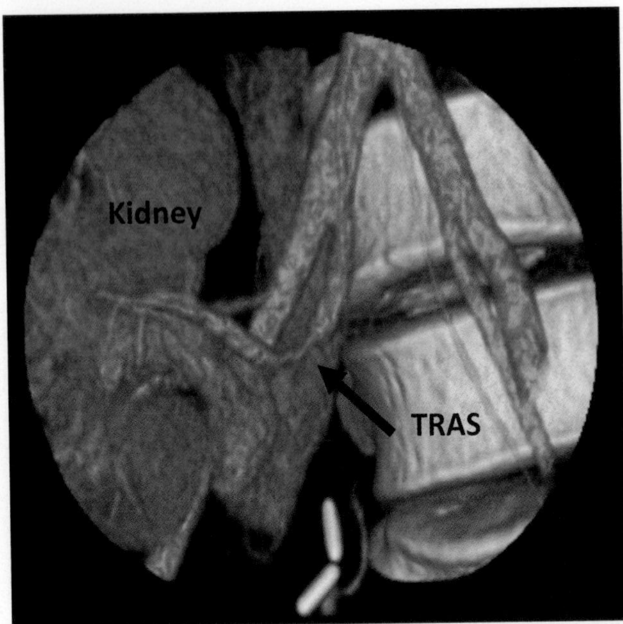

FIGURE 28-23 ■ Computed tomography scan with vascular contrast and three-dimensional reconstruction showing transplant renal artery stenosis (TRAS) distal to anastomosis to the internal iliac artery 2 months after living donor kidney transplantation. The stenosis is likely due to intimal fibrosis.

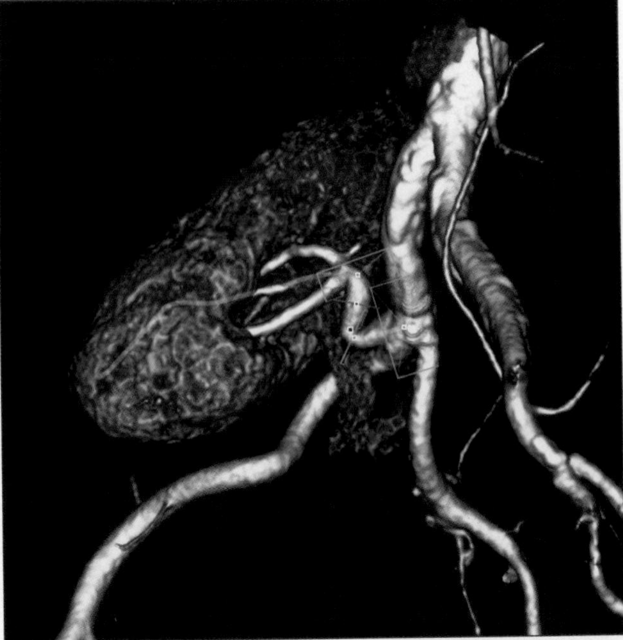

FIGURE 28-24 ■ Computed tomography angiogram with vascular reconstruction of a left-sided deceased donor kidney anastomosed to the bifurcation of the right common iliac artery. It demonstrates two kinks, one near the anastomosis and a lesser kink closer to the hilum.

anastomoses.[37] Progressive anastomotic stenosis, particularly involving the end of the renal artery, as is the case for living donor kidneys, probably represents fibrosis and intimal hyperplasia in response to damage to the renal artery at the time of donation or implantation surgery, or an intimal flap (Figure 28-23).

Kinking or twisting of the renal artery of the heterotopic positioned kidney at time of wound closure probably occurs more frequently than appreciated by transplant surgeons. The kink occurs either at the apex of the curve of the artery or near the anastomosis where the artery is comparatively fixed in position, or both (Figure 28-24). A twist in the transplant renal artery is more likely to be seen nearer the hilum of the kidney.

The long and more diffuse stenoses tend to occur later and have been attributed to immune-mediated endothelial injury with progressive intimal proliferation, particularly if concentric in nature. Multiple stenoses, often associated with renal artery branching, probably fit into the same category (Figure 28-25). The reported temporal association with vascular rejection and subsequent stenosis is inconclusive.[58] A single-center study of 27 patients with TRAS showed a significant association by multivariate analysis with cytomegalovirus (CMV) infection and delayed graft function.[4] CMV infection is thought to trigger endothelial damage. It has a similar role in the development of cardiac allograft vasculopathy. An example of stenosis that could be attributed to CMV is demonstrated in Figure 28-26. The recipient presented with severe hypertension requiring three antihypertensive agents, elevated creatinine, CDUS findings of elevated peak systolic velocities (PSVs) in both branches, fever, and CMV viremia. With reduced immunosuppression and prolonged use of antiviral agents, hypertension resolved and CDUS findings returned to normal 3 months later.

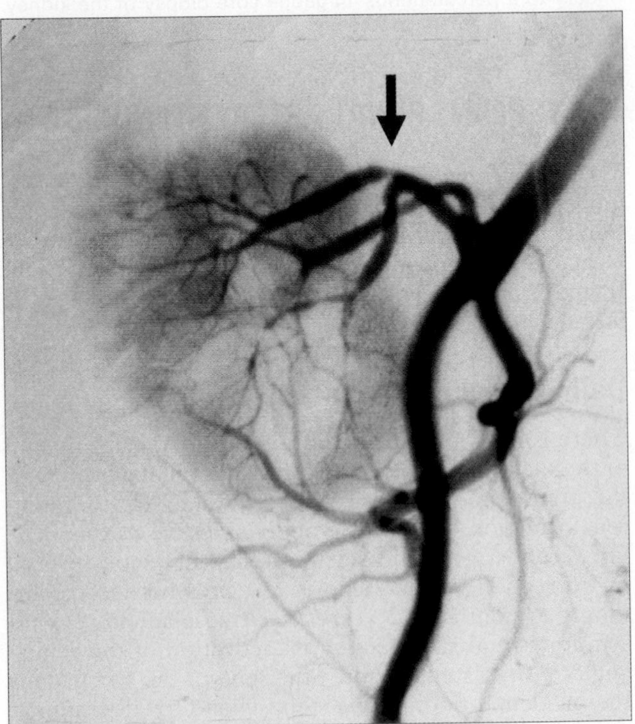

FIGURE 28-25 ■ Angiogram demonstrating multiple stenoses of the renal artery branches (arrow) in a kidney transplanted 2 years previously and complicated by rejection.

Atherosclerosis, occurring either de novo or already present in the donor renal artery (Figure 28-27), is an uncommon cause of TRAS. Equally, an arterial stenosis or obstruction anywhere in the arterial tree upstream from the transplanted kidney can produce the

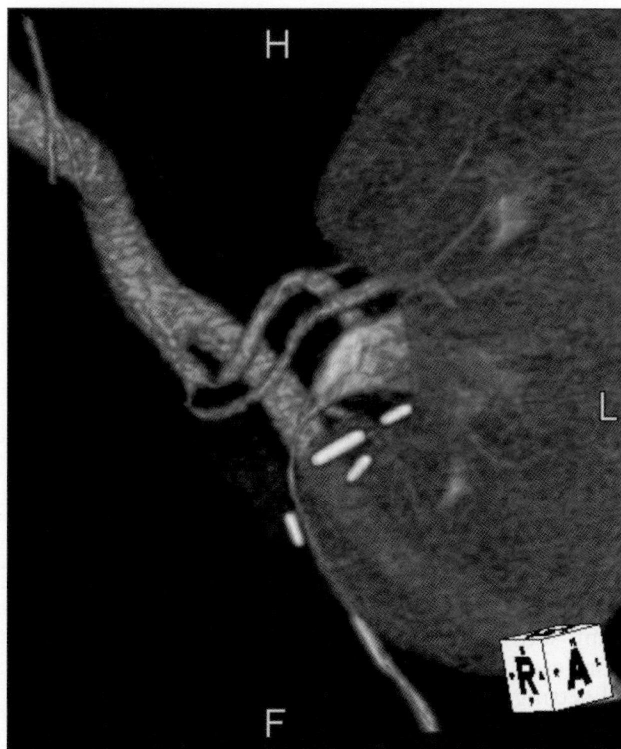

FIGURE 28-26 ■ Computed tomography angiogram with vascular reconstruction of a living donor kidney demonstrating stenoses in both main renal artery branches 3 months after transplantation. The main renal artery is anastomosed to the internal iliac artery.

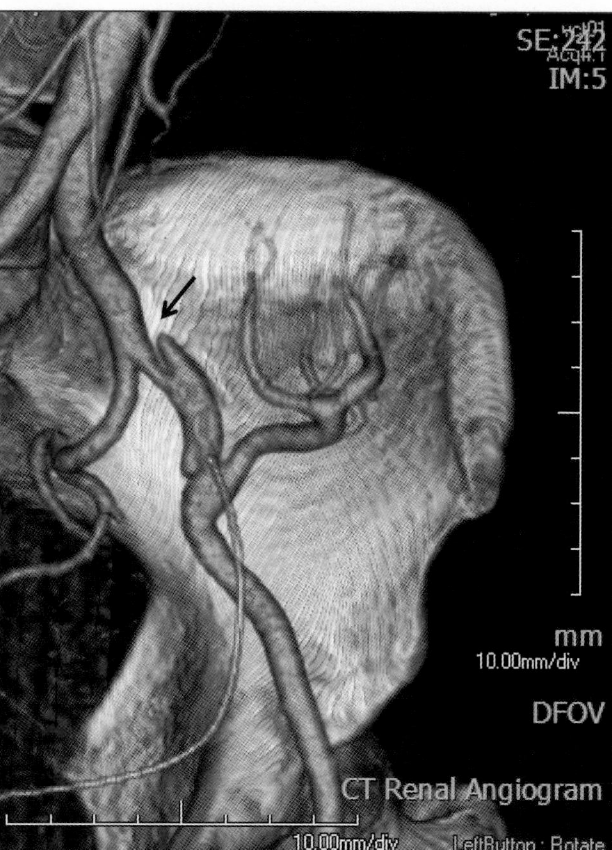

FIGURE 28-27 ■ Computed tomography angiogram of kidney transplant anastomosed to the left external iliac artery (EIA) in a patient with poor kidney function 2 weeks after transplantation and hypertension. It demonstates an intimal flap (arrow) of the proximal EIA consistent with a vascular clamp injury at time of surgery. It was subsequently managed with an endovascular stent. A less significant second intimal injury is noted adjacent to the anastomosis below.

same clinical presentation as TRAS. Many transplant recipients, particularly smokers and older patients with maturity-onset diabetes, have progressive diffuse arterial disease at time of successful transplantation. A stenosis can be precipitated by a vascular clamp injuring an already diseased iliac artery at the time of transplant surgery (Figure 28-28). Of clinical relevance in this setting is the combined history of progressive claudication symptoms and worsening hypertension. An iliofemoral bruit may be present together with a weak or absent femoral pulse, as demonstrated in Figure 28-29.

Pathophysiology – "One Kidney, One Clip"

In 1934, Goldblatt and colleagues[16] published their seminal study on the hypertensive effect of partial reduction of the blood flow to a kidney in dogs by applying a silver clip to one of the two renal arteries. They proposed the existence of a pressor substance released by the ischemic kidney. Over the next 25 years, others subsequently defined the renin–angiotensin system, with renin being the hormone released from the ischemic kidney.[5] Elevated renin levels are found in the venous blood of the ischemic kidney. Its pressor effect follows the release of angiotensin by enzymatic processes from the circulating substrate, angiotensinogen, an octapeptide with wide-ranging effects, including vasoconstriction, renal sodium retention, aldosterone secretion, and hypertrophy of myocardium and arteries.[14] Blood pressure is driven by the direct pressor effect of angiotensin II, with excess salt and water

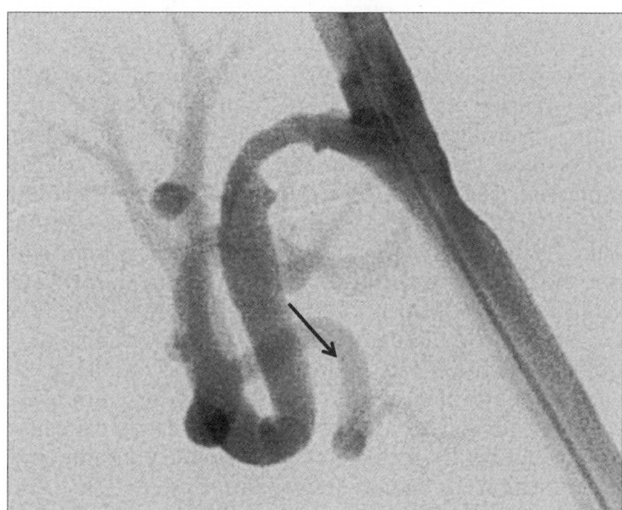

FIGURE 28-28 ■ Angiography demonstrating a transplant renal artery stenosis in a deceased donor right-sided kidney about 6 months after transplantation. At time of transplantation, the atheromatous aortic patch with a tight orifice stenosis had been excised. Pressure measurements at time of angiography identified a mean systolic drop of 24 mmHg across the stenosis.

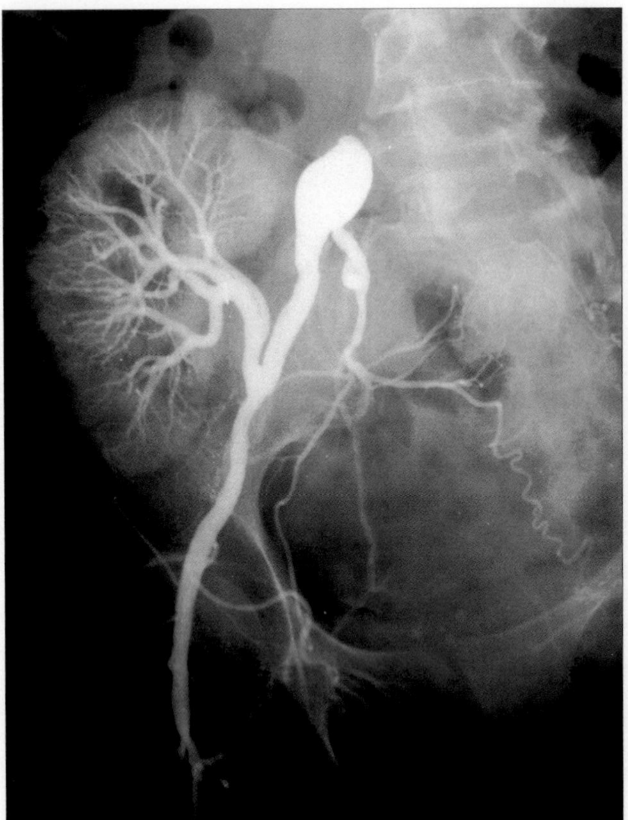

FIGURE 28-29 ■ Angiogram shows occlusion of an aneurysmal right common iliac artery proximal to the kidney transplant. At the time of angiography and before proximal arterial bypass surgery, the patient had been receiving hemodialysis for 2 months. After bypass surgery, normal kidney transplant function returned.

excreted by the non-ischemic good kidney, and is treated by inhibitors of the renin–angiotensin system. This does not apply in the kidney transplant setting.

An analogous situation to the transplanted kidney with a hemodynamically significant renal artery stenosis was the effect of applying one clip to the renal artery in a dog with one kidney ("one kidney, one clip"). Hypertension also results from the balance between the angiotensin-dependent system and volume-dependent mechanisms based on salt and water retention which otherwise would be excreted by a normal contralateral kidney. The perfusion pressure to the single ischemic kidney is maintained by the high circulating volume and not the direct pressor effect of angiotensin. Renal vein renin levels are near normal and sufficient to maintain the elevated circulating volume, and with it, normal glomerular filtration rate and renal function. In the presence of renin–angiotensin system inhibitors, however, the drive for salt and water retention is removed, causing reduction in perfusion to the solitary kidney and deterioration in kidney transplant dysfunction. The diagnosis of TRAS is often made by observation of rapid deterioration in function with the introduction of renin–angiotensin system inhibitors.

Dogs have been used to determine the minimal degree of renal arterial stenosis needed to cause hypertension. In an exceptional publication in 1992, Imanishi et al.[20] demonstrated clearly the relationship between the degree of stenosis and the ability of the kidney to autoregulate its blood flow. In anesthetized dogs, they constricted the left renal artery concentrically using a radiolucent device and evaluated the stenosis by cine angiography. With the kidney either innervated or denervated, systemic blood pressure began to increase when the stenosis was more than 70% of the diameter of the renal artery. Renal blood flow decreased when the stenosis was more than 75% of the diameter. In an equally impressive canine study using magnetic resonance imaging (MRI) and an implanted inflatable arterial cuff and flow probe, Schoenberg et al.[51] demonstrated that stenoses of 30–80% gradually reduced downstream early systolic peak velocity, but only minimally affected peak mean flow. At 50% stenosis, the mean pressure decrease across the stenosis was recorded at about 10 mmHg, and at 80%, 28 mmHg. At a stenosis of 90%, mean flow was decreased by greater than 50%.

An equivalent study in humans is unlikely. However, extrapolation of Imanishi's findings into the transplant setting would explain why TRAS of 60% or more can be clinically insignificant. Also, in the clinical setting, it should be possible to learn more about the relationship between the magnitude of the pressure gradient across a TRAS required to achieve better blood pressure control after correction of that stenosis by angioplasty. Results could be correlated with spiral CT angiography assessment of the cross-sectional area of the stenosis before angioplasty. Such a study has not been reported.

Imaging

Contrast angiography has long been the "gold standard" investigation of TRAS. The 1975 reporting of Hamburger's 14-year experience from 1959 of TRAS concluded that angiography was so valuable that it should be performed at routine intervals in all transplant recipients.[27] Although angiography still might be the "gold standard," CDUS examination has become the imaging modality to enable routine surveillance of transplant renal arteries. It provides an instantaneous assessment of intrarenal vasculature and a global impression of transplant perfusion.

There are two ultrasound approaches to the diagnosis of TRAS. The extrarenal approach involves scanning the renal artery from the hilum to the anastomosis and beyond to the proximal iliac artery. The PSV is measured along the whole course of these vessels. A hemodynamically significant stenosis has a PSV of greater than 2.5 m/s.[53] The degree of stenosis and the site of maximum PSV can be reported with a high degree of accuracy in the hands of an experienced ultrasonographer (Figure 28-30). Secondary spectral findings of downstream turbulence and spectral broadening increase the confidence of the diagnosis of TRAS. A prolonged acceleration time and a ratio of >3.0 between renal and iliac artery PSV increase the diagnostic accuracy. However, the technique is operator-dependent and time-consuming. The unpredictable course of transplant renal artery makes it difficult to

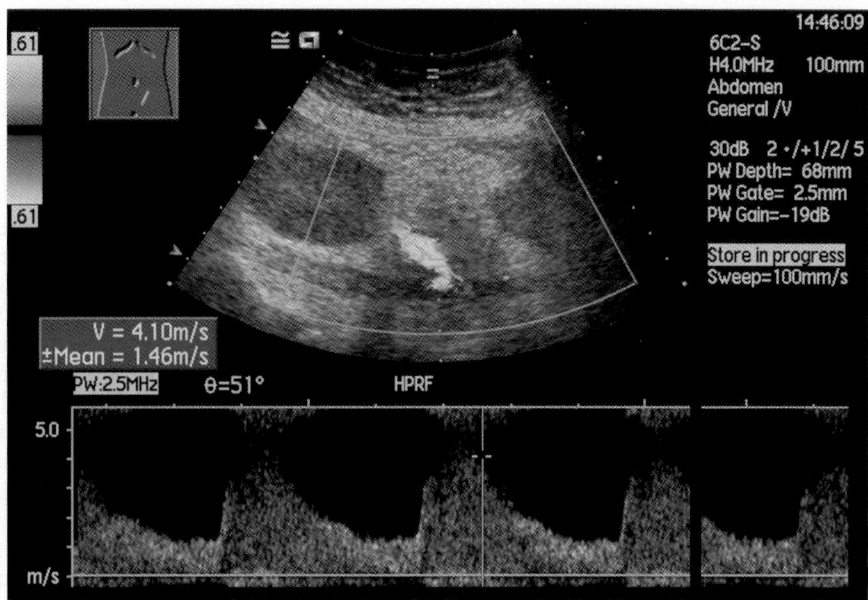

FIGURE 28-30 ■ Color Doppler ultrasound scanning of a kidney transplant demonstrating peak systolic velocity in the main renal artery of 4.10 m/s, diagnostic of transplant renal artery stenosis.

obtain the accurate angle of correction necessary for precise spectral quantification. Distinguishing a focal stenosis from a tortuous renal artery can be problematic, and reporting can err on the side of false-positive findings. A careful diagram and direct communication with the ultrasonographer can increase the value of the report.

The intrarenal approach has the advantage of being less operator-dependent, more reproducible, and easy to perform. It relies on the intrarenal downstream assessment of the effects of a TRAS. The early systolic peak is flattened and delayed, the so-called parvus-tardus pattern. It is associated with a low resistive index of 0.5 (Figure 28-31). The intrarenal technique is specific but not sensitive and can only diagnose high-grade stenoses of greater than 75%. It cannot localize the stenosis. Hence, the preferred approach is to combine both, but the request may not be well received in a busy general hospital ultrasound laboratory at short notice. Nevertheless, the routine evaluation for TRAS at designated time points after transplantation has merit.

Having identified a TRAS by CDUS examination, the next decision is whether to proceed with vascular contrast studies. The decision is not difficult if graft loss is imminent. The risk of contrast nephropathy in an already compromised kidney can be reduced by adequate hydration with normal saline before and after injection of contrast material.[38] Multislice helical CT permits accurate

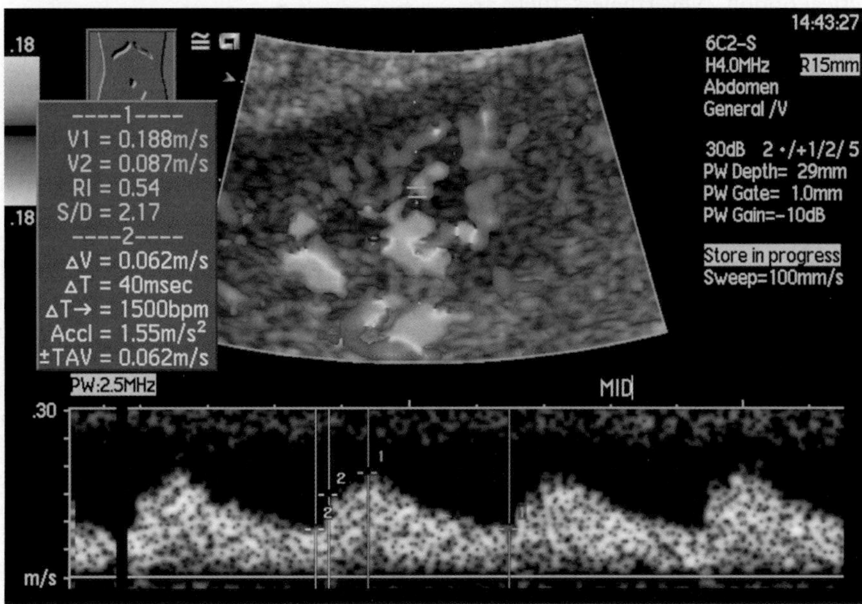

FIGURE 28-31 ■ Color Doppler ultrasound scanning of a kidney transplant demonstrating arterial waveform of the intrarenal arcuate artery, showing the features of parvus tardus, also indicative of transplant renal artery stenosis. Note the low resistance index of 0.54.

assessment of the site and degree of TRAS and provides valuable imaging for planning subsequent intervention. Advocates claim that helical CT requires less volume of iodinated vascular contrast medium than formal angiography and less toxicity with intravenous infusion of contrast. Protection of the transplanted kidney is recommended at all times when vascular contrast medium is injected, regardless of renal function and contrast volume. The alternative is to perform helical CT or MRI with gadolinium, a non-iodinated contrast medium. However, reports of nephrogenic systemic sclerosis with use of gadolinium are concerning, definition is less satisfactory because of its lower density, and therapeutic intervention is impossible. Good screening images nevertheless can be achieved, as shown in Figure 28-15 of a torted intraperitoneal kidney.

Conventional angiography remains the gold standard investigation because of the quality of definition, the ability to measure pressure gradients across the stenosis, and the potential to intervene at the same visit to the angiography suite. The contralateral femoral artery approach is used for kidneys transplanted to the internal iliac artery by end-to-end technique. Otherwise, an ipsilateral approach is used to complete an aortoiliac run using 20–30 mL of iodinated vascular contrast medium, a step avoided by helical CT or MRI images. Selective runs are performed with oblique or other views as necessary using about 10 mL of contrast medium with each run. False-negative examinations can occur if insufficient views are obtained. To this extent, multislice helical CT angiography with reconstructions has advantages over conventional angiography.

Conservative Treatment

If extrarenal CDUS demonstrates TRAS in the order of 60%, kidney transplant function is satisfactory, and the recipient is not hypertensive or has easily treated hypertension, continued observation with repeat ultrasound examination is a practical option. Nevertheless, there are no reports of the long-term safety of this line of management, and the natural history of a 60% TRAS is unknown. Anecdotal evidence suggests this is probably safe for a kinked transplant renal artery, particularly if there is no deterioration of kidney function.[9] However, based on the previously described canine studies demonstrating reduction in kidney perfusion, one is more nervous about continued observation of a stenosis of >70% on CDUS examination, irrespective of acceptable transplant function. Such a stenosis would be more susceptible to occlusion in the presence of periods of dehydration or cardiovascular instability, and intervention should be considered.

Angioplasty and Stenting

Percutaneous transluminal angioplasty (PTA) is recognized as the initial treatment of choice for TRAS.[24] Technical success has been reported as greater than 80%, but with clinical success, as judged by reduction in blood pressure and improvement of renal function, being considerably less. Intervention has inherent risks, and it can be argued that, unless a significant pressure drop exists across the TRAS, PTA should not be undertaken. However, there is not an agreed mean pressure drop beyond which intervention is warranted. The canine studies of Schoenberg et al.[51] suggest the figure should be >10 mmHg.

In the presence of a satisfactory radiological result and no improvement in clinical parameters, other underlying causes of hypertension and graft pathology should be sought. To this extent, PTA could be performed as an investigation of exclusion if the complication rates were acceptable. As with other forms of interventional angiography, most of the complications relate to puncture site problems in the groin. Local clinician skill may dictate the wisdom of this line of management and the success of interventional angiography is likely influenced by cooperative decision making by the radiologist and transplant surgeon. Increasingly, with newer premounted stents deployed by balloons, complications leading to graft loss are unusual.[24] Equally, it can be argued that, when thrombosis does complicate PTA, an experienced interventional radiologist using urokinase and further stenting usually benefits the recipient much faster and more efficaciously than the surgeon who must find an emergency operating room and rapidly undertake a difficult dissection and vascular reconstruction (Figure 28-32).

The restenosis rates are reported to be 10–60% and are probably influenced by cause of the stenosis, length of follow-up, and use of stents.[24,34] Data on long-term effects of PTA on kidney allograft survival after PTA are scarce and understandably are based on observational studies.[15] For ethical reasons, a randomized trial might only be feasible in patients with stable function and blood pressure control, with the measure of success of the procedure based on graft survival. Such a trial is unlikely as it would need to be multicenter and take a decade or more to complete.

Surgical Correction

Historically, correction of TRAS by surgery is seen as a difficult operation, with graft loss rates of 20%.[6,27] Surgery is therefore, and perhaps unfairly, viewed as the last resort or rescue therapy for cases unsuitable for PTA. Sometimes there is no alternative but surgery, as the following examples demonstrate. The limiting factors for surgical correction of TRAS are access to the artery, availablity of arterial inflow alternatives, and the resultant warm ischemia time. A heparinized kidney allograft might tolerate warm ischemia of 30 minutes or more because of the pre-existing diminished blood flow and the presence of a collateral flow, albeit with increasing risk of ATN and cortical necrosis as the minutes tick away.

The surgical approach will depend on the cause. Easiest is removal of a factor that might be causing the kink together with release of fibrous tissue surrounding the kink. An example is demonstrated in Figure 28-33 of a sheep farmer with large polycystic kidneys who presented 6 months after transplantation with a hypertensive crisis and rapidly deteriorating graft function a day

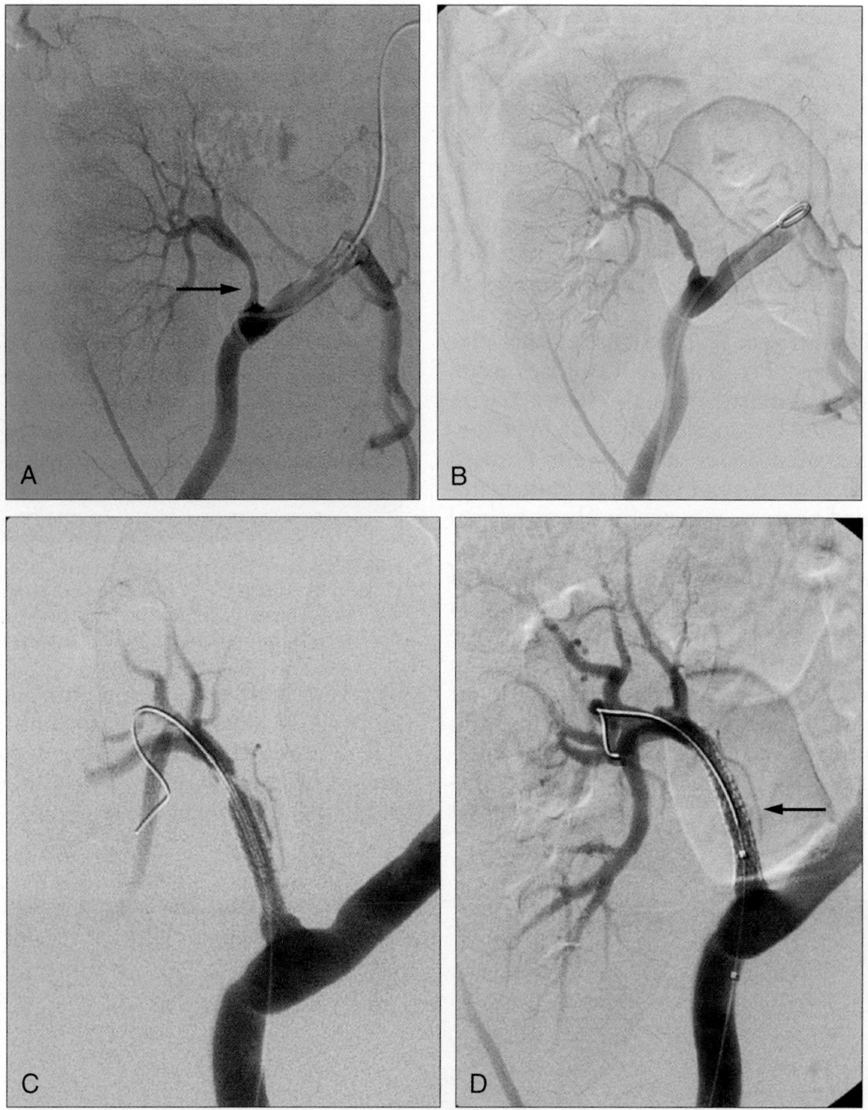

FIGURE 28-32 ■ (A) Angiogram of a kidney transplant 3 months after transplantation. The mean arterial pressure gradient across the stenosis (arrow) in this symptomatic patient was 16 mmHg. (B) Appearance of the renal artery 24 hours after percutaneous transluminal angioplasty. (C) Appearance of transplant renal artery after insertion of a self-expanding stent. (D) After additional more distal stent. The transplant eventually failed 6 years later as a result of chronic allograft nephropathy.

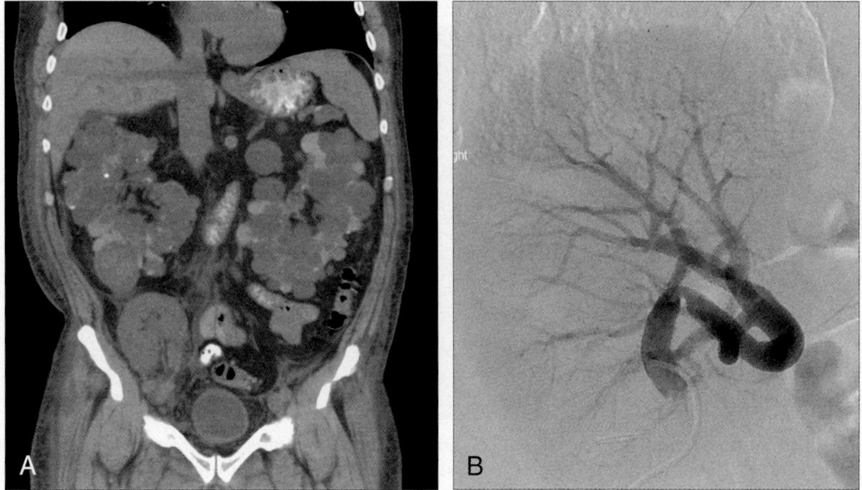

FIGURE 28-33 ■ (A) Computed tomography scan (coronal view) demonstrating large polycystic kidneys, one of which is directly above a right-sided deceased donor kidney transplant in the right iliac fossa. The hilum of the transplant is directed inferolaterally. (B) Digital subtraction angiogram of the transplant renal artery demonstrating marked kinking that was able to be corrected by excision of the right polycystic kidney and mobilization of the artery.

after manually moving a couple of tonnes of animal feed. The ipilateral polycystic kidney above was excised and the kinked transplant artery fully mobilized. Graft function rapidly returned to baseline, as did antihypertensive medication requirement.

Another option is excision of the stenosis with direct anastomosis to adjacent iliac artery, an example of which is used to correct the TRAS illustrated in Figure 28-24 and demonstrated in Figure 28-34. Interposition grafting with long saphenous vein or recipient internal iliac artery may be necessary. Preserved ABO blood group compatible deceased donor artery can also be used, with the United Network for Organ Sharing guidelines recommending that deceased donor artery grafts be used within 7 days of donation. Use of synthetic graft material is usually avoided because of concerns about intimal hyperplasia.

An infrequently used option is autotransplantation of the kidney after back table reconstruction of a complex arterial problem. Figure 28-35 illustrates one such case in which deceased donor vessels were used to replace an aneurysmal transplant renal artery. The original donor kidney came from an 8-year-old child with brain death resulting from rupture of an intracerebral artery aneurysm. The recipient was 14 years old at the time of transplantation and presented 6 years later with sudden onset of severe graft dysfunction after introduction of an angiotensin II blocking agent to control hypertension. The TRAS was caused by kinking secondary to distortion caused by the enlarging aneurysm, off which came four branches of the renal artery.

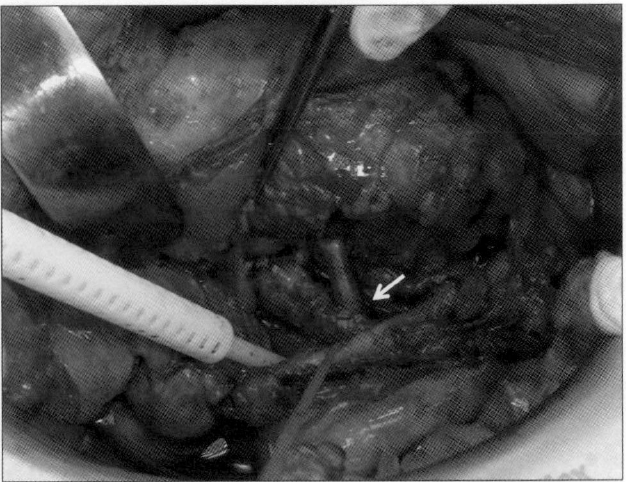

FIGURE 28-34 ■ The transplant renal artery stenosis caused by kinking in Figure 28-24 has been corrected surgically by ligating the renal artery, excising the kink, and reanastomosis (arrow) to the more proximal common iliac artery.

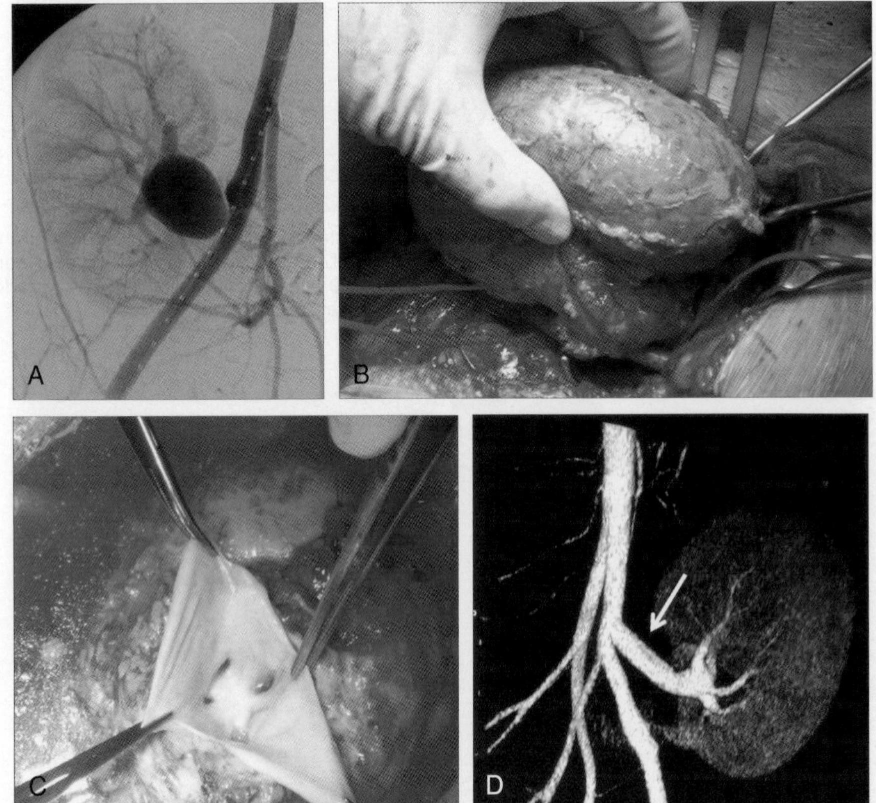

FIGURE 28-35 ■ (A) Digital subtraction angiogram shows a 4-cm aneurysm of the transplant renal artery of a right-sided donor kidney 6 years after transplantation into a 14-year-old boy. Note the kinking of the artery proximal to the aneurysm. The donor kidney came from an 8-year-old child who sustained brain death after bleeding from a cerebral artery aneurysm. (B) Complete mobilization of the kidney transplant, before removal for ex situ reconstruction of the renal artery using cadaver donor vessels. (C) View of the inside of the thin-walled aneurysm showing four branches with takeoff from the aneurysm of the transplanted renal artery. (D) Computed tomography angiogram with oblique view of arterial reconstruction 2 weeks after replacement of the transplant renal artery and vein with deceased donor iliac vessels and autotransplantation.

LYMPHOCELE

A lymphocele is a collection of lymph that accumulates in a non-epithelialized cavity in the postoperative field. After kidney transplantation, a lymphocele occurs after division of recipient lymphatics accompanying the iliac vessels. The incidence and frequency of detection have increased with the routine surveillance of the kidney transplant by CDUS and the introduction of mTOR inhibitors as part of maintenance immunosuppression regimens.[41] Lymphoceles are usually innocuous and asymptomatic but can equally cause dramatic presentations as a result of external pressure on the transplant and its adjacent structures, or when complicated by infection involving the transplant wound. The best approach to treatment of a symptomatic lymphocele is not well defined.

Incidence

Considering the frequency with which iliac vessels are exposed during routine vascular operations and the rarity of lymphatic complications, it came as a surprise to surgeons when the severity of lymphatic leakage after renal transplantation was first appreciated.[32] Early reports after kidney transplantation, based on clinical presentation, estimated the incidence to be around 2%. The advent of ultrasound for routine graft surveillance caused the figure to be revised to about 50%, although accepting that most lymphatic collections remain subclinical and resolve spontaneously.[44]

Etiology

An obvious suspected source of lymphatic leakage after kidney transplantation would be the graft itself, and occasionally this may be the case. A normal kidney has well-developed lymphatic drainage that is generally left unligated when transplanted. However, studies of injected radiopaque dyes and radiolabeled substances showed that most lymphoceles originate from iliac vessel lymphatics of the recipient (Figure 28-36). It is estimated that 300 mL of lymph per day passes through the external iliac lymph channels. Why the transplant kidney lymphatics contribute so little, if any, to the presence of a lymphocele remains unexplained.

Meticulous ligation of even the smallest lymphatic trunk with non-absorbable or slowly absorbed ligature material during mobilization of the iliac vessels is crucial in the prevention of lymphoceles (Figure 28-37). The author's observation is that more surgical care than usual is required when encountering large, fleshy external iliac lymph nodes. Use of high suction wound drains also might encourage open lymphatics to remain open. Based on their own experience, Sansalone et al. proposed that lymphoceles could be preventable if the vascular anastomoses were to the common iliac vessels, where fewer lymphatics and lymph nodes are encountered during dissection.[50]

The only differences between a routine retroperitoneal vascular procedure on the iliac vessels and kidney transplantation are the physical presence of the kidney, an alloimmune response, and immunosuppression. Potentially, the kidney can create areas of dead space, particularly near the upper or lower pole, and into which open lymph channels can, and do, drain. Immunosuppression may also have a role in preventing the normal healing processes from sealing the lymphatic vessels and is the more

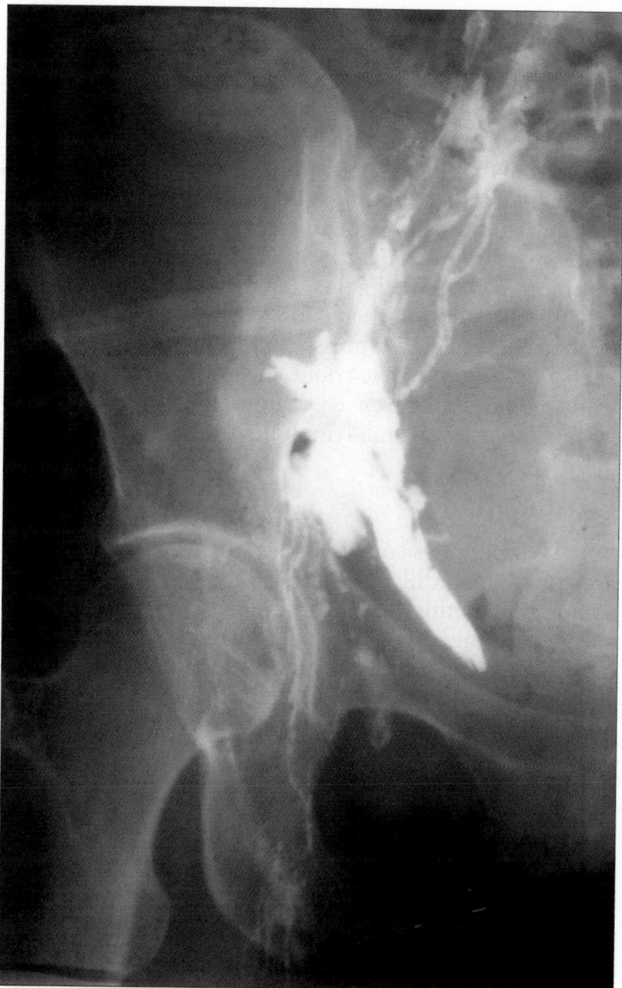

FIGURE 28-36 ■ Lymphangiogram shows leakage of lymph from external iliac lymph channels causing a lymphocutaneous fistula through the transplant wound.

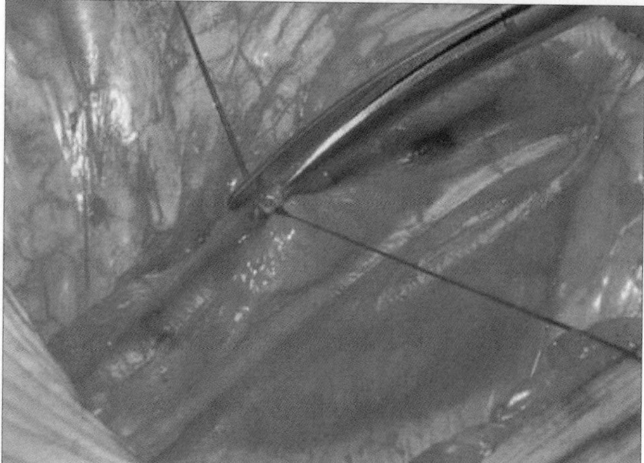

FIGURE 28-37 ■ Division of external iliac lymphatics after ligation with absorbable suture material.

likely explanation for the difference in the transplant setting. Macrophage function is adversely affected by steroids, and there is some evidence that the incidence of lymphoceles has decreased since the introduction of low-dose steroid regimens. The more recent strong association of mTOR inhibitors with problematic lymphoceles is attributed to their powerful antifibroblastic activity, particularly in obese patients being treated for rejection (body mass index >30 kg/m^2).[41,55] Lymphoceles are more common in obese recipients, possibly because the lymph channels are more difficult to identify during dissection of the iliac vessels. Aggressive use of diuretics also has been implicated, but it could equally be they are more likely to be used in an edematous transplant recipient with greater lower-limb lymph flow.

Presentation

Small lymphoceles containing less than 100 mL of lymph are usually clinically silent and found on routine ultrasonography within days of transplantation and often resolve spontaneously with time. Larger collections may become apparent clinically and usually do so at 1 week to 6 months after transplantation, with a peak incidence after hospital discharge towards the end of the first month.[44] Most are situated adjacent to the lower pole of the kidney and posterolateral to the transplant ureter, as illustrated in Figure 28-38. Although intralymphocele fluid pressure measurements have not been reported, they must be considerable. The most common presentation is sleep disturbance owing to urinary frequency as a result of compression of the bladder. They can be associated with a sense of fullness in the pelvis and ipsilateral painless leg edema is often present. The timing of clinical presentation of a lymphocele soon after removal of a transplant ureteric stent 1–2 months after transplantation can be anticipated with clinical concern of deteriorating renal function due to compression of the ureter.

A lymphocutaneous fistula can develop between a lymphocele through an infected transplant wound. A less common presentation is as a DVT resulting from compression of the external iliac vein (see Figure 28-17). Bladder outlet obstruction has also been described.[19]

Diagnosis

CDUS examination is the key to diagnosis. It can distinguish a lymphocele from hematoma collection on the basis of characteristic homogeneity and distinctive shape and position.[1] Most lymphoceles are adjacent to, but clearly separate from, the bladder. They can be multilocular and multiple in number (Figure 28-39) and, if in doubt, findings can be confirmed by the passage of a urinary catheter and repeat ultrasound. The examination also may show hydronephrosis with obstruction of the ureter with dilated calyces. Diagnosis can be further confirmed by ultrasound- or CT-guided drainage, allowing biochemical and cytological analysis of the fluid. If emptied, resolution of the hydronephrosis is seen. The use of vascular contrast medium helps with localization of the ureter in the excretory phase.

Treatment

Unnecessary intervention of small and symptom-free collections may lead to infective complications. For symptomatic lymphoceles, a systematic review of retrospective studies has suggested an algorithm that begins with

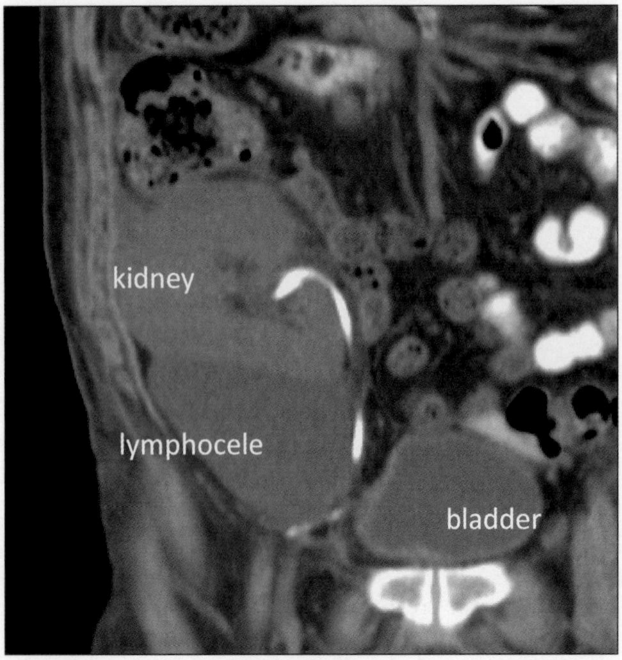

FIGURE 28-38 ■ Computed tomography scan (coronal view) demonstrating a lymphocele situated inferolateral to the kidney transplant and stented transplanted ureter.

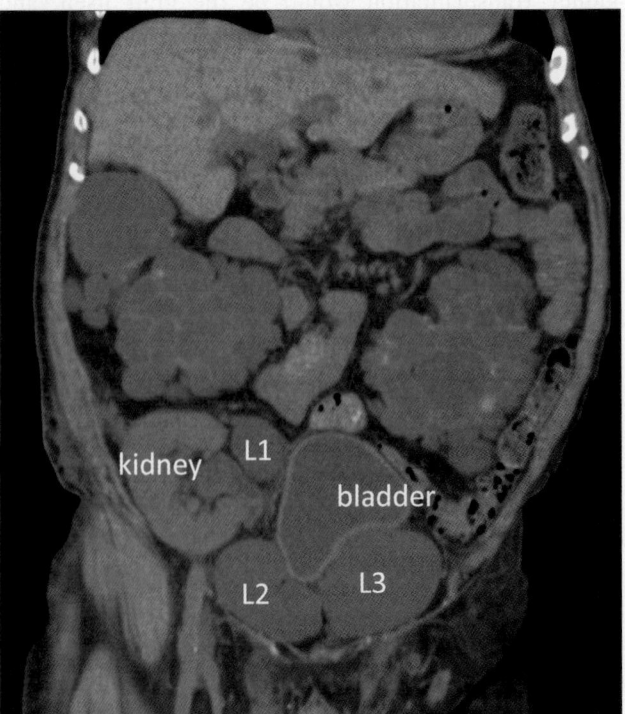

FIGURE 28-39 ■ Computed tomography scan (coronal view) demonstrating three lymphoceles (L) compressing bladder and kidney transplant in a patient with polycystic kidneys.

ultrasound- or CT-guided drainage both to confirm the diagnosis and to provide initial treatment.[30] The possible urgency of the situation is resolved by relief of urinary obstruction and restoration of kidney transplant function. About half the time, simple aspiration will be curative. It may be repeated on several occasions, although the likelihood of spontaneous resolution becomes small after three aspirations followed by recurrence.[44] Every aspiration brings a small risk of infection. Symptoms and signs can recur within days.

Prolonged external drainage through a percutaneously inserted catheter has been advocated by some authors and is possible in an outpatient setting (Figure 28-40). Injection of sclerosants has been described. Injection of povidone-iodine in association with external drainage has been claimed to be effective, with a low failure rate.[48] The drawback of prolonged drainage is that it is up to 30 days before drainage ceases, during which time the risk of infection remains. Of further concern is the observation of acute renal failure as a result of the direct nephrotoxic effect of povidone-iodine.[33] This treatment option is also poorly tolerated by the transplant recipient.

If simple percutaneous aspiration fails, a recent systematic review recommends a simple surgical procedure, namely fenestration of the lymphocele, the principle of which is to drain the potential 300 mL/day of lymph production into the peritoneal cavity, where it is absorbed by the peritoneum. This operation of choice has been called incorrectly "marsupialization" – it is correctly described as "fenestration." It can be done either laparoscopically or by open surgery through a lower midline abdominal incision and a transperitoneal approach to the lymphocele. Depending on its relationship to the kidney transplant, the previous wound can be reopened to achieve access. The same systematic review identified laparoscopic surgery as having a lower recurrence rate of 8% and a need for conversion to open surgery of 12%.[30] The least invasive surgical technique is a laparoscopic approach.[30,52] A planning CT scan is obtained to provide information about the position and presence of loculi. To facilitate

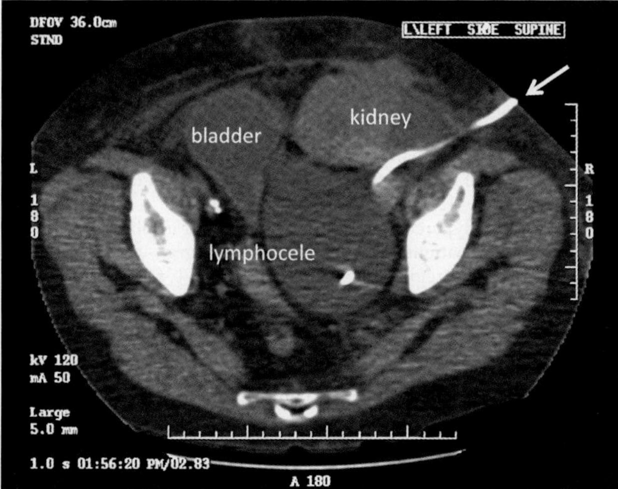

FIGURE 28-40 ■ Computed tomography scan with axial view of lymphocele with percutaneous drain (arrow) below the lower pole of the kidney transplant. Note displacement to the right and compression of the bladder.

localization, surgery is scheduled when the lymphocele cavity is full, and not the day after drainage. The surgeon ensures that the recipient has an indwelling catheter and the bladder is empty. The lymphocele is usually seen bulging into the peritoneal cavity. Localization with intraoperative ultrasound can be of assistance, particularly in obese patients and deeply situated lymphoceles. It is sometimes easy to confuse the swelling made by the extraperitoneal kidney with that made by the lymphocele. The role of intraoperative ultrasound in avoiding confusion is encouraged.[30] An opening between the lymphocele and the peritoneal cavity is made, taking care to avoid damage to any structures that may be running between the wall of the collection and the peritoneum, particularly the ureter. The most difficult lymphocele position to treat is one situated deep in the pelvis and lateral to transplant artery and vein. These are more safely treated by an open operative approach.

To avoid recurrence, various authors have recommended maneuvers such as excision of a 5-cm disc of the wall of the lymphocele, oversewing the edges, and mobilizing the omentum, which is then stitched down into the cavity.[7] Routine fenestration at the end of the transplant operation could potentially be performed but seems an unnecessary procedure with the added risk of small-bowel herniation.[60]

Lymphocutaneous Fistula

The most challenging lymphatic complication to manage is a fistula draining about 300 mL/day from a divided external iliac chain lymphatic and a transplant wound infected with a multiresistant organism. They present invariably in the first weeks after transplantation, typically in obese patients with diabetes and a surgical wound infection. Wound healing is slow and, as a result, skin sutures or staples tend to be left in place for longer than the norm and provide a portal of entry for bacteria. Prolonged use of appropriate antibiotics and free drainage are usually attempted optimistically, along with all possible measures that might improve wound healing, including reduction in steroid immunosuppression.

In these situations, the transplant wound can be reopened, and a large peritoneal fenestration created. Sometimes it is possible to see the offending leaking lymphatic channel at the base of the lymphocele cavity, usually anterior to the external iliac artery. Suture ligation is invariably successful. The risk of this procedure is introduction of antibiotic-resistant infection to the peritoneal cavity. The muscle wall is closed with large absorbable interrupted sutures. If need be, it may be possible to use a vacuum dressing to facilitate closure of subcutaneous tissues. In the meantime, the transplant recipient has been hospitalized for several months and is likely to require rehabilitation because of loss of muscle bulk. An unintended positive outcome from this scenario may be weight loss because of enforced hospitalization.

There are also lessons for the transplant surgeon from this almost inevitable scenario, illustrated in Figure 28-41. Obesity at time of transplantation surgery has become more commonplace and dictates the need for preventive strategies to reduce the risk of lymphatic and coexisting wound

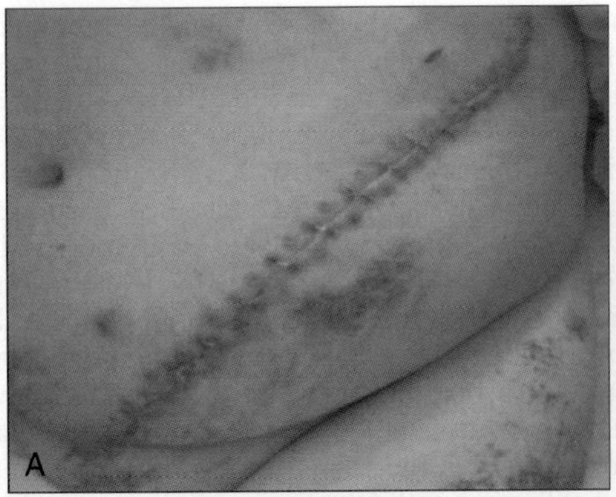

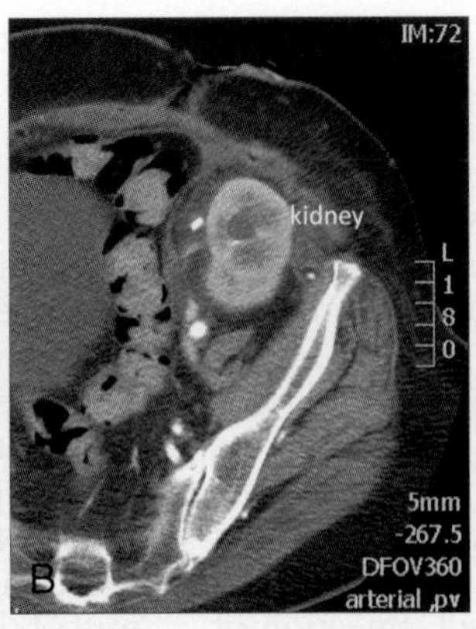

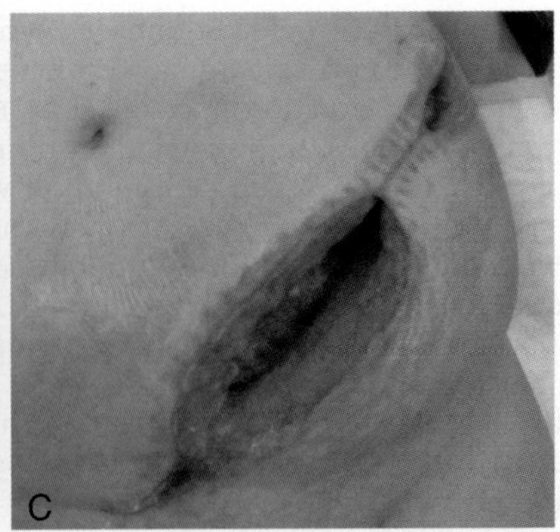

FIGURE 28-41 ■ Left iliac fossa kidney transplant in an obese diabetic recipient. (A) Surgical wound closed with skin staples, 2 weeks after surgery. (B) Arterial phase of computed tomography angiogram with axial view demonstrating a kidney transplant in the left iliac fossa surrounded by lymphatic fluid in continuity with an infected open wound. (C) Transplant wound 4 months after transplantation.

complications. Immunosuppression can be modified by minimizing steroid and lymphocyte-depleting antibodies and avoiding the use of mTor inhibitors for at least 1 month after the operation. The incision should be in a line of skin creases and, if possible, the rectus abdominis muscle preserved. Lymphatic division should be kept to a minimum. Ligation where necessary should be meticulous and nonabsorbable ligatures used and consideration might be given to creating a small peritoneal window before wound closure. Suction drainage can potentially be avoided, although can still be of value overnight if placed in the subcutaneous layer only. Finally, use of staples for wound closure should be avoided, with preference given to apposition of Scarpa's fascia to eliminate wound dead space and use of an absorbable monofilament suture for subcuticular skin closure.

CONCLUSIONS

Vascular and lymphatic complications are relatively common, but their incidence can be reduced by meticulous attention to detail during removal of the kidney(s), back table inspection and preparation, preparation of the implantation site in the recipient, and the technique of implantation.

REFERENCES

1. Akbar SA, Jafri SZ, Amendola MA, et al. Complications of renal transplantation. Radiographics 2005;25(5):1335–56.
2. Allen RD, Michie CA, Murie JA, et al. Deep venous thrombosis after renal transplantation. Surg Gynecol Obstet 1987;164:137–42.
3. Arrazola L, Sutherland DE, Sozen H, et al. May-Thurner syndrome in renal transplantation. Transplantation 2001;71:698–702.
4. Audard V, Matignon M, Hemery F, et al. Risk factors and long-term outcome of transplant renal artery stenosis in adult recipients after treatment by percutaneous transluminal angioplasty. Am J Transplant 2006;6:95–9.
5. Basso N, Terragno NA. History about the discovery of the renin-angiotensin system. Hypertension 2001;38:1246–9.
6. Bruno S, Remuzzi G, Ruggenenti P, et al. Transplant renal artery stenosis. J Am Soc Nephrol 2004;15:134–41.
7. Bry J, Hull D, Bartus SA, et al. Treatment of recurrent lymphoceles following renal transplantation. Remarsupialization with omentorplasty. Transplantation 1990;49:477–80.
8. Burke 3rd GW, Ciancio G, Figueiro J, et al. Hypercoagulable state associated with kidney-pancreas transplantation. Thromboelastogram-directed anti-coagulation and implications for future therapy. Clin Transplant 2004;18:423–8.
9. Buturovic-Ponikvar J. Renal transplant artery stenosis. Nephrol Dial Transplant 2003;18(Suppl. 5):v74–7.
10. Carter JT, Freise CE, McTaggart RA, et al. Laparoscopic procurement of kidneys with multiple renal arteries is associated with increased ureteral complications in the recipient. Am J Transplant 2005;5:1312–8.
11. Casserly LF, Dember LM. Thrombosis in end-stage renal disease [see comment]. Semin Dial 2003;16:245–56.
12. Friedman GS, Meier-Kriesche HU, Kaplan B, et al. Hypercoagulable states in renal transplant candidates: impact of anticoagulation upon incidence of renal allograft thrombosis. Transplantation 2001;72:1073–8.
13. Gao J, Ng A, Shih G, et al. Intrarenal color duplex ultrasonography: a window to vascular complications of renal transplants. J Ultrasound Med 2007;26:1403–18.
14. Garovic VD, Textor SC. Renovascular hypertension and ischemic nephropathy. Circulation 2005;112:1362–74.
15. Ghazanfar A, Tavakoli A, Augustine T, et al. Management of transplant renal artery stenosis and its impact on long-term allograft survival: a single-centre experience. Nephrol Dial Transplant 2011;26:336–43.
16. Goldblatt H, Lynch J, Hanzal RE, et al. Studies on experimental hypertension, I: The production of persistent elevation of systolic blood pressure by means of renal ischaemia. J Exp Med 1934;59:347–79.
17. Hsu TH, Su LM, Ratner LE, et al. Demographics of 353 laparoscopic renal donor and recipient pairs at the Johns Hopkins Medical Institutions. J Endourol 2003;17:393–6.
18. Hurst FP, Abbott KC, Neff RT, et al. Incidence, predictors and outcomes of transplant renal artery stenosis after kidney transplantation: analysis of USRDS. Am J Nephrol 2009;30:459–67.
19. Hwang EC, Kang TW, Koh YS, et al. Post-transplant lymphocele: an unusual cause of acute urinary retention mimicking urethral injury. Int J Urol 2006;13:468–70.
20. Imanishi M, Akabane S, Takamiya M, et al. Critical degree of renal arterial stenosis that causes hypertension in dogs. Angiology 1992;43:833–42.
21. Irish A. Hypercoagulability in renal transplant recipients. Identifying patients at risk of renal allograft thrombosis and evaluating strategies for prevention. Am J Cardiovasc Drugs 2004;4:139–49.
22. Johnson DW, Mudge DW, Kaisar MO, et al. Deceased donor renal transplantation – does side matter? Nephrol Dial Transplant 2006;21:2583–8.
23. Kanchanabat B, Siddins M, Coates T, et al. Segmental infarction with graft dysfunction: an emerging syndrome in renal transplantation? Nephrol Dial Transplant 2002;17:123–8.
24. Kobayashi K, Censullo ML, Rossman LL, et al. Interventional radiologic management of renal transplant dysfunction: indications, limitations, and technical considerations. Radiographics 2007;27:1109–30.
25. Kujovich JL. Thrombophilia and thrombotic problems in renal transplant patients. Transplantation 2004;77:959–64.

26. Kusyk T, Verran D, Stewart G, et al. Increased risk of hemorrhagic complications in renal allograft recipients receiving systemic heparin early posttransplantation. Transplant Proc 2005;37:1026–8.
27. Lacombe M. Arterial stenosis complicating renal allotransplantation in man: a study of 38 cases. Ann Surg 1975;181:283–8.
28. Leonardou P, Gioldasi S, Zavos G, et al. Mycotic pseudoaneurysms complicating renal transplantation: a case series and review of literature. J Med Case Rep 2012;6:59.
29. Lucewicz A, Isaacs A, Allen RDM, et al. Torsion of intraperitoneal kidney transplant. ANZ J Surg 2012;82:299–302.
30. Lucewicz A, Wong G, Lam VWT, et al. Management of primary symptomatic lymphocele after kidney transplantation: a systematic review. Transplantation 2011;92:663–73.
31. Mackinnon B, Fraser E, Simpson K, et al. Is it necessary to stop antiplatelet agents before a native renal biopsy? Nephrol Dial Transplant 2008;23:3566–70.
32. Madura JA, Dunbar JD, Cerilli GJ, et al. Perirenal lymphocele as a complication of renal homotransplantation. Surgery 1970;68:310–3.
33. Manfro RC, Comerlato L, Berdichevski RH, et al. Nephrotoxic acute renal failure in a renal transplant patient with recurrent lymphocele treated with povidone-iodine irrigation. Am J Kidney Dis 2002;40:655–7.
34. Marini M, Fernandez-Rivera C, Cao I, et al. Treatment of transplant renal artery stenosis by percutaneous transluminal angioplasty and/or stenting: study in 63 patients in a single institution. Transplant Proc 2011;43:2205–7.
35. Mathis AS, Shah NK. Exaggerated response to heparin in a post-operative renal transplant recipient with lupus anticoagulant undergoing plasmapheresis. Transplantation 2004;77:957–8.
36. Melamed ML, Kim HS, Jaar BG, et al. Combined percutaneous mechanical and chemical thrombectomy for renal vein thrombosis in kidney transplant recipients. Am J Transplant 2005;5:621–6.
37. Morris PJ, Yadav RV, Kincaid-Smith P, et al. Renal artery stenosis in renal transplantation. Med J Aust 1971;1:1255–7.
38. Pannu N, Manns B, Lee H, et al. Systematic review of the impact of N-acetylcysteine on contrast nephropathy [see comment]. Kidney Int 2004;65:1366–74.
39. Parrott NR, Forsythe JL, Matthews JN, et al. Late perfusion. A simple remedy for renal allograft primary nonfunction. Transplantation 1990;49:913–5.
40. Paulson WD, Moist L, Lok CE, et al. Vascular access surveillance: an ongoing controversy. Kidney Int 2012;81:132–42.
41. Pengel LH, Liu LQ, Morris PJ, et al. Do wound complications or lymphoceles occur more often in solid organ transplant recipients on mTOR inhibitors? A systematic review of randomized controlled trials. Transpl Int 2011;24:1216–30.
42. Pengelly A, Snow J, Mills SY, et al. Short-term study on the effects of rosemary on cognitive function in an elderly population. J Med Food 2012;15:10–7.
43. Penny MJ, Nankivell BJ, Disney AP, et al. Renal graft thrombosis: a survey of 134 consecutive cases. Transplantation 1994;58:565–9.
44. Pollak R, Veremis SA, Maddux MS, et al. The natural history of and therapy for perirenal fluid collections following renal transplantation. J Urol 1988;140:716–20.
45. Ram Reddy C, Ram R, Swarnalatha G, et al. "True" mycotic aneurysm of the anastomotic site of the renal allograft artery. Exp Clin Transplant 2012;10:398–402.
46. Ramirez PJ, Gohh RY, Kestin A, et al. Renal allograft loss due to proximal extension of ileofemoral deep venous thrombosis. Clin Transplant 2002;16:310–3.
47. Richardson AJ, Higgins RM, Jaskowski AJ, et al. Spontaneous rupture of renal allografts: the importance of renal vein thrombosis in the cyclosporin era. Br J Surg 1990;77:558–60.
48. Rivera M, Marcen R, Burgos J. Treatment of posttransplant lymphocele with povidone-iodine sclerosis: long-term follow-up. Nephron 1996;74:324–7.
49. Robertson AJ, Nargund V, Gray DW, et al. Low dose aspirin as prophylaxis against renal-vein thrombosis in renal-transplant recipients. Nephrol Dial Transplant 2000;15:1865–8.
50. Sansalone CV, Aseni P, Minetti E, et al. Is lymphocele in renal transplantation an avoidable complication? Am J Surg 2000;179:182–5.
51. Schoenberg SO, Bock M, Kallinwoski F, et al. Correlation of hemodynamic impact and morphologic degree of renal artery stenosis in a canine model. J Am Soc Nephrol 2000;11:2190–8.
52. Smyth GP, Beitz G, Eng MP, et al. Long-term outcome of cadaveric renal transplant after treatment of symptomatic lymphocele. J Urol 2006;176:1069–72.
53. Thalhammer C, Aschwanden M, Mayr M, et al. Colour-coded duplex sonography after renal transplantation. Ultraschall Med 2007;28:6–21, quiz 25.
54. Vacher-Coponat H, McDonald S, Clayton P, et al. Inferior early posttransplant outcomes for recipients of right versus left deceased donor kidneys: an ANZDATA registry analysis. Am J Transplant 2013;13:399–405.
55. Vitko S, Margreiter R, Weimar W, et al. Three-year efficacy and safety results from a study of everolimus versus mycophenolate mofetil in de novo renal transplant patients. Am J Transplant 2005;5:2521–30.
56. Voiculescu A, Schmitz M, Hollenbeck M, et al. Management of arterial stenosis affecting kidney graft perfusion: a single-centre study in 53 patients. Am J Transplant 2005;5:1731–8.
57. Wheatley K, Ives N, Gray R, et al. Revascularization versus medical therapy for renal-artery stenosis. N Engl J Med 2009;361:1953–62.
58. Wong W, Fynn SP, Higgins RM, et al. Transplant renal artery stenosis in 77 patients – does it have an immunological cause? Transplantation 1996;61:215–9.
59. Wuthrich RP, Cicvara-Muzar S, Booy C, et al. Heterozygosity for the factor V Leiden (G1691A) mutation predisposes renal transplant recipients to thrombotic complications and graft loss. Transplantation 2001;72:549–50.
60. Zaontz MR, Firlit CF. Pelvic lymphocele after pediatric renal transplantation: a successful technique for prevention. J Urol 1988;139:557–9.

CHAPTER 29

UROLOGICAL COMPLICATIONS AFTER KIDNEY TRANSPLANTATION

Daniel Shoskes • Juan Antonio Jiménez

CHAPTER OUTLINE

Urological complications are inevitable in renal transplantation. Their incidence and impact on graft survival can however be minimized. This chapter reviews the types of urological complications that may occur, maneuvers to prevent them, when to suspect and how to diagnose them, and treatments to maximize long-term outcome. Retrospective series quote an incidence of urological complications of 1–15%.[14,19,24,26] The incidence depends on many factors, in particular duration of follow-up and how broadly urological complications are defined. Some studies include hematuria, urinary tract infection, and urinary retention; others are confined to ureteric strictures or leaks. This chapter discusses the following urological complications: ureteral leak, ureteral obstruction, urinary calculi, urinary retention, erectile dysfunction, and urologic cancers.

URETERAL COMPLICATIONS

Ureteral leaks and obstructions are the result of technical errors, ischemia, external compression, or intraluminal blockage (e.g., ureteral stone). Unlike the native ureter, which derives its blood supply from renal and pelvic sources, the transplant ureter is supplied only by branches of the anastomosed renal artery, and therefore, the distal segment of the ureter is the most ischemic. To overcome this, the renal allograft is placed into the pelvis, which minimizes the length of the transplant ureter. During organ procurement, care should be taken to preserve the ureteral blood supply by removing the ureter along with a significant margin of periureteral tissue. Likewise, during the back table preparation of the kidney, the perirenal fat bordered by the ureter and lower pole of the kidney (the "golden triangle") should be preserved, as demonstrated in Figure 29-1. When encountered, lower-pole renal artery branches should be preserved or repaired, as they are commonly the end artery supplying the ureter. Ureteral complications may be more common in kidneys with multiple ureters,[10] and in such cases, small upper-pole arteries should be preserved as well.

Ureteral Leak

Ureteral leaks are reported in 1–3% of renal transplants.[14,26] The two most common causes are surgical error and ureteral ischemia with resultant necrosis. Technical errors include misplacement of ureteral sutures, unrecognized ureteral transection or renal pelvis laceration, and insufficient ureteral length, placing tension on the anastomosis. Other rare causes of urine leaks include outflow obstruction (as caused by a blocked Foley catheter or urinary retention) with disruption of the ureterovesical anastomosis, acute ureteral obstruction with perforation through a renal calyx, and extrusion of a ureteral stent. Leaks resulting from technical errors often occur within the first 24 hours, whereas leaks resulting from ischemia and necrosis usually occur within the first 14 days. However, kidneys with delayed graft function may not have an evident leak until suitable diuresis ensues.

Because the risk factors for ureteral leak are known, the incidence can be reduced by preventive measures. Preservation of periureteral tissue is essential, especially in living donors procured laparoscopically. Whereas the early experience with laparoscopic donor nephrectomy was associated with high rates of urinary leaks, improvements in surgical techniques have led to a decline in the rate to be almost as good as open donors.[18] A ureter that appears compromised at the time of surgery or fails to become pink and bleed after reperfusion should be cut as proximally as necessary to reach well-perfused tissue. This may necessitate an alternative technique to achieve urinary continuity, either by anastomosis to the ipsilateral native ureter or by an extension technique of the bladder, such as a psoas hitch or Boari flap (see later).

The clinical presentation of ureteral leaks can be obvious or subtle. The clearest clinical scenario is a patient

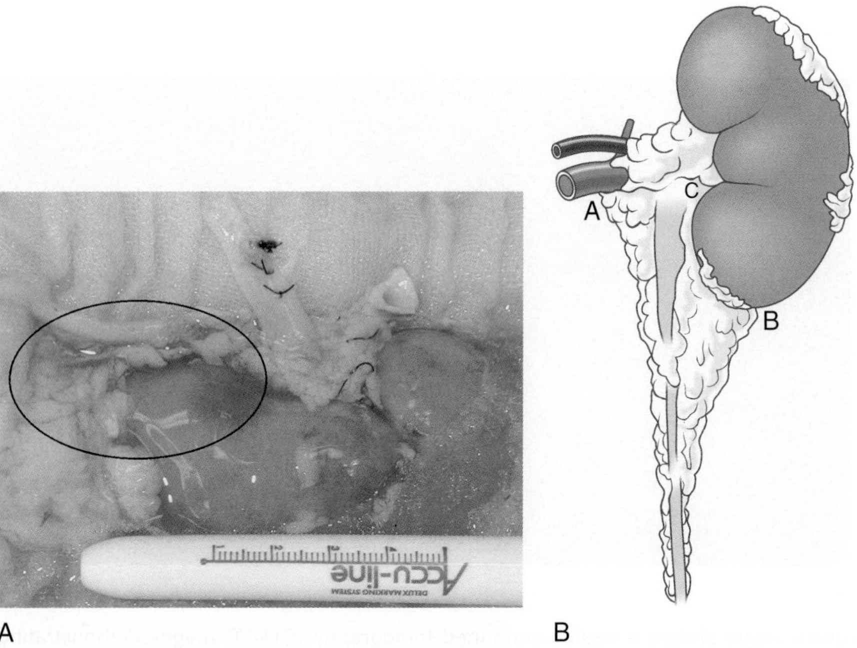

FIGURE 29-1 ■ (A) Cadaveric donor kidney after back table bench preparation. Note the preservation of the tissue between the lower pole of the kidney and the ureter (circled), which typically contains the blood supply to the ureter and must be preserved. (B) The golden triangle (as outlined by A, B, and C). Dissection in this area should be avoided during removal and preparation of the kidney for transplantation.

with excellent recovery of renal function whose urine output suddenly decreases or stops completely, associated with drainage of fluid through the wound or increased drain output. More often, however, confounding factors, including high urine output produced by the native kidneys, delayed graft function that may limit urine output, and a pre-existing lymphocele or seroma make the presentation more subtle. Urine leak should be part of the differential diagnosis in the early posttransplant period whenever there is poor urine output, a new fluid collection, new wound drainage, or delayed graft function. Any new fluid drainage or aspirated fluid collection should be sent for creatinine measurement, and the value should be compared with serum. Several imaging studies may be diagnostic. A ^{99m}Tc-MAG-3 renogram may show tracer outside the anatomical confines of the urinary tract but can be indeterminate, a cystogram may show the leak, particularly if it is located at the ureterovesical junction, and an ultrasound or computed tomography (CT) scan may show a fluid collection, but not its source. For more precise diagnosis and localization of a urinary leak, single photon emission CT (SPECT)/CT fusion imaging can be performed (Figure 29-2).

Management of a ureteral leak can be endoscopic or operative. In a patient with an indwelling ureteral stent and no Foley catheter, replacing the catheter often resolves the leak, unless the entire distal ureter is necrotic. If this is effective, the catheter should remain in place for at least 2 weeks, followed by a confirmatory cystogram prior to catheter removal. If no ureteral stent was placed, treatment modalities include stenting or immediate surgical exploration. Placement of a retrograde stent in a transplant ureter can be technically challenging because of the ectopic position of the ureteric orifice and lack of periureteral supports. Furthermore, percutaneous nephrostomy with antegrade stent placement can be challenging because of the lack of hydronephrosis with urine leaks. In the case of ureteral necrosis, it is preferable to explore and repair these leaks early.

Multiple surgical approaches exist to repair a ureteral leak depending on the location and extent of ureteral necrosis. Regardless of the technique, we prefer to use a three-way Foley catheter connected to irrigation that can intermittently fill and empty the bladder to identify the leak better. If the ureter is well perfused and a leak at the ureterovesical junction is due to a technical problem with the anastomosis, the leak can be repaired by placing additional interrupted sutures. If the distal portion of the ureter is necrotic, it should be resected back to healthy tissue. If the ureteral loss is minor, a simple reimplant of the transplant ureter is sufficient. Because a urine leak often results in local inflammation and tissue edema, all ureteral repairs or reimplantations should be performed over a stent.

If a tension-free anastomosis cannot be achieved due to limited ureteral length, several options are available (Table 29-1). With a psoas hitch, the bladder is brought closer to the ureter by mobilizing its attachments, in particular, by severing the contralateral obliterated umbilical artery. The bladder is incised transversely and reconfigured by closing the bladder incision in line with the ureter, displacing the bladder toward the transplant ureter (Figure 29-3).[15] The bladder, now elongated in the direction of the ureter, is fixed to the ipsilateral psoas muscle to allow a tension-free ureteral reimplant. This technique, however, may not provide sufficient length in a small bladder, as is found in long-standing oliguric patients. Alternatively, or in addition to the psoas hitch, a Boari flap of bladder can be created to bridge the gap for an anastomosis either to the transplant ureter or to the transplant renal pelvis (Figure 29-4).[6]

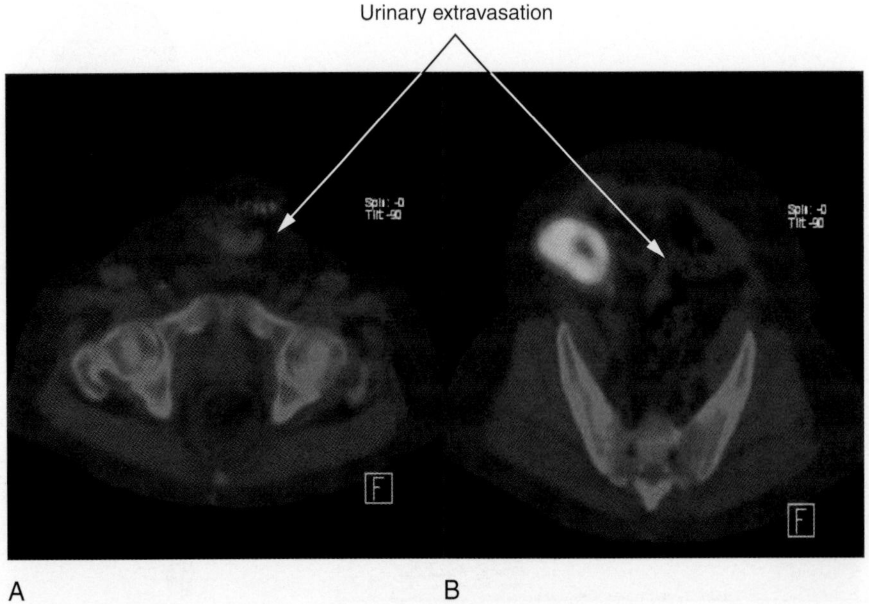

FIGURE 29-2 ■ (A, B) Fusion single photon emission computed tomography (CT)/CT images demonstrating a urine leak (arrows) outside confines of the urinary bladder.

TABLE 29-1 Surgical Techniques to Bridge the Gap between Transplant Ureter and Bladder

Technique	Advantages	Disadvantages
Direct reanastomosis	Simple, quick	Limited by length of well-perfused ureter
Psoas hitch	Bladder reconfigured, no loss of bladder volume	Must mobilize bladder, limited distance for small bladder
Boari flap	Can bridge large distance, well vascularized	Loss of bladder volume
Ureteroureterostomy	Simple, bladder not entered, well vascularized	Ureter may be absent or atretic
Pyelovesicostomy	No need for donor or recipient ureter	May be difficult to reach, especially if renal pelvis is anterior (e.g., left kidney in right iliac fossa), free reflux
Ileal ureter	Can bridge large gap, large lumen in event of stone formation	Need for bowel anastomosis, free reflux

Because a Boari flap reduces the total bladder volume, its use may be inappropriate in the atrophied bladder of a previously anuric patient. The preferred technique here is to anastomose the ipsilateral ureter, if present, to either the transplant ureter or the allograft renal pelvis (Figure 29-5). Typically, the proximal native ureter can be tied off without the need for ipsilateral native nephrectomy.[9] The advantages of this technique include excellent ureteral blood supply, a large segment of native ureter that can be repositioned without tension, and no compromise of bladder volume. If native urothelium is unavailable, an ileal ureter can bridge the bladder and transplant renal pelvis (see Chapters 11 and 12).[23]

Ureteral Stenosis

Stenosis of the transplant ureter occurs in approximately 3% of transplant recipients.[24] The obstruction can be extraluminal (compression from a lymphocele or spermatic cord), intrinsic (ureteral ischemia), or intraluminal (renal stone, fungal ball, sloughed renal papilla, or foreign body). Ureteral stenosis may occur months or years after an otherwise successful transplant. Risk factors for late ureteral stenosis include advanced donor age, delayed graft function, and kidneys with more than two arteries.[11] Recently, the emergence of human polyomavirus (BK virus) can produce ureteritis and ultimately ureteral stenosis.[4] Although ureteral stenting at the time of transplant reduces the incidence of early stenosis, it has no impact on the rate of late ureteral stenosis.[22]

The clinical presentation of ureteral stenosis can vary according to its location, degree, and speed of onset. Most commonly, ureteral stenosis is gradual and asymptomatic, with an unexplained increase in serum creatinine and the discovery of hydronephrosis on ultrasound. Pain over the allograft is rare, unless the obstruction is sudden and high-grade. Hydronephrosis is not always synonymous with obstruction, however. Dilation of the renal pelvis and calices can occur without obstruction in the setting of prior obstruction (e.g., long-standing ureteropelvic junction obstruction in the donor), reflux, or loss of renal cortex parenchyma, such as in chronic allograft nephropathy. Patients with new-onset hydronephrosis should also be screened for urinary retention by checking a post-void residual volume.

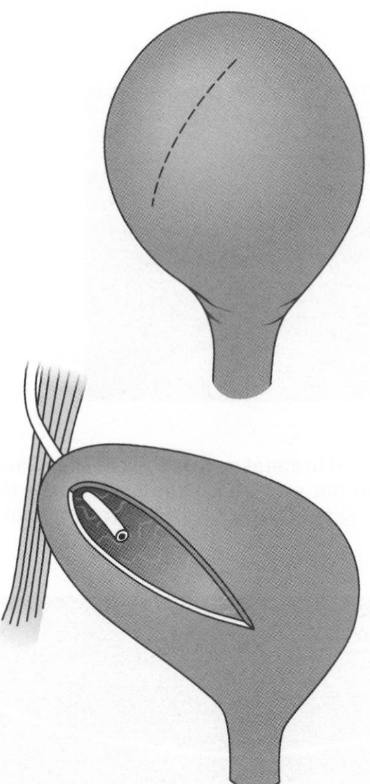

FIGURE 29-3 ■ A psoas hitch can provide 5cm of additional length. The contralateral peritoneal bladder attachments are divided to bring the bladder closer to the ureter. The bladder is incised transversely, and the ureter is reimplanted with a submucosal tunnel superolateral to the dome of the bladder. The bladder is then tacked down to the fascia of the ipsilateral psoas muscle. A double-J ureteral stent is placed, and the bladder is closed in two layers.

After discovering hydronephrosis, two further confirmatory tests include a diuretic ^{99m}Tc-MAG-3 renogram or a percutaneous antegrade nephrostogram (Figure 29-6). A diuretic renogram suggests obstruction if the clearance curve shows pelvicaliceal hold-up, especially after diuretic administration.[17] False-negative results can occur in patients with poor renal function, and false-positive results can occur with bladder outlet obstruction or vesicoureteral reflux. Antegrade pyelography is the preferred test when obstruction is strongly suspected. A hydronephrotic transplant kidney is easily accessible with a small spinal needle to inject contrast medium.[2] If obstruction is confirmed, the needle can be converted to a nephrostomy tube over a wire, and antegrade stenting can be performed immediately or after the renal function and ureteral edema improve.

Endoscopic management of transplant ureteral strictures is preferable to surgery, which can be difficult when done months or years after the original transplant surgery. The stricture can be accessed in an antegrade or retrograde fashion. If a stent does not pass easily over a wire, the stricture can be balloon-dilated or an endoureterotomy can be performed with a laser or an Accucise cutting balloon. The endoscopic approach is successful in about 50–65% of cases; however, recurrent strictures may result from inadequate primary therapy or failure due to extensive ischemia. Although patients with recurrent strictures can be mangaged with long-term indwelling ureteral stents, recurrent strictures are best treated with an open approach. When the site of obstruction is identified and the diseased segment of ureter is excised, the operative approach is similar to that for a ureteral leak (e.g., psoas hitch, Boari flap, ureteropyelostomy, pyelocystostomy, or ileal ureter). Successful treatment of transplant ureteral stenosis is critical, as long-term graft survival is improved.[11]

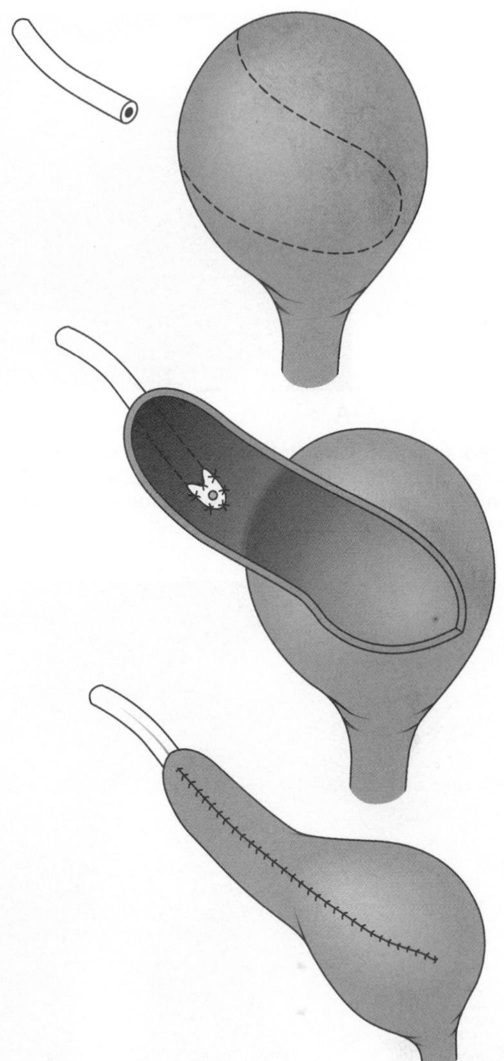

FIGURE 29-4 ■ A Boari flap can provide 10–15cm of additional length. The bladder is mobilized as in the psoas hitch. A full-thickness U-shaped bladder flap is created. The length of the flap varies depending on the length of the gap that needs to be bridged. To assure adequate blood supply, the base of the flap should be at least 2cm greater than the apex, and the width of the flap should be three to four times the diameter of the ureter. The ureter is then anastomosed with a submucosal tunnel or in an end-to-end fashion with the flap. A double-J ureteral stent is placed, and the bladder flap is closed in two layers. For a tension-free anastomosis, the tip of the flap can be secured to the ipsilateral psoas muscle.

USE OF PROPHYLACTIC URETERAL STENTS

The routine use of ureteral stents (Figure 29-7) at the time of kidney transplantation is controversial. Table 29-2 lists the pros and cons. As reported in some series, stents

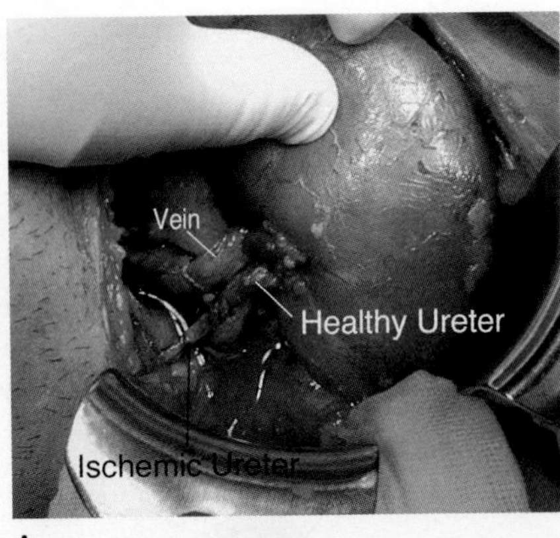

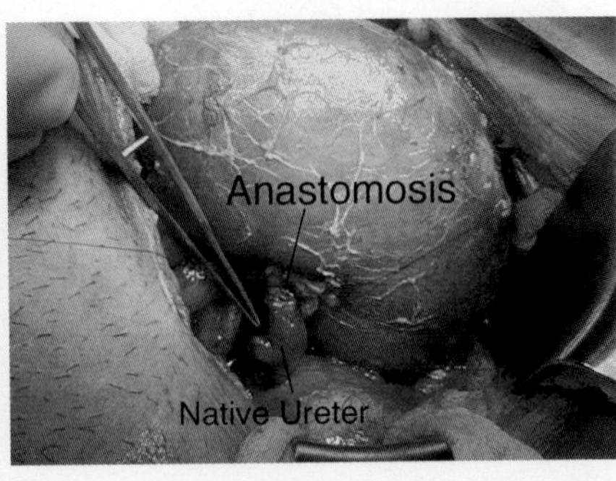

FIGURE 29-5 ■ Repair of transplant ureteral necrosis by ureteroureterostomy. (A) Distal ureteral necrosis. Note the distal ureter, proximal ureter, and accumulation of urine in the wound. (B) After repair. The native ureter was transected and rotated to the proximal transplant ureter. The anastomosis was made end-to-end over a double-J stent using 5-0 PDS suture. The proximal native ureter was tied off without native nephrectomy.

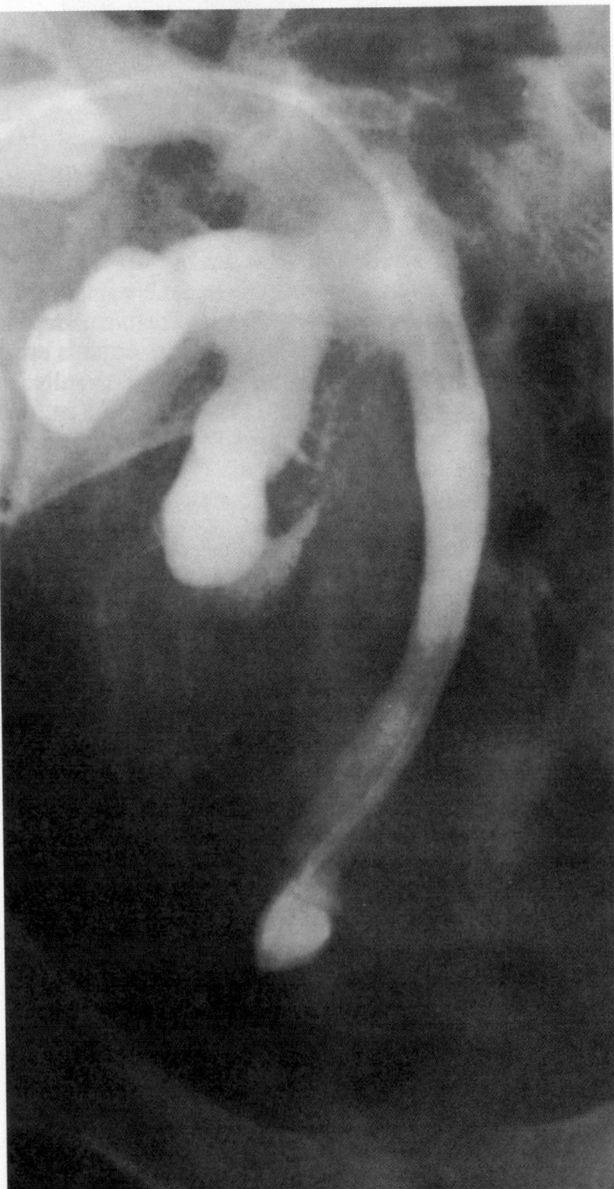

FIGURE 29-6 ■ Antegrade nephrostogram in a transplanted kidney showing an obstructed distal ureter.

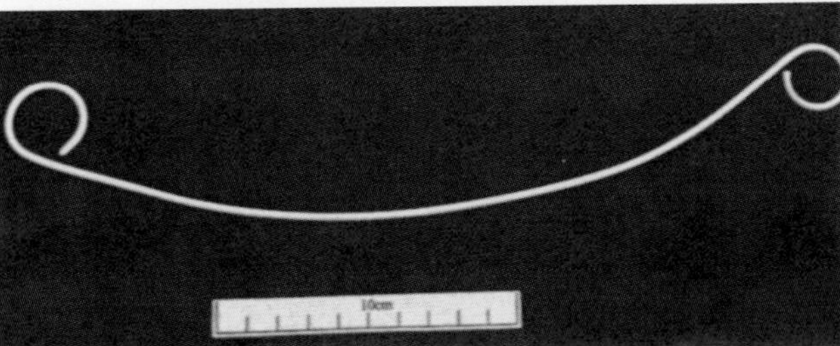

FIGURE 29-7 ■ Double-J ureteral stent.

TABLE 29-2 Advantages and Disadvantages of Routine Prophylactic Ureteral Stenting in Renal Transplants

Advantages	Disadvantages
Reduction in ureteric complications	95% of patients have unnecessary stent
Urine leak easier to manage	Increased risk of urinary tract infection
Cost-effective	Risk of stent migration or stone encrustation
	No evidence for patient or graft survival benefit
	Patient discomfort from bladder spasm

can reduce the incidence of ureteral leaks and early ureteral stenosis,[22] while making the early management of leaks easier. Other reports, including prospective randomized trials, demonstrated no utility for prophylactic stenting.[8] Mangus and Haag performed a meta-analysis of 49 published studies, including randomized controlled trials, and demonstrated a significant reduction in ureteric complications with stents (from 9% to 1.5%; $P < 0.0001$).[13] A review in the Cochrane Register of Controlled Trials demonstrated the relative risk of major urological complications with stents to be 0.24 (95% confidence interval 0.07–0.77; $P = 0.02$).[29] Although the optimal duration of prophylactic stenting has not been determined, for most centers it is typically for 2–6 weeks. Urinary tract infections in stented patients can be reduced

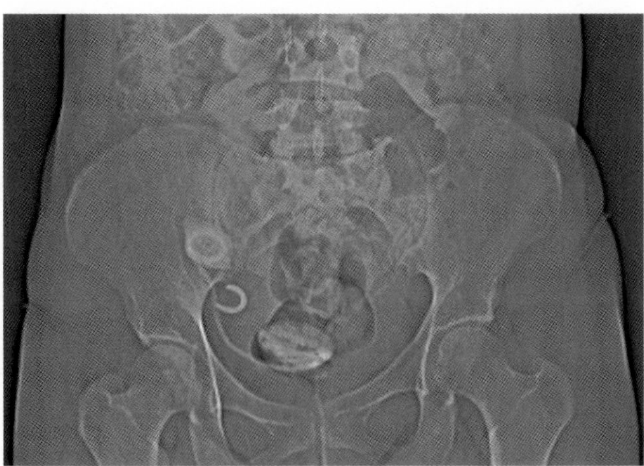

FIGURE 29-8 ■ Plain radiograph of an encrusted, retained stent. The patient had stent placement at the time of transplant, but moved to another country before the stent was removed. The patient presented to our institution 2 years later with stones in the kidney and bladder.

with the administration of routine antibiotic prophylaxis. If a ureteral stent is placed, the patient's chart should be flagged and the patient should be told to return for stent removal. Especially in busy programs, the danger exists that a stent may be forgotten and remain in place for several months or years until the patient presents with a retained, calcified stent (Figure 29-8).

URINARY CALCULI IN TRANSPLANT RECIPIENTS

The incidence of nephrolithiasis in renal transplant recipients ranges from 1% to 5%.[3,12] In the United States, only 1 in 1000 transplanted patients had a hospital admission for stones, with the strongest risk factors being female sex and prior history of stone disease.[1] As more centers transplant kidneys from living donors with known asymptomatic renal stones, this incidence may increase. Other causes of stones include the use of non-absorbable suture in the urinary tract, foreign bodies such as a retained stent, persistent urinary tract infection, ileal conduit diversion, and incomplete bladder emptying. Metabolic evaluation of transplant recipients who form stones most commonly reveals hypocitraturia, hyperparathyroidism, hypophosphatemia, and hypercalcemia. Hypocitraturia has been linked with the use of calcineurin inhibitors.[25]

Because the transplanted kidney is denervated, the clinical presentation of transplant nephrolithiasis is varied and includes pain over the graft site, gross hematuria, and reduced or absent urine output. Asymptomatic stones may be discovered during routine imaging or as part of a workup of elevated creatinine, and stone number and location are best delineated by non-contrast CT scan. Urine culture should be collected from all patients with kidney stones. If a patient presents with anuria, emergent intervention with percutaneous nephrostomy is indicated. Bladder calculi also should be evaluated by cystoscopy to prevent outflow obstruction.

The treatment of stones in a transplanted kidney is similar to that of native kidneys, with the exception that percutaneous approaches are easier due to the location of the kidney in the pelvis. Most often, small stones pass spontaneously without intervention. Larger obstructing stones can be treated with extracorporeal shockwave lithotripsy, antegrade or retrograde ureteroscopic stone extraction (with laser lithotripsy if necessary), or, rarely, open surgery.[3] When a stone is identified in a living donor, the kidney with the stone should be selected for transplantation, and the stone can be successfully removed by back table ureteroscopy or ultrasound-guided nephrolithotomy.

URINARY RETENTION

After renal transplantation, urinary retention may be due to bladder outlet obstruction or an acontractile detrusor muscle. In previously anuric patients, these problems may not be identified until after the Foley catheter is removed. Patients with a flaccid bladder usually have a prior history of voiding dysfunction or a neurogenic bladder. When bladder pathology is suspected, urodynamics with pressure flow studies and cystoscopy should be performed to characterize the bladder and bladder neck, and the patient should be instructed to perform intermittent self-catheterization, which is safe and effective in transplant recipients.

Bladder outlet obstruction after transplantation is almost exclusively seen in men and may be due to urethral stricture, benign prostatic hyperplasia, bladder calculus, or bladder neck contracture. Anuric men with benign prostatic hyperplasia should not be offered surgical treatment prior to transplantation because transurethral prostatic surgery in a "dry urethra" has a high incidence of stricture formation. After transplant, therapy for men with significant bladder outlet obstruction from benign prostatic hyperplasia should begin with an alpha-blocker alone or in combination with a 5α-reductase inhibitor. Men in retention despite medical therapy should start intermittent self-catheterization and delay definitive endoscopic prostatic surgery for at least 3 months posttransplant. Although transurethral resection of the prostate can be done in the immediate posttransplantation period, significant morbidity[20] and mortality[24] have been reported.

ERECTILE DYSFUNCTION

With an aging transplant population, erectile dysfunction is a prevalent and increasingly identified concern, occurring in up to 53% of male transplant recipients.[21] Factors contributing to erectile dysfunction are often the same factors responsible for renal failure, including diabetes, vasculopathy, and hypertension (owing to its medical treatment). Dialysis patients often have an elevated serum prolactin level which decreases testosterone levels, resulting in low libido and erectile dysfunction. This may account partly for the 20% of patients whose erectile dysfunction improves after transplant.[21]

Although the internal iliac artery is less commonly used for the renal artery anastomosis, it should be avoided in men receiving a second transplant, as the risk of developing vasculopathic impotence can be as high as 25% in this situation.[27]

Given the multifactorial nature of erectile dysfunction in this population, there is limited value in an extensive workup beyond measuring testosterone and prolactin levels. Transplant patients tolerate phosphodiesterase-5 inhibitor therapy well, with sildenafil demonstrating good efficacy and no impact on calcineurin levels.[30] For patients who fail oral therapy, intracorporeal injection of agents such as prostaglandin E_1 or papaverine is effective. Alternatively, inflatable penile prostheses are safe and effective in transplant patients, and the risk of prosthesis infection and erosion is no higher despite the immunocompromised state and poor tissue healing. Risk of device malfunction and damage to the prosthesis, however, is higher in transplant patients who receive a traditional three-piece model with a retroperitoneal fluid reservoir, owing to the need for multiple retroperitoneal surgeries. The Ambicor two-piece prosthesis should be considered in these patients because it lacks a fluid reservoir.[5] Patients being evaluated for transplant with a known penile prosthesis or artificial urinary sphincter should have preoperative imaging performed (Figure 29-9) to confirm the existence and laterality of a fluid reservoir, and the contralateral side should be chosen for allograft placement.

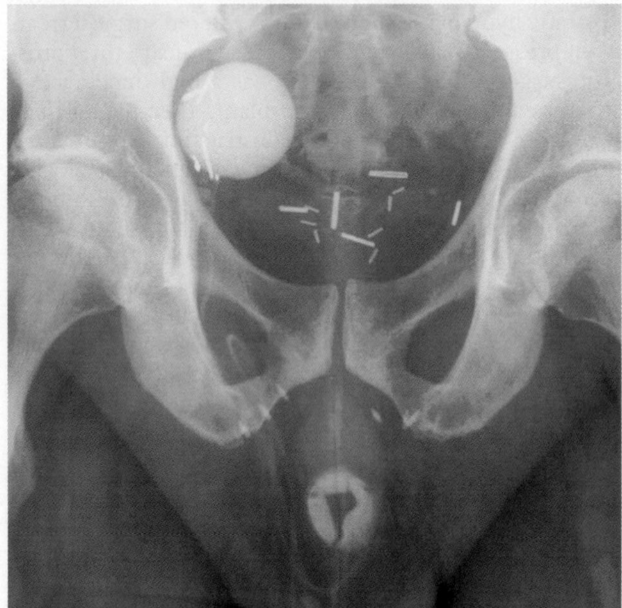

FIGURE 29-9 ■ Plain radiograph of a patient with an artificial urinary sphincter. Note the position of the fluid reservoir containing radiopaque contrast in the lower right pelvis, where it could be damaged during transplant recipient dissection. A traditional three-component inflatable penile prosthesis would have a similar reservoir but would be filled with saline and be radiolucent. Pretransplant imaging with a non-contrast computed tomography scan can confirm the location and direct the incision to the contralateral side.

UROLOGIC MALIGNANCIES

Organ transplantation is associated with an elevated risk of certain cancers, especially within the first 6 years of transplantation. Urologic malignancies in renal transplant recipients can occur as de novo tumors, recurrences, or unrecognized transmitted donor malignancies (see Chapter 35). Immunosuppression, infection with oncogenic viruses, and loss of T-suppressor function are known risk factors for malignant transformation. These cancers tend to be more aggressive and have poorer outcomes in transplant patients than in the general population.[16] Urothelial cell carcinoma is the most common type of bladder cancer. Immunosuppression with cyclophosphamide or glucocorticoids is an additional risk factor.[7,28] Kidney cancer may occur in the transplanted kidney or the patient's native kidneys. The risk of renal cell carcinoma in the native kidneys is elevated, especially if patients had prolonged dialysis before transplant. Radical nephrectomy is performed for tumors of the native kidneys, and nephron-sparing surgery should be attempted for masses in the allograft. The risk of developing prostate cancer is not elevated in renal transplant patients; however, morbidity may be increased, so age-appropriate screening with a digital rectal exam and prostate-specific antigen should be performed annually. Curative therapy for pelvic urologic malignancies, whether with radiation or surgery, puts the transplant ureter at risk for damage, and the presence of the allograft can limit treatment of the ipsilateral pelvic lymph nodes.

REFERENCES

1. Abbott KC, Schenkman N, Swanson SJ, et al. Hospitalized nephrolithiasis after renal transplantation in the United States. Am J Transplant 2003;3:465–70.
2. Bach D, Grutzner G, Kniemeyer HW, et al. Diagnostic value of antegrade pyelography in renal transplants: a comparison of imaging modalities. Transplant Proc 1993;25:2619.
3. Challacombe B, Dasgupta P, Tiptaft R, et al. Multimodal management of urolithiasis in renal transplantation. BJU Int 2005;96:385–9.
4. Coleman DV, Mackenzie EF, Gardner SD, et al. Human polyomavirus (BK) infection and ureteric stenosis in renal allograft recipients. J Clin Pathol 1978;31:338–47.
5. Cuellar DC, Sklar GN. Penile prosthesis in the organ transplant recipient. Urology 2001;57:138–41.
6. del Pizzo JJ, Jacobs SC, Bartlett ST, et al. The use of bladder for total transplant ureteral reconstruction. J Urol 1998;159:750–2, discussion 752–753.
7. Dietrich K, Schned A, Fortuny J, et al. Glucocorticoid therapy and risk of bladder cancer. Br J Cancer 2009;101:1316–20.
8. Dominguez J, Clase CM, Mahalati K, et al. Is routine ureteric stenting needed in kidney transplantation? A randomized trial. Transplantation 2000;70:597–601.
9. Gallentine ML, Wright Jr FH. Ligation of the native ureter in renal transplantation. J Urol 2002;167:29–30.
10. Haferkamp A, Dorsam J, Mohring K, et al. Ureteral complications in renal transplantation with more than one donor ureter. Nephrol Dial Transplant 1999;14:1521–4.
11. Karam G, Hetet JF, Maillet F, et al. Late ureteral stenosis following renal transplantation: risk factors and impact on patient and graft survival. Am J Transplant 2006;6:352–6.
12. Khositseth S, Gillingham KJ, Cook ME, et al. Urolithiasis after kidney transplantation in pediatric recipients: a single center report. Transplantation 2004;78:1319–23.
13. Mangus RS, Haag BW. Stented versus nonstented extravesical ureteroneocystostomy in renal transplantation: a metaanalysis. Am J Transplant 2004;4:1889–96.

14. Mangus RS, Haag BW, Carter CB. Stented Lich-Gregoir ureteroneocystostomy: case series report and cost-effectiveness analysis. Transplant Proc 2004;36:2959–61.
15. Mathews R, Marshall FF. Versatility of the adult psoas hitch ureteral reimplantation. J Urol 1997;158:2078–82.
16. Miao Y, Everly JJ, Gross TG, et al. De novo cancers arising in organ transplant recipients are associated with adverse outcomes compared with the general population. Transplantation 2009;87:1347–59.
17. Nankivell BJ, Cohn DA, Spicer ST, et al. Diagnosis of kidney transplant obstruction using Mag3 diuretic renography. Clin Transplant 2001;15:11–8.
18. Philosophe B, Kuo PC, Schweitzer EJ, et al. Laparoscopic versus open donor nephrectomy: comparing ureteral complications in the recipients and improving the laparoscopic technique. Transplantation 1999;68:497–502.
19. Praz V, Leisinger HJ, Pascual M, et al. Urological complications in renal transplantation from cadaveric donor grafts: a retrospective analysis of 20 years. Urol Int 2005;75:144–9.
20. Reinberg Y, Manivel JC, Sidi AA, et al. Transurethral resection of prostate immediately after renal transplantation. Urology 1992;39:319–21.
21. Russo D, Musone D, Alteri V, et al. Erectile dysfunction in kidney transplanted patients: efficacy of sildenafil. J Nephrol 2004;17:291–5.
22. Sansalone CV, Maione G, Aseni P, et al. Advantages of short-time ureteric stenting for prevention of urological complications in kidney transplantation: an 18-year experience. Transplant Proc 2005;37:2511–5.
23. Shokeir AA, Shamaa MA, Bakr MA, et al. Salvage of difficult transplant urinary fistulae by ileal substitution of the ureter. Scand J Urol Nephrol 1993;27:537–40.
24. Shoskes DA, Hanbury D, Cranston D, et al. Urological complications in 1000 consecutive renal transplant recipients. J Urol 1995;153:18–21.
25. Stapenhorst L, Sassen R, Beck B, et al. Hypocitraturia as a risk factor for nephrocalcinosis after kidney transplantation. Pediatr Nephrol 2005;20:652–6.
26. Streeter EH, Little DM, Cranston DW, et al. The urological complications of renal transplantation: a series of 1535 patients. BJU Int 2002;90:627–34.
27. Taylor RM. Impotence and the use of the internal iliac artery in renal transplantation: a survey of surgeons' attitudes in the United Kingdom and Ireland. Transplantation 1998;65:745–6.
28. Tuttle TM, Williams GM, Marshall FF. Evidence for cyclophosphamide-induced transitional cell carcinoma in a renal transplant patient. J Urol 1988;140:1009–11.
29. Wilson CH, Bhatti AA, Rix DA, et al. Routine intraoperative ureteric stenting for kidney transplant recipients. Cochrane Database Syst Rev 2005;4:CD004925.
30. Zhang Y, Guan DL, Ou TW, et al. Sildenafil citrate treatment for erectile dysfunction after kidney transplantation. Transplant Proc 2005;37:2100–3.

CHAPTER 30

CARDIOVASCULAR DISEASE IN RENAL TRANSPLANTATION

Emily P. McQuarrie • Alan G. Jardine

CHAPTER OUTLINE

INTRODUCTION

A successful renal transplant is the most effective way of reducing the incidence of cardiovascular disease (CVD) and cardiovascular (CV) mortality in patients with end-stage renal disease (ESRD). The risk of CVD in renal transplant recipients (RTR) is approximately one-fifth of that of patients receiving maintenance hemodialysis[8,29,57] for whom the overall risk of CVD is approximately 10–20 times that of the general population. Moreover, premature CVD is a leading cause of graft failure – "death with a functioning graft." These observations are well established, and illustrated in Figure 30-1. However, the pattern of CVD, the underlying mechanisms, and their management are more complex than in the general population.[57]

There are specific problems relating to CVD in RTR. The first is that there are limited epidemiological data and very few clinical trials in RTRs on which to base our understanding. Secondly, a detailed description of CVD in this population must also include analysis of CVD in patients with progressive chronic kidney disease (CKD) and patients with ESRD receiving maintenance dialysis, who carry with them to transplantation the burden of accumulated CV risk. Moreover, some transplant recipients may spend multiple periods on maintenance dialysis between transplants, and this adds further to the complexity of accumulated CV risk. Thirdly, there are aspects of CVD in transplantation that are unique to this population; specifically, the influence of immunosuppressive agents, and the complications of transplantation. Finally, there is the nature of CVD itself and whether the predominant issue is of coronary heart disease (CHD) or whether there are other pathophysiological processes; also whether it is appropriate to use risk factor relationships and therapeutic strategies derived from the general population.[8,57]

BACKGROUND: CVD IN CKD

Over the last decade, the recognition that CKD is associated with increased CV risk has resulted in the widespread reporting of estimated glomerular filtration rate (eGFR) and its acceptance as a CV risk equivalent.[113] As GFR declines, the risk of CVD increases progressively, with the highest risk being in ESRD. In early CKD the pattern of CVD is probably similar to the general population, with an increased risk of lipid-dependent coronary artery disease (CAD). In more advanced CKD, there is a disproportionate increase in deaths due to heart failure and sudden, presumed arrhythmic deaths. The latter pattern is more akin to that seen in advanced heart failure

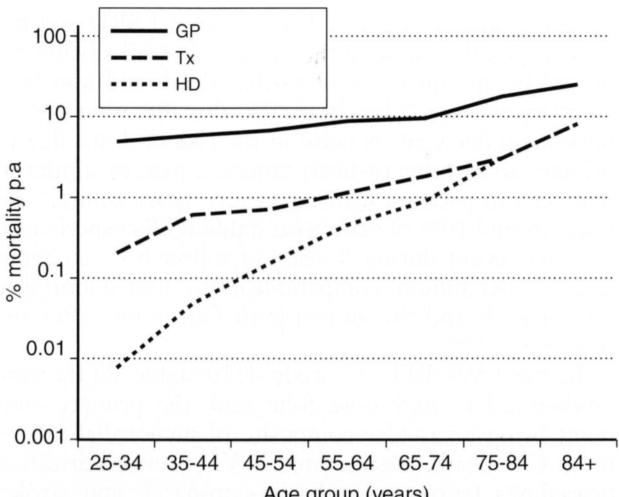

FIGURE 30-1 ■ Percentage cardiovascular mortality per annum (p.a.) by age group in the general population (GP), renal transplant population (Tx), and hemodialysis population (HD). The figure demonstrates the vastly increased cardiovascular risk in patients on hemodialysis; this risk is improved in patients who are transplanted, but not back to baseline. (Derived from the USRDS. Foley RN, Parfrey PS, Sarnak MJ. Clinical epidemiology of cardiovascular disease in chronic renal disease. Am J Kidney Dis 1998;32:S112-S9.)

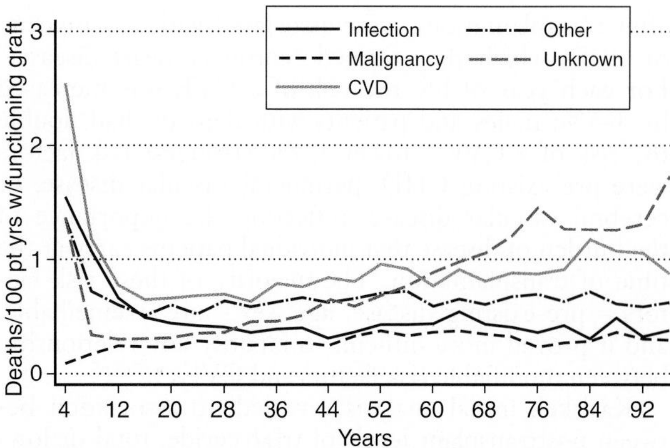

FIGURE 30-2 ■ Deaths per 100 patient years, in a renal transplant population, showing cause of death with time following transplantation surgery. The data include first-time kidney-only transplant recipients, age 18 and older, and transplanted between 1997 and 2006, who died with a functioning graft (n=14 169). CVD, cardiovascular disease. (Data from the USRDS annual report 2008; www.usrds.org.)

than to that of CHD.[57] In both ESRD and advanced heart failure, total serum cholesterol levels are low, markers of inflammation are elevated, and the conventional relationship between lipids and total CV events (CVE) is lost (or even reversed). Moreover, treatment strategies proven in the general population – specifically statins – have little or no effects in these patient groups,[16,26,112,114,138] presumably reflecting the low proportion of the overall CV burden which is due to cholesterol-dependent coronary disease.

The determinants of excess CVD in advanced CKD include vascular calcification, elevated phosphate, hypertension, inflammation, and malnutrition – bone mineral disease and intravascular volume overload.[8,57] Vascular stiffness and hypertension lead to the development of uremic cardiomyopathy,[28] the most common form of which is extreme left ventricular hypertrophy (LVH) with fibrosis, which promotes the development of systolic dysfunction and sudden arrhythmic death.[76] Overall, the pattern of CVD in ESRD, its pathogenesis, and the implications for treatment are markedly different from the general population and, although the risk of CHD is increased, the disproportionate increase is in sudden death and death due to heart failure.

Thus, potential transplant recipients carry with them the burden of accumulated CV risk – conventional and non-conventional – to the posttransplant period. Following transplantation surgery, there is an abrupt increase in overall (and CV) events and mortality, particularly in the perioperative period (Figure 30-2). This falls progressively and survivors beyond the first few months have a mortality rate approximately half that of patients receiving maintenance dialysis.[144]

Once transplanted, there are specific risk factors. Dyslipidemia and hypertension are both common after transplantation, affecting the vast majority of patients. Lipid levels rise in the weeks after transplantation,[44] reflecting improved wellbeing, diet, and immunosuppressive agents. Immunosuppressive agents also contribute to hypertension and to the development of diabetes (new-onset diabetes after transplantation (NODAT)). These, together with the level of posttransplant renal function and pre-existing CVD and risk, contribute to the overall level of CV risk following transplantation.[8,57]

EPIDEMIOLOGY AND NATURE OF POSTTRANSPLANT CVD

Several registries and longitudinal follow-up studies have examined the natural history and determinants of CVD in RTR. In looking at these data it is important to consider ongoing developments to immunosuppressive therapy, the increasing age of transplant recipients, and the use of kidneys from extended criteria donors (where the expectations for graft function are less good). Each of these is likely to influence the pattern of CVD in RTR in the future. A second issue is the description of CVEs. End-points recorded in registries may be inaccurate and investigators in clinical trials often pool CV end-points, with the assumption that they share common pathophysiological mechanisms, and thus are likely to respond to the same interventions. With the atypical mix of events and pathophysiology in RTR one cannot rely on these assumptions.[8,47,57] A final issue, that is often ignored, is that of "competing risk," where an individual risk factor may contribute to more than one adverse outcome. In transplant recipients, for example, smoking may increase the risk of infection, malignancy, and CVD, thus diminishing the apparent effect on any single outcome.[47]

The best-established studies are those of Kasiske and colleagues, who reported longitudinal follow-up of over 1000 RTRs in a single US center.[63,65] These studies demonstrated the high prevalence of CVEs and CV mortality in RTR. They confirmed that conventional CV risk factors, including age, sex, smoking status, and the presence of diabetes mellitus (either pre-existing or developing after transplantation), were associated with a composite of CVEs which they termed "coronary heart disease." For each year of life the risk of a CVE was increased by 3–5%; males and patients with diabetes had double the risk of a CVE. However, the strongest risk factors were pre-existing CHD, peripheral vascular disease, or cerebral vascular disease, reflecting the importance of the burden of disease that individual patients carry at the time of transplantation. The majority of these risk factors – pre-existing disease, age, sex – are irremediable, and it proved more difficult to identify any relationship between modifiable risk factors and CVEs.[8,57,63,65]

Kasiske's initial analysis revealed no association between posttransplant levels of triglyceride, total or low-density lipoprotein (LDL) cholesterol, and CVE in RTR.[65] However, a subsequent larger analysis[63] did show an association of risk with hyperlipidemia, with very high levels of total cholesterol being associated with an increased risk of long-term CVE. However, the lack of a clear, progressive relationship between lipid levels and CVEs, in keeping with the pattern seen in ESRD,[73] provides support for the notion that CVD in RTR differs from the traditional atherosclerotic model.[8,57] There are similar large single-center studies from Europe which have reported similar findings.[133]

Although epidemiological studies in RTR are limited, long-term follow-up of clinical trials provides additional data, with the added benefit that end-points are externally validated and more accurate than registry data.[13,41,43,56,140] Both the ALERT (Assessment of LEscol in Renal Transplantation[41,43,56]) and, more recently, the FAVORIT (Folic Acid for Vascular Outcome Reduction in Transplantation[13,140]) studies have been used to provide data on CVEs collected during follow-up of potential interventions in large populations of RTR. In the ALERT study[43] 2100 stable RTRs were randomized to receive placebo or fluvastatin (40–80 mg/day) and followed for up to 8 years.[41,43] When these data are compared with studies of statin therapy in non-transplant populations, at comparable, high risk of CVEs, there are clear differences. Patients with dyslipidemia and a history of CAD are likely to have further coronary events; the risk of cardiac death is approximately one-third that of a non-fatal event.[16,112,114] In contrast, patients with ESRD receiving maintenance dialysis[26,138] are much more likely to suffer cardiac death than a non-fatal coronary event. RTRs occupy a position intermediate between ESRD and the general population, with the increase in CVEs being reflected by an equal risk of cardiac death and non-fatal coronary events.[41,43] It is likely that this alteration in proportions reflects an increase in the risk of death due to primary arrhythmia or heart failure, a pattern similar to that seen in patients with congestive heart failure.[33] Of note, around 10% of otherwise stable RTRs experienced a cardiac event during 5 years of follow-up – an event rate (2% per annum) comparable to the annual mortality rate of RTR and the annual graft failure rate after the first year.[41,43,140]

In the FAVORIT[13,140] study 4110 stable RTRs were randomized to high-dose folic acid, the primary end-point being a vascular composite of myocardial infarction, CV death, resuscitated CVD, revascularization procedures (coronary and non-coronary), and stroke. Given the above analyses, and the potentially disparate nature of the pooled end-points, it is perhaps not surprising that there was no benefit of the intervention, that LDL cholesterol had no relationship with the composite outcome, and that the main determinants were age, pre-existing CVD, diabetes, systolic blood pressure, and low eGFR.[13,140] Table 30-1 shows the atypical relationship between risk factors and CVEs in this population.

A recent prospective multinational study – the PORT study (Patient Outcomes in Renal Transplantation[55,101]) – followed 23 575 adult RTRs for a median of 4.5 years. CVD disease was defined as a composite of proven myocardial infarction, coronary intervention, and cardiac death. The overall cumulative incidence was 3.1%, 5.2%, and 7.6% at 1, 3, and 5 years after transplantation. In the first year the distribution of events was non-fatal myocardial infarction (49%), coronary intervention (38%), and cardiac death (13%); beyond 1 year the corresponding values were 39%, 38%, and 23%. Conventional modifiable CV risk factors were very poor predictors of cardiac events, and varied with time after transplantation. Early events were predicted by age, male sex, history of cancer or diabetes, obesity, pre-existing CV disease (CHD, peripheral vascular disease, cerebrovascular disease), deceased donor transplant, and time on dialysis prior to transplantation. Conventional risk factors such as smoking, hypercholesterolemia, and hypertension were not significant, although they did correlate with a past history of CVD. Later events were dependent on poor graft function

TABLE 30-1 Data on Risk Factors for Myocardial Infarction and Sudden Cardiac Death from the FAVORIT Study[140]

	RR	Confidence Interval	*P*
Age	1.13	(1.08, 1.19)	<0.0001
Diabetes	2.30	(1.90, 2.80)	<0.0001
Smoking (current)	1.38	(1.05, 1.82)	0.07
Cardiovascular disease	2.06	(1.71, 2.48)	<0.0001
Low-density lipoprotein	1.01	(0.98, 1.04)	0.41
Systolic blood pressure	1.17	(1.11, 1.23)	<0.0001
Diastolic blood pressure	0.89	(0.81, 0.98)	0.02
Body mass index	0.91	(0.84, 0.98)	0.02
Lymphoproliferative disease	0.84	(0.70, 1.01)	0.07

RR, relative risk of event with 95% confidence intervals for age in years, diabetes (presence or absence of), cigarette smoking, pre-existing cardiovascular disease, blood pressure, and body mass index with levels of significance.

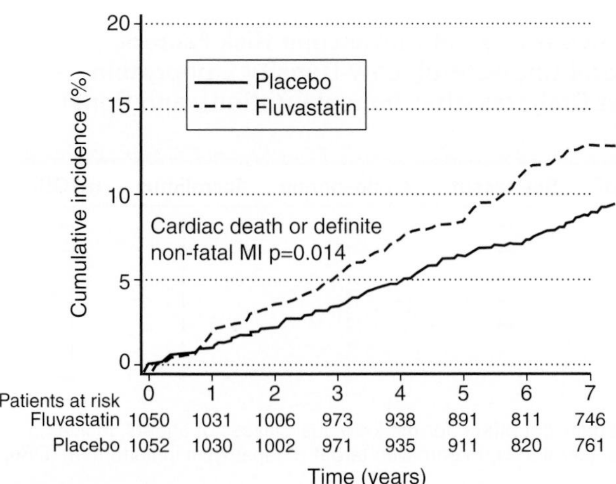

FIGURE 30-3 ■ Kaplan–Meier curves of time to cardiac death and non-fatal acute myocardial infarction (MI) in the ALERT study (with extended follow-up) of fluvastatin 40–80 mg/day versus placebo in 2100 renal transplant recipients. Statin therapy was associated with a reduction in cardiac death and non-fatal MI during 8 years of follow-up (P=0.014, log rank test). (Data from Holdaas H, Fellstrom B, Cole E, et al. Long-term cardiac outcomes in renal transplant recipients receiving fluvastatin: the ALERT extension study. Am J Transplant 2005;5:2929–36.)

(low eGFR; and factors that adversely influence graft function such as acute rejection, delayed graft function, and posttransplant lymphoproliferative disease), and the development of NODAT and race.

Some of the differences in the analyses above may be explained by pooling end-points. The ALERT study also allows us to examine the relationship between risk factors and individual CVE (e.g., acute myocardial infarction (aMI) or cardiac death) (Figure 30-3), and to examine relationships masked by pooling of CVE with different determinants.[56,121] In a multivariate analysis, the leading potentially remediable determinants of aMI (in addition to age, gender, and pre-existing diabetes) were lipid levels. As in the general population, all major serum lipid subfractions were associated with aMI: total and LDL cholesterol, and triglyceride with an increased risk; HDL cholesterol with reduced risk.[56] In contrast, no lipid subfraction was significantly associated with cardiac death, the main determinants of which were low eGFR and LVH, particularly when associated with subendocardial ischemia (LVH with "strain") and pulse pressure.[56] These observations strongly support the established literature on "uremic cardiomyopathy" and suggest that severe LVH, driven by renal dysfunction, hypertension, and the presence of LVH at the time of transplantation, may lead to increased risk of death due to heart failure or arrhythmia – with or without coexistent coronary disease.

The key message from these observations is that RTRs do suffer from CAD (fatal and non-fatal myocardial infarction), the determinants of which are the same as the general population. However, cardiac death is perhaps a greater problem, the determinants of which are LVH, vascular stiffness, and hypertension. Studies by other investigators, including Abbott[1] and Rigatto,[108] support these findings, and underscore the observation that non-coronary events such as heart failure are common. In addition, they demonstrated that specific transplant risk factors including graft dysfunction (specifically graft failure) were associated with an approximately threefold increase in CVEs, including heart failure. Anemia proved to be a risk factor for the development of heart failure, although with improved anemia management a relationship with hemoglobin is now difficult to confirm.[25,27,57,108]

NOVEL AND TRANSPLANT-SPECIFIC RISK FACTORS

In the general population, the limited predictive ability of conventional CV risk factors has led to the search for novel risk factors and potential therapeutic targets. The presence of inflammation has become a central mechanism, with the recognition that inflammatory cells are involved in atherosclerosis and that circulating markers of inflammation, such as C-reactive protein, can identify patients at increased risk of atherosclerotic vascular disease who may benefit from established treatments. In RTRs there are similar initiatives. Markers of inflammation and circulating inhibitors of endothelial function[2,3] have been studied in transplantation and are associated with an increased risk of CVD. Patients with simple features of inflammation, such as low albumin, are at higher risk.[2,133] There are also transplant-specific risk factors, including those factors which contribute to poor graft function. These include the occurrence and severity of acute rejection episodes, delayed graft function, chronic rejection, cytomegalovirus infection, and other factors.[25,27,57]

SPECIFIC RISK FACTORS AND MANAGEMENT

In this section we will cover individual CV risk factors, their role, and their management. As noted above, it is important to realize that transplantation is one phase in the course of progressive renal disease. Patients bring with them to transplantation accumulated risk, much of which is irremediable. For example, vascular stiffness and calcification which develop in advanced CKD contribute to hypertension following transplantation. Moreover, nearly all of the immunosuppressive drugs which have revolutionized the management of transplant recipients have effects on CV risk factors – some good, such as higher GFR; others potentially bad, such as hypertension and dyslipidemia. The pattern of effects of immunosuppressive agents is shown in Table 30-2[8,57], and discussed in more detail below.

HYPERTENSION AND UREMIC CARDIOMYOPATHY

Hypertension is an almost invariable accompaniment of renal transplantation – a consequence of pre-existing hypertension at the time of transplantation and the effects of immunosuppressive agents. In general, hypertension is a consequence of two mechanisms: increased vascular resistance and increased intravascular volume. In CKD,

TABLE 30-2 Effects of Immunosuppressive Agents in Conventional Cardiovascular Risk Factors, Including Hypertension, Left Ventricular Hypertrophy, Total Cholesterol, Low-Density Lipoprotein Cholesterol, Triglycerides, Diabetes Mellitus (New-Onset Diabetes After Transplantation), and Renal Function

Cardiovascular Risk Factors	Steroids	Azathioprine/MMF	Belatacept	Cyclosporine	Tacrolimus	mTORi
Hypertension	↑	↔	↔	↑	↑	↔
Left ventricular hypertrophy	↑	↔	↔	↑	↑	↔
Total cholesterol	↑	↔	↔	↑	↑	↑
Low-density lipoprotein	↑	↔	↔	↑	↑	↑
Triglycerides	↑	↔	↔	↑	↑	↑
Diabetes mellitus	↑	↔	↔	↑	↑	↑
Renal function	↔	↔	↔	↓	↓	↔

The arrows indicate an adverse or beneficial effect, or the absence of any significant effect, for the individual classes of agents, including corticosteroids, azathioprine/mycophenolate mofetil (MMF), cyclosporine, tacrolimus, mammalian target of rapamycin inhibitors (mTORi), and newer biologic agents.

as GFR declines, salt and water excretion are impaired, and volume-dependent mechanisms assume greater importance; following transplantation the contribution of volume-dependent mechanisms will similarly depend on the level of graft function.[57,74,102]

The majority of RTRs with hypertension receive antihypertensive medication and, of these, the majority require more than one agent.[21,74,102,130] In keeping with the general population, the choice of agent requires an understanding of the mechanisms involved but is also driven by the need to treat comorbid disease – for example, beta-blockers for patients with symptomatic angina, and blockers of the renin–angiotensin system for patients with proteinuria.[21,68] There is evidence of increased or inappropriate activation of vasoconstrictor mechanisms in RTRs, including the sympathetic nervous system, the renin–angiotensin system, and endothelin both in humans and experimental animals.[74,85,102,106] These, coupled with evidence of impaired endothelium-dependent vascular relaxation,[3,74,85,102,106] shift the balance towards vasoconstriction. The mechanisms underlying these phenomena are less well understood. Corticosteroids are associated with hypertension in other clinical conditions and have two principal actions – to promote retention of salt and water due to actions of corticosteroids on the kidney,[136] and to enhance sympathetic activity, leading to increased vascular tone.[136] Calcineurin inhibitors (CNIs) cause hypertension through direct renal sodium retention and increased vasoconstrictor tone as well as indirectly via renal impairment, as a consequence of the nephrotoxic effects of CNI.[49,74,102]

There are few prospective trials of antihypertensive treatment in RTRs.[70,99] Specifically, no trials have been completed to assess antihypertensive therapy and "hard" CV outcomes; the one large-scale trial of angiotensin receptor blockade was stopped early due to the low event rate.[99] Similarly, there are no trials which have assessed specific blood pressure targets. However, there are many short-term studies that have examined the effects of individual antihypertensive agents which have demonstrated that the commonly used agents – angiotensin receptor blockers, angiotensin-converting enzyme (ACE) inhibitors, and calcium channel blockers – have antihypertensive effects comparable to those seen in other populations.[21,74,102] Dihydropyridine calcium channel antagonists – such as nifedipine and amlodipine – may attenuate the nephrotoxic effects of CNI[74,102,136] and have been favored in the early phases following transplantation. Blockers of the renin–angiotensin system may have specific benefits in patients with proteinuria[99] and LVH, although the uptake has been slow because of concerns about the possible adverse effects in patients with undiagnosed, functional stenosis of the single transplant renal artery.[32]

The best evidence for the importance of managing hypertension and treatment targets comes from the European Registry. Opelz and colleagues[88,89] examined the impact of blood pressure measurements recorded at outpatient clinics in patients with a functioning transplant 1 year after transplantation. These data show that blood pressure, albeit not independently from graft function, is a major determinant of long-term patient and graft survival. Moreover, this effect was seen even at levels below which one would label the patient as being hypertensive such that patients with a systolic blood pressure of 130 mmHg had a substantially worse graft outcome than patients with a systolic blood pressure of 120 mmHg. Subsequent analyses which examined CV disease, specifically, identified an important relationship between blood pressure across the range from "normal" to hypertensive and the development of posttransplant CV disease (Figure 30-4).[88,89]

Epidemiological studies, which include the placebo arms of interventional trials in transplant recipients, have confirmed that hypertension is associated with CVEs[56,140] – specifically stroke, cardiac death, and heart failure – rather than non-fatal coronary events. Hypertension was the strongest determinant of cardiac death in the ALERT study.[56] The most significant blood pressure parameters in these studies were systolic blood pressure and pulse pressure, both markers associated with vascular stiffness.

A consistent finding in RTR is that hypertension is associated with manifestations of end-organ damage in RTRs – specifically proteinuria and LVH.[94,98] Elevated blood pressure is the major determinant of LVH in patients with ESRD,[116] including transplant recipients, and LVH is strongly associated with poor outcome[56] in RTRs. The pathophysiology of LVH in CKD (uremic cardiomyopathy) is marked by the presence of subendocardial ischemia and myocardial fibrosis.[76,126] Fibrosis leads to

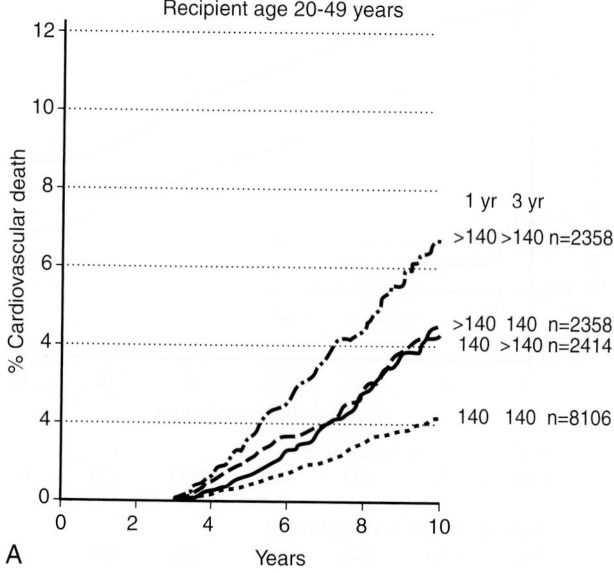

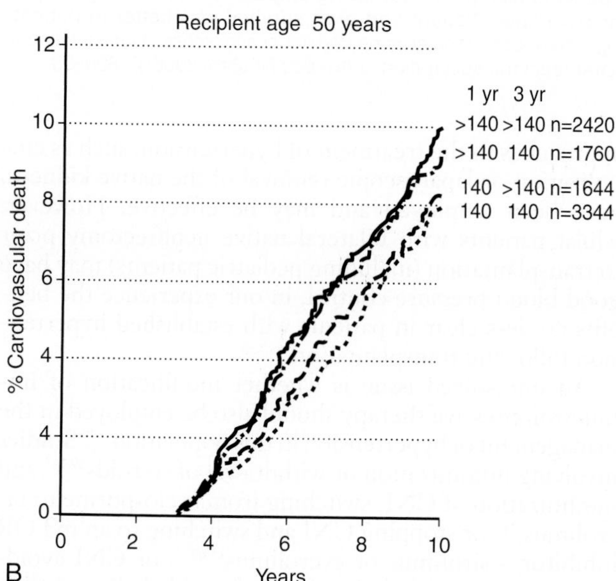

FIGURE 30-4 ■ (A, B) Kaplan–Meier curves of cumulative incidence of cardiovascular events by systolic blood pressure (mmHg) at 1 and 3 years of follow-up, in two age groups from the Collaborative Transplant Study. In both age groups, having a systolic blood pressure <140 mmHg, as compared with above 140 mmHg, at both 1 and 3 years of follow-up was associated with a reduced incidence of cardiovascular events. (Data from Opelz G, Dohler B. Collaborative Transplant Study. Improved long-term outcomes after renal transplantation associated with blood pressure control. Am J Transplant 2005;5:2725–31.

aberrant conduction (and is associated with markers of aberrant conduction and arrhythmogenicity, such as prolonged QT interval and abnormal T-wave alternans,[95] which provide the likely link to fatal arrhythmias and sudden cardiac death.[57] Arrhythmias may be spontaneous or complicate otherwise minor ischemic episodes. These observations identify hypertension, LVH, and electrocardiographic abnormalities as markers of adverse outcome in RTR, and as potential targets for intervention.[57] The less common manifestation of uremic dilated cardiomyopathy (with systolic dysfunction) may be a sequel of LVH or may be associated with (often silent) CHD.[10,57,76]

These cardiac abnormalities develop, primarily, during the time patients spend with advanced CKD, and on maintenance dialysis programs, and are highly prevalent in transplant recipients.[116] Whilst there are studies which suggest that the manifestations of uremic cardiomyopathy may improve following transplantation,[131] with apparent regression of LVH and improved systolic function, these studies may not reflect the true situation. Echocardiographic analyses are highly dependent on chamber diameters (e.g., in the estimation of LV mass[76,98]) which are, in turn, dependent on hydration status. Whilst patients with advanced CKD and treated by dialysis have a tendency to volume overload, this resolves following successful transplantation. Thus, intravascular volume is normalized, correcting artefactual overestimation of LV mass and systolic dysfunction and, whereas echocardiographic studies have shown improved cardiac structure and function after transplantation, studies that use volume-independent technology (specifically cardiac magnetic resonance imaging) have failed to show similar improvement.[97] Long-term risks associated with the various manifestations of uremic cardiomyopathy in patients receiving maintenance dialysis are carried forward in patients who undergo transplantation.[28,79,97] Following transplantation, there are limited data on uremic cardiomyopathy, restricted to LVH, suggesting that effective blood pressure control and the avoidance of CNI may reduce LVH.[82,93] A series of small short-term studies suggests that the use of dihydropyridine calcium antagonists,[82] inhibitors of mammalian target of rapamycin (mTOR[93]), sirolimus or everolimus in place of CNI, or CNI withdrawal[7] is associated with regression – or lack of progression – of LVH in RTRs.

OTHER SURROGATES: VASCULAR STIFFNESS AND CALCIFICATION

LVH is one consequence of progressive CKD, and ESRD, and the associated metabolic and physiological changes. However, there are other vascular abnormalities associated with adverse prognosis in RTR.[7,50,53] These include vascular calcification and vascular stiffness (secondary to calcification or vascular hypertrophy). These contribute to the development of systolic hypertension (in particular) and also to the development of LVH. Moreover, they are also linked to adverse CV outcomes in RTR, with coronary artery calcification at time of transplantation also being predictive of cardiac events.[109] These measures provide potential short-term surrogate end-points for trials of CV interventions in this patient group.[50,53]

CHOICE OF ANTIHYPERTENSIVE AGENT

Most classes of antihypertensive agent have been used and have some efficacy in RTR.[21,74,102] There has been a tendency to avoid effective ACE inhibitors and angiotensin receptor blockers because of the risk of undiagnosed

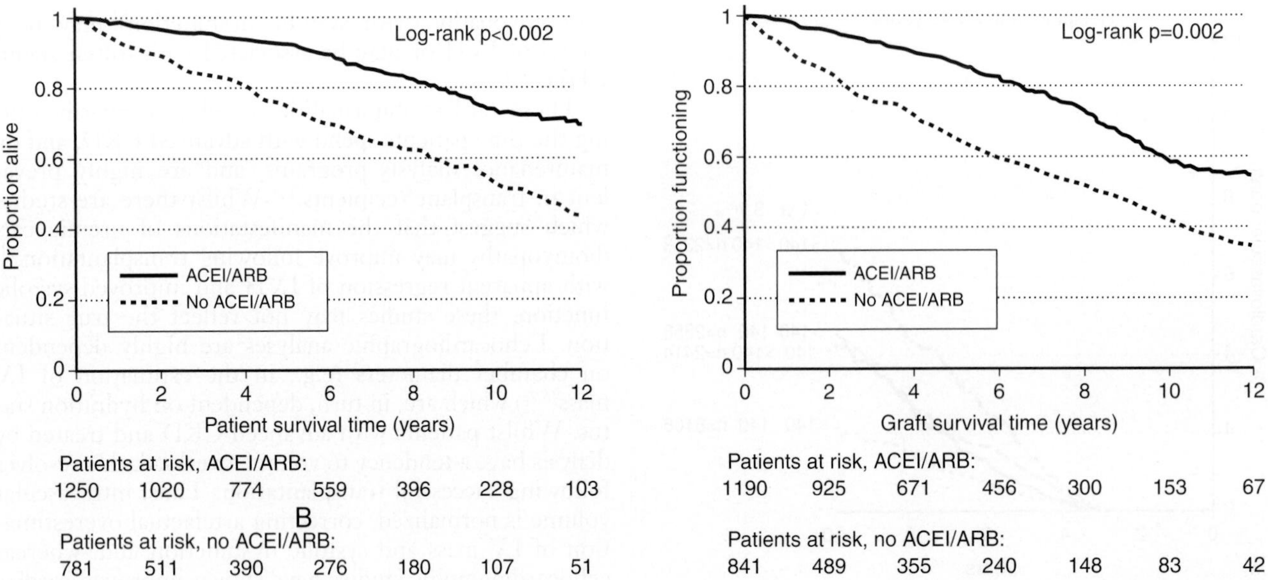

FIGURE 30-5 ■ A retrospective analysis of patient and graft survival in patients taking and not taking angiotensin-converting enzyme inhibitors (ACEI) or angiotensin receptor blockers (ARB), adjusted for covariates. Patient and graft survival was better in patients prescribed ACEI/ARB. (Data from Heinze G, Mitterbauer C, Regele H, et al. Angiotensin-converting enzyme inhibitor or angiotensin II type 1 receptor antagonist therapy is associated with prolonged patient and graft survival after renal transplantation. J Am Soc Nephrol 2006;17:889–99.

renal artery stenosis[68,74,102] in the transplanted kidney, and the possibility of precipitating acute renal failure. However, a carefully conducted retrospective analysis from Austria, performed by Oberbauer and colleagues, showed that patients treated with ACE inhibitors or angiotensin receptor blockers fared better with respect to both graft function and patient survival (Figure 30-5[37]). Although a similar analysis performed by Opelz et al., on a highly selected subgroup of the European Renal Registry, failed to show a similar trend,[90] there has been a progressive increase in the use of these agents over recent years (Figure 30-6[101]). Short-term studies of renin–angiotensin system blockade, or dihydropyridine calcium antagonists, have shown efficacy in both blood pressure reduction and the added potential regression of LVH.[82] Caution should be exerted with regard to hyperkalemia in the context of ACE inhibition and CNI.[68]

The single published long-term CV outcome study in RTR[99] set out to compare the angiotensin receptor blocker candesartan with conventional therapy. Although the study demonstrated the safety of this agent, and superior effects on reduction of proteinuria, the trial was discontinued because the event rate was too low, and the study unlikely to deliver a result.

Overall, dihydropyridine calcium antagonists are often favored in the early posttransplant period, and when CNI nephrotoxicity is suspected.[68] Of the other types of calcium antagonists, diltiazem is associated with increased cyclosporine levels, and this has limited its use, although it has been exploited in some circumstances to reduce the cost of cyclosporine. ACE inhibitors and angiotensin receptor blockers are favored when proteinuria is an issue.[74,68,99,102] Exclusion of transplant renal artery stensosis is often performed before starting ACE inhibitors and is probably a counsel of perfection, as the benefits of intervention in transplant renal artery stenosis are uncertain in this population, as in other patient groups. More radical approaches to the treatment of hypertension, such as embolization or laparoscopic removal of the native kidneys, have been employed and may be effective. However, whilst patients with bilateral native nephrectomy prior to transplantation (including pediatric patients) may have good blood pressure control, in our experience the benefits are less clear in patients with established hypertension following transplantation.[68,120]

An unresolved issue is whether modification of immunosuppressive therapy should also be employed in the management of hypertension in this population.[124] Studies involving minimization or withdrawal of steroids[69,145] and minimization of CNI, switching from cyclosporine to tacrolimus,[111] or stopping CNI and switching to an mTOR inhibitor – sirolimus or everolimus[15,60] – or CNI avoidance using co-stimulation blockade with belatacept[71,132] have all shown a substantial reduction in blood pressure, similar to that achieved by antihypertensive therapy. As noted above, the use of inhibitors of mTOR, in place of CNI, may be associated with regression of LVH.[93] However, it is our experience that clinicians and patients are reluctant to modify immunosuppression to achieve blood pressure control; modification of immunosuppression is driven by rejection episodes, and the desire to minimize the nephrotoxic effects of CNI (or other causes of poor graft function).

Most clinics use standard "office-based" blood pressure measurements, using a standard sphygmomanometer. In our experience, it is unusual for these measurements to be made with the rigor that is often recommended – for example, using repeated measurements, with the patient seated after a period of rest – and it has been suggested that ambulatory,[35,105] or home monitoring[6,105] may be more informative. In patients with essential hypertension these methods are recommended for patients with resistant hypertension, or where "white coat" syndrome is suspected. In transplant recipients ambulatory recordings

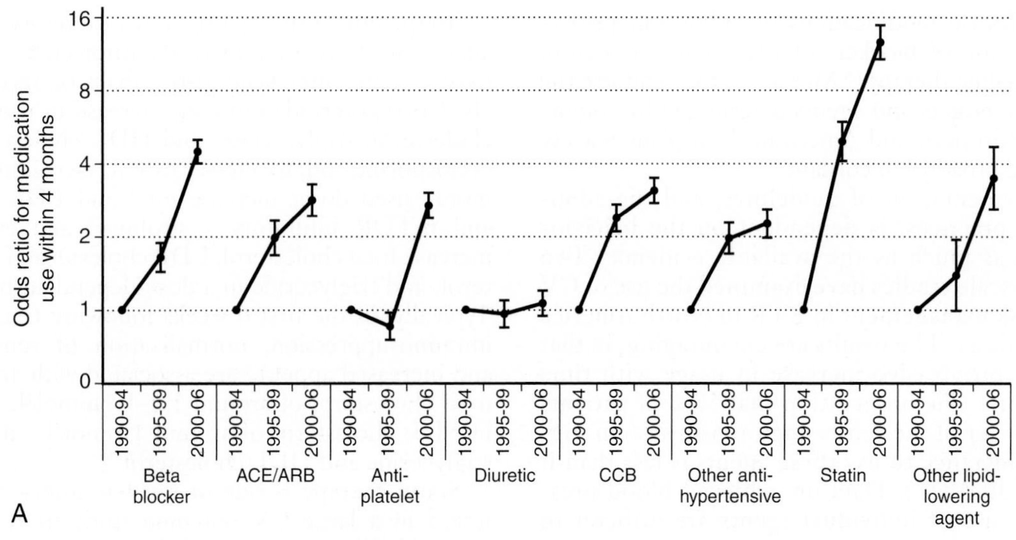

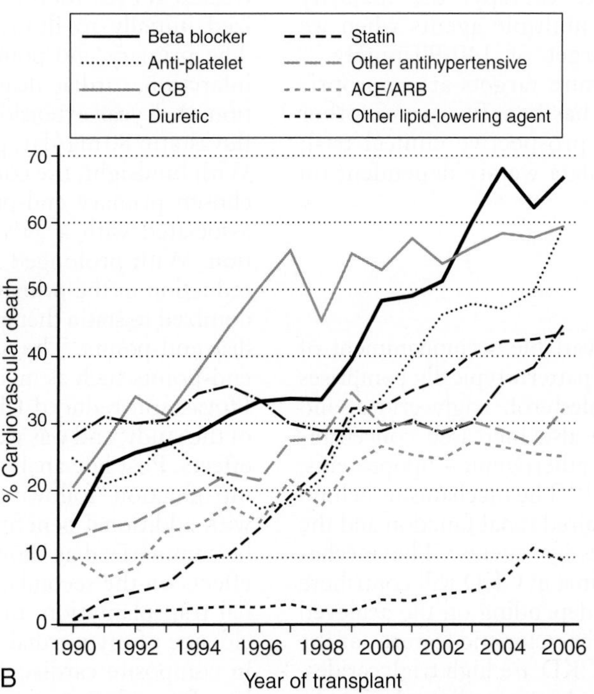

FIGURE 30-6 ■ Graph demonstrating the use of cardioprotective medications in the PORT study, documenting changes in prescription over time posttransplant. (A) Adjusted odds ratios for CVD medication use in the first 4 months posttransplant in more recent eras. (B) Model adjusted for age, sex, race, and primary cause of renal failure. ACE/ARB, angiotensin-converting enzyme inhibitors/angiotensin II receptor blockers; CCB, calcium channel blockers. (Data from Pilmore HL, Skeans MA, Snyder JJ, et al. Cardiovascular disease medications after renal transplantation: results from the Patient Outcomes in Renal Transplantation study. Transplantation 2011;91:542–51.)

are associated with prognosis and loss of diurnal profile, or loss of the "nocturnal dip," confers additional prognostic information.[52] These methods should be used in patients with poor blood pressure control, and may give additional information in clinical trials.

GUIDELINES AND OBSERVED PATTERNS OF USAGE

There are numerous guidelines on the management of hypertension following transplantation.[68] Whilst these are based on the evidence discussed in this chapter, they also draw on the practical expertise of the guideline committees. In the absence of studies which have addressed appropriate targets for blood pressure control in RTR, they have endorsed targets derived from observational studies, such as that of Opelz,[88,89] and targets taken from other populations, specifically those with CKD. Thus, the targets are arbitrary and are not aimed, for example, at regression of LVH, or specific reversal of proteinuria. The recently published Kidney Disease Improving Global Outcomes (KDIGO) guidelines suggest a target of 130/80 mmHg in patients with diabetes or proteinuria, the use of lifestyle modifications including salt restriction, and the use of blockers of the renin–angiotensin system as first-line therapy.[68] Moreover, they endorse the use of specific targets and agents determined by comorbidity. The European and American Transplant Society guidelines are broadly concordant.[36]

The implementation of guidelines, and the adoption of new practices, is dependent on the behavior of clinicians as much as the available evidence. Two recent large-scale studies have examined the use of CV drugs and risk management in RTR in North America and in Australasia. The results are encouraging, in that they show a progressive increase in usage with time in recent years. The observation that 50% of patients receive a blocker of the renin–angiotensin system suggests that reluctance to use these agents is less than it was (Figure 30-6[32,101]). Data on achieved blood pressure and the use of individual agents are difficult to obtain. In our own center, a proportion of patients remain uncontrolled despite therapy; the majority of those controlled require multiple agents when we considered an historical target of 140/90 mmHg.[130] Whether or not blood pressure targets are appropriate, and whether one agent has benefits over another require to be assessed in a prospective clinical trial; in the absence of objective data we are dependent on available registry data.

DYSLIPIDEMIA

Dyslipidemia is almost an invariable accompaniment of renal transplantation.[8,57] The pattern typically comprises elevated total and LDL cholesterol, triglycerides, and HDL cholesterol. There are also increased concentrations of intermediate – highly atherogenic – lipoproteins, including small dense LDL.[45,134] The mechanisms behind this dyslipidemia include impaired renal function and the influences of immunosuppressive agents. The mechanisms which lead to dyslipidemia in CKD will contribute to a varying degree in RTR, depending on the achieved level of renal function. The characteristic features of the dyslipidemia associated with CKD are high triglycerides, low HDL cholesterol, elevated intermediate-density lipoprotein (IDL) cholesterol and a neutral effect on LDL and total plasma cholesterol.[134] There are qualitative changes in lipoproteins, notably failure of maturation and excess of triglyceride-rich, atherogenic lipoproteins.[134] The main underlying mechanisms, expertly delineated and reviewed by Vaziri,[134] are reduced activity of lipoprotein lipase, and hepatic lipase, which contribute to impaired clearance of IDL and increased triglyceride concentrations in circulating lipoproteins and chylomicrons. Activity of HMG-CoA reductase is not altered by CKD but is increased in the presence of nephritic-range proteinuria, resulting in increased cholesterol biosynthesis. There are other more minor enzymatic defects as well as lipoprotein receptors, reduction of which impairs clearance of atherogenic lipoproteins; the most notable are reduced activity or expression of the LDL and very-low-density lipoprotein receptor, which impairs clearance of lipoproteins.[134]

To the effects of impaired renal excretory function are added the effects of individual antirejection agents which have specific, often synergistic effects on serum lipid levels. Corticosteroids cause an increase in total and LDL cholesterol, triglycerides, and HDL cholesterol; CNI – cyclosporine and, to a lesser extent, tacrolimus – at commonly used doses increase total and LDL cholesterol; and mTOR inhibitors – sirolimus and everolimus – increase total cholesterol, LDL cholesterol, HDL cholesterol, and triglyceride in a dose-dependent manner.[45,64,83] Typically, in the first 6 weeks following transplantation, immunosuppression, normalization of renal function, and increased appetite are associated with an increase in total cholesterol of around 1.0–1.5 mmol/L, an increase in LDL cholesterol of around 1 mmol/L, and increased triglyceride and HDL cholesterol.[44]

Statin therapy is one of the few interventions to be tested in a large CV outcome study in RTR.[41,43] The main ALERT trial studied 2100 stable, cyclosporine-treated RTRs, followed for up to 6 years, and randomized initially to fluvastatin 40–80 mg daily or placebo. The primary end-point was a composite of myocardial infarction, cardiac death, stroke, and coronary intervention. A 2-year extension, where all patients were offered fluvastatin 80 mg/day, prolonged follow-up to 8 years.[41,43] With hindsight, the core study was underpowered for the chosen primary end-point, although statin therapy was associated with a 35% reduction in myocardial infarction. With prolonged follow-up, there was a significant reduction in the primary end-point in those patients randomized to statin therapy, and to a variety of individual cardiac end-points. The main effect was on lipid-dependent end-points such as myocardial infarction (Figure 30-3[43]). Fluvastatin reduced LDL by 1 mmol/L for the duration of the study, and was well tolerated, with placebo-like side effects. Post hoc analyses of this study revealed that early introduction following transplantation was associated with additional benefit.[42] Overall, the ALERT study can be summarized as showing that fluvastatin has beneficial effects on the secondary dyslipidemia associated with renal transplantation, that this translates into reduced incidence of myocardial infarction (with a lesser reduction in composite cardiac end-points), and that to maximize benefits early initiation of therapy is important.

Fluvastatin is not metabolized by CYP3A4, an enzyme inhibited by CNIs. In patients receiving CNI, use of statins metabolized by CYP3A4 (specifically simvastatin, lovastatin, and, to a lesser extent, atorvastatin) is associated with increased statin levels, and with increased efficacy and side effects.[58] An important, underappreciated message is that, with the exception of fluvastatin and pravastatin, statins should be started at very low dose and monitored cautiously in CNI-treated RTR. A study of fluvastatin at the time of transplantation (SOLAR[44]), which proved that the pleiotropic effects of statins on lymphocyte function do not reduce the risk of acute rejection in RTR, showed no increase in adverse effect. Thus, of the available statins, there is most evidence for the safety of fluvastatin, particularly in the perioperative period.[41,43,44]

Recently, the SHARP study examined the use of simvastatin plus ezetimibe on dyslipidemia and outcomes in 9000 patients with CKD, including 3000 on maintenance dialysis. Although medication was not continued in patients who received transplants, there was an overall benefit in the incidence of atherosclerotic CVEs that lends support to the use of statin-based therapy for patients with progressive CKD, including those who will ultimately receive transplants.[9] This study adds to the ALERT dataset, and is consistent with Registry data and retrospective, uncontrolled studies.[19]

The use of statins has been adopted by guidelines for minimizing CV risk in RTR.[1,86] These guidelines have tended to adopt lipid targets from the general population (LDL cholesterol for adult patients of 2.6 mmol/L), as there are inadequate data on targets specific for the transplant population. Of interest, however, the most recent KDIGO guidelines (www.kdigo.org) on lipid lowering in CKD have proposed that it is more important to establish patients on statin therapy than to achieve a target and have not recommended a target-driven approach in this patient population (including RTR). Although there is a strong rationale for statin use, a report suggests much lower uptake of therapy in RTR compared to other high-risk populations.[32] However, there is a pattern of increasing use that suggests that transplant clinicians may simply be cautiously following the trend in other patient groups (Figure 30-6[101]).

One reason for the slow adoption of statin therapy and CV risk management in RTR is the inherent relationship between immunosuppression and dyslipidemia; the expectation is that posttransplant reduction of immunosuppression will correct dyslipidemia. Many studies have investigated the short-term impact of modification of immunosuppressive therapy alone on hyperlipidemia in transplant recipients, including steroid withdrawal or avoidance[69,145] or CNI withdrawal, switch, or minimization.[111] The only study to compare directly modification of immunosuppression with the initiation of lipid-lowering therapy is the study of Wissing and colleagues.[142] In this study patients were switched from cyclosporine-based therapy to tacrolimus-based therapy, and this was compared to the addition to atorvastatin. Although tacrolimus-based therapy was associated with a reduction in total LDL cholesterol and triglycerides, patients on cyclosporine and atorvastatin had lipid levels comparable to those on tacrolimus and atorvastatin combined. Thus, modification of the CNI provided no additional benefit to statin therapy. Additionally, the fact that some components of the dyslipidemia – e.g., hypertriglyceridemia – are insensitive to statin therapy, and that both atherogenic and potentially protective lipid subfractions (HDL cholesterol) are increased with immunosuppression has heightened reluctance to use statins. Most clinicians and patients are reluctant to change immunosuppression primarily on the basis of dyslipidemia, without data to support long-term outcomes with this strategy.

Finally, there is very little, other than hypothetical reasoning, and considerable negative information, on the use of alternative lipid-lowering agents, specifically fibrates and nicotinic acid derivatives, in transplantation. At present, their use is not encouraged by guidelines, and any use – particularly as add-on therapy – should be carefully monitored.[86]

RENAL FUNCTION

In the general population, renal dysfunction (CKD) has evolved as a risk factor for CV disease. Whilst statistically an independent risk factor, CKD is associated with dyslipidemia and hypertension. The "independent" impact of renal dysfunction may reflect the presence of, as yet poorly defined, "uremic toxins," or factors known to be associated with renal impairment, such as hyperphosphatemia or elevated FGF-23.[78,125] These same factors are likely to play a role in the pathophysiology of CVD in RTR with suboptimal levels of renal function. Until recently, renal function has not been reported routinely as an outcome of trials of immunosuppression in renal transplantation, where the primary outcome is limited to the incidence of acute rejection, graft and patient survival. Recent major trials have reported mean (or other summary measures of) serum creatinine levels (or estimated GFR). This neglects the fact that mean levels are of relevance to populations and not to individuals,[24] and does not include proteinuria, or other renal factors associated with poor graft outcomes. Improved reporting of renal outcomes in trials of transplantation is important, specifically, to permit long-term graft and patient outcomes (see below[123]).

Nonetheless, graft function has emerged as a strong determinant of graft and patient survival, and of CV risk in transplant recipients. Post hoc analyses of the two largest CV outcome trials in RTR – FAVORIT and ALERT[56,140] – have shown renal function to predict the risk of graft loss and of patient outcomes. Figure 30-7 shows the relationship between GFR and outcomes in the FAVORIT study.[140] These data show the importance of achieving good graft function in RTR. The available data support the use of low-dose tacrolimus in combination with mycophenolic acid/mycophenolate and corticosteroids (with anti-interleukin-2 receptor antibodies) as the most effective primary immunosuppressive strategy to produce optimal graft function. The SYMPHONY study[24] compared cyclosporine and tacrolimus-based immunosuppressive regimens with sirolimus as an adjunct agent. Low-dose tacrolimus (with a target blood level of 4–7 ng/mL) in combination with mycophenolate mofetil and corticosteroids was the best-tolerated and most effective regimen, lending strong support to the established pattern of use in the clinical community. Moreover, the achieved level of renal function was best in this group, with a mean eGFR of 65.4 mL/min compared with 56.7–59.4 mL/min in the other groups.[24] These outcomes persisted 3 years after transplantation,[23] albeit with lesser differences. CNI minimization, for example, by switching to an mTOR inhibitor (sirolimus or everolimus) has been examined in a variety of trials, incorporating a switch from CNI-based to mTOR inhibitor-based therapy at various time points from 7 weeks to years after transplantation.[14,15,46,60,84] Although this strategy has been associated with an increased risk of acute rejection

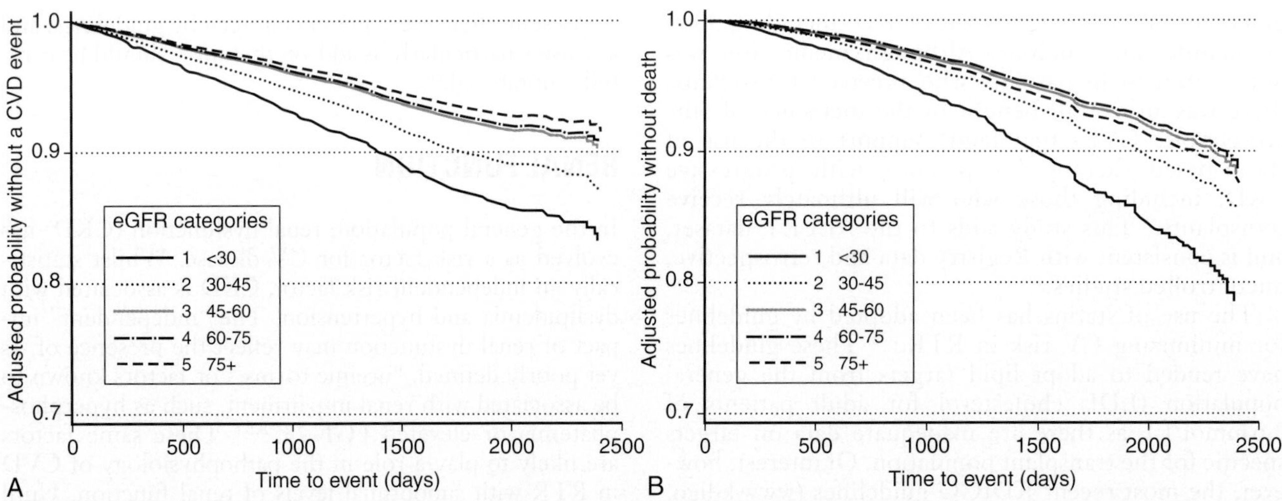

FIGURE 30-7 ■ **Impact of renal function on long-term cardiovascular event (A) and patient death risk (B) from the FAVORIT trial. Patients were stratified into five groups based on estimated glomerular filtration rate (eGFR), demonstrating that patients with poorer renal function are at increased risk of adverse events. CVD, cardiovascular disease.** (Data from Bostom AG, Carpenter MA, Kusek JW, et al. Homocysteine-lowering and cardiovascular disease outcomes in kidney transplant recipients: primary results from the Folic Acid for Vascular Outcome Reduction in Transplantation trial. Circulation 2011;123:1763–70; Weiner DE, Carpenter MA, Levey AS, et al. Kidney function and risk of cardiovascular disease and mortality in kidney transplant recipients: the FAVORIT trial. Am J Transplant 2012;12:2437–45.)

and the side effects limit the general applicability, renal function is generally improved following early protocol-driven switching.

More recently, the trials of belatacept, a co-stimulation blocker, in place of CNI in standard recipients (BENEFIT[71,132]) or recipients at risk of suboptimal graft function (BENEFIT-EXT[71,132]) have shown a similar pattern of increased risk of acute rejection, but better graft function, associated with reduced incidence of dyslipidemia and hypertension. In the post hoc analyses of the ALERT study, renal function was one of the main determinants of CV risk, regardless of whether an arbitrary cut-off was used (serum creatinine 200 µmol/L), or renal function was used as a continuous variable.[25,27] Patients whose grafts failed were at highest risk of CVEs. When risk of specific CVEs was analyzed, renal dysfunction was a stronger risk factor for cardiac death than were nonfatal atheromatous coronary events,[25,27,56] the latter being more dependent on lipid levels.

Several other analyses lend support to the impact of graft function on CVEs after transplantation.[27,80,140] These highlight the underlying importance of rejection episodes, cytomegalovirus infection, BK virus nephropathy, and drug-induced nephrotoxicity, which contribute to graft dysfunction and may show association with CVD in univariate analyses.[56,63,65] Strategies to limit the impact of graft dysfunction on CV risk will necessarily address the underlying factors, and are thus the strategies we employ to maximize graft survival and minimize rejection.

SMOKING

In the general population cigarette smoking is highly associated with the development of CVD. Studies in RTR have shown that smoking is associated with all-cause mortality, with CVEs, with graft loss, and more rapid progression of chronic transplant glomerulopathy.[5,51,56,67] Although the early studies by Kasiske et al.[65] failed to identify smoking as an independent risk factor, subsequent analyses have shown smoking to be associated with increasing risk. Smoking status is a good example of a risk factor that tends to be inaccurately reported by patients[56] and, since it is a risk factor for "competing outcomes" – such as respiratory infection, malignancy, and non-CV death – conventional survival analyses may underestimate the true impact of smoking on CV disease.[47] As yet, there are no studies of smoking cessation, although this strategy is strongly endorsed in published guidelines.[68]

NEW-ONSET DIABETES AFTER TRANSPLANTATION

Diabetes is the leading cause of ESRD, with the major increase being in the incidence of ESRD due to type 2 diabetes. As a consequence, the prevalence of diabetes amongst transplant recipients has increased in recent years. Moreover, we have become increasingly aware of the importance of posttransplant diabetes (or NODAT) and its long-term consequences. NODAT occurs against the background development of age-related type 2 diabetes in the population of patients with ESRD awaiting transplantation, and may be viewed as accelerating that process by increasing insulin resistance and, to a lesser extent, reducing insulin secretion.[40,139]

The reported incidence of NODAT varies from 3% to 20% of patients. It is more common in older patients, in patients who are overweight, of African or Asian origin, or who have a history of stress-induced diabetes (associated with surgery, use of corticosteroids, or pregnancy[107,146]). It occurs primarily in the first few months after transplantation (Figure 30-8[146]), the incidence thereafter returning to the age-related rate. The main contributory factor is the

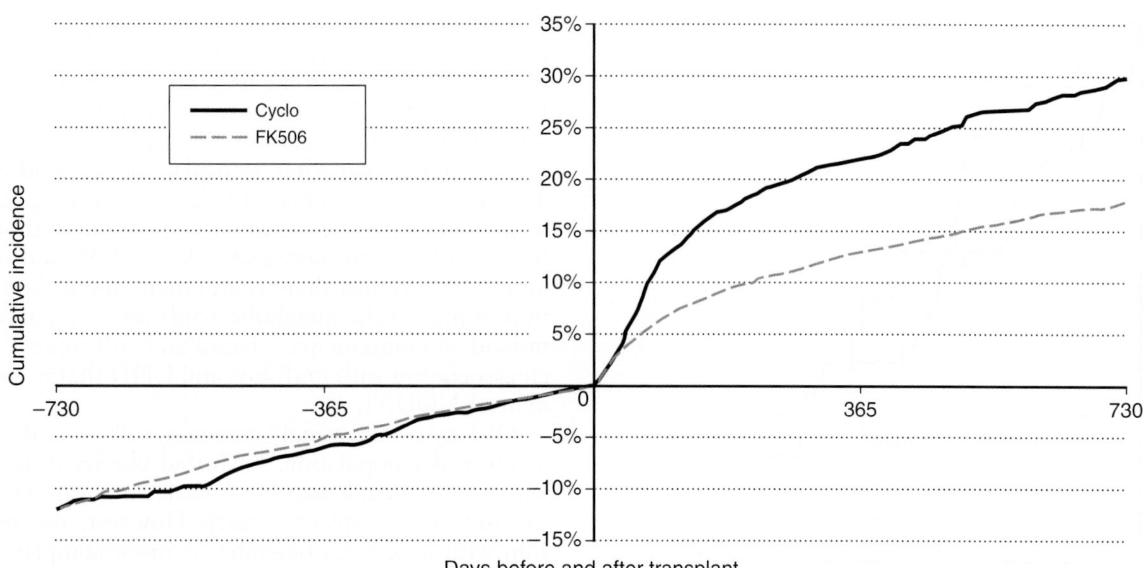

Sample size		Days before transplant			Days after transplant		
		−730	−365	−1	1	365	730
Type of calcineurin inhibitor	Cyclosporine	1776	3954	5867	6014	5521	2551
	Tacrolimus	471	911	1260	929	835	302

Note: The incremental incidence of diabetes for cyclosporine was 9.4% at 1 year and 8.4% at 2 years. The incremental incidence of diabetes for tacrolimus was 15.4% at 1 year and 17.7% at 2 years.

FIGURE 30-8 ■ **Data on the cumulative risk of diabetes in the 2 years prior to transplantation, and 2 years after transplantation, in renal transplant recipients taking cyclosporine (Cyclo)- or tacrolimus (FK506)-based immunosuppression. Patients prescribed tacrolimus are at increased risk.** (Data from Woodward RS, Schnitzler MA, Baty J, et al. Incidence and cost of new onset diabetes mellitus among U.S. wait-listed and transplanted renal allograft recipients. Am J Transplant 2003;3:590–8.)

use of corticosteroids which cause insulin resistance, and which are associated with the development of diabetes in other patient groups.[62,107,146] Minimization of steroid dose reduces the risk of NODAT and may reverse diabetes and restore insulin sensitivity.[81] CNI can also contribute to the development of diabetes; tacrolimus is more diabetogenic than cyclosporine. This reflects the role of tacrolimus-specific, intracellular FK-binding proteins on insulin secretion,[39,48,146] and is probably the common mechanism through which inhibitors of mTOR promote the development of NODAT.[61] Minimization of corticosteroids or tacrolimus or switching from tacrolimus to cyclosporine are both appropriate therapeutic measures.[48,146] Despite these measures, however, many patients require insulin or oral hypoglycemic agents. An alternative strategy is to avoid tacrolimus and/or steroids in patients at high risk for the development of posttransplant diabetes mellitus. This strategy may be of particular relevance in older patients where rejection is less of an issue than in younger patients.[62] Such an approach has few advocates, largely as a consequence of the availability of management strategies for diabetes and the failure to recognize the long-term consequences of NODAT.

The importance of individual mechanisms – insulin resistance and reduced insulin secretion – was explored in a study by van Hooff[48] where patients with NODAT had the steroid dose reduced followed by minimization of tacrolimus. This resulted in increased insulin sensitivity followed by a sequential increase in insulin secretion.[48] The DIRECT study compared cyclosporine- and tacrolimus-based regimens in de novo transplantation and showed conclusively, in a study with NODAT as the primary endpoint, that tacrolimus-based therapy was associated with a higher incidence of NODAT, and of NODAT that required pharmacological management. Moreover, the study confirmed that tacrolimus use, compared with cyclosporine, was associated with reduced insulin secretion.[135]

Previously viewed as a nuisance, NODAT is now known to have long-term implications for patients, and is associated with a two- to threefold increase in all-cause mortality and CVEs.[18,107,141] Figure 30-9 shows data from our own unit on the impact of NODAT, with outcomes beyond 7 years after transplantation that are comparable between patients with ESRD due to diabetic nephropathy and those who developed NODAT.[107] Data from Hjelmesaeth and colleagues in Norway[40] and from Kasiske's studies in the United States[67] have shown that CV disease is the major cause of death; the risk is increased threefold in patients developing NODAT. Recent studies that highlight the importance of NODAT have also shown that the risk to the patients far outweighs the risk associated with acute rejection in the first year after

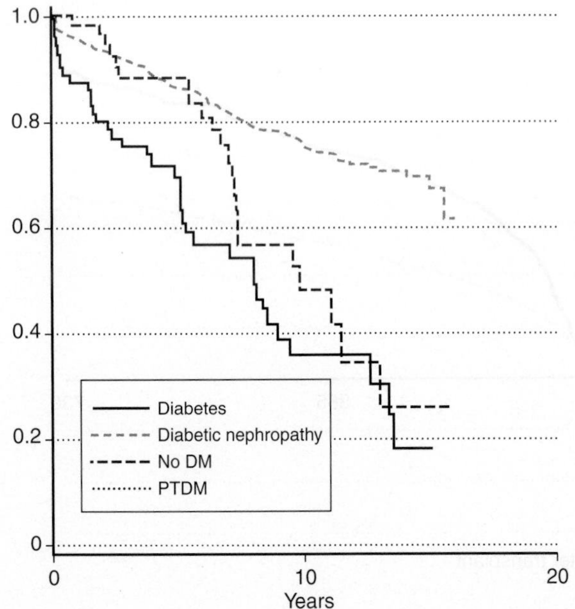

FIGURE 30-9 ■ Long-term survival of renal transplant recipients without diabetes (- - - - -), with diabetes at the time of transplantation (diabetic nephropathy, ———), and those who developed posttransplant diabetes mellitus (PTDM, ...), demonstrating an increased cardiovascular risk, matching those with pre-existing diabetes, in patients with PTDM. (Data from Revanur VK, Jardine AG, Kingsmore DB, et al. Influence of diabetes mellitus on patient and graft survival in recipients of kidney transplantation. Clin Transplant 2001;15:89–94.)

transplantation.[141] Thus, strategies to limit the incidence and impact of NODAT have emerged as a major target in the prevention of CVD. Guidelines have endorsed regular screening,[11] with the use of oral glucose tolerance tests (if practical) and regular fasting glucose measurements in transplant follow-up to identify patients with NODAT, and its precursor, impaired glucose tolerance. Studies, again from Hjaelmesaeth and colleagues,[81] have shown that minimization of steroids (with rapid tapering to 5 mg prednisolone daily) can reverse NODAT and impaired glucose tolerance in a large proportion of patients. Steroid-free regimens are associated with reduced incidence of NODAT and may be preferred in patients at high risk of developing NODAT; as may the use of cyclosporine rather than tacrolimus.[135,141] The management of NODAT is similar to that of type 2 diabetes in the general population. A proportion of patients who develop severe hypoglycemia, particularly early after transplantation, require insulin as primary therapy (although it may not be required in the long term, if immunosuppression is tailored appropriately), whereas those with milder hyperglycemia may be managed with diet and oral agents.[141] The available guidelines concur on the importance of monitoring for long-term complications of diabetes and early involvement of diabetic services.[141]

OBESITY AND THE METABOLIC SYNDROME

The metabolic syndrome is defined as the presence of three of the following: hyperglycemia, hypertriglyceridemia, low HDL cholesterol, hypertension, and high body mass index. As one would predict, given the high prevalence of diabetes and the individual components, the metabolic syndrome is common in RTR.[11,20,22,54] Data from the PORT study[54] report a prevalence of 40% in the second year after transplantation and 35% in the fourth year after transplantation. Studies have demonstrated an increased risk of developing diabetes in patients with the metabolic syndrome without diabetes, and also an increased risk of CVD, and of graft loss.[11,20,22,54] Whilst there is argument about the relative importance of the metabolic syndrome compared to its individual components,[22] Israni and colleagues[54] report an association with graft loss and CHD that is independent of NODAT.

Obesity is increasingly common, reflecting the trends in the wider population.[103] Morbid obesity is associated with a higher incidence of technical complications around the time of transplant surgery. However, the relationship with long-term outcomes is more complex. There is a non-linear relationship between weight and all-cause mortality, reflecting the impact of comorbidity, whilst obese patients exhibit a progressive increase in CV risk. Some centers have employed weight reduction surgery[77] as part of the workup for inclusion on to the waiting list for transplantation, although whether this improves patient outcomes remains to be established.

OTHER RISK FACTORS AND INTERVENTIONS

There are other strategies for the prevention of CV risk in the general population. Patients with ESRD have very poor exercise capacity, which should improve following transplantation. However, exercise and improvement in objective measures of exercise capacity (such as VO_{2max}) may require active encouragement in transplant recipients who often find barriers to engagement in exercise, both physical and psychological, which are related to protracted disability and ill health. There are several studies which have shown the association of poor exercise capacity with adverse CV outcomes following transplantation,[59,92,110] and a small interventional study which showed potential benefits, albeit without significant modification of conventional CV factors.[91] Exercise and weight loss are part of the general advice recommended in guidelines about post-transplant management.[36,68]

Novel factors which are associated with CVD in the general population, including C-reactive protein, inflammation, oxidative stress, hyperhomocystinemia, and elevated serum phosphate, have not been widely studied in RTR. However, in the recent past there have been studies showing association of a wide variety of biomarkers with CV and related outcomes. These include circulating inhibitors of nitric oxide,[2,3] elevated phosphate, FGF-23, osteoprotegerin,[34,78,125,127,143] oxidative stress,[4,129] endothelin,[104] paraoxonase,[128] and hyperuricemia.[17] Whether these are independent markers and therapeutic targets remains to be resolved. In addition to exercise there is interest in functional factors, such as depression, which are associated with outcome and are potentially remediable.[147]

SCREENING

Clearly, with CVD in RTR being a common cause of morbidity, mortality, and graft loss posttransplant and with considerations relating to equitable distribution of organs, interest has focused on screening patients for CVD prior to transplantation. The aims of this approach are to identify patients for whom the risk of transplantation outweighs the risks associated with maintenance dialysis.[31,96,137] In reality, there are very few patients for whom successful transplantation would not offer a survival advantage,[144] and the decision on whether to list someone for transplantation is largely subjective.[96] CV screening in some form is performed in most units with the aim of identifying CAD that can be corrected prior to transplantation.[31,96,137] Whilst this seems a laudable aim and one which may benefit patients regardless of whether they are ultimately transplanted, in the United Kingdom cardiologists have become reluctant to recommend coronary revascularization in asymptomatic patients in the light of the COURAGE trial, which showed no benefit over medical therapy.[12] Moreover, the high prevalence of calcified lesions makes coronary revascularization challenging.[75] In our own center, the delay to wait-listing inherent in a screening program did not benefit patients and those with coronary disease were less likely to be listed and unlikely to undergo coronary intervention. One consistent observation in screening programs is that the intervention rate is low – around 5% of all those screened ultimately undergo revascularization.[96]

Thus, there is little to support routine screening of asymptomatic patients based on the available literature, and a general view that a trial of screening is required but unlikely to be performed. In the absence of these data, some form of screening is popular. This generally involves echocardiography or some assessment of left ventricular structure and function, together with a "stress test" to look for reversible ischemia.[31,137] Conventional exercise tests are difficult to interpret due to a high prevalence of electrocardiographic abnormalities in patients receiving maintenance dialysis and poor exercise capacity. Pharmacological stress tests are commonly performed, with echocardiography or nuclear imaging, to look for regions of reversible ischemia.[31,137] Coronary angiography, with or without intervention, is typically reserved for those with positive non-invasive tests or who are at particularly high risk.[31,96,137] A trial to test the benefits of CV screening prior to transplantation has been proposed.[66]

INTERVENTION AND SECONDARY PREVENTION

Just as the likelihood of intervention after screening is low, there is concern that RTRs are less likely to receive intervention for aMI (thrombolysis or primary revascularization) or secondary preventions (high-dose statin therapy, antiplatelet agents, plus blockade of the renin–angiotensin system) proven in the general population. This is particularly true in patients with advanced CKD, but beyond the early postoperative period the general consensus, endorsed in guidelines, is that RTRs should receive the same intervention and management as the general population.[66] Data in the population with CKD do suggest that there is increasing use of primary revascularization in this population, albeit lagging behind the general population. It may be prudent to delay the introduction of new treatments in high-risk populations, such as RTRs at higher risk of complications, and so the reported pattern of introduction probably reflects cautious practice.

The data in Figure 30-10, collated by Henry and Herzog[38] in the United States, show that RTRs have a substantial risk of mortality following coronary interventions, but a risk that is considerably better than that of patients receiving maintenance dialysis. The PORT study,[101] which examined the use of CV risk medications, suggests that the use of risk factor medications (Figure 30-6), including those used for secondary prevention, has increased year by year, with the pattern of adoption and use following that in the general population. A similar pattern of increasing use has been reported by Lentine and colleagues[72] for secondary prevention following myocardial infarction and in other populations.[32]

Overall, the message for RTR is that patients should not be denied revascularization and secondary prevention for CAD. Although there does appear to be an increase in mortality, compared to non-transplant recipients, associated with revascularization procedures (specifically bypass surgery and vein grafting) the mortality risk is much less than that associated with patients with ESRD receiving dialysis.

OTHER CARDIOVASCULAR CONDITIONS

In this chapter, we have focused on CHD and the common patterns of CVD and risk that affect RTR. However, RTRs are also at increased risk of the common valvular conditions and arrhythmias. There are limited data on their incidence and management. Calcific aortic stenosis is common in patients with ESRD and progresses more rapidly in parallel with the development of vascular calcification.[10,117] The incidence of infective endocarditis is increased, reflecting the higher prevalence of valvular abnormalities and concomitant immunosuppression.[118] The management of valvular disease and endocarditis in RTR is the same as in the general population. Again, the risk associated with valve replacement is higher in RTR but better than that of patients with ESRD receiving maintenance dialysis.[10,117]

Recent data suggest that the risk of developing atrial fibrillation is increased in CKD, including RTR, and associated with CV risk.[87] RTRs are likely to benefit from rate control and anticoagulant therapy and there is no reason to withhold this therapy, proven in other populations.

PREDICTING CARDIOVASCULAR RISK

In the general population we predict CV risk based on established factors and calculations. The most commonly used is the Framingham risk factor calculator, or its derivatives. This has not proved appropriate for patients

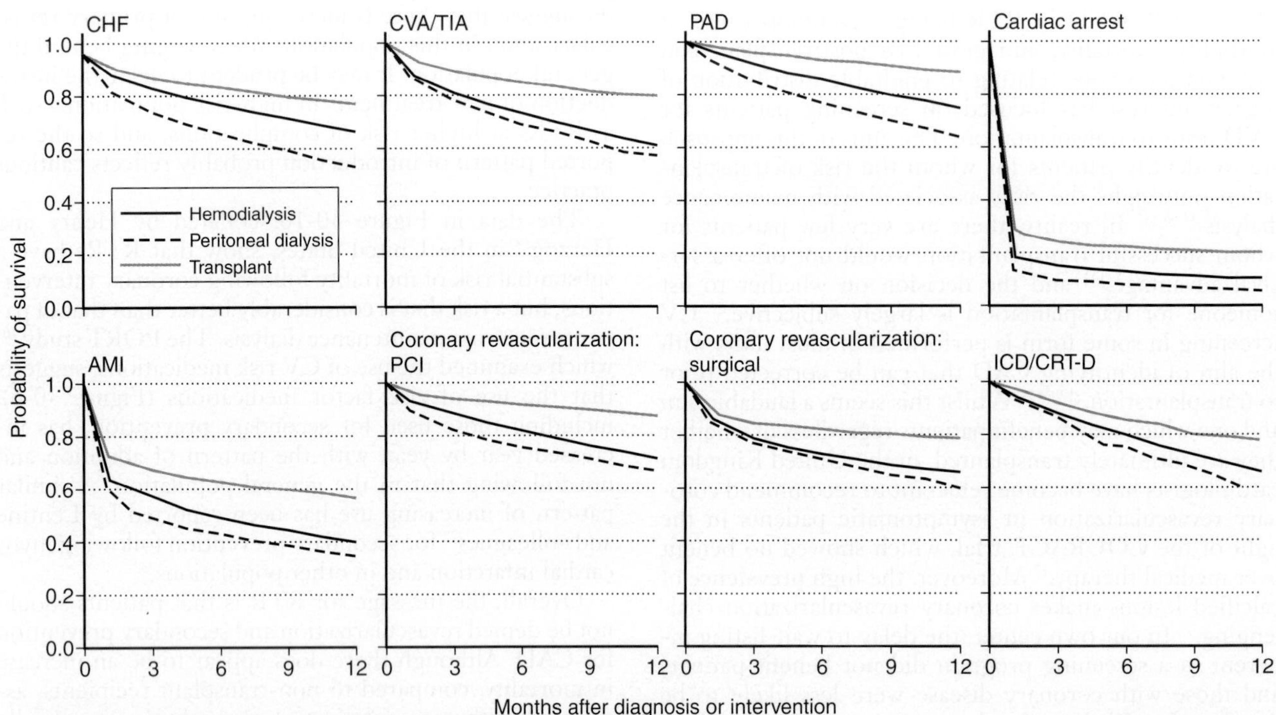

FIGURE 30-10 ■ **Mortality for individual cardiac interventions for patients with end-stage renal disease (ESRD), subdivided by modality. In all cases, patients with a transplant have better outcomes. CHF, congestive heart failure; CVA/TIA, cerebrovascular accident/transient ischemic attack; PAD, peripheral arterial disease; AMI, acute myocardial infarction; PCI, percutaneous coronary intervention; ICD/CRT-D, implantable cardiodefibrillator/cardiac resynchronization device.** (Data from Henry TD, Herzog CA. Bad kidneys are bad for the heart. Catheter Cardiovasc Interv 2012;80:358–60.)

with CKD, including transplant recipients,[63,65,119] reflecting the atypical nature of CVD. Recently, using data from the ALERT study, we have derived a CV risk factor calculator from data in RTR.[122,123] There are limitations – notably, that all patients were treated with cyclosporine – and it has yet to be independently verified. However, it performed well on internal validation. The factors included in the calculator are: age, diabetes, LDL cholesterol, serum creatinine, smoking status, pre-existing CHD, and the number of transplants. The details of the calculator are shown in Figure 30-11. Prospective collection of risk factor data and validation within existing datasets should allow the derivation of more accurate calculators for transplant recipients in the future.

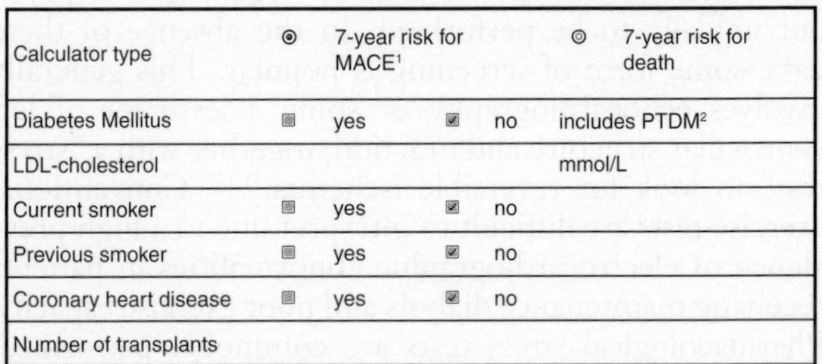

Calculator type	◉ 7-year risk for MACE¹		◎ 7-year risk for death
Diabetes Mellitus	yes	no	includes PTDM²
LDL-cholesterol			mmol/L
Current smoker	yes	no	
Previous smoker	yes	no	
Coronary heart disease	yes	no	
Number of transplants			
Creatinine		◉ µmol/L	◎ mg/dL
Age			years
7-year risk for MACE			

MACE¹ - major adverse cardiac event
PTDM¹ - post transplant diabetes mellitus

The use of this calculator requires clinical judgement and depends on context

FIGURE 30-11 ■ **Cardiovascular risk calculator for renal transplant recipients.** (Data from Soveri I, Holme I, Holdaas H, et al. A cardiovascular risk calculator for renal transplant recipients. Transplantation 2011;94:57–62. Access online at: http://www.anst.uu.se/insov254/calculator/.)

TRIAL END-POINTS

Clinical trials of immunosuppression in transplantation have, for the most part, concentrated on graft-specific end-points and the current favored Food and Drug Administration end-point of acute rejection, graft loss, death, or loss to follow-up, and to short timescales of up to 12 months. Whilst these are dictated by the need to develop drugs in a timely manner, they fail to address long-term patient-specific issues, and ignore observations that, for example, the development of NODAT has a greater negative impact on patient survival than an acute rejection episode.[123,141]

One way to address the importance of CV disease in transplantation would be to include CVEs in trial design, perhaps as a part of a patient-specific composite end-point. Such a strategy would probably require larger trials, with longer follow-up, that might limit the applicability of this design. An alternative approach is to model the expected CV effects of a particular immunosuppressive strategy, based on data available at earlier time points. For example, two recent studies have attempted to predict long-term outcomes based on short-term data.[115,123] Whilst the validity of this approach requires to be established, reporting of accurate risk factor data – blood pressure, lipid levels, renal function, and NODAT – should be a minimum requirement of trials in transplantation.

CONCLUSION

In writing this chapter we reviewed previous editions of this textbook, specifically the chapter by Professor Tony Raine in the fourth edition, that is now almost 20 years old. His review focused on atherosclerotic CV disease and highlighted the need for trials of lipid-lowering therapy. In the intervening 20 years we have completed trials of lipid-lowering therapy in transplant recipients and patients with CKD, including patients who received transplants. These have shown that statins are effective in the prevention of atherosclerotic events but that atherosclerotic coronary disease is only one component of the complex accelerated CV disease in this population. We have made much less progress on the prevention or treatment of uremic cardiomyopathy, and other complications of hypertension in RTR, and a trial of antihypertensive therapy and blood pressure targets is still required. There have been major changes in immunosuppression over the last 20 years, and we now have a spectrum of agents with differing immunosuppressive actions and side effect profiles. This may permit tailoring of immunosuppression to minimize the risk of long-term complications – including CV disease risk – but, at present, the clinical community continues to focus on rejection and immunological risk when selecting immunosuppressive strategies. A future change in the design and conduct of clinical trials in transplantation to recognize the importance of the major "end-points" for patients – CVD, malignancy and infection, as well as rejection and graft survival – might focus attention on the importance of immunosuppressive choice.

Regardless, and despite the increasing age of transplant recipients, their increasing comorbidity, and other changes to the transplant population that may have been predicted to worsen outcome, there has been a progressive reduction in CVD in the transplant population (Figure 30-12[100]). This follows the pattern of CVD across the developed world, reflecting improved understanding of CVD and lifestyle improvements, and may reflect the improved management of RTR in general, together with the progressive uptake of cardioprotective mechanisms. It is an encouraging observation and provides a positive point on which to finish. However, the absolute rate of CVD remains high and must remain a priority for those involved in renal transplantation. Given the accrued burden of risk that many patients have at the time of transplantation, the most important message is the need to consider the prevention of posttransplant CVD when one first encounters a patient with progressive primary renal disease at the renal clinic.

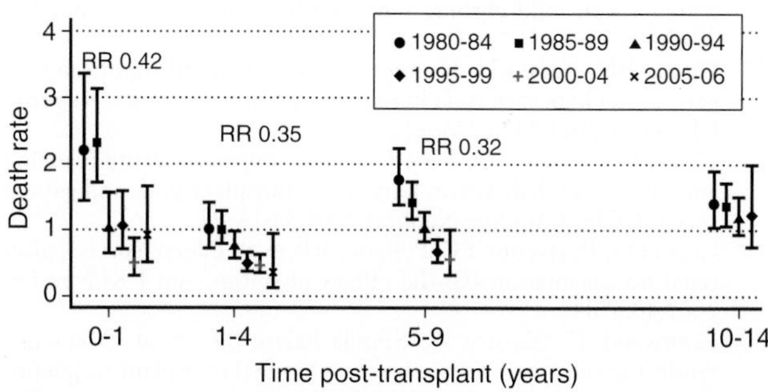

FIGURE 30-12 ■ Changing pattern of cardiovascular disease (CVD) survival in the ANZDATA Registry by era. Cardiovascular survival can be seen to have improved over the eras studied. RR, relative risk. (Data from Pilmore H, Dent H, Chang S, et al. Reduction in cardiovascular death after kidney transplantation. Transplantation 2010;89:851–7.)

REFERENCES

1. Abbott KC, Hypolite IO, Hshieh P, et al. Hospitalized congestive heart failure after renal transplantation in the United States. Ann Epidemiol 2002;12:115–22.
2. Abedini S, Holme I, März W, et al. Inflammation in renal transplantation. Clin J Am Soc Nephrol 2009;4:1246–54.
3. Abedini S, Meinitzer A, Holme I, et al. Asymmetrical dimethylarginine is associated with renal and cardiovascular outcomes and all-cause mortality in renal transplant recipients. Kidney Int 2010;77:44–50.
4. Abedini S, Norby GE, Holme I, et al. Inflammation-associated graft loss in renal transplant recipients. Nephrol Dial Transplant 2011;26:3756–61.
5. Agarwal PK, Hellemons ME, Zelle DM, et al. Smoking is a risk factor for graft failure and mortality after renal transplantation. Am J Nephrol 2011;34:26–31.
6. Agena F, Prado Edos S, Souza PS, et al. Home blood pressure (BP) monitoring in kidney transplant recipients is more adequate to monitor BP than office BP. Nephrol Dial Transplant 2011;26:3745–9.
7. Bachelet-Rousseau C, Kearney-Schwartz A, Frimat L, et al. Evolution of arterial stiffness after kidney transplantation. Nephrol Dial Transplant 2011;26:3386–91.
8. Baigent C, Burbury K, Wheeler D. Premature cardiovascular disease in chronic renal failure. Lancet 2000;356:147–52.
9. Baigent C, Landray MJ, Reith C, et al. The effects of lowering LDL cholesterol with simvastatin plus ezetimibe in patients with chronic kidney disease (Study of Heart and Renal Protection): a randomised placebo-controlled trial. Lancet 2011;377:2181–92.
10. Bakri K, Goldsmith DJ. Accelerated progression of calcific aortic stenosis in dialysis patients: what we still need to learn. Nephron Clin Pract 2003;94:c27–8.
11. Bayer ND, Cochetti PT, Anil Kumar MS, et al. Association of metabolic syndrome with development of new-onset diabetes after transplantation. Transplantation 2010;90:861–6.
12. Boden WE, O'Rourke RA, Teo KK, et al. Optimal medical therapy with or without PCI for stable coronary disease. N Engl J Med 2007;356:1503–16.
13. Bostom AG, Carpenter MA, Kusek JW, et al. Homocysteine-lowering and cardiovascular disease outcomes in kidney transplant recipients: primary results from the folic acid for vascular outcome reduction in transplantation trial. Circulation 2011;123:1763–70.
14. Budde K, Becker T, Arns W, et al. Everolimus-based, calcineurin-inhibitor-free regimen in recipients of de-novo kidney transplants: an open-label, randomised, controlled trial. Lancet 2011;377:837–47.
15. Campistol JM, de Fijter JW, Nashan B, et al. Everolimus and long-term outcomes in renal transplantation. Transplantation 2011;92:S3–26.

16. Chonchoi M, Cook M, Kjekshus J, et al. Simvastatin for secondary prevention of all-cause mortality and major coronary events in patients with mild chronic renal insufficiency. Am J Kidney Dis 2007;49:373–82.
17. Chung BH, Kang SH, Hwang HS, et al. Clinical significance of early-onset hyperuricemia in renal transplant recipients. Nephron Clin Pract 2011;117:c276–83.
18. Cole EH, Johnston O, Rose CL, et al. Impact of acute rejection and new-onset diabetes on long-term transplant graft and patient survival. Clin J Am Soc Nephrol 2008;3:814–21.
19. Cosio FG, Pesavento TE, Pelletier RP, et al. Patient survival after renal transplantation III: the effects of statins. Am J Kidney Dis 2002;40:63843.
20. Courivaud C, Kazory A, Simula-Faivre D, et al. Metabolic syndrome and atherosclerotic events in renal transplant recipients. Transplantation 2007;83:1577–81.
21. Cross NB, Webster AC, Masson P, et al. Antihypertensives for kidney transplant recipients: systematic review and meta-analysis of randomized controlled trials. Transplantation 2009;88:7–18.
22. de Vries AP, Bakker SJ, van Son WJ, et al. Metabolic syndrome is associated with impaired long-term renal allograft function; not all component criteria contribute equally. Am J Transplant 2004;4:1675–83.
23. Ekberg H, Bernasconi C, Tedesco-Silva H, et al. Calcineurin inhibitor minimization in the Symphony study: observational results 3 years after transplantation. Am J Transplant 2009;9: 1876–85.
24. Ekberg H, Tedesco-Silva H, Demirbas A, et al. Reduced exposure to calcineurin inhibitors in renal transplantation. N Engl J Med 2007;357:2562–75.
25. Fellstrom B, Holdaas H, Jardine AG, et al. Risk factors for reaching renal endpoints in the Assessment of Lescol in Renal Transplantation (ALERT) trial. Transplantation 2005;79:205–12.
26. Fellstrom BC, Jardine AG, Schmieder RE, et al. Rosuvastatin and cardiovascular events in patients undergoing hemodialysis. N Engl J Med 2009;360:1395–407.
27. Fellstrom B, Jardine AG, Soveri I, et al. Renal dysfunction is a strong and independent risk factor for mortality and cardiovascular complications in renal transplantation. Am J Transplant 2005;5:1986–91.
28. Foley RN, Parfrey PS, Harnett JD, et al. The prognostic importance of left ventricular geometry in uremic cardiomyopathy. J Am Soc Nephrol 1995;5:2024–31.
29. Foley RN, Parfrey PS, Sarnak MJ. Clinical epidemiology of cardiovascular disease in chronic renal disease. Am J Kidney Dis 1998;32:S112–9.
30. Fox CS, Muntner P, Chen AY, et al. Use of evidence-based therapies in short-term outcomes of ST-segment elevation myocardial infarction and non-ST-segment elevation myocardial infarction in patients with chronic kidney disease: a report from the National Cardiovascular Data Acute Coronary Treatment and Intervention Outcomes Network Registry. Circulation 2010;121:357–65.
31. Galvão De Lima JJ, Wolff Gowdak LH, de Paula FJ, et al. The role of myocardial scintigraphy in the assessment of cardiovascular risk in patients with end-stage chronic kidney disease on the waiting list for renal transplantation. Nephrol Dial Transplant 2012;27:2979–84.
32. Gaston RS, Kasiske BL, Fieberg AM, et al. Use of cardioprotective medications in kidney transplant recipients. Am J Transplant 2009;9:1811–5.
33. Gissi-HF Investigators, Tavazzi L, Maggioni AP, et al. Effect of rosuvastatin in patients with chronic heart failure (the GISSI-HF trial): a randomised, double-blind, placebo-controlled trial. Lancet 2008;372:1231–9.
34. Gungor O, Kismali E, Sisman AR, et al. The relationships between serum sTWEAK, FGF-23 levels, and carotid atherosclerosis in renal transplant patients. Ren Fail 2013;35:77–81.
35. Haydar AA, Covic A, Jayawardene S, et al. Insights from ambulatory blood pressure monitoring: diagnosis of hypertension and diurnal blood pressure in renal transplant recipients. Transplantation 2004;77:849–53.
36. Heemann U, Abramowicz D, Spasovski G, et al. Endorsement of the kidney disease improving global outcomes (KDIGO) guidelines on kidney transplantation: a European renal best practice (ERBP) position statement. Nephrol Dial Transplant 2011;26:2099–106.
37. Heinze G, Mitterbauer C, Regele H, et al. Angiotensin-converting enzyme inhibitor or angiotensin II type 1 receptor antagonist therapy is associated with prolonged patient and graft survival after renal transplantation. J Am Soc Nephrol 2006;17:889–99.
38. Henry TD, Herzog CA. Bad kidneys are bad for the heart. Catheter Cardiovasc Interv 2012;80:358–60.
39. Hjelmesaeth J, Hagen LT, Asberg A, et al. The impact of short-term ciclosporin a treatment on insulin secretion and insulin sensitivity in man. Nephrol Dial Transplant 2007;22:1743–9.
40. Hjelmesaeth J, Hartmann A, Leivestad T, et al. The impact of early-diagnosed new-onset post-transplantation diabetes mellitus on survival and major cardiac events. Kidney Int 2006;69:588–95.
41. Holdaas H, Fellstrom B, Cole E, et al. Long-term cardiac outcomes in renal transplant recipients receiving fluvastatin: the ALERT extension study. Am J Transplant 2005;5:2929–36.
42. Holdaas H, Fellström B, Jardine AG, et al. Beneficial effect of early initiation of lipid-lowering therapy following renal transplantation. Nephrol Dial Transplant 2005;20:974–80.
43. Holdaas H, Fellstrom B, Jardine AG, et al. Effect of fluvastatin on cardiac outcomes in renal transplant recipients: a multicentre, randomised, placebo-controlled trial. Lancet 2003;361:2024–31.
44. Holdaas H, Jardine AG, Wheeler DC, et al. Effect of fluvastatin on acute renal allograft rejection: a randomized multicenter trial. Kidney Int 2001;60:1990–7.
45. Holdaas H, Kobashigawa JA, Fellstrom B, et al. Special transplant populations: transplant recipients. In: Ballantyne CM, editor. Clinical lipidology. Philadelphia: Elsevier; 2008. p. 486–99.
46. Holdaas H, Rostaing L, Serón D, et al. Conversion of long-term kidney transplant recipients from calcineurin inhibitor therapy to everolimus: a randomized, multicenter, 24-month study. Transplantation 2011;92:410–8.
47. Holme I, Fellstrom BC, Jardine AG, et al. Model comparisons for competing risks and recurrent events for graft failure in renal transplant recipients. Clin J Am Soc Nephrol 2013;8:241–7.
48. Hooff JP, Christiaans MH, van Duijnhoven EM. Tacrolimus and post-transplant diabetes mellitus in renal transplantation. Transplantation 2005;79:1465–9.
49. Hoorn EJ, Walsh SB, McCormick JA, et al. Pathogenesis of calcineurin inhibitor-induced hypertension. J Nephrol 2012;25:269–75.
50. Hornum M, Clausen P, Idorn T, et al. Kidney transplantation improves arterial function measured by pulse wave analysis and endothelium-independent dilatation in uraemic patients despite deterioration of glucose metabolism. Nephrol Dial Transplant 2011;26:2370–7.
51. Hurst FP, Altieri M, Patel PP, et al. Effect of smoking on kidney transplant outcomes: analysis of the United States Renal Data System. Transplantation 2011;92:1101–7.
52. Ibernon M, Moreso F, Sarrias X, et al. Reverse dipper pattern of blood pressure at 3 months is associated with inflammation and outcome after renal transplantation. Nephrol Dial Transplant 2012;27:2089–95.
53. Ignace S, Utescu MS, De Serres SA, et al. Age-related and blood pressure-independent reduction in aortic stiffness after kidney transplantation. J Hypertens 2011;29:130–6.
54. Israni AJ, Snyder JJ, Skeans MA, et al. Clinical diagnosis of metabolic syndrome: predicting new-onset diabetes, coronary heart disease and allograft failure late after kidney transplantation. Transpl Int 2012;25:748–57.
55. Israni AK, Snyder JJ, Skeans MA, et al. Predicting coronary heart disease after kidney transplantation: Patient Outcomes in Renal Transplantation (PORT) study. Am J Transplant 2010;10:338–53.
56. Jardine AG, Fellstrom B, Logan JO, et al. Cardiovascular risk and renal transplantation: post hoc analyses of the assessment of lescol in renal transplantation (ALERT) study. Am J Kidney Dis 2005;46:529–36.
57. Jardine AG, Gaston RS, Fellstrom BC, et al. Prevention of cardiovascular disease in adult recipients of kidney transplants. Lancet 2011;378:1419–27.
58. Jardine A, Holdaas H. Fluvastatin in combination with cyclosporin in renal transplant recipients: a review of clinical and safety experience. J Clin Pharm Ther 1999;24:397–408.
59. Johansen KL, Painter P. Exercise in individuals with CKD. Am J Kidney Dis 2012;59:126–34.

60. Johnson RW, Kreis H, Oberbauer R, et al. Sirolimus allows early cyclosporine withdrawal in renal transplantation resulting in improved renal function and lower blood pressure. Transplantation 2001;72:777–86.
61. Johnston O, Rose CL, Webster AC, et al. Sirolimus is associated with new-onset diabetes in kidney transplant recipients. J Am Soc Nephrol 2008;19:1411–8.
62. Joss N, Staatz CE, Thomson AH, et al. Predictors of new onset diabetes after renal transplantation. Clin Transplant 2007;21:136–43.
63. Kasiske BL, Chakkera HA, Roel J. Explained and unexplained ischemic heart disease risk after renal transplantation. J Am Soc Nephrol 2000;11:1735–43.
64. Kasiske BL, de MA, Flechner SM, et al. Mammalian target of rapamycin inhibitor dyslipidemia in kidney transplant recipients. Am J Transplant 2008;8:1384–92.
65. Kasiske BL, Guijarro C, Massy ZA, et al. Cardiovascular disease after renal transplantation. J Am Soc Nephrol 1996;7:158–65.
66. Kasiske BL, Israni AK, Snyder JJ, et al. Design considerations and feasibility for a clinical trial to examine coronary screening before kidney transplantation (COST). Am J Kidney Dis 2011;57:908–16.
67. Kasiske BL, Klinger D. Cigarette smoking in renal transplant recipients. J Am Soc Nephrol 2000;11:753–9.
68. KDIGO clinical practice guideline for the care of kidney transplant recipients. Am J Transplant 2009;9(Suppl. 3):S1–155.
69. Knight SR, Morris PJ. Steroid avoidance or withdrawal after renal transplantation increases the risk of acute rejection but decreases cardiovascular risk. A meta-analysis. Transplantation 2010;89:1–14.
70. Knoll GA, Cantarovitch M, Cole E, et al. The Canadian ACE-inhibitor trial to improve renal outcomes and patient survival in kidney transplantation – study design. Nephrol Dial Transplant 2008;23:354–8.
71. Larsen CP, Grinyó J, Medina-Pestana J, et al. Belatacept-based regimens versus a cyclosporine A-based regimen in kidney transplant recipients: 2-year results from the BENEFIT and BENEFIT-EXT studies. Transplantation 2010;90:1528–35.
72. Lentine KL, Villines TC, Xiao H, et al. Cardioprotective medication use after acute myocardial infarction in kidney transplant recipients. Transplantation 2011;91:1120–6.
73. Liu Y, Coresh J, Eustace JA, et al. Association between cholesterol level and mortality in dialysis patients. JAMA 2004;291:451–9.
74. Mangray M, Vella JP. Hypertension after kidney transplant. Am J Kidney Dis 2011;57:331–41.
75. Maréchal C, Coche E, Goffin E, et al. Progression of coronary artery calcification and thoracic aorta calcification in kidney transplant recipients. Am J Kidney Dis 2012;59:258–69.
76. Mark PB, Johnston N, Groenning BA, et al. Redefinition of uremic cardiomyopathy by contrast-enhanced cardiac magnetic resonance imaging. Kidney Int 2006;69:1839–45.
77. Marszałek R, Ziemia ski P, Lisik W, et al. Bariatric surgery as a bridge for kidney transplantation in obese subjects. Ann Transplant 2012;17:108–12.
78. Mazzaferro S, Pasquali M, Pugliese F, et al. Distinct impact of vitamin D insufficiency on calcitriol levels in chronic renal failure and renal transplant patients: a role for FGF23. J Nephrol 2012;25:1108–18.
79. McGregor EM, Jardine AG, Dargie HJ, et al. Echocardiographic abnormalities and survival following renal transplantation. Nephrol Dial Transplant 1998;13:1499–505.
80. Meier-Kriesche HU, Baliga R, Kaplan B. Decreased renal function is a strong risk factor for cardiovascular death after renal transplantation. Transplantation 2003;75:1291–5.
81. Midtvedt K, Hjelmesaeth J, Hartmann A, et al. Insulin resistance after renal transplantation: the effect of steroid dose reduction and withdrawal. J Am Soc Nephrol 2004;15:3233–9.
82. Midtvedt K, Ihlen H, Hartmann A, et al. Reduction of left ventricular mass by lisinopril and nifedipine in hypertensive renal transplant recipients: a prospective randomized double-blind study. Transplantation 2001;72:107–11.
83. Miller LW. Cardiovascular toxicities of immunosuppressive agents. Am J Transplant 2002;2:807–18.
84. Mjörnstedt L, Sørensen SS, von Zur Mühlen B, et al. Improved renal function after early conversion from a calcineurin inhibitor to everolimus: a randomized trial in kidney transplantation. Am J Transplant 2012;12:2744–53.
85. Morris STW, McMurray JJV, Rodger RSC, et al. Endothelial dysfunction in renal transplant recipients maintained on cyclosporin. Kidney Int 2000;57:1100–6.
86. National Kidney Foundation. K/DOQI clinical practice guidelines for managing dyslipidemias in chronic kidney disease. Am J Kidney Dis 2003;41:S1–92.
87. Nelson SE, Shroff GR, Li S, et al. Impact of chronic kidney disease on risk of incident atrial fibrillation and subsequent survival in Medicare patients. J Am Heart Assoc 2012;1:e002097.
88. Opelz G, Döhler B. Collaborative Transplant Study. Improved long-term outcomes after renal transplantation associated with blood pressure control. Am J Transplant 2005;5:2725–31.
89. Opelz G, Ritz E. Association of chronic kidney graft failure with recipient blood pressure. Kidney Int 1998;53:217–22.
90. Opelz G, Zeier M, Laux G, et al. No improvement of patient or graft survival in transplant recipients treated with angiotensin-converting enzyme inhibitors or angiotensin II type 1 receptor blockers: a collaborative transplant study report. J Am Soc Nephrol 2006;17:3257–62.
91. Painter PL, Hector L, Ray K, et al. A randomized trial of exercise training after renal transplantation. Transplantation 2002;74:42–8.
92. Painter PL, Hector L, Ray K, et al. Effects of exercise training on coronary heart disease risk factors in renal transplant recipients. Am J Kidney Dis 2003;42:362–9.
93. Paoletti E, Cannella G. Regression of left ventricular hypertrophy in kidney transplant recipients: the potential role for inhibition of mammalian target of rapamycin. Transplant Proc 2010;42:S41–3.
94. Pascual J, Pérez-Sáez MJ, Mir M, et al. Chronic renal allograft injury: early detection, accurate diagnosis and management. Transplant Rev 2012;26:280–90.
95. Patel RK, Mark PB, Halliday C, et al. Microvolt T-wave alternans in end-stage renal disease patients – associations with uremic cardiomyopathy. Clin J Am Soc Nephrol 2011;6:519–27.
96. Patel RK, Mark PB, Johnston N, et al. Prognostic value of cardiovascular screening in potential renal transplant recipients: a single-center prospective observational study. Am J Transplant 2008;8:1673–83.
97. Patel RK, Mark PB, Johnston N, et al. Renal transplantation is not associated with regression of left ventricular hypertrophy: a magnetic resonance study. Clin J Am Soc Nephrol 2008;3:1807–11.
98. Patel RK, Oliver S, Mark PB, et al. Determinants of left ventricular mass and hypertrophy in hemodialysis patients assessed by cardiac magnetic resonance imaging. Clin J Am Soc Nephrol 2009;4:1477–83.
99. Philipp T, Martinez F, Geiger H, et al. Candesartan improves blood pressure control and reduces proteinuria in renal transplant recipients: results from SECRET. Nephrol Dial Transplant 2010;25:967–76.
100. Pilmore H, Dent H, Chang S, et al. Reduction in cardiovascular death after kidney transplantation. Transplantation 2010;89:851–7.
101. Pilmore HL, Skeans MA, Snyder JJ, et al. Cardiovascular disease medications after renal transplantation: results from the Patient Outcomes in Renal Transplantation study. Transplantation 2011;91:542–51.
102. Ponticelli C, Cucchiari D, Graziani G. Hypertension in kidney transplant recipients. Transpl Int 2011;24:523–33.
103. Potluri K, Hou S. Obesity in kidney transplant recipients and candidates. Am J Kidney Dis 2010;56:143–56.
104. Raina A, Horn ET, Benza RL. The pathophysiology of endothelin in complications after solid organ transplantation: a potential novel therapeutic role for endothelin receptor antagonists. Transplantation 2012;94:885–93.
105. Prasad RGV. Ambulatory blood pressure monitoring in solid organ transplantation. Clin Transplant 2012;26:185–91.
106. Recio-Mayoral A, Banerjee D, Streather C, et al. Endothelial dysfunction, inflammation and atherosclerosis in chronic kidney disease – a cross-sectional study of predialysis, dialysis and kidney-transplantation patients. Atherosclerosis 2011;216:446–51.
107. Revanur VK, Jardine AG, Kingsmore DB, et al. Influence of diabetes mellitus on patient and graft survival in recipients of kidney transplantation. Clin Transplant 2001;15:89–94.
108. Rigatto C, Parfrey P, Foley R, et al. Congestive heart failure in renal transplant recipients: risk factors, outcomes, and relationship with ischemic heart disease. J Am Soc Nephrol 2002;13:1084–90.

109. Roe P, Wolfe M, Joffe M, et al. Inflammation, coronary artery calcification and cardiovascular events in incident renal transplant recipients. Atherosclerosis 2010;212:589–94.
110. Rosas SE, Reese PP, Huan Y, et al. Pretransplant physical activity predicts all-cause mortality in kidney transplant recipients. Am J Nephrol 2012;35:17–23.
111. Rostaing L, Sánchez-Fructuoso A, Franco A, et al. Conversion to tacrolimus once-daily from ciclosporin in stable kidney transplant recipients: a multicenter study. Transpl Int 2012;25:391–400.
112. Sacks FM, Pfeffer MA, Moye LA, et al. The effect of pravastatin on coronary events after myocardial infarction in patients with average cholesterol levels. Cholesterol and Recurrent Events Trial Investigators. N Engl J Med 1996;335:1001–9.
113. Sarnak MJ, Levey AS, Schoolwerth AC, et al. Kidney disease as a risk factor for development of cardiovascular disease: a statement from the American Heart Association Councils on Kidney in Cardiovascular Disease, High Blood Pressure Research, Clinical Cardiology, and Epidemiology and Prevention. Circulation 2003;108:2154–69.
114. Scandinavian Simvastatin Survival Study (4S). Randomised trial of cholesterol lowering in 4444 patients with coronary heart disease. Lancet 1994;344:1383–9.
115. Schnitzler MA, Lentine KL, Axelrod D, et al. Use of 12-month renal function and baseline clinical factors to predict long-term graft survival: application to BENEFIT and BENEFIT-EXT trials. Transplantation 2012;9:172–81.
116. Shamseddin MK, Knoll GA. Posttransplantation proteinuria: an approach to diagnosis and management. Clin J Am Soc Nephrol 2011;6:1786–93.
117. Sharma A, Gilbertson DT, Herzog CA. Survival of kidney transplantation patients in the United States after cardiac valve replacement. Circulation 2010;121:2733–9.
118. Shroff GR, Skeans M, Herzog CA. Outcomes of renal transplant and waiting list patients with bacterial endocarditis in the United States. Nephrol Dial Transplant 2008;23:2381–5.
119. Silver SA, Huang M, Nash MM, et al. Framingham risk score and novel cardiovascular risk factors underpredict major adverse cardiac events in kidney transplant recipients. Transplantation 2011;92:183–9.
120. Skauby MH, Øyen O, Hartman A, et al. Kidney transplantation with and without simultaneous bilateral native nephrectomy in patients with polycystic kidney disease: a comparative retrospective study. Transplantation 2012;94:383–8.
121. Soveri I, Holdaas H, Jardine A, et al. Renal transplant dysfunction – importance quantified in comparison with traditional risk factors for cardiovascular disease and mortality. Nephrol Dial Transplant 2006;21:2282–9.
122. Soveri I, Holme I, Holdaas H, et al. A cardiovascular risk calculator for renal transplant recipients. Transplantation 2011;94:57–62.
123. Soveri I, Snyder J, Holdaas H, et al. The external validation of the cardiovascular risk equation for renal transplant recipients. Applications to BENEFIT and BENEFIT-EXT Trials. Transplantation 2013;95:142–7.
124. Srinivas TR, Meier-Kriesche HU. Minimizing immunosuppression, an alternative approach to reducing side effects: objectives and interim result. Clin J Am Soc Nephrol 2008;3(Suppl. 2):S101–16.
125. Stevens KK, Morgan IR, Patel RK, et al. Serum phosphate and outcome at one year after deceased donor renal transplantation. Clin Transplant 2011;25:E199–204.
126. Stewart GA, Gansevoort RT, Mark PB, et al. Electrocardiographic abnormalities and uremic cardiomyopathy. Kidney Int 2005;67:217–26.
127. Svensson M, Dahle DO, Mjøen G, et al. Osteoprotegerin as a predictor of renal and cardiovascular outcomes in renal transplant recipients: follow-up data from the ALERT study. Nephrol Dial Transplant 2012;27:2571–5.
128. Sztanek F, Seres I, Harangi M, et al. Decreased paraoxonase 1 (PON1) lactonase activity in hemodialyzed and renal transplanted patients. A novel cardiovascular biomarker in end-stage renal disease. Nephrol Dial Transplant 2012;27:2866–72.
129. Turkmen K, Tonbul HZ, Toker A, et al. The relationship between oxidative stress, inflammation, and atherosclerosis in renal transplant and end-stage renal disease patients. Ren Fail 2012;34:1229–37.
130. Tutone VK, Mark PB, Stewart GA, et al. Hypertension, antihypertensive agents and outcomes following renal transplantation. Clin Transplant 2005;19:181–92.
131. Vaidya OU, House JA, Coggins TR, et al. Effect of renal transplantation for chronic renal disease on left ventricular mass. Am J Cardiol 2012;110:254–7.
132. Vanrenterghem Y, Bresnahan B, Campistol J, et al. Belatacept-based regimens are associated with improved cardiovascular and metabolic risk factors compared with cyclosporine in kidney transplant recipients (BENEFIT and BENEFIT-EXT studies). Transplantation 2011;91:976–83.
133. Vanrenterghem YFC, Claes K, Montagnino G, et al. Risk factor for cardiovascular events after successful renal transplantation. Transplantation 2008;85:209–16.
134. Vaziri ND. Dyslipidaemia of chronic renal failure: the nature, mechanisms and potential consequences. Am J Physiol Renal Physiol 2006;290:F262–72.
135. Vincenti F, Friman S, Scheuermann E, et al. Results of an international, randomized trial comparing glucose metabolism disorders and outcome with cyclosporine versus tacrolimus. Am J Transplant 2007;7:1506–14.
136. Walker BR. Glucocorticoids and cardiovascular disease. Eur J Endocrinol 2007;157:545–59.
137. Wang LW, Fahim MA, Hayen A, et al. Cardiac testing for coronary artery disease in potential kidney transplant recipients. Cochrane Database Syst Rev 2011;12:CD008691.
138. Wanner C, Krane V, Marz W, et al. Atorvastatin in patients with type 2 diabetes mellitus undergoing hemodialysis. N Engl J Med 2005;353:238–48.
139. Wauters RP, Cosio FG, Suarez Fernandez ML, et al. Cardiovascular consequences of new-onset hyperglycemia after kidney transplantation. Transplantation 2012;94:377–82.
140. Weiner DE, Carpenter MA, Levey AS, et al. Kidney function and risk of cardiovascular disease and mortality in kidney transplant recipients: the FAVORIT trial. Am J Transplant 2012;12:2437–45.
141. Wilkinson A, Davidson J, Dotta F, et al. Guidelines for the treatment and management of new-onset diabetes after transplantation. Clin Transplant 2005;19:291–8.
142. Wissing KM, Unger P, Ghisdal L, et al. Effect of atorvastatin therapy and conversion to tacrolimus on hypercholesterolemia and endothelial dysfunction after renal transplantation. Transplantation 2006;82:771–8.
143. Wolf M, Molnar MZ, Amaral AP, et al. Elevated fibroblast growth factor 23 is a risk factor for kidney transplant loss and mortality. J Am Soc Nephrol 2011;22:956–66.
144. Wolfe RA, Ashby VB, Milford EL, et al. Comparison of mortality in all patients on dialysis, patients on dialysis awaiting transplantation, and recipients of a first cadaveric transplant. N Engl J Med 1999;341:1725–30.
145. Woodle ES, First MR, Pirsch J, et al. A prospective, randomized, double-blind, placebo-controlled multicenter trial comparing early (7 day) corticosteroid cessation versus long-term, low-dose corticosteroid therapy. Ann Surg 2008;248:564–77.
146. Woodward RS, Schnitzler MA, Baty J, et al. Incidence and cost of new onset diabetes mellitus among U.S. wait-listed and transplanted renal allograft recipients. Am J Transplant 2003;3:590–8.
147. Zelle DM, Dorland HF, Rosmalen JG, et al. Impact of depression on long-term outcome after renal transplantation: a prospective cohort study. Transplantation 2012;94:1033–40.

CHAPTER 31

INFECTION IN KIDNEY TRANSPLANT RECIPIENTS

Jay A. Fishman

CHAPTER OUTLINE

OVERVIEW

Successful management of infections in kidney transplant recipients is complicated by factors related to the immune status of the host and the epidemiology of infection.[57] Transplant recipients are susceptible to a broad spectrum of infectious pathogens while manifesting diminished signs and symptoms of invasive infection. Thus, the diagnosis of infection is more difficult in transplantation than in immunologically normal individuals. The interactions between infection, immunosuppression, and immune function play out in a complex environment in which multiple simultaneous processes, such as infection and graft rejection, may contribute to the clinical presentation. Immunocompromised patients tolerate invasive, established infection poorly with high morbidity and mortality, lending urgency to the need for an early, specific diagnosis to guide antimicrobial therapy. Given the T-lymphocyte dysfunction inherent to transplant immunosuppression, viral infections in particular are increased. These viral infections not only contribute to graft dysfunction, graft rejection, and systemic illness but also enhance the risk for other opportunistic infections (e.g., *Pneumocystis* and *Aspergillus*) and virally mediated cancers.

RISK OF INFECTION

The risk of infection in a kidney transplant recipient is determined by the interaction of two key factors:

1. The epidemiological exposures of the patient, including the timing, intensity, and virulence of the organisms experienced.
2. The patient's "net state of immunosuppression," a conceptual measure of all the factors that contribute to the host's risk for infection.[16,24]

The importance of any infectious exposure is determined by the ability of the host to "deal" effectively with the pathogen. Thus, the diabetic is at greater risk for bacterial skin infections than is a non-diabetic with calcineurin inhibitor therapy. An understanding of the risk factors for each transplant recipient allows the development of differential diagnoses for infectious syndromes, and the development of preventive strategies (prophylaxis, vaccination) appropriate to each individual's risk for infection.[3,4]

Epidemiological Exposures

Epidemiologic exposures of importance can be divided into four overlapping categories: (1) donor-derived infections; (2) recipient-derived infections; (3) community-derived exposures; and (4) nosocomial exposures (Table 31-1).

Donor-Derived Infections

Infections derived from donor tissues and activated in the recipient are uncommon, but have been recognized as among the important infectious exposures in transplantation. Some of these infections are latent (e.g., viral, parasitic), whereas others are the result of active infection (e.g., sepsis) in the donor at the time of procurement. Common pathogens and endemic organisms causing significant morbidity in potential recipients form the basis of screening paradigms for organ donors.[10,23,25,31,41]

Most types of infection have been recognized in transplant recipients at some point. Bacteremic or fungemic infections (e.g., *Staphylococcus aureus*, *Candida* species, Gram-negative bacteria) in donors at the time of donation can cause local (abscess) or systemic (bacteremic) infections, and may selectively adhere to anastomotic sites (vascular, urinary) to produce leaks or mycotic aneurysms. Some viral infections are ubiquitous, including cytomegalovirus (CMV) and Epstein–Barr virus (EBV), and are associated with particular syndromes and morbidity in the immunocompromised population (see section on selected infections of importance). The greatest risk of these infections is to seronegative (immunologically naïve) recipients who receive infected grafts from seropositive donors (latent viral infection). Some viruses demonstrate accelerated progression (lymphocytic choriomeningitis, lymphocytic choriomeningitis virus (LCMV), rabies) in transplant recipients. Latent infections, such as tuberculosis, toxoplasmosis, or strongyloidiasis, may activate from grafts many years after the initial, often unrecognized exposures.

Donor screening for transplantation is limited by the available technology and by the time available within which organs from deceased donors must be used.[25,31] At present, routine evaluation of donors relies on antibody detection (serological) tests for common infections. As a result, some active infections remain undetected because seroconversion may not occur during acute infection. These limitations suggest that, to achieve the benefits of transplantation, some organs are implanted carrying unidentified pathogens. This risk is exhibited by clusters of donor-derived *Trypanosoma cruzi* (Chagas' disease), rabies virus, West Nile virus, and LCMV infections in organ transplant recipients. Molecular assays for donor screening (e.g., for human immunodeficiency virus (HIV), hepatitis B virus (HBV), hepatitis C virus (HCV)) have the capacity to reduce the "window period" between exposure and development of a positive microbiological assay (nucleic acid test (NAT) instead of seroconversion) with some risk for false-positive assays given heightened NAT sensitivity.

Given the risk of transmission of infection from the organ donor to the recipient, certain infections should be considered relative contraindications to organ donation. Because kidney transplantation is typically elective surgery, it is reasonable to avoid donation from individuals with unexplained fever, rash, or infectious syndromes, including meningitis or encephalitis. Common criteria for exclusion of organ donors are listed in Table 31-2.

TABLE 31-1 Significant Epidemiological Exposures Relevant to Transplantation

Donor-Derived
Viral
Herpesvirus group (CMV, EBV, HHV-6, HHV-7, HHV-8, HSV)
Hepatitis viruses (HBV, HCV)
Retroviruses (HIV, HTLV-I/II)
Others (rabies, LCMV, West Nile)
Bacteria
Gram-positive and Gram-negative bacteria (*Staphylococcus*, *Pseudomonas*, Enterobacteriaceae)
Mycobacteria (tuberculous and non-tuberculous)
Nocardia asteroides
Fungi
Candida species
Aspergillus
Endemic fungi (*Cryptococcus neoformans*)
Geographic fungi (*Histoplasma capsulatum*, *Coccidioides immitis*, *Blastomyces dermatitidis*)
Parasites
Toxoplasma gondii
Trypanosoma cruzi
Nosocomial Exposures*
Methicillin-resistant *Staphylococcus aureus*
Vancomycin-resistant enterococci
ESBL Gram-negative bacilli
Aspergillus species
Non-*albicans Candida* species
Community Exposures*
Foodborne and water-borne (*Listeria monocytogenes*, *Salmonella*, *Cryptosporidium*, hepatitis A, *Campylobacter*)
Respiratory viruses (RSV, influenza, parainfluenza, adenovirus, metapneumovirus)
Common viruses, often with exposure to children (coxsackievirus, parvovirus, polyomavirus, papillomavirus)
Atypical respiratory pathogens (*Legionella*, *Mycoplasma*, *Chlamydia*)
Geographic fungi and *Cryptococcus*, *Pneumocystis jiroveci*
Parasites (often distant) (*Strongyloides stercoralis*, *Leishmania*, *Toxoplasma gondii*, *Trypanosoma cruzi*, *Naegleria fowleri*)

*Colonization and infection of the recipient in advance of transplantation may occur due to these potential pathogens.

CMV, cytomegalovirus; EBV, Epstein–Barr virus; ESBL, extended-spectrum beta-lactamase; HBV, hepatitis B virus; HCV, hepatitis C virus; HHV, human herpesvirus; HIV, human immunodeficiency virus; HSV, herpes simplex virus; HTLV, human T-cell lymphotropic virus; LCMV, lymphocytic choriomeningitis virus; RSV, respiratory syncytial virus.

Recipient-Derived Exposures

Recipient-derived exposures generally reflect colonization or latent infections that reactivate during immunosuppression. Certain common infections are recognized during the evaluation of the transplant candidate, including HBV, HCV, and HIV. It is necessary to obtain a

TABLE 31-2 Common Infectious Exclusion Criteria for Organ Donors*

Central Nervous System Infection
Unknown infection of central nervous system (encephalitis, meningitis)
Herpes simplex encephalitis or other encephalitis
History of JC virus infection
West Nile virus infection
Cryptococcal infection of any site
Rabies
Creutzfeldt–Jakob disease
Other fungal or viral encephalitis
Untreated bacterial meningitis (requires proof of cure)
Disseminated and Untreated Infections
HIV (serological or molecular) (may be considered for HIV-positive recipient?)
HSV (with active viremia), acute EBV (mononucleosis)
Serological or molecular evidence of HTLV-I/HTLV-II
Active hepatitis A (may consider non-viremic HBV and HCV-infected donors for appropriate recipients)
Parasitic infections (*Trypanosoma cruzi, Leishmania donovani, Strongyloides stercoralis, Toxoplasma gondii*)
Infections Difficult to Treat on Immunosuppression
Active tuberculosis
SARS
Untreated pneumonia
Untreated bacterial or fungal sepsis (e.g., candidemia)
Untreated syphilis
Multisystem organ failure due to overwhelming sepsis, gangrenous bowel

*These must be considered in the context of the individual donor/recipient.

EBV, Epstein–Barr virus; HBV, hepatitis B virus; HCV, hepatitis C virus; HIV, human immunodeficiency virus; HSV, herpes simplex virus; HTLV, human T-cell lymphotropic virus; SARS, severe acute respiratory syndrome.

careful history of prior infections, travel, and exposures to guide preventive strategies and empirical therapies. Notable among these infections are mycobacterial infection (including tuberculosis), strongyloidiasis, viral infections (herpes simplex virus (HSV) and varicella-zoster virus (VZV) or shingles), histoplasmosis, coccidioidomycosis, and paracoccidiomycosis (Figure 31-1). Vaccination status should be evaluated (tetanus, HBV, childhood vaccines, influenza, pneumococcus); vaccines not previously administered should be considered in advance of transplantation as live virus vaccines are contraindicated after transplantation (Table 31-3). Dietary habits also should be considered, including the use of well water (*Cryptosporidium*), uncooked meats (*Salmonella, Listeria*), and unpasteurized dairy products (*Listeria*).

Community Exposures

Common exposures in the community are often related to contaminated food and water ingestion; exposure to infected family members or coworkers; or exposures related to hobbies, travel, or work. Infection caused by common respiratory viruses (influenza, parainfluenza, respiratory syncytial virus (RSV), adenovirus, and metapneumovirus) and by more atypical pathogens (HSV) carry risk for viral pneumonia and increased risk for bacterial or fungal superinfections. Community (contact or transfusion-associated) exposure to CMV and EBV may produce severe primary infection in the non-immune host. Recent and remote exposures to endemic, geographically restricted systemic mycoses (*Blastomyces dermatitidis, Coccidioides immitis*, and *Histoplasma capsulatum*) and *Mycobacterium tuberculosis* can result in localized pulmonary, systemic, or metastatic infection. Asymptomatic *Strongyloides stercoralis* infection may activate more than 30 years after initial exposure due to immunosuppressive therapy (Figure 31-1). Such reactivation can result in either a diarrheal illness and parasite migration with hyperinfestation syndrome (characterized by hemorrhagic enterocolitis, hemorrhagic pneumonia, or both) or disseminated infection with accompanying (usually) Gram-negative bacteremia or meningitis. Gastroenteritis secondary to *Salmonella, Cryptosporidium*, and a variety

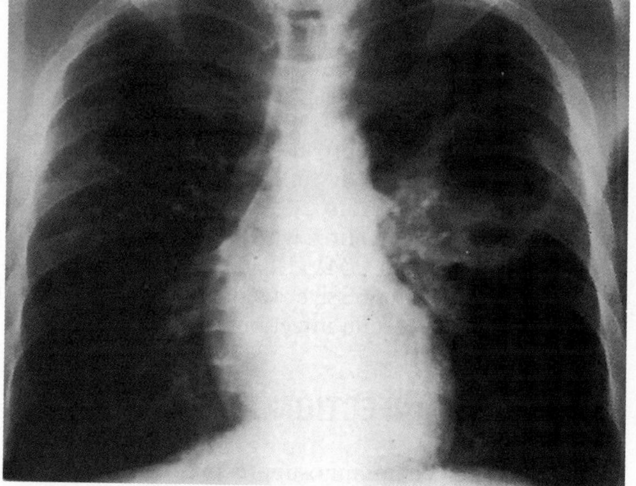
A

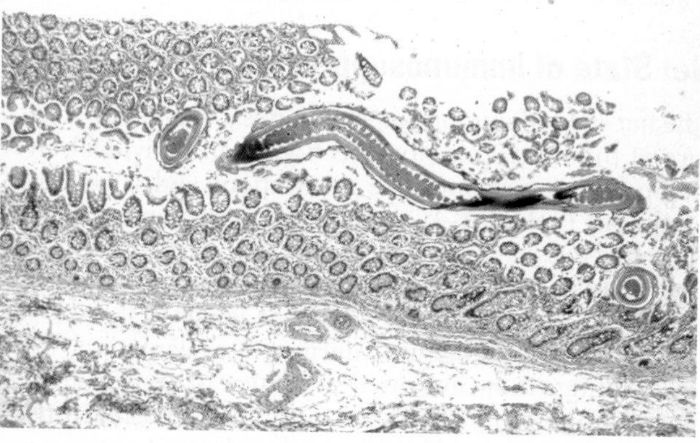
B

FIGURE 31-1 ■ Simultaneous *Pneumocystis* pneumonia and bacterial lung abscess secondary to co-infection by *Strongyloides stercoralis* in a Vietnamese kidney transplant recipient. (A) Chest radiograph shows a lung abscess secondary to *Enterobacter* species. Bronchoscopic examination also revealed simultaneous *Pneumocystis carinii* (*jiroveci*) and *S. stercoralis* infections. Migration of *Strongyloides* across the wall of the gastrointestinal tract during immunosuppression (hyperinfection) is associated with systemic signs of "sepsis" and central nervous system infection (parasitic and bacterial). (B) *S. stercoralis* from the lung of the same patient.

TABLE 31-3 Vaccinations to Consider Before Transplantation*

Measles/mumps/rubella (MMR)
Diphtheria/tetanus/pertussis (DTP)
Poliovirus
Haemophilus influenzae b (Hib)
Hepatitis B
Pneumococcus
Influenza
Varicella

*Live virus vaccinations are generally precluded in immunosuppressed hosts.

of enteric viruses can result in persistent infection, with more severe and prolonged diarrheal disease and an increased risk of primary or secondary blood stream invasion and metastatic infection.

Nosocomial Exposures

Nosocomial infections are of increasing importance. Organisms with significant antimicrobial resistance are present in most medical centers, including enterococci that are resistant to vancomycin, linezolid and/or quinupristin/dalfopristin, methicillin-resistant staphylococci, Gram-negative bacteria producing extended-spectrum beta-lactamases (ESBL), and fluconazole-resistant *Candida* species (Table 31-1). A single case of nosocomial *Aspergillus* infection in an immunocompromised host in the absence of a clear epidemiologic exposure should be viewed as a failure of infection control practices. Antimicrobial misuse and inadequate infection control practices have caused increased rates of *Clostridium difficile* colitis. Outbreaks of infections secondary to *Legionella* have been associated with hospital plumbing and contaminated water supplies or ventilation systems. Nosocomial spread of *Pneumocystis jiroveci* between immunocompromised patients has been suggested by a number of case series.[52] Respiratory viral infections may be acquired from medical staff and should be considered among the causes of fever and respiratory decompensation in hospitalized or institutionalized, immunocompromised individuals. Each nosocomially acquired infection should be investigated to ascertain the source and prevent subsequent infections.

Net State of Immunosuppression

The net state of immunosuppression is a qualitative measure of the risk factors for infection in an individual, including immunosuppressive medications and iatrogenic conditions (Table 31-4). Among the most important are the following:

1. The specific immunosuppressive therapy, including dose, duration, and sequence of agents (Table 31-5)
2. Technical difficulties during transplantation, resulting in an increased incidence of leaks (blood, lymph, urine) and fluid collections, devitalized tissue, poor wound healing, and prolonged use of surgical drainage catheters
3. Prolonged instrumentation, including airway intubation and use of vascular access devices (e.g., dialysis catheters)
4. Prolonged use of broad-spectrum antibiotics
5. Renal or hepatic dysfunction, or both (in addition to graft dysfunction)
6. Presence of infection with an immunomodulating virus, including CMV, EBV, HBV, HCV, or HIV.

Specific immunosuppressive agents are associated with increased risk for certain infections (Table 31-5).

TABLE 31-4 Factors Contributing to the Net State of Immunosuppression

Immunosuppressive therapy: type, temporal sequence, intensity, cumulative dose
Prior therapies (chemotherapy and antimicrobials)
Mucocutaneous barrier integrity (catheters, lines, drains)
Neutropenia, lymphopenia (often drug-induced)
Underlying immunodeficiencies
• Autoimmune diseases
• Hypogammaglobulinemia from proteinuria or drug therapy
• Complement deficiencies
• Other disease states (HIV, lymphoma/leukemia)
Metabolic conditions (uremia, malnutrition, diabetes, cirrhosis)
Viral infections (CMV, hepatitis B and C, RSV)
Graft rejection and treatment
Cancer/cellular proliferation

CMV, cytomegalovirus; HIV, human immunodeficiency virus; RSV, respiratory syncytial virus.

TABLE 31-5 Immunosuppression and Common Infections

Agent	Common Infections/Effects
Antilymphocyte globulins (lytic) and alloimmune response	Activation of latent viruses, fever, cytokines
Anti-CD20 antibody	Unknown so far
Plasmapheresis	Encapsulated bacteria
Costimulatory blockade	Unknown so far
Corticosteroids	Bacteria, *Pneumocystis jiroveci*, hepatitis B and C
Azathioprine	Neutropenia, papillomavirus (?)
Mycophenolate mofetil	Early bacterial infection, B cells, late CMV (?)
Calcineurin inhibitors	Enhanced viral replication (absence of immunity), gingival infection, intracellular pathogens
mTOR inhibitors	Poor wound healing, idiosyncratic pneumonitis syndrome
Belatacept	Posttransplant lymphoproliferative disorder

CMV, cytomegalovirus.

TIMELINE OF INFECTION

With standardized immunosuppressive regimens, specific infections that occur most often vary in a predictable pattern depending on the time elapsed since transplantation (Figure 31-2). This is primarily a reflection of changing risk factors over time, including surgery and hospitalization, tapering of immunosuppression, acute and chronic

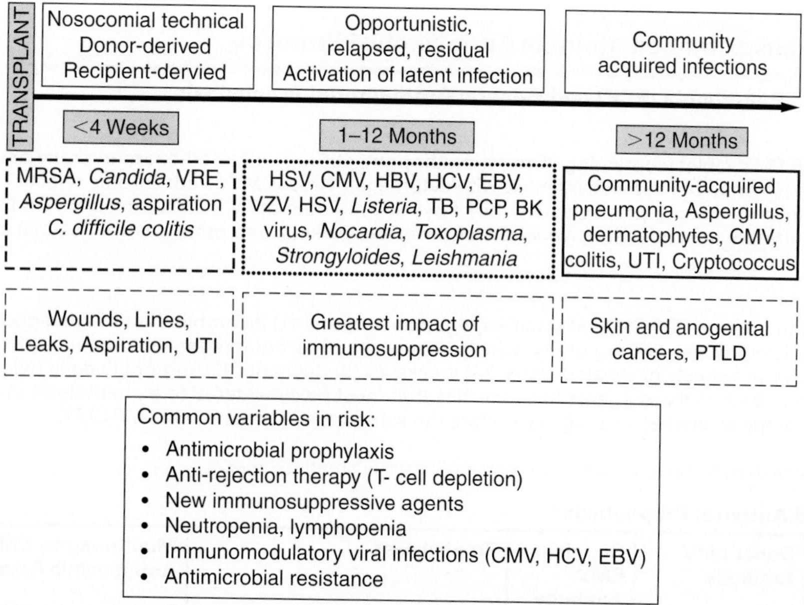

FIGURE 31-2 ■ The timeline of posttransplantation infections. Infection after transplantation tends to occur in a predictable pattern based on the epidemiologic exposure of the host and the nature of immune deficits. Patients with infections falling outside the usual patterns suggest unusual exposures or excessive immunosuppression. CMV, cytomegalovirus; EBV, Epstein–Barr virus; HBV, hepatitis B virus; HCV, hepatitis C virus; HSV, herpes simplex virus; MRSA, methicillin-resistant *Staphylococcus aureus*; PCP, *Pneumocystis jiroveci* pneumonia; PTLD, posttransplant lymphoproliferative disorder; TB, tuberculosis; UTI, urinary tract infection; VRE, vancomycin-resistant enterococcus; VZV, varicella-zoster virus.

rejection, and exposure to infections in the community.[57] The predicted pattern of infection changes with alterations in the immunosuppressive regimen (pulse-dose steroids or intensification for graft rejection), intercurrent viral infections, neutropenia (drug toxicity), graft dysfunction, or significant epidemiological exposures (travel or food). The timeline remains a useful starting point for the differential diagnosis of infection after transplantation, although it is altered by the introduction of new immunosuppressive agents and patterns of use, including reduced use of corticosteroids and calcineurin inhibitors, increased use of antibody-based (induction) therapies or sirolimus, routine antimicrobial prophylaxis, improved molecular assays, antimicrobial resistance, transplantation in HIV-infected and HCV-infected individuals, and broader epidemiological exposures from work or travel.

Figure 31-2 shows three overlapping periods of risk for infection after transplantation, each associated with differing patterns of common pathogens, as follows:

1. The perioperative period to approximately 4 weeks after transplantation, reflecting surgical and technical complications and nosocomial exposures
2. The period 1 to 6–12 months after transplantation (depending on the rapidity of taper of immunosuppression, the use of antilymphocyte "induction" therapy, and deployment of prophylaxis), reflecting intensive immunosuppression with viral activation and opportunistic infections
3. The period beyond the first year after transplantation, reflecting community-acquired exposures and some unusual pathogens based on the level of maintenance immunosuppression.

The timeline can be used in a variety of ways: (1) to establish a differential diagnosis for a transplant patient suspected to have infection; (2) to provide a clue to the presence of an excessive environmental hazard for the individual, either within the hospital or in the community; and (3) to serve as a guide to the design of preventive antimicrobial strategies. Infections occurring outside the usual period or of unusual severity suggest either excessive epidemiological hazard or excessive immunosuppression.

The prevention of infection must be linked to the risk for infection at various times after transplantation. Table 31-6 outlines some of the routine preventive strategies from the Massachusetts General Hospital. Such strategies serve only to delay the onset of infection in the face of epidemiological pressure. The use of antimicrobial prophylaxis, vaccines, and behavioral modifications (e.g., routine hand washing or advice against digging in gardens without masks) may result only in a "shift to the right" of the infection timeline, unless the intensity of immunosuppression is reduced or immunity develops.

First Phase (0–4 Weeks after Transplantation)

During the first month after transplantation, three types of infection occur. The first type is infection or colonization present in the recipient before transplantation which emerges in the setting of surgery and immunosuppression. Pretransplantation pneumonia and vascular access infections are common examples of this type of infection. Colonization of the recipient with resistant organisms that infect intravenous catheters or surgical drains also is common (e.g., methicillin-resistant *Staphylococcus aureus*). All infection should be controlled or eradicated to the degree possible before transplantation.

The second type of early infection is donor-derived. This type may be nosocomially derived (resistant Gram-negative bacilli and *S. aureus* or *Candida* species) secondary to systemic infection in the donor (e.g., line infection)

TABLE 31-6 Renal Transplantation: Routine Antimicrobial Protocols

Pneumocystis jiroveci Pneumonia (PCP) and General Antibacterial Prophylaxis

REGIMEN

One single-strength TMP-SMX tablet (containing 80 mg trimethoprim, 400 mg sulfamethoxazole) orally daily for a minimum of 4–6 months posttransplantation. Patients infected with cytomegalovirus (CMV), with chronic rejection, or with recurrent infections are maintained on lifelong prophylaxis. A thrice-weekly regimen of TMP-SMX prevents PCP, but does not prevent other infections (e.g., urinary tract infection, *Nocardia, Listeria, Toxoplasma*, and other gastrointestinal and pulmonary infections).

ALTERNATIVE REGIMEN

For patients proven not to tolerate TMP-SMX, alternative regimens include: (1) a combination of atovaquone, 1500 mg orally daily with meals, plus levofloxacin, 250 mg orally daily (or equivalent fluoroquinolone without anaerobic activity); (2) pentamidine, 300 mg intravenously or inhaled every 3–4 weeks; or (3) dapsone, 100 mg orally daily twice weekly, with or without pyrimethamine. Each of these agents has toxicities that must be considered (e.g., hemolysis in G6PD-deficient hosts with dapsone). None of these alternative programs offers the same broad protection of TMP-SMX.

G6PD, glucose-6-phosphate dehydrogenase; TMP-SMX, trimethoprim/sulfamethoxazole.

Cytomegalovirus and Antiviral Prophylaxis*

T-Cell Depletion (induction)?	Donor CMV Antibody	Recipient CMV Antibody	Prophylaxis*	Monitoring by CMV Viral Load or Antigenemia Assays
Yes	+	+	Valganciclovir po x 6 mos	After completion of prophylaxis based on intensity of immunosuppression. For symptoms, or monthly x 3 months from 6-9 mos
		+		
	+	-		
	-	-	Acyclovir, Famciclovir, or Valacyclovir (ACV/Fam/ValACV) x 6 mos	
No	+	+	Valganciclovir po x 3 mos	Monthly x 3 months from 3-6 mos
	-	+		
	+	-		
	-	-	ACV/Fam/ValACV x 3 mos	If clinically indicated
Intensified suppression for treatment of graft rejection	Either D^+ or R^+		Valganciclovir po x 2-3 mos	For symptoms or monthly x 3
	-	-	ACV/Fam/ValACV x 2-3 mos	

*First dose of ganciclovir is generally intravenous but valganciclovir may be used if taking oral medications. All antiviral agents adjusted for renal function. For abnormal renal function, formal creatinine clearance measurement may be indicated. The dose of antiviral therapy is generally not reduced for neutropenia. Consider other options first. CMV, cytomegalovirus. D^+/R^-, donor seropositive, recipient seronegative.

Antifungal Prophylaxis

Mucocutaneous candidiasis can be prevented with oral clotrimazole or nystatin 2–3 times per day during corticosteroid therapy or in the face of broad-spectrum antibacterial therapy and in diabetic transplant patients. Fluconazole, 200 mg/day for 10–14 days, is used to treat prophylaxis failures. Routine prophylaxis with fluconazole is used for pancreas and kidney–pancreas transplants. Other prophylaxis is determined based on the presence or absence of colonization or other risk factors for fungal infection.

or contamination during the organ procurement process. Rarely, infections transmitted from donor to recipient may emerge earlier than predicted (e.g., tuberculosis, histoplasmosis). Most recent clusters of donor-derived infection have been due to unfortunate timing – a donor who acquired acute infection (HIV, West Nile virus, rabies) prior to death due to unrelated causes.

The third and most common source of infection in the early period is related to the surgical procedure of transplantation. These infections include surgical wound infections, pneumonia (aspiration), bacteremia secondary to vascular access or surgical drainage catheters, urinary tract infections, and infections of fluid collections – leaks of vascular or urinary anastomoses or of lymphoceles. These are nosocomial infections and, as such, may carry the same antimicrobial-resistant pathogens observed in non-immunosuppressed patients undergoing comparable surgery. Given immunosuppression, the signs of infection may be subtle, however, and the severity or duration usually is greater. Thus, bowel perforation may be clinically silent marked only by a rising white blood cell count or graft dysfunction. The technical skill of the surgeons and meticulous postoperative care (i.e., wound care and proper maintenance and timely removal of endotracheal tubes, vascular access devices, and drainage catheters) are the determinants of risk for these infections. Another common infection is *Clostridium difficile* colitis.

Limited perioperative antibiotic prophylaxis (i.e., from a single dose to 24 hours of an antibiotic such as cefazolin or amoxicillin-clavulanate) is usually adequate with additional coverage required for known risk factors (e.g., prior colonization with methicillin-resistant *S. aureus*).

For pancreas transplantation, additional perioperative prophylaxis against yeasts is common using fluconazole, mindful of potential increases in sirolimus and calcineurin inhibitor levels when used with azole antifungal agents.

Opportunistic infections are notable for their absence in the first month after transplantation, even though the daily doses of immunosuppressive drugs may be greatest during this time. The implication of this observation is important. It suggests that it is not the daily dose of immunosuppressive drugs that is important but rather the cumulative dose of these drugs – the "area under the curve" – that determines the true state of immunosuppression. The net state of immunosuppression is not great enough to support the occurrence of opportunistic infections, unless an exposure has been excessive. The occurrence of a single case of opportunistic infection in this period should trigger an epidemiological investigation for an environmental hazard.

Second Phase (1–12 Months after Transplantation)

The second phase of infection was originally 1–3 months, but has been altered by two main factors. These include: successful use of prophylaxis or monitoring programs against CMV and the herpesviruses, against *Pneumocystis* and urinary tract infections, and for HBV; and intensification of immunosuppression using more potent agents or antibody-based therapies with prolonged effects on immune function (Table 31-6). Infection in the transplant recipient 1–12 months after transplantation has one of three causes:

1. Infection from the perisurgical period, including relapsed *C. difficile* colitis, inadequately treated pneumonia, or infection related to a technical problem (e.g., a urine leak, lymphocele, ureteric stricture, hematoma). Fluid collections in this setting generally require drainage.
2. Viral infections including CMV, HSV, shingles (VZV), human herpesvirus (HHV)-6 or HHV-7, EBV, hepatitis (HBV, HCV), and HIV. This group of viruses is unique. These infections are lifelong and tissue-associated, and are often transmitted with the allograft from seropositive donors. These viruses are systemically immunosuppressive, predisposing to opportunistic infection or acceleration of other infections (HCV) and predispose to graft rejection. The herpesviruses are prominent given the importance of T-cell function in antiviral control and the disproportionate degree of T-cell inhibition by most immunosuppressive regimens. Other common viral pathogens of this period include BK polyomavirus (in association with allograft dysfunction or polyomavirus-associated nephropathy (PVAN)) and community-acquired respiratory viruses (adenovirus, influenza, parainfluenza, respiratory syncytial virus, metapneumovirus). Superinfection of virally infected hosts is common.
3. Opportunistic infections secondary to *Pneumocystis jiroveci*, *Listeria monocytogenes*, *Toxoplasma gondii*, *Nocardia*, *Aspergillus*, and other agents.

In this period, the stage also is set for the emergence of a subgroup of patients – the "chronic ne'er do well" – the patient who requires higher than average immunosuppression to maintain graft function or who has prolonged, untreated viral infections and other opportunistic infections, which predict long-term susceptibility to other infections (third phase, discussed below). Such patients may benefit from prolonged (lifelong) prophylaxis (antibacterial, antifungal, antiviral, or a combination) to prevent life-threatening infection.

The specific opportunistic infections that occur reflect the specific immunosuppressive regimen used, individual epidemiology, and the presence or absence of immunomodulating viral infection. Viral pathogens (and rejection) are responsible for most febrile episodes that occur in this period. During this period, anti-CMV strategies and trimethoprim/sulfamethoxazole prophylaxis are effective in decreasing the risk of infection. Trimethoprim/sulfamethoxazole prophylaxis effectively prevents *Pneumocystis* pneumonia and reduces the incidence of urinary tract infection and urosepsis, *Listeria monocytogenes* meningitis, *Nocardia* species infection, and *T. gondii*.

Third Phase (>6–12 Months after Transplantation)

Recipients who underwent tranplantation more than 6–12 months previously can be divided into three groups in terms of infection risk. Most transplant recipients (70–80%) have a technically good procedure with satisfactory allograft function, reduced immunosuppression, and absence of chronic viral infection. These patients resemble the general community in terms of infection risk, with community-acquired respiratory viruses constituting their major risk. Occasionally, such patients develop primary CMV infection (socially acquired) or infections related to underlying diseases (e.g., skin infections in diabetes). A second group of patients has chronic viral infection, which may produce end-organ damage (e.g., BK polyomavirus leading to fibrosis, HCV leading to cryoglobulinemia and cirrhosis, CMV with chronic graft rejection) or malignancy (e.g., posttransplantation lymphoproliferative disease (PTLD) secondary to EBV, skin or anogenital cancer related to papillomaviruses). In the absence of specific and effective antiviral therapy, these patients often suffer graft rejection as a result of reduced intensity of immunosuppression.

A third group of patients has unsatisfactory allograft function, and suffers the ravages of renal dysfunction, often despite intensified immunosuppression used to preserve graft function. More recently, this has been the result of underlying disease progression (atherosclerosis, IgA or diabetes), calcineurin inhibitor toxicity, or humoral as well as cellular graft rejection. As a result, these patients are overimmunosuppressed relative to the risk for infection. These patients may benefit from lifetime maintenance trimethoprim/sulfamethoxazole prophylaxis and often fluconazole prophylaxis. In this group, one also should consider organisms more often associated with immune dysfunction of acquired immunodeficiency syndrome (AIDS) (*Bartonella*, *Rhodococcus*, *Cryptosporidium*, and microsporidia) and invasive fungal pathogens (*Aspergillus*, *Zygomycetes*, and Dematiaceae or pigmented molds). Even minimal clinical signs or symptoms warrant careful evaluation in this group of "high-risk" patients.

ASSESSMENT OF INFECTIOUS DISEASES IN RECIPIENTS AND POTENTIAL DONORS BEFORE TRANSPLANTATION

Guidelines for pretransplant screening have been the subject of several publications, including a consensus conference of the Immunocompromised Host Society, the American Society for Transplantation Clinical Practice Guidelines for the evaluation of kidney transplant candidates, and the American Society of Transplant Surgeons Clinical Practice Guidelines for the evaluation of living kidney transplant donors.[3,13,31,34,38,43–45,71–73,78,79]

Transplant Donor

Deceased Donor Evaluation

A crucial feature in screening of deceased organ donors is time limitation. A useful organ must be procured and implanted before some microbiologic assessments have been completed. Major infections must be excluded, and appropriate cultures and samples must be obtained for future reference. As a result, bacteremia or fungemia may not be detected until after the transplantation has been performed. Such infections generally have not resulted in transmission of infection as long as the infection has been adequately treated in terms of use of antimicrobial agents to which the organism is susceptible and time. In recipients of tissues from 95 bacteremic donors, a mean of 3.8 days of effective therapy after transplantation seemed adequate to prevent transmission of susceptible pathogens. Longer courses of therapy in the recipient are preferred, targeting known donor-derived pathogens.[17,26] Bacterial meningitis must be treated with antibiotics that penetrate the cerebrospinal fluid before organ procurement. Individuals with unidentified and untreated causes of meningoencephalitis or sepsis should not be used as organ donors. Donor-derived infections due to *Candida* species have resulted from contamination or candidemia at the time of procurement.[57,58] These require susceptibility testing of the isolate and prolonged treatment (2–4 weeks) with effective agents to avoid pyelonephritis, abscess formation, mycotic aneurysm, or fungemia in the recipient. Vascular involvement by *Candida* species in the recipient requires at least 6 weeks of therapy. Certain acute infections (CMV, HSV, EBV, HIV, and HCV) may be undetected in the period before antibody formation. Viral nucleic acid detection assays are preferred for sensitivity. Likewise, the donor's clinical, social, and medical histories are essential to reducing the risk of such infections. In the presence of known infection, such infections must be treated before procurement if possible. Several more recent clusters of donor-derived infection have shown the risk for infection secondary to previously unrecognized pathogens, including lymphocytic choriomeningitis virus, Chagas' disease, and HSV, in addition to other, more common pathogens. Major exclusion criteria are outlined in Table 31-2.

Living Donor Evaluation

In contrast to the above-described scenario, the living donor procedure should be considered elective, and the evaluation should be completed and infections should be treated before such procedures. An interim history must be taken at the time of surgery to assess the presence of new infections since the initial donor evaluation. Intercurrent infections (flu-like illness, headache, confusion, myalgias, cough) might be the harbinger of important infection (West Nile virus, severe acute respiratory syndrome (SARS), *Trypanosoma cruzi*). Live donors undergo a battery of serological tests (Table 31-7), purified protein derivative (PPD) skin test or tuberculosis interferon-γ release assay, and, if indicated, chest radiograph. The testing must be individualized, based on unique risk factors (e.g., travel). Of particular importance to the kidney transplant recipient is the exclusion of urinary tract infections (including yeasts) and bacteremia at the time of donation. Recent recommendations of the US Public Health Service suggest rescreening of potential donors within 7 days of donation using NAT for HIV, HCV, and HBV.

Special Infectious Risks and Organ Procurement

Tuberculosis. *Mycobacterium tuberculosis* from the donor represented approximately 4% of reported posttransplant tuberculosis cases in a review of 511 patients by Singh and Paterson.[66,75] Much higher rates occur in endemic regions.[54] Active disease should be excluded in PPD-positive donors with chest radiograph, sputum cultures, and chest computed tomography (CT) if the chest radiograph is abnormal. Urine acid-fast bacillus cultures may be useful in a PPD-positive kidney donor. Isoniazid prophylaxis of the recipient should be considered for untreated PPD-positive donors.[23] Factors favoring prophylaxis include a donor from an endemic region, use of a high-dose steroid regimen, or high-risk social environment.

TABLE 31-7 Cerebrospinal Fluid Analysis in Transplantation

Opening pressure
Cell count with differential
Glucose and total protein concentrations
Gram stain and bacterial culture
India ink (or other fungal stain) and fungal culture
Viral culture
Cryptococcal polysaccharide antigen
Histoplasma polysaccharide antigen (if indicated)
Coccidioides immitis complement fixation antibodies (if indicated)
Nucleic acid detection (in clinical context)

- Herpes simplex virus 1 and 2
- Varicella-zoster virus
- Epstein–Barr virus
- Cytomegalovirus
- Human herpesvirus 6
- JC virus
- Enterovirus
- *Toxoplasma gondii*

Cytology and flow cytometry

Parasites. Chagas' disease (*Trypanosoma cruzi*) has been transmitted by transplantation in endemic areas and more recently in the United States.[10,17,48,74] Schistosomiasis and infection by *Strongyloides stercoralis* are generally recipient-derived issues. Though common, malaria and leishmaniasis have been rarely transmitted with allografts.

Viral Infections Other than Cytomegalovirus. EBV infection is a major risk factor for the development of PTLD. The risk is greatest in the EBV-seronegative recipient of an EBV-seropositive allograft (i.e., donor seropositive, recipient seronegative (D^+/R^-)). This situation is most common in pediatric transplant recipients and in adults co-infected with CMV or receiving greater intensity of immunosuppression, notably with T-cell depletion and possibly with belatacept. Monitoring should be considered for at-risk individuals using a quantitative molecular assay (e.g., polymerase chain reaction) for EBV.[2,28,29,47,56,66,81] EBV also is a cofactor for other lymphoid malignancies.

VZV screening should be used to identify seronegative individuals (no history of chickenpox or shingles) for vaccination before transplantation. HSV screening is performed by most centers despite the use of antiviral prophylaxis during the posttransplant period. VZV serological status is particularly important in children who may be exposed at school (for antiviral or VZV immunoglobulin prophylaxis) and in adults with atypical presentations of infection (pneumonia or gastrointestinal disease).[61] Other herpesviruses also may reactivate, with HHV-6 and HHV-7 serving as cofactors for CMV and fungal infections and, in endemic regions, Kaposi's sarcoma-associated herpesvirus (HHV-8) causing malignancy, notably in endemic regions in South America and surrounding the Mediterranean basin.

HBV surface antigen (HBsAg) and HBV core antibody (HBcAb) are used for screening purposes (see Chapter 32 for detailed discussion).[1,43,49,71] A positive HBV surface antibody titer indicates either vaccination or prior infection. HBcAb-IgM positivity suggests active HBV infection, whereas IgG positivity suggests a more remote or persistent infection. The HBsAg-negative, HBcAb-IgG-positive donor will have viral DNA in the liver but may be appropriate as a kidney donor for HBV-infected or vaccinated renal recipients; quantitative viral assays for HBV should be obtained to guide further therapy. The presence of HBsAg-negative, HBcAb-IgG-positive assays may be a false-positive result or reflect true, latent HBV infection.

HCV infection generally progresses more rapidly with immunosuppression and with CMV co-infection (see Chapter 32 for detailed discussion). HCV-seropositive kidney transplant candidates are more likely to develop cirrhosis and complications of liver failure. Therapies for HCV infection are limited, with the side effects of standard therapies (pegylated interferon-α and ribavirin) increased in the transplant population. Newer protease inhibitors and other agents are available and efficacy in the immunosuppressed host under investigation. Management involves monitoring disease progression by quantitative molecular viral assays for HCV RNA with intermittent liver biopsy. Management is likely to change as newer HCV antiviral agents become available (see Chapter 32).

The use of HIV-infected donors for HIV-infected recipients is precluded in the United States but is under study in South Africa and elsewhere. The progression of untreated recipient HIV infection is rapid. Based on current criteria, donors may be excluded based on historical evidence of risk factors significant for HIV infection and confirmatory testing.

Human T-cell lymphotropic virus I (HTLV-I) is endemic in the Caribbean and parts of Asia (Japan) and can progress to HTLV-I-associated myelopathy/tropical spastic paraparesis or to adult T-cell leukemia/lymphoma. HTLV-II is similar to HTLV-I serologically, but it is less clearly associated with disease. Use of organs from such donors is generally avoided; however serologic testing does not distinguish between the two types of virus. Donor screening for HTLV in the United States is now voluntary.[29,35,55,76]

West Nile virus is a flavivirus associated with viral syndromes and meningoencephalitis and may be transmitted by blood transfusion and organ transplantation.[7,36,46,59,72] Routine screening of donors is not advocated other than in areas with endemic infection. Donors with unexplained changes in mental status or recent viral illness with neurologic signs should be avoided.

Transplant Recipient

The pretransplant period is useful for obtaining travel, animal, environmental, and exposure histories; updating immunizations; and counseling of the recipient regarding travel, food, and other infection risks.[15] Ongoing infection must be eradicated before transplantation. Two forms of infection pose a special risk – blood stream infection related to vascular access (including that for dialysis), and pneumonia, which puts the patient at high risk for subsequent lung infection with nosocomial organisms. Several other infections are commonly encountered and should be treated and cleared before transplantation. Infected ascites or peritoneal dialysis fluid also must be cleared before surgery. Urinary tract infection must be eliminated with antibiotics with or without nephrectomy. Similarly, skin disease threatens the integrity of a primary defense against infection and should be corrected even if doing so requires the initiation of immunosuppression before transplantation (e.g., the initiation of immunosuppression to treat psoriasis or eczema). Finally, a history of more than one episode of diverticulitis should initiate an evaluation to determine whether sigmoid colectomy should be done before transplantation.

Among important considerations in transplant recipients are strongyloidiasis, tuberculosis, and AIDS. *Strongyloides* hyperinfestation syndrome (hemorrhagic enterocolitis, pneumonia, Gram-negative or mixed bacteremia, or meningitis) may emerge more than 30 years after transplantation. Empirical pretransplantation therapy of *Strongyloides*-seropositive recipients (ivermectin) prevents such infections.

The incidence of active tuberculous disease and the occurrence of disseminated infection secondary to *Mycobacterium tuberculosis* are higher in the transplant recipient than in the general population. Active tuberculous disease must be eradicated before transplantation. The major antituberculous drugs are potentially hepatotoxic, and significant drug interactions are common between antituberculosis agents and immunosuppressive agents. In patients with active infection, from endemic regions or with high-risk exposures, tuberculosis therapy should be initiated in all PPD-positive individuals before transplantation. Some judgment may be used as to the optimal timing of treatment in individuals without evidence of active or pleuropulmonary disease. Patients at greater risk of tuberculosis infection or exposure include individuals with prior history of active tuberculosis or significant signs of old tuberculosis on chest radiograph, recent tuberculin reaction conversion, known exposure to active disease, protein-calorie malnutrition, cirrhosis, other immunodeficiency, or living exposures (e.g., in a shelter or other group housing).

For many patients receiving antiretroviral therapy, HIV infection has been converted from a progressively fatal disease to a chronic infection controlled by complex regimens of antiviral agents or highly active antiretroviral therapy (HAART). HAART has been associated with reduced viral loads, improved $CD4^+$ lymphocyte counts, and reduced susceptibility to opportunistic infections. In the pre-HAART era, organ transplantation generally was associated with a rapid progression to AIDS. Prolonged disease-free survival with HAART has led, however, to a reconsideration of this policy. Kidney transplantation in HIV has been associated with good outcomes in individuals with controlled HIV infection and in the absence of HCV co-infection.[8,12,20,59,70,68,80] Management requires experience with immunosuppressive agents and various HAART regimens. The main hurdle is the drug interactions between protease inhibitors and calcineurin inhibitors and the need for full immusuppression despite HIV infection.

SELECTED INFECTIONS OF IMPORTANCE

General Considerations

The spectrum of infection in the immunocompromised host is quite broad. Given the toxicity of antimicrobial agents and the need for rapid interruption of infection, early, specific diagnosis is essential in this population. Advances in diagnostic modalities (e.g., CT or magnetic resonance imaging, molecular microbiologic techniques) may greatly assist in this process. The need for invasive diagnostic tools cannot be overemphasized, however. Given the diminished immune responses of the host, and the frequency of multiple simultaneous processes, invasive diagnosis is often required for specific microbiological diagnosis, to minimize side effects of therapy, and to improve clinical responses. The initial, empiric therapy is broad by necessity, with a rapid narrowing of the antimicrobial spectrum as data become available.

Among the decisions in anti-infective therapy is whether to reduce the intensity of immunosuppression, with the understanding that the risk of such an approach is graft rejection. For latent viral infections or tuberculosis, activation should be seen as evidence of excessive immunosuppression relative to the host's immune function. In contrast, for intercurrent bacterial or fungal infections, reductions in immunosuppression should be reconsidered when resolution of infection is demonstrated. The specific reduction chosen may depend on the organisms isolated, e.g., corticosteroids and bacterial infections. Similarly, reversal of some immune deficits (e.g., neutropenia, hypogammaglobulinemia) may be possible with adjunctive therapies (e.g., colony-stimulating factors or antibody). Co-infection with virus (CMV) is common and requires additional therapy. The adverse effects of reduced immune suppression during infection are best demonstrated in patients with cryptococcal meningitis in whom a "rebound" of inflammatory responses may result in worsening symptoms and hydrocephalus. This reflects the immune reconstitution and inflammatory syndrome (IRIS) seen with any patient in whom immune deficits are reversed in the face of ongoing inflammation.

Viral Pathogens

Cytomegalovirus

Invasive infection due to CMV has become less common due to the availability of effective antiviral therapies and diagnostic and monitoring assays for the virus (Table 31-6). However, even latent infection or low-level replication has important implications for transplant outcomes and strategies used to prevent (universal versus pre-emptive therapy with monitoring) and treat infection vary between centers. The manifestations of CMV infection have been traditionally termed "direct" and "indirect" effects. More accurate terms might be "viremic/cytopathic" effects and "cellular/immunologic" effects. The common direct effects or clinical syndromes include:

- "CMV syndrome": viremia associated with fever and neutropenia syndrome with variable features of infectious mononucleosis, including hepatitis, nephritis, lymphadenitis, leukopenia, and/or thrombocytopenia
- Pneumonitis – often difficult to distinguish from apparently benign secretion
- Gastrointestinal invasion with esophagitis, colitis, gastritis, ulcers, bleeding, or perforation
- Hepatitis, pancreatitis, myocarditis, or chorioretinitis
- Meningoencephalitis
- Hemolytic uremic syndrome or microangiopathic thrombosis.

With the exception of chorioretinitis, the direct clinical manifestations of CMV infection usually occur 1–6 months after transplantation in the absence of prophylaxis. Viremia and symptomatic infections are rare during effective antiviral prophylaxis and have generally been delayed until after cessation of prophylaxis or develop in association with intensification of immunosuppression (e.g., for rejection). Chorioretinitis occurs at low levels of viral replication and generally later in the posttransplant course.

The cellular and immunologic effects of CMV infection (discussed below) are the result of the suppression of a variety of host defense mechanisms and predispose to secondary invasion by *P. jiroveci*, *Candida*, and *Aspergillus* species, and other bacterial and fungal pathogens. CMV infection also contributes to the risk for graft rejection, PTLD, acceleration of HCV co-infection, HHV-6 and HHV-7 infections, and increased risk for death.

Patterns of Transmission. Transmission of CMV in the transplant recipient occurs in one of three patterns: primary infection, reactivation infection, and superinfection.

Primary CMV Infection. The greatest risk for infection is in the setting of primary CMV infection when seronegative individuals receive grafts from latently infected, seropositive donors (D^+R^-), with subsequent reactivation of the virus with systemic dissemination. Over 50% of these patients become viremic in the absence of prophylaxis, often without symptoms. Many will become viremic after the cessation of antiviral, prophylaxis with symptomatic "late infection" occurring in up to a third of recipients previously treated with prophylaxis. Primary CMV infection may also occur in seronegative individuals after transfusion or sexual contacts in the community. This disease may be severe. The allograft may be a privileged site for viral replication because the major histocompatibility complex (MHC)-restricted, virus-specific, cytotoxic T cells have a decreased ability to eliminate virally infected cells in the presence of MHC mismatch between donor and recipient.

Reactivation CMV Infection. In reactivation infection, seropositive individuals reactivate endogenous virus after transplantation (D^+ or D^-, R^+). When conventional immunosuppressive therapy is used without antilymphocyte antibody "induction" treatment, approximately 10–15% experience direct infectious disease syndromes in the absence of prophylaxis with a higher rate, up to 50%, following T-cell depletion therapies.

CMV Superinfection. Virus derived from the donor may be reactivated in the setting of an allograft from a seropositive donor transplanted into a seropositive recipient (D^+R^+). Blood transfusions, even if leukocyte-reduced, have a low rate (~4%) of transmission of CMV infection. This observation gains importance in patients requiring significant transfusion in the perioperative setting.

Pathogenesis of Infection. CMV activation occurs as the result of multiple factors, including the intensity of immunosuppression (notably pulsed-dose corticosteroids), the amount of virus in the graft, the use of lytic T-cell-depleting therapies, co-infections, notably with other herpesviruses (HHV-6 and HHV-7), and graft rejection. These events share features of inflammation and fever, endothelial activation and injury, and secretion of proinflammatory cytokines, including tumor necrosis factor-α that activates intracellular NF-κB. NF-κB translocates to the cell nucleus to activate the CMV major immediate-early promoter/enhancer and viral replication.

The risk for viral activation in the setting of intensified immunosuppression for graft rejection must be linked to prophylaxis, notably in the CMV serostatus D^+/R^- combination. The alloimmune response carries both the effects of injury to the graft that is generally the site of greatest viral load and systemic inflammation. Thus, a bidirectional linkage exists between CMV replication and graft rejection. In an interesting study, Reinke et al.[67] showed that 17 of 21 patients for whom biopsy revealed evidence of "late acute rejection" demonstrated a response to antiviral therapy. Further, Lowance et al.[56] demonstrated that the prevention of CMV infection also resulted in a lower incidence of graft rejection.

The cellular and immunological effects of CMV ("indirect effects") may be as important to the immunocompromised host as is invasive viral infection. The mechanisms for these effects are complex and relate to viral strategies to evade the host's antiviral responses to allow human CMV-infected antigen-presenting cells to travel throughout the host to spread virus.

Diagnosis. Clinical management of CMV, including prevention and treatment, is based on an understanding of the causes of CMV activation and the available diagnostic techniques.[22] CMV cultures generally are too slow and insensitive for clinical utility. A positive CMV culture (or shell vial culture) derived from respiratory secretions or urine is of little diagnostic value – many immunosuppressed patients secrete CMV in the absence of invasive disease. Serological tests are useful before transplantation to predict risk but are of little value after transplantation in defining clinical disease, including measurements of anti-CMV IgM levels, as seroconversion is generally delayed. Seroconversion to CMV provides evidence that the patient has developed some degree of immunity and appears to correlate with T-cell function as well as antibodies.

Quantitation of the intensity of CMV infection has been linked to the risk for infection in transplant recipients.[6,8,14,32,40,41,49] Two types of quantitative assays have been developed: molecular and antigen detection assays.[6] The antigenemia assay is a semiquantitative fluorescent assay in which circulating neutrophils are stained for CMV early antigen (pp65) that is taken up non-specifically as a measure of the total viral burden in the body. The molecular assays (direct DNA polymerase chain reaction, hybrid capture, amplification assays) are highly specific and sensitive for the detection of viremia.[37,53] The most commonly used assays include plasma-based polymerase chain reaction testing and the whole-blood hybrid capture assay. Whole-blood and plasma-based assays cannot be directly compared and assays performed by different laboratories are often discordant. World Health Organization standards have been created to use in the harmonization of assays between centers. The highest viral loads often are associated with tissue-invasive disease, with the lowest in asymptomatic CMV infection. Viral loads in the CMV syndrome vary. Either assay can be used in management.

The advent of quantitative assays for the diagnosis and management of CMV infection has allowed non-invasive diagnosis in many patients with two important exceptions:

1. Neurological disease, including chorioretinitis
2. Gastrointestinal disease, including invasive colitis and gastritis.

In these syndromes, the CMV assays are often negative. For the diagnosis of gastrointestinal CMV disease the demonstration of CMV inclusions in tissues and/or immunohistology for CMV antigens remains essential. The central role of assays is illustrated by the approach to the management of CMV risk (Table 31-6). The schedule for screening is linked to the risk for infection. In the high-risk patient (D⁺/R⁺ or R⁺ with antilymphocyte globulin), after the completion of prophylaxis, monthly screening is performed to ensure the absence of infection for 3–6 months. In the patient being treated for CMV infection, the assays provide an end-point for therapy and the initiation of prophylaxis.

Cytomegalovirus prevention. Prevention of CMV infection must be individualized for immunosuppressive regimens and the patient (Table 31-6).[27,40,47,50,60,62,65] Two strategies are commonly used for CMV prevention – universal prophylaxis and pre-emptive therapy. Universal prophylaxis involves giving antiviral therapy to all at-risk patients beginning at or immediately after transplantation for a defined period. In pre-emptive therapy, quantitative assays are used to monitor patients at predefined intervals (generally weekly for weeks 1–12) to detect early disease. Positive assays result in therapy. Pre-emptive therapy incurs extra costs for monitoring and coordination of outpatient care, while reducing the cost of drugs and the inherent toxicities. Prophylaxis has the possible advantage of not only preventing CMV infection during the period of greatest risk but also diminishing infections secondary to HHV-6, HHV-7, and EBV. The indirect effects of CMV (i.e., graft rejection, opportunistic infection) also may be reduced by routine prophylaxis. In practice, neither universal prophylaxis nor pre-emptive therapy is perfect. Many centers use a combination of both approaches: universal prophylaxis for the highest-risk recipients (D⁺/R⁻ and R⁺ with T-cell depletion), and pre-emptive therapy for others. Infrequently, breakthrough disease and ganciclovir resistance have been observed with both approaches.[1]

Given the risk for invasive infection, patients at risk for primary infection (CMV D⁻/R⁻) and seropositive patients receiving depleting anti-T-lymphocyte antibodies are generally given prophylaxis for 3–6 months after transplantation. Other groups are candidates for pre-emptive therapy if an appropriate monitoring system is in place, and patient compliance is good. Current data support the use of universal prophylaxis (not pre-emptive therapy), however, in the prevention of indirect effects of CMV infection, including PTLD, opportunistic infections, allograft rejection, and mortality.[1,42] Increasingly, "late" disease has been observed after the completion of prophylaxis.[38,39] Thus, monitoring may be useful after prophylaxis. The rate of late disease varies but is thought to be as high as 17–37% in D⁺/R⁻ recipients. This observation has suggested the value of 6 months of prophylaxis in D⁺/R⁻ renal recipients (the IMPACT study).

Options for CMV prophylaxis include valganciclovir (900 mg orally once daily), oral ganciclovir (1 g three times daily), intravenous ganciclovir (5 mg/kg once daily), or high-dose oral valacyclovir (2 g four times daily) – each corrected for renal function. Valganciclovir and ganciclovir are associated with neutropenia; however, dose reduction risks breakthrough viremia and the emergence of viral resistance. Prophylaxis should be reinitiated during treatments with antilymphocyte therapies. Given changing renal function after transplantation and the costs of medication, many regimens employ lower doses of valganciclovir. Such regimens should be coupled to monitoring to assure efficacy. After the completion of treatment for CMV disease (see below), many centers initiate a course of secondary prophylaxis (1–3 months). An alternative is a period of virologic monitoring for this period.

Treatment. The standard of care for treating invasive CMV disease is 2–4 weeks of intravenous ganciclovir (5 mg/kg twice daily, with dosage adjustments for renal dysfunction) until a quantitative assay for CMV is negative.[40,47,62] In patients with mild to moderately severe symptoms, valganciclovir (900 mg po twice daily corrected for renal function) may be used as an alternative. In symptomatic patients slow to respond to therapy and who are seronegative, the addition of 3 months of CMV hyperimmune globulin in seronegative individuals (150 mg/kg/dose iv monthly) may be useful, but is costly and of uncertain benefit. Relapse does occur, primarily in seronegative patients, in those with high viral burdens, if not treated to the achievement of a negative quantitative assay, and in some with gastrointestinal disease treated with oral regimen. Repeat endoscopy should be considered to ensure the clearance of infection. In practice, it is reasonable to initiate therapy with intravenous ganciclovir, monitor weekly to assure a response, and treat until monitoring is negative. Such patients may benefit from 2–4 months of oral valganciclovir (900 mg daily based on creatinine clearance) administered as secondary prophylaxis after the completion of intravenous therapy. This approach has resulted in rare symptomatic relapses and has been associated uncommonly with the emergence of antiviral resistance. It may be worth measuring a formal creatinine clearance to assure adequate dosing.

The incidence of ganciclovir resistance in CMV is generally low.[5,11,13] The risk for resistance is greatest in D⁺/R⁻ recipients, with higher viral loads, who received inadequate dosing of prophylactic or therapeutic ganciclovir, more intensive immunosuppression including antilymphocyte antibody induction, and with prolonged antiviral prophylaxis. Clinically, the patient's viral load or clinical syndrome fails to respond to appropriate therapy, including a reduction in immunosuppression over 10–14 days. Genetic resistance testing is useful in managing resistant CMV infection; mutations in the viral UL97 (thymidine kinase) or UL54 (DNA polymerase) genes can confer ganciclovir resistance.[32,51] Some of the common mutations in the UL97 gene respond to higher doses of intravenous ganciclovir. Combined mutations

(UL97 and UL54) may manifest high-level resistance to ganciclovir. Alternative therapies are available in intravenous form only. These include foscarnet and cidofovir. Foscarnet is active against many ganciclovir-resistant strains of CMV, although associated with marked magnesium and potassium wasting, seizures (notably with calcineurin inhibitor therapy), and some renal toxicity. Cidofovir may also be used, but often incurs significant nephrotoxicity and ocular toxicity. Liposomal cidofovir is under investigation. UL54 mutations may cause resistance to foscarnet and to cidofovir depending on the nature of the mutation. Multiple courses of antiviral therapy may be needed to cure resistant CMV infection. Given the toxicity of available medications, several investigational drugs are under study that may alter recommended therapies for antiviral-resistant CMV. Combination therapy (ganciclovir and foscarnet) may be useful, as is the addition of hyperimmune globulins. Most centers try to reduce overall immunosuppression during the course of therapy. Alternative agents include the dihydroorotate dehydrogenase inhibitors (leflunamide) approved for immunosuppression in treatment of rheumatological diseases with useful, incidental activity against CMV (and possibly BK polyomavirus).

Epstein–Barr Virus

EBV is a ubiquitous herpesvirus that infects B lymphocytes.[2,29,30,66] In immunosuppressed transplant recipients, primary EBV infection (and relapses in the absence of antiviral immunity) causes a mononucleosis-type syndrome, generally manifesting as a lymphocytosis (B cell) with or without lymphadenopathy or pharyngitis. Meningitis, hepatitis, and pancreatitis also are observed. Remitting-relapsing EBV infection is common in children and may reflect the interplay between evolving antiviral immunity and immunosuppression. Regardless of its mode of expression, this syndrome should suggest relative overimmunosuppression.

EBV also plays a central role in the pathogenesis of PTLD.[14,47,55,53,59,70] PTLD represents a spectrum of disease from benign B-cell mononucleosis-like syndrome to monomorphic B-cell lymphoma as well as tumors of T-cell, natural killer cell, and null-cell origins (Figure 31-3). The most clearly defined risk factor for PTLD is primary EBV infection, which increases the risk for PTLD by 10–76-fold. PTLD may occur in the absence of EBV infection or in seropositive patients and the role of EBV in the pathogenesis of the non-B-cell tumors is less clear. Other risk factors include CMV co-infection, T-cell depletion therapy, duration of immunosuppression, and, in adults, older age. Posttransplant non-Hodgkin's lymphoma is a common complication of solid-organ transplantation. Lymphomas constitute 15% of tumors among adult transplant recipients (51% in children) with mortality of 40–60%. Many deaths are associated with allograft failure after withdrawal of immunosuppression during treatment of malignancy.

Compared with the general population, PTLD has increased extranodal involvement, poor response to conventional therapies, and poor outcomes. The spectrum of disease is broad and ranges from benign polyclonal, B-cell, infectious mononucleosis-like disease to malignant, monoclonal lymphoma.[80] Most disease is of B-cell origin, although T-cell, natural killer cell, and null cell tumors are described. EBV-negative PTLD has been

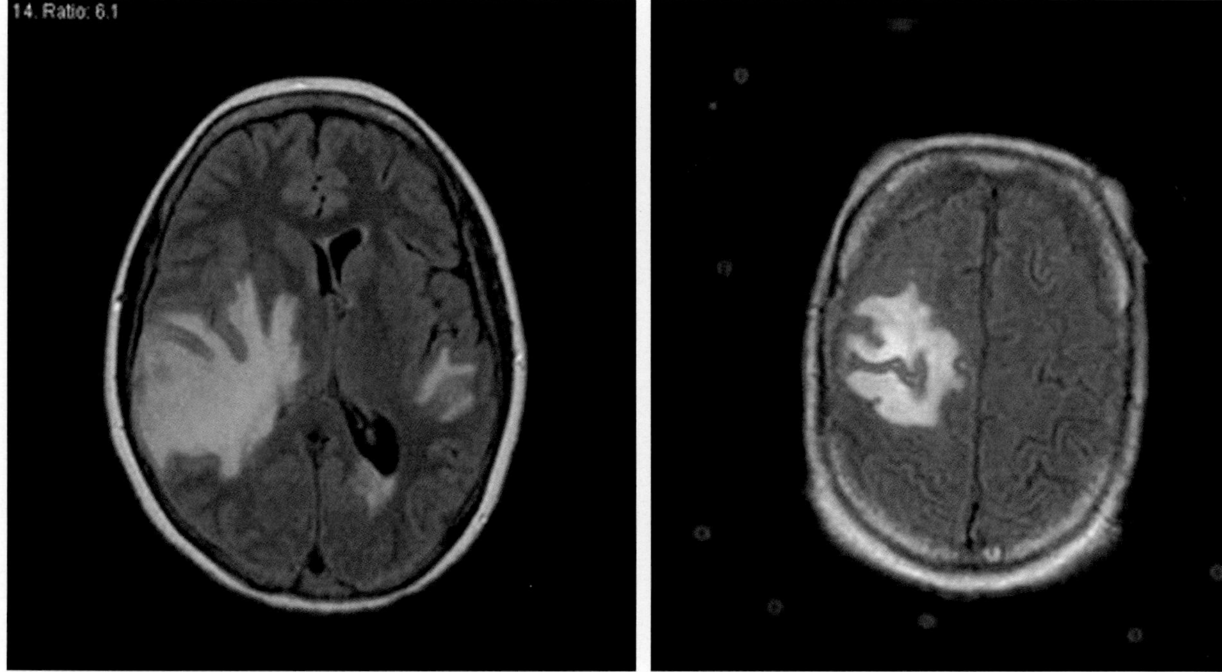

FIGURE 31-3 ■ (A) Central nervous system lymphoma with positive staining for Epstein–Barr virus (posttransplantation lymphoproliferative disorder) in a 63-year-old man 6 years status post renal transplantation. (B) Acute stroke syndrome in a 65-year-old man with progressive multifocal leukoencephalopathy.

described, and T-cell PTLD has been shown in allografts thought to have rejection or other viral infection. PTLD late (>1–2 years) after transplantation is more often EBV-negative in adults.

The clinical presentations of EBV-associated PTLD vary widely and include:

- Unexplained fever (fever of unknown origin) with viremia
- A mononucleosis-type syndrome, with fever and malaise, with or without pharyngitis or tonsillitis (often diagnosed incidentally in tonsillectomy specimens); often no lymphadenopathy is observed
- Gastrointestinal bleeding, obstruction, or perforation
- Abdominal mass lesions
- Infiltrative disease of the allograft
- Hepatocellular or pancreatic dysfunction
- Central nervous system (CNS) mass lesions.

Diagnosis. Serological testing is not useful for the diagnosis of acute EBV infection or PTLD in transplantation. Quantitative EBV viral load testing is required for the diagnosis and management of PTLD.[2,5,20,28,29,66,72,74] Serial assays are more useful in an individual patient than specific viral load measurements. These assays are not standardized and cannot be directly compared between centers. Some data suggest that assays using unfractionated whole blood are preferable to plasma samples for EBV viral load surveillance. The diagnosis of PTLD may be suggested by the presence of a compatible clinical syndrome with demonstration of EBV viral load. EBV viral load in whole blood and plasma appear to be similar but some controversy exists with respect to preferred sample type. Viral load monitoring is non-standardized and results may not be compared between clinical laboratories. Trends in individual patients over time using a single assay are most useful. The demonstration of EBV-specific nucleic acids in tissues may diagnose EBV-associated PTLD. RNA in situ hybridization against EBV-encoded small nuclear RNAs is more sensitive than the detection of viral DNA. The EBV latent antigens EBNA-1, EBNA-2, and LMP-1 can be detected by immunohistochemistry.

Management. Clinical management depends on the stage of disease. In the polyclonal form, particularly in children, re-establishment of immune function may suffice to cause PTLD to regress. At this stage, it is possible that antiviral therapy might have some utility given the viremia and role of EBV, and of CMV if present, as an immunosuppressive agent. With the progression of disease to extranodal and monoclonal malignant forms, reduction in immunosuppression may be useful, but alternative therapies are often required. In kidney transplantation, the failure to regress with significant reductions in immunosuppression may suggest the need to sacrifice the allograft for patient survival. Combinations of anti-B-cell therapy (anti-CD20, rituximab), chemotherapy (CHOP: cyclophosphamide, hydroxydaunomycin, vincristine, prednisone), irradiation especially for CNS tumors, or adoptive immunotherapy with stimulated T cells have been used.[15,26,28,30]

Polyomaviruses

Polyomaviruses have been identified in transplant recipients in association with nephropathy and ureteral obstruction (BK virus), and in association with demyelinating disease of the brain (JC virus) similar to progressive multifocal leukoencephalopathy (PML) of AIDS. Adult levels of seroprevalence are 65–90%. BK virus resides in latency in renal tubular epithelial cells. JC virus also has been isolated from renal tissues but seems to have preferred tropism for neural tissues. Reactivation occurs with immunodeficiency and immunosuppression and tissue injury (e.g., ischemia-reperfusion).

BK Polyomavirus Infection. BK virus is associated with a range of clinical syndromes in immunocompromised hosts, including viruria and viremia, ureteral ulceration and stenosis, and hemorrhagic cystitis.[22,34,40,42,58,60,61,63,77,80] Active infection of renal allografts has been associated with progressive loss of graft function ("BK nephropathy") in approximately 4% (range 1–8%) of kidney transplant recipients; this is referred to as PVAN. BK nephropathy is rarely recognized in recipients of extrarenal organs. The clinical presentation of disease is usually as sterile pyuria, reflecting shedding of infected tubular and ureteric epithelial cells. These cells contain sheets of virus and are detected by urine cytology as "decoy cells." In some cases, the patient presents with diminished renal allograft function or with ureteric stenosis and obstruction. In such patients, the etiologies of decreased renal function must be carefully evaluated (e.g., mechanical obstruction, drug toxicity, pyelonephritis, rejection, thrombosis, recurrent disease), and choices must be made between increasing immunosuppression to treat suspected graft rejection or reducing immunosuppression to allow the immune system to control infection. Patients with BK nephropathy treated with increased immunosuppression have a high incidence of graft loss. Reduced immunosuppression may stabilize renal allograft function but risks graft rejection.

Risk factors for BK nephropathy are poorly defined. Some studies have implicated high-dose immunosuppression (particularly T-cell depletion, tacrolimus, and mycophenolate mofetil), pulse-dose steroids for treatment of graft rejection, ischemia-reperfusion injury, increased number of HLA mismatches between donor and recipient, and the intensity of viremia in the pathogenesis of disease. The role of specific immunosuppressive agents has not been confirmed. The greatest incidence of BK nephropathy is at centers with the most intensive immunosuppressive regimens.

Screening, Prevention, and Diagnosis. BK virus infection is generally asymptomatic. Renal tubular cell injury in PVAN is reflected in a rising serum creatinine. Most centers have developed screening programs to document early disease. The use of urine cytology to detect the presence of infected decoy cells in the urine has approximately 100% sensitivity for BK virus infection but a low (29%) predictive value.[64] Detection of urine BK virus by electron microscopy, urine BK viral (DNA) loads greater than 7 log gEq/mL or BK virus VP1 gene mRNA of >6 log copies/ng total urine RNA are useful diagnostically. Patients with BK nephropathy have higher plasma viral loads (>7700 BK virus copies per mL of plasma, $P<0.001$, 50% positive predictive value, 100% negative predictive value) when compared to patients without such disease.[34]

A high serum BK viral load is considered a basis for reduction in immunosuppression, especially if serum creatinine has risen. However, the diagnosis should be made by demonstration of BK virus cytopathic changes with cellular infiltration consistent with the diagnosis of interstitial nephritis in the allograft and by immunohistology for BK virus proteins, or by in situ hybridization for BK virus nucleic acids in a renal biopsy. There is a semiquantitative scoring system for histologic changes of PVAN. For immunohistochemistry, cross-reacting antibodies against the large T-antigen of the simian virus 40 or antibodies against BK virus VP1 or agnoprotein have been used. PVAN is characterized by intranuclear polyomavirus inclusion bodies in tubular epithelial and/or glomerular cells. Fibrosis is often prominent, occasionally with calcification. PVAN is often focal, with false-negative biopsies in some cases. Graft rejection may accompany PVAN, and complicates both diagnosis and management.

Recommendations regarding screening for BK virus infection vary, but generally suggest testing once every 3 months during the first 2 years after transplantation, and at least annually for years 2–5.[33,34] A urinary test for BK virus (cytology for decoy cells or urine BK virus loads over 7 log gEq/mL) is adequate for screening. Patients with high urinary BK viral loads require testing for plasma BK virus DNA. Screening can also be performed using plasma BK virus DNA loads. For patients with plasma BK viral DNA loads of >4 log10 gEq/mL on duplicate testing 2–3 weeks apart, a presumptive diagnosis of PVAN should be made and immunosuppression reduced (see below). If screening is performed by plasma viral load, the interval between screening assays should be reduced to monthly for the first 6 months posttransplant. This reflects reduced time before permanent renal injury in patients with circulating viremia compared with urinary excretion.

Treatment. There is no accepted treatment for PVAN other than reduction in the intensity of immune suppression. It is useful to monitor the response to such maneuvers using plasma viral load measurements. Despite controversy, it is reasonable to reduce dosing of both calcineurin inhibitors and antimetabolites in a stepwise fashion while monitoring BK virus plasma loads. Given the toxicity of calcineurin inhibitors for tubular cells, the role of injury in the activation of BK virus, as well as the need for anti-BK T-cell activity, these agents should be included in initial reductions. General targets include tacrolimus trough levels of <6 ng/mL, cyclosporine trough levels <150 ng/mL, sirolimus trough levels of <6 ng/mL, and/or mycophenolate mofetil daily dose equivalents of ≤1000 mg. Regardless of the approach, renal function (at least 1–2 times per week), drug levels, and viral loads (alternate weeks) must be monitored carefully during reductions. Rebiopsy may be needed for poor responses.

The use of adjunctive antiviral therapies remains controversial. Some centers advocate the use of cidofovir for BK nephropathy in low doses (0.25–1 mg/kg every 2 weeks). Significant renal toxicity may be observed with this agent. Leflunomide, an immunosuppressant used in rheumatoid arthritis, and fluoroquinolones have some anti-BK activity. Use of these agents should prompt consultation with clinicians expert in this area. Repletion of serum immunoglobulins and treatment with intravenous immunoglobulins have also been used with anecdotal success in some patients.

Retransplantation has been successful in PVAN patients with failed allografts, possibly as a reflection of immunity developing subsequent to reduction in immune suppression. Most centers allow retransplantation after immunosuppression has been discontinued for some period (6 months) and BK virus is undetectable in blood and low in urine. Surgical removal of the allograft does not protect against future BK infection or PVAN but may be needed if immunosuppression cannot be reduced (double transplants, allosensitization) and/or elevated viral loads persist. In the future, measurements of BK virus-specific cellular immunity after discontinuation of immunosuppression may help to determine the optimal time for retransplantation.

JC Virus

Infection of the CNS by JC polyomavirus has been observed uncommonly in transplant recipient as PML (Figure 31-3). This infection may present with focal neurologic deficits or seizures as well as more slowly progressive neurologic lesions and may progress to death following extensive demyelination. PML may be confused with calcineurin neurotoxicity; both may respond to a reduction in drug levels. No proven therapies exist, although reduction of immunosuppression is commonly employed, on analogy to immune reconstitution in AIDS patients with PML.

Fungal Infections

In addition to the endemic mycoses, transplant recipients are at risk for opportunistic infections with a variety of fungal agents, the most important of which are *Candida*, *Aspergillus*, and *Cryptococcus neoformans*.

Candida

The most common fungal pathogen in transplant patients is *Candida*, with more than 50% being of non-*albicans* strains. Mucocutaneous candidal infection (e.g., oral thrush, esophageal infection, cutaneous infection at intertriginous sites, candidal vaginitis) is most common in diabetics, with high-dose steroid therapy, and during broad-spectrum antibacterial therapy. These infections are usually treatable through correction of the underlying metabolic abnormality and topical therapy with clotrimazole or nystatin (Table 31-6). Thrush also may complicate viral (HSV, CMV) or toxic (drugs including mycophenolate mofetil) esophagitis. Optimal management of candidal infection occurring in association with the presence of vascular access catheters, surgical drains, and bladder catheters requires removal of the foreign body and systemic antifungal therapy with fluconazole or echinocandin.

A special problem in kidney transplant recipients is candiduria, including in asymptomatic patients. Notably in individuals with poor bladder function, obstructing fungal balls can develop at the ureteropelvic junction, resulting in obstructive uropathy, ascending pyelonephritis, and the possibility of systemic dissemination. A single positive culture result for *Candida* species from a blood specimen necessitates systemic antifungal therapy; this finding carries a significant risk of dissemination or invasion in this population.

Aspergillus

Invasive aspergillosis is a medical emergency in the transplant recipient, with the portal of entry being the lungs and sinuses in more than 90% of patients and the skin in most of those remaining. The predominant species depends on the clinical center and prior exposures to soil and construction sites. The pathological hallmark of invasive aspergillosis is blood vessel invasion, which accounts for the three clinical characteristics of this infection – tissue infarction, hemorrhage, and systemic dissemination with metastatic invasion. Early in the course of transplantation, CNS involvement with fungal infection is most often due to *Aspergillus*; 1 year or later after transplantation, other fungi (*Zygomycetes*, dematiaceous fungi) become more prominent. The drug of choice for documented *Aspergillus* infection is voriconazole, despite its significant interactions with calcineurin inhibitors and rapamycin. Liposomal amphotericin is an equally effective alternative, and combination therapies are under study. Surgical debridement is usually essential for successful clearance of such invasive infections.

Central Nervous System Infections and Cryptococcus neoformans

CNS infection in the transplant recipient may result from a broad spectrum of organisms. Infections are often metastatic to the CNS from the blood stream and lungs. Viral etiologies include CMV (nodular angiitis), HSV meningoencephalitis, JC virus (progressive multifocal leukoencephalopathy), and VZV. Local epidemiology (West Nile virus, Eastern equine encephalitis) also must be considered. Common bacterial infections in addition to the pneumococcus include Lyme disease, *Listeria monocytogenes*, tuberculosis, *Nocardia*, and occasionally *Salmonella*. Brain abscess and epidural abscess have been observed and may be particularly problematic when secondary to methicillin-resistant *Staphylococcus aureus*, penicillin-resistant *Pneumococcus*, and quinolone-resistant streptococci. As noted earlier, fungi may be metastatic from lungs (*Aspergillus* and *Cryptococcus*) but also may spread from sinuses (Mucoraceae), skin (Dematiaceae), and the blood stream (*Histoplasma* and *Pseudallescheria/Scedosporium*, *Fusarium*). Parasites include *Toxoplasma gondii* and *Strongyloides stercoralis*.

Given the spectrum of etiologies, precise diagnosis is essential (Table 31-7). A reasonable empirical regimen would treat *Pneumococcus* and *Haemophilus influenzae* (ceftriaxone and vancomycin), *Listeria* (ampicillin), *Cryptococcus* (fluconazole or amphotericin), and HSV (acyclovir) while awaiting data (lumbar puncture, blood cultures, and radiographic studies). Non-infectious etiologies, including calcineurin inhibitor toxicity, lymphoma, and metastatic cancer, should be included in the differential diagnosis. Molecular assays (HSV) and biopsy (for non-infectious etiologies) may be needed for diagnosis.

Cryptococcus neoformans. Cryptococcal infection is rarely seen in the transplant recipient until more than 6 months after transplantation. In the relatively intact transplant recipient, the most common presentation of cryptococcal infection is that of an asymptomatic pulmonary nodule, often with active organisms present. In the "chronic ne'er-do-well" patient, pneumonia and meningitis are common, with skin involvement at sites of tissue injury (catheters) and in prostate or bone also reported.

Cryptococcosis should be suspected in transplant recipients who present with unexplained headaches (especially when accompanied by fevers), decreased state of consciousness, failure to thrive, or unexplained focal skin disease (which requires biopsy for culture and pathological evaluation) more than 6 months after transplantation. Diagnosis is often achieved by serum cryptococcal antigen detection, but all such patients should have lumbar puncture for cell counts, culture, India ink preparation, and cryptococcal antigen studies (Figure 31-4). Initial treatment is best with liposomal amphotericin and 5-flucytosine (monitoring serum levels) followed by high-dose fluconazole until the cryptococcal antigen is cleared from blood and cerebrospinal fluid. Lifetime prophylaxis is needed. IRIS may require adjunctive use of corticosteroids during the acute phase of CNS cryptococcal infection. IRIS or scarring may cause obstruction with increased cerebrospinal fluid pressure and hydrocephalus.

Strongyloides stercoralis. *S. stercoralis* infection may activate over 30 years after initial exposure with immunosuppressive therapy. Such reactivation can result in either diarrheal illness or parasite migration with hyperinfestation syndrome (characterized by hemorrhagic

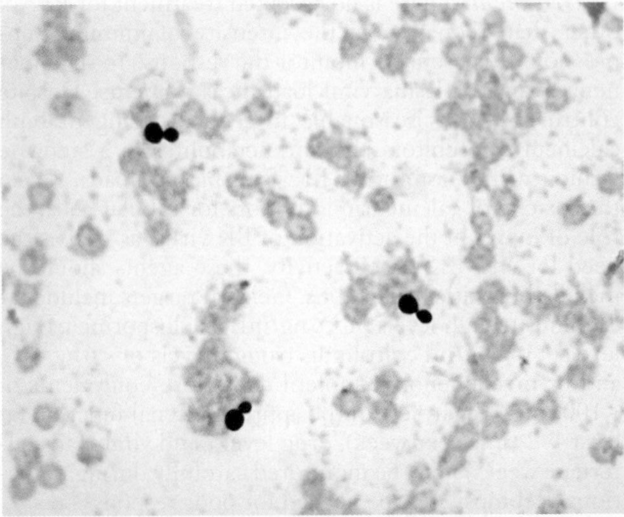

FIGURE-31-4 ■ *Cryptococcus neoformans* meningitis – India ink preparation of cerebrospinal fluid from a 53-year-old man 16 months after renal transplantation.

enterocolitis, hemorrhagic pneumonia, or both) or disseminated infection with accompanying (usually) Gram-negative bacteremia or meningitis. Patients from tropical areas and the southeastern United States should be screened with *Strongyloides* IgG serology prior to transplantation, and should be treated with ivermectin pre-emptively if seropositive.

Pneumocystis and Fever with Pneumonitis

The spectrum of potential pathogens of the lungs in the transplant recipient is broad. Some general concepts are worth consideration. As for all infections in transplantation, invasive diagnostic techniques are often necessary for specific microbiological diagnosis. This avoids unnecessary toxicities of antimicrobial agents and selection of optimal therapy. The depressed inflammatory response of the immunocompromised transplant patient may greatly modify or delay the appearance of a pulmonary lesion on radiograph. Focal or multifocal consolidation of acute onset is likely to be caused by bacterial infection. Similar multifocal lesions with subacute to chronic progression are more likely secondary to fungi, tuberculosis, or nocardial infections. Large nodules are usually a sign of fungal or nocardial infection, particularly if they are subacute to chronic in onset. Subacute disease with diffuse abnormalities, either of the peribronchovascular type or miliary micronodules, are usually caused by viruses (especially CMV) or *Pneumocystis*.[54,75] Additional clues can be found by examining pulmonary lesions for cavitation, which suggests necrotizing infection as may be caused by fungi (*Aspergillus* or Mucoraceae), *Nocardia*, *Staphylococcus*, and certain Gram-negative bacilli, most commonly *Klebsiella pneumoniae* and *Pseudomonas aeruginosa*.[35,76]

CT of the chest is useful when the chest radiograph is negative or when the radiographic findings are subtle or non-specific. CT also is essential to the definition of the extent of the disease process, to the discernment of the possibility of simultaneous processes (superinfection), and to the selection of the optimal invasive technique to achieve pathological diagnosis.

***Pneumocystis* Pneumonia.** The risk of infection with *Pneumocystis jiroveci* pneumonia (PCP) is greatest in the first 6 months after transplantation and during periods of increased immunosuppression.[18,19,52,54,57,75] In patients not receiving trimethoprim/sulfamethoxazole (or alternative drugs) as prophylaxis, most transplant centers report an incidence of *Pneumocystis* pneumonia of approximately 10% in the first 6 months after transplantation. There is a continued risk of infection in three overlapping groups of transplant recipients: (1) recipients who require higher than normal levels of immunosuppression for prolonged periods because of poor allograft function or chronic rejection; (2) recipients with chronic CMV infection; and (3) recipients undergoing treatments that increase the level of immunodeficiency, such as cancer chemotherapy or neutropenia secondary to drug toxicity. The expected mortality secondary to *Pneumocystis* pneumonia is increased in patients on cyclosporine compared with other immunocompromised hosts.

The hallmark of infection resulting from PCP is the presence of marked hypoxemia, dyspnea, and cough with a paucity of physical or radiological findings. In the transplant recipient, *Pneumocystis* pneumonia is generally acute to subacute in development. Atypical *Pneumocystis* infection (radiographically or clinically) may be seen in patients who have coexisting pulmonary infections or who develop disease while receiving prophylaxis with second-choice agents (e.g., pentamidine or atovaquone). Patients outside the usual period of greatest risk for *P. carinii* (*jiroveci*) pneumonia may present with indolent disease, which may be radiographically confused with heart failure. In such patients, diagnosis often has to be made by invasive procedures. The role of rapamycin therapy in the clinical presentation is unknown. Numerous patients have been identified with interstitial pneumonitis while receiving rapamycin.[3,9] This syndrome may occur in the presence or absence of concomitant infections (adenovirus, respiratory syncytial virus, *Pneumocystis*).

Diagnosis, Therapy, and Prophylaxis. The characteristic hypoxemia of *Pneumocystis* pneumonia produces a broad alveolar-arterial partial pressure of oxygen gradient. The level of serum lactate dehydrogenase is elevated in most patients with *Pneumocystis* pneumonia (>300 IU/mL). Many other diffuse pulmonary processes also increase serum lactate dehydrogenase levels, however. No diagnostic pattern exists for *Pneumocystis* pneumonia on routine chest radiograph. The chest radiograph may be entirely normal or develop the classic pattern of perihilar and interstitial ground-glass infiltrates (Figure 31-1). Chest CT scans are more sensitive to the diffuse interstitial and nodular pattern than routine radiographs. The clinical and radiological manifestations of *P. carinii* (*jiroveci*) pneumonia are virtually identical to the manifestations of CMV. The clinical challenge is to determine whether both pathogens are present. Significant extrapulmonary disease is uncommon in the transplant recipient. Bronchoalveolar lavage may be helpful.

Early therapy with trimethoprim/sulfamethoxazole is preferred; few kidney transplant patients tolerate full-dose trimethoprim/sulfamethoxazole for prolonged periods.[21,52,69] This reflects the elevation of creatinine by trimethoprim (competing for secretion in the kidney), and the toxicity of sulfa agents for the renal allograft. Hydration and the gradual initiation of therapy may help. Alternative therapies are less desirable but have been used with success, including intravenous pentamidine, atovaquone, clindamycin with primaquine or pyrimethamine, and trimetrexate. Although a reduction in the intensity of immunosuppression is generally considered a part of anti-infective therapy in transplantation, the use of short courses of adjunctive steroids with a gradual taper is generally useful.

The importance of preventing *Pneumocystis* infection cannot be overemphasized.[19,52,68,69] Low-dose trimethoprim/sulfamethoxazole is well tolerated and should be used in the absence of concrete data showing true allergy or interstitial nephritis. Alternative prophylactic strategies, including dapsone, atovaquone, and inhaled or intravenous pentamidine, are less effective than trimethoprim/sulfamethoxazole but are useful in patients with significant allergy to sulfa drugs. Trimethoprim/sulfamethoxazole is the most effective agent for prevention of infection caused by *P. carinii (jiroveci)*. The advantages of trimethoprim/sulfamethoxazole include increased efficacy; lower cost; availability of oral preparations; and possible protection against other organisms, including *T. gondii*, *Isospora belli*, *Cyclospora cayetanensis*, *Nocardia asteroides*, and common urinary, respiratory, and gastrointestinal bacterial pathogens. Alternative agents lack this spectrum of activity.

Urinary Tract Infection

The majority of urinary tract infections occur in the first year after kidney transplantation. A subset of patients have recurrent disease and may suffer pyelonephritis or bacteremia. Urinary tract infection beyond 6 months after transplantation is associated with reduced renal graft survival and increased mortality. The risk of urinary tract infection after kidney transplantation is increased in women, with prolonged bladder catheterization, with increased intensity of immunosuppression, in recipients of deceased donor grafts, and, possibly, with vesicoureteral reflux. The risk for vesicoureteral reflux is dependent in part on the technical approach to implantation of the ureter taken in surgery. The risk for candiduria in particular is increased in patients who have received prior antimicrobial therapy, with neurogenic bladder, with indwelling urethral catheters, and in intensive care units. Most kidney transplant recipients with bacteriuria are asymptomatic, while pain with pyelonephritis represents transmural infection with local inflammation outside the denervated allograft causing what is perceived as allograft tenderness.

The major causative organisms include Gram-negative bacilli (*Escherichia coli*, *Klebsiella*, *Pseudomonas*, *Enterobacter*, *Proteus*) as well as Gram-positives (largely enterococci) and fungi (*Candida* species). Each of these groups may manifest important antimicrobial resistance; therapy should be based on susceptibility pattern determinations. Therapy should be guided by the presence or absence of structural abnormalities (obstruction, delayed bladder emptying) as well as by the microbiology of infection. Thus, imaging (ultrasound to exclude hydronephrosis) as well as cultures should be obtained in patients with upper tract infection. Initial empiric therapy should include antimicrobial agents not used previously for prophylaxis and, where possible, not used in prior episodes of infection given the risk for development antimicrobial resistance. The spectrum of agents can be narrowed based on susceptibility data. Short-course therapy is not recommended for treatment of uncomplicated urinary tract infection after transplantation. The resolution of infection should be demonstrated (7-day minimum with effective agents) and upper tract disease (at least 2–3 weeks of therapy) and may require intravenous therapy initially. Asymptomatic candiduria should be treated in patients with renal allografts (although data are limited) with fluconazole (200 mg orally per day for 7–14 days). Upper tract disease with *Candida* species should suggest obstruction and requires more intensive therapy (fluconazole 400 mg daily for 3–4 weeks). The echinocandins are not useful for the treatment of most urinary tract infections as they achieve poor concentrations in the urinary tract. Removal of stents and catheters is generally required for resolution of urinary tract infection.

The prevention of urinary tract infections has been dramatically altered by the routine use of trimethoprim/sulfamethoxazole, which has the advantage of prevention of *Pneumocystis* pneumonia as well as urinary tract infections and other infections. Trimethoprim/sulfamethoxazole given for 6 months to 1 year post kidney transplantation is generally effective in the absence of instrumentation or obstruction. Few recent studies address whether the changing ecology of bacteria have reduced the efficacy of prophylaxis. In patients intolerant of trimethoprim/sulfamethoxazole, a fluoroquinolone may be used with the addition of another agent against PCP (atovaquone, dapsone).

CONCLUSIONS

Transplant infectious disease is increasingly characterized by the ability to monitor and prevent infection based on prophylaxis, new antimicrobial agents, and vaccination. Despite significant advances, infection poses a life-threatening challenge for many recipients. In the future, increased availability of pathogen-specific immune function tests, enhanced screening of donors and recipients, and a better understanding of risk factors such as genetic polymorphisms should combine with advances in transplant immunosuppression to reduce risks of infection still further.

REFERENCES

1. Ahn HJ, Kim MS, Kim YS, et al. Clinical outcome of renal transplantation in patients with positive pre-transplant hepatitis B surface antigen. J Med Virol 2007;79(11):1655–63.
2. Allen U, Preiksaitis J. Epstein–Barr virus and posttransplant lymphoproliferative disorder in solid organ transplant recipients. Am J Transplant 2009;9(Suppl. 4):S87–96.
3. Avery RK. Recipient screening prior to solid-organ transplantation. Clin Infect Dis 2002;35(12):1513–9.
4. Avery RK, Ljungman P. Prophylactic measures in the solid-organ recipient before transplantation. Clin Infect Dis 2001;33(Suppl. 1):S15–21.
5. Boivin G, Goyette N, Gilbert C, et al. Absence of cytomegalovirus-resistance mutations after valganciclovir prophylaxis, in a prospective multicenter study of solid-organ transplant recipients. J Infect Dis 2004;189(9):1615–8.
6. Caliendo AM, St George K, Kao SY, et al. Comparison of quantitative cytomegalovirus (CMV) PCR in plasma and CMV antigenemia assay: clinical utility of the prototype AMPLICOR CMV MONITOR test in transplant recipients. J Clin Microbiol 2000;38(6):2122–7.
7. Capobianchi MR, Sambri V, Castilletti C, et al. Retrospective screening of solid organ donors in Italy, 2009, reveals unpredicted circulation of West Nile virus. Euro Surveill 2010;15(34).
8. Centers for Disease Control and Prevention. HIV transmitted from a living organ donor – New York city, 2009. MMWR Morb Mortal Wkly Rep 2011;60(10):297–301.
9. Champion L, Stern M, Israel-Biet D, et al. Brief communication: sirolimus-associated pneumonitis: 24 cases in renal transplant recipients. Ann Intern Med 2006;144(7):505–9.
10. Chin-Hong PV, Schwartz BS, Bern C, et al. Screening and treatment of Chagas disease in organ transplant recipients in the United States: recommendations from the Chagas in transplant working group. Am J Transplant 2011;11(4):672–80.
11. Chou S, Lurain NS, Thompson KD, et al. Viral DNA polymerase mutations associated with drug resistance in human cytomegalovirus. J Infect Dis 2003;188(1):32–9.
12. Coffin CS, Stock PG, Dove LM, et al. Virologic and clinical outcomes of hepatitis B virus infection in HIV-HBV coinfected transplant recipients. Am J Transplant 2010;10(5):1268–75.

13. Couzi L, Helou S, Bachelet T, et al. High incidence of anti-cytomegalovirus drug resistance among D+R− kidney transplant recipients receiving preemptive therapy. Am J Transplant 2012;12:202–9.
14. Emery VC, Sabin CA, Cope AV, et al. Application of viral-load kinetics to identify patients who develop cytomegalovirus disease after transplantation. Lancet 2000;355(9220):2032–6.
15. Fischer SA, Avery RK. Screening of donor and recipient prior to solid organ transplantation. Am J Transplant 2009;9(Suppl. 4):S7–18.
16. Fishman JA. Infection in solid-organ transplant recipients. N Engl J Med 2007;357(25):2601–14.
17. Fishman JA. *Pneumocystis carinii* and parasitic infections in transplantation. Infect Dis Clin North Am 1995;9(4):1005–44.
18. Fishman JA. Prevention of infection due to *Pneumocystis carinii*. Antimicrob Agents Chemother 1998;42(5):995–1004.
19. Fishman JA. Prevention of infection caused by *Pneumocystis carinii* in transplant recipients. Clin Infect Dis 2001;33(8):1397–405.
20. Fishman JA. Transplantation for patients infected with human immunodeficiency virus: no longer experimental but not yet routine. J Infect Dis 2003;188(10):1405–11.
21. Fishman JA. Treatment of infection due to *Pneumocystis carinii*. Antimicrob Agents Chemother 1998;42(6):1309–14.
22. Fishman JA, Emery V, Freeman R, et al. Cytomegalovirus in transplantation – challenging the status quo. Clin Transplant 2007;21(2):149–58.
23. Fishman JA, Issa NC. Infection in organ transplantation: risk factors and evolving patterns of infection. Infect Dis Clin North Am 2010;24(2):273–83.
24. Fishman JA, Rubin RH. Infection in organ-transplant recipients [see comment]. N Engl J Med 1998;338(24):1741–51.
25. Fishman JA, Strong DM, Kuehnert MJ. Organ and tissue safety workshop 2007: advances and challenges. Cell Tissue Bank 2009;10(3):271–80.
26. Freeman RB, Giatras I, Falagas ME, et al. Outcome of transplantation of organs procured from bacteremic donors. Transplantation 1999;68(8):1107–11.
27. Gane E, Saliba F, Valdecasas GJ, et al. Randomised trial of efficacy and safety of oral ganciclovir in the prevention of cytomegalovirus disease in liver-transplant recipients. The Oral Ganciclovir International Transplantation Study Group. Lancet 1997;350(9093):1729–33.
28. Green M. Management of Epstein–Barr virus-induced post-transplant lymphoproliferative disease in recipients of solid organ transplantation. Am J Transplant 2001;1(2):103–8.
29. Green M, Mazariegos GV. Persistent detection of Epstein–Barr virus DNA after pediatric liver transplantation: unclear risks and uncertain responses. Liver Transpl 2008;14(8):1077–80.
30. Green M, Michaels MG. Loads, lungs, and lymphoproliferative disorders: role of Epstein–Barr virus and limitations of what we know. Transpl Infect Dis 2010;12(4):281–3.
31. Grossi PA, Fishman JA, the AST Infectious Disease Community of Practice. Donor-derived infections in solid organ transplant recipients. Am J Transplant 2009;9(Suppl. 4):S19–26.
32. Hakki M, Chou S. The biology of cytomegalovirus drug resistance. Curr Opin Infect Dis 2011;24(6):605–11.
33. Hirsch HH, Mohaupt M, Klimkait T. Prospective monitoring of BK virus load after discontinuing sirolimus treatment in a renal transplant patient with BK virus nephropathy. J Infect Dis 2001;184(11):1494–5, author reply 1495-6.
34. Hirsch HH, Randhawa P. BK virus in solid organ transplant recipients. Am J Transplant 2009;9(Suppl. 4):S136–46.
35. Huang RC, Fishman JA. Screening of deceased organ donors: no easy answers. Transplantation 2011;91(2):146–9.
36. Humar A. Screening for West Nile virus: more uncertainty. Am J Transplant 2004;4(8):1217–8.
37. Humar A, Gregson D, Caliendo AM, et al. Clinical utility of quantitative cytomegalovirus viral load determination for predicting cytomegalovirus disease in liver transplant recipients. Transplantation 1999;68(9):1305–11.
38. Humar A, Lebranchu Y, Vincenti F, et al. The efficacy and safety of 200 days valganciclovir cytomegalovirus prophylaxis in high-risk kidney transplant recipients. Am J Transplant 2010;10(5):1228–37.
39. Humar A, Limaye AP, Blumberg EA, et al. Extended valganciclovir prophylaxis in D+/R− kidney transplant recipients is associated with long-term reduction in cytomegalovirus disease: two-year results of the IMPACT study. Transplantation 2010;90(12):1427–31.
40. Humar A, Snydman D. Cytomegalovirus in solid organ transplant recipients. Am J Transplant 2009;9(Suppl. 4):S78–86.
41. Ison MG, Nalesnik MA. An update on donor-derived disease transmission in organ transplantation. Am J Transplant 2011;11(6):1123–30.
42. Kalil AC, Levitsky J, Lyden E, et al. Meta-analysis: the efficacy of strategies to prevent organ disease by cytomegalovirus in solid organ transplant recipients [see comment]. Ann Intern Med 2005;143(12):870–80.
43. Kamar N, Rostaing L, Selves J, et al. Natural history of hepatitis C virus-related liver fibrosis after renal transplantation. Am J Transplant 2005;5(7):1704–12.
44. Kasiske BL, Cangro CB, Hariharan S, et al. The evaluation of renal transplantation candidates: clinical practice guidelines. Am J Transplant 2001;1(Suppl. 2):3–95.
45. Kasiske BL, Ravenscraft M, Ramos EL, et al. The evaluation of living renal transplant donors: clinical practice guidelines. Ad Hoc Clinical Practice Guidelines Subcommittee of the Patient Care and Education Committee of the American Society of Transplant Physicians. J Am Soc Nephrol 1996;7(11):2288–313.
46. Kiberd BA, Forward K. Screening for West Nile virus in organ transplantation: a medical decision analysis. Am J Transplant 2004;4(8):1296–301.
47. Kotton CN, Kumar D, Caliendo AM, et al. International consensus guidelines on the management of cytomegalovirus in solid organ transplantation. Transplantation 2010;89(7):779–95.
48. Kotton CN, Ryan ET, Fishman JA. Prevention of infection in adult travelers after solid organ transplantation. Am J Transplant 2005;5(1):8–14.
49. Levitsky J, Doucette K. Viral hepatitis in solid organ transplant recipients. Am J Transplant 2009;9(Suppl. 4):S116–30.
50. Lowance D, Neumayer HH, Legendre CM, et al. Valacyclovir for the prevention of cytomegalovirus disease after renal transplantation. International Valacyclovir Cytomegalovirus Prophylaxis Transplantation Study Group [see comments]. N Engl J Med 1999;340(19):1462–70.
51. Lurain NS, Chou S. Antiviral drug resistance of human cytomegalovirus. Clin Microbiol Rev 2010;23(4):689–712.
52. Martin SI. Fishman JA, the AST Infectious Disease Community of Practice. Pneumocystis pneumonia in solid organ transplant recipients. Am J Transplant 2009;9(Suppl. 4):S227–33.
53. Mazzulli T, Drew LW, Yen-Lieberman B, et al. Multicenter comparison of the digene hybrid capture CMV DNA assay (version 2.0), the pp 65 antigenemia assay, and cell culture for detection of cytomegalovirus viremia. J Clin Microbiol 1999;37(4):958–63.
54. Munoz P, Rodriguez C, Bouza E. *Mycobacterium tuberculosis* infection in recipients of solid organ transplants. Clin Infect Dis 2005;40(4):581–7.
55. Nalesnik MA. The diverse pathology of post-transplant lymphoproliferative disorders: the importance of a standardized approach. Transpl Infect Dis 2001;3(2):88–96.
56. Opelz G, Dohler B. Lymphomas after solid organ transplantation: a collaborative transplant study report. Am J Transplant 2004;4(2):222–30.
57. Pappas PG, Silveira FP. Candida in solid organ transplant recipients. Am J Transplant 2009;9(Suppl. 4):S173–9.
58. Patel R, Portela D, Badley AD, et al. Risk factors of invasive Candida and non-Candida fungal infections after liver transplantation. Transplantation 1996;62(7):926–34.
59. Paya CV, Fung JJ, Nalesnik MA, et al. Epstein–Barr virus-induced posttransplant lymphoproliferative disorders. ASTS/ASTP EBV-PTLD task force and the mayo clinic organized international consensus development meeting. Transplantation 1999;68(10):1517–25.
60. Paya C, Humar A, Dominguez E, et al. Efficacy and safety of valganciclovir vs. oral ganciclovir for prevention of cytomegalovirus disease in solid organ transplant recipients. Am J Transplant 2004;4(4):611–20.
61. Pergam SA, Limaye AP. Varicella zoster virus (VZV) in solid organ transplant recipients. Am J Transplant 2009;9(Suppl. 4):S108–15.
62. Preiksaitis JK, Brennan DC, Fishman J, et al. Canadian society of transplantation consensus workshop on cytomegalovirus management in solid organ transplantation final report. Am J Transplant 2005;5(2):218–27.
63. Ramos E, Drachenberg CB, Wali R, et al. The decade of polyomavirus BK-associated nephropathy: state of affairs. Transplantation 2009;87(5):621–30.

64. Randhawa P, Vats A, Shapiro R. Monitoring for polyomavirus BK and JC in urine: comparison of quantitative polymerase chain reaction with urine cytology. Transplantation 2005;79(8):984–6.
65. Razonable RR, Brown RA, Humar A, et al. Herpesvirus infections in solid organ transplant patients at high risk of primary cytomegalovirus disease. J Infect Dis 2005;192(8):1331–9.
66. Razonable RR, Paya CV. Herpesvirus infections in transplant recipients: current challenges in the clinical management of cytomegalovirus and Epstein–Barr virus infections. Herpes 2003;10(3):60–5.
67. Reinke P, Fietze E, Ode-Hakim S, et al. Late-acute renal allograft rejection and symptomless cytomegalovirus infection. Lancet 1994;344:1737–8.
68. Rodriguez M, Fishman JA. Prevention of infection due to *Pneumocystis* spp. in human immunodeficiency virus-negative immunocompromised patients. Clin Microbiol Rev;17(4):770-782.
69. Rodriguez M, Sifri CD, Fishman JA. Failure of low-dose atovaquone prophylaxis against *Pneumocystis jiroveci* infection in transplant recipients. Clin Infect Dis 2004;38(8):e76–8.
70. Roland ME, Barin B, Carlson L, et al. HIV-infected liver and kidney transplant recipients: 1- and 3-year outcomes. Am J Transplant 2008;8(2):355–65.
71. Rostaing L, Weclawiak H, Izopet J, et al. Treatment of hepatitis C virus infection after kidney transplantation. Contrib Nephrol 2012;176:87–96.
72. Rowe DT, Qu L, Reyes J, et al. Use of quantitative competitive PCR to measure Epstein–Barr virus genome load in the peripheral blood of pediatric transplant patients with lymphoproliferative disorders. J Clin Microbiol 1997;35(6):1612–5.
73. Schaffner A. Pretransplant evaluation for infections in donors and recipients of solid organs. Clin Infect Dis 2001;33(Suppl. 1):S9–14.
74. Schwartz BS, Paster M, Ison MG, et al. Organ donor screening practices for *Trypanosoma cruzi* infection among US Organ Procurement Organizations. Am J Transplant 2011;11(4): 848–51.
75. Singh N, Paterson DL. *Mycobacterium tuberculosis* infection in solid-organ transplant recipients: impact and implications for management. Clin Infect Dis 1998;27(5):1266–77.
76. Tanabe K, Kitani R, Takahashi K, et al. Long-term results in human T-cell leukemia virus type 1-positive renal transplant recipients. Transplant Proc 1998;30(7):3168–70.
77. Tsai DE, Douglas L, Andreadis C, et al. EBV PCR in the diagnosis and monitoring of posttransplant lymphoproliferative disorder: results of a two-arm prospective trial. Am J Transplant 2008;8(5):1016–24.
78. US PHS guideline for preventing transmission of HIV through transplantation of human tissue and organs. MMWR Morb Mortal Wkly Rep 1994;43(RR8):1–17. Available online at: http://www.cdc.gov/mmwr/PDF/RR/RR4308.pdf.
79. US Public Health Service. (Draft) Public Health Service guideline for reducing transmission of human immunodeficiency virus (HIV), hepatitis B virus (HBV), and hepatitis C virus (HCV) through solid organ transplantation. In: Services, editor. vol. 76/Notices 58517. Federal Register CDC 2011: [Docket No. CDC–2011–0011].
80. Yao F, Seed C, Farrugia A, et al. The risk of HIV, HBV, HCV and HTLV infection among musculoskeletal tissue donors in Australia. Am J Transplant 2007;7(12):2723–6.
81. Young L, Alfieri C, Hennessy K, et al. Expression of Epstein–Barr virus transformation-associated genes in tissues of patients with EBV lymphoproliferative disease. N Engl J Med 1989;321(16):1080–5.

CHAPTER 32

LIVER DISEASE AMONG RENAL TRANSPLANT RECIPIENTS

Adnan Said • John P. Rice • Nasia Safdar • Jennifer T. Wells • Michael R. Lucey

CHAPTER OUTLINE

OVERVIEW OF INCIDENCE AND CLINICOPATHOLOGICAL ASSOCIATIONS

Theoretically, the spectrum of liver disease in renal transplant recipients should mimic the spectrum of disease seen in society. It is axiomatic that renal transplant recipients are at risk for all the acute and chronic liver disorders seen in the non-transplant population. Surveys of the prevalence of chronic liver injury in otherwise healthy subjects suggest that the burden of unrecognized liver disease in the apparently healthy community is high. A study by Ioannou et al.[115] used the National Health and Nutrition Examination Survey (NHANES) conducted between 1999 and 2002 to assess the prevalence of elevated serum transaminase activities in a cohort of 6823 American adults. The prevalence of elevated alanine aminotransferase (ALT) was 8.9%, a result that is more than double that of previously available estimates in similar populations. Recently, another NHANES study of American adolescents identified the presence of an elevated ALT, defined as a value above 30 U/mL, in 8.0% of the population.[95] Risk factors for an elevated ALT included higher waist circumference, body mass index, fasting blood glucose, and fasting triglycerides.

These studies indicate the potential hazards in estimating the likely prevalence of liver disease in a special population such as recipients of renal transplantation in the absence of good data. The rise in non-alcoholic steatohepatitis, the recognition of chronic hepatitis C virus (HCV), and possible changing use of alcohol mean that a contemporary assessment of the spectrum of liver disease might be quite different from previous reports, and in one country compared to another.[148] Consequently, it should be noted that there have been no comprehensive attempts to characterize liver disease in renal transplant recipients since Allison et al.[7] examined the prevalence and nature of chronic liver disease among 538 patients with functioning renal allografts managed in Scotland between 1980 and 1989. The authors reported that biochemical evidence of liver dysfunction was observed in 37 patients (7%), 19 (4%) of whom were seropositive for HCV. The work of Allison et al. is most likely an underestimate given that it was undertaken just as HCV infection was discovered, and, as will be discussed below, HCV prevalence in renal transplant cohorts has been reported to be as high as 40%.

In the subsequent sections of this chapter we will discuss in more detail some liver disorders which appear to occur in greater frequency in renal transplant recipients compared with the background population. In some circumstances, such as autosomal dominant polycystic disease, the liver and kidney disorder are part of the same underlying disease. In other patients in whom renal failure coexists with liver disease, the two conditions are acquired separately. Chronic infections with hepatotropic viruses (HBV and HCV) fall into this category. We will consider liver diatheses that are consequences of the inherent risks of the transplant process, including drug-related injury secondary to immunosuppressant medications or hepatic manifestations of opportunistic infections secondary to immunosuppression.

COMBINED LIVER AND KIDNEY DISEASES

Polycystic Disease

Autosomal dominant polycystic disease is a condition arising from mutations in two distinct genes that result in the development of the renal and liver cysts. Mutations in *AD-PKD1* account for up to 90% adult-onset combined kidney and liver polycystic disease and mutations in *AD-PKD2* account for the majority of the remainder.[74,197] Patients with mutations in *PKD2* tend to have later onset of disease and approximately 16 years of increased life expectancy compared with patients who have mutations in *PKD1*, but otherwise the natural history is identical. Renal cystic disease associated with autosomal dominant polycystic disease may develop renal failure that requires hemodialysis or renal transplantation. The severity of hepatic cystic disease correlates with both the severity of renal cystic disease and the degree of renal dysfunction.

Hepatic cysts are lined with secretory biliary epithelium. The cysts are first noted after puberty and increase in prevalence with age.[18] Hepatic cyst prevalence is correlated with renal cyst volume.[18] The lifetime risk for expression of hepatic cysts is equal in male and female holders of the genetic defect, but hepatic cysts tend to be larger and more numerous in women, possibly due to the influence of estrogen on hepatic cyst growth.[215]

Symptoms due to hepatic cysts in adult-onset autosomal dominant polycystic disease are the result of a compartment disorder in which the abdominal cavity is unable to accommodate the cystic mass. Patients with massive hepatic cysts can experience abdominal pain, early satiety, or dyspnea (Figure 32-1). These "bulk" symptoms may be so troubling as to warrant liver transplantation. In addition, uncommon complications, such as cyst rupture, infection, torsion, or hemorrhage, can occur.[47] Hepatic function and portal hemodynamics are usually normal. Biliary obstruction, portal hypertension, ascites, variceal hemorrhage, and encephalopathy are rare features of autosomal dominant polycystic disease.

There is no good medical therapy for the abdominal symptoms associated with autosomal dominant polycystic disease. Agents such as somatostatin and sirolimus have been tried without much success.[142] For women with symptomatic cysts, stopping oral contraceptive or hormone replacement therapy should be considered, but data on efficacy are anecdotal. There are many procedures described to ameliorate the discomfort associated with liver cysts. Cyst aspiration under sonographic guidance may

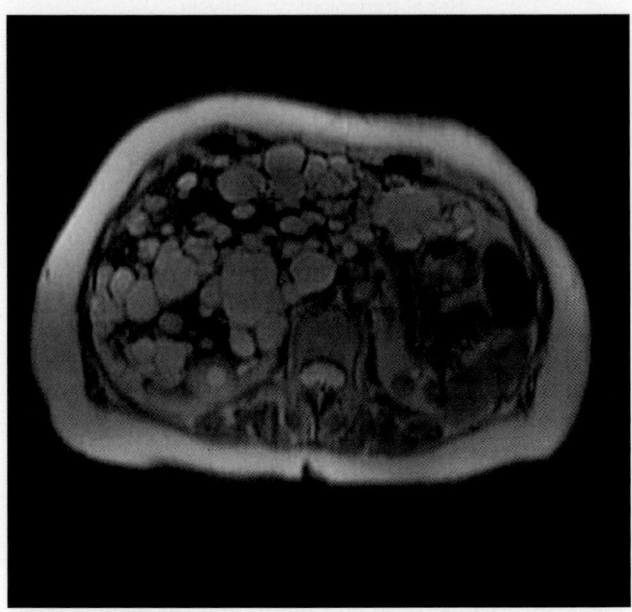

FIGURE 32-1 ■ The liver has innumerable cysts, ranging from small to large, in a patient with autosomal dominant polycystic liver/kidney disease.

provide temporary relief, but the cysts inevitably recur. Continuous or intermittent drainage through a permanent percutaneous catheter should be strongly discouraged as it runs the risk of converting a sterile cyst into a pyogenic abscess. Surgical approaches include open or laparoscopic cyst fenestration, hepatic resection, and liver transplantation.

Autosomal recessive polycystic kidney disease (ARPKD) is caused by mutations in the *PKHD-1* gene which encodes the protein fibrocystin.[233] Congenital hepatic fibrosis (CHF), due to ductal plate malformation of the developing biliary system, is invariably present in patients with ARPKD.[129] Clinical presentation is related to age. Renal disease predominates in patients that present neonatally. Hepatic manifestations predominate in older children and adults, although overlap is common.[129] The predominant manifestations of CHF are the development of portal hypertension, dilation of the intrahepatic bile ducts (also known as Caroli's syndrome), and vascular anomalies. Variceal formation and hemorrhage, splenomegaly, and thrombocytopenia are common.[129] Dilation of the intrahepatic bile ducts can result in recurrent bile stasis and cholangitis. Finally, anomalies of portal venous anatomy are frequent. Treatment for CHF is focused on prevention of variceal hemorrhage and promotion of adequate biliary drainage to prevent cholangitis.[241]

Drug-Induced Hepatotoxicity

Drug-induced liver injury (DILI) can have a wide spectrum of severity ranging from asymptomatic elevations of liver enzymes to acute liver failure. With rare exceptions, the serum biochemical and liver histological patterns are not diagnostic of drug-related injury. Rather, DILI is often diagnosed based upon a combination of temporal relationship to a particular drug use, exclusion of other pathology (such as viral hepatitis), and knowledge of common pattern of liver test abnormalities associated with particular dr ugs.[11,41,131,156,179] Improvement of liver tests with discontinuation of the offending medications offers further evidence of DILI, but improvement may take weeks.

The severity of drug-related injury may be predicted by the degree of impairment of hepatic function. In particular the presence of jaundice in association with elevated aminotransferases (known as "Hy's rule") is often an ominous sign of significant hepatocellular injury and risk of progression to liver failure.[11,41,156,179,149] In the two largest series to date, mortality or liver transplantation from idiosyncratic (excluding acetaminophen) drug reactions occurred in 11.7% and 15% of cases.[11,41]

The mechanisms of drug injury are multiple as well. Toxic metabolites produced by detoxification of medications through the liver, most commonly via the cytochrome P-450 mechanisms, may contribute to dose-related hepatotoxicity such as seen with acetaminophen.[131,235] Other medications may have immunologic mechanisms of injury that are not dose-related and considered idiosyncratic.[131,179,235] Most patients present asymptomatically or with non-specific symptoms. Occasionally, a hypersensitivity reaction of fever, lymphadenopathy and leukocytosis, often with eosinophilia, may be seen.[49,133] Liver test abnormalities are variable. The most common pattern is acute hepatocellular injury with elevations of aminotransferases greater than twofold normal with lesser elevations of alkaline phosphatase; however, cholestasis and bile duct loss (e.g., amoxicillin-clavulinic acid toxicity) and bland fibrosis (methotrexate) are also seen.[11,41,157]

In transplant patients the opportunities for drug-related hepatotoxicity abound due to the use of multiple medications, many of which are metabolized via the same pathways in the liver, thereby increasing the risk of accumulation of hepatotoxic metabolites. Common medication classes used in transplant that have been implicated in DILI include immunosuppressive medications,[73,154,180] antibiotics,[11,41] antihyperlipidemics,[11,41] and drugs for hypertension and diabetes.[11,41] In addition, numerous herbal and non-prescription agents have also been implicated in the development of DILI. Finally, more than one agent may be implicated as the etiology for DILI in a given patient.[41] Table 32-1 shows some common medications that stimulate or block the cytochrome P-450 system within the liver and may influence the serum concentrations of other drugs and their metabolites.

The main treatment for DILI is withdrawal of the offending drug. There are few therapies that have been shown to improve outcomes in clinical trial. Two exceptions are *N*-acetylcysteine for acetaminophen toxicity and L-carnitine for valproic acid toxicity.[26,192] Corticosteroids are of unproven benefit. In cases that progress to liver failure, liver transplantation should be considered.[192]

TABLE 32-1 **Medications that Stimulate or Inhibit the Cytochrome P-450 System and can Influence the Level of Other Medications (Such as Cyclosporine)**

Medications that Stimulate Cytochrome P-450 and Can Decrease the Level of Calcineurin Inhibitor
Trimethoprim-sulfamethoxazole
Isoniazid
Nafcillin
Phenytoin
Carbamazepine
Omeprazole
Medications that Inhibit Cytochrome P-450 and Can Increase the Level of Calcineurin Inhibitor
Diltiazem
Fluconazole
Tetracycline
Tacrolimus
Sex hormones
Metoclopramide

SPECIFIC IMMUNOSUPPRESSIVE AGENTS IN RENAL TRANSPLANTATION AND HEPATOTOXICITY

Azathioprine

Azathioprine is an antimetabolite agent that inhibits purine synthesis. It is the prodrug of 6-mercaptopurine (6-MP) and inhibits DNA and RNA synthesis. A broad range of hepatotoxicity has been associated with the use of azathioprine in renal transplant recipients, although it is considered rare.[61,64,73,158,165,168] The pathogenesis of azathioprine hepatotoxicity is multifactorial, resulting from endothelial damage,[103] direct hepatotoxicity,[12] and interlobular bile duct injury.[112] In addition, serum levels of the 6-MP metabolite 6-methylmercaptopurine ribonucleotide have been associated with the development of hepatotoxicity.[214]

The most severe manifestation of azathioprine toxicity is sinusoidal obstruction syndrome (SOS), previously known as veno-occlusive disease. The hallmark of SOS is obliteration and fibrosis of the central hepatic venule and sinusoidal congestion.[165] SOS is manifested by jaundice, ascites, hepatomegaly, weight gain, and elevated liver enzymes (typically alkaline phosphatase with minimal increases in aminotransferases). In the first few months after kidney transplantation it can present with asymptomatic hyperbilirubinemia and elevated liver enzymes, but progresses to jaundice, hepatomegaly, and ascites after the first year.[184] The diagnosis can be made clinically, but is often difficult to make. In the hematopoietic stem cell population, SOS is diagnosed by two of the three criteria being met: serum bilirubin greater than 2 mg/dL, hepatomegaly or right upper quadrant pain, and sudden weight gain of 2% body weight.[168] However, these criteria were established in the hematopoietic stem cell transplant population and not validated in solid-organ transplantation. Doppler ultrasound is useful for documenting ascites and hepatomegaly, and ruling out biliary obstruction or infiltrative processes. Liver biopsy can be used to help make a diagnosis, as can measurement of the wedged hepatic venous portal gradient (HVPG).[191,216] Poor outcomes are associated with higher bilirubin, degree of weight gain, aminotransferase elevation, and HVPG elevation.[191] With cessation of azathioprine SOS has rarely been reported to regress.[136] Specific therapy for SOS, including defibrotide, heparin, ursodeoxycholic acid, and prostaglandin E_1, has produced mixed results.[191] Transjugular intrahepatic portosystemic shunt and liver transplantation have been reported in small series and case reports, respectively.[15,105] Other vascular diseases of the liver have also been attributed to azathioprine, including peliosis hepatis (dilated blood-filled cavities within the liver), presumably secondary to endothelial injury within the liver, leading to sinusoidal dilation. Nodular regenerative hyperplasia can be associated with peliosis. Veno-occlusive disease is rarely seen as well and by the time it appears, portal hypertension with complications of ascites and variceal hemorrhage are often present.[32]

Azathioprine-induced hepatitis has been reported more frequently in kidney transplant recipients with chronic viral hepatitis. In one study of 1035 transplant recipients, 21 fulfilled the criteria for azathioprine hepatitis with jaundice at presentation. Viral hepatitis markers (HCV, HBV, or both) were present in all 20 that were tested. The jaundice disappeared and liver enzymes normalized in all within 4–12 weeks of azathioprine discontinuation or dose reduction. Rechallenge with azathioprine was performed in four patients, with recurrence of jaundice in all cases.[188] In some of these patients histological findings were more consistent with azathioprine toxicity than viral hepatitis with intrahepatic cholestasis, centrilobular hepatocellular necrosis and vascular lesions. Most did have chronic liver disease secondary to viral hepatitis on histology (18/21).

Some have suggested that patients with viral hepatitis and associated chronic inflammation have reduced catabolism and higher levels of toxic azathioprine metabolites in the liver, with resultant increases in rates of fibrosis and cirrhosis as well as hepatotoxicity.[188] Other potential mechanisms include accelerated course of viral hepatitis due to the use of more potent immunosuppressive regimens (prednisone–azathioprine–cyclosporine) with improvements occurring due to withdrawal of immunosuppression. These theories are difficult to prove. Nevertheless, in transplanting patients with viral hepatitis it is a good policy to use minimal immunosuppression (single or dual regimens rather than triple regimens) to minimize acceleration of viral hepatitis-associated liver disease.

Calcineurin Inhibitor-Induced Hepatotoxicity

Cyclosporine and tacrolimus are immunosuppressive medications that belong to the class of calcineurin inhibitors.[34,182] Cyclosporine-induced hepatotoxicity is uncommon and the mechanisms of cyclosporine toxicity are incompletely understood. Cyclosporine is metabolized via the cytochrome P-450 system and interactions with medications that inhibit or stimulate this pathway can result in increased or decreased cyclosporine levels respectively, thereby increasing the risk of hepatotoxicity.[93] Cyclosporine-induced decrease in bile flow can result from reduced bile acid secretion and is associated with risk of bile duct stones and sludge formation in 2–5% of transplant recipients.[153] Rarely, increases in aminotransferases have occurred, mostly in the first 90 days, and these respond to reduction in doses. Persistent elevations in aminotransferases are rare and occur in less than 5–10% of renal transplant recipients.[101,190] Transient elevations of bilirubin or aminotransferases are more common, occur early (within the first 3 months posttransplantation), and are reversible with dose reductions or discontinuation.[153] Among renal transplant recipients without pre-existing liver disease, azathioprine-treated patients had a higher incidence of posttransplant chronic liver disease compared with cyclosporine-treated patients.[173]

Tacrolimus has a similar immunosuppressive mechanism of action to cyclosporine.[34] In liver transplant recipients it is associated with fewer episodes of acute rejection, need for salvage immunosuppressive therapy or ductopenic rejection than cyclosporine. The overall patient and graft survival rates are similar to those seen with cyclosporine.[190]

Similar to cyclosporine, tacrolimus levels were higher in HCV-positive renal transplant recipients, presumably secondary to impaired cytochrome P-450-related metabolism of tacrolimus.[161] Unlike cyclosporine, tacrolimus is not associated with reductions in bile flow and choledocholithiasis. Also tacrolimus was associated with less hyperbilirubinemia (0.3%) as compared to cyclosporine (3.3%) in renal transplant recipients in a large comparative trial.[164] Elevations in aminotransferases are generally mild, even with supratherapuetic levels,[107] and reversible with dose reduction.

Sirolimus

Sirolimus (rapamycin) is an mTOR inhibitor which is structurally related to tacrolimus. Sirolimus-induced hepatotoxicity is uncommon. Elevations of aminotransferases with non-specific histological changes have been reported.[118,181] The liver test abnormalities have resolved with discontinuation of sirolimus. Sirolimus hepatotoxicity has been better described in liver transplant recipients. Of 10 patients treated with sirolimus, two had sinusoidal congestion and one had eosinophilia consistent with a drug-related allergic reaction. Increases in aminotransferases were mild and normalized in all patients by 1 month.[180] Another recent study analyzed a cohort of 97 patients treated with sirolimus-based immunosuppression post liver transplant.[186] Surprisingly, 61 patients discontinued treatment due to adverse effects, including 21 patients that discontinued treatment due to hepatotoxicity.[186] Cyclosporine, but not tacrolimus, can interfere with sirolimus pharmacokinetics, and caution must be exercised when combining these agents.

Mycophenolate Mofetil, Mycophenolic Acid

Mycophenolate mofetil is an ester of mycophenolic acid that is readily absorbed. It inhibits purine synthesis by non-competitively inhibiting a key enzyme in the de novo purine pathway, inosine monophosphate dehydrogenase. Hepatotoxicity is exceedingly uncommon but has been reported in isolated cases.[154]

Monoclonal Antibodies

Monoclonal antibodies have been used as induction immunosuppression in kidney transplantation. Use of alemtuzumab (Campath) (anti-CD52 humanized antibody) has been shown to accelerate hepatic fibrosis in HCV-infected transplant recipients and should generally be avoided in solid-organ recipients with chronic viral hepatitis.[163] Anti-Cd3 antibodies are used less often now for salvage of refractory rejection but have rarely been associated with severe hepatitis and elevation of aminotransferases up to 20-fold.[99] Cytokine-mediated reactions presumably can cause the occasional hepatotoxicity seen with anti-Cd3 antibodies. The interleukin-2 receptor antibody basiliximab has only been reported to cause hepatotoxicity in case reports in children.[87]

T-Cell Costimulatory Inhibitor

Belatacept is a fusion protein designed to inhibit T-cell activation by blocking the costimulatory pathway. Belatacept binds CD80 and CD86 on antigen-presenting cells with high affinity, preventing T-cell activation. To date, there have been no reports of hepatotoxicity related to belatacept.

HEPATITIS VIRUSES ASSOCIATED WITH RENAL TRANSPLANTATION

Hepatitis B Virus

Viral Structure and Proteins

The hepatitis B virus is a hepatotropic enveloped, partially double-stranded DNA virus which is a member of the hepadnavirus family.[209] The core of the virus comprises an RNA-dependent DNA polymerase plus a partially double-stranded DNA. After entry into the hepatocyte, the HBV enters the nucleus and forms what is known as covalently closed circular DNA (cccDNA). This DNA is produced by repair of the gapped virion DNA and is the likely source of the transcripts used to produce the viral proteins. The genome of the HBV encodes four different genes. The C gene encodes core protein, the P gene encodes the hepatitis B polymerase, the S gene encodes three different polypeptides of the envelope (pre S1, pre S2 and S), and the X gene encodes proteins potentially involved in transactivation of viral replication.

The hepatitis B viral antigens consist of the hepatitis B core antigen (HBcAg) and a subunit of the core called the hepatitis B e antigen (HBeAg). HBeAg is released in high concentrations in the plasma during viral replication and is an indirect marker of active viral replication. The envelope protein is referred to as the hepatitis B surface antigen (HBsAg) and is likely responsible for viral binding to the hepatocyte. HBsAg is released in excess in the serum in individuals with chronic hepatitis B infection. Its presence in individuals 6 months after exposure to HBV defines the presence of chronic hepatitis B infection.

Presently, there are eight distinct genotypes of HBV. The prevalence of these distinct genotypes varies geographically. While there is growing evidence that HBV genotype may have implications for treatment success, seroconversion, severity of liver disease, and development of hepatocellular carcinoma (HCC), current management does not change with HBV genotype and thus is not routinely determined.[135]

Tests for Detection of Hepatitis B (Table 32-2)

HBV can cause acute and chronic infections. Acute infection is associated with acute hepatitis characterized by inflammation and hepatocellular necrosis. The diagnosis rests on detecting HBsAg in the serum of a patient with clinical and laboratory evidence of acute hepatitis. Patients with a silent, self-limiting infection are able to produce protective antibody (HBsAb) and ultimately clear the virus. These patients are negative for HBsAg but positive for HBsAb and HBcAb.

Chronic HBV infection is accompanied by evidence of hepatocellular injury and inflammation and is associated with chronic hepatitis. The diagnosis is made by showing persistently elevated serum transaminases and HBsAg in the serum at least 6 months after exposure to HBV infection.[135]

TABLE 32-2 **Commonly Used Tests for Detection of Hepatitis B Infection and their Interpretation**

HBsAg	Anti-HBs	Anti-HBc	Interpretation
+	–	–	Early acute infection
+	–	+	Acute or chronic infection
–	+	+	Cleared HBV infection – immune
–	+	–	Vaccine response – immune

HBsAg, hepatitis B surface antigen; HBc, hepatitis B core; HBV, hepatitis B virus.

Epidemiology of HBV

Routes of Transmission. Hepatitis B is widespread worldwide with over a billion individuals estimated to be carrying the virus. Areas of high incidence include China, South-East Asia and sub-Saharan Africa.[144,189] Worldwide, over 350 million people have chronic HBV infection, and in the United States alone over 1 million individuals are estimated to have chronic infection.[169] HBV is transmitted via perinatal, parenteral, or sexual exposure; transmission via the feco-oral route does not occur. In countries with a high prevalence of hepatitis B infection the route of transmission is mainly vertical, at childbirth or, to a lesser degree, horizontally among household contacts in the first decade of life. In countries with a lower prevalence of hepatitis B infection, the majority of infections occur in adulthood and are transmitted sexually and to a lesser extent by intravenous drug use.[6]

Natural History of HBV Infection. Hepatitis B can result either in a self-limited acute infection or progress to chronic liver disease. Progression to chronic hepatitis B infection after acute infection depends upon the age of exposure to the virus. The risk of developing chronic HBV infection is over 90% for vertically acquired (mother-to-child) virus. The risk of chronic HBV infection after exposure in young children (<5 years old) is 25–30%. Clinically symptomatic infection is rare in children. Conversely, transmission in adulthood is associated with clinically apparent hepatitis in over 30% of individuals (>90%).[6,169] Acute infection in adults when clinically apparent is often associated with jaundice and elevated aminotransferases with liver histology revealing portal inflammation, interface hepatitis, and lobular inflammation. Eventually, often over several weeks, the jaundice resolves and aminotransferases are more modestly elevated. Eventually, over 80% of non-immune-suppressed adults who develop acute hepatitis B will not progress to chronic infection (HBsAg-negative, HBsAb-positive, HBcAb-positive). However, in dialysis patients, exposure to acute HBV results in chronic infection in the majority of non-vaccinated individuals (80%), likely due to their immune-compromised state and inability to mount protective antibody and T-cell responses.[94]

The natural history of chronic hepatitis B infection depends upon the age at which infection occurs. After perinatally transmitted infection there is an immune-tolerant phase in which high levels of viral replication (with high serum HBV DNA levels) are accompanied by only minimal injury on liver biopsy and normal serum liver enzymes. The immune-tolerant phase can last from the first up to the third decade of life, after which transition occurs to the immune clearance phase.[135] In this phase immune activity against HBV is noted by elevated levels of liver enzymes and decreasing HBV DNA. Immune clearance can fail and lead to recurrent phases of HBV replication accompanied by surges of serum HBV DNA and aminotransferases which increase the risk of fibrosis progression toward cirrhosis and HCC. Some patients can further enter into the "inactive carrier state" with disappearance of the HBeAg from serum and development of anti-HBe antibodies. These patients have detectable HBsAg and may have low levels of HBV viremia, but aminotransferases are normal or near-normal and there is little to no necroinflammation on liver biopsy. Even in the inactive carrier state, patients can revert to HBeAg positivity and develop evidence of chronic hepatitis. Therefore, they require lifelong follow-up. In addition, some patients remain HBeAg-negative, but develop evidence of ongoing chronic hepatitis marked by HBV viremia, elevated aminotransferases, and ongoing necroinflammation on liver biopsy.[27,135] Most of these patients are felt to have virus with a mutation in the precore or core promoter region of the viral genome. Serum HBsAg positivity is lost infrequently.

The outcomes of chronic HBV infection vary from an inactive carrier state to cirrhosis and its attendant complications, such as variceal hemorrhage, ascites, and encephalopathy. Risk for liver disease progression is increased in older patients, patients with higher HBV DNA levels, in patients co-infected with human immunodeficiency virus (HIV), HCV, or HDV, and with concomitant toxin exposures such as alcohol, smoking, or aflatoxin.[135,240] In addition, the risk of HCC is elevated in chronic HBV, even in the absence of cirrhosis.

Hepatitis B Infection in Patients Awaiting Renal Transplant on Dialysis

The incidence and prevalence of hepatitis B infection among patients awaiting renal transplantation have declined in recent decades, in large measure due to hepatitis B vaccination of patients on dialysis as well as improved infection control measures during dialysis. Prior to hepatitis B vaccination, 3–10% of patients on dialysis developed this disease,[242] with even higher incidences reported from countries with a high prevalence of HBV infection. Presently, about 1% of patients on dialysis in the United States are infected with the HBV, with a higher prevalence seen in developing countries.[45,88,232]

HBV vaccination is important for the prevention of HBV transmission during hemodialysis. One case-control study demonstrated a 70% reduction in risk of acquiring HBV among hemodialysis patients that underwent HBV vaccination.[170] Universal vaccination of dialysis patients, although recommended, is not universally undertaken. One survey of 12 centers from 11 countries showed routine vaccination of non-immune subjects in only 66.7% (8 of 12) of centers.

Vaccination has a lower response rate in end-stage renal disease patients, with 50–60% of dialysis patients developing adequate titers of anti-HBs antibodies.[178,213] Similarly, success of HBV vaccination correlates with glomerular filtration rate and thus "earlier" vaccination is more successful.[58] Despite lower rates of anti-HBs development, there is some evidence that vaccination confers protective T-cell responses and there are reduced rates of HBV infection even if anti-HBs antibodies are not detected in vaccinated dialysis patients.[3]

There are several additional strategies to improve the success of HBV vaccination, including intramuscular injections, doubling of vaccine dose, giving additional booster doses, and prompt revaccination in non-responders.[76] Non-response is defined as an antiHBs antibody titer less than 10 IU/L 1–2 months post series completion.[195] Annual testing of anti-HBs titers should be undertaken with boosters given whenever the anti-HBs titer falls under 10 IU/L.

Clinical and histological outcomes in dialysis patients with HBV infection are generally similar to those seen in immunocompetent individuals. The majority of these individuals do not die from liver disease. In one study of dialysis patients in which 30% were infected with HBV, less than 5% died from liver disease. This may be due to the presence of other comorbidities (competing causes of mortality) in dialysis patients such as cardiovascular disease or infections as well as insufficient length of follow-up.[122] The impact of antiviral therapy on the natural history of chronic HBV infection on hemodialysis patients has not been studied.

Pretransplant Management of Hepatitis B-Positive Dialysis Patients

Liver enzymes (aminotransferases) do not accurately reflect the stage of liver disease in patients with chronic viral hepatitis and end-stage renal disease. Patients with chronic HBV on dialysis should undergo liver biopsy for accurate assessment of liver fibrosis (staging) prior to renal transplantation. Patients with cirrhosis on the biopsy should be considered for a combined liver–kidney transplant when portal hypertension develops.

Criteria for antiviral therapy in non-transplant patients include evidence of chronic necroinflammation of the liver, evidenced by an elevated ALT and aspartate aminotransferase (AST) in the setting of HBeAg positivity or in the setting of an elevated serum HBV DNA in HBeAg-negative patients.[135] However in patients undergoing renal transplantation there is increased risk of reactivation of viral replication as well as increased viral replication after transplantation with exposure to immunosuppressive agents. In addition, HBV-positive renal allograft recipients have worse outcomes in terms of liver disease and renal allograft function (discussed below). Therefore, it is prudent to start antiviral therapy prior to renal transplantation for patients with evidence of active viral replication. This includes patients with positivity for HBsAg as well as any detectable viral load.

Posttransplant Prognosis in Hepatitis B-Infected Recipients

Post renal transplantation, hepatitis B-infected recipients are generally felt to have decreased survival compared to non-infected recipients, although this finding is controversial. In one study of 1250 renal allograft recipients, with a median follow-up of 125 months, cirrhosis occurred in 30% and renal allograft survival was reduced compared to recipients not infected with chronic hepatitis B.[94] Overall mortality was not different between HBV-positive and HBV-negative recipients in this study. A study of 51 renal transplant recipients with chronic hepatitis B infection found reduced patient survival and a higher incidence of death due to liver failure in the hepatitis B group (44%) compared to non-hepatitis-infected controls (0.6%).[172] In multivariable analysis in the hepatitis B group the presence of hepatitis B antigen was not an independent predictor of death; patient age, serum creatinine, and proteinuria at 3 months after transplant were independent predictors of reduced patient survival.[172]

Other large studies have found significant reductions in long-term patient and graft survival in HBsAg-positive kidney transplant recipients as compared to non-infected renal transplant recipients. In a cohort of 128 renal transplant recipients infected with HBV, the 10-year survival was 55% compared to 80% in non-HBV-infected renal transplant recipients.[166] Age at transplant and presence of cirrhosis were independent prognostic factors for survival in this study. Another study found a significant difference in long-term survival between hepatitis B-positive recipients as compared to recipients without chronic viral hepatitis[14] with a relative risk (RR) of mortality of 2.36 for 42 HBsAg-positive recipients. Finally, a meta-analysis that included 6050 renal transplant recipients found increased mortality (RR of death with HBsAg positivity 2.49) associated with chronic hepatitis B infection as well as reduced graft survival (RR of graft loss 2.49).[80,81]

Differences in outcome between studies may result from small numbers in some studies, length of follow-up, heterogeneity of patient characteristics such as age at transplant, replicative state of hepatitis B, presence or absence of cirrhosis at time of transplant, and the confounding effect of antiviral therapy for hepatitis B. Studies with larger numbers, longer follow-up and with matched case-control design and multivariate analysis have tended to show a reduction in patient and graft survival associated with chronic hepatitis B infection in renal transplant recipients.

Several studies have documented the progression of fibrosis in HBsAg-positive kidney transplant recipients after transplant. In a study of 151 HBsAg-positive kidney transplant recipients, 28% had a histologic diagnosis of cirrhosis a mean of 66 months post transplant.[94] HCV co-infection was the only identifiable risk factor for fibrosis progression. More recently, a cohort of 55 HBsAg-positive kidney transplant recipients underwent liver biopsy at a mean of 5 years after transplantation. On logistic regression, the only risk factor for the development of cirrhosis was time interval between kidney transplant and liver biopsy.[167]

In rare cases viral replication may become uncontrolled in the setting of immunosuppression after renal transplantation. In this state the virus may become directly cytopathic and lead to a state of hepatocellular failure with profound cholestasis. The liver biopsy is characteristic with hepatocyte ballooning, cholestasis, and perisinusoidal fibrosis. This condition is called fibrosing cholestatic hepatitis, and was first described in liver transplant recipients infected with HBV.[60] Once established, the prognosis is poor, even with antiviral therapy. Pre-emptive suppressive antiviral therapy is the judicious strategy to prevent this feared outcome. In rare cases suppression of viral replication with long-term antiviral therapy has resulted in salvage of liver and graft function (discussed below).

The natural history of chronic HBV infection in kidney transplant recipients in the era of antiviral therapy is less well studied. A recent, small study of 63 HBsAg-positive kidney transplant recipients revealed an improved 20-year mortality (83% versus 34%, P=0.006) in patients treated with antiviral therapy.[238]

De Novo HBV Infection after Kidney Transplantation

Development of de novo hepatitis B after renal transplantation can be associated with rapid viral replication and progression of liver disease.[83] The hepatitis B serologic and virologic status of the donor and recipient are important risk factors that predict development of de novo hepatitis B infection after renal transplantation. The highest risk of de novo hepatitis exists in recipients who are nonimmune for hepatitis B (HBsAb-negative) and receive an organ from HBsAg/HBeAg-positive donors. The risk of transmission from an HBcAb-positive-only donor (HBsAg-negative, HBcAb-positive, negative serum HBV DNA donor) to a hepatitis B-negative recipient also exists, although it is reduced compared to that seen in liver transplant recipients.[62,90] It is important to note that isolated HBcAb positivity could represent an early, acute HBV infection or possibly a longstanding, chronic infection with low-level HBV viremia. Determination of donor IgM HBcAb should be performed in patients with an isolated positive HBcAb. Positive titers for IgM suggest a recent infection and should be considered high risk for transmission of HBV to the recipient. HBV DNA should also be determined in the isolated HBcAb-positive donor with consideration of HBV prophylaxis for the recipient.

The risk of the de novo HBV infection is considerably reduced if the recipient is positive for HBsAb, although the risk is not completely eliminated. In one series where HBcAb-positive-only donors were used for recipients with a prior history of hepatitis B or HBV vaccination, none developed clinically evident hepatitis B, although 27% did develop HBcAb and/or HBsAb positivity after transplant.[155] In a more recent study from Italy, 344 patients received anti-HBcAb-positive allografts and no recipient developed HBsAg positivity, including 62 patients that had not undergone HBV vaccination.[62] Finally, a cohort of 46 patients that received an anti-HBcAb-positive donor kidney were followed for 36 months posttransplant.[4] Anti-HBsAb-positive (immunized) recipients received no prophylaxis. Naïve patients received 1 year of lamivudine prophylaxis. No patients developed evidence of HBV viremia or development of HBsAg.[4]

Ultimately, prevention of de novo hepatitis B in renal transplant recipients is best achieved by universal vaccination of all dialysis patients. Alternatively organs from HBsAg-positive donors can be offered only to recipients with pre-existing HBV infection or those individuals who have been successfully vaccinated for HBV. Use of HBcAb-positive donors is often center-specific. If such organs are used, posttransplant usage of prophylaxis with antiviral medication or hepatitis B immune globulin should be considered, especially in patients without evidence of HBV immunity.

Antiviral Therapy of Chronic Hepatitis B in Renal Transplant Candidates/Recipients (*Table 32-3*)

Data regarding the optimal timing of antiviral therapy for HBV in renal transplant candidates are scarce. The risks of liver disease progression and severe hepatitis B reactivation posttransplant have to be weighed against the risk of antiviral toxicity and viral resistance developing. However, with the development of the newer-generation antinucleos(t)ide analogues entecavir and tenofovir (see below), the risk of viral resistance is much lower than with lamivudine or adefovir. Data for antiviral therapy posttransplant have mostly been performed using lamivudine. In one trial, the efficacy of lamivudine in preventing viral replication after renal transplantation was compared in HBsAg-positive recipients using three strategies: pre-emptive lamivudine therapy (HBV DNA-positive recipients, received lamivudine therapy 0–9 months before renal transplant, n=7); prophylactic lamivudine therapy (HBV DNA-negative, received lamivudine therapy before transplant, n=3); salvage therapy (HBV DNA-positive, advanced hepatic dysfunction after transplant, received lamivudine after transplant after hepatic dysfunction, n=6).[105] HBV DNA disappeared in all recipients in all groups on therapy. The recurrence rate of HBV viremia was 10% (1/10) in the pre-emptive and prophylactic group compared to 42% (11/25) in a non-lamivudine-treated group. In the group treated for hepatic dysfunction HBV DNA disappeared in all six cases but recurred in 50% (3/6) while on lamivudine. In another trial of lamivudine therapy, HBV DNA levels were measured and lamivudine was started before renal transplantation if the HBV DNA rose to more than 2.83 × 108 copies/mL alone or to >2.83 × 107 copies/mL with elevated AST/ALT from 1996 to 2000 (so-called de novo group).[42] This strategy was compared to pre-emptive use of lamivudine for patients who had undergone transplantation before 1996 (when lamivudine became commercially available) and thus received therapy later after transplantation than the de novo group. Even though suppression of HBV DNA and normalization of aminotransferases were achieved in all patients, the survival of the de novo treated group was comparable to that of HBsAg-negative controls whereas HBsAg-positive patients who were transplanted before 1996 and received pre-emptive therapy with rising HBV DNA after renal transplantation had a higher risk of overall (RR 9.7) and liver-related mortality (RR 68.0).

TABLE 32-3 **Selected Pretransplant and Posttransplant (Non-Liver) Studies of Antiviral Therapy in HBV Patients**

Study	Patient Population	Number In Study	HBV Antiviral Therapy	Duration of Therapy	HBV DNA Suppression	HBeAg Seroconversion to anti-HBe	Virologic Breakthrough
Pretransplant							
Fontaine et al. 2004[92]	Dialysis patients	5	Lamivudine 10 mg daily in 3, 50 mg thrice weekly in 2	12 months (7–28)	5/5	1/5	2/5 (at months 7, 18 of lamivudine)
Duarte et al. 1995[70]	Dialysis patients	2	Interferon-α 3 mU thrice weekly	3 months	2/2	2/2	None
Posttransplant							
Fontaine et al. 2004[92]	Post-renal transplant patients with HBV infection	26	Lamivudine 100 mg/day	16.5 months (4–31)	26/26 undetectable	6/26	8/26
Fontaine et al. 2005[91]	Post kidney transplantation with lamivudine-resistant HBV	11	Adefovir 10 mg/day	15 months (3–19)	Median change −5.6 log copies/mL (−2.2 to −7.7)	0/6 that were initially HBeAg⁺	Not detected
Han et al. 2001[105]	Post kidney transplantation with HBV (HBsAg⁺)	Group 1: After developing recurrent hepatic dysfunction after renal transplant (6) Group 2: Pre-emptive or prophylactic treatment for HBsAg-positive recipients beginning before renal transplantation (10)	Lamivudine 100 mg/day	Group 1: Follow-up 15–60 months Group 2: Follow-up 9–30 months	On treatment Group 1: 6/6 On treatment Group 2: 11/11	Group 1: 0/6 Group 2: 0/11	Group 1: 3/6 Group 2: 1/10
Chan et al. 2002[42]	Post kidney transplantation with HBV (HBsAg⁺)	Period II: Post 1996. De novo pre-emptive therapy before renal transplantation and continued after transplantation (11) Period I: pre-1996. Pre-emptive therapy after renal transplantation	Lamivudine 100 mg/day	Period I: 36.3 ±11.4 months Period II: 27.6 ± 14.5 months	26/26 undetectable	Not mentioned. 3/14 HBeAg⁺ patients became undetectable	11 (40.7%) became lamivudine-resistant at 9.5–24 months after starting treatment

Continued on following page

TABLE 32-3 **Selected Pretransplant and Posttransplant (Non-Liver) Studies of Antiviral Therapy in HBV Patients (Continued)**

Study	Patient Population	Number In Study	HBV Antiviral Therapy	Duration of Therapy	HBV DNA Suppression	HBeAg Seroconversion to anti-HBe	Virologic Breakthrough
Posttransplant							
Puchhammer-Stockl et al. 2000[193]	Post kidney transplantation with HBV (HBsAg$^+$)	11	Lamivudine 100 mg/day in 7, reduced dose in 4 per renal function	> 12 months	HBV undetectable in 10/11 undetectable by PCR	Not reported	Lamivudine resistance in 5/11 from 9–15 months after starting lamivudine
Thabut et al. 2004[225]	Post kidney transplantation with HBV (HBsAg$^+$)	14	Lamivudine 100 mg/day	Median duration 64.5 months (6–93)	11/11 undetectable on treatment	None of 4 HBeAg$^+$ patients	Lamivudine resistance with virologic breakthrough in 8/14 patients from 9–24 months after starting lamivudine
Chan et al. 2004[43]	Post kidney transplantation with HBV (HBsAg$^+$)	29	Lamivudine 100 mg/day	56.7 ± 12.5 months	29/29 undetectable on treatment initially	5/15 who were HBeAg$^+$	14/29 (48%) developed lamivudine resistance (10–35 months after starting treatment)
Fabrizi et al. 2004[75]	Post kidney transplantation with HBV (HBsAg$^+$)	184 (meta-analysis of 14 studies)	Lamivudine 50–150 mg/day	Variable	91% HBV DNA undetectable	27% in 4 of 14 studies	18% in 8 of 14 studies
Kamar et al. 2008[126]	Posttransplantation with lamivudine or adefovir-resistant HBV (HBsAg$^+$)	10 (8 kidney)	Entecavir 0.5 mg/day titrated to 1.0 mg/day after 1 month	Median 16.5 months	5/8 kidney recipients developed undetectable HBV DNA	Not reported	Not reported

HBeAg, hepatitis B e antigen; HBsAg, hepatitis B surface antigen; HBV, hepatitis B virus; PCR, polymerase chain reaction.

More recently, a meta-analysis of 14 clinical trials using lamivudine in kidney transplant recipients demonstrated that HBV DNA clearance occurred in 91% and normalization of ALT occurred in 81% of treated patients.[78]

Antiviral therapy should thus be offered to all hepatitis B-positive (HBsAg-positive) kidney transplant recipients, including those on the waiting list. This recommendation applies even to surface antigen-positive patients with a negative HBV DNA. The optimal duration of therapy is yet to be determined and in an immunocompromised host may need to be indefinite. Cessation of antiviral therapy in the immunocompromised host is associated with an increased risk of flare of liver disease and, rarely, decompensated liver disease in both the transplant recipient and patients without organ transplantation.[42,150]

Specific Antiviral Agents for HBV Used in Renal Transplant Recipients

Lamivudine. The cytosine analogue lamivudine has been the most extensively studied antiviral for HBV. A dose of 100 mg/day has been shown to be highly effective in suppression of HBV replication and normalization of aminotransferases in over 80% of individuals.[78,79,134,200] Cessation of antiviral therapy has been associated with virologic and clinical relapse.[200]

The major drawback with lamivudine is the high rate of viral resistance. The risk of resistance increases with duration of lamivudine therapy. In a meta-analysis of 14 clinical trials (184 recipients) of lamivudine after renal transplantation, the majority of recipients had HBV DNA clearance (91%) and biochemical normalization (81%) and the risk of lamivudine resistance was 18%.[79] Although HBeAg loss was higher with prolonged therapy, the resistance was also higher, thereby limiting its efficacy. Given the high risk of viral resistance, lamivudine is no longer preferred as first-line therapy for HBV.[135]

Adefovir. Adefovir dipivoxil, an oral prodrug of adefovir, is a nucleotide analogue of adenosine monophosphate. Adefovir therapy has demonstrated efficacy in treatment-naïve and lamivudine-resistant patients with HBV.[104,162,188] Standard adefovir dosage is 10 mg/day. The dose should be adjusted based on glomerular filtration rate. In patients with renal transplant it has been used in small studies, mostly reported in lamivudine-resistant recipients. In one study of 11 renal transplant recipients, there was a significant reduction in HBV DNA after initiation of adefovir with a median decline of 5.5 log in HBV DNA after 12 months of therapy. No virologic breakthrough was observed and no significant changes in creatinine occurred.[91] Adefovir resistance is much less common than with lamivudine, even after prolonged therapy.[104]If adefovir is used in patients with lamivudine resistance, lamivudine should continue to be administered and dual therapy continued indefinitely.

The principal drawback to adefovir therapy is the risk of nephrotoxicity. In a recent study of 11 renal transplant recipients with chronic HBV, adefovir therapy was associated with an increased serum creatinine and increased proteinuria at 2-year follow-up. In addition, there was evidence for proximal tubular dysfunction with adefovir usage.[125,116] Given the risk of nephrotoxicity, adefovir should be used with caution in kidney transplant recipients.

Entecavir. Entecavir, an analogue of 2′-deoxyguanosine, is a nucleoside analogue with potent activity against HBV replication. In a randomized, controlled trial of HBeAg-positive non-transplant patients, 48 weeks' treatment with entecavir, dosed at 0.5 mg/day, resulted in higher rates of histologic, virologic (undetectable HBV DNA), and biochemical (normalization of ALT) response when compared to lamivudine 100 mg/day.[46]

Unlike lamivudine, resistance to entecavir is low in treatment-naïve patients. In phase III trial data, viral breakthrough was only seen in 3.6% of treatment-naïve patients at 96 weeks of entecavir therapy.[54] However, entecavir should be used with caution in patients with lamivudine resistance or viral breakthrough while on lamivudine therapy. In a study of non-transplant patients on 5 years of entecavir therapy for chronic HBV, entecavir resistance developed in 51% of patients with documented lamivudine resistance.[224]

Data regarding entecavir usage in kidney transplant recipients are sparse. In a study where 10 transplant recipients (8 kidney) with adefovir or lamivudine resistance were treated with entecavir, mean HBV DNA levels decreased and HBV DNA clearance was achieved in 50%.[126]

Despite the lack of data in transplant recipients, entecavir should be considered a first-line treatment for kidney transplant candidates and recipients with chronic HBV that have no concern for lamivudine resistance.

Tenofovir. Tenofovir disoproxil fumarate is a nucleotide analogue originally approved for therapy against HIV. Tenofovir is structurally similar to adefovir, but less nephrotoxic, allowing for higher dosing and a more potent antiviral effect. In randomized, controlled trials of non-transplant patients with chronic HBV, tenofovir has been shown to be an effective antiviral against HBV. In a phase III trial of tenofovir versus adefovir in HBeAg-positive patients, after 48 weeks of therapy a greater proportion of tenofovir-treated patients achieved a negative HBV DNA (76% versus 13%), ALT normalization (68% versus 54%), and surface antigen loss (3% versus 0%).

Tenofovir resistance appears rare. In the original phase III clinical trials, no patients had virus with genotypic evidence of mutations known to cause tenofovir resistance. Unlike entecavir, tenofovir is effective in the setting of lamivudine resistance. In a randomized trial of HIV/HBV-co-infected patients known to be lamivudine-resistant, both adefovir and tenofovir were found to be efficacious in decreasing HBV DNA at 48 weeks.[188] Tenofovir should be used with caution in cases of known adefovir resistance.

Data regarding tenofovir in transplant recipients are scarce. A recent study of seven transplant (three kidney) patients with chronic HBV treated with tenofovir showed a decline in HBV DNA during treatment, with three patients achieving serum DNA clearance.[59] Despite the lack of data in kidney transplant recipients, tenofovir should be considered a first-line agent for the treatment of chronic HBV in kidney transplant candidates and recipients.

Interferon. Use of interferon is associated with an unacceptably high risk of precipitating renal allograft rejection, sometimes irreversibly, despite salvage immunosuppressive therapy. Its use in the renal transplant recipient should thus be avoided with the availability of other antiviral agents for hepatitis B.[71,177]

Treatment of Fibrosing Cholestatic Hepatitis B in Renal Transplant Recipients

Fibrosing cholestatic hepatitis B is a histological and clinical variant of hepatitis B characterized by hepatocyte ballooning, cholestasis, minimal inflammation, periportal fibrosis, and massive viral replication (Figure 32-2). This was first described in HBV-infected recipients of liver allografts but has also been subsequently described in other immunosuppressed states.[124] Patients often develop rapidly progressive liver failure and spontaneous recovery is rare. Lamivudine has been reported to be useful in case reports, resulting in successful resolution of the severe acute hepatitis and hepatic failure associated with this condition.[44] With appropriate antiviral therapy, fibrosing cholestatic HBV should occur extremely infrequently.

Summary

In summary, chronic HBV infection in kidney transplant candidates and recipients has become less common in developed countries. This decrease in prevalence and incidence of new cases can be attributed to improved public health efforts, particularly infection control measures during hemodialysis and widespread HBV immunization. All patients with chronic kidney disease should be immunized against HBV. HBV vaccination is more successful at higher glomerular filtration rate and therefore should ideally be administered well before the onset of hemodialysis.

All patients who are candidates or who have undergone kidney transplantation and are positive for HBsAg should undergo a liver biopsy and be given antiviral therapy to decrease the risk of liver disease progress or a severe HBV exacerbation after initiation of immunosuppression. Tenofovir and entecavir should be considered first-line antiviral therapy due to their potency and tolerability, and the low risk of resistance development.

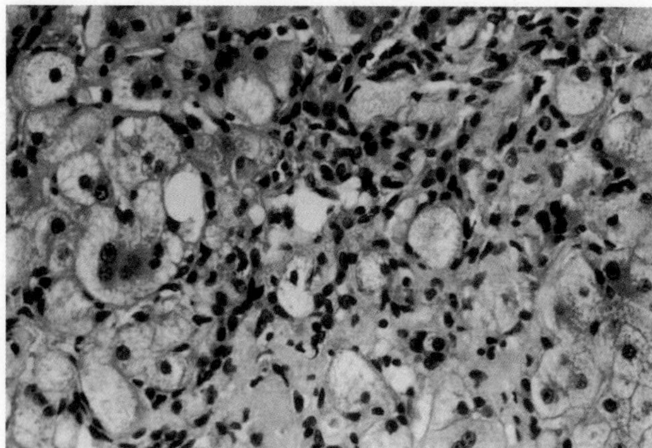

FIGURE 32-2 ■ Perisinusoidal fibrosis and hepatocyte ballooning without inflammatory infiltration. Characteristic histologic appearance of fibrosing cholestatic hepatitis B.

Hepatitis C Virus

Viral Structure

The discovery of hepatitis A and B between the years of 1967 and 1973[86] was a medical breakthrough; however it left many unanswered questions. For the next 16 years, patients with non-A non-B hepatitis became increasingly recognized as having a form of chronic liver disease. In 1989, Choo et al.[51] published the first account of the HCV, which was further described as a single-stranded, enveloped, positive-sense RNA virus. It is classified in the Flaviviridae family.

HCV Species

HCV can be thought of as a spectrum of similar viruses. Seven HCV genotypes with several distinct subtypes have been identified throughout the world.[139] Within a genotype or subtype, the genome of HCV is highly mutable due to the lack of efficient proofreading capabilities. As the virus replicates over time, selective pressures from the immune system and/or antiviral treatments cause the viral populations to evolve. These mutant versions of genotypes are called quasispecies. The heterogeneity of this virus is what allows it to evade immunologic detection and elimination and, thus far, prevent development of a vaccine.

Epidemiologic studies on the HCV genotypes demonstrate significant regional variation. Genotype 1 is found worldwide though it is by far the most common (60–70% of isolates) in the United States, Europe,[117] Japan, and Taiwan. While less common, genotypes 2 and 3 are also found in these areas, with genotypes 4, 5, and 6 being rarely encountered. Genotype 3 is predominant in India, the Far East, and Australia.[110,123] Genotype 4 is present in North Africa and the Middle East, with a particularly high incidence in Egypt. Genotype 5 has been most frequently detected in South Africa whereas genotype 6 has been rather isolated to Hong Kong.[243]

The significance of viral genotypes is not entirely clear, but important clinical differences have been shown. Amoroso et al.[10] followed patients with acute viral hepatitis and found that those infected with genotype 1 developed chronic infection at a significantly higher rate when compared to those with genotypes 2 and 3. Regarding the genotypic sensitivities to treatment, there is ample evidence that genotypes 2, 3, and 5[104,147] are more responsive to interferon-based treatments than genotypes 1 and 4.[66,104] Finally, one of the two newly approved NS3/4A protease inhibitors, telaprevir, demonstrated activity against genotype 1 and 2 virus, but not genotype 3 virus.[98]

Clinical Manifestations of Hepatitis C Infection in Immunocompetent Hosts

In general, HCV is a chronic infection and its acute form often goes unrecognized. Twenty to 30% of patients with acute HCV have symptoms 2–12 weeks after exposure.[227,234] The symptoms are generally mild and include lethargy, nausea, vomiting, jaundice, and anorexia. Serum aminotransferases can range from two- to 10-fold above normal. Rarely, acute HCV can lead to acute hepatic failure,[84] though this is exceedingly uncommon. Diagnosis of acute HCV is made by testing for HCV RNA, which can be identified in serum a few days to weeks after exposure.[84,141] Anti-HCV antibodies are typically not detected for weeks to months after exposure and may not develop in immune-compromised individuals.[100]

Chronic HCV develops in about 85% of those who are exposed. In the majority of patients, the clinical course is remarkably non-specific. Fatigue and non-specific arthralgias are common complaints and typically improve with eradication of the virus.[35] Studies have estimated 20–35% of patients will have progression of liver disease to cirrhosis over 20–30 years.[166] A study by Cacoub et al.[35] found that 38% of HCV patients presented with at least one clinical extrahepatic manifestation. The associated findings include hematologic disorders such as cryoglobulinemia and lymphoma as well as porphyria cutanea tarda and other rashes. Dry eyes and mouth, pruritus, renal disease including membranoproliferative glomerulonephritis (MPGN), and diabetes are often present.

Incidence/Prevalence and Transmission of Hepatitis C in Renal Transplant Patients

It is estimated that 180 million people are infected with HCV worldwide, with 4 million people in the United States thought to be HCV antibody carriers. Among those with anti-HCV antibodies, about 80% are viremic.[13] The principal risk factors for HCV infection are transfusion of unscreened blood products and intravenous drug use. With the development of blood donor screening in the 1990s, transfusion-related HCV transmission is now exceedingly rare.[67] Other risk factors for HCV transmission include nosocomial transmission, including via hemodialysis and occupational exposure. Transmission of HCV via hemodialysis and occupationally is less frequent with the use of improved universal precautions. Sexual transmission is to be rare.

The prevalence of HCV in patients with chronic kidney disease is higher than in the general population, particularly in patients on hemodialsysis. HCV prevalence in hemodialysis units across seven countries was reported in the Dialysis Outcomes and Practice Patterns Study and showed a mean HCV prevalence of 13.5% with a range between the countries of 2.6–22.9%. HCV prevalence is higher in Japan, Italy, and Spain and lower in Germany and the United Kingdom. The United States had a 14% HCV prevalence and a hemodialysis seroconversion rate of 2.5% per 100 patient years.[89] However, in the United States, there is high variability in the prevalence of chronic HCV among hemodialysis units based on location.[217] Historically, blood products were the major contributor to infection in these patients. As mentioned above, in the past decade this method of transmission has been virtually eliminated with reliable screening methods[68,135] and decreased transfusion requirements directly related to the increased use of hematopoeitic growth factors.[68,109] Despite these improvements, studies show de novo infections do occur in dialysis units, though clearly identifiable risk factors have not been reproducibly demonstrated.[63]

Given the prevalence of chronic HCV among patients on hemodialysis, a significant number of patients on the renal transplant waiting list are infected with HCV. Accurate data regarding infection rates in this transplant-associated population are complicated by several factors, including the insidious and indolent nature of the disease in the setting of uremia,[82] regional variations of the HCV genome, the use of non-standardized diagnostic methods,[33,109] and the absence of good prospective, well-powered studies. Risk factors for HCV among transplant candidates include length of time on hemodialysis, exposure to blood products prior to universal screening, and the prevalence of chronic HCV infection in the dialysis center.

Allograft Transmission of HCV

As transplant waiting lists soar to record levels, programs of all organ types are faced with decisions regarding the use of extended criteria (previously called marginal) donor organs, including those positive for HCV antibody. Historically, allocation of HCV-positive organs has been restricted to HCV-positive recipients. This recommendation is based on evidence that transplantation of HCV-positive organs into HCV-negative recipients is a risk factor for poorer outcomes in renal transplant patients.[1,202] In contrast, outcome data regarding kidney transplantation from anti-HCV-positive antibody-positive donors to HCV-positive recipients are mixed. Recipient wait time may be substantially reduced and there appears to be no effect on short-term mortality.[5,159,171] Similarly, registry studies have shown that kidney transplantation from deceased anti-HCV antibody-positive donors has a survival advantage compared to staying on dialysis for HCV-positive recipients.[1]

Currently, the Kidney Disease Improving Global Outcomes practice guidelines[132] recommend restricting the use of allografts from HCV-infected donors to HCV-infected recipients.[162]

Impact of Pretransplant HCV on Posttransplant Outcomes (Table 32-4)

Patient and Graft Survival. Some controversy exists regarding the impact of pretransplant HCV infection on the outcome of renal transplantation. Initially, studies of short follow-up periods suggested that neither patient nor graft survival was altered posttransplant despite a logarithmic

TABLE 32-4 **Outcomes in HCV-Positive Recipients (Compared to HCV-Negative Recipients) Undergoing Renal Transplantation**

Type of Transplant	Outcome
Renal transplant	Decreased long-term patient survival (follow-up >10 years) Decreased graft survival De novo or recurrent glomerulopathy Cirrhosis Posttransplant diabetes

HCV, hepatitis C virus.

increase in HCV RNA levels.[130,162,185,219] Orloff et al.[185] reported the liver biopsy findings at 3–7 years after kidney transplantation in HCV-positive subjects. Twelve percent of these had chronic active hepatitis, 50% showed mild hepatitis, and 38% had normal histology. Furthermore, hepatitis C conferred no adverse effect on patient or graft survival. Lee et al.[145] agreed that HCV infection did not reduce renal allograft or patient survival; however they identified more liver disease and a greater prevalence of life-threatening sepsis in the HCV-infected recipient population.[162]

In contrast, studies with more lengthy follow-up after transplantation have found decreased patient and/or graft survival in HCV-positive renal transplant recipients.[28,106,146,166,187] Periera et al.[187] compared the prevalence of posttransplantation liver disease and graft and patient survival in HCV-positive and -negative kidney transplant recipients. Among recipients who were HCV-positive prior to transplantation, the RR of posttransplantation liver disease was 5.0, of graft loss was 1.3, and death was 3.3. There was a significant increase in death due to sepsis with an RR of 9.9. Similarly, Hanafusa et al.[106] found clinically significant hepatitis in 55% of HCV-positive kidney transplant recipients. They also found a significant decline in the 20-year survival in the HCV-positive patients compared to the HCV-negative cohort (64% versus 88%). In a meta-analysis of observational studies after renal transplantation that included eight studies, the presence of HCV antibody was an independent risk factor for death and graft failure after renal transplant (RR for death 1.79, 95% CI 1.57–2.03) and for renal graft failure 1.56 (95% CI 1.35–1.80). HCC and liver cirrhosis were more frequent causes of mortality in HCV-positive than HCV-negative recipients.[81]

Despite the finding that graft and overall survival are probably decreased in kidney transplant recipients with chronic HCV infection, overall mortality has been shown to be improved with transplantation over long-term dialysis and therefore HCV infection should not be considered a contraindication to consideration of kidney transplantation.[25,213]

Most studies regarding posttransplant HCV outcomes are directed to chronically infected recipients, usually subjects who acquired HCV during hemodialysis. However the subset of solid-organ transplant recipients who become infected with HCV in the perioperative period have a markedly different course. Delladetsima et al.[65] followed 17 such patients by biochemical and histologic markers for a mean of 7 years. Six (35%) patients died a median of 6 years posttransplant due to fibrosing cholestatic hepatitis, vanishing bile duct syndrome, cirrhosis, miliary tuberculosis, myocardial infarction. Overall the yearly fibrosis progression rate was five times that of age-matched immunocompetent HCV-infected patients.[221] These studies suggest that HCV acquired at the time of transplantation may have a particularly aggressive course.

HCV and Posttransplant Diabetes in the Renal Transplant Recipient

The association of diabetes mellitus and HCV has become increasingly apparent both in the immune-competent HCV population and particularly after solid-organ transplantation in HCV-infected patients. The overall incidence of posttransplant diabetes mellitus (PTDM) has been reported to vary from 10% to 54% and has shown similar long-term effects as diabetes mellitus types 1 and 2, with cardiac and renal dysfunction in a significant proportion.[81] Yildiz et al.[239] reported a case-controlled study of 43 renal transplant recipients with PTDM in which 72% were HCV-infected, compared with a prevalence of 37% in the recipients without PTDM (P=0.002).[207] This association was further observed by Bloom et al.,[24] where PTDM occurred more frequently in HCV-positive than HCV-negative patients (39.4% versus 9.8%; P=0.0005). Their data further found that among the HCV-positive patients there was an eight times increased incidence of PTDM in those treated with tacrolimus (58%) when compared to cyclosporine (7.7%)

HCV and Posttransplant Nephropathy

Posttransplant renal disease is common among HCV-positive recipients of any organ. While the causes of renal injury after transplantation are multifactorial in nature, chronic allograft nephropathy among renal transplant recipients and nephrotoxicity due to calcineurin inhibitors are the most common etiologies. Kidney transplant recipients with chronic HCV infection are at risk for additional immune-mediated nephropathies, with MPGN being the most common, followed by membranous nephropathy, minimal change disease, and renal thrombotic microangiopathy. These may be recurrent or present de novo. MPGN has been reported in 45% of HCV-positive renal transplant recipients who underwent renal biopsy for worsening renal function. In the HCV-negative group, the incidence was only 5.9%.[169] De novo disease was found in 18% of the MPGN patients and chronic renal allograft nephropathy was similar in both HCV-positive and negative recipients.[56]

Immunosuppressive Strategies in Renal Transplant Patients Infected with HCV

No studies have been performed to determine optimal immunosuppressive regimens in renal transplant recipients infected with HCV. Viral replication is increased with the use of immunosuppressive agents, but the impact on patient survival, progression of liver disease, and graft function is unknown. As mentioned previously, studies have clearly demonstrated tacrolimus as an additive risk in HCV patients for the development of posttransplant diabetes mellitus.[229] In addition, as mentioned previously, in liver transplant recipients cyclosporine may have an anti-HCV effect and improve the probability of successful HCV treatment.[40,210] However, there are no data regarding cyclosporine effects on HCV in kidney transplant recipients. Similarly, although corticosteroid boluses have been shown to increase HCV viral load dramatically and decrease time to HCV recurrence in liver transplant recipients,[162] there are no data in kidney transplant recipients. Finally, while poor outcomes have been reported with antibody induction in HCV-positive liver transplant recipients, there are no data on kidney transplant recipients.

In the absence of data, few recommendations can be made regarding immunosuppression strategy in HCV-infected kidney transplant recipients. Given the permissive effects of immunosuppression on HCV replication, a reasonable goal is to provide the minimum dose of immunosuppression to prevent rejection.

Hepatitis C Antiviral Therapy (Table 32-5)

Pretransplant Antiviral Therapy. Eradication of HCV prior to transplantation has several theoretical benefits. HCV is associated with worse patient and graft survival as well as increased risk of PTDM and de novo glomerulopathy. Eradication of HCV pretransplant might mitigate some of these adverse outcomes.[57,114,127] Furthermore, interferon therapy posttransplantation is associated with reduced treatment response rates, a greater incidence of organ rejection, and impairment of renal function.[19,201] Thus it would be best if treatment could be undertaken before embarking on the solid-organ transplant.

Results of treatment of HCV in dialysis patients vary, with sustained virologic rates (SVR) ranging from 16% to 68%.[79] These rates are not significantly different from that seen in the non-end-stage renal disease population and in many reports are higher than in patients with normal renal function. This may due to higher circulating levels of interferon in patients on dialysis[199] or lower viral loads in patients on hemodialysis.[79]

The standard of care for HCV treatment has evolved over the years from standard interferon monotherapy, to standard interferon plus the antiviral ribavirin, to pegylated interferon and ribavirin, to, most recently, the addition of direct-acting antivirals.

Most studies report treatment regimens including interferon monotherapy administered for 6–12 months. Interferon side effects in the dialysis population vary but appear to be more frequent than in the non-end-stage renal disease (ESRD) patient. Discontinuation rates are as high as 51% compared to studies of non-ESRD patients where dropout rates are approximately 20%. Two meta-analyses revealed treatment dropout rates much higher (17–30%) than in the non-hemodialysis population (3–10%).[77,204] Ribavirin is renally excreted and its use has generally been avoided in dialysis patients. Discontinuation due to severe hemolytic anemia may occur despite doses as low as 200 mg thrice a week in dialysis patients.[222] However, some pilot studies have reported ribavirin use in addition to interferon in patients on dialysis.[30] In this study, lower doses of ribavirin were used (170–300 mg/day) along with use of erythropoietin and iron and monitoring of ribavirin levels. A sustained virologic response was seen in one of the six patients treated and there was no evidence that adding ribavirin in dialysis patients provided any added therapeutic benefit. Another small, uncontrolled study showed an SVR rate of 66% in patients treated with standard interferon and ribavirin.[175] Longer-term and larger studies with pre-emptive hematopoietic growth factors are needed to improve tolerance and measure virologic response.

Weekly pegylated interferon-α has been shown to be more effective than conventional interferon in achieving SVR in patients with normal renal function. While there is considerable clinical experience using pegylated interferon monotherapy in dialysis patients with chronic HCV, data regarding safety and efficacy are limited. In one study, 16 patients were randomized to 0.5 μg/kg/week versus 1.0 μg/kg/week of pegylated interferon-α_{2b} for 48 weeks. Sustained viral response was 40% in the 1.0 μg/kg group and 22% in the 0.5 μg/kg group. Adverse effects, primarily hypertension and infection, led to discontinuation of therapy in 56% of the subjects (5/9) in the 1.0 μg/kg group and in 28% (2/7) of the 0.5 μg/kg group.[203] Additional studies have shown highly variable rates of response and dropout.[55,176] It is also important to note that response rates using pegylated interferon may not be better than with standard interferon in dialysis patients since the half-life of regular interferon is increased in patients on dialysis. Further, prospective studies are needed to better determine the pharmacokinetics, efficacy, and tolerability of pegylated interferon-α in patients on hemodialysis.

Studies using the combination of pegylated interferon with ribavirin are limited. In patients with normal renal function, the combination of pegylated interferon-α and ribavirin results in an enhanced SVR rate when compared to standard interferon and ribavirin.[96,104,162] The largest pilot study treated 35 patients with chronic HCV with mixed genotypes. Ribavirin was dosed at 200 mg/day and trough levels were measured to guide treatment. Thirty patients completed therapy and 97% achieved an SVR.[151] These results have not been replicated to date. More data on safety, tolerability, efficacy, and pharmacokinetics of combination therapy are needed in dialysis patients before routine use and doses can be recommended.

Long-term maintenance of response is generally good after a successful virologic response pretransplant and after renal transplant. Casanovas-Taltavull et al.[38] reported that, of 14 dialysis patients that received interferon, 9 were HCV RNA-negative at the time of transplant and 8 of the 9 remained HCVRNA-negative at long-term follow-up of 41 ± 28 months. Persistent biochemical normalization after renal transplantation is seen in the majority of interferon-treated patients.

Interferon therapy is therefore associated with reasonable response rates in dialysis patients with frequent maintenance of response after renal transplantation. Given the lower patient and graft survival rates after renal transplantation in HCV-positive compared to HCV-negative patients, interferon should be considered for renal transplant candidates infected with HCV and demonstrating active viral replication. A liver biopsy should be performed to assess underlying activity and stage of HCV-related liver disease. This information can help guide expected response rates as well as aggressiveness of therapy. Those with advanced fibrosis and/or cirrhosis need to be considered for a dual-organ transplant.

Protease Inhibitors. Recently, the US Food and Drug Administration approved two new medications for the treatment of chronic HCV genotype 1 – boceprevir and telaprevir. Both agents are direct antiviral agents with activity against the NS3/4A serine protease, a critical protein in viral replication and assembly. Both agents are used in combination with pegylated interferon-α

TABLE 32-5 **Selected Pretransplant and Posttransplant (Non-Liver) Studies of Antiviral Therapy in HCV Patients**

Study	Patient Population	N	Antiviral Therapy	Follow-up After Therapy	ETVR	SVR	Biochemical Response	Histological Response	Side Effects/ Discontinuation	Outcome After Transplant
Pretransplant										
Casanovas-Taltavull et al. 1995[39]	Dialysis patients	10	IFN 3 mU 3/week, tapering to 1.5 mU 3/week for 1 year	6 months	1/10	2/10	9/10		IFN stopped in 3	4 of 5 maintained normal renal function, 1 had acute vascular rejection
Huraib et al. 2001[114]	Renal transplant candidates	30	15 patients – IFN 3 mU 3/week for 1 year, 11 had renal transplant (group A) 15 patients: no antiviral therapy; 10 had transplant (group B)	12 months		4/11			Minimal or no dose adjustment	HAI at 1 year after transplant lower in group A (1.19) than in group B (5.5)
Benci et al. 1998[21]	Dialysis patients	10	IFN 1 mU 3/week, for relapsers 3 mU 3/week, 1 year total therapy	6 months		3/10			IFN stopped in 1	
Morales et al. 1995[171]	Dialysis patients	19 received IFN, 17 controls	IFN 3 mU 3/week for 6 months	3–33 months	14/19	8/19			IFN stopped in 10/19	3 remained HCV RNA negative and 1 relapsed
Casanovas-Taltavull et al. 2001[38]	Dialysis patients	29	IFN 3 mU 3/week for 6 months and 1.5 mU 3/week for 6 months	41± 28 months	23/28	18/28	18/28		IFN stopped in 7/29	8 remained HCV RNA-negative and 1 relapsed
Bruchfeld et al.[29]	Dialysis patients	6	PEG-IFN-α_{2a} 135 μg/week or PEGα-2b 50 μg/week plus ribavirin titrated to trough of 10–15 μmol/L	Variable	6/6	3/6			Treatment stopped in 2/6	2 patients transplanted and remain negative
Liu et al. 2009[151]	Dialysis patients-prior IFN relapsers	35	PEG-IFN-α_{2a} 135 μg/week plus ribavirin 200 mg/day	Unknown	91%	60% (52% genotype 1)			Discontinuation in 17%	NA
Posttransplant										
Yap et al.[238]	Acute de novo HCV infection after renal transplant	4	IFN 3 mU 3/week+ ribavirin 1000–1200 mg/day for 48 weeks	15–42 mos	3/4	3/4	3/4		Dose-dependent hemolysis, no renal dysfunction	

Rostaing et al. 1995[201]	Renal transplant recipients with HCV	15 treated (group A) and 15 controls (group B)	IFN 3 mu 3/week for 6 months	12 months	4/14	0/14	10/14		Renal failure in 5/14, renal function recovered in only 2 despite steroid pulse
Lee et al. 2001[145]	Renal transplant recipients with HCV	11	IFN 1 mu 3/week+ribavirin 600 mg/day for 48 weeks	NR	5/11	3/11	10/11		IFN stopped in 3, 1 with acute graft failure
Fontaine et al. 2004[92]	Renal transplant recipients with HCV	13	Ribavirin 724 ± 224 mg/day for 22.6 ± 13.3 months	22.6 ± 13 months	0/13	0/13	Decrease in mean AST from 128 to 53	Metavir activity score decreased from 2.46 ±0.78 to 1.23 ± 1.01	1 patient required erythropoietin
Kamar et al. 2003[128]	Renal transplant recipients with HCV	16 received ribavirin (group A) and 32 controls (group B)	Ribavirin starting at 1000 mg/day adjusted to hemoglobin. 1 year therapy	12 months	0/16	0/16	Decrease in mean ALT from 85 to 48	No improvement in inflammation and fibrosis. Improvement in proteinuria	3 cases ribavirin stopped despite erythropoietin therapy
Durlik et al. 1998[71]	Renal transplant recipients (7 with HCV alone, 6 HBV alone and 2 HBV, HCV, HDV)	15	IFN 3 mu 3/week for 6 months	3–53 months			ALT improved in all (normal in 50%)		Rejection in 5/15, 4 lost grafts (3 from irreversible rejection)
Thervet et al. 1994[226]	Renal transplant recipients with HBV, HCV, or both	13	IFN 3 mu 3/week for 6 months	3–26 months			AST, ALT improved significantly on therapy, returned to previous levels after end of treatment		IFN stopped in 7, acute renal failure in 2 patients (1 chronic rejection)
Tokumoto et al. 1996[228]	Renal transplant recipients with HCV	6	IFN 10 mu daily for 2 weeks then 5–10 mu 3/week for 22 weeks	17–27 months	3/6	3/6	6/6 normalized AST, ALT		1 with renal failure (acute vascular rejection)

ALT, alanine aminotransferase; AST, aspartate aminotransferase; ETVR, end of treatment virologic response, defined as undetectable HCV RNA at end of therapy; HAI, hospital-acquired infection; hepatitis B virus; HCV, hepatitis C virus; HDV; HAI, hepatic activity index; IFN, interferon; PEG-IFN, pegylated interferon; SVR, sustained virologic response, defined as undetectable HCV RNA 6 months after the end of therapy.

and ribavirin (triple therapy) and neither is approved for HCV genotypes other than genotype 1. Both agents have shown substantial improvement in the probability of SVR achievement.[17,188]

There have been no studies evaluating triple therapy in patients with chronic kidney disease or on hemodialysis.

Posttransplant Antiviral Therapy for Hepatitis C

Posttransplantation interferon therapy is generally contraindicated in organ transplant recipients other than liver allografts. The reluctance to treat HCV posttransplant is due to a low probability of success and evidence to suggest that interferon therapy can precipitate renal failure and organ rejection.[201] For this reason we recommend that interferon therapy should be limited to patients with severe recurrence of HCV, such as fibrosing cholestatic hepatitis C, or in the setting of well-constructed, appropriately powered clinical trials.

Hepatitis E

HEV is a non-enveloped, single-strand RNA virus of the family Hepaviridae.[102] HEV is considered endemic in developing countries and is spread via fecal–oral transmission, similarly to hepatitis A (HAV).[20] In immunocompetent patients, HEV has a clinical course similar to HAV, manifested by an acute, sometimes icteric, self-limited illness without the potential for chronicity.

However, in recent years, zoonotic transmission (frequently from a swine vector) of HEV in industrialized countries has become increasingly recognized. In France, anti-HEV antibodies are present in 16.6% of blood donors and 6–16% of renal transplant recipients.[126,160] In addition, chronic hepatitis due to HEV infection has been reported in immunocompromised patients, including liver and kidney transplant recipients.[97,126] Thus, chronic HEV infection should be considered in kidney transplant recipients with unexplained liver test abnormalities.

There is no effective vaccination available for HEV. Current recommendations for HEV prevention focus primarily on proper hygiene and consumption of properly cooked food. Blood-borne transmission of HEV is felt to be rare.

There are no data on the natural history of HEV infection on kidney transplant recipients. Similarly, there are very limited data on treatment for chronic HEV. Pegylated interferon-α has been used in liver transplant recipients, but caution should be used in renal transplant recipients due to the known risk of allograft loss.[127] Ribavirin has also been used in kidney transplant recipients with chronic HEV infection. Kamar et al.[127] published a series of six kidney transplant recipients with chronic HEV hepatitis treated with ribavirin at a dose of 600–800 mg/day. All patients achieved serum viral clearance at 3 months. Four patients achieved a durable response after cessation of ribavirin.[127] Larger studies are needed to determine optimal dose and duration of ribavirin therapy for chronic HEV.

HEPATOCELLULAR CARCINOMA AFTER RENAL TRANSPLANTATION

In the setting of immunosuppression, loss of tumor surveillance can lead to higher risk for various malignancies. HCC is likely more common after renal transplantation (incidence 1.4–4%) than in the general population (incidence 0.005–0.015%).[119,152,183,198] This risk is particularly true for renal transplant recipients infected with chronic HBV or HCV. In areas endemic for HBV, HCC is the most common tumor after renal transplantation (20–45%).[48,50] Recently, Hoffman et al.[111] published data on the development of de novo HCC in transplant recipients. Using US registry data of over 200 000 transplant recipients, the incidence of HCC in non-liver transplant recipients was 6.5 per 100 000 person-years. HBV and HCV infection were independently predictive of the development of de novo HCC. Estimated survival was worse than that expected for similar-stage tumors in non-transplanted populations.[48,198] Since outcomes after HCC are poor, preventive measures are important, including: vaccination of renal transplant waiting list patients for HBV, antiviral therapy for HCV and HBV in the dialysis population, continued antiviral treatment for HBV in the renal transplant recipient, exclusion of patients with ESRD and cirrhosis from isolated kidney transplantation, and in select cases consideration of these patients for combined liver transplantation.

Renal transplant recipients infected with HBV/HCV and uncontrolled viral replication or with advanced fibrosis/cirrhosis should be entered in an HCC surveillance protocol. Current American Association for the Study of Liver Diseases guidelines recommend surveillance with ultrasound with or without α-fetoprotein every 6 months.[31]

SYSTEMIC INFECTIONS RESULTING IN HEPATITIS AND LIVER DISEASE

A number of systemic infections have hepatitis as part of the clinical manifestation. Foremost among these are infections caused by herpesviruses, which are major pathogens in organ transplantation. Other infections primarily involving the liver are also reviewed.

Liver Abscess

Pyogenic liver abscess does not represent a specific liver disease but is a final common pathway of many pathologic processes. The incidence of pyogenic liver abscess ranges from 8 to 20 cases per 100 000 hospital admissions[121]; a population-based study reported 2.3 cases per 100 000 persons per year.[130] A recent population-based study found no increased risk of pyogenic liver abscess in renal transplant recipients.[130]

Abscesses may be classified by presumed route of hepatic invasion: (1) biliary tree; (2) portal vein; (3) hepatic artery; (4) direct extension from contiguous focus of infection; and (5) penetrating trauma.[121] Approximately 50% of pyogenic liver abscesses are cryptogenic.[194] The microbiology of pyogenic liver abscess is variable and depends on the route of infection. Most infections are polymicrobial, with enteric facultative and anerobic bacteria being the most common agents. *Candida* species should also be suspected as a pathogen in pyogenic abscesses, accounting for 22% of abscesses in one series.[113]

While fever and constitutional symptoms are frequent, only one in 10 patients presents with the classic triad of fever, jaundice, and right upper quadrant tenderness. Although liver function tests are abnormal in most patients, the elevation is usually modest. Radiographic imaging using magnetic resonance imaging, computed tomography, or ultrasonography is essential to making the diagnosis. Microbiologic diagnosis rests upon obtaining purulent material from the abscess cavity, which should be sent for Gram stain and culture. In general, treatment consists of antimicrobial therapy for 3–4 weeks and drainage of the abscess. Some investigators have reported success with treatment of small abscesses with antibiotic therapy alone; however most patients will require some form of abscess drainage.[36] Drainage may be achieved by percutaneous aspiration with or without placement of a drainage catheter. Generally, abscesses larger than 5 cm require placement of a catheter. Endoscopic drainage via endoscopic retrograde cholangiopancreatography has been reported to be successful in cases where the abscess communicates with the biliary tree.[212] Finally, surgical drainage may be needed in cases with multifocal abscesses, heavily loculated abscesses, or unsuccessful percutaneous drainage.

Amebiasis is a far less common cause of liver abscess in the United States but one that must be considered in patients living in or traveling to countries where the prevalence of amebiasis is high. There is a marked male predominance and amebic liver abscesses are usually solitary.[218] Clinical signs and symptoms and liver test abnormalities do not help to distinguish amebic from pyogenic liver abscesses. Serology for antibodies to *Entamoeba histolytica* is useful to determine current or past infection. Following confirmation of an abscess on imaging, if amebic rather than pyogenic liver abscess is suspected, treatment with metronidazole for 10 days is necessary. Renal transplant recipients travelling to areas endemic for amebiasis should be counseled to avoid ingestion of potentially contaminated food and water, such as fresh produce that cannot be adequately cooked.[138] Boiling water before use is essential to destroy the cysts of *E. histolytica* which are not killed by low-dose iodine or chlorine tablets.

Mycobacterial Infection

Tuberculosis is an important cause of morbidity and mortality among renal transplant recipients. The risk of active tuberculosis is at least 50-fold higher in renal transplant recipients compared to non-transplant patients; most reactivation disease has been reported to occur in the first year following transplantation.[2,207] Liver involvement with tuberculosis remains rare; when present, it is usually associated with pulmonary or gastrointestinal involvement with tuberculosis. Three patterns of tuberculous liver involvement have been reported[8]: (1) diffuse involvement of the liver in association with tuberculosis at other body sites; (2) miliary involvement of the liver with no other known organ involvement (granulomatous hepatitis); and (3) focal lesion in the liver, either an abscess or a tuberculoma.[220,38] Constitutional symptoms and fever are common but non-specific. A modest degree of transaminase and alkaline phosphatase elevation is common. Imaging followed by tissue staining for acid-fast bacilli and culture for mycobacteria are required to confirm the diagnosis.

Viral Infections

Herpesviruses

The herpesviruses include cytomegalovirus (CMV), Epstein–Barr virus (EBV), herpes simplex virus, human herpesvirus 6 and 7 and varicella-zoster virus (VZV). The herpesvirus family is responsible for considerable morbidity and mortality in transplant recipients. In particular, CMV remains a major health threat following solid-organ transplantation. All the herpesviruses have the ability to remain latent in tissues after acute infection. Liver involvement frequently is a part of the clinical presentation of herpesvirus-related diseases.

Cytomegalovirus

CMV is one of the most important pathogens in transplant recipients.[137,138] Unlike the other herpesviruses, such as herpes simplex virus and VZV, which remain latent in highly restricted areas of the body, once acquired, latent CMV can be found in multiple body sites.

After transplantation, approximately 50% of transplant patients excrete CMV in body secretions (e.g., saliva and urine) at some point.[162] In addition, over 60% of patients develop antigenemia within the first 100 days after transplantation.[205]

Hepatitis is a major clinical manifestation of CMV disease. In the immunocompetent patient, the disease is usually mild and self-limiting, although rare cases of fulminant CMV hepatitis have been described.[211] In the transplant recipient, CMV hepatitis is a more severe illness, usually with other organ involvement or disseminated disease, and is not uncommon. In a series of 97 renal transplant recipients with CMV disease, half had evidence of CMV hepatitis; the severity of hepatitis was greater in primary disease than in cases of reactivation.[206]

In an autopsy series of four immunocompromised patients with overwhelming CMV infection, Ten Napel et al. showed that liver cell damage was extensive but inflammatory infiltration was less prominent than in immunocompetent patients with CMV infection.[223] Intracellular CMV inclusion bodies were found in the hepatocytes, vascular endothelium, and bile epithelium. Given the significant morbidity and mortality of CMV infection, including CMV hepatitis, in solid-organ transplant recipients, prevention and treatment of CMV infection posttransplant are of utmost importance. The diagnosis and treatment of CMV infection and strategies for CMV prophylaxis in kidney transplant recipients are covered in Chapter 31.

Epstein–Barr Virus

EBV, a member of the human gamma herpesvirus family, is a ubiquitous pathogen. More than 90% of the world's population is infected.[23] The virus is shed intermittently into saliva[237] and is believed to be transmitted through close contact with oral secretions. EBV infection may present as primary or secondary infection (reactivation). Childhood disease is usually asymptomatic. Infection acquired in adolescence or young adulthood frequently causes the clinical syndrome of acute infectious mononucleosis, characterized by fever, pharyngitis, and lymphadenopathy in 75% of patients.[72] A non-specific hepatitis is common in acute infectious mononucleosis. Jaundice is apparent in 5–9% of patients. Liver function test abnormalities peak with acute illness and return to normal over 1–2 months. In instances where liver biopsies have been obtained, minimal swelling and vacuolization of hepatocytes can be seen accompanied by a lymphocytic or monocytic infiltrate in portal regions.[69]

EBV establishes latency[16] and may reactivate later; the risk of reactivation is especially high in immunosuppressed patients. Primary infection with EBV following transplantation may manifest as a febrile illness with constitutional signs and symptoms.

EBV has a central role in the pathogenesis of posttransplant lymphoproliferative disorder (PTLD),[231] although not all PTLD is caused by EBV.

The diagnosis and treatment of EBV and PTLD are discussed in Chapter 31.

Herpes Simplex Virus

Herpes simplex virus (HSV) is an alpha herpesvirus with a genome consisting of a linear, double-stranded DNA molecule.[236] The two types of HSV – HSV-1 and HSV-2 – have 50% sequence homology. In the US population, seroprevalence rates range from 56% to 60% for HSV-1 and from 15% to 18% for HSV-2. First episodes of HSV, or primary infection, are frequently accompanied by systemic signs and symptoms and have a longer duration of symptoms.[9] The virus esablishes latency in ganglia, and may reactivate. Immunocompromised patients have been found to have more severe primary infections and more frequent reactivations.[230] In renal transplant recipients, the incidence of HSV infection has been reported to be 30–50% in the absence of prophylaxis.[120,208] The risk of HSV reactivation is highest in the first 3 months posttransplant due to the higher level of immunosuppression needed during this period. Oral acyclovir for prophylaxis against HSV has greatly reduced the incidence of HSV infection.[120,208]

Hepatitis with HSV has been well described in the general population as well as the renal transplant population. Kusne et al.[140] reported a series of 12 cases of HSV hepatitis which developed a median of 18 days after solid-organ transplantation. The clinical features included fever, herpetic stomatitis, and abdominal pain, usually in association with disseminated disease. Clinical features associated with mortality included bacteremia, hypotension, disseminated intravascular coagulation, and gastrointestinal bleeding. HSV hepatitis was associated with 67% mortality in this patient population.

Conclusive diagnosis of HSV hepatitis rests on demonstration of viral involvement of liver tissue. Histologically, hepatocytes have enlarged "ground-glass" nuclei with chromatin margination. Due to the high mortality associated with HSV hepatitis, transplant recipients who present with fever, progressive transaminase elevation, and abdominal symptoms with or without evidence of cutaneous herpes simplex infection should prompt consideration of HSV hepatitis and treatment with intravenous acyclovir.

Varicella-Zoster Virus

VZV is another herpesvirus that causes two distinct diseases – varicella and herpes zoster. Primary infection with VZV causes varicella in susceptible hosts. Children generally develop mild disease when compared to adults or immunosuppressed patients. While only 0.1% of varicella infections develop in this population, 25% of varicella-related deaths occur in this patient population.

Hepatic involvement with varicella is uncommon but has been described in transplant recipients. A study assessing clinical features of liver transplant patients with varicella hepatitis showed that the most common presenting features were cutaneous vesicular lesions, fever, and acute abdominal or back pain. The rash may not be apparent at the time of hepatic involvement, however, and the diagnosis of varicella hepatitis may be delayed. In case reports, high-dose acyclovir (10 mg/kg every 8 hours) has been shown to treat varicella hepatitis successfully.

Like all herpesviruses, VZV establishes latency and may subsequently reactivate.[53] Reactivation of latent VZV typically results in a localized skin infection known as herpes zoster or shingles.

Disseminated zoster in transplant patients can be a severe, prolonged illness with hepatitis as a prominent manifestation. In a case series of four renal transplant recipients that developed primary (1) or reactivation VZV infection (3), all four had multiorgan involvement and three of the four developed hepatitis.[85] In general, primary varicella infection is a more severe illness than reactivated disease. Fehr et al.[85] reviewed all cases of herpes zoster in renal transplant recipients and found 34 reported cases, most of which were primary infections. Analysis of these cases showed that disseminated intravascular coagulation and hepatitis occurred in half of the cases and pneumonitis in 29% of patients. The overall mortality was 34%, although it appears to have decreased over time from 53% to 22%

Treatment of disseminated zoster in transplant patients should be undertaken promptly with high-dose acyclovir.

Human Herpesviruses 6 and 7

Human herpesvirus 6 (HHV-6) and HHV-7 are ubiquitous lymphotrophic herpesviruses and were initially isolated from patients with lymphoproliferative disorders.[37] Seroprevalence surveys have found that HHV-6 infection occurs in the majority of children by age 3 years, and the prevalence in adults is greater than 90%.

The major childhood clinical syndrome caused by HHV-6 primary infection is exanthem subitum.

Infection in immune-competent adults is usually benign, presenting as fever with lymphadenopathy or an infectious mononucleosis-like syndrome. HHV-6 infection posttransplant has been frequently reported in kidney transplant recipients.[143,174] Typically, HHV-6 reactivation is asymptomatic, even in kidney transplant patients. However, symptomatic and even fatal HHV-6 infections have been reported in the kidney transplant population. Hepatitis has been rarely reported in both the immune-competent and transplant populations.[52,108,189] There are no controlled trials of antiviral therapy for HHV-6 or HHV-7 infection. According to the American Society of Transplantation Infectious Disease Community of Practice guidelines, intravenous ganciclovir or foscarnet is first-line therapy for active disease.[196]

REFERENCES

1. Abbott KC, Lentine KL, Bucci JR, et al. The impact of transplantation with deceased donor hepatitis C-positive kidneys on survival in wait-listed long-term dialysis patients. Am J Transplant 2004;4(12):2032–7.
2. Agarwal SK, Gupta S, Dash SC, et al. Prospective randomised trial of isoniazid prophylaxis in renal transplant recipient. Int Urol Nephrol 2004;36(3):425–31.
3. Aguilar P, Renoult E, Jarrosson L, et al. Anti-HBs cellular immune response in kidney recipients before and 4 months after transplantation. Clin Diagn Lab Immunol 2003;10(6):1117–22.
4. Akalin E, Ames S, Sehgal V, et al. Safety of using hepatitis B virus core antibody or surface antigen-positive donors in kidney or pancreas transplantation. Clin Transplant 2005;19(3):364–6.
5. Ali MK, Light JA, Barhyte DR, et al. Donor hepatitis C virus status does not adversely affect short-term outcomes in HCV+ recipients in renal transplantation. Transplantation 1998;66(12):1694–7.
6. Allain JP. Epidemiology of hepatitis B virus and genotype. J Clin Virol 2006;36(Suppl. 1):S12–7.
7. Allison MC, Mowat A, McCruden EA, et al. The spectrum of chronic liver disease in renal transplant recipients. Q J Med 1992;83(301):355–67.
8. Alvarez SZ. Hepatobiliary tuberculosis. J Gastroenterol Hepatol 1998;13(8):833–9.
9. Amir J. Clinical aspects and antiviral therapy in primary herpetic gingivostomatitis. Paediatr Drugs 2001;3(8):593–7.
10. Amoroso P, Rapicetta M, Tosti ME, et al. Correlation between virus genotype and chronicity rate in acute hepatitis C. J Hepatol 1998;28(6):939–44.
11. Andrade RJ, Lucena MI, Fernandez MC, et al. Drug-induced liver injury: an analysis of 461 incidences submitted to the Spanish registry over a 10-year period. Gastroenterology 2005;129(2):512–21.
12. Arber N, Zajicek G, Nordenberg J, et al. Azathioprine treatment increases hepatocyte turnover. Gastroenterology 1991;101(4):1083–6.
13. Armstrong GL, Wasley A, Simard EP, et al. The prevalence of hepatitis C virus infection in the United States, 1999 through 2002. Ann Intern Med 2006;144(10):705–14.
14. Aroldi A, Lampertico P, Montagnino G, et al. Natural history of hepatitis B and C in renal allograft recipients. Transplantation 2005;79(9):1132–6.
15. Azoulay D, Castaing D, Lemoine A, et al. Transjugular intrahepatic portosystemic shunt (TIPS) for severe veno-occlusive disease of the liver following bone marrow transplantation. Bone Marrow Transplant 2000;25(9):987–92.
16. Babcock GJ, Decker LL, Volk M, et al. EBV persistence in memory B cells in vivo. Immunity 1998;9(3):395–404.
17. Bacon BR, Gordon SC, Lawitz E, et al. Boceprevir for previously treated chronic HCV genotype 1 infection. N Engl J Med 364(13):1207–17.
18. Bae KT, Zhu F, Chapman AB, et al. Magnetic resonance imaging evaluation of hepatic cysts in early autosomal-dominant polycystic kidney disease: the Consortium for Radiologic Imaging Studies of Polycystic Kidney Disease cohort. Clin J Am Soc Nephrol 2006;1(1):64–9.
19. Baid S, Tolkoff-Rubin N, Saidman S, et al. Acute humoral rejection in hepatitis C-infected renal transplant recipients receiving antiviral therapy. Am J Transplant 2003;3(1):74–8.
20. Balayan MS, Andjaparidze AG, Dubois F, et al. Evidence for a virus in non-A, non-B hepatitis transmitted via the fecal–oral route. Intervirology 1983;20(1):23–31.
21. Benci A, Caremani M, Menchetti D, et al. Low-dose leukocyte interferon-alpha therapy in dialysed patients with chronic hepatitis C. Curr Med Res Opin 1998;14(3):141–4.
22. Deleted in proof.
23. Biggar RJ, Henle G, Bocker J, et al. Primary Epstein–Barr virus infections in African infants. II. Clinical and serological observations during seroconversion. Int J Cancer 1978;22(3):244–50.
24. Bloom RD, Rao V, Weng F, et al. Association of hepatitis C with posttransplant diabetes in renal transplant patients on tacrolimus. J Am Soc Nephrol 2002;13(5):1374–80.
25. Bloom RD, Sayer G, Fa K, et al. Outcome of hepatitis C virus-infected kidney transplant candidates who remain on the waiting list. Am J Transplant 2005;5(1):139–44.
26. Bohan TP, Helton E, McDonald I, et al. Effect of L-carnitine treatment for valproate-induced hepatotoxicity. Neurology 2001;56(10):1405–9.
27. Bortolotti F, Guido M, Bartolacci S, et al. Chronic hepatitis B in children after e antigen seroclearance: final report of a 29-year longitudinal study. Hepatology 2006;43(3):556–62.
28. Breitenfeldt MK, Rasenack J, Berthold H, et al. Impact of hepatitis B and C on graft loss and mortality of patients after kidney transplantation. Clin Transplant 2002;16(2):130–6.
29. Bruchfeld A, Lindahl K, Reichard O, et al. Pegylated interferon and ribavirin treatment for hepatitis C in haemodialysis patients. J Viral Hepat 2006;13(5):316–21.
30. Bruchfeld A, Stahle L, Andersson J, et al. Ribavirin treatment in dialysis patients with chronic hepatitis C virus infection – a pilot study. J Viral Hepat 2001;8(4):287–92.
31. Bruix J, Sherman M. Management of hepatocellular carcinoma: an update. Hepatology 53(3):1020–2.
32. Buffet C, Cantarovitch M, Pelletier G, et al. Three cases of nodular regenerative hyperplasia of the liver following renal transplantation. Nephrol Dial Transplant 1988;3(3):327–30.
33. Bukh J, Wantzin P, Krogsgaard K, et al. High prevalence of hepatitis C virus (HCV) RNA in dialysis patients: failure of commercially available antibody tests to identify a significant number of patients with HCV infection. Copenhagen Dialysis HCV Study Group. J Infect Dis 1993;168(6):1343–8.
34. Busuttil RW, Lake JR. Role of tacrolimus in the evolution of liver transplantation. Transplantation 2004;77(Suppl. 9):S44–51.
35. Cacoub P, Renou C, Rosenthal E, et al. Extrahepatic manifestations associated with hepatitis C virus infection. A prospective multicenter study of 321 patients. The GERMIVIC Groupe d'Etude et de Recherche en Medecine Interne et Maladies Infectieuses sur le Virus de l'Hepatite C. Medicine (Baltimore) 2000;79(1):47–56.
36. Calvo-Romero JM, Lima-Rodriguez EM. Favourable outcome of multiple pyogenic liver abscesses with conservative treatment. Scand J Infect Dis 2005;37(2):141–2.
37. Campadelli-Fiume G, Mirandola P, Menotti L. Human herpesvirus 6: an emerging pathogen. Emerg Infect Dis 1999;5(3):353–66.
38. Casanovas-Taltavull T, Baliellas C, Sesé E, et al. Efficacy of interferon for chronic hepatitis C virus-related hepatitis in kidney transplant candidates on hemodialysis: results after transplantation. Am J Gastroenterol 2001;96(4):1170–7.
39. Casanovas Taltavull T, Baliellas C, Benasco C, et al. Interferon may be useful in hemodialysis patients with hepatitis C virus chronic infection who are candidates for kidney transplant. Transplant Proc 1995;27(4):2229–30.
40. Cescon M, Grazi GL, Cucchetti A, et al. Predictors of sustained virological response after antiviral treatment for hepatitis C recurrence following liver transplantation. Liver Transpl 2009;15(7):782–9.
41. Chalasani N, Fontana RJ, Bonkovsky HL, et al. Causes, clinical features, and outcomes from a prospective study of drug-induced liver injury in the United States. Gastroenterology 1934;135(6):1924–34, e1-4.

42. Chan TM, Fang GX, Tang CS, et al. Preemptive lamivudine therapy based on HBV DNA level in HBsAg-positive kidney allograft recipients. Hepatology 2002;36(5):1246–52.
43. Chan TM, Tse KC, Tang CS, et al. Prospective study on lamivudine-resistant hepatitis B in renal allograft recipients. Am J Transplant 2004;4(7):1103–9.
44. Chan TM, Wu PC, Li FK, et al. Treatment of fibrosing cholestatic hepatitis with lamivudine. Gastroenterology 1998;115(1):177–81.
45. Chandra M, Khaja MN, Hussain MM, et al. Prevalence of hepatitis B and hepatitis C viral infections in Indian patients with chronic renal failure. Intervirology 2004;47(6):374–6.
46. Chang TT, Gish RG, de Man R, et al. A comparison of entecavir and lamivudine for HBeAg-positive chronic hepatitis B. N Engl J Med 2006;354(10):1001–10.
47. Chauveau D, Fakhouri F, Grunfeld JP, et al. Liver involvement in autosomal-dominant polycystic kidney disease: therapeutic dilemma. J Am Soc Nephrol 2000;11(9):1767–75.
48. Chiang YJ, Chen CH, Wu CT, et al. De novo cancer occurrence after renal transplantation: a medical center experience in Taiwan. Transplant Proc 2004;36(7):2150–1.
49. Chitturi S, George J. Hepatotoxicity of commonly used drugs: nonsteroidal anti-inflammatory drugs, antihypertensives, antidiabetic agents, anticonvulsants, lipid-lowering agents, psychotropic drugs. Semin Liver Dis 2002;22(2):169–83.
50. Chok KS, Lam CM, Li FK, et al. Management of hepatocellular carcinoma in renal transplant recipients. J Surg Oncol 2004;87(3):139–42.
51. Choo QL, Kuo G, Weiner AJ, et al. Isolation of a cDNA clone derived from a blood-borne non-A, non-B viral hepatitis genome. Science 1989;244(4902):359–62.
52. Clark DA. Human herpesvirus 6 and human herpesvirus 7: emerging pathogens in transplant patients. Int J Hematol 2002;76(Suppl. 2):246–52.
53. Cohen JI, Brunell PA, Straus SE, et al. Recent advances in varicella-zoster virus infection. Ann Intern Med 1999;130(11):922–32.
54. Colonno RJ, Rose R, Baldick CJ, et al. Entecavir resistance is rare in nucleoside naive patients with hepatitis B. Hepatology 2006;44(6):1656–65.
55. Covic A, Maftei ID, Mardare NG, et al. Analysis of safety and efficacy of pegylated-interferon alpha-2a in hepatitis C virus positive hemodialysis patients: results from a large, multicenter audit. J Nephrol 2006;19(6):794–801.
56. Cruzado JM, Carrera M, Torras J, et al. Hepatitis C virus infection and de novo glomerular lesions in renal allografts. Am J Transplant 2001;1(2):171–8.
57. Cruzado JM, Casanovas-Taltavull T, Torras J, et al. Pretransplant interferon prevents hepatitis C virus-associated glomerulonephritis in renal allografts by HCV-RNA clearance. Am J Transplant 2003;3(3):357–60.
58. DaRoza G, Loewen A, Djurdjev O, et al. Stage of chronic kidney disease predicts seroconversion after hepatitis B immunization: earlier is better. Am J Kidney Dis 2003;42(6):1184–92.
59. Daude M, Rostaing L, Sauné K, et al. Tenofovir therapy in hepatitis B virus-positive solid-organ transplant recipients. Transplantation 91(8): 916–20.
60. Davies SE, Portmann BC, O'Grady JG, et al. Hepatic histological findings after transplantation for chronic hepatitis B virus infection, including a unique pattern of fibrosing cholestatic hepatitis. Hepatology 1991;13(1):150–7.
61. de Boer NK, Mulder CJ, van Bodegraven AA, et al. Nodular regenerative hyperplasia and thiopurines: the case for level-dependent toxicity. Liver Transpl 2005;11(10):1300–1.
62. De Feo TM, Grossi P, Poli F, et al. Kidney transplantation from anti-HBc+ donors: results from a retrospective Italian study. Transplantation 2006;81(1):76–80.
63. De Vos JY, Elseviers M, Pancirová A, et al. European practice in haemodalysis: results of the EPD. EDTNA ERCA J 2006;32(1):20–3.
64. Degott C, Rueff B, Kreis H, et al. Peliosis hepatitis in recipients of renal transplants. Gut 1978;19(8):748–53.
65. Delladetsima I, Psichogiou M, Sypsa V, et al. The course of hepatitis C virus infection in pretransplantation anti-hepatitis C virus-negative renal transplant recipients: a retrospective follow-up study. Am J Kidney Dis 2006;47(2):309–16.
66. Derbala M, Amer A, Bener A, et al. Pegylated interferon-alpha 2b-ribavirin combination in Egyptian patients with genotype 4 chronic hepatitis. J Viral Hepat 2005;12(4):380–5.
67. Dodd RY, Notari EPt, Starmer SL, et al. Current prevalence and incidence of infectious disease markers and estimated window-period risk in the American Red Cross blood donor population. Transfusion 2002;42(8):975–9.
68. Donahue JG, Munoz A, Ness PM, et al. The declining risk of post-transfusion hepatitis C virus infection. N Engl J Med 1992;327(6):369–73.
69. Drebber U, Kasper HU, Krupacz J, et al. The role of Epstein–Barr virus in acute and chronic hepatitis. J Hepatol 2006;44(5):879–85.
70. Duarte R, Huraib S, Said R, et al. Interferon-alpha facilitates renal transplantation in hemodialysis patients with chronic viral hepatitis. Am J Kidney Dis 1995;25(1):40–5.
71. Durlik M, Gaciong Z, Rowinska D, et al. Long-term results of treatment of chronic hepatitis B, C and D with interferon-alpha in renal allograft recipients. Transpl Int 1998;11(Suppl. 1):S135–9.
72. Ebell MH. Epstein–Barr virus infectious mononucleosis. Am Fam Physician 2004;70(7):1279–87.
73. Eisenbach C, Goeggelmann C, Flechtenmacher C, et al. Severe cholestatic hepatitis caused by azathioprine. Immunopharmacol Immunotoxicol 2005;27(1):77–83.
74. Everson GT, Taylor MR, Doctor RB. Polycystic disease of the liver. Hepatology 2004;40(4):774–82.
75. Fabrizi F, Bunnapradist S, Martin P. HBV infection in patients with end-stage renal disease. Semin Liver Dis 2004;24(Suppl. 1): 63–70.
76. Fabrizi F, Dixit V, Messa P, et al. Intradermal vs intramuscular vaccine against hepatitis B infection in dialysis patients: a meta-analysis of randomized trials. J Viral Hepat 18(10):730–7.
77. Fabrizi F, Dulai G, Dixit V, et al. Meta-analysis: interferon for the treatment of chronic hepatitis C in dialysis patients. Aliment Pharmacol Ther 2003;18(11–12):1071–81.
78. Fabrizi F, Dulai G, Dixit V, et al. Lamivudine for the treatment of hepatitis B virus-related liver disease after renal transplantation: meta-analysis of clinical trials. Transplantation 2004;77(6):859–64.
79. Fabrizi F, Martin P, Bunnapradist S, et al. Treatment of chronic viral hepatitis in patients with renal disease. Gastroenterol Clin North Am 2004;33(3):655–70, xi.
80. Fabrizi F, Martin P, Dixit V, et al. Hepatitis C virus antibody status and survival after renal transplantation: meta-analysis of observational studies. Am J Transplant 2005;5(6):1452–61.
81. Fabrizi F, Martin P, Dixit V, et al. HBsAg seropositive status and survival after renal transplantation: meta-analysis of observational studies. Am J Transplant 2005;5(12):2913–21.
82. Fabrizi F, Poordad FF, Martin P. Hepatitis C infection and the patient with end-stage renal disease. Hepatology 2002;36(1): 3–10.
83. Fairley CK, Mijch A, Gust ID, et al. The increased risk of fatal liver disease in renal transplant patients who are hepatitis Be antigen and/or HBV DNA positive. Transplantation 1991;52(3):497–500.
84. Farci P, Alter HJ, Shimoda A, et al. Hepatitis C virus-associated fulminant hepatic failure. N Engl J Med 1996;335(9):631–4.
85. Fehr T, Bossart W, Wahl C, et al. Disseminated varicella infection in adult renal allograft recipients: four cases and a review of the literature. Transplantation 2002;73(4):608–11.
86. Feinstone SM, Kapikian AZ, Purceli RH. Hepatitis A: detection by immune electron microscopy of a viruslike antigen associated with acute illness. Science 1973;182(4116):1026–8.
87. Ferrajolo C, Capuano A, Verhamme KM, et al. Drug-induced hepatic injury in children: a case/non-case study of suspected adverse drug reactions in VigiBase. Br J Clin Pharmacol 70(5): 721–728.
88. Finelli L, Miller JT, Tokars JI, et al. National surveillance of dialysis-associated diseases in the United States, 2002. Semin Dial 2005;18(1):52–61.
89. Fissell RB, Bragg-Gresham JL, Woods JD, et al. Patterns of hepatitis C prevalence and seroconversion in hemodialysis units from three continents: the DOPPS. Kidney Int 2004;65(6):2335–42.
90. Fong TL, Bunnapradist S, Jordan JS, et al. Impact of hepatitis B core antibody status on outcomes of cadaveric renal transplantation: analysis of united network of organ sharing database between 1994 and 1999. Transplantation 2002;73(1):85–9.
91. Fontaine H, Vallet-Pichard A, Chaix ML, et al. Efficacy and safety of adefovir dipivoxil in kidney recipients, hemodialysis patients, and patients with renal insufficiency. Transplantation 2005;80(8):1086–92.

92. Fontaine H, Vallet-Pichard A, Chaix ML, et al. Histopathologic efficacy of ribavirin monotherapy in kidney allograft recipients with chronic hepatitis C. Transplantation 2004;78(6):853–7.
93. Formea CM, Evans CG, Karlix JL, et al. Altered cytochrome p450 metabolism of calcineurin inhibitors: case report and review of the literature. Pharmacotherapy 2005;25(7):1021–9.
94. Fornairon S, Pol S, Legendre C, et al. The long-term virologic and pathologic impact of renal transplantation on chronic hepatitis B virus infection. Transplantation 1996;62(2):297–9.
95. Fraser A, Longnecker MP, Lawlor DA, et al. Prevalence of elevated alanine aminotransferase among US adolescents and associated factors: NHANES 1999-2004. Gastroenterology 2007;133(6):1814–20.
96. Fried MW, Shiffman ML, Reddy KR, et al. Peginterferon alfa-2a plus ribavirin for chronic hepatitis C virus infection. N Engl J Med 2002;347(13):975–82.
97. Gerolami R, Moal V, Colson P. Chronic hepatitis E with cirrhosis in a kidney-transplant recipient. N Engl J Med 2008;358(8):859–60.
98. Ghany MG, Nelson DR, Strader DB, et al. An update on treatment of genotype 1 chronic hepatitis C virus infection: 2011 practice guideline by the American Association for the Study of Liver Diseases. Hepatology 2011;54(4):1433–44.
99. Go MR, Bumgardner GL. OKT3 (muromonab-CD3) associated hepatitis in a kidney transplant recipient. Transplantation 2002;73(12):1957–9.
100. Gourishankar S, McDermid JC, Jhangri GS, et al. Herpes zoster infection following solid organ transplantation: incidence, risk factors and outcomes in the current immunosuppressive era. Am J Transplant 2004;4(1):108–15.
101. Groth CG, Backman L, Morales JM, et al. Sirolimus (rapamycin)-based therapy in human renal transplantation: similar efficacy and different toxicity compared with cyclosporine. Sirolimus European Renal Transplant Study Group. Transplantation 1999;67(7):1036–42.
102. Guu TS, Liu Z, Ye Q, et al. Structure of the hepatitis E virus-like particle suggests mechanisms for virus assembly and receptor binding. Proc Natl Acad Sci U S A 2009;106(31):12992–7.
103. Haboubi NY, Ali HH, Whitwell HL, et al. Role of endothelial cell injury in the spectrum of azathioprine-induced liver disease after renal transplant: light microscopy and ultrastructural observations. Am J Gastroenterol 1988;83(3):256–61.
104. Hadziyannis SJ, Sette Jr H, Morgan TR, et al. Peginterferon-alpha2a and ribavirin combination therapy in chronic hepatitis C: a randomized study of treatment duration and ribavirin dose. Ann Intern Med 2004;140(5):346–55.
105. Han DJ, Kim TH, Park SK, et al. Results on preemptive or prophylactic treatment of lamivudine in HBsAg(+) renal allograft recipients: comparison with salvage treatment after hepatic dysfunction with HBV recurrence. Transplantation 2001;71(3):387–94.
106. Hanafusa T, Ichikawa Y, Kishikawa H, et al. Retrospective study on the impact of hepatitis C virus infection on kidney transplant patients over 20 years. Transplantation 1998;66(4):471–6.
107. Hardwick LL, Batiuk TD. Severe prolonged tacrolimus overdose with minimal consequences. Pharmacotherapy 2002;22(8):1063–6.
108. Harma M, Hockerstedt K, Lautenschlager I. Human herpesvirus-6 and acute liver failure. Transplantation 2003;76(3):536–9.
109. Hinrichsen H, Leimenstoll G, Stegen H, et al. Prevalence and risk factors of hepatitis C virus infection in haemodialysis patients: a multicentre study in 2796 patients. Gut 2002;51(3):429–33.
110. Hissar SS, Goyal A, Kumar M, et al. Hepatitis C virus genotype 3 predominates in North and Central India and is associated with significant histopathologic liver disease. J Med Virol 2006;78(4):452–8.
111. Hoffmann CJ, Subramanian AK, Cameron AM, et al. Incidence and risk factors for hepatocellular carcinoma after solid organ transplantation. Transplantation 2008;86(6):784–90.
112. Horsmans Y, Rahier J, Geubel AL. Reversible cholestasis with bile duct injury following azathioprine therapy. A case report. Liver 1991;11(2):89–93.
113. Huang CJ, Pitt HA, Lipsett PA, et al. Pyogenic hepatic abscess. Changing trends over 42 years. Ann Surg 1996;223(5):600–7 discussion, 607–609.
114. Huraib S, Iqbal A, Tanimu D, et al. Sustained virological and histological response with pretransplant interferon therapy in renal transplant patients with chronic viral hepatitis C. Am J Nephrol 2001;21(6):435–40.
115. Ioannou GN, Boyko EJ, Lee SP. The prevalence and predictors of elevated serum aminotransferase activity in the United States in 1999–2002. Am J Gastroenterol 2006;101(1):76–82.
116. Izzedine H, Kheder-Elfekih R, Housset P, et al. Adefovir dipivoxil-induced acute tubular necrosis and Fanconi syndrome in a renal transplant patient. AIDS 2009;23(4):544–5.
117. Jacobson, McHutchison JG, Dusheiko G, et al. Telaprevir for previously untreated chronic hepatitis C virus infection. N Engl J Med 364(25):2405–16.
118. Jacques J, Dickson Z, Carrier P, et al. Severe sirolimus-induced acute hepatitis in a renal transplant recipient. Transpl Int 23(9): 967–70.
119. Jeng LB, Huang CC, Lai MK, et al. Hepatocellular carcinoma after kidney transplantation. Transplant Proc 1999;31(1–2):1273–4.
120. Jirasiritham S, Sumethkul V, Chiewsilp P, et al. Prevention of recurrent herpes infection after renal transplantation by low-dose oral acyclovir. Transplant Proc 1994;26(4):2125–6.
121. Johannsen EC, Sifri CD, Madoff LC. Pyogenic liver abscesses. Infect Dis Clin North Am 2000;14(3):547–63, vii.
122. Josselson J, Kyser BA, Weir MR, et al. Hepatitis B surface antigenemia in a chronic hemodialysis program: lack of influence on morbidity and mortality. Am J Kidney Dis 1987;9(6): 456–61.
123. Kaba S, Dutta U, Byth K, et al. Molecular epidemiology of hepatitis C in Australia. J Gastroenterol Hepatol 1998;13(9):914–20.
124. Kairaitis LK, Gottlieb T, George CR. Fatal hepatitis B virus infection with fibrosing cholestatic hepatitis following renal transplantation. Nephrol Dial Transplant 1998;13(6):1571–3.
125. Kamar N, Huart A, Tack I, et al. Renal side effects of adefovir in hepatitis B virus-(HBV) positive kidney allograft recipients. Clin Nephrol 2009;71(1):36–42.
126. Kamar N, Milioto O, Alric L, et al. Entecavir therapy for adefovir-resistant hepatitis B virus infection in kidney and liver allograft recipients. Transplantation 2008;86(4):611–4.
127. Kamar N, Sandres-Saune K, Selves J, et al. Long-term ribavirin therapy in hepatitis C virus-positive renal transplant patients: effects on renal function and liver histology. Am J Kidney Dis 2003;42(1):184–92.
128. Kamar N, Toupance O, Buchler M, et al. Evidence that clearance of hepatitis C virus RNA after alpha-interferon therapy in dialysis patients is sustained after renal transplantation. J Am Soc Nephrol 2003;14(8):2092–8.
129. Kamath BM, Piccoli DA. Heritable disorders of the bile ducts. Gastroenterol Clin North Am 2003;32(3):857–75, vi.
130. Kaplan GG, Gregson DB, Laupland KB. Population-based study of the epidemiology of and the risk factors for pyogenic liver abscess. Clin Gastroenterol Hepatol 2004;2(11):1032–8.
131. Kaplowitz N. Drug-induced liver injury. Clin Infect Dis 2004;38(Suppl. 2):S44–8.
132. KDIGO clinical practice guideline for the care of kidney transplant recipients. Am J Transplant 2009;9(Suppl. 3):S1–155.
133. Kelly BD, Heneghan MA, Bennani F, et al. Nitrofurantoin-induced hepatotoxicity mediated by CD8+ T cells. Am J Gastroenterol 1998;93(5):819–21.
134. Kletzmayr J, Watschinger B, Müller C, et al. Twelve months of lamivudine treatment for chronic hepatitis B virus infection in renal transplant recipients. Transplantation 2000;70(9):1404–7.
135. Knudsen F, Wantzin P, Rasmussen K, et al. Hepatitis C in dialysis patients: relationship to blood transfusions, dialysis and liver disease. Kidney Int 1993;43(6):1353–6.
136. Kohli HS, Jain D, Sud K, et al. Azathioprine-induced hepatic veno-occlusive disease in a renal transplant recipient: histological regression following azathioprine withdrawal. Nephrol Dial Transplant 1996;11(8):1671–2.
137. Kotton CN, Fishman JA. Viral infection in the renal transplant recipient. J Am Soc Nephrol 2005;16(6):1758–74.
138. Kotton CN, Ryan ET, Fishman JA. Prevention of infection in adult travelers after solid organ transplantation. Am J Transplant 2005;5(1):8–14.
139. Kuiken C, Simmonds P. Nomenclature and numbering of the hepatitis C virus. Methods Mol Biol 2009;510:33–53.

140. Kusne S, Schwartz M, Breinig MK, et al. Herpes simplex virus hepatitis after solid organ transplantation in adults. J Infect Dis 1991;163(5):1001–7.
141. Lai ME, Mazzoleni AP, Argiolu F, et al. Hepatitis C virus in multiple episodes of acute hepatitis in polytransfused thalassaemic children. Lancet 1994;343(8894):388–90.
142. Lau JY, Davis GL, Brunson ME, et al. Hepatitis C virus infection in kidney transplant recipients. Hepatology 1993;18(5):1027–31.
143. Lautenschlager I, Razonable RR. Human herpesvirus-6 infections in kidney, liver, lung, and heart transplantation: review. Transpl Int 2012;25:493–502.
144. Lavanchy D. Hepatitis B virus epidemiology, disease burden, treatment, and current and emerging prevention and control measures. J Viral Hepat 2004;11(2):97–107.
145. Lee WC, Shu KH, Cheng CH, et al. Long-term impact of hepatitis B, C virus infection on renal transplantation. Am J Nephrol 2001;21(4):300–6.
146. Legendre C, Garrigue V, Le Bihan C, et al. Harmful long-term impact of hepatitis C virus infection in kidney transplant recipients. Transplantation 1998;65(5):667–70.
147. Legrand-Abravanel F, Sandres-Saune K, Barange K, et al. Hepatitis C virus genotype 5: epidemiological characteristics and sensitivity to combination therapy with interferon-alpha plus ribavirin. J Infect Dis 2004;189(8):1397–400.
148. Leon DA, McCambridge J. Liver cirrhosis mortality rates in Britain, 1950 to 2002. Lancet 2006;367(9511):645.
149. Lewis JH. 'Hy's law', the 'Rezulin Rule', and other predictors of severe drug-induced hepatotoxicity: putting risk-benefit into perspective. Pharmacoepidemiol Drug Saf 2006;15(4):221–9.
150. Liaw YF, Chien RN. Case report: dramatic response to lamivudine therapy following corticosteroid priming in chronic hepatitis B. J Gastroenterol Hepatol 1999;14(8):804–6.
151. Liu CH, Liang CC, Liu CJ, et al. Pegylated interferon alpha-2a plus low-dose ribavirin for the retreatment of dialysis chronic hepatitis C patients who relapsed from prior interferon monotherapy. Gut 2009;58(2):314–6.
152. Llovet JM, Burroughs A, Bruix J. Hepatocellular carcinoma. Lancet 2003;362(9399):1907–17.
153. Lorber MI, Van Buren CT, Flechner SM, et al. Hepatobiliary complications of cyclosporine therapy following renal transplantation. Transplant Proc 1987;19(1 Pt 2):1808–10.
154. Loupy A, Anglicheau D, Mamzer-Bruneel MF, et al. Mycophenolate sodium-induced hepatotoxicity: first report. Transplantation 2006;82(4):581.
155. Madayag RM, Johnson LB, Bartlett ST, et al. Use of renal allografts from donors positive for hepatitis B core antibody confers minimal risk for subsequent development of clinical hepatitis B virus disease. Transplantation 1997;64(12):1781–6.
156. Maddrey WC. Drug-induced hepatotoxicity: 2005. J Clin Gastroenterol 2005;39(4 Suppl. 2):S83–9.
157. Malatjalian DA, Ross JB, Williams CN, et al. Methotrexate hepatotoxicity in psoriatics: report of 104 patients from Nova Scotia, with analysis of risks from obesity, diabetes and alcohol consumption during long term follow-up. Can J Gastroenterol 1996;10(6):369–75.
158. Malekzadeh MH, Grushkin CM, Wright HT, et al. Hepatic dysfunction after renal transplantation in children. J Pediatr 1972;81(2):279–85.
159. Mandal AK, Kraus ES, Samaniego M, et al. Shorter waiting times for hepatitis C virus seropositive recipients of cadaveric renal allografts from hepatitis C virus seropositive donors. Clin Transplant 2000;14(4 Pt 2):391–6.
160. Mansuy JM, Abravanel F, Calot JP, et al. Acute hepatitis E in south-west France over a 5-year period. J Clin Virol 2009;44(1):74–7.
161. Manzanares C, Moreno M, Castellanos F, et al. Influence of hepatitis C virus infection on FK 506 blood levels in renal transplant patients. Transplant Proc 1998;30(4):1264–5.
162. Marcellin P, Heathcote EJ, Buti M, et al. Tenofovir disoproxil fumarate versus adefovir dipivoxil for chronic hepatitis B. N Engl J Med 2008;359(23):2442–55.
163. Marcos A, Eghtesad B, Fung JJ, et al. Use of alemtuzumab and tacrolimus monotherapy for cadaveric liver transplantation: with particular reference to hepatitis C virus. Transplantation 2004;78(7):966–71.
164. Margreiter R. Efficacy and safety of tacrolimus compared with ciclosporin microemulsion in renal transplantation: a randomised multicentre study. Lancet 2002;359(9308):741–6.
165. Marubbio AT, Danielson B. Hepatic veno-occlusive disease in a renal transplant patient receiving azathioprine. Gastroenterology 1975;69(3):739–43.
166. Mathurin P, Mouquet C, Poynard T, et al. Impact of hepatitis B and C virus on kidney transplantation outcome. Hepatology 1999;29(1):257–63.
167. Matos CA, Perez RM, Lemos LB, et al. Factors associated with the intensity of liver fibrosis in renal transplant patients with hepatitis B virus infection. Eur J Gastroenterol Hepatol 2007;19(8):653–7.
168. McDonald GB, Sharma P, Matthews DE, et al. Venocclusive disease of the liver after bone marrow transplantation: diagnosis, incidence, and predisposing factors. Hepatology 1984;4(1):116–22.
169. Meyers CM, Seeff LB, Stehman-Breen CO, et al. Hepatitis C and renal disease: an update. Am J Kidney Dis 2003;42(4):631–57.
170. Miller ER, Alter MJ, Tokars JI, et al. Protective effect of hepatitis B vaccine in chronic hemodialysis patients. Am J Kidney Dis 1999;33(2):356–60.
171. Morales JM, Campistol JM, Castellano G, et al. Transplantation of kidneys from donors with hepatitis C antibody into recipients with pre-transplantation anti-HCV. Kidney Int 1995;47(1):236–40.
172. Morales JM, Dominguez-Gil B, Sanz-Guajardo D, et al. The influence of hepatitis B and hepatitis C virus infection in the recipient on late renal allograft failure. Nephrol Dial Transplant 2004;19(Suppl. 3):iii72–6.
173. Moreno F, Morales JM, Colina F, et al. Influence of long-term cyclosporine therapy on chronic liver disease after renal transplantation. Transplant Proc 1990;22(5):2314–6.
174. Morris DJ, Littler E, Arrand JR, et al. Human herpesvirus 6 infection in renal-transplant recipients. N Engl J Med 1989;320(23):1560–1.
175. Mousa DH, Abdalla AH, Al-Shoail G, et al. Alpha-interferon with ribavirin in the treatment of hemodialysis patients with hepatitis C. Transplant Proc 2004;36(6):1831–4.
176. Mukherjee S, Gilroy RK, McCashland TM, et al. Pegylated interferon for recurrent hepatitis C in liver transplant recipients with renal failure: a prospective cohort study. Transplant Proc 2003;35(4):1478–9.
177. Munoz de Bustillo E, Ibarrola C, Andrés A, et al. Hepatitis-B-virus-related fibrosing cholestatic hepatitis after renal transplantation with acute graft failure following interferon-alpha therapy. Nephrol Dial Transplant 1998;13(6):1574–6.
178. Nainan OV, Alter MJ, Kruszon-Moran D, et al. Hepatitis C virus genotypes and viral concentrations in participants of a general population survey in the United States. Gastroenterology 2006;131(2):478–84.
179. Navarro VJ, Senior JR. Drug-related hepatotoxicity. N Engl J Med 2006;354(7):731–9.
180. Neff GW, Ruiz P, Madariaga JR, et al. Sirolimus-associated hepatotoxicity in liver transplantation. Ann Pharmacother 2004;38(10):1593–6.
181. Niemczyk M, Wyzgal J, Perkowska A, et al. Sirolimus-associated hepatotoxicity in the kidney graft recipient. Transpl Int 2005;18(11):1302–3.
182. O'Grady JG, Burroughs A, Hardy P, et al. Tacrolimus versus microemulsified ciclosporin in liver transplantation: the TMC randomised controlled trial. Lancet 2002;360(9340):1119–25.
183. Oldakowska-Jedynak M, Durlik M, Paczek L, et al. Hepatocellular carcinoma development in renal allograft recipients. Transplant Proc 2000;32(6):1363–4.
184. Olsen TS, Fjeldborg O, Hansen HE. Portal hypertension without liver cirrhosis in renal transplant recipients. APMIS Suppl 1991;23:13–20.
185. Orloff SL, Stempel CA, Wright TL, et al. Long-term outcome in kidney transplant patients with hepatitis C (HCV) infection. Clin Transplant 1995;9(2):119–24.
186. Panaro F, Piardi T, Gheza F, et al. Causes of sirolimus discontinuation in 97 liver transplant recipients. Transplant Proc 43(4):1128–31.

187. Periera BJ, Wright TL, Schmid CH, et al. The impact of pretransplantation hepatitis C infection on the outcome of renal transplantation. Transplantation 1995;60(8):799–805.
188. Peters MG, Andersen J, Lynch P, et al. Randomized controlled study of tenofovir and adefovir in chronic hepatitis B virus and HIV infection: ACTG A5127. Hepatology 2006;44(5):1110–6.
189. Pilmore H, Collins J, Dittmer I, et al. Fatal human herpesvirus-6 infection after renal transplantation. Transplantation 2009;88(6):762–5.
190. Pirsch JD, Miller J, Deierhoi MH, et al. A comparison of tacrolimus (FK506) and cyclosporine for immunosuppression after cadaveric renal transplantation. FK506 Kidney Transplant Study Group. Transplantation 1997;63(7):977–83.
191. Plessier A, Rautou PE, Valla DC, et al. Management of hepatic vascular diseases. J Hepatol 56 (Suppl):S25-S38.
192. Polson J, Lee WM. AASLD position paper: the management of acute liver failure. Hepatology 2005;41(5):1179–97.
193. Puchhammer-Stockl E, Mandl CW, Kletzmayr J, et al. Monitoring the virus load can predict the emergence of drug-resistant hepatitis B virus strains in renal transplantation patients during lamivudine therapy. J Infect Dis 2000;41:2063.
194. Rahimian J, Wilson T, Oram V, et al. Pyogenic liver abscess: recent trends in etiology and mortality. Clin Infect Dis 2004;39(11):1654–9.
195. Rangel MC, Coronado VG, Euler GL, et al. Vaccine recommendations for patients on chronic dialysis. The Advisory Committee on Immunization Practices and the American Academy of Pediatrics. Semin Dial 2000;13(2):101–7.
196. Razonable RR, Zerr DM. HHV-6, HHV-7 and HHV-8 in solid organ transplant recipients. Am J Transplant 2009;9(Suppl. 4):S100–3.
197. Reed B, McFann K, Kimberling WJ, et al. Presence of de novo mutations in autosomal dominant polycystic kidney disease patients without family history. Am J Kidney Dis 2008;52(6):1042–50.
198. Ridruejo E, Mando OG, Davalos M, et al. Hepatocellular carcinoma in renal transplant patients. Transplant Proc 2005;37(5):2086–8.
199. Rostaing L, Chatelut E, Payen JL, et al. Pharmacokinetics of alphaIFN-2b in chronic hepatitis C virus patients undergoing chronic hemodialysis or with normal renal function: clinical implications. J Am Soc Nephrol 1998;9(12):2344–8.
200. Rostaing L, Henry S, Cisterne JM, et al. Efficacy and safety of lamivudine on replication of recurrent hepatitis B after cadaveric renal transplantation. Transplantation 1997;64(11):1624–7.
201. Rostaing L, Izopet J, Baron E, et al. Treatment of chronic hepatitis C with recombinant interferon alpha in kidney transplant recipients. Transplantation 1995;59(10):1426–31.
202. Roth D, Zucker K, Cirocco R, et al. Transmission of hepatitis C virus by kidney transplantation: impact of perfusion techniques and course of viremia post transplant. Pediatr Nephrol 1995;9 (Suppl.):S29–34.
203. Russo MW, Ghalib R, Sigal S, et al. Randomized trial of pegylated interferon alpha-2b monotherapy in haemodialysis patients with chronic hepatitis C. Nephrol Dial Transplant 2006;21(2):437–43.
204. Russo MW, Goldsweig CD, Jacobson IM, et al. Interferon monotherapy for dialysis patients with chronic hepatitis C: an analysis of the literature on efficacy and safety. Am J Gastroenterol 2003;98(7):1610–5.
205. Sagedal S, Hartmann A, Nordal KP, et al. Impact of early cytomegalovirus infection and disease on long-term recipient and kidney graft survival. Kidney Int 2004;66(1):329–37.
206. Sagedal S, Nordal KP, Hartmann A, et al. A prospective study of the natural course of cytomegalovirus infection and disease in renal allograft recipients. Transplantation 2000;70(8):1166–74.
207. Sayiner A, Ece T, Duman S, et al. Tuberculosis in renal transplant recipients. Transplantation 1999;68(9):1268–71.
208. Seale L, Jones CJ, Kathpalia S, et al. Prevention of herpesvirus infections in renal allograft recipients by low-dose oral acyclovir. JAMA 1985;254(24):3435–8.
209. Seeger C, Mason WS. Hepatitis B virus biology. Microbiol Mol Biol Rev 2000;64(1):51–68.
210. Selzner N, Renner EL, Selzner M, et al. Antiviral treatment of recurrent hepatitis C after liver transplantation: predictors of response and long-term outcome. Transplantation 2009;88(10):1214–21.
211. Serna-Higuera C, Gonzalez-Garcia M, Milicua JM, et al. Acute cholestatic hepatitis by cytomegalovirus in an immunocompetent patient resolved with ganciclovir. J Clin Gastroenterol 1999;29(3):276–7.
212. Serste T, Bourgeois N, Vanden Eynden F, et al. Endoscopic drainage of pyogenic liver abscesses with suspected biliary origin. Am J Gastroenterol 2007;102(6):1209–15.
213. Sezer S, Ozdemir FN, Guz G, et al. Factors influencing response to hepatitis B virus vaccination in hemodialysis patients. Transplant Proc 2000;32(3):607–8.
214. Shaye OA, Yadegari M, Abreu MT, et al. Hepatotoxicity of 6-mercaptopurine (6-MP) and azathioprine (AZA) in adult IBD patients. Am J Gastroenterol 2007;102(11):2488–94.
215. Sherstha R, McKinley C, Russ P, et al. Postmenopausal estrogen therapy selectively stimulates hepatic enlargement in women with autosomal dominant polycystic kidney disease. Hepatology 1997;26(5):1282–6.
216. Shulman HM, Gooley T, Dudley MD, et al. Utility of transvenous liver biopsies and wedged hepatic venous pressure measurements in sixty marrow transplant recipients. Transplantation 1995;59(7):1015–22.
217. Sivapalasingam S, Malak SF, Sullivan JF, et al. High prevalence of hepatitis C infection among patients receiving hemodialysis at an urban dialysis center. Infect Control Hosp Epidemiol 2002;23(6):319–24.
218. Stanley Jr SL. Amoebiasis. Lancet 2003;361(9362):1025–34.
219. Stempel CA, Lake J, Kuo G, et al. Hepatitis C – its prevalence in end-stage renal failure patients and clinical course after kidney transplantation. Transplantation 1993;55(2):273–6.
220. Subramanyam SG, Kilpadi AB, Correa M, et al. Hepatic TB: four cases and a review of the literature. Trop Doct 2006;36(2):121–2.
221. Sypsa V, Touloumi G, Tassopoulos NC, et al. Reconstructing and predicting the hepatitis C virus epidemic in Greece: increasing trends of cirrhosis and hepatocellular carcinoma despite the decline in incidence of HCV infection. J Viral Hepat 2004;11(4):366–74.
222. Tan AC, Brouwer JT, Glue P, et al. Safety of interferon and ribavirin therapy in haemodialysis patients with chronic hepatitis C: results of a pilot study. Nephrol Dial Transplant 2001;16(1):193–5.
223. Ten Napel HH, Houthoff HJ, The TH. Cytomegalovirus hepatitis in normal and immune compromised hosts. Liver 1984;4(3):184–94.
224. Tenney DJ, Rose RE, Baldick CJ, et al. Long-term monitoring shows hepatitis B virus resistance to entecavir in nucleoside-naive patients is rare through 5 years of therapy. Hepatology 2009;49(5):1503–14.
225. Thabut D, Thibault V, Bernard-Chabert B, et al. Long-term therapy with lamivudine in renal transplant recipients with chronic hepatitis B. Eur J Gastroenterol Hepatol 2004;16(12):1367–73.
226. Therret E, Pol S, Legendre C, et al. Low-dose recombinant leukocyte interferon-alpha treatment of hepatitis C viral infection in renal transplant recipients. A pilot study. Transplantation 1994;58(5):625–8.
227. Thimme R, Oldach D, Chang KM, et al. Determinants of viral clearance and persistence during acute hepatitis C virus infection. J Exp Med 2001;194(10):1395–406.
228. Tokumoto T, Tanabe K, Tokumoto T, et al. Effect of interferon (IFN-alpha) for prevention of hepatitis C transmission from a seropositive donor to a seronegative recipient in renal transplantation. Transplant Proc 1996;28(3):1503–4.
229. van Duijnhoven EM, Christiaans MH, van Duijnhoven EM, et al. Glucose metabolism in the first 3 years after renal transplantation in patients receiving tacrolimus versus cyclosporine-based immunosuppression. J Am Soc Nephrol 2002;13(1):213–20.
230. Walker DP, Longson M, Mallick NP, et al. A prospective study of cytomegalovirus and herpes simplex virus disease in renal transplant recipients. J Clin Pathol 1982;35(11):1190–3.
231. Walker RC, Marshall WF, Strickler J, et al. Pretransplantation assessment of the risk of lymphoproliferative disorder. Clin Infect Dis 1995;20(5):1346–53.

232. Wang C, Sun J, Zhu B, et al. Hepatitis B virus infection and related factors in hemodialysis patients in China – systematic review and meta-analysis. Ren Fail 32(10):1255–64.
233. Ward CJ, Hogan MC, Rossetti S, et al. The gene mutated in autosomal recessive polycystic kidney disease encodes a large, receptor-like protein. Nat Genet 2002;30(3):259–69.
234. Wasley A, Alter MJ. Epidemiology of hepatitis C: geographic differences and temporal trends. Semin Liver Dis 2000;20(1):1–16.
235. Watkins PB, Seeff LB. Drug-induced liver injury: summary of a single topic clinical research conference. Hepatology 2006;43(3):618–31.
236. Whitley RJ, Kimberlin DW, Roizman B. Herpes simplex viruses. Clin Infect Dis 1998;26(3):541–53, quiz 554–5.
237. Yao QY, Rickinson AB, Epstein MA, et al. Oropharyngeal shedding of infectious Epstein-Barr virus in healthy virus-immune donors. A prospective study. Chin Med J (Engl) 1985;98(3):191–6.
238. Yap DY, Tang CS, Yung S, et al. Long-term outcome of renal transplant recipients with chronic hepatitis B infection-impact of antiviral treatments. Transplantation 90(3):325–30.
239. Yildiz A, Sever MS, Turkmen A, et al. Tuberculosis after renal transplantation: experience of one Turkish Centre. Nephrol Dial Transplant 1998;13(7):1872–5.
240. Yim HJ, Lok AS. Natural history of chronic hepatitis B virus infection: what we knew in 1981 and what we know in 2005. Hepatology 2006;43(2 Suppl. 1):S173–81.
241. Yonem O, Bayraktar Y. Clinical characteristics of Caroli's syndrome. World J Gastroenterol 2007;13(13):1934–7.
242. Younossi ZM, Braun WE, Protiva DA, et al. Chronic viral hepatitis in renal transplant recipients with allografts functioning for more than 20 years. Transplantation 1999;67(2): 272–5.
243. Zein NN. Clinical significance of hepatitis C virus genotypes. Clin Microbiol Rev 2000;13(2):223–35.

CHAPTER 33

NEUROLOGICAL COMPLICATIONS AFTER KIDNEY TRANSPLANTATION

Andria L. Ford • Katie D. Vo • Jin-Moo Lee

CHAPTER OUTLINE

Neurological disease commonly arises as a complication of kidney transplantation. Benign to life-threatening neurological disease may be encountered hours to years after transplantation. Neurological consultation may be obtained for a variety of reasons, including altered mental status, new-onset seizures, sudden hemiplegia, or slowly progressive numbness and tingling. Diagnosis and treatment are best undertaken in conjunction with a neurologist acquainted with transplantation. Diagnostic confusion can be caused by the residue of prior neurological disease, the coexistence of multiple diagnoses, and the suppression of normal inflammatory responses by immunosuppressive therapies.

Over the years, as surgical techniques have been refined, and immunosuppressants have been improved, transplant complications have declined. An early, large retrospective study found the neurological complication rate to be 30% over an 18-year period.[2] Two more recent studies found lower rates of 8% and 10% over a 26-year period and a 19-year period, respectively.[52,95] Neurological complications may be underdiagnosed, however. In a prospective brain magnetic resonance imaging (MRI) study, 30% of 187 renal transplant patients had abnormal neuroradiological findings.[4]

Neurological disease can result from the disease process underlying renal failure. Therefore, symptoms should not be ascribed to the transplant when they may have been extant before the procedure. This chapter discusses the most commonly encountered pre-existing neurological syndromes. When one suspects de novo neurological disease in a renal transplant patient, it is helpful to localize the area of neurological dysfunction broadly into central nervous system (CNS) or peripheral nervous system (PNS) dysfunction and to assess the timing of complication onset (acute, subacute, or chronic), to aid in differential diagnosis.

NEUROLOGICAL DISEASE PRECEDING RENAL TRANSPLANTATION

Diseases that underlie kidney failure often cause coincidental injury to the nervous system, which may not be discovered until long after transplantation. Patients with longstanding uremia frequently have signs of chronic PNS toxicity. Additionally, dialysis has been associated with at least two forms of CNS neurological disturbance – dialysis dysequilibrium syndrome and dialysis dementia.[18]

Systemic Disease

Disease processes that cause renal insufficiency commonly cause progressive injury to the nervous system. These underlying disease processes include diabetes mellitus, hypertension, autoimmune diseases such as systemic lupus erythematosus, and human immunodeficiency virus (HIV). Diabetes and hypertension predispose patients to small-vessel disease. Ischemic strokes may manifest with acute neurological deficits or may occur subclinically, with gradual accumulation of cognitive deficits. Diabetes is known for its effects on the peripheral nerves as well, primarily causing a painful sensory neuropathy. Systemic lupus erythematosus is associated with cognitive dysfunction, headache, seizures, chorea, cerebrovascular events, myelopathy, polyneuropathy, and mononeuropathy.[79] Other autoimmune disorders may disturb the nervous system similarly.[18] HIV is capable of numerous neurological syndromes; the most common are dementia, vacuolar myelopathy, and sensory neuropathies.[69]

Uremia

Acute and chronic uremia produce characteristic neurological syndromes. Acutely, an increase in blood urea nitrogen (BUN) produces an encephalopathy characterized by fluctuating level of consciousness, seizures, and prominent asterixis accompanied by diffuse weakness.[29] Chronic uremia may cause milder symptoms and signs, such as anorexia, insomnia, restlessness, and mild asterixis.[84] Uremic encephalopathy correlates less with levels of BUN and more with rate of increase, with rapid BUN accumulation causing a more severe alteration in consciousness.[93] The mechanism underlying the encephalopathy is not well established but may be secondary to abnormalities in brain energy usage, accumulation of toxic organic acids in the CNS, or direct toxic effects of parathyroid hormone in the CNS.[18,66]

Chronic uremia as seen in end-stage renal disease is a well-known cause of a length-dependent, axonal, symmetrical, sensorimotor polyneuropathy that is partially reversible with correction of renal function.[15] Autonomic neuropathy leads to postural hypotension, sudomotor abnormalities, impotence, and gastrointestinal disturbances. The autonomic impairment may be partially responsible for significant blood pressure lability seen frequently during dialysis.[57]

Dialysis Dysequilibrium Syndrome and Dialysis Dementia

Dialysis dysequilibrium syndrome was first recognized in the 1960s when patients were rapidly dialyzed over short periods. Today, dialysis is performed slowly and intermittently, and the syndrome is seen in a milder form when a patient initiates dialysis. Dialysis dysequilibrium syndrome is characterized by headache, irritability, restless legs, agitation, somnolence, confusion, seizures, muscle cramps, and nausea. These symptoms may stabilize or improve with long-term dialysis. The syndrome is thought to be caused by increased intracranial pressure and cerebral edema from the osmotic gradient that develops between the plasma and brain during rapid dialysis.[18]

Independently of vascular risk factors, patients with chronic kidney disease have an increased risk of developing dementia compared to the general population.[97] Dialysis dementia is a progressive encephalopathy thought to be related to aluminum intoxication; this is less commonly seen because aluminum-rich dialysate is not widely used and because dietary aluminum intake is restricted.[29,64] A more recent study, however, could not confirm an association of aluminum concentration or use of aluminum-containing phosphate binders and carrying a diagnosis of dementia, but did find age, black race, low educational attainment, cerebrovascular disease, diabetes, malnutrition, and anemia to be independent predictors of dementia.[59]

APPROACH TO THE RENAL TRANSPLANT PATIENT WITH NEUROLOGICAL DISEASE

Although a few neurological illnesses may occur at any time after transplantation, most problems are likely to occur as immediate, subacute, or chronic complications of transplantation. Within each time period, neurological syndromes may be divided into central and peripheral etiologies. CNS dysfunction localizes to any abnormality of the brain or spinal cord. PNS dysfunction localizes to the nerve roots, peripheral nerves, or muscle.

Central Nervous System Dysfunction

Encephalopathy

CNS illness often manifests as altered mental status, also known as encephalopathy. The hallmark of encephalopathy is reduced attention span with a decreased or fluctuating level of consciousness. Patients typically are disoriented to varying degrees, with poor awareness of their environment and circumstances surrounding their illness. The etiologies are numerous, ranging from infection to metabolic derangement to multiple embolic strokes. CNS dysfunction may occur in the absence of encephalopathy; this is seen with focal seizures or neurological deficits from a stroke or mass lesion.

Seizures

A seizure is a symptom of CNS dysfunction, and an underlying etiology should be sought. Seizures are common after transplantation, estimated to occur in 6–36% of posttransplant patients.[35,38,70] In a review of 119 renal transplants in children, 17% of the children had seizures over a period of 10 years. Most occurred less than 55 days after transplant.[7] The etiologies included hypertensive encephalopathy, fever with infection, and acute allograft rejection. Of the patients with posttransplant seizures, 25% had a history of seizures before transplantation.

Seizures are classified as being either partial in origin – electrical focus in one region of the brain – or generalized – electrical abnormality coming from the entire brain. An electroencephalogram may help define the patient's seizure type. Routine electrolytes, magnesium, and drug levels of cyclosporine and tacrolimus should be obtained. If brain imaging by MRI is unrevealing for a mass lesion, spinal fluid should be examined for signs of increased intracranial pressure, infection, inflammation, abnormal cytology, and, with complaints of severe headache, subarachnoid hemorrhage.

Treatment of seizures is best directed toward correction of the underlying abnormality. While awaiting these treatments to take effect, benzodiazepines can be used on a short-term basis; however, these can cause sedation, which may compromise the neurological examination of an already encephalopathic patient. Multiple antiepileptic medications can be tried if a patient is at risk of developing more seizures. The cytochrome P-450-inducing anticonvulsants (phenytoin, carbamazepine, and phenobarbital) may affect immunosuppressive agents metabolized by the liver. The clearance of cyclosporine and corticosteroids is increased in the presence of these anticonvulsants.[61] Levetiracetam may be preferable because of its minimal effects on the liver. Isolated seizures in the setting of organ transplantation rarely lead to epilepsy, and long-term anticonvulsant therapy is seldom needed.[7,62]

Peripheral Nervous System Dysfunction

PNS illness encompasses any neurological abnormality affecting: (1) the nerve roots exiting the spinal cord, known as radiculopathy; (2) the peripheral nerves, known as neuropathy; and (3) the muscle, termed myopathy. Disease affecting the nerve roots may cause weakness, numbness, and pain, as in the case of Guillain–Barré syndrome. The peripheral nerves typically are affected in a length-dependent fashion causing slowly progressive numbness and tingling. A focal nerve may be compressed during surgery, however, causing an asymmetric weakness and numbness in the distribution of that nerve. Myopathy may manifest with cramps, myalgias, and weakness of proximal muscles and is typically symmetrical. Difficulty with standing from a seated position and walking up stairs are common complaints.

IMMEDIATE NEUROLOGICAL COMPLICATIONS

Neurological complications that occur within days of renal transplantation have characteristic etiologies, which help with the differential diagnostic possibilities. We have categorized these complications into disorders involving the CNS and disorders involving the PNS (as described earlier).

Central Nervous System Dysfunction

Hypoxic-Ischemic Insult and Perioperative Sedation

In the immediate postoperative period, transplant patients may exhibit behavioral changes ranging from a mild confusional state to severe encephalopathy. Acute confusional states often are related to a global hypoxic-ischemic insult. Neuroimaging with computed tomography (CT) or MRI may aid with this diagnosis. In the absence of evidence of ischemia, other causes (see later) should be explored. In patients with renal or hepatic failure, poor metabolism and excretion of anesthetics and other sedating medications should be considered. Altered mental status occurring 2–5 days after surgery may be the result of intensive care unit (ICU) psychosis, which may resolve with neuroleptics or environmental reorientation.[62]

Electrolyte Imbalance

Electrolyte abnormalities are common after transplantation. If sodium decreases to less than approximately 120 mEq/L, generalized tonic-clonic seizures and worsening mental status from cerebral edema may occur.[6] Hypomagnesemia may also cause seizures. Although anticonvulsants may help, treatment is best achieved by correcting the electrolyte imbalance. The sodium should be corrected slowly (≤10 mEq/L over 24 hours) because rapid correction can lead to central pontine myelinolysis, also known as osmotic demyelination syndrome, as discussed subsequently.

Rejection Encephalopathy

The term rejection encephalopathy has been used to describe an episode of acute graft rejection that is accompanied by altered mental status.[7] The entity was initially proposed based on a case series of 13 patients who exhibited a reversible acute neurological syndrome that coincided with severe acute rejection of the transplanted kidney.[40] The majority of these patients were <20 years old and developed various combinations of seizures, headache, confusion, disorientation, and irritability, and one had papilledema. Acute rejection was defined by the presence of graft swelling and tenderness, fever, weight gain, and hypertension. Patients with encephalopathy had a greater increase in serum creatinine compared to patients without encephalopathy. No differences were noted between the groups when comparing blood pressure or rate of increase of blood pressure. There were no differences in serum electrolytes, weight gain or fluid retention, or type of immunosuppressant in the two groups. The patients in this cohort had an excellent prognosis with no residual sequelae.[39,40] It is unclear whether rejection encephalopathy should be regarded as a direct consequence of graft rejection or a reflection of the accumulation of metabolic and physiological insults occurring during severe graft rejection and its treatment.

Hypertensive Encephalopathy

Hypertensive encephalopathy has been reported after transplantation. The diagnosis should be considered when other causes of altered mental status have been excluded. Sometimes the entity, also called malignant hypertension, is accompanied by papilledema and seizures.[7] It is thought to be the cause of death in some patients, especially in children after renal transplantation.[95,112] Hypertensive encephalopathy is associated with posterior leukoencephalopathy and has characteristic findings on MRI (discussed below under Subacute Neurological Complications: Cyclosporine). The MRI abnormalities are often reversible after blood pressure is controlled.

Infection

Despite immunosuppressant doses being high during this period, CNS infection within 1 month of transplantation is uncommon. When infections are present, it suggests that the infection may have been present before transplantation, was acquired from the donated organ, or was related to the surgery itself, such as the presence of an indwelling catheter.[85] These infections are usually due to common pathogens found in the general, non-immunosuppressed population.[25,45]

Central Pontine Myelinolysis

Central pontine myelinolysis, also known as osmotic demyelination syndrome, is rare in renal transplant recipients, occurring more frequently after liver transplantation (Figure 33-1).[56,80] It usually occurs within 10 days of transplantation and is seen after rapid correction of chronic hyponatremia.[74,101] Patients develop symmetrical limb weakness with extensor plantar responses over hours to days. Facial and bulbar musculature may be paralyzed. In severe cases, a locked-in state develops, in which the patient remains fully conscious but no voluntary movements are possible apart from vertical eye movements, a state that may be misinterpreted as coma. Death and chronic disability are common, and full recovery is rare. To prevent this disorder, it is recommended that serum sodium correction should not exceed 10 mEq/L in 24 hours.[80,123,124]

Peripheral Nervous System Dysfunction

Peripheral nerve injuries during renal transplantation are uncommon, with estimates between 2% and 5%.[2,18,98] The most common sites involved are the femoral nerve, lateral femoral cutaneous nerve, the lumbosacral plexus, and the ulnar nerve. Nerve damage is thought to occur by several mechanisms, including ischemia, compression from malpositioning a pharmacologically paralyzed patient, compression by local hematoma formation, or stretching of the nerve owing to prolonged retraction.

Femoral Neuropathy

Acute femoral neuropathy may complicate renal transplantation in 0.1–3% of patients.[113] In one Chinese

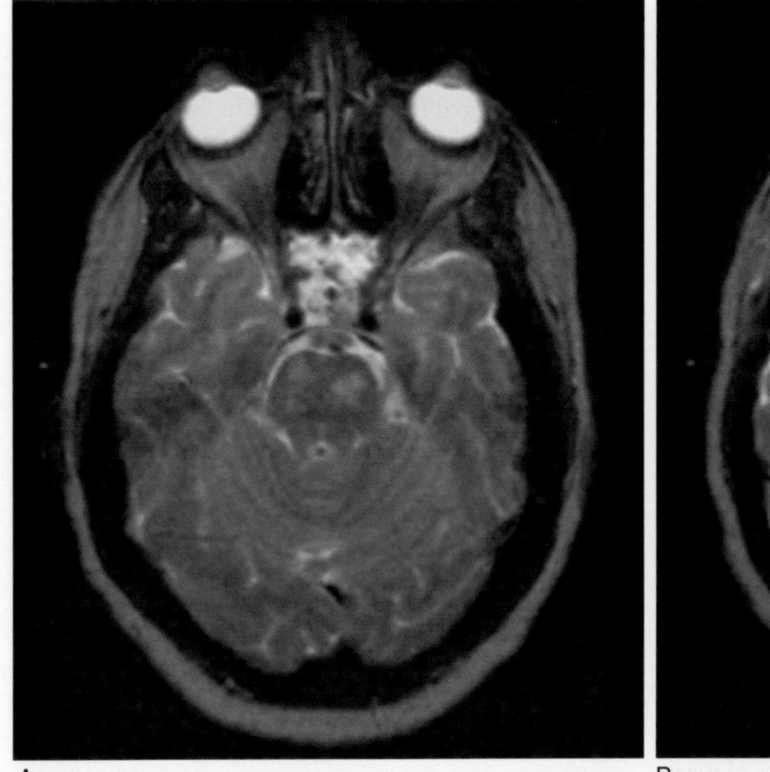

A

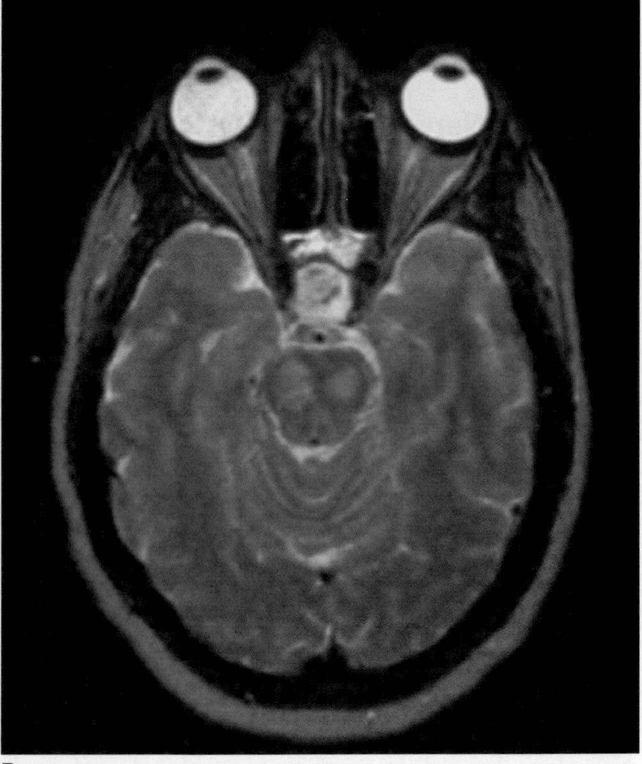

B

FIGURE 33-1 ■ Central pontine myelinolysis. A 52-year-old woman with end-stage renal disease on hemodialysis presents with 2 days of progressive lethargy and tetraparesis. (A, B) Axial T2-weighted magnetic resonance images of the brain show bilateral pontine signal hyperintensity consistent with the diagnosis of central pontine myelinolysis. The patient had gradual and complete improvement of her weakness.

retrospective study the incidence varied significantly based on the mode and duration of the iliac artery anastomosis.[63] Femoral neuropathy is typically noticed within 24–48 hours after surgery but may not be apparent until the patient attempts to walk. Nerve damage may occur from stretching of the nerve secondary to self-retaining retractors.[114] Another mechanism is ischemia to the femoral nerve during anastomosis of the graft renal artery to the internal iliac artery by a "steal phenomenon."[51] On neurological examination, patients exhibit unilateral weakness of knee extension; loss of the patellar reflex; and decreased sensation on the anterior-medial aspect of the thigh, knee, and calf. Neuropathic changes on nerve conduction studies and electromyography typically are seen 1 week after injury. Compressive femoral neuropathies usually resolve entirely, but this takes several months and can be incomplete.[71,91,92,102,114,125] The lateral femoral cutaneous nerve is often exposed and retracted during transplantation and was injured in 2.4% of patients in one series.[102] Injury to this nerve causes numbness over the lateral aspect of the thigh.

Lumbosacral Plexopathy

Lumbosacral plexopathy occurs when the internal iliac artery is used for revascularization of the graft, particularly in diabetic patients.[43] Postoperatively, the patient complains of buttock pain and demonstrates weakness of ankle dorsiflexion, ankle eversion, and sometimes proximal leg weakness. Recovery occurs, but may be incomplete.

Ulnar Neuropathy

Ulnar neuropathy may occur from mechanical trauma at the elbow, from the weight of the patient and physician on the adducted arm, and from the blood pressure cuff compressing the cubital fossa. Arms with and without an arteriovenous fistula seem to be affected equally.[126] Patients with diabetes seem to be more susceptible.[96] Patients may have sensory complaints in the medial aspect of the hand, including the ring and little fingers.

SUBACUTE NEUROLOGICAL COMPLICATIONS

Within weeks of renal transplantation, many of the neurological complications are related to immunosuppression directed at the transplanted kidney. Central dysfunction from calcineurin inhibitors often manifests as altered mental status that may be accompanied by seizures. The severe manifestations of calcineurin inhibitor toxicity usually develop within the first 3 months of therapy and have been reduced with the use of a microemulsion preparation that allows for steadier absorption.[120]

PNS dysfunction from immunosuppressants manifests as symmetrical paresthesias or as myopathy. Another category of a PNS dysfunction that occurs weeks after transplantation is Guillain–Barré syndrome, which can be life-threatening if not diagnosed quickly and appropriately managed.

Central Nervous System Dysfunction

Tacrolimus

Tacrolimus is frequently the first-line immunosuppressant agent utilized after renal transplant. Studies of liver transplant recipients have shown neurotoxic side effects, however, in 20–30% of patients.[75,122] Tacrolimus and cyclosporine were compared in a prospective unblinded randomized trial of 400 patients after renal transplantation. The tacrolimus group reported higher rates of all neurological side effects; tremor was significantly greater than in the cyclosporine group at 54% versus 34%, as were paresthesias at 23% versus 15%.[89] Side effects usually occur within the first months of therapy and are more common at higher doses. Generalized seizures, tremor, ataxia, encephalopathy, nightmares, and agitation have occurred, most resolving with dose reduction.

Confusion, coma, cortical blindness, cerebellar syndromes, hemiplegias, and flaccid quadriparesis all have been described in tacrolimus and cyclosporine recipients. The multifocal disorder including various combinations of these features has been termed reversible posterior leukoencephalopathy (RPLE) and is also known as posterior reversible encephalopathy syndrome; this is a clinical-radiological syndrome with other etiologies such as malignant hypertension and pre-eclampsia.[103,109] A prospective brain MRI study was performed in 187 kidney transplant recipients and 29 liver transplant recipients. In the patients who received a kidney transplant, 1.6% had findings consistent with RPLE (two with cyclosporine toxicity and one with tacrolimus toxicity), whereas 20.1% of liver transplant recipients met criteria for the diagnosis.[4] Classically, the posterior white matter is involved; however, it is now known to affect the frontal lobes and gray matter as well (Figure 33-2).

The neurological syndrome and brain imaging abnormalities usually resolve within 2 weeks of stopping the offending agent or after dosage reduction if blood levels were particularly high. Although the syndrome is usually reversible, a small percentage of patients progress to death or have incomplete recovery.[107] Cortical blindness is a rare complication and is usually completely reversible with reduction or withdrawal of the medication.[34] The mechanism of RPLE is thought to be related to disruption of the blood–brain barrier, possibly mediated by astroglial cellular effects on endothelial permeability.[32]

Cyclosporine

Cyclosporine-related neurological side effects are more common in liver transplant recipients, possibly as a result of associated hypocholesterolemia and hyponatremia.[2,28] In renal transplant patients, cyclosporine was estimated to be responsible for approximately 20% of neurological complications; however, given cyclosporine is often no longer the first-line agent, these percentages are being shared with tacrolimus.[12,54,83] These side effects range from tremor and paresthesias to a serious leukoencephalopathy. Limb tremor is the most common side effect of cyclosporine. It is a fine tremor in the upper extremities that is most prominent while holding hands in posture, typically seen within the first 3 months.[54,120] Many

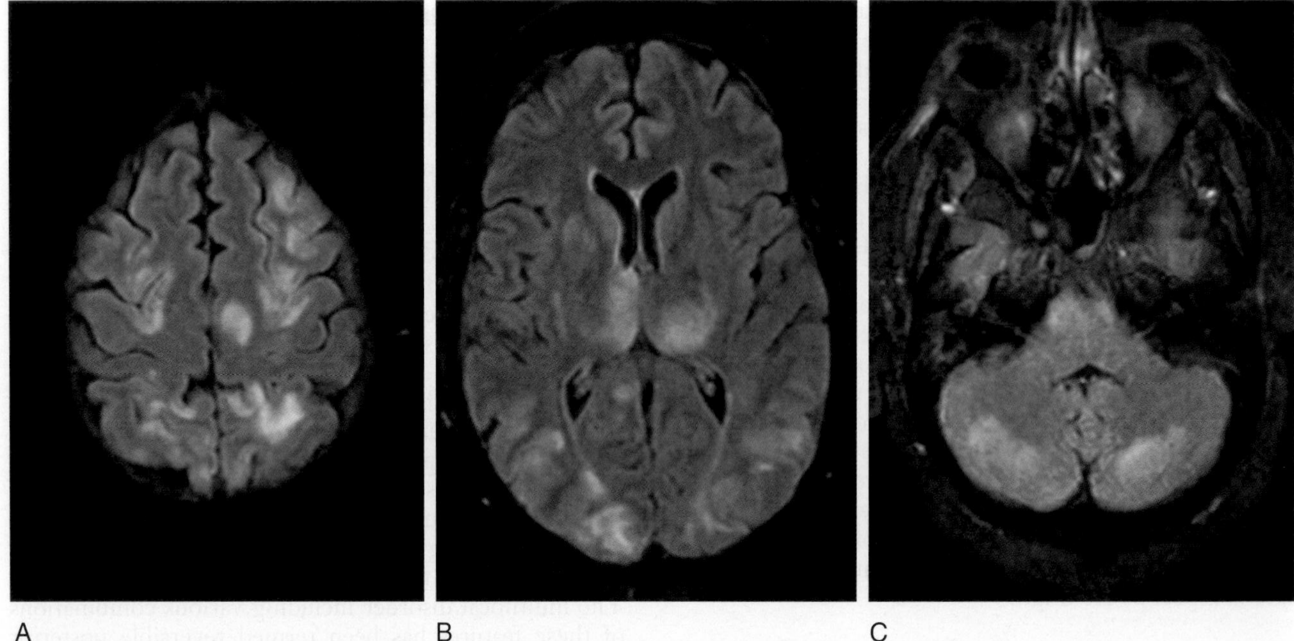

FIGURE 33-2 ■ Reversible posterior leukoencephalopathy secondary to cyclosporine toxicity. A 45-year-old woman with a history of non-Hodgkin's lymphoma had undergone a matched unrelated donor bone marrow transplant 1 month previously. Over 24 hours, she developed altered mental status and generalized tonic-clonic seizures. Cyclosporine was found to be at a toxic blood level of 806 ng/mL. (A–C) Axial fluid-attenuated inversion recovery magnetic resonance images of the brain show abnormal hyperintense signal in the cortex and subcortical white matter of the occipital and parietal lobes and cerebellum bilaterally. There is extension into the frontal lobes (A), deep gray matter of the basal ganglia and thalami (B), and pons (C). Cyclosporine was discontinued, and the patient was given tacrolimus. She had no further seizures, and her mental status returned to normal.

instances of tremor and paresthesias are not sufficiently troublesome to warrant reducing effective immunosuppressive therapy. A lower-extremity pain syndrome has been associated with cyclosporine and renal transplant patients, termed calcineurin inhibitor pain syndrome. Nine patients on cyclosporine developed severe pain in their feet in one study. MRI showed bone marrow edema in the painful bones.[41]

A leukoencephalopathy similar to that caused by tacrolimus can be seen on MRI.[49,50,106] This syndrome usually manifests with occipital headache, nausea, and vomiting, followed by seizures and visual disturbances. Cyclosporine blood levels may be high, although not invariably, and the disorder resolves with dosage reduction.

FKB12 Ligands: Sirolimus and Everolimus

When encountering neurotoxicity due to cyclosporine or tacrolimus, newer, less neurotoxic agents known as the FKBP12 ligands – sirolimus and everolimus – may be tried; however, these have also been associated with RPLE in a few case reports.[14,67,111]

Monoclonal Antibodies

Since OKT3 is no longer available for clinical use, other monoclonal antibodies have been studied and have not demonstrated neurotoxicity thus far in renal transplant patients, although alemtuzumab has been associated with sensorimotor polyneuropathy and myelitis and rituxumab has been associated with progressive multifocal leukoencephalopathy (PML) in other non-solid and solid-organ transplants, respectively.[21,23,116]

Steroids

High-dose steroid therapy may cause mood alteration in the form of mania and depression and occasionally causes psychosis requiring anxiolytics and antipsychotics if the steroid dosage cannot be reduced safely. Such psychiatric disturbances have been associated with greater incidence of immunosuppressant non-compliance leading to higher rates of transplant rejection.[1] Epidural spinal lipomatosis is a well-described but uncommon complication in the posttransplant population, related to the use of steroids for immunosuppression.[108]

Peripheral Nervous System Dysfunction

Cyclosporine

Limb paresthesias are common in patients taking cyclosporine. Many patients report burning sensation of the limbs, but clinical and electrophysiological evaluation usually does not reveal evidence of peripheral neuropathy. If neuropathy is present in such patients, it is usually attributable to prolonged uremia before transplantation or other predisposing conditions. Whether cyclosporine alone causes neuropathy is debatable.[117]

Tacrolimus

A severe demyelinating sensorimotor peripheral neuropathy has been associated with tacrolimus use in liver transplant patients. Whether this neuropathy also occurs in renal transplant recipients receiving tacrolimus is unknown.[16]

Steroids

Steroids have long been associated with myopathy, but the prevalence has not been well established. Steroid myopathy does not seem to be dose-dependent, occurring with acute and long-term use.[5,55] Current study of steroid-induced myopathy is in the context of ICU patients who are receiving steroids and neuromuscular-blocking paralytic agents. It does not seem to be related to length of ICU stay.[13] One prospective study followed 281 liver transplants and identified four patients who developed acute quadriplegic myopathy postoperatively. These four patients were receiving typical steroid doses. All had significantly higher intraoperative complications and required longer ICU and hospital stays than the average transplant patient. Muscle pathology showed loss of myosin in the thick muscle fibers. All patients had improvement and were able to walk but had mild persistent proximal weakness at long-term follow-up.[73]

Guillain–Barré Syndrome

Subacute tetraparesis caused by Guillain–Barré syndrome has followed renal transplantation and is associated with transmitted cytomegalovirus (CMV) infection or reactivation of latent CMV infection.[9,37] In some cases, the patient is CMV-negative.[17] One renal transplant patient with Guillain–Barré syndrome was found to have bacteremia with *Campylobacter jejuni*, a common prodromal infection in non-transplant Guillain–Barré syndrome patients.[65] Guillain–Barré syndrome typically manifests as an ascending paralysis over 2–3 days with areflexia, often accompanied by a mild ascending sensory loss. It may progress quickly to involve the respiratory muscles, requiring intubation. Nerve conduction studies show a proximal demyelinating polyneuropathy. Treatment is with total plasma exchange or intravenous immuneglobulin.[68] Although many patients have full recovery within months, others may have permanent neurological deficits in the form of weakness and sensory loss.[33]

CHRONIC NEUROLOGICAL COMPLICATIONS

There are few PNS complications that begin months after renal transplantation. The most common chronic CNS complications are infection and stroke. Infection can occur at any time after transplantation, but risk increases significantly at 1 month after the transplant operation.[63] Ischemic and hemorrhagic strokes may occur at any time but are typically seen many months after transplantation. Primary CNS lymphoma can occur during this time, often manifesting several months after transplantation but in most cases within 1 year.

Infection (see Chapter 31)

At some point after transplantation, 5–10% of transplant patients develop a CNS infection, with 44–77% of the infections resulting in death.[25] An Indian cohort of 792 renal allograft recipients found that CNS infections constituted most neurological complications, accounting for 39% of brain dysfunction.[95] CNS infection can be divided into four categories based on clinical presentation: (1) meningitis, including acute bacterial and insidious fungal infections; (2) encephalitis or meningoencephalitis; (3) focal brain abscess; and (4) progressive dementia.

Meningitis

A non-immunosuppressed patient with acute meningitis presents with fever, nuchal rigidity, headache, and confusion; meningitis progresses quickly to death if untreated over 24–48 hours. CNS infection in transplant patients may be difficult to diagnose because immunosuppressant therapy minimizes the symptoms and signs that would normally develop from meningeal inflammation. Transplant patients with advanced CNS infections may present with few clinical signs of infection.

Listeria monocytogenes is the most common cause of acute and subacute bacterial meningitis in transplant patients. Other common pathogens include *Haemophilus influenzae*, *Neisseria meningitidis*, and *Streptococcus pneumoniae*. Fever and headache most commonly develop over 1 to several days. Focal neurological deficits, impaired consciousness, and meningismus are encountered in less than half of cases.[90] *Listeria* may occur at any time after transplantation but rarely within the first month.[45] Analysis of cerebrospinal fluid (CSF) shows pleocytosis, increased protein, and normal or reduced glucose concentration. Gram stain may be positive in less than one-third of the cases.[77] CSF cultures positive for *Listeria* may develop late, and blood cultures may reveal the organism first.[31,105] Confirmation of the diagnosis may prove difficult in patients with non-meningitic *Listeria*. The most common non-meningitic form of CNS listeriosis is a meningoencephalitis, which manifests with ataxia and multiple cranial nerve abnormalities, such as oculomotor weakness or dysarthria.[31] *Listeria* may manifest as a focal brain abscess with a higher mortality rate. Twenty-five percent of these patients also have meningitis, and almost all patients become bacteremic.[31]

In a patient with subacute or chronic meningeal symptoms, such as low-grade fevers and mild headache, fungi are the most common etiological agent and are associated with 70% mortality. In the Indian cohort described earlier, of the 31 renal allograft patients who had CNS infection, cryptococcal meningitis occurred in 12, mucormycosis in 6, and aspergillosis in 1 patient.[95]

Cryptococcus neoformans meningitis usually develops more than 6 months after engraftment with insidious clinical progression.[120] Clinical presentation of cryptococcal meningitis in transplant recipients includes encephalopathy (64%), nausea and vomiting (50%), fever (46%), headache (46%), nuchal rigidity (14%), visual loss (7%), and seizures (4%). The duration of symptoms before the diagnosis of meningitis was 17 days (range 2–30 days).[115] Culturing the organism from CSF may take weeks, and immunological detection of CSF cryptococcal antigen is recommended as a quick, reliable diagnostic method. Brain imaging in transplant patients with cryptococcal meningitis may be normal or reveal non-specific results.[115] Antifungal treatment with intravenous amphotericin B or fluconazole or both may eradicate the infection without necessitating a reduction in immunosuppression that might jeopardize graft survival.[45,119]

Mycobacterium tuberculosis infection affects 2–3% of renal transplant recipients which spreads to the CNS in about 50% of patients.[53] CSF examination reveals positive staining for acid-fast bacilli. Treatment typically includes rifampin, as one of four antibiotics, which induces hepatic enzymes and thus can decrease cyclosporine levels. Other chronic meningeal infections are *Strongyloides stercoralis*, *Coccidioides immitis*, and *Histoplasma capsulatum*.

Encephalitis

Transplant recipients may acquire viral encephalitis (also called meningoencephalitis) due to primary infection, from a donor who carried the virus, or from reactivation of a latent virus. Patients may exhibit prominent confusion and difficulty forming new memories. Cranial neuropathies are common with brainstem involvement. Headache and fever are only variably present. Proven CMV encephalitis is rare in transplant recipients but when seen may be associated with retinitis.[10] Brain MRI may show white-matter abnormalities or meningeal enhancement, or may be normal. The CSF should be sent for CMV polymerase chain reaction, which reliably indicates CMV infection in the CNS.[24] Making the diagnosis is important because of the prospect for treatment with ganciclovir or foscarnet and the need to reduce the immunosuppressant drug regimen.[119]

Varicella-zoster virus is a common posttransplant infection that affects many organs and causes brainstem encephalitis. Other offending agents that produce encephalitis include *Toxoplasma gondii*, human herpesvirus-6, *S. stercoralis*, and *Cryptococcus neoformans*.[58] West Nile virus has the potential to cause a severe meningoencephalitis in transplant recipients. It has been transmitted by the organ donor and acquired naturally in communities where the virus is endemic.[22,30]

Focal Brain Infections

Cerebral abscesses in transplant recipients are usually due to aspergillosis or less often due to candidal abscess, cryptococcosis, nocardiosis, toxoplasmosis, mucormycosis, or listeriosis. *Aspergillus fumigatus* usually occurs at 3 months post renal transplantation with a mean incidence of 0.7% in kidney transplant recipients.[100] Aspergillosis in the CNS usually causes sudden focal neurological deficits or seizures. The stroke-like onset of symptoms reflects invasion of cerebral blood vessels by fungus with distal embolization. There is evidence of disseminated disease in one-third of cases, most commonly involving the lung.[11,100] Head CT or MRI may show single or multiple lesions with little mass effect or contrast enhancement. Lung or cerebral biopsy is required for diagnosis. The mortality rate in transplant recipients with invasive aspergillosis ranges from 74% to 92%.[100] Downward deterioration is rapid, and most patients die despite antifungal therapy.[11,45]

A brain abscess from *Nocardia asteroides* is frequently disseminated from a pulmonary focus. Clusters of patients with nocardial infection may occur in transplant units.[8] Associated subcutaneous lesions may be palpable, and biopsy specimens can be obtained. *Toxoplasmosis gondii* is a rare CNS infection in renal transplant recipients. It commonly occurs as multiple progressive mass lesions but also may cause diffuse encephalopathy or meningoencephalitis.[78,110] Imaging studies may not always lead to the diagnosis. The presence of multiple ring-enhancing lesions is characteristic, but this also is seen in other focal infections and neoplasms.[4] Mucormycosis is common in transplanted diabetics and nearly always fatal.[95] It starts in the paranasal sinuses, producing periorbital edema and proptosis, and subsequently may invade the intracavernous carotid artery, leading to cerebral artery emboli and strokes.[20]

Progressive Dementia

PML is a rare and fatal condition producing widespread demyelination within the CNS. Initially described in patients with acquired immunodeficiency syndrome, PML was eventually identified in many immunosuppressed individuals. It is caused by polyomavirus infection, usually JC virus but sometimes SV40 or BK virus.[88] The clinical presentation is insidious, with progressive dementia, blindness, or bilateral weakness. The diagnosis is suggested by the history in conjunction with brain MRI, which shows diffuse subcortical white-matter T2 hyperintensity without mass effect or contrast enhancement. Definitive diagnosis requires tissue showing demyelination and identification of virus particles in enlarged oligodendrocyte nuclei by electron microscopy.[60] Although JC virus DNA is detected in the CSF of 90% of patients with PML, a negative polymerase chain reaction result cannot reliably be used to rule out infection.[36] A French study found JC virus DNA in 7% of 103 renal transplant recipients and none developed PML; however these patients were followed for 1 year only.[72] Patients die within months to 1 year after a relentlessly progressive decline and currently there is no effective treatment.

Stroke (see Chapter 28)

Stroke competes with infection as the most frequent neurological complication of kidney transplantation, but it is the most frequent cause of neurological illness among chronic complications.[3,95] A review of 403 patients who received one kidney graft between 1979 and 2000 found a stroke prevalence of 8% at 10 years, one-third of which were cerebral hemorrhages. The mean age was 50 years (range 23–63 years). The mean time from transplant to stroke was 49 months. Three risk factors were identified as predictors of stroke: diabetic neuropathy, peripheral vascular disease, and age older than 40.[81] Another large retrospective review found a posttransplant stroke prevalence of 9.5%, with most occurring more than 6 months after transplantation.[3]

In a single-center study of 1600 kidney transplants between 1983 and 2002, 105 patients died, and 60.3% died with a functioning graft. Stroke was the second greatest cause of death at 17%, preceded only by infection, which accounted for 24% of deaths. After stroke, the most frequent causes were cardiovascular disease at 16%, malignant neoplasm at 15%, and hepatic failure at 11%.[99] A retrospective study looking at causes of death from renal transplantation from 1970 to 1999 found that the percentage of deaths from stroke increased over the years from 2.4% to 8% as the percentage of graft rejection at death decreased.[46]

Ischemic Stroke

Various risk factors contribute to the increase in stroke after transplantation.[3] Age older than 40 years places a transplant recipient at particular risk.[3,47] One study noted an increased risk in patients whose renal failure originally was due to hypertension.[47] This association was not found in another survey, however, which noted a clear association of ischemic stroke with underlying polycystic renal disease, a condition in which hypertension is common.[3]

Hyperlipidemia occurs in renal failure and persists to some degree after transplantation, likely contributing to accelerated atherosclerosis.[47] Long-term steroid therapy may accelerate atherosclerosis.

Ischemic stroke usually manifests with abrupt onset of a focal neurological deficit, such as hemiparesis, speech disturbance, clumsiness, or visual field cut. Head CT does not typically show signs of stroke in the first 24 hours after stroke, unless the stroke is particularly large. Brain MRI may show restricted diffusion 30 minutes after the onset of an ischemic event.

Potentially reversible stroke risk factors include hypertension, hyperlipidemia, smoking, and diabetes mellitus. The fungal infections aspergillosis and mucormycosis can present as stroke after hyphal invasion of cerebral arteries with distal embolization. Cerebral vasculitis has been reported in immunosuppressed transplant recipients.[94]

Hemorrhagic Stroke

A retrospective study by the Mayo Clinic identified 10 cases of intracerebral hemorrhage among 1573 patients who received a renal transplant between 1966 and 1998. Six of the 10 patients died. The interval from renal transplantation to intracerebral hemorrhage ranged from 12 to 114 months (average 57 months). All patients with intracerebral hemorrhage had poorly controlled hypertension. Patients with polycystic kidney disease had a 10-fold increased risk of developing a hemorrhage, and patients with diabetes mellitus had a fourfold increased risk. Most cerebral hemorrhages were catastrophic and fatal but overall were responsible for only 1% of the deaths after renal transplantation.[121]

Primary Central Nervous System Lymphoma

Non-Hodgkin's lymphoma is the second most common neoplasia occurring after solid-organ transplantation, although it is less common in renal transplant patients compared to other transplanted organs.[86] In two very large studies of renal transplantation, 0.7–1.4% of patients developed non-Hodgkin's lymphoma. Of those, 22% had CNS involvement and 11% were diagnosed with primary CNS lymphoma, with 5-year survival ranging from 38% to 80%.[19,82,87] Younger age and having received OKT3 were associated with greater risk of developing lymphoma, whereas having been treated with mycophenolate mofetil or azathioprine was associated with a lower risk.[19] Primary CNS lymphoma typically occurs within 1 year of transplantation, with a median interval of 9 months (range 5.5–46 months).[44] In a study of 25 patients who developed primary CNS lymphoma after renal transplantation, the mean age at diagnosis was 46 years. The diagnosis was made 4–264 months after transplant (median of 18 months).[104]

Patients may present with a single lesion or multifocal lesions; the latter are seen 33–72% of the time.[76,104,119] The lesions are often supratentorial and periventricular in location. Cerebral lymphoma can invade the meninges, but malignant meningitis more often reflects spread from a systemic primary. Two risk factors have been identified in the development of primary CNS lymphoma: (1) the intensity of immunosuppressive regimen; and (2) Epstein–Barr virus seropositivity.[48,118] Epstein–Barr virus is suspected to play a causative role in cerebral lymphoma, based on serum antibody responses, immunostaining, and DNA hybridization studies of biopsy specimens.[42]

Patients usually present with neurological deficits that worsen over several weeks. In a French study of 25 patients with primary CNS lymphoma after renal transplantation, the most common presenting symptom was a focal neurological deficit in 84%, either an isolated deficit or associated with seizures or increased intracranial pressure.[104] Headache is a late symptom, often reflecting increased intracranial pressure or meningeal involvement.[44] Less frequent presentations include malignant meningitis, spinal cord lesions, and visual disturbance from ocular deposits.[44]

In immunocompetent patients, brain MRI shows primary CNS lymphoma lesions as homogeneously enhancing with gadolinium. In transplant patients, the lesions may show homogeneous, heterogeneous, or no enhancement (Figure 33-3). Ring enhancement may be easily mistaken for glioblastoma multiforme or abscess. In primary CNS lymphoma, the CSF may have modestly elevated protein levels and low glucose but often does not show the presence of lymphomatous cells.[104] With diffuse lymphomatous involvement of the meninges, multiple cytological specimens may be required before histological confirmation is forthcoming.

A suspected diagnosis of primary CNS lymphoma should be confirmed by prompt neurosurgical biopsy. High-dose steroid therapy before obtaining the biopsy specimen may interfere with the reliability of histological diagnosis.[27] Resection of the tumor does not seem to enhance long-term survival, and there is substantial morbidity after attempts to resect a deep-seated tumor.[27]

The outcome of posttransplant primary CNS lymphoma is poor. In a large study of non-Hodgkin's lymphoma in 145 000 deceased donor kidney transplants, of patients diagnosed with primary CNS lymphoma, 38% had a 5-year survival.[82] Most commonly, initial treatment is with reduction of immunosuppressive therapy; however, this rarely results in clinical remission alone. There are many treatment options, including intraventricular infusion of monoclonal antibodies, chemotherapy, and radiotherapy, each of which yields only 50% clinical remission. In the French cohort of 25 patients, the median survival across all treatment regimens was 26 months. An improved median survival of 42 months was reported when

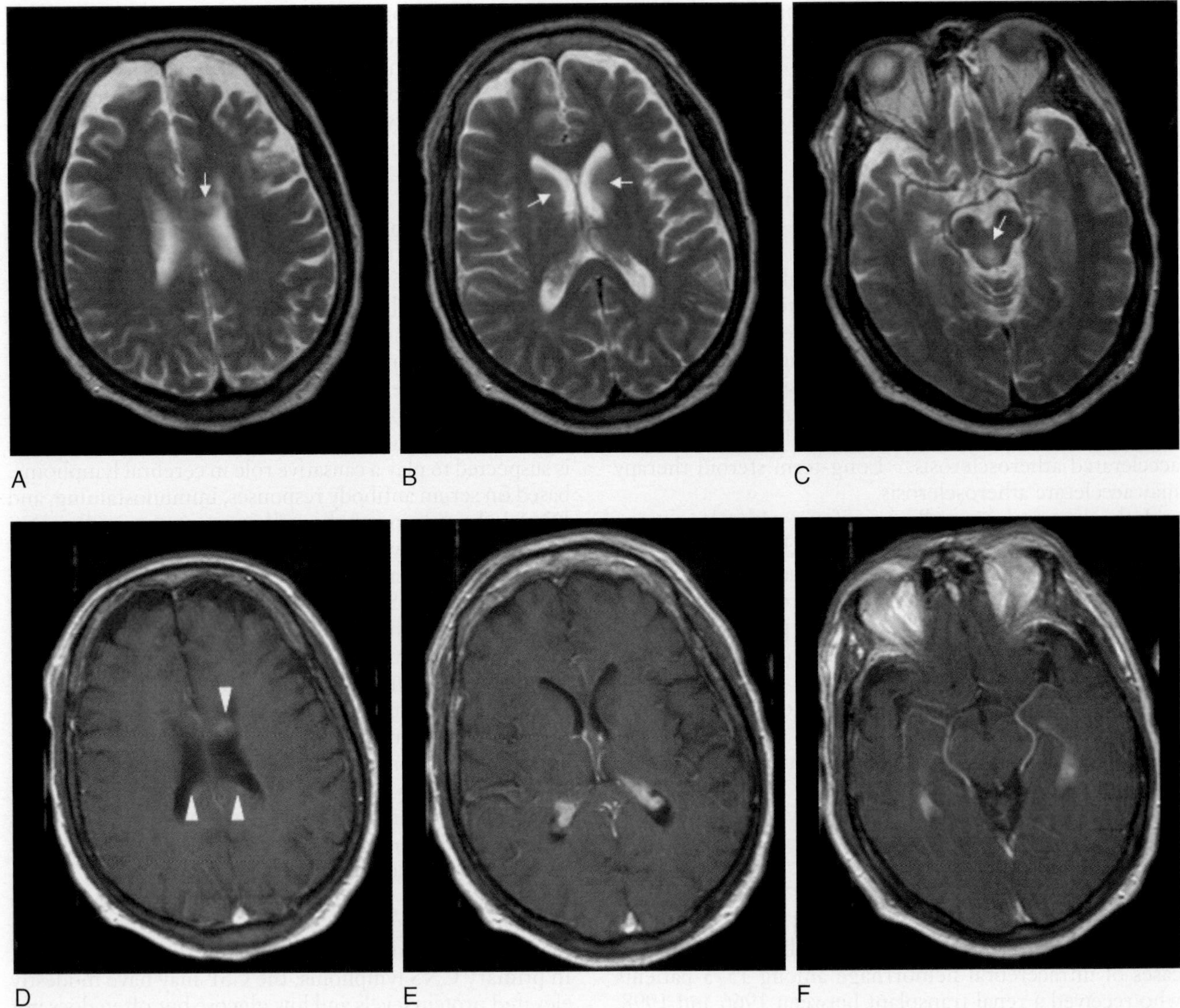

FIGURE 33-3 ■ Primary central nervous system lymphoma. A 56-year-old man with a history of deceased donor renal transplant developed lethargy and altered mental status 1 year after transplantation. Cerebrospinal fluid cytology showed monomorphic large B cells consistent with primary central nervous system lymphoma. (A–C) Axial T2-weighted magnetic resonance images of the brain show regions of hyperintensity (arrows) in the corpus callosum (A), bilateral caudate (B), and periaqueductal region of the midbrain (C). (D–F) Contrast-enhanced axial T1-weighted magnetic resonance images show subtle enhancement of the lesions of the corpus callosum (arrowheads in D) with no enhancement of the lesions in the caudate and midbrain. The patient was treated with intrathecal methotrexate and later died as a result of sepsis.

high-dose cytosine arabinoside and intrathecal methotrexate were combined with radiotherapy.[27] Intravenous methotrexate before radiotherapy produces tumor response in 85% of patients, but this combined therapy carries a high risk of leukoencephalopathy in a few years, causing dementia, ataxia, and incontinence, especially in older patients.[26] Optimal treatment regimens for primary CNS lymphoma are currently being sought, and patients should be managed by an oncologist experienced in this area.

SUMMARY

Neurological problems are major contributors to morbidity and mortality in transplant recipients. Many problems occur months or years after engraftment and may never come to the attention of the transplant surgeon. It is helpful to approach a patient with neurological disease by broadly localizing disease to the CNS or PNS. In the immediate postoperative period, encephalopathy with or without seizures may occur secondary to a variety of conditions. Compressive femoral neuropathy may occur as a perioperative neurological complication. Weeks after the transplantation, the most common neurological problems are related to immunosuppressant drugs, which may induce encephalopathy, tremor, neuropathy, or myopathy. Guillain–Barré syndrome is seen rarely. Chronic neurological complications tend to be caused by CNS infection, stroke, or primary CNS lymphoma.

REFERENCES

1. Abbott KC, Agodoa LY, O'Malley PG. Hospitalized psychoses after renal transplantation in the United States: incidence, risk factors, and prognosis. J Am Soc Nephrol 2003;14:1628–35.
2. Adams DH, Ponsford S, Gunson B, et al. Neurological complications following liver transplantation. Lancet 1987;1:949–51.
3. Adams Jr HP, Dawson G, Coffman TJ, et al. Stroke in renal transplant recipients. Arch Neurol 1986;43:113–5.
4. Agildere AM, Basaran C, Cakir B, et al. Evaluation of neurologic complications by brain MRI in kidney and liver transplant recipients. Transplant Proc 2006;38:611–8.
5. Argov Z. Drug-induced myopathies. Curr Opin Neurol 2000;13:541–5.
6. Armour A. Dilutional hyponatraemia: a cause of massive fatal intraoperative cerebral oedema in a child undergoing renal transplantation. J Clin Pathol 1997;50:444–6.
7. Awan AQ, Lewis MA, Postlethwaite RJ, et al. Seizures following renal transplantation in childhood. Pediatr Nephrol 1999;13:275–7.
8. Baddour LM, Baselski VS, Herr MJ, et al. Nocardiosis in recipients of renal transplants: evidence for nosocomial acquisition. Am J Infect Control 1986;14:214–9.
9. Bale Jr JF, Rote NS, Bloomer LC, et al. Guillain–Barré-like polyneuropathy after renal transplant: possible association with cytomegalovirus infection. Arch Neurol 1980;37:784.
10. Bamborschke S, Wullen T, Huber M, et al. Early diagnosis and successful treatment of acute cytomegalovirus encephalitis in a renal transplant recipient. J Neurol 1992;239:205–8.
11. Beal MF, O'Carroll CP, Kleinman GM, et al. Aspergillosis of the nervous system. Neurology 1982;32:473–9.
12. Bechstein WO. Neurotoxicity of calcineurin inhibitors: impact and clinical management. Transpl Int 2000;13:313–26.
13. Bird SJ, Rich MM. Critical illness myopathy and polyneuropathy. Curr Neurol Neurosci Rep 2002;2:527–33.
14. Bodkin CL, Eidelman BH. Sirolimus-induced posterior reversible encephalopathy. Neurology 2007;68:2039–40.
15. Bolton CF. Peripheral neuropathies associated with chronic renal failure. Can J Neurol Sci 1980;7:89–96.
16. Bronster DJ, Yonover P, Stein J, et al. Demyelinating sensorimotor polyneuropathy after administration of FK506. Transplantation 1995;59:1066–8.
17. Bulsara KR, Baron PW, Tuttle-Newhall JE, et al. Guillain–Barré syndrome in organ and bone marrow transplant patients. Transplantation 2001;71:1169–72.
18. Burn DJ, Bates D. Neurology and the kidney. J Neurol Neurosurg Psychiatry 1998;65:810–21.
19. Caillard S, Dharnidharka V, Agodoa L, et al. Posttransplant lymphoproliferative disorders after renal transplantation in the United States in era of modern immunosuppression. Transplantation 2005;80:1233–43.
20. Carbone KM, Pennington LR, Gimenez LF, et al. Mucormycosis in renal transplant patients – a report of two cases and review of the literature. Q J Med 1985;57:825–31.
21. Carson KR, Evens AM, Richey EA, et al. Progressive multifocal leukoencephalopathy after rituximab therapy in HIV-negative patients: a report of 57 cases from the research on adverse drug events and reports project. Blood 2009;113:4834–40.
22. Centers for Disease Control and Prevention. West Nile virus infection in organ donor and transplant recipients – Georgia and Florida, 2002. JAMA 2002;288:1465–6.
23. Clatworthy MR, Friend PJ, Calne RY, et al. Alemtuzumab (Campath-1h) for the treatment of acute rejection in kidney transplant recipients: long-term follow-up. Transplantation 2009;87:1092–5.
24. Cohen BA. Prognosis and response to therapy of cytomegalovirus encephalitis and meningomyelitis in aids. Neurology 1996;46:444–50.
25. Conti DJ, Rubin RH. Infection of the central nervous system in organ transplant recipients. Neurol Clin 1988;6:241–60.
26. DeAngelis LM. Primary central nervous system lymphoma. J Neurol Neurosurg Psychiatry 1999;66:699–701.
27. DeAngelis LM, Yahalom J, Heinemann MH, et al. Primary CNS lymphoma: combined treatment with chemotherapy and radiotherapy. Neurology 1990;40:80–6.
28. de Groen PC, Aksamit AJ, Rakela J, et al. Central nervous system toxicity after liver transplantation. The role of cyclosporine and cholesterol. N Engl J Med 1987;317:861–6.
29. Delanty N, Vaughan CJ, French JA. Medical causes of seizures. Lancet 1998;352:383–90.
30. DeSalvo D, Roy-Chaudhury P, Peddi R, et al. West Nile virus encephalitis in organ transplant recipients: another high-risk group for meningoencephalitis and death. Transplantation 2004;77:466–9.
31. Doganay M. Listeriosis: clinical presentation. FEMS Immunol Med Microbiol 2003;35:173–5.
32. Dohgu S, Kataoka Y, Ikesue H, et al. Involvement of glial cells in cyclosporine-increased permeability of brain endothelial cells. Cell Mol Neurobiol 2000;20:781–6.
33. El-Sabrout RA, Radovancevic B, Ankoma-Sey V, et al. Guillain–Barré syndrome after solid organ transplantation. Transplantation 2001;71:1311–6.
34. Esterl Jr RM, Gupta N, Garvin PJ. Permanent blindness after cyclosporine neurotoxicity in a kidney-pancreas transplant recipient. Clin Neuropharmacol 1996;19:259–66.
35. Estol CJ, Lopez O, Brenner RP, et al. Seizures after liver transplantation: a clinicopathologic study. Neurology 1989;39:1297–301.
36. Ferrante P, Caldarelli-Stefano R, Omodeo-Zorini E, et al. Comprehensive investigation of the presence of JC virus in aids patients with and without progressive multifocal leukoencephalopathy. J Med Virol 1997;52:235–42.
37. Garcia Alvarez T, Garcia Herrera A, Mazuecos Blanca A, et al. Guillain–Barré syndrome in kidney transplant. Nefrologia 2010;30:260–1.
38. Gilmore RL. Seizures and antiepileptic drug use in transplant patients. Neurol Clin 1988;6:279–96.
39. Gross ML, Pearson R, Sweny P, et al. Rejection encephalopathy. Proc Eur Dial Transplant Assoc 1981;18:461–4.
40. Gross ML, Sweny P, Pearson RM, et al. Rejection encephalopathy. An acute neurological syndrome complicating renal transplantation. J Neurol Sci 1982;56:23–34.
41. Grotz WH, Breitenfeldt MK, Braune SW, et al. Calcineurin-inhibitor induced pain syndrome (CIPS): a severe disabling complication after organ transplantation. Transpl Int 2001;14:16–23.
42. Hanto DW, Gajl-Peczalska KJ, Frizzera G, et al. Epstein–Barr virus (EBV) induced polyclonal and monoclonal B-cell lymphoproliferative diseases occurring after renal transplantation. Clinical, pathologic, and virologic findings and implications for therapy. Ann Surg 1983;198:356–69.
43. Hefty TR, Nelson KA, Hatch TR, et al. Acute lumbosacral plexopathy in diabetic women after renal transplantation. J Urol 1990;143:107–9.
44. Hochberg FH, Miller DC. Primary central nervous system lymphoma. J Neurosurg 1988;68:835–53.
45. Hooper DC, Pruitt AA, Rubin RH. Central nervous system infection in the chronically immunosuppressed. Medicine (Baltimore) 1982;61:166–88.
46. Howard RJ, Patton PR, Reed AI, et al. The changing causes of graft loss and death after kidney transplantation. Transplantation 2002;73:1923–8.
47. Ibels LS, Stewart JH, Mahony JF, et al. Deaths from occlusive arterial disease in renal allograft recipients. Br Med J 1974;3:552–4.
48. Jamil B, Nicholls K, Becker GJ, et al. Impact of acute rejection therapy on infections and malignancies in renal transplant recipients. Transplantation 1999;68:1597–603.
49. Jarosz JM, Howlett DC, Cox TC, et al. Cyclosporine-related reversible posterior leukoencephalopathy: MRI. Neuroradiology 1997;39:711–5.
50. Jeruss J, Braun SV, Reese JC, et al. Cyclosporine-induced white and grey matter central nervous system lesions in a pediatric renal transplant patient. Pediatr Transplant 1998;2:45–50.
51. Jog MS, Turley JE, Berry H. Femoral neuropathy in renal transplantation. Can J Neurol Sci 1994;21:38–42.
52. Jost L, Nogues M, Davalos M, et al. Neurological complications of renal transplant. Medicina (B Aires) 2000;60:161–4.
53. Kaaroud H, Beji S, Boubaker K, et al. Tuberculosis after renal transplantation. Transplant Proc 2007;39:1012–3.

54. Kahan BD, Flechner SM, Lorber MI, et al. Complications of cyclosporine-prednisone immunosuppression in 402 renal allograft recipients exclusively followed at a single center for from one to five years. Transplantation 1987;43:197–204.
55. Kanda F, Okuda S, Matsushita T, et al. Steroid myopathy: pathogenesis and effects of growth hormone and insulin-like growth factor-i administration. Horm Res 2001;56(Suppl. 1):24–8.
56. Kato T, Hattori H, Nagato M, et al. Subclinical central Pontine myelinolysis following liver transplantation. Brain Dev 2002;24:179–82.
57. Knox DL, Hanneken AM, Hollows FC, et al. Uremic optic neuropathy. Arch Ophthalmol 1988;106:50–4.
58. Kotton CN, Fishman JA. Viral infection in the renal transplant recipient. J Am Soc Nephrol 2005;16:1758–74.
59. Kurella M, Mapes DL, Port FK, et al. Correlates and outcomes of dementia among dialysis patients: the dialysis outcomes and practice patterns study. Nephrol Dial Transplant 2006;21:2543–8.
60. Kwak EJ, Vilchez RA, Randhawa P, et al. Pathogenesis and management of polyomavirus infection in transplant recipients. Clin Infect Dis 2002;35:1081–7.
61. Lake KD. Management of drug interactions with cyclosporine. Pharmacotherapy 1991;11:110S–8S.
62. Lee JM, Raps EC. Neurologic complications of transplantation. Neurol Clin 1998;16:21–33.
63. Li QS, Huo WQ, Nie ZL, et al. Acute femoral neuropathy following renal transplantation: a retrospective, multicenter study in China. Transplant Proc 2010;42:1699–1703.
64. Lockwood AH. Neurologic complications of renal disease. Neurol Clin 1989;7:617–27.
65. Maccario M, Tarantino A, Nobile-Orazio E, et al. *Campylobacter jejuni* bacteremia and Guillain–Barré syndrome in a renal transplant recipient. Transpl Int 1998;11:439–42.
66. Mahoney CA, Arieff AI. Uremic Encephalopathies: clinical, biochemical, and experimental features. Am J Kidney Dis 1982;2:324–36.
67. Maramattom BV, Wijdicks EF. Sirolimus may not cause neurotoxicity in kidney and liver transplant recipients. Neurology 2004;63:1958–9.
68. Mazzoni A, Pardi C, Bortoli M, et al. Plasma exchange for polyradiculoneuropathy following kidney transplantation: a case report. Transplant Proc 2004;36:716–7.
69. McArthur JC, Brew BJ, Nath A. Neurological complications of HIV infection. Lancet Neurol 2005;4:543–55.
70. McEnery PT, Nathan J, Bates SR, et al. Convulsions in children undergoing renal transplantation. J Pediatr 1989;115:532–6.
71. Meech PR. Femoral neuropathy following renal transplantation. Aust N Z J Surg 1990;60:117–9.
72. Mengelle C, Kamar N, Mansuy JM, et al. JC virus DNA in the peripheral blood of renal transplant patients: a 1-year prospective follow-up in France. J Med Virol 2011;83:132–6.
73. Miro O, Salmeron JM, Masanes F, et al. Acute quadriplegic myopathy with myosin-deficient muscle fibres after liver transplantation: defining the clinical picture and delimiting the risk factors. Transplantation 1999;67:1144–51.
74. Monseu G, Flament-Durand J. Pathogenesis of central Pontine myelinolysis. A clinical and pathological description of three cases. Pathol Eur 1971;6:75–94.
75. Mueller AR, Platz KP, Bechstein WO, et al. Neurotoxicity after orthotopic liver transplantation. A comparison between cyclosporine and FK506. Transplantation 1994;58:155–70.
76. Murray K, Kun L, Cox J. Primary malignant lymphoma of the central nervous system. Results of treatment of 11 cases and review of the literature. J Neurosurg 1986;65:600–7.
77. Mylonakis E, Hohmann EL, Calderwood SB. Central nervous system infection with *Listeria monocytogenes*. 33 years' experience at a general hospital and review of 776 episodes from the literature. Medicine (Baltimore) 1998;77:313–36.
78. Nasser QJ, Power RE, Eng MP, et al. Toxoplasmosis after a simultaneous pancreas and kidney transplantation. Transplant Proc 2004;36:2843–4.
79. Nived O, Sturfelt G, Liang MH, et al. The ACR nomenclature for CNS lupus revisited. Lupus 2003;12:872–6.
80. Norenberg MD, Leslie KO, Robertson AS. Association between rise in serum sodium and central pontine myelinolysis. Ann Neurol 1982;11:128–35.
81. Oliveras A, Roquer J, Puig JM, et al. Stroke in renal transplant recipients: epidemiology, predictive risk factors and outcome. Clin Transplant 2003;17:1–8.
82. Opelz G, Dohler B. Lymphomas after solid organ transplantation: a collaborative transplant study report. Am J Transplant 2004;4:222–30.
83. O'Sullivan DP. Convulsions associated with cyclosporin A. Br Med J (Clin Res Ed) 1985;290:858.
84. Palmer CA. Neurologic manifestations of renal disease. Neurol Clin 2002;20:23–34, v.
85. Patchell RA. Neurological complications of organ transplantation. Ann Neurol 1994;36:688–703.
86. Penn I. Neoplastic complications of transplantation. Semin Respir Infect 1993;8:233–9.
87. Penn I, Porat G. Central nervous system lymphomas in organ allograft recipients. Transplantation 1995;59:240–4.
88. Perrons CJ, Fox JD, Lucas SB, et al. Detection of polyomaviral DNA in clinical samples from immunocompromised patients: correlation with clinical disease. J Infect 1996;32:205–9.
89. Pirsch JD, Miller J, Deierhoi MH, et al. A comparison of tacrolimus (fk506) and cyclosporine for immunosuppression after cadaveric renal transplantation. FK506 Kidney Transplant Study Group. Transplantation 1997;63:977–83.
90. Pollock SS, Pollock TM, Harrison MJ. Infection of the central nervous system by *Listeria monocytogenes*: a review of 54 adult and juvenile cases. Q J Med 1984;53:331–40.
91. Pontin AR, Donaldson RA, Jacobson JE. Femoral neuropathy after renal transplantation. S Afr Med J 1978;53:376–8.
92. Probst A, Harder F, Hofer H, et al. Femoral nerve lesion subsequent to renal transplantation. Eur Urol 1982;8:314–6.
93. Raskin NH. Neurological complications of renal failure. New York: Churchill Livingstone; 1995.
94. Rothenberg RJ. Isolated angiitis of the brain. Case in a renal transplant recipient. Am J Med 1985;79:629–32.
95. Sakhuja V, Sud K, Kalra OP, et al. Central nervous system complications in renal transplant recipients in a tropical environment. J Neurol Sci 2001;183:89–93.
96. Schady W, Abuaisha B, Boulton AJ. Observations on severe ulnar neuropathy in diabetes. J Diabetes Complications 1998;12:128–32.
97. Seliger SL, Siscovick DS, Stehman-Breen CO, et al. Moderate renal impairment and risk of dementia among older adults: the cardiovascular health cognition study. J Am Soc Nephrol 2004;15:1904–11.
98. Sharma KR, Cross J, Santiago F, et al. Incidence of acute femoral neuropathy following renal transplantation. Arch Neurol 2002;59:541–5.
99. Shimmura H, Tanabe K, Tokumoto T, et al. Analysis of cause of death with a functioning graft: a single-center experience. Transplant Proc 2004;36:2026–9.
100. Singh N, Paterson DL. Aspergillus infections in transplant recipients. Clin Microbiol Rev 2005;18:44–69.
101. Singh N, Yu VL, Gayowski T. Central nervous system lesions in adult liver transplant recipients: clinical review with implications for management. Medicine (Baltimore) 1994;73:110–8.
102. Sisto D, Chiu WS, Geelhoed GW, et al. Femoral neuropathy after renal transplantation. South Med J 1980;73:1464–6.
103. Small SL, Fukui MB, Bramblett GT, et al. Immunosuppression-induced leukoencephalopathy from tacrolimus (FK506). Ann Neurol 1996;40:575–80.
104. Snanoudj R, Durrbach A, Leblond V, et al. Primary brain lymphomas after kidney transplantation: presentation and outcome. Transplantation 2003;76:930–7.
105. Stamm AM, Dismukes WE, Simmons BP, et al. Listeriosis in renal transplant recipients: report of an outbreak and review of 102 cases. Rev Infect Dis 1982;4:665–82.
106. Stein DP, Lederman RJ, Vogt DP, et al. Neurological complications following liver transplantation. Ann Neurol 1992;31:644–9.
107. Stott VL, Hurrell MA, Anderson TJ. Reversible posterior leukoencephalopathy syndrome: a misnomer reviewed. Intern Med J 2005;35:83–90.
108. Tobler WD, Weil S. Epidural lipomatosis and renal transplantation. Surg Neurol 1988;29:141–4.
109. Torocsik HV, Curless RG, Post J, et al. FK506-induced leukoencephalopathy in children with organ transplants. Neurology 1999;52:1497–500.

110. Townsend JJ, Wolinsky JS, Baringer JR, et al. Acquired toxoplasmosis. A neglected cause of treatable nervous system disease. Arch Neurol 1975;32:335–43.
111. Tsagalou EP, Anastasiou-Nana MI, Margari ZJ, et al. Possible everolimus-induced, severe, reversible encephalopathy after cardiac transplantation. J Heart Lung Transplant 2007;26:661–4.
112. van der Voort van Zyp NC, Davin JC, Idu M, et al. Kidney transplant survival rates and surgical complications in kidney transplants in children; experiences in the Emma Children's hospital AMC. Ned Tijdschr Geneeskd 2005;149:584–8.
113. Van Veer H, Coosemans W, Pirenne J, et al. Acute femoral neuropathy: a rare complication after renal transplantation. Transplant Proc 2010; 42:4384–8.
114. Vaziri ND, Barton CH, Ravikumar GR, et al. Femoral neuropathy: a complication of renal transplantation. Nephron 1981;28:30–1.
115. Vilchez RA, Fung J, Kusne S. Cryptococcosis in organ transplant recipients: an overview. Am J Transplant 2002;2:575–80.
116. Vo AA, Lukovsky M, Toyoda M, et al. Rituximab and intravenous immune globulin for desensitization during renal transplantation. N Engl J Med 2008;359:242–51.
117. Walker RW, Brochstein JA. Neurologic complications of immunosuppressive agents. Neurol Clin 1988;6:261–78.
118. Walker RC, Paya CV, Marshall WF, et al. Pretransplantation seronegative Epstein-Barr virus status is the primary risk factor for posttransplantation lymphoproliferative disorder in adult heart, lung, and other solid organ transplantations. J Heart Lung Transplant 1995;14:214–21.
119. Watson AJ, Russell RP, Cabreja RF, et al. Cure of cryptococcal infection during continued immunosuppressive therapy. Q J Med 1985;55:169–72.
120. Wijdicks EF. Neurotoxicity of immunosuppressive drugs. Liver Transpl 2001;7:937–42.
121. Wijdicks EF, Torres VE, Schievink WI, et al. Cerebral hemorrhage in recipients of renal transplantation. Mayo Clin Proc 1999;74:1111–2.
122. Wijdicks EF, Wiesner RH, Dahlke LJ, et al. FK506-induced neurotoxicity in liver transplantation. Ann Neurol 1994;35:498–501.
123. Wright DG, Laureno R, Victor M. Pontine and extrapontine myelinolysis. Brain 1979;102:361–85.
124. Wszolek ZK, McComb RD, Pfeiffer RF, et al. Pontine and extrapontine myelinolysis following liver transplantation. Relationship to serum sodium. Transplantation 1989;48:1006–12.
125. Yazbeck S, Larbrisseau A, O'Regan S. Femoral neuropathy after renal transplantation. J Urol 1985;134:720–1.
126. Zylicz Z, Nuyten FJ, Notermans SL, et al. Postoperative ulnar neuropathy after kidney transplantation. Anaesthesia 1984;39:1117–20.

CHAPTER 34

NON-MALIGNANT AND MALIGNANT SKIN LESIONS IN KIDNEY TRANSPLANT PATIENTS

Aoife Lally • Sasha Nicole Jenkins • Fiona Zwald

CHAPTER OUTLINE

INTRODUCTION

Cutaneous disorders in kidney transplant recipients are common and well recognized, with most attention naturally focused on malignant cutaneous disease. Non-malignant cutaneous diseases are predominantly infectious or iatrogenic in nature (Table 34-1). However, inflammatory cutaneous disease and benign cutaneous tumors are also seen. The range of benign cutaneous changes identified in this population is illustrated in Figure 34-1, which shows findings from a recent study from Oxford.[70] As compliance with immunosuppressive medications is crucial to graft survival, it is important that cutaneous disease which may cause functional or aesthetic problems affecting quality of life[94] is addressed so that adherence with immunosuppressive drugs is maintained.

There is a similar profile of drug-related cutaneous side effects in kidney transplant recipients of all racial groups, but the consequences of immunosuppression differ

TABLE 34-1 **Summary of Studies of Benign Cutaneous Diseases in Renal Transplant Recipients**

Study	Country	No. of Patients	Time Posttransplant (Months)	Mean Age (Years)	IS Regimen	Cutaneous Infection	Cutaneous Iatrogenic Effects
Haim et al. 1973[54]	Israel	35	7–48	29	Prednisolone Azathioprine	39 infections: • Bacterial 10 • Viral 8 • Fungal 21	–
Koranda et al. 1974[68]	United States	200	3–108	30	Prednisolone Azathioprine	• Bacterial 4 • Viral warts 86 • Viral other 96 • Fungal 50	Cushingoid: • Purpura 200 • Acne 126 • Striae 116 • KP 110 • Hirsutism 98 • Hair loss 108
Bergfeld and Roenigk 1978[11]	United States	215	N/A	N/A	Prednisolone Azathioprine	• Bacterial 59 • Viral 40 (viral warts 8) • Fungal 34	• Steroid acne 12 • Purpura fulminans 1
Bencini et al. 1983[9]	Italy	105	1–132 Mean=40	35	Prednisolone Azathioprine	107 infections in 74 RTRs: • Bacterial 16 • Viral 38 • Fungal 53	• Cushingoid 55
Bencini et al. 1986[10]	Italy	67	1–17 Mean=3.2	35	Cyclosporine Steroid (low dose)	26 RTRs • Bacterial 8 • Viral 16 • Fungal 8	54 RTRs • Hypertrichosis 40 • Epidermal cysts 19 • Gum hypertrophy 14 • Steroid acne 10 • Sebaceous hyperplasia 7
Brown et al. 1988[22]	Northern Ireland	223	24–252 Mean=79	36	Prednisolone Azathioprine	• Viral warts 52	• Acne and purpura "common"
Blohme and Larko 1990[14]	Sweden	98	120–276	50	Azathioprine Prednisolone Cyclosporine (5)	• Viral warts 54 • Fungal 7	• Steroid effects 21
Bunney et al. 1990[23]	Scotland	162	N/A	45	Cyclosporine (94) Azathioprine (68)	• Warts 22/94, 20/68 • Fungal 8/94, 8/68	• Hypertrichosis 8/94 • Gum hypertrophy 1/94 • Acne 12/94, 6/68
Lugo-Janer et al. 1991[81]	Puerto Rico	82	1–165 Mean=35	35	Azathioprine Prednisolone Cyclosporine	63 RTRs • Bacterial 14 • Viral 26 • Fungal 100	55 RTRs • Cushingoid 54 • Acne 25 • Hypertrichosis 27 • KP 27 • Gingival hyperplasia 16
Menni et al. 1991[93]	Italy Children	32	1–96 Mean=32	13	Azathioprine Prednisolone Cyclosporine	• Bacterial 2 • Viral 6 • Fungal 2	• Gingival hyperplasia 26 • Hypertrichosis 23 • Acne 5

Continued on following page

TABLE 34-1 **Summary of Studies of Benign Cutaneous Diseases in Renal Transplant Recipients** (Continued)

Study	Country	No. of Patients	Time Posttransplant (Months)	Mean Age (Years)	IS Regimen	Cutaneous Infection	Cutaneous Iatrogenic Effects
Strumia et al. 1992[132]	Italy	53	Up to 240	44	Azathioprine Prednisolone Cyclosporine (29)	• Bacterial 1 • Viral warts 15 • Fungal 37	52 RTRs
Hepburn et al. 1994[57]	New Zealand	52	3–258 Mean=116	44	Azathioprine Prednisolone Cyclosporine (15)	• Bacterial 1 • Viral warts 39 • Fungal 5	• Acne 2 • Hypertrichosis 1
Chugh et al. 1994[31]	India	157	1–23	36	Azathioprine Prednisolone Cyclosporine	• Bacterial 11 • Viral 35 • Fungal 117	• Cushingoid 133 • Acne 94 • Hypertrichosis 65 • Gum hypertrophy 2
Barba et al. 1996[6]	Italy	285	N/A	45	Azathioprine Prednisolone Cyclosporine	• Bacterial 15 • Viral warts 88 • Fungal 65	• Cushingoid 139 • Hypertrichosis 98 • Acne 27
Seckin et al. 1998[117]	Turkey	80	1.5–240 Mean=49	35	Azathioprine Prednisolone Cyclosporine	69 patients • Bacterial 14 • Viral 44 • Fungal 47 • Parasitic 2	78 patients • Hypertrichosis 61 • Cushingoid 64 • Acne 29 • Gingival hyperplasia 32
Euvrard et al. 2001[42]	France Children (all solid-organ recipients)	145	1–120	? All <18	Azathioprine Prednisolone Cyclosporine Tacrolimus (18) MMF (14)	102 patients • Bacterial 9 • Viral 103 • Fungal 25	• Striae 8 • Acne 8 (21 teenagers with acne vulgaris) • Hypertrichosis 14 • Gingival hyperplasia 8
Mahe et al. 2005[84]	France	80	18 months of sirolimus	48	Sirolimus (first 36, switch 44) Prednisolone MMF Azathioprine Tacrolimus	79/80 adverse cutaneous events, 6/80 stopped sirolimus because of skin ifections: bacterial 3, viral 27, fungal 13	• Pilosebaceous unit: acne 37, scalp folliculitis 21 • Aphthous ulceration 48, epistaxis 48, nail disorders 59 • Skin fragility 25, xerosis 32, edemas 44
Lally et al. 2011[70]	Oxford, England	308	Mean=128	51	Azathioprine Prednisolone Cyclosporine MMF Tacrolimus Sirolimus	• Bacterial 83 • Viral 118 • Fungal 56	• Hypertrichosis 207 • Gingival hyperplasia 84 • Sebaceous hyperplasia 77 • Striae 56 • Acne 37

IS, immunosuppression; KP, keratosis pilaris; MMF, mycophenolate mofetil; No., number; N/A, not available; RTRs, renal transplant recipients.

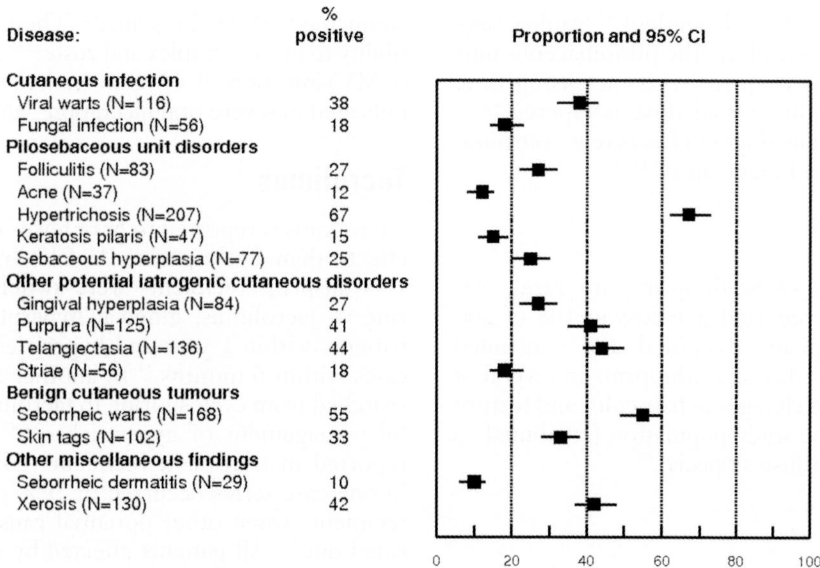

FIGURE 34-1 ■ Prevalence of benign cutaneous disease among kidney transplant recipients from Oxford (n=308).

markedly with racial group, skin type, and geographical location. In patients of northern European ancestry, the dominant long-term problem is non-melanoma skin cancer (NMSC), which is particularly burdensome in patients living in areas with high levels of ambient ultraviolet (UV) exposure. In tropical and subtropical areas, infections predominate, and Kaposi's sarcoma is seen.

DRUG SIDE EFFECTS

Over the last decade or so, immunosuppressive regimes in transplant recipients have moved away from combinations of prednisolone, azathioprine, and cyclosporine to regimens predominantly based on combinations of mycophenolate mofetil and tacrolimus with or without prednisolone. mTOR inhibitors such as sirolimus are also increasingly being used. These changes to immunosuppressive regimens have an impact on the iatrogenic cutaneous effects observed in this population. As transplant recipients are often on a number of medications in addition to their immunosuppressive drugs, it must also be taken into consideration that non-immunosuppressive medications may play a role in the etiology of some cutaneous signs seen in this population. The role played by immunosuppressive agents in the pathogenesis of cutaneous malignancy will be discussed later in the chapter. Findings from studies looking at iatrogenic cutaneous effects are summarized in Table 34-1 and we outline below the major cutaneous findings generally attributed to individual immunosuppressive agents.

Corticosteroids

Most transplant immunosuppression regimens include corticosteroids at some stage. Cutaneous effects of corticosteroid use are well recognized and cushingoid effects, including redistribution of body fat, purpura, striae, telangiectasia, and thinning of the skin, are observed in kidney transplant recipients.[6,9,14,31,68,81,117] Corticosteroids stimulate the pilosebaceous unit, possibly through an androgen-mediated mechanism, and this is responsible for the appearance of hirsutism and steroid acne. Steroid acne resembles acne vulgaris (Figure 34-2), affecting only androgen-dependent areas of skin bearing sebaceous glands (i.e., face, chest, back, and upper arms), but with predominant monomorphic papulopustules and a paucity of open comedones (blackheads). Severe forms of acne also may occur, with deep-seated inflammatory nodulocystic lesions capable of scarring. Acne is more common in younger kidney transplant recipients[70,81] and in studies of children posttransplantation is only seen in adolescents,[42,93] suggesting that hormonal factors may be important. However, in general drug-induced cutaneous changes tend to be most severe in younger

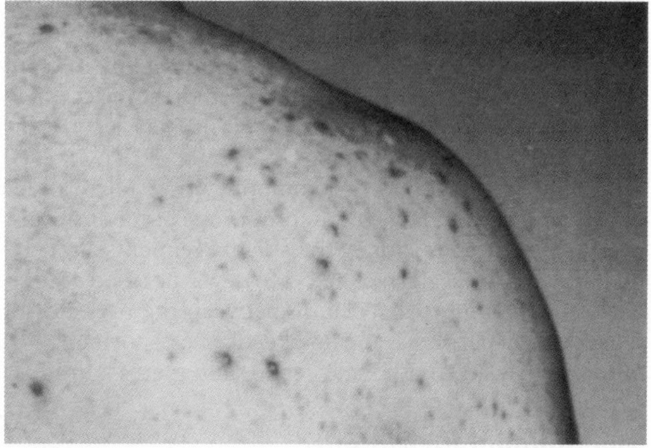

FIGURE 34-2 ■ Steroid acne with monomorphic inflamed lesions and few comedones.

children and seem to be dose-dependent.[42] Studies suggest that the effects of steroids on the pilosebaceous unit (e.g., acne) become less frequent with increasing time posttransplantation as the steroid dose is tapered,[9,31,81] whereas other chronic cushingoid effects (e.g., purpura, friable skin) persist for a longer time.[9,14,81]

Azathioprine

Cutaneous side effects of azathioprine are rarely reported. Koranda et al. reported hair loss in 108 of 200 (54%) transplant recipients examined and concluded that diffuse alopecia was due to azathioprine in several of these cases.[68] In addition changes in hair color and texture were seen in 22% of the study population (attributed to azathioprine-induced diffuse alopecia).[68]

Cyclosporine

With changes to immunosuppression regimens, far fewer transplant recipients are now exposed to cyclosporine posttransplantation. However cutaneous side effects of this drug are worth outlining as the skin is one of the major sites of accumulation of cyclosporine.[96] The commonest cyclosporine-induced mucocutaneous effects are hypertrichosis (affecting up to 100% of those taking this drug[78]) and gingival hyperplasia (affecting 2–81%[6,93]). Hypertrichosis does not appear to be an androgen-mediated side effect because cyclosporine-induced hypertrichosis is not confined to androgen-dependent areas of skin[95] and is independent of sex hormone levels.[78] Hypertrichosis is more common the longer that transplant recipients are exposed to cyclosporine.[10,70]

Other disorders of the pilosebaceous unit, including acne and epidermoid cysts, have been reported in cyclosporine-treated individuals. Clearance of prednisolone is reduced during cyclosporine therapy[98] and this may further potentiate the effects these drugs have on the pilosebaceous unit. In addition there have been case reports of acne keloidalis nuchae[5,28] and hypertrophic pseudofolliculitis barbae[73,74] in patients taking cyclosporine.

Gingival hyperplasia is more common with increasing time posttransplantation[10] and younger transplant recipients exposed to cyclosporine.[34,93] The changes may be more severe in patients with poor oral hygiene,[137] although they also occur in otherwise healthy mouths.[10] Similar gingival hyperplasia may be produced by calcium channel blockers such as nifedipine and the effect may be synergistic.[70,124] Gingival hyperplasia may also occur secondary to phenytoin intake.[80]

Sebaceous hyperplasia, commonly observed in older individuals not on any immunosuppressive medications, was first reported in kidney transplant recipients after the introduction of cyclosporine.[10] However detailed studies have since found no association between the presence of sebaceous hyperplasia and intake of cyclosporine,[36,70,114] but it is associated with male gender and increasing age.[70]

Mycophenolate Mofetil

Mycophenolate mofetil seems to have a low incidence of skin side effects, with fewer side effects documented compared with azathioprine.[123] There is increased susceptibility to herpes simplex and zoster[136] and cytomegalovirus (CMV) infections.[142] Mycophenolate mofetil has also been indicated in severe oral ulceration[49] and onycholysis.[111]

Tacrolimus

Tacrolimus is reported to have fewer mucocutaneous side effects than cyclosporine.[24,25,47,126] In one study, where 15 transplant recipients were switched from cyclosporine to tacrolimus, gingival hyperplasia resolved in all patients within 1 year and hypertrichosis resolved in all cases within 6 months.[24] In another study, patients were switched from cyclosporine to tacrolimus for the successful management of hypertrichosis.[47] Alopecia has been reported in transplant recipients taking tacrolimus and in one case series occurred in 29% of kidney transplant recipients when other potential causes of alopecia were ruled out.[135] All patients affected by clinically significant alopecia in this study were female.

Sirolimus

Cutaneous side effects in kidney transplant recipients receiving sirolimus were characterized in a study by Mahe et al.[84] Disorders of the pilosebaceous unit were frequently observed, with acneiform eruptions being the most common – observed in 46%. Among the males, acne was more frequent in patients with a history of severe acne vulgaris. Scalp folliculitis was often seen in combination with acne and males were affected more commonly than females. There was no correlation between the daily dose of sirolimus, the blood trough level of sirolimus, and the development of acne. Chronic edema was seen in 55% and angioedema in 15%. Of note, a trigger for these reported episodes of angioedema was identified in all but one patient. Mucous membrane pathologies were also very common. Aphthous ulceration was significantly associated with sirolimus therapy and was observed in 60% of the population studied. Alopecia of the scalp was observed in 11% and hypertrichosis was seen in 16%. During the 3-month period after completion of the study, 12% of patients had to stop sirolimus secondary to cutaneous effects, including hidradenitis suppurativa, severe acne, severe limb edema, and aphthous ulceration.

Management of Drug Side Effects

Many drug side effects require no specific treatment and tend to improve as doses are lowered to maintenance levels. Most cutaneous effects of immunosuppressive medication result in aesthetic problems. However compliance is often an issue, particularly in young kidney transplant recipients, therefore it is important to tackle cosmetic side effects appropriately. With changes to immunosuppression regimens, mucocutaneous effects such as gingival hyperplasia and hypertrichosis are less commonly observed now. Acne remains a significant problem for many transplant recipients however. First-line treatment for drug-induced acne is the use of topical agents. More severe cases require oral antibiotics such as a tetracycline, given as a 3–12-month course. In severe cases, isotretinoin is given at a dose of 0.5 or 1 mg/kg for a minimum of 4 months, although cheilitis, paronychia, and effects on lipids are sometimes troublesome.

INFECTIONS

The state of non-specific immunosuppression posttransplantation renders this group susceptible to many bacterial, viral, fungal, and parasitic infections. Infection rates depend on the duration and intensity of immunosuppression and geographic location (Table 34-1). Types of infection identified are also dependent on study design, with incidence studies better placed to detect acute infections (e.g., herpes simplex virus (HSV)) and prevalence studies better at identifying chronic infections (e.g., viral warts).

Bacterial Infections

Wound infections,[11,68] abscesses,[11,31,68] folliculitis,[6,9,10,11,31,59,63,81,84,93,132] impetigo,[9,42,59,63] cellulitis,[11,54,84] and erysipelas[6,7,54,59] are all observed in immunosuppressed transplant recipients. A retrospective analysis of skin infection in a transplant population found that impetigo was common in the first year posttransplant and folliculitis more common thereafter.[59] This study found that men were more likely to get folliculitis and women more likely to be infected with erysipelas and impetigo.[59] A more recent study has also found that folliculitis is up to six times more likely in males and also more common in younger transplant recipients.[70] In addition to age, time since transplantation, and gender, exposure to UV may be another risk factor for the development of bacterial infection.[133]

As in immunocompetent subjects, group A streptococci and *Staphylococcus aureus* are the commonest causative organisms. However the possibility of unusual pathogens should be borne in mind as atypical opportunistic cutaneous infections are unsurprisingly observed in kidney transplant recipients.[11,31,42,52,54,57,68,81] In view of the risk of serious infection, antibiotic treatment should be started promptly on clinical grounds, but only after obtaining appropriate specimens for bacteriological confirmation.

Viral Infections

The predominant groups of viruses affecting skin posttransplantation are the herpesviruses and the human papillomaviruses (HPV). Molluscum contagiosum due to poxvirus has also been reported in transplant populations.[42,133]

Herpesviruses

Reactivation of latent HSV and herpes zoster virus (HZV) infections may occur in kidney transplant recipients due to their immunosuppressed state. Rates of herpetic infection recorded by studies depend on whether lesions found by examination of study participants are recorded (3–17%)[9,10,54,81] or recall of infection by patient or review of clinical notes is used (13–39%).[20,68,128,132] In other studies where the method of data collection is unclear, rates of herpetic infection range from 3% to 11%.[11,31,117] More extensive disease with an atypical clinical appearance is often seen in kidney transplant recipients.[9,10,11,20] Consequently HZV does not always present with blisters or eroded areas in a dermatomal distribution and more generalized lesions are often observed. Prompt treatment with systemic antiviral therapy is recommended as generalized cutaneous disease or systemic dissemination may occur.

Herpetic infection does not appear to be related to duration of exposure to immunosuppression and can occur at any time posttransplantation.[10,81,127] Short-term exposure to UV appears to play a role in the etiology of herpetic infections, with HSV being more common in the spring and HZV more common in the summer.[133]

Human herpesvirus type 8 causes Kaposi's sarcoma and is commonest in patients from the Mediterranean, Middle East, and parts of Africa (see Chapter 35). Cutaneous CMV has been reported in transplant recipients[11] and can give rise to non-specific cutaneous findings, including ulceration.[61] Oral hairy leukoplakia, originally described in patients infected with human immunodeficiency virus (HIV), may be seen and is associated with opportunistic Epstein–Barr virus (EBV) infection.[66]

Human Papillomaviruses

Papillomaviruses are small non-enveloped DNA viruses that infect mucosal and cutaneous epithelia. Almost 100 types affecting humans (HPV) have been described to date, based on isolation of complete genomes.[62] The heterogeneous group of HPV includes the causative organisms for common warts, plantar warts, flat warts, and genital warts. HPV is a known oncovirus and its potential association with cutaneous squamous cell carcinoma (SCC) is discussed later in this chapter.

Viral warts due to infection with human HPV are common in kidney transplant recipients. Overall rates of infection reported vary from 6% to 90%.[54,76] Viral warts are usually multiple[9,14,20,22,57,76,92] and may be of cosmetic concern to transplant recipients.[128] They also tend to be resistant to treatment in transplant populations.[20,22] Common warts are the most frequent clinical type (Figure 34-3). Other clinical types observed in kidney transplant recipients include flat warts, unusual wart lesions with a pityriasis versicolor-like appearance, plantar warts,[83] and genital warts.[6,23,113] Warts presenting on severely sun-damaged skin may be difficult to distinguish clinically from other keratotic lesions, including solar keratoses, and SCC. All these lesions may coexist.

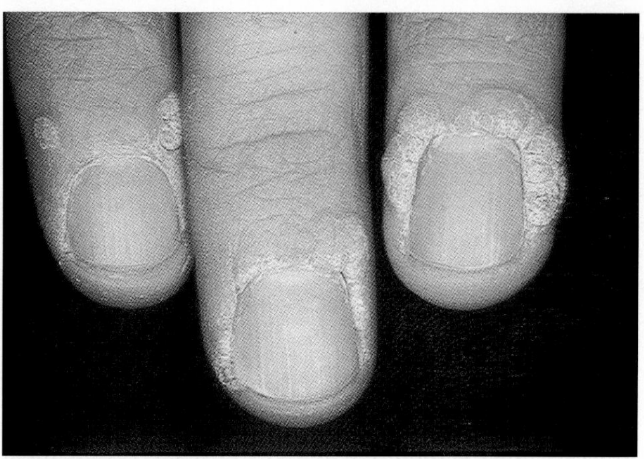

FIGURE 34-3 ■ Extensive common warts on the hands of a kidney transplant recipient.

In kidney transplant recipients, several factors (in addition to HPV infection) are thought to be important in their etiology and these include length of time exposed to immunosuppression, age at transplantation, and UV exposure. Viral warts tend to be more common in those transplanted for longer. Studies report that warts do not occur until 8 months,[68] 1 year,[128] or much later posttransplantation.[9,10,14,57,70,81,82] An Italian study observed warts in 9.7% of patients less than 3 years after transplantation and in 53% of those 9 years or more posttransplantation.[6] A French study found that age of transplantation was important for the development of viral warts, with time interval from transplantation to development of viral warts significantly shorter for patients receiving grafts after the age of 10 years.[42] Viral warts have been found more often in kidney transplant recipients with a high level of sun exposure[20,57,92] and fairer skin type.[92] Warts are more likely to occur on sun-exposed sites[6,70,81,92] and sun protection reduces the numbers of warts observed.[6] Although warts predominate on sun-exposed skin, they are not confined to these sites and in children 50% of warts are plantar.[42]

Viral warts have been reported as a risk factor for the development of cutaneous malignancy,[17,108,120] but studies by Hepburn et al.,[57] Blohme and Larko,[13] and Jensen et al. (in heart transplant recipients)[63] found no such association between viral warts and skin cancer.

Management of Cutaneous Viral Warts

If there is doubt regarding the clinical diagnosis, particularly when multiple warty lesions present on sun-damaged skin, biopsy may be helpful. However some lesions appear to be mixed histologically, with dysplasia often coexisting with viral changes in a single lesion.[12] Treating the warts rarely results in cure. Over-the-counter wart paints or gels may be of variable benefit and duct tape has been used with some reported improvement.[48] Cryosurgery using liquid nitrogen is rarely effective and repeated treatments are required as recurrence is common. Curettage may be undertaken for bulky lesions and filiform lesions. Topical treatments such as 5-fluorouracil (5-FU) and imiquimod may also be used. Success with topical or intralesional cidofovir has also been reported.[15] Lasers may be used in the treatment of warts (CO_2 and Nd:YAG), but pain, scarring, and cost are limiting factors with this therapy.

Fungal Infections

Reported frequencies of cutaneous fungal infections in kidney transplant recipients range from 7%[14] to 75%.[31] Pityriasis versicolor (5–59%),[6,9,23,31,46,52,68,81,82,84,93,117,132] onychomycosis (1.5–52%),[11,31,52,68,81,84,115,132] candidiasis (1–46%),[9,10,11,31,52,54,81,82,84,132] and deeper fungal infections, such as mucormycosis and *Cryptococcus* (1–3%),[11,31,54] have all been described in transplant populations. Factors such as gender,[81] time since transplantation,[9,81,117,132] immunosuppressive medication,[52] skin type,[91] tropical environment,[31] and UV exposure[133] may be associated with cutaneous fungal infection in kidney transplant recipients. The literature suggests that cutaneous fungal infections are more common in kidney transplant recipients in tropical and subtropical countries[31,81] (Table 34-1).

Pityriasis Versicolor

The *Malassezia* group of yeast-like fungi (previously known as *Pityrosporum*) produces a distinctive eruption with multiple minimally scaly macular lesions widely scattered over the trunk and upper arms, known as pityriasis versicolor (Figure 34-4). The macules may be hyperpigmented or hypopigmented and usually are asymptomatic, apart from their appearance. The diagnosis is made clinically and topical therapy is usually employed, with oral itraconazole rarely being used. Relapses are common. Persistence of hypopigmentation for many months is common and does not imply failure of treatment, although lesions with scaling usually harbor fungus.

Dermatophyte Infections

The skin of patients who are chronically immunosuppressed is more frequently colonized with potentially pathogenic fungi than that of healthy control subjects.[68,121] Common sites for fungal infections in kidney transplant patients are feet, scalp, and nails (Figure 34-5). Skin infections may be clinically typical (i.e., annular lesions with scaling at the margins), but more atypical presentations, including extensive skin involvement, Majocchi's granuloma, or atypical nodular lesions have been reported.[11,37,118] Whenever fungal infection is a possibility, skin scrapings, skin biopsy, and/or nail clippings should be

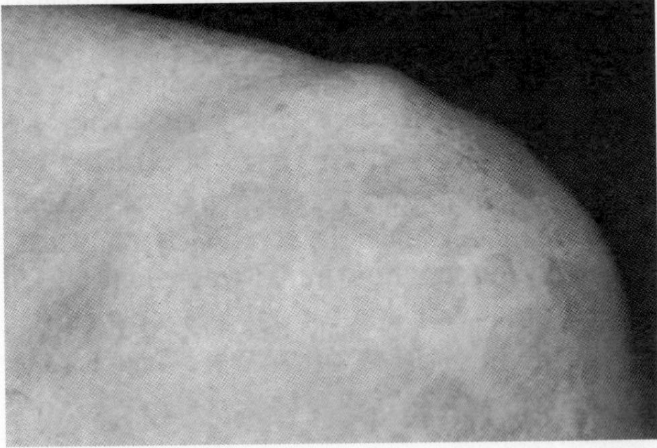

FIGURE 34-4 ■ Pityriasis versicolor: pigmented macular lesions with superficial scaling over the shoulder region.

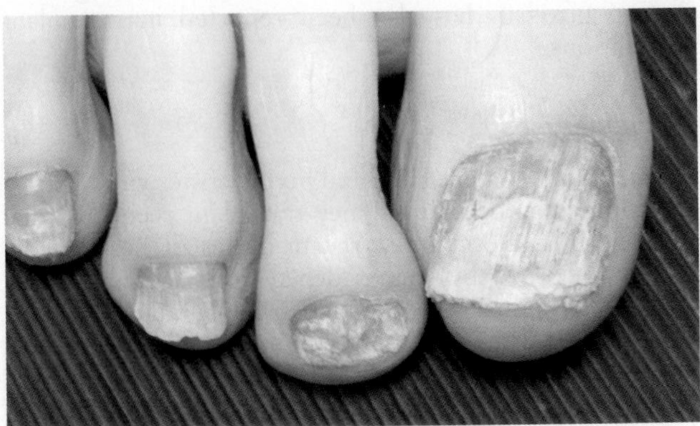

FIGURE 34-5 ■ Fungal nail infection (onychomycosis) affecting toenails.

sent for microscopy and fungal culture. Topical imidazoles and terbinafine are used in the treatment of localized dermatophyte infection of skin. Extensive, nodular, and granulomatous infections all require systemic treatment. Nail infections respond only to prolonged systemic treatment, but topical nail preparations may suppress the infection. If oral antifungal therapy is required, close liaison with the transplant physicians should take place as alteration of immunosuppressive medication doses and monitoring of drug levels are often necessary.

Candida

Infections by *Candida albicans* usually are superficial and localized, although skin lesions also may accompany systemic candidiasis. The yeast thrives in moist intertriginous sites, such as the inframammary folds, groin, vulva, and digital web spaces, producing the familiar well-demarcated glazed erythema, satellite lesions, and curdy plaques. Vesicles and superficial pustules occasionally may be present. Obesity, diabetes, and occlusion (e.g., under rings) are additional predisposing factors. Angular cheilitis and stomatitis are other common presentations.[54] Chronic paronychia, with a tender heaped-up nail fold, usually is associated with *C. albicans* infection, although other *Candida* species (e.g., *C. parapsilosis*) may be found. Frequent hand wetting and loss of the protective cuticle are important predisposing factors. Culture of *Candida* from skin swabs and nail clippings helps confirm the clinical diagnosis. Where possible, topical therapy should be employed and once again oral agents are only used in liaison with transplant physicians.

Parasitic Infestations

Scabies is rarely described in the transplant literature but rates of 3%[117] to 12%[141] have been reported. Scabies may present with the typical clinical picture of intense generalized pruritus with burrows and other lesions that characteristically favor the hands, feet, and genitals but spare the head and neck. Scabies can however be atypical and difficult to diagnose in immunosuppressed individuals and may present with a wide variety of clinical features, including facial and scalp involvement or a flexural predilection,[4,140] and exceptionally heavy mite infections are possible, producing widespread scaling mimicking chronic eczema (Norwegian or crusted scabies).[37,145] More than one application of a scabicide (e.g., permethrin 5%) to the whole body, including the head, is required to achieve cure. All contacts must be treated simultaneously to prevent reinfection.

INFLAMMATORY AND NON-INFLAMMATORY CUTANEOUS FINDINGS

Kidney transplant recipients usually have a long history of renal failure and dialysis treatment and therefore skin changes that occur posttransplantation may replace or be superimposed upon the skin changes from preceding periods. Many cutaneous conditions that present during dialysis, such as prurigo and xerosis, may improve.[132] There is, however, a paucity of information in the literature regarding prevalence of inflammatory or non-inflammatory benign cutaneous findings in transplant recipients.

Seborrheic Dermatitis

Seborrheic dermatitis (seborrheic eczema) presents with erythema, pruritus, and scaling and affects 1–3% of the immunocompetent population.[53] The etiology of this condition is not fully understood. *Malassezia* (previously *Pityrosporum*) yeasts are thought to play a role. Seborrheic dermatitis is a well-recognized manifestation of immunosuppression in HIV infection, occurring in 30–83% of this immunosuppressed population.[46,125] The reported incidence in kidney transplant recipients is lower, at 4–14%,[6,14,71,81] but higher than other inflammatory dermatoses such as psoriasis or eczema.[71] Seborrheic dermatitis is more common in males and those transplanted for longer.[71]

Treatment is with topical steroids in combination with antiyeast preparations, for example, hydrocortisone and clotrimazole or miconazole for the face and skin folds, and these or more potent steroids for less delicate skin areas.

Eczemas

In contrast with seborrhoeic eczema, other endogenous eczemas, such as atopic eczema, pompholyx eczema, and discoid eczema, have been rarely reported in kidney transplant recipients.[11,81,84] Atopic eczema in children has been reported to improve or disappear completely post-transplantation.[42] This is unsurprising given the fact that immunosuppressive agents, such as azathioprine, cyclosporine and mycophenolate mofetil, may be used in the management of severe/treatment-resistant eczemas.

Psoriasis

Pre-existing psoriasis often ceases to be a problem after transplantation because of the immunosuppressive medications.[10,42] If psoriasis is persistent posttransplantation and does not respond to simple topical measures, increasing the dose of immunosuppressive medication should be considered. Phototherapy should be avoided because of photocarcinogenesis. Pustular psoriasis has been reported following transplantation[33] and one individual taking sirolimus as part of an immunosuppression regimen developed psoriasis.[84]

Seborrheic Keratoses

Seborrheic keratoses (seborrheic warts or basal cell papillomas) are benign warty growths with a variety of clinical appearances that are common in the immunocompetent population, particularly with increasing age. They have been observed in transplant recipients,[6,23,57,68,84,117] and are more common with increasing age and in those transplanted for longer when potential confounding factors are allowed for.[72] However it is unclear whether they are more common in this population. Their importance lies

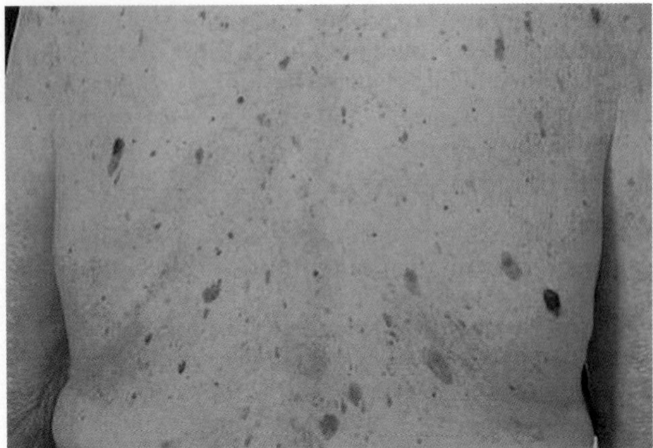

FIGURE 34-6 ■ Seborrheic keratoses on the trunk of a male patient, illustrating the number and variation in shape, size, and color that may be observed in these lesions.

in their frequent confusion by non-dermatologists with dysplastic lesions and there is a possible association with NMSC risk.[72] Seborrheic keratoses vary in color from skin-colored to deep brown or black (Figure 34-6). They are raised plaques with an irregular warty surface and may have a greasy appearance. These warts are usually multiple and vary in size from a few millimeters to a few centimeters. They do not require any treatment but are removed easily by curettage, which also allows histological confirmation of the diagnosis, or they may be treated with cryosurgery.

Skin Tags

Skin tags (fibroepithelial polyps) are pedunculated benign lesions that vary in size and color. They are frequently multiple and often seen together with seborrheic keratoses. They are commonly seen in patients with diabetes mellitus and those with an increased body mass index and this association has also been identified in kidney transplant recipients.[70] Euvrard et al. found multiple minute skin tags on the neck and axillary folds of 5.5% of a pediatric transplant population[42] and a more recent study of adult transplant recipients identified skin tags in a third of those examined.[70] Skin tags can be a major cosmetic problem (Figure 34-7) and if indicated may be removed by snip excision.

Other Benign Cutaneous Changes

Epidermoid cysts have been reported in studies of kidney transplant recipients with a prevalence of 4–28%.[6,10,81,117] Corticosteroids or cyclosporine may play a role in the etiology of epidermoid cysts through their influence on the pilosebaceous unit. Eruptive melanocytic nevi have been reported posttransplantation.[2,42,90] In one study, melanocytic nevi were reported to increase in number in 11 of 145 (8%) pediatric transplant recipients.[42] This increase was progressive and occurred after the age of 7, regardless of age of transplantation. Pyogenic granulomas have also been observed in pediatric transplant recipients (9/145, 6%).[42]

Cutaneous changes, such as xerosis and friable skin, are difficult to define and quantify but are frequently mentioned in studies that look at posttransplantation populations.[6,10,14,31,81,84,93] Numbers are often small and it is not possible to link all cutaneous findings in transplant recipients to the process of transplantation as they may be present independently of immunosuppressive medications.

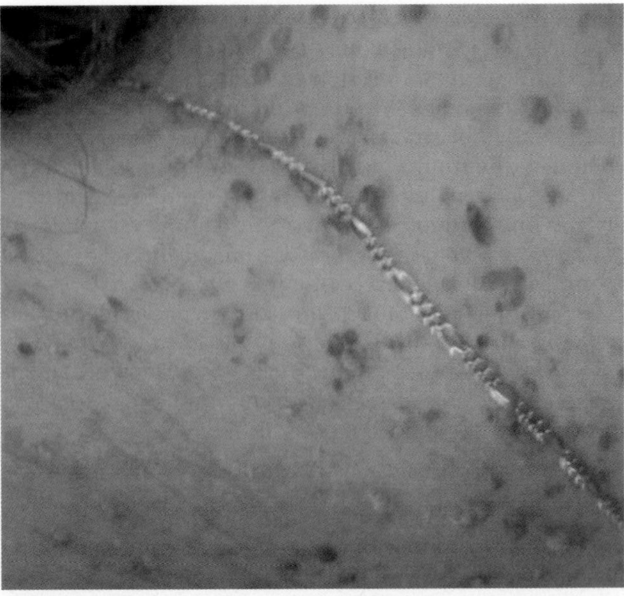

FIGURE 34-7 ■ Extensive skin tags on the neck of a kidney transplant recipient.

Nail Changes

Nail disorders of many kinds are commonly observed in transplant recipients. A comprehensive review of 205 kidney transplant recipients found nail pathology in 57%.[115] However, leukonychia was the only nail disease more common in transplant recipients than in hemodialysis patients or controls.[115] Prevalence of nail pathologies in this study increased with age and longer duration of immunosuppression but was not influenced by different immunosuppressive regimens. Other series have identified onychopathies in 7–74% of transplant recipients examined.[6,10,84,93,132] These included leukonychia,[10,132] fragile nails,[84,93,132] trachyonychia,[132] half-and-half nails,[10] and splinter hemorrhages.[84]

PREMALIGNANT AND MALIGNANT SKIN CONDITIONS

Advances in the management of kidney transplantation recipients have led to improved survival. According to the survival data from the scientific registry of transplant recipients, the 5-year survival for kidney transplants is about 85%.[116] As a result of improved survival, kidney transplant recipients face many consequences of being on long-term immunosuppression, including an increased risk of developing premalignant and malignant skin cancers. In fact, skin cancers are the most common malignancy posttransplantation, comprising almost 40% of posttransplant malignancies.[146] In addition to the increased risk of developing skin cancers in transplant recipients, the tumors also tend to behave more aggressively than in non-transplant patients.

The most frequent cutaneous malignancies in transplant recipients are NMSC, with SCC and basal cell carcinomas (BCC) representing about 90–95% of the total in multiple reported cohorts.[64,144] Although the incidence of both types of malignancies is increased, the rate of SCC is disproportionately higher. Transplant recipients are also at increased risk for developing other premalignant and malignant cutaneous conditions, including actinic keratosis (AK), Bowen's disease, malignant melanoma,[102] Kaposi's sarcoma, and Merkel cell carcinoma.[67] In addition, there have been cases of atypical fibroxanthoma (AFX),[89] lymphoma, and angiosarcoma[1] arising in transplant recipients.

In the immunocompetent population, BCC is the more common type of NMSC. However, in the transplant population the ratio is reversed, with the ratio of SCC to BCC at least 4:1.[40,139] Although the risk of BCC is increased 10-fold to 16-fold, SCC occurs at an increased frequency of 65 times that of the general population.[77,146] In addition, the majority of transplant patients usually develop multiple tumors over their lifetime. The time period between transplantation and development of a skin cancer varies from a few months to up to 20 years, depending on the time after transplantation and the level of sun exposure and skin type. In a retrospective study of 1098 kidney transplant recipients in Queensland, Australia, 45% developed at least one SCC by 10 years posttransplantation and 70% by 20 years.[18] In a comprehensive review of transplant recipients in Oxford, 19.1% of patients developed at least one malignancy, with 64% of those patients having more than one skin cancer.[16] In this study, the cumulative incidence of skin cancer reached 61% at 20 years after transplantation.[16] About 25% of transplant patients will develop a second SCC within 13 months and 50% within 3.5 years.[100] The increased incidence of SCC in transplant recipients is such that the diagnosis of a first SCC has been shown to be predictive of the development of additional NMSC within 5 years.[43] Due to longer duration of immunosuppression and younger average age at transplantation, kidney transplant recipients tend to develop more individual tumors during their lifetime.[43]

NMSCs typically arise on sun-exposed skin in areas of field cancerization. Field cancerization is the term referred to extensive areas of actinic damage, especially the forearms and dorsal hands (commonly known as transplant hands – Figure 34-8), with multiple keratotic lesions, including AK, Bowen's disease, and keratoacanthomas. The distribution of SCC is more commonly located on the head, neck, and dorsum of hands, while BCCs typically develop on the head, neck, and trunk.[55]

Transplant recipients are at a fivefold increase in the risk of malignant melanoma, and accounts for 6.2% of posttransplantation skin cancers in adults and 15% in children.[60,102] The mean duration of transplantation to the development of melanoma is 5 years.[40] The risk factors for the development of melanoma in transplant recipients are similar to those of the general population, including fair complexion, light hair and eyes, tendency to freckle, and large number of nevi, the latter being important in children with kidney transplants.[24,40] In a recent study of melanoma in transplant patients, the overall survival rate of patients with a history of transplantation was worse, regardless of Breslow thickness or Clark level, compared to expected survival rates derived from cases reported in the Surveillance, Epidemiology, and End Results Program. In addition, immunosuppressed organ transplant recipients with thicker melanoma (Breslow thickness of 1.51–3.00 mm or Clark level III of IV) had a significantly poorer malignant melanoma cause-specific survival rate.[21]

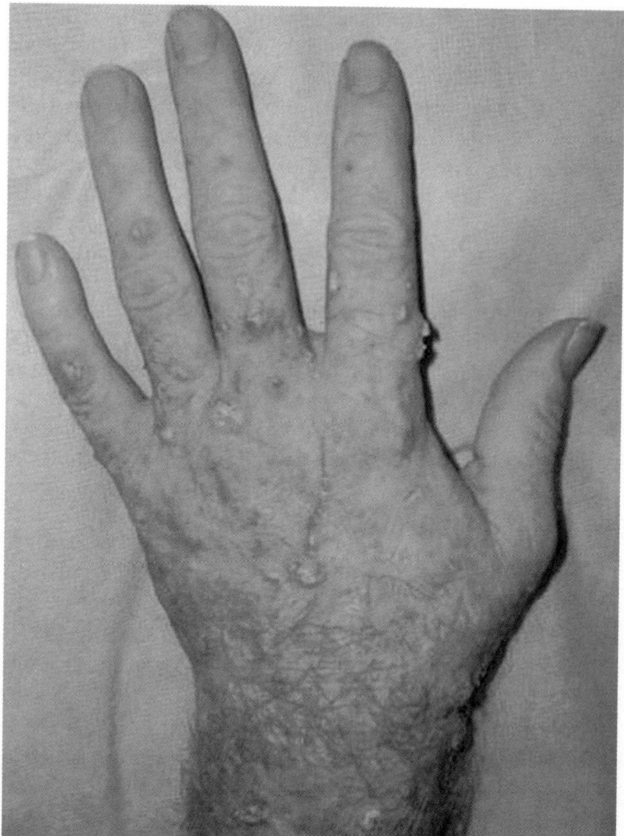

FIGURE 34-8 ■ Field cancerization on the hands, also known as transplant hands.

The risk of skin cancers in the pediatric (<18 years old) transplant population is also increased compared to the general pediatric population. In a Dutch pediatric kidney transplant recipient population, the standardized risk for development of NMSC was found to be 222-fold higher.[41] Skin cancers typically arise 12–15 years after transplantation, at an average age of 26–28 years.[41] SCCs are also more common than BCCs in the pediatric transplant recipient population. In one series, NMSC spread to lymph nodes was more common in pediatric transplant recipients compared to adults.[101]

Premalignant Skin Tumors

Actinic Keratosis

AK manifests as scaly, erythematous papules arising on sun-exposed skin, commonly on the face, dorsal hands, and balding scalp, usually 1–3 mm. In transplant recipients, AK can coalesce, leading to field cancerization. Actinic cheilitis occurs when AKs coalesce on the lower lip, also common in transplant recipients. Histologically, they represent atypical keratinocytes in the basal portion of the epidermis with evidence of solar damage. The major risk factor for development of AKs is long-term exposure to UV light, especially in the UVB spectrum (290–320 nm).[86] Emerging evidence suggests that HPV, particularly beta PV, also plays a role in the development of AKs.[19]

Although there are no population-based studies to determine the true prevalence of AKs in transplant patients, the prevalence of AKs at a single center in France was found to be 54%.[44]

They are considered to represent one end of a spectrum of cutaneous neoplasia on which SCCs represent the opposite, most severe end of the spectrum. In transplant recipients, AKs tend to appear 2–6 months after transplantation. They are usually multiple, recur after treatment, and evolve more rapidly into SCC compared to immunocompetent patients. Thus, AKs require early treatment and close follow-up, usually every 6 months.[129]

Bowen's Disease

Normally manifesting as well-defined scaly plaques on sun-exposed surfaces of the skin, Bowen's disease is SCC in situ, representing a true malignancy. The annual incidence of Bowen's disease in one kidney transplant group in the United Kingdom was 2.52%,[109] while the incidence was 16.3% in a kidney transplant population in Australia.[29] Due to the potential to become invasive, Bowen's disease should be recognized and treated early.

Porokeratosis

Porokeratosis can present clinically in a variety of lesions, all unified by classic histology. The most common presentation of porokeratosis in transplant recipients is disseminated superficial actinic porokeratosis (DSAP).[58] DSAP presents with multiple small (1–2 cm) circular plaques with central atrophy and a peripheral keratotic raised rim, distributed over sun-exposed surfaces, commonly involving the extremities. Porokeratosis of Mibelli presents as a single well-demarcated circular plaque that slowly expands in a centripetal fashion with central atrophy and raised border. Other variants, including linear porokeratosis, punctate porokeratosis, and porokeratosis of the palms and soles, have also been described.[79,134]

In one series of kidney transplant patients in Spain, 10.68% developed porokeratosis, with a mean time to development of 3.5 years.[58] In another series of kidney transplant, 8% developed porokeratosis by 15 years.[100] In these studies, none of the lesions evolved into SCC. Despite this favorable prognosis, there has been a case report documenting the development of a fatal SCC within a chronic porokeratosis in a kidney transplant recipient.[122] Thus, sufficient evidence exists of the potential progression of a porokeratosis to SCC in kidney transplant patients to warrant total body skin exams.

Malignant Skin Tumors

Keratoacanthoma

A variant of a SCC, keratoacanthomas typically arise rapidly on sun-exposed skin. Typical lesions present as a firm, dome-shaped tumor with a central keratin core, and can often be ulcerated. Due to the central core, they are often referred to as "crateriform." In immunocompetent patients, these lesions can often regress. However, any rapidly growing skin lesion in a transplant patient should be biopsied, and treated aggressively if pathology suggests a keratoacanthoma.[131]

Squamous Cell Carcinoma

SCCs are the most frequent type of skin cancer in transplant patients. Due to the varied clinical presentations, recognition of any suspicious lesion warrants biopsy for further investigation. In transplant patients, SCCs present as enlarging, raised, keratotic lesions on an indurated, erythematous base. They are often tender, and can become ulcerated (Figure 34-9). SCCs can be aggressive, metastasizing to the lymph nodes, and can cause death. The risk of local recurrence is 13.4%, usually during the

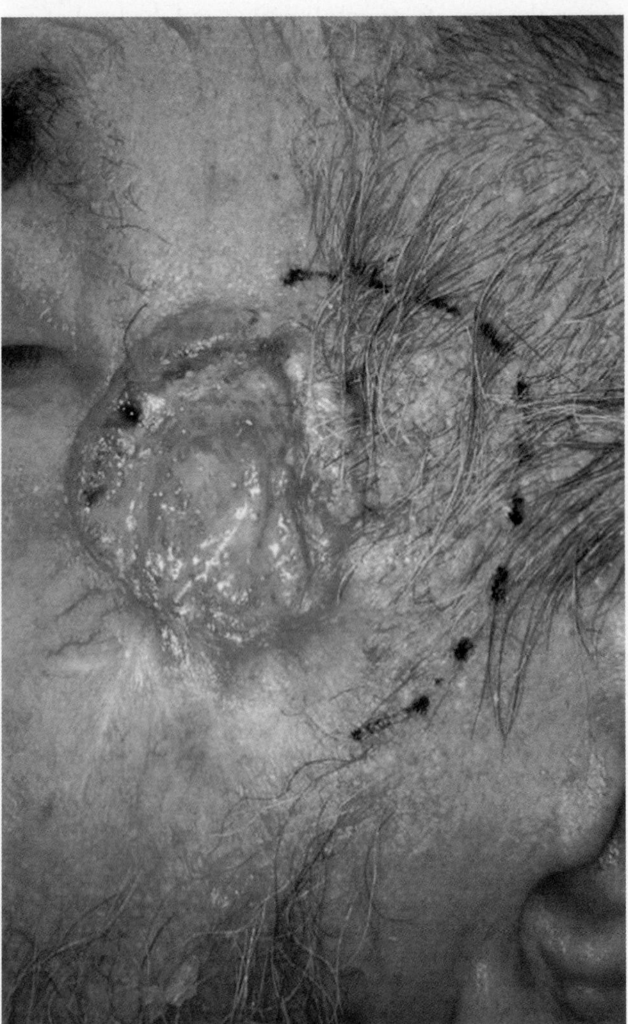

FIGURE 34-9 ■ Squamous cell carcinoma on the left temple.

TABLE 34-2 High-Risk Features of Squamous Cell Carcinoma in Organ Transplant Patients

Large size (>2 cm)
Multiple squamous cell carcinomas
High-risk location (ear, lips, over parotid gland, scalp, or temple)
In-transit metastatic lesion
Recurrence
Histology
Poorly differentiated
- Perineural invasion
- Deep invasion

From Zwald F, Brown M. Skin cancer in solid organ transplant recipients: advances in therapy and management: Part 2. Management of skin cancer in solid organ transplant recipients. J Am Acad Dermatol 2011;65:263–79.

first 6 months of excision.[144] The risk of metastasis of SCC in the general population is 0.5–5%. The risk increases to 8% for organ transplant recipients.[119]

High-risk clinical features of SCC include size >2 cm and location of ear and lip.[45] High-risk clinical and histological features of SCC are found in Table 34-2.[147] Invasive SCCs commonly occur on the head and neck in transplant patients, especially the lip.[100] After treatment, patients should be regularly followed for recurrence.

Basal Cell Carcinoma

Unlike SCCs in transplant patients, BCCs have a less varied clinical presentation, although BCC has distinct clinical subtypes.[131] The nodular variant of BCC presents as a flesh-colored pearly papule with a characteristic rolled border, often with central ulceration and overlying telangiectases. The superficial BCC presents as an enlarging erythematous plaque with minimal overlying scale and a scalloped border. A morpheaform variant, or scar-like, BCC appears as an indurated, atrophic plaque with ill-defined borders. In some cases, BCC can contain hyperpigmentation. Although BCCs are often locally aggressive and rarely metastasize, follow-up is still necessary after treatment.

Malignant Melanoma

The subtypes of melanoma are derived from clinicopathologic features rather than outcome, and include the following: superficial spreading, lentigo maligna, nodular, and acral lentiginous. All variants, with the exception of amelanotic melanoma, present as changing pigmented lesions. The "ABCDE" acronym summarizes the clinical features of melanoma: asymmetry, border irregularity, color variation, diameter more than 6 mm, and/or evolution (i.e., change in size, color, shape, surface texture, or symptoms).[85,131] Loss of color should also raise suspicion. Due to the fact that melanomas can arise de novo or within pre-existing nevus, total body skin examination is important. Any suspicious lesion should be biopsied, and treatment is based upon the pathology (Breslow depth ± ulceration or mitoses) and lymph node involvement of melanoma.

Merkel Cell Carcinoma

Merkel cell carcinoma is a rare, but highly aggressive, neoplasm of neuroendocrine origin with a tendency to distant metastatic spread. Many of these lesions present on the head and neck. Lesions present as dome-shaped pinkish-red to bluish-brown papules or nodules, often with overlying telangiectases. They often grow rapidly and frequently ulcerate. Usually, at the time of diagnosis, they are less than 2 cm in size but can demonstrate satellite lesions, a sign of in-transit spread to lymph nodes.[131,146]

Atypical Fibroxanthoma and Undifferentiated Pleomorphic Sarcoma

AFX is a rare spindle cell neoplasm that presents as a solitary asymptomatic pink to red nodule, usually arising on the head and neck. AFX is considered to be an indeterminate lesion, a less aggressive superficial variant of undifferentiated pleomorphic sarcoma, previously known as malignant fibrous histiocytoma. Both AFX and undifferentiated pleomorphic sarcoma have a higher rate of local recurrence and metastasis in immunocompromised organ transplant patients.[89] Treatment should be aggressive, with Mohs micrographic surgery (MMS) or wide local excision (with 2-cm margins) followed by wide-field adjuvant radiation therapy.[89]

Risk Factors and Pathogenesis

Risk factors for the development of skin cancer in organ transplant recipients include Fitzpatrick skin type I–III, cumulative sun exposure, propensity to sunburn, and intensity and duration of immunosuppression (Table 34-3).[146] Genetic factors, infection with HPV, history of lymphoma or leukemia, and previous history of voriconazole use are additional factors that contribute to the pathogenesis of skin cancer.

Skin Phototype and Ultraviolet Exposure

As in the general population, the majority of skin cancers arise on sun-exposed skin because the major risk factor for developing skin cancers is UV exposure.[7] Increased age

TABLE 34-3 Risk Factors for Development of Skin Cancer in Organ Transplant Patients

Fitzpatrick skin type I–III
Increasing age at transplantation
Duration and level of immunosuppression
Type of organ transplant (heart/lung > kidney > liver)
Previous transplant
Squamous cell carcinoma before transplant
History of lymphoma pre-/posttransplant
Pretransplant end-organ disease (e.g., rheumatoid arthritis, systemic lupus erythematosus, or autoimmune hepatitis)
Liver transplant recipients with psoriasis on previous biologic therapy/psoralen plus ultraviolet A light phototherapy

From Zwald F, Brown M. Skin cancer in solid organ transplant recipients: advances in therapy and management: Part 1. Epidemiology of skin cancer in solid organ transplant recipients. J Am Acad Dermatol 2011;65:253–61.

is also correlated with the development of skin cancers, most likely due to the greater total UV radiation exposure in the elderly.[59] The use of adopting sun-protective behaviors has shown to decrease the development of SCC in transplant patients.[43] Chronic sun exposure causes AK and SCC, while intermittent high-dose exposure causes melanoma and BCC.

UV radiation, particularly UVB (290–320 nm), produces mutagenesis through induction of DNA byproducts as well as immune function dysregulation. The major target for UV-induced damage is p53 tumor suppressor gene, and causes dipyrimidine cyclobutane dimers. UV radiation reduces the number of Langerhans cells and impairs their antigen-presenting capacity. The stimulation of keratinocytes and macrophages to produce certain cytokines, such as interleukin (IL)-10, is also induced by UV exposure. The combination of DNA damage and reactive oxygen species and cytokine production produces an environment for tumor formation and progression.[110]

Immunosuppressive Drugs

Although immunosuppressive drugs are critical to transplant graft survival, chronic immunosuppression accelerates the development of skin cancers through direct oncogenic effect, impaired immunosurveillance, and inability to correct precancerous changes. The incidence of skin cancer is directly proportional to the dosage, duration, and even type of immunosuppression.[146]

Azathioprine photosensitizes human skin to UVA radiation. The skin of patients who are taking azathioprine contains 6-thioguanine, which is a strong UVA chromophore, resulting in abnormal photosensitivity, production of reactive oxygen species, and accelerated photocarcinogensis.[104,146] Studies have shown that tacrolimus and cyclosporine, both calcineurin inhibitors, produce their tumorigenesis via expression of transforming growth factor-β as well as decreased tumor surveillance via decreased production of IL-2.[75] Increased risk of skin cancer has also been connected to patients receiving induction therapy with antithymocyte globulin, OKT3, or monoclonal anti-IL-2 receptor antibodies.[51,146]

Multiple studies have shown that patients receiving triple immunosuppression (with cyclosporine, prednisone, and azathioprine or sirolimus) were at higher risk of developing skin cancers compared to patients on dual therapy (prednisone and azathioprine or sirolimus).[27]

Human Papillomavirus

HPV is a known oncovirus, causing carcinogenesis of anogenital malignancies. There have been studies to confirm its role in the development of SCC.[130] The exact mechanism of pathogenesis of HPV in NMSC is uncertain at this point. Although transplant patients have been shown to have an increased quantity of low- and medium-risk HPV types in SCC, there is also a high prevalence of HPV infection in non-lesional areas as well.[56,130,146]

HPV-encoded oncoproteins E6 and E7 are associated with malignant transformation of cells. In a study of transplant patients, E6 and E7 transcripts of HPVs 8, 9, and 15 were found in AK and SCC.[35] A recent study found that HPV (beta PV genus type) 36, 5, 9, and 24 were associated with an increased risk of SCC in transplant patients.[107] More research is necessary to elucidate the exact mechanism further and the role of HPV in the carcinogenesis of NMSC.

Genetic Factors

Mutations in the p53 tumor suppressor gene are the most commonly found mutation detected in organ transplant patients. A common polymorphism at exon 72 leading to either a proline or arginine has been described in some studies to correlate with an increased risk of development of SCC in kidney transplant patients, and in other studies to have no association.[26,97] Although no single factor is causative in skin cancer carcinogenesis in transplant patients, interactions of some mechanisms with known environmental factors can lead to an increased risk.

Voriconazole

In transplant patients who develop invasive aspergillosis, voriconazole, a second-generation antifungal, is an approved treatment. In addition, voriconazole is used off-label for long-term prophylaxis against invasive fungal infections in solid-organ transplant patients. One of the side effects of voriconazole is photosensitivity, resulting in reversible sunburn-like erythema on sun-exposed sites. However, recent studies have suggested that transplant patients on voriconazole have an increased risk of developing SCC skin cancer, suggesting that voriconazole-induced photosensitivity may be carcinogenic.[32,88]

The mechanism by which voriconazole photosensitivity occurs is unclear. Chronic voriconazole-associated photosensitivity could potentially accelerate UV radiation-induced skin damage, thus promoting the development of skin cancer. Cytochrome P-450 enzymes CYP2C19, CYP2C9, and CYP3A4 metabolize voriconazole. Homozygous polymorphisms in CYP2C19 result in higher serum voriconazole levels. Studies are needed to determine if the pharmacokinetics, host genetic factors, and relationship with UV exposure are factors in increased risk of SCC in voriconazole use. Thus, strict photoprotective behaviors and careful consideration of long-term voriconazole use are required in organ transplant patients at risk for skin cancer.[32,39,146]

Management

The dermatologic management of transplant patients requires a multidisciplinary approach, with involvement of the dermatologist, transplant team, medical and surgical oncologist, and radiation oncologist. Evaluation should begin before transplantation with a baseline total body skin examination and education of their increased risk of skin cancer development. Daily application of broad-spectrum sunscreen (containing both UVA and UVB coverage), wide-brimmed hats, long sleeves, and avoidance of sun tanning should be encouraged.

Frequent skin exams are necessary in patients with multiple skin cancers, and patients should be educated regarding monitoring their skin for any new or changing

TABLE 34-4 Follow-up Intervals for Total Body Skin Examination for Solid-Organ Transplantation

Patient Risk Factor	Interval for Total Body Skin Examination (No. of Months)
No skin cancer/field disease	12
Field disease	3–6
One non-melanoma skin cancer	3–6
Multiple non-melanoma skin cancers	3
High-risk squamous cell carcinoma or melanoma	3
Metastatic squamous cell carcinoma or melanoma	1–3

From Zwald F, Brown M. Skin cancer in solid organ transplant recipients: advances in therapy and management: Part 2. Management of skin cancer in solid organ transplant recipients. J Am Acad Dermatol 2011;65:263–79.

lesions (Table 34-4). Patients should be educated on performing skin exams, as well as palpating draining lymph nodes in high-risk patients. Any suspicious lesion should be biopsied and treated promptly.

Topical Therapy

Field cancerization becomes a treatment dilemma in patients with organ transplants. A patient might have one clinically apparent tumor arising in a surrounding area of precancerous lesions, all of which have malignant potential. Treatment of these entire areas can be difficult with excision or ablative techniques. New developments in the treatment of field cancerization include cyclical implementation of topical therapies and photodynamic therapy (PDT). If lesions persist despite these efforts, a skin biopsy is necessary to rule out underlying skin cancer.

Topical 5-Fluorouracil. 5-FU is a chemotherapeutic agent that inhibits pyrimidine metabolism and DNA synthesis. Applied topically to affected skin twice daily, 5-FU can be used to decrease the size and number of lesions in transplant patients.[103] Common side effects include erythematous inflammation and patient discomfort. One of the main benefits of 5-FU is that the patient can apply it at home. Topical 5-FU can be even more effective under occlusion, especially on thick keratotic lesions on the lower extremities or upper extremities with Unna boot wraps changed weekly. The use of 5-FU should be avoided in patients taking nucleoside analogues (brivudin and sorivudin) because of systemic toxicity of 5-FU.

Topical Imiquimod. Imiquimod is a non-specific immune modulator that has been shown to be safe and effective in the treatment of AK in transplant patients. Imiquimod 5% cream is typically used three to five times per week for 16 weeks, and it can also be applied at home by the patient. Studies have demonstrated its efficacy, with clearance rates up to 62%.[138] Patients using this treatment method should look for inflammation. If no inflammation is present, application under occlusion can be tried. However, if there is still no inflammation, then treatment should be changed to another agent.

Photodynamic Therapy

PDT is another treatment modality for areas of field cancerization. PDT involves the use of an exogenously administered precursor of photosensitizer protoprohyrin IX synthesis (usually either aminolevulinic acid or methyl aminolevulinate) that is activated by light, producing reactive oxygen species and destroying tumor cells. PDT has been effective in the treatment of AK and superficial NMSC in transplant patients.[106,143,147] PDT must be administered under physician supervision in a clinic setting. Common side effects are pain and erythema.

Capecitabine

Capecitabine, a prodrug of 5-deoxy-5-fluorouridine, is metabolized by the liver to 5-FU. Initially used for the treatment of metastatic breast and colon cancer, the use of systemic 5-FU has been shown to be beneficial in reducing the development of precancerous and cancerous lesions in organ transplant patients.[38,147] In a recent retrospective review performed at the University of Minnesota, 15 organ transplant patients who were given low-dose capecitabine had lower rates of developing NMSC and AK compared to the period prior to capecitabine treatment. However, grade 3 and 4 toxicities were common, causing discontinuation.[65] Prospective studies are needed to determine the long-term efficacy and safety of lower doses.

Systemic Retinoids

Retinoid derivatives, such as acitretin, have been shown to be effective in the suppression of SCC development, including reduction in AKs and SCCs.[8,50] Indications for the initiation of systemic retinoids in organ transplant patients are the following: development of multiple SCCs per year (5–10/year); development of multiple SCCs in high-risk locations (head/neck); patients with a history of lymphoma/leukemia and SCCs; a single SCC with high metastatic risk; metastatic SCC; explosive SCC development; and eruptive keratoacanthomas.[69]

Low-dose acitretin 10 mg therapy should be started to minimize side effects with slow titration by 10-mg increments at 2–4-week intervals to the target dose of 20–25 mg daily. Side effects are dose-related, with dry eyes and mouth being the most common, while dry skin and pruritus are less common. Acitretin is a known teratogen (pregnancy category X) and its use should be carefully considered in childbearing women who wish to conceive in 3 years. Severe hyperlipidemia that is refractory to standard treatment is a contraindication. Lab monitoring must be performed frequently, including a baseline pregnancy test, complete blood count, fasting lipid panel, liver panel, and serum creatinine.

Chemoprevention with oral retinoids is a lifelong treatment. When the medication is discontinued, a rebound effect occurs that is difficult to control. Patients can experience the eruption of multiple aggressive SCCs over a relatively short period of time. Thus, reduction of the dosage of acitretin is usually successful at maintaining patient compliance while still benefiting from chemoprevention.[147]

Altering the Immunosuppressive Regimen

Given that the type, duration, and intensity of immunosuppressive therapy is associated with an increased risk of skin cancer, adjusting the immunosuppression regimen to the least amount of immunosuppression necessary to support graft survival is beneficial to reducing the risk of development of skin cancers. Expert consensus survey by the International Transplant Skin Cancer Collaborative and the Skin Cancer in Organ Transplant Patients Europe supports the modification of immunosuppression in transplant patients with numerous or life-threatening NMSCs and melanoma.[99] Patients at high risk for metastases from SCC or patients with 5–10 high-risk SCCs per year are candidates for immunosuppressive therapy modification.

Modification of immunosuppressive therapy can be done in multiple ways in collaboration with the transplant team. Either reduction in the total dosage of the immunosuppressive medication, or in cases of triple therapy regimens, discontinuing one agent (usually azathioprine) can reduce the overall risk of skin cancer. Recent studies have shown that mammalian target of rapamycin (mTOR) inhibitors, such as sirolimus and everolimus, may confer a decreased risk of skin cancer development in posttransplant patients relative to traditional calcineurin inhibitors.[75,87] A recently published randomized control trial, CONVERT, showed that patients who were transitioned to sirolimus after 2 years posttransplant had a statistically significant reduction in the number of NMSCs compared to patients who stayed on calcineurin inhibitors.[3] Currently, there are multiple ongoing randomized control trials to evaluate the role of the antineoplastic effects of sirolimus in transplant patients. Although there has been evidence to support the safety of conversion to sirolimus, the frequency of side effects, such as ulcers, edema, acneiform eruptions, hyperlipidemia, thrombocytopenia, and delayed wound healing, may offset the use of sirolimus.[75]

Surgery

Surgical treatment of premalignant and malignant skin lesions can be performed through cryosurgery, electrodesiccation and curettage (ED&C), standard surgical excision, and MMS.

Premalignant skin lesions, such as warts and AKs, can be treated with liquid nitrogen. Any lesion that is not responding to aggressive cryosurgery should be biopsied. ED&C is performed under local anesthesia, and involves a histological sample with destruction to the base of the lesion. ED&C can be used in the treatment of hyperkeratotic AK, Bowen's disease, and superficial BCCs, and SCC in situ, or in patients with multiple lesions, where ED&C is easier to tolerate.[147]

In patients with biopsy-proven skin cancer, MMS or excision with clear surgical margins is the treatment of choice. Patients with high-risk SCC should be treated and monitored aggressively (Table 34-2). In these patients, MMS is the standard treatment, allowing for tissue conservation where needed with high cure rates. In cases of high-risk SCC, preoperative evaluation with computed tomography (CT) or magnetic resonance imaging (MRI) may be required to evaluate deep extension or nodal involvement. Adjuvant therapy with either node dissection and/or radiation therapy for high-risk SCC should also be considered, especially if perineural invasion is present, even in the absence of clinically palpable lymphadenopathy. Patients with metastatic SCC to the lymph nodes portend a poor prognosis. Treatment of these patients requires surgery with parotidectomy with or without neck dissection in operable patients along with adjuvant radiation therapy to improve local and regional control.[129,147] Patients should be followed closely, with frequent positron emission tomography CT or MRI. The use of radiation therapy in transplant patients is outlined in Table 34-5.[147]

TABLE 34-5 Indications for Radiation Therapy in the Treatment of Squamous Cell Carcinomas in Organ Transplant Recipients

Non-surgical candidates
Adjuvant therapy for incomplete tumor resection
Adjuvant therapy for lymph node involvement
Adjuvant therapy for perineural tumor involvement

The role of chemotherapy in the treatment of high-risk SCC remains unclear.[147] However, therapy targeting epidermal growth factor receptors, such as cetuximab, is being explored in the treatment of SCC in clinical trials.[105]

In-transit metastases of high-risk SCC in transplant patients present as rapidly enlarging subcutaneous nodules with no epidermal extension in close proximity to the primary or recurrent tumor. Treatment of these lesions is individualized, but usually requires surgical excision followed by adjuvant radiation therapy.[30,147]

Role of Sentinel Lymph Node Biopsy

Surgical staging of the primary nodal basin achieved by sentinel lymph node biopsy (SLNB) has been shown to be a prognostic factor in melanoma. There are emerging data that SLNB may have a role in high-risk SCC. SLNB may accurately detect subclinical lymph node metastasis in patients, potentially allowing for the earliest possible therapeutic lymphadenopathy if the SLNB was positive.[112,147] Prospective studies are needed to determine which risk factors predict nodal and distant metastases, and thus which patients would warrant an SLNB.

SUMMARY

Given that organ transplant patients are at increased risk for developing skin cancers, a multidisciplinary approach is necessary in caring for these patients. Early and aggressive treatment of skin cancers is necessary. Education regarding sun-protective behaviors is essential, as well as counseling patients on self-exams and early treatment of new or changing skin lesions. Initiation of chemoprophylaxis is also important in the management of organ transplant patients. Baseline total body skin exams should be performed. Regularly scheduled skin exams can lessen the morbidity associated with skin cancer, as well as improve overall quality of life in the posttransplantation period.[147]

REFERENCES

1. Ahmed I, Hamacher KL. Angiosarcoma in a chronically immunosuppressed renal transplant recipient: report of a case and review of the literature. Am J Dermatopathol 2002;24(4):330–5.
2. Alaibac M, Piaserico S, Rossi CR, et al. Eruptive melanocytic nevi in patients with renal allografts: report of 10 cases with dermoscopic findings. J Am Acad Dermatol 2003;49:1020.
3. Alberu J, Pascoe MD, Campistol JM, et al. Lower malignancy rates in renal allograft recipients converted to sirolimus-based, calcineurin inhibitor-free immunotherapy: 24-month results from the CONVERT trial. Transplantation 2011;92(3):303–10.
4. Anolik MA, Rudolph RI. Scabies simulating Darier disease in an immunosuppressed host. Arch Dermatol 1976;112:73.
5. Azurdia RM, Graham RM, Weismann K, et al. Acne keloidalis in caucasian patients on cyclosporin following organ transplantation. Br J Dermatol 2000;143:465.
6. Barba A, Tessari G, Boschiero L, et al. Renal transplantation and skin diseases: review of the literature and results of a 5-year follow-up of 285 patients. Nephron 1996;73:131.
7. Bavinck JN, De Boer A, Vermeer BJ, et al. Sunlight, keratotic skin lesions and skin cancer in renal transplant recipients. Br J Dermatol 1993;129(3):242–9.
8. Bavinck JN, Tieben LM, Van der Woude FJ, et al. Prevention of skin cancer and reduction of keratotic skin lesions during acitretin therapy in renal transplant recipients: a double-blind, placebo-controlled study. J Clin Oncol 1995;13(8):1933–8.
9. Bencini PL, Montagnino G, De Vecchi A, et al. Cutaneous manifestations in renal transplant recipients. Nephron 1983;34:79.
10. Bencini PL, Montagnino G, Sala F, et al. Cutaneous lesions in 67 cyclosporin-treated renal transplant recipients. Dermatologica 1986;172:24.
11. Bergfeld WF, Roenigk Jr HH. Cutaneous complications of immunosuppressive therapy. A review of 215 renal transplant patients. Cutis 1978;22:169.
12. Blessing K, McLaren KM, Benton EC, et al. Histopathology of skin lesions in renal allograft recipients – an assessment of viral features and dysplasia. Histopathology 1989;14:129.
13. Blohme I, Larko O. Premalignant and malignant skin lesions in renal transplant patients. Transplantation 1984;37:165.
14. Blohme I, Larko O. Skin lesions in renal transplant patients after 10–23 years of immunosuppressive therapy. Acta Derm Venereol 1990;70:491.
15. Bonatti H, Aigner F, De Clercq E, et al. Local administration of cidofovir for human papilloma virus associated skin lesions in transplant recipients. Transpl Int 2007;20:238.
16. Bordea C, Wojnarowska F, Millard PR, et al. Skin cancers in renal-transplant recipients occur more frequently than previously recognized in a temperate climate. Transplantation 2004;77(4):574–9.
17. Bouwes Bavinck JN, Euvrard S, Naldi L, et al. Keratotic skin lesions and other risk factors are associated with skin cancer in organ-transplant recipients: a case-control study in The Netherlands, United Kingdom, Germany, France, and Italy. J Invest Dermatol 2007;127:1647.
18. Bouwes Bavinck JN, Hardie DR, Green A, et al. The risk of skin cancer in renal transplant recipients in Queensland, Australia. A follow-up study. Transplantation 1996;61(5):715–21.
19. Bouwes Bavinck JN, Neale RE, Abeni D, et al. Multicenter study of the association between betapapillomavirus infection and cutaneous squamous cell carcinoma. Cancer Res 2010;70(23):9777–86.
20. Boyle J, MacKie RM, Briggs JD, et al. Cancer, warts, and sunshine in renal transplant patients. A case-control study. Lancet 1984;1:702.
21. Brewer JD, Christenson LJ, Weaver AL, et al. Malignant melanoma in solid transplant recipients: collection of database cases and comparison with surveillance, epidemiology, and end results data for outcome analysis. Arch Dermatol 2011;147(7):790–6.
22. Brown JH, Hutchison T, Kelly AM, et al. Dermatologic lesions in a transplant population. Transplantation 1988;46:530.
23. Bunney MH, Benton EC, Barr BB, et al. The prevalence of skin disorders in renal allograft recipients receiving cyclosporin a compared with those receiving azathioprine. Nephrol Dial Transplant 1990;5:379.
24. Busque S, Demers P, Saint-Louis G, et al. Hypertrichosis and gingival hypertrophy regression in renal transplants following the substitution of cyclosporin by tacrolimus. Ann Chir 1999;53:687.
25. Busque S, Demers P, St-Louis G, et al. Conversion from neoral (cyclosporine) to tacrolimus of kidney transplant recipients for gingival hyperplasia or hypertrichosis. Transplant Proc 1998;30:1247.
26. Cairey-Remonnay SHO, Mougin C, Algros MP, et al. TP53 polymorphism of exon 4 at codon 72 in cutaneous squamous cell carcinoma and benign epithelial lesions of renal transplant recipients and immunocompetent individuals: lack of correlation with human papillomavirus status. J Invest Dermatol 2002;118(6):1026–31.
27. Campistol JM, Eris J, Oberbauer R, et al. Sirolimus therapy after early cyclosporine withdrawal reduces the risk for cancer in adult renal transplantation. J Am Soc Nephrol 2006;17(2):581–9.
28. Carnero L, Silvestre JF, Guijarro J, et al. Nuchal acne keloidalis associated with cyclosporin. Br J Dermatol 2001;144:429.
29. Carroll RP, Ramsay HM, Fryer AA, et al. Incidence and prediction of nonmelanoma skin cancer post-renal transplantation: a prospective study in Queensland, Australia. Am J Kidney Dis 2003;41(3):676–83.
30. Carucci JA, Martinez JC, Zeitouni NC, et al. In-transit metastasis from primary cutaneous squamous cell carcinoma in organ transplant recipients and nonimmunosuppressed patients: clinical characteristics, management, and outcome in a series of 21 patients. Dermatol Surg 2004;30(4 Pt 2):651–5.
31. Chugh KS, Sharma SC, Singh V, et al. Spectrum of dermatological lesions in renal allograft recipients in a tropical environment. Dermatology 1994;188:108.
32. Clancy CJ, Nguyen MH. Long-term voriconazole and skin cancer: is there cause for concern? Curr Infect Dis Rep 2011;13(6):536–43.
33. Coulson IH, Evans CD, Holden CA. Generalized pustular psoriasis after renal transplantation – failure to suppress with cyclosporin A. Clin Exp Dermatol 1988;13:416.
34. Daley TD, Wysocki GP, Day C. Clinical and pharmacologic correlations in cyclosporine-induced gingival hyperplasia. Oral Surg Oral Med Oral Pathol 1986;62:417.
35. Dang C, Koehler A, Forschner T, et al. E6/E7 expression of human papillomavirus types in cutaneous squamous cell dysplasia and carcinoma in immunosuppressed organ transplant recipients. Br J Dermatol 2006;155(1):129–36.
36. de Berker DA, Taylor AE, Quinn AG, et al. Sebaceous hyperplasia in organ transplant recipients: shared aspects of hyperplastic and dysplastic processes? J Am Acad Dermatol 1996;35:696.
37. Dymock RB. Skin diseases associated with renal transplantation. Australas J Dermatol 1979;20:61.
38. Endrizzi BT, Lee PK. Management of carcinoma of the skin in solid organ transplant recipients with oral capecitabine. Dermatol Surg 2009;35(10):1567–72.
39. Epaulard O, Leccia MT, Blanche S, et al. Phototoxicity and photocarcinogenesis associated with voriconazole. Med Mal Infect 2011;41(12):639–45.
40. Euvrard S, Kanitakis J, Claudy A. Skin cancers after organ transplantation. N Engl J Med 2003;348(17):1681–91.
41. Euvrard S, Kanitakis J, Cochat P, et al. Skin cancers following pediatric organ transplantation. Dermatol Surg 2004;30(4 Pt 2): 616–21.
42. Euvrard S, Kanitakis J, Cochat P, et al. Skin diseases in children with organ transplants. J Am Acad Dermatol 2001;44:932–9.
43. Euvrard S, Kanitakis J, Decullier E, et al. Subsequent skin cancers in kidney and heart transplant recipients after the first squamous cell carcinoma. Transplantation 2006;81(8):1093–100.

44. Euvrard S, Kanitakis J, Pouteil-Noble C, et al. Comparative epidemiologic study of premalignant and malignant epithelial cutaneous lesions developing after kidney and heart transplantation. J Am Acad Dermatol 1995;33(2 Pt 1):222–9.
45. Farasat S, Yu SS, Neel VA, et al. A new American Joint Committee on Cancer staging system for cutaneous squamous cell carcinoma: creation and rationale for inclusion of tumor (T) characteristics. J Am Acad Dermatol 2011;64(6):1051–9.
46. Farthing CF, Staughton RC, Rowland Payne CM. Skin disease in homosexual patients with acquired immune deficiency syndrome (AIDS) and lesser forms of human T cell leukaemia virus (HTLV III) disease. Clin Exp Dermatol 1985;10:3.
47. Fernando ON, Sweny P, Varghese Z. Elective conversion of patients from cyclosporine to tacrolimus for hypertrichosis. Transplant Proc 1998;30:1243.
48. Focht 3rd DR, Spicer C, Fairchok MP. The efficacy of duct tape vs cryotherapy in the treatment of verruca vulgaris (the common wart). Arch Pediatr Adolesc Med 2002;156:971.
49. Garrigue V, Canet S, Dereure O, et al. Oral ulcerations in a renal transplant recipient: a mycophenolate mofetil-induced complication? Transplantation 2001;72:968.
50. George R, Weightman W, Russ GR, et al. Acitretin for chemoprevention of non-melanoma skin cancers in renal transplant recipients. Australas J Dermatol 2002;43(4):269–73.
51. Geusau A, Dunkler D, Messeritsch E, et al. Non-melanoma skin cancer and its risk factors in an Austrian population of heart transplant recipients receiving induction therapy. Int J Dermatol 2008;47(9):918–25.
52. Gulec AT, Demirbilek M, Seckin D, et al. Superficial fungal infections in 102 renal transplant recipients: a case-control study. J Am Acad Dermatol 2003;49:187.
53. Gupta AK, Madzia SE, Batra R. Etiology and management of seborrheic dermatitis. Dermatology 2004;208:89.
54. Haim S, Friedman-Birnbaum R, Better OS, et al. Skin complications in immunosuppressed patients: follow-up of kidney recipients. Br J Dermatol 1973;89:169.
55. Hartevelt MM, Bavinck JN, Kootte AM, et al. Incidence of skin cancer after renal transplantation in the Netherlands. Transplantation 1990;49(3):506–9.
56. Harwood CA, Surentheran T, Sasieni P, et al. Increased risk of skin cancer associated with the presence of epidermodysplasia verruciformis human papillomavirus types in normal skin. Br J Dermatol 2004;150(5):949–57.
57. Hepburn DJ, Divakar D, Bailey RR, et al. Cutaneous manifestations of renal transplantation in a New Zealand population. N Z Med J 1994;107:497.
58. Herranz P, Pizarro A, De Lucas R, et al. High incidence of porokeratosis in renal transplant recipients. Br J Dermatol 1997;136(2):176–9.
59. Hogewoning AA, Goettsch W, van Loveren H, et al. Skin infections in renal transplant recipients. Clin Transplant 2001;15:32.
60. Hollenbeak CS, Todd MM, Billingsley EM, et al. Increased incidence of melanoma in renal transplantation recipients. Cancer 2005;104(9):1962–7.
61. Horn TD, Hood AF. Cytomegalovirus is predictably present in perineal ulcers from immunosuppressed patients. Arch Dermatol 1990;126:642.
62. IARC. Monographs on the evaluation of the carcinogenic risk to humans, human papillomaviruses. IARC Monographs on the Evaluation of Carcinogenic Risks to Humans, vol. 90. 2007.
63. Jensen P, Clausen OP, Geiran O, et al. Cutaneous complications in heart transplant recipients in Norway 1983–1993. Acta Derm Venereol 1995;75:400.
64. Jensen P, Moller B, Hansen S. Skin cancer in kidney and heart transplant recipients and different long-term immunosuppressive therapy regimens. J Am Acad Dermatol 2000;42(2 Pt 1):307.
65. Jirakulaporn T, Endrizzi B, Lindgren B, et al. Capecitabine for skin cancer prevention in solid organ transplant recipients. Clin Transplant 2011;25(4):541–8.
66. Kanitakis J, Euvrard S, Lefrancois N, et al. Oral hairy leukoplakia in a HIV-negative renal graft recipient. Br J Dermatol 1991;124:483.
67. Koljonen V, Kukko H, Tukiainen E, et al. Incidence of Merkel cell carcinoma in renal transplant recipients. Nephrol Dial Transplant 2009;24(10):3231–5.
68. Koranda FC, Dehmel EM, Kahn G, et al. Cutaneous complications in immunosuppressed renal homograft recipients. JAMA 1974;229:419.
69. Kovach BT, Sams HH, Stasko T. Systemic strategies for chemoprevention of skin cancers in transplant recipients. Clin Transplant 2005;19(6):726–34.
70. Lally A, Casabonne D, Imko-Walczuk B, et al. Prevalence of benign cutaneous disease among Oxford renal transplant recipients. J Eur Acad Dermatol Venereol 2011;25:462.
71. Lally A, Casabonne D, Newton R, et al. Seborrhoeic dermatitis among Oxford renal transplant recipients. J Eur Acad Dermatol Venereol 2009;161:78–84.
72. Lally A, Casabonne D, Waterboer T, et al. Association of seborrhoeic warts with skin cancer in renal transplant recipients. J Eur Acad Dermatol Venereol 2010;24:302.
73. Lally A, Wojnarowska F. Hypertrophic pseudofolliculitis in white renal transplant recipients. Clin Exp Dermatol 2007;32:268.
74. Lear J, Bourke JF, Burns DA. Hyperplastic pseudofolliculitis barbae associated with cyclosporin. Br J Dermatol 1997; 136:132.
75. Leblanc Jr KG, Hughes MP, Sheehan DJ. The role of sirolimus in the prevention of cutaneous squamous cell carcinoma in organ transplant recipients. Dermatol Surg 2011;37(6):744–9.
76. Leigh IM, Glover MT. Skin cancer and warts in immunosuppressed renal transplant recipients. Recent Results Cancer Res 1995;139:69.
77. Lindelof B, Sigurgeirsson B, Gabel H, et al. Incidence of skin cancer in 5356 patients following organ transplantation. Br J Dermatol 2000;143(3):513–9.
78. Lindholm A, Pousette A, Carlstrom K, et al. Ciclosporin-associated hypertrichosis is not related to sex hormone levels following renal transplantation. Nephron 1988;50:199.
79. Lorenz GE, Ritter SE. Linear porokeratosis: a case report and review of the literature. Cutis 2008;81(6):479–83.
80. Lucchesi JA, Cortelli SC, Rodrigues JA, et al. Severe phenytoin-induced gingival enlargement associated with periodontitis. Gen Dent 2008;56:199.
81. Lugo-Janer G, Sanchez JL, Santiago-Delpin E. Prevalence and clinical spectrum of skin diseases in kidney transplant recipients. J Am Acad Dermatol 1991;24:410.
82. Lugo-Janer GJ, Pedraza R, Morales Otero LA, et al. Superficial mycosis in renal transplant recipients. Transplant Proc 1991;23:1787.
83. Lutzner M, Croissant O, Ducasse MF, et al. An unusual wart-like skin lesion found in a renal allograft recipient. Arch Dermatol 1981;117:43.
84. Mahe E, Morelon E, Lechaton S, et al. Cutaneous adverse events in renal transplant recipients receiving sirolimus-based therapy. Transplantation 2005;79:476.
85. Markovic SN, Erickson LA, Rao RD, et al. Malignant melanoma in the 21st century, part 1: epidemiology, risk factors, screening, prevention, and diagnosis. Mayo Clin Proc 2007;82(3):364–80.
86. Marks R, Rennie G, Selwood TS. Malignant transformation of solar keratoses to squamous cell carcinoma. Lancet 1988;1(8589):795–7.
87. Martinez JC, Otley CC, Stasko T, et al. Defining the clinical course of metastatic skin cancer in organ transplant recipients: a multicenter collaborative study. Arch Dermatol 2003;139(3):301–6.
88. McCarthy KL, Playford EG, Looke DF, et al. Severe photosensitivity causing multifocal squamous cell carcinomas secondary to prolonged voriconazole therapy. Clin Infect Dis 2007;44(5):e55–6.
89. McCoppin HH, Christiansen D, Stasko T, et al. Clinical spectrum of atypical fibroxanthoma and undifferentiated pleomorphic sarcoma in solid organ transplant recipients: a collective experience. Dermatol Surg 2012;38(2):230–9.
90. McGregor JM, Barker JN, MacDonald DM. The development of excess numbers of melanocytic naevi in an immunosuppressed identical twin. Clin Exp Dermatol 1991;16:131.
91. McLelland J, Chu AC. Fungal infection in renal transplant patients. Br J Dermatol 1988;118:734.
92. McLelland J, Rees A, Williams G, et al. The incidence of immunosuppression-related skin disease in long-term transplant patients. Transplantation 1988;46:871.

93. Menni S, Beretta D, Piccinno R, et al. Cutaneous and oral lesions in 32 children after renal transplantation. Pediatr Dermatol 1991;8:194.
94. Moloney FJ, Keane S, O'Kelly P, et al. The impact of skin disease following renal transplantation on quality of life. Br J Dermatol 2005;153:574.
95. Mortimer PS, Thompson JF, Dawber RP, et al. Hypertrichosis and multiple cutaneous squamous cell carcinomas in association with cyclosporin A therapy. J R Soc Med 1983;76:786.
96. Neiderberger W., Lemaire M., Maurer G., et al. (eds): Distribution and binding of cyclosporin in blood and tissues. In: Kahan BD, editor. Cyclosporin. Orlando, FL: Grune & Stratton; 1984. p. 203.
97. O'Connor DP, Kay EW, Leader M, et al. p53 codon 72 polymorphism and human papillomavirus associated skin cancer. J Clin Pathol 2001;54(7):539–42.
98. Ost L. Impairment of prednisolone metabolism by cyclosporine treatment in renal graft recipients. Transplantation 1987;44:533.
99. Otley CC, Berg D, Ulrich C, et al. Reduction of immunosuppression for transplant-associated skin cancer: expert consensus survey. Br J Dermatol 2006;154(3):395–400.
100. Otley C, Stasko T. Skin disease in organ transplantation. New York: Cambridge University Press; 2008.
101. Penn I. De novo malignancy in pediatric organ transplant recipients. J Pediatr Surg 1994;29(2):221–6, discussion 227–8.
102. Penn I. Malignant melanoma in organ allograft recipients. Transplantation 1996;61(2):274–8.
103. Perrett CM, McGregor JM, Warwick J, et al. Treatment of post-transplant premalignant skin disease: a randomized intrapatient comparative study of 5-fluorouracil cream and topical photodynamic therapy. Br J Dermatol 2007;156(2):320–8.
104. Perrett CM, Walker SL, O'Donovan P, et al. Azathioprine treatment photosensitizes human skin to ultraviolet A radiation. Br J Dermatol 2008;159(1):198–204.
105. Phase III randomized study of adjuvant intensity-modulated radiotherapy with versus without cetuximab in patients with locally advanced resected squamous cell carcinoma of the head and neck. ClinicalTrials.gov identifier: NCT00956007. Available online at: http://clinicaltrials.gov/ct2/show/NCT00956007 [accessed 20.03.12].
106. Piaserico S, Belloni Fortina A, Rigotti P, et al. Topical photodynamic therapy of actinic keratosis in renal transplant recipients. Transplant Proc 2007;39(6):1847–50.
107. Proby CM, Harwood CA, Neale RE, et al. A case-control study of betapapillomavirus infection and cutaneous squamous cell carcinoma in organ transplant recipients. Am J Transplant 2011;11(7):1498–508.
108. Ramsay HM, Fryer AA, Reece S, et al. Clinical risk factors associated with nonmelanoma skin cancer in renal transplant recipients. Am J Kidney Dis 2000;36:167–76.
109. Ramsay HM, Reece SM, Fryer AA, et al. Seven-year prospective study of nonmelanoma skin cancer incidence in U.K. renal transplant recipients. Transplantation 2007;84(3):437–9.
110. Rangwala S, Tsai KY. Roles of the immune system in skin cancer. Br J Dermatol 2011;165(5):953–65.
111. Rault R. Mycophenolate-associated onycholysis. Ann Intern Med 2000;133:921.
112. Ross AS, Schmults CD. Sentinel lymph node biopsy in cutaneous squamous cell carcinoma: a systematic review of the English literature. Dermatol Surg 2006;32(11):1309–21.
113. Rudlinger R, Smith IW, Bunney MH, et al. Human papillomavirus infections in a group of renal transplant recipients. Br J Dermatol 1986;115:681.
114. Salim A, Reece SM, Smith AG, et al. Sebaceous hyperplasia and skin cancer in patients undergoing renal transplant. J Am Acad Dermatol 2006;55:878.
115. Saray Y, Seckin D, Gulec AT, et al. Nail disorders in hemodialysis patients and renal transplant recipients: a case-control study. J Am Acad Dermatol 2004;50:197.
116. Scientific Registry of Transplant Recipients. OPTN / SRTR 2010 Annual Data Report. 2011. Available online at: http://www.srtr.org/annual_reports/2010/ [accessed 02.04.12].
117. Seckin D, Gulec TO, Demirag A, et al. Renal transplantation and skin diseases. Transplant Proc 1998;30:802.
118. Sequeira M, Burdick AE, Elgart GW, et al. New-onset Majocchi's granuloma in two kidney transplant recipients under tacrolimus treatment. J Am Acad Dermatol 1998;38:486.
119. Sheil AG, Disney AP, Mathew TH, et al. De novo malignancy emerges as a major cause of morbidity and late failure in renal transplantation. Transplant Proc 1993;25(1 Pt 2):1383–4.
120. Shuttleworth D, Marks R, Griffin PJ, et al. Dysplastic epidermal change in immunosuppressed patients with renal transplants. Q J Med 1987;64:609.
121. Shuttleworth D, Philpot CM, Salaman JR. Cutaneous fungal infection following renal transplantation: a case control study. Br J Dermatol 1987;117:585.
122. Silver SG, Crawford RI. Fatal squamous cell carcinoma arising from transplant-associated porokeratosis. J Am Acad Dermatol 2003;49(5):931–3.
123. Simmons WD, Rayhill SC, Sollinger HW. Preliminary risk–benefit assessment of mycophenolate mofetil in transplant rejection. Drug Saf 1997;17:75.
124. Slavin J, Taylor J. Cyclosporin, nifedipine, and gingival hyperplasia. Lancet 1987;2:739.
125. Smith KJ, Skelton HG, Yeager J, et al. Cutaneous findings in HIV-1-positive patients: a 42-month prospective study. Military Medical Consortium for the Advancement of Retroviral Research (MMCARR). J Am Acad Dermatol 1994;31:746.
126. Spencer CM, Goa KL, Gillis JC. Tacrolimus. An update of its pharmacology and clinical efficacy in the management of organ transplantation. Drugs 1997;54:925.
127. Spencer ES, Andersen HK. Clinically evident, non-terminal infections with herpesviruses and the wart virus in immunosuppressed renal allograft recipients. Br Med J 1970;1:251.
128. Spencer ES, Andersen HK. Viral infections in renal allograft recipients treated with long-term immunosuppression. Br Med J 1979;2:829.
129. Stasko T, Brown MD, Carucci JA, et al. Guidelines for the management of squamous cell carcinoma in organ transplant recipients. Dermatol Surg 2004;30(4 Pt 2):642–50.
130. Stockfleth E, Nindl I, Sterry W, et al. Human papillomaviruses in transplant-associated skin cancers. Dermatol Surg 2004;30(4 Pt 2):604–9.
131. Stoff B, Salisbury C, Parker D, et al. Dermatopathology of skin cancer in solid organ transplant recipients. Transplant Rev (Orlando) 2010;24(4):172–89.
132. Strumia R, Perini L, Tarroni G, et al. Skin lesions in kidney transplant recipients. Nephron 1992;62:137.
133. Termorshuizen F, Hogewoning AA, Bouwes Bavinck JN, et al. Skin infections in renal transplant recipients and the relation with solar ultraviolet radiation. Clin Transplant 2003;17:522.
134. Touraud JP, Dalac S, Collet E, et al. Punctate porokeratosis in a renal transplant recipient. Clin Exp Dermatol 2003;28(3):329–30.
135. Tricot L, Lebbe C, Pillebout E, et al. Tacrolimus-induced alopecia in female kidney–pancreas transplant recipients. Transplantation 2005;80:1546.
136. Triemer HL, Pearson TC, Odom KL, et al. Analysis of a single-center experience with mycophenolate mofetil based immunosuppression in renal transplantation. Clin Transplant 2000;14:413.
137. Tyldesley WR, Rotter E. Gingival hyperplasia induced by cyclosporin-A. Br Dent J 1984;157:305.
138. Ulrich C, Bichel J, Euvrard S, et al. Topical immunomodulation under systemic immunosuppression: results of a multicentre, randomized, placebo-controlled safety and efficacy study of imiquimod 5% cream for the treatment of actinic keratoses in kidney, heart, and liver transplant patients. Br J Dermatol 2007;157(Suppl. 2):25–31.
139. Ulrich C, Schmook T, Sachse MM, et al. Comparative epidemiology and pathogenic factors for nonmelanoma skin cancer in organ transplant patients. Dermatol Surg 2004;30(4 Pt 2):622–7.
140. Venning VA, Millard PR. Recurrent scabies with unusual clinical features in a renal transplant recipient. Br J Dermatol 1992;126:204.
141. Vijayakumar R, Fernando E, Rajendran S, et al. Dermatological manifestations in renal transplant recipients. Transplant Proc 1998;30:3136.
142. Wang K, Zhang H, Li Y, et al. Safety of mycophenolate mofetil versus azathioprine in renal transplantation: a systematic review. Transplant Proc 2004;36:2068.

143. Wennberg AM, Stenquist B, Stockfleth E, et al. Photodynamic therapy with methyl aminolevulinate for prevention of new skin lesions in transplant recipients: a randomized study. Transplantation 2008;86(3):423–9.
144. Winkelhorst JT, Brokelman WJ, Tiggeler RG, et al. Incidence and clinical course of de-novo malignancies in renal allograft recipients. Eur J Surg Oncol 2001;27(4):409–13.
145. Wolf R, Wolf D, Viskoper RJ, et al. Norwegian-type scabies mimicking contact dermatitis in an immunosuppressed patient. Postgrad Med 1985;78:228.
146. Zwald FO, Brown M. Skin cancer in solid organ transplant recipients: advances in therapy and management: part I. Epidemiology of skin cancer in solid organ transplant recipients. J Am Acad Dermatol 2011;65(2):253–61 quiz 262.
147. Zwald FO, Brown M. Skin cancer in solid organ transplant recipients: advances in therapy and management: part II. Management of skin cancer in solid organ transplant recipients. J Am Acad Dermatol 2011;65(2):263–79, quiz 280.

CHAPTER 35

Cancer in Dialysis and Kidney Transplant Patients

John F. Thompson • Angela C. Webster

CHAPTER OUTLINE

For dialysis patients and kidney transplant recipients, the risk of malignancy is considerably greater than for the general population. This chapter discusses all aspects of cancer in dialysis and transplant patients with the exception of skin malignancy, which is one of the greatest cancer risks they face, but which is considered separately in Chapter 34.

CANCER IN DIALYSIS PATIENTS

Soon after the first reports of cancer arising de novo in kidney transplant recipients,[21,77] it was suggested that patients on dialysis programs, many awaiting transplantation, also were at heightened risk of cancer development.[59] The reasons were not immediately apparent. Subsequent reports confirmed that the incidence of malignancy is considerably greater in patients on dialysis than in the population at large. However, most of these cancers affected the renal tract, either directly or indirectly, and this led to some uncertainty over whether dialysis patients were more susceptible to malignancies that did not affect the renal tract. It is now clear that there is indeed an overall increase in the incidence of malignancy in patients with chronic renal failure.[34,53,59,64,91,95] Rarely, renal failure may be a consequence of malignancies such as those arising in lung or colon because they lead to glomerulopathy.[25] It has been suggested that this glomerular disease in cancer patients could be a result of tumor-associated antigens. Nephrotic syndrome is most often associated with Hodgkin's disease. Malignant disease of the kidney or ureter can impair renal function by causing obstruction, and occasionally renal dysfunction results from a treatment-related nephropathy secondary to radiation or drugs.

Magnitude of the Cancer Risk in Dialysis Patients

Some of the most comprehensive long-term data on the development of malignancy in dialysis patients and kidney transplant recipients are available from the Australia and New Zealand Dialysis and Transplant (ANZDATA) registry. This registry has collected information on all patients in Australia and New Zealand who have been treated with dialysis or received a kidney transplant since

1963. Although there are several much larger registries in the world, the completeness of the information contained in the ANZDATA registry sets it apart from most others.

In the 2009 ANZDATA report,[101] the incidence of cancer in 33 772 patients treated with dialysis and following a first kidney transplant in Australia and New Zealand between 1982 and 2005 was reported. From this information, which represented 90 504 person-years of follow-up during dialysis treatment and 120 121 person-years of follow-up after a first transplant, the cancer risk for each group was able to be calculated by comparing the incidence of each cancer type with that in the general population. To compare the risk of cancer at different sites, the observed number of incident cancer diagnoses notified to ANZDATA was compared with the expected number of cancer diagnoses in the general population. Indirect standardization was used, standardizing for differences in age, sex, and calendar year, to calculate standardized incidence ratios (SIR) with their 95% confidence intervals (CI). SIR can be interpreted as relative risk (RR), where a SIR value of 1 is risk equal to that of the general population of similar age and sex, living in an equivalent time period in the same country, and a SIR of 2 is double the risk. For the general population, cancer incidence data were obtained from the Australian National Cancer Statistics Clearing House. This database does not contain information on non-melanoma skin cancer (NMSC), because reporting of NMSC is not mandatory in Australia. Although the number of dialysis and transplant patients who developed NMSC is available in the ANZDATA registry, the increased risk compared with the general population could therefore not be ascertained.

The results of the ANZDATA analysis of cancer in dialysis and transpant patients are summarized in Table 35-1. It is apparent that, when considering cancer risk by cancer site, the pattern of increased risk is varied. For many cancers there is a slight increase in risk among dialysis patients, with a somewhat greater increase following transplantation. Examples of this include cancers arising in the lung and colon. For several other cancers, however, the risk increase after transplantation is more marked; most of these are known or

TABLE 35-1 Risk of Cancer Following Commencement of Dialysis and After a First Kidney Transplant, Australia and New Zealand, 1982–2005

		On Dialysis		*Posttransplant*	
Cancer Site	**ICD-O Code**	**Observed**	**SIR (95% CI)**	**Observed**	**SIR (95% CI)**
Head and neck	C01–14	26	1.25 (0.82–1.83)	66	4.45 (3.44–5.66)
Esophagus	C15	22	1.61 (1.01–2.44)	28	4.29 (2.85–6.20)
Stomach	C16	34	1.20 (0.83–1.68)	16	1.24 (0.71–2.01)
Small intestine	C17	8	2.99 (1.29–5.90)	4	2.56 (0.70–6.56)
Colorectal	C18–20	169	1.16 (0.99–1.34)	127	1.72 (1.43–2.04)
Anus	C21	4	1.70 (0.46–4.36)	18	12.4 (7.4–19.7)
Liver	C22	23	2,85 (1.91–4.27)	19	4.43 (2.67–6.91)
Gallbladder	C23–24	9	1.21 (0.55–2.29)	8	2.35 (1.02–4.63)
Pancreas	C25	22	0.95 (0.60–1.44)	15	1.44 (0.81–2.37)
Nasal cavity, sinuses	C30–31	4	2.50 (0.68–6.40)	7	7.09 (2.85–14.6)
Larynx	C32	8	0.86 (0.37–1.68)	12	2.07 (1.07–3.62)
Trachea, bronchus, lung	C33–34	201	1.63 (1.41–1.87)	115	1.96 (1.62–2.35)
Other thoracic organs	C37–38	13	17.70 (9.42–30.3)	8	15.2 (6.57–30.0)
Bone and articular cartilage	C40–41	3	2.64 (0.55–7.73)	5	4.90 (1.59–11.4)
Melanoma of skin	C43	107	1.41 (1.16–1.71)	180	3.11 (2.67–3.60)
Mesothelioma	C45	11	1.71 (0.86–3.07)	3	0.98 (0.20–2.86)
Kaposi's sarcoma	C46	8	10.99 (4.75–21.7)	23	25.5 (16.2–38.3)
Peritoneum, other connective and soft tissue	C47–49	3	0.67 (0.14–1.97)	9	2.91 (1.33–5.53)
Breast (female)	C50	116	2.57 (2.13–3.08)	81	2.35 (1.89–2.92)
Female gynecological	C51–58	183	10.00 (8.63–11.6)	231	18.0 (15.7–20.4)
Penis	C60	1	2.47 (0.06–13.7)	9	37.4 (17.1–71.0)
Prostate	C61	100	1.30 (1.05–1.57)	54	1.72 (1.30–2.25)
Testis	C62	1	1.03 (0.03–5.72)	4	1.96 (0.54–5.03)
Other male genital	C63	1	8.23 (0.20–45.9)	1	14.7 (0.37–82.1)
Kidney	C64	173	8.30 (7.11–9.63)	122	9,76 (8.10–11.7)
Other urinary tract	C65–66, C68	33	6.38 (4.39–8.95)	46	19.6 (14.3–26.1)
Bladder	C67	135	3.77 (3.16–4.46)	93	6.19 (5.00–7.58)
Eye	C69	0	0.00 (0.00–1.53)	6	3.80 (1.39–8.36)
Brain	C71	21	1.69 (1.05–2.59)	12	1.33 (0.69–2.32)
Other central nervous system	C70, C72	1	1.96 (0.05–10.9)	4	9.06 (2.47–23.2)
Thyroid	C73	35	5.89 (4.10–8.19)	30	4.82 (3.25–6.89)
Other endocrine	C74–75	5	10.1 (3.29–23.7)	4	9.38 (2.56–24.0)
All lymphoma	C81–85, C96	58	1.56 (1.18–2.02)	266	11.4 (10.1–12.9)
Multiple myeloma	C90	96	7.60 (6.15–9.28)	15	2.48 (1.39–4.09)
Leukemias	C91–95	23	0.88 (0.56–1.32)	32	2.39 (1.63–3.37)

ICD-O, International Classification of Diseases for Oncology; SIR, standardized incidence ratio; CI, confidence interval.

Adapted from Webster AC, Wong G, McDonald SP. Chapter 10, Cancer. ANZDATA Registry Report 2009. 32nd annual report. Adelaide, South Australia: Australia and New Zealand Dialysis and Transplant Registry (http://www.anzdata.org.au), 2010.

postulated to have a viral etiology – for example, carcinoma of the cervix, lymphoma, and Kaposi's sarcoma.

It is more difficult to obtain comprehensive data on the incidence of malignancy in dialysis patients treated in other countries. In Japan, a nation with a large population of patients on long-term dialysis, an analysis of deaths caused by cancer (including renal tract tumors) revealed that the RR of cancer mortality for dialysis patients was greatly increased compared with the general population (male RR 2.48; female RR 3.99).[38]

To examine the question of malignancy in dialysis patients, a major international study was undertaken by Stewart and coworkers,[90] involving analysis of pooled data for patients who received dialysis for end-stage kidney disease (ESKD) between 1980 and 1994. A cohort of 834884 patients treated in the United States, Europe, Australia, and New Zealand was assembled. The observed frequency of cancer among these patients during 2 045 035 person-years of follow-up was compared with the frequency of cancer in the respective background populations. Patients with NMSC were excluded. It was found that the overall risk of cancer was increased in patients with ESKD, and that the distribution of tumor types in dialysis patients resembled the pattern seen after transplantation. The excess risk was largely ascribed to effects on the kidney and bladder of underlying renal or urinary tract disease, or to loss of renal function. Also considered likely to be responsible was an increased susceptibility to viral carcinogenesis.

During the short mean follow-up of 2.5 years in this study, 3% of the study population developed cancer. The expected number of individuals developing cancer in the population at large was lower, so that the SIR was 1.18. In younger patients (<35 years old), the risk of cancer was considerably higher (SIR 3.68), and this risk gradually decreased with increasing age. Particularly high risks were observed for cancer of the kidney (SIR 3.60), the bladder (SIR 1.50), and the thyroid and other endocrine organs (SIR 2.28). Excess numbers of cancers occurred in several organs in which viruses have been suspected as causative carcinogenic agents, whereas cancers of the lung, colon and rectum, prostate, breast, and stomach were not consistently increased.

Reasons for the Increased Risk of Cancer in Dialysis Patients

Patients maintained on dialysis are potentially at risk of cancer for several reasons. These include the presence of chronic infection (especially in the urinary tract), a depressed immune system, previous treatment with immunosuppressive or cytotoxic drugs, nutritional deficiencies, and altered DNA repair mechanisms.[96] In addition, the underlying disease leading to renal failure, the persistent metabolic changes associated with it, and the development of certain complications such as acquired renal cystic disease may predispose to cancer. Some forms of genitourinary disease are known to predispose to renal, ureteric, or bladder tumors. The risk of renal cancer is increased in patients with inherited or acquired cystic disease of the kidney[45,57]; the risk of renal cell cancer associated with acquired cystic disease seems to be the total duration of renal impairment, rather than the duration of dialysis treatment.[71] Other conditions predisposing to cancer include Balkan nephropathy and analgesic nephropathy, both of which are associated with a high risk of developing tumors of the renal pelvis and ureter.[17,54]

An interesting observation is that the increased risk of some cancer types is rapidly reversed when immunosuppression is reduced or withdrawn after kidney transplant failure. These cancer types include Kaposi's sarcoma, non-Hodgkin lymphoma, melanoma, and lip cancer. However, the risk of cancer at other sites remains significantly elevated after iatrogenic immunosuppression is ceased. These cancer types include leukemia, lung cancer, and cancers related to ESKD.[97]

The Particular Problem of Renal Tract Malignancy in Patients with End-Stage Kidney Disease

Pathology studies have shown that renal tumors are more common in the pretransplant ESKD population than had previously been reported on the basis of radiological imaging.[19] A large study undertaken by Maisonneuve and colleagues[56] was important because most previous studies had been too small to detect potentially important findings on less common types of tumors or small increases in risk, or to study the relationship between cancer and the various causes of renal failure or the method of dialysis treatment (hemodialysis or peritoneal dialysis). The study confirmed an overall increased risk of cancer in patients with ESKD. Generally, the types of cancer developing in patients with ESKD were similar to the cancer types observed with increased frequency in transplant recipients. Most common were cancers of the urinary tract, but cancers of the tongue, liver, lower genital tract in women, external genitalia in men, and thyroid, also lymphomas and multiple myeloma, were observed to have an increased incidence. In seeking to explain their findings, the authors of this study suggested that viral infections were likely to be important as causative agents for some of the tumors.

Viral infections occur in about 10% of patients after transplantation.[26] The frequency of viral infections in dialysis patients is poorly documented, but there is no doubt that ESKD patients have a greater than normal exposure to hepatitis B and C viruses,[67] and this probably accounts for the observed excess of liver cancer. Human papillomavirus (HPV) is thought to play a role in the development of cancers of the tongue, cervix, vagina, vulva, and penis.[6,18] In dialysis and transplant patients, the increased risk of developing lymphomas is thought likely to be due to activation of dormant Epstein–Barr virus (EBV).[104,108] A possible explanation for the observed increase in risk of thyroid tumors is the repeated imaging of the neck to investigate secondary hyperparathyroidism. In support of this hypothesis is the observation that the frequency of thyroid tumors increases with duration on dialysis.

An important point to emerge from the study by Maisonneuve and colleagues[56] is that the risk of cancer was not related to the type of dialysis. It was concluded that the uremic state, rather than any treatment-related phenomenon, was likely to be the cause of the increased risk.

The uremia is thought likely to lead to an impairment of immunity, perhaps by interfering with DNA repair mechanisms or by causing a reduction in antioxidant defense. Chronic infections and inflammatory processes, potentially associated with the development of malignancies, are more common in patients with renal failure. A final point to consider is that any degree of renal impairment could lead to the accumulation of carcinogenic compounds.[96]

In the previously mentioned study by Stewart and coworkers,[90] it also was concluded that dialysis itself conferred no additional risk of cancer other than by prolonging exposure to the uremic state. These authors reported that, in the dialysis population, the risk of developing cancer of the kidney or bladder was relatively (but not absolutely) greater at younger ages, and in women rather than men. They found that the dialysis population exhibited a risk of cancers of the kidney and urinary tract over and above the heightened risk of cancer seen in many other sites. They reported that there was no excess risk of kidney cancer in patients with ESKD due to polycystic disease, and noted that primary renal disease accounted for almost all of the excess risk of urothelial cancer, whether in the bladder or elsewhere in the urinary tract. They determined that the carcinogenic potential of acquired renal cystic disease was greater than that of primary (hereditary) polycystic renal disease. They reported that the SIR for kidney cancer increased significantly with time on dialysis, whereas the SIR for bladder cancer progressively decreased.[90]

Screening for Cancer in Dialysis Patients

Some authors have suggested that routine cancer screening of patients on long-term dialysis is not cost-effective.[15,35,43] Others have argued, however, that although general cancer screening is not cost-effective in dialysis patients, selective screening in younger patients and for known cancer types is warranted. Parathyroid cancer is a good example, and this condition should be suspected in dialysis patients if rapid changes in serum parathyroid hormone levels are observed.[78] Careful and regular screening for premalignant and malignant skin lesions is another good example; this is likely to be of particular value in countries such as Australia, where frequent exposure to intense solar ultraviolet (UV) radiation is almost inevitable. Ishikawa and associates[39] proposed that screening is valuable in the detection of renal cell cancer, and pointed out that survival is best in young patients with a short duration of dialysis, and when the renal cell cancer is detected by screening, rather than by direct reporting of symptoms. Satoh and coworkers[83] likewise suggested that early diagnosis of renal cell cancer by regular imaging of patients with ESKD who are on dialysis would result in an improved outcome. Wong and colleagues assessed the cost-effectiveness of breast cancer screening in women on dialysis,[105] and pointed out that cost-effectiveness analyses can help put expectations from screening programs into context. They found that screening resulted in an absolute reduction in breast cancer mortality of 0.1%, with a net gain in life expectancy of only 1.3 days. The total incremental cost to screen and save one extra cancer death approximated A$403 000 per life saved from breast cancer.

Management of Cancer in Dialysis Patients

If malignancy does develop in a patient on dialysis, the condition should be treated with current standard therapy. For dialysis patients who have surgical treatment for malignancy, postoperative complications are, however, much higher than usual, as would be expected.[16] If surgery is not considered appropriate, chemotherapy may be possible, but individual drug dosage adjustments are likely to be required.[11] Treatment with radioactive iodine can be undertaken for thyroid cancer in patients on dialysis, but dosage adjustment is necessary because iodine is cleared mainly by the kidneys or by the dialysis process.[36]

CANCER IN KIDNEY TRANSPLANT RECIPIENTS

The magnitude of the cancer problem in kidney transplant recipients is apparent from the SIR values reported in Table 35-1. The risk increases steadily from the time of transplantation, with the rate of increase very much dependent on the age of the patient at the time of transplantation. This is clearly demonstrated in Figure 35-1 and Table 35-2.[99] Long-term data from the ANZDATA registry indicate that a total of 1642 (10.8%) of 15 183 kidney transplant recipients developed cancer. The cancer rates were similar to those in non-transplant people 20–30 years older. Risk was inversely related to age (SIR 15–30 for children, 2 if >65 years). Females aged 25–29 had rates equivalent to those of women aged 55–59 in the general population. The age trend for lymphoma, colorectal cancer, and breast cancer risk was similar: melanoma showed less variability across age cohorts; prostate cancer showed no risk increase. Within the transplanted population, risk was affected by age differently for each sex (P=0.007). It was increased by prior malignancy (hazard ratio (HR) 1.40; CI 1.3–1.89) and white race (HR 1.36, CI 1.12–1.89), but reduced by diabetic ESKD (HR 0.67, CI 0.50–0.89). As well as demonstrating how absolute risk differs across patient groups, Figure 35-1 allows the risk of cancer developing after transplantation to be estimated, based on clinical details known at the time of transplantation. For example, men aged 45–54 surviving 10 years have cancer risks varying from 1 in 13 (non-white, no prior cancer, diabetic ESKD) to 1 in 5 (white, prior cancer, ESKD from another cause).

The risk of cancer development is particularly great in patients who are older when they first undergo transplantation. For men who are less than 35 years of age at the time of first kidney transplantation, the adjusted risk of developing cancer (excluding NMSC) after 10 years is 4.2, whereas for men who are 55 years of age or older at the time of transplantation, it is 24.6. For women, the corresponding risk values after 10 years are 5.8 and 20.9. The overall results of this analysis are shown in Table 35-2.

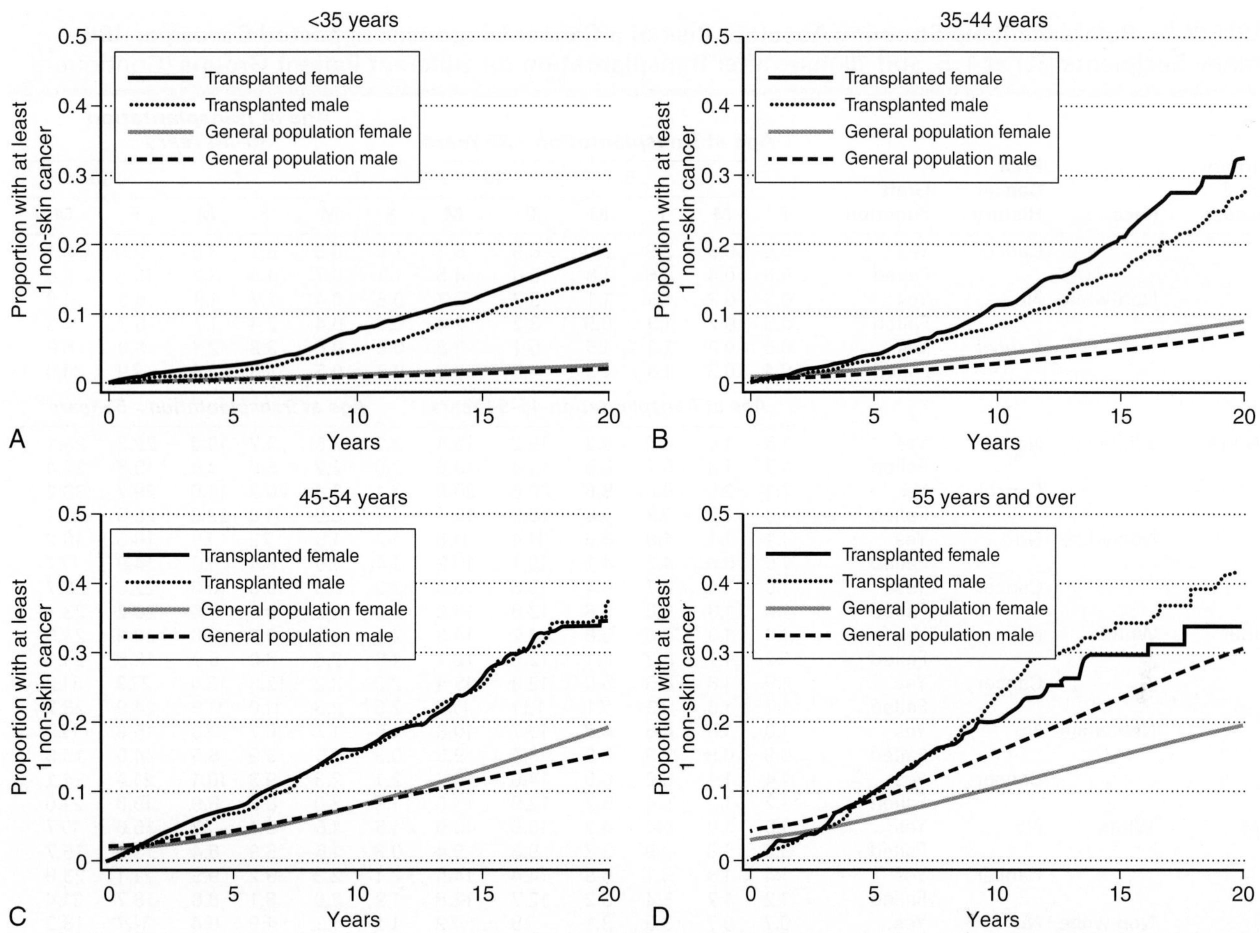

FIGURE 35-1 ■ **Cumulative risk of cancer (excluding non-melanocytic skin and lip cancer) in kidney transplant recipients by age at transplantation, with expected cumulative risk for a comparable general population of the same age and sex. (A) <35 years; (B) 35–44 years; (C) 45–54 years; (D) 55 years and over.** (Adapted from Webster AC, Craig JC, Simpson JM, et al. Identifying high risk groups and quantifying absolute risk of cancer after kidney transplantation: a cohort study of 15183 recipients. Am J Transplant 2007;7:2140–51.)

TABLE 35-2 **Reference Table Showing Absolute Risk of a Cancer Diagnosis: Expected Cases per 100 Kidney Recipients (%) at 1, 5, and 10 Years after Transplantation for Different Patient Groups***

Primary Renal Disease	Race	Prior Cancer History	Graft Function	*Age at Transplantation <35 Years* 1 F	1 M	5 F	5 M	10 F	10 M	*Age at Transplantation 35–44 Years* 1 F	1 M	5 F	5 M	10 F	10 M
GN/IgA	White	No	Yes	0.7	0.5	3.0	2.1	7.3	5.2	1.2	0.8	5.4	3.6	12.7	9.5
			Failed	0.6	0.4	2.7	1.9	6.4	4.8	1.1	0.8	4.7	3.4	11.2	8.5
		Cancer	Yes	0.9	0.7	4.2	3.0	10.0	7.5	1.2	1.2	7.4	5.3	17.3	13.2
			Failed	0.8	0.6	3.7	2.6	8.8	6.6	1.5	1.1	6.5	4.7	15.3	11.7
	Non-white	No	Yes	0.5	0.4	2.1	1.6	5.2	4.0	0.8	0.6	3.7	2.8	9.3	7.2
			Failed	0.4	0.3	2.0	1.3	4.7	3.4	0.8	0.5	3.5	2.5	8.4	6.4
		Cancer	Yes	0.7	0.5	3.1	2.2	7.5	5.6	1.3	0.9	5.5	4.0	13.0	9.9
			Failed	0.6	0.4	2.7	1.9	6.6	4.9	1.1	0.5	4.8	3.5	11.5	8.8
Other	White	No	Yes	0.6	0.4	2.8	2.0	6.8	4.9	1.1	0.8	5.0	3.6	11.9	9.0
			Failed	0.6	0.4	2.5	1.7	6.0	4.4	1.0	0.7	4.4	3.1	10.4	7.9
		Cancer	Yes	0.9	0.6	3.9	2.8	9.4	7.0	1.6	1.1	6.9	4.9	16.2	12.3
			Failed	0.7	0.5	3.4	2.4	8.2	6.1	1.4	0.9	6.1	4.4	14.3	10.9
	Non-white	No	Yes	0.5	0.3	2.1	1.5	5.0	3.7	0.8	0.6	3.7	2.6	8.9	6.7
			Failed	0.4	0.3	1.8	1.3	4.4	3.3	0.7	0.5	3.2	2.3	7.8	5.9
		Cancer	Yes	0.7	0.5	2.9	2.0	7.0	5.2	1.2	0.8	5.1	3.7	12.2	9.2
			Failed	0.6	0.4	2.5	1.8	6.1	4.6	1.0	0.7	4.5	3.2	10.7	8.1
DM	White	No	Yes	0.5	0.3	2.1	1.4	5.0	3.6	0.8	0.6	3.7	2.6	8.8	6.6
			Failed	0.4	0.3	1.8	1.3	4.4	3.2	0.7	0.5	3.2	2.3	7.7	5.8

Continued on following page

TABLE 35-2 Reference Table Showing Absolute Risk of a Cancer Diagnosis: Expected Cases per 100 Kidney Recipients (%) at 1, 5, and 10 Years after Transplantation for Different Patient Groups (Continued)

				Age at Transplantation <35 Years						***Age at Transplantation 35–44 Years***					
				1		**5**		**10**		**1**		**5**		**10**	
Primary Renal Disease	**Race**	**Prior Cancer History**	**Graft Function**	**F**	**M**	**F**	**M**	**F**	**M**	**F**	**M**	**F**	**M**	**F**	**M**
		Cancer	Yes	0.6	0.5	2.9	2.0	6.9	5.1	1.1	0.8	5.1	3.6	12.0	9.1
			Failed	0.6	0.4	2.5	1.8	6.0	4.5	1.0	0.7	4.4	3.2	10.6	8.0
	Non-white	No	Yes	0.3	0.2	1.5	1.1	3.7	2.7	0.6	0.4	2.7	1.9	6.5	4.9
			Failed	0.3	0.2	1.3	0.9	3.2	2.4	0.5	0.4	2.4	1.7	5.7	4.3
		Cancer	Yes	0.5	0.3	2.1	1.5	5.1	3.8	0.8	0.6	3.8	2.7	9.0	6.8
			Failed	0.4	0.3	1.8	1.3	4.5	3.3	0.7	0.5	3.3	2.4	7.9	6.0
				Age at Transplantation 45–54 Years						***Age at Transplantation ≥55 Years***					
GN/IgA	White	No	Yes	1.5	1.4	6.5	6.2	15.2	15.4	2.2	2.5	9.7	10.6	22.3	25.1
			Failed	1.3	1.3	5.7	5.5	13.4	13.6	2.0	2.2	8.6	9.3	19.8	22.4
		Cancer	Yes	2.1	2.0	9.0	8.6	20.6	20.8	3.1	3.4	20.3	14.0	29.7	33.2
			Failed	1.8	1.7	7.9	7.6	18.3	18.4	2.7	3.0	11.8	12.9	26.5	30.1
	Non-white	No	Yes	1.1	1.1	4.8	4.6	11.4	11.6	1.7	1.8	7.2	7.9	16.9	19.2
			Failed	1.0	0.9	4.2	4.1	10.1	10.2	1.4	1.6	6.4	7.0	14.9	17.1
		Cancer	Yes	1.5	1.4	6.7	6.4	15.6	15.8	2.3	2.5	10.0	10.8	22.8	25.7
			Failed	1.3	1.3	5.8	5.6	13.8	14.0	2.0	2.2	8.8	9.6	20.2	23.1
Other	White	No	Yes	1.4	1.3	6.0	5.8	14.2	14.3	2.1	2.3	9.1	9.8	20.9	23.5
			Failed	1.2	1.1	5.3	5.1	12.5	12.7	1.8	2.0	8.0	8.7	18.5	21.1
		Cancer	Yes	1.9	1.8	8.3	8.0	19.3	19.4	2.9	3.2	12.5	13.4	27.9	31.2
			Failed	1.7	1.6	7.3	7.1	17.1	17.2	2.5	2.8	11.0	11.9	24.9	28.2
	Non-white	No	Yes	1.0	1.0	4.5	4.3	10.7	10.8	1.5	1.7	6.7	7.3	15.8	17.9
			Failed	0.9	0.9	3.9	3.8	9.4	9.5	0.3	1.5	5.9	6.5	14.0	15.9
		Cancer	Yes	1.4	1.4	6.2	6.0	14.6	14.7	2.1	2.3	9.3	10.1	21.4	24.1
			Failed	1.2	1.2	5.4	5.2	12.9	13.0	1.9	2.0	8.2	8.9	19.0	21.6
DM	White	No	Yes	1.0	1.0	4.4	4.2	10.5	10.6	1.5	1.6	6.7	7.2	15.6	17.7
			Failed	0.9	0.8	3.9	3.7	9.3	9.4	0.3	1.5	5.9	6.4	13.8	15.7
		Cancer	Yes	1.4	1.3	6.1	5.9	14.4	14.5	2.1	2.3	9.2	9.9	21.1	23.9
			Failed	1.2	1.2	5.4	5.2	12.7	12.8	1.9	2.0	8.1	8.8	18.7	21.4
	Non-white	No	Yes	0.7	0.7	3.3	3.1	7.9	7.9	1.1	1.2	4.9	5.4	11.7	13.3
			Failed	0.6	0.6	2.9	2.8	6.9	7.0	1.0	1.1	4.3	4.7	10.3	11.9
		Cancer	Yes	1.0	1.0	4.5	4.4	10.8	10.9	1.6	1.7	6.8	7.4	16.0	18.1
			Failed	0.9	0.9	4.0	3.8	9.5	9.6	1.4	1.5	6.0	6.5	14.1	16.2

GN/IgA, glomerulonephritis/immunoglobulin A; DM, diabetes mellitus.

*Based on a table originally published in Webster AC, et al. Am J Transplant 2007;7(9):2140–51. © 2007 The American Society of Transplantation and the American Society of Transplant Surgeons and Blackwell Publishing. All rights reserved.

From this table it is possible to give an estimate of a patient's risk of developing a cancer (excluding NMSC) according to gender and age at transplantation. This information allows clinicians to identify patient groups at higher risk of developing malignancy and may be useful for pretransplant counseling when informed consent is being obtained. Vajdic and colleagues[95] report in detail the ANZDATA registry data relating to the risk of cancer after kidney transplantation.

Transmission of Cancer from the Donor

Early in the history of kidney transplantation, it became apparent that cancer in the transplanted organ or at other sites occurred frequently in recipients who received apparently normal kidney allografts from cancer-affected donors.[58,63,72] It was soon recognized that organs retrieved from such donors could harbor malignant cells that had the potential to proliferate in the recipient, causing death.[58,63] Although most patients with a transplanted cancer ultimately die of the malignancy, early experiences showed that cure occasionally could be achieved by stopping the patient's immunosuppressive therapy with a view to precipitating rejection of the transplanted organ and the cancer, and then removing the allograft.[61,103]

Because of the almost universally disastrous results of transplanting organs from a donor known to have cancer other than a primary brain tumor or an NMSC, such individuals are generally excluded as potential organ donors. This exclusion applies to both cadaver and living donors. Selection criteria for cadaveric and living donors are discussed in detail in Chapters 6 and 7.

Despite all efforts to avoid the situation, kidneys occasionally are transplanted from donors who are subsequently discovered to have primary or metastatic malignancies. There is general consensus that these renal grafts should be removed as soon as possible, with reinstatement of dialysis. All potential recipients must be made aware of the possibility that malignancy might be transferred with the donor organ, and this risk should be included in informed consent documentation.

If a transplant recipient develops cancer, particularly if it is soon after transplantation, the possibility that it is a malignancy transferred from the donor always needs to be considered. The other recipients of organs from the same donor should therefore be investigated as soon as possible and monitored carefully.

Development of De Novo Cancers in Kidney Transplant Recipients

Several aspects of this problem have already been discussed in the section of this chapter dealing with cancer development in dialysis patients. Early reports of de novo cancers arising in immunosuppressed transplant recipients undoubtedly underestimated the long-term risk.[55] These estimates were based on single-center and registry reports, which indicated that malignancies (excluding NMSCs) arose in 2–8% of transplant recipients. Even more recent estimates of risk also are likely to be serious underestimates because transplant recipient populations on which the incidence of cancer is based are biased by the large numbers of recently transplanted patients compared with the small number of long-surviving patients. A large study in the United States that attempted to determine the incidence of malignancy in kidney transplant recipients reported only the cancer rates in the first, second, and third years after transplantation.[42]

When incidence figures are determined on the basis of the number of years since transplantation, a different picture emerges, with reports of 34–50% of immunosuppressed transplant recipients developing cancer if they are followed for 20 years or more after transplantation.[28,65,88] Long-term data from the ANZDATA registry reveal that, in recipients of cadaver kidneys transplanted 30 years earlier, the incidence of skin cancer is 75%, and the incidence of non-skin cancer is 33%, with some form of cancer (either skin or non-skin cancer) developing in 80% of patients overall.[87] Transplant registry data from other countries also show a substantial risk of cancer development in kidney transplant recipients, which steadily increases as the time since transplantation lengthens.[1,8,10]

Reasons for the Increased Risk of Cancer in Transplant Patients

Numerous mechanisms are likely to contribute to the increased risk of cancer in immunosuppressed allograft recipients. Some of these are undoubtedly the same as the mechanisms responsible for the development of malignancy in patients with ESKD on dialysis. In transplant recipients, however, the dominant factors are believed to be impaired immune surveillance for neoplastic cells and depressed antiviral immune activity.

Impaired Immune Surveillance

Over a century ago, Ehrlich (1909) proposed that abnormal cells arise frequently in normal individuals as a result of somatic mutation, viral infection, or some other mechanism. If these abnormal cells are not eliminated, they have the potential to become autonomous and to develop into a malignant process. Based on the assumption that the immune system is important in eliminating such abnormal cells,[92] it was logical to make the further assumption that any impairment of immune surveillance could result in cancer.[12,44]

Several pieces of evidence support the importance of immune surveillance in protection against cancer in humans. One is the observed increase in cancer incidence with increasing age. Another is the well-documented increase in cancer incidence that occurs in congenital and acquired immunodeficiency states,[46] particularly in patients with human immunodeficiency virus (HIV).[30] Particularly powerful additional evidence comes from experience with human transplantation, including the transfer of malignancy to immunosuppressed transplant recipients, the increased incidence of de novo cancer in these individuals, and studies showing that the immunosuppression can lead to tumor recurrence.[27]

The mechanisms by which immunosuppressive agents lead to the development of cancer are complex. It is likely that the type, extent, and duration of immunosuppressive therapy have a role to play. Immunosuppressive agents may act as potentiating agents for other oncogenic stimuli, such as oncogenic viruses, chemical carcinogens, and UV light. Immunosuppressive agents with powerful antilymphocyte activity, including calcineurin inhibitors, antilymphocyte globulin, antithymocyte globulin, and anti-T-cell antibodies, may potentiate the effects of oncogenic viruses by eliminating T lymphocytes or impairing their normal function. In early studies, a clear potentiating effect of antilymphocyte globulin on cancer development was observed when the agent was used in conjunction with oncogenic viruses[3,51] or chemical carcinogens.[4,14,81]

Oncogenic Viruses

Viruses that have oncogenic properties have long been recognized in experimental studies.[3,84] Organ transplant recipients are particularly susceptible to viral infections, some of which are known to be potentially oncogenic in humans. These include EBV, cytomegalovirus, herpes simplex, herpes zoster, hepatitis B, hepatitis C, and HPV. The fact that the most common types of cancer occurring in transplant recipients are those in which oncogenic viruses are known to be causative is unlikely to be coincidental. Viral oncogenesis is considered to play a role in the development of most posttransplant lymphomas and lymphoproliferative disorders, cancers of the skin and cervix, and hepatomas.[23] The rapidity with which some malignancies occur after transplantation also is consistent with the concept that viral oncogenesis is involved because the start of immunosuppression is likely to produce very rapid viral transformation.

Chronic Antigenic Stimulation and Immune Regulation

It has been suggested that the continuing presence of foreign allograft antigens in a recipient may be important in cancer causation. This possibility is supported by evidence that chronic lymphoid stimulation results in a high incidence of malignant lymphomas.[89] The mechanism may be a direct consequence of protracted antigenic stimulation of the lymphoreticular system, with continued stimulation of lymphoid tissue leading to hyperplasia and ultimately to neoplasia.

Environmental Factors

A range of factors could account for the observed regional variations in the pattern of cancers that occur in patients transplanted at different centers around the world. A striking example of environmental effect is the association between the development of skin cancer in white transplant recipients and solar UV exposure. This association undoubtedly accounts for the high incidence of skin cancer in kidney transplant recipients in Australia and New Zealand (see Chapter 34). Exposure to UV light also can cause immunosuppression that may influence the development of other forms of cancer, such as non-Hodgkin's lymphoma.[5,70] Other factors that might predispose to the development of malignancy include viral infections encountered by patients before or after transplantation and local practices in viral infection prevention, detection, and therapy. Such factors operate against a background of general influences, such as age, gender, and genetic diversity, and depend on the length of time after transplantation. The complex interactions of such factors determine the incidence and pattern of posttransplant malignancy for each individual transplant center.

Direct Neoplastic Action of Immunosuppressive Drugs

The immunosuppressive drugs used to prevent and treat rejection in transplant recipients (see Chapters 15–22) generally have the effect of increasing the risk of cancer. This is consistent with the concept that malignancies arise when immune surveillance is impaired. Paradoxically, some of these immunosuppressive drugs also may have antineoplastic properties.[31]

Calcineurin Inhibitors (Cyclosporine and Tacrolimus). There is now a considerable body of experimental and clinical evidence that cyclosporine and tacrolimus promote rather than induce the development of cancer. The effect seems to be due to aberrant production of cytokines that regulate tumor growth, metastasis, and angiogenesis.[31] There also is evidence, however, that cyclosporine inhibits multidrug resistance in cancer cells,[94] and that it can even be combined with cytotoxic drugs such as paclitaxel to inhibit tumor growth in some cases.[52]

Mammalian Target of Rapamycin Inhibitors (mTORi). The basis for the immunosuppressive activity of these agents is their action in blocking interleukin-2 stimulation of lymphocyte proliferation. There is accumulating evidence that mTORi have antineoplastic properties,[50,82] and there have been several reports that the incidence of posttransplant malignancy is markedly lower in patients who receive sirolimus-based immunosuppression or sirolimus in association with calcineurin inhibitors compared with patients receiving calcineurin inhibitor therapy alone.[13,31,60] In a recent multicenter, randomized, controlled trial, sirolimus was substituted for calcineurin inhibitors in kidney transplant recipients who had cutaneous squamous cell carcinomas, and a marked reduction in the incidence of new squamous cell carcinomas was observed.[24] The trial data suggested that the earlier conversion to sirolimus occurred after an initial diagnosis of cutaneous squamous cell carcinoma, the greater the efficacy in terms of preventing the development of new squamous cell carcinomas.

Corticosteroids. Corticosteroids have anti-inflammatory and immunosuppressive properties, and their effects on the immune system are complex. Although they have been used clinically for several decades, their exact mechanisms of action are still not clearly understood. Their primary effects seem to be a result of inhibition of the production of T-cell lymphokines, which are needed to amplify macrophage and lymphocyte responses. They also cause lymphopenia as a result of redistribution of lymphocytes from the vascular compartment into lymphoid tissues, and they inhibit the migration of monocytes.

Corticosteroids such as prednisone and prednisolone have been used as part of most immunosuppressive regimens since human organ transplantation began, but their role in the causation of cancer in transplant recipients has been difficult to assess and remains unclear because almost always they have been used in conjunction with other immunosuppressive therapy. Although there is some experimental evidence that corticosteroids increase the risk of malignancy,[98] and it is known that there is an increased incidence of Kaposi's sarcoma in patients receiving them for long periods,[93] corticosteroids also are used in combination with other drugs to treat certain types of cancer, including lymphomas.

Azathioprine. Azathioprine disrupts the synthesis of DNA and RNA, causing immunosuppression by interfering with lymphocyte proliferation. When used as a single agent to treat autoimmune diseases, azathioprine is associated with an increased risk of lymphomas and an increased risk of a wide range of solid neoplasms, including squamous cell carcinomas, urinary bladder tumors, breast carcinomas, and brain tumors. In a follow-up study of 1000 kidney transplant recipients, it was found that patients who received azathioprine had a lower cumulative incidence of tumors after transplantation than patients who received cyclosporine.[62] It was unclear, however, whether this was due to the drugs themselves or to the overall intensity of the immunosuppression.

Mycophenolate Mofetil. Mycophenolate mofetil was originally developed as an antineoplastic agent.[102] Its main mode of action as an immunosuppressant is through blockage of the de novo purine synthesis pathway.[2] Preliminary analysis of data from large transplant registries suggests that the rate of development of cancer in patients receiving mycophenolate mofetil is lower than the rate in patients receiving other immunosuppressive therapies, but longer follow-up is required before firm conclusions can be drawn.

Lymphocyte-Depleting Agents. Although a common pathway for many immunosuppressive agents used in organ transplantation seems to be the suppression of lymphocyte proliferation, some agents are known or are thought to act by causing the death of lymphocytes. Examples are antilymphocyte globulin and antithymocyte globulin, both polyclonal antibodies; the monoclonal antibody muromonab (OKT3), which is directed against the CD3 antigen complex found on all mature human T cells; and antilymphocyte antibodies, such as the anti-CD25 antibodies basiliximab and daclizumab, which are highly specific interleukin-2 receptor blockers. After administration of these agents, the total lymphocyte count decreases as lymphocytes, especially T cells, are lysed after antibody binding and complement deposition on the cell surface, inactivated by binding to T-cell receptors, or cleared from the circulation and deposited in the reticuloendothelial system. Overall, lymphatic depletion is thought to increase the risk of malignancy by reducing the effectiveness of an individual's immune surveillance.

Types of Cancer in Kidney Transplant Recipients

The cancers that occur in kidney transplant recipients, with a distribution that differs considerably from that in the general population, have already been discussed in the section of this chapter dealing with cancer in dialysis patients, and details are given in Table 35-1. However, some cancer types that occur in kidney transplant recipients warrant special mention.

Skin Malignancies

NMSCs are the most common malignancies in kidney transplant recipients, in whom they can be very aggressive. They represent a particular problem in parts of the world where predominantly white populations are exposed regularly to high-intensity solar UV light. Skin malignancies in transplant recipients are discussed in detail in Chapter 34.

Posttransplant Lymphoproliferative Disorder

Posttransplant lymphoproliferative disorder (PTLD) is a spectrum of major, life-threatening lymphoproliferative diseases occurring in the posttransplant setting. The majority of PTLD is of B-cell origin and is associated with several risk factors, the most significant being EBV infection. The term EBV-associated PTLD includes all clinical syndromes of EBV-associated lymphoproliferation, ranging from uncomplicated posttransplant infectious mononucleosis to true malignancies that contain clonal chromosomal abnormalities.[68,79] Classification has changed over time, with the most recent suggested by the World Health Organization.[40] EBV-associated malignancies affect approximately 1–2% of all kidney transplant recipients.[86] There is a bimodal distribution of timing of occurrence after transplantation, with a peak of cases occurring in the first 2 years and a second peak occurring between 5 and 10 years after transplantation. However, the incidence of non-EBV-positive PTLD remains far higher than the incidence of lymphoma in non-immunocompromised subjects.

A marked increase in the incidence of PTLD in kidney transplant recipients was reported after the introduction of cyclosporine[76] and tacrolimus.[66] This raised concern that the drugs themselves might have a specific role in lymphoma causation; however, registry reports from different countries suggest that this is not the case.[69,87] It is now generally believed that PTLD and malignant lymphomas are an inevitable consequence of effective immunosuppressive therapy regardless of the particular immunosuppressive agents used. The effect of EBV infection, whether as a primary event or as a reactivation of a previous infection, is thought to be mediated by B-lymphocyte proliferation secondary to inhibition of the T-cell-dominated immune responses produced by powerful immunosuppression.[32] The T-cell-suppressive, B-cell-stimulatory cytokine interleukin-10 has been implicated.[7]

It has been known for over 40 years that EBV is linked to the development of Burkitt's lymphoma[33] and to nasopharyngeal carcinoma. EBV is ubiquitous, with 95% of the adult population in most countries having serological evidence of prior exposure. The possibility of reactivation is high if immunosuppression is excessive. In children who undergo transplantation, approximately 50% are likely to be EBV-negative at the time, resulting in susceptibility to primary infection from a virus-positive graft or blood transfusion.[22]

The frequency with which lymphomas occurring in transplant recipients involve the central nervous system is notable. In approximately 40% of lymphomas in transplant recipients, the brain or spinal cord is involved compared with 2% of such malignancies in the general population. These lymphomas involving the central nervous system are frequently multicentric.

Kaposi's Sarcoma

Kaposi's sarcoma is an angioproliferative disorder that requires infection with human herpesvirus, also known as Kaposi's sarcoma-associated herpesvirus, for its development. Genetic predisposition has an important role as well, and Kaposi's sarcoma occurs more frequently in immunosuppressed transplant recipients of Italian, Greek, Jewish, Arabic, and African ancestry,[74] no matter where these patients are resident when they receive their transplant. The incidence of Kaposi's sarcoma in any transplant population depends largely on the proportion of patients with Mediterranean heritage in that population. In countries such as the United States and Australia, Kaposi's sarcoma affects approximately 0.25% of renal allograft recipients, contributing 2–3% of all cancers. In Japan, Kaposi's sarcoma is extremely rare,[37] whereas it is common in the Middle East, affecting approximately 5% of recipients in Saudi Arabia, and constituting 40–70% of all posttransplant cancers.[80] Men are affected three times as frequently as women, and almost 50% of cases occur within the first year after transplantation.[74] The role of immunosuppression in the development of Kaposi's sarcoma is supported by the fact that withdrawal of immunosuppression sometimes results in complete remission.[74]

Kaposi's sarcoma developing in transplant recipients tends to be multicentric. Of transplant patients with this condition, 60% have involvement of the skin or the oropharyngolaryngeal mucosa or both.[75] In these sites, the lesions appear as circumscribed purplish macules or as granulomas that fail to heal. The remaining patients have visceral disease, particularly involving the gastrointestinal tract or the respiratory system. Approximately 40% of patients with non-visceral lesions have complete or partial remission after cessation or reduction of immunosuppressive therapy, although with reduced immunosuppression, more than 50% of these patients lose their grafts to rejection. Patients with visceral involvement usually fail to respond to any form of therapy. There is some evidence from case series that mTORi may provide effective therapy[9,29] (see Chapter 19).

Time of Cancer Presentation

In non-immunosuppressed individuals, known carcinogens, such as tobacco, UV light, and ionizing radiation, have long latent periods between exposure and the development of malignancy. In immunosuppressed kidney transplant recipients, the process of oncogenesis is greatly accelerated. In Australia, the mean time of appearance for lymphomas, Kaposi's sarcoma, and malignancy of the endocrine glands is approximately 6 years after transplantation; for cancer affecting the respiratory tract it is 8 years; for breast cancer, genitourinary system cancers, and leukemia it is 9 years; and for cancer of the alimentary tract it is 10 years.[87]

Management of Cancer in Kidney Transplant Recipients

Localized non-skin malignancies should be treated by standard surgical excision, with adjuvant radiotherapy or chemotherapy as considered appropriate. If complete surgical excision is possible, it is usually considered reasonable to continue immunosuppressive therapy. If metastatic disease is present or develops, however, most clinicians withdraw immunosuppression, arrange excision of metastases if these appear to be single or localized, institute chemotherapy if surgical removal is impossible, and remove the allograft when rejection occurs. As expected, survival rates are lower in transplant recipients than they are in the general population.

The treatment of PTLD is an evolving area and management varies significantly according to the type of lymphoproliferative disease present. In general, reduction of immunosuppression on diagnosis is instituted, but the optimal immunosuppression reduction to ensure regression of disease is unknown, and decisions are usually based on the severity of the disease in combination with the health risk associated with possible loss of the allograft. Although there is currently no evidence of the efficacy of antiviral therapy for treatment of PTLD, antiviral agents such as ganciclovir are commonly used for EBV-associated PTLD. Patients with monoclonal malignancies can be treated with chemotherapy, commonly CHOP (cyclophosphamide, doxorubicin, vincristine, prednisolone), For patients who have PTLD that expresses CD20^{+}, chemotherapy is usually administered in conjunction with rituximab. There have been no published randomized studies comparing different chemotherapy regimens in PTLD and a choice is generally made based upon physician experience and side effect profile. Novel therapies of adoptive immunotherapy are under investigation. EBV-seropositive allogeneic donor lymphocyte infusions have been used successfully, as has infusion of in vitro-generated autologous and allogeneic EBV-specific cytotoxic T lymphocytes, with the aim of reconstituting EBV-specific T-cell immunity. Localized lymphoma may be suitable for debulking surgical excision.

TRANSPLANTATION IN PATIENTS WITH A HISTORY OF CANCER

In general, for potential transplant recipients with a prior history of cancer, a recurrence-free waiting period of 2–5 years before transplantation is recommended; however this must be individualized based on patient and tumor characteristics.[41,49] In an early review of the problem, Penn[73] reported patients with non-renal malignancies who had been treated before transplantation. Of 119 patients with tumors involving the breast or a variety of internal organs, 18 (14%) developed recurrence or metastasis, mostly from tumors of the breast, bladder, or large bowel. Although recurrence generally was less likely to occur with greater time from treatment of the cancer to transplantation, 28% of the recurrences occurred in patients who had been treated an average of 7 years before transplantation. There were 22 patients with prior lymphatic malignancies, and the disease persisted or recurred in 50%. Most of the recurrences were in patients who had multiple myeloma. Nine of the 11 patients were not being treated or were not in remission at the time of transplantation, or the existing malignancies had not been recognized. Generally, recurrences did not occur in patients treated more than 2 years before transplantation or who were in remission at the time of transplantation.

Previously treated melanoma presents a particular problem because in non-immunosuppressed patients this disease can recur more than 25 years after apparently successful treatment,[85] indicating that in some cases the disease persists but is controlled by the individual's immune defenses. The risks of recurrence of melanoma after transplantation are considerable, and if transplantation is contemplated, screening with a sensitive test such as a positron emission tomography scan should be performed before proceeding, although microscopic metastatic disease will not be detected using this test or any other investigation presently available.

Currently, most clinicians consider it reasonable to offer transplantation to patients with ESKD without wait time after treatment of low-grade cancers such as NMSC, in situ cancer of the cervix, in situ bladder cancer, and all non-invasive papillary tumors of the bladder. For patients who have had other cancers treated successfully, guidelines advise deferring transplantation for at least 2 years. A wait of 5 years following treatment is advised for melanoma, breast cancer with regional node involvement, bilateral disease, or inflammatory histology, and colorectal carcinoma other than in situ Dukes A or B1 disease.

PREVENTION AND EARLY DETECTION OF CANCER IN KIDNEY TRANSPLANT RECIPIENTS

As indicated earlier, all reasonable measures should be taken to exclude malignancy in every potential recipient before offering transplantation. The known risks of cigarette smoking should be explained, and appropriate advice should be given about sun protection, particularly in geographic areas where there is a high risk of skin malignancy. Pretransplant dermatological assessment is advisable, and existing skin lesions should be treated. In female patients, pretransplant gynecological assessment should be mandatory, and any abnormality of the uterine cervix should be treated adequately before transplantation. Pretransplant viral studies should be undertaken, including tests for hepatitis B, hepatitis C, cytomegalovirus, HIV, EBV, herpes simplex, and herpes zoster. Donor viral studies also should be routine to avoid or at least document viral transmission. After transplantation, the use of prophylactic antiviral agents may be considered for patients who are judged to be at high risk for viral infection, such as cytomegalovirus-negative or EBV-negative recipients who receive organs from donors positive for these viruses, or for recipients receiving high-dose immunosuppression to treat rejection (see Chapter 29). By preventing or controlling infections, it is hoped that the risk of post-transplant malignancy will be reduced.

As kidney transplant recipients are at higher risk of cancer at most sites, and cancer after transplantation causes considerable morbidity and mortality, participation in cancer screening programs is appealing. However, the survival benefits demonstrasted in an otherwise healthy general population may not be assumed in a kidney transplant population. The role of infections in carcinogenesis may offer opportunity to intervene to reduce risk. Although immunization against infections known to have oncogenic potential may seem an obvious preventive strategy for transplant recipients, achieving a protective immune response following vaccination is not always possible. People on dialysis have a reduced response to vaccination, with a lower antibody titer and an inability to maintain adequate antibody titers over time.[20] Antibody response after transplantation is usually even worse, particularly in the first posttransplant year, when the burden of iatrogenic immunosuppression is most intense.

Because early diagnosis offers the best chance of effective treatment, clinicians caring for kidney transplant recipients must be constantly alert to the possibility of cancer development. Regular clinical review by transplant clinicians is essential, with periodic gynecological review of female recipients, and careful dermatological surveillance for all recipients considered to be at risk of developing skin malignancy.

Health economic evaluations can offer insights into the likely effectivness of screening programs. For female recipients, the recommended policy of annual screening for cervical cancer using conventional cytology is cost-effective. The replacement of conventional cytology with liquid-based cytology is likely to provide minimal survival benefit but incur considerable additional cost. Assuming the reported trial-based vaccine efficacy in HPV-naïve women, a program of HPV vaccination before kidney transplantation may not be cost-effective.[107]

When considering screening for colorectal cancer, transplant recipients have both a higher risk and a worse prognosis than the general population. Economic evaluation suggests that colorectal cancer screening using annual fecal occult blood testing may be cost-effective in kidney transplant recipients, if at least 50% of recipients participate. Annual and biennial fecal occult blood testing is the only screening modality that has been shown in randomized controlled trials to reduce colorectal cancer-specific mortality in the general population. However, without a randomized controlled trial in the kidney transplant population assessing the benefits and harms of colorectal cancer screening, uncertainties will always exist.[106]

Considering screening for breast and prostate cancer in kidney recipients, neither is likely to produce the magnitude of benefit seen in the general population, principally because fewer years of life are likely to be lost to cancer, due to competing risks for morbidity and mortality. Only those non-diabetic transplant recipients at elevated risk of cancer are likely to see benefit from screening of the magnitude measured in the general population.[47]

SURVIVAL IN KIDNEY TRANSPLANT RECIPIENTS WHO DEVELOP CANCER

Whether overall mortality rates for specific cancer types are different in transplant populations compared to the general population is not entirely clear. Analysis of the United States Renal Data System showed that the standardized mortality ratios were very high in younger transplant recipients and low in older transplant recipients, although there was no overall increase.[48] The authors suggested that competing risks of death from other causes dampen the impact of immunosuppression-induced malignancy in the older transplant population. Cardiovascular mortality is the most important cause of death, particularly in patients with diabetes and those with a prior cardiac history. Consistent with this hypothesis, older age, diabetes, and prior history of congestive heart failure and stroke were independently associated with lower cancer mortality. The higher cancer standardized mortality ratios in younger patients also support this hypothesis, as patients in this group have longer projected life expectancies (lower competing risks of death) with greater cumulative risks of succumbing to their malignancy. The authors also suggested that early cancer mortality might be delayed because pretransplant screening eliminates potential recipients with serious cancers; this was based on the finding that death rates were lower in the most recently transplanted patients, increasing after year 5 posttransplantation.

Analysis using the ANZDATA registry compared death rates among four groups: (1) those with a transplant but no cancer; (2) those with a transplant and cancer; (3) those with cancer but no transplant; and (4) those with neither transplant nor cancer (i.e., the general population) between 1988 and 2005.[100] Death rates

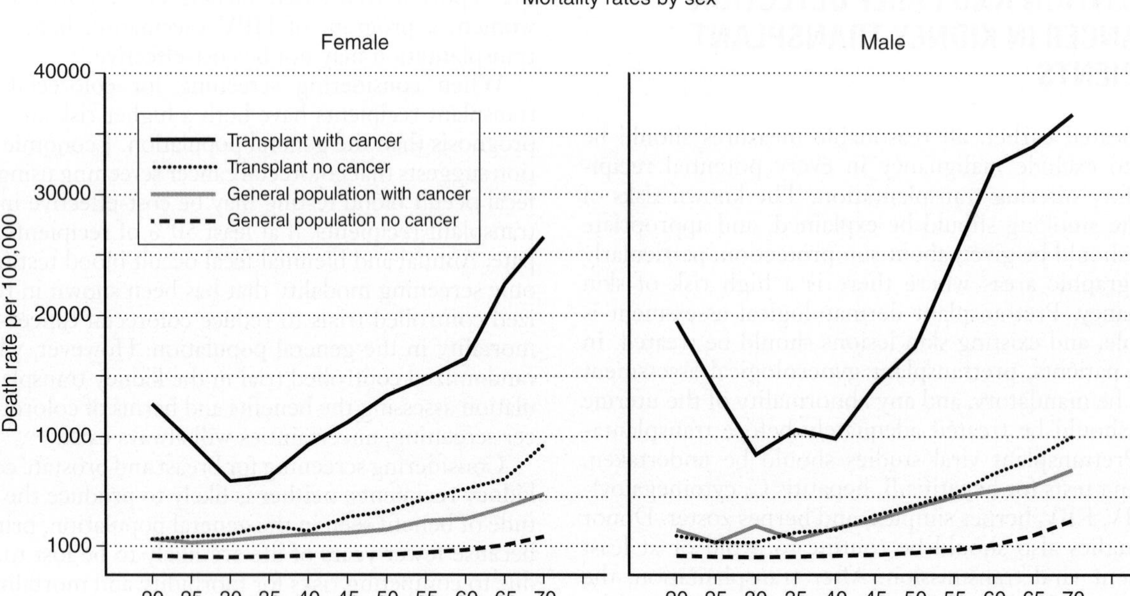

FIGURE 35-2 ■ Mortality rates with and without cancer after transplantation. Death rates indirectly standardized by age, sex, and calendar year for people in Australia and New Zealand, 1988–2005. (From Webster AC, Wong G. Chapter 10, Cancer. ANZDATA Registry Report 2008. 31st annual report. Adelaide, South Australia: Australia and New Zealand Dialysis and Transplant Registry (http://www.anzdata.org.au), 2009.)

were compared, after applying indirect standardization by age, sex, and calendar year. The results are shown in Figure 35-2. As expected, there were differences in survival for men and for women. Death rates for people with a transplant and no cancer were similar to those with cancer but no transplant, and these death rates are similar to those of people 30 years older from the general population with neither a transplant nor cancer. Between 1963 and 2006 there were 15 183 transplant recipients, with a mean follow-up of 9.0 years, and a total 135 968 years of risk. During follow-up 1642 (10.8%) developed at least one cancer and 6479 (42.7%) died. Within the transplant population, older age and male sex increased the risk of death (transplanted >55 years versus <35 years HR 4.47, 4.15–4.83; male versus female HR 1.09, 1.04–1.15), as did diabetic ESKD (versus glomerulonephritis HR 1.78, 1.61–1.96) and graft failure (HR 3.81, 3.62–4.01), but white racial background was protective (HR 0.79, 0.73–0.85). After allowing for these effects, a cancer diagnosis increased the risk of early death more than fourfold (HR 4.12, 3.84–4.43).

An alternative way to consider cancer-related mortality in the transplant population is to examine relative survival. This is calculated as the ratio of observed compared to expected survival in the general population of the same age and sex, over the same time period. A ratio of 1 indicates survival equivalent to the general population; ratios <1 indicate lower survival (higher mortality) compared to the general population. Work from the ANZDATA registry considered expected survival for transplant patients with breast or colorectal cancer compared to transplant recipients without cancer, and compared it with people in the general population diagnosed with breast or colorectal cancer. The relative survival analysis standardized for any differences in mortality attributable to age, sex, calendar year, and country (Australia or New Zealand) among the populations.[101]

Relative survival for people with breast cancer is shown in Figure 35-3. The effect of comorbidity with a kidney transplant and breast cancer was pronounced overall and for all age subgroups, with poorer relative survival compared with the transplant alone and the breast cancer alone groups. This is reported in Figure 35-3. For example, a woman aged 50–59 with breast cancer experiences 14% excess mortality compared with expected background mortality in the general population, a woman of the same age with a transplant experiences 16% excess mortality, and a woman with both a transplant and a breast cancer experiences 48% excess mortality.

Relative survival for people with colorectal cancer is shown in Figure 35-3. Survival differed by age and sex (shown in Figure 35-3). For males >55 years, the 5-year relative survival was 0.79 with a transplant alone, 0.57 with colorectal cancer alone, but 0.27 with transplant plus colorectal cancer (73% excess mortality compared to general population expectations). Women with both a transplant and colorectal cancer had a marked excess mortality compared to men, and to women with cancer alone or a transplant alone.

CONCLUSIONS

The great success of dialysis and transplantation programs over the past several decades has meant that large numbers of patients are surviving for much longer than previously. However, this has meant that the problem of malignancy developing in dialysis and transplant patients has steadily increased, because of their prolonged survival. Those caring for these patients must therefore

Age	Colorectal				Breast		
	<55 years		55 and over		<50 years	50–59	60 and over
Sex	Male	Female	Male	Female	Female		
Cancer alone	0.61	0.63	0.57	0.57	0.83	0.86	0.81
Transplant alone	0.92	0.91	0.79	0.81	0.91	0.84	0.81
Transplant and cancer	0.55	0.30	0.27	0.21	0.72	0.52	0.62

A

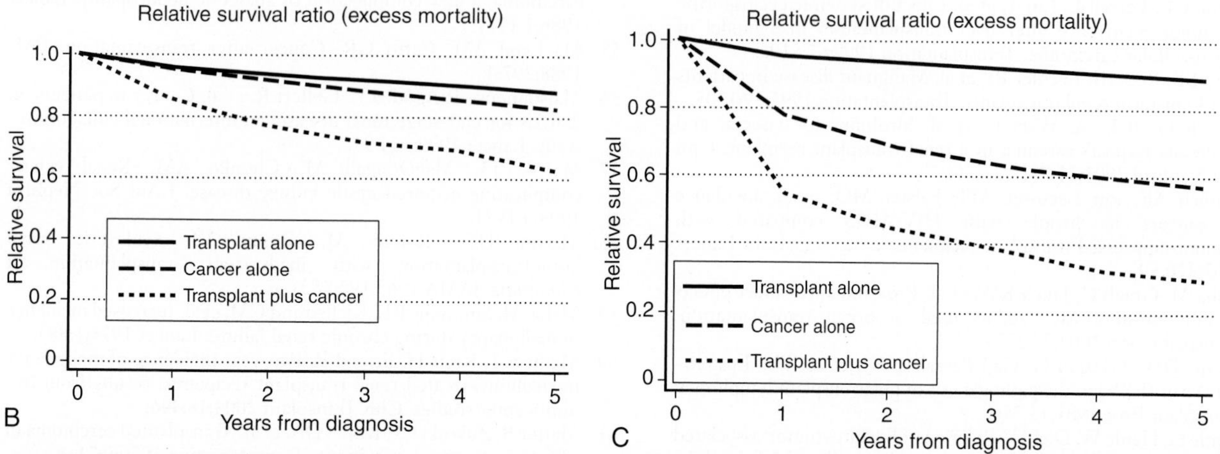

FIGURE 35-3 ■ Relative survival (excess mortality) for people with colorectal cancer or breast cancer. (A) Five-year relative survival for transplant recipients with and without breast or colorectal cancer, and people without transplants with breast or colorectal cancer, compared with expected survival in the general population. (B) Relative survival for female transplant recipients with and without breast cancer, and women with breast cancer alone. (C) Relative survival for transplant recipients with and without colorectal cancer, and people with colorectal cancer alone.

be ever vigilant for the earliest evidence of malignancy, allowing treatment to be initiated promptly. As well, routine screening for the most common malignancies should be considered, and patients should receive appropriate education about symptoms and signs that will allow early detection of malignancies that they are likely to be able to recognize themselves (such as skin cancers). In the future, modification of immunosuppressive drug regimens and the new immunosuppressive strategies may reduce the incidence of posttransplant malignancies. The prevention or control of the viral infections that are clearly related to the development of some of these malignancies may also assist in reducing their incidence.

REFERENCES

1. Adami J, Gabel H, Lindelof B, et al. Cancer risk following organ transplantation: a nationwide cohort study in Sweden. Br J Cancer 2003;89:1221.
2. Allison AC. Mechanisms of action of mycophenolate mofetil. Lupus 2005;14(Suppl. 1):s2.
3. Allison AC, Berman LD, Levey RH. Increased tumour induction by adenovirus type 12 in thymectomized mice and mice treated with anti-lymphocyte serum. Nature 1967;215:185.
4. Balner H, Dersjant H. Increased oncogenic effect of methylcholanthrene after treatment with anti-lymphocyte serum. Nature 1969;224:376.
5. Bentham G. Association between incidence of non-Hodgkin's lymphoma and solar ultraviolet radiation in England and Wales. BMJ 1996;312:1128.
6. Beutner KR, Tyring S. Human papillomavirus and human disease. Am J Med 1997;102:9.
7. Birkeland SA, Bendtzen K, Moller B, et al. Interleukin-10 and posttransplant lymphoproliferative disorder after kidney transplantation. Transplantation 1999;67:876.
8. Birkeland SA, Lokkegaard H, Storm HH. Cancer risk in patients on dialysis and after renal transplantation. Lancet 2000;355:1886.
9. Boratynska M, Watorek E, Smolska D, et al. Anticancer effect of sirolimus in renal allograft recipients with de novo malignancies. Transplant Proc 2007;39:2736.
10. Brunner FP, Landais P, Selwood NH. Malignancies after renal transplantation: the EDTA-ERA registry experience. European Dialysis and Transplantation Association-European Renal Association. Nephrol Dial Transplant 1995;10(Suppl. 1):74.
11. Budakoglu B, Abali H, Uncu D, et al. Good tolerance of weekly irinotecan in a patient with metastatic colorectal cancer on chronic hemodialysis. J Chemother 2005;17:452.
12. Burnet FM. Immunological aspects of malignant disease. Lancet 1967;1:1171.
13. Campistol JM, Eris J, Oberbauer R, et al. Sirolimus therapy after early cyclosporine withdrawal reduces the risk for cancer in adult renal transplantation. J Am Soc Nephrol 2006;17:581.
14. Cerilli GJ, Treat RC. The effect of antilymphocyte serum on the induction and growth of tumour in the adult mouse. Transplantation 1969;8:1865.
15. Chertow GM, Paltiel AD, Owen Jr WF, et al. Cost-effectiveness of cancer screening in end-stage renal disease. Arch Intern Med 1996;156:1345.
16. Ciriaco P, Casiraghi M, Melloni G, et al. Pulmonary resection for non-small-cell lung cancer in patients on hemodialysis: clinical outcome and long-term results. World J Surg 2005;29:1516.
17. Cuckovic C, Djukanovic L, Jankovic S, et al. Malignant tumors in hemodialysis patients. Nephron 1996;73:710.
18. de Villiers EM, Weidauer H, Otto H, et al. Papillomavirus DNA in human tongue carcinomas. Int J Cancer 1985;36:575.
19. Denton MD, Magee CC, Ovuworie C, et al. Prevalence of renal cell carcinoma in patients with ESRD pre-transplantation: a pathologic analysis. Kidney Int 2002;61:2201.
20. Dinits-Pensy M, Forrest GN, Cross AS, et al. The use of vaccines in adult patients with renal disease. Am J Kidney Dis 2005; 46:997.
21. Doak PB, Montgomerie JZ, North JD, et al. Reticulum cell sarcoma after renal homotransplantation and azathioprine and prednisone therapy. BMJ 1968;4:746.
22. Dunn SP, Krueger LJ. Immunosuppression of paediatric liver transplant recipients: minimising the risk of posttransplant lymphoproliferative disorders. Transplant Immunol Lett 1998;14:5.

23. el-Sabrout R, Gruber SA. Etiology and pathogenesis of posttransplant tumors: new insights into viral oncogenesis. Ann Transplant 1997;2:67.
24. Euvrard S, Morelon E, Rostaing L, et al. Sirolimus and secondary skin-cancer prevention in kidney transplantation. N Engl J Med 2012;367:329.
25. Fer MF, McKinney TD, Richardson RL, et al. Cancer and the kidney: complications of neoplasms. Am J Med 1981;71:704.
26. Fishman JA, Rubin RH. Infection in organ-transplant recipients. N Engl J Med 1998;338:1741.
27. Freise CE, Ferrell L, Liu T, et al. Effect of systemic cyclosporine on tumor recurrence after liver transplantation in a model of hepatocellular carcinoma. Transplantation 1999;67:510.
28. Gaya SB, Rees AJ, Lechler RI, et al. Malignant disease in patients with long-term renal transplants. Transplantation 1995;59:1705.
29. Gheith O, Bakr A, Wafa E, et al. Sirolimus for visceral and cutaneous Kaposi's sarcoma in a renal-transplant recipient. Clin Exp Nephrol 2007;11:251.
30. Grulich AE, van Leeuwen MT, Falster MO, et al. Incidence of cancers in people with HIV/AIDS compared with immunosuppressed transplant recipients: a meta-analysis. Lancet 2007;370:59.
31. Guba M, Graeb C, Jauch KW, et al. Pro- and anti-cancer effects of immunosuppressive agents used in organ transplantation. Transplantation 2004;77:1777.
32. Hanto DW, Frizzera G, Gajl-Peczalska KJ, et al. The Epstein–Barr virus (EBV) in the pathogenesis of posttransplant lymphoma. Transplant Proc 1981;13:756.
33. Henle G, Henle W, Diehl V. Relation of Burkitt's tumor-associated herpes-type virus to infectious mononucleosis. Proc Natl Acad Sci U S A 1968;59:94.
34. Herr HW, Engen DE, Hostetler J. Malignancy in uremia: dialysis versus transplantation. J Urol 1979;121:584.
35. Holley JL. Preventive medical screening is not appropriate for many chronic dialysis patients. Semin Dial 2000;13:369.
36. Holst JP, Burman KD, Atkins F, et al. Radioiodine therapy for thyroid cancer and hyperthyroidism in patients with end-stage renal disease on hemodialysis. Thyroid 2005;15:1321.
37. Hoshida Y, Tsukuma H, Yasunaga Y, et al. Cancer risk after renal transplantation in Japan. Int J Cancer 1997;71:517.
38. Iseki K, Osawa A, Fukiyama K. Evidence for increased cancer deaths in chronic dialysis patients. Am J Kidney Dis 1993; 22:308.
39. Ishikawa I, Honda R, Yamada Y, et al. Renal cell carcinoma detected by screening shows better patient survival than that detected following symptoms in dialysis patients. Ther Apher Dial 2004;8:468.
40. Jaffe ES, Harris NL, Stein H, et al, editors. World health organization classification of tumours: pathology and genetics of tumours of haematopoietic and lymphoid tissues. Lyons: IARC; 2001.
41. Kasiske BL, Cangro CB, Hariharan S, et al. The evaluation of renal transplantation candidates: clinical practice guidelines. Am J Transplant 2001;1(Suppl. 2):3.
42. Kasiske BL, Snyder JJ, Gilbertson DT, et al. Cancer after kidney transplantation in the United States. Am J Transplant 2004;4:905.
43. Kausz AT, Guo H, Pereira BJ, et al. General medical care among patients with chronic kidney disease: opportunities for improving outcomes. J Am Soc Nephrol 2005;16:3092.
44. Keast D. Immunosurveillance and cancer. Lancet 1970;2:710.
45. Keith DS, Torres VE, King BF, et al. Renal cell carcinoma in autosomal dominant polycystic kidney disease. J Am Soc Nephrol 1994;4:1661.
46. Kersey JH, Spector BD, Good RA. Immunodeficiency and cancer. Adv Cancer Res 1973;18:211.
47. Kiberd BA, Keough-Ryan T, Clase CM. Screening for prostate, breast and colorectal cancer in renal transplant recipients. Am J Transplant 2003;3:619.
48. Kiberd BA, Rose C, Gill JS. Cancer mortality in kidney transplantation. Am J Transplant 2009;9:1868.
49. Knoll G, Cockfield S, Blydt-Hansen T, et al. Canadian society of transplantation consensus guidelines on eligibility for kidney transplantation. CMAJ 2005;173:1181.
50. Law BK. Rapamycin: an anti-cancer immunosuppressant? Crit Rev Oncol Hematol 2005;56:47.
51. Law LW, Ting RC, Allison AC. Effects of antilymphocyte serum on induction of tumours and leukemia by murine sarcoma virus. Nature 1968;220:61.
52. Lin HL, Lui WY, Liu TY, et al. Reversal of Taxol resistance in hepatoma by cyclosporin A: involvement of the PI-3 kinase-AKT 1 pathway. Br J Cancer 2003;88:973.
53. Lindner A, Farewell VT, Sherrard DJ. High incidence of neoplasia in uremic patients receiving long-term dialysis. Cancer and long-term dialysis. Nephron 1981;27:292.
54. Lornoy W, Becaus S, de Vleeschouwer M, et al. Renal cell carcinoma, a new complication of analgesic nephropathy. Lancet 1986;1:1271.
55. MacLeod AM, Catto GR. Cancer after transplantation. BMJ 1988;297:4.
56. Maisonneuve P, Agodoa L, Gellert R, et al. Cancer in patients on dialysis for end-stage renal disease: an international collaborative study. Lancet 1999;354:93.
57. Marple JT, MacDougall M, Chonko AM. Renal cancer complicating acquired cystic kidney disease. J Am Soc Nephrol 1994;4:1951.
58. Martin DC, Rubini M, Rosen VJ. Cadaveric renal homotransplantation with inadvertent transplantation of carcinoma. JAMA 1965;192:752.
59. Matas AJ, Simmons RL, Kjellstrand CM, et al. Increased incidence of malignancy during chronic renal failure. Lancet 1975;1:883.
60. Mathew T, Kreis H, Friend P. Two-year incidence of malignancy in sirolimus-treated renal transplant recipients: results from five multicenter studies. Clin Transplant 2004;18:446.
61. Matter B, Zukoski CF, Killen DA, et al. Transplanted carcinoma in an immunosuppressed patient. Transplantation 1970;9:71.
62. McGeown MG, Douglas JF, Middleton D. One thousand renal transplants at Belfast City Hospital: post-graft neoplasia 1968–1999, comparing azathioprine only with cyclosporin-based regimes in a single centre. Clin Transpl 2000;193.
63. McPhaul JJ, McIntosh DA, Hall W. Tissue transplantation still vexes. N Engl J Med 1965;272:105.
64. Miach PJ, Dawborn JK, Xipell J. Neoplasia in patients with chronic renal failure on long-term dialysis. Clin Nephrol 1976;5:101.
65. Montagnino G, Lorca E, Tarantino A, et al. Cancer incidence in 854 kidney transplant recipients from a single institution: comparison with normal population and with patients under dialytic treatment. Clin Transplant 1996;10:461.
66. Newell KA, Alonso EM, Whitington PF, et al. Posttransplant lymphoproliferative disease in pediatric liver transplantation. Interplay between primary Epstein–Barr virus infection and immunosuppression. Transplantation 1996;62:370.
67. Niu MT, Coleman PJ, Alter MJ. Multicenter study of hepatitis C virus infection in chronic hemodialysis patients and hemodialysis center staff members. Am J Kidney Dis 1993;22:568.
68. Nourse JP, Jones K, Gandhi MK. Epstein–Barr virus-related post-transplant lymphoproliferative disorders: pathogenetic insights for targeted therapy. Am J Transplant 2011;11:888.
69. Opelz G, Henderson R. Incidence of non-Hodgkin lymphoma in kidney and heart transplant recipients. Lancet 1993;342:1514.
70. Otley CC. Non-Hodgkin lymphoma and skin cancer: a dangerous combination. Australas J Dermatol 2006;47:231.
71. Peces R, Martinez-Ara J, Miguel JL, et al. Renal cell carcinoma co-existent with other renal disease: clinico-pathological features in pre-dialysis patients and those receiving dialysis or renal transplantation. Nephrol Dial Transplant 2004;19:2789.
72. Penn I. Development of cancer as a complication of clinical transplantation. Transplant Proc 1977;9:1121.
73. Penn I. Kaposi's sarcoma in immunosuppressed patients. J Clin Lab Immunol 1983;12:1.
74. Penn I. Sarcomas in organ allograft recipients. Transplantation 1995;60:1485.
75. Penn I. Some contributions of transplantation to our knowledge of cancer. Transplant Proc 1980;12:676.
76. Penn I, Brunson ME. Cancers after cyclosporine therapy. Transplant Proc 1988;20:885.
77. Penn I, Hammond W, Brettschneider L, et al. Malignant lymphomas in transplantation patients. Transplant Proc 1969;1:106.
78. Pineda E, Perez-Ordonez B, Dackiw A, et al. Parathyroid carcinoma should be suspected in dialysis patients with rapid changes in serum parathormone levels. Perit Dial Int 2005;25:93.

79. Preiksaitis JK, Keay S. Diagnosis and management of posttransplant lymphoproliferative disorder in solid-organ transplant recipients. Clin Infect Dis 2001;33(Suppl. 1):S38.
80. Qunibi W, Akhtar M, Sheth K, et al. Kaposi's sarcoma: the most common tumor after renal transplantation in Saudi Arabia. Am J Med 1988;84:225.
81. Rabbat AG, Jeejeebhoy HF. Heterologous antilymphocyte serum (ALS) hastens the appearance of methylcholanthrene-induced tumours in mice. Transplantation 1970;9:164.
82. Rao RD, Buckner JC, Sarkaria JN. Mammalian target of rapamycin (mTOR) inhibitors as anti-cancer agents. Curr Cancer Drug Targets 2004;4:621.
83. Satoh S, Tsuchiya N, Habuchi T, et al. Renal cell and transitional cell carcinoma in a Japanese population undergoing maintenance dialysis. J Urol 2005;174:1749.
84. Schwartz RS, Beldotti L. Malignant lymphomas following allogenic disease: transition from an immunological to a neoplastic disorder. Science 1965;149:1511.
85. Shaw HM, Rivers JK, McCarthy SW, et al. Cutaneous melanomas exhibiting unusual biologic behavior. World J Surg 1992;16:196.
86. Sheil AG. Cancer report 2001. In: Ross GR, editor. ANZDATA registry report 2001. Adelaide, South Australia: Australia and New Zealand Dialysis and Transplant Registry; 2001. p. 84.
87. Sheil AGR. Cancer report 1997. In: Disney APS, editor. The twentieth annual report: Australia and New Zealand dialysis and transplant registry. Adelaide, South Australia: Queen Elizabeth Hospital; 1997. p. 138.
88. Slavis SA, Novick AC, Steinmuller DR, et al. Outcome of renal transplantation in patients with a functioning graft for 20 years or more. J Urol 1990;144:20.
89. Smithers DW, Field EO. Immunosuppression and cancer. Lancet 1969;1:672.
90. Stewart JH, Buccianti G, Agodoa L, et al. Cancers of the kidney and urinary tract in patients on dialysis for end-stage renal disease: analysis of data from the United States, Europe, and Australia and New Zealand. J Am Soc Nephrol 2003;14:197.
91. Sutherland GA, Glass J, Gabriel R. Increased incidence of malignancy in chronic renal failure. Nephron 1977;18:182.
92. Thomas L. Cellular and humoral aspects of the hypertensive states. London: Cassell; 1959.
93. Trattner A, Hodak E, David M, et al. The appearance of Kaposi sarcoma during corticosteroid therapy. Cancer 1993; 72:1779.
94. Twentyman PR, Fox NE, White DJ. Cyclosporin A and its analogues as modifiers of adriamycin and vincristine resistance in a multi-drug resistant human lung cancer cell line. Br J Cancer 1987;56:55.
95. Vajdic CM, McDonald SP, McCredie MR, et al. Cancer incidence before and after kidney transplantation. JAMA 2006;296:2823.
96. Vamvakas S, Bahner U, Heidland A. Cancer in end-stage renal disease: potential factors involved [editorial]. Am J Nephrol 1998;18:89.
97. van Leeuwen MT, Webster AC, McCredie MR, et al. Effect of reduced immunosuppression after kidney transplant failure on risk of cancer: population based retrospective cohort study. BMJ 2010;340:c570.
98. Walker SE, Anver MR, Schechter SL, et al. Prolonged lifespan and high incidence of neoplasms in NZB/NZW mice treated with hydrocortisone sodium succinate. Kidney Int 1978;14:151.
99. Webster AC, Craig JC, Simpson JM, et al. Identifying high risk groups and quantifying absolute risk of cancer after kidney transplantation: a cohort study of 15,183 recipients. Am J Transplant 2007;7:2140.
100. Webster AC, Wong G. Cancer. ANZDATA registry report 2008. 31st Annual report. Adelaide, South Australia: Australia and New Zealand Dialysis and Transplant Registry; 2008.
101. Webster AC, Wong G. Cancer. ANZDATA registry report 2009. 32nd Annual report. Adelaide, South Australia: Australia and New Zealand Dialysis and Transplant Registry; 2009.
102. Williams RH, Lively DH, DeLong DC, et al. Mycophenolic acid: antiviral and antitumor properties. J Antibiot 1968;21:463.
103. Wilson RE, Hager EB, Hampers CL, et al. Immunologic rejection of human cancer transplanted with a renal allograft. N Engl J Med 1968;278:479.
104. Winkelspecht B, Mueller-Lantzsch N, Kohler H. Serological evidence for reactivation of EBV infection due to uraemic immunodeficiency. Nephrol Dial Transplant 1997;12:2099.
105. Wong G, Howard K, Chapman JR, et al. Cost-effectiveness of breast cancer screening in women on dialysis. Am J Kidney Dis 2008;52:916.
106. Wong G, Howard K, Craig JC, et al. Cost-effectiveness of colorectal cancer screening in renal transplant recipients. Transplantation 2008;85:532.
107. Wong G, Howard K, Webster A, et al. The health and economic impact of cervical cancer screening and human papillomavirus vaccination in kidney transplant recipients. Transplantation 2009;87:1078.
108. Yamamoto T, Nakajima Y, Yamamoto M, et al. Epstein–Barr virus activity in patients on chronic hemodialysis. Nephron 1995;70:449.

CHAPTER 36

Pancreas and Kidney Transplantation for Diabetic Nephropathy

Angelika C. Gruessner • Rainer W.G. Gruessner

CHAPTER OUTLINE

Type 1 diabetes, which most commonly manifests in childhood, continues to represent a therapeutic challenge. Secondary diabetes complications, observed in 30–50% of patients who live more than 20 years after onset of the disease, result in poor quality of life (QOL), premature death, and considerable healthcare costs.[79] The principal determinant of the risk of devastating diabetes complications is the total lifetime exposure to elevated blood glucose levels.[17] Establishing safe and effective methods of achieving and maintaining normoglycemia would have substantial implications for the health and QOL of individuals with diabetes.

The Diabetes Control and Complications Trial (DCCT) showed that, given a qualified diabetes care team and intensive insulin treatment control, near-normalization of glycemia could be achieved and sustained for several years. Such a near-perfect level of treatment would increase a patient's burden of day-to-day diabetes management, be difficult to implement for many patients, require more attention and medical services than are routinely available in clinical practice,[10] and be accompanied by an increased frequency of severe hypoglycemia.[17] Currently, the only way to restore sustained normoglycemia without the associated risk of hypoglycemia is to replace the patient's glucose-sensing and insulin-secreting pancreatic islet beta cells either by the transplantation of a vascularized pancreas[121] or by the infusion of isolated pancreatic islets.[113] The tradeoff is the need for immunosuppression to prevent rejection of allogeneic tissue, and, for this reason, most pancreas or islet transplant recipients have been adults, but the potential for application earlier in the course of the disease exists, particularly in diabetic children already on immunosuppression for other indications.[4]

By the mid-1990s, more than 1500 pancreas transplants were being done annually worldwide (Figure 36-1), as reported to the International Pancreas Transplant Registry (IPTR).[36] By 2005, about 25 000 vascularized

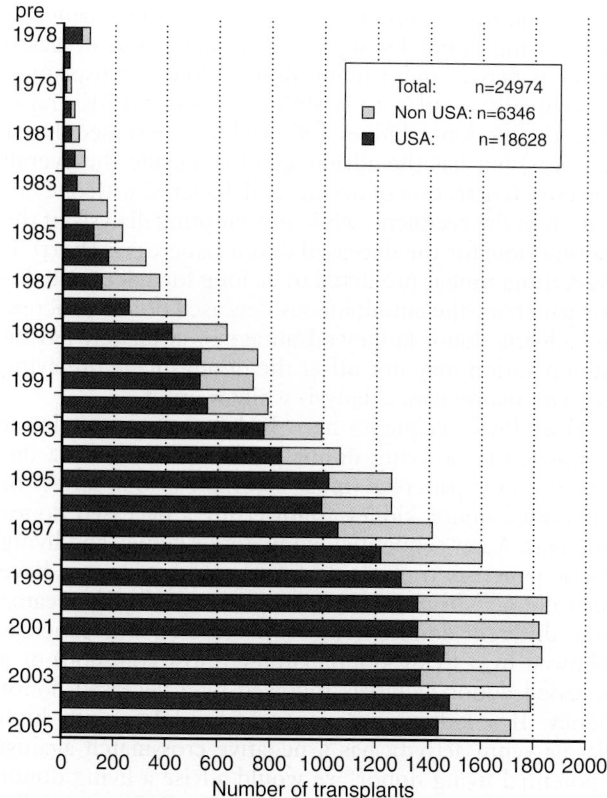

FIGURE 36-1 ■ Annual number of US and non-US pancreas transplants reported to the International Pancreas Transplant Registry, 1978–2005.

pancreas transplants had been performed, approximately three-fourths in the United States, with very large series at some centers.[126] Most were done to establish insulin independence in patients with de novo type 1 diabetes mellitus, but enteric drainage pancreas transplants have been used to correct endocrine and exocrine deficiency after total pancreatectomy in some patients[40,43] and from diseases such as cystic fibrosis in other patients.[112]

More than 120 institutions in the United States and nearly the same number outside the United States have performed pancreas transplants.[36] The IPTR was founded in 1980 to analyze the cases.[120] In 1987, reporting of US cases became obligatory through the United Network for Organ Sharing (UNOS), and annual reports have been made since then.[35–37]

HISTORY

The first clinical pancreas transplant was performed in 1966 by Kelly and Lillehei, simultaneously with a kidney transplant, in a uremic diabetic patient at the University of Minnesota.[53] Shortly thereafter, a few institutions around the world began to perform pancreas transplants, as detailed in a comprehensive history in another book.[125]

The success rate (long-term insulin independence) with pancreas transplantation was initially low, but it increased considerably in the 1980s, leading to increased application (Figure 36-1). Innovations in surgical techniques and in immunosuppression were responsible for the improved success rates.

The first pancreas transplant was a duct-ligated segmental (body and tail) graft,[53] but this approach was associated with multiple complications. In a series of 13 more pancreas transplants between 1966 and 1973 at the University of Minnesota,[61,62] Lillehei and colleagues devised the whole pancreas–duodenal transplant technique to the iliac vessels with enteric drainage via a duodenoenterostomy to native small bowel, which is now a routine at most centers. The initial results were not as good as today, however, and several surgeons devised alternative techniques during the 1970s and early 1980s.[125] Dubernard and colleagues[22] in Lyons, France, introduced duct injection of a synthetic polymer as a method to block secretions and cause fibrosis in the exocrine pancreas of a segmental graft with sparing of the endocrine component, and many pioneering centers adopted this technique, although it is little used today. Gliedman and associates[30] introduced urinary drainage via a ureteroductostomy for segmental grafts, and Sollinger and coworkers[106] later modified this approach with direct anastomosis of a duodenal patch of a whole-pancreas graft to the recipient bladder. Nghiem and Corry[83] did further modification of urinary drainage, retaining a bubble of duodenum for duodenocystostomy as Lillehei and associates[62] had done for duodenoenterostomy.

From the early 1980s until the mid-1990s, the bladder drainage technique with duodenocystostomy was the predominant technique for pancreas transplants. The bladder drainage technique had a low acute complication rate and was helpful in monitoring for rejection by detection of a decline in urine amylase activity, but chronic complications, such as recurrent urinary tract infections or dehydration from fluid loss via the exocrine secretions, were common. In the mid-1990s, a switch occurred, and enteric drainage, as described by Lillehei and colleagues[62] and never totally out of fashion,[109,126] overtook bladder drainage as the predominant technique. In addition, portal rather than systemic venous drainage began to be used by some groups for enteric drainage whole-pancreas duodenal transplants.[99] Portal venous drainage was originally introduced by Calne in 1984[14] for segmental pancreas grafts as a more physiological technique and was applied by several groups sporadically over the years.[125]

With advances in immunosuppression, including the introduction of cyclosporine by Calne and associates in 1979,[15] tacrolimus by Starzl and coworkers in 1989,[110] and mycophenolate mofetil by Sollinger in 1995,[105] bladder drainage had become less important for monitoring for rejection. In recipients of simultaneous pancreas and kidney (SPK) transplants from the same donor, the kidney could be monitored for rejection episodes (elevation of serum creatinine) as a surrogate marker for pancreas rejection before there was sufficient pancreas damage to cause hyperglycemia. In solitary pancreas transplants, serum creatinine could not be used as a marker for rejection, however, and in such cases bladder drainage remained useful and continues to be applied.[125]

INDICATIONS AND CATEGORIES

Indications

A pancreas transplant is performed to treat diabetes mellitus, most commonly in conjunction with a kidney transplant for patients with kidney failure or dysfunction secondary to diabetic nephropathy (see Recipient Categories, below). For such patients, the decision to undergo a pancreas transplant is not difficult. Because they are already candidates for a kidney transplant, they would require lifelong immunosuppression. The only significant additional risk of a pancreas transplant is the surgical risk associated with the operative procedure. The options available for such patients include undergoing both transplants simultaneously (from a deceased or a living donor or a combination of both) or undergoing the two transplants sequentially (usually the kidney transplant first, followed weeks or months later by the pancreas transplant). Which option is best depends on the individual patient's medical status, the availability of donors, and personal preference. These options are discussed in more detail later.

For diabetic patients with preserved kidney function, the decision to undergo a pancreas transplant must balance the risks of long-term immunosuppression with risks of long-term insulin therapy. The decision is easiest for patients with brittle diabetes who have rapid fluctuations in blood glucose levels, frequent episodes of diabetic ketoacidosis, or significant hypoglycemic unawareness.[46] For such patients, a successful pancreas transplant becomes a life-saving procedure. Even for patients with less severe diabetes, a pancreas transplant can improve QOL markedly and, to some extent, halt progression of secondary complications of diabetes.

Recipient Categories

Diabetic pancreas transplant recipients can be divided into two broad classifications: (1) patients with nephropathy to such a degree that they also undergo a kidney transplant, either simultaneously or sequentially; and (2) patients, usually without end-stage renal disease, who undergo only a pancreas transplant. Within these two broad classifications are several recipient categories. The traditional categories are as follows:

1. SPK transplant
2. Pancreas after kidney (PAK) transplant (in the interval between the two transplants, the recipient would be in the kidney transplant alone (KTA) category)
3. Pancreas transplant alone (PTA)
4. Kidney after pancreas (KAP) transplant (in the interval between the two transplants, the recipient would be in the PTA category).

Worldwide, in most SPK transplants, both organs have come from the same donor, and the donor has been a deceased donor,[35] but at the University of Minnesota, from 1994 through 2002, 10% were from a living donor.[126] Other centers have done living donor, same donor SPK transplants as well.[5] For some SPK transplants, each organ has come from different donors, and transplants have been done with a simultaneous deceased donor pancreas and a living donor kidney.[41,124] A simultaneous deceased donor pancreas and a living donor kidney transplant is conceptually similar to a different donor PAK transplant (living donor kidney followed by a deceased donor pancreas) but has the advantage of achieving the overall objective (correction of uremia and diabetes) with one operation in the recipient, while pre-empting dialysis (if the waiting time for the deceased donor pancreas is short). If the waiting time is predicted to be long for a deceased donor pancreas, the simultaneous deceased donor pancreas and a living donor kidney advantage of ultimately having one operation may not offset the disadvantage of having to go on maintenance dialysis while waiting.

Most PAK recipients have had two deceased donor organs, either a living donor kidney followed by a deceased donor pancreas (most common in our series) or a deceased donor kidney followed by a deceased donor pancreas. A few sequential living donor kidney and living donor pancreas transplants from different donors have been done.[126] In most KAP recipients, each organ came from different donors, either a deceased donor pancreas followed by a living donor kidney (most common) or a deceased donor pancreas followed by a deceased donor kidney. If a kidney and pancreas candidate with high plasma renin activity has a negative crossmatch against a potential living donor, we would advise a living donor KTA with subsequent placement on the PAK waiting list or a living donor, same donor SPK transplant if a suitable donor is willing to give both organs.

If a PTA candidate with moderately advanced nephropathy (e.g., glomerular filtration rate of 60 mL/min or less) has an identified living donor for a kidney in case one is needed, a deceased donor pancreas transplant can be done first, knowing that if the native kidneys deteriorate a living donor kidney can be added pre-emptively as uremic symptoms appear. If the candidate does not have a living donor for a kidney, a judgment has to be made about the value of correcting diabetes at the possible expense of accelerating the decline in kidney function by exposure to calcineurin inhibitors. At the University of Minnesota,[126] as has been done elsewhere,[60] such patients are placed on calcineurin inhibitors before transplantation. If kidney function deteriorates acutely, the drug is stopped and the patient is placed on the waiting list for a deceased donor SPK transplant; the wait may be long, but the zero-HLA mismatch lottery gives a chance of a pre-emptive transplant, even before reaching the glomerular filtration rate level (20 mL/min) that confers eligibility for waiting time points. Not all PTA patients with moderately advanced nephropathy experience progressive deterioration of kidney function while on calcineurin inhibitors. For some patients, their native kidney morphology improves after correction of the diabetic state.[27]

In the University of Minnesota experience with more than 400 PTA recipients, about 4% went on to have a KAP within 1 year, and 10% had a KAP within 5 years of pancreas transplant.[126] Only 6% of the KAP recipients at the University of Minnesota were on dialysis at the time of kidney transplant.[126] About half of the KAP recipients had a functioning pancreas at the time of kidney transplant. About one-third of the KAP transplants at the

University of Minnesota have been done in conjunction with a pancreas retransplant (SPK); most patients in this subgroup had rejected the PTA graft because calcineurin inhibitor levels were kept low in an attempt to preserve native kidney function. By adding a normal kidney to the pancreas retransplant, adequate calcineurin inhibitor levels can be maintained to prevent rejection.

KAP recipients with functioning pancreas grafts underwent kidney transplant to obviate early uremic symptoms and chronic fatigue and to obtain the full benefit of immunosuppression. This strategy has been highly effective. At 1 year, graft survival rates in KAP recipients of a solitary kidney are 96%.[126] Two-thirds of the KAP transplants of a solitary kidney were from a living donor, greatly facilitating the process. Even for PTA candidates with moderately advanced nephropathy who tolerate pretransplant calcineurin inhibitors with minimal early deterioration, early identification of potential living donors for a kidney is encouraged so that the KAP option can be expedited whenever appropriate.

In contrast to the subgroup of PTA recipients whose native kidney function deteriorated to the point where a KAP was done, there is a subgroup of PTA recipients with moderately advanced nephropathy (per pretransplant native kidney biopsy specimens) whose lesions completely or partially resolve 5–10 years after transplantation.[27] These PTA recipients were probably spared from a kidney transplant; based on their original biopsy findings, progressive deterioration would have been predicted had they remained diabetic.

The native kidney function of some PTA candidates is in a gray zone. Diabetic nephropathy may be moderately advanced, but uremic symptoms are absent or minimal. Some such candidates are extremely sensitive to the nephrotoxic effect of calcineurin inhibitors.[60] At the University of Minnesota, all PTA candidates are placed on calcineurin inhibitors before transplantation and then monitored for kidney function and side effects. If kidney function declines substantially and symptoms appear, the calcineurin inhibitor is stopped, and the patient becomes a candidate for a kidney transplant, ideally from a living donor. If no living donor is available, the candidate is placed on the waiting list for a deceased donor SPK transplant.

The patient would remain on the PTA list if his or her diabetes is extremely labile, recognizing that the interval until dialysis if necessary could be shortened by reintroduction of a calcineurin inhibitor at the time of a PTA. Such an extreme approach is prompted by the fact that, in the United States under the UNOS system, waiting time points for a deceased donor kidney (KTA, SPK, or KAP) do not accumulate until the candidate's creatinine clearance is 20 mL/min or less. Many candidates for a deceased donor SPK transplant have a creatinine clearance greater than 20 mL/min when initially evaluated.

Diabetic patients referred as potential PTA candidates encompass a broad range of kidney function. Patients with a creatinine clearance of 100 mL/min or better are at low risk for calcineurin inhibitor-induced reduction of kidney function to the point where a kidney transplant is indicated. Some patients with a creatinine clearance of 50–60 mL/min are sensitive to calcineurin inhibitors, while others are resistant, and some have kidneys with the capacity to stabilize functionally and improve morphologically after a PTA.[27] For patients in the gray zone, the findings on native kidney biopsy specimens, kidney function while on calcineurin inhibitors, and availability of living donors are our three main guides to selecting the treatment plan: PTA or simultaneous or sequential kidney and pancreas transplants.

ALLOCATION

The allocation scheme must accommodate candidates for a solitary pancreas transplant and candidates for a deceased donor kidney transplant. In some organ procurement organizations, usually single-center organizations, SPK candidates are given priority over KTA candidates when the pancreas and a kidney from a deceased donor are suitable for transplantation. Some organ procurement organizations have no, or few, solitary PTA candidates listed. In such organizations, the local use of deceased donor pancreata depends on whether SPK candidates are given priority over KTA candidates (diabetic and non-diabetic). If priority is given to SPK candidates, theoretically, half of the kidneys would go to uremic diabetics (even though they comprise less than half of the combined SPK and KTA list). The result would be shorter kidney waiting times for patients with diabetic nephropathy than for patients with other causes of end-stage renal disease. The proportion of uremic diabetic patients who are listed for an SPK transplant (versus KTA) approaches 100% in some organ procurement organizations, so virtually all KTA candidates are non-diabetic.

In practice, not all deceased kidney donors are judged to have a pancreas suitable for transplantation. Even with the extreme policy of full priority of SPK over KTA candidates for a kidney from deceased donors with a suitable pancreas, less than half of the locally procured deceased kidneys are transplanted in SPK recipients. With such a policy, waiting times are shorter for diabetic SPK (versus non-diabetic or diabetic KTA) candidates. About 25% of kidney transplant candidates are diabetic, so in organ procurement organizations with an extreme policy the pancreata from all deceased donors with a suitable pancreas tend to be used.

At the other end of the spectrum are organ procurement organizations (usually multicenter) that give no priority to SPK candidates. In such organizations, the kidneys are allocated to the two highest-ranked suitable candidates on the specific list generated for a deceased donor. The donor pancreas is used locally for an SPK candidate but only if that candidate is one of the two highest-ranked suitable candidates for the kidney. Other organ procurement organizations have allocation schemes that fall between the extremes.

Compared with non-diabetic kidney transplant candidates, uremic diabetics have a high mortality rate while waiting for transplants (6% per year according to UNOS). This fact provides one rationale for including medical priority in a deceased kidney allocation scheme (as is the case in liver and heart allocation); a pancreas allocation scheme that gives full priority to SPK candidates in effect incorporates medical priority.

Meanwhile, living donors are needed to compensate for the shortage of deceased donors. Rejection rates have declined for deceased and living donor recipients, so the main incentive to use living donors is to eliminate the waiting time and high mortality rate in certain candidates while waiting. As more diabetics are listed for deceased donor pancreas transplant, the waiting time is expected to approach or exceed that for deceased donor kidneys, and the incentive to use living donors for pancreas transplant is expected to increase. Incentives to use living donors for segmental pancreas transplants have included the ability to induce an insulin-independent and dialysis-free state with one operation (SPK), and the elimination or reduction of waiting time for candidates in any category (PAK, PTA, and SPK) who have a high potential for a long wait on the deceased donor transplant list (e.g., because of high plasma renin activity). When diabetic candidates for pancreas transplants with low plasma renin activity are waiting 2–4 years for a deceased donor, the incentive to take the pancreas living donor option increases, as has happened for kidney transplants.

Methods to screen potential pancreas living donors for suitability have been developed. Briefly, volunteers are suitable to be hemipancreas donors if they have a body mass index less than 28 kg/m^2 (to minimize the need for increased insulin secretion to compensate for obesity), no history of gestational diabetes, and normal glucose tolerance with a threefold increase in first-phase blood insulin concentration on intravenous arginine and glucose stimulation. Living donors who meet these criteria retain normal glucose tolerance post donation; any changes in glucose or insulin levels would be no greater in magnitude than the changes in creatinine clearance that are seen after kidney donation.

Islet autograft cases show the potential to increase the efficiency of islet preparation and transplantation from deceased donors by duplicating, as nearly as possible, ideal conditions (very short preservation time, elimination of purification process with reduced tissue volume from half of a pancreas). The cases also show the potential to transplant more than one recipient with islets from one pancreas. The precedent for splitting a deceased pancreas for transplantation as immediately vascularized grafts (head and tail) into two diabetic recipients goes back to 1988[127] and preceded the use of split deceased liver transplants.[23]

SPECIFIC RISK FACTORS

The preceding sections outlined algorithms for pancreas transplants in general diabetic and uremic diabetic patients. Some candidates have risk factors that require special consideration, however. Jehovah's Witnesses do not allow blood transfusions. Most pancreas transplants are done without substantial blood loss, but, as is true for any major surgery, some patients may need transfusions. The Jehovah's Witnesses we have transplanted all have survived the operation,[49] but they faced an above-average risk.

Chronic viral infection (e.g., human immunodeficiency virus (HIV) or hepatitis C virus (HCV)) also pose additional risks for allograft candidates. With modern HIV therapeutic agents, infected patients have been successfully transplanted.[59] HIV-positive diabetics should be considered for pancreas transplantation according to clinical indications. HCV can recur in liver allograft recipients, but overall outcomes have been good. In kidney allograft recipients, HCV does not seem to progress more than in renal failure patients on dialysis.[111] HCV-positive uremic diabetic patients have had SPK or PAK transplants in our program; the incidence of progressive liver disease was no different from that of non-diabetic KTA recipients. We see no reason to withhold pancreas transplantation from asymptomatic HCV-positive diabetics.

The age of pancreas transplant recipients theoretically has no limits. Analyses of pancreas transplant outcome by recipient age have shown that the rejection rate is lower for recipients who are more than 45 years old.[35,126] In the PTA category, patient survival rate at 1 year is nearly 100% in the group older than 45 years, and graft survival rate is significantly higher than in younger recipients. This finding is consistent with studies showing a blunting of primary immune responses as individuals age. In the older group, the main risk factor to address is cardiovascular disease. Candidates should be screened for coronary artery disease; if present, it should be corrected before pancreas transplant, even if asymptomatic.[64]

Pancreas transplants have been done in diabetic children (<18 years old).[4] Pediatric SPK recipients have had less rejection than pediatric PTA recipients.[4] In the early experience, juvenile PTA recipients had more frequent or severe rejection episodes than adults. The immunosuppressive regimen for pediatric patients must be more aggressive than that for adults. Living donors are particularly attractive for pancreas transplants in children because the rejection rates for all types of organ allografts are lower than with deceased donors. Obtaining a sufficient beta-cell mass should nearly always be possible with parental donors of pediatric recipients.

Diabetic patients with exocrine deficiency as a result of a total pancreatectomy for benign disease (usually chronic pancreatitis) also are special cases. Ideally, pancreatectomized patients should have had diabetes prevented by an islet autograft (if they were non-diabetic before the total pancreatectomy). Some become diabetic from the chronic pancreatitis before the pancreatectomy, however. Others have an insufficient yield of autologous islets to prevent diabetes. Still others have had the pancreatectomy at institutions not offering islet autotransplants. The combination of diabetes and exocrine deficiency poses a special problem. Erratic food absorption coupled with exogenous insulin predisposes to hypoglycemic events. Such patients would benefit most from an enteric drainage pancreas transplant so that exocrine and endocrine deficiencies are corrected.

Some patients with severe exocrine deficiency from chronic pancreatitis are not diabetic. Some are pain-free, and exocrine deficiency is the sole problem. Oral enzyme therapy usually improves food absorption but not in all. Enteric drainage pancreas transplants have abolished steatorrhea and the need for oral enzyme therapy in some patients with exocrine deficiency.[40,112] There is a rationale to treat exocrine deficiency by enteric drainage pancreas transplant in patients with serious nutritional problems. We have done so by adding a second enteric drainage pancreas transplant in a totally pancreatectomized patient whose initial bladder drainage pancreas transplant corrected only diabetes.[126] For technical reasons, a conversion from bladder drainage to enteric drainage could not be done, so the steatorrhea and malabsorption persisted despite heavy administration of pancreatic enzymes orally. The enzyme deficiency was solved by the enteric drainage pancreas transplant, leaving the functioning bladder drainage graft in place.[126]

PROCEDURE

Surgical Techniques

The pretransplant evaluation does not differ substantially from that which is undertaken for diabetic kidney transplant recipients. Examination of the cardiovascular system is most important because significant coronary artery disease may be present without symptoms. Non-invasive testing may not identify such disease, so coronary angiography is performed routinely. In PTA candidates, detailed neurological, ophthalmological, metabolic, and renal function testing may be needed to assess the degree of progression of secondary complications. When patients are placed on a waiting list, their medical condition should be reassessed yearly or more frequently.

As mentioned in the history section, a variety of techniques have been used for management of the exocrine secretions and venous drainage of pancreas transplants. Most pancreas grafts are procured from multiorgan deceased donors, and because the liver and pancreas share the origins of their arterial blood supply, a whole-organ pancreas graft usually requires a reconstruction.[11,66] The tail of the pancreas is supplied by the splenic artery originating from the celiac axis, and the head of the pancreas is supplied by the pancreaticoduodenal arcades originating from the superior mesenteric artery and the hepatic artery. Because the latter goes with the liver, along with the celiac axis, the usual approach is to attach an arterial Y-graft of the donor iliac vessels, with anastomosis of the hypogastric artery to the graft splenic artery and the external iliac artery to the graft superior mesenteric artery, leaving the common iliac artery of the Y-graft for anastomosis to the recipient arterial system, usually the right common iliac artery. The portal vein of the pancreas graft can be anastomosed to the recipient's common iliac vein (usually after the hypogastric veins have been doubly ligated and divided) or vena cava, or to the recipient's superior mesenteric vein.

When venous drainage is to the recipient's iliac vein, the whole-pancreas graft can be oriented with the head directed into the pelvis or into the upper abdomen. When directed cephalad, enteric drainage is the only option. When directed caudally, the duodenum can be anastomosed to either the bladder (Figure 36-2) or the bowel (Figure 36-3). Figure 36-2, showing the bladder drainage technique, also depicts a kidney transplant to the left iliac vessels, but, as mentioned, enteric drainage is more common than bladder drainage (Figure 36-4).

With the bladder drainage technique, the anastomosis may be hand-sewn or performed with an end-to-end

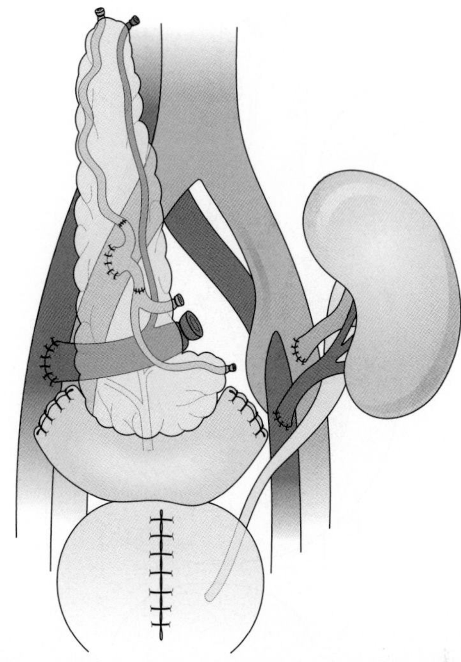

FIGURE 36-2 ■ Simultaneous pancreas–kidney (SPK) transplantation using a whole pancreas–duodenal graft from a deceased donor with systemic venous drainage to the right iliac vein and bladder drainage of the pancreas exocrine secretions via a duodenocystostomy. The pancreas and the kidney are placed intraperitoneally through a midline incision. The donor splenic artery, supplying the pancreatic tail, and the donor superior mesenteric artery, supplying the pancreatic head, have been joined by a Y-graft constructed from the donor common/external/internal iliac artery complex during a benchwork procedure, and the base of the Y-graft is anastomosed to the recipient common iliac artery. The mid-duodenum is anastomosed to the posterior dome of the bladder, and the duodenal stumps are oversewn. The kidney graft could be from a living donor or the same deceased donor as the pancreas graft, but in either case it is preferentially placed to the left iliac vessels so that the right side, with its more superficial vessels, can be used for the pancreas transplant. In this illustration, the donor ureter was implanted into the bladder using the Politano-Leadbetter technique via an anterior cystotomy, a technique that also allows the duodenocystostomy to be performed with an end-to-end anastomosis stapler with internal oversewing of the anastomotic line using an absorbable suture to cover the staples, followed by closure of the cystotomy. When enteric drainage is used for an SPK transplant, however, an external ureterocystoneostomy is usually done. (From Gruessner RWG, Sutherland DER, editors. Transplantation of the pancreas. New York: Springer-Verlag; 2004. Color plate xiv.)

anastomosis (EEA) stapler brought through the distal duodenum (which is subsequently stapled closed) for connection to the post of the anvil projected through the posterior bladder via an anterior cystostomy (Figure 36-2). The inner layer is reinforced with a running absorbable suture for hemostasis and for burying the staples under the mucosa.

With the enteric drainage–systemic venous drainage technique, the anastomosis also may be hand-sewn in a side-to-side fashion (Figure 36-3); stapled in a side-to-side fashion, including using an EEA stapler inserted into the distal graft duodenum with the post projected through the side for connection to the anvil inserted into recipient bowel through an enterotomy closed around the post with a pursestring; or hand-sewn in an end-to-side fashion. The enteric anastomosis can be done directly to

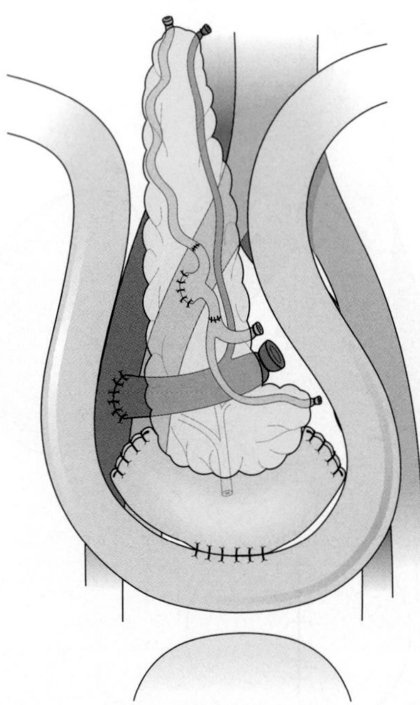

FIGURE 36-3 ■ Whole pancreas–duodenal transplantation from a deceased donor with systemic venous drainage and enteric drainage of graft exocrine secretions to a proximal loop of recipient jejunum. In this case, a side-to-side stapled or hand-sewn duodenojejunostomy is illustrated. The pancreas with its vascular anastomosis (donor Y-graft to recipient common iliac artery, donor portal vein to recipient common iliac vein) is implanted in the standard fashion on the right side of the pelvis. (From Gruessner RWG, Sutherland DER, editors. Transplantation of the pancreas. New York: Springer-Verlag; 2004. Color plate XVII.)

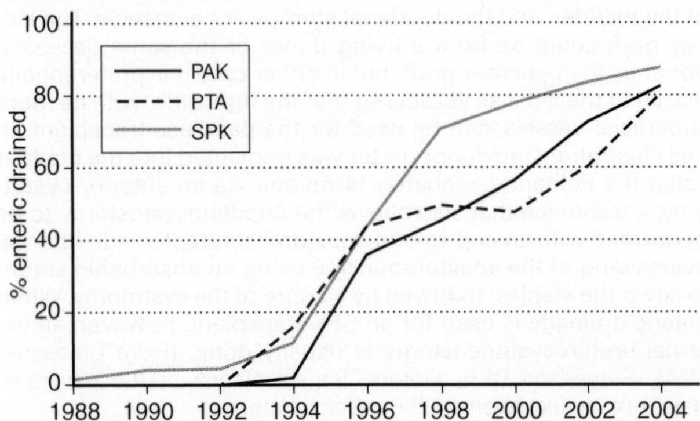

FIGURE 36-4 ■ Percentage of enteric drainage pancreas transplants performed in the United States from 1988 through 2004 by recipient category. PAK, pancreas after kidney transplant; PTA, pancreas transplant alone; SPK, simultaneous pancreas–kidney.

the most convenient proximal small-bowel loop of the recipient (depicted) or to a Roux-en-Y segment of recipient bowel that is created at the time. Outcome analyses (see later) do not show any statistical advantage to creation of a Roux-en-Y loop.

For portal drainage of the pancreas graft venous effluent (Figures 36-5 and 36-6), the head and duodenum of the graft are oriented cephalad, and the graft portal vein is anastomosed directly to the recipient superior mesenteric vein. In Figure 36-5, the pancreas graft is ventral to the recipient small-bowel mesentery so that the venous anastomosis is to the ventral side of the

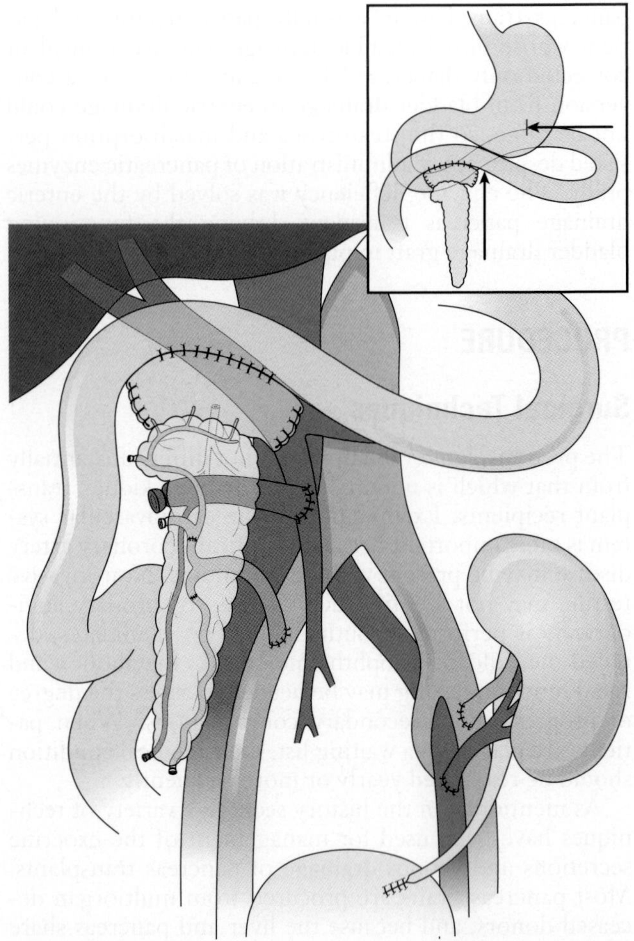

FIGURE 36-5 ■ Whole pancreas–duodenal transplantation from a deceased donor with portal venous drainage via an end-to-side anastomosis to the recipient superior mesenteric vein accessed below its confluence with the splenic vein. Drainage of exocrine secretions is via a side-to-side duodenojejunostomy, about 40–80 cm distal to the ligament of Treitz. Note the cephalad position of the pancreatic head when portal venous drainage is done, as opposed to the caudal orientation possible with systemic venous drainage, no different than that needed when bladder drainage is done. In this illustration, the pancreas graft overlies the root of the small-bowel mesentery, with the duodenal segment below the transverse colon, and the arterial Y-graft anastomosed to the recipient common iliac artery through a mesenteric tunnel. A retroperitoneal approach under the right colon also is possible, in which case the arterial Y-graft can be anastomosed directly to the recipient iliac artery, but the enteric anastomosis must be via a Roux-en-Y limb of recipient bowel brought through the mesentery. If a kidney is simultaneously transplanted to the left iliac vessels, the ureter can be implanted into the bladder using the extravesical ureterocystoneostomy (Lich) technique, as illustrated. (From Gruessner RWG, Sutherland DER, editors. Transplantation of the pancreas. New York: Springer-Verlag; 2004. Color plate xx.)

superior mesenteric vein, and the arterial Y-graft must be brought through a window of mesentery for anastomosis to the recipient's aorta or common iliac artery. The graft duodenum is anastomosed to recipient small bowel by the same techniques described for systemic venous drainage, with or without (depicted) a Roux-en-Y loop of recipient bowel.

An alternative approach for portal venous drainage of the pancreas graft effluent is to place the pancreas

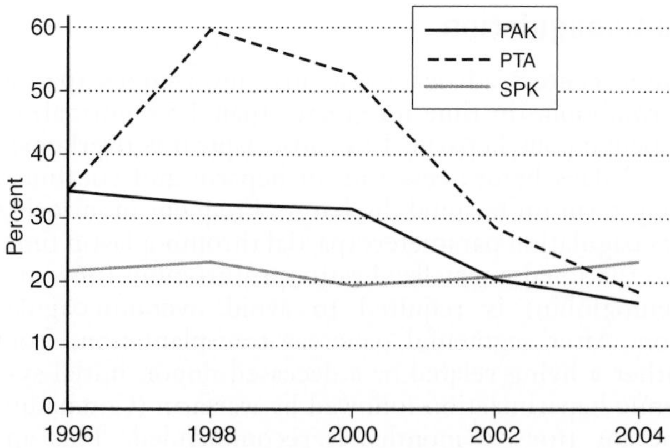

FIGURE 36-6 ■ Percentage of portal drainage in enteric drainage pancreas transplants performed in the United States from 1996 through 2004 by recipient category. PAK, pancreas after kidney transplant; PTA, pancreas transplant alone; SPK, simultaneous pancreas–kidney.

retroperitoneally by reflecting the right colon to the left and exposing the dorsal surface of the superior mesenteric vein, as described by Boggi and coworkers.[12,13] The arterial Y-graft can be anastomosed directly to the right common iliac artery, but this approach mandates creation of a Roux-en-Y limb of recipient bowel to bring through the small bowel or transverse colon mesentery for a graft duodenoenterostomy.

Other techniques can be used, including duct injection for a segmental graft. Segmental grafts are rarely used, except in the few cases of living donor pancreas transplants,[5,39,123] and most of these have the exocrine secretions managed by a ductoenterostomy to a Roux-en-Y limb of recipient bowel or by ductocystostomy (depicted) to the recipient's bladder (Figure 36-7). Segmental pancreas transplants from living donors, with or without a kidney transplant, are particularly useful in candidates who would otherwise have a long wait for a deceased donor organ, such as candidates with a high level of HLA antibodies but with a negative crossmatch to a living volunteer. More details are given on the variety of surgical techniques in pancreas donors (deceased and living) and recipients in a book dedicated to pancreas transplantation.[8]

Immunosuppression

Immunosuppression management of pancreas transplant recipients is similar to that of recipients of other solid-organ transplants, including kidney transplants, which most pancreas recipients also receive. Induction immunosuppression with anti-T-cell monoclonal or polyclonal-depleting or non-depleting agents may be used or reserved for rejection episodes. Maintenance immunosuppression usually consists of a combination of a calcineurin inhibitor (cyclosporine or tacrolimus) with the dosage and blood levels adjusted to minimize nephrotoxicity and an antiproliferative agent (mycophenolate mofetil or sirolimus), with or without prednisone. Steroid-free regimens are common for all organ transplants, including the pancreas.[51]

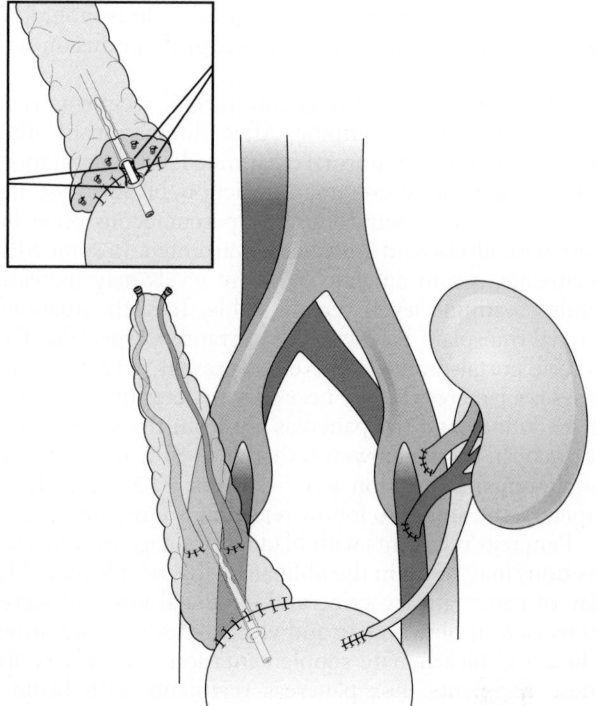

FIGURE 36-7 ■ Living donor segmental (body and tail) pancreas transplantation to right iliac vessels (systemic venous drainage) and bladder drainage of exocrine secretions through a ductocystostomy via an intraperitoneal approach. The donor splenic artery and splenic vein are anastomosed end-to-side to the recipient external iliac artery and vein, after ligation and division of all hypogastric veins to bring the main vein as superficial as possible. The splenic artery anastomosis is lateral and proximal to the splenic vein anastomosis. A two-layer ductocystostomy is constructed. The pancreatic duct is approximated to the urothelial layer (inner layer) using interrupted 7-0 absorbable sutures over a stent (inset). If a kidney is transplanted simultaneously, the donor ureter is implanted into the bladder using the extravesical ureterocystoneostomy (Lich) technique. (From Gruessner RWG, Sutherland DER, editors. Transplantation of the pancreas. New York: Springer-Verlag; 2004. Color plate xvi.)

MANAGEMENT

Intraoperative Care

Blood glucose is monitored hourly and may be controlled with an insulin drip. At the time of organ reperfusion, adequate volume status and blood pressure are imperative to avoid graft hypoperfusion. Before revascularization, diuretics are frequently given to promote early kidney graft function in SPK recipients (using furosemide) and reduce pancreas graft swelling (using mannitol, 0.25–1 g/kg). On completion of the procedure, the abdomen is copiously irrigated with antimicrobial solutions (e.g., containing bacitracin and amphotericin).

Postoperative Care

In the initial postoperative period, serum glucose levels are followed closely, and an intravenous insulin infusion is continued as needed to maintain the serum glucose at 80–110 mg/dL. Persistent elevation or acute increase in the serum glucose to more than 200 mg/dL requires immediate evaluation with Doppler ultrasonography or radionuclide scanning to assess graft perfusion and function.

The sentinel sign of rejection in SPK recipients is an increase in serum creatinine. After elimination of other possibilities for an abnormal creatinine level (dehydration, calcineurin toxicity, ureteral obstruction, bladder dysfunction, or vascular compromise), a percutaneous renal biopsy with ultrasound guidance is warranted. In some SPK recipients, serum amylase or lipase levels may increase, while creatinine levels remain stable. In such situations, a renal transplant biopsy is still warranted, especially if an enteric portal-drained pancreas is present.[103] Only in rare cases is a pancreas biopsy necessary to determine rejection if the kidney and the pancreas are from the same donor. It has been shown, however, that in an SPK recipient one organ remains rejection-free.[45,65,129] For PTA and PAK recipients, the ability to follow rejection is more difficult.

Pancreas recipients with bladder drainage exocrine secretions may result in the obligatory loss of at least 1–2 L/day of pancreatic exocrine and duodenal mucosal secretions rich in bicarbonate and electrolytes into the urine. Fluid and bicarbonate supplementation is necessary for these recipients. For pancreas recipients with bladder drainage of exocrine secretions, urinary amylase levels can be monitored.[89–91] Studies have shown that urinary amylase levels expressed in units per hour are more consistent compared with measurements in units per liter and lead to more accurate assessment of pancreas graft function. An analysis of a 12-hour or 24-hour urine collection in which urinary amylase levels have declined 50% or more from baseline suggests rejection or pancreatitis. When confronted with this situation, further evaluation and probable biopsy are warranted, whether percutaneously via ultrasound or computed tomography guidance, or transcystoscopically, assisted by ultrasound guidance.[1,7,48]

The development of hematuria in bladder drainage pancreas recipients also warrants further evaluation and may necessitate the initiation of continuous bladder irrigation through a three-way Foley catheter to prevent obstructive thrombus formation. Cystoscopy is usually necessary to determine the etiology or remove the clot or both. Urethritis or cystitis owing to enzymatic irritation, the most common cause of hematuria, may resolve with increased bicarbonate supplementation.[107] Enteric conversion may be required for refractory irritation; however, such an extreme intervention is rarely required in the early postoperative period.[108] Bleeding from the duodenal–bladder anastomosis may arise, especially when a stapled anastomosis is performed. This complication can be avoided by oversewing the staple line at the time of the anastomosis. If a problem does develop, staples can be removed cystoscopically, although enteric conversion ultimately may be required to alleviate the bleeding.

Serum amylase and lipase levels provide additional means for following pancreas function, especially for enterically drained grafts.[47,117] These markers lack the sensitivity and specificity of urinary amylase, however. Serum human anodal trypsinogen has been shown to complement serum amylase and lipase levels in the determination of graft dysfunction.[20,86] Few laboratories are equipped to monitor this factor, however.

Anticoagulation

Some centers advocate low-dose intravenous (partial thromboplastin time no greater than 1.5× normal) or subcutaneous heparin. Low-dose aspirin is overlapped for 2 days before cessation of heparin and continued long term on hospital discharge. Frequent monitoring of coagulation parameters (partial thromboplastin time, international normalized ratio, prothrombin time, and hemoglobin) is required to avoid overanticoagulation. After segmental pancreas transplantation, from either a living related or a deceased donor, initial systemic heparinization followed by warfarin (Coumadin) therapy (for ≤6 months) is recommended. This approach is mandated by the more narrow caliber of the vascular anastomoses and the associated higher risk of thrombosis.[5,41]

Antimicrobial Prophylaxis

The literature clearly shows that early infection results in the highest incidence of graft loss and in serious patient morbidity and mortality.[6,24,84,88] Various single agents or combinations are available and should be given over the first 24–48 hours after transplantation. Recipients with positive urine cultures (from preoperative specimens) or positive intraoperative duodenal stump cultures should have antibiotic coverage for 3–7 days. Retrospective studies have shown that pancreas recipients are at high risk for losing a second pancreatic allograft to the same infectious agent when their first graft was lost to infection. A detailed microbial history of an individual transplant candidate is imperative so that appropriate antibiotic coverage can be initiated intraoperatively.

Because of the duodenal anastomosis in pancreas transplantation and the potential contamination of the operative field with small-bowel contents, many centers also recommend antifungal prophylaxis with fluconazole. Calcineurin inhibitor serum levels must be monitored closely when azoles are administered because of decreased metabolism of the immunosuppressant and resultant higher systemic concentrations. As shown in several articles (referenced earlier), fungal infections result in the highest rates of graft loss and patient mortality.

Cytomegalovirus prophylaxis is recommended for any positive combination of a donor–recipient pair.[29,52] Controversy exists as to whether negative-to-negative combinations require prophylaxis. When antilymphocyte therapy is used, cytomegalovirus prophylaxis is almost always administered. Ganciclovir and, more recently, valganciclovir are presently the antiviral agents of choice in pancreas transplantation and can be initiated intravenously or per nasogastric tube in the immediate postoperative period, and then orally when the patient tolerates a diet. Patients intolerant to ganciclovir may tolerate valaciclovir, which provides adequate prophylaxis against cytomegalovirus infection in renal-only transplantation.[63] The efficacy of valganciclovir in pancreas transplantation is currently under investigation. Most centers begin trimethoprim/sulfamethoxazole immediately postoperatively and continue long-term prophylaxis against *Pneumocystis carinii* and *Nocardia* infections.

PANCREAS TRANSPLANT OUTCOMES

Changes over Time of Pancreas Transplant Outcomes

The changes of outcomes with deceased donor pancreas transplantation according to recipient categories, surgical technique, and immunosuppression protocol for US cases as reported to UNOS are summarized here. From December 16, 1966, to December 31, 2005, about 25 000 pancreas transplants were reported to the IPTR, including more than 18 000 from the United States and almost 6000 from outside the United States. The annual number of US and non-US cases reported is shown in Figure 36-1. The annual number of US pancreas transplants from 1988 through 2005 for those identified by major recipient category (SPK, PAK, and PTA) is shown in Figure 36-8. Most have been SPK transplants, but the number of PAK and PTA transplants has increased significantly in recent years. In 2005, of the 1367 pancreas transplants in which a major recipient category was designated, 896 were SPK (66%), 339 were PAK (25%), and 132 were PTA (10%). In the PAK category there has been a significant change in the percentage of recipients whose kidney came from a living donor from 37% for 1988–1989 to 70% for 2004–2005.

Recipient age at the time of transplant increased significantly over time from mid-30s to early 40s. This trend can be seen in all three categories. Reporting of the diabetes type also began in 1994. The percentages of recipients labeled as having type 2 diabetes mellitus has continuously increased and in 2004–2005 was 7% for SPK recipients.

Figure 36-4 shows the changes in duct management over the years. Fewer than 10% of all pancreas transplants were done using enteric drainage before 1995–1996. Since then, the proportion of pancreas transplants that were managed by enteric drainage has steadily increased. Of the 2004–2005 pancreas transplants, 88% in the SPK, 83% in the PAK, and 80% in the PTA categories were enteric drainage.

Portal vein drainage of the pancreas graft venous effluent for enteric drainage transplants has been done since the early 1980s but not in large numbers until the mid-1990s. The proportion of enteric drainage transplants with portal drainage has varied by category and year (Figure 36-6). Although the proportion of enteric drainage SPK transplants with portal drainage has been constant at around 20% since 1994, the proportion in the PAK category has decreased steadily from the high-water mark of 35% in 1994–1995. In 1998–1999 (peak era), 60% of all enteric drainage PTA cases had portal drainage, but the proportion has since declined as well. In 2004–2005, 23% of enteric drainage SPK, 17% of enteric drainage PAK, and 18% of enteric drainage PTA cases had portal drainage.

There has been a progressive decline in the degree to which pancreas recipients have been matched for HLA, more so in the SPK than in the PTA and PAK categories (Figure 36-9). For 2004–2005 cases, 58% of SPK recipients were mismatched for five or six HLA at the A, B, and DR loci (out of a possible six). A high proportion of solitary pancreas recipients in the latest era also were highly mismatched, however. In 2004–2005, 47% of PAK and 38% of PTA recipients were mismatched for five or six antigens.

Besides the changes in maintenance immunosuppression from cyclosporine to predominantly tacrolimus and from azathioprine to predominantly mycophenolate mofetil during the years 1994 and 1996, a change in the usage of anti-T-cell agents for induction therapy has occurred over time. In all three categories, the proportion of recipients given induction therapy was the lowest between 1990 and 1993 but thereafter increased significantly. In 2004–2005, more than 80% of all patients received some sort of anti-T-cell induction therapy.

Improvements in Pancreas Transplant Outcomes by Era

The results of US primary deceased donor pancreas transplants analyzed by 2-year intervals are given to show changes in outcome over time. Long-term and short-term patient survival rates improved constantly over the

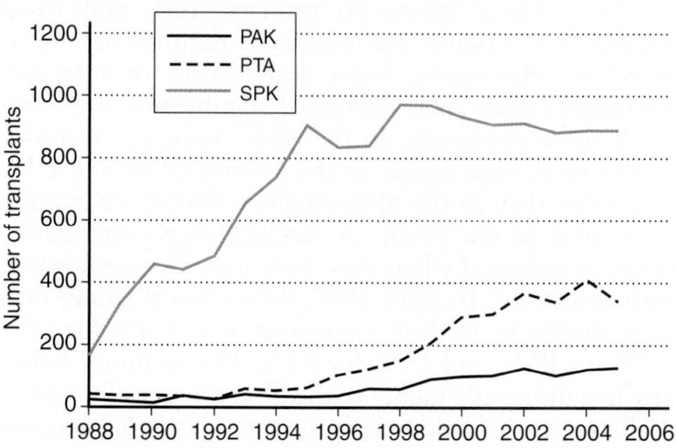

FIGURE 36-8 ■ Number of pancreas transplants performed annually in the United States from 1988 through 2005 by recipient category. PAK, pancreas after kidney transplant; PTA, pancreas transplant alone; SPK, simultaneous pancreas–kidney.

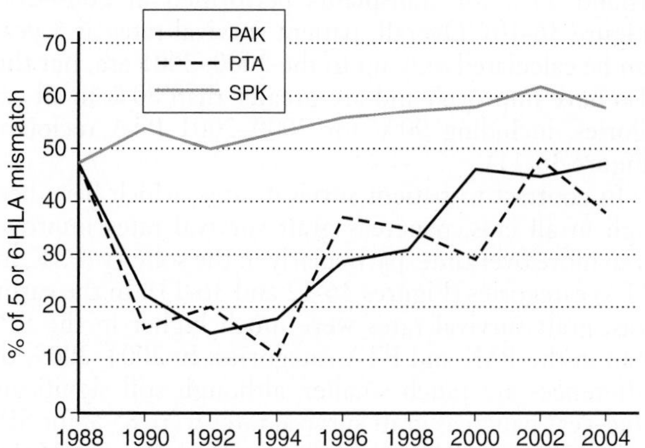

FIGURE 36-9 ■ Percentage of US pancreas transplant recipients mismatched for five or six human leukocyte antigen (HLA)-A, HLA-B, and HLA-DR donor antigens, by category and era, in 2-year intervals, 1988 through 2005. PAK, pancreas after kidney transplant; PTA, pancreas transplant alone; SPK, simultaneous pancreas–kidney.

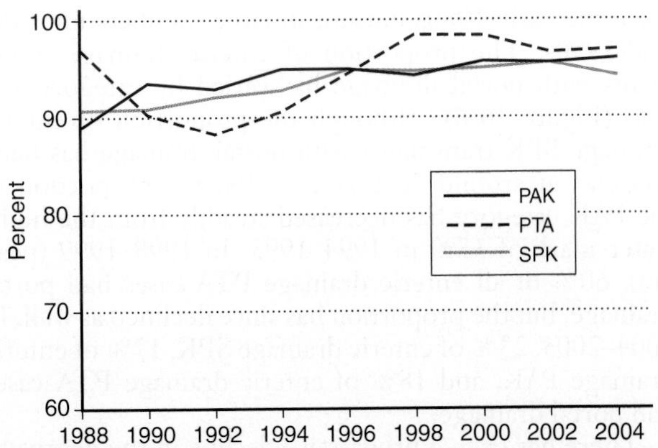

FIGURE 36-10 ■ Patient 1-year survival rates for US deceased donor primary pancreas transplant recipients by category and era, in 2-year intervals, 1988 through 2005. PAK, pancreas after kidney transplant; PTA, pancreas transplant alone; SPK, simultaneous pancreas–kidney.

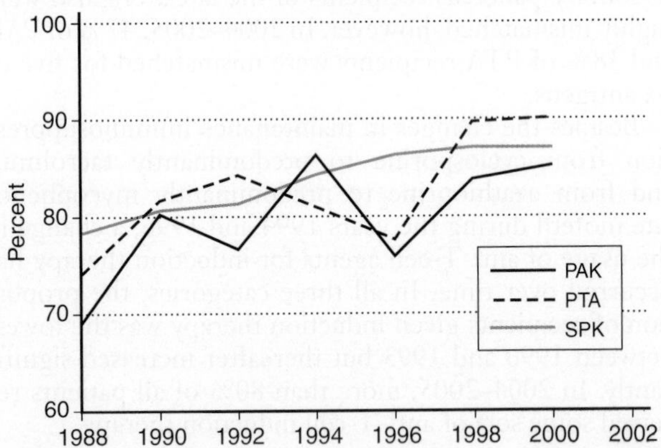

FIGURE 36-11 ■ Patient 5-year survival rates for US deceased donor primary pancreas transplant recipients by category and era, in 2-year intervals, 1988 through 2005. PAK, pancreas after kidney transplant; PTA, pancreas transplant alone; SPK, simultaneous pancreas–kidney.

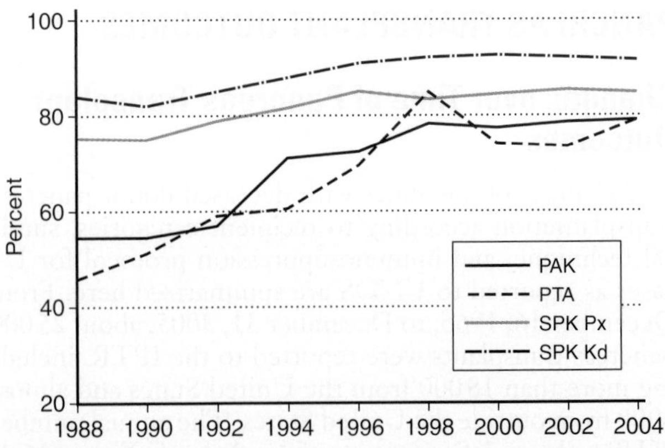

FIGURE 36-12 ■ Pancreas and simultaneous pancreas–kidney (SPK) 1-year graft survival rates for US deceased donor primary pancreas transplant recipients by category and era, in 2-year intervals, 1988 through 2005. Kd, kidney; PAK, pancreas after kidney transplant; PTA, pancreas transplant alone; Px, pancreas.

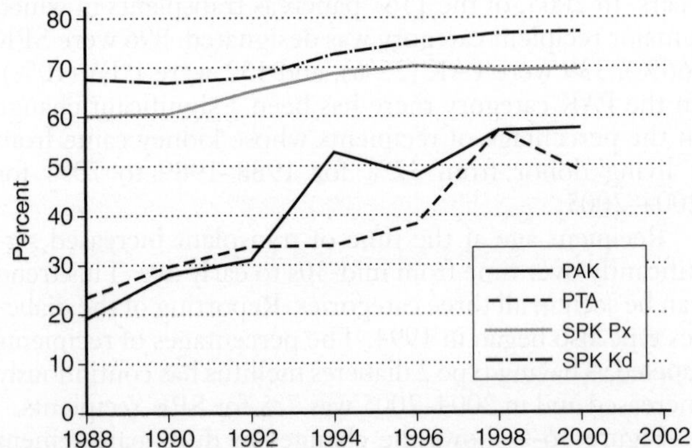

FIGURE 36-13 ■ Pancreas and simultaneous pancreas–kidney (SPK) 5-year graft survival rates for US deceased donor primary pancreas transplant recipients by category and era, in 2-year intervals, 1988 through 2005. Kd, kidney; PAK, pancreas after kidney transplant; PTA, pancreas transplant alone; Px, pancreas.

years in all three categories (Figures 36-10 and 36-11). Survival rates at 1 year have been greater than 90% in all recipient categories since the earliest era and are now around 95% for transplants performed in 2004–2005 (Figure 36-10). Overall, patient survival rates at 5 years can be calculated only up to the 2000–2001 era, but they also have improved and are greater than 80% in all categories, including 90% for 2000–2001 PTA recipients (Figure 36-11).

In contrast to patient survival rates, which have been high in all eras, pancreas graft survival rates improved even more over time, particularly in the solitary (PAK and PTA) categories (Figures 36-12 and 36-13). In the earlier eras, graft survival rates were much higher in the SPK than in the PAK and PTA categories. In 2004–2005, the differences are much smaller, although still significant. One-year pancreas graft survival rates were 85% for SPK versus 79% for PAK and 78% for PTA (Figure 36-12). One-year kidney graft survival rates in the SPK category also improved significantly for many years, reaching 92% in 1998–1999 but plateauing since then.

Graft survival rates at 5 years can be calculated only for the years preceding 2000–2001, but in the solitary categories (PAK and PTA) they more than doubled to 57% for PAK and 49% for PTA in 2000–2001 (Figure 36-13). For that era, in SPK recipients, the 5-year pancreas graft survival reached 70%, and the kidney graft survival reached 77%.

The technical failures are primarily early graft losses attributed to vascular thrombosis or removal because of bleeding, anastomotic leaks, pancreatitis, or infection. Technical failure rates decreased significantly over time in all three categories. In the early years, the technical failure rates were higher in the solitary (PAK and PTA) categories than in the SPK category, which, we hypothesize, may be due partly to misclassifying some thromboses as technical when they were actually secondary to early rejections. In 2004–2005, the technical failure rates were similar in all three categories, with 6.4% for SPK, 8.9% for PAK, and 3.9% for PTA. The technical failure rate is significantly higher in the SPK category for enteric drainage versus bladder drainage transplants, 6.5% versus 3.2% in the 2002–2003 era ($P = 0.02$).[37]

The improvement in pancreas graft survival rates is due not only to a decline in the technical failure rate but also to declines in the rejection loss rates (Figure 36-14).

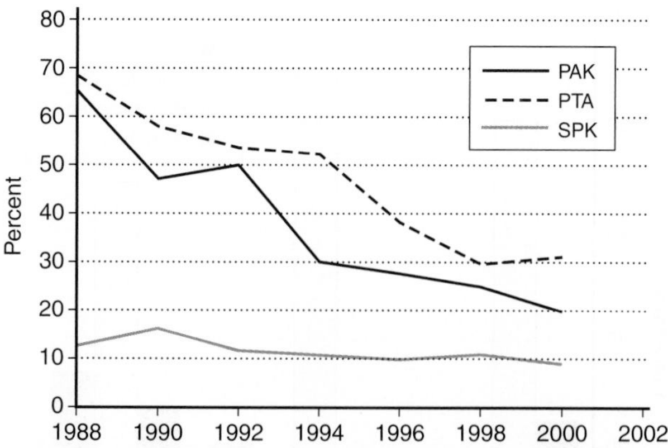

FIGURE 36-14 ■ Immunological 5-year graft loss rates for US deceased donor primary pancreas transplants by recipient category and era, in 2-year intervals, 1988 through 2005. PAK, pancreas after kidney transplant; PTA, pancreas transplant alone; SPK, simultaneous pancreas–kidney.

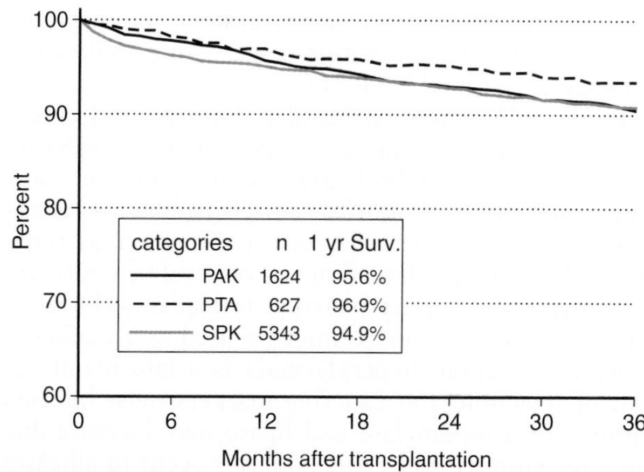

FIGURE 36-15 ■ Patient survival rates for 2000–2005 US deceased donor primary transplants by recipient category. PAK, pancreas after kidney transplant; PTA, pancreas transplant alone; SPK, simultaneous pancreas–kidney.

The rejection loss rates at 1 year declined fourfold to fivefold from the earliest to the most recent years, and in 2004–2005 were 5.4% for PAK, 11% for PTA, and 2% for SPK. The decline in the long-term rejection loss rates in the solitary (PAK and PTA) categories were more than halved from the years 1988–1989 and were 20% for PAK and 31% for PTA in the latest era for which a calculation can be made, 2000–2001 (Figure 36-14).

Pancreas Transplant Outcome for Contemporary (2000–2005) US Cases

Current outcomes with deceased donor pancreas transplantation according to recipient categories, surgical technique, and immunosuppression protocol for US cases as reported to UNOS from January, 2000, to December, 2005, are summarized here. During this period, greater than 7500 pancreas transplants were reported to UNOS, including greater than 5300 SPK transplants, greater than 1600 PAK transplants, and greater than 600 PTAs.

The primary transplant patient survival rates in the three recipient categories are shown in Figure 36-15. At 1 year, 94.9% of the SPK, 95.6% of the PAK, and 96.9% of the PTA recipients were alive; at 3 years, 90.8% of the SPK, 90.2% of the PAK, and 93.4% of the PTA recipients were alive ($P > 0.06$). The highest patient survival rate was in the PTA category, presumably because this group had less advanced complications before transplantation.

The primary pancreas graft survival rates in the three recipient categories are shown in Figure 36-16. At 1 year, 84.7% of the SPK, 78% of the PAK, and 75.9% of the PTA recipients were insulin-independent; at 3 years, 77.7% of the SPK, 65.6% of the PAK, and 59.9% of the PTA recipients were insulin-independent ($P<0.0001$). The highest pancreas graft survival rates are in the SPK category, presumably because the kidney graft (usually from the same donor as the pancreas) can be used to detect rejection episodes earlier than in the other categories, where only the pancreas can be monitored. Support for this hypothesis comes from registry data showing no significant differences in graft technical failure rates between categories but large differences in rejection loss rates.

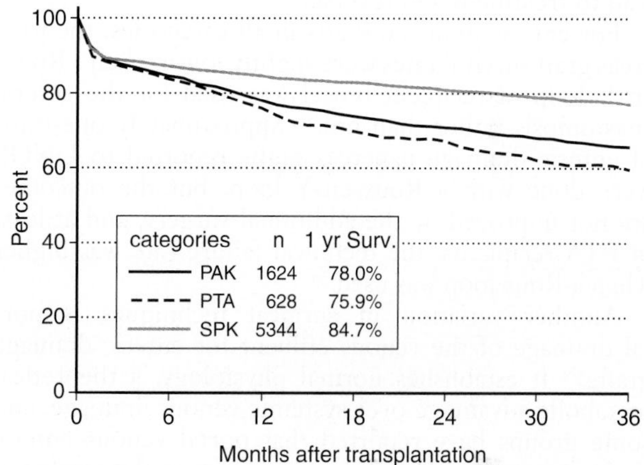

FIGURE 36-16 ■ Pancreas graft functional survival rates (insulin independence) for 2000–2005 US deceased donor primary transplants by recipient category. PAK, pancreas after kidney transplant; PTA, pancreas transplant alone; SPK, simultaneous pancreas–kidney.

Of the primary pancreas grafts between 2000 and 2005, 8% failed for technical reasons, with thrombosis being the biggest risk for technical loss (5%). Infection, pancreatitis, and anastomotic leak constituted the rest. There were no significant differences between categories in regard to technical losses.

In regard to management of pancreatic duct exocrine secretions for cases between 2000 and 2004, enteric drainage predominated for SPK transplants (81%); for PAK and PTA, the proportion of cases that were enteric drainage was slightly lower (67% and 56%). Overall, the technical failure rate was slightly higher with enteric drainage than with bladder drainage (8% versus 6%). Pancreas graft survival rates were not significantly different, however, for enteric drainage versus bladder drainage transplants in any of the categories: at 1 year, 85% ($n = 3047$) versus 79% ($n = 707$) for SPK; 77% ($n = 733$) versus 80% ($n = 364$) for PAK; and 72% ($n = 238$) versus 79% ($n = 184$) for PTA cases. For PTA cases between 2000 and 2005, the failure rate from rejection for technically successful grafts was 8% ($n = 185$) for bladder drainage, 10%

($n = 250$) for enteric drainage with systemic drainage, and 13% ($n = 101$) for enteric drainage with portal venous drainage at 1 year (P NS 0.71).

In the SPK category, bladder drainage and enteric drainage would be expected to give similar results because in most cases both grafts come from the same donor, and monitoring of serum creatinine serves as a surrogate marker for rejection in the pancreas transplant, allowing easy detection and reversal by treatment. In contrast, for solitary pancreas transplants (PAK and PTA), serum creatinine cannot be used as a marker of pancreas rejection; hyperglycemia is a late manifestation of rejection, and exocrine markers must be used. Although serum amylase and lipase may increase during a rejection episode, this does not occur in all cases, but for bladder drainage grafts, a decrease in urine amylase eventually always accompanies rejection (100% sensitive, although it is not specific), and nearly always precedes hyperglycemia, so a rejection episode is more likely to be diagnosed in a bladder drainage graft and lead to treatment and reversal.

For enteric drainage grafts in all categories, the pancreas graft survival rates were slightly lower when a Roux-en-Y loop of recipient bowel was used for the enteric anastomosis rather than not.[36] Approximately one-third of enteric drainage pancreas grafts reported to UNOS were done with a Roux-en-Y loop, but the outcomes are not improved by the additional surgery, and at least in PTA recipients, the technical failure rate was higher when a Roux loop was used.[36]

Another variation in surgical techniques is portal drainage of the venous effluent for enteric drainage grafts.[99] It establishes normal physiology, a theoretical metabolic advantage over systemic venous drainage, and some groups have reported that portal venous–enteric drainage grafts are less prone to rejection than systemic venous–enteric drainage grafts.[87,116] The registry analysis shows that portal venous drainage was used for one-fifth of enteric drainage transplants, but there were no significant differences in pancreas graft survival versus systemic venous–enteric drainage transplants in any of the categories: at 1 year, 85% ($n = 610$) versus 85% ($n = 2437$) for SPK; 78% ($n = 168$) versus 77% ($n = 564$) for PAK; and 71% ($n = 85$) versus 72% ($n = 153$) for PTA enteric drainage cases.

In regard to immunosuppression, according to the latest registry analysis, anti-T-cell agents were used for induction therapy in about three-fourths of US pancreas recipients in each category between 2000 and 2005 (Figure 36-17). The agents available can be divided into two groups: (1) T-cell-depleting polyclonal (e.g., antithymocyte gammaglobulin (Atgam), antithymocyte globulin (Thymoglobulin)) or monoclonal (e.g., OKT3, alemtuzumab (Campath)) antibodies; or (2) non-depleting (monoclonal anti-CD25-directed, daclizumab, or basiliximab) antibodies.

The most frequently used regimen for maintenance immunosuppression (two-thirds of the recipients in each category) was tacrolimus and mycophenolate mofetil in combination (Figure 36-18), with or without prednisone (Figure 36-19). In recipients of primary deceased donor pancreas grafts given anti-T-cell agents for induction and tacrolimus and mycophenolate mofetil for maintenance immunosuppression, the 1-year graft survival rates in the SPK, PAK, and PTA categories were 87% ($n = 2728$), 80% ($n = 817$), and 79% ($n = 328$). Sirolimus was

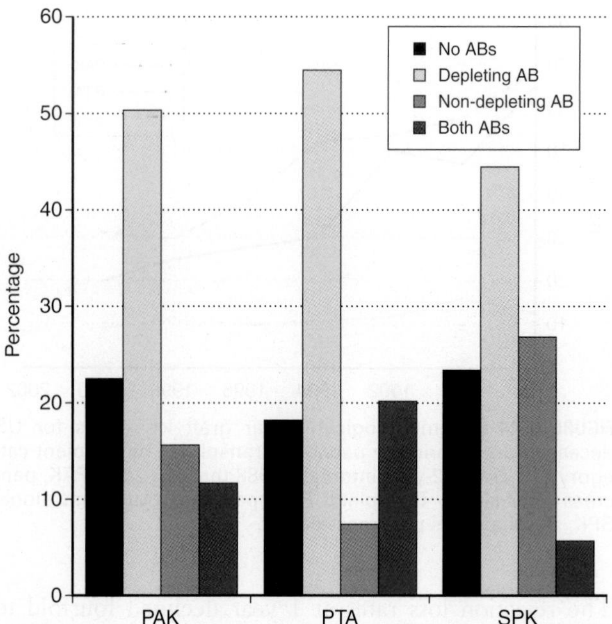

FIGURE 36-17 ■ Frequency distribution of use of and type of anti-T-cell antibody (AB) induction therapy by recipient category for US deceased donor primary pancreas transplants, 2000–2005 cases. PAK, pancreas after kidney transplant; PTA, pancreas transplant alone; SPK, simultaneous pancreas–kidney.

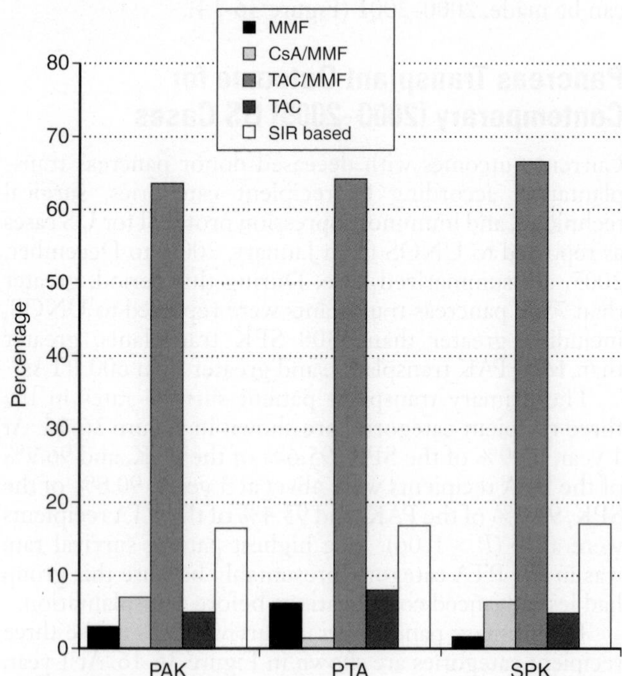

FIGURE 36-18 ■ Frequency distribution of use of and type of major maintenance immunosuppressive protocols by recipient category for US deceased donor primary pancreas transplants, 2000–2005 cases. CsA, cyclosporine; MMF, mycophenolate mofetil; PAK, pancreas after kidney transplant; PTA, pancreas transplant alone; SIR, sirolimus; SPK, simultaneous pancreas–kidney; TAC, tacrolimus.

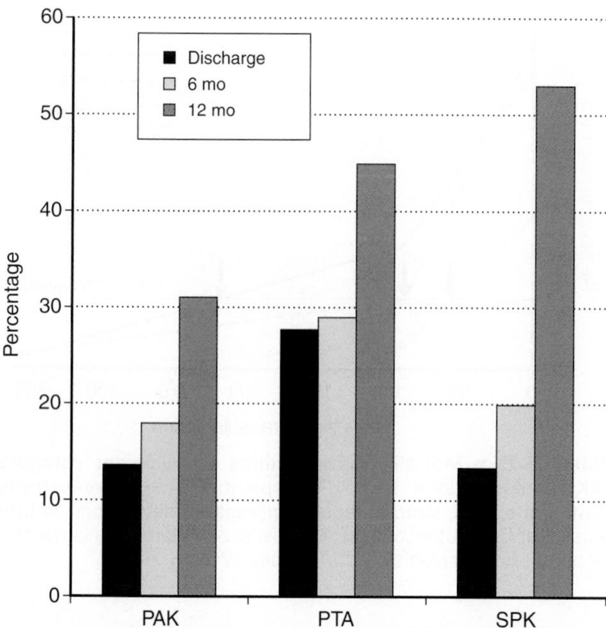

FIGURE 36-19 ■ Frequency distribution of patients off steroids by recipient category for US deceased donor primary pancreas transplants, 2000–2005 cases. PAK, pancreas after kidney transplant; PTA, pancreas transplant alone; SPK, simultaneous pancreas–kidney.

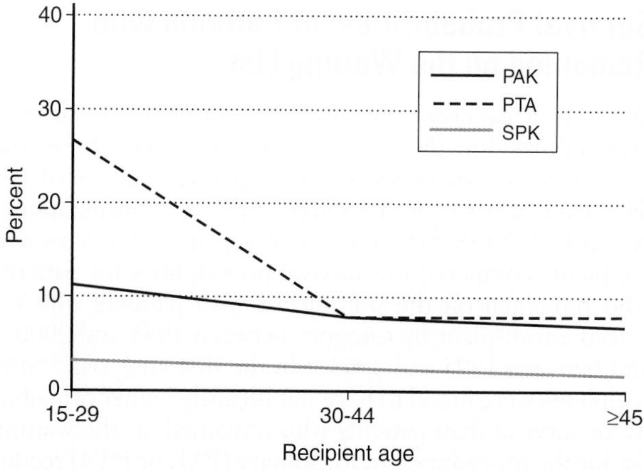

FIGURE 36-20 ■ Immunological graft loss rates at 1 year for US deceased donor primary pancreas transplant recipients by age and category, 2000–2004 cases. PAK, pancreas after kidney transplant; PTA, pancreas transplant alone; SPK, simultaneous pancreas–kidney.

used as a maintenance immunosuppressive drug in about one-sixth of recipients in each category with comparable outcomes. The 1-year pancreas graft survival rates in the SPK, PAK, and PTA categories were 90% (n = 527), 84% (n = 170), and 82% (n = 79).

Outcome by Recipient and Donor Risk Factors

In regard to the logistics of pancreas transplantation, registry data[37] showed a slight increase in technical failure rates and a slight decrease in graft survival rates with increasing preservation time. In the SPK category, 1-year pancreas graft survival rates were 86% with 4–7 hours of preservation versus 81% with 28–31 hours of preservation. HLA matching had virtually no impact on SPK graft survival rates, but matching at least at the class I loci had a beneficial effect in the PAK and the PTA categories.

In regard to pancreas recipient age, the registry analysis of 2000–2004 cases showed an effect on outcome mainly in PTA recipients, with rejection more likely in the youngest recipients (Figure 36-20). In the PAK category, all recipients were older than 20 years, and in analysis of rejection rates by decade of age, at 1 year the rates varied from 4% to 7%; in the SPK category, the rejection rate at 1 year was 2–4% in the various age groups older than 20 years but 0% for recipients younger than 20 years (n = 4). In contrast, in the PTA category, the rejection rate at 1 year was 50% for recipients younger than 20 years (n = 14) and 13% for recipients 20–29 years old (n = 39); for PTA recipients older than age 30, the 1-year rejection loss rates were 4–6%, similar to the other two recipient categories.

The young non-uremic diabetic patient is highly immunocompetent and more prone to reject a pancreas graft, consistent with an earlier analysis of outcomes in US pediatric pancreas transplant recipients from 1988 to 1999.[68] In that analysis, of slightly more than 8000 pancreas transplants, only 49 were in recipients younger than 21 years old (<1%): 36 in the SPK, two in the PAK, and 13 in the PTA category; all were deceased donor pancreas transplants except for two PTA segmental grafts from living donors. Fewer than half of the pediatric pancreas recipients were younger than 19 years old. In the PTA recipients, the 1-year graft survival rate was only 15%, with all but one loss being from rejection in less than 1 year. The registry data do not include the indications for a PTA in the pediatric recipients, but presumably they had extremely labile diabetes justifying placement on immunosuppression in an attempt to gain control. In the pediatric SPK recipients, the 1-year patient, pancreas, and kidney graft survival rates were 96%, 78%, and 71%, outcomes comparable to that of adult SPK recipients for the entire period. Of the pediatric SPK recipients, most had a renal disease other than diabetic nephropathy.

In regard to donor age, in the registry analysis of 2000–2004 primary deceased donor pancreas transplants, graft survival rates in all recipient categories tended to be highest with younger donors and lowest with older donors, principally because technical failure rates increased with increasing donor age.[37] Only 3.4% of all donors were 50 years old or older, and those donors were also mainly used in SPK.

With respect to outcome measures other than insulin independence – prevention and reversal of secondary complications, improvement in QOL, expansion of lifespan, and reduction of healthcare costs per quality-adjusted life-year – these all have been positively shown in type 1 diabetic pancreas transplant recipients.[21,27,32,82,114,132,137] In patients with labile diabetes and hypoglycemic unawareness, a pancreas transplant can resolve an otherwise intractable and life-threatening problem.[54,80,96]

Survival Probabilities for Patients who Remained on the Waiting List

Whether a pancreas transplant has an effect on survival probabilities for the diabetic patients selected for the procedure is controversial. Two separate analyses of US data from the Organ Procurement and Transplantation Network/UNOS for pancreas transplant candidates and recipients compared the survival probabilities for patients who remained on the waiting list with patients who received a transplant by category between 1995 and 2000[134] and between 1995 and 2003.[44] In the first analysis,[134] SPK recipients were found to have significantly higher probability of survival than patients who remained on the waiting list for the procedure, but for solitary (PAK or PTA) recipients, just the opposite was the case. There is an explanation for the different results between the two studies. In the second analysis (Figures 36-21 and 36-22),[44] multiple listings were eliminated. However, in the first study, they were not. By eliminating the multiple listings, patients were counted only once – from the first date of listing – increasing the accuracy of the waiting list mortality calculations.

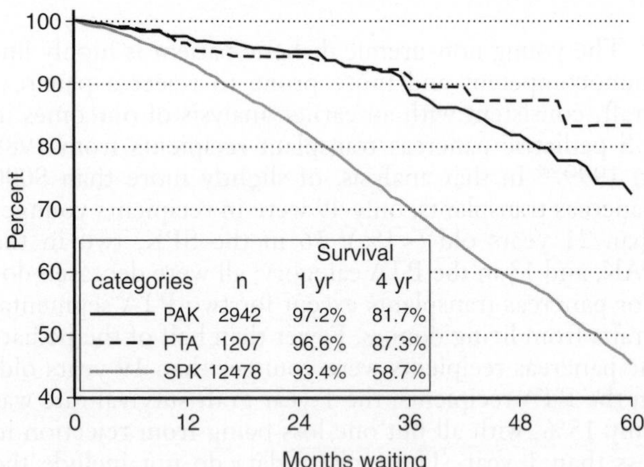

FIGURE 36-21 ■ Patient survival rates on the pancreas waiting lists for 1995–2003 US deceased donor primary transplants by recipient category. PAK, pancreas after kidney transplant; PTA, pancreas transplant alone; SPK, simultaneous pancreas–kidney. (Modified from Gruessner RW, Sutherland DE, Gruessner AC. Mortality assessment for pancreas transplants. Am J Transplant 2004;4:2018.)

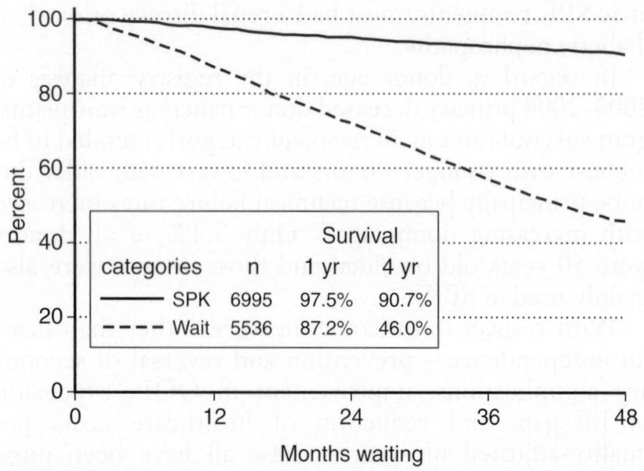

FIGURE 36-22 ■ Patient survival rates on the pancreas waiting lists and after pancreas transplants for 1995–2003 US deceased donor primary transplants in the simultaneous pancreas–kidney (SPK) category. (Modified from Gruessner RW, Sutherland DE, Gruessner AC. Mortality assessment for pancreas transplants. Am J Transplant 2004;4:2018.)

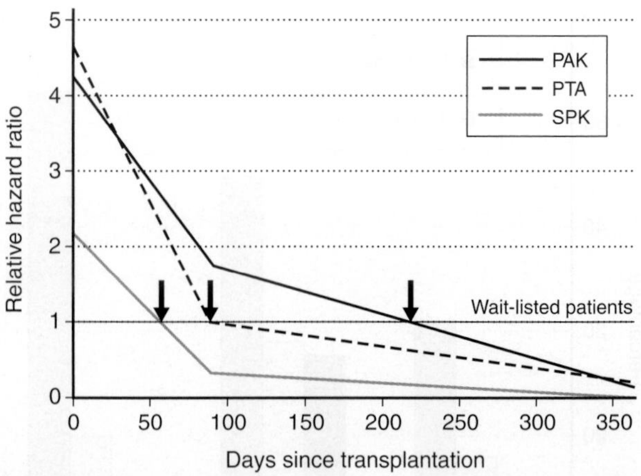

FIGURE 36-23 ■ Mortality hazard ratios by recipient category. PAK, pancreas after kidney transplant; PTA, pancreas transplant alone; SPK, simultaneous pancreas–kidney. (Modified from Gruessner RW, Sutherland DE, Gruessner AC. Mortality assessment for pancreas transplants. Am J Transplant 2004;4:2018.)

Figure 36-23 shows hazard ratios of death among transplant recipients compared with patients who remained on the waiting list in the second study. For all categories, the hazard ratio in the early posttransplant period was greater than 1 because the surgical procedure itself increases the mortality hazard. In all three recipient categories, the hazard ratio was significantly decreased, however. Pancreas transplantation does not entail a higher risk than staying on exogenous insulin for patients on the waiting list and may improve survival probabilities for solitary and SPK recipients.

Expected Life-Year Gains from an Extra Deceased Donor

Understanding the additional life-years given to patients by deceased organ donors is necessary because substantial investments are being proposed to increase organ donation. Data were drawn from the US Scientific Registry of Transplant Recipients. All patients placed on the wait list as eligible to receive or receiving a deceased donor solid-organ transplant between 1995 and 2002 were studied.[100] The average expected gain in life-years for kidney–pancreas waitlisted patients from an extra deceased organ donor was 12.9 life-years. Average benefit given average frequency of transplants in 2002 was 1.9 life-years.

PANCREAS RETRANSPLANTS

The following data are from the University of Minnesota. In a series of pancreas transplants from 1978 to 2005 ($n = 1835$), 321 (17%) were retransplants (14% second transplants, 2.5% third transplants, 0.5% fourth transplants); all but three were from deceased donors. From 1985 to 2005, 53 deceased donor SPK retransplants (38 second transplants) were performed. The overall 1-year pancreas graft survival rate was 62% for all SPK retransplants together and 66% for second SPK transplants only; at 3 years, survival rates were 45% for all and 52% for second transplants only. From 1978 to 2005, 163 deceased donor PAK retransplants (135 second transplants) were done. From 1994 to 2005 cases combined, the 1-year graft survival rate for deceased donor PAK retransplants with second, third, and fourth transplants included (n = 117) was 67% and for second transplants only (n = 99) was 65%; at 3 years, survival rates were 51% for all and 50% for second transplants only. From 1978 to 2005, there were 99 deceased donor PTA retransplants (86 second transplants). From 1998 to 2005 cases combined, the 1-year graft survival rate for deceased donor PAK retransplants with second, third, and fourth transplants included (n = 49) was 67% and for second transplants only (n = 43) was 66%; at 3 years, survival rates were 50% for all and 48% for second transplants only.

LIVING DONOR PANCREAS TRANSPLANTS

The following data are from the University of Minnesota. Nearly all of the living donor solitary (PAK and PTA) pancreas transplants were done from 1978 to 1994. All but two of the living donor SPK transplants (n = 38) were done from 1994 to 2005.[126]

Living donor SPK transplants started in March 1994.[42] Of the 38 donors, 6 were HLA-identical siblings, 25 were HLA-mismatched relatives, and 7 were unrelated. Two donors were ABO-incompatible; antibody reduction was successfully accomplished with plasmapheresis,[67] and both grafts are currently functioning at more than 6 years. In the overall series of 38 living donor SPK transplants, the 1-, 5-, and 10-year patient survival rates were 100%, 100%, and 84%; the 1-, 5-, and 10-year segmental pancreas graft survival rates (technical failures included, death with functioning graft counted as a graft failure) were 84%, 70%, and 60%; and the 1-, 5-, and 10-year kidney graft survival rates are 100%, 86%, and 67%. We used duct injection technique in four living donor SPK transplants – the first two SPK segmental pancreas grafts (one still functioning at >12 years; one failed at >10 years) and in two later cases (one pancreas failed at 4 months, the kidney is still functioning at >10 years; in the other case, both grafts are functioning at >1 year). We used enteric drainage in two cases (both organs are functioning at >2 and >7 years) and bladder drainage in the other 32.

A comparison of outcomes from 1994 to 2005 cases combined was made for primary living donor SPK (n = 36) versus primary deceased donor SPK (n = 324) transplants (Table 36-1). The patient survival rates were significantly higher (P = 0.01 Wilcoxon and P = 0.03 log rank) in the living donor versus deceased donor cases – at 1, 3, and 7 years after transplantation, 100%, 100%, and 95% in living donor versus 90%, 86%, and 79% in deceased donor recipients. Pancreas graft survival rates were not significantly different between the living donor and deceased donor SPK recipients – at 1, 3, and 7 years after transplantation, 86%, 78%, and 67% in living donor versus 78%, 74%, and 62% in deceased donor cases. Kidney graft survival rates were marginally significantly higher (P = 0.09 Wilcoxon, P = 0.19 log rank) in living donor versus deceased donor SPK recipients – at 1, 3, and 7 years after transplantation, 100%, 91%, and 79% in living donor versus 87%, 86%, and 67% in deceased donor cases.

QUALITY-OF-LIFE STUDY

At University of Minnesota, from 1985 to 2003, 316 SPK, 204 PAK, and 98 PTA recipients enrolled in a prospective study of QOL changes after pancreas transplantation.[126] For QOL assessment, we used four dimensions of the Karnofsky index: status of health, management of life, life satisfaction, and health satisfaction. Each recipient's response was recorded on a scale of 1 (low) to 5 (high) for each parameter. A total score was calculated from the sum of the four parameters (maximum score possible, 20). The impact of a successful or failed transplant was assessed by the changes in scores from baseline in annual follow-up evaluations.

The baseline (before pancreas transplant) median total scores were significantly higher ($P < 0.0001$) in the PAK (13.3) than in the SPK (11.3) and PTA (10.9) candidates. The ranges of baseline scores for the two midquarters in each recipient category are provided in Table 36-2. The mean baseline scores in these eras were 9.5 ± 2.6 (n = 109), 12.3 ± 3.9 (n = 131), and 13 ± 3.7 (n = 62) for SPK (P = 0.0001); 10.9 ± 2.6 (n = 32), 13.9 ± 3.3 (n = 82), and

TABLE 36-1 **Primary Simultaneous Pancreas–Kidney Transplantation Living Donor Versus Deceased Donor Outcomes from 1994 to 2005**

	Patient Survival (%)		***Pancreas GSR (%)***		***Kidney GSR (%)***	
Years Post Transplantation	**LD**	**DD**	**LD**	**DD**	**LD**	**DD**
1	100	90	86	78	100	87
3	100	86	78	74	91	86
5	100	85	74	69	86	73
7	95	79	67	62	79	67
10	79	72	67	55	65	57
	P = 0.01/0.03		P = 0.31/0.41		P = 0.09/0.19	

P = Wilcoxon/log-rank tests.
DD, deceased donor; GSR, graft survival rate; LD, living donor.

TABLE 36-2 **Pretransplant Baseline Quality-of-Life Scores* from 1985 to 2003: Pancreas Transplant Recipient Study Patients (Range of Middle Two Quartiles)**

Category (*n*)	Q1	Median	Q2
SPK (316)	8.4	11.3	14.6
PAK (204)	11.7	13.3	15.9
PTA (98)	8.1	10.9	13.4

Q1 = highest sum in first quartile; Q2 = highest sum in third quartile.

PAK, pancreas after kidney; PTA, pancreas transplant alone; SPK, simultaneous pancreas–kidney.

*Scores are summation of four parameters from Karnofsky index: status of health, management of life, life satisfaction, and health satisfaction.

15.2 ± 2.8 (*n* = 46) for PAK (*P* = 0.0001); and 9.9 ± 2.9 (*n* = 26), 10.3 ± 3.6 (*n* = 30), and 12.7 ± 3.3 (*n* = 24) for PTA (*P* = 0.009) candidates. Possibly, diabetic patients are coming to pancreas transplantation in better health condition than in the past.

It is not the absolute QOL score but rather the change (Δ) in score from the pretransplant baseline to the posttransplant evaluation that is important. The total score Δ for each recipient category according to graft function at 1 year is shown in Tables 36-3 and 36-4. SPK recipients were divided into four groups by graft status: (1) both grafts had sustained function (*n* = 130); (2) the pancreas had sustained function, but the kidney graft failed (*n* = 5); (3) the kidney graft had sustained function, but the pancreas graft failed (*n* = 24); or (4) both grafts failed (*n* = 2).

At 1 year after transplantation, the mean increase from baseline in total QOL scores was highly significant (*P* = 0.0001) in the SPK recipients with both grafts functioning but not in recipients with a functioning pancreas but a failed kidney. In recipients with a functioning kidney, but a failed pancreas graft, there was virtually no change from baseline. Only two recipients in whom both grafts failed completed the follow-up

TABLE 36-3 **One-Year Posttransplant Mean (±SD) Change (Δ) in Quality-of-Life Scores from Pretransplant Baseline in Simultaneous Pancreas–Kidney Recipients According to Graft Function or Failure**

	Graft Status (n)		
	Pancreas Fxn, Pancreas Fail, Kidney Fxn (24)	**Pancreas Fxn, Kidney Fxn (130), Kidney Fail (2)**	**Pancreas Fail, Kidney Fail (5)**
Quality-of-life score change	5.2 ± 4.0	2.4 ± 1.5	0.2 ± 3.7
P value	≤0 0.0001 NA	0.12	>0.5

Fail, failure; Fxn, function; NA, not applicable.

TABLE 36-4 **One-Year Posttransplant Mean (±SD) Change (Δ) in Mean Quality-of-Life Score from Pretransplant Baseline in Solitary Pancreas after Kidney Transplant Recipients with Functioning or Failed Grafts**

	Graft Status	
	Functioning	**Failed**
PAK (*n*)	3.7 ± 4.1 (55)	0.9 ± 2.5 (16)
P value	0.0001	0.009
PTA (*n*)	5.9 ± 4.2 (25)	2.8 ± 4.8 (12)
P value	0.0001	0.07

PAK, pancreas after kidney; PTA, pancreas transplant alone.

evaluation at 1 year. The total score did not change in one; it was lower compared with the pretransplant baseline in the other. The results in the SPK recipients in whom only one graft failed suggest that achieving insulin independence improves QOL more than becoming dialysis-free. At 1 year, the mean total QOL score increased significantly (*P* = 0.0001) from baseline in PAK recipients with sustained graft function (*n* = 55) (but not in recipients with failed grafts (*n* = 16) (Table 36-4). At 1 year, the mean total QOL score increased significantly (*P* = 0.0001) from baseline in PTA recipients with sustained graft function (*n* = 25) but not in recipients with failed grafts (*n* = 12) (Table 36-4).

LONG-TERM QUALITY OF LIFE

The increase in mean total points from pretransplant baseline was sustained in succeeding years in patients with functioning grafts. At 2 years, the mean increases were 4.3 ± 0.8 points for SPK (*n* = 100), 3.7 ± 5.6 for PAK (*n* = 32), and 6.4 ± 4.3 for PTA (*n* = 8) (*P* = 0.0001). For 50 SPK study patients who completed the evaluation at 4 years, the mean increase in total points from baseline was 6.2 ± 4.6 (*n* = 50) (*P* = 0.0001). Overall, our study showed that diabetic patients who become insulin-independent perceive their QOL as having improved despite immunosuppression. The data presented here are original and complement past QOL studies, done by independent investigators,[31–34,136,137] of the Minnesota pancreas recipients.

METABOLIC STUDIES

Formal metabolic studies of the Minnesota pancreas recipients and living donors have been conducted since the inception of our program[128] and are still ongoing.[98] The initial studies were very basic: 24 metabolic profiles of glucose and insulin values before and after meals, and standard oral or intravenous glucose tolerance tests in pancreas recipients who were insulin-independent as a result of a functioning graft.[128] The profiles usually resembled those of non-diabetic individuals, or at least those of non-diabetic kidney allograft recipients, with or without portal drainage of the graft venous effluent.[122] The metabolic profile and glucose tolerance test studies were used to compare posttransplant endocrine function by duration of pancreas graft preservation[76] and to compare function in recipients who did or did not have reversible rejection episodes.[72] Metabolic profile and glucose tolerance test results were similar regardless of preservation time or occurrence of rejection episodes in recipients with sustained insulin independence; short-term[73] and long-term[74] glycosylated hemoglobin levels[75] were normal. More sophisticated metabolic studies using new methods were introduced[94] and carried out by a series of fellows and associate faculty members in the Division of Endocrinology.[2,18,19,50,54,55,94,101,102,130] These studies not only examined pancreatic graft beta-cell function but also alpha-cell function, glucose counterregulatory mechanisms, and the impact of the site of venous drainage (systemic or portal) of a pancreas graft.

Diem and colleagues[18] were the first to establish systemic venous drainage as the principal cause of systemic venous hyperinsulinemia after pancreas transplantation. A smaller portion of the hyperinsulinemia could be attributed to recipients' glucocorticoid use. Despite this metabolic abnormality, virtually all measures of carbohydrate metabolism in the fasting state and after a mixed meal remained normal.[50]

Possible adverse effects of immunosuppressive drugs on beta-cell function and glucose tolerance also were studied. Many of the drugs are known to interfere with insulin synthesis or secretion, or action. Teuscher and coworkers[130] assessed insulin secretory reserve in pancreas transplant recipients by measuring glucose potentiation of arginine-induced insulin secretion and observed abnormally low insulin responses. Because diminished insulin secretory reserve also was observed in non-diabetic kidney recipients, the immunosuppressive drugs were the likely causes of this metabolic abnormality. A similar defect was observed in psoriasis patients treated with cyclosporine but not in arthritis patients treated with glucocorticoids; cyclosporine was the likely cause of diminished insulin secretory reserve.[130] Despite the hyperinsulinemia consequent to systemic drainage and glucocorticoids, and despite the diminished insulin secretory reserve attributable to cyclosporine, we have reported normal levels of fasting plasma glucose and hemoglobin A_{1c} in a group of pancreas recipients followed for 10–18 years.[97]

Defective glucagon and epinephrine counterregulatory responses to hypoglycemia are serious consequences of type 1 diabetes. These abnormalities can lead to dangerous levels of hypoglycemia that incapacitate patients and seriously compromise their QOL. This scenario is worsened because such patients lose normal symptom recognition of hypoglycemia, which prevents them from taking early corrective measures. Studies by Diem and colleagues[19] showed that a successful pancreas transplant restores normal glucagon responses. Later studies by Kendall and associates[56] concluded that the transplanted pancreas, rather than the alpha cells in the native pancreas, provided the restored glucagon response. Barrou and colleagues[3] used isotopic infusions and hypoglycemic clamp methodology to show that the restored glucagon response normalized hepatic glucose production during hypoglycemia. Kendall and associates[54] showed that a successful pancreas transplant partially restored epinephrine response during hypoglycemia. More importantly, these studies also documented that recipients of a successful pancreas transplant re-establish normal symptom recognition.

More recently, Paty and coworkers[85] have shown that restored hypoglycemic counterregulation is stable in pancreas recipients with functioning grafts for at least two decades after transplantation. The effect of the occurrence of posttransplant obesity in pancreas recipients was studied, and a detrimental effect on metabolism was shown similar to that in the general population.[95]

Although most of our pancreas transplants were from deceased donors, nearly 10% were segmental grafts from living donors. The metabolic responsitivity of the transplanted hemipancreas is generally indistinguishable from that of whole-pancreas grafts. Donors of the pancreatic segments generally maintain normal glucose levels, but follow-up studies of the donors (before we established our current criteria to be a living donor) show that about 25% had metabolic evidence of acquired glucose intolerance several years after donation.[55] Studies by Seaquist and Robertson[102] established that beta-cell and alpha-cell responses were compromised in hemipancreatectomized donors during measurements of insulin secretory reserve. Later studies by Seaquist and colleagues[101] showed that hemipancreatectomy also was associated with elevated circulating levels of proinsulin, presumably owing to release of immature insulin granules in which cleavage of C peptide from proinsulin was not yet complete.

The results of these studies prompted us to modify our criteria to be a living donor. Now, all living donors must have a body mass index less than 28 kg/m², in addition to having normal glucose tolerance test results, and plasma insulin levels must increase by 300% within 1–2 minutes after intravenous stimulation with glucose or arginine. Living donors who meet these criteria have so far remained euglycemic and insulin-independent, but they need to be carefully studied over time. More recent studies of living hemipancreatectomized donors and their recipients during the second decade after surgery have shown a relationship between the development of obesity and occurrence of diabetes,[95] and the potential for weight gain in donors and recipients must be taken into account when selecting living donors and recipients for hemipancreatectomy and segmental pancreas transplantation. Most living segmental pancreas donors retain normal hormonal responses to metabolic challenges, however.[98]

STUDIES OF DIABETIC SECONDARY COMPLICATIONS

Formal studies on the course of pre-existing diabetic secondary complications after pancreas transplantation were initiated.[118,119] Until the multicenter DCCT[17] was completed in 1993, the best evidence that a constant euglycemic state mitigated the progression of secondary complications was from studies at the University of Minnesota[9,57,81,92,133] and those of others.[104,135] These studies were done by faculty from ophthalmology,[92] pediatric nephrology,[9,27] and neurology.[57,80–82] The failure rate of pancreas transplants was high, generating a control group for these studies. Recipients were studied at baseline, and subsequently divided into two groups: (1) recipients with early pancreas graft failure (<3 months), and (2) recipients with sustained graft function for more than 1 year.

Retinopathy

Ramsay and colleagues[92] studied solitary pancreas recipients. Retinopathy and visual acuity were quantitated before and serially after transplantation. Most candidates had advanced proliferative retinopathy. At 2 years after transplantation, the incidence of progression to a higher grade of retinopathy was the same (approximately 30%) in the eyes of recipients with versus without graft function. After 3 years, no further progression occurred in the recipients with functioning grafts. Seventy percent with failed transplants advanced to a higher grade by 5 years, however. Only a few recipients had no retinopathy at the pretransplant baseline examination, but disease has not emerged in the subgroup with continuously functioning pancreas grafts.

Nephropathy

Studies of diabetic nephropathy focused on disease recurrence or on preventing it in the kidney grafts of diabetic KTA, SPK, or PAK recipients[9,71,77] and on disease progression, stabilization, or regression of disease in the native kidneys of PTA recipients.[27,28] Mauer and associates[69–71] documented the recurrence of diabetic nephropathy (vascular lesions[69] and an increase in glomerular and tubular basement membrane and mesangial matrix[71]) in nearly half of kidneys transplanted without a pancreas in uremic diabetic recipients.[70]

Initial evidence that a successful pancreas transplant can influence the course of diabetic nephropathy came from kidney allograft biopsy studies in PAK recipients by Bilous and colleagues.[9] At the time of the pancreas transplant, 1–7 years (mean 4 years) after the kidney transplant, the graft glomerular mesangial volume was moderately increased and glomerular basement membrane was moderately thickened. There was no progression; there was regression of glomerular lesions in follow-up biopsy specimens obtained 2–10 years later (mean 4.5 years). These findings contrasted with the findings in the KTA recipients in whom progressive diabetic glomerulopathy occurred,[70] leading to kidney graft failure and the need for a kidney retransplant in some recipients.[78]

The most dramatic and surprising findings came from studies by Fioretto and colleagues[27,28] of native kidneys in PTA recipients. Baseline biopsy specimens of native kidneys were obtained in most of the PTA recipients.[25] Follow-up biopsy samples in some showed cyclosporine-induced lesions that were associated with a progressive decline in kidney function, independent of the diabetic lesions already present.[26,77,131] The diabetic kidney lesions were distinct. In eight PTA recipients who were non-uremic at the time of the pancreas transplant, but who had mild to moderately advanced lesions of diabetic nephropathy at baseline, 10-year follow-up biopsy specimens showed that glomerular basement membrane and tubular basement membrane thickness and mesangial fractional volume of the glomerulus had decreased and returned to normal.[27] In follow-up studies, Fioretto and colleagues[28] also showed remodeling of renal interstitial and tubular lesions in the kidneys of the pancreas transplant recipients. Although these studies were in patients with diabetic nephropathy, the fact that structural lesions could be reversed shows in principle that the kidney has the capacity for remodeling if the environmental perturbations responsible for the lesions originally are removed, having implications for renal disease in general, and not just that secondary to diabetes.

Although it takes at least 5 years of normoglycemia, a pancreas transplant can reverse the lesions of diabetic nephropathy. Such reversal does not guarantee normal function because independent damage to the kidney may occur from the calcineurin inhibitors needed to prevent pancreas rejection[26] – hence the need for attempts to develop effective non-nephrotoxic immunosuppressive regimens.[38] Nearly all patients with early diabetic nephropathy would benefit from a pancreas transplant if successful.

Neuropathy

As with the eye and kidney, our pancreas recipients had baseline neurological studies with serial follow-up.[57,82,92] More than 80 of our recipients had symptomatic neuropathy, and more than 90% had an abnormal neurologic examination at baseline.[58] Kennedy and associates[57] showed significant improvement in motor and sensory indices and autonomic function 1–4 years after transplantation; we concluded that progression of diabetic neuropathy is halted, and that an improvement is possible with sustained normoglycemia.

Navarro and coworkers[81] found mortality rates were higher in patients with autonomic dysfunction or abnormal nerve conduction studies compared with patients with minimal disease. The mortality rate also was high in non-transplanted diabetic patients with neuropathy. In neuropathic patients with a successful pancreas transplant, the mortality rate was significantly lower, however, even if neuropathy improved only minimally.[80] The combination of diabetes and severe neuropathy is lethal; correction of diabetes improves survival even if neuropathy persists. Navarro and coworkers[82] did follow-up studies at 10 years of diabetic pancreas recipients. In control patients (patients with a failed transplant), neuropathy progressively worsened, whereas in recipients with sustained graft function, the improvement in neuropathy was sustained.

SUMMARY

Pancreas transplantation should be in the armamentarium of every transplant center for the treatment of diabetic patients. Likewise, every endocrinologist should consider pancreas transplantation in the treatment of patients in whom type 1 diabetes is complicated by hypoglycemia-associated autonomic failure[16] or progressive microvascular complications or both. Continued clinical research on pancreas transplantation is needed to identify the most appropriate recipient population, the optimal timing of transplant in the course of diabetes, and the most suitable donor tissue and transplant protocol for a given patient. Pancreas transplantation needs to be made as economical as possible.[115] Studies such as those done in pancreas–kidney transplant recipients showed the efficiency in the treatment of complicated diabetes.[21] Currently, pancreas transplantation has a well-defined clinical role for diabetic patients, and it is expected to remain an important option in the treatment of diabetes.

REFERENCES

1. Allen RD, Wilson TG, Grierson JM, et al. Percutaneous biopsy of bladder-drained pancreas transplants. Transplantation 1991;51:1213.
2. Barrou B, Barrou Z, Gruessner A, et al. Probability of retaining endocrine function (insulin independence) after definitive loss of exocrine function in bladder-drained pancreas transplants. Transplant Proc 1994;26:473.
3. Barrou Z, Seaquist ER, Robertson RP. Pancreas transplantation in diabetic humans normalizes hepatic glucose production during hypoglycemia. Diabetes 1994;43:661.
4. Bendel-Stenzel MR, Kashtan CE, Sutherland DE, et al. Simultaneous pancreas-kidney transplant in two children with hemolytic-uremic syndrome. Pediatr Nephrol 1997;11:485.
5. Benedetti E, Dunn T, Massad MG, et al. Successful living related simultaneous pancreas-kidney transplant between identical twins. Transplantation 1999;67:915.
6. Benedetti E, Gruessner AC, Troppmann C, et al. Intra-abdominal fungal infections after pancreatic transplantation: incidence, treatment, and outcome. J Am Coll Surg 1996;183:307.
7. Benedetti E, Najarian JS, Gruessner AC, et al. Correlation between cystoscopic biopsy results and hypoamylasuria in bladder-drained pancreas transplants. Surgery 1995;118:864.
8. Benedetti E, Sileri P, Kandaswamy R, et al. Surgical aspects of pancreas transplantation. In: Gruessner RWG, Sutherland DER, editors. Transplantation of the pancreas. New York: Springer-Verlag; 2004. p. 111–78.
9. Bilous RW, Mauer SM, Sutherland DE, et al. The effects of pancreas transplantation on the glomerular structure of renal allografts in patients with insulin-dependent diabetes. N Engl J Med 1989;321:80.
10. Bloomgarden ZT. American Diabetes Association postgraduate course, 1996: treatment and prevention of diabetes. Diabetes Care 1996;19:784.
11. Boggi U, Vistoli F, Del Chiaro M, et al. A simplified technique for the en bloc procurement of abdominal organs that is suitable for pancreas and small-bowel transplantation. Surgery 2004;135:629.
12. Boggi U, Vistoli F, Del Chiaro M, et al. Retroperitoneal pancreas transplantation with portal-enteric drainage. Transplant Proc 2004;36:571.
13. Boggi U, Vistoli F, Signori S, et al. A technique for retroperitoneal pancreas transplantation with portal-enteric drainage. Transplantation 2005;79:1137.
14. Calne RY. Paratopic segmental pancreas grafting: a technique with portal venous drainage. Lancet 1984;1:595.
15. Calne RY, Rolles K, White DJ, et al. Cyclosporin A initially as the only immunosuppressant in 34 recipients of cadaveric organs: 32 kidneys, 2 pancreases, and 2 livers. Lancet 1979;2:1033.
16. Cryer PE. Banting lecture. Hypoglycemia: the limiting factor in the management of IDDM. Diabetes 1994;43:1378.
17. Diabetes Control and Complications Trial Research Group. The effect of intensive treatment of diabetes on the development and progression of long-term complications in insulin-dependent diabetes mellitus. N Engl J Med 1993;329:977.
18. Diem P, Abid M, Redmon JB, et al. Systemic venous drainage of pancreas allografts as independent cause of hyperinsulinemia in type I diabetic recipients. Diabetes 1990;39:534.
19. Diem P, Redmon JB, Abid M, et al. Glucagon, catecholamine and pancreatic polypeptide secretion in type I diabetic recipients of pancreas allografts. J Clin Invest 1990;86:2008.
20. Douzdjian V, Cooper JL, Abecassis MM, et al. Markers for pancreatic allograft rejection: comparison of serum anodal trypsinogen, serum amylase, serum creatinine and urinary amylase. Clin Transplant 1994;8:79.
21. Douzdjian V, Ferrara D, Silvestri G. Treatment strategies for insulin-dependent diabetics with ESRD: a cost-effectiveness decision analysis model. Am J Kidney Dis 1998;31:794.
22. Dubernard JM, Traeger J, Neyra P, et al. A new method of preparation of segmental pancreatic grafts for transplantation: trials in dogs and in man. Surgery 1978;84:633.
23. Emond JC, Whitington PF, Thistlethwaite JR, et al. Transplantation of two patients with one liver: analysis of a preliminary experience with 'split-liver' grafting. Ann Surg 1990;212:14.
24. Everett JE, Wahoff DC, Statz C, et al. Characterization and impact of wound infection after pancreas transplantation. Arch Surg 1994;129:1310.
25. Fioretto P, Mauer SM, Bilous RW, et al. Effects of pancreas transplantation on glomerular structure in insulin-dependent diabetic patients with their own kidneys. Lancet 1993;342:1193.
26. Fioretto P, Steffes MW, Mihatsch MJ, et al. Cyclosporine associated lesions in native kidneys of diabetic pancreas transplant recipients. Kidney Int 1995;48:489.
27. Fioretto P, Steffes MW, Sutherland DE, et al. Reversal of lesions of diabetic nephropathy after pancreas transplantation. N Engl J Med 1998;339:69.
28. Fioretto P, Sutherland DE, Najafian B, et al. Remodeling of renal interstitial and tubular lesions in pancreas transplant recipients. Kidney Int 2006;69:907.
29. Fishman JA, Rubin RH. Infection in organ-transplant recipients. N Engl J Med 1998;338:1741.
30. Gliedman ML, Gold M, Whittaker J, et al. Clinical segmental pancreatic transplantation with ureter-pancreatic duct anastomosis for exocrine drainage. Surgery 1973;74:171.
31. Gross CR, Kangas JR, Lemieux AM, et al. One-year change in quality-of-life profiles in patients receiving pancreas and kidney transplants. Transplant Proc 1995;27:3067.
32. Gross CR, Limwattananon C, Matthees BJ. Quality of life after pancreas transplantation: a review. Clin Transplant 1998;12:351.
33. Gross CR, Zehrer CL. Health-related quality of life outcomes of pancreas transplant recipients. Clin Transplant 1992;6:165.
34. Gross CR, Zehrer CL. Impact of the addition of a pancreas to quality of life in uremic diabetic recipients of kidney transplants. Transplant Proc 1993;25:1293.
35. Gruessner AC, Sutherland DER. Pancreas transplant outcomes for United States (US) and non-US cases as reported to the United Network for Organ Sharing (UNOS) and the International Pancreas Transplant Registry (IPTR) as of October 2002. In: Cecka JM, Terasaki PI, editors. Clinical transplants 2002. Los Angeles: UCLA Immunogenetics Center; 2003. p. 41–77.
36. Gruessner AC, Sutherland DER. Pancreas transplant outcomes for United States (US) and non-US cases as reported to the United Network for Organ Sharing (UNOS) and the International Pancreas Transplant Registry (IPTR) as of May 2003. In: Cecka JM, Terasaki PI, editors. Clinical transplants 2003. Los Angeles: UCLA Immunogenetics Center; 2004. p. 21–51.
37. Gruessner AC, Sutherland DE. Pancreas transplant outcomes for United States (US) and non-US cases as reported to the United Network for Organ Sharing (UNOS) and the International Pancreas Transplant Registry (IPTR) as of June 2004. Clin Transplant 2005;19:433.
38. Gruessner RW, Kandaswamy R, Humar A, et al. Calcineurin inhibitor- and steroid-free immunosuppression in pancreas-kidney and solitary pancreas transplantation. Transplantation 2005;79:1184.
39. Gruessner RW, Kendall DM, Drangstveit MB, et al. Simultaneous pancreas-kidney transplantation from live donors. Ann Surg 1997;226:471.
40. Gruessner RW, Manivel C, Dunn DL, et al. Pancreaticoduodenal transplantation with enteric drainage following native total pancreatectomy for chronic pancreatitis: a case report. Pancreas 1991;6:479.
41. Gruessner RW, Sutherland DE. Simultaneous kidney and segmental pancreas transplants from living related donors – the first two successful cases. Transplantation 1996;61:1265.
42. Gruessner RW, Sutherland DE, Drangstveit MB, et al. Pancreas transplants from living donors: short- and long-term outcome. Transplant Proc 2001;33:819.
43. Gruessner RW, Sutherland DE, Dunn DL, et al. Transplant options for patients undergoing total pancreatectomy for chronic pancreatitis. J Am Coll Surg 2004;198:559.

44. Gruessner RW, Sutherland DE, Gruessner AC. Mortality assessment for pancreas transplants. Am J Transplant 2004;4:2018.
45. Gruessner RWG, Najarian JS, Gruessner A, et al. Comparison of rejection in clinical transplantation of pancreas alone or associated with kidney transplant. In: Touraine JL, Traeger J, Betuel H, et al., editors. Transplantation and clinical immunology: multiple transplants. Amsterdam: Excerpta Medica; 1991. p. 47–54.
46. Hering BJ, Kandaswamy R, Harmon JV, et al. Transplantation of cultured islets from two-layer preserved pancreases in type 1 diabetes with anti-CD3 antibody. Am J Transplant 2004;4:390.
47. Hesse UJ, Sutherland DE. Influence of serum amylase and plasma glucose levels in pancreas cadaver donors on graft function in recipients. Diabetes 1989;38(Suppl. 1):1.
48. Jones JW, Nakhleh RE, Casanova D, et al. Cystoscopic transduodenal pancreas transplant biopsy: a new needle. Transplant Proc 1994;26:527.
49. Kandaswamy R, Ramcharan T, Matas A, et al. Kidney and kidney-pancreas transplants in Jehovah's Witnesses – a single-center experience with 50 transplants. Acta Chir Aust 2001;33(Suppl. 174):3.
50. Katz H, Homan M, Velosa J, et al. Effects of pancreas transplantation on postprandial glucose metabolism. N Engl J Med 1991;325:1278.
51. Kaufman DB, Leventhal JR, Koffron AJ, et al. A prospective study of rapid corticosteroid elimination in simultaneous pancreas-kidney transplantation: comparison of two maintenance immunosuppression protocols: tacrolimus/mycophenolate mofetil versus tacrolimus/sirolimus. Transplantation 2002;73:169.
52. Kaufman DB, Parker M, Leventhal J, et al. Multivariate analysis of the impact of CMV in simultaneous pancreas-kidney transplantation in the mycophenolate mofetil/tacrolimus era. Transplantation 2000;69(Suppl.):S271.
53. Kelly WD, Lillehei RC, Merkel FK, et al. Allotransplantation of the pancreas and duodenum along with the kidney in diabetic nephropathy. Surgery 1967;61:827.
54. Kendall DM, Rooney DP, Smets YF, et al. Pancreas transplantation restores epinephrine response and symptom recognition during hypoglycemia in patients with long-standing type I diabetes and autonomic neuropathy. Diabetes 1997;46:249.
55. Kendall DM, Sutherland DE, Najarian JS, et al. Effects of hemipancreatectomy on insulin secretion and glucose tolerance in healthy humans. N Engl J Med 1990;322:898.
56. Kendall DM, Teuscher AU, Robertson RP. Defective glucagon secretion during sustained hypoglycemia following successful islet allo- and autotransplantation in humans. Diabetes 1997;46:23.
57. Kennedy WR, Navarro X, Goetz FC, et al. Effects of pancreatic transplantation on diabetic neuropathy. N Engl J Med 1990;322:1031.
58. Kennedy WR, Navarro X, Sutherland DE. Neuropathy profile of diabetic patients in a pancreas transplantation program. Neurology 1995;45:773.
59. Kuo PC, Stock PG. Transplantation in the HIV+ patient. Am J Transplant 2001;1:13.
60. Lane JT, Ratanasuwan T, Mack-Shipman R, et al. Cyclosporine challenge test revisited: does it predict outcome after solitary pancreas transplantation? Clin Transplant 2001;15:28.
61. Lillehei RC, Ruix JO, Aquino C, et al. Transplantation of the pancreas. Acta Endocrinol Suppl 1976;205:303.
62. Lillehei RC, Simmons RL, Najarian JS, et al. Pancreatico-duodenal allotransplantation: experimental and clinical experience. Ann Surg 1970;172:405.
63. Lowance D, Neumayer HH, Legendre CM, et al. Valacyclovir for the prevention of cytomegalovirus disease after renal transplantation. International Valacyclovir Cytomegalovirus Prophylaxis Transplantation Study Group. N Engl J Med 1999;340:1462.
64. Manske CL, Wang Y, Rector T, et al. Coronary revascularisation in insulin-dependent diabetic patients with chronic renal failure. Lancet 1992;340:998.
65. Margreiter R, Klima G, Bosmuller C, et al. Rejection of kidney and pancreas after pancreas-kidney transplantation. Diabetes 1989;38(Suppl. 1):79.
66. Marsh CL, Perkins JD, Sutherland DE, et al. Combined hepatic and pancreaticoduodenal procurement for transplantation. Surg Gynecol Obstet 1989;168:254.
67. Matsumoto S, Kandaswamy R, Sutherland DE, et al. Clinical application of the two-layer (University of Wisconsin solution/ perfluorochemical plus O2) method of pancreas preservation before transplantation. Transplantation 2000;70:771.
68. Mauer M, Gruessner A. Pediatric pancreas transplantation in the USA 1988–2000. Pediatr Transplant 2000;4(Suppl. 2):157.
69. Mauer SM, Barbosa J, Vernier RL, et al. Development of diabetic vascular lesions in normal kidneys transplanted into patients with diabetes mellitus. N Engl J Med 1976;295:916.
70. Mauer SM, Goetz FC, McHugh LE, et al. Long-term study of normal kidneys transplanted into patients with type I diabetes. Diabetes 1989;38:516.
71. Mauer SM, Steffes MW, Connett J, et al. The development of lesions in the glomerular basement membrane and mesangium after transplantation of normal kidneys to diabetic patients. Diabetes 1983;32:948.
72. Morel P, Brayman KL, Goetz FC, et al. Long-term metabolic function of pancreas transplants and influence of rejection episodes. Transplantation 1991;51:990.
73. Morel P, Chau C, Brayman K, et al. Quality of metabolic control at 2 to 12 years after a pancreas transplant. Transplant Proc 1992;24:835.
74. Morel P, Goetz FC, Moudry-Munns K, et al. Long-term glucose control in patients with pancreatic transplants. Ann Intern Med 1991;115:694.
75. Morel P, Goetz F, Moudry-Munns K, et al. Serial glycosylated hemoglobin levels in diabetic recipients of pancreatic transplants. Transplant Proc 1990;22:649.
76. Morel P, Moudry-Munns K, Najarian JS, et al. Influence of preservation time on outcome and metabolic function of bladder-drained pancreas transplants. Transplantation 1990;49:294.
77. Morel P, Sutherland DE, Almond PS, et al. Assessment of renal function in type I diabetic patients after kidney, pancreas, or combined kidney-pancreas transplantation. Transplantation 1991;51:1184.
78. Najarian JS, Kaufman DB, Fryd DS, et al. Long-term survival following kidney transplantation in 100 type I diabetic patients. Transplantation 1989;47:106.
79. Nathan DM. Long-term complications of diabetes mellitus. N Engl J Med 1993;328:1676.
80. Navarro X, Kennedy WR, Aeppli D, et al. Neuropathy and mortality in diabetes: influence of pancreas transplantation. Muscle Nerve 1996;19:1009.
81. Navarro X, Kennedy WR, Loewenson RB, et al. Influence of pancreas transplantation on cardiorespiratory reflexes, nerve conduction, and mortality in diabetes mellitus. Diabetes 1990;39:802.
82. Navarro X, Sutherland DE, Kennedy WR. Long-term effects of pancreatic transplantation on diabetic neuropathy. Ann Neurol 1997;42:727.
83. Nghiem DD, Corry RJ. Technique of simultaneous renal pancreatoduodenal transplantation with urinary drainage of pancreatic secretion. Am J Surg 1987;153:405.
84. Papalois BE, Troppmann C, Gruessner AC, et al. Long-term peritoneal dialysis before transplantation and intra-abdominal infection after simultaneous pancreas-kidney transplantations. Arch Surg 1996;131:761.
85. Paty BW, Lanz K, Kendall DM, et al. Restored hypoglycemic counterregulation is stable in successful pancreas transplant recipients for up to 19 years after transplantation. Transplantation 2001;72:1103.
86. Perkal M, Marks C, Lorber MI, et al. A three-year experience with serum anodal trypsinogen as a biochemical marker for rejection in pancreatic allografts: false positives, tissue biopsy, comparison with other markers, and diagnostic strategies. Transplantation 1992;53:415.
87. Philosophe B, Farney AC, Schweitzer EJ, et al. Superiority of portal venous drainage over systemic venous drainage in pancreas transplantation: a retrospective study. Ann Surg 2001;234:689.
88. Pirsch JD, Odorico JS, D'Alessandro AM, et al. Posttransplant infection in enteric versus bladder-drained simultaneous pancreas-kidney transplant recipients. Transplantation 1998;66:1746.
89. Powell CS, Lindsey NJ, Nolan MS, et al. Urinary amylase as a marker of rejection in duct to ureter drained pancreas grafts. Transplant Proc 1987;19:1023.
90. Prieto M, Sutherland DE, Fernandez-Cruz L, et al. Experimental and clinical experience with urine amylase monitoring for early diagnosis of rejection in pancreas transplantation. Transplantation 1987;43:73.
91. Prieto M, Sutherland DE, Fernandez-Cruz L, et al. Urinary amylase monitoring for early diagnosis of pancreas allograft rejection in dogs. J Surg Res 1986;40:597.

92. Ramsay RC, Goetz FC, Sutherland DE, et al. Progression of diabetic retinopathy after pancreas transplantation for insulin-dependent diabetes mellitus. N Engl J Med 1988;318:208.
93. Rayhill SC, Kirk AD, Odorico JS, et al. Simultaneous pancreas-kidney transplantation at the University of Wisconsin. In: Cecka JM, Terasaki PI, editors. Clinical transplants 1995. Los Angeles: UCLA Tissue Typing Laboratory; 1996. p. 261–9.
94. Robertson RP. Seminars in medicine of the Beth Israel Hospital, Boston: pancreatic and islet transplantation for diabetes – cures or curiosities? N Engl J Med 1992;327:1861.
95. Robertson RP, Lanz KJ, Sutherland DE, et al. Relationship between diabetes and obesity 9 to 18 years after hemipancreatectomy and transplantation in donors and recipients. Transplantation 2002;73:736.
96. Robertson RP, Sutherland DE, Kendall DM, et al. Metabolic characterization of long-term successful pancreas transplants in type I diabetes. J Invest Med 1996;44:549.
97. Robertson RP, Sutherland DE, Lanz KJ. Normoglycemia and preserved insulin secretory reserve in diabetic patients 10–18 years after pancreas transplantation. Diabetes 1999;48:1737.
98. Robertson RP, Sutherland DE, Seaquist ER, et al. Glucagon, catecholamine, and symptom responses to hypoglycemia in living donors of pancreas segments. Diabetes 2003;52:1689.
99. Rosenlof LK, Earnhardt RC, Pruett TL, et al. Pancreas transplantation: an initial experience with systemic and portal drainage of pancreatic allografts. Ann Surg 1992;215:586.
100. Schnitzler MA, Whiting JF, Brennan DC, et al. The life-years saved by a deceased organ donor. Am J Transplant 2005;5:2289.
101. Seaquist ER, Kahn SE, Clark PM, et al. Hyperproinsulinemia is associated with increased beta cell demand after hemipancreatectomy in humans. J Clin Invest 1996;97:455.
102. Seaquist ER, Robertson RP. Effects of hemipancreatectomy on pancreatic alpha and beta cell function in healthy human donors. J Clin Invest 1992;89:1761.
103. Shapiro R, Jordan ML, Scantlebury VP, et al. Renal allograft rejection with normal renal function in simultaneous kidney/pancreas recipients: does dissynchronous rejection really exist? Transplantation 2000;69:440.
104. Solders G, Tyden G, Persson A, et al. Improvement of nerve conduction in diabetic neuropathy: a follow-up study 4yr after combined pancreatic and renal transplantation. Diabetes 1992;41:946.
105. Sollinger HW. Mycophenolate mofetil for the prevention of acute rejection in primary cadaveric renal allograft recipients. U.S. Renal Transplant Mycophenolate Mofetil Study Group. Transplantation 1995;60:225–32.
106. Sollinger HW, Cook K, Kamps D, et al. Clinical and experimental experience with pancreaticocystostomy for exocrine pancreatic drainage in pancreas transplantation. Transplant Proc 1984;16:749.
107. Sollinger HW, Messing EM, Eckhoff DE, et al. Urological complications in 210 consecutive simultaneous pancreas-kidney transplants with bladder drainage. Ann Surg 1993;218:561.
108. Sollinger HW, Sasaki TM, D'Alessandro AM, et al. Indications for enteric conversion after pancreas transplantation with bladder drainage. Surgery 1992;112:842.
109. Starzl TE, Iwatsuki S, Shaw Jr BW, et al. Pancreaticoduodenal transplantation in humans. Surg Gynecol Obstet 1984;159:265.
110. Starzl TE, Todo S, Fung J, et al. FK 506 for liver, kidney, and pancreas transplantation. Lancet 1989;2:1000.
111. Stempel CA, Lake J, Kuo G, et al. Hepatitis C – its prevalence in end-stage renal failure patients and clinical course after kidney transplantation. Transplantation 1993;55:273.
112. Stern RC, Mayes JT, Weber Jr FL, et al. Restoration of exocrine pancreatic function following pancreas-liver-kidney transplantation in a cystic fibrosis patient. Clin Transplant 1994;8:1.
113. Stock PG, Bluestone JA. Beta-cell replacement for type I diabetes. Annu Rev Med 2004;55:133.
114. Stratta RJ. The economics of pancreas transplantation. Graft 2000;3:19.
115. Stratta RJ, Cushing KA, Frisbie K, et al. Analysis of hospital charges after simultaneous pancreas-kidney transplantation in the era of managed care. Transplantation 1997;64:287.
116. Stratta RJ, Shokouh-Amiri MH, Egidi MF, et al. A prospective comparison of simultaneous kidney-pancreas transplantation with systemic-enteric versus portal-enteric drainage. Ann Surg 2001;233:740.
117. Stratta RJ, Sollinger HW, Groshek M, et al. Differential diagnosis of hyperamylasemia in pancreas allograft recipients. Transplant Proc 1990;22:675.
118. Sutherland DER. Effect of pancreas transplantation on secondary complications of diabetes. In: Dubernard JM, Sutherland DER, editors. International handbook of pancreas transplantation. Boston: Kluwer Academic Publishers; 1989. p. 257–89.
119. Sutherland DER. Effect of pancreas transplants on secondary complications of diabetes: review of observations at a single institution. Transplant Proc 1992;24:859.
120. Sutherland DER. International human pancreas and islet transplant registry. Transplant Proc 1980;12(Suppl. 2):229.
121. Sutherland DER. Pancreas and islet transplant population. In: Gruessner RWG, Sutherland DER, editors. Transplantation of the pancreas. New York: Springer-Verlag; 2004. p. 91–102.
122. Sutherland DER, Goetz FC, Moudry KC, et al. Use of recipient mesenteric vessels for revascularization of segmental pancreas grafts: technical and metabolic considerations. Transplant Proc 1987;19:2300.
123. Sutherland DER, Goetz FC, Najarian JS. Pancreas transplants from related donors. Transplantation 1984;38:625.
124. Sutherland DER, Gores PF, Farney AC, et al. Evolution of kidney, pancreas, and islet transplantation for patients with diabetes at the University of Minnesota. Am J Surg 1993;166:456.
125. Sutherland DER, Gruessner RWG. History of pancreas transplantation. In: Gruessner RWG, Sutherland DER, editors. Transplantation of the Pancreas. New York: Springer-Verlag; 2004. p. 39–68.
126. Sutherland DER, Gruessner RWG, Dunn DL, et al. Lessons learned from more than 1000 pancreas transplants at a single institution. Ann Surg 2001;233:463.
127. Sutherland DER, Morel P, Gruessner RW. Transplantation of two diabetic patients with one divided cadaver donor pancreas. Transplant Proc 1990;22:585.
128. Sutherland DER, Najarian JS, Greenberg BZ, et al. Hormonal and metabolic effects of a pancreatic endocrine graft: vascularized segmental transplantation in insulin-dependent diabetic patients. Ann Intern Med 1981;95:537.
129. Tesi RJ, Henry ML, Elkhammas EA, et al. The frequency of rejection episodes after combined kidney-pancreas transplant – the impact on graft survival. Transplantation 1994;58:424.
130. Teuscher AU, Seaquist ER, Robertson RP. Diminished insulin secretory reserve in diabetic pancreas transplant and nondiabetic kidney transplant recipients. Diabetes 1994;43:593.
131. Troppmann C, Gruessner RW, Matas AJ, et al. Results with renal transplants performed after previous solitary pancreas transplants. Transplant Proc 1994;26:448.
132. Tyden G, Bolinder J, Solders G, et al. Improved survival in patients with insulin-dependent diabetes mellitus and end-stage diabetic nephropathy 10 years after combined pancreas and kidney transplantation. Transplantation 1999;67:645.
133. van der Vliet JA, Navarro X, Kennedy WR, et al. The effect of pancreas transplantation on diabetic polyneuropathy. Transplantation 1988;45:368.
134. Venstrom JM, McBride MA, Rother KI, et al. Survival after pancreas transplantation in patients with diabetes and preserved kidney function. JAMA 2003;290:2817.
135. Wilczek HE, Jaremko G, Tyden G, et al. Pancreatic graft protects a simultaneously transplanted kidney from developing diabetic nephropathy: a 1- to 6-year follow-up study. Transplant Proc 1993;25:1314.
136. Zehrer CL, Gross CR. Prevalence of "low blood glucose" symptoms and quality of life in pancreas transplant recipients. Clin Transplant 1993;7:312.
137. Zehrer CL, Gross CR. Quality of life of pancreas transplant recipients. Diabetologia 1991;34(Suppl. 1):S145.

CHAPTER 37

RENAL TRANSPLANTATION IN CHILDREN

Pamela Winterberg • Barry Warshaw

CHAPTER OUTLINE

INTRODUCTION

Kidney transplantation is the preferred treatment for end-stage renal disease (ESRD) in children and confers improved survival,[194] skeletal growth,[229] heath-related quality of life,[262] and neuropsychological development[216] compared to dialysis.

The medical and surgical care of ESRD and kidney transplantation in children poses unique challenges.[12] Growth and neurocognitive development are impaired during CKD and are a unique focus of pediatric nephrology care. The diagnosis of ESRD in children creates an extra burden for caretakers and siblings. Therefore, treatment of ESRD and kidney transplant in the pediatric population focuses on family-centered care and often utilizes a multidisciplinary approach. Psychological development is also addressed as children acquire the skills and attitudes needed to live an independent life as an adult.

Children who receive kidney transplants have longer expected remaining lifetimes than adults at the time of kidney transplant.[315] Therefore, it is particularly important to maximize graft function and survival in this population. Children are also undergoing immune system development and maturation at the time of transplant. This, coupled with longer survival time, underscores the importance of optimizing exposure to long-term immunosuppression.

The number of children receiving kidney transplants every year is small, and even the largest centers in the United States rarely transplant more than 30 children per year. Therefore, it has been extremely important to maintain national and international databases to identify areas for research and improvement in outcomes among pediatric kidney transplant recipients.

There are two databases for pediatric kidney transplantation in wide use in North America. The United Network for Organ Sharing (UNOS) collects information for every kidney transplant in the United States within the Organ Procurement and Transplantation Network (OPTN). Wait list, demographic, and survival statistics from this database are reported annually through the Scientific Registry of Transplant Recipients (SRTR) report. Although this registry also contains pediatric recipients, there are several pediatric-specific variables (growth, for example) that are not reported in this registry. In 1987, the North American Pediatric Renal Trials and Collaborative Studies (NAPRTCS) began a voluntary registry that included up to 159 medical centers in the United States, Canada, and Mexico. By 2010, the registry contained information for 11 603 kidney transplants in 10 632 children.[232]

Other databases around the world have also been used to study risk factors and trends in pediatric kidney transplantation. The Canadian Pediatric End-Stage Renal Disease database has been constructed by linking registry data with administrative data from their universal healthcare delivery system to study outcomes for children with ESRD in Canada.[272] The European Renal Association-European Dialysis and Transplant Association (ERA-EDTA) registry collects data from national and regional registries from 30 European and Mediterranean countries with individual patient data from 26 national and regional registries and aggregate data from 19 national registries.[317] The Australia and New Zealand Dialysis and Transplant Registry (ANZDATA) collects data on all dialysis and transplant patients, including children, in Australia and New Zealand.[195] In 2004, the Latin American Pediatric Nephrology Association (ALANEPE) began collecting prospective data on children receiving kidney transplants at 31 centers in 14 Latin American countries in the first Latin American Registry of Pediatric Renal Transplantation.[173]

Most figures and statistical references in this chapter are from the SRTR and NAPRTCS databases, but we also cite literature from studies of other registries around the world.

EPIDEMIOLOGY OF END-STAGE RENAL DISEASE IN CHILDREN

Incidence

The incidence and prevalence of ESRD have been increasing health concerns worldwide[335] over the past two decades, but especially in the developed countries. The United States had 113 000 new cases of ESRD in 2009 (adjusted incidence rate: 355 new cases per million population) with a prevalence of over 570 000 ESRD patients, including those with a functioning graft (prevalence rate: 1738 ESRD cases per million population).[315] The incidence and prevalence of ESRD in children represent a very small fraction, less than 2%, of the overall ESRD population in the United States (Table 37-1). Unlike the adult ESRD population, the incidence rate of ESRD in children has been relatively stable, with about 10–15% increase since 1990 (14 per million in 1990, 15.5 per million in 2009) compared to a 150% increase in the incidence in adults over the same time period (overall incidence rate of 220/million in 1990 versus 355/million in 2009).

Although chronic kidney disease (CKD) has become a global health issue,[335] estimates of worldwide incidence and prevalence have been limited by lack of national registries and surveys in most of the world, varying definitions of ESRD, and differences in timing of referral to subspecialists. The median incidence of ESRD in children worldwide has been estimated at 9 cases per million age population.[128]

TABLE 37-1 Unadjusted Incidence Rates of End-Stage Renal Disease in Children by Age Groups

Age Group (Years)	Incident Rate (Per Million Population)
0–4	14.6
5–9	7.0
10–14	13.4
15–19	27.1
Overall (0–19)	15.7

Data (incidence in 2010) from National Institutes of Health, National Institute of Diabetes and Digestive Kidney Diseases. 2011. *USRDS 2011 Annual Data Report: Atlas of Chronic Kidney Disease and End-Stage Renal Disease in the United States.* Bethesda, MD: National Institutes of Health, National Institute of Diabetes and Digestive and Kidney Diseases.

Etiology

Diabetic nephropathy and hypertensive nephropathy are the most common causes of ESRD in adults, but are rare in childhood. Rather, the most common causes of ESRD in children are congenital, cystic, and hereditary disease, which account for 35% of incident cases.[315] Glomerulonephritis is the second most common etiology, accounting for 23% of new cases, predominantly due to focal segmental glomerulosclerosis (FSGS). Secondary glomerulonephritis and vasculitis account for 11% of new cases, of which lupus nephritis is most common (Table 37-2). The underlying etiology of ESRD also varies by age of presentation. The congenital and structural diseases are more common in the young age groups, while glomerulonephritis is the leading cause in adolescents[231] (Figure 37-1).

Overall, the male-to-female ratio for incident ESRD is 1.2 (57% of new cases are male), but is highest in the youngest patients, who predominantly suffer from congenital disorders (roughly 3:1 male-to-female ratio), some of which only occur in males (i.e., obstruction due to posterior urethral valves). In contrast, secondary glomerulonephritis, especially lupus nephritis, is more common in females (1:4 male-to-female ratio).[315] Finally, the majority of patients with hereditary and structural etiologies are Caucasian, while FSGS and secondary glomerulonephritis affect more patients of African American decent.

The industrialized nations (North America, Europe, Japan, Australia, New Zealand) have a similar distribution of etiologies as US Renal Data System (USRDS) data presented above, except for a lower proportion of cases due to glomerulonephritis in European registries, likely due to differences in racial distribution.[208]

TABLE 37-2 Common Etiologies of End-Stage Renal Disease (ESRD) in Children: Percentage of Incident Cases

Cystic/Hereditary/Congenital Diseases	**34.8%**
Renal hypoplasia, dysplasia, oligonephronia	11.8
Polycystic, autosomal recessive	2.2
Hereditary nephritis, Alport's syndrome	2.2
Ureteropelvic junction/ureterovesical junction obstruction	1.6
Other congenital obstructive uropathy	7.4
Prune-belly syndrome	1.4
Glomerulonephritis (GN)	**23.1%**
Focal glomerular sclerosis	12.3
Not histologically examined	4.2
Secondary GN/Vasculitis	**11.3%**
Lupus erythematosus (systemic lupus erythematosus nephritis)	6.1
Hemolytic-uremic syndrome	2.2
Interstitial Nephritis/Pyelonephritis	**5.7%**
Chronic pyelonephritis/reflux nephropathy	3.1
Hypertensive/Large-Vessel Disease	**4.9%**
Neoplasms/Tumors	**2.2%**
Tubular Necrosis (without Recovery)	**2.1%**

Data (*n*=6633 incident ESRD patients 2005–2009) from National Institutes of Health, National Institute of Diabetes and Digestive Kidney Diseases. 2011. *USRDS 2011 Annual Data Report: Atlas of Chronic Kidney Disease and End-Stage Renal Disease in the United States.* Bethesda, MD: National Institutes of Health, National Institute of Diabetes and Digestive and Kidney Diseases.

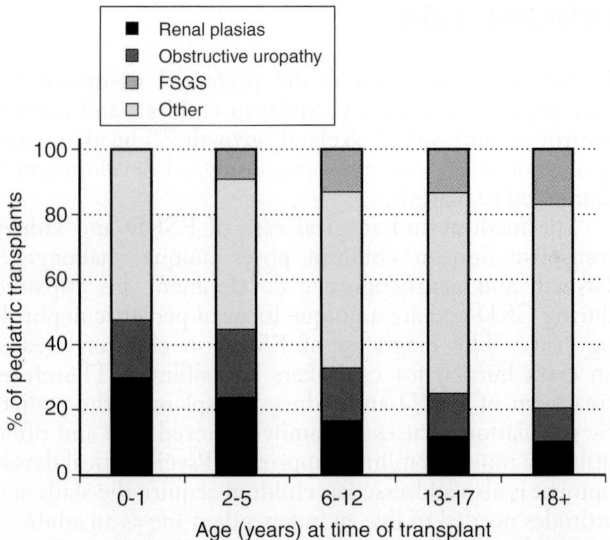

FIGURE 37-1 ■ Etiology of end-stage renal disease by age at the time of transplant. FSGS, focal segmental glomerulosclerosis. (Data from North American Pediatric Renal Trials and Collaborative Studies. 2008. *NAPRTCS 2008 Annual Report: Renal Transplantation, Dialysis, and Chronic Renal Insufficiency.* Available online at: https://web.emmes.com/study/ped/annlrept/annlrept.html (accessed 9/24/2012).)

In the developing world, single-center studies and survey reports suggest some differences. Overall, congenital anomalies of the kidney and urinary tract are still the most prevalent, similar to industrialized nations. In Turkey and the Middle East, there is a higher proportion of uropathies reported rather than hypoplasia/dysplasia.[8,27,217] There are also higher rates of genetic disease in this region thought to be due to the high rate of consanguineous marriages.[215] Various reports from South America, the Caribbean, South East Asia, and India indicate chronic glomerulonephritis as a leading cause of CKD in children, thought to be due to endemic bacterial, viral, and parasitic infections that are known to cause kidney disease in those regions.[10,128,209]

ACCESS TO TRANSPLANTATION

In the United States, roughly 850 children receive kidney transplants each year, comprising only 5% of the total number of kidney transplants. Children under the age of 18 years represent 1.2% of total patients listed for kidney transplant in the United States (1144 children versus 84 614 adults listed as of the end of 2009). Of the pediatric patients on the waiting list in 2009, 72% were over the age of 11 years.[245] Data from the SRTR indicate that the total number of kidney transplants in children in the United States increased by 30% between the years of 2000 and 2009 (Figure 37-2).

The transplant community has consistently supported timely access of deceased donor kidneys to pediatric recipients. As a result, children have the highest rates of kidney transplantation for all age groups (51.6 per 100 person-years on wait list for deceased donor compared to 12.0 per 100 person-years for adults). In 2009, 29% of ESRD patients under age 19 years were transplanted within 1 year of being declared end-stage,[315] and over 80% of children waitlisted had received a kidney transplant by 5 years after ESRD declaration.[225]

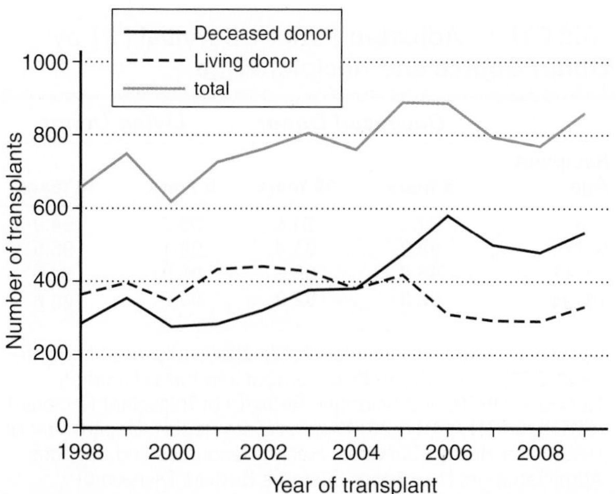

FIGURE 37-2 ■ Trends in living donor kidney transplant for pediatric recipients. (Data from Organ Procurement and Transplantation Network (OPTN) and Scientific Registry of Transplant Recipients (SRTR). OPTN / SRTR 2010 Annual Data Report. Department of Health and Human Services, Health Resources and Services Administration, Healthcare Systems Bureau, Division of Transplantation, 2011. Available online at: http://srtr.transplant.hrsa.gov/annual_reports/2010 (accessed 9/24/2012).)

Historically, living related donor transplants were more common in children than deceased donor transplants.[245] This was likely driven by parents' understanding of the benefit of living donation for their child. However, the rate of living donor transplants in children has been declining since 2002 (Figure 37-2). Children under the age of 5 years are slightly more likely to receive a living donor transplant (51% of transplants in this age group during 2007–2009 were from living donors), while children over 11 years old are more likely to receive a kidney from a deceased donor (65% of transplants in this age group were from deceased donors during 2007–2009).[245] Of the 5846 living donor transplants in the NAPRTCS database, 79% are from parents (the majority from mothers).[232]

In 2005, the UNOS enacted an updated policy to improve access of deceased donor kidneys from young adult donors (<35 years old) for pediatric recipients (referred to hereafter as the SHARE 35 policy). Under this policy, recipients under the age of 18 years receive priority for kidneys from donors under 35 years old, except for zero-mismatch, renal/non-renal allocation, and highly sensitized (panel-reactive antibodies or PRA >80%) adult recipients.

Median wait times for recipients under 18 years old decreased from 11.2 months in 1998 to 6.8 months in 2009, but most of the gain was realized for patients with O blood type.[2,245] The most recent SRTR report indicates that the longest wait time continues to be for children with blood type B (median 10.7 months in 2008 compared to 6.6 months for type A, 5.5 months for type AB, and 8.0 months for type O).[245]

The SHARE 35 policy also appears to have lessened some of the racial disparities seen in access to kidneys for pediatric recipients, especially for Hispanics (median wait times decreased from 370 days for Hispanics to 169 days; for blacks from 219 to 129 days, and for whites from 163 to 100 days).[11]

The absolute number and proportion of deceased donor kidney transplants in pediatric recipients increased following institution of the SHARE 35 policy from 40–50% during 1998–2005 to 61–65% during 2006–2009 and was accompanied by a decrease in the absolute number of living donor transplants.[5,245] It is unclear at this time if the trend in fewer living donor transplants is a direct consequence of the policy change or possibly due to more prevalent comorbidities in parents (obesity and diabetes in particular) that preclude them from donating, as the downward trend in living related donor transplants predates the policy (Figure 37-2).

Although the average donor age decreased from 25–26 years prior to SHARE 35 to 20–21 years after SHARE 35, pediatric recipients also received more kidneys with 5–6 mismatched human leukocyte antigen (HLA) loci.[5,245] The long-term consequences of these trends on overall graft survival in children will need future study.

Organ allocation in the United Kingdom prioritizes access to young donors for pediatric recipients but also prioritizes the degree of HLA matching for children.[152,192] Some European countries report higher rates of living donor kidney transplant in children.[317] Japan has very few kidney transplants in comparison to ESRD prevalence (1136 transplants per 264 473 prevalent ESRD patients in 2007), with 83% of them from living donors. Access to deceased donor kidney transplantation is very limited in Japan (82 deceased donor kidney transplants performed between 1997 and 2008) due to cultural and legal barriers.[312]

Access to transplantation for pediatric recipients in the developing world is limited by healthcare access. Donor sources vary greatly depending on the availability of an organ allocation program within the country; therefore, the majority of transplants in the developing world are from living donors. The age range of recipients varies by country, with most performing transplants in children over 7 years of age. In general, the countries that perform transplants in children under 7 years of age also have access to deceased donor sources, suggesting a more developed healthcare delivery system, with access to the specialized surgical and supportive care required by smaller recipients.[264]

TIMING OF TRANSPLANTATION

Transplantation is initially considered when renal replacement therapy is imminent. Due to increased risk of graft loss and mortality in infants and children under 2 years of age, most pediatric centers perform transplants in children once they achieve a weight above 10–15 kg. Reports from a few centers have described successful transplant outcomes in children under 15 kg.[131,204,274] Infants and young children with ESRD frequently have delayed growth, so often a child will be greater than 2 years old before achieving the threshold size and weight for the transplant center.

From 2007–2009, nearly 30% of kidney transplants in children were performed prior to initiation of dialysis (i.e., pre-emptively). Half of these were from deceased donors. An additional 28% of pediatric kidney transplant recipients were on dialysis for less than 1 year at the time of transplant.[245]

There is conflicting evidence for a benefit of pre-emptive transplant for patient and graft survival in pediatric transplant recipients.[159,273,291,321] Time on dialysis prior to transplant continues to be a risk factor for decreased graft survival,[43,199] although some recent analyses suggest short times on dialysis (less than 2 years) in children may not have as big an effect.[168,273] Increasing time with ESRD during childhood is also associated with impaired growth and development and can result in disruption of education. Accordingly, pre-emptive transplant may have quality-of-life benefits to children beyond graft survival.[127]

PATIENT AND GRAFT SURVIVAL

Patient survival for pediatric kidney transplant is excellent, with overall 3-year survival of 98% reported in NAPRTCS (era 1996–2010). When broken down by age of recipient, the youngest (under 2 years old) have historically had the highest mortality following transplant. Three-year survival for this group has improved in the more recent era from 90% for living related donor transplanted 1987–1995 to 96% transplanted 1996–2007, and from 79% to 93% for deceased donor transplants in the same time periods.[232] Survival for all pediatric ages at 5 years are equal or superior to adults, and at 10 years even exceeds that seen for young adults aged 18–34 years[245] (Table 37-3). Patient survival has significantly improved for deceased donor transplants in children from 90% 5-year survival for transplants performed 1987–1995 (early era) to 96% for the more recent era (1996–2007) in the NAPRTCS database. Some improvement has also been seen for children receiving living donor transplants, with 5-year survival improving from 95% in the early era to 97% in the more recent era.[232]

The most common causes of death in children following transplant are infection (28.5%), cardiopulmonary disease (14.7%), cancer/malignancy (11.3%), and dialysis-related complications (3.1%). Of the deaths reported in the NAPRTCS database (n=573), 47.5% died with a functioning graft.[232]

TABLE 37-3 Adjusted Patient Survival (%) by Donor Source and Recipient Age

Recipient Age	Deceased Donor 5 Years	Deceased Donor 10 Years	Living Donor 5 Years	Living Donor 10 Years
1–5	94.1	91.4	95.7	94.8
6–11	98.2	93.4	99.1	95.5
12–17	95.0	85.3	96.9	91.5
18–34	92.9	82.2	95.8	88.6

Data (5-year cohort transplanted 2003–2008; 10-year transplanted 1998–2008) from Organ Procurement and Transplantation Network (OPTN) and Scientific Registry of Transplant Recipients (SRTR). OPTN / SRTR 2010 Annual Data Report. Department of Health and Human Services, Health Resources and Services Administration, Healthcare Systems Bureau, Division of Transplantation, 2011. Available online at: http://srtr.transplant.hrsa.gov/annual_reports/2010 (accessed 9/24/2012).

Data from the USRDS consistently show lower mortality rates for children receiving kidney transplants compared to children on dialysis.[315] The adjusted relative risk for mortality for children receiving renal replacement therapy decreases with increasing age. The highest mortality for both dialysis and transplant was in the 0–5-year-old age group, but transplant still provided extra survival benefit. Gillen et al.[110] analyzed USRDS data and found that children who had received a kidney transplant had a lower mortality rate (13.1 deaths/1000 patient years) than children remaining on the wait list (17.6 deaths/1000 patient years). Unlike similar studies in adults,[336] there was no significant excess mortality within the first 6 months posttransplant.

Historically, graft survival rates in children were inferior to adults. However, in the past 15 years, graft survival in children of all ages now rivals the rates seen in adults. Graft survival improved dramatically for children during the 1980s and 1990s, but little progress has been made since 2000 (Figure 37-3). When broken down by age, the

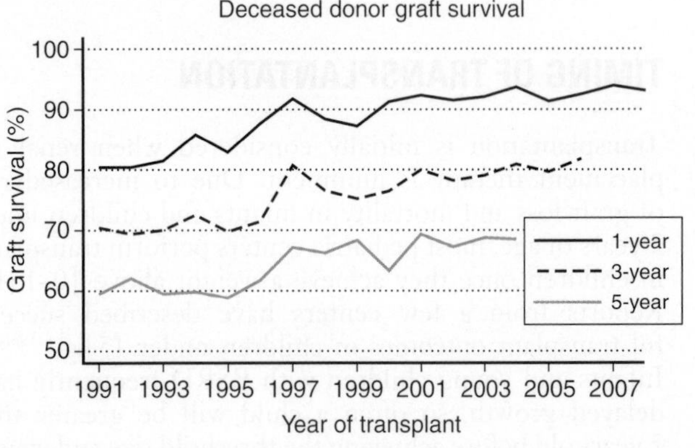

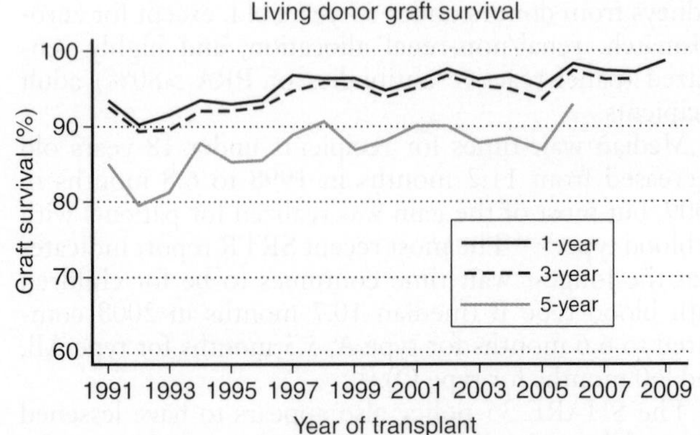

FIGURE 37-3 ■ Graft survival for deceased donor (left panel) and living donor (right panel) transplants in recipients under 19 years old. (Data from Organ Procurement and Transplantation Network (OPTN) and Scientific Registry of Transplant Recipients (SRTR). OPTN / SRTR 2010 Annual Data Report. Department of Health and Human Services, Health Resources and Services Administration, Healthcare Systems Bureau, Division of Transplantation, 2011. Available online at: http://srtr.transplant.hrsa.gov/annual_reports/2010 (accessed 9/24/2012).)

TABLE 37-4 **Adjusted Graft Survival (%) by Donor Source and Recipient Age**

	Deceased Donor			*Living Donor*		
Recipient Age	**1 Year**	**5 Years**	**10 Years**	**1 Year**	**5 Years**	**10 Years**
1–5	89.9	78.7	63.9	96.0	91.4	80.6
6–11	95.6	76.7	54.2	97.8	86.7	66.8
12–17	94.4	67.3	41.7	95.5	76.6	53.5
18–34	92.3	71.4	48.7	96.8	80.8	60.6

Data (1-year cohort was transplanted 2007–2008; 5-year cohort transplanted 2003–2008; 10-year transplanted 1998–2008) from Organ Procurement and Transplantation Network (OPTN) and Scientific Registry of Transplant Recipients (SRTR). OPTN / SRTR 2010 Annual Data Report. Department of Health and Human Services, Health Resources and Services Administration, Healthcare Systems Bureau, Division of Transplantation, 2011. Available online at: http://srtr.transplant.hrsa.gov/annual_reports/2010 (accessed 9/24/2012), tables 5.8a and 5.8d.

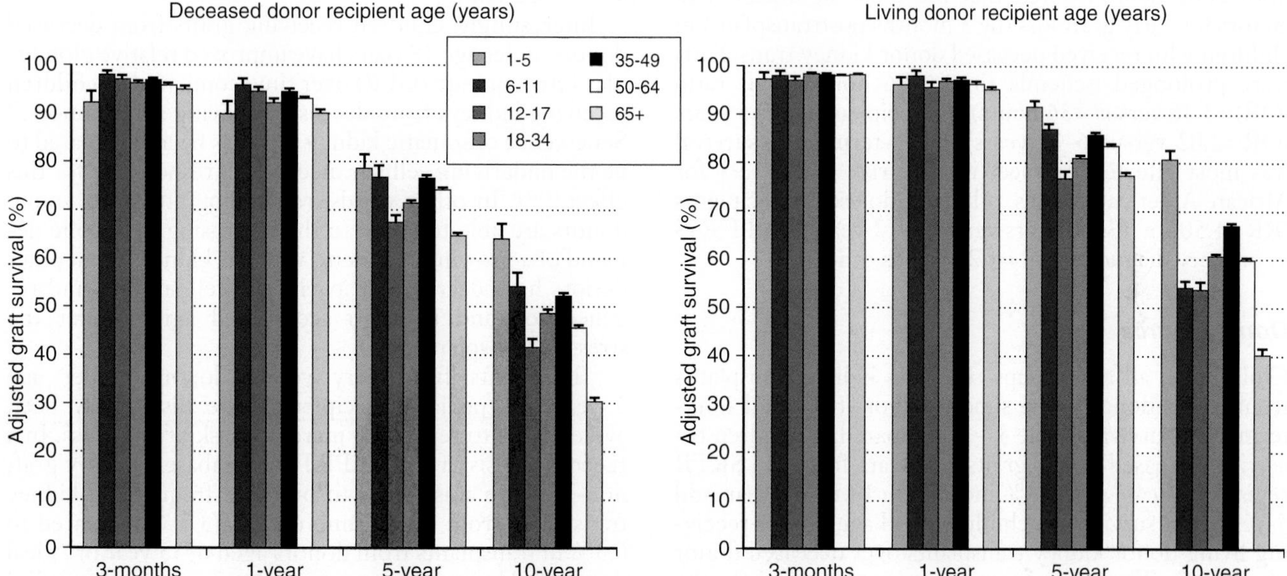

FIGURE 37-4 ■ **Adjusted graft survival for deceased donor (left panel) and living donor (right panel) kidney transplants by age of recipient.** (Data from Organ Procurement and Transplantation Network (OPTN) and Scientific Registry of Transplant Recipients (SRTR). OPTN / SRTR 2010 Annual Data Report. Department of Health and Human Services, Health Resources and Services Administration, Healthcare Systems Bureau, Division of Transplantation, 2011. Available online at: http://srtr.transplant.hrsa.gov/annual_reports/2010 (accessed 9/24/2012), tables 5.8a and 5.8d.)

youngest recipients (1–5 years old) have the worst 1-year graft survival rate for deceased donors, but the highest long-term survival for both deceased and living donor transplants of any age (Table 37-4). The adolescent age group has the worst long-term graft survival of all age groups (Figure 37-4).

Incidence and Causes of Graft Failure

Of 11 603 transplants in the NAPRTCS database, 2920 (or 25%) have failed, including 300 patients who have lost two or more grafts since the study start in 1987. Of first transplants, 25% have failed, while 35% of the 971 subsequent transplants have failed. The most common causes of graft loss are represented in Figure 37-5. Of the transplants since 2000, the most common cause of graft failure was chronic rejection (41%), followed by acute rejection (10%). While vascular thrombosis continues to be an important cause of graft failure (7%), the proportion of grafts lost to this event has decreased in the more recent era (2000–2007). Other causes of graft loss reported include

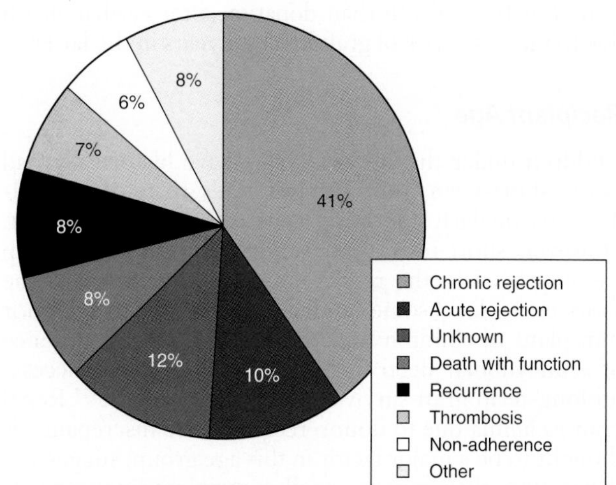

FIGURE 37-5 ■ **Causes of graft loss in pediatric renal transplant recipients 2000–2010.** (Data from North American Pediatric Renal Trials and Collaborative Studies. 2010. *NAPRTCS Annual Transplant Report.* Available online at: https://web.emmes.com/study/ped/annlrept/annlrept.html (accessed 9/24/2012).)

recurrence of primary renal disease (8%), non-adherence (6%), primary non-function (2.2%), infection (1.8%), and malignancy (1.3%). Approximately 12% of reported graft failures had unknown causes in the database, and death with a functioning graft represented 10% of graft losses.[232]

Prognostic Factors Influencing Graft Survival

The following factors have been found to be important determinants of short-term and long-term graft survival in pediatric kidney transplants. Some of these factors are more predictive of short-term survival while others have an effect on long-term graft survival. For example, an analysis of the UNOS database from 1995 until 2002 demonstrated that the most significant risk factors for early graft loss (by 3 months posttransplant) in children who received deceased donor kidney transplants were prolonged ischemia time (>36 hours; odds ratio (OR)=3.38 versus <36 hours) and recipient age 2–5 years (OR=2.02 versus 6–12 years). Long-term graft survival was most affected by race (relative risk (RR)=1.93 for African American versus others), adolescent recipients (RR=1.50 for 13–20 years versus 6–12 years), and FSGS as primary diagnosis (RR=1.27 versus others).[139]

Donor Source

Children in all age groups receiving kidney transplants from living donors have superior short-term and long-term graft survival (Table 37-4) compared to children receiving deceased donor grafts.[62,309] Data from the SRTR registry indicate a 10–20% increase in 1-year, 3-year, and 5-year graft survival for children of all age groups receiving living donor kidney transplants over deceased donor transplants. The effect is even more pronounced for the youngest recipients[322] (Figure 37-4). The improved outcomes for living donor kidney transplants are thought to be due to reduced cold ischemia time, improved HLA matching, and improved preoperative preparation of the recipient. Finally, for deceased donor kidneys, outcomes are superior for pediatric recipients of grafts from donation after brain death than donation after cardiac death due to increased risk of graft loss by 4 years in the latter.[316]

Recipient Age

Children under the age of 2 years have historically had lower short-term graft survival rates than older children, particularly following deceased donor transplant. However, short-term graft survival for this age group has improved in the recent era.[116,232] In contrast to the short-term data, some studies suggest deceased donor transplant in children under 2 years old, in the absence of acute tubular necrosis (ATN), has the most successful long-term graft survival of any age group.[156,274] Renal graft ischemia due to donor–recipient size discrepancy is thought to be a major factor in this age group, suggesting that graft perfusion in the smallest recipients may serve as a modifiable risk factor.[221]

Although children aged 2–5 years have the lowest short-term graft survival of all ages after deceased donor transplant, they have the potential for the best long-term graft survival for both deceased and living donor kidneys (Figure 37-4).[10,238]

Long-term graft survival for adolescent children is the lowest for any age group, with 76.6% 5-year and 53.5% 10-year adjusted graft survival[315] (Figure 37-4). Worse outcomes in this group are attributed to higher rates of rejection.[176]

Donor Age

Multiple reports in the literature indicate that donation from young adults improves graft survival.[130,177,236,244] The "ideal" donor age derived from these analyses has been determined to be above 6 years old and less than 45–50 years old.

Interestingly, children receiving grafts from deceased donors under age 18 years have improved relative glomerular filtration rate (GFR) over time compared to children receiving kidneys from deceased or living adult donors.[78] Senescence of somatic kidney cells has been postulated to be the underlying cellular mechanism responsible for this effect.[125,201] In other words, renal allografts from young donors are able to adapt to the increasing metabolic demand of a growing recipient, whereas kidneys from older donors have decreased capacity for cell survival and regeneration and undergo accelerated aging under the stress of transplantation.

Transplants from very young donors (under age 5 years) to pediatric recipients have historically been avoided due to reports of increased risk of graft loss. In a recent analysis of the NAPRTCS database, primary graft non-function was found to be more frequent in kidney transplants from very young donors (3.7% compared to 0.3% in transplants from donors aged 6–35 year or "ideal donors"). However, longer term, the 3-year graft survival and estimated GFR (eGFR) of functioning grafts from very young donors was equivalent to ideal donors.[217]

Recipient Race

African American children have worse long-term graft survival than all other races.[10,241] African American children are also more likely to be older at the time of transplant, receive fewer living donor transplants, and have longer duration of dialysis prior to transplant. After controlling for 19 variables, including age, primary diagnosis, pre-emptive transplant, rejection experience, HLA-B mismatch, immunosuppression, and gender, Omoloja et al.[241] report that black patients still had higher risk for graft failure (hazard ratio=1.6, 95% confidence interval (CI) 1.46–1.86).

Although FSGS, which is a suggested risk factor for decreased graft survival due to recurrent disease, is more common among African American children receiving kidney transplants, a recent analysis found equally poor allograft survival among black children with FSGS and those with other causes of renal failure (after adjusting for recipient age, donor source, HLA zero mismatch, and acute rejection).[137]

HLA Matching

Although the ideal situation would be donation from an HLA-identical sibling, this has occurred in only

3.4% of pediatric living donor transplants reported in NAPRTCS.[232] Most live kidney donations come from haplo-identical parents. An analysis of NAPRTCS in 2000 suggested that a six-antigen-matched deceased donor kidney had equivalent graft survival and rejection rates as haplo-identical living donor transplants.[304] However, long-term graft survival (5 years) was actually 10% better for the children who received sixantigen-matched deceased donor kidneys.

There is some evidence that donation from a sibling with non-inherited maternal antigens confers survival benefit[42,205] for the graft and may be due to bidirectional immune regulation[57] between donor and recipient immune cells. Grafts from mothers in these studies had poorer outcomes. This has particular relevance for pediatrics, since mothers represent the majority of parental donors.[232]

There is debate as to the impact of degree of HLA mismatch on acute rejection and graft survival.[243] In 2004, Su et al. reported a diminishing risk of rejection over time by degree of six-antigen HLA mismatch via analysis of the UNOS database for deceased donor transplants from 1995 through 1998.[296] They concluded that modern immunosuppressive therapy has decreased the contribution of HLA mismatch to graft survival. In response, an analysis of the Collaborative Transplant Study (the majority of recipients were European), published in 2007 by Opelz and Dohler, concluded that HLA mismatch continues to have a significant effect on both the need for posttransplant rejection treatment and graft survival.[243] Children comprised about 5% of the transplant recipients in both of these studies. A more recent analysis of 9029 pediatric recipients in the Collaborative Transplant Study found a hierarchical relationship for an effect of increasing mismatches at the A-, B-, and DR-loci on graft survival.[244]

Similarly, there are inconsistent findings on the role of HLA-DR matching and graft survival.[108] In 2008, Gritsch et al. reported that children in the United States receiving zero HLA-DR mismatched deceased donor kidneys had comparable 5-year graft survival to children who had received one or two DR mismatched kidneys.[121] A recent analysis of European pediatric kidney transplants[244] found that, while two HLA-DR mismatches were associated with lower graft survival in children receiving transplants from 1988 to 1997, this effect was not seen in the more recent era (1998–2007). They did, however, describe a disturbing association of HLA-DR double mismatch with increased risk of developing non-Hodgkin's lymphoma.[244] This interesting finding needs to be validated in additional cohorts of pediatric kidney transplant recipients.

Children in the United States receive fewer zero-mismatched kidneys than adults (3% of pediatric recipients versus 8% of adults) under the current allocation policy. As mentioned earlier, an increasing proportion of deceased donor transplants in children (54% from 2007 to 2009) are mismatched at more than five HLA loci.[5,245] The impact on long-term graft survival under the new policy will need to be studied to determine whether the earlier access to young donors outweighs the risk of increasingly mismatched histocompatibility.

The risk of sensitization associated with increasing HLA mismatch has also been debated.[121] As stated earlier, children have longer expected remaining lifetimes following transplantation, and increased expectancy for multiple transplants. Therefore, the risk of sensitization from mismatched primary transplants may have a negative impact on this population if it becomes a barrier to subsequent transplant. The most recent analysis of the SRTR database by Meier-Kriesche and colleagues concluded that children and African American recipients are at increased risk of becoming highly sensitized after their first kidney transplant.[200]

Presensitization

NAPRTCS reported that more than five transfusions significantly increased the frequency of delayed graft function (defined as dialysis in the first transplant week) and graft failure (relative hazard (RH)=1.22, P=0.016 for living donor transplants and RH=1.25, P<0.001 for deceased donor transplants). This effect was presumed to be due to increased sensitization. The practice of donor-specific blood transfusion has fallen out of favor in the recent era given lower rejection rates on the newer immunosuppression regimens. In the NAPRTCS database, the percentage of patients without prior transfusion increased from 17% at study start (1987) to an average of 66% from 2006 to 2009.[232] This is likely due to increased use of erythropoietin to treat anemia during ESRD and increased awareness of the risk of sensitization from repeated blood transfusions. Of the children on the US wait list in 2009, 82% had PRA <10%.

Delayed Graft Function and Technical Factors

Graft survival is significantly worse in the presence of ATN requiring early dialysis. ATN is reported in 5% of index living donor and 16% of index deceased donor transplants in the NAPRTCS registry. Among deceased donor grafts with function at 1 week posttransplant, 56% of children with ATN had a functioning graft at 5 years versus 75% of children without ATN.[232]

Native nephrectomy may be undertaken in small children at the time of transplant to control excessively high urine output or for other specific indications. Of the children receiving transplants followed in the NAPRTCS registry, 22% underwent nephrectomy. The NAPRTCS report indicates that native nephrectomy was associated with a significantly increased risk for ATN. This finding could relate to prolongation of operative time and cold ischemia time, increased third spacing of fluid, more complex postoperative fluid management, and increased risk of poor graft perfusion.

Thrombosis remains a significant cause of graft failure in children, accounting for 7% of all graft losses reported in NAPRTCS since the year 2000. Overall, technical causes of graft loss (vascular thrombosis, primary nonfunction, and others) contributed to 13% of all graft failures reported in NAPRTCS since 1987, suggesting that these events occur in about 3% of pediatric transplants.[232] Several studies of pediatric transplant registries in the United Kingdom, Ireland, and the Netherlands reported similar rates of thrombosis. Risk factors for graft thrombosis in children include recipient age <6 years, donor age <6 years, cold ischemia time >24 hours, and history of peritoneal dialysis.[160,197,223]

Induction Therapy

Early (1987–1996) retrospective analysis of the NAPRTCS database found an increased risk of rejection for patients who did not receive induction therapy (either monoclonal or polyclonal); however, the effect has been lost in the more recent era (1996–2010). When assessing factors that influence graft survival, induction therapy is now of only borderline significance in the NAPRTCS registry.[232] Moreover, a prospective controlled study found no benefit to OKT3 induction compared to cyclosporine.[30] A recent analysis of OPTN/UNOS data by Sampaio and colleagues also concluded that induction therapy was not associated with reduced rejection episodes or with improvement in the 3-year graft survival for pediatric kidney transplant recipients.[269]

Transplant Center Volume

An analysis of the NAPRTCS registry in 1999 showed that centers performing an average of 10 or more pediatric kidney transplants per year had improved graft survival at 3 months compared to centers that perform fewer than 5 per year (which comprised 63% of the centers entering data in the registry). The improvement in graft survival in the higher-volume centers was attributed to significantly lower rates of graft thrombosis and ATN. [281]

CONTRAINDICATIONS TO TRANSPLANTATION

Children with ESRD have fewer comorbid conditions that might mitigate against major surgery or use of immunosuppressive medications than adults, so that the risks of kidney transplantation are often greatly outweighed by the benefits. Therefore, most children with ESRD are eventually referred for transplant. According to the USRDS,[315] about 30% of prevalent ESRD patients aged 1–17 years in the United States are listed for transplant.

There are few absolute contraindications to kidney transplant in children. Situations that might not be appropriate for referral or listing include active or untreated malignancy, active or untreated infection, and multiple or progressive medical conditions with overall poor prognosis for recovery (e.g., severe brain injury or multiorgan failure). Transplant is considered following a reasonable disease-free period for children with prior malignancies.

Mild, isolated mental retardation is not a contraindication to transplant per se, as improvement in neurocognitive development has been seen following transplant.[202] Children with devastating neurological dysfunction may not benefit appreciably from transplant, but the potential for rehabilitation, self-care, and parental preferences should be considered. Finally, issues with medical compliance or unstable family situations can delay consideration for kidney transplant.

RECURRENCE OF ORIGINAL DISEASE

Recurrent disease is a significant cause of graft loss in children (Figure 37-5). For example, children with hemolytic-uremic syndrome (HUS), FSGS, or oxalosis had the worst overall graft half-life of 5.6 years in a single-center study of pediatric transplants between 1984 and 1997 at the University of Minnesota.[322] Recurrence in the transplanted kidney can occur with primary glomerulonephritis, secondary glomerulonephritis, and metabolic diseases.

Primary Glomerulonephritis

Focal Segmental Glomerulosclerosis

FSGS recurs in 20–60% of children with nephrotic syndrome undergoing renal transplant and is the most common cause of graft loss due to recurrence.[98,99,138,232,302] Earlier age of nephrotic syndrome diagnosis[283] (between 6 and 15 years), rapid progression to ESRD[63,302] (within 3 years of diagnosis), and mesangial proliferation on native kidney biopsy[283] have been associated with an increased risk of FSGS recurrence in children undergoing kidney transplant. Similarly to adults,[1] white and Hispanic children with FSGS in the NAPRTCS database were found to have increased risk for recurrence compared to black children.[302]

In an analysis of USRDS data, the impact of FSGS recurrence on graft loss was more significant in children than in adults.[1] Children with recurrent FSGS following living donor transplant had graft survival equivalent to children without FSGS receiving deceased donor transplant in an analysis of NAPRTCS.[25] This observation has led to reservation about offering living donor transplants, especially from first-degree relatives, to children suspected to be at high risk of FSGS recurrence. In contrast, a study of adult transplants in the USRDS registry found lower death-censored graft loss for patients with FSGS receiving living donor transplants compared to those receiving deceased donor transplants.[58] It is unclear if the findings of increased graft loss in children with FSGS receiving living donor transplants are due to the use of related donors who may be carriers for genetic mutations underlying FSGS.

Higher rates of ATN in both living donor and deceased donor transplants have been reported in children with FSGS compared to children with other causes of ESRD.[25] It has been suggested that the increased rate of ATN, possibly due to early FSGS recurrence, plays a role in the decreased graft survival for children with FSGS.[24] This observation influenced some centers to offer living donor transplant (which have lower rates of ATN in general) with pretransplant plasmapheresis to try to prevent rapid FSGS recurrence and improve graft survival; however, the use of plasmapheresis pretransplant has not proven consistently beneficial in small trials.[115,118]

Genetic forms of FSGS were historically considered to be at low risk for recurrence. Some groups have demonstrated low rates of recurrence (3%) for patients with homozygous[331] and compound heterozygous podocin (NPHS2) mutations.[154] Although Bertelli et al. found patients with NPHS2 mutations to have similar rates of recurrence (5 of 13, or 38%) as non-mutation carriers (12 of 27, or 48%),[33] the majority of this effect was seen in patients with simple heterozygous mutation (3 of 4 patients with heterozygous mutation recurred, compared to 2 of 9 patients with homozygous mutation).

Recurrence of FSGS often presents early following kidney transplantation in children, with a reported median time to recurrence of 6–14 days,[63,302] though heavy proteinuria often can be detected within hours following transplant. It is usually characterized by nephrotic-range proteinuria (protein/creatinine ratio >2 mg/mg) and hypoalbuminemia, but can present as complete nephrotic syndrome, including anasarca and hypercholesterolemia. Whereas recurrent disease typically presents within the first 2 years following transplant, the presentation of nephrotic syndrome after 2 years is generally considered to be secondary to calcineurin inhibitor (CNI) toxicity, chronic rejection, or de novo disease.

Biopsies early following recurrence often demonstrate normal histology on light microscopy with effacement of podocyte foot processes on electron microscopy.[46,55,295] Later biopsies have characteristic segmental lesions of FSGS with endocapillary proliferation and foam cell accumulation and can progress to glomerular sclerosis and interstitial fibrosis.[46,55] Patients achieving complete and sustained remission of proteinuria do not typically demonstrate FSGS on biopsy.[46]

The pathophysiology of idiopathic FSGS in native kidneys and recurrent FSGS following transplant remains unclear. It is likely a multifactorial process involving cytokines secreted by T cells,[174,337] a humoral factor that alters podocyte cytoskeletal structure,[129,288] and a balance between circulating permeability factors and inhibitors of such factors.[107] Recurrence of nephrotic syndrome in children with NPHS2 mutations does not appear to be due to antipodocin antibodies.[26] Further study is needed to clarify the pathogenesis of recurrence in this population.

A circulating factor has been proposed to cause increased albumin permeability of the slit diaphragm during FSGS recurrence, but the identity, source, and pathologic effects of such a factor are yet to be fully elucidated.[49,288,289] Bioassays of albumin permeability have had conflicting results in predicting FSGS recurrence[63] and have not proven to be specific or highly predictive of response to therapy or long-term renal outcome in patients with nephrotic syndrome.[49,308] Furthermore, demonstration of a neutralizing effect of normal serum[287] or urine from nephrotic patients[48] on albumin permeability suggests that loss or deficiency of a natural inhibitor may play a role.

Recently, Wei et al. identified serum soluble urokinase receptor (suPAR) as a circulating factor capable of causing FSGS.[332] Two-thirds of the patients with FSGS in this study had elevated serum suPAR concentrations compared to healthy controls and patients with other glomerular diseases. Furthermore, patients who had FSGS recurrence following transplant had the highest serum concentrations of suPAR, suggesting that this could be developed into a clinically predictive test. Prospective studies are needed to validate the predictive value of suPAR concentrations for FSGS recurrence.

The treatment of recurrent FSGS is not well established. The most commonly reported therapies for recurrent FSGS are plasmapheresis or protein A immunoadsorption therapy. A recent review of the literature found that 49 of 70 children (70%) receiving plasmapheresis for FSGS recurrence achieved partial or full remission.[255] Early detection of recurrence and initiation of plasmapheresis appear to provide the best results.[257] However, these studies likely overrepresent the benefit of plasmapheresis given small sample sizes and the use of only historical groups for comparison in a few of the studies or no comparison group in others. In general, it is recommended that children at risk should have daily monitoring of protein/creatinine ratios in the early posttransplant period to allow rapid detection of FSGS recurrence and early initiation of treatment.

Some centers perform plasmapheresis either before a planned living donor transplant or in the perioperative period of deceased donor transplant.[115] It is unclear if this practice offers any benefit over early detection and treatment of established recurrence.[118]

High-dose cyclosporine has shown efficacy in achieving complete or partial remission of recurrent nephrotic syndrome in children.[261,266] The antiproteinuric effect of CNIs has been postulated to be due to T-cell suppression and inhibition of cytokine secretion thought to be injurious to podocytes,[174] as well as to a direct effect on the stabilization of the podocyte cytoskeleton.[49,86] The alkylating agent, cyclophosphamide, has also been reported to be efficacious in some children with recurrent FSGS, usually in combination with plasmapheresis.[55,63] Reduction in proteinuria has also been reported with the use of angiotensin blockade,[138,210] either alone or in conjunction with plasmapheresis.

Finally, there have been anecdotal cases reporting prolonged remission from proteinuria in children with recurrent FSGS following plasmapheresis and B-cell depletion with rituximab.[134,136] This was first reported for a child who incidentally achieved remission of FSGS recurrence following rituximab therapy to treat posttransplant lymphoproliferative disease (PTLD).[253] The true value of this approach remains to be established.

Congenital Nephrotic Syndrome

Congenital nephrotic syndrome (CNS) by definition occurs within the first 3 months of life and is most commonly due to mutations in the NPHS1 gene encoding nephrin, a major structural component of the slit diaphragm. Infants with CNS are frequently born prematurely, have an enlarged placenta, and present with nephrotic-range proteinuria, anasarca, and hypoalbuminemia. Secondary causes (i.e., neonatal cytomegalovirus (CMV), congenital rubella, human immunodeficiency virus (HIV), hepatitis B, toxoplasmosis, syphilis, and infantile lupus) should be excluded. The genetics of CNS are proving more complex in recent years with the identification of additional genetic mutations (including genes previously only associated with FSGS).[31]

Recurrence of nephrotic syndrome has been reported in 25% of children with CNS due to homozygous Finmajor mutations in nephrin (NPHS1) with mean time to recurrence of 12 months posttransplant (range of 5 days to 2 years). Antinephrin antibodies have been implicated in a majority of these children.[249,327] There is one report of a child with compound heterozygous NPSH1 mutation who had recurrence but no detectable antinephrin antibodies.[294]

Vascular thrombosis and death from infection (with a functional graft) have been described more often in children with CNS following transplant compared to children with other primary diseases.[163] Hypercoagulability due to urinary losses of antithrombin III along with younger age at the time of transplant likely contribute to the increased risk of these complications.

Diffuse mesangial sclerosis (DMS) can also present as nephrotic syndrome in early infancy and is associated with mutations of the Wilms' tumor suppressor gene 1 (WT1). Denys–Drash syndrome consists of progressive glomerulopathy (DMS) and male pseudohermaphroditism (although genotypic females have also been described) and is due to heterozygous mutations within exon 8 or 9 of WT1.[228] Children with Denys–Drash syndrome are at increased risk of developing Wilms' tumor; therefore, bilateral nephrectomy is often performed once they develop ESRD. Frasier syndrome presents with normal female genitalia with streak gonads, XY karyotype, and progressive glomerulopathy (DMS on histology) and is due to splice mutations within exon 9 of WT1.[166] Children with Frasier syndrome are at risk of developing gonadoblastoma and therefore should undergo oopherectomy. There have also been reports of isolated DMS in children with WT1 mutations without other syndromic features[147] who may not be at risk for malignancy.

Other than one report of recurrent MPGN in a child with Denys–Drash,[227] no other studies report recurrence of nephrotic syndrome in children with WT1 mutations undergoing kidney transplant.[233] Overall, children with Denys–Drash have comparable patient and graft survival as children with other causes of ESRD.[232]

Alport's Syndrome

Alport's syndrome (AS) is a clinically and genetically heterogeneous nephropathy characterized by glomerular basement membrane (GBM) defects due to alterations in the type IV collagen matrix. AS presents with persistent microscopic hematuria and proteinuria that can progress to renal failure and is often associated with sensorineural hearing loss and ocular abnormalities. It is the prototype of inherited nephritis and accounts for 2% of children with ESRD in the United States. The most common, and severe, form is inherited in an X-linked recessive pattern and is associated with early progression to ESRD (50% of boys by age 25 years). Autosomal recessive and autosomal dominant forms have also been described.

The genetics of X-linked AS was defined over 20 years ago as a mutation in the gene encoding the α5 chain of type IV collagen (COL4A5). Patients with mutations resulting in a truncated protein (i.e., large rearrangement, premature stop, or frameshift mutations) tend to progress to ESRD earlier (50% by age 19 years).[122] Female carriers of COL4A5 mutation are considered to have a less severe course, but some do develop ESRD in late adulthood.[149] Development of hearing loss and progression of proteinuria appear predictive of a more severe course in female carriers. Evaluation of potential living donors, especially female relatives, should include evaluation for hematuria and proteinuria, as the heterozygous carrier state carries a risk of developing ESRD following donation.[123]

Autosomal recessive forms involving mutations in the α3 (COL4A3) and α5 (COL4A4) chains have also been described. Rare autosomal dominant mutations in COL4A3 and COL4A4 have also been reported with less severe renal disease, fewer cases of hearing loss, and absence of reported ocular changes.[150,188,318]

Although AS itself does not recur, development of de novo anti-GBM disease has been reported to occur in approximately 3–5% of AS males within the first year following transplant.[40,44] Late occurrence has also been described.[67]

Antibodies are generated against the type IV collagen α5 or α3 chains.[52,328] Patients with mutations resulting in complete absence or severe truncation of these proteins appear to be at highest risk of developing anti-GBM antibodies. It should be noted that the anti-GBM antibodies in these patients are specific for different epitopes of the non-collagenous domains of the α3α4α5(IV) collagen network than the Goodpasture's alloepitope, and therefore may not be detectable in the serum using the clinically available enzyme-linked immunosorbent assay used to diagnose spontaneous anti-GBM nephritis in Goodpasture's disease.

Early reports described rapidly progressive anti-GBM disease with nearly 90–100% graft loss.[64,240] With better recognition of this entity, reports of subclinical anti-GBM (i.e., demonstration of linear IgG deposits along the GBM in transplant biopsies without graft dysfunction) suggest a broader spectrum of clinical disease.[44,254] Despite the poor graft outcome described during anti-GBM nephritis in AS, the severe form does not occur frequently enough to impact overall graft survival statistics for AS patients.[114,124] Chronic rejection is the most common cause of graft loss in this population. Patients who have lost a prior graft to anti-GBM disease are at higher risk of recurrence following a subsequent transplant, although some have reported successful retransplantation.[40]

Membranoproliferative Glomerulonephritis

Membranoproliferative glomerulonephritis (MPGN) describes a pattern of glomerular injury with common histologic features of glomerular capillary wall thickening (membrano-) and hypercellularity in the glomerular tufts (-proliferative). MPGN was historically classified into three morphologic types: type I, with presence of immune deposits in the subendothelial and mesangial areas; type II, with electron-dense deposits within the basement membrane; and type III, with complex GBM formation with subendothelial and subepithelial electron-dense deposits that are bridged by intramembranous deposits. MPGN can be primary (or idiopathic, most commonly in children) or secondary to infectious and autoimmune disease. A unifying characteristic of all types of MPGN is hypocomplementemia (low C3). MPGN type II, known as dense deposit disease (DDD), is now considered a separate entity from MPGN types I and III, since it has unique pathogenic and clinical features.[326] Therefore DDD is addressed in the next section of this chapter.

Historic reports characterizing the transplant outcomes for patients with MPGN typically combined patients with MPGN type I and type II in their analyses. More recent reports separate the two groups. Disease recurrence for MPGN type I is estimated to be 20–30%.[13,213]

A recent analysis of UNOS data showed MPGN type I has a significant negative impact on graft survival compared to other forms of glomerulonephritis, and a significant, but modest, negative effect compared to other causes of ESRD.[14] Disease recurrence was the most common cause of graft loss (14.5%) for patients with MPGN type I in this study. Graft loss has been reported in about 50% of patients with recurrent MPGN type I.[213] Low complement levels (C3) at the time of transplant[186,213] and younger age at time of transplant[213] have been associated with increased risk of recurrence. A recent report of serial protocol biopsies identified that some patients have asymptomatic recurrence of MPGN I.[186]

Recurrent MPGN presents with hematuria, progressive proteinuria, and deteriorating graft function. Low or low-normal C3 levels have been reported.

Treatment of recurrent MPGN type I is not well established. Case reports and small case series suggest that cyclophosphamide combined with CNIs and steroids,[45,181] plasmapheresis combined with steroids,[218,278] and plasmapheresis combined with rituximab[252] may be beneficial.

Dense Deposit Disease (Formerly MPGN II)

As mentioned earlier, MPGN type II or DDD is now considered to have a pathophysiology distinct from the other forms of MPGN.[15] DDD is characterized by the deposition of electron-dense deposits within the GBM and is associated with uncontrolled activation of the alternative pathway of the complement cascade. Most patients are diagnosed between the ages of 5 and 15 years and about 50% progress to ESRD within 10 years. It is a rare disease, representing 0.8% of children reported in the NAPRTCS transplant registry.[232]

Uncontrolled activation of the alternative complement pathway in DDD is caused by stabilization of the C3 convertase, C3bBb. C3bBb is normally stabilized by properidin and inhibited by factor H. Approximately 80% of patients with DDD have an autoantibody, called C3 nephritic factor, that stabilizes C3bBb and prevents its normal degradation. Other causes include deficiency of factor H,[76] or presence of an inhibitory autoantibody against factor H,[203] the natural inhibitor of C3bBb.

An analysis of the NAPRTCS database showed significantly worse 5-year graft survival (50.0%) for children with MPGN type II compared to the database as a whole (74.3%).[38] The most common cause of graft failure in children with MPGN type II was recurrent disease (14.7% of graft losses). Of the children with MPGN II who had posttransplant biopsies (n=18) in the registry, 67% had recurrent MPGN type II. No correlation was found between pretransplant presentation or C3 levels with the risk of recurrence or graft loss.[38] In a single-center, retrospective study, MPGN type II was reported to recur in 60% of children while the rate of graft loss was similar to other children transplanted at that center.[219] Finally, an analysis of the UNOS database, including children and adults, reported graft loss due to recurrence in 30% of patients with MPGN type II, and significantly worse graft survival compared to patients with other forms of glomerulonephritis.[14]

Similar to MPGN type I, there is no established treatment of posttransplant recurrence of DDD. Non-specific treatments using angiotensin blockade, steroids, anticoagulation, or antiplatelet therapy have been reported in the literature with variable success. In patients with deficiency in factor H, plasma infusion can be used to correct the deficiency. Plasmapheresis has been reported to remove the C3 nephritic factor.[96] More recently, the use of an anti-C5 antibody (eculizumab) has been proposed to block the downstream effects of uncontrolled C3 convertase activity, but the clinical utility, long-term implications, and identification of patients who would benefit most from this therapy still need to be defined.[193,324]

Secondary Glomerulonephritis

IgA and Henoch–Schönlein Purpura

Histological recurrence in adult transplant recipients with IgA nephropathy has been reported to be 30–35%.[126,246,256] Transplant patients with abnormal urinalysis (hematuria or proteinuria) are more likely to show histological evidence of recurrence. The role of recurrence in graft loss is variable in these reports. As high as 40–50% of patients with recurrence have been reported to have graft failure in some single-center studies[155,256]; however, a recent analysis of patients in East Asia found that chronic rejection had a larger effect on long-term graft survival rate in patients with IgA nephropathy.[126]

Histologic recurrence of Henoch–Schönlein purpura (HSP) nephritis has been reported in as high as 70% of patients within 2 years following transplant,[305] with clinically evident recurrence (hematuria, moderate proteinuria, and hypertension) in 15–35%.[126,255] Long-term graft survival, however, does not appear to be greatly affected by recurre nce.[126,157,305] An analysis of adolescents and young adults in the UNOS database revealed graft loss due to recurrent disease in 13.6% of patients with HSP.[270]

Hemolytic-Uremic Syndrome

HUS accounts for approximately 2–2.5% of children with ESRD in the United States.[226,232] HUS is characterized by the clinical triad of microangiopathic hemolytic anemia, thrombocytopenia, and renal failure and can be due to secondary causes (infectious, drug-induced, autoantibodies) or primary genetic defects in complement regulatory components that lead to persistent activation of the alternative pathway of the complement cascade.

The most common cause of HUS in children (accounting for approximately 90% of cases) is associated with colitis due to Shiga toxin-producing bacteria (*Escherichia coli*, *Shigella dysenteriae*, others). Epidemiological studies estimate that 5–10% of children with Shiga toxin-producing *E. coli* (STEC) infections develop HUS, with children under the age of 5 years carrying the highest risk.[119,184] Of the children who develop HUS, about two-thirds develop oligoanuric renal failure.[133] In a meta-analysis of long-term prognosis (>1 year) following diarrhea-associated HUS, death or ESRD occurred in 10–15% of children with HUS.[101] The presence of anuria or prolonged oliguria has been associated with higher risk for long-term sequelae, including CKD, proteinuria, and hypertension in as many as 30% of HUS survivors.[234,285] The risk of developing HUS and the severity of renal failure appear to vary among different serotypes of STEC.[170] The risk of disease recurrence following transplant in this particular group appears to be very low (<1%) and graft survival is similar to children with non-glomerular primary disease.[89,182]

Infections with bacteria other than STEC, including *Shigella dysenteriae* and *Citrobacter* sp. that produce Shiga or Shiga like toxins, have also been implicated in the etiology of HUS in children. Furthermore, urinary tract infections (UTIs) with STEC have also been found in children with HUS presenting without diarrhea.

Finally, invasive *Streptococcus pneumoniae* infections have also been linked with a rare, but severe, form of HUS that has higher rates of progression to ESRD than the classical diarrhea-associated disease. Cases typically have large bacterial burden with empyema and bacteremia, but cases with meningitis or pericarditis have also been described.[20] Bacterial neuraminidase exposes a crypt antigen known as the Thomsen-Freidenrich (or T-) antigen on erythrocytes, platelets, and endothelium and is thought to play a role in endothelial activation and subsequent microvascular thrombus formation. T-antigen exposure can be confirmed on patient erythrocytes using the lectin *Arachis hypogaea*. Recurrence of pneumococcal HUS following transplantation has not been reported for these patients.

HUS that cannot be associated with infection (often referred to as atypical HUS) accounts for 5–10% of all cases in children and carries a higher risk to progress to ESRD without treatment. Genetic or acquired disorders of complement regulation are identified in about 60–70% of these cases. They also have higher risk of recurrence and graft loss posttransplant. Therefore, identifying these cases is paramount for both pre-emptive treatment to prevent progression to ESRD and planning for successful transplantation.

In recent years, a clear link has been established between disordered regulation of the alternative pathway of the complement system and atypical HUS. Mutations have been described in three important regulatory proteins of the alternative pathway: complement factor H (CFH: 20–30% of atypical HUS registry cases),[76,230] complement factor I (CFI: 2–12%),[34,103] and membrane cofactor protein (MCP: 10–15%).[340] Gain-of-function mutations in genes encoding complement factor B (CFB: 1–2%) and complement C3 (10%) and loss-of-function mutations in thrombomodulin (THBD gene) have also been associated with atypical HUS. Finally, autoantibodies to factor H[77] are detectable in 5–10% of patients with atypical HUS, but up to 40% of these patients also carry a mutation in CFH, CFI, MCP, or C3.[212]

Atypical HUS is increasingly recognized as a complex, polygenic disease. First, incomplete penetrance is common in most of these mutations, suggesting that "multiple hits" contribute to a predisposition to atypical HUS. Second, various polymorphisms in genes encoding CFH, MCP, CFH-related protein (CFHR1), and C4b-binding protein (C4b-BP) have been associated with atypical HUS.[82] Furthermore, bigenic abnormalities have been described in about 10% of patients; therefore mutational analysis of all complement components is recommended during the workup of patients suspected to have atypical HUS.[82,334] Finally, cases of de novo thrombotic microangiopathy following kidney transplant in patients with non-HUS causes of ESRD have also been found retrospectively to have CFH or CFI mutations.[175]

Historically, studies on the outcomes of children with HUS have used simple delineation of cases based on the presence or absence of prodromal diarrhea. This delineation is not always straightforward clinically, for Shiga toxin-related cases may present without diarrhea and 20–30% of cases of atypical HUS are preceded by a diarrheal illness (including STEC infection).[282] Furthermore, as mentioned previously, there are non-diarrheal bacterial infections associated with HUS (STEC UTI and *Pneumococcus*). A recent guideline has been published in an effort to standardize diagnostic workup and treatment for children with atypical HUS.[17] Children without diarrheal prodrome or pneumococcal infection, or those with recent diarrhea and certain clinical characteristics associated with increased risk of genetic predisposition (Box 37-1), should undergo full diagnostic evaluation for cause of HUS, including investigation for Shiga toxin-producing bacteria as well as mutational analysis.

Recurrence following transplant can present as graft thrombosis or graft failure with hematological signs of HUS (microangiopathic hemolytic anemia and thrombocytopenia). The risk of recurrence following transplant varies depending on the genetic mutation identified. Approximately 80% of patients with factor H or factor I mutations develop HUS recurrence posttransplant with high rates of graft loss (80–100%) within 1 year of recurrence.[39,183] In theory, patients with isolated mutations in the membrane-bound MCP protein should not develop recurrent HUS since the allograft would have wild-type, functional MCP protein. A recent analysis of the International Registry of Recurrent and Familial HUS/TTP (thrombotic thrombocytopenic purpura) included 3 patients with documented MCP mutations, all with excellent graft function at 3–13 years posttransplant.[230] However, HUS recurrence has been reported in a few patients with MCP mutation. Possible explanations include endothelial microchimerism in which endothelial cells of recipient origin (expressing the mutated form of MCP) repopulate the transplanted kidney,[95] or additional, undiagnosed, genetic susceptibility of the recipient (in circulating or fluid-phase complement components). Living donation is not advised for children with potential

BOX 37-1 Suggested Evaluation of Children with Hemolytic-Uremic Syndrome (HUS)

Risk factors that should prompt a diagnostic workup for atypical HUS, even if diarrhea is present, include:
- Age of onset under 6 months old
- Insidious onset
- Relapse of HUS or a suspected previous case of HUS
- Previous unexplained anemia
- Non-synchronous family history of HUS
- Presentation with severe hypertension
- Presentation of HUS posttransplant (for any organ)

Diagnostic workup includes:
- Serum/plasma C3 level (although normal values do not exclude inherited disorders of complement regulation)
- Plasma/serum concentration of factor H and factor I
- Antifactor H antibody titers
- Membrane cofactor protein (MCP: CD46) surface expression on mononuclear leukocytes by flow cytometry
- Gene mutation analysis for factor H, factor I, MCP, factor B and C3
- Plasma vWF protease activity (ADAMTS13)
- Homocysteine and methylmalonic acid levels (plasma and urine) to evaluate for defects in cobalamin metabolism

Adapted from Ariceta G, Besbas N, Johnson S, et al. 2009. Guideline for the investigation and initial therapy of diarrhea-negative hemolytic uremic syndrome. Pediatr Nephrol 24; 687–696.

atypical HUS given the high risk of recurrence and the uncertain effects of gene–gene interactions even from related donors found not to carry the same mutation as the recipient.

Plasma therapy has historically been the cornerstone of treatment for children with atypical HUS with CFH mutations. Infusion of fresh frozen plasma can provide functional factor H, factor I, and C3 for patients with deficiencies in these factors while plasma exchange withdraws anti-CFH antibodies and mutated forms of factor H.

Pre-emptive plasma exchange initiated prior to and continuing for some time following transplant has been successful in preventing atypical HUS recurrence in a small number of patients with CFH mutation, but delayed recurrence can occur with tapering of therapy or during infections (especially CMV infection).[183] Furthermore, several patients with CFH or CFI mutations have been reported to have graft loss following HUS recurrence despite plasma exchange, although these cases did not receive pre-emptive plasma exchange. Finally, patients with MCP mutation do not appear to benefit from plasma therapy.

Although CNIs have been associated with de novo HUS following solid-organ transplant, avoidance of CNIs has not been shown to affect the risk of recurrence in genotyped patients with atypical HUS.[39,93,95]

Liver transplant alone or in combination with kidney transplant has been reported for children with factor H mutation with the rationale that the transplanted liver would provide wild-type factor H. While early attempts resulted in acute thrombotic events and high mortality rates, several centers in Europe have reported improved outcomes with ancillary plasma exchange and anticoagulation therapies. However, the risk of morbidity and mortality has limited the use of this approach.

Finally, the use of the anti-C5 monoclonal antibody, eculizumab, to prevent membrane attack complex formation holds promise for both the prevention and treatment of recurrence in children with atypical HUS undergoing renal transplantation.[6,333,341] Moreover, the use of eculizumab may prevent progression to ESRD and obviate the need for renal transplantation.[51,112] Optimal dosage and interval between eculizumab infusions remain to be fully defined, and the high cost of this agent may limit access. While studies of long-term outcomes are not available, a requirement for lifelong therapy is anticipated.

Membranous Nephropathy

Membranous nephropathy is rare in children, so risk of recurrence in children following transplant is not clear. Only 47 (of a total of 10 632) children have been reported in the NAPRTCS transplant registry from 1987 to 2009 with the diagnosis of membranous nephropathy.[232]

Systemic Lupus Erythematosus (SLE)

Data on lupus nephritis recurrence in children are scarce. This is likely owing to the late presentation of recurrence, which for most patients who are transplanted as adolescents would occur in adulthood. An analysis of the NAPRTCS registry reported similar patient and graft survival for children with SLE compared to matched controls.[22] There was an increased incidence of recurrent rejection episodes in SLE patients receiving living donor transplants, for which there is no current explanation.

c-ANCA and p-ANCA-positive Glomerulonephritis

Pauci-immune glomerulonephritis associated with antineutrophil cytoplasmic antibody with cytoplasmic (c-ANCA) or perinuclear (p-ANCA) staining patterns are a rare cause of ESRD in children. Recurrence rates of the small-vessel vasculitides in the adult literature are low, at about 5–6%,[255] and recurrence of granulomatosis with polyangiitis (or GPA; formerly known as Wegener's granulomatosis) is rare. Average time to recurrence is 31 months, but can occur within weeks to many years following transplant. Graft loss due to recurrence has been reported in 2–7% of adults transplanted with diagnosis of small-vessel vasculitides.

Renal recurrence is often heralded by microscopic hematuria and proteinuria with focal or diffuse pauci-immune necrotizing glomerulonephritis seen on biopsy. The ANCA pattern or titers at the time of transplant do not appear to be predictive of disease recurrence. Similar to SLE, a waiting period of 6–12 months of inactive disease is recommended prior to transplant. Persistently positive ANCA serologies, however, should not preclude transplant since they are not an accurate marker of disease activity. There are anecdotal reports of the use of cyclophosphamide, corticosteroids, mycophenolate, and plasmapheresis for treatment of recurrence in patients with GPA and p-ANCA-associated glomerulonephritis.[255]

Metabolic Disease

Primary Hyperoxaluria Type I (Oxalosis)

Primary hyperoxaluria type I (PH1, also known as oxalosis) is a rare autosomal recessive disorder caused by a defect in hepatic alanine:glyoxylate aminotransferase (AGT) which catalyzes the conversion of glycoxylate to glycine. AGT deficiency results in overproduction of oxalate, resulting in massive renal excretion of insoluble calcium oxalate, leading to nephrolithiasis and nephrocalcinosis. As GFR declines with progressive renal involvement, oxalate accumulates and results in systemic oxalosis. More than 100 different mutations have been described and there is considerable phenotypic heterogeneity, even within family members with identical mutations.

The most severe form presents in infancy with renal failure necessitating dialysis. In children with less severe presentation and early diagnosis, conservative management with pyridoxine (thought to reduce oxalate production in a subset of B6-responsive patients), increased fluid intake, and citrate treatment might delay the progression of kidney disease.[85] Some centers advocate for preemptive liver transplant or combined liver–kidney transpl ant.[84,251,279] The use of hemodialysis prior to transplant has also been advocated to reduce systemic oxalate levels to mitigate injury to the allograft. Data from the NAPRTCS registry indicate poor patient and graft survival for children with oxalosis following kidney-only transplant with high rates of recurrence and death from sepsis.[232] Recent longitudinal studies from Europe suggest improved outcomes in recent years with the best outcomes in children who were diagnosed early and underwent combined kidney–liver transplant.[32]

Nephropathic Cystinosis

Cystinosis is a rare autosomal recessive disease due to a defect in the lysosomal cystine transporter (encoded by the cystinosin gene), resulting in intracellular accumulation of cystine, proximal tubule dysfunction (renal Fanconi syndrome), and progressive kidney disease. Since the development of the cystine-depleting drug cysteamine, progression to ESRD may be delayed. While nephropathic cystinosis does not recur posttransplant, protocol biopsies have shown interstitial deposition of cystine crystals without apparent clinical consequences. Graft survival rates for children with cystinosis are comparable to others in the NAPRTCS registry.[171,232] Extrarenal manifestations of continued cystine accumulation (i.e., visual impairment, hypothyroidism, endocrine pancreatic insufficiency, and myopathy) have become more apparent as the lifespan of patients with cystinosis increases and likely are postponed by continued cysteamine treatment posttransplant.[102]

PRETRANSPLANT EVALUATION

Evaluation of Potential Living Donor

Evaluation of a potential living donor (see Chapter 7) for a pediatric recipient is no different than that for an adult recipient. Living donors are evaluated for comorbid conditions that would either increase their own risk for developing ESRD or impact the recipient (i.e., certain viral infections). Adult-sized kidneys from living donors have excellent potential for long-term graft survival in pediatric recipients. Live donation from a sibling is also considered, but most programs do not routinely accept donors under the age of 18 years on ethical grounds. There have been exceptional cases, however, that required court consent. Although the ideal situation would be donation from an HLA-identical sibling, most live kidney donations for pediatric recipients come from haplo-identical parents.

Evaluation of Recipient

Many similarities exist in the medical evaluation of potential pediatric and adult transplant recipients (see Chapter 4). However, certain conditions occur more frequently in children, so the medical evaluation of pediatric recipients has a slightly different emphasis. The following section describes the common medical, surgical, and psychological issues taken into consideration during the pretransplant evaluation of a pediatric patient.

Medical Evaluation of Issues Related to ESRD

Cardiovascular Disease. Hypertension is a common problem in children with CKD. Chronic fluid overload can result in left ventricular hypertrophy and dilated cardiomyopathy. Impaired systolic function following transplant can impair perfusion of the allograft, increasing the risk of delayed graft function and impacting graft survival. Therefore, aggressive management of persistent hypertension, including intensified dialysis treatment and optimization of pharmacotherapy in children on dialysis, is paramount to successful transplant outcomes. Among hypertensive or other at-risk patients, echocardiography at the time of pretransplant evaluation and periodically thereafter (semi-annual to annual basis) can identify patients at highest risk for cardiovascular morbidity. Bilateral nephrectomy is sometimes required to control recalcitrant hypertension in children with elevated blood pressures despite multiple antihypertensive medications and optimized fluid management (see section below).

GN of Unknown Etiology. The underlying cause of ESRD should be identified in preparation for transplant in order to anticipate the risk of recurrence. Children with unknown cause of ESRD suspected to be due to glomerulonephritis should undergo a thorough evaluation to delineate the underlying etiology. Complement levels (C3 and C4), antinuclear antibody, ANCA, and anti-double-stranded DNA (anti-dsDNA) titers should be performed. As mentioned in the previous section, children suspected of having HUS as a cause of ESRD should be evaluated for atypical forms of HUS, including mutational analysis and complement levels (Box 37-1). Finally, identifying a hereditary disease as the cause of ESRD also aids in the evaluation of potential living donors.

Nephrotic Syndrome. Typically, heavy proteinuria diminishes as children with nephrotic syndrome approach ESRD. Active nephrotic syndrome with hypoalbuminemia at the time of transplant can complicate postoperative fluid management because of increased third spacing, thereby increasing the risk of electrolyte derangement, graft hypoperfusion, thromboembolic events, and delayed graft function. Continued heavy proteinuria from native kidneys may also mask early FSGS recurrence posttransplant. Native nephrectomies have been utilized at some centers to minimize this confounding variable.

Some centers also perform pre-emptive unilateral[191] or bilateral nephrectomy in children with CNS with short-term peritoneal dialysis in preparation for transplantation.[162] This allows normalization of serum albumin and IgG levels, resolution of hypercoagulability, and optimization of nutrition with concomitant improvement in growth prior to transplant. Another approach includes "medical nephrectomy" via the use of renin–angiotensin system blockade and prostaglandin inhibitors to effectively reduce GFR and minimize proteinuria with or without unilateral nephrectomy.[167,180]

Renal Osteodystrophy. Aggressive treatment of secondary hyperparathyroidism, renal osteodystrophy, and adynamic bone disease with vitamin D analogs and calcimimetics is vitally important for children with ESRD to optimize growth and anemia management prior to transplant. In general, secondary hyperparathyroidism improves following transplant, but it can often take several months to a year for parathyroid hormone (PTH) levels to normalize completely. Persistent hyperparathyroidism following kidney transplant can result in hypercalcemia and limits growth potential. The risk of developing persistent hyperparathyroidism after transplant is attributed to hyperplasia of the parathyroid gland. Over time, uncontrolled secondary hyperparathyroidism can lead to nodular transformation and monoclonal growth, resulting in tertiary hyperparathyroidism (resistant to vitamin D therapy). In this severe case partial parathyroidectomy is often needed to improve PTH levels. Ideally, pediatric transplant candidates should have intact PTH levels within the Kidney Disease Outcomes Quality Initiative target range for CKD stage 5 (200–300 pg/mL); however, transplant may proceed safely despite higher PTH levels provided serum calcium and phosphorus levels are under acceptable control.

Nutrition and Growth. Poor feeding is a prominent feature of uremia in young children, and many children with ESRD require gastrostomy tube placement for supplemental nutrition to optimize growth. As mentioned previously, most centers prefer pediatric patients to achieve a weight of 10–15 kg prior to kidney transplant, and infants on dialysis may not reach this goal prior to 2 years of age. The use of recombinant human growth hormone (rhGH) in children with ESRD has been shown to promote "catch-up growth" in children with linear growth delay secondary to renal failure. Optimized nutrition will also promote healing from transplant surgery.

Evaluation of Extrarenal Disease

Infections. Pediatric transplant candidates should be free from active infection to prevent infectious complications posttransplant. Subclinical infections of the dialysis access site, skin, teeth, sinuses, and urinary tract should be excluded prior to transplantation. Risk of tuberculosis infection (latent or active) should be screened for by history (including personal or close contacts with signs/symptoms of tuberculosis, recent immigration or travel to an endemic region), physical exam, chest X-ray, and purified protein derivative skin testing. HIV screening is required.

Urinary tract infections. Many children with ESRD have abnormal urinary tract anatomy, bladder outlet obstruction, or vesicoureteral reflux that places them at increased risk for recurrent UTI. Indeed, UTI is the most common bacterial infection in children awaiting kidney transplant. Aggressive antibiotic treatment and prophylaxis are helpful in suppressing UTI in most children. However, pre-emptive nephrectomy is sometimes undertaken to control recalcitrant pyelonephritis or to reduce the risk of urosepsis in children with recurrent UTI, particularly in the context of severe vesicoureteral reflux.

Cytomegalovirus (CMV). The incidence of CMV infection increases with age, so young children are more likely to be CMV-naïve at the time of transplant than adults. Anti-CMV IgM and IgG titers as well as CMV polymerase chain reaction (PCR) should be obtained at the time of pretransplant evaluation to plan for CMV prophylaxis following transplant. If initial studies are negative, repeat studies at the time of transplant can confirm immunological naiveté in the recipient. Donor CMV titers are also indicated to stratify the risk for developing posttransplant CMV disease.

Epstein–Barr Virus (EBV). Similar to CMV, many children undergoing evaluation for kidney transplant are naïve to EBV exposure. Primary EBV infection posttransplant increases the risk of PTLD. Anti-EBV IgM and IgG titers as well as EBV PCR should be assessed at the time of evaluation and, if initially negative, repeated at the time of transplant to confirm seronegativity and absence of infection.

Hepatitis B and C. Annual screening for hepatitis B and hepatitis C infection remains standard of care for children on dialysis. Prevalence of hepatitis C remains high for children with ESRD, with around 20% of children receiving hemodialysis testing positive for HCV antibodies[153] or viral antigens and nucleic acid.[207] Longer time on hemodialysis, but not the number of transfusions received, has been associated with higher risk of HCV infection in children and adolescents.[207] Children undergoing evaluation for transplant should have hepatitis B and hepatitis C testing along with serum aminotransferase levels to exclude the presence of active infection prior to transplant.

Immunization Status. Routine childhood immunizations should be completed prior to kidney transplant.[3] Live attenuated virus vaccines (i.e., measles, mumps, rubella and varicella vaccines) are generally contraindicated in immunosuppressed patients due to the increased risk of disseminated disease by the vaccine virus strain. Therefore, children awaiting transplant should receive live virus vaccination at least 1–2 months prior to transplant. Other, non-live virus vaccinations (i.e., hepatitis A, tetanus, diphtheria, acellular pertussis or Tdap, expanded 13-valent pneumococcal, meningococcal, and human papillomavirus) should also be administered prior to transplant since the immunosuppressant therapy to prevent rejection can impair immunological response to these vaccines. Children awaiting transplant should also receive annual influenza vaccination. Antibody titers against hepatitis B, hepatitis A, measles, mumps, rubella, and varicella should be evaluated to determine if booster vaccination is needed within 6 months of transplant.[104,258]

Hemostasis. As mentioned earlier, thrombosis is a significant cause of graft loss in very young recipients. However, identifying children at highest risk for this complication has been difficult. Retrospective studies have identified the following risk factors for graft thrombosis in pediatric recipients: recipient age under 5 years, history of peritoneal dialysis,[237] high urine output pretransplant, young donor age (<5 years old), and prolonged cold ischemia times (>24 hours).[145,320] Central venous lines are the most common vascular access for children receiving hemodialysis, and line-associated thrombosis is a common event in this patient population. Data linking prior history of catheter-associated thrombosis in children on dialysis with risk of graft thrombosis following transplant are not established.

There are few data on the prevalence of inherited hypercoagulability that may predispose some children to graft thrombosis. In adults, inheritance of factor V Leiden or prothrombin (G20210A) mutations significantly increases the risk of graft thrombosis. Adults with SLE, especially in the presence of detectable antiphospholipid antibody or β_2-glycoprotein-1, are at particularly high risk of thromboembolic events.[145] There are insufficient data to determine the risk of posttransplant thrombosis in patients with hyperhomocystinemia or 5,10-methylene tetrahydrofolate reductase (MTHFR) polymorphisms.

Children with a history of recurrent thrombotic events, or a strong family history of thrombophilia, should undergo coagulation workup to determine if chronic anticoagulation therapy is warranted. Evaluation of hypercoagulability includes measurement of prothrombin time, partial thromboplastin time, platelet count, fibrinogen, antithrombin III level, protein C and protein S levels, and activated protein C resistance (to monitor factor V Leiden). Adolescents with a history of SLE should be screened for antiphospholipid antibody, anticardiolipin antibody, and β_2-glycoprotein-1. Further workup including mutational analysis in other genes associated with inherited thrombophilia should be undertaken under the advice of a pediatric hematologist.

Prior Malignancy. In general, children with ESRD do not need to be screened for malignancy, but a prior history of malignancy warrants additional evaluation. Wilms' tumor is the most common malignancy resulting in ESRD in children. A waiting period of 2 years has resulted in excellent outcomes with low risk of recurrence following transplant.[165] A recent subanalysis of the NAPRTCS registry reported 5-year patient survival of 93% and graft survival of 82% for 56 patients with Wilms' tumor listed as the primary diagnosis.[232] Kidney transplant in children with a history of other extrarenal malignancies is generally considered after a recurrence-free period of 2–5 years.

Surgical Evaluation

Children undergoing kidney transplant evaluation often need multiple surgical interventions, including bladder augmentation, placement of Mitrofanoff continent urinary diversion, vesicostomy closure, gastrostomy tube placement, or native nephrectomy prior to or at the time of transplant. Therefore, it is vital that a surgical plan be established amongst pediatric surgeons, transplant surgeons, and urologists prior to kidney transplant in children in order to coordinate surgical approaches and spare or maintain the vascular supplies that are unique for each procedure.

Vascular Evaluation. The abdominal vasculature should be assessed for patency in preparation for transplant surgery. Children with a prior history of femoral lines (including dialysis catheters) or inflammatory conditions of the abdomen (such as multiple abdominal surgeries or recurrent peritonitis) are at increased risk of thrombosis of the inferior vena cava (IVC) or iliac vessels, thereby complicating vascular anastomosis of the graft. Magnetic resonance venogram and computed tomography angiography are sensitive techniques for assessing IVC patency as well as providing a detailed anatomic survey of abdominal vasculature. In patients at lower risk of thrombosis, Doppler ultrasound is useful to screen for IVC and iliac vein patency, but may be dependent on operator expertise, especially in small children.

Urological Evaluation. As mentioned earlier, nearly 25% of children receiving kidney transplants have underlying urological abnormalities, including lower tract obstruction, vesicoureteral reflux, or bladder dysfunction. Therefore, pediatric urologists play an important role in the management of these patients prior to and following transplantation.[7]

All children under consideration for kidney transplant should have a renal ultrasound to evaluate for hydronephrosis, hydroureter, and bladder wall thickening. In cases where excessive urine production is suspected, a 24-hour urine collection should be obtained, if possible, for determination of urinary volume.

A voiding cystourethrogram should be performed in select children undergoing evaluation for kidney transplant, including those with a history of urological causes of ESRD, history of UTIs, hydronephrosis on ultrasound, or signs (e.g., thickened bladder wall on ultrasound) or symptoms suggestive of dysfunctional voiding.[290] Low-grade reflux (grade I–II) has not been associated with adverse graft outcomes.

Urodynamic studies are indicated for selected children with urinary tract abnormalities to assess bladder capacity, compliance, voiding pressure, leak point pressure, and postvoid residual (see Chapter 12). Early, aggressive treatment of neurogenic or dysfunctional bladder is critical as elevated bladder pressures have been associated with increased risk of developing reflux into the transplanted kidney[21] and worse graft survival.[4] Medical management of neurogenic bladder often includes anticholinergic therapy combined with intermittent catheterization and should be continued following transplant. Children with a history of posterior urethral valves should be assessed for persistent anatomic obstruction following valve ablation or have a neourethra (e.g., Mitrofanoff) that can be intermittently catheterized following transplant to prevent lower urinary tract obstruction posttransplant.

In some cases, poor bladder compliance persists despite appropriate medical management, necessitating bladder augmentation with small-bowel or colon segments prior to transplant. However, otherwise healthy but small-capacity, defunctionalized bladders in children with oliguric ESRD do not require augmentation in order to achieve excellent graft outcomes.[9,267] Typically, urological correction should be undertaken 3–6 months prior to transplant to allow for adequate healing prior to immunosuppression.[263]

Native Nephrectomy. The most common indications for native nephrectomy in children undergoing kidney transplant are excessive urine output, high-grade vesicoureteral reflux with recurrent or recalcitrant pyelonephritis, continued heavy proteinuria (see Congenital Nephrotic Syndrome section, above), uncontrolled hypertension, and risk of renal malignancy.[83,105] Multiple-drug-dependent hypertension, especially that requiring treatment with minoxidil, may also be an indication for native nephrectomies.

Excessive urine output (>20 mL/kg/24 hours) has been associated with an increased risk of renal transplant thrombosis in children.[320] Furthermore, high urine output following the immediate posttransplant period (>4 L/day) can complicate fluid management for small children for whom it would be difficult to consume such large volumes to avoid hypovolemia.[169]

Early UTI following transplant has been associated with increased risk of graft loss.[70] Therefore, nephrectomy of a native kidney with severe reflux (grade 3 or 4) should be considered to reduce the risk for early UTI or urosepsis following transplant.[36,83]

Pre-emptive native nephrectomy has been advocated for certain patients for which the underlying renal disease results in continued urinary losses of electrolytes (i.e., for Bartter's syndrome)[53] or heavy proteinuria (i.e., FSGS or CNS)[105] complicating the optimal nutritional and medical management of children prior to transplant. Reduction in heavy proteinuria due to FSGS following nephrectomy may reduce the risk of thrombotic events by correcting the hypercoagulable state and allow for earlier recognition of recurrent FSGS following transplant. As mentioned earlier, children with CNS may benefit from improved nutrition and reduced risk for infection following nephrectomy. Finally, children with autosomal recessive polycystic kidney disease often require unilateral or bilateral nephrectomy of rapidly enlarging kidneys to allow for both improved respiratory status and adequate space in the abdomen for a future kidney graft.

Many centers, including ours, perform pretransplant native nephrectomies for patients on dialysis with recalcitrant hypertension with good short-term results, including achievement of age-normative blood pressures and a reduction in the number and dosage of antihypertensive medications. The underlying pathophysiology for this situation appears to be complex. Fluid overload certainly contributes; however some children continue to have significant hypertension despite aggressive treatment of fluid overload and maximal doses of multiple antihypertensive medications. Studies in rats that received syngeneic kidney transplants after 5/6 nephrectomy were shown to have persistent hypertension despite normal renal function and absence of rejection or exposure to steroids or CNIs.[60] Interestingly, removal of the diseased native kidney achieved normalization of blood pressures in these rats. The presence of high renin production and activation of the sympathetic nervous system from diseased native kidneys have been theorized to contribute to persistent hypertension in this setting.

The efficacy of bilateral nephrectomy in improving blood pressure control for children on dialysis or preventing posttransplant hypertension has not been extensively studied. Reportsfrom our center involving unilateral or bilateral nephrectomy of diseased kidneys have shown good results during short-term follow-up.[19] Similarly, children with multicystic dysplastic kidney disease or reflux nephropathy resulting in a unilateral poorly functioning kidney have been reported to have resolution of hypertension or diminution of antihypertensive medications following nephrectomy.[280] However, a recent retrospective study did not demonstrate an effect of bilateral nephrectomy on the risk of posttransplant hypertension or left ventricular hypertrophy.[50] Prospective longitudinal studies are needed to evaluate whether bilateral nephrectomy for hypertension improves long-term cardiovascular morbidity in children receiving kidney transplant.

Children with disorders related to mutations in the WT1 gene, such as Denys–Drash syndrome and Frasier syndrome, are at increased risk for developing Wilms' tumor over time. Therefore, bilateral nephrectomy is considered once they approach ESRD.[18]

The surgical approach to nephrectomy (retroperitoneal or transperitoneal; open or laparoscopic) should be based on the center's expertise as the risk of vascular and bowel injuries is low for both approaches.[79,161] Although a recent report from Italy suggests that renal embolization in children may be a minimally invasive alternative to nephrectomy for indications other than risk of malignancy,[47] we have observed unacceptable morbidity from this procedure and would not recommend this approach.

Neurodevelopment

Developmental Delay. It is increasingly recognized that children with CKD have higher rates of neurocognitive delays. Factors that have been associated with increased risk for neurocognitive deficits include longer duration of CKD, increased severity of disease (i.e., advanced stages of CKD), and younger onset of disease.[292]

Children with onset of ESRD in infancy can have significant developmental delay due to uremia. In the absence of structural brain abnormalities, psychomotor delay can improve following transplant, with many infants regaining normal developmental milestones.[202] Although overall neurodevelopmental outcomes are favorable following transplant, in a prospective study of neurodevelopmental outcomes in children undergoing kidney transplant prior to age 5 years,[260] children who were born prematurely and had multiple hypertensive crises or seizures during dialysis were found to have lower IQ and need for special education following transplant. This study suggests that identification of susceptible children and prevention of hypertension-related morbidity may allow for optimal neurodevelopmental outcome for young children following kidney transplant.

Other infants needing dialysis in the first year of life may have structural neurological abnormalities resulting from insults associated with premature birth or anoxic/ischemic injury (e.g., hypoxic ischemic encephalopathy, periventricular leukomalacia following intraventricular hemorrhage, or microcephaly). Children with structural neurological abnormalities can present with hypotonia, spasticity, myoclonus, severe cognitive delays, and seizures. Children with severe mental retardation may not respond well to the constraints of ESRD care where the need for multiple, and often painful, procedures can be confusing and uncomfortable. In such situations the potential for rehabilitation, self-care, and parental preferences should be considered during joint decision making between the medical team and family/caregivers in determining whether long-term dialysis or transplantation should be pursued.

Seizures. Seizure disorder requiring anticonvulsant therapy is present in about 5% of pediatric transplant recipients.[232] Adequate seizure control should be obtained prior to transplantation, preferably with anticonvulsants that do not interfere with the metabolism of commonly used immunosuppressant medications. Phenytoin (Dilantin), barbiturates, and carbamazepine can significantly reduce serum levels of CNIs and prednisone. Newer anticonvulsants may not interfere with immunosuppressant drug levels, but it is prudent to check for updates in drug–drug interactions when planning for transplant.

Psychosocial Issues

Psychoemotional Status. A multidisciplinary approach with involvement of physicians, child psychologists, and child life specialists is important for the preparation of children and their families for kidney transplantation. Children with emotional or psychiatric disorders often require additional mental health resources, including psychiatric care. Acquisition of coping skills, problem-solving skills, and behavior modification can improve a child's experience with the inherent complexity of dialysis or transplantation medical care. Pharmacotherapy for depression, bipolar disorder, and attention deficit hyperactivity disorder are important adjunctive therapies. Reduced clearance with impaired renal function, clearance by dialysis, and interference with the metabolism of immunosuppressive medications should be considered when selecting psychotropic medications in children with ESRD. Most selective serotonin reuptake inhibitors do not interfere with immunosuppressive medications.

Non-adherence. Suspected non-adherence contributes to approximately 44% of graft losses and 23% of late acute rejection episodes reported in the literature for adolescent kidney transplant recipients.[74] Patterns of medication and dialysis treatment compliance should be assessed for every child undergoing evaluation for kidney transplant to identify patients at high risk for non-adherence posttransplant. Social, behavioral, and psychiatric interventions should be initiated prior to transplant for those patients with identified or anticipated issues with non-compliance. Identification and nurturing of psychosocial support systems and frequent medical and social work follow-up are often required to prepare the pediatric candidate for transplantation. Again, the best chance of rehabilitation and preparation for transplant is achieved when there is close coordination between medical and mental health providers. It is also of particular importance for the transplant and dialysis medical teams to maintain close communication as the recipient prepares for transplant.

Evaluation Updates

Pediatric candidates for kidney transplant should be re-evaluated at regular intervals (generally every 6–12 months) to identify any changes in their medical condition or psychosocial status that alters the risk of commencing with transplantation. A simplified version of the initial medical evaluation is appropriate for update visits.

PERIOPERATIVE MANAGEMENT OF PEDIATRIC RENAL TRANSPLANT RECIPIENTS

Preoperative Management

Children presenting for imminent kidney transplant surgery should be clinically stable without signs of active infection. A final set of laboratory studies is obtained to evaluate for any electrolyte or metabolic derangements that require dialysis or medical treatment prior to anesthesia induction.

Intravascular volume status is important prior to transplant surgery as children with hypovolemia (especially those with high urine output) are at increased risk of graft thrombosis[320] and graft hypoperfusion, leading to ATN. Therefore, if dialysis treatment is indicated prior to surgery, excessive fluid removal should be avoided. Similarly, children with residual urine output should receive intravenous fluids to maintain intravascular volume (e.g., fluid volume replacement to equal urinary output) while oral intake is restricted awaiting surgery.

Subclinical infections of skin, dialysis access site, peritoneal fluid, and urinary tract should be screened for with a thorough history, physical exam, urinalysis, and urine culture if indicated, peripheral white blood cell count with differential, blood cultures (for those with indwelling venous catheters), and peritoneal cell count and culture (for those maintained on peritoneal dialysis). A recent episode of peritonitis or peritoneal dialysis catheter exit site infection does not preclude transplantation, but the child should complete 10–14 days of antibiotics and have a negative peritoneal fluid culture off antibiotics prior to transplant.

As mentioned earlier, CMV and EBV serologies should be repeated if previous results revealed immunological naiveté. Final crossmatch is performed within 1 week prior to living donor kidney transplant or in the hours preceding deceased donor transplant.

Intraoperative Management

Small children can present operative challenges given the relatively large size of an adult kidney graft. Children weighing over 30 kg are often treated surgically as small adults with graft placement in the standard extraperitoneal pelvic location and vascular anastomoses to the common iliac artery and vein. However, in small children (usually less than 20 kg), intra-abdominal placement may be preferable with vascular anastomoses to the infrarenal aorta and IVC. The surgical approach should be individualized with appropriate matching of blood vessel size and attention to expected circulatory volume requirements.

Intraoperative management of the pediatric kidney transplant recipient is focused on achieving optimal graft perfusion and preventing complications arising from underlying ESRD. Typically, a central venous catheter is inserted for close monitoring of central venous pressures. Central venous pressures should be maintained at 8–12 cm H_2O and mean arterial pressures above 70 mmHg via infusion of crystalloid or 5% albumin prior to clamp release to ensure adequate perfusion to the adult-sized transplanted kidney.[268]

It is important to recognize the challenge this can pose in children under 30 kg as a kidney graft from an adult can sequester 150–250 mL of blood, which can represent well over 10% of a small child's total circulating volume. In infants, up to 50% of cardiac output is directed to perfusion of an adult-sized kidney graft. Transfusion with packed red blood cells is often necessary in the smallest recipients to avoid severe anemia. In addition, continuous dopamine infusion at 2–3 μg/kg/min is often necessary, especially in infants, to maintain higher mean arterial pressures, and is continued for 24–48 hours postoperatively to allow the graft to accommodate slowly to lower mean arterial pressure in the recipient. Finally, mannitol (1 g/kg) with or without furosemide (1 mg/kg) is often administered prior to clamp removal to facilitate diuresis.

Blood gases and lactate levels should be monitored intraoperatively since clamping of the aorta or iliac artery can result in lactic acid accumulation, metabolic acidosis, and vasoconstriction. Occasionally, calcium channel antagonists such as verapamil[185] or papaverine are injected into the arterial anastomosis to overcome arterial spasm that impairs graft perfusion.

For most immunosuppression protocols, intravenous methylprednisolone sodium succinate (Solu-Medrol) is administered at the beginning of the surgical case. In addition, many pediatric transplant centers use intravenous biological agents for induction therapy, and these are also administered intraoperatively.

Postoperative Management

Children are monitored in the intensive care unit setting for the immediate postoperative period (see Chapter 14). In the first 2–3 days, the postoperative management continues to focus primarily on optimizing graft perfusion and mitigating the effects of fluid overload (e.g., electrolyte derangements and hypertension). As mentioned earlier, small children often require dopamine infusion for 24–48 hours posttransplant to maintain graft perfusion and allow gradual accommodation of the graft to the lower mean arterial pressures of the recipient.

Fluid management in small children requires fastidious care due to their small size and potentially very large posttransplant urine volumes. Urinary losses are replaced in equal volumes with intravenous 0.45% or 0.9% sodium chloride infusion for the first 24–48 hours. Dextrose should be withheld from the initial intravenous fluids given for urine replacement in order to avoid hyperglycemia and osmotic diuresis. Replacement of insensible water losses should be administered as a separate infusion with dextrose-containing crystalloid. Hypokalemia and hypophosphatemia may develop in the first few postoperative days. Potassium and/or phosphate salts can be added to the replacement fluids as appropriate.

As the kidney graft regains urinary concentrating ability, urine output declines to levels that are more reasonably achievable as daily oral intake. Urine replacement with intravenous crystalloid can be discontinued at that time, and intake goals of 150–200% of calculated maintenance needs should be started by mouth. Children with intra-abdominal graft placement are susceptible to prolonged postoperative ileus[224] due to displacement of the colon and intestines with an adult-sized graft occupying almost the entire right side of the abdomen. These children often require continuation of maintenance intravenous fluids beyond the first few days until they can tolerate oral fluids and nutrition.

Hypertension is commonly observed in children following transplant. In some instances, elevated blood pressures improve with adequate analgesia. Fluid overload can also contribute to postoperative hypertension and often improves once spontaneous mobilization of fluid occurs. Aggressive treatment of hypertension is typically not recommended to avoid sudden changes in mean arterial pressure and decreased graft perfusion. This being said, children who were on multiple antihypertensive medications prior to transplant may need reinstitution of at least some of their previous medications to avoid severe hypertension and the accompanying adverse effects.

Goals for hospital discharge of the pediatric transplant recipient include adequate oral fluid intake to prevent hypovolemia (and subsequent graft hypoperfusion), stable immunosuppression regimen, completion of family and caregiver education, access to medications, and arrangement of outpatient follow-up.

IMMUNOSUPPRESSIVE PROTOCOLS AND DRUGS

Several other chapters in this book are devoted to a detailed discussion of the various classes of immunosuppressant medications used for induction, maintenance, and treatment of rejection following kidney transplantation (see Chapters 15–22). Therefore, this chapter will discuss pediatric-specific issues related to various immunosuppressant medications and trends in immunosuppressant protocols following kidney transplantation in children.

Infants and small children cannot swallow pills and therefore frequently require special formulations of immunosuppressive medications (i.e., compounded solutions). Furthermore, it has become increasingly recognized that the metabolism of these medications undergoes maturation in children so pharmacokinetics can vary by age. Therefore, children with kidney transplants may require a different dosing schedule than that published in the adult literature. Finally, fewer clinical trials of new immunosuppressant medications have included children, so there are often limited data on safety and efficacy in the pediatric population. Consequently, most of the immunosuppressant medications used to prevent or treat rejection in pediatric kidney transplant recipients are not approved by the US Food and Drug Administration for use in children and therefore are administered as "off-label" use.

Induction Therapy Agents

Figure 37-6 illustrates the trends in the use of induction antibodies for pediatric kidney transplants reported in the NAPRTCS registry. Induction therapy of some form was reported for approximately 50–60% of transplant recipients in the NAPRTCS registry over the past 10 years.

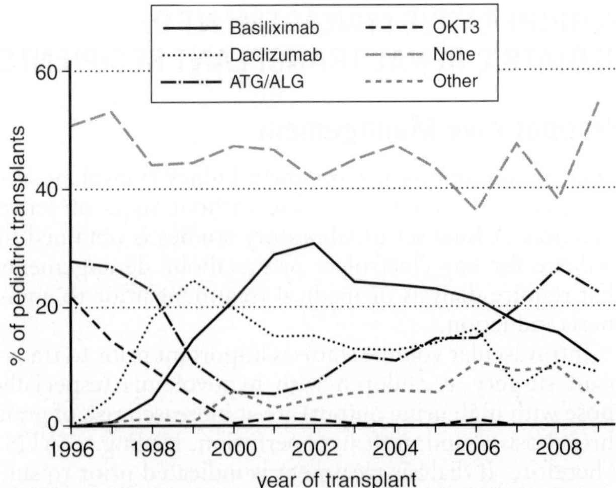

FIGURE 37-6 ■ Trends in induction immunosuppression for pediatric kidney transplants in North America. ATG, antithymocyte globulin; ALG, antilymphocyte globulin. (Data from North American Pediatric Renal Trials and Collaborative Studies. 2010. *NAPRTCS Annual Transplant Report*. Available online at: https://web.emmes.com/study/ped/annlrept/annlrept.html (accessed 9/24/2012).)

Although adult trials have demonstrated decreased rates of rejection using induction therapy, there are no controlled trials in pediatrics to verify the benefits of this practice.

Initial retrospective studies of the NAPRTCS registry consistently showed an increased risk for acute rejection for children who did not receive induction therapy.[303] However, a randomized, prospective multicenter trial found no improvement in the rate of acute rejection or graft failure for children receiving induction with muromunab-CD3 (also known as OKT3) compared to continuous cyclosporine infusion.[30] Furthermore, a recent retrospective analysis of pediatric recipients in the UNOS registry found no difference in the number of rejection episodes or 3-year graft survival for children receiving polyclonal rabbit antithymocyte globulin (rATG) or monoclonal anti-IL-2Ra antibody compared to no induction (all were discharged with triple immunosuppressive maintenance therapy, including a CNI, antimetabolite, and steroids).[269]

Lymphocyte-Depleting Agents

OKT3. The first monoclonal drug available in this class was the lymphocyte-depleting drug, muromunab-CD3 (or OKT3). Administration of OKT3 was complicated by severe symptoms of cytokine release, often referred to as the "first-dose effect." Use of OKT3 for children undergoing kidney transplant fell out of favor in the late 1990s with the availability of alternative depleting agents that were better tolerated. The manufacturer of OKT3 voluntarily withdrew it from the US market due to decreased demand.

Antithymocyte Globulin. Polyclonal ATGs are the most commonly used induction therapy for patients reported in the NAPRTCS registry, accounting for 22% of patients reported in 2009. There are two preparations in use: one derived from the immunization of rabbits (rATG or Thymoglobulin, Genzyme) and one from the immunization of horses (hATG or Atgam, Upjohn). In Europe, a similar polyclonal antibody derived from rabbit serum is available from Fresenius. Due to the sclerosing nature of these formulations, they are administered via central venous catheter. Although ATG formulations are better tolerated than OKT3, they still carry the risk of severe cytokine release and anaphylaxis; accordingly, premedication with corticosteroids, acetaminophen, and antihistamine 30–60 minutes prior to infusion is recommended.

Thymoglobulin is typically administered at 1–2 mg/kg/day in daily doses for 5 days as induction therapy. Some centers stop Thymoglobulin doses once therapeutic CNI levels are achieved. Furthermore, intermittent therapy based on peripheral CD3+ lymphocyte counts has been suggested to reduce cumulative dose with low rate of acute rejection in high-risk adult kidney transplant recipients,[250] but this practice has not been validated in children. Atgam is typically dosed at 10–15 mg/kg daily for 5–10 days. The median duration of ATG/antilymphocyte globulin treatment reported in the NAPRTCS registry is 5 days.[232]

Single-center, retrospective studies report adequate immunological graft survival rates following rATG and triple immunosuppression with 10-year follow-up.[61,239] A small study in pediatric kidney transplant recipients suggested greater T-cell depletion following 5 days of Thymoglobulin compared to Atgam.[56,88] However, a direct comparison of patient outcomes between Thymoglobulin and Atgam has not been reported in pediatric recipients.

Concerns have been raised regarding an increased risk of PTLD associated with depletional induction therapy, especially with high doses of OKT3 or Thymoglobulin.[56,88] However, long-term exposure to CNIs and murine target of rapamycin (mTOR) inhibitors or possibly the balance between B-cell and T-cell depletion may be more relevant determinants of PTLD risk.[87,164]

Alemtuzumab. Alemtuzumab (or Campath-1H) is a monoclonal antibody directed at CD52-positive T cells and B cells. The use of alemtuzumab induction in adult kidney transplant recipients along with reduced doses of CNI and mycophenolate mofetil (MMF) and without long-term steroids has had encouraging results in small series.[247] However, pharmacokinetic data and long-term outcomes in children receiving alemtuzumab induction are still limited. Bartosh et al. first described the use of alemtuzumab in 4 high-risk pediatric kidney transplant recipients.[23] They reported similar prolonged lymphocyte depletion and increased risk of developing anti-HLA antibodies in the absence of CNI, as had been reported in adults. Since then, ongoing trials of alemtuzumab induction in low-risk pediatric kidney transplant recipients has allowed for steroid-free immunosuppression and reduced CNI exposure.[68,242,286] The optimal dose of alemtuzumab in pediatric recipients is still unclear. The Pittsburgh group reports a single dose 0.4–0.5 mg/kg for induction,[300] and the prospective phase II trial (PC-01) utilizes two doses (on day −1 and day +1) of 0.3 mg/kg (with a maximum dose of 20 mg).[68]

A longitudinal study of the immune profile and development of anti-HLA antibodies in children receiving alemtuzumab induction was recently published.[68] This study was part of a multicenter clinical trial of alemtuzumab induction (PC-01 trial, mentioned above) with initial maintenance of tacrolimus and MMF followed by conversion to sirolimus and MMF at 2–3 months for low-risk children receiving living donor kidney transplants (n=35). The cumulative hazard of developing circulating anti-HLA antibodies in children (roughly 33% at 24 months posttransplant) was higher than that reported in the adult literature (15–20% at 1–5 years). However, development of anti-HLA antibodies in this study was not associated with a decline in renal function or histological changes on 2-year surveillance biopsy. Long-term follow-up of these patients will be needed to assess the potential benefits of this immunosuppressive regimen in children.

Non-Depleting Agents

Anti-IL2RA Antibodies. There have been two high-affinity monoclonal antibodies against the inducible α-chain of the interleukin-2 receptor (IL2-ra or CD25) in use for the prevention of allograft rejection in children. Basiliximab (Simulect, Novartis) is a chimeric antibody approved for the prevention of acute rejection in pediatric kidney transplant recipients and is generally given in two doses (10 mg for children <35 kg and 20 mg for children >35 kg) on days 0 and 4 posttransplant. Daclizumab (Zenapax, Roche), which was recently withdrawn from the US market, is a humanized antibody and is administered at a dose of 1 mg/kg every 14 days for five doses beginning within 24 hours of transplant. This dosing regimen in 61 pediatric kidney transplant recipients resulted in serum levels predicted to provide saturation of the Tac subunit of IL-2 receptors for approximately 90 days posttransplant.[297]

Anti-IL2-ra antibody induction is overall well tolerated in children. There is one report, however, of two children who developed non-cardiogenic pulmonary edema in the absence of delayed graft function.[75]

Basiliximab is commonly combined with triple-therapy immunosuppression with CNI, MMF, and prednisone.[235] Standard-dose daclizumab has also been used in conjunction with triple immunosuppression, while a protocol of steroid avoidance utilized extended-dose daclizumab (given for 6 months posttransplant).[276]

Maintenance Therapy

Figure 37-7 illustrates the trends in maintenance immunosuppression for children receiving kidney transplants in the United States over the past decade, as reported by the SRTR. There are several different immunosuppression protocols in use in children. As reported in the NAPRTCS registry from 2005 to 2010, the most common maintenance regimen, utilized in 63% of deceased donor and 55% of living donor transplants, includes triple therapy with tacrolimus, MMF, and prednisone.[232] Overall trends include decreased usage of cyclosporine and azathioprine and increased use of tacrolimus and mycophenolate.

Corticosteroids

Corticosteroids have long played a key role in the prevention of rejection following solid-organ transplant. Data from the SRTR report, as illustrated in Figure 37-7, indicate that the use of prednisone for maintenance immunosuppression in pediatric kidney transplant recipients has been declining over the past decade. Nearly 40% of children in 2009 were discharged from the hospital following kidney transplant on a maintenance regimen that did not include steroids.[245] This trend likely reflects a shifting focus on reducing the off-target side effects of long-term glucocorticoid exposure, including impaired linear growth, reduced bone density, hypertension, glucose intolerance, and risk for avascular necrosis of the femoral head. Furthermore, the undesirable cosmetic effects of long-term corticosteroid use, including cushingoid facial features and acne, likely contribute to non-adherence, particularly in adolescent patients.

Steroid-Based Regimens. Steroids continue to be utilized as a maintenance immunosuppression therapy in the majority of children receiving kidney transplantation. The use of more potent immunosuppressant medications, namely tacrolimus and MMF, has allowed for overall reduction of prednisone dose used for prevention of rejection and mitigation of steroid side effects. The most recent NAPRTCS transplantation report indicates that children transplanted in the most recent era and maintained on triple therapy with prednisone, tacrolimus, and MMF received lower mean daily prednisone dosing compared to the historical regimens that incorporated cyclosporine and/or azathioprine (cyclosporine/azathioprine/prednisone or cyclosporine/MMF/prednisone).[232]

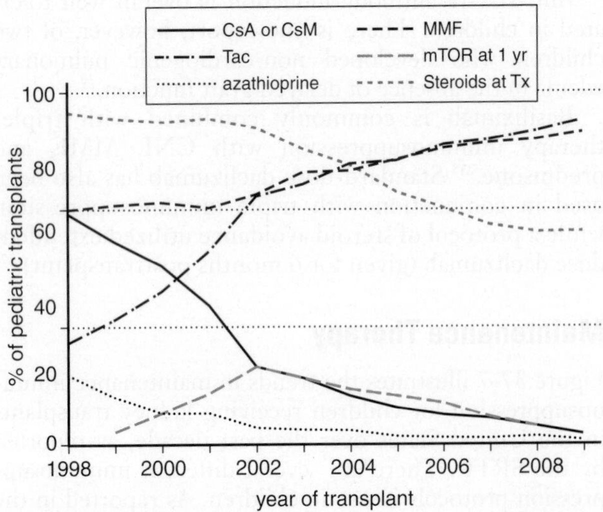

FIGURE 37-7 ■ Trends in maintenance immunosuppression for pediatric kidney transplants in the United States. (Data from Organ Procurement and Transplantation Network (OPTN) and Scientific Registry of Transplant Recipients (SRTR). OPTN / SRTR 2010 Annual Data Report. Department of Health and Human Services, Health Resources and Services Administration, Healthcare Systems Bureau, Division of Transplantation, 2011. Available online at: http://srtr.transplant.hrsa.gov/annual_reports/2010 (accessed 9/24/2012).)

Although reduction of corticosteroid dose has been demonstrated to improve hypertension, bone and joint complications, and cataracts, this strategy has not been shown to address the suppression of linear growth in children effectively.[97] Alternate-day administration of equivalent cumulative prednisone dose has been suggested as a strategy to allow catch-up growth without compromising graft survival.[41,148] This regimen, however, may be more cumbersome for the patient and family and more prone to non-adherence.

More recently, studies of immunosuppressant protocols to minimize glucocorticoid exposure in pediatric kidney transplant recipients have focused on either steroid withdrawal (early or late) or total steroid avoidance.[323] The following paragraphs will summarize the major studies reporting these approaches in children.

Steroid Withdrawal (Late). Initial reports of late steroid withdrawal were concerning for increased risk of rejection and allograft loss.[158] More recently, however, a multicenter, randomized, open-label study in children with low immunological risk compared late steroid withdrawal (greater than 1 year posttransplant) to continuous steroid treatment and maintenance therapy with cyclosporine microemulsion and mycophenolate, with similar rates of acute rejection observed between groups and stable graft function at 2 years following steroid withdrawal.[135] The patients who underwent late steroid withdrawal benefited from superior longitudinal growth, less frequent hypertension, reduction in the number of antihypertensive medications, and improved carbohydrate and lipid metabolism compared to the patients remaining on steroids (5 mg/m^2 prednisone daily). This study suggests that withdrawal of steroids in select, stable pediatric transplant recipients receiving CNI therapy and MMF is safe and may mitigate the metabolic and cardiovascular side effects of prolonged steroid use. Of note, the effect on growth observed in this study was more pronounced and occurred earlier in prepubertal patients, but even the pubertal patients had significant improvement in mean standardized height after 24 months following withdrawal of steroids.

Valid concerns have arisen regarding excessive immunosuppression with newer agents in protocols designed to minimize exposure to steroids.[189] This was poignantly exemplified by the early termination of the only randomized, double-blinded, controlled study of late steroid withdrawal (commencing at 6 months) in pediatric kidney transplant recipients due to an unacceptably high rate of PTLD.[196] Patients in this study received intensified early immunosuppression with basiliximab induction and maintenance with prednisone, cyclosporine, or tacrolimus, and sirolimus followed by randomization either to undergo complete steroid withdrawal (gradually over 6 months if they had no clinical or histological evidence of rejection on a 6-month protocol biopsy) or to continue low-dose steroids. There were no differences in acute rejection episodes in the two groups, and the steroid withdrawal group had superior 3-year allograft survival.[29] However, the high rate of complications (most notably of PTLD) led to the early termination of this study and recommendations against the routine use of this potent immunosuppressant protocol in children.

Steroid Withdrawal (Early). Several case series of early steroid withdrawal (within 5–7 days posttransplant) have been reported with similar rates of acute rejection and graft survival compared to historic or non-randomized controls receiving long-term steroids.

Chavers et al. reported a prospective, non-randomized study of rapid steroid withdrawal over the first 6 days posttransplant in 21 children utilizing 5–7 days of Thymoglobulin induction with cyclosporine and MMF maintenance.[54] Compared to 39 age-matched controls transplanted over the same time period who received standard prednisone doses, the group undergoing rapid discontinuation of prednisone had similar rates of acute rejection and graft survival at 2 years.[54] Although mean height standard deviation scores for the rapid discontinuation of prednisone group were significantly improved, there was no difference observed in the incidence of hypercholesterolemia, hypertriglyceridemia, glucose intolerance, or obesity.

The TWIST study was a multicenter, randomized, open-label trial to evaluate the effect of daclizumab induction (2 doses) with tacrolimus, MMF, and rapid steroid withdrawal (by day 5) compared to triple therapy with tacrolimus, MMF, and standard-dose prednisone (no induction) on growth and steroid-related metabolic complications in pediatric kidney transplant recipients.[120] The end point of the study was relatively short, at 6 months. Patient survival, graft survival, and renal function over this short time period were comparable between the two groups. The group receiving rapid steroid withdrawal had improved lipid and glucose metabolic profiles. Prepubertal patients in the steroid withdrawal group had significantly improved catch-up growth at 6 months posttransplant compared to patients remaining on steroids.

Finally, Tan and colleagues reported their 4-year experience with induction therapy utilizing a single dose of alemtuzumab and two perioperative doses of methylprednisolone (day −1 as premedication for alemtuzumab infusion and intraoperatively prior to graft reperfusion) followed by tacrolimus monotherapy in 42 low-immunological-risk pediatric living donor kidney transplant recipients.[300] A subset of these patients were also able to tolerate weaning of tacrolimus to every-other-day dosing. They reported excellent graft survival (97.6% at 1 year and 85.4% at 2–4 years) and low cumulative risk of acute cellular rejection (0% at 1 year and 4.8% at 4 years) using this approach. Furthermore, they reported no episodes of antibody-mediated rejection, CMV infection, BK nephropathy, or PTLD. Furthermore, this group has previously reported increased estimated GFR and a greater increase in height Z-score at 1 year for 15 preadolescent children receiving tacrolimus monotherapy.[80] A low incidence (7.7%) of posttransplant diabetes was also reported.[286]

Steroid Avoidance. Early results of a single-center trial of complete steroid avoidance using an extended (up to 6 months) induction with daclizumab and maintenance therapy with tacrolimus and MMF were very encouraging, with significant improvement in growth, low rates of rejection, and decreased rates of hypertension, posttransplant diabetes, and hyperlipidemia compared to historical controls receiving steroids.[178,277]

Longer-term results (3-year follow-up) in unsensitized pediatric kidney transplant recipients were recently reported for a multicenter, randomized trial comparing steroid-free and steroid-based immunosuppression with concomitant tacrolimus, MMF, and standard-dose daclizumab (steroid-based) or extended daclizumab induction (steroid-free).[276] There was no difference in biopsy-proven acute rejection or 3-year graft survival between the two groups. Patients receiving the steroid-free regimen had lower systolic blood pressures and lower cholesterol levels at 3 years. While overall height Z-score change after 3 years was not statistically different between the groups, recipients under the age of 5 years receiving the steroid-free regimen had significantly improved linear growth. The cumulative incidence of antibody-mediated rejection was numerically higher in the steroid-free group (6.7% versus 2.9%) but did not reach statistical significance.[222] A significant increase in chronic histological damage was observed over time, without difference between the steroid-free and steroid-based groups. The same group has also reported a steroid-free protocol using Thymoglobulin induction (rather than extended daclizumab) in a small series of high-immunological-risk pediatric recipients, resulting in equivalent rates of rejection, but increased rates of subclinical viremia compared to the daclizumab protocol.[179]

In 2008 Roche announced voluntary withdrawal of daclizumab in all countries where it was licensed due to decreased market demand. Several trials of steroid avoidance or early steroid withdrawal using basiliximab induction have been reported in adult kidney transplant recipients, but it remains to be seen how the pediatric protocol with extended daclizumab treatment would be altered to utilize basiliximab.

Calcineurin Inhibitors

As mentioned earlier, nearly 90% of pediatric kidney transplants reported by SRTR receive CNIs at the time of hospital discharge (see Chapter 17). Tacrolimus has for the most part replaced cyclosporine in the United States.

Historically, dosing of cyclosporine in children was complicated by variable gastrointestinal absorption of oil-based formulations and a higher rate of metabolism in young children necessitating higher mg/kg and more frequent dosing (up to thrice daily). The introduction of the microemulsion formulations enhanced bioavailability and reduced variability in serum drug levels. Therapeutic monitoring of cyclosporine in children commonly utilizes trough measurements as correlation of C2 levels with drug efficacy or toxicity is not well established in children or well accepted by patients and families due to the requirement of multiple, painful blood draws. The side effect profile of cyclosporine in children is similar to that in adults. The undesirable cosmetic effects of hypertrichosis and gingival hypertrophy are particularly distressful for adolescent recipients, possibly contributing to dangerous non-adherence. Hypercholesterolemia and hypertriglyceridemia are also common.

Tacrolimus therapy is typically initiated in the first few days posttransplant once serum creatinine falls by 50% of pretransplant level. Average tacrolimus doses for the first few months following transplant are 0.1–0.15 mg/kg/dose twice daily.[232] Information on tacrolimus pharmacokinetics in the pediatric population is limited and has primarily been studied in pediatric liver transplant recipients.[65] In general, therapeutic drug monitoring of tacrolimus is considered to have good correlation between trough levels and drug exposure. However, abbreviated sampling for area under the concentration–time curve can be helpful in cases where low or appropriate trough levels accompany signs of toxicity.

Many centers using triple immunosuppressive therapy with tacrolimus, MMF, and prednisone have high initial tacrolimus trough goals (in the range of 10–15 ng/mL) for the first 1–2 weeks posttransplant with decreasing goals over the subsequent 4–6 months. The median tacrolimus level (via immunoassay) reported in the NAPRTCS registry at 12 months posttransplant is 6 ng/mL.[232]

Tacrolimus is primarily metabolized by the liver via the CYP3A system. Drug interactions related to inducers or inhibitors of CYP3A can be expected to affect drug levels. Diarrhea, a common problem in children, can dramatically increase tacrolimus serum levels. Therefore, tacrolimus drug levels should be monitored closely during diarrheal illness (and dosage adjusted accordingly) to avoid toxicity, and rechecked as diarrhea improves to ensure continued therapeutic levels.

The most common side effects seen in children treated with long-term tacrolimus therapy include impaired glucose tolerance, posttransplant diabetes, tremor, alopecia, and mild sleep disturbances. In contrast to cyclosporine, tacrolimus rarely causes the cosmetic side effects mentioned earlier. There are a few studies of protocols to minimize exposure to CNIs in pediatric kidney transplant recipients; most report using alemtuzumab induction. As mentioned earlier, the Pittsburgh group has reported excellent graft survival and function in 42 consecutive pediatric kidney transplant recipients over 4 years with alemtuzumab induction (or Thymoglobulin) and low-dose tacrolimus monotherapy.[300] Results of a National Institutes of Health-sponsored multicenter, single-arm, prospective phase II trial of alemtuzumab induction followed by tacrolimus withdrawal in pediatric recipients of living donor kidney transplants are also anticipated.[68]

mTOR Inhibitors

Inhibitors of mTOR have a side effect profile unique from the CNIs, including lower risk for diabetes, neoplasm, and nephrotoxicity, and therefore offer an attractive alternative for protocols that seek to minimize CNI exposure (see Chapter 19). As demonstrated in Figure 37-7, mTOR inhibitors are not commonly administered to pediatric kidney transplant recipients in the United States. Most data on the use of mTOR inhibitors in pediatric kidney transplant recipients have been with sirolimus.

A shorter drug half-life for sirolimus in children, especially prepubertal children, dictates twice-daily dosing, in contrast to once-daily dosing described in adults. Furthermore, the optimal target trough level has yet to be fully defined in children. The most common side effects reported for sirolimus in pediatric patients include recurrent aphthous ulcers, impaired wound healing, and proteinuria. Mild testosterone deficiency needs further evaluation in the adolescent group. Adverse effects, especially aphthous ulcers, are reportedly more significant at higher trough levels (>9 ng/mL).[211]

Conversion from CNI to mTOR inhibitor has been suggested to improve GFR. In a retrospective study of pediatric kidney transplant recipients converted from cyclosporine to sirolimus due to biopsy-proven chronic allograft nephropathy (CAN), patients with mild CAN (grade I) had improved estimated GFR at 3 months and stable proteinuria. However, patients with more advanced CAN did not benefit from the conversion in terms of renal function. While there was no increase in the rate of acute rejection or graft loss following conversion to sirolimus, there was a trend of increased adverse effects, including infection and nephrotic-range proteinuria.[144]

We reported our single-center experience with conversion from tacrolimus to sirolimus at 3 months posttransplant in stable, low-risk pediatric kidney transplant recipients.[142] Patients with stable serum creatinine levels and surveillance biopsy without evidence of acute rejection, including borderline histology, were eligible for conversion to sirolimus. Additional exclusion criteria included a history of nephrotic syndrome as the etiology of ESRD, second renal transplant, and biopsy-proven BK nephropathy. Actuarial 5-year graft survival was 91% for those patients who remained on sirolimus (78% of the patients undergoing conversion). Acute rejection occurred in 13% in the 12 months following conversion. Aphthous ulcers and BK viremia were the most common complications.

The antiproliferative and antiangiogenic actions of sirolimus have the potential to alter growth plate function and thereby impair linear growth in children. Furthermore, inhibition of mTOR has been demonstrated to disrupt intracellular signaling of the insulin-like growth factor (IGF)-1 axis in chondrocytes and therefore might interfere with the effects of endogenous or exogenous growth hormone. However, retrospective investigations of the effect of sirolimus therapy on linear growth in pediatric kidney transplant recipients have resulted in conflicting conclusions.[117,143]

Antimetabolites

MMF has largely replaced azathioprine in the United Statse for pediatric kidney transplant adjunctive maintenance therapy (see Chapter 18). Over 85% of pediatric kidney transplant patients in the United States are discharged on a regimen that includes MMF. As mentioned earlier, the incorporation of MMF into standard immunosuppression regimens has facilitated the use of lower corticosteroid doses following transplantation. MMF has also proven useful in steroid-free protocols where it is combined with tacrolimus or sirolimus. Furthermore, it is used in combination with sirolimus and corticosteroids in CNI-sparing protocols.

The most common, and troublesome, side effects during MMF use in children include leukopenia and diarrhea. MMF dosage reduction is often first tried for these undesirable effects. Enteric-coated tablets can also be tried for gastrointestinal disturbance. Therapeutic drug monitoring of MMF in children (via mycophenolic acid or levels) has been criticized due to high inter- and intra-individual variability.[306,339] The metabolism of MMF may be enhanced by corticosteroids, and the bioavailability can be decreased by cyclosporine or antacids containing magnesium or aluminum hydroxides. Pharmacokinetics are reported to vary based on age, with young children requiring higher doses to achieve comparable mycophenolic acid area under the curve.[90] For patients receiving tacrolimus, MMF is typically started at 250–400 mg/m^2/dose twice daily, but some have advocated for higher doses (500 mg/m^2 dosed BID) for children under the age of 2 years.[90] When used alone, MMF is recommended at 600 mg/m^2/dose.

ACUTE REJECTION IN PEDIATRIC TRANSPLANTATION

As mentioned earlier, acute rejection accounts for 10% of graft losses reported in the NAPRTCS registry.[232] With modern immunosuppressive therapy, rates of acute rejection in pediatric kidney transplant recipients have decreased. According to the most recent NAPRTCS report, 13.2% of pediatric kidney transplants reported in the registry between 2007 and 2010 have had at least one rejection episode, in contrast to overall rates of 24% for 2003–2006 and 32% from 1999 to 2002. Deceased donor kidney transplant recipients had higher rates of rejection (15.2% compared to 10.3% of living donors). Historically, nearly half of pediatric kidney transplant recipients experienced acute rejection within the first 12 months following transplant. However, in the most recent NAPRTCS cohort (2007–2010), the majority of children have a rejection-free first year, with only 8.6% of living donor recipients and 16.6% of deceased donor recipients reported to have rejection within the first 12 months.

Chronic allograft rejection is a leading cause of graft loss in children (Figure 37-5). As with adults, late episodes of acute rejection and multiple episodes of acute rejection are associated with worse long-term allograft survival.

Diagnosis of Acute Rejection

The diagnosis of acute rejection is not always straightforward in pediatric kidney transplant recipients. Small children who have adult-sized allografts have a large renal reserve relative to their muscle mass. Therefore, a small increase in serum creatinine can represent significant renal dysfunction. Children with acute rejection can present with low-grade fever and mild hypertension, but can also be asymptomatic.

The differential diagnosis for elevated serum creatinine in pediatric kidney transplant recipients is similar to adults and includes hypovolemia, CNI toxicity, UTI, urinary obstruction, BK nephropathy, and acute rejection. Renal biopsy is the gold standard to diagnose rejection and is well tolerated by children using sedation. Diagnosis of rejection based on biopsy has become standard of care in children (so-called biopsy-proven rejection). Urinalysis and urine culture, viral PCR (BK, CMV, EBV), and renal ultrasound studies should be performed in a timely manner prior to biopsy. Intravenous crystalloid is also administered to eliminate prerenal azotemia as a possible etiological or confounding factor in raising the serum creatinine level.

The role of protocol biopsy in pediatric kidney transplant is not well established.[140] Protocols of steroid or CNI minimization often rely on protocol biopsies to survey for early pathology (i.e., subclinical rejection) that might benefit from intensified immunosuppression or evidence of drug toxicity that might benefit from dose reduction. However, not all pediatric centers perform regularly scheduled surveillance biopsies.

Treatment of Acute Rejection

There are few controlled trials in children to guide the treatment of acute allograft rejection. As with adults, high-dose corticosteroids are the first-line treatment in children with suspected or biopsy-proven acute rejection. Intravenous methylprednisolone succinate is typically administered at 10–30 mg/kg/dose for 3–5 consecutive doses. A taper of oral corticosteroids back down to maintenance doses over 3–5 days is used by some, but not all, pediatric transplant centers. It is not uncommon for the serum creatinine to increase slightly during the first few days of steroid pulse. In addition, serum creatinine may not return to baseline levels for several days following completion of the pulse, but typically a trend of decreasing creatinine is suggestive of a response to therapy.

Severe Rejection

Severe rejection or steroid-resistant rejection has historically been treated with lymphocyte-depleting antibodies (e.g., Thymoglobulin). Alemtuzumab has also been reported to be effective in some cases of refractory cellular rejection.[314]

Research in the past decade has identified an additional role for B cells during acute cellular rejection, even in the absence of identifiable antibody-mediated rejection. B cells are postulated to contribute to cellular rejection via antigen presentation, activation of dendritic cells, and by providing co-stimulatory help to T cells. B-cell transcript signatures[275] and dense B-cell infiltrates in biopsies of pediatric kidney transplant recipients have been associated with poor graft survival[311] and are predictive of graft loss.[220]

A recent prospective, randomized, open-label trial compared standard treatment with pulse steroids and Thymoglobulin with anti-CD20 monoclonal antibody therapy (rituximab) for treatment of biopsy-proven acute cellular rejection with B-cell infiltrate.[338] Patients receiving rituximab therapy had significantly increased recovery of graft function and improvement in rejection scores on biopsy at 6 and 12 months following treatment compared to those receiving standard therapy, despite higher rejection grade and greater number of patients with humoral rejection randomized to the rituximab treatment group.

Antibody-Mediated Rejection

Antibody-mediated rejection in pediatrics can be treated with intravenous immunoglobulin (IVIG), plasmapheresis, or rituximab,[35] but the efficacy of these approaches is variable. Successful use of the proteasome inhibitor, bortezomib (Velcade, Millennium Pharmaceuticals), for treatment of antibody-mediated rejection has been reported for adult kidney transplant[59] and pediatric heart[214] and multivisceral[146] transplant recipients. A case series of 10 consecutive kidney transplant patients with humoral rejection (including several adolescent patients) who were administered bortezomib in combination with plasmapheresis and IVIG reported a trend toward improved graft survival (6 of 10 patients with functioning graft at 18 months) compared to historical controls who received rituximab with plasmapheresis and IVIG (1 of 10 with functioning graft at 18 months).[325]

LONG-TERM MANAGEMENT POSTTRANSPLANT

The success of kidney transplantation in children with ESRD now results in 10-year patient survival of 80–95%. Therefore, the long-term management of these patients is focused on maintaining good quality of life and minimizing significant long-term side effects of immunosuppression. Outpatient management of pediatric kidney transplant recipients includes identifying and reducing the cardiovascular and metabolic effects of long-term immunosuppressive therapy, preventing infection and chronic rejection, ensuring good long-term quality of life, and managing a smooth transition into adulthood.

Hypertension and Cardiovascular Disease

Children with ESRD have increased cardiovascular mortality relative to their peers and cardiovascular disease accounts for nearly 40% of deaths among pediatric ESRD patients.[194,248] High prevalence of traditional cardiovascular risk factors, including hypertension (50–75% of uremic children) and hyperlipidemia (70–90% of children on dialysis), accompanies ESRD in childhood. Although kidney transplantation leads to a dramatic improvement in renal function and elimination of many traditional risk factors, cardiovascular disease still accounts for over one-third of the cause of death for patients who received kidney transplant prior to age 21 years.[94]

According to the 2010 NAPRTCS transplantation report, a substantial number of pediatric kidney transplant recipients receive antihypertensive medications during long-term follow-up. The use of antihypertensive medications is highest in the immediate posttransplant period, with 83% of deceased donor and 78% of living donor recipients at the time of transplant. The rates decrease similarly for both groups over time, with 70% of deceased donor recipients and 58% of living donor recipients reportedly receiving antihypertensive medications at 5 years posttransplant.

In addition to the concerns for long-term cardiovascular risk associated with uncontrolled hypertension, a retrospective analysis of pediatric kidney transplant recipients in Cincinnati has also suggested that systolic hypertension independently predicts poor long-term allograft survival.[206] Nocturnal hypertension is relatively common in pediatric kidney transplant recipients. Furthermore, a recent cross-sectional study reported masked hypertension and nocturnal hypertension in a significant portion of pediatric kidney transplant recipients with stable graft function, suggesting the use of ambulatory blood pressure monitoring may be a beneficial tool to identify patients with hidden cardiovascular risk factors.

The development of obesity and/or posttransplant diabetes with tacrolimus and/or corticosteroids is another risk factor for cardiovascular morbidity and mortality. Hypercholesterolemia and hypertriglyceridemia were more commonly seen in the era of cyclosporine use. Weight gain should be monitored closely following transplant to identify children early who are at risk for obesity, as weight gain and increases in body mass index in the first 3 months following transplant are likely to be persistent. Collaboration with pediatric dieticians can be helpful in educating patients and their families about heart-healthy dietary habits, especially since many of the severe dietary restrictions placed on children during ESRD are suddenly lifted following transplant.

In addition, semiannual screening for hypercholesterolemia, hypertriglyceridemia, and impaired glucose tolerance is suggested. Lifestyle modification, including dietary changes and increased physical activity, are typically preferred for young children with hyperlipidemia. The use of 3-hydroxy-3-methylgultaryl-coenzyme A (HMG-CoA) reductase inhibitors (statins) is generally considered safe and effective in children over the age of 8 years; however, there are few data on long-term safety.[37]

Infections After Transplantation

While modern immunosuppression regimens (CNI, MMF, and steroids) have reduced the rate of acute rejection, infectious complications have become more frequent. In particular, pediatric transplant recipients are at increased risk for developing virus-related complications due to immunological naiveté.

Viral Infections

Cytomegalovirus. CMV remains an important opportunistic pathogen following kidney transplant in children. The development of improved diagnostic methods and effective prophylaxis regimens has decreased the mortality previously associated with CMV disease, but morbidity remains high. Rates of CMV infection in pediatric kidney transplant recipients have historically been reported to be as high as 75%. The reported incidence of CMV disease is between 5% and 30%, with disease onset typically within the first 2 months posttransplant.[265]

Valgancyclovir has been demonstrated to be safe and effective for the prevention and treatment of CMV disease in children following solid-organ transplant.[172] Doses for prophylaxis are typically 15 mg/kg (maximum 900 mg/dose) dosed daily, while treatment doses are dosed twice daily. Valgancyclovir dosing should be adjusted for GFR under 60 mL/min/1.73 m^2. CMV-negative recipients of CMV-negative donor kidneys (D–/R–) have the lowest risk (<5%) of developing CMV disease and often do not receive prophylaxis. CMV-positive recipients (R+) are at intermediate risk and are recommended to receive 12 weeks of prophylaxis, although some centers use 2–4 weeks' prophylaxis followed by surveillance and pre-emptive therapy. Finally, the highest-risk group is that of CMV-negative recipients of CMV-positive grafts (D+/R–). Prophylaxis is generally recommended for this highest-risk group for at least 100 days, but some centers extend the period of prophylaxis to 6 months. CMV infection or disease can occur once prophylaxis is discontinued.

Epstein–Barr Virus. Rates of PTLD are higher in children than adults, with just over 2% of pediatric transplant recipients reported to have PTLD by 4 years posttransplant.[245] PTLD in children is often associated with EBV infection, and children who are immunologically naïve to EBV at the time of transplant are at highest risk of developing PTLD.[73] Of the pediatric transplant patients reported in the SRTR from 2005 to 2009, 30–40% were seronegative for EBV at the time of transplant.

PTLD, or its precursor, EBV-related lymphoid hyperplasia, often presents as adenotonsillar hypertrophy in children,[284] but can also develop in the gastrointestinal tract (presenting as chronic diarrhea), peripheral lymph nodes (presenting with lymphadenopathy or frank lymphoma), or within the renal allograft, leading to graft failure. Central nervous system involvement is also described and can be fatal. Therefore, prevention and early recognition of PTLD are essential.

Children who were seronegative for EBV at the time of transplant should be monitored with peripheral blood EBV viral PCR to detect increasing viral load prior to the development of PTLD.[307] The majority of patients will respond to a reduction in immunosuppression, but sometimes anti-B-cell antibodies (e.g., rituximab), T-cell therapy, or chemotherapy are required.[71,72,100,113]

Polyomavirus. The incidence of BK virus nephropathy in pediatric kidney transplant recipients is estimated to be 4.6%.[293] BK virus infection (e.g., viremia) can occur early (within the first month) or late (several years) following kidney transplant in children.[141] Definitive diagnosis of BK nephropathy is obtained only by renal biopsy. Children with BK nephropathy are at greater risk for graft loss.[141]

Prospective monitoring for BK viremia using PCR assays to detect viral DNA with pre-emptive lowering of immunosuppression has been suggested as an effective approach.[111,141,259] BK virus-specific cellular immunity has been associated with viral clearance and underscores the approach of reducing T-cell suppression.[111,310] Other options include treatment with IVIG, cidofovir, or leflunamide, although the efficacy of these is not proven in pediatrics.[16]

Bacterial Infections

UTI are the most common infectious complication following kidney transplant in children, occurring in 15–33% of patients.[151,190] According to the NAPRTCS registry, at 1 year posttransplant antibiotics for UTI prophylaxis are prescribed for 55% of patients with renal dysplasia, 65% of patients diagnosed with reflux nephropathy, and 68% of those with obstructive uropathy.[232] Recurrent UTI has been associated with faster deterioration in graft function in children.[132]

Risk factors for febrile UTI include anatomical abnormalities, dysfunctional bladder, presence of foreign material (e.g., urinary catheter or stents), and baseline immunosuppression. Parenteral antibiotics are indicated for febrile UTI in pediatric transplant patients.

Lower Urinary Tract Symptoms

Even children with non-urological etiologies to their ESRD have been reported to have lower urinary tract symptoms following transplant, including increased bladder capacity, incomplete bladder emptying, night-time or daytime incontinence, and UTIs.[319] Children with dysfunctional voiding can benefit from pelvic floor training and timed voiding to avoid graft damage and dysfunction.[187] Anticholinergic therapy and intermittent catheterization should be continued as medical management of neurogenic bladder following transplantation.

Growth

Impaired linear growth in children with CKD is multifactorial and is mainly due to disturbances in the axis involving growth hormone, IGF, and IGF-binding protein. Despite satisfactory renal function following transplant, spontaneous catch-up growth is often insufficient.

Determinants of growth following transplant include age at the time of transplant, exposure to glucocorticoids, allograft function, and administration of rhGH. Children under the age of 6 years have increased growth rates following transplant compared to older children.[301] Glucocorticoids induce hyporesponsiveness to the action of growth hormone[198,313] and young children on steroid-free immunosuppression protocols have been demonstrated to have improved linear growth compared to children receiving prednisone-based immunosuppression. eGFR at 30 days posttransplant is predictive of long-term height Z-score, with those recipients who have an eGFR <60 mL/min/1.73 m^2 having reduced height Z-score.[81,91] The degree of growth stunting prior to transplant is also predictive of final adult height.[81] Finally, rhGH is effective in improving the growth velocity[92] and increased final adult height[109] of children following kidney transplant.

Non-Adherence in Pediatric Transplantation

Non-adherence is a major problem in pediatric kidney transplant. A recent systematic review estimated that non-adherence accounts for an estimated 44% of graft losses and 23% of late acute rejection episodes.[74] Overall prevalence of non-adherence across 16 studies involving pediatric kidney transplant patients was 31% (weighted mean across 16 studies). Adolescent patients were at higher risk, with weighted mean prevalence of non-adherence of 43% in the same review.

The use of self-reporting of missed doses likely under-represents the true incidence as patients and families are often reluctant to report non-adherence. Missed clinic appointments and schedule tests are also common forms of non-adherence reported for pediatric solid-organ transplant patients.[69] Factors associated with non-adherence include lack of supervision in taking medications, family conflicts, miscommunication between parents and the medical team, and numbers of medications and fastidious schedules of dosing.[66]

Adolescent Issues

Adolescence is an important transition period between childhood and adulthood characterized by a quest for independence and autonomy. This rapidly changing and volatile developmental period places adolescent transplant recipients at increased risk for medication non-adherence, acute rejection episodes, and graft loss.[74,176] Medical management of this population can be challenging and may require specialized, multidisciplinary approaches to improve outcomes.

Psychosocial Development

The adolescent strives to establish an identity independently from parents and other adult authority figures and this can result in oppositional and defiant behaviors. The need for independence coupled with a sense of invulnerability and evolving capacity for abstract thought can result in illogical thinking and risk-taking behaviors. Beyond the normal psychological conflicts present during adolescence, transplant recipients are exposed to additional psychosocial stress related to their chronic illness. Developmental delay, issues with body image from drug side effects, difficulty interacting with peers, fastidious schedules required of immunosuppressant medication regimens, symptoms of posttraumatic stress, and family disruption due to financial burden or role strain may all exacerbate psychosocial difficulties in the transplanted adolescent. Collaboration with psychologists, psychiatrists, and social workers may be beneficial in the early identification and intensified treatment of high-risk individuals.

Puberty

Onset of puberty is an important milestone during adolescence. There are few reports describing puberty and sexual maturity in children following kidney transplant, with most focusing on pubertal growth velocity. The majority of children achieve normal puberty following transplant, but many may have a delayed onset and shortened duration of pubertal growth spurt.[299] In general, onset of puberty is often delayed in children who have delayed bone age compared to their chronological age.[106]

Sexuality and Body Image

Sexuality-related issues, including prevention of sexually transmitted diseases and family planning, also need to be addressed with teenage patients. Adolescent female transplant recipients have successfully become pregnant while receiving cyclosporine or tacrolimus. The effect of contraception on the metabolism of immunosuppressant medications needs to be considered when counseling adolescent girls about pregnancy prevention. In addition, the teratogenicity of certain immunosuppressant medications (notably MMF and CNIs) and antihypertensive medications (e.g., angiotensin-converting enzyme inhibitors) should be explained to the adolescent female and her family.

Teenagers also need to balance their developing sexuality with changes in body image following transplant. It is difficult for teenagers to accept the cosmetic side effects of immunosuppressant medications, including weight gain, cushingoid features, acne, and gum hypertrophy. The accompanying psychological stress and impact on self-image for teenagers can provide a dangerous disincentive to adhere to medication regimens.

Transitional Care

Several reports have demonstrated a high risk of graft failure, particularly at the time of transfer from pediatric to adult care.[271,329] It is increasingly recognized for other chronic conditions (e.g., survivors of pediatric cancer) that adolescents and young adults (aged 14–29 years) are more vulnerable to adverse outcomes and probably deserve a different approach to healthcare delivery than that used for younger children or older adults.[298] The identification of strategies to facilitate transition to adult healthcare delivery systems and improve outcomes for adolescent transplant recipients has become a priority for the pediatric transplant community.[28,330]

Transition is a process that includes a purposeful, planned effort to prepare the patient to move from pediatric care that is caregiver-directed to adult care that requires disease self-management. Although the timing should be individualized, there is a growing consensus that preparation for transition should begin early (between 10 and 14 years of age). There is significant variability in the attainment of the skills needed to accomplish successful transition and therefore transfer to an adult unit may not be optimally decided based solely on a patient's age.

Critical milestones for patients to achieve a successful transfer to adult care include: (1) the understanding and ability to describe the underlying cause of ESRD and need for transplant; (2) awareness of the long- and short-term implications of transplant on their overall health; (3) comprehension of the impact of their condition on their reproductive health; (4) demonstration of a sense of responsibility for their own healthcare; (5) capacity to provide most self-care independently; and (6) an expressed readiness to move into adulthood.[28,330]

The application of transitional care has been described in a variety of forms, ranging from having adult providers meet the patient prior to transfer, having a pediatric team member accompany patients to their first adult clinic visit, overlapping or alternating visits between pediatric and adult teams, to fully shared adolescent/young adult transplant clinics. Mechanisms to monitor and assess the readiness for transfer have been described but are not standardized. Furthermore, there are still significant systems issues (insurance coverage, healthcare policies, resource allocations) to overcome.

There is a need for longitudinal analyses of the outcomes of children who are transitioned to adult care. A great opportunity exists to form collaborative efforts between pediatric and adult transplant communities to improve outcomes for this high-risk population.

REFERENCES

1. Abbott KC, Sawyers ES, Oliver Iii JD, et al. Graft loss due to recurrent focal segmental glomerulosclerosis in renal transplant recipients in the United States. Am J Kidney Dis 2001;37:366–73.
2. Abraham EC, Wilson AC, Goebel J. Current kidney allocation rules and their impact on a pediatric transplant center. Am J Transplant 2009;9:404–8.
3. Abuali MM, Arnon R, Posada R. An update on immunizations before and after transplantation in the pediatric solid organ transplant recipient. Pediatr Transplant 2011;15:770–7.
4. Adams J, Mehls O, Wiesel M. Pediatric renal transplantation and the dysfunctional bladder. Transpl Int 2004;17:596–602.
5. Agarwal S, Oak N, Siddique J, et al. Changes in pediatric renal transplantation after implementation of the revised deceased donor kidney allocation policy. Am J Transplant 2009;9:1237–42.
6. Al-Akash SI, Almond PS, Savell Jr VH, et al. Eculizumab induces long-term remission in recurrent post-transplant HUS associated with C3 gene mutation. Pediatr Nephrol 2011;26:613–9.
7. Alam S, Sheldon C. Urological issues in pediatric renal transplantation. Curr Opin Urol 2008;18:413–8.
8. Al-Eisa A, Naseef M, Al-Hamad N, et al. Chronic renal failure in Kuwaiti children: an eight-year experience. Pediatr Nephrol 2005;20:1781–5.
9. Alexopoulos S, Lightner A, Concepcion W, et al. Pediatric kidney recipients with small capacity, defunctionalized urinary bladders receiving adult-sized kidney without prior bladder augmentation. Transplantation 2011;91:452–6.
10. Ali E-TA, Abdelraheem M, Mohamed R, et al. Chronic renal failure in Sudanese children: aetiology and outcomes. Pediatr Nephrol 2009;24:349–53.
11. Amaral S, Patzer RE, Kutner N, et al. Racial disparities in access to pediatric kidney transplantation since share 35. J Am Soc Nephrol 2012;23:1069–77.
12. Andreoli SP, Brewer ED, Watkins S, et al. American Society of Pediatric Nephrology position paper on linking reimbursement to quality of care. J Am Soc Nephrol 2005;16:2263–9.
13. Andresdottir MB, Assmann KJ, Hoitsma AJ, et al. Recurrence of type I membranoproliferative glomerulonephritis after renal transplantation: analysis of the incidence, risk factors, and impact on graft survival. Transplantation 1997;63:1628–33.
14. Angelo JR, Bell CS, Braun MC. Allograft failure in kidney transplant recipients with membranoproliferative glomerulonephritis. Am J Kidney Dis 2011;57:291–9.
15. Appel GB, Cook HT, Hageman G, et al. Membranoproliferative glomerulonephritis type II (dense deposit disease): an update. J Am Soc Nephrol 2005;16:1392–403.
16. Araya CE, Garin EH, Neiberger RE, et al. Leflunomide therapy for BK virus allograft nephropathy in pediatric and young adult kidney transplant recipients. Pediatr Transplant 2010;14:145–50.
17. Ariceta G, Besbas N, Johnson S, et al. Guideline for the investigation and initial therapy of diarrhea-negative hemolytic uremic syndrome. Pediatr Nephrol 2009;24:687–96.
18. Auber F, Jeanpierre C, Denamur E, et al. Management of Wilms tumors in Drash and Frasier syndromes. Pediatr Blood Cancer 2009;52:55–9.
19. Baez-Trinidad LG, Lendvay TS, Broecker BH, et al. Efficacy of nephrectomy for the treatment of nephrogenic hypertension in a pediatric population. J Urol 2003;170:1655–7, discussion 1658.
20. Banerjee R, Hersh AL, Newland J, et al. *Streptococcus pneumoniae*-associated hemolytic uremic syndrome among children in North America. Pediatr Infect Dis J 2011;30:736–9.
21. Barrero R, Fijo J, Fernandez-Hurtado M, et al. Vesicoureteral reflux after kidney transplantation in children. Pediatr Transplant 2007;11:498–503.
22. Bartosh SM, Fine RN, Sullivan EK. Outcome after transplantation of young patients with systemic lupus erythematosus: a report of the North American pediatric renal transplant cooperative study. Transplantation 2001;72:973–8.
23. Bartosh SM, Knechtle SJ, Sollinger HW. Campath-1H use in pediatric renal transplantation. Am J Transplant 2005;5:1569–73.
24. Baum MA. Outcomes after renal transplantation for FSGS in children. Pediatr Transplant 2004;8:329–33.
25. Baum MA, Stablein DM, Panzarino VM, et al. Loss of living donor renal allograft survival advantage in children with focal segmental glomerulosclerosis. Kidney Int 2001;59:328–33.
26. Becker-Cohen R, Bruschi M, Rinat C, et al. Recurrent nephrotic syndrome in homozygous truncating NPHS2 mutation is not due to anti-podocin antibodies. Am J Transplant 2007;7:256–60.
27. Bek K, Akman S, Bilge I, et al. Chronic kidney disease in children in Turkey. Pediatr Nephrol 2009;24:797–806.
28. Bell LE, Bartosh SM, Davis CL, et al. Adolescent transition to adult care in solid organ transplantation: a consensus conference report. Am J Transplant 2008;8:2230–42.
29. Benfield MR, Bartosh S, Ikle D, et al. A randomized double-blind, placebo controlled trial of steroid withdrawal after pediatric renal transplantation. Am J Transplant 2010;10:81–8.
30. Benfield MR, Tejani A, Harmon WE, et al. A randomized multicenter trial of OKT3 mAbs induction compared with intravenous cyclosporine in pediatric renal transplantation. Pediatr Transplant 2005;9:282–92.
31. Benoit G, Machuca E, Antignac C. Hereditary nephrotic syndrome: a systematic approach for genetic testing and a review of associated podocyte gene mutations. Pediatr Nephrol 2010;25:1621–32.
32. Bergstralh EJ, Monico CG, Lieske JC, et al. Transplantation outcomes in primary hyperoxaluria. Am J Transplant 2010;10:2493–501.
33. Bertelli R, Ginevri F, Caridi G, et al. Recurrence of focal segmental glomerulosclerosis after renal transplantation in patients with mutations of podocin. Am J Kidney Dis 2003;41:1314–21.
34. Bienaime F, Dragon-Durey MA, Regnier CH, et al. Mutations in components of complement influence the outcome of factor I-associated atypical hemolytic uremic syndrome. Kidney Int 2010;77:339–49.
35. Billing H, Rieger S, Ovens J, et al. Successful treatment of chronic antibody-mediated rejection with IVIG and rituximab in pediatric renal transplant recipients. Transplantation 2008;86:1214–21.
36. Bouchot O, Guillonneau B, Cantarovich D, et al. Vesicoureteral reflux in the renal transplantation candidate. Eur Urol 1991;20:26–8.
37. Braamskamp MJ, Wijburg FA, Wiegman A. Drug therapy of hypercholesterolaemia in children and adolescents. Drugs 2012;72:759–72.
38. Braun MC, Stablein DM, Hamiwka LA, et al. Recurrence of membranoproliferative glomerulonephritis type II in renal allografts: the North American Pediatric Renal Transplant Cooperative Study experience. J Am Soc Nephrol 2005;16:2225–33.
39. Bresin E, Daina E, Noris M, et al. Outcome of renal transplantation in patients with non-Shiga toxin-associated hemolytic uremic syndrome: prognostic significance of genetic background. Clin J Am Soc Nephrol 2006;1:88–99.
40. Browne G, Brown PA, Tomson CR, et al. Retransplantation in Alport post-transplant anti-GBM disease. Kidney Int 2004;65:675–81.
41. Broyer M, Guest G, Gagnadoux MF. Growth rate in children receiving alternate-day corticosteroid treatment after kidney transplantation. J Pediatr 1992;120:721–5.

42. Burlingham WJ, Grailer AP, Heisey DM, et al. The effect of tolerance to noninherited maternal HLA antigens on the survival of renal transplants from sibling donors. N Engl J Med 1998;339:1657–64.
43. Butani L, Perez RV. Effect of pretransplant dialysis modality and duration on long-term outcomes of children receiving renal transplants. Transplantation 2011;91:447–51.
44. Byrne MC, Budisavljevic MN, Fan Z, et al. Renal transplant in patients with Alport's syndrome. Am J Kidney Dis 2002;39:769–75.
45. Cahen R, Trolliet P, Dijoud F, et al. Severe recurrence of type I membranoproliferative glomerulonephritis after transplantation: remission on steroids and cyclophosphamide. Transplant Proc 1995;27:1746–7.
46. Canaud G, Dion D, Zuber J, et al. Recurrence of nephrotic syndrome after transplantation in a mixed population of children and adults: course of glomerular lesions and value of the Columbia classification of histological variants of focal and segmental glomerulosclerosis (FSGS). Nephrol Dial Transplant 2010;25:1321–8.
47. Capozza N, Collura G, Falappa P, et al. Renal embolization as an alternative to surgical nephrectomy in children. Transplant Proc 2007;39:1782–4.
48. Carraro M, Zennaro C, Candiano G, et al. Nephrotic urine prevents increased rat glomerular albumin permeability induced by serum from the same patient with idiopathic nephrotic syndrome. Nephrol Dial Transplant 2003;18:689–93.
49. Cattran D, Neogi T, Sharma R, et al. Serial estimates of serum permeability activity and clinical correlates in patients with native kidney focal segmental glomerulosclerosis. J Am Soc Nephrol 2003;14:448–53.
50. Cavallini M, Di Zazzo G, Giordano U, et al. Long-term cardiovascular effects of pre-transplant native kidney nephrectomy in children. Pediatr Nephrol 2010;25:2523–9.
51. Cayci FS, Cakar N, Hancer VS, et al. Eculizumab therapy in a child with hemolytic uremic syndrome and CFI mutation. Pediatr Nephrol 2012;27:2321–31.
52. Charytan D, Torre A, Khurana M, et al. Allograft rejection and glomerular basement membrane antibodies in Alport's syndrome. J Nephrol 2004;17:431–5.
53. Chaudhuri A, Salvatierra Jr O, Alexander SR, et al. Option of pre-emptive nephrectomy and renal transplantation for Bartter's syndrome. Pediatr Transplant 2006;10:266–70.
54. Chavers BM, Chang YC, Gillingham KJ, et al. Pediatric kidney transplantation using a novel protocol of rapid (6-day) discontinuation of prednisone: 2-year results. Transplantation 2009;88:237–41.
55. Cheong HI, Han HW, Park HW, et al. Early recurrent nephrotic syndrome after renal transplantation in children with focal segmental glomerulosclerosis. Nephrol Dial Transplant 2000;15:78–81.
56. Cherikh WS, Kauffman HM, Mcbride MA, et al. Association of the type of induction immunosuppression with posttransplant lymphoproliferative disorder, graft survival, and patient survival after primary kidney transplantation. Transplantation 2003;76:1289–93.
57. Choi JY, Kwon OJ, Kang CM. The effect of donor–recipient relationship on long-term outcomes of living related donor renal transplantation. Transplant Proc 2012;44:257–60.
58. Cibrik DM, Kaplan B, Campbell DA, et al. Renal allograft survival in transplant recipients with focal segmental glomerulosclerosis. Am J Transplant 2003;3:64–7.
59. Clatworthy MR, Friend PJ, Calne RY, et al. Alemtuzumab (Campath-1H) for the treatment of acute rejection in kidney transplant recipients: long-term follow-up. Transplantation 2009;87:1092–5.
60. Coffman TM, Himmelstein S, Best C, et al. Post-transplant hypertension in the rat: effects of captopril and native nephrectomy. Kidney Int 1989;36:35–40.
61. Colleen Hastings M, Wyatt RJ, Lau KK, et al. Five years' experience with thymoglobulin induction in a pediatric renal transplant population. Pediatr Transplant 2006;10:805–10.
62. Dale-Shall AW, Smith JM, Mcbride MA, et al. The relationship of donor source and age on short- and long-term allograft survival in pediatric renal transplantation. Pediatr Transplant 2009;13:711–8.
63. Dall'amico R, Ghiggeri G, Carraro M, et al. Prediction and treatment of recurrent focal segmental glomerulosclerosis after renal transplantation in children. Am J Kidney Dis 1999;34:1048–55.
64. Dehan P, Van Den Heuvel LPWJ, Smeets HJM, et al. Identification of post-transplant anti-α5(IV) collagen alloantibodies in X-linked Alport syndrome. Nephrol Dial Transplant 1996;11:1983–8.
65. Del Mar Fernandez De Gatta M, Santos-Buelga D, Dominguez-Gil A, et al. Immunosuppressive therapy for paediatric transplant patients: pharmacokinetic considerations. Clin Pharmacokinet 2002;41:115–35.
66. Delucchi A, Gutierrez H, Arrellano P, et al. Factors that influence nonadherence in immunosuppressant treatment in pediatric transplant recipients: a proposal for an educational strategy. Transplant Proc 2008;40:3241–3.
67. De Sandes-Freitas TV, Holanda-Cavalcanti A, Mastroianni-Kirsztajn G, et al. Late presentation of Alport posttransplantation anti-glomerular basement membrane disease. Transplant Proc 2011;43:4000–1.
68. De Serres SA, Mfarrej BG, Magee CN, et al. Immune profile of pediatric renal transplant recipients following alemtuzumab induction. J Am Soc Nephrol 2012;23:174–82.
69. Dew MA, Dabbs AD, Myaskovsky L, et al. Meta-analysis of medical regimen adherence outcomes in pediatric solid organ transplantation. Transplantation 2009;88:736–46.
70. Dharnidharka VR, Agodoa LY, Abbott KC. Effects of urinary tract infection on outcomes after renal transplantation in children. Clin J Am Soc Nephrol 2007;2:100–6.
71. Dharnidharka VR, Araya CE. Post-transplant lymphoproliferative disease. Pediatr Nephrol 2009;24:731–6.
72. Dharnidharka VR, Gupta S. PTLD treatment: reducing the chemotherapy burden through addition of rituximab. Pediatr Transplant 2010;14:10–1.
73. Dharnidharka VR, Lamb KE, Gregg JA, et al. Associations between EBV serostatus and organ transplant type in PTLD risk: an analysis of the SRTR National Registry Data in the United States. Am J Transplant 2012;12:976–83.
74. Dobbels F, Ruppar T, De Geest S, et al. Adherence to the immunosuppressive regimen in pediatric kidney transplant recipients: a systematic review. Pediatr Transplant 2010;14:603–13.
75. Dolan N, Waldron M, O'Connell M, et al. Basiliximab induced non-cardiogenic pulmonary edema in two pediatric renal transplant recipients. Pediatr Nephrol 2009;24:2261–5.
76. Dragon-Durey MA, Fremeaux-Bacchi V, Loirat C, et al. Heterozygous and homozygous factor h deficiencies associated with hemolytic uremic syndrome or membranoproliferative glomerulonephritis: report and genetic analysis of 16 cases. J Am Soc Nephrol 2004;15:787–95.
77. Dragon-Durey M-A, Loirat C, Cloarec S, et al. Anti-factor H autoantibodies associated with atypical hemolytic uremic syndrome. J Am Soc Nephrol 2005;16:555–63.
78. Dubourg L, Cochat P, Hadj-Aissa A, et al. Better long-term functional adaptation to the child's size with pediatric compared to adult kidney donors. Kidney Int 2002;62:1454–60.
79. El-Ghoneimi A, Abou-Hashim H, Bonnard A, et al. Retroperitoneal laparoscopic nephrectomy in children: at last the gold standard? J Pediatr Urol 2006;2:357–63.
80. Ellis D, Shapiro R, Moritz M, et al. Renal transplantation in children managed with lymphocyte depleting agents and low-dose maintenance tacrolimus monotherapy. Transplantation 2007;83:1563–70.
81. Englund MS, Tyden G, Wikstad I, et al. Growth impairment at renal transplantation – a determinant of growth and final height. Pediatr Transplant 2003;7:192–9.
82. Esparza-Gordillo J, Jorge EGD, Buil A, et al. Predisposition to atypical hemolytic uremic syndrome involves the concurrence of different susceptibility alleles in the regulators of complement activation gene cluster in 1q32. Hum Mol Genet 2005;14:703–12.
83. European best practice guidelines for renal transplantation. Section IV: long-term management of the transplant recipient. IV.11 Paediatrics (specific problems). Nephrol Dial Transplant 2002;17(Suppl. 4):55–8.
84. Eytan Mor MD, Weismann I. Current treatment for primary hyperoxaluria type 1: when should liver/kidney transplantation be considered. Pediatr Transplant 2009;13:805–7.
85. Fargue S, Harambat J, Gagnadoux MF, et al. Effect of conservative treatment on the renal outcome of children with primary hyperoxaluria type 1. Kidney Int 2009;76:767–73.

86. Faul C, Donnelly M, Merscher-Gomez S, et al. The actin cytoskeleton of kidney podocytes is a direct target of the antiproteinuric effect of cyclosporine A. Nat Med 2008;14:931–8.
87. Faull RJ, Hollett P, Mcdonald SP. Lymphoproliferative disease after renal transplantation in Australia and New Zealand. Transplantation 2005;80:193–7.
88. Fernberg P, Edgren G, Adami J, et al. Time trends in risk and risk determinants of non-Hodgkin lymphoma in solid organ transplant recipients. Am J Transplant 2011;11:2472–82.
89. Ferraris JR, Ramirez JA, Ruiz S, et al. Shiga toxin-associated hemolytic uremic syndrome: absence of recurrence after renal transplantation. Pediatr Nephrol 2002;17:809–14.
90. Filler G, Foster J, Berard R, et al. Age-dependency of mycophenolate mofetil dosing in combination with tacrolimus after pediatric renal transplantation. Transplant Proc 2004;36:1327–31.
91. Fine RN, Martz K, Stablein D. What have 20 years of data from the North American Pediatric Renal Transplant Cooperative Study taught us about growth following renal transplantation in infants, children, and adolescents with end-stage renal disease? Pediatr Nephrol 2010;25:739–46.
92. Fine RN, Stablein D, Cohen AH, et al. Recombinant human growth hormone post-renal transplantation in children: a randomized controlled study of the NAPRTCS. Kidney Int 2002;62:688–96.
93. Florman S, Benchimol C, Lieberman K, et al. Fulminant recurrence of atypical hemolytic uremic syndrome during a calcineurin inhibitor-free immunosuppression regimen. Pediatr Transplant 2002;6:352–5.
94. Foster BJ, Dahhou M, Zhang X, et al. Change in mortality risk over time in young kidney transplant recipients. Am J Transplant 2011;11:2432–42.
95. Fremeaux-Bacchi V, Arzouk N, Ferlicot S, et al. Recurrence of HUS due to CD46/MCP mutation after renal transplantation: a role for endothelial microchimerism. Am J Transplant 2007; 7:2047–51.
96. Fremeaux-Bacchi V, Weiss L, Brun P, et al. Selective disappearance of C3NeF IgG autoantibody in the plasma of a patient with membranoproliferative glomerulonephritis following renal transplantation. Nephrol Dial Transplant 1994;9:811–4.
97. Fryer JP, Benedetti E, Gillingham K, et al. Steroid-related complications in pediatric kidney transplant recipients in the cyclosporine era. Transplant Proc 1994;26:91–2.
98. Fuentes GM, Meseguer CG, Carrion AP, et al. Long-term outcome of focal segmental glomerulosclerosis after pediatric renal transplantation. Pediatr Nephrol 2010;25:529–34.
99. Fujisawa M, Iijima K, Ishimura T, et al. Long-term outcome of focal segmental glomerulosclerosis after Japanese pediatric renal transplantation. Pediatr Nephrol 2002;17:165–8.
100. Gallego S, Llort A, Gros L, et al. Post-transplant lymphoproliferative disorders in children: the role of chemotherapy in the era of rituximab. Pediatr Transplant 2010;14:61–6.
101. Garg AX, Suri RS, Barrowman N, et al. Long-term renal prognosis of diarrhea-associated hemolytic uremic syndrome: a systematic review, meta-analysis, and meta-regression. JAMA 2003;290:1360–70.
102. Geelen JM, Monnens LA, Levtchenko EN. Follow-up and treatment of adults with cystinosis in the Netherlands. Nephrol Dial Transplant 2002;17:1766–70.
103. Geelen J, Van Den Dries K, Roos A, et al. A missense mutation in factor I (IF) predisposes to atypical haemolytic uraemic syndrome. Pediatr Nephrol 2007;22:371–5.
104. Genc G, Ozkaya O, Aygun C, et al. Vaccination status of children considered for renal transplants: missed opportunities for vaccine preventable diseases. Exp Clin Transplant 2012;10:314–8.
105. Ghane Sharbaf F, Bitzan M, Szymanski KM, et al. Native nephrectomy prior to pediatric kidney transplantation: biological and clinical aspects. Pediatr Nephrol 2012;27:1179–88.
106. Ghanem ME, Emam ME, Albaghdady LA, et al. Effect of childhood kidney transplantation on puberty. Fertil Steril 2010;94:2248–52.
107. Ghiggeri GM, Artero M, Carraro M, et al. Glomerular albumin permeability as an in vitro model for characterizing the mechanism of focal glomerulosclerosis and predicting post-transplant recurrence. Pediatr Transplant 2004;8:339–43.
108. Ghoneim MA, Refaie AF. Is matching for human leukocyte antigen-DR beneficial in pediatric kidney transplantation? Nat Clin Pract Nephrol 2009;5:70–1.
109. Gil S, Vaiani E, Guercio G, et al. Effectiveness of rhGH treatment on final height of renal-transplant recipients in childhood. Pediatr Nephrol 2012;27:1005–9.
110. Gillen DL, Stehman-Breen CO, Smith JM, et al. Survival advantage of pediatric recipients of a first kidney transplant among children awaiting kidney transplantation. Am J Transplant 2008;8:2600–6.
111. Ginevri F, Azzi A, Hirsch HH, et al. Prospective monitoring of polyomavirus BK replication and impact of pre-emptive intervention in pediatric kidney recipients. Am J Transplant 2007;7:2727–35.
112. Giordano M, Castellano G, Messina G, et al. Preservation of renal function in atypical hemolytic uremic syndrome by eculizumab: a case report. Pediatrics 2012;130:e1385–8.
113. Giraldi E, Provenzi M, Fiocchi R, et al. Fludarabine, cyclophosphamide, doxorubicin (FCD), and rituximab: a remission induction therapy for aggressive pediatric post-transplant lymphoproliferative disease (PTLD). Pediatr Blood Cancer 2011; 57:324–8.
114. Gobel J, Olbricht CJ, Offner G, et al. Kidney transplantation in Alport's syndrome: long-term outcome and allograft anti-GBM nephritis. Clin Nephrol 1992;38:299–304.
115. Gohh RY, Yango AF, Morrissey PE, et al. Preemptive plasmapheresis and recurrence of FSGS in high-risk renal transplant recipients. Am J Transplant 2005;5:2907–12.
116. Goldsmith PJ, Asthana S, Fitzpatrick M, et al. Transplantation of adult-sized kidneys in low-weight pediatric recipients achieves short-term outcomes comparable to size-matched grafts. Pediatr Transplant 2010;14:919–24.
117. Gonzalez D, Garcia CD, Azocar M, et al. Growth of kidney-transplanted pediatric patients treated with sirolimus. Pediatr Nephrol 2011;26:961–6.
118. Gonzalez E, Ettenger R, Rianthavorn P, et al. Preemptive plasmapheresis and recurrence of focal segmental glomerulosclerosis in pediatric renal transplantation. Pediatr Transplant 2011; 15:495–501.
119. Gould LH, Demma L, Jones TF, et al. Hemolytic uremic syndrome and death in persons with *Escherichia coli* O157:H7 infection, foodborne diseases active surveillance network sites, 2000–2006. Clin Infect Dis 2009;49:1480–5.
120. Grenda R, Watson A, Trompeter R, et al. A randomized trial to assess the impact of early steroid withdrawal on growth in pediatric renal transplantation: the TWIST study. Am J Transplant 2010;10:828–36.
121. Gritsch HA, Veale JL, Leichtman AB, et al. Should pediatric patients wait for HLA-DR-matched renal transplants? Am J Transplant 2008;8:2056–61.
122. Gross O, Netzer KO, Lambrecht R, et al. Meta-analysis of genotype–phenotype correlation in X-linked Alport syndrome: impact on clinical counselling. Nephrol Dial Transplant 2002;17:1218–27.
123. Gross O, Weber M, Fries JW, et al. Living donor kidney transplantation from relatives with mild urinary abnormalities in Alport syndrome: long-term risk, benefit and outcome. Nephrol Dial Transplant 2009;24:1626–30.
124. Gumber MR, Kute VB, Goplani KR, et al. Outcome of renal transplantation in Alport's syndrome: a single-center experience. Transplant Proc 2012;44:261–3.
125. Halloran PF, Melk A. Renal senescence, cellular senescence, and their relevance to nephrology and transplantation. Adv Nephrol Necker Hosp 2001;31:273–83.
126. Han SS, Sun HK, Lee JP, et al. Outcome of renal allograft in patients with Henoch–Schönlein nephritis: single-center experience and systematic review. Transplantation 2010;89:721–6.
127. Harada H, Seki T, Nonomura K, et al. Pre-emptive renal transplantation in children. Int J Urol 2001;8:205–11.
128. Harambat J, Van Stralen KJ, Kim JJ, et al. Epidemiology of chronic kidney disease in children. Pediatr Nephrol 2012;27:363–73.
129. Hattori M, Akioka Y, Chikamoto H, et al. Increase of integrin-linked kinase activity in cultured podocytes upon stimulation with plasma from patients with recurrent FSGS. Am J Transplant 2008;8:1550–6.

130. Heidotting NA, Ahlenstiel T, Kreuzer M, et al. The influence of low donor age, living related donation and pre-emptive transplantation on end-organ damage based on arterial hypertension after paediatric kidney transplantation. Nephrol Dial Transplant 2012;27:1672–6.
131. Herthelius M, Celsi G, Edstrom Halling S, et al. Renal transplantation in infants and small children. Pediatr Nephrol 2012;27:145–50.
132. Herthelius M, Oborn H. Urinary tract infections and bladder dysfunction after renal transplantation in children. J Urol 2007;177:1883–6.
133. Hickey CA, Beattie TJ, Cowieson J, et al. Early volume expansion during diarrhea and relative nephroprotection during subsequent hemolytic uremic syndrome. Arch Pediatr Adolesc Med 2011;165:884–9.
134. Hickson LJ, Gera M, Amer H, et al. Kidney transplantation for primary focal segmental glomerulosclerosis: outcomes and response to therapy for recurrence. Transplantation 2009;87:1232–9.
135. Hocker B, Weber LT, Feneberg R, et al. Improved growth and cardiovascular risk after late steroid withdrawal: 2-year results of a prospective, randomised trial in paediatric renal transplantation. Nephrol Dial Transplant 2010;25:617–24.
136. Hristea D, Hadaya K, Marangon N, et al. Successful treatment of recurrent focal segmental glomerulosclerosis after kidney transplantation by plasmapheresis and rituximab. Transpl Int 2007;20:102–5.
137. Huang K, Ferris ME, Andreoni KA, et al. The differential effect of race among pediatric kidney transplant recipients with focal segmental glomerulosclerosis. Am J Kidney Dis 2004;43: 1082–90.
138. Hubsch H, Montane B, Abitbol C, et al. Recurrent focal glomerulosclerosis in pediatric renal allografts: the Miami experience. Pediatr Nephrol 2005;20:210–6.
139. Hwang AH, Cho YW, Cicciarelli J, et al. Risk factors for short- and long-term survival of primary cadaveric renal allografts in pediatric recipients: a UNOS analysis. Transplantation 2005;80:466–70.
140. Hymes LC, Greenbaum L, Amaral SG, et al. Surveillance renal transplant biopsies and subclinical rejection at three months post-transplant in pediatric recipients. Pediatr Transplant 2007;11:536–9.
141. Hymes LC, Warshaw BL. Polyomavirus (BK) in pediatric renal transplants: evaluation of viremic patients with and without BK associated nephritis. Pediatr Transplant 2006;10:920–2.
142. Hymes LC, Warshaw BL. Five-year experience using sirolimus-based, calcineurin inhibitor-free immunosuppression in pediatric renal transplantation. Pediatr Transplant 2011;15:437–41.
143. Hymes LC, Warshaw BL. Linear growth in pediatric renal transplant recipients receiving sirolimus. Pediatr Transplant 2011;15:570–2.
144. Ibanez JP, Monteverde ML, Diaz MA, et al. Sirolimus in chronic allograft nephropathy in pediatric recipients. Pediatr Transplant 2007;11:777–80.
145. Irish A. Hypercoagulability in renal transplant recipients. Identifying patients at risk of renal allograft thrombosis and evaluating strategies for prevention. Am J Cardiovasc Drugs 2004;4:139–49.
146. Island ER, Gonzalez-Pinto IM, Tsai HL, et al. Successful treatment with bortezomib of a refractory humoral rejection of the intestine after multivisceral transplantation. Clin Transpl 2009;465–9.
147. Ito S, Takata A, Hataya H, et al. Isolated diffuse mesangial sclerosis and Wilms tumor suppressor gene. J Pediatr 2001;138:425–7.
148. Jabs K, Sullivan EK, Avner ED, et al. Alternate-day steroid dosing improves growth without adversely affecting graft survival or long-term graft function. A report of the North American Pediatric Renal Transplant Cooperative Study. Transplantation 1996;61:31–6.
149. Jais JP, Knebelmann B, Giatras I, et al. X-linked Alport syndrome: natural history and genotype–phenotype correlations in girls and women belonging to 195 families: a "European Community Alport Syndrome Concerted Action" study. J Am Soc Nephrol 2003;14:2603–10.
150. Jefferson JA, Lemmink HH, Hughes AE, et al. Autosomal dominant Alport syndrome linked to the type IV collage alpha 3 and alpha 4 genes (COL4A3 and COL4A4). Nephrol Dial Transplant 1997;12:1595–9.
151. John U, Everding AS, Kuwertz-Broking E, et al. High prevalence of febrile urinary tract infections after paediatric renal transplantation. Nephrol Dial Transplant 2006;21:3269–74.
152. Johnson RJ, Fuggle SV, Mumford L, et al. A New UK 2006 National Kidney Allocation Scheme for deceased heart-beating donor kidneys. Transplantation 2010;89:387–94.
153. Jonas MM, Zilleruelo GE, Larue SI, et al. Hepatitis C infection in a pediatric dialysis population. Pediatrics 1992;89:707–9.
154. Jungraithmayr TC, Hofer K, Cochat P, et al. Screening for NPHS2 mutations may help predict FSGS recurrence after transplantation. J Am Soc Nephrol 2011;22:579–85.
155. Kamal Aziz A, Mousson C, Berthoux F, et al. Renal transplantation outcome in selected recipients with IgA nephropathy as native disease: a bicentric study. Ann Transplant 2012;17:45–51.
156. Kamel MH, Rampersad A, Mohan P, et al. Cadaveric kidney transplantation in children<or =20 kg in weight: long-term single-center experience. Transplant Proc 2005;37:685–6.
157. Kanaan N, Mourad G, Thervet E, et al. Recurrence and graft loss after kidney transplantation for Henoch–Schönlein purpura nephritis: a multicenter analysis. Clin J Am Soc Nephrol 2011;6:1768–72.
158. Kasiske BL, Chakkera HA, Louis TA, et al. A meta-analysis of immunosuppression withdrawal trials in renal transplantation. J Am Soc Nephrol 2000;11:1910–7.
159. Kasiske BL, Snyder JJ, Matas AJ, et al. Preemptive kidney transplantation: the advantage and the advantaged. J Am Soc Nephrol 2002;13:1358–64.
160. Keller AK, Jorgensen TM, Jespersen B. Identification of risk factors for vascular thrombosis may reduce early renal graft loss: a review of recent literature. J Transplant 2012;2012:793461.
161. Kim C, Mckay K, Docimo SG. Laparoscopic nephrectomy in children: systematic review of transperitoneal and retroperitoneal approaches. Urology 2009;73:280–4.
162. Kim MS, Primack W, Harmon WE. Congenital nephrotic syndrome: preemptive bilateral nephrectomy and dialysis before renal transplantation. J Am Soc Nephrol 1992;3:260–3.
163. Kim MS, Stablein D, Harmon WE. Renal transplantation in children with congenital nephrotic syndrome: a report of the North American Pediatric Renal Transplant Cooperative Study (NAPRTCS). Pediatr Transplant 1998;2:305–8.
164. Kirk AD, Cherikh WS, Ring M, et al. Dissociation of depletional induction and posttransplant lymphoproliferative disease in kidney recipients treated with alemtuzumab. Am J Transplant 2007;7:2619–25.
165. Kist-Van Holthe JE, Ho PL, Stablein D, et al. Outcome of renal transplantation for Wilms' tumor and Denys-Drash syndrome: a report of the North American Pediatric Renal Transplant Cooperative Study. Pediatr Transplant 2005;9:305–10.
166. Klamt B, Koziell A, Poulat F, et al. Frasier syndrome is caused by defective alternative splicing of WT1 leading to an altered ratio of WT1 +/–KTS splice isoforms. Hum Mol Genet 1998;7:709–14.
167. Kovacevic L, Reid CJ, Rigden SP. Management of congenital nephrotic syndrome. Pediatr Nephrol 2003;18:426–30.
168. Kramer A, Stel VS, Geskus RB, et al. The effect of timing of the first kidney transplantation on survival in children initiating renal replacement therapy. Nephrol Dial Transplant 2012;27: 1256–64.
169. Kravarusic D, Sigalet DL, Hamiwka LA, et al. Persistent post-transplant polyuria managed by bilateral native-kidney laparoscopic nephrectomy. Pediatr Nephrol 2006;21:880–2.
170. Krogvold L, Henrichsen T, Bjerre A, et al. Clinical aspects of a nationwide epidemic of severe haemolytic uremic syndrome (HUS) in children. Scand J Trauma Resusc Emerg Med 2011;19:44.
171. Langlois V, Geary D, Murray L, et al. Polyuria and proteinuria in cystinosis have no impact on renal transplantation. A report of the North American Pediatric Renal Transplant Cooperative Study. Pediatr Nephrol 2000;15:7–10.
172. Lapidus-Krol E, Shapiro R, Amir J, et al. The efficacy and safety of valganciclovir vs. oral ganciclovir in the prevention of symptomatic CMV infection in children after solid organ transplantation. Pediatr Transplant 2010;14:753–60.
173. Latin American registry of pediatric renal transplantation 2004–2008. Pediatr Transplant 2010;14:701–8.
174. Le Berre L, Godfrin Y, Perretto S, et al. The Buffalo/Mna rat, an animal model of FSGS recurrence after renal transplantation. Transplant Proc 2001;33:3338–40.

175. Le Quintrec M, Lionet A, Kamar N, et al. Complement mutation-associated de novo thrombotic microangiopathy following kidney transplantation. Am J Transplant 2008;8:1694–701.
176. Levine MH, Reese PP, Wood A, et al. Inferior allograft outcomes in adolescent recipients of renal transplants from ideal deceased donors. Ann Surg 2012;255:556–64.
177. Lezaic V, Naumovic R, Stanic M, et al. Factors affecting graft function in pediatric and adult recipients of adult live donor kidney transplants. Pediatr Transplant 2007;11:906–13.
178. Li L, Chang A, Naesens M, et al. Steroid-free immunosuppression since 1999: 129 pediatric renal transplants with sustained graft and patient benefits. Am J Transplant 2009;9:1362–72.
179. Li L, Chaudhuri A, Chen A, et al. Efficacy and safety of thymoglobulin induction as an alternative approach for steroid-free maintenance immunosuppression in pediatric renal transplantation. Transplantation 2010;90:1516–20.
180. Licht C, Eifinger F, Gharib M, et al. A stepwise approach to the treatment of early onset nephrotic syndrome. Pediatr Nephrol 2000;14:1077–82.
181. Lien YH, Scott K. Long-term cyclophosphamide treatment for recurrent type I membranoproliferative glomerulonephritis after transplantation. Am J Kidney Dis 2000;35:539–43.
182. Loirat C, Niaudet P. The risk of recurrence of hemolytic uremic syndrome after renal transplantation in children. Pediatr Nephrol 2003;18:1095–101.
183. Loirat C, Noris M, Fremeaux-Bacchi V. Complement and the atypical hemolytic uremic syndrome in children. Pediatr Nephrol 2008;23:1957–72.
184. Lopez EL, Contrini MM, Glatstein E, et al. An epidemiologic surveillance of Shiga-like toxin-producing *Escherichia coli* infection in Argentinean children: risk factors and serum Shiga-like toxin 2 values. Pediatr Infect Dis J 2012;31:20–4.
185. Lopez-Neblina F, Jimenez H, Finkelstein London I, et al. Transoperative renal intraarterial verapamil in kidney transplantation decreases acute tubular necrosis. Transplant Proc 1999;31:3030.
186. Lorenz EC, Sethi S, Leung N, et al. Recurrent membranoproliferative glomerulonephritis after kidney transplantation. Kidney Int 2010;77:721–8.
187. Luke PP, Herz DB, Bellinger MF, et al. Long-term results of pediatric renal transplantation into a dysfunctional lower urinary tract. Transplantation 2003;76:1578–82.
188. Marcocci E, Uliana V, Bruttini M, et al. Autosomal dominant Alport syndrome: molecular analysis of the COL4A4 gene and clinical outcome. Nephrol Dial Transplant 2009;24:1464–71.
189. Marks SD, Trompeter RS. Steroid preservation: the rationale for continued prescribing. Pediatr Nephrol 2006;21:305–7.
190. Martin-Pena A, Cordero E, Fijo J, et al. Prospective study of infectious complications in a cohort of pediatric renal transplant recipients. Pediatr Transplant 2009;13:457–63.
191. Mattoo TK, Al-Sowailem AM, Al-Harbi MS, et al. Nephrotic syndrome in 1st year of life and the role of unilateral nephrectomy. Pediatr Nephrol 1992;6:16–8.
192. Mayer G, Persijn GG. Eurotransplant kidney allocation system (ETKAS): rationale and implementation. Nephrol Dial Transplant 2006;21:2–3.
193. Mccaughan JA, O'rourke DM, Courtney AE. Recurrent dense deposit disease after renal transplantation: an emerging role for complementary therapies. Am J Transplant 2012;12:1046–51.
194. Mcdonald SP, Craig JC. Long-term survival of children with end-stage renal disease. N Engl J Med 2004;350:2654–62.
195. Mcdonald SP, Russ GR, Kerr PG, et al. ESRD in Australia and New Zealand at the end of the millennium: a report from the ANZDATA registry. Am J Kidney Dis 2002;40:1122–31.
196. Mcdonald RA, Smith JM, Ho M, et al. Incidence of PTLD in pediatric renal transplant recipients receiving basiliximab, calcineurin inhibitor, sirolimus and steroids. Am J Transplant 2008;8:984–9.
197. Mcdonald RA, Smith JM, Stablein D, et al. Pretransplant peritoneal dialysis and graft thrombosis following pediatric kidney transplantation: a NAPRTCS report. Pediatr Transplant 2003;7:204–8.
198. Mehls O, Himmele R, Homme M, et al. The interaction of glucocorticoids with the growth hormone-insulin-like growth factor axis and its effects on growth plate chondrocytes and bone cells. J Pediatr Endocrinol Metab 2001;14(Suppl. 6):1475–82.
199. Meier-Kriesche HU, Kaplan B. Waiting time on dialysis as the strongest modifiable risk factor for renal transplant outcomes: a paired donor kidney analysis. Transplantation 2002;74:1377–81.
200. Meier-Kriesche HU, Scornik JC, Susskind B, et al. A lifetime versus a graft life approach redefines the importance of HLA matching in kidney transplant patients. Transplantation 2009;88:23–9.
201. Melk A, Schmidt BM, Braun H, et al. Effects of donor age and cell senescence on kidney allograft survival. Am J Transplant 2009;9:114–23.
202. Mendley SR, Zelko FA. Improvement in specific aspects of neurocognitive performance in children after renal transplantation. Kidney Int 1999;56:318–23.
203. Meri S, Koistinen V, Miettinen A, et al. Activation of the alternative pathway of complement by monoclonal lambda light chains in membranoproliferative glomerulonephritis. J Exp Med 1992;175:939–50.
204. Mickelson JJ, Macneily AE, Leblanc J, et al. Renal transplantation in children 15 Kg or less: the British Columbia Children's Hospital experience. J Urol 2006;176:1797–800.
205. Miles CD, Schaubel DE, Liu D, et al. The role of donor–recipient relationship in long-term outcomes of living donor renal transplantation. Transplantation 2008;85:1483–8.
206. Mitsnefes MM, Khoury PR, Mcenery PT. Early posttransplantation hypertension and poor long-term renal allograft survival in pediatric patients. J Pediatr 2003;143:98–103.
207. Molle ZL, Baqi N, Gretch D, et al. Hepatitis C infection in children and adolescents with end-stage renal disease. Pediatr Nephrol 2002;17:444–9.
208. Mong Hiep TT, Ismaili K, Collart F, et al. Clinical characteristics and outcomes of children with stage 3–5 chronic kidney disease. Pediatr Nephrol 2010;25:935–40.
209. Mong Hiep TT, Janssen F, Ismaili K, et al. Etiology and outcome of chronic renal failure in hospitalized children in Ho Chi Minh City, Vietnam. Pediatr Nephrol 2008;23:965–70.
210. Montagnino G, Tarantino A, Banfi G, et al. Double recurrence of FSGS after two renal transplants with complete regression after plasmapheresis and ACE inhibitors. Transpl Int 2000;13:166–8.
211. Monteverde ML, Ibanez J, Balbarrey Z, et al. Conversion to sirolimus in pediatric renal transplant patients: a single-center experience. Pediatr Transplant 2012;16:582–8.
212. Moore I, Strain L, Pappworth I, et al. Association of factor H autoantibodies with deletions of CFHR1, CFHR3, CFHR4, and with mutations in CFH, CFI, CD46, and C3 in patients with atypical hemolytic uremic syndrome. Blood 2010;115:379–87.
213. Moroni G, Casati C, Quaglini S, et al. Membranoproliferative glomerulonephritis type I in renal transplantation patients: a single-center study of a cohort of 68 renal transplants followed up for 11 years. Transplantation 2011;91:1233–9.
214. Morrow WR, Frazier EA, Mahle WT, et al. Rapid reduction in donor-specific anti-human leukocyte antigen antibodies and reversal of antibody-mediated rejection with bortezomib in pediatric heart transplant patients. Transplantation 2012;93:319–24.
215. Mortazavi F, Rafiee A. Etiology of pediatric chronic kidney diseases in north-west of Iran. Pak J Biol Sci 2010;13:456–9.
216. Motoyama O, Kawamura T, Aikawa A, et al. Head circumference and development in young children after renal transplantation. Pediatr Int 2009;51:71–4.
217. Moudgil A, Martz K, Stablein DM, et al. Good outcome of kidney transplants in recipients of young donors: a NAPRTCS data analysis. Pediatr Transplant 2011;15:167–71.
218. Muczynski KA. Plasmapheresis maintained renal function in an allograft with recurrent membranoproliferative glomerulonephritis type I. Am J Nephrol 1995;15:446–9.
219. Muller T, Sikora P, Offner G, et al. Recurrence of renal disease after kidney transplantation in children: 24 years of experience in a single center. Clin Nephrol 1998;49:82–90.
220. Muorah MR, Brogan PA, Sebire NJ, et al. Dense B cell infiltrates in paediatric renal transplant biopsies are predictive of allograft loss. Pediatr Transplant 2009;13:217–22.
221. Naesens M, Kambham N, Concepcion W, et al. The evolution of nonimmune histological injury and its clinical relevance in adult-sized kidney grafts in pediatric recipients. Am J Transplant 2007;7:2504–14.
222. Naesens M, Salvatierra O, Benfield M, et al. Subclinical inflammation and chronic renal allograft injury in a randomized

trial on steroid avoidance in pediatric kidney transplantation. Am J Transplant 2012;12:2730–43.

223. Nagra A, Trompeter RS, Fernando ON, et al. The effect of heparin on graft thrombosis in pediatric renal allografts. Pediatr Nephrol 2004;19:531–5.
224. Najarian JS, Frey DJ, Matas AJ, et al. Renal transplantation in infants. Ann Surg 1990;212:353–65 discussion 366–367.
225. National Institutes of Health, National Institute of Diabetes and Digestive and Kidney Diseases. USRDS 2008 annual data report: atlas of chronic kidney disease and end-stage renal disease in the United States. Bethesda, MD: National Institutes of Health, National Institute of Diabetes and Digestive and Kidney Diseases; 2008.
226. National Institutes of Health, National Institute of Diabetes and Digestive Kidney Diseases. USRDS 2011 annual data report: atlas of chronic kidney disease and end-stage renal disease in the united states. Bethesda, MD: National Institutes of Health, National Institute of Diabetes and Digestive and Kidney Diseases; 2011.
227. Neuhaus TJ, Arnold W, Gaspert A, et al. Recurrence of membranoproliferative glomerulonephritis after renal transplantation in Denys-Drash. Pediatr Nephrol 2011;26:317–22.
228. Niaudet P, Gubler MC. WT1 and glomerular diseases. Pediatr Nephrol 2006;21:1653–60.
229. Nissel R, Brazda I, Feneberg R, et al. Effect of renal transplantation in childhood on longitudinal growth and adult height. Kidney Int 2004;66:792–800.
230. Noris M, Caprioli J, Bresin E, et al. Relative role of genetic complement abnormalities in sporadic and familial aHUS and their impact on clinical phenotype. Clin J Am Soc Nephrol 2010;5:1844–59.
231. North American Pediatric Renal Trials and Collaborative Studies. NAPRTCS 2008 annual report: renal transplantation, dialysis, and chronic renal insufficiency. 2008. Available online at: https://web.emmes.com/study/ped/annlrept/annlrept.html [accessed 24.09.12].
232. North American Pediatric Renal Trials and Collaborative Studies. NAPRTCS annual transplant report. 2010. Available online at: https://web.emmes.com/study/ped/annlrept/annlrept.html [accessed 24.09.12].
233. Nso Roca AP, Pena Carrion A, Benito Gutierrez M, et al. Evolutive study of children with diffuse mesangial sclerosis. Pediatr Nephrol 2009;24:1013–9.
234. Oakes RS, Kirkham JK, Nelson RD, et al. Duration of oliguria and anuria as predictors of chronic renal-related sequelae in post-diarrheal hemolytic uremic syndrome. Pediatr Nephrol 2008;23:1303–8.
235. Offner G, Toenshoff B, Hocker B, et al. Efficacy and safety of basiliximab in pediatric renal transplant patients receiving cyclosporine, mycophenolate mofetil, and steroids. Transplantation 2008;86:1241–8.
236. Oien CM, Reisaeter AV, Leivestad T, et al. Living donor kidney transplantation: the effects of donor age and gender on short- and long-term outcomes. Transplantation 2007;83:600–6.
237. Ojo AO, Hanson JA, Wolfe RA, et al. Dialysis modality and the risk of allograft thrombosis in adult renal transplant recipients. Kidney Int 1999;55:1952–60.
238. Ojogho O, Sahney S, Cutler D, et al. Superior long-term results of renal transplantation in children under 5 years of age. Am Surg 2002;68:1115–9.
239. Olaitan OK, Zimmermann JA, Shields WP, et al. Long-term outcome of intensive initial immunosuppression protocol in pediatric deceased donor renal transplantation. Pediatr Transplant 2010;14:87–92.
240. Oliver TB, Gouldesbrough DR, Swainson CP. Acute crescentic glomerulonephritis associated with antiglomerular basement membrane antibody in Alport's syndrome after second transplantation. Nephrol Dial Transplant 1991;6:893–5.
241. Omoloja A, Mitsnefes M, Talley L, et al. Racial differences in graft survival: a report from the North American Pediatric Renal Trials and Collaborative Studies (NAPRTCS). Clin J Am Soc Nephrol 2007;2:524–8.
242. Ona ET, Danguilan RA, Africa J, et al. Use of alemtuzumab (Campath-1H) as induction therapy in pediatric kidney transplantation. Transplant Proc 2008;40:2226–9.
243. Opelz G, Dohler B. Effect of human leukocyte antigen compatibility on kidney graft survival: comparative analysis of two decades. Transplantation 2007;84:137–43.
244. Opelz G, Dohler B. Pediatric kidney transplantation: analysis of donor age, HLA match, and posttransplant non-Hodgkin lymphoma: a collaborative transplant study report. Transplantation 2010;90:292–7.
245. Organ procurement and transplantation network (OPTN) and scientific registry of transplant recipients (SRTR). OPTN / SRTR 2010 annual data report. Department of Health and Human Services, Health Resources and Services Administration, Healthcare Systems Bureau, Division of Transplantation; 2011. Available online at: http://srtr.transplant.hrsa.gov/annual_reports/2010 [accessed 24.09.12].
246. Ortiz F, Gelpi R, Koskinen P, et al. IgA nephropathy recurs early in the graft when assessed by protocol biopsy. Nephrol Dial Transplant 2012;27:2553–8.
247. Ortiz J, Palma-Vargas J, Wright F, et al. Campath induction for kidney transplantation: report of 297 cases. Transplantation 2008;85:1550–6.
248. Parekh RS, Carroll CE, Wolfe RA, et al. Cardiovascular mortality in children and young adults with end-stage kidney disease. J Pediatr 2002;141:191–7.
249. Patrakka J, Ruotsalainen V, Reponen P, et al. Recurrence of nephrotic syndrome in kidney grafts of patients with congenital nephrotic syndrome of the Finnish type: role of nephrin. Transplantation 2002;73:394–403.
250. Peddi VR, Bryant M, Roy-Chaudhury P, et al. Safety, efficacy, and cost analysis of thymoglobulin induction therapy with intermittent dosing based on CD3+ lymphocyte counts in kidney and kidney-pancreas transplant recipients. Transplantation 2002;73:1514–8.
251. Perera MT, Sharif K, Lloyd C, et al. Pre-emptive liver transplantation for primary hyperoxaluria (PH-I) arrests long-term renal function deterioration. Nephrol Dial Transplant 2011;26:354–9.
252. Perez-Saez MJ, Toledo K, Navarro MD, et al. Recurrent membranoproliferative glomerulonephritis after second renal graft treated with plasmapheresis and rituximab. Transplant Proc 2011;43:4005–9.
253. Pescovitz MD, Book BK, Sidner RA. Resolution of recurrent focal segmental glomerulosclerosis proteinuria after rituximab treatment. N Engl J Med 2006;354:1961–3.
254. Peten E, Pirson Y, Cosyns JP, et al. Outcome of thirty patients with Alport's syndrome after renal transplantation. Transplantation 1991;52:823–6.
255. Ponticelli C, Moroni G, Glassock RJ. Recurrence of secondary glomerular disease after renal transplantation. Clin J Am Soc Nephrol 2011;6:1214–21.
256. Ponticelli C, Traversi L, Feliciani A, et al. Kidney transplantation in patients with IgA mesangial glomerulonephritis. Kidney Int 2001;60:1948–54.
257. Pradhan M, Petro J, Palmer J, et al. Early use of plasmapheresis for recurrent post-transplant FSGS. Pediatr Nephrol 2003; 18:934–8.
258. Prelog M, Pohl M, Ermisch B, et al. Demand for evaluation of vaccination antibody titers in children considered for renal transplantation. Pediatr Transplant 2007;11:73–6.
259. Puliyanda DP, Toyoda M, Traum AZ, et al. Outcome of management strategies for BK virus replication in pediatric renal transplant recipients. Pediatr Transplant 2008;12:180–6.
260. Qvist E, Pihko H, Fagerudd P, et al. Neurodevelopmental outcome in high-risk patients after renal transplantation in early childhood. Pediatr Transplant 2002;6:53–62.
261. Raafat RH, Kalia A, Travis LB, et al. High-dose oral cyclosporin therapy for recurrent focal segmental glomerulosclerosis in children. Am J Kidney Dis 2004;44:50–6.
262. Riano-Galan I, Malaga S, Rajmil L, et al. Quality of life of adolescents with end-stage renal disease and kidney transplant. Pediatr Nephrol 2009;24:1561–8.
263. Riley P, Marks SD, Desai DY, et al. Challenges facing renal transplantation in pediatric patients with lower urinary tract dysfunction. Transplantation 2010;89:1299–307.
264. Rizvi SA, Zafar MN, Lanewala AA, et al. Challenges in pediatric renal transplantation in developing countries. Curr Opin Organ Transplant 2009;14:533–9.
265. Robinson L-G, Hilinski J, Graham F, et al. Predictors of cytomegalovirus disease among pediatric transplant recipients within one year of renal transplantation. Pediatr Transplant 2002;6:111–8.

266. Salomon R, Gagnadoux MF, Niaudet P. Intravenous cyclosporine therapy in recurrent nephrotic syndrome after renal transplantation in children. Transplantation 2003;75:810–4.
267. Salvatierra Jr O, Sarwal M, Alexander S, et al. A new, unique and simple method for ureteral implantation in kidney recipients with small, defunctionalized bladders. Transplantation 1999;68:731–8.
268. Salvatierra Jr. O, Singh T, Shifrin R, et al. Successful transplantation of adult-sized kidneys into infants requires maintenance of high aortic blood flow. Transplantation 1998;66:819–23.
269. Sampaio MS, Poommipanit N, Kuo HT, et al. Induction therapy in pediatric kidney transplant recipients discharged with a triple drug immunosuppressive regimen. Pediatr Transplant 2010;14:770–8.
270. Samuel JP, Bell CS, Molony DA, et al. Long-term outcome of renal transplantation patients with Henoch–Schönlein purpura. Clin J Am Soc Nephrol 2011;6:2034–40.
271. Samuel SM, Nettel-Aguirre A, Hemmelgarn BR, et al. Graft failure and adaptation period to adult healthcare centers in pediatric renal transplant patients. Transplantation 2011;91:1380–5.
272. Samuel SM, Tonelli MA, Foster BJ, et al. Overview of the Canadian pediatric end-stage renal disease database. BMC Nephrol 2010;11:21.
273. Samuel SM, Tonelli MA, Foster BJ, et al. Survival in pediatric dialysis and transplant patients. Clin J Am Soc Nephrol 2011;6:1094–9.
274. Sarwal MM, Cecka JM, Millan MT, et al. Adult-size kidneys without acute tubular necrosis provide exceedingly superior long-term graft outcomes for infants and small children: a single center and UNOS analysis. United Network for Organ Sharing. Transplantation 2000;70:1728–36.
275. Sarwal M, Chua MS, Kambham N, et al. Molecular heterogeneity in acute renal allograft rejection identified by DNA microarray profiling. N Engl J Med 2003;349:125–38.
276. Sarwal MM, Ettenger RB, Dharnidharka V, et al. Complete steroid avoidance is effective and safe in children with renal transplants: a multicenter randomized trial with three-year follow-up. Am J Transplant 2012;12:2719–29.
277. Sarwal MM, Vidhun JR, Alexander SR, et al. Continued superior outcomes with modification and lengthened follow-up of a steroid-avoidance pilot with extended daclizumab induction in pediatric renal transplantation. Transplantation 2003;76:1331–9.
278. Saxena R, Frankel WL, Sedmak DD, et al. Recurrent type I membranoproliferative glomerulonephritis in a renal allograft: successful treatment with plasmapheresis. Am J Kidney Dis 2000;35:749–52.
279. Scheinman JI. Liver transplantation in oxalosis prior to advanced chronic kidney disease. Pediatr Nephrol 2010;25:2217–22.
280. Schlomer BJ, Smith PJ, Barber TD, et al. Nephrectomy for hypertension in pediatric patients with a unilateral poorly functioning kidney: a contemporary cohort. J Pediatr Urol 2011;7:373–7.
281. Schurman SJ, Stablein DM, Perlman SA, et al. Center volume effects in pediatric renal transplantation. A report of the North American Pediatric Renal Transplant Cooperative Study. Pediatr Nephrol 1999;13:373–8.
282. Sellier-Leclerc AL, Fremeaux-Bacchi V, Dragon-Durey MA, et al. Differential impact of complement mutations on clinical characteristics in atypical hemolytic uremic syndrome. J Am Soc Nephrol 2007;18:2392–400.
283. Senggutuvan P, Cameron JS, Hartley RB, et al. Recurrence of focal segmental glomerulosclerosis in transplanted kidneys: analysis of incidence and risk factors in 59 allografts. Pediatr Nephrol 1990;4:21–8.
284. Shapiro NL, Strocker AM, Bhattacharyya N. Risk factors for adenotonsillar hypertrophy in children following solid organ transplantation. Int J Pediatr Otorhinolaryngol 2003;67:151–5.
285. Sharma AP, Filler G, Dwight P, et al. Chronic renal disease is more prevalent in patients with hemolytic uremic syndrome who had a positive history of diarrhea. Kidney Int 2010;78:598–604.
286. Shapiro R, Ellis D, Tan HP, et al. Alemtuzumab pre-conditioning with tacrolimus monotherapy in pediatric renal transplantation. Am J Transplant 2007;7:2736–8.
287. Sharma R, Sharma M, Mccarthy ET, et al. Components of normal serum block the focal segmental glomerulosclerosis factor activity in vitro. Kidney Int 2000;58:1973–9.
288. Sharma M, Sharma R, Mccarthy ET, et al. The focal segmental glomerulosclerosis permeability factor: biochemical characteristics and biological effects. Exp Biol Med (Maywood) 2004;229:85–98.
289. Sharma M, Sharma R, Reddy SR, et al. Proteinuria after injection of human focal segmental glomerulosclerosis factor. Transplantation 2002;73:366–72.
290. Singer JS, Zaid U, Gritsch HA, et al. Selective use of voiding cystourethrography in children undergoing renal transplant evaluation. J Urol 2009;182:1158–62.
291. Sinha R, Marks SD. Comparison of parameters of chronic kidney disease following paediatric preemptive versus non-preemptive renal transplantation. Pediatr Transplant 2010;14:583–8.
292. Slickers J, Duquette P, Hooper S, et al. Clinical predictors of neurocognitive deficits in children with chronic kidney disease. Pediatr Nephrol 2007;22:565–72.
293. Smith JM, Dharnidharka VR, Talley L, et al. BK virus nephropathy in pediatric renal transplant recipients: an analysis of the North American Pediatric Renal Trials and Collaborative Studies (NAPRTCS) registry. Clin J Am Soc Nephrol 2007;2:1037–42.
294. Srivastava T, Garola RE, Kestila M, et al. Recurrence of proteinuria following renal transplantation in congenital nephrotic syndrome of the Finnish type. Pediatr Nephrol 2006;21:711–8.
295. Stokes MB, De Palma J. Post-transplantation nephrotic syndrome. Kidney Int 2006;69:1088–91.
296. Su X, Zenios SA, Chakkera H, et al. Diminishing significance of HLA matching in kidney transplantation. Am J Transplant 2004;4:1501–8.
297. Swiatecka-Urban A. Anti-interleukin-2 receptor antibodies for the prevention of rejection in pediatric renal transplant patients: current status. Paediatr Drugs 2003;5:699–716.
298. Tai E, Buchanan N, Townsend J, et al. Health status of adolescent and young adult cancer survivors. Cancer 2012;118:4884–91.
299. Tainio J, Qvist E, Vehmas R, et al. Pubertal development is normal in adolescents after renal transplantation in childhood. Transplantation 2011;92:404–9.
300. Tan HP, Donaldson J, Ellis D, et al. Pediatric living donor kidney transplantation under alemtuzumab pretreatment and tacrolimus monotherapy: 4-year experience. Transplantation 2008;86:1725–31.
301. Tejani A, Fine R, Alexander S, et al. Factors predictive of sustained growth in children after renal transplantation. The North American Pediatric Renal Transplant Cooperative Study. J Pediatr 1993;122:397–402.
302. Tejani A, Stablein DH. Recurrence of focal segmental glomerulosclerosis posttransplantation: a special report of the North American Pediatric Renal Transplant Cooperative Study. J Am Soc Nephrol 1992;2:S258–63.
303. Tejani AH, Stablein DM, Sullivan EK, et al. The impact of donor source, recipient age, pre-operative immunotherapy and induction therapy on early and late acute rejections in children: a report of the North American Pediatric Renal Transplant Cooperative Study (NAPRTCS). Pediatr Transplant 1998;2:318–24.
304. Tejani A, Sullivan EK. Do six-antigen-matched cadaver donor kidneys provide better graft survival to children compared with one-haploidentical living-related donor transplants? A report of the North American Pediatric Renal Transplant Cooperative Study. Pediatr Transplant 2000;4:140–5.
305. Thervet E, Aouizerate J, Noel LH, et al. Histologic recurrence of Henoch–Schönlein purpura nephropathy after renal transplantation on routine allograft biopsy. Transplantation 2011;92:907–12.
306. Tonshoff B, David-Neto E, Ettenger R, et al. Pediatric aspects of therapeutic drug monitoring of mycophenolic acid in renal transplantation. Transplant Rev (Orlando) 2011;25:78–89.
307. Toyoda M, Moudgil A, Warady BA, et al. Clinical significance of peripheral blood Epstein–Barr viral load monitoring using polymerase chain reaction in renal transplant recipients. Pediatr Transplant 2008;12:778–84.
308. Trachtman H, Greenbaum LA, Mccarthy ET, et al. Glomerular permeability activity: prevalence and prognostic value in pediatric patients with idiopathic nephrotic syndrome. Am J Kidney Dis 2004;44:604–10.
309. Traynor C, Jenkinson A, Williams Y, et al. Twenty-year survivors of kidney transplantation. Am J Transplant 2012;12:3289–95.
310. Trydzenskaya H, Sattler A, Muller K, et al. Novel approach for improved assessment of phenotypic and functional

characteristics of BKV-specific T-cell immunity. Transplantation 2011;92:1269–77.

311. Tsai EW, Rianthavorn P, Gjertson DW, et al. CD20+ lymphocytes in renal allografts are associated with poor graft survival in pediatric patients. Transplantation 2006;82:1769–73.
312. Tsukamoto Y. End-stage renal disease (ESRD) and its treatment in Japan. Nephrol Dial Transplant 2008;23:2447–50.
313. Ulinski T, Cochat P. Longitudinal growth in children following kidney transplantation: from conservative to pharmacological strategies. Pediatr Nephrol 2006;21:903–9.
314. Upadhyay K, Midgley L, Moudgil A. Safety and efficacy of alemtuzumab in the treatment of late acute renal allograft rejection. Pediatr Transplant 2012;16:286–93.
315. U.S. Renal Data System. USRDS 2011 annual data report: atlas of chronic kidney disease and end-stage renal disease in the United States. Bethesda, MD: National Institutes of Health, National Institute of Diabetes and Digestive Kidney Diseases; 2011. Available online at: http://www.usrds.org/atlas11.aspx [accessed 24.09.12].
316. Van Arendonk KJ, James NT, Locke JE, et al. Late graft loss among pediatric recipients of DCD kidneys. Clin J Am Soc Nephrol 2011;6:2705–11.
317. Van De Luijtgaarden MWM, Noordzij M, Wanner C, et al. Renal replacement therapy in Europe – a summary of the 2009 ERA–EDTA registry annual report. Clin Kidney J 2012;5:109–19.
318. Van Der Loop FT, Heidet L, Timmer ED, et al. Autosomal dominant Alport syndrome caused by a COL4A3 splice site mutation. Kidney Int 2000;58:1870–5.
319. Van Der Weide MJ, Cornelissen EA, Van Achterberg T, et al. Lower urinary tract symptoms after renal transplantation in children. J Urol 2006;175:297–302 discussion 302.
320. Van Lieburg AF, De Jong MC, Hoitsma AJ, et al. Renal transplant thrombosis in children. J Pediatr Surg 1995;30:615–9.
321. Vats AN, Donaldson L, Fine RN, et al. Pretransplant dialysis status and outcome of renal transplantation in North American children: a NAPRTCS Study. North American Pediatric Renal Transplant Cooperative Study. Transplantation 2000;69:1414–9.
322. Vats A, Gillingham K, Matas A, et al. Improved late graft survival and half-lives in pediatric kidney transplantation: a single center experience. Am J Transplant 2002;2:939–45.
323. Vidhun JR, Sarwal MM. Corticosteroid avoidance in pediatric renal transplantation. Pediatr Nephrol 2005;20:418–26.
324. Vivarelli M, Pasini A, Emma F. Eculizumab for the treatment of dense-deposit disease. N Engl J Med 2012;366:1163–5.
325. Waiser J, Budde K, Schutz M, et al. Comparison between bortezomib and rituximab in the treatment of antibody-mediated renal allograft rejection. Nephrol Dial Transplant 2012;27:1246–51.
326. Walker PD, Ferrario F, Joh K, et al. Dense deposit disease is not a membranoproliferative glomerulonephritis. Mod Pathol 2007;20:605–16.
327. Wang SX, Ahola H, Palmen T, et al. Recurrence of nephrotic syndrome after transplantation in CNF is due to autoantibodies to nephrin. Exp Nephrol 2001;9:327–31.
328. Wang XP, Fogo AB, Colon S, et al. Distinct epitopes for anti-glomerular basement membrane alport alloantibodies and Goodpasture autoantibodies within the noncollagenous domain of alpha3(IV) collagen: a Janus-faced antigen. J Am Soc Nephrol 2005;16:3563–71.
329. Watson AR. Non-compliance and transfer from paediatric to adult transplant unit. Pediatr Nephrol 2000;14:469–72.
330. Watson AR, Harden P, Ferris M, et al. Transition from pediatric to adult renal services: a consensus statement by the International Society of Nephrology (ISN) and the International Pediatric Nephrology Association (IPNA). Pediatr Nephrol 2011;26:1753–7.
331. Weber S, Gribouval O, Esquivel EL, et al. NPHS2 mutation analysis shows genetic heterogeneity of steroid-resistant nephrotic syndrome and low post-transplant recurrence. Kidney Int 2004;66:571–9.
332. Wei C, El Hindi S, Li J, et al. Circulating urokinase receptor as a cause of focal segmental glomerulosclerosis. Nat Med 2011;17:952–60.
333. Weitz M, Amon O, Bassler D, et al. Prophylactic eculizumab prior to kidney transplantation for atypical hemolytic uremic syndrome. Pediatr Nephrol 2011;26:1325–9.
334. Westra D, Volokhina E, Van Der Heijden E, et al. Genetic disorders in complement (regulating) genes in patients with atypical haemolytic uraemic syndrome (aHUS). Nephrol Dial Transplant 2010;25:2195–202.
335. White SL, Chadban SJ, Jan S, et al. How can we achieve global equity in provision of renal replacement therapy? Bull World Health Organ 2008;86:229–37.
336. Wolfe RA, Ashby VB, Milford EL, et al. Comparison of mortality in all patients on dialysis, patients on dialysis awaiting transplantation, and recipients of a first cadaveric transplant. N Engl J Med 1999;341:1725–30.
337. Yap HK, Cheung W, Murugasu B, et al. Th1 and Th2 cytokine mRNA profiles in childhood nephrotic syndrome: evidence for increased IL-13 mRNA expression in relapse. J Am Soc Nephrol 1999;10:529–37.
338. Zarkhin V, Li L, Kambham N, et al. A randomized, prospective trial of rituximab for acute rejection in pediatric renal transplantation. Am J Transplant 2008;8:2607–17.
339. Zhao W, Fakhoury M, Deschenes G, et al. Population pharmacokinetics and pharmacogenetics of mycophenolic acid following administration of mycophenolate mofetil in de novo pediatric renal-transplant patients. J Clin Pharmacol 2010;50:1280–91.
340. Zuber J, Le Quintrec M, Sberro-Soussan R, et al. New insights into postrenal transplant hemolytic uremic syndrome. Nat Rev Nephrol 2011;7:23–35.
341. Zuber J, Quintrec ML, Krid S, et al. Eculizumab for atypical hemolytic uremic syndrome recurrence in renal transplantation. Am J Transplant 2012;12:3337–54.

CHAPTER 38

Kidney Transplantation in Developing Countries

M. Rafique Moosa

CHAPTER OUTLINE

PREAMBLE

On October 31, 2011 the world population reached a staggering 7 billion people. Over 80% of humanity is resident in so-called developing countries and this proportion is set to increase inexorably (Figure 38-1). The World Bank classifies countries into three major categories depending on their economic performance. Based on 2010 gross national income (GNI, formerly referred to as gross national product – GNP) per capita, the groups are: low income, \$1005 or less; lower middle income, \$1006–\$3975; upper middle income, \$3976–\$12 275; and high income, \$12 276 or more. Countries in the middle- and low-income economies are considered to be "developing" countries. This classification is one of convenience, not one reflecting the state or rate of development. The world currently faces major new challenges such as global warming, rising energy costs, and a crippling global economic recession. These challenges invariably tend to impact more heavily on developing countries. In addition, the health and welfare of the populace of these countries are often further compromised by the lack of access to basic facilities, such as potable water, sanitation, and electricity, as well as cultural and societal constraints, such as low literacy rates, poverty, and poor governance, not to mention natural and man-made disasters.

The health challenges faced by developing countries also differ, with greater emphasis on communicable diseases. However, it has become increasingly apparent that non-communicable diseases are accounting for a greater proportion of disease globally, but especially in developing countries – a fact not yet fully appreciated by greater society or indeed governments. It has

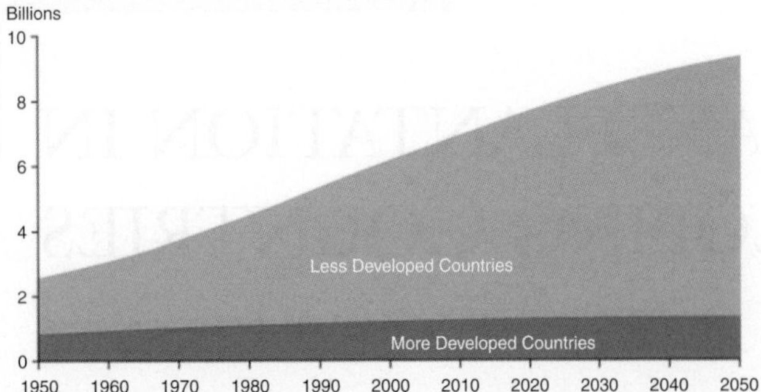

FIGURE 38-1 ■ Growth of the world population in different world regions. Over 80% of the world's population lives in developing countries, with this proportion set to increase rapidly over the coming decades. (Reproduced with permission from United Nations Population Division, World population prospects 2010, The 2010 revision, medium variant (2011). Geneva: United Nations.)

been estimated that chronic non-communicable diseases account for 60% of deaths globally, and 80% of these chronic disease deaths occur in developing countries.[57] The numbers dying from non-communicable diseases is double the numbers that succumb to infectious diseases (including human immunodeficiency virus/acquired immunodeficiency syndrome (HIV/AIDS), tuberculosis, and malaria), maternal and perinatal conditions, and nutritional deficiencies, combined. Of great import too is that the brunt of non-communicable diseases is borne by the poorest in the community. The rising burden of non-communicable diseases manifests with an increase in the number of deaths, among others, from chronic kidney disease (Figure 38-2).[145] The main reason for the surge in kidney disease is the rampant epidemic of diabetes mellitus in developing countries and the aging of the world population.[147,266] The diabetes pandemic is threatening developing countries more than developed countries; it is estimated that within the next generation the number of people with diabetes will increase by 88% in Latin America, 98% in Africa, and 91% in Asia, compared with 18% in Europe. By 2030 more than 80% of diabetics will be from developing countries. Type 2 diabetes mellitus has now overtaken glomerulonephritis as the major cause of end-stage kidney failure in both the developed and developing world.[15]

For most patients with irreversible kidney failure in developing countries, kidney transplantation is the only viable therapeutic option. The demand for kidney transplantation has grown inexorably as the number of patients with end-stage kidney disease (ESKD) has escalated rapidly worldwide. It has been estimated that between 2001 and 2010, the number of patients on dialysis worldwide had doubled to more than 2 million, and the aggregate cost of treatment during this decade would be greater than US $1 trillion.[137] Although the powerful economies of the developed countries permit almost universal access to renal replacement treatment for their populace, the struggling economies of developing countries fail to provide even basic medical care. The diagnosis of ESKD for the majority of patients in developing countries is a death sentence. The high cost of dialysis limits this form of treatment to a privileged few, making a successful kidney transplant a greater necessity than in rich countries.

Globally, the growing discrepancy between the number of patients with ESKD and the number who receive transplants continues to grow at an alarming rate. Of all the transplants performed worldwide, fewer than 10% are performed in developing countries, which rely heavily, and in some cases exclusively, on living related donors. Access to and the rate of transplantation vary considerably; however, demand exists even among the poorest nations.[124]

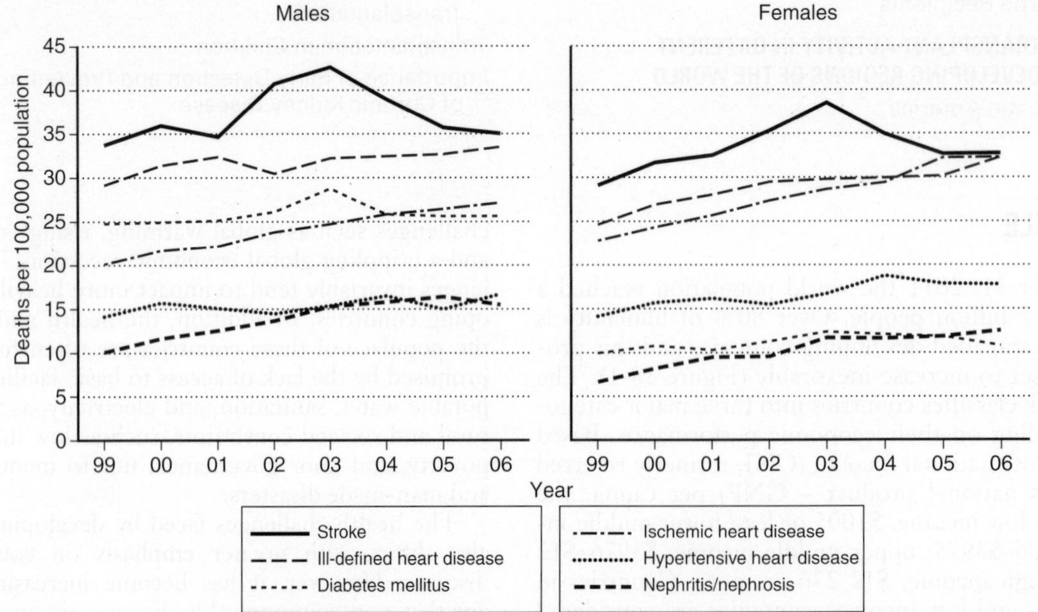

FIGURE 38-2 ■ Death rate per 100 000 population from cardiovascular and related diseases in 15–64-year-old male and female South Africans, 1999–2006. In this report from South Africa the mortality from kidney disease increased by an alarming 67% over a mere 7 years. The progressive increase in deaths from kidney disease parallels the increase in diabetes. (Reproduced with permission from Mayosi BM, Flisher AJ, Lalloo UG, et al. The burden of non-communicable diseases in South Africa. Lancet 2012;374:934–947.)

"Transplant tourism" has been burgeoning since the 1990s and has become an important factor in the medical economies of several developing countries, such as Peru, South Africa, India, the Philippines, Iraq, China, Russia, and Turkey.[222] However, these practices have attracted international criticism, and condemnation of organ trafficking and all forms of commerce in organs.[181] Another major challenge facing transplant specialists, especially in sub-Saharan Africa, is the HIV pandemic that is decimating large swathes of people. Not only is HIV infection adding to the burden of chronic kidney disease, it is also compromising access to deceased donor organs because it affects the most vulnerable group – the young adult, the main source of donor organs.[250] Paradoxically, antiretroviral therapy, while significantly reducing mortality, does herald an increase in the aging population with HIV, and its accompanying burden of non-communicable diseases, including chronic kidney disease.[149]

END-STAGE KIDNEY DISEASE IN DEVELOPING COUNTRIES

The Burden

ESKD has become a major public health challenge. Worldwide, the growing number of patients with ESKD has exceeded all initial predictions by a substantial margin.[69] Most of the increase has occurred in developing countries[93] and estimates place the number of patients on dialysis worldwide at over 2 million, having grown at an annual rate of 7%.[69] In the absence of formal registries, the true incidence in individual developing countries is difficult to determine with any degree of certainty. Estimates put the incidence of ESKD at 48–240 per 1 million population (pmp) in developing countries compared with 88.9–338 pmp in the developed regions of North America,[151] Europe, and the Asia-Pacific region.[174] ESKD in developing countries seems to be at least as common, if not more common, compared with developed countries. The main reason for the dramatic increase in ESKD is the high incidence of diabetes, alluded to earlier, and the aging of the world population. The highest incidence of ESKD has been reported from Mexico, with Morelos and Jalisco having rates of 419 pmp and 597 pmp respectively. Over one-half of these patients have diabetes. In Taiwan, the prevalence of ESKD reached 2447 pmp in 2009 compared to 1811 pmp in the United States.[259] ESKD represents only a fraction of the total chronic disease burden borne by the population: for every patient with stage 5 disease there are 50 with milder forms of the disease.[49] Several other factors aggravate the challenges faced by developing countries. Despite increasing urbanization, the majority of the population of developing countries resides in rural areas with very limited access to healthcare facilities and almost none to renal replacement treatment. It is almost certain that large numbers of patients with kidney failure die without receiving any treatment. In addition, the vast majority of patients present very late and consequently have a grim prognosis.[201] In the United States 43% of ESKD patients had not seen a nephrologist when they commence dialysis[259]; in India 90% of patients had never seen a nephrologist.[126]

The Patient

The typical ESKD patient commencing treatment in a developing country is considerably younger and more likely to be male. The mean age of patients may be as young as 30 years in some countries, compared to the 62.6 years of patients commencing treatment in 2009 in the United States, with the incidence rising most rapidly in patients older than 75 years.[259] In contrast to other developing countries, the mean age of patients receiving hemodialysis in China is 51.5 years.[94] As the population of the world's most populous nation ages and diabetes takes its toll, the mean age will no doubt increase too. The marked male predominance in the incidence of renal replacement therapy is also characteristic of developing countries. In the United States, men account for 53% of patients started on treatment. In developing countries, men account for up to 93% of patients receiving treatment and reflect social and cultural factors in paternalistic societies that favor men, who often are the sole breadwinners. [198]

The Causes (Figure 38-3)

If the incidence of ESKD is difficult to establish because of the lack of registry data, the etiology of ESKD in developing countries is even more problematic. While there are regional differences in the etiology of chronic kidney disease, it is becoming apparent that one disease is on the increase throughout the world and rapidly taking its toll both in developed and developing countries. Diabetic nephropathy, the leading cause of ESKD in Australasia, Europe, and North America, is also the main cause of ESKD in developing countries such as India, Malaysia, Turkey, and several Latin American countries. Among Mexicans, diabetes affects 25% of individuals aged 25–40 years, while in Puerto Rico diabetic nephropathy accounts for 65% of ESKD.[50,267] In the Middle Eastern countries of Egypt, Kuwait, Lebanon, and Saudi Arabia, diabetes is also a common cause of ESKD.[229] In developing countries infectious diseases such as HIV, hepatitis B and C virus, schistosomiasis, and tuberculosis continue to take a heavy toll on kidneys.[24,229]. In India, North Africa, and some Middle Eastern countries, sickle cell anemia, environmental factors, analgesic abuse, and traditional medicines are imporant causes of ESKD.[24,126] In addition, distinct diseases occur in certain regions: the Afro-Asian stone belt extends from the east rim of Africa across the Middle East, reaching South Asia.[199] In the Mediterranean basin familial Mediterranean fever causes amyloidosis that recurs in the transplanted kidney.[201] Again, in contrast to the experience elsewhere, in a recent report from China, diabetic nephropathy accounted for only 15% of ESKD, and chronic glomerulonephritis for 46%.[274]

The Resources

In developing countries the minority of patients with ESKD receive dialysis. This is starkly reflected in a

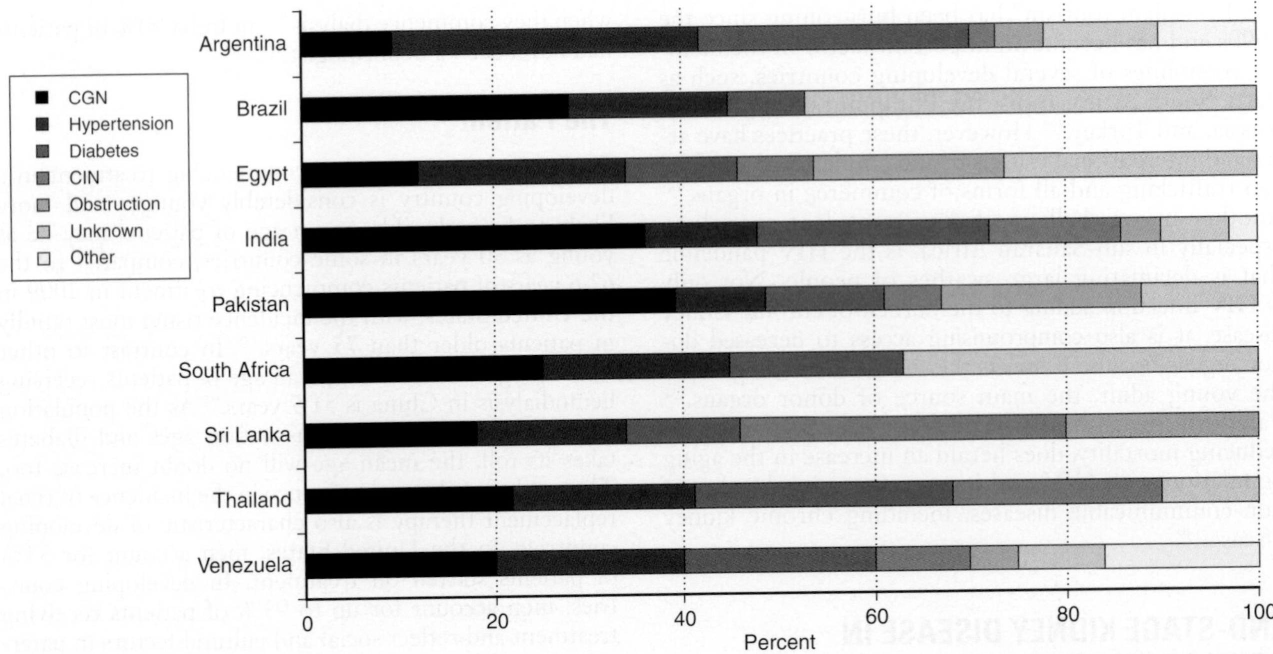

FIGURE 38-3 ■ **Causes of end-stage kidney disease (ESKD) in developing countries. Diabetes is poised to dominate the incidence of ESKD globally. Hypertension and diabetes together account for some two-thirds of all ESKD. CGN, chronic glomerulonephritis; CIN, chronic interstitial nephritis.** (Data from Jha V, Chugh KS. Economics of ESRD in developing countries. In: El Nahas M (ed.) Kidney diseases in the developing world and ethnic minorities. London: Taylor and Francis, 2005, pp. 39–57.)

report that less than 10% of Indian patients with ESKD received renal replacement treatment and 70% of these had succumbed within 3 months, unable to sustain the costs of treatment.[217] This epitomizes the reality facing patients and their caregivers in developing countries with their heavy burden of ESKD, where only those able to pay receive dialysis treatment. Despite the comparable incidence of ESKD, the prevalence of renal replacement treatment strongly favors developed countries. The prevalence of treatment is proportionate to the economic strength of individual countries (Figure 38-4). Of all patients on dialysis treatment worldwide, 52% are being treated in just four countries (United States, Japan, Brazil, and Germany) that constitute merely 11% of the world population.[93] By contrast, less than 1% of patients with ESKD in sub-Saharan Africa receive dialysis treatment.[19]

The cost of dialysis varies from country to country. In most developing countries the high cost of dialysis compared to available healthcare funds means that the dialysis is seldom a priority for national governments. The emerging economies of most developing countries generally spend less than 5% of GNI on health. Beside budgetary constraints, the lack of adequate infrastructure and, more importantly, lack of adequately skilled personnel

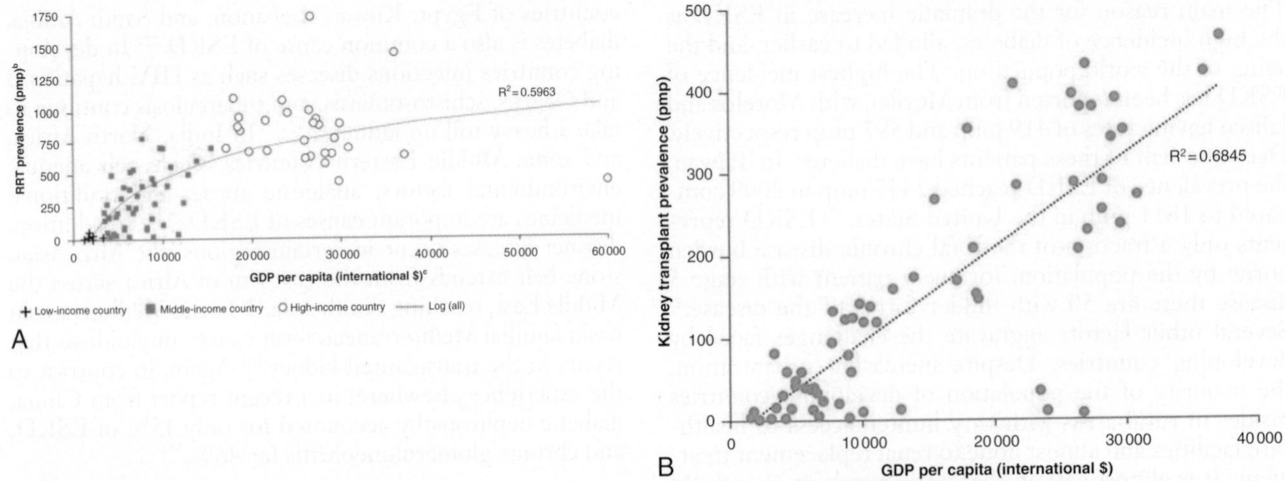

FIGURE 38-4 ■ **(A) Correlation between renal replacement therapy (RRT) and gross domestic product (GDP) per capita. Access to renal replacement is a function of the economic strength of individual countries: where there is greater access, the richer the country. Patients from low-income countries have virtually no access to any treatment. (B) A similar correlation exists with kidney transplants performed in individual countries.** (Reproduced with permission from White SL, Chadban SJ, Jan S, et al. How can we achieve global equity in provision of renal replacement therapy? Bull WHO 2008;86:229–237.)

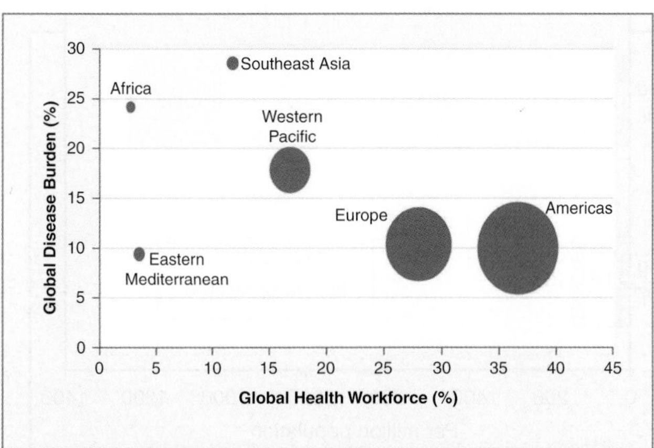

FIGURE 38-5 ■ Distribution of the global healthcare workforce in relation to the disease burden. The size of the circles represents the health expenditure in the six World Health Organization regions. Africa, with almost 25% of the global disease burden, has less than 5% of the healthcare workforce and spends the least on healthcare. (From Taylor AL, Hwenda L, Larsen B-I, et al. Stemming the brain drain – a WHO global code of practice on international recruitment of health personnel. N Engl J Med 2011;365:2348–2351.)

are major limiting factors. The uneven distribution of the global health workforce and the migration of skilled staff from developing countries aggravate the situation (Figure 38-5). Despite these challenges, even some of the poorer countries are initiating dialysis programs, albeit on a restricted basis. These initiatives are often launched with the effort of dedicated individuals supported by international organizations such as the International Society of Nephrology. In order to ensure some fairness and equity in the allocation of dialysis, some countries have so-called Life or Death Committees that decide on who should be offered renal replacement treatment.[159] While this is a fairer way of distributing scarce resources, many inherent dangers may compromise the process. When transplants are done, it is crucially important that the timing of transplantation be optimized, graft function maximized, and costs and complications minimized.

DIALYSIS IN DEVELOPING COUNTRIES (Figure 38-6)

The management of ESKD poses complex medical, social, political, ethical, and economic challenges for patients and communities in developing nations. Dialysis is a highly resource-intensive treatment that few governments are able to afford. Because of insufficient government support, chronic dialysis is poorly organized, lacks clear policies, and is largely unsustainable, because of the need for out-of-pocket payments by patients or their supporters. At less than 20 persons pmp the lowest treatment rates in the world prevail in sub-Saharan Africa (with the exception of South Africa, that has a treatment rate of 70 pmp). Several countries in sub-Saharan Africa are unable to offer any dialysis therapy.[163] In other parts of Africa, treatment rates range from 8.7 pmp in Kenya to 670 pmp in Tunisia.[16] Dialysis in most of Africa is privately funded with only a few states (such as Mali, Mauritius, and South Africa) subsidizing the cost of treating a limited number of patients.[163] In many developing countries around the world, ESKD patients and their families are in the main unable to sustain the costs of chronic dialysis beyond the first few months following initiation. In a recent report from Nigeria, less than 2% of patients initiated on dialysis were still receiving treatment 1 year later.[12] On the Indian subcontinent, the estimated incidence of ESKD is 232 pmp but less than 10% of all patients with ESKD receive any form of renal replacement therapy. Of these, only 6% are still on dialysis after 12 months.[126] The current practice is to limit the frequency of dialysis sessions to 1–2 times weekly, depending on affordability and the patient's symptoms, while dialyzer reuse is the rule.[111] The situation is better in North Africa and the Middle East, with average dialysis rates of 171 pmp and 140 pmp respectively.[25] In Asia, the dialysis rate is 70 pmp. Of the developing regions, Latin America is faring best, with the prevalence of dialysis treatment 320 pmp.[93] The political and economic emancipation of the former communist bloc countries in Central and Eastern Europe has resulted in a significant increase in the prevalence of treatment, with an average rate of 220 pmp, ranging from 500 pmp in Slovenia to 77 pmp in Lithuania.[150,212]

Hemodialysis

Globally, hemodialysis is the preferred mode of dialysis despite the many advantages of peritoneal dialysis in the developing countries setting.[93] In developing countries dialysis facilities are inadequate and mostly in the private sector using refurbished machines that are poorly maintained. Water quality is often substandard with very high aluminum content resulting in excessive blood and bone aluminum levels.[73] Infections are a major cause of morbidity and the second most common cause of mortality (after cardiac causes) among patients on dialysis due to overcrowding, malnutrition, and the use of temporary catheters. *Staphylococcus aureus* is the most common pathogen (60%), of which 35% are methicillin-resistant.[113] Hepatitis B and C virus infections continue to be important causes of hepatitis because of ineffective screening of patients, frequent blood transfusions, and poor infection prevention measures.[113] Malnutrition, which may be present in 77% of patients with ESKD in developing countries, is aggravated by cultural practices that promote restriction of dietary animal protein intake and by inadequate dialysis that results in loss of appetite.[1,161] Besides high costs, the initiation of hemodialysis programs is restricted by lack of trained staff; many infrastrucure issues taken for granted in developed countries pose significant challenges to the provision of hemodialysis in developing countries, including a reliable source of electricity, and adequate technical support and maintenance.[23,73,146] As their financial situation worsens, many patients reduce the frequency of treatment, which results in progressive uremia and ultimately death.[113] In developing countries a greater proportion of the population lives in rural areas far from existing dialysis centers; because of the expense and work disruption, patients attend infrequently for treatment, which ultimately leads to poor outcome on dialysis. The lack of access to ancillary treatment, such as erythropoietin and iron, also contributes

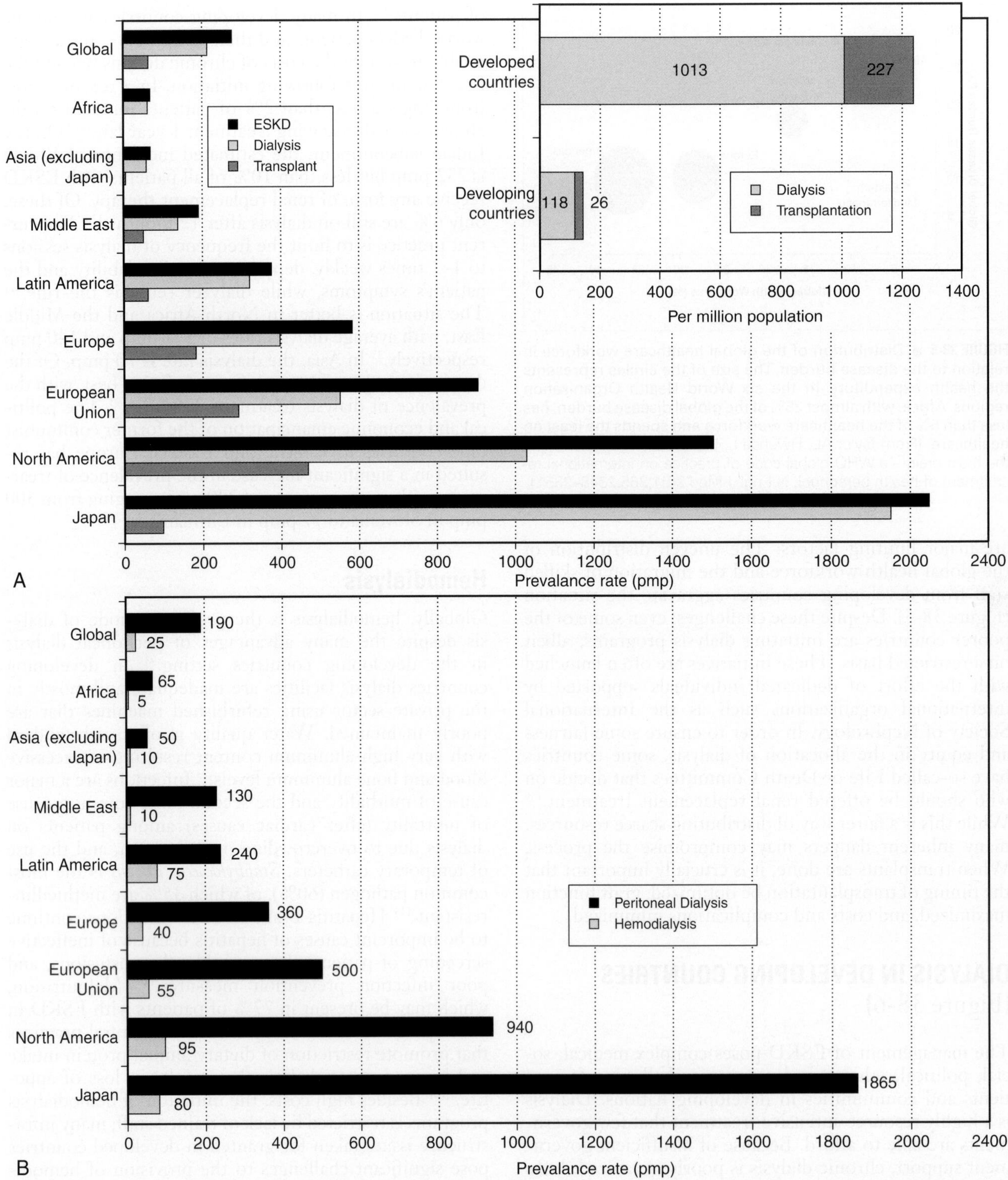

FIGURE 38-6 ■ **(A) Prevalence of treatment in different world regions. Note the low transplant activity in Japan despite the leading end-stage kidney disease (ESKD) prevalence. Inset: The relative overall renal replacement activity in developed and developing regions in 2001. (B) Hemodialysis is by far the more popular choice of dialysis. See text for more detailed discussions.** (Drawn using data from: Grassmann A, Gioberge S, Moeller S, et al. ESRD patients in 2004: global overview of patient numbers, treatment modalities and associated trends. Nephrol Dial Transplant 2005;20:2587–2593; Rizvi SAH, Naqvi SAA, Ahmed E. Renal transplantation in developing countries. In: El Nahas M (ed.) Kidney diseases in the developing world and ethnic minorities. New York: Taylor and Francis, 2005, pp. 211–245.)

to poor outcome; in a survey reported in 2002, less than 25% of patients received erythropoietin therapy, and often the dose was suboptimal.[23] Late referral of patients with ESKD also is an important consideration in the outcome of dialysis. Despite these challenges the mean annual survival of patients on hemodialysis in several developing countries was comparable to results in the west, indicating that treatment of an adequate quality can be

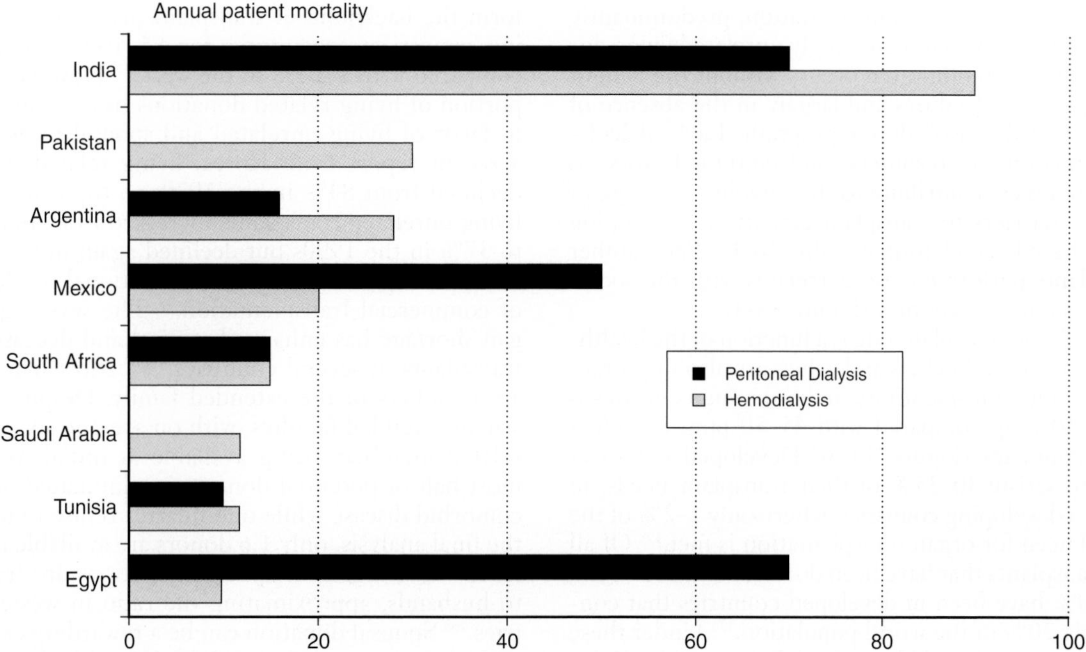

FIGURE 38-7 ■ Mortality of patients on dialysis. The outcome of patients on peritoneal dialysis is particularly dismal in some developing countries. Reasons for the poor outcomes include the high peritonitis rates, poor nutrition, poor patient selection, poor adherence, and the late presentation of patients.[138] (Drawn using data from Barsoum RS. End-stage renal disease in North Africa. Kidney Int Suppl 2003;(83):S111–S114.)

achieved.[23] The annual survival rates in dialysis patients from Central and Eastern Europe has especially improved and now approach those of their western counterparts, ranging from 91% in Romania to 81% in the Czech Republic.[150,211]

Peritoneal Dialysis

Peritoneal dialysis is an efficient form of renal replacement therapy that is often the preferred form of treatment in many countries.[171] Globally, only 11% of ESKD patients received peritoneal dialysis in 2004, down from 14% in 1997.[91,92] Countries like Mexico and Republic of Korea have significantly greater numbers of patients on peritoneal dialysis, with the former approaching 75% of its prevalent dialysis population.[91] Advantages of peritoneal dialysis are that it is more physiological than intermittent hemodialysis, requires less stringent dietary and fluid restrictions, does not require expensive equipment, is more appropriate for certain categories of patients, such as diabetics and children, and after initial training only requires intermittent hospital visits. Peritoneal dialysis offers patients greater independence and mobility, and may allow breadwinners to return to work.[126] It can also be performed in remote regions with limited facilities. Organizationally, it does not require the major capital expenditure associated with setting up a hemodialysis unit and it it possible to service large numbers of patients, even in remote areas. Peritoneal dialysis would be an ideal form of renal replacement treatment in a developing country setting. The chief reason for its limited use is the high cost of treatment in developing countries because peritoneal dialysis solutions have to be imported.[23] It may be 1.5–3 times more expensive than hemodialysis, precluding its widespread use.[113] Although peritoneal dialysis holds tremendous promise, failure to ensure adequate standards of care can result in dismal outcomes. In developing countries, the dose of treatment is related to available resources, and many patients are unable to afford the standard three to four exchanges per day. As residual renal function fails, patients become increasingly uremic and succumb (Figure 38-7). The introduction of new connection technology, such as the Y-system and twin-bag system, has resulted in a significant reduction in acute peritonitis rates.[241] Automated peritoneal dialyis (APD) has been responsible for the increase in the numbers of patients on peritoneal dialysis in many developed countries (with up to 62% of patients in the United States on peritoneal dialysis receiving APD). The penetration of APD into developing countries has been tempered by economic and infracture considerations. In Mexico and Korea, the two developing countries with the largest populations of peritoneal dialysis patients, 21% and 5% of patients, respectively, were treated on APD.[93]

KIDNEY TRANSPLANTATION

A kidney transplant is the treatment of choice for patients with ESKD, with pre-emptive transplantation being the ideal option. However, even in first-world settings only 5.3% of patients received pre-emptive transplants.[253] For a patient from a developing country, a successful kidney transplant carries a lower cost, and offers a better quality of life, a superior prognosis, and the opportunity to be economically active.[267] For patients from those countries where the option of dialysis may not exist, a successful transplant is the sole hope for survival. A striking feature of renal replacement therapy programs in developing countries is the emphasis, and in some cases exclusive reliance, on living donor transplantation, predominantly related living donors but increasingly unrelated living donors.[217] Transplantation often occurs without the benefit of backup dialysis facilities and largely in the absence of an established deceased donor program. Lack of legislation, infrastrucure, resources, and cultural factors, as well as ignorance, contribute to the ongoing shortage of organs.[5,196] Barriers to transplant activity in developing countries have been identified (Table 38-1). The number of transplants performed also correlates with the socioeconomic status of a country (Figure 38-4).

Although the transplant rate is a function of the healthcare system, cultural beliefs and values are also important barriers.[259] The transplant rate in developing countries is less than 10 pmp compared with 45–50 pmp in industrialized countries (Figure 38-6). Developed countries are able to satisfy 30–35% of their transplant needs, in contrast to developing countries, where only 1–2% of the estimated need for organ transplantation is met.[198] Of all kidney transplants that have been done around the world, almost 90% have been in developed countries that constitute only 20% of the world population.[126] Under these circumstances, trade in kidneys from living unrelated donors has flourished.

Donors

Kidneys for transplantation may be derived from living or deceased donors (Figure 38-8). Living donors may be related, spouses, or unrelated; deceased donors may be heartbeating or non-heartbeating. Living donors still form the backbone of transplant programs in developing countries, accounting for 85–100% of donations compared with 1–25% in the west.[198] However, the proportion of living related donations has steadily declined in favor of living unrelated and spousal transplants. In a recent report from Korea, living related transplants declined from 84% in the 1970s to 61% in the 2000s; living unrelated transplants increased from 14% (1970s) to 37% in the 1990s but declined again in the 2000s to 19%, perhaps reflecting the international condemnation of commercial transplantation.[47] The severe global organ shortage has enhanced spousal and deceased donor transplants in several countries.[47,207] Most living donors are members of the extended family. Despite the large size of extended families, with on average six genetically related members being available at initial workup, almost half of potential donors are eliminated because of comorbid disease while one-quarter refuse to donate. In the final analysis, only 1.6 donors are available per recipient.[108] Two-thirds of spousal donations are from wives to husbands, approximating the ratio in western countries.[168] Spousal donation can be a rewarding experience, with donors expressing satisfaction with their decision and improvement in family relationships.[175] The results of spousal transplants also are superior to the results of parental and living unrelated donors.[207,271] With the exception of some Latin American countries, deceased donor transplants are limited in most developing countries for a variety of reasons, including religious and cultural issues. After some initial resistance, most religious commentators, including Islamic, Christian, Hindu, Judaic, and Buddhist, support solid-organ transplantation. Saudi Arabia is an excellent example of a conservative Muslim country that has implemented a deceased donor program successfully. The growth of the deceased donor program in Latin America is another example of what can be achieved with the combined effort of the medical community and governmental involvement.[273] The United States is the only country that performs more deceased donor transplants than Brazil, which reached an absolute number of 3400 in 2001.[273] The critical shortage of organs means expanded criteria donors (ECDs) are being used increasingly. Several developed countries report good results with the use of kidneys from non-heartbeating donors but it is a source that is yet to be explored by developing countries.

TABLE 38-1 Factors Contributing to Poor Transplantation Rates in Developing Countries

Governmental
Inadequate funding and other resources
Skills shortage
Inadequate legislation
Inadequate health infrastructure
Inadequate public awareness campaigns and education
Inadequate deceased donor transplant programs

Societal
Poverty
Illiteracy (especially among women)
Lack of access to potable water and sanitation
Cultural constraints
Deceased donor shortage
Transplant tourism

Environmental
Poor nutrition
Human immunodeficiency virus (HIV) pandemic
Tuberculosis

Healthcare professionals
Apathy and ignorance in respect of organ donation
Lack of team spirit
Lack of planning for organ procurement

Posttransplant
Out-of-pocket payments for ongoing immunosuppression
Posttransplant infections

See text for discussion.

Barriers to Transplantation Programs

A range of obstacles hinder the development of transplant programs in developing countries. Challenges vary from country to country and are listed in Table 38-1.

Resources and Infrastructure

Poorer countries are in general battling communicable diseases such as malaria, HIV/AIDS, and tuberculosis that have a major impact on the health of its population. Health authorities tend to prioritize these diseases over chronic kidney failure, which is seen as affecting a relatively small proportion of the population, is expensive to treat, and requires vast resources.[5] The lack of technical

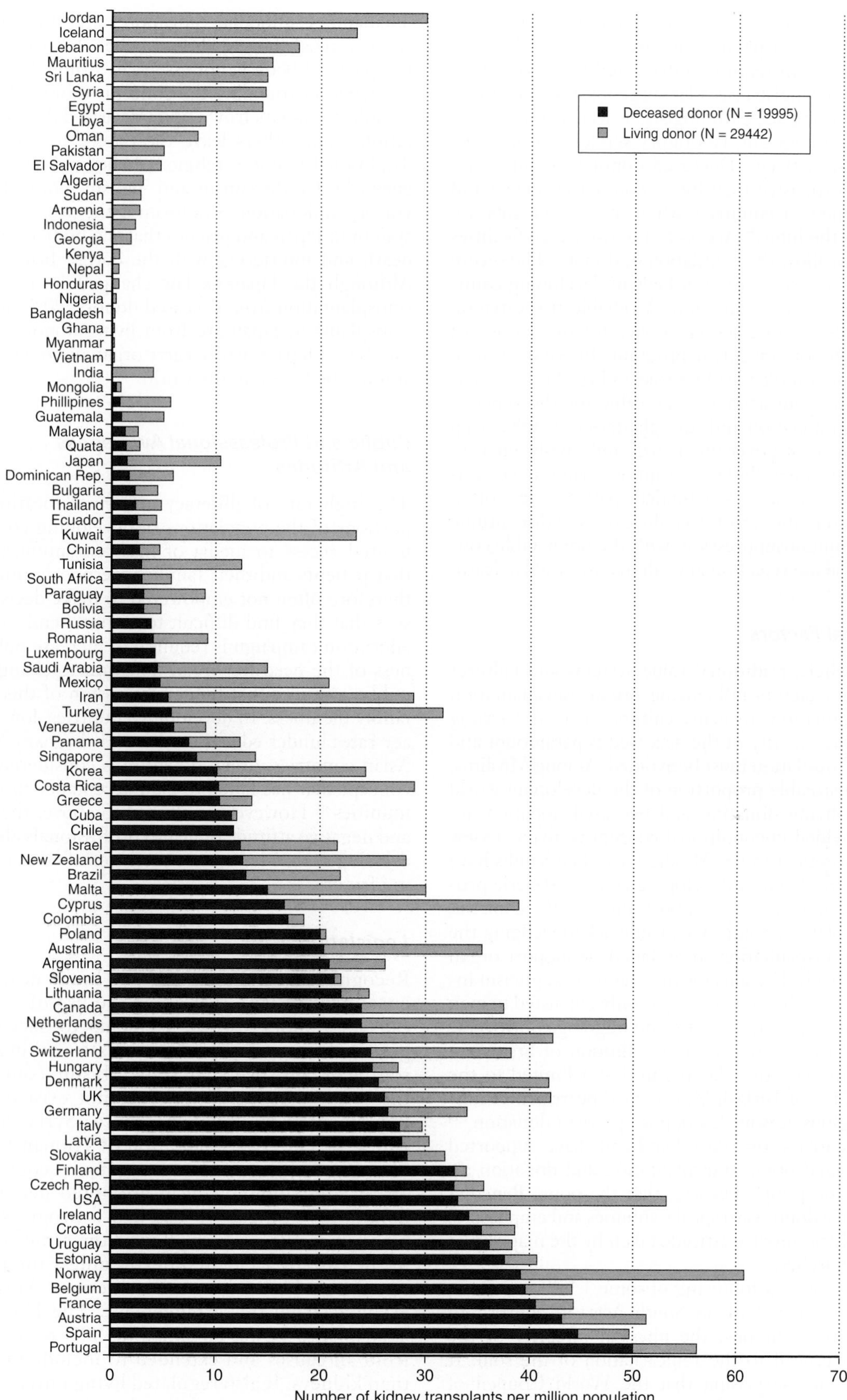

FIGURE 38-8 ■ Transplant activity in different countries in 2009 ordered from lowest to highest rates of kidney transplantation involving deceased donors. Developing countries rely more heavily, and in many cases, exclusively on living organ donors. The number of countries transplanting has increased and even some of the poorer countries are initiating transplant programs, emphasizing the growing global demand. (Reproduced with permission from Delmonico FL, Dominguez-Gil B, Matesanz R, et al. A call for government accountability to achieve national self-sufficiency in organ donation and transplantation. Lancet 2011;378:1414–1418.)

and medical expertise is an even greater challenge to the development of transplant programs. A successful kidney transplant program requires a dedicated team consisting of surgeons (urologists, vascular surgeons, transplant surgeons), nephrologists, pathologists, as well as the backup of a good radiology and laboratory service, not to mention a dialysis service.[5] Deceased donor programs tend to be more expensive than living donor transplants and are constrained in countries where health budgets are stretched to the limit.[44] Access to intensive care facilities is required to allow the ventilation of donors. The severe shortage of intensive care unit beds in developing countries can be a major limitation. A reliable tissue-typing laboratory also is an essential service for the success of a deceased donor transplant program. In Saudi Arabia, the government took a leading role and established a national procurement agency responsible for the supervision of organ donation and transplantation, emphasizing the importance of government will and involvement.[230] Governments generally fail to support maintenance immunosuppression and self-funded patients are often forced, by economic reality, to reduce or even discontinue the costly immunosuppression, with the predictable consequence of acute rejection and, almost invariably, death.

Sociological Factors

Religious beliefs, traditional value systems and cultures are important factors influencing organ transplantation and organ donation. In many cultures there is a strong belief that the sanctity of the deceased is paramount and any form of mutilation must be avoided. Among Muslims, who form a sizeable proportion of the developing world population, living donation and deceased donation are allowed provided unconditional consent is given, a view especially prevalent in the Middle East. The Saudis have been at the forefront of developing active cadaveric programs, enacting laws to support these.[89] By contrast, Muslim scholars in South Asia, while acknowledging the benefit of transplantation, have failed to support organ donation actively. Reasons for the ongoing skepticism include belief that the human body is only entrusted to man and may not be interfered with, and ongoing controversy with regard to the concept and definition of brainstem death.[172] However, this skepticism is not limited to the lay public: 21% of Turkish Muslim healthcare professionals had religious reasons for opposing organ donation.[254] Christian scholars, on the other hand, have supported and encouraged organ transplantation and donation almost since inception. The fact that the pope, Benedict XVI, carried a donor card speaks volumes and emphasizes the generally permissive attitude taken by the majority of Christian churches.

Hinduism, with a following of some 1 billion people, is the predominant faith in South Asia. In contrast to the Abrahamic religions, the physical integrity of the body is not crucial to the reincarnation of the soul. It is therefore not surprising that the World Council of Hindus stated, "Organ donation is an integral part of our living." Similarly, Sikhs believe the soul is eternal but that the physical body is not crucial to the cycle of rebirth. Buddhism, practiced in much of Asia, especially Thailand, Cambodia, Singapore, and Vietnam, is also characterized by rebirth and belief that the integrity of the physical body is not essential, although there is ambivalence surrounding the concept of brain death. Some Buddhist scholars frown upon deceased donor transplantation while others leave the choice to the individual. Traditional Chinese religious beliefs are strongly influenced by Confucianism and Taoism, both of which favor organ donation. Shintoism is the predominant belief system in Japan and teaches that the body is impure after death and interfering with the corpse brings bad luck. Although the Japanese law changed in 1997 to allow transplantation from deceased donors, 90% of all kidney transplants in Japan are from living donors. Today, the number of Japanese who carry organ donor cards remains among the lowest in the world.[172]

Public and Professsional Awareness and Attitudes

The high rate of illiteracy and rural location of large portions of the populations of developing countries and limited access to media of mass communication mean that patients and their families are poorly informed and therefore often not empowered to make decisions on issues that they find difficult to comprehend. A concerted education campaign is required to increase public awareness of the need for organ donation to change negative public attitudes that hinder discussion of this subject by family members. In developing countries, low adult literacy rates hinder education drives.[217] In many South-East Asian countries, organ donation is considered a western concept that has failed to gain acceptance in these communities.[41] However, as alluded to above, the ignorance and negative attitude of health professionals also need addressing as they have been been identified as major limiting factors.[254]

Legislation

Recognition of the concept of brain death and the enactment of laws that allow the use of organs from cadaver donors are key elements to successful programs. The concept of brain death continues to be a source of controversy in some Muslim countries, with the result that legislation does not exist or is poorly implemented in Egypt, Morocco, Syria, Sudan, and Libya.[227] The Transplantation of Human Organs Act of India banned trade in organs, recognized brain death, and simultaneously promoted deceased organ donation.[166] Singapore has had a progressive law in place since 1987, which allowed the removal of organs in the case of accidental death, unless the person had opted out during his or her lifetime. Muslims were excluded from this arrangement. The Human Organ Transplant Act was amended in 2004 to include death from all causes and extended to include organs other than kidneys. It also regulated living unrelated donors. Pakistan, the center of illegal trade in organs, passed the Transplantation of Human Organs and Human Tissue Ordinance of 2007 into law in March 2010, after considerable international and national pressure.

The law shares all the key components of the corresponding Indian act. Early indications are that the promulgation is already having an impact but it remains to be seen if this will be sustained.[193] The exceptional achievements of Saudi Arabia in addressing all aspects, including legislative, have been alluded to above.

Organ Trafficking and Transplant Tourism

One of the most serious threats to the image of transplantation in the world and global transplant programs is the scourge of organ trafficking. The World Health Organization (WHO) has estimated that 5–10% of all kidney transplant occurring globally are commercial transplants with patients from more affluent countries seeking organs from donors in economically deprived countries.[67] This practice is on the increase, driven on the one hand by the steadily increasing waiting times for kidneys in rich countries – the waiting time for kidneys in the United States now exceeds 3 years and is projected to increase.[107] On the other hand, vendors in developing countries who live in abject poverty view sale of an organ as an opportunity to improve themselves financially. Both parties, but especially the vendors, are mercilessly exploited by unscrupulous middlemen who prey on the vulnerability of both parties.[107] Syndicates comprising doctors, brokers, technicians, and hospitals service this lucrative market. The lay press as well as academic publications are replete with accounts of impropriety.[36,107] These networks function with impunity in the absence of national legislative and regulatory frameworks or, where these do exist, are blatantly flouted in corrupt environments.[5] Countries such as India, Pakistan, and Turkey have developed notoriety as "kidney bazaars,"[107] but the country that has become the leading destination for transplant tourism is China. In 2006, 11 000 transplants were performed with organs harvested from judicially executed prisoners.[33] The macabre practice had developed into a well-organized industry servicing the domestic need but also catered for the increasingly lucrative foreign market.[264] As the Chinese health services became increasingly market-driven, managers were under pressure to generate additional sources of income; this coupled with the steadily improving medical services rapidly transformed the country into a transplant mecca.[264] However, following an international outcry and ahead of the Olympic Games the Chinese government adopted the Human Transplantation Act in 2007 which expressly outlawed commerce in organs (see below). This had the effect of immediately halving foreign transplants.[33]

The Vendors

The profile of organ vendors (also labeled commercial living donors) is similar in all countries where organ trafficking occurs.[34] They are generally male, illiterate, unemployed, and living below the poverty line. The decision to resort to organ donation is often triggered by a personal financial crisis. Studies from Egypt, India, Iran, Pakistan, and the Philippines have all documented similar negative health, economic, social, and psychological consequences.[34,170,223,272] Between 48% and 98% of commercial donors reported detrimental health consequences. Sadly, the sale not only fails to ameliorate the poverty or improve the economic/financial situation – the main motivation for the donation – but the majority of donors declare a deterioration in their personal circumstances because they were often unable to return to a competitive labor market. In Egypt, 81% of donors had depleted the funds arising from vending within 5 months; in India, 75% of donors remained impoverished. Beside the economic and health consequences donors also suffer emotionally and socially. Vendors are stigmatized and ostracized by their communities. There is a significant increase in marital conflict and divorce rates soar following donation. The experience leaves donors with such severe emotional distress that very few would ever recommend the sale of kidney to reduce poverty.[34,170,223,272]

Global concern has culminated in several statements by august conferences that include the Madrid Resolution, the Declaration of Istanbul, and the 63rd World Health Assembly Resolution. The WHO has urged individual countries to develop national self-sufficiency with regard to their organs needs by mobilizing resources from within their own population. Self-sufficiency would include strategies to increase the donor pool and preventive programs to reduce the burden of kidney disease.[60] While these efforts, driven by advocates for change, are commendable, it remains to be seen how successful they are going to be in the face of the strong market and other forces that drive the practice, and other arguments championing donor autonomy.

The Recipients

The reported outcomes of commercial transplants are variable, with some studies, usually with small data sets, reporting poorer outcomes compared with international benchmarks; in others reported patient and graft survival rates are comparable to local standards.[236] A recent in-depth review of commercial kidney transplants found that, while some studies reported good patient and graft survival, the results in the main were inferior to those obtained in the United States. Of greater concern, though, was the number of serious infections, including malaria, HIV, hepatitis B and C, tuberculosis, and cytomegalovirus (CMV).[214]

TRANSPLANT ACTIVITY IN DIFFERENT DEVELOPING REGIONS OF THE WORLD

No country in the world can claim to have sufficient donors to meet its transplantation needs. At best, 45–50% of the prevalent ESKD population has functioning grafts in developed countries. In developing countries, the situation is considerably worse, but significant growth has occurred in many regions. Growth in transplant activity has been particularly good in the former Soviet bloc countries, the Middle East, and Latin America, but renal replacement treatment has lagged in Africa and Asia.

Latin America

Latin America comprises 20 countries, including Mexico, Central and South American countries, and the Hispanic Caribbean Islands. It is economically, socially, and racially a heterogeneous region, which is manifested in widely differing wealth and health indicators. Latin America is recognized as the most unequal region in the world, undermining economic development and contributing to poverty, one of the region's most pressing social challenges. But economic giants in the region Brazil and Mexico are predicted to be among the top five world economies by 2050, after China, the United States, and India. The incidence of ESKD in this region has increased progressively and was 188 pmp in 2006.[55] There are variations in the incidence of ESKD within the region, with Mexico having the highest (345.9 pmp) and Paraguay the lowest (12.6 pmp) (Figure 38-9). In common with the trends elsewhere in the world, the incidence of diabetic nephropathy has increased, and together with hypertension accounts for almost two-thirds of all ESKD in this region (Figure 38-10). The annual growth in ESKD patients is almost sevenfold greater than the population growth of Latin America.[56] The second reason for the dramatic increase in ESKD (in common with developed countries) has been the aging of the incident population, with patients older than 65 years accounting for 38% of patients starting treatment in 2001 compared with 20% a decade previously. The number of patients over 75 years increased from 5% to 25% in the same time period.[56] Hemodialysis is the most prevalent form of renal replacement treatment, with the exception of Mexico, where peritoneal dialysis is the leading treatment (Figure 38-10).

Argentina pioneered kidney transplantation in Latin America in 1957 and this region is the fastest growing in terms of number of transplants and progress with deceased organ donation (Figure 38-9). Since the first transplant in 1957, a cumulative total of over 107 000 kidney transplants had been performed by 2006, with Brazil and Mexico performing 62% of these. There has been an impressive improvement in the transplantation rate from 3.7 pmp in 1987 to 15 pmp in 2005.[55] The first country to promulgate transplantation laws was Brazil in 1968 and since then almost all countries have adopted progressive and ethical laws enabling organ harvesting and organ allocation and prohibiting commerce.[152] Eight countries in the region have adopted presumed consent laws for organ retrieval.[152] In 2001, the region with 8.5% of the world population performed 12.7% of all kidney transplants.[80] The Latin American Dialysis and Renal Transplant Registry, created in 1991, represents 20 countries with a regional population of 544 million and recorded 8224 kidney transplants in 2006. The majority of transplants are from living donors but deceased donor kidney transplants have increased, and in at least eight countries these exceed living donor transplants. The overall deceased donor rate in Latin America was 2.5 pmp in 2001 but averaged 10 pmp in Uruguay, Puerto Rico, Chile, and Cuba.[80] Part of the success of the deceased donor program has been ascribed to the introduction in 2001 of the Punta Cana Group, formed by the Latin American transplant coordinators and based on the "Spanish model." The potential donor pool is 60–100 pmp per year, the donor notification rate ranges from 4.3 to 47 pmp, and the effective donor rate from 1 to 18 pmp. However, with an estimated kidney waiting list of some 72 000, there is a need to improve further.[152]

The treatment of ESKD places an enormous economic burden on countries. Different public healthcare funding models exist, ranging from full coverage by government to very restricted coverage.[152] This region spends 6.4% of GNI on health. Although this is second only to Organization for Economic Cooperation and Development countries, this amount is still 10 times less than that spent by industrialized nations.[205] In Brazil, the government bears the cost of a kidney transplant of US $10 000 as well as the cost of triple therapy (cyclosporine, azathioprine, and steroids); it also allows the use of mycophenolate mofetil (MMF) and tacrolimus.[273] In Mexico, the treatment prevalence rate among the poor was 166 pmp compared with 939 pmp among the insured; the transplant rate was 7.5 pmp and 72 pmp among the poor and insured respectively.[81] The inequities in coverage and access exemplified here are a reality in much of the developing world and require creative solutions.

Asia

The first kidney transplant in Asia was performed in 1956 in Japan[176] but the leading nations in this area are India and China (see Table 38-3, below).[43] The Asia-Pacific region probably represents the most diverse social, cultural, economic, and ethnic spectrum of all the areas of the developing world. The true incidence and etiology of ESKD in this region are unknown because of the absence of regional or national registries. In one of the first population-based studies of its kind, Modi and Jha reported the age-adjusted incidence of ESKD of 232 pmp in Southern India.[153] In keeping with trends elsewhere in the world, the inexorable increase in the incidence of ESKD parallels the increase in diabetes, that accounted for 41–44% of ESKD. Hypertension with diabetes together account for almost two-thirds of all ESKD.[59] Part of this region also falls in the Afro-Asian stone belt that stretches across North Africa and the Middle East to South Asia, in which nephrolithiasis is a small but important preventable cause of ESKD. In the hospital-based component of the report, stone disease accounted for almost 10% of ESKD.[59] There has been speculation on the possible role of maternal malnutrition, which is rife in this region, and the subsequent development of chronic kidney disease in children. An unusual form of tubulointerstitial nephritis has been described in Sri Lankan farmers that shares several features with Chinese herbal nephropathy and Balkan nephropathy; it is postulated to be caused by environmental toxins.[111]

The mean age of the Indian patients recently reported was 47 years and 58% were male.[153] Kidney disease thus affects economically active individuals in the prime of their lives. Two-thirds of the population reside in rural areas because the economies are agriculture-based. In urban areas, large numbers live in slums and in abject poverty. The majority of ESKD patients

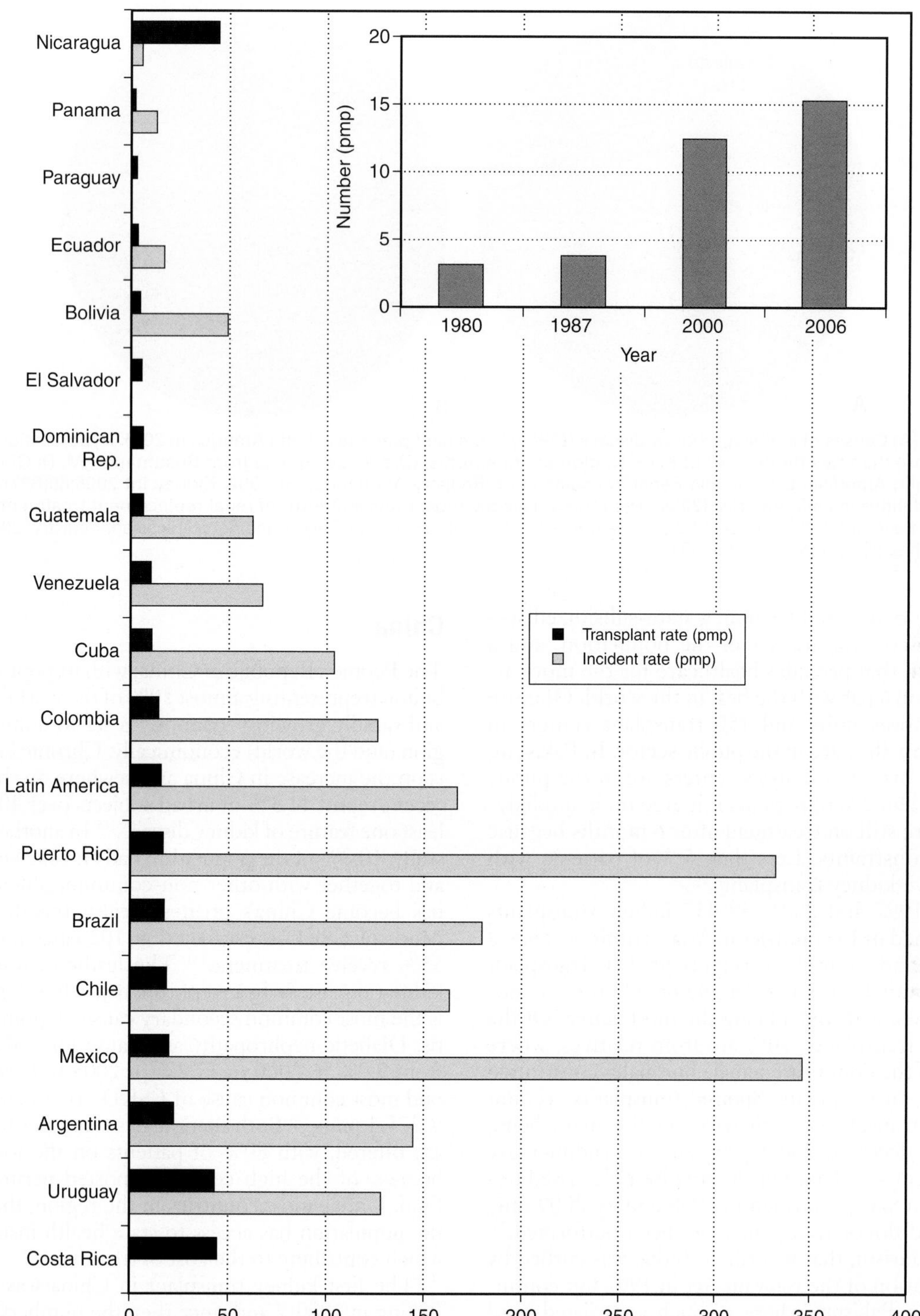

FIGURE 38-9 ■ The incidence of renal replacement treatment in Latin America in 2006. Brazil performs the greatest number of transplants in the region, accounting for 40% of all activity. No data available for Honduras. No incidence data for Costa Rica, El Salvador, Guatemala, Panama, or Puerto Rico. Inset: Transplant activity in the region since 1980. Kidney transplant activity has grown steadily over 26 years. (Drawn using data from Cusumano AM, Gonzalez Bedat MC, Garcia-Garcia G, et al. Latin American Dialysis and Renal Transplant Registry: 2008 report (data 2006). Clin Nephrol 2010;74 (Suppl. 1):S3–S8; Garcia VD, Garcia CD, Santiago-Delpin EA. Organ transplants in Latin America. Transplant Proc 2003;35:1673–1674.)

present late with advanced complications. Limited expenditure on health by governments (most countries in this region spend less than 1.5% of GNI on health) means inadequate healthcare services, especially in rural areas. Beside the lack of capital resources, other challenges include the lack of government policies for the management of chronic diseases and the shortage of skilled personnel. Access to treatment of ESKD is inextricably linked to the level of economic development of individual countries. In the region, India has been the most prolific in developing new dialysis units. In common with many other countries, healthcare in India is

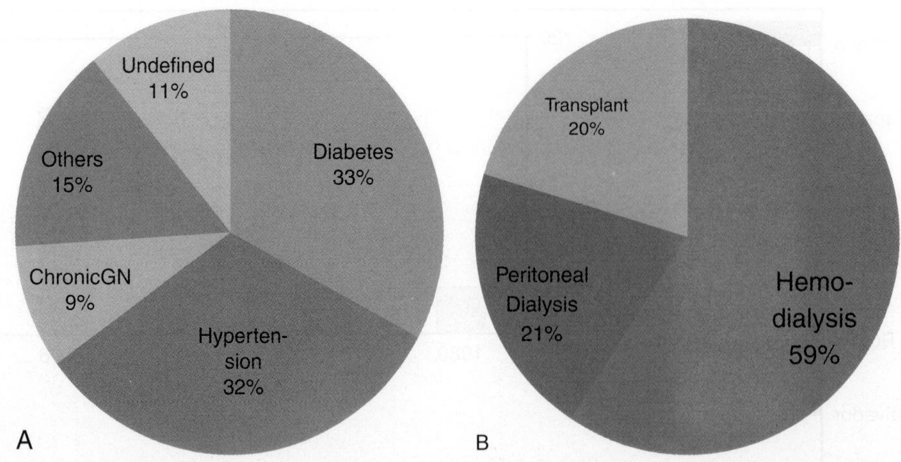

FIGURE 38-10 ■ (A) Causes of end-stage kidney disease (ESKD) in incident patients in Latin America in 2001. Hypertension and diabetes account for more than two-thirds of all ESKD. GN, glomerulonephritis. (Drawn using data from Cusumano AM, Di Gioia C, Hermida O, et al. The Latin American Dialysis and Renal Transplantation Registry Annual Report 2002. Kidney Int 2005;68(S97):S46–S52.) (B) Treatment modalities in Latin America (2006). Hemodialysis is the most prevalent form of renal replacement treatment. (Drawn using data from Cusumano AM, Gonzalez Bedat MC, Garcia-Garcia G, et al. Latin American Dialysis and Renal Transplant Registry: 2008 report (data 2006). Clin Nephrol 2010;74 (Suppl. 1):S3–S8.)

provided in a two-tiered fashion: a state-subsidized system which serves the masses of the population, and a private system that provides healthcare for the more affluent and is on a par with the best in the world. Of more than 750 dialysis units and 150 transplant centers in India, less than 20% are in the public sector. In Pakistan, only 30% of over 195 dialysis centers are in the public sector. Less than 2% of patients initiated on hemodialysis in India are still on treatment after 6 months because of funding constraints. Less than 5% of patients with ESKD receive kidney transplants.[203]

Between 1997 and 2001, 49 437 kidney transplants were performed in 13 countries in Asia[175]; of these, 59.5% were living donor transplants (Figure 38-11). Transplant activity in South-East Asia is largely based on living donor transplants, with India being the most active. Of the living donor transplants, 70% are from relatives, where two-thirds of the donors are female but males constituted over 83% of all recipients. Spousal transplants account for 20% of transplants, with wives in the main being donors. The deceased donor programs are rudimentary or non-existent – in Pakistan the first local deceased donor transplant was performed in 1998 and by 2009 only four deceased donor transplants had been performed.[203] Transplant tourism, that was rife in India, was curbed by the promulgation of the relevant Act in 1997 but continued openly in Pakistan where no such act existed until 2010, when the Pakistani Parliament passed a law outlawing commerce in organs. The act seems to have effectively curbed commercial kidney transplants, as it did in India.[203] Despite the active transplant program in India, there are other challenges facing patients and their caregivers in India: although kidney transplants performed in public hospitals carry no cost to patients, patients have to purchase their own immunosuppressive drugs. Because of the high costs, patients are often forced to discontinue the more expensive calcineurin inhibitors, with a high risk of graft loss due to acute rejection.[111] The relative costs of renal replacement treatment in India are shown in Table 38-2.

China

The People's Republic of China, with its population of 1.35 billion (representing almost 20% of the world's population) and rapidly growing economy, is set to dominate this region (and the world) economically. Chronic kidney disease is on the increase in China as elsewhere on the globe; in a recent report 11.3% of urban subjects over 40 years had at least one feature of kidney disease.[268] In another even larger study, 10.8% of the population had chronic kidney disease, and together with other non-communicable diseases, this has become China's greatest health threat.[275] The incidence of ESKD is estimated at 102 cases pmp, of whom 55% receive treatment.[133] The leading cause of chronic kidney disease is IgA nephropathy, while lupus nephritis is the most common secondary cause of glomerulonephritis. Diabetic nephropathy as a cause for ESKD increased from 9.9% in 2000 to 17.2% in 2005 to become the second most common cause of ESKD. Treatment prevalence is 275.4 pmp.[270] Both hemodialysis and peritoneal dialysis are offered, with 80% of patients on the former, largely because of the high cost of imported peritoneal dialysis fluid. Unlike most countries in the region, the majority of the population has access to state health insurance funds, which contribute to the cost of treatment.[133]

The first kidney transplant in China was perfomed in Beijing in 1960[132] and since then the numbers have rapidly escalated (Figure 38-11). Access to healthcare has dramatically increased and reached near-universal coverage in a very short time, escalating from 29.7% in 2003 to 95.7% in 2011![68] However, funding for transplants is not provided by the government and this remains a major barrier to transplantation; for patients on medical insurance, the sum of US$12 000 is available in the first year. Locally produced cyclosporine is used with steroids and MMF to achieve 1-year graft survival rates in excess of 80%.[133] The principal sources of kidneys are brain-dead donors (see section on Organ Trafficking and Transplant Tourism, above). The Chinese government introduced new legislation in 2007 to curb the rampant commercialism in organ transplantation.

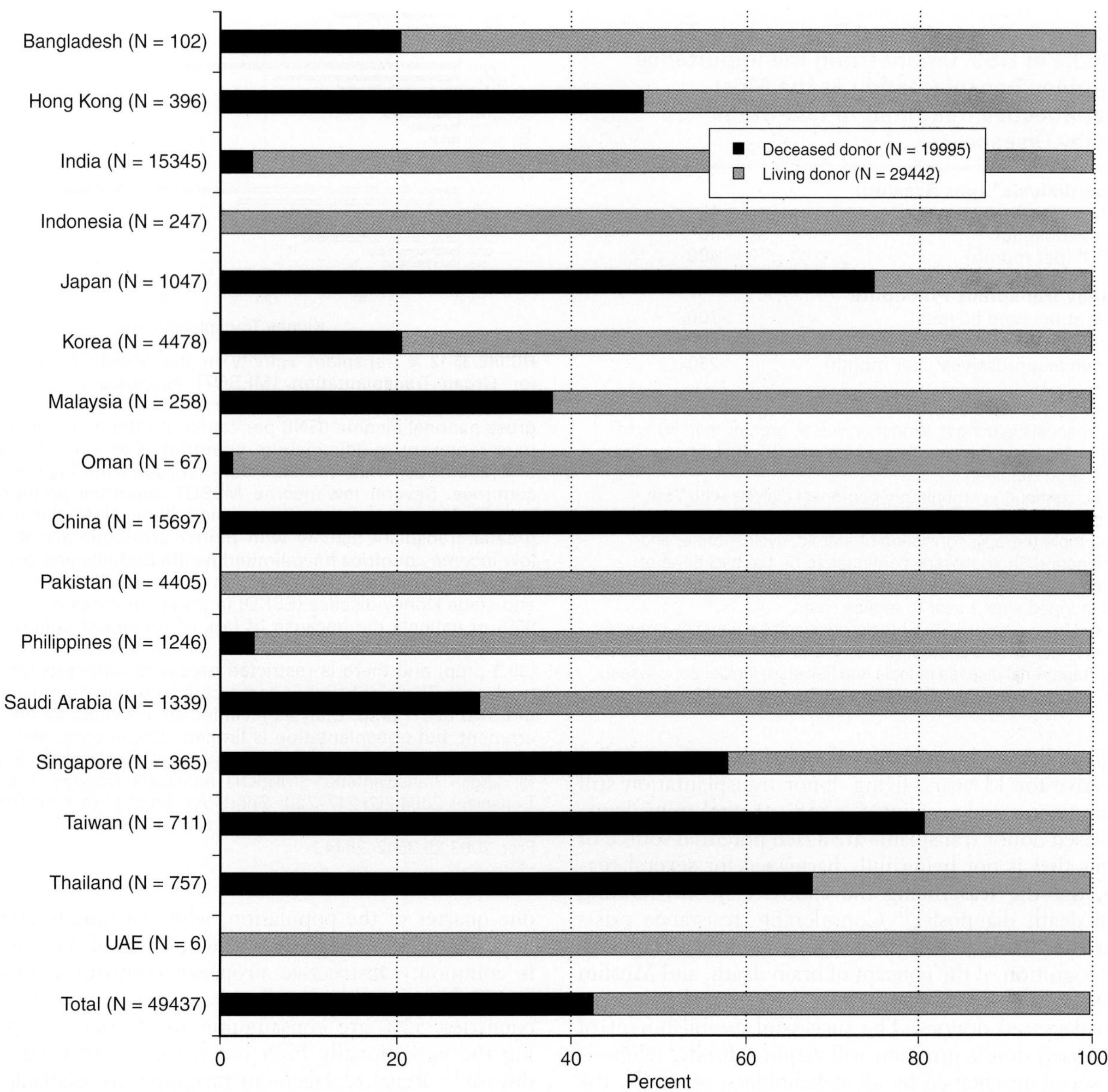

FIGURE 38-11 ■ **Kidney transplant activity in Asian countries (1997–2001). Living donors remain the main source of kidneys in this region, accounting for almost 60% of all transplants. The People's Republic of China performs the greatest number of transplants but organs are predominantly from individuals undergoing judicial executions. The largest numbers of conventional transplants are performed in India and these are almost exclusively living donor transplants.** (Drawn using data from Ota K. Current status of organ transplants in Asian countries. Transplant Proc 2004;36:2535–2538.)

This required transplant centers to be accredited and the number of units plummeted from 600 to a mere 163 that were approved to perform kidney transplants.[235,255]

The annual number of kidney transplants has increased in Asia over the years, but great potential remains for further growth. This growth can be achieved through legal and social acceptance of the brain death concept, the establishment of organ procurement organizations, and, most importantly, education of the public and healthcare providers through systematic support from the authorities.

Middle East and Afro-Arab Region

Kidney transplantation in the region has followed fairly distinct patterns historically. Initially, deceased donor kidney transplants were undertaken in Europe and North America. Local living related transplant programs were then established, followed by local experience with imported cadaver kidneys. During this period, commercialized living unrelated donor transplantation in neighboring countries thrived. The region has seen considerable progress, with almost all Middle Eastern countries now having successful transplant programs, including several with active deceased donor programs. The introduction of cyclosporine and, more importantly, the issuance of the Amman Declaration in 1986 gave new impetus to transplant programs. Despite this, the programs currently yield only 9 kidney transplants pmp, while there is an estimated average of 200 patients pmp who require kidney transplants.[228] All countries in this region, with the exception of Egypt, Iran, and Iraq, have adopted laws that permit use of organs from deceased donors and

TABLE 38-2 **Cost of Renal Replacement Therapy in India in US$, Emphasizing the Importance of Kidney Transplantation as the Most Cost-Effective Treatment of End-Stage Kidney Disease**

Hemodialysis* (per Session)	
State-subsidized hospital	10
Private hospital	40
CAPD¶ (per month)	400
Kidney Transplant Procedure	
State-subsidized hospital	700
Private hospital	6000
Immunosuppressives† (per month)	250

*Most patients are dialysed only twice weekly, reuse of dialyzers after manual cleaning is almost universal, greater than 50% of haemodialysis units use acetate, and only 30–40% of patients can afford erythropoietin.

†CAPD, continuous ambulatory peritoneal dialysis with Y-set, performing three exchanges per week.

¶Basic triple therapy, consisting of steroid, cyclosporine, and azathioprine. Triple therapy continues to be the backbone of immunosuppressive protocols, although the cyclosporine is often discontinued after 1 year to reduce costs.

Adapted from Agarwal SK. Chronic kidney disease and its prevention in India. Kidney Int 2005;68(S98):S41–S45; and Sakhuja V, Kohli HS. End-stage renal disease in India and Pakistan: incidence, causes, and management. Ethn Dis 2006;16(2 Suppl 2):S2–S3.

regulate living donations.[144] Despite these laws being operative for 15 years, living donor transplantation still predominates and accounts for 85% of total transplants. Deceased donor transplants are a rich potential source of organs that is not being fully harnessed for several reasons, not the least being the controversy surrounding brain death diagnosis.[228] Considerable resistance exists from the Muslim medical community notwithstanding the reognition of the concept of brain death, and Muslim clergy passing edicts that permit the retrieval of organs from deceased donors. The successful establishment of a deceased donor program will require, firstly, religious and social acceptance by all stakeholders; secondly, the requisite legal framework; and finally, government commitment.[228] Saudi Arabia has led the way in deceased donor transplants that now comprise 30% of all transplants. In Turkey and Kuwait, deceased donor organs account for 25% of kidney transplants while Iran has steadily increased its proportion of deceased donor transplants from 0.4% in 2002 to 31% in 2008.[71]

The Middle East Society for Organ Transplantation (MESOT) registry, established in 1987, documents transplant activity in the region; MESOT also promotes public awareness of transplantation and scientific cooperation.[144,228] The Registry represents over 29 countries from the Middle East, North Africa, and neighboring states, comprising a total population of 635 million.[84,228] The number of patients receiving kidney transplants is only 9 pmp; the regional ESKD incidence ranges from 34 to 200 pmp.[144] Economically, the region is divided into three income groups with transplant activity related to economic activity (Figure 38-12). The most common cause of ESKD is diabetes mellitus; it accounts for 45% of new ESKD in Saudi Arabia, 46.8% in Lebanon, 21.2% in Kuwait, and 35% in Egypt. Hypertension affects approximately

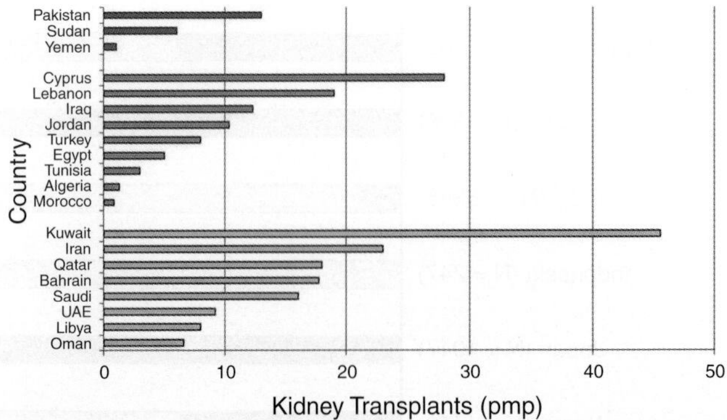

FIGURE 38-12 ■ Transplant activity in the Middle East Society for Organ Transplantation (MESOT) countries in 2003. The countries depicted by red bars are low-income countries with gross national income (GNI) per capita of $100–1200; the green bars represent middle-income countries with GNI per capita of $1200–5000, while the blue bars represent the high-income countries. Several low-income MESOT countries perform no transplants and are not represented here. Note the overall greater transplant activity with higher economic activity. The low-income countries have limited health budgets and small or non-existent dialysis and transplant programs. The incidence of end-stage kidney disease (ESKD) in these countries is 101 pmp; 95% of patients die because of lack of treatment options. The medium-income countries have a similar incidence of ESKD (99.3 pmp) and there is restricted access to renal replacement treatment. The eight high-income countries have an incidence of ESKD of 111 pmp. Dialysis facilities are provided by the government, but transplantation is limited. (Drawn using data from: Masri MA, Haberal MA, Shaheen FA, et al. Middle East Society for Organ Transplantation (MESOT) Transplant Registry. Exp Clin Transplant 2004;2(2):217–220; Ghods AJ. Should we have live unrelated donor renal transplantation in MESOT countries? Transplant Proc 2003;35:2542–2544.)

one-quarter of the population, while chronic interstitial nephritis due to analgesic abuse and herbal medications is common. Obstructive uropathy constitutes 40% of ESKD in certain Arab countries. Of all unions in Arab countries, 52% are consanguineous marriages, explaining the exceptionally high incidence of inherited renal disease.[231] Renal replacement programs are available but limited. Only one-half of patients are started on dialysis treatment, and because of limited transplant activity, these patients remain permanently on dialysis, placing an enormous burden on already strained health budgets.[84]

There are three predominant models of transplantation and organ donation in the MESOT region. In the Saudi model, a quasi-government organization is responsible for all aspects of organ donation, from increasing awareness in the medical fraternity and public education to organ procurement and allocation.[228] This organization has enjoyed considerable success, as evidenced by a remarkable increase in the number of transplant centers and organs transplanted.[230] Iran performs the largest number of kidney transplants in this region, of which 77% are from living unrelated donors.[144] The Iranian model allows for living unrelated donors to be compensated by the recipient or a charitable organization, and the cost of the transplant is borne by the government. The model has been so successful that the waiting list for kidney transplantation in Iran has been eliminated.[86] However, the feedback from donors clearly indicates that much remains to be done to improve the process of donation.[230] Improvements suggested are that all compensation be made by the government, and that compensation of living donors be substantial and "life-changing."[86] This model yields 17 donors pmp but may not be applicable to multiethnic populations and several ethical issues remain unresolved. Finally, the Pakistani model pioneered by the Sind Institute of Urology and Transplantation involves community and government partnership in the care of patients, in which the latter contributes 40–50% toward the cost of the transplant and the community the remainder. The center averages 110 kidney transplants per year. The free supply of medication to the patient is an important factor in the success of the initiative. The program prides itself on its transparency, accountability, and high quality of its care.[198]

Sub-Saharan Africa

Sub-Saharan Africa comprises 47 countries and includes 70% of the world's poorest nations. In 2007 it had a population of 800 million people and, of these, 41% lived in extreme poverty, surviving on less than $1 a day.[163] It also has a double burden of disease – infections and parasitic diseases killed 5.5 million people, and HIV/AIDS 2 million in 2005; this is compounded by the growing threat of non-communicable diseases which in the same year accounted for 2.4 million deaths.[164] This region is the epicenter of the world's HIV/AIDS pandemic; comprising only 11.6% of the world population, it has two-thirds of all HIV cases. Health authorities are under pressure to fight this scourge, with the result that other areas of healthcare, such as renal replacement therapy, are neglected. AIDS has reduced life expectancy in this region to 46 years. The lack of registries in sub-Saharan Africa makes it difficult to establish the prevalence and etiology of ESKD in this region. The estimated prevalence of ESKD is 200–300 pmp.[164] ESKD is possibly three to four times more common than in economically advanced countries.[163] Hypertension and chronic glomerulonephritis are the most prevalent causes of chronic kidney disease while HIV-associated kidney disease accounts for 6–48.5% of CKD.[164] A recent report suggests that diabetes is, as elsewhere in the developing world, likely to become an ever-increasing problem[165] and currently is responsible for some 25% of CKD cases.[159] Chronic kidney disease affects relatively younger patients in the age range 20–50 years compared to developed countries where chronic kidney disease affects the middle-aged to elderly. Resources are very limited, with several countries having no specialist nephrologists and very limited access to renal replacement therapy. The dialysis rate in sub-Saharan Africa is less than 20 pmp, the lowest renal replacement therapy rate in the world, with several countries offering none at all. Of 1.8 million people on dialysis worldwide in 2004, less than 5% were in sub-Saharan Africa.[164]

Of all the developing regions, sub-Saharan Africa has the lowest transplant rate, averaging less than 5 pmp.[163] Only five countries in sub-Saharan Africa perform kidney transplants on a regular basis, namely South Africa, Mauritius, Ghana, Kenya, and Nigeria.[20,164] The majority of transplants in sub-Saharan Africa are living donor transplants, with the exception of South Africa. South Africa has the most active transplant programs, performing some 240 transplants annually, of which 80% are deceased donor transplants (Figure 38-13). Transplant activity in this region is severely compromised by religious and social constraints, lack of resources (including personnel), and other health priorities alluded to earlier, while deceased donor transplants lack the relevant legal framework. Renal replacement treatment is privately funded in the main, with only a few goverments, such as those of South Africa, Mali, and Mauritius, assisting indigent patients.[164]

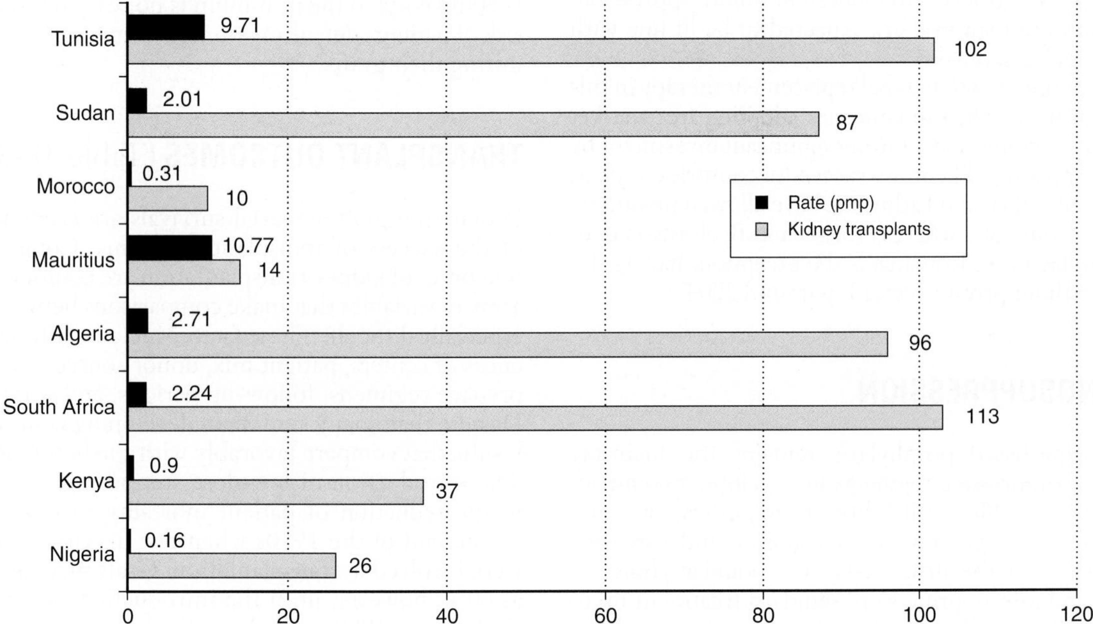

FIGURE 38-13 ■ **Kidney transplant activity in selected African countries in 2010. Compared to data from earlier years, the total number of transplants is declining in several countries.** (Drawn using data from: Global observatory on donation and transplantation. Organ donation and transplantation: Activities, laws and organization 2010 [online], 2012. http://www.transplant-observatory.org/Data%20Reports/2010%20Report%20final.pdf; Naicker S. Burden of end-stage renal disease in sub-Saharan Africa. Clin Nephrol 2010;74 (Suppl. 1): S13–S16.)

Central and Eastern Europe

The sociopolitical and economic landscape of this region has changed dramatically over the past few decades. With the collapse of communism and the economic reforms that embraced the free-market system there has been dramatic improvements in the welfare of these states, including healthcare. Of all developing regions, Central and Eastern Europe has shown the most growth in prevalent renal replacement treatment in recent years. This region constitutes 18 countries with more than 330 million inhabitants. The epidemiology of ESKD is also changing. The main cause of ESKD is still chronic glomerulonephritis followed by interstitial kidney disease.[136] Diabetes is accounting for an ever-increasing proportion of ESKD, averaging 10–14%, but in the Czech Republic, it accounts for 32% of all dialyzed patients.[209] Another important epidemiological observation is the aging of the population, which may explain the increase in hypertensive renal disease.[210]

Although dialysis has increased dramatically by over 50%, the rate of increase of transplantation has been less spectacular: since 1990, the number of transplant units in the region has increased by 148%, but the number of kidney transplants by only 44%. The Baltic states, Poland, Lithuania, and Romania, have experienced the best progress in dialysis facilities.[211] The region performs on average 22 transplants pmp, ranging from 1.5 to 54.5 pmp (Figure 38-14). Deceased donors are the main source of kidneys but Bosnia-Herzegovina, Macedonia, Romania, and Serbia perform mainly living donor transplants for religious and cultural reasons.[209] The deceased donor program has failed to grow significantly for a variety of reasons. The growth in dialysis is commendable but the lack of a commensurate growth in transplantation can overwhelm available dialysis resources rapidly. The results of kidney transplants in the region have yet to be analyzed, but with access to modern immunosuppression, patient and graft survival are expected to be in line with international outcomes.[209]

Much of the growth in renal replacement therapy in this region can be ascribed to countries adopting free-market systems of economy and allowing significant investment by private companies. The more successful countries, such as Hungary, Slovakia, and Lithuania, have allowed private facilities to proliferate, whereas Russia and Byelorussia have no private facilities. Romania is the exception, having developed without private-sector input until 2004.[209]

IMMUNOSUPPRESSION

Cyclosporine-based prophylaxis remains the mainstay of immunosuppressive regimens in developing countries (Figure 38-15). The availability of safe, efficacious, and cheaper generic versions of cyclosporine and extensive experience with the drug make it a popular choice.[169] Steroids and azathioprine were standard treatment up to the early 1980s, and are still used in some living related donor transplants with very good matches. Acute rejection is treated with pulses of methylprednisolone and resistant rejection with polyclonal/monoclonal antibodies.[233] Antibodies are used occasionally in induction, especially in high-risk patients, such as the elderly.[169,245] In most developing countries immunosuppresive costs are not state-subsidized, which means patients and their families have to bear the full costs of the agents; not many can afford to do so and this represents a barrier to successful long-term graft survival.[127]

In Latin America, there has been a shift in immunosuppression from cyclosporine-based therapy to regimens increasingly using MMF and tacrolimus. In addition, the full spectrum of biological antisera is used in the induction and treatment of rejection. Sirolimus is the only newer agent that has failed to gain widespread acceptance.[221] In other parts of the developing world, costs limit the use of MMF and tacrolimus. If chronic allograft nephropathy is diagnosed, some centers substitute MMF for azathioprine and reduce the dose of cyclosporine.[169] Globally, tacrolimus has replaced cyclosporine as the calcinerin inhibitor of choice but in most developing countries, because of cost considerations and a lower incidence of diabetes mellitus following transplantation, cyclosporine is still favored. In India, interestingly, tacrolimus is cheaper than cyclopsorine and, combined with steroids and azathioprine, is first-line treatment. Azathioprine is preferred to MMF mainly because of its cost-effectiveness and comparable outcomes to MMF. The use of interleukin-2 receptor antibodies is also limited to patients that represent a high immunological risk or where a steriod-free regimen is planned.[127] In developing countries proliferation signal inhibitors, such as sirolimus, enjoyed limited use because of high costs and long-term studies have shown sirolimus/MMF to be inferior to tacrolimus/MMF combinations.[244]

It is crucially important that in developing countries the cheapest immunosuppressive regimen that provides optimal immunosuppression is used. Running the tight balance between optimizing immunosupression while keeping costs to the minimum is not easy but reduces the risk of patients defaulting on treatment and thus compromising their grafts.

TRANSPLANT OUTCOMES (Table 38-3)

Patient and graft actuarial survivals are crude indicators of the success of transplant programs. Comparisons of outcomes of kidney transplantation are confounded by an array of variables that make comparisons between regions especially difficult. These factors include differing experiences of centers, patient mix, donor source, immunosuppressive regimens, follow-up periods, and compliance.[105] Despite that, many centers in developing countries boast results that compare favorably with the best in the world. The introduction of low-dose steroid regimens resulted in the reduction of patient mortality to less than 10% by the end of the 1970s when few developing countries were involved in transplantation. Graft survival remained at 60%, however, until the introduction of cyclosporine in the early 1980s, which resulted in dramatic improvements in 1-year graft survival rates.[160]

The best outcomes are achieved with living related kidney transplantation, followed by spousal

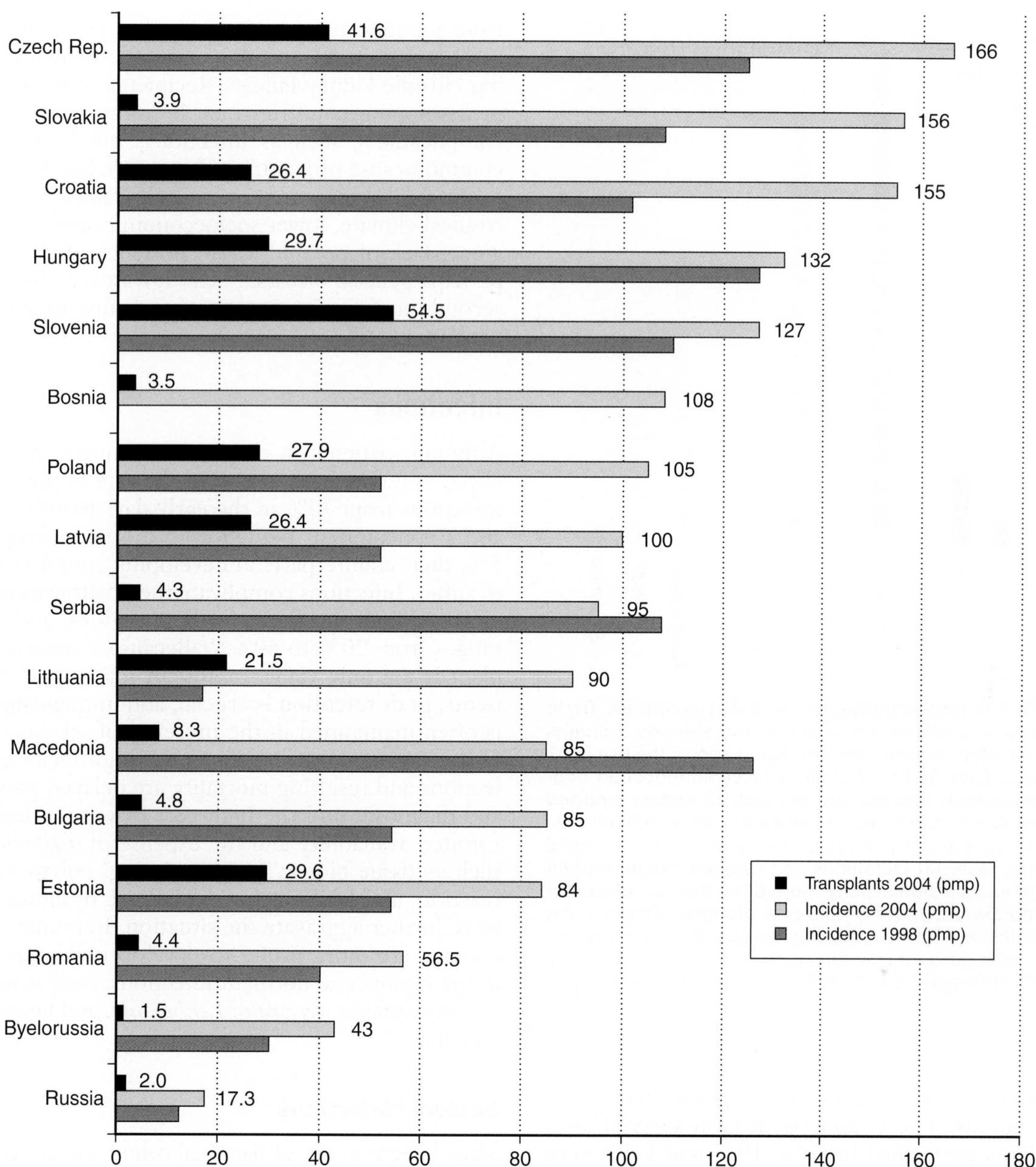

FIGURE 38-14 ■ Change in the incidence rates of dialysis over 6 years, and transplant rates in 2004 in Central and Eastern European (CEE) countries. All the countries, with two exceptions, showed a significant uptake of dialysis. Poland leads, with a total of 1067 kidney transplants in 2004 but, relative to the size of the population, Slovenia and the Czech Republic performed the best; significant increases were shown by the Baltic countries, Hungary and Poland. In the remaining CEE countries, the progress in transplantation has been disappointing, with Byelorussia and Russia having the worst transplant rates. Russia has been least successful in developing facilities and has actually seen a decline in transplant numbers. (Drawn using data from Rutkowski B. Availability of renal replacement therapy in Central and Eastern Europe. Ethnicity Dis 2009;19:18–22; Rutkowski B. Highlights of the epidemiology of renal replacement therapy in Central and Eastern Europe. Nephrol Dial Transplant 2006;21:4–10.)

transplantation, living unrelated transplantation, and deceased donor transplantation. Living unrelated transplants yield results that are superior to deceased donor transplantation despite histoincompatibility.[225] Indeed, living unrelated transplantation boasts results comparable to living related transplantation,[240] although long-term results significantly favor better HLA matching.[38] Commercial transplantation, on the other hand, has a poorer outcome, possibly due to suboptimal preparation of recipients, suboptimal perioperative care, and immunosuppression.[5] Significant morbidity was reported in most studies of commercially transplanted recipients, but these studies were uncontrolled. Infection was the most commonly reported complication and the most common cause of mortality; surgical problems were also common. These patients were more likely to acquire unusual and/or potentially fatal complications such as malaria, invasive fungal infections, septicemia, HIV infection, and hepatitis.[214,240]

Actuarial graft survival averaged 88% at 1 year (Table 38-3) and decreased progressively with longer follow-up. Graft survivals in HLA-identical donor transplants of 95% at 5 years have been reported, whereas survival in HLA-haploidentical and poorly matched donor transplants was equally impressive, with 5-year survival rates of 90%.[120,197] Latin America has the most

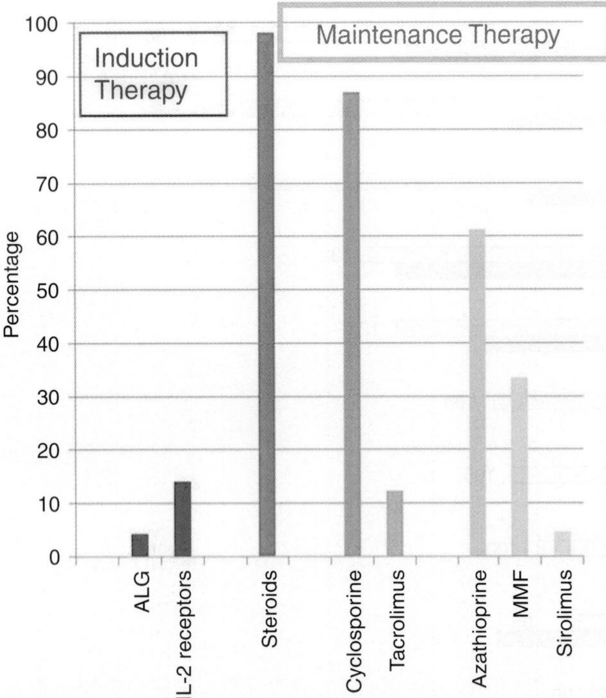

FIGURE 38-15 ■ Immunosuppression in Asian countries. Triple therapy, including calcineurin inhibitor and steroids, remains popular in developing countries. The figure shows the use in 17 Asian centers. Only 18.4% of patients received induction therapy with an antibody preparation, although 13 centers reported using interleukin-2 (IL-2) receptor antibodies. Of all transplants, 80% were living donor transplants. The recipients of deceased donor organs received tacrolimus and mycophenolate mofetil (MMF) maintenance significantly more often than cyclosporine and azathioprine. ALG, antilymphocyte globulin. (Drawn using data from Vathsala A. Immunosuppression use in renal transplantation from Asian transplant centers: A preliminary report from the Asian Transplant Registry. Transplant Proc 2004;36:1868–1870.)

active deceased donor transplant program among developing regions. The 1- and 3-year graft survival rates of transplants performed between 1987 and 1997 were 74% and 60%.[173] Of the newer programs, both that of Saudi Arabia and India have reported very good results (Table 38-3). With the severe shortage of donor organs, countries are resorting increasingly to the use of ECD. Goplani et al. report the successful use of ECD in India, with 1-year graft survival rate an impressive 86%.[90] From Korea, Jeong et al. also reported 1-year graft survival of ECD recipients comparable to standard criteria donors, although the estimated glomerular filtration rate at 1 year was lower in the former.[110] The unique Iranian program of living unrelated transplantation yields good long-term results: 1-year graft survival rates of 87% compare favorably with the 89% of living related transplants (Table 38-3).

POSTTRANSPLANT COMPLICATIONS

Optimal immunosuppression in the transplanted patient is a delicate balance between maximizing graft survival and minimizing complications. Most complications arise from immunosuppression, but other posttransplant diseases may occur as a result of the underlying disease causing chronic kidney failure. Recipients of renal allografts in developing countries may be more prone to certain complications, such as infections, which are the most common cause of posttransplant mortality. Contributing to the risk for infections are protein-calorie malnutrition, tropical climate, lower socioeconomic status, lack of hygiene, lack of potable water, presence of parasites, and perhaps genetic factors.[197] Cardiovascular disease is the second most common cause of mortality in transplanted patients.

Infections

Although patients in developed countries have experienced a dramatic reduction in the rate of posttransplant infections from 70% in the early days to 40% currently, and a concomitant reduction in mortality from 40% to 5%, their counterparts in developing countries continue to suffer. Infections complicate the posttransplant course of 50–75% of recipients in these regions, and mortality ranges from 20% to 60%.[112] Because a successful transplant is the only viable treatment for most of these patients, graft retention is crucial, and immunosuppression is often maintained in the presence of serious infection. Other factors contributing to the high incidence of infections and resulting mortality are delayed presentation and diagnosis, and the high cost of vital antimicrobials. Limited availability and the expense of diagnostic tools, such as tissue biopsy, antigen testing, polymerase chain reaction, and facilities for the culture of unusual organisms, further aggravate the situation. Immunosuppressed patients are more prone to develop infections endemic to the region, and dormant infections, such as tuberculosis, *Strongyloides stercoralis*, *Leishmania*, and herpesviruses, may flare.[112]

Bacterial Infections

Most infections are of bacterial origin and are commonly encountered in the early postoperative periods. The urinary tract and lungs are the most common sites infected, with the former predominating by far (42% versus 6%).[185] Pneumonia (excluding tuberculosis) occurred in 16% of 110 South African renal allograft recipients at a mean of 3 months posttransplantation,[66] comparable to the 18% reported from the Indian subcontinent.[112] Causative organisms range from community-acquired *Streptococcus pneumoniae* and *Haemophilus influenzae* to dreaded multidrug-resistant nosocomial organisms.[112] With appropriate intervention, patients with lung infections respond very well. However, *Pneumocystis joveci*, fungal infections, and CMV infections are all possibilities and, in one-third of cases, more than a single organism has been identified. Thus, and because early appropriate therapy is important, an aggressive diagnostic approach, including invasive procedures such as bronchalveolar lavage, is justified.[119] Co-trimoxazole in the first few months after transplantation is recommended prophylaxis for *P. joveci* pneumonia. The classic symptoms of urinary tract infection are almost consistently absent, with the diagnosis being made on the

TABLE 38-3 **Outcomes of Kidney Transplantation in Adults and Children in Selected Developing Countries**

Country (Period)	No. of Transplants	Donor Type	Immuno-suppression*	% Survival (at Year Indicated)		Reference
				Patient	Graft	
Bangladesh	68	LRD	Aza	–	96(1)+81(3)	192
(1982–1992)	26	LURD	CsA[†]			
Brazil	687	LRD	NS	–		88,224
(1970–1989)	60	LURD	CsA (42%)	–	70(1),49(5)	
(1987–1989)	239	CD	CsA (75%)	—	76(2)	
	1051	LD		89(2)	61(2)	
	467	CD		80(2)		
	45	?				
Chile (1983–2003)[‡]	100	CD/LRD	CNI/MMF/IL-2	96(1),96(5)	89(1),73(5)	61
China 2002	2016	LDT	–		83(1),66(5),48(10)	186
(1999–2004)	2575	DD	CNI		94(1);72(5),54(10)	247
Egypt (1976–1995)[‡]	216	LRD	CsA	98(1), 88(5)	93(1),73(5)	75
(1994)	45	LRD	Aza (good matches)	92(1),86(5)	89(1),73(5)	22
(1992)	130	LURD(C)	CsA	88(1),80(4)	86(1),58(4)	21
	15	CD	CsA			
	30	LRD	CsA			
	124	LURD(C)	CsA			
(1976–2001)	82	Pre-emptive	Aza/CsA	95(1),88(5)	94(1),81(5)	74
(1983–1988)	1197	LD	Aza/Csa	96(1),88(5)	92(1),74(5)	83
20-year	130	LD	Aza	89(1),76(5),61(10)	85(1),70(5),52(10)	
	239	LD	Aza/CsA	96(1),85(5),73(10)	92(1),72(5),51(10)	
Hungary (1983–2001)	1825(Cc)	CD	CNI	98(1),85(5),74(10)	89(1),76(5),57(10)	130
	93 (Gy)	CD	CNI	95(1),88(5),82(10)	79(1),54(5),34(10)	130
India	153	LRD	Aza	–	83(1)	251
(1985–1988)	303	LURD(C)	CsA	–	83(1)	
(1981–1989)	144	LRD	Aza	53(10)	47(10)	2
(1995–2001)	100	CD	NS	86(1),80(2)	82(1),74(2)	239
(1991–2005) [‡]	90	LRD	CsA	95(1),87(5)	98(1),85(5)	200
(1994–2004)[‡]	39	LRD	CsA[†]	89(1),70(3)	89(1),50(5)	95
(1995–2008) [‡]	45	LRD	CNI/MMF/Aza	95(1),88(5),77(10)	91(1),80(5),75(10)	242
(1984–1996)[‡]	63	LRD	CsA	92(1),90(3)	88(1),86(3)	148
(2006–2009)	160	CD	MMF/CNI (ATG)	80(1),77(2),75(3)	92(1),88(2),88(3)	96
(2006–2009)	29	ECD	MMF/CNI/(ATG)	90(1)	86(1)	90
Iran (1985–2003)[‡]	278	LRD/LURD	CsA/Aza/MMF	92(1),74(5)	89(1),67(5)	177
(1986–2000)	478	LRD[§]	CsA/MMF	93(1),84(5),	89(1),82(5),70(10)	85
	942	LURD	CsA/MMF	73(10) overall	87(1),64(5),44(10)	
(1996–1999)	207	LD	CsA	94(1),90(3),77(10)	89(1),83(3),54(10)	123
(1992–2002)	242	LURD?	–	–	87(1),84(5),71(7)	99
(? –2003)	61	Spousal	CsA/Aza/MMF	97(1),93(3)	91(1),86(3)	207
	433	LRD		96(1),92(3)	91(1),85(3)	
	427	LURD		93(1),91(3)	87(1),82(3)	
	118	CD		93(1),92(3)	88(1),84(3)	
	1039	Overall		94(1),92(3)	88(1),84(3)	

Continued on following page

TABLE 38-3 **Outcomes of Kidney Transplantation in Adults and Children in Selected Developing Countries** (Continued)

Country (Period)	No. of Transplants	Donor Type	Immuno-suppression*	% Survival (at Year Indicated) Patient	Graft	Reference
Iraq (1979–1999)	182	LD	Csa/Aza	83(1),80(5)	84(1),64(5)	8
Korea (1979–1996)	1500	LD/CD	Aza/CsA	91(5),80(10)	81(5),61(10)	179
(1997–2011)						110
Kuwait (1985–1990)	53	LURD(C)	NS	90(2)	90(2)	118
(1993–1998)	151	LRD	CsA(MMF)	94(1),92(5)	89(1),85(5)	220
(1996–2004)	158	CD	NS	93(1),89(7)	81(1),75(7)	219
	402	LRD	NS	97(1),95(5)	95(1),91(5)	
Latin America	5347	CD	CsA*	NS	74(1),60(3)	173
(1987–1997)		LRD	CsA*	NS	86(1),74(3)	
Mexico	282	LRD	CsA 1984†	86(1),68(5)	77(1),60(5)	29
(1967–1991)	10	LURD	(Aza in HLA-identical			
	46	CD	LRD)			
Macedonia (2004)	16	LURD(C)	CsA/Aza/MMF	78(1),70(5)	78(1),33(5)	106
	14	LURT	As above	100(1),86(5)	100(1),78(5)	
Myanmar (Burma)	21	LRD	CsA	95(1)	95(1)	252
(1997–2003)						
Pakistan (2002)	1000	LRD	CsA 1990	95(1), 85(5)	90(1), 75(5)	198
(1992–2000)	711	LRD	CsA/MMF	90(1),78(5)	90(1),75(5)	169
(1986–1999)‡	75	LRD	CsA	90(1),75(5)	88(1),65(5)	202
(1997 – 2007)	180	LRD	CsA/Aza/MMF		94(1),80(5)	204
	126	LURD(C)			86(1),45(5)	204
Philippines	1024	LRD	CsA† (1983)	90(1)	90(1)	135
(1969–1992)		CAD	CsA†	75(1),71(3)	62(1),56(3)	
Saudi Arabia (1999)	~2,500	LRD	CsA	96(1)	90(1)	7
(1991–1996)	910	CD	CsA	95(1)	78(1)	9
(1987–1996)	60	LURD(C)	CsA	94(1),81(3)	93(1),60(5)	11
(2003 – 2007)	LD	172	CsA	99(1),93(5),86(10)	97(1),86(5),70(10)	232
	CD	188	CsA (ATG)	98(1),94(5),91(10)	86(1),72(5),58(10)	
	CD	524	CNI/MMF/Sir	97(1),92(5)	88(1), 80(5)	

Singapore	47	LRD	CsA	95(1),88(7)	86(1),77(7)	263
(1985–1992)	157	CD	CsA		98(1),92(6)	
Slovenia	83	CD	CsA	91(1),88(3)	73(1),73(3)	121
(1986–1991)	65	LRD	CsA	95(1),93(5)	90(1),90(3)	
South Africa	542	CD	Aza/CsA	81(1),60(5)	50(1) Aza, 72(1)CsA	155
(1976–1999)						
(1984–2003)‡	282	LRD/CD	CsA	97(1),84(5),68(10)	82(1),44(5),23(10)	183
Sri Lanka	105	LRD	CsA†	71(1),47(4)	71(1),47(4)	234
(1985–1992)						
Taiwan	~1,000	LRD	NS	92(1)	82(1)	131
(1968–1992)		CD				
Thailand	46	CD/LRD		96(1),88(5)	98(1),84(5)	246
(1996 – 2000)‡						
Tunisia (1986–2005)	330	LRD/CD	CsA/Aza	NS	85(1),30(5),16(15)	31
Turkey (1975–2004)‡	80	LRD/CD	CNI/MMF/Aza	98(1), 90(5)	91(1), 67(5)	76
(1985–1989)	80	LURD	NS	95(1–3)	80(1–3)	58
(1975–1993)	766	LRD	CsA (1985)	Aza: 60(10)	Aza: 42(10)	98
	230	CD	CsA	CsA: 87(1),72(5)	CsA: 66(1),37(5)	
(1985–1992)	391	LRD	DST+Aza or+CsA	DST 98(1)	92(1)	100
				DST 94(1)	72(1)	
(1992–1999)	115	LURD(C)	CsA	90(2),80(5)	84(2),66(5)	226
	NS	LRT	NS	90(2),85(5)	86(2),78(5)	
(1991–1995)	127	LURD(C)	CsA	93(1),92(5)	83(1),57(5)	48
UAE/Oman	130	LURD(C)	CsA	82(1),81(3.75)	77(1),75(3.75)	218
(1984–1988)						
Venezuela	NS	All	NS	NS	83(1),50(10)	28
(2002)		LRT	NS	NS	90(1),64(10)	

*Regimen predominantly used.
†Cyclosporine discontinued at 3–12 months.
‡Pediatric cases.
§HLA-identical matched donor.
ATG, antithymocyte globulin; Aza, azathioprine; Cc, Caucasian; CD, deceased donor; CNI, calcineurin inhibitor; CsA, cyclosporine as part of triple or dual therapy; DST, donor-specific blood transfusion; ECD, expanded criteria donor; Gy, gypsy; IL-2, interleukin-2; LD, living donor; LRD, living related donor; LURD, living unrelated donor; LURD(C), commercial living unrelated donor; MMF, mycophenolate mofetil; NS, not specified; Sir, sirolimus.

presence of bacteriuria.[184,257] The most common organisms isolated are *Escherichia coli* and *Klebsiella*. Although the response to antibiotic treatment is good, relapses are frequent. Organisms resistant to commonly employed antibiotics are prevalent. Their eradication is often problematic because these organisms respond only to expensive and parenteral antibiotics that are impractical to use.

Tuberculosis. In developing countries, the incidence of tuberculosis posttransplantation is considerably higher than in industrialized countries; malnutrition, overcrowding, HIV/AIDS, poverty, and illiteracy contribute to this high incidence.[158] On the Indian subcontinent, up to 15% of kidney transplant patients[116,215] develop tuberculosis compared with 1.7% in the United Kingdom.[101] In Turkey, tuberculosis is 8.5 times more common than in the general population.[37]

The interval between development of tuberculosis posttransplantation ranges from 1 month to 10 years, but 50–80% occur within 1 year of transplantation.[77] Transplant recipients who have had treatment for acute rejection with steroids or monoclonal/polyclonal antibodies are at greater risk of tuberculosis.[14,26] The disease manifests with the classic symptoms of cough, fever, night sweats, and weight loss,[26] but the classic features of tuberculosis are often obscured by immunosuppression.[140,158] Transplant patients are prone to developing extrapulmonary and disseminated forms of tuberculosis; these may account for 12–46% of all cases of posttransplant tuberculosis. The mortality of disseminated tuberculosis is high in transplant recipients in developing countries – almost 40% compared with 11% in the isolated form.[189]

The diagnosis of tuberculosis, especially extrapulmonary forms, may be challenging, and a high index of suspicion is required in the appropriate setting.[51] Radiologically, the typical apical cavitatory disease in pulmonary tuberculosis is absent in 90% of cases, showing pulmonary opacification or effusions instead. Diagnosis of pulmonary tuberculosis is most commonly made by examination of the sputum for acid/alcohol-fast bacilli using appropriate staining techniques and culture, although the latter is time-consuming and expensive. The diagnostic yield can be enhanced by bronchoscopy and bronchoalveolar lavage.[115] The HIV/AIDS pandemic has thrown into sharp focus the urgent need for improved methods of diagnosing tuberculosis. A concerted global effort has yielded several promising diagnostic tests, some of which have already been endorsed by the WHO.[64] The tuberculin skin test has limited diagnostic value in developing countries, where tuberculosis is endemic, and most of the population has been exposed to the tubercle bacillus.[189] Most kidney transplant patients are anergic.[26] For extrapulmonary forms, bone marrow biopsy and liver biopsy should be considered.[126]

The treatment of tuberculosis in kidney transplant recipients poses no less challenge, mainly because of drug–drug interactions. Most recipients receive triple immunosuppressive therapy, and rifampicin and isoniazid are the mainstays of antituberculous treatment. Rifampicin and, to a lesser extent, isoniazid are potent inducers of the liver cytochrome P-450 enzyme system, markedly enhancing the elimination of calcineurin inhibitors and steroids. The dose of steroids needs doubling, but calcineurin inhibitor doses may need to be increased severalfold to maintain therapeutic blood levels. The cost of treatment is increased, as is the risk of acute rejection.[167] Patients with renal allografts who develop tuberculosis respond well to conventional therapy.[37] The duration of therapy is determined by the choice of drugs. If the combination of isoniazid and rifampicin is used with another agent, usually pyrazinamide, 6 months of therapy is adequate, although some centers treat for 9 months.[112] If a rifampicin-free regimen is used, treatment should be continued for a minimum of 9–12 months and possibly extended to 18 months.[260] With prolonged therapy, compliance is a potential problem, and multidrug resistance is an ever-increasing concern. Directly observed therapy, pioneered in developing countries, has ensured the success of intermittent therapy where other techniques have failed.[125] The use of isoniazid chemoprophylaxis is controversial but a recent systematic review and meta-analysis of four randomized controlled studies clearly suggests a benefit to the use of isoniazid in endemic countries and in high-risk patients. Importantly, the risk of hepatotoxicity is not increased. In the absence of more robust randomized controlled studies this is currently the strongest evidence in support of isoniazid chemoprophylaxis.[53] The development of drug resistance remains a concern.

Protozoan Infections

Malaria. Malaria, caused by *Plasmodium*, is the most common parasitic infection in developing countries and occurs in kidney transplant patients after the bite of an infected mosquito, the transfusion of infected blood,[35] or rarely, from an infected kidney.[42] Most reported cases have occurred in recipients of living unrelated transplants who received their grafts in India and were diagnosed when they returned home after transplantation.[258] Patients respond well to standard antimalarial treatment, and the prognosis is good.[258] There generally are no contraindications to the use of malaria chemoprophylaxis in kidney transplant patients. Patients traveling to malaria-endemic areas should be advised that personal protection measures are the most important to prevent malaria.[74]

Chagas' Disease. American trypanosomiasis (Chagas' disease) is endemic in South America, where an estimated 16–18 million people are infected with the extracellular protozoan *Trypanosoma cruzi*. The infection has been transmitted with donor organs.[39] Liberalization of use of organs from donors with Chagas' disease was controversially instituted in the late 1980s in Argentina and disease occurred in 19% of uninfected kidney recipients. Reactivation occurred in 22% of chagasic recipients 1 to 29 months after transplantation. Patients responded well to benznidazole, the specific therapy available. In view of the low transmission rate and availability of effective treatment, the use of organs from potential seropositive donors should not be excluded.[194]

Visceral Leishmaniasis (Kala-Azar). Visceral leishmaniasis caused by *Leishmania donovani* is endemic in parts of India, Africa, and South-West Asia. Full-blown visceral leishmaniasis manifests clinically with fever, weight loss, hepatosplenomegaly, cytopenia, and hypergammaglobulinemia, although it is suspected that most human infections are subclinical. Patients develop clinical features of disease 3 months to 8 years after transplantation and manifest typically with the full-blown clinical picture of the disease. Diagnosis is confirmed by bone marrow aspirate or serology. The treatment of choice is sodium stibogluconate for 20–30 days.[112]

Helminthic Infestations

Schistosomiasis. Schistosomiasis is a major public health problem in many parts of the developing world. Patients with urinary schistosomiasis can be transplanted successfully. Graft and patient survivals are comparable with controls, even with prolonged follow-up,[139] but urological complications occur in 15% of schistosomal patients.[238] Patients with schistosomiasis require 67% more cyclosporine to achieve the same blood levels as uninfected recipients because intestinal disease impairs absorption of cyclosporine.[139] Schistosomal reinfection occurs in approximately one-quarter of patients, but this does not have an impact on graft function if the disease is adequately treated. These patients may be at increased risk of bladder carcinoma, and cystoscopy should be part of long-term follow-up.[237]

Strongyloidiasis. Strongyloidiasis is an intestinal nematode infestation endemic in South-East Asia, sub-Saharan Africa, and Central and South America. It is an uncommon but potentially devastating disease in immunosuppressed patients. Because of the organism's capacity to multiply repeatedly within the host without external reinfection, a state of hyperinfestation may occur years after exposure. In recipients, this hyperinfestation may take a fulminant course.[243] Eosinophilia should alert the clinician to the possibility of *Strongyloides* infestation. In severely ill patients, supportive treatment may be needed, in addition to specific therapy with thiabendazole or mebendazole. *Strongyloides* may be transmitted with a kidney graft.[35]

Fungal Infections

Invasive fungal infections complicate the course of 1.4–10% of patients after kidney transplantation, with a high mortality of 60–100%.[45,165] The most commonly encountered pathogens are opportunistic organisms, such as *Candida* and *Cryptococcus*, but more recently there has been an increase in infection by angioinvasive *Aspergillus* and *Mucor*. Infections rarely have been caused by geographically restricted mycoses, such as histoplasmosis.[79] Almost two-thirds of systemic fungal infections in the tropics occur more than 12 months posttransplantation, contradicting Rubin's timetable, which suggests that most fungal infections occur within 6 months. The most common risk factors for the development of these infections are diabetes mellitus and CMV infection and clinically manifest as fever unresponsive to antibiotics.[117]

Systemic candidiasis, the most common invasive fungal infection in patients after kidney transplantation in developing countries, manifests most commonly with clinical features of pyelonephritis affecting the graft.[45] Prolonged urinary catheterization, use of broad-spectrum antibiotics, and diabetes enhance the risk of infection. The diagnosis can be confirmed with culture of *Candida* in blood or urine.

Cryptococcus is common in kidney transplant recipients in the tropics and presents most commonly with features of meningitis; India ink staining of cerebrospinal fluid shows the presence of the organism. Dissemination to other organs, such as the skin and eye, can occur. The diagnosis is confirmed on positive latex agglutination test or culture of the organism from cerebrospinal fluid, blood, or urine.[112]

Rhinocerebral mucormycosis typically manifests with cavernous sinus thrombosis; approximately 70% of kidney transplant patients who develop mucormycosis are also diabetic. Aspergillosis is an uncommon but serious fungal infection that carries a very high mortality in renal allograft recipients. It also most commonly manifests as a necrotizing pneumonia or disseminated infection.[112]

Amphotericin B is the drug of choice for fungal infections because it controls infections sooner, although fluconazole is less toxic. Fluconazole also increases cyclosporine levels.[79] Liposomal amphotericin B is less nephrotoxic but more expensive.

Viral Infections

Herpesvirus Infections. The herpes group of viruses takes an immense toll on kidney transplant patients in developing countries.[109] The main culprit is CMV, which occurs in 60–90% of recipients in the first year posttransplantation. Of these, about one-third develop overt disease, and 28% die as a result of CMV-related complications.[52,142] Reactivation and de novo infection are the two epidemiological patterns of CMV infection recognized. Transmission of CMV from an infected donor to an unexposed recipient may occur. Symptomatic CMV disease occurs in the first 4 months posttransplantation when immunosuppression is most intense. It also may predispose to other opportunistic fungal and bacterial infections. In developing countries, the clinical diagnosis may be confounded by coinfection with hepatitis viruses, tuberculosis, and fungal infections.[191] The treatment of CMV infection is with intravenous ganciclovir. Oral valganciclovir is available for prophylaxis but is prohibitively expensive. Diagnosed and treated early, CMV infection has a good outcome.

Hepatitis Infections. The prevalence of hepatitis B virus (HBV) and hepatitis C virus (HCV) infections, which are usually acquired before transplantation, ranges from 12% to 53% for HBV and 4% to 68% for HCV in the dialysis populations of developing countries. The prevalence in transplant patients is higher than in the general population.[78] However, the prevalence of HBV is declining as blood product usage has diminished and because of HBV vaccination. Immunosuppression causes rampant viral replication and, in early reports, acute hepatitis occurred in 60% of HBV recipients, with high mortality owing to acute liver failure.[208] The presence of chronic liver disease is associated with a poorer outcome, and a liver biopsy before transplantation is invaluable in guiding management of patients. In terms of prognosis, recent studies of the long-term outcome of hepatitis virus-infected patients indicate 10-year patient and graft survivals are compromised, although 5-year survival rates are comparable to those of uninfected patients, with HBV patients doing worse than HCV patients. HBV patients had poorer graft and patient outcomes regardless of whether or not they had evidence of viral replication, such as HBeAg and HBV DNA.[256]

The introduction of lamivudine heralded a new era in the treatment of HBV kidney transplant patients.[256] The use of lamivudine in HBV patients after transplantation resulted in a dramatic improvement in patient survival by a factor of almost 10,[40] as well as improving graft survival, making it comparable to HBV-negative patients.[4] The emergence of resistance and expense are major limiting factors in the use of this agent in developing countries.[180,256] Interferon should be avoided in transplant patients because of the risk of acute rejection, which may be irreversible.[256]

Other Viral Infections. HIV infection has reached epidemic proportions worldwide and is particularly rampant in developing countries. Of the 40 million people infected with HIV worldwide, greater than 95% live in developing countries. HIV infection was generally considered a contraindication to kidney transplantation, but there are encouraging reports of graft and patient survival rates, comparable to other high-risk patients.[129,187] Although the patients tolerate the combination of antiretroviral drugs and immunosuppressives well, the risk of acute rejection is high.[129,206] Evidence suggests that in HIV/AIDS patients who develop associated ESKD, survival is better following transplantation than on dialysis.[129] An interesting report from South Africa documented the successful transplantation of kidneys from HIV-infected donors to HIV-infected patients.[46] Patients can acquire HIV as a result of organ transplantation either from unscreened blood products or from a contaminated kidney, usually following commercial transplants. Organ transplantation accounted for 1.5% of all cases of HIV infection in Saudi Arabia.[10]

Polyomavirus (BK virus)-induced nephropathy is a novel disease that occurs in approximately 5%[102] of all cases in developed countries and results in graft loss in 50% of affected patients.[65,261] The infection is associated with excessive immunosuppression.[32,103] It mimics acute rejection, except that it occurs 10–13 months after transplantation.[190,261] It can be diagnosed with confidence only on histology, although the presence of decoy cells in urine provides a valuable clue.[190] Its prevalence in developing countries is uncertain. In a report from Korea, BK virus infection occurred in 4.7% of all patients. All the patients who developed disease were receiving tacrolimus and MMF treatment, suggesting a role for the intensity of immunosuppression.[104] Based on anecdotal cases and a better understanding of the interaction between the virus and the immune system, the primary therapeutic recommendation is reduction of immunosuppression.[17]

Malignancies (Figure 38-16)

Malignancies are an important complication of kidney transplantation, occurring in 1–25% of renal allograft recipients. With patients surviving longer, the risks of malignancies increases, and malignancies are the third most common cause of mortality after infections and cardiovascular disease.[198] The overall incidence of posttransplant malignancies is lower in developing countries; this could be related to the shorter duration of follow-up in developing countries that have relatively new transplant programs, younger patients, and lower intensity of immunosuppression in programs that perform predominantly living related transplants.[157] The pattern of malignancies in developed and developing countries also differs.

Kaposi's Sarcoma

Kaposi's sarcoma is the most common malignancy in kidney transplant patients in most developing countries, accounting for 80% of all malignancies in transplant recipients.[97] The mean time to the development of Kaposi's sarcoma is 21 months, but it may occur within a few months. The disease typically affects skin but lesions also may occur in the oropharynx and conjunctivae.[277] Visceral involvement has a grave prognosis.[156] Human herpesvirus-8 has been causally linked to all forms of Kaposi's sarcoma.[265] Reduction in immunosuppression should be

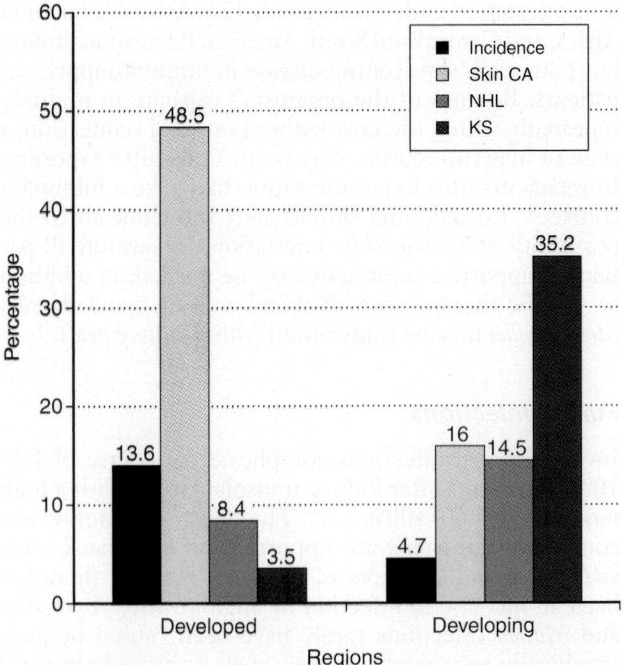

FIGURE 38-16 ■ The overall incidence and pattern of malignancies in developed and developing countries. The most common malignancy in western countries is that of skin and lip, while the most common malignancy in developing regions is Kaposi's sarcoma (KS). The reason for this difference may be geographical or ethnic/genetic factors. Black and white patients in the same geographical region have patterns of cancer (CA) that epitomize that seen in the west and developing countries, emphasizing the importance of ethnogenicity. NHL, non-Hodgkin's lymphoma. (Reproduced with permission from Moosa MR. Racial and ethnic variations in incidence and pattern of malignancies after kidney transplantation. Medicine (Baltimore) 2005;84:12–22.)

the first line of treatment and has been highly effective in improvement of lesions without compromising the graft.[70,156] Sirolimus, with its antiproliferative properties, is increasingly used to treat Kaposi's sarcoma in kidney transplant recipients, and there are now reports from developing countries of both cutaneous and visceral disease being successfully treated.[154,277]

Posttransplantation Lymphoproliferative Disease

Posttransplantation lymphoproliferative disease (PTLD) is a spectrum of abnormal hyperplastic and neoplastic lymphocyte growths from a benign self-limited form of lymphoproliferation to aggressive, widely disseminated disease.[188] Approximately 85–90% of these growths are of B-cell origin,[182] and 90–95% contain the Epstein–Barr virus.[188] Patients with PTLD have different histological findings, have a more aggressive clinical course (more extranodal disease, especially intestinal involvement), respond poorly to conventional treatment for lymphoma, and have a poorer prognosis (70% mortality) compared with immunocompetent individuals who develop lymphomas.[188] Globally, non-Hodgkin's lymphoma is the second most common posttransplant malignancy after skin and lip cancers. In developing countries, posttransplant lymphomas are more common than in industrialized countries, accounting for 14.5% of malignancies in developing countries and 8.5% of malignancies in industrialized countries.[157] These lymphomas are the major cause of cancer-related mortality and morbidity after transplantation.[18,157] In reports from developing countries, the latent period from transplantation to the diagnosis of PTLD was comparatively longer (range 2.6–7 years).[188,276] The latent period under cyclosporine and OKT3 monoclonal antibody was shorter.[188]

SPECIAL CONSIDERATIONS IN TRANSPLANTATION

Pregnancy and Contraception after Kidney Transplantation

Pregnancy is uncommon in women on dialysis, and when it occurs, is associated with a high rate of complications and fetal wastage.[141] Correction of the uremic state by a functioning renal allograft restores fertility in women of reproductive age, and may result in a high number of unwanted pregnancies. In recent reports from China, and Iran, 15% and 29% respectively of women reported having unwanted pregnancies.[82,204] In contrast to the pregnancy rates of 2–3% in western countries,[134] reported pregnancy rates in women of childbearing age in developing countries range from 14% (Brazil),[213] 27% (Morocco),[30] 31% (Oman),[6] to 55% in the Middle East.[128] With care, pregnancy can be undertaken successfully after kidney transplantation, with live birth rates (74%) and miscarriage rates (14%) superior to those of that of the general US population.[62] On the other hand, gestational diabetes, eclampsia, cesarean section, and preterm delivery rates are higher than in the general population (Figure 38-17).[62] Infections, predominantly of the urinary tract, can occur in 86% of pregnancies.[248] Graft and patient survivals are comparable to controls,[213,248] even after repeated pregnancies.[178] Available information suggests that pregnancy after successful kidney transplantation is safe if the patient has normal renal function and delays conception for 1 year posttransplantation. Careful management by a multidisciplinary team is essential. However, it is not uncommon for patients to be unaware of the return of the reproductive capacity, which may culminate in unwanted pregnancies, and female patients should be advised on effective contraception until they are ready to conceive.[122,269]

Transplantation in Children

A well-functioning renal allograft is the best treatment for a child with ESKD – perhaps even more so than in an adult.[95] However, children in developing countries constitute less than 5% of all renal allograft recipients.[242] The incidence of ESKD is 7 per 1 million child population in these countries, similar to or slightly higher than that reported from developed countries.[72] The causes of ESKD in children are most commonly chronic glomerulonephritis, chronic interstitial nephritis, and congenital abnormalities.[200] Resources in developing countries for treating uremic children with dialysis are severely limited and prioritized for the care of adults. Transplantation offers the recipient the opportunity of a better quality of life, improved growth and psychomotor development, and the re-establishment of psychosocial functioning. With the low incidence of deceased donor transplantation in developing countries, living related donor transplantation is the main option.[95] Mothers are the donors in more than two-thirds of cases.[95,242] Cyclosporine forms the basis of immunosuppression in developing countries[202] but induction with interleukin-2 antagonists significantly reduces rejection episodes.[200] Outstanding 1- and 5-year actuarial graft survival rates of 94% and of 73%, respectively, have been reported from Egypt (Table 38-3). In general, however, the results in developing countries are inferior, bearing testimony to the challenges of undertaking this complex multidisciplinary intervention in a resource-constrained environment.[200]

Importance of Early Detection and Prevention of Chronic Kidney Disease

Kidney transplantation is not only the best biological replacement for an irreversibly damaged kidney but also the most economical. Kidney transplantation is considerably cheaper to perform in developing countries, but in contrast to developed countries, where the state contributes significantly to the costs, patients are personally responsible for all costs in most developing countries (see above). In these countries, the annual cost of renal replacement is more than 10-fold the GNI per capita compared with twice the GNI per capita in the United States.[126] With ESKD escalating worldwide, a paradigm shift was required, especially in developing countries that bear the brunt of the disease burden. Whereas emphasis was on treatment in the previous decades, the 21st

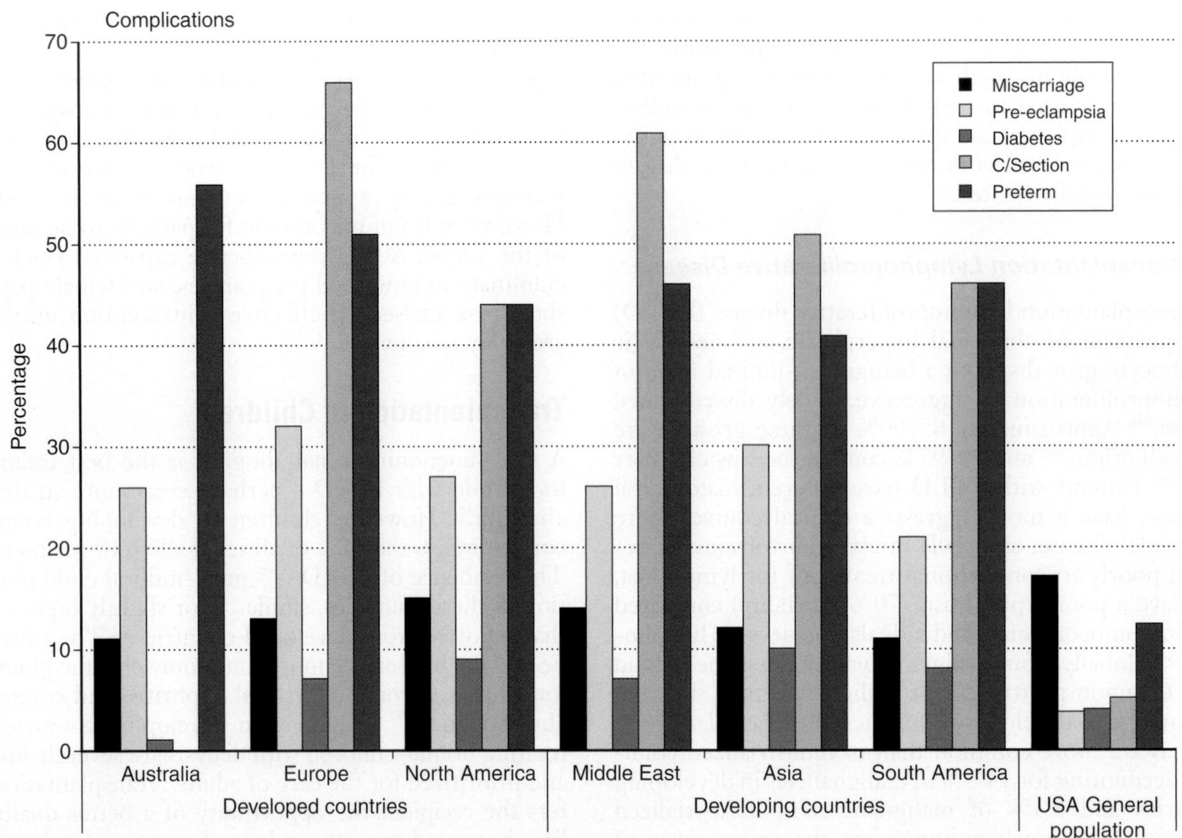

FIGURE 38-17 ■ **Pregnancy after kidney transplantation in various regions compared with the US population. Pregnancy is very successful but is associated with significantly increased maternal and fetal morbidity. The most common complication is pre-eclampsia, which is 5–10 times greater than in women in the general population. The cesarean section (C/section) rate is especially increased, although the miscarriage rate is lower. The risk of eclampsia is significantly increased.** (Drawn using data from: Deshpande NA, James NT, Kucirka LM, et al. Pregnancy outcomes in kidney transplant recipients: a systematic review and meta-analysis. Am J Transplant 2011;11:2388–2404; Kukla A, Issa N, Ibrahim HN. Pregnancy in renal transplantation: Recipient and donor aspects in the Arab world. Arab J Urol 2012; 10: 175–181.)

century ushered in a renewed interest in the early detection and prevention of chronic kidney disease. Adding to the urgency was the recognition that proteinuria and chronic kidney disease were also risk factors for cardiovascular disease, having a major impact on the overall health of the population.[195] While the importance of this strategy was recognized by all developing regions,[13,54,231] very few actually have chronic kidney disease prevention programs and, where they do occur, they are often rudimentary.[13] The Bellagio Declaration suggested screening and treatment should focus on cost-effective interventions that all countries could afford. Screening includes blood pressure and detection of albuminuria.[63] Primary prevention consists of lifestyle modifications, such as weight reduction, exercise, smoking cessation, and dietary changes, combined with tight control of blood pressure and diabetes mellitus.[27] For patients with established chronic kidney disease, in addition to these measures pharmacological agents, including angiotensin-converting enzyme inhibitors, angiotensin receptor blockers, and non-dihydropyridine calcium channel blockers, should be considered.[147] Screening and intervention programs require considerable human and financial resources but the excellent results achieved by Mani, who implemented a prevention program in India, using volunteers and at very low cost, could serve as a model for other regions to emulate.[143]

REFERENCES

1. Abraham G, Varsha P, Mathew M, et al. Malnutrition and nutritional therapy of chronic kidney disease in developing countries: the Asian perspective. Adv Ren Replace Ther 2003;10(3):213–21.
2. Agarwal SK, Dash SC, Mehta SN, et al. Results of renal transplantation on conventional immunosuppression in second decade in India: a single centre experience. J Assoc Physicians India 2002;50:532–6.
3. Agarwal SK. Chronic kidney disease and its prevention in India. Kidney Int 2005;68(S98):S41–5.
4. Ahn HJ, Kim MS, Kim YS, et al. Clinical outcome of renal transplantation in patients with positive pre-transplant hepatitis B surface antigen. J Med Virol 2007;79(11):1655–63.
5. Akoh J. Renal transplantation in developing countries. Saudi J Kidney Dis Transpl 2011;22(4):637–50.
6. Al Hassani MK, Sharma U, Mohsin P, et al. Pregnancy in renal transplantation recipients: outcome and complications in 44 pregnancies. Transplant Proc 1995;27(5):2585.
7. Al Khader AA. Cadaveric renal transplantation in the kingdom of Saudi Arabia. Nephrol Dial Transplant 1999;14(4):846–50.
8. Al-Taee IKS, Al-Shamaa I. Longterm follow-up of renal transplant recipients – a single centre experiece in Iraq. Saudi J Kidney Dis Transpl 2005;16(1):40–5.
9. Al-Wakeel J, Mitwalli AH, Tarif N, et al. Living unrelated renal transplant: outcome and issues. Saudi J Kidney Dis Transpl 2000;11:553–8.
10. Alrajhi AA, Halim MA, Al Abdely HM. Mode of transmission of HIV-1 in Saudi Arabia. AIDS 2004;18(10):1478–80.
11. Alshaibani K, Raza S, Alfurayh O, et al. The kidney transplant program at King Faisal Specialist Hospital and Research Center; results of the last ten years. Transplant Proc 1998;30:3103–5.

12. Arije A, Kadiri S, Akinkugbe OO. The viability of hemodialysis as a treatment option for renal failure in a developing economy. Afr J Med Med Sci 2000;29(3–4):311–4.
13. Arogundade FA, Barsoum RS. CKD prevention in sub-Saharan Africa: a call for governmental, nongovernmental, and community support. Am J Kidney Dis 2008;51(3):515–23.
14. Aslani J, Einollahi B. Prevalence of tuberculosis after renal transplantation in Iran. Transplant Proc 2001;33(5):2804–5.
15. Atkins RC. The changing patterns of chronic kidney disease: the need to develop strategies for prevention relevant to different regions and countries. Kidney Int Suppl 2005;98:S83–5.
16. Ayodele OE, Alebiosu CO. Burden of chronic kidney disease: an international perspective. Adv Chronic Kidney Dis 2010;17(3):215–24.
17. Babel N, Volk HD, Reinke P. BK polyomavirus infection and nephropathy: the virus-immune system interplay. Nat Rev Nephrol 2011;7(7):399–406.
18. Bakr MA, Sobh M, El-Agroudy A, et al. Study of malignancy among Egyptian kidney transplant recipients. Transplant Proc 1997; 29(7):3067–70.
19. Bamgboye EL. Hemodialysis: management problems in developing countries, with Nigeria as a surrogate. Kidney Int Suppl 2003;83:S93–5.
20. Bamgboye EL. Barriers to a functional renal transplant program in developing countries. Ethn Dis 2009;19(1 Suppl. 1):S1–9.
21. Barsoum RS. Renal transplantation in a developing country. Afr J Health Sci 1994;1(1):30–6.
22. Barsoum RS. End-stage renal disease in the developing world. Artif Organs 2002;26(9):735–6.
23. Barsoum RS. Overview: end-stage renal disease in the developing world. Artif Organs 2002;26(9):737–46.
24. Barsoum RS. End-stage renal disease in North Africa. Kidney Int Suppl 2003;83:S111–4.
25. Barsoum RS. Chronic kidney disease in the developing world. N Engl J Med 2006;354(10):997–9.
26. Basiri A, Moghaddam SMM, Simforoosh N, et al. Preliminary report of a nationwide case-control study for identifying risk factors of tuberculosis following renal transplantation. Transplant Proc 2005;37(7):3041–4.
27. Bello AK, Nwankwo E, El Nahas AM. Prevention of chronic kidney disease: a global challenge. Kidney Int Suppl 2005;68(98):S11–7.
28. Bellorin-Font E, Milanes CL, Rodriguez-Iturbe B. End-stage renal disease and its treatment in Venezuela. Artif Organs 2002;26(9):747–9.
29. Bordes-Aznar J, Peña JC, Herrera-Accosta J, et al. Twenty-four-year experience in kidney transplantation at one single institution in Mexico City. Transplant Proc 1992;24(5):1794–5.
30. Bouattar T, Hakim H, Rhou H, et al. Pregnancy in renal transplant recipients. Transplant Proc 2009;41(5):1586–8.
31. Boubaer K, Bouabid B, Bardi R, et al. Immunological factors and renal allograft survival for more than 15 years: a single centre study from Tunisia. Saudi J Kidney Dis Transpl 2006;17(1):70–6.
32. Bressollette-Bodin C, Coste-Burel M, Hourmant M, et al. A prospective longitudinal study of BK virus infection in 104 renal transplant recipients. Am J Transplant 2005;5(8):1926–33.
33. Budiani-Saberi DA, Delmonico FL. Organ trafficking and transplant tourism: a commentary on the global realities. Am J Transplant 2008;8(5):925–9.
34. Budiani-Saberi D, Mostafa A. Care for commercial living donors: the experience of an NGO's outreach in Egypt. Transpl Int 2011;24(4):317–23.
35. Cantarovich F, Vazquez M, Garcia WD, et al. Special infections in organ transplantation in South America. Transplant Proc 1992;24(5):1902–8.
36. Carvajal D. Trafficking investigations put surgeon in spotlight. New York Times 2-10-2011;, 1-30-2012.
37. Cavusoglu C, Cicek-Saydam C, Karasu Z, et al. *Mycobacterium tuberculosis* infection and laboratory diagnosis in solid-organ transplant recipients. Clin Transplant 2002;16(4):257–61.
38. Cecka JM. The UNOS Scientific Renal Transplant Registry – ten years of kidney transplants. Clin Transpl 1997;1–14.
39. Centers for Disease Control, Prevention. Chagas disease after organ transplantation – United States, 2001. MMWR Morb Mortal Wkly Rep 2002;51(10):210–2.
40. Chan TM, Fang GX, Tang CS, et al. Preemptive lamivudine therapy based on HBV DNA level in HBsAg-positive kidney allograft recipients. Hepatology 2002;36(5):1246–52.
41. Cheng IK. Special issues related to transplantation in Hong Kong. Transplant Proc 1992;24(6):2423–5.
42. Chiche L, Lesage A, Duhamel C, et al. Posttransplant malaria: first case of transmission of *Plasmodium falciparum* from a white multiorgan donor to four recipients. Transplantation 2003;75(1):166–8.
43. Chugh KS. Five decades of Indian nephrology: a personal journey. Am J Kidney Dis 2009;54(4):753–63.
44. Chugh KS, Jha V. Commerce in transplantation in Third World countries. Kidney Int 1996;49(5):1181–6.
45. Chugh KS, Sakhuja V, Jain S, et al. High mortality in systemic fungal infections following renal transplantation in third-world countries. Nephrol Dial Transplant 1993;8(2):168–72.
46. Chugh KS, Jha V. Problems and outcomes of living unrelated donor transplants in the developing countries. Kidney Int 2000;57(S74):S131–5.
47. Chung BH, Jung MH, Bae SH, et al. Changing donor source pattern for kidney transplantation over 40 years: a single-center experience. Korean J Intern Med 2010;25(3):288–93.
48. Colakoglu M, Yenicesu M, Akpolat T, et al. Nonrelated living-donor kidney transplantation: medical and ethical aspects. Nephron 1998;79(4):447–51.
49. Coresh J, Astor BC, Greene T, et al. Prevalence of chronic kidney disease and decreased kidney function in the adult US population: Third National Health and Nutrition Examination Survey. Am J Kidney Dis 2003;41(1):1–12.
50. Correa-Rotter R, Gonzalez-Michaca L. Early detection and prevention of diabetic nephropathy: a challenge calling for mandatory action for Mexico and the developing world. Kidney Int Suppl 2005;98:S69–75.
51. Coutts II, Jegarajah S, Stark JE. Tuberculosis in renal transplant patients. Br J Dis Chest 1979;73(2):141–8.
52. Çuhadaroglu S, Tokyay R, Velidedeoglu E, et al. The incidence of cytomegalovirus infection in kidney recipients. Transplant Proc 1992;24(5):1924–5.
53. Currie AC, Knight SR, Morris PJ. Tuberculosis in renal transplant recipients: the evidence for prophylaxis. Transplantation 2010;90(7):695–704.
54. Cusumano AM, Gonzalez Bedat MC. Chronic kidney disease in Latin America: time to improve screening and detection. Clin J Am Soc Nephrol 2008;3(2):594–600.
55. Cusumano AM, Gonzalez Bedat MC, Garcia-Garcia G, et al. Latin American Dialysis and Renal Transplant Registry: 2008 report (data 2006). Clin Nephrol 2010;74(Suppl. 1):1S3–S8.
56. Cusumano AM, Di Gioia C, Hermida O, et al. The Latin American Dialysis and Renal Transplantation Registry Annual Report 2002. Kidney Int 2005;68(S97):S46–52.
57. Daar AS, Singer PA, Persad DL, et al. Grand challenges in chronic non-communicable diseases. Nature 2007;450(7169):494–6.
58. Daar AS. Organ donation – world experience; the Middle East. Transplant Proc 1991;23:2505–7.
59. Dash SC, Agarwal SK. Incidence of chronic kidney disease in India. Nephrol Dial Transplant 2006;21(1):232–3.
60. Delmonico FL, Dominguez-Gil B, Matesanz R, et al. A call for government accountability to achieve national self-sufficiency in organ donation and transplantation. Lancet 2011;378(9800):1414–8.
61. Delucchi A, Ferrario M, Varela M, et al. Pediatric renal transplantation: a single center experience over 14 years. Pediatr Transplant 2006;10(2):193–7.
62. Deshpande NA, James NT, Kucirka LM, et al. Pregnancy outcomes in kidney transplant recipients: a systematic review and meta-analysis. Am J Transplant 2011;11(11):2388–404.
63. Dirks JH, de Zeeuw D, Agarwal SK, et al. Prevention of chronic kidney and vascular disease: toward global health equity – the Bellagio 2004 Declaration. Kidney Int Suppl 2005;98:S1–6.
64. Dorman SE. New diagnostic tests for tuberculosis: bench, bedside, and beyond. Clin Infect Dis 2010;50(Suppl. 3):S173–7.
65. Drachenberg CB, Beskow CO, Cangro CB, et al. Human polyoma virus in renal allograft biopsies: morphological findings and correlation with urine cytology. Hum Pathol 1999;30(8):970–7.
66. Edelstein CL, Jacobs JC, Moosa MR. Pulmonary complications in 110 consecutive renal transplant recipients. S Afr Med J 1995;85(3):160–3.
67. Editorial. Legal and illegal organ donation. Lancet 2007;369(9577):1901.

68. Editorial. What can be learned from China's health system? Lancet 2012;379(9818):777.
69. Eggers PW. Has the incidence of end-stage renal disease in the USA and other countries stabilized? Curr Opin Nephrol Hypertens 2011;20(3).
70. Einollahi B. Kaposi sarcoma after kidney transplantation. Iran J Kidney Dis 2007;1(1):2–11.
71. Einollahi B. Is the annual number of deceased donor kidney transplantations in Iran lower than the Middle Eastern countries? Transplant Proc 2009;41(7):2718–9.
72. Eke FU, Eke NN. Renal disorders in children. Pediatr Nephrol 1994;8383–6.
73. Ekrikpo UE, Udo AI, Ikpeme EE, et al. Haemodialysis in an emerging centre in a developing country: a two year review and predictors of mortality. BMC Nephrol 2011;1250.
74. el Agroudy AE, Donia AF, Bakr MA, et al. Preemptive living-donor kidney transplantation: clinical course and outcome. Transplantation 2004;77(9):1366–70.
75. El Husseini AA, Foda MA, Bakr MA, et al. Pediatric live-donor kidney transplantation in Mansoura Urology & Nephrology Center: a 28-year perspective. Pediatr Nephrol 2006;21(10):1464–70.
76. Emiroglu R, Moray G, Sevmis S, et al. Long-term results of pediatric kidney transplantation at one center in Turkey. Transplant Proc 2005;37(7):2951–3.
77. Ergun I, Ekmekci Y, Sengul S, et al. *Mycobacterium tuberculosis* infection in renal transplant recipients. Transplant Proc 2006;38(5):1344–5.
78. Fehr T, Ambuhl PM. Chronic hepatitis virus infections in patients on renal replacement therapy. Nephrol Dial Transplant 2004;19(5):1049–53.
79. Gandhi BV, Bahadur MM, Dodeja H, et al. Systemic fungal infections in renal diseases. J Postgrad Med 2005;51(Suppl. 1): S30–6.
80. Garcia VD, Garcia CD, Santiago-Delpin EA. Organ transplants in Latin America. Transplant Proc 2003;35(5):1673–4.
81. Garcia-Garcia G, Monteon-Ramos JF, Garcia-Bejarano H, et al. Renal replacement therapy among disadvantaged populations in Mexico: a report from the Jalisco Dialysis and Transplant Registry (REDTJAL). Kidney Int Suppl 2005;68(97):S58–61.
82. Ghazizadeh S, Lessan-Pezeshki M, Khatami M, et al. Unwanted pregnancy among kidney transplant recipients in Iran. Transplant Proc 2005;37(7):3085–6.
83. Gheith OA, Bakr MA, Fouda MA, et al. Steroid and azathioprine versus steroid, cyclosporine, and azathioprine therapies in primary haplo-identical living donor kidney transplantation: twenty-year experience. Iran J Kidney Dis 2008;2(1):34–9.
84. Ghods AJ. Should we have live unrelated donor renal transplantation in MESOT countries? Transplant Proc 2003;35(7): 2542–4.
85. Ghods AJ. Renal transplantation in Iran. Nephrol Dial Transplant 2002;17(2):222–8.
86. Ghods AJ, Savaj S. Iranian model of paid and regulated living-unrelated kidney donation. Clin J Am Soc Nephrol 2006;1(6):1136–45.
87. Global observatory on donation, transplantation. Organ donation and transplantation: activities, laws and organization 2010. 2012. Available online at http://www.transplant-observatory.org/Data%20 Reports/2010%20Report%20final.pdf [accessed 30.01.12].
88. Goldani JC, Bianchini AC, Mattos A, et al. Renal transplantation in the state of Rio Grande do Sul, Brazil. Transplant Proc 1991;23(5):2541.
89. Golmakani MM, Niknam MH, Hedayat KM. Transplantation ethics from the Islamic point of view. Med Sci Monit 2005;11(4):RA105–9.
90. Goplani KR, Firoz A, Ramakrishana P, et al. Deceased donor organ transplantation with expanded criteria donors: a single-center experience from India. Transplant Proc 2010;42(1):171–4.
91. Grapsa E. Is the underutilization of peritoneal dialysis in relation to hemodialysis, as renal replacement therapy, justifiable worldwide? Yes or no. Hippokratia 2011;15(Suppl. 1):13–5.
92. Grassmann A, Gioberge S, Moeller S, et al. End-stage renal disease: global demographics in 2005 and observed trends. Artif Organs 2006;30(12):895–7.
93. Grassmann A, Gioberge S, Moeller S, et al. ESRD patients in 2004: global overview of patient numbers, treatment modalities and associated trends. Nephrol Dial Transplant 2005;20(12):2587–93.
94. Guanyu W, Nan C, Jiaqi Q, et al. Nephrology, dialysis and transplantation in Shanghai, 1999. Nephrol Dial Transplant 2000;15(7):961–3.
95. Gulati S, Kumar A, Sharma RK, et al. Outcome of pediatric renal transplants in a developing country. Pediatr Nephrol 2004;19(1): 96–100.
96. Gumber MR, Kute VB, Goplani KR, et al. Deceased donor organ transplantation: a single center experience. Indian J Nephrol 2011;21(3):182–5.
97. Haberal AN, Suren D, Demirhan B, et al. Evaluation of posttransplantation malignancies compared with de novo tumors. Transplant Proc 2007;39(4):1057–62.
98. Haberal M, Demirag A, Cohen B, et al. Cadaver kidney transplantation in Turkey. Transplant Proc 1995;27(5):2768–9.
99. Haghighi AN, Rahbar K, Fasihi F, et al. Characteristics of hemodialysis patients who underwent renal transplantation in Tehran, Iran: a 10-year follow-up study. Transplant Proc 2003;35(7):2584–5.
100. Hamaloglu E, Tokyay R, Arslan G, et al. Living related donor transplantation at a Turkish center. Transplant Proc 1992;24(5):1848–9.
101. Higgins RM, Cahn AP, Porter D, et al. Mycobacterial infections after renal transplantation. Q J Med 1991;78(286):145–53.
102. Hirsch HH, Brennan DC, Drachenberg CB, et al. Polyomavirus-associated nephropathy in renal transplantation: interdisciplinary analyses and recommendations. Transplantation 2005;79(10):1277–86.
103. Howell DN, Smith SR, Butterly DW, et al. Diagnosis and management of BK polyomavirus interstitial nephritis in renal transplant recipients. Transplantation 1999;68(9):1279–88.
104. Hwang EA, Kang MJ, Han SY, et al. Viral infection following kidney transplantation: long-term follow-up in a single center. Transplant Proc 2004;36(7):2118–9.
105. Isaacs RB, Nock SL, Spencer CE, et al. Racial disparities in renal transplant outcomes. Am J Kidney Dis 1999;34(4):706–12.
106. Ivanovski N, Popov Z, Cakalaroski K, et al. Living-unrelated (paid) renal transplantation – ten years later. Transplant Proc 2005;37(2):563–4.
107. Jafar TH. Organ trafficking: global solutions for a global problem. Am J Kidney Dis 2009;54(6):1145–57.
108. Jawad F, Hussain Z, Ahmed E, et al. Problems of donor selection in a living related renal transplant program. Transplant Proc 1998;30(7):3643.
109. Jenkins FJ, Rowe DT, Rinaldo Jr CR. Herpesvirus infections in organ transplant recipients. Clin Diagn Lab Immunol 2003;10(1):1–7.
110. Jeong JC, Kim MG, Ro H, et al. Kidney transplantation using expanded criteria donors in Korea. Transplant Proc 2012;44(1):54–6.
111. Jha V. Current status of chronic kidney disease care in southeast Asia. Semin Nephrol 2009;29(5):487–96.
112. Jha V, Chugh KS. Posttransplant infections in the tropical countries. Artif Organs 2002;26(9):770–7.
113. Jha V, Chugh KS. The practice of dialysis in the developing countries. Hemodial Int 2003;7239–49.
114. Jha V, Chugh KS. Economics of ESRD in developing countries. In: El Nahas M, editor. Kidney diseases in the developing world and ethnic minorities. London: Taylor and Francis; 2005. p. 39–57.
115. Jha V, Sakhuja V, Gupta D, et al. Successful management of pulmonary tuberculosis in renal allograft recipients in a single center. Kidney Int 1999;56(5):1944–50.
116. John GT, Shankar V, Abraham AM, et al. Risk factors for post-transplant tuberculosis. Kidney Int 2001;60(3):1148–53.
117. John GT, Shankar V, Talaulikar G, et al. Epidemiology of systemic mycoses among renal-transplant recipients in India. Transplantation 2003;75(9):1544–51.
118. Johny KV, Nesim J, Namboori N, et al. Values gained and lost in live unrelated renal transplantation. Transplant Proc 1990;22(3):915–7.
119. Kalra V, Agarwal SK, Khilnani GC, et al. Spectrum of pulmonary infections in renal transplant recipients in the tropics: a single center study. Int Urol Nephrol 2005;37(3):551–9.
120. Kamel G, Stephan A, Salme P, et al. Renal transplantation: the Lebanese experience. Transplant Proc 1993;25:2356–7.

121. Kandus A, Buturovic PJ, Malovrh M, et al. Kidney transplantation in Slovenia from 1986 through 1991. Transplant Proc 1992;24(6):2430–1.
122. Karkar A. Pregnancy and contraceptive issues in renal transplant recipients. Saudi J Kidney Dis Transpl 2008;19(2):165–73.
123. Kayedi M, Golbabaie M, Najafi I, et al. Renal transplantation in Iran: a single-center study. Transplant Proc 2001; 33(5):2646–7.
124. Kazim E, Al-Rukmani M, Fernandez SN, et al. Buying a kidney: the easy way out? Transplant Proc 1992;24(5):2112–3.
125. Khatri GR, Frieden TR. Controlling tuberculosis in India. N Engl J Med 2002;347(18):1420–5.
126. Kher V. End-stage renal disease in developing countries. Kidney Int 2002;62(1):350–62.
127. Kher V, Pokhariyal S. Optimizing immuosuppressive regimens in the developing world: issues of cost vs quality. J Nephrol Renal Transplant 2009;2(1):136–45.
128. Kukla A, Issa N, Ibrahim HN. Pregnancy in renal transplantation: recipient and donor aspects in the Arab world. Arab J Urol 2012;10:175–81.
129. Kumar MS, Sierka DR, Damask AM, et al. Safety and success of kidney transplantation and concomitant immunosuppression in HIV-positive patients. Kidney Int 2005;67(4):1622–9.
130. Langer RM, Hidvegi M, Jaray J. Significant differences in the efficacy of kidney transplantation between Hungarian Caucasians and gypsies. Transplant Proc 2005;37(2):729–30.
131. Lee CJ. Organ transplantation in Taiwan. Transplant Proc 1992;24(5):1824–7.
132. Li L. End-stage renal disease in China. Kidney Int 1996;49(1):287–301.
133. Lin S. Nephrology in China: a great mission and momentous challenge. Kidney Int Suppl 2003;83:S108–10.
134. Lindheimer MD, Katz AI. Pregnancy in the renal transplant patient. Am J Kidney Dis 1992;19:173–6.
135. Liquete RMOR, Ona ET. Transplant practices in the Philippines. Transplant Proc 1992;24(5):1809–10.
136. Locatelli F, D'Amico M, Cernevskis H, et al. The epidemiology of end-stage renal disease in the Baltic countries: an evolving picture. Nephrol Dial Transplant 2001;16(7):1338–42.
137. Lysaght MJ. Maintenance dialysis population dynamics: current trends and long-term implications. J Am Soc Nephrol 2002;13(Suppl. 1):S37–40.
138. Mactier R. Peritonitis is still the achilles' heel of peritoneal dialysis. Perit Dial Int 2009;29(3):262–6.
139. Mahmoud KM, Sobh MA, el Agroudy AE, et al. Impact of schistosomiasis on patient and graft outcome after renal transplantation: 10 years' follow-up. Nephrol Dial Transplant 2001; 16(11):2214–21.
140. Malhotra KK, Dash SC, Dhawan IK, et al. Tuberculosis and renal transplantation – observations from an endemic area of tuberculosis. Postgrad Med J 1986;62(727):359–62.
141. Malik GH, Al Harbi A, Al Mohaya S, et al. Pregnancy in patients on dialysis – experience at a referral center. J Assoc Physicians India 2005;53937–41.
142. Mancilla E, Alberu J, Alessio-Robles L, et al. Prevalence of clinically overt cytomegalovirus disease in kidney transplant patients. Transplant Proc 1992;24(5):1919–20.
143. Mani MK. Prevention of chronic renal failure at the community level. Kidney Int Suppl 2003;83:S86–9.
144. Masri MA, Haberal MA, Shaheen FA, et al. Middle East Society for Organ Transplantation (MESOT) Transplant Registry. Exp Clin Transplant 2004;2(2):217–20.
145. Mayosi BM, Flisher AJ, Lalloo UG, et al. The burden of non-communicable diseases in South Africa. Lancet 2012;374(9693):934–47.
146. McLigeyo SO, Otieno LS, Kinuthia DM, et al. Problems with a renal replacement programme in a developing country. Postgrad Med J 1988;64(756):783–6.
147. Meguid EN, Bello AK. Chronic kidney disease: the global challenge. Lancet 2005;365(9456):331–40.
148. Mehrotra S, Gopalakrishnan G, Chacko KN, et al. Paediatric renal transplantation – a 15 year experience. Asian J Surg 2002;25(3):198–202.
149. Mills EJ, Barnighausen T, Negin J. HIV and aging – preparing for the challenges ahead. N Engl J Med 2012;366(14): 1270–3.
150. Mircescu G, Capsa D, Covic M, et al. Nephrology and renal replacement therapy in Romania – transition still continues (Cinderella story revisited). Nephrol Dial Transplant 2004; 19(12):2971–80.
151. Mitka M. Kidney failure rates end 20-year climb. JAMA 2005;294(20):2563.
152. Mizraji R, Alvarez I, Palacios RI, et al. Organ donation in Latin America. Transplant Proc 2007;39(2):333–5.
153. Modi GK, Jha V. The incidence of end-stage renal disease in India: a population-based study. Kidney Int 2006;70(12):2131–3.
154. Mohsin N, Budruddin M, Pakkyara A, et al. Complete regression of visceral Kaposi's sarcoma after conversion to sirolimus. Exp Clin Transplant 2005;3(2):366–9.
155. Moosa MR. The long-term outcome of kidney transplantation in patients under cyclosporine – a developing country experience. Clin Transplant 2004;18(3):267–73.
156. Moosa MR. Kaposi's sarcoma in kidney transplant recipients: a 23-year experience. Q J Med 2005;98(3):205–14.
157. Moosa MR. Racial and ethnic variations in incidence and pattern of malignancies after kidney transplantation. Medicine (Baltimore) 2005;84(1):12–22.
158. Moosa MR, Bouwens C. Tuberculosis in renal allograft recipients: the South African experience. Transplant Rev 1997;11(2):84–94.
159. Moosa MR, Kidd M. The dangers of rationing dialysis treatment: the dilemma facing a developing country. Kidney Int 2006;70(6):1107–14.
160. Morris PJ. Transplantation – a medical miracle of the 20th century. N Engl J Med 2004;351(26):2678–80.
161. Naicker S. Nutritional problems associated with end-stage renal disease in the developing world. Artif Organs 2002;26(9):757–9.
162. Naicker S. End-stage renal disease in sub-Saharan and South Africa. Kidney Int Suppl 2003;83:S119–22.
163. Naicker S. End-stage renal disease in sub-Saharan Africa. Ethn Dis 2009;19(1 Suppl. 1):S1–5.
164. Naicker S. Burden of end-stage renal disease in sub-Saharan Africa. Clin Nephrol 2010;74(Suppl. 1):S13–6.
165. Nampoory MR, Khan ZU, Johny KV, et al. Invasive fungal infections in renal transplant recipients. J Infect 1996;33(2): 95–101.
166. Naqvi A, Rizvi A. Renal transplantation in Pakistan. Transplant Proc 1995;27(5):2778.
167. Naqvi A, Rizvi A, Hussain Z, et al. Developing world perspective of posttransplant tuberculosis: morbidity, mortality, and cost implications. Transplant Proc 2001;33(1–2):1787–8.
168. Naqvi AA. Ethical issues in renal transplantation in developing countries. J Pak Med Assoc 1995;45(9):233–4.
169. Naqvi SAA. Immunosuppression strategies in developing countries. Transplant Proc 2002;34(6):2083–4.
170. Naqvi SAA, Ali B, Mazhar F, et al. A socioeconomic survey of kidney vendors in Pakistan. Transpl Int 2007;20(11):934–9.
171. Oeopoulos DG. The optimization of continuous ambulatory peritoneal dialysis. Kidney Int 1999;55:1131–49.
172. Oliver M, Woywodt A, Ahmed A, et al. Organ donation, transplantation and religion. Nephrol Dial Transplant 2011;26(2):437–44.
173. Opelz G. Factors influencing kidney graft survival in Latin America. Transplant Proc 1999;31(7):2951–4.
174. Ota K. Strategies for increasing transplantation in Asia and prospects of organ sharing: the Japanese experience. Transplant Proc 1998;30:3650–2.
175. Ota K. Current status of organ transplantations in Asian countries. Transplant Proc 2003;35(1):8–11.
176. Ota K, Teraoka S, Kawai T. Transplantation in Asia: organ transplantation in Japan. Transplant Proc 1995;27:1463–5.
177. Otukesh H, Basiri A, Simfrosh N, et al. Outcome of pediatric renal transplantation in Labfi Nejad Hospital, Tehran, Iran. Pediatr Nephrol 2006;21(10):1459–63.
178. Owda A, Abdalla A, Al Sulaiman M, et al. No evidence of functional deterioration of renal graft after repeated pregnancies – a report on three women with 17 pregnancies. Nephrol Dial Transplant 1998;13(5):1281–4.
179. Park K, Kim Y-S, Kim S-I, et al. Single center experience of 1500 kidney transplants. Transplant Proc 1998;30:3088–9.
180. Park SK, Yang WS, Lee YS, et al. Outcome of renal transplantation in hepatitis B surface antigen-positive patients after introduction of lamivudine. Nephrol Dial Transplant 2001;16(11):2222–8.

181. Participants in the International Summit on Transplant Tourism and Organ Trafficking Convened by The Transplantation Society and International Society of Nephrology in Istanbul TA. The Declaration of Istanbul on organ trafficking and transplant tourism. Clin J AmSoc Nephrol 2008;3(5):1227–31.
182. Penn I. The problem of cancer in organ transplant recipients: an overview. Transplant Sci 1994;4(1):23–32.
183. Pitcher GJ, Beale PG, Bowley DM, et al. Pediatric renal transplantation in a South African teaching hospital: A 20-year perspective. Pediatr Transplant 2006;10(4):441–8.
184. Pourmand G, Pourmand M, Salem S, et al. Posttransplant infectious complications: a prospective study on 142 kidney allograft recipients. Urol J 2006;3(1):23–31.
185. Pourmand G, Salem S, Mehrsai A, et al. Infectious complications after kidney transplantation: a single-center experience. Transpl Infect Dis 2007;9(4):302–9.
186. Qi J, Min Z, Zhu Y, et al. Cadaver renal transplantation and multivariate analysis for graft survival: a clinical review of 2 016 cases. Zhonghua Wai Ke Za Zhi 2002;40(4):241–7.
187. Qiu J, Terasaki PI, Waki K, et al. HIV-positive renal recipients can achieve survival rates similar to those of HIV-negative patients. Transplantation 2006;81(12).
188. Quintanilla ML, Lome MC, Schwarzmann F, et al. Post-transplantation lymphoproliferative disorders in Mexico: an aggressive clonal disease associated with Epstein–Barr virus type A. Mod Pathol 1998;11(2):200–8.
189. Qunibi WY, Al-Sibai BM, Taher S, et al. Mycobacterial infection after renal transplantation – report of 14 cases and review of the literature. Q J Med 1990;77(282):1039–60.
190. Ramos E, Drachenberg CB, Papadimitriou JC, et al. Clinical course of polyoma virus nephropathy in 67 renal transplant patients. J Am Soc Nephrol 2002;13(8):2145–51.
191. Rao M, Finny GJ, Abraham P, et al. Cytomegalovirus infection in a seroendemic renal transplant population: a longitudinal study of virological markers. Nephron 2000;84(4):367–73.
192. Rashid HU, Hossain RM, Khanam A. Outcome of acute renal failure in adults in a teaching hospital in Bangladesh. Ren Fail 1993;15(5):603–7.
193. Raza M, Skordis-Worrall J. Pakistan's kidney trade: an overview of the 2007 'Transplantation of Human Organs and Human Tissue Ordinance'. To what extent will it curb the trade? J Pak Med Assoc 2012;62(1):85–9.
194. Riarte A, Luna C, Sabatiello R, et al. Chagas' disease in patients with kidney transplants: 7 years of experience 1989–1996. Clin Infect Dis 1999;29(3):561–7.
195. Ritz E, McClellan WM. Overview: increased cardiovascular risk in patients with minor renal dysfunction: an emerging issue with far-reaching consequences. J Am Soc Nephrol 2004;15(3):513–6.
196. Rizvi SA, Naqvi A. The need to increase transplantation activity in developing countries. Transplant Proc 1995;27(5):2739–40.
197. Rizvi SA, Naqvi SA, Hussain Z, et al. Factors influencing renal transplantation in a developing country. Transplant Proc 1998;30(5):1810–1.
198. Rizvi SA, Naqvi SA, Hussain Z, et al. Renal transplantation in developing countries. Kidney Int Suppl 2003;83:S96–100.
199. Rizvi SA, Naqvi SA, Hussain Z, et al. The management of stone disease. BJU Int 2002;89(Suppl. 1):62–8.
200. Rizvi SA, Zafar MN, Lanewala AA. Challenges in pediatric renal transplantation in developing countries. Curr Opin Organ Transplant 2009;14(5):533–9.
201. Rizvi SAH, Naqvi SAA, Ahmed E. Renal transplanation in developing countries. In: El Nahas M, editor. Kidney diseases in the developing world and ethnic minorities. New York: Taylor and Francis; 2005. p. 211–45.
202. Rizvi SAH, Naqvi SAA, Hussain Z, et al. Living-related pediatric renal transplants: a single-center experience from a developing country. Pediatr Transplant 2002;6(2):101–10.
203. Rizvi SAH, Naqvi SAA, Zafar MN, et al. A renal transplantation model for developing countries. Am J Transplant 2011;11(11):2302–7.
204. Rizvi SAH, Naqvi SAA, Zafar MN, et al. Commercial transplants in local Pakistanis from vended kidneys: a socio-economic and outcome study. Transpl Int 2009;22(6):615–21.
205. Rodriguez-Iturbe B, Bellorin-Font E. End-stage renal disease prevention strategies in Latin America. Kidney Int Suppl 2005;98:S30–6.
206. Roland ME, Barin B, Carlson L, et al. HIV-infected liver and kidney transplant recipients: 1- and 3-year outcomes. Am J Transplant 2008;8(2):355–65.
207. Roozbeh J, Mehdizadeh AR, Izadfar MA, et al. Comparison of spousal with other donor groups: study of a single center. Transplant Proc 2006;38(2):562–3.
208. Roy DM, Thomas PP, Dakshinamurthy KV, et al. Long-term survival in living related donor renal allograft recipients with hepatitis B infection. Transplantation 1994;58(1):118–9.
209. Rutkowski B. Availability of renal replacement therapy in central and eastern Europe. Ethn Dis 2009;19(1):18–22.
210. Rutkowski B. Changing pattern of end-stage renal disease in central and eastern Europe. Nephrol Dial Transplant 2000;15(2):156–60.
211. Rutkowski B. Highlights of the epidemiology of renal replacement therapy in central and eastern Europe. Nephrol Dial Transplant 2006;21(1):4–10.
212. Rutkowski R, Ciocalteu A, Djukanovic L, et al. Central and Eastern Europe Advisory Board in chronic renal failure. Evolution of renal replacement therapy in Central and Eastern Europe seven years after political and economic liberation. Nephrol Dial Transplant 1998;13:860–4.
213. Saber LT, Duarte G, Costa JA, et al. Pregnancy and kidney transplantation: experience in a developing country. Am J Kidney Dis 1995;25(3):465–70.
214. Sajjad I, Baines LS, Patel P, et al. Commercialization of kidney transplants: a systematic review of outcomes in recipients and donors. Am J Nephrol 2008;28(5):744–54.
215. Sakhuja V, Jha V, Varma PP, et al. The high incidence of tuberculosis among renal transplant recipients in India. Transplantation 1996;61(2):211–5.
216. Sakhuja V, Kohli HS. End-stage renal disease in India and Pakistan: incidence, causes, and management. Ethn Dis 2006; 16(2 Suppl. 2):S2–3.
217. Sakhuja V, Sud K. End-stage renal disease in India and Pakistan: burden of disease and management issues. Kidney Int Suppl 2003;(83)S115–8.
218. Salahudeen AK, Woods HF, Pingle A, et al. High mortality among recipients of bought living-unrelated donor kidneys. Lancet 1990;336:725–8.
219. Samhan M, Al Mousawi M, Hayati H, et al. Results in 158 consecutive cadaveric renal transplantations. Transplant Proc 2005;37(7):2965–6.
220. Samhan M, Lao M, Nampoory MRN, et al. Results of 151 renal transplants in Kuwait. Transplant Proc 1999;31(8):3113–5.
221. Santiago Delpin EA, Duro GV. The 11th report of the Latin American Transplant Registry: 62,000 transplants. Transplant Proc 2001;33(1–2):1986–8.
222. Scheper-Hughes N. Keeping an eye on the global traffic in human organs. Lancet 2003;361(9369):1645–8.
223. Schieppati A, Remuzzi G. Chronic renal diseases as a public health problem: epidemiology, social, and economic implications. Kidney Int Suppl 2005;98:S7–10.
224. Sesso R, Ancao MS, Draibe SA, et al. Survival analysis of 1563 renal transplants in Brazil: report of the Brazilian Registry of Renal Transplantation. Nephrol Dial Transplant 1990;5(11):956–61.
225. Sesso R, Josephson MA, Ancao MS, et al. A retrospective study of kidney transplant recipients from living unrelated donors. J Am Soc Nephrol 1998;9(4):684–91.
226. Sever MS, Kazancioglu R, Yildiz A, et al. Outcome of living unrelated (commercial) renal transplantation. Kidney Int 2001;60(4):1477–83.
227. Shaheen FA. Organ donation in the Middle East countries. Ethn Dis 2009;19(1 Suppl. 1):S1–7.
228. Shaheen FA. Organ donation in the Middle East countries. Ethn Dis 2009;19(1 Suppl. 1):S1–7.
229. Shaheen FA, Al Khader AA. Preventive strategies of renal failure in the Arab world. Kidney Int Suppl 2005;98:S37–40.
230. Shaheen FA, Souqiyyeh MZ. How to improve organ donation in the MESOT countries. Ann Transplant 2004;9(1):19–21.
231. Shaheen FAM, Al Khader AA. Preventive strategies of renal failure in the Arab world. Kidney Int Suppl 2005;98:S37–40.
232. Shaheen MF, Shaheen FAM, Attar B, et al. Impact of recipient and donor nonimmunologic factors on the outcome of deceased donor kidney transplantation. Transplant Proc 2010;42(1):273–6.
233. Sharma RK, Kumar A, Kumar J, et al. Low-dose ATG is effective in treatment of acute rejection episodes. Transplant Proc 2003;35(1):225–6.

234. Sheriff R, de Abrew K, Jayasekara G, et al. Living related donor kidney transplantation in Sri Lanka. Transplant Proc 1992;24(5):1816–7.
235. Shi BY, Chen LP. Regulation of organ transplantation in China: difficult exploration and slow advance. JAMA 2011;306(4):434–5.
236. Shimazono Y. The state of the international organ trade: a provisional picture based on integration of available information. Bull World Health Organ 2007;85(12):955–62.
237. Shokeir AA. Renal transplantation: the impact of schistosomiasis. BJU Int 2001;88(9):915–20.
238. Shokeir AA, Bakr MA, el Diasty TA, et al. Urological complications following live donor kidney transplantation: effect of urinary schistosomiasis. Br J Urol 1992;70(3):247–51.
239. Shroff S, Navin S, Abraham G, et al. Cadaver organ donation and transplantation – an Indian perspective. Transplant Proc 2003;35(1):15–7.
240. Simforoosh N, Basiri A, Fattahi MR, et al. Living unrelated versus living related kidney transplantation: 20 years' experience with 2155 cases. Transplant Proc 2006;38(2):422–5.
241. Singh N, Gupta S, Chandra J, et al. Chronic ambulatory peritoneal dialysis (CRPD) – an initial Indian experience. J Indian Med Assoc 2005;103:22–6.
242. Sinha A, Hari P, Guleria S, et al. Outcome of pediatric renal transplantation in north India. Pediatr Transplant 2010;14(7):836–43.
243. Soman R, Vaideeswar P, Shah H, et al. A 34-year-old renal transplant recipient with high-grade fever and progressive shortness of breath. J Postgrad Med 2002;48(3):191–6.
244. Srinivas TR, Schold JD, Guerra G, et al. Mycophenolate mofetil/sirolimus compared to other common immunosuppressive regimens in kidney transplantation. Am J Transplant 2007;7(3):586–94.
245. Stephan A, Barbari A, Karam A, et al. Updating renal transplantation therapies in developing countries. Transplant Proc 2002;34(6):2475–7.
246. Sumboonnanonda A, Lumpaopong A, Kingwatanakul P, et al. Pediatric kidney transplantation in Thailand: experience in a developing country. Transplant Proc 2008;40(7):2271–3.
247. Tan J, Qiu J, Lu T, et al. Thirty years of kidney transplantation in two Chinese centers. Clin Transpl 2005;203–7.
248. Tan PK, Tan AS, Tan HK, et al. Pregnancy after renal transplantation: experience in Singapore General Hospital. Ann Acad Med Singapore 2002;31(3):285–9.
249. Taylor AL, Hwenda L, Larsen B-I, et al. Stemming the brain drain – a WHO global code of practice on international recruitment of health personnel. N Engl J Med 2011;365(25):2348–51.
250. The International Society of Nephrology. A briefing on the global impact of kidney disease. 2011. Available online at: http://cdn.theisn.org/images/stories/WHO_CKD_Brochure_LR.pdf.
251. Thiagarajan CM, Reddy KC, Shunmugasundaram D, et al. The practice of unconventional renal transplantation (UCRT) at a single centre in India. Transplant Proc 1990;22(3):912–4.
252. Thin NNKS. An audit and comparative analysis of the kidney transplantation programme in Burma. Int J Surg 2004;2(2):84–7.
253. Thiruchelvam PT, Willicombe M, Hakim N, et al. Renal transplantation. BMJ 2011;343d:7300.
254. Topbas M, Can G, Can MA, et al. Outmoded attitudes toward organ donation among Turkish health care professionals. Transplant Proc 2005;37(5):1998–2000.
255. Trey T, Halpern A, Singh MA. Organ transplantation and regulation in China. JAMA 2011;306(17):1863–4.
256. Tsai MC, Chen YT, Chien YS, et al. Hepatitis B virus infection and renal transplantation. World J Gastroenterol 2010;16(31):3878–87.
257. Tsai M-K, Lee P-H, Hu R-H, et al. Infectious complications in renal transplant recipients: a 10-year review of cyclosporine-based immunosuppression. Transplant Proc 1998;30(7):3125–6.
258. Turkmen A, Sever MS, Ecder T, et al. Posttransplant malaria. Transplantation 1996;62(10):1521–3.
259. U.S. Renal Data System. USRDS 2011 Annual Data Report. Atlas of Endstage Renal Disease in the United States. U.S. Renal Data System, Bethesda, MD: National Institutes of Diabetes and Digestive and Kidney Disease; 2011.
260. Vachharajani T, Abreo K, Phadke A, et al. Diagnosis and treatment of tuberculosis in hemodialysis and renal transplant patients. Am J Nephrol 2000;20(4):273–7.
261. Vasudev B, Hariharan S, Hussain SA, et al. BK virus nephritis: risk factors, timing, and outcome in renal transplant recipients. Kidney Int 2005;68(4):1834–9.
262. Vathsala A. Immunosuppression use in renal transplantation from Asian transplant centers: A preliminary report from the Asian Transplant Registry. Transplant Proc 2004;36(7):1868–70.
263. Vathsala A, Woo KT, Lim CH. Renal transplantation in Singapore. Transplant Proc 1992;24(5):1819–20.
264. Watts J. China introduces new rules to deter human organ trade. Lancet 2007;369(9577):1917–8.
265. Weiss RA, Whitby D, Talbot S, et al. Human herpesvirus type 8 and Kaposi's sarcoma. J Natl Cancer Inst Monogr 1998;23:51–4.
266. White SL, Cass A, Atkins RC, et al. Chronic kidney disease in the general population. Adv Chronic Kidney Dis 2005;12(1):5–13.
267. White SL, Chadban SJ, Jan S, et al. How can we achieve global equity in provision of renal replacement therapy? Bull World Health Organ 2008;86(3):229–37.
268. Xie Y, Chen X. Epidemiology, major outcomes, risk factors, prevention and management of chronic kidney disease in China. Am J Nephrol 2008;28(1):1–7.
269. Xu L, Yang Y, Shi JG, et al. Unwanted pregnancy among Chinese renal transplant recipients. Eur J Contracept Reprod Health Care 2011;16(4):270–6.
270. Yao Q, Zhang W, Qian J. Dialysis status in China: a report from the Shanghai Dialysis Registry (2000–2005). Ethn Dis 2009; 19(1 Suppl. 1):S1–6.
271. Yoon HE, Song JC, Hyoung BJ, et al. Comparison of long-term outcomes between spousal transplants and other living unrelated donor transplants: single-center experience. Nephron Clin Pract 2009;113(4):c241–9.
272. Zargooshi J. Iranian kidney donors: motivations and relations with recipients. J Urol 2001;165(2):386–92.
273. Zatz R, Romao JE, Noronha IL. Nephrology in Latin America, with special emphasis on Brazil. Kidney Int 2003;63(S83):S131–4.
274. Zhang AH, Cheng LT, Zhu N, et al. Comparison of quality of life and causes of hospitalization between hemodialysis and peritoneal dialysis patients in China. Health Qual Life Outcomes 2007;549.
275. Zhang L, Wang F, Wang L, et al. Prevalence of chronic kidney disease in China: a cross-sectional survey. Lancet 2012;379(9818):815–22.
276. Ziarkiewicz-Wroblewska B, Gornicka B, Suleiman W, et al. Posttransplant lymphoproliferative disorder: morphological picture and diagnostic difficulties. Transplant Proc 2006;38(1):168–72.
277. Zmonarski SC, Boratynska M, Rabczynski J, et al. Regression of Kaposi's sarcoma in renal graft recipients after conversion to sirolimus treatment. Transplant Proc 2005;37(2):964–6.

CHAPTER 39

RESULTS OF RENAL TRANSPLANTATION

Rachel E. Patzer • Stuart J. Knechtle

CHAPTER OUTLINE

INTRODUCTION

Outcome data for renal transplantation in the United States represent one of the best available examples of medical care supported by a local and national database to allow evidence-based decisions in the field. According to requirements directed by the United Network for Organ Sharing (UNOS), a federal government-authorized body, all transplant centers must submit transplant data to the Scientific Registry of Transplant Recipients (SRTR), where such data are collated and analyzed on a center-specific basis and cumulative national basis. Much of the data from the United States summarized in this chapter is substantially derived from the 2010 SRTR report on kidney and pancreas transplant outcomes,[79] which is available in published form in the *American Journal of Transplantation* and online at http://www.blackwell-synergy.com/loi/ajt.

The massive amount of data in the 2010 SRTR report has been reduced to that which is included in this chapter for the purpose of greater usefulness and readability. The source of the data is acknowledged in figures and tables. In addition, other data have been added to supplement the SRTR report, including United States Renal Data System (USRDS) surveillance data, individual center reports and multicenter trial data, data from Europe through the Collaborative Transplant Study (CTS), and the Australia and New Zealand Dialysis and Transplant (ANZDATA) Registry. These data inform decisions regarding patient access and outcomes and organ allocation. These data refer to transplantation in the western world; results from less well-developed countries are discussed in Chapter 38.

RENAL FAILURE TREATMENTS – DIALYSIS VERSUS TRANSPLANTATION

Renal failure is known to increase mortality from cardiovascular disease and from causes directly resulting from renal failure itself, including fluid and electrolyte imbalance and uremia.[28] Although dialysis addresses the immediately life-threatening complications of renal failure, it does not provide the fluid and electrolyte homeostasis comparable to a well-functioning kidney.

Several additional metabolic functions of the kidney, such as vitamin D synthesis and erythropoietin synthesis, also are not regulated appropriately in the absence of a well-functioning kidney. This reality is reflected by the well-documented finding that patients with end-stage renal disease (ESRD) have improved survival with transplantation compared with dialysis therapy.[22,49,79,94,108,112,119] Patients who receive dialysis have an expected remaining lifetime of 5.9 years, compared to 16.4 years for transplant recipients.[109] In addition, kidney transplantation is cost-effective compared with dialysis and offers improved quality of life.[25,51,89,108] Studies have shown an increasing cardiovascular risk proportional to the increase in serum creatinine, suggesting that renal failure at least correlates with, if not causes, accelerated vascular and metabolic defects that predispose to cardiovascular death. Dialysis patients are known to experience accelerated atherosclerosis,[41,53,117] and several inflammatory and atherogenic factors may account for this.[34,54,110,113,120] Given these facts, it is not surprising that analysis of USRDS data revealed that longer time on the wait list for renal transplantation correlates with poorer death-censored graft survival after renal transplantation (Figure 39-1). While there is a clear advantage of receiving a kidney transplant prior to ever starting dialysis,[85] i.e., pre-emptive renal transplantation, this practice is not widely adopted. In 2009, 16% of incident ESRD patients underwent pre-emptive transplantation, whereas the remaining patients started dialysis.[109]

The better outcomes of patients with pre-emptive transplants and with shorter time on dialysis underscore the importance of early referral and evaluation for renal transplantation. However, there are a number of barriers that patients face in accessing early transplantation, including organ allocation policies and delayed referral to nephrology care or transplant centers. In the United States, these barriers are particularly apparent for African Americans versus whites: African Americans have a lower rate of accessing each step of the kidney transplant process, including referral, evaluation, wait listing, and transplant receipt.[75,76,116] Patients with ESRD benefit from transplantation as early as possible to maximize their potential for long survival after transplantation.

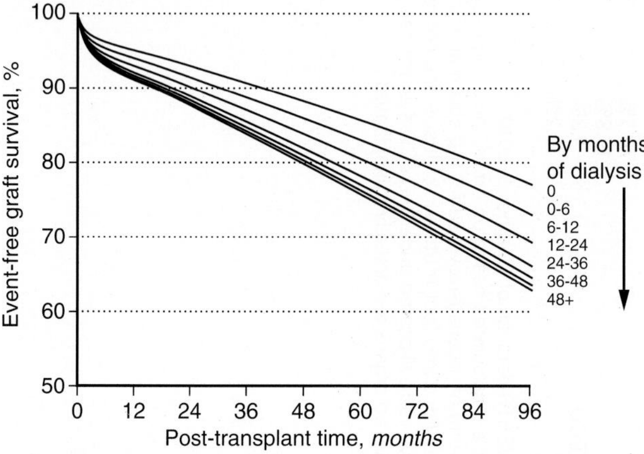

FIGURE 39-1 ■ Death-censored graft survival estimated by Cox proportional hazard analysis in the United States. (From Meier-Kriesche HU, Port FK, Ojo AO, et al. Effect of waiting time on renal transplant outcome. Kidney Int 2000;58:1311.)

KIDNEY DONATION

In the United States, the total number of deceased and live kidney transplants increased 34.1% from 1998 to 2006, but decreased 1.8% from 2006 to 2009. Kidney donation from deceased donors increased overall from 2000 to 2009, although donation rates remained fairly stable from 2005 to 2009, at 25.1 per million population in 2009. The number of kidneys transplanted from living donors decreased from 2005 to 2008, but increased 7% from 2008 to 2009, resulting in a total of 6388 donors in 2009.[97] In contrast, in Europe, there is wide variation in deceased donor rates between countries. Deceased donation has generally remained stagnant or even decreased over recent years, with the exception of Spain, Austria, and Belgium, where donor rates are the highest in the world following the introduction of presumed consent (opt-out) policies.[11,84] There has been a steady increase in living donors but overall not approaching the rate in the United States.

Expanded Criteria Donors

Expanded criteria donors (ECDs) are defined as all deceased donors older than age 60 or deceased donors between ages 50 and 59 who have two of the following three criteria: (1) a history of hypertension; (2) death caused by cerebrovascular accident; and (3) creatinine greater than 1.5 mg/dL at the time of procurement. ECDs have increased throughout the world in recent years. In 1998, ECD kidneys accounted for 13.6% of deceased donors; in 2009, ECD kidneys comprised 15.0% of the donor pool but 22.1% of the organs recovered (Table 39-1).[97] Outcomes for ECD kidney transplants are addressed later.

Donation after Cardiac Death

Donation after cardiac death (DCD) can yield either ECD or standard criteria donors (SCD). DCD has increased substantially since 2000: DCD/SCD represented 10.8% and DCD/ECD represented 1.1% of all organ donors in the United States in 2009.[97] DCD kidneys are kidneys procured after cessation of cardiac activity (in Europe, often referred to as non-heart-beating donors); this also is discussed in Chapters 6 and 9. Growth in DCD donors for kidney transplantation represents the largest increase in a type of donor kidney available for recipients in the United States. The ethics and methods of DCD recovery have been discussed at length by D'Alessandro and colleagues,[12] and single-center experiences have resulted in outcomes not significantly different from SCD kidney transplantation.[10] Several larger retrospective studies have compared short- and long-term outcomes of DCD versus SCD and ECD donors and found equivalent patient and graft survival at 5 years.[20,88] In a large UNOS registry study that examined more than 75 000 transplant recipients, results suggest that DCD kidneys from donors less than 50 years old have equivalent graft survival to SCD kidneys.[52] The use of DCD donors, normal practice in the early days of transplantation, was pioneered in the

TABLE 39-1 Deceased Donor Characteristics, 1999–2009

	Year									
Donor Category	**2000**	**2001**	**2002**	**2003**	**2004**	**2005**	**2006**	**2007**	**2008**	**2009**
Total	5489	5528	5638	5753	6325	6700	7178	7241	7188	7248
Standard criteria donor (SCD)	4289	4317	4358	4278	4588	4637	4961	4846	4718	4744
Expanded criteria donor (ECD)	1088	1052	1097	1222	1365	1531	1593	1637	1638	1605
Donation after cardiac death, non-ECD (DCD non-ECD)	101	140	154	202	305	432	521	640	714	785
ECD-DCD	11	19	29	51	67	100	103	118	118	114
Total (%)	100.0%	100.0%	100.0%	100.0%	100.0%	100.0%	100.0%	100.0%	100.0%	100.0%
SCD	78.1%	78.1%	77.3%	74.4%	72.5%	69.2%	69.1%	66.9%	65.6%	65.5%
ECD	19.8%	19.0%	19.5%	21.2%	21.6%	22.9%	22.2%	22.6%	22.8%	22.1%
DCD non-ECD	1.8%	2.5%	2.7%	3.5%	4.8%	6.4%	7.3%	8.8%	9.9%	10.8%
ECD-DCD	0.2%	0.3%	0.5%	0.9%	1.1%	1.5%	1.4%	1.6%	1.6%	1.6%

From OPTN/SRTR data, as of October 1, 2010.
Percentages are calculated based on totals, including missing and unknown cases.
Includes donors of organs recovered for transplant and not used, as well as those transplanted.
Donors are divided into four mutually exclusive and complete categories. All donors meeting the criteria for expanded criteria donors for kidney are classified as ECD, regardless of whether the kidneys were allocated under the ECD system, falling into either the ECD or the ECD-DCD category. Non-ECDs include all other donors, including SCDs and DCD non-ECDs.
Not all recovered organs are actually transplanted.

modern era by Kootstra's team at Maastricht some years ago,[46,47] and continued at the University of Wisconsin as the shortage of kidneys grew.[10]

Recipient Pool

At the end of 2009, there were 84 614 patients awaiting renal transplantation in the United States. New registrations for kidney transplantation in 2009 numbered 33 215 (Table 39-2). From 1998 to 2006, transplants increased 34%, including a 26% increase in the number of deceased donor transplants and a 51% increase in living donor transplants. However, from 2006 to 2009, the number of transplants declined 1.8%, including a 2.1% decline in deceased donors and a 1.8% decline in living donor transplants. The largest demographic increase in this population was in the 50–64-year-old age range.[97] Since 2003, the age group with the greatest percentage increase in registration for renal transplantation comprised patients 65 years old and older. For pediatric patients in the United States, access to the deceased donor waiting list and transplantation has increased since the introduction of the Organ Procurement and Transplantation Network (OPTN) Share 35 policy in 2005 that preferentially offers organs from deceased donors younger than 35 years of age to children less than 18 years; however, this has also resulted in a decline in the use of living donor transplants for this population.[70] Factors contributing to the increase of older patients on the waiting list include the aging general population of the United States, the increased incidence of ESRD with aging, and improvements in transplantation outcomes in the elderly. This disproportion between the increase in the waiting list and the number of patients receiving a transplant is similar throughout the western world. In developing countries, where access to deceased donor transplantation is low, the disparity between need and provision of kidneys is even greater.

TABLE 39-2 **Kidney Transplant Waiting List Activity Among Adult Patients**

	2007	2008	2009
Listings at start of year	68 754	74 501	79 161
Listings added during year	31 988	32 097	33 215
Listings removed during year	26 241	27 437	27 762
Listings at end of year	74 501	79 161	84 614
Removal reason			
Deceased donor transplant	11 796	11 828	11 765
Living donor transplant	4369	4572	5065
Patient died	5041	5306	5412
Patient refused transplant	266	259	307
Transferred to another center	1581	1510	1401
Condition improved, transplant not needed	121	133	132
Too sick to transplant	992	1243	1475
Changed to kidney–pancreas list	266	243	221
Other	1809	2343	1984

The racial representation on the United States wait list includes 38% white and 35% African American, with the remaining 27% comprising an increasing percentage of Hispanics, Asians, and others.[97] Gender representation remains unchanged, with males accounting for 58.5% and females 41.5% of the waiting list. The proportion of patients undergoing retransplantation in 2009 was 11.0% of living donor and 12.7% of deceased donor transplants. The length of time on the waiting list continues to increase, with 29.7% of active patients at the end of 2009 having waited 3 years or more, compared with 14% at the end of 1995.[97]

Glomerular disease, diabetes, and hypertension are the most common primary diseases among adult waiting list patients, at 30% (diabetes), 26% (hypertension), and 15% (glomerular disease) (see Chapters 3 and 4). Diabetes is likely to remain the most common diagnosis of patients awaiting renal transplantation in the United States; in most European countries, diabetes is not the major cause of renal failure in patients on the waiting list. The median time from listing to transplantation was considerably different among ethnic minorities and whites. For registrants added to the waiting list in 2005, the median time to transplant was 4.42 years for African Americans, 4.35 years for Hispanics, 4.3 years for Asians, and 2.02 years for whites.[97] Reasons for these racial disparities in waiting times have been addressed in several publications[27] and relate to human leukocyte antigen (HLA) typing and antigen representation in the donor population,[4,38,48] poverty,[75,91] social networks,[3] patient preferences,[6] or provider bias.[5]

ABO blood groups significantly influence median time to transplant, with blood group B registrants waiting the longest, or 4.18 years for registrants listed in 2009. Blood group AB registrants had the shortest waiting time, at 1.28 years. Patients with a previous organ transplant wait nearly twice as long as registrants awaiting their first kidney transplant,[68] owing to sensitization and presence of comorbidities.

Death on the waiting list for children 11–17 years old was approximately half that of children <6 years old (Table 39-3). As expected, death on the waiting list increases with increasing age, although death rates for patients younger than age 50 have decreased over the past 10 years. Death rates for patients 65 years old and older are nearly four times the rate for patients 18–34 years old.[97]

TABLE 39-3 **Pretransplant Mortality Rates Among Patients Wait-Listed for a Kidney Transplant**

	Age Group (Years)						
Year	**<6**	**6–10**	**11–17**	**18–34**	**35–49**	**50–64**	**65+**
1998	6.8	3.5	2.8	3.7	6.1	9.2	11.6
2000	5.5	3.7	2.4	3.5	5.8	9.3	12.8
2002	5.3	2.6	4.2	3.3	5.6	9.1	12.3
2004	5.4	3.2	3.0	3.1	5.2	8.6	12.7
2006	6.0	1.1	1.8	2.8	4.9	8.2	11.4
2008	3.4	0.7	1.8	2.6	4.3	7.1	10.2

Data from OPTN/SRTR, as of May 4, 2009.

In the United States, there were a total of 15 964 adult kidney transplant recipients in 2009, of which 62.1% were deceased donor and 37.9% were living donor transplants. Characteristics of transplant recipients are given in Table 39-4.

Factors Influencing Outcome

Many factors influence the outcome of renal transplantation, as illustrated by an earlier analysis of consecutive deceased donor kidney transplants in the United Kingdom between 1994 and 1998.[64] Factors such as HLA matching, donor age, cause of death, and cold ischemia time were found to have a significant impact on outcome. This section looks at these factors and others that influence outcome.

Donor Age

Analysis of 5-year outcomes by Gjertson[31] showed that donor age was the most important factor governing the survival rates of living donor and deceased donor renal transplants. Logistic regression analysis of OPTN/UNOS Registry data from 1996 to 2003 was used to calculate the impact of 21 prognostic factors in 85 270 recipients whose grafts survived beyond 1 year and were followed for 5 years. This result underscores the importance of the quality of the donor kidney with respect to long-term function. The European data from the CTS shows the same impact of donor age on graft outcome (Figure 39-2). Donor age was identified as the most important predictor of 3-year graft failure or patient mortality among the UK Transplant Registry.[115]

Recipient Age

Since the first report of an acceptable outcome to renal transplantation in the elderly[71] and the widespread introduction of cyclosporine-based immunosuppressive protocols, all units adopted a much more liberal approach to the selection of elderly recipients for transplantation. The results of renal transplantation in the elderly (arbitrarily defined as >55, >60, or >65 years old in various reports) have continued to confirm the validity of such policies (Figure 39-3). Patients aged 65 years and older represent nearly half of the ESRD population in the United States.[109] Although there is a higher mortality rate among elderly patients in the early years after transplantation, which is reflected by a poorer graft survival, rejection is less common than in younger patients and rarely a major problem.[42] Pulmonary embolism and infection are the two major causes of death in this age group. It is unusual for a graft to be lost through irreversible rejection.

Bearing in mind the shortage of deceased donor kidneys for renal transplantation, it is important to select elderly patients who are relatively low-risk recipients[67,95] and to use lower levels of immunosuppression. Nyberg and coworkers[67] pointed out that some of their elderly patients lost muscular strength after transplantation, which they did not regain, emphasizing that rehabilitation after transplantation is not as good as that in the younger patient. The study by Wolfe and associates,[119] referred to earlier, points out that older patients have a survival advantage with a transplant compared with survival on dialysis. This study confirmed the same suggestion from an earlier Canadian study.[93] A more recent analysis from the SRTR examined the outcome of renal transplantation in patients on the waiting list who were 70 years old or older, the fastest-growing group in the United States.[81] This analysis showed that transplantation offered a significant reduction in mortality compared with dialysis.

Obesity

Obesity has reached epidemic proportions in the United States, reaching a prevalence in 2007–2008 of over 30% of the adult population.[111] Based on body mass index (BMI) criteria, defining obesity as BMI greater than or equal to 30, 32.2% of men and 35.5% of women are obese.[27,40] Between 1987 and 2001, renal transplant patients classified as obese increased by 11.6%.[29] Obesity in renal transplantation is a risk factor for wound infections,[32,78] delayed graft function,[62] acute rejection,[32,59] increased radiographic monitoring, and need for biopsy,[32,43] and is associated with worse graft survival (Figure 39-4).[32,59] Although analysis of USRDS data by Meier-Kriesche and associates[59] suggested a higher risk of patient death after renal transplantation in the obese, a subsequent study by Gore and colleagues[32] showed that comorbidities, including hypertension, diabetes, and hyperlipidemia, accounted for the increased risk of death in obese patients. Donor obesity does not seem to have an impact on recipient outcomes. Voluntary weight loss and bariatric surgery before renal transplantation[1] may achieve significant long-term weight loss and relief of comorbidities in obese patients anticipating renal transplantation.

Race

In the United States, graft and survival outcomes are best for individuals of Asian background; outcomes are worst for African Americans. In 2009, 5-year graft survival for deceased donor transplantation was 74.8% (±0.4%) for Caucasians and 66.3% (±0.5%) for African Americans. Much effort has been expended on determining why these differences exist. Biologic factors, such as increased immunologic risk and lower absorption of immunosuppressants among recipients[45] or the presence of APOL1 gene variants in African American donors,[82] are hypothesized to play a role. Potentially modifiable factors, such as distrust of the healthcare system, transportation barriers, poorer adherence to medications, and ability to pay for immunosuppressant drugs[24] may also influence access to and quality of posttransplant follow-up care. An analysis of an experience of deceased donor transplantation from the University of Alabama, where more than half the recipients are African American, has shown a continuing improvement in graft survival in the non-African American population and in the African American population with the use of more potent immunosuppressive regimens. Long-term graft survival remains inferior, however, and the authors suggest that their data reinforce the importance of non-immunological variables, such as

TABLE 39-4 **Characteristics of Adult Kidney Transplant Patients, 2009**

		All		***Deceased***		***Living***	
		n	**%**	**n**	**%**	**n**	**%**
Age (years)	18–34	2208	13.8	1000	10.1	1208	20.0
	35–49	4541	28.4	2643	26.7	1898	31.4
	50–64	6556	41.1	4363	44.0	2193	36.2
	65+	2659	16.7	1906	19.2	753	12.4
Gender	Female	6322	39.6	3969	40.0	2353	38.9
	Male	9642	60.4	5943	60.0	3699	61.1
Race	White	8525	53.4	4530	45.7	3995	66.0
	Black	4105	25.7	3259	32.9	846	14.0
	Hispanic	2259	14.2	1376	13.9	883	14.6
	Asian	874	5.5	602	6.1	272	4.5
	Other/unknown	201	1.3	145	1.5	56	0.9
Primary cause of disease	Diabetes	3921	24.6	2581	26.0	1340	22.1
	Hypertension	3931	24.6	2759	27.8	1172	19.4
	Glomerulonephritis	3060	19.2	1676	16.9	1384	22.9
	Cystic kidney disease	2070	13.0	1126	11.4	944	15.6
	Other cause	2982	18.7	1770	17.9	1212	20.0
Blood type	A	5954	37.3	3646	36.8	2308	38.1
	B	2096	13.1	1294	13.1	802	13.3
	AB	768	4.8	534	5.4	234	3.9
	O	7146	44.8	4438	44.8	2708	44.7
PRA	<10%	11 257	70.5	6666	67.3	4591	75.9
	10%+	3667	23.0	2631	26.5	1036	17.1
	Unknown	1040	6.5	615	6.2	425	7.0
History of renal replacement therapy	Pre-emptive transplant	2639	16.5	905	9.1	1734	28.7
	<1 year	2169	13.6	687	6.9	1482	24.5
	<3 years	4056	25.4	2536	25.6	1520	25.1
	<5 years	2856	17.9	2371	23.9	485	8.0
	5+ years/unknown	4244	26.6	3413	34.4	831	13.7
Insurance	Private	6270	39.3	2677	27.0	3593	59.4
	Medicare	8729	54.7	6581	66.4	2148	35.5
	Other	965	6.0	654	6.6	311	5.1
HLA mismatches with donor	0	1264	7.9	787	7.9	477	7.9
	1	371	2.3	87	0.9	284	4.7
	2	1391	8.7	405	4.1	986	16.3
	3	2904	18.2	1301	13.1	1603	26.5
	4	3594	22.5	2630	26.5	964	15.9
	5	4221	26.4	3117	31.4	1104	18.2
	6	2089	13.1	1516	15.3	573	9.5
	Unknown	130	0.8	69	0.7	61	1.0
Kidney transplant history	First transplant	14 037	87.9	8653	87.3	5384	89.0
	Subsequent transplant	1927	12.1	1259	12.7	668	11.0
DCD status*	Non-DCD			8633	87.1		
	DCD			1279	12.9		
SCD/ECD status*	SCD			7892	79.6		
	ECD			2020	20.4		
Total		15 964	100.0	9912	100.0	6052	100.0

*For deceased donor transplant only.
HLA, human leukocyte antigen; DCD, donation after cardiac death; SCD, standard criteria donor; ECD, expanded criteria donor; PRA, panel-reactive antibody.

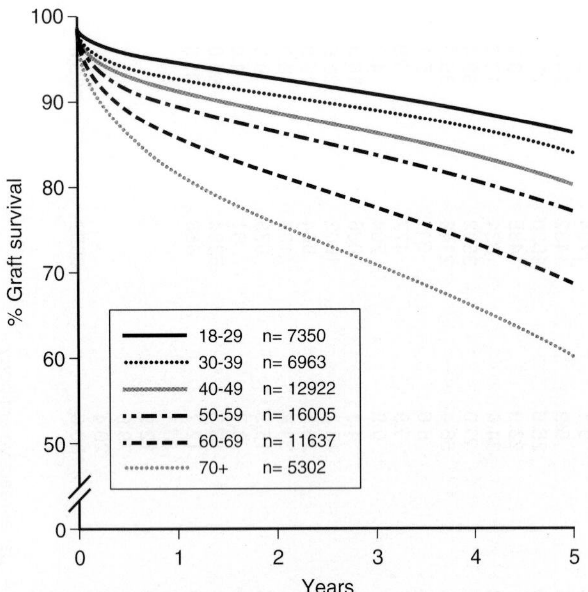

FIGURE 39-2 ■ **Impact of donor age on graft outcome. Donor age and graft survival of first cadaver kidney transplants, 1997–2010, in Europe.** (Data from Collaborative Transplant Study. Available online at: http://www.ctstransplant.org.)

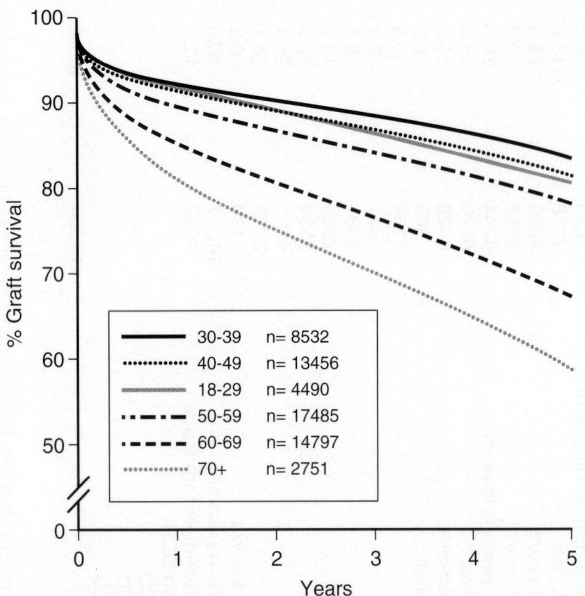

FIGURE 39-3 ■ **Impact of recipient age on graft outcome. Recipient age and graft survival of first cadaver kidney transplants, 1997–2010, in Europe.** (Data from Collaborative Transplant Study. Available online at: http://www.ctstransplant.org.)

time on dialysis before transplantation, diabetes, and access to medical care.[21]

In support of this hypothesis, a study by Pallet and coworkers[73] of black recipients transplanted between 1987 and 2003 in France suggested that there was not a difference between white and black recipients. The authors suggest that the origin of the difference is not so much genetic, immunological, or pharmacological as it is related to universal access to immunosuppressive drugs (i.e., compliance, and social and economic factors). A study by Lunsford and associates[55] from the University

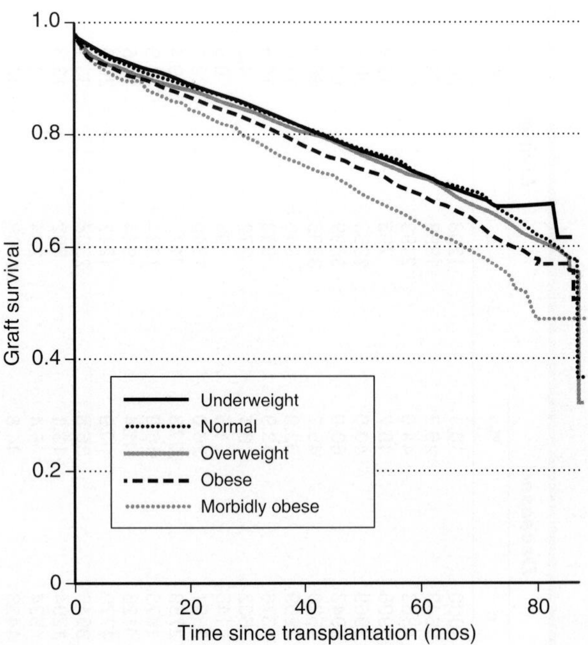

FIGURE 39-4 ■ **Graft survival after renal transplantation stratified by recipient body mass index at the time of transplantation.** (From Gore JL, Pham PT, Danovitch GM, et al. Obesity and outcome following renal transplantation. Am J Transplant 2006;6:357–63.)

of South Carolina suggested that, from a study of 333 patients awaiting transplantation, of which 61% were African American, African Americans are less accepting of their renal failure and more likely to deny the need for renal transplantation than their counterparts. Similar to the findings for African Americans, Press and colleagues[80] have reported that Hispanics also have a higher rate of graft failure compared with whites after adjustment for poverty and other covariates, and that poverty, but not race or ethnicity, is related to functional status after renal transplantation.

HLA Mismatch and Prior Sensitization

There continues to be an advantage of receiving a well-matched kidney, meaning fewer donor–recipient HLA mismatches, as illustrated by the CTS registry data (Figure 39-5) (see Chapter 10). In the United States, 7.9% of kidney transplant recipients in 2009 received a zero-mismatched kidney versus 12% in 1995.[97] Transplants into patients with four or more HLA antigen mismatches in 2009 accounted for 73% of deceased donor, non-ECD transplants, reflecting decreased emphasis on HLA matching in allocation policy and increased accrued waiting time emphasis.

In other words, most recipients in the United States of deceased donor kidneys are not well matched, if defined as at least three of six matches or fewer than four mismatches. An analysis of UNOS data in 2004 suggested that the impact of HLA compatibility on graft outcome has diminished in recent years with the advent of more potent immunosuppression.[103] Opelz and Dohler[69] analyzed CTS data in two decades, 1985–1994 and 1995–2004, and in more recent years have found that the influence of HLA on graft survival remains strong.

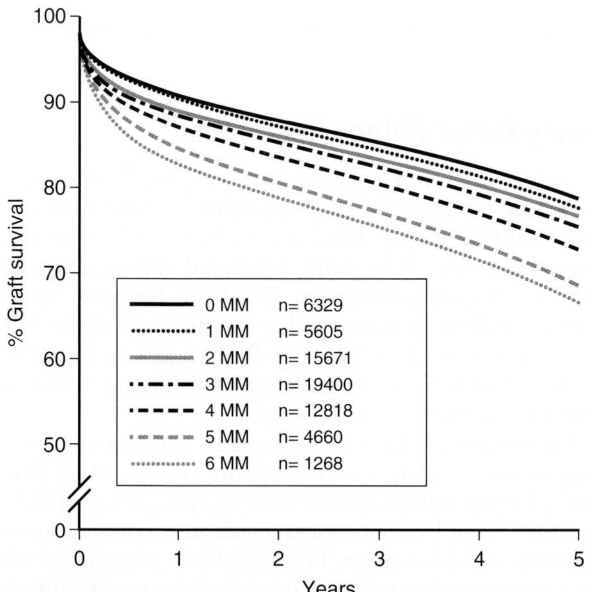

FIGURE 39-5 ■ Human leukocyte antigen (HLA)-A, HLA-B, and HLA-DR mismatches and first cadaver kidney transplants, 1985–2010. MM, HLA mismatches. (Data from Collaborative Transplant Study. Available online at: www.ctstransplant.org.)

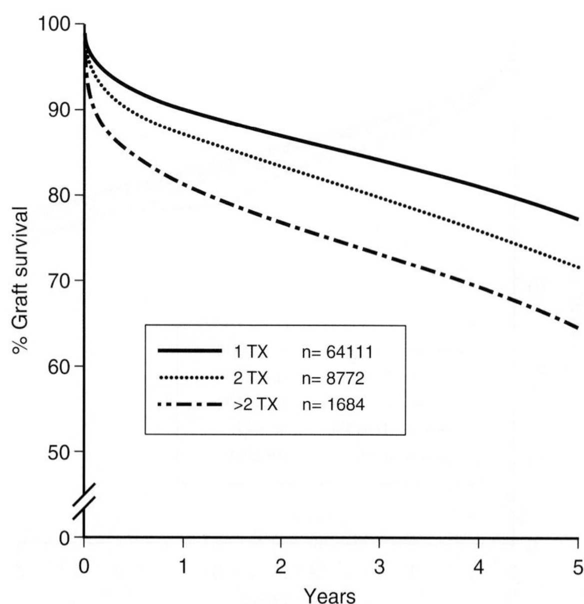

FIGURE 39-6 ■ Number of cadaver kidney transplants (TX) and graft survival, 1985–2010. (Data from Collaborative Transplant Study. Available online at: www.ctstransplant.org.)

Between 1998 and 2009, the percentage of deceased donor, non-ECD kidney transplants into recipients with a panel-reactive antibody frequency of 80% or greater at the time of transplant increased from 2.2% to 8.1%.[97] Highly sensitized patients, as measured by a high panel-reactive antibody percentage, are receiving transplants much more frequently, perhaps owing to the better definition of antibodies and the development of immunosuppressive strategies to aid in such cases in the United States. Nevertheless, in 2009, 15.9% of wait-listed patients had a panel-reactive antibody greater than 80%. National data for success of these strategies are still lacking. Center data suggest that desensitization strategies may provide greater benefit than waiting for a compatible organ (Montgomery RA, et al. NEJM 2011;365:318-26). In Europe, the acceptable mismatch strategy, which is based on the precise definition of antibodies in the recipient, is used more often (see Chapter 10).

The available data continue to support the benefit of more HLA matches compared with less, although it also can be argued that even a poorly matched kidney transplant is preferable to dialysis when measured by outcome analysis. Primary renal transplants have better outcomes than retransplants overall, again well illustrated by the CTS registry data (Figure 39-6). Living donor transplants that are HLA-identical continue to have better outcomes, followed by haploidentical living donor transplants and deceased donor grafts (Figure 39-7).

Cold Ischemia Time

The percentage of kidney transplants completed with cold ischemic times of less than 12 hours in the United States (see Chapter 9). The shifts in overall percentages of kidneys transplanted with shorter cold ischemia times reflect the value of short preservation times. Most kidneys are now transplanted in less than 31 hours of the time of procurement. Regardless of the choice of preservation solution or cold storage versus machine perfusion, shorter preservation tends to be an advantage in graft function and survival; this is well illustrated by the CTS data (Figure 39-8). The University of Wisconsin preservation solution is the dominant choice worldwide for kidney preservation and, at least in the CTS European data, is associated with the best graft outcome (Figure 39-9).[69] For ECD kidneys, longer cold ischemia time is a risk factor for delayed graft function but does not appear to affect graft survival.[44]

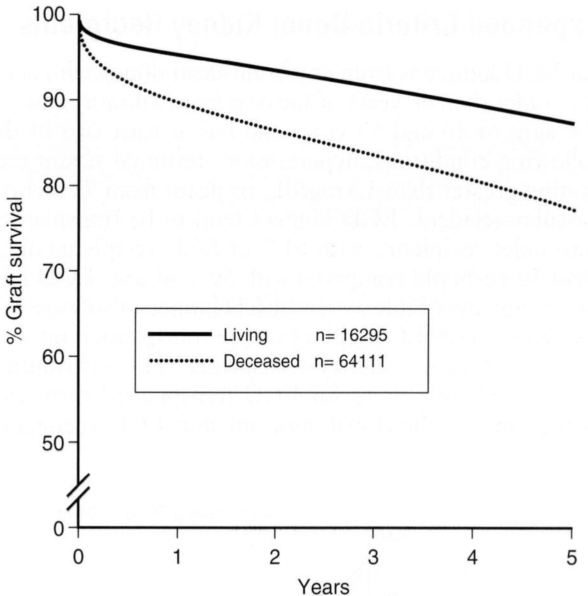

FIGURE 39-7 ■ Relationship of donor type and graft survival of first kidney transplant recipients, 1985–2010. (Data from Collaborative Transplant Study. Available online at: http://www.ctstransplant.org.)

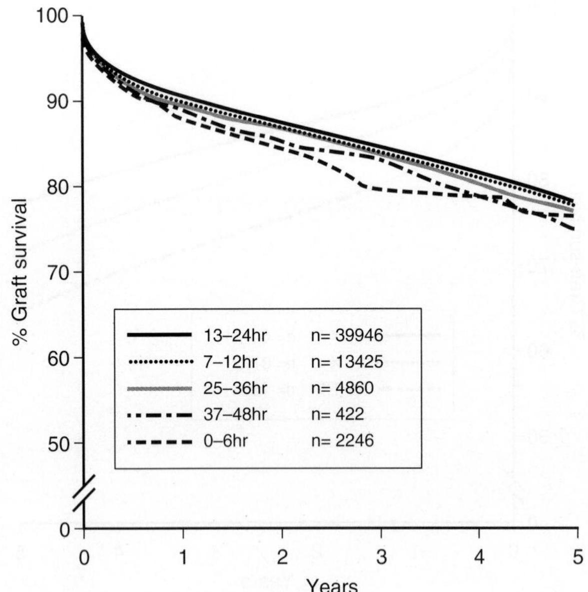

FIGURE 39-8 ■ Cold ischemia time and graft survival of first cadaver kidney transplants, 1990–2010, in Europe. (Data from Collaborative Transplant Study. Available online at: http://www.ctstransplant.org.)

Expanded Criteria Donor Kidney Recipients

An ECD kidney is from any brain-dead donor who is either older than 60 years of age or is from a donor between the ages of 50 and 59 years and has at least two of the following conditions: hypertension, terminal serum creatinine greater than 1.5 mg/dL, or death from a cerebrovascular accident. ECD kidneys tend to be transplanted into older recipients, with 81% of ECD recipients older than 50 years old compared with 50% of non-ECD kidney recipients (Table 39-4).[97] ECD kidneys also were less likely than non-ECD kidneys to be transplanted into recipients of repeat kidney transplants. The distribution of cold ischemia times for ECD transplanted recipients is the same as the distribution for non-ECD recipients, with cold ischemia time of less than 31 hours for approximately 80%.

Living Donor Kidney Recipients

Living donor kidney recipients comprised 36% of all transplants in 2009[25] were predominantly white (66%) in 2009. Of 6388 living donations in 2009, 50% were from related donors, 22% from unrelated directed donors, 13% from spouses/partners, 8% from distantly related donors, and the remaining due to paired donation (4%) or other donors (4%).[97] Living donor age is an important predictor of long-term graft survival among recipients who are less than 50 years of age.[66]

Pre-emptive kidney transplants in patients not yet on dialysis increased from 605 patients (17.9% of all living donor kidney transplants) in 1995 to 2192 patients (32.1% in 2009),[33] and living donor transplants accounted for the majority of this increase. This trend is in accordance with data showing elevated creatinine to be a significant cardiovascular risk factor and a risk factor for mortality.[28] Data also show enhanced patient and graft survival for patients undergoing pre-emptive renal transplantation compared with patients transplanted while on dialysis.[60] However, pre-emptive transplantation prior to estimated glomerular filtration rate $<15\ mL/min/1.73\ m^2$ does not appear to offer any patient or graft survival benefit.[33]

Immunosuppression

In the United States, induction immunosuppression with an antibody at the time of transplantation was used for 83% of kidney recipients in 2009 compared with 27% of recipients in 1995.[97] In 2009, a T-cell-depleting antibody was used for 58% of kidney transplants, 21% received interleukin-2 receptor antagonist, and 3.6% received both agents (Figure 39-10). Maintenance steroid use decreased from 94% of recipients in 2001 to 74% in 2005 and 65.7% in 2009. Tacrolimus was used in 87.8% of recipients in 2009 and cyclosporine in 5.7% at the time

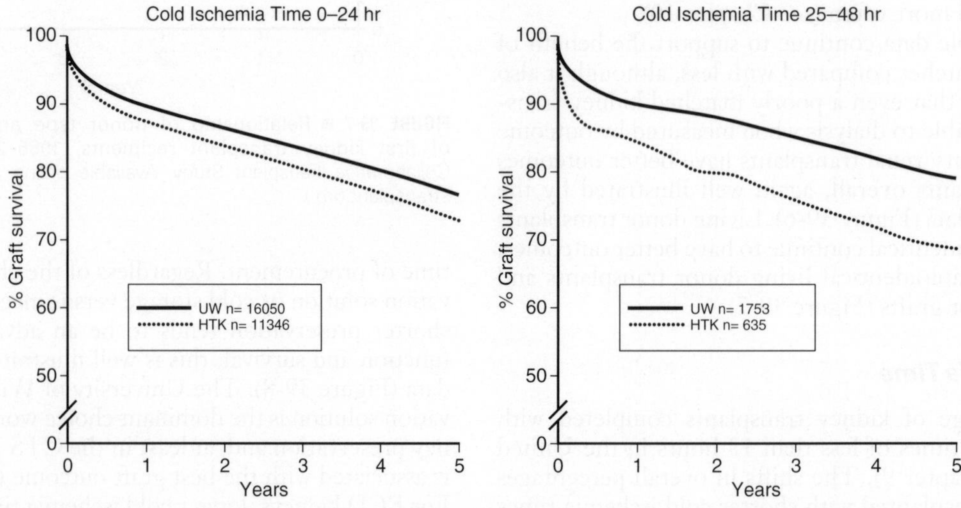

FIGURE 39-9 ■ Preservation solution and graft survival of first cadaver kidney transplants, 1997–2010, in Europe. HTK, histidine-tryptophan-ketoglutarate solution; UW, University of Wisconsin. (Data from Collaborative Transplant Study. Available online at: http://www.ctstransplant.org.)

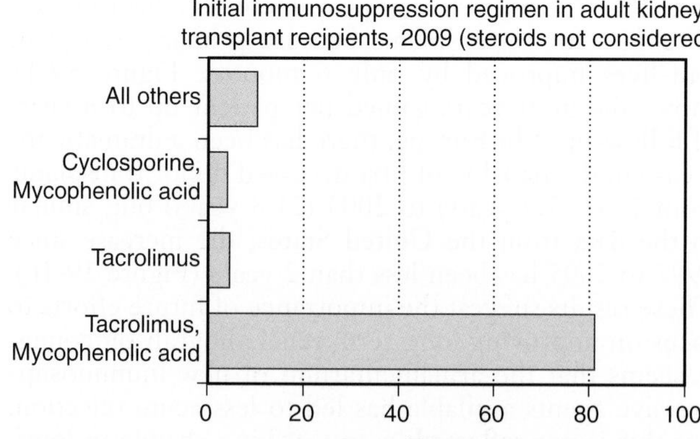

FIGURE 39-10 ■ **Immunosuppression agents used for induction in kidney transplantation, 2009.** (Data from OPTN/SRTR Annual Report, 2010. Available online at: http://www.srtr.org/annual_reports/2010.)

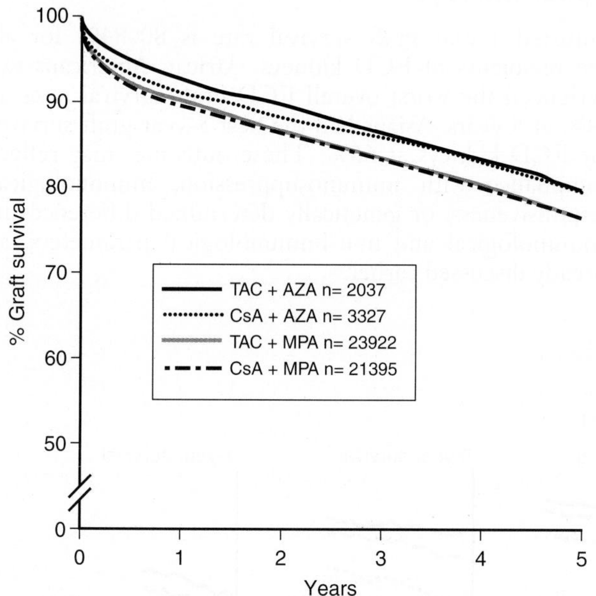

FIGURE 39-11 ■ **Trends in immunosuppression maintenance regimens, 1-year post transplant for kidney transplantation, 1999–2010, in Europe. AZA, azathioprine; CsA, cyclosporine; MPA, mycophenolic acid; TAC, tacrolimus.** (Data from Collaborative Transplant Study. Available online at: http://www.ctstransplant.org.)

of discharge; this represents a substantial shift from cyclosporine to tacrolimus over the past 15 years and continued reliance on calcineurin inhibitors as the backbone of renal transplant immunosuppression. Mycophenolate mofetil was used in 89.9% of cases in 2009 at the time of discharge. Three percent of patients received sirolimus at the time of discharge, and 6.5% received sirolimus during the first year. Figure 39-11 summarizes US trends in maintenance immunosuppression for kidney transplants.

In contrast, in Europe, the use of antibody induction is less prevalent than in the United States, although the use of an interleukin-2 receptor antibody for induction is becoming more common. In the CTS European database between 1998 and 2005, 36% of patients had induction with only an antibody (Figure 39-12). Similarly, there has been a swing toward tacrolimus from cyclosporine for primary maintenance therapy, but not to the same extent

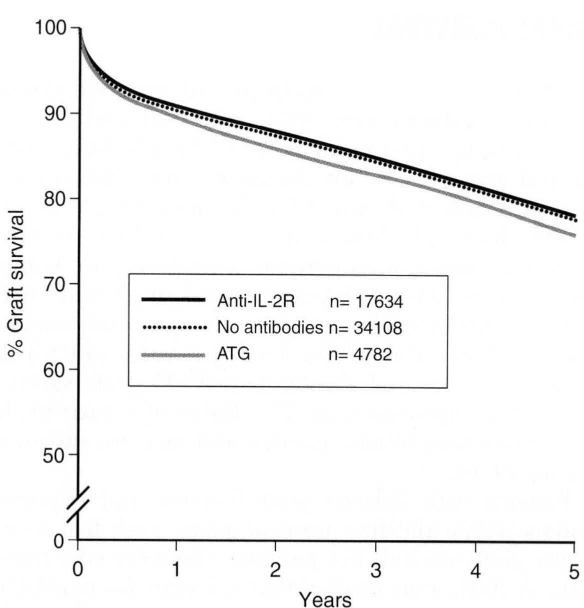

FIGURE 39-12 ■ **Prophylactic antibody induction with OKT3, antithymocyte globulin (ATG), and anti-interleukin-2 receptor (IL-2R) and graft survival of first cadaver kidney transplants, 1998–2005, in Europe.** (Data from Collaborative Transplant Study. Available online at: http://www.ctstransplant.org.)

as in the United States. There has been a marked change, however, from azathioprine to mycophenolate mofetil. Data are available from Europe with respect to incidence of rejection by 1 year, with approximately 20% of patients with deceased donor or one-haploypte-related kidneys treated (http://www.CTStransplant.org).

Adherence (Compliance) with Immunosuppressive Treatment

Non-adherence is defined as "deviation from the prescribed medication regimen sufficient to influence adversely the regimen's intended effect," according to a 2010 Consensus Conference on Nonadherence. The importance of non-adherence with immunosuppression, often resulting in rejection and graft loss, began to attract attention in the 1980s.[90,96] Butler and colleagues[8] performed a systematic review of the frequency and impact of non-adherence to immunosuppressive drugs after renal transplantation and pointed out that non-adherence is common, and that the odds of graft loss are sevenfold greater in non-adherent patients than in adherent patients. In a more recent meta-analysis of 72 kidney transplant studies representing 25 different countries within North America, Europe, Asia, Australia, and South America, Dew et al. identified that the rate of non-adherence of immunosuppressant medications was 35.6 cases (±2.3) per 100 person years.[16] The prevalence of non-adherence is more common among adolescents compared to other age groups, and has been reported in the range of 30–53%.[19,83] The gold standard for measuring non-adherence is direct observation that medication was consumed[26]; however, in practice, this is difficult to achieve. Combining several measures of adherence, such as self-report, assays, and clinician report, results in the best results (72% sensitivity and 42% specificity) compared to electronic monitoring.[92]

GRAFT SURVIVAL

Graft survival rates for recipients of deceased donor, non-ECD kidneys were 92% at 1 year and 70% at 5 years (Figure 39-13 and Table 39-5). The best 5-year survival rate of 78% for deceased donor kidneys was seen in Asians with non-ECD kidneys. One-year and 5-year deceased donor, non-ECD kidney survival rates were superior in patients with polycystic kidney disease, with poorer 5-year survival in patients with diabetes, hypertension, nephrosclerosis, and vascular diseases. Since the 1990s, 1-year, 3-year, and 5-year unadjusted deceased donor, non-ECD graft survival rates have improved only 2%. Rates of return to dialysis according to age, gender, and race are shown in Figure 39-14.

Patients with delayed graft function and requiring dialysis within the first posttransplant week had worse 5-year graft survival. For patients who received a transplant in 2004, graft survival rate at 5 years for non-ECD kidneys was 54% if dialysis was needed in the first week versus 74% if dialysis was not needed.

Chronic rejection and death with a functioning graft are the main causes of late graft loss (see Chapters 27 and 31).[74]

Analysis of renal transplant half-lives based on Kaplan–Meier analysis using the US SRTR data showed that half-lives improved overall by 2 years between 1988 and 1995.[61] Most of this improvement was due to better outcomes for retransplants because primary transplant half-lives improved by only 6 months. Figure 39-15 shows the graft years gained per patient up to 8 years of follow-up.[61] In Europe, there has been a dramatic increase in the half-life of first deceased donor transplants from 1982 (7.9 years) to 2005 (21.8 years) but, similar to the data from the United States, the increase since 1997 to 2005 has been less than 2 years (Figure 39-16). These results suggest the importance of future efforts to focus on improving long-term renal allograft outcomes. It seems that the armamentarium of new immunosuppressive agents available has led to less acute rejection, but this is not reflected in any striking change in long-term graft survival.

Graft Survival for Expanded Criteria Donor Kidneys

Adjusted 1-year graft survival rate is 80–84% for all age recipients of ECD kidneys. African Americans experienced the worst overall ECD graft survival rates at 44% at 5 years. Asians had the best 5-year graft survival for ECD kidneys at 66%. These outcomes may reflect compliance with immunosuppression, immunological responsiveness, or genetically determined differences in immunological and non-immunological parameters, as already discussed earlier.

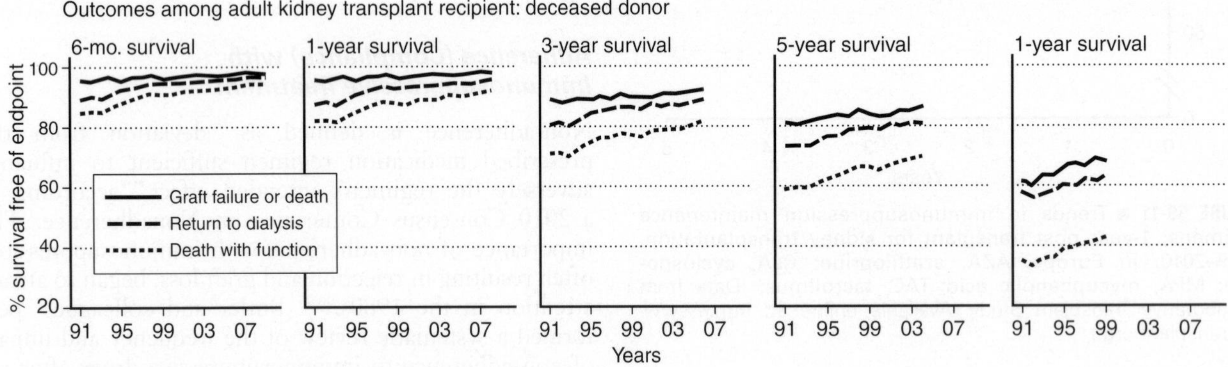

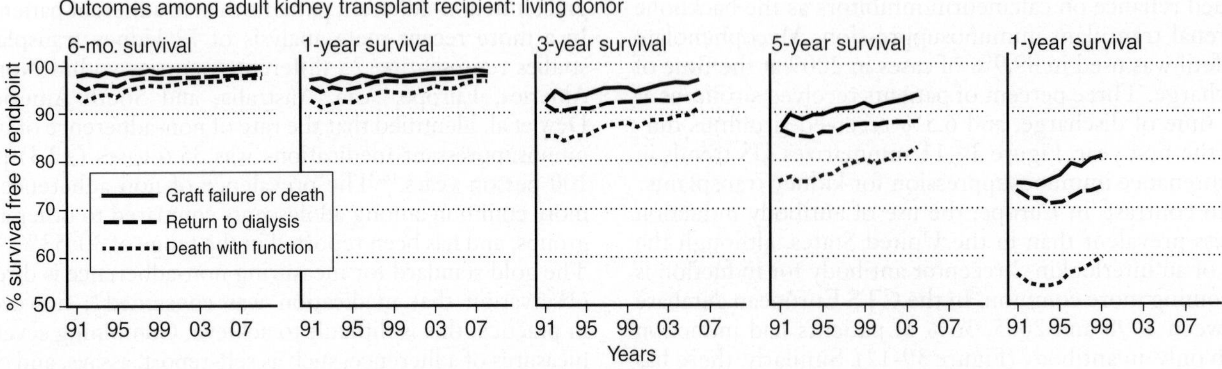

FIGURE 39-13 ■ Graft survival outcomes among adult kidney transplant recipients, by donor type, 1990–2009. (From 2010 OPTN/SRTR Annual Report. Available online at: http://www.srtr.org/annual_reports/2010.)

TABLE 39-5 **Adjusted Graft Survival, Deceased Donor Non-Expanded Criteria Donor Kidney Transplants: Survival at 3 Months, 1 Year, 3 Years, and 5 Years in the United States**

	6-Month Survival			*1-Year Survival*			*3-Year Survival*			*5-Year Survival*			*10-Year Survival*		
	Graft Failure or Death	Return to Dialysis	Death with Function	Graft Failure or Death	Return to Dialysis	Death with Function	Graft Failure or Death	Return to Dialysis	Death with Function	Graft Failure or Death	Return to Dialysis	Death with Function	Graft Failure or Death	Return to Dialysis	Death with Function
1991	84.7	89.3	95.6	82.0	87.5	94.4	70.7	80.4	88.8	59.1	73.4	81.0	35.2	57.6	61.3
1992	85.3	90.1	95.3	82.2	88.1	93.9	70.6	80.7	88.1	58.8	73.5	80.5	33.6	56.3	60.2
1993	84.8	89.2	95.6	81.6	87.1	94.2	70.1	79.9	88.3	59.2	73.3	81.2	35.9	57.1	63.6
1994	86.4	90.2	96.3	83.2	88.5	94.5	72.5	82.0	88.9	60.7	74.3	82.1	36.7	58.4	63.6
1995	87.9	92.2	95.6	85.0	90.6	94.0	74.3	84.0	88.8	62.6	76.1	82.6	39.1	60.0	66.0
1996	89.2	92.8	96.2	86.3	91.2	94.8	76.1	84.8	89.9	63.9	76.9	83.5	39.9	60.0	67.3
1997	90.6	94.1	96.4	87.8	92.7	94.7	76.3	85.8	89.1	65.0	78.4	83.3	40.7	61.9	66.6
1998	91.1	94.1	96.9	88.3	92.5	95.5	77.6	85.9	90.5	66.2	78.1	85.2	41.8	61.7	68.7
1999	90.8	94.4	96.2	87.6	92.6	94.7	77.4	86.3	89.8	66.4	79.1	84.2	42.7	63.5	68.2
2000	90.8	94.4	96.2	87.3	92.6	94.4	76.7	85.7	89.7	65.7	78.9	83.6			
2001	91.7	94.9	96.6	88.6	93.2	95.2	78.3	87.4	89.7	67.2	80.8	83.5			
2002	91.8	94.7	96.9	88.9	93.1	95.5	78.4	86.6	90.7	68.1	80.1	85.3			
2003	92.1	95.1	96.9	89.0	93.4	95.3	79.0	87.2	90.6	69.3	81.4	85.4			
2004	92.4	95.2	97.1	89.7	93.6	95.8	79.2	87.0	91.1	70.0	81.2	86.4			
2005	92.9	95.6	97.2	89.9	93.9	95.7	80.6	88.2	91.5						
2006	93.3	95.8	97.3	90.5	94.1	96.2	81.9	88.7	92.3						
2007	93.9	96.1	97.7	91.4	94.7	96.5									
2008	94.2	96.1	97.9	92.0	94.8	96.9									
2009	94.4	96.4	97.8												

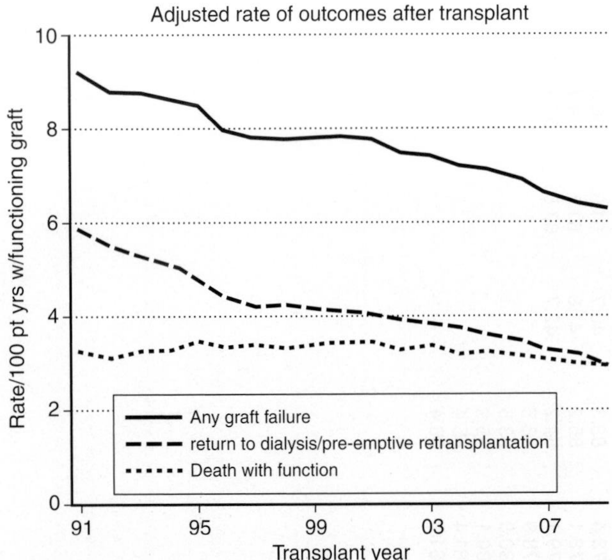

FIGURE 39-14 ■ Rates of graft failure, death with a functioning graft, and return to dialysis or pre-emptive retransplant, adjusted for age, gender, and race. (From 2011 ADR USRDS. Available online at: http://www.usrds.org/adr.htm.)

Graft Survival among Living Donor Recipients (Table 39-6)

Monozygotic Twins

Monozygotic twins are the ideal donor and recipient because of their genetic identity for major and minor histocompatibility antigens. Transplantation between identical twins has not been uniformly successful, however, because failures occur as a result of technical problems or recurrent glomerulonephritis. Tilney and coworkers[37,107] reviewed the results of 28 identical twin transplants at the Peter Bent Brigham Hospital, where the first successful pioneering transplant between identical twins was performed in 1954. Two deaths occurred within 2 weeks of transplantation – one from infarction of the kidney and one from septicemia secondary to a perinephric infection. Seven other patients developed recurrent nephritis at 6 months to 10 years after transplantation; 5 patients died of the recurrent disease because of lack of maintenance dialysis to which these patients could be returned. An analysis of the Brigham experience of 30 identical twin transplants,[35,106] in which follow-up lasted 27 years, showed a 25-year patient survival rate of around 65% and a graft survival rate of around 55%. Eight of the 11 graft failures were due to recurrent nephritis, occurring 3 months to 20 years after

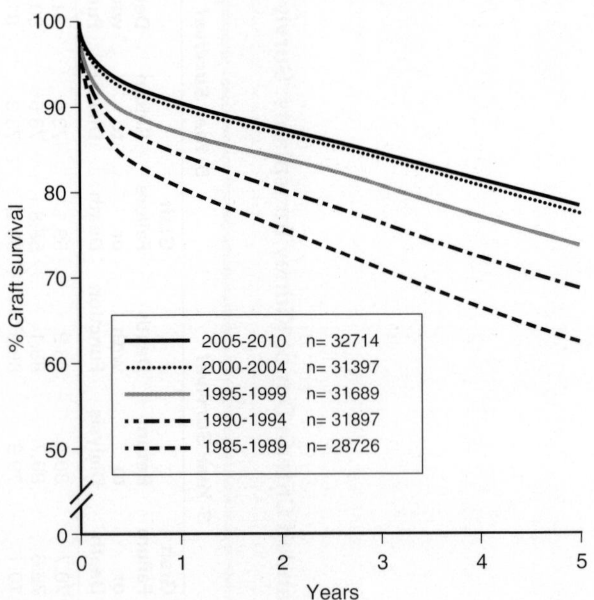

FIGURE 39-16 ■ Graft survival of first cadaver kidney transplants in Europe according to transplant year. (Data from Collaborative Transplant Study. Available online at: http://www.ctstransplant.org.)

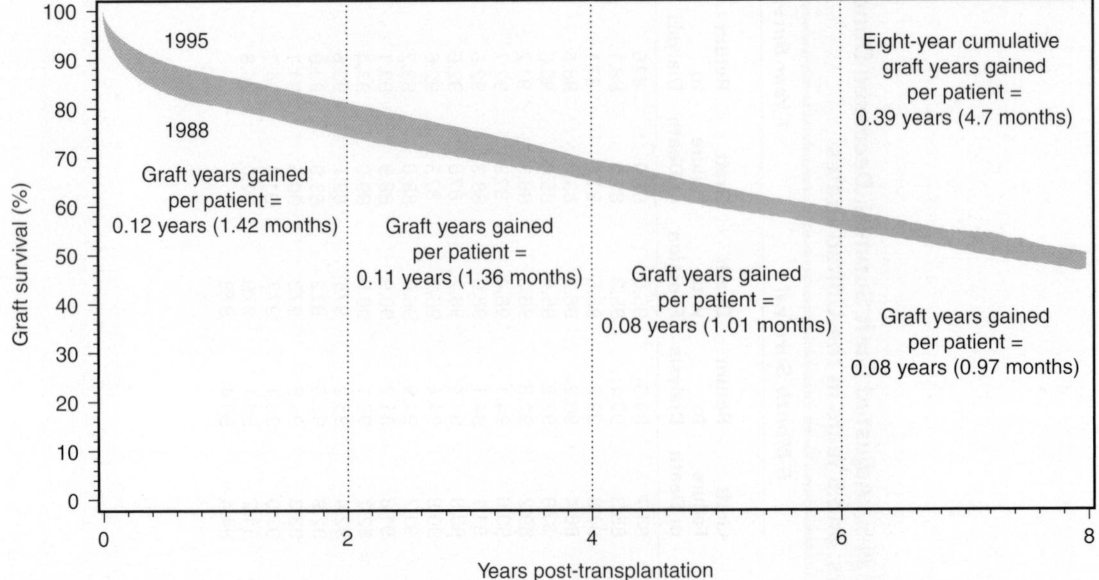

FIGURE 39-15 ■ Increased cumulative graft years per patient in deceased donor transplant recipients. Kaplan–Meier survival curves from transplants in 1988 and 1995. (Data from Meier-Kriesche HU, Schold JD, Kaplan B. Long-term renal allograft survival: have we made significant progress or is it time to rethink our analytic and therapeutic strategies? Am J Transplant 2004;4:1289.)

TABLE 39-6 **Adjusted Graft Survival, Living Donor Kidney Transplants: Survival at 3 Months, 1 Year, 3 Years, and 5 Years in the United States**

	6-Month Survival			*1-Year Survival*			*3-Year Survival*			*5-Year Survival*			*10-Year Survival*		
	Graft Failure or Death	Return to Dialysis	Death with Function	Graft Failure or Death	Return to Dialysis	Death with Function	Graft Failure or Death	Return to Dialysis	Death with Function	Graft Failure or Death	Return to Dialysis	Death with Function	Graft Failure or Death	Return to Dialysis	Death with Function
1991	93.9	96.1	97.8	92.6	95.6	96.8	85.0	91.6	92.3	75.7	86.3	86.7	56.4	74.0	75.2
1992	92.6	94.8	98.0	91.4	94.3	97.2	85.3	90.4	94.7	76.7	85.4	89.7	54.3	71.9	74.9
1993	93.8	96.0	97.9	91.9	95.2	96.5	84.3	90.5	93.0	75.7	85.4	88.4	53.9	71.8	74.6
1994	94.1	95.9	98.4	92.5	95.0	97.6	85.3	91.1	93.5	75.7	84.8	89.2	53.7	71.0	75.7
1995	93.5	95.6	97.9	92.3	95.0	97.2	85.2	91.0	93.7	77.0	85.9	89.6	54.2	71.1	76.5
1996	94.8	96.5	98.3	93.6	95.8	97.8	86.3	91.4	94.5	77.4	85.7	90.5	56.6	71.9	79.2
1997	95.3	96.9	98.3	93.9	96.4	97.4	87.5	92.1	95.1	78.9	87.0	90.8	57.2	73.2	78.6
1998	96.0	97.3	98.7	94.4	96.5	97.9	87.6	92.1	95.2	79.5	87.5	91.0	58.3	73.4	80.1
1999	95.8	97.3	98.5	94.3	96.5	97.8	87.9	92.3	95.3	80.2	87.6	91.8	59.6	74.4	80.8
2000	96.0	97.3	98.7	94.1	96.3	97.7	87.1	92.1	94.5	79.5	87.5	91.0			
2001	95.9	97.3	98.6	94.3	96.5	97.8	87.9	92.5	95.0	80.0	87.4	91.6			
2002	96.4	97.6	98.8	94.9	96.7	98.1	88.4	92.7	95.4	81.0	88.0	92.1			
2003	96.7	97.6	99.0	95.4	97.0	98.4	88.5	92.4	95.8	81.2	87.9	92.5			
2004	96.8	97.7	99.0	95.3	96.8	98.4	89.3	92.9	96.1	82.5	88.5	93.2			
2005	96.7	97.6	99.0	95.4	96.9	98.4	89.6	93.2	96.2						
2006	97.3	98.1	99.2	96.2	97.4	98.7	90.9	94.0	96.7						
2007	97.7	98.3	99.3	96.7	97.8	98.8									
2008	97.5	98.2	99.2	96.5	97.7	98.8									
2009	97.7	98.3	99.3												

transplantation. Generally, the recipients remained in excellent health; cardiovascular disease took its toll as time progressed, primarily in the more elderly recipients.

The European Dialysis and Transplantation Association registry has reported 41 renal transplants between monozygotic twins. Glomerulonephritis was the original cause of renal failure in 24 of these patients. Of 41 patients, 36 were alive with functioning grafts 12–174 months after transplantation. Two grafts failed from recurrent disease, two grafts failed from de novo glomerulonephritis, and one recipient died in a traffic accident.[29] One donor developed renal failure secondary to the same glomerulonephritis as in the original recipient. There seems to be a case for using some immunosuppression in identical twin recipients when the original disease is a type of glomerulonephritis with a high recurrence rate (see Chapter 4), but how much and what type of immunosuppression should be used are uncertain. There are no data concerning outcome of renal transplants in monozygotic twins in this situation in the cyclosporine era.

Family Donors

One-year graft survival in the United States is 93% among patients 65 years old and older and 95% among recipients in the 1–5-year-old age group. As with deceased donor recipients, the best 5-year graft survival rates among living donor recipients occur in patients whose ESRD was secondary to polycystic kidney disease, and the worst outcomes are noted in patients with diabetes, hypertension, nephrosclerosis, and vascular disease. These data underscore that the ideal donor is a living donor owing to superior recipient outcomes.

Graft survival was 5% lower in patients with a panel-reactive antibody of 80% or greater. Graft survival in patients requiring dialysis within the first posttransplant week for recipients of living donors was 65% compared with 97% for patients who did not require dialysis. This finding reflects the fact that technical problems with the transplant are usually responsible for the need for dialysis in the first week after a living donor renal transplant and portend a poor outcome.

Paired Kidney Donation and Living Unrelated Donor Outcomes

Outcomes for recipients of paired kidney donation or living unrelated renal transplants are superior to deceased donor renal transplantation and continue to increase in number, with over 550 paired kidney transplants done in the United States in 2010.[98]

KIDNEY-ALONE VERSUS KIDNEY–PANCREAS TRANSPLANTATION FOR DIABETES

OPTN data have documented superior graft survival for simultaneous kidney–pancreas (SPK) recipients with type 1 diabetes mellitus compared with patients receiving a kidney transplant alone (see Chapter 36).[56] Half-life of kidneys in SPK patients was 9.6 years compared with 6.3 years in patients with kidneys alone. These results may be related to selection of more ideal donors for patients receiving SPK. Graft survival for living donor kidneys in type 1 diabetes mellitus was nearly equivalent to SPK transplants in the Wisconsin experience.[100] The International Pancreas Transplant Registry collected data on 18 159 US pancreas transplants performed from 1978 to 2005 with follow-up to 2011. Five-, 10-, and 20-year graft function showed 80%, 68%, and 45%, respectively, for SPK transplants.[36] Recipient selection also may favor the better outcome of SPK patients because stricter criteria (healthier patients) are generally selected for SPK transplantation compared with kidney-alone transplantation. Nevertheless, successful pancreas transplantation may prevent recurrence of diabetic nephropathy. These findings apply to SPK transplants and have not been shown for sequential kidney and pancreas transplants.

CANCER RISK

Cancer risk is discussed at length in Chapters 34 and 35 and is one of the major long-term complications of renal transplantation. US and Australia–New Zealand databases show an increased risk of malignancies after kidney transplantation,[9,93] with the greatest increase in cancers caused by viruses. The risk is highest for non-melanoma skin cancers and posttransplant lymphoproliferative disease, with the latter linked to Epstein–Barr virus infection and induction with antithymocyte globulin/OKT3. In the United States-based Transplant Center Match Study, which was a large, population-based study of solid-organ transplant recipients (n=175 732) during 1987–2008 from SRTR linked with 13 state and regional cancer registries, there was a twofold increased risk of cancer among all solid-organ transplant recipients compared to the general population. The increased risk was observed for 32 different malignancies, including both infection-related and unrelated cancers. Among kidney transplant recipients, the standardized incidence ratio (SIR: observed/expected cases) was significantly higher than expected for non-Hodgkin lymphoma (SIR 6.05; 95% confidence interval (CI) 5.59–6.54), kidney cancer (SIR 6.66; 95% CI 6.12–7.23), lung cancer (SIR 1.46; 95% CI 1.34–1.59).[23] Two antiproliferative agents, sirolimus and mycophenolate mofetil, may be associated with a lower incidence of posttransplant lymphoproliferative disease (Table 39-7), but follow-up of the relevant studies is no longer than 1 year. Robson and colleagues[85a] conducted an observational cohort study of mycophenolate mofetil using data from the OPTN/UNOS and CTS database with a follow-up of 3 years. This study showed no increased risk of posttransplant lymphoproliferative disease in patients receiving mycophenolate mofetil, and suggested that there may be a lower risk in some populations.

PREGNANCY AFTER RENAL TRANSPLANTATION

Among women of childbearing age, ESRD is associated with a 10-fold decrease in fertility rate compared to the general population.[114] A well-functioning renal transplant usually reverses infertility associated with ESRD and permits

TABLE 39-7 **Incidence of Posttransplant Lymphoproliferative Disease from Registration Trials (Phase III) of Commonly Used Immunosuppressive Agents**

Study	Follow-Up (Years)	Antibody Induction	Concurrent Immunosuppression	Arms	Patients (No.)	PTLD (%)
US, Pirsch, 1999	3	ATG/OKT3	Aza/Pred	TAC	205	2.4
				CsA	207	2.9
US, Vincenti, 2002	5	ATG/OKT3	Aza/Pred	TAC	205	3.4
				CsA	207	2.9
MMF						
US, Sollinger, 1995	0.5	ATG	CsA/Pred	Aza	164	0
				MMF 2 g	165	0.6
				MMF 3 g	166	1.2
Tricontinental,* 1998	3	NA	CsA/Pred	Aza	162	0.6
				MMF 2 g	171	1.2
				MMF 3 g	164	1.8
SRL						
US, Kahan, 2000	1	None	CsA/Pred	Aza	159	0.6
				SRL 2 mg	281	0.4
				SRL 5 mg	269	0.7
Europe,* Groth, 1999†	1	None	Aza/Pred	CsA	41	0
				SRL	42	0
Europe,* Kreis, 2000†	1	None	MMF/Pred	CsA	38	0
				SRL	40	0
Bas						
Nashan, 1997	1	None	CsA/Pred	Bas	193	0.5
				PBO	187	0.5
Bela						
Vincenti, 2005	3	Simulect	MMF	Bela MI	219	0.5
				Bela LI	226	0.4
				Cyclosporine	221	0

ATG, antithymocyte globulin; Aza, azathioprine; Bas, basiliximab; Bela LI, belatacept less intensive; Bela MI, belatacept more intensive; CsA, cyclosporine; MMF, mycophenolate mofetil; NA, not available; OKT3, muromonab-CD3 antilymphocyte antibody preparations; PBO, placebo; Pred, prednisone; PTLD, posttransplant lymphoproliferative disease; SRL, sirolimus; TAC, tacrolimus.
*North America, Europe, and Australia.
†Phase II studies.

reproductive function to recover.[14] The most important prognostic factor for a good outcome to pregnancy in renal transplant patients is good renal function and absent or well-managed hypertension.[99,105] As in women with normal native kidneys, during pregnancy, glomerular filtration rate may increase even in transplant recipients with a single kidney.[13]

Data from combined US, continental European, and UK transplant registries on pregnancies in kidney transplant recipients (Figure 39-17) show a marked increase over 15 years in pregnancies, including pregnancies beyond the first trimester.[57] The combined databases report more than 2000 live births to women with organ transplants (of all types) as of 2006. In a systematic review and meta-analysis including 50 studies from 25 countries of 4706 pregnancies among 3570 kidney transplant recipients, overall birth rate was higher than the general population (73.5% versus 66.7%) and miscarriage rate was lower (14.0% versus 17.1%). In aggregate, a total of 4.2% of patients experienced an acute rejection episode and 5.3% experienced graft loss at 1 year posttransplant, and results were similar across countries. However, the incidence of pregnancy complications, including preeclampsia (27.0%), gestational diabetes (8.0%), cesarean section (56.9%), and preterm delivery (45.6%), were higher than in the general US population. Risks for complications were lower among those with lower mean maternal ages, and shorter time interval (<2 years) between transplantation and pregnancy.[15] A consensus conference in 2003 advised that conception is safe after the first posttransplant year if the graft is functioning well and no rejection episodes have occurred in the year before conception.[58] Pregnancies after transplantation should be handled as high-risk, however, with close prenatal monitoring. Cesarean delivery is indicated only for obstetrical reasons.[14] Because calcineurin inhibitors have significantly improved graft survival, it is most attractive to continue calcineurin inhibitor therapy during pregnancy, albeit with close monitoring of drug levels and renal function.[60] Few data exist on the impact of immunosuppressive drug therapy on the fetus and newborn. Despite reduction of T- and B-cell counts in newborns, these counts have been reported to normalize within a few months, and there is no reported increase in incidence of infection or autoimmune disease in these children.[18,104] The long-term consequences of in utero exposure to immunosuppression are unknown.[2,7,30,72] Of 48 children of recipients of solid-organ transplants followed for a mean of 5.2 years, no structural or developmental abnormalities were noted, despite a premature birth rate of 56%.[118]

RENAL TRANSPLANTATION IN HUMAN IMMUNODEFICIENCY VIRUS-POSITIVE PATIENTS

Human immunodeficiency virus (HIV) seropositivity is no longer considered a contraindication to renal transplantation at some centers, based on encouraging

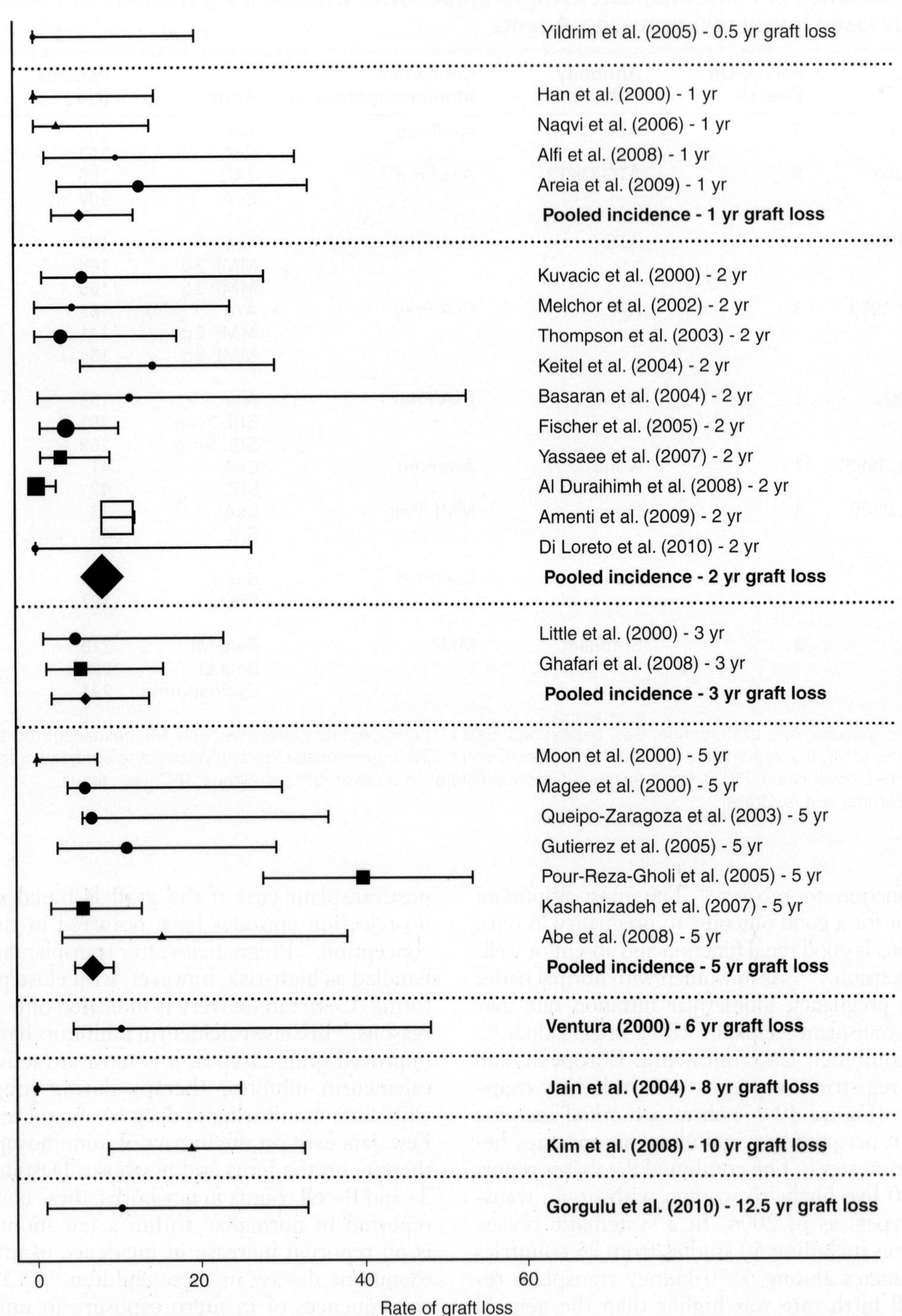

Figure 39-17 ■ **Postpregnancy graft loss among kidney transplant recipients.** (Reprinted from Deshpande NA, James NT, Kucirka LM, et al. Pregnancy outcomes in kidney transplant recipients: a systematic review and meta-analysis. Am J Transplant 2011;11:2388–404.)

results in a number of patients transplanted to date. In the era of highly active antiretroviral therapy, patients have markedly extended survival, and graft survival rates comparable to the rates of HIV-negative patients have been reported (Table 39-8).[77,87,101] Patients treated with protease inhibitors require far less calcineurin inhibitor therapy to achieve target blood levels, as reported by Stock and colleagues.[102] Despite low CD4 counts, HIV-positive recipients may be prone to acute rejection and particularly antibody-mediated rejection.[86] Nevertheless, few opportunistic infections were reported. Among a larger, more recent cohort of 150 HIV-infected kidney transplant recipients, patient survival at 1 and 3 years was 94.6±2.0% and 88.2%±3.8%, respectively.

Inclusion criteria for HIV-positive patients being considered for renal transplantation have included: (1) a CD4 count greater than 200 cells/mL for the previous 6 months; (2) undetectable HIV RNA for 3–6 months;

TABLE 39-8 **Rates of Patient Survival and Graft Survival at 1 and 3 Years among HIV-Infected Kidney Transplant Recipients and Patients in the Scientific Registry of Transplant Recipients (SRTR) Database**

	Patient Survival		***Graft Survival***	
Population	**1 Year % (95% CI)**	**3 Years % (95% CI)**	**1 Year % (95% CI)**	**3 Years % (95% CI)**
Study patients	94.6 (88.9–97.4)	99.2 (78.3–93.8)	90.4 (83.9–94.3)	73.7 (61.9–82.4)
SRTR Comparison				
Age≥65 years	91.8 (91.1–92.4)	79.5 (78.0–80.9)	88.3 (87.5–89.1)	74.4 (72.9–75.9)
Overall	96.2 (96.0–96.4)	90.6 (90.2–91.0)	92.5 (92.3–92.8)	82.8 (82.3–83.3)

CI, confidence interval; HIV, human immunodeficiency virus.
Data from Stock PG, Barin B, Murphy B, et al. Outcomes of kidney transplantation in HIV-infected recipients. N Engl J Med 2010; 362:2004–14.

(3) no prior opportunistic infections or neoplasm except for drug-sensitive esophageal conditions; (4) antiretroviral therapy stable for at least 3 months or off therapy and able to maintain undetectable HIV RNA; and (5) no signs of significant wasting. Although the published experience is small, good outcomes have been achieved in such patients undergoing renal transplantation.

PREVALENCE OF PEOPLE LIVING WITH A FUNCTIONING KIDNEY TRANSPLANT

The number of people in the United States living with a functioning kidney transplant doubled between 1995 and 2004. At the end of 1995 there were 50 529 people with a functioning kidney transplant and 3156 people living with a functioning kidney–pancreas transplant. By the beginning of 2005, there were 101 440 people with a functioning kidney transplant and 7213 people with a functioning kidney–pancreas transplant. Based on 2004 data from the USRDS, kidney and kidney–pancreas recipients living with a functioning kidney transplant represented 18% of all end-stage renal failure patients in 1995 and 21% of all end-stage renal failure patients in 2002.[109]

The longest surviving recipients of a kidney transplant with a functioning graft are 9 patients with more than 40 years' graft survival from the University of Colorado, Denver. More than 100 patients have been reported with greater than 25 years' graft survival.[9] At least 8 patients with living donor kidney transplants have experienced greater than 20 years' graft survival without continuing immunosuppression long term.[9] In other words, such patients have clinically shown immunological tolerance for a prolonged period.

LONG-TERM OUTCOMES OF RENAL TRANSPLANTATION

Kidney allograft survival has increased substantially over the last several decades, with 92.0% 1-year survival for patients transplanted with deceased donors and 96.5% for patients transplanted with living donors in 2008. Meier-Kriesche and colleagues recently reported that the improvements in overall graft survival are primarily attributed to improvements in short-term graft survival. The graft half-life for deceased donor transplants increased from 6.6 years in 1989 to 8 years in 1995, and 8.8 years in 2005. Among living donor recipients, graft half-life was nearly unchanged from 11.4 years to 11.9 years from 1989 to 2005, respectively.[50] The CTS European data (see Figure 39-16) is compatible, with similar 5-year graft survival reported from 2000–2004 to 2005–2010.

Nevertheless, the availability of more potent immunosuppression over the last 10 years is not yet reflected in improved long-term outcomes. There continues to be a dire need for therapy and diagnostics that translate into better long-term success. This goal depends on: (1) better ways to improve patient survival, perhaps through better cardiovascular health management and reduced risk of malignancy; (2) immunosuppressive strategies that better preserve renal function and reduce chronic rejection; and (3) better monitoring and early diagnosis of renal transplant dysfunction.

QUALITY OF LIFE

Although, traditionally, outcomes have been measured in terms of graft and patient survival because the goal of kidney transplantation is to restore normal kidney function and prolong life, measurements of the quality of life after renal transplantation focus in more detail on the impact of a successful kidney transplant on parameters such as physical function, physical pain, general health, vitality, social functioning, and mental health. Because the immunosuppression associated with renal transplantation has an extensive list of associated side effects, how these affect overall quality of life can be measured.

Neipp and colleagues[65] reported on the quality of life in adult renal transplant recipients more than 15 years after transplantation. This single-center study of 139 patients found that 29% were employed, 7% were seeking employment, 58% were retired, and 5% were homemakers. Using a 36-item health survey, a validated quality-of-life survey, and a kidney transplant questionnaire, the authors reported on eight aspects of the health of these patients. In contrast to retired and unemployed patients, employed recipients reported a significantly improved health-related quality of life, including physical functioning, physical pain, general health, vitality, social functioning, mental health, physical symptoms, fatigue, uncertainty and fear, and emotional health. All of these parameters

TABLE 39-9 **Prevalence of Sexual Problems in Renal Replacement Therapy Patients Compared with a Control Group**

	Prevalence in Treatment Group	
	Men (%)	Women (%)
Control	8.7	14.9
Hemodialysis	62.9	75
Peritoneal dialysis	69.8	66.7
Kidney transplant	48.3	44.4

From Habwe VQ. Posttransplantation quality of life: more than graft function. Am J Kidney Dis 2006;47:S98. Data from Diemont WL, Vruggink PA, Meuleman EJ, et al. Sexual dysfunction after renal replacement therapy. Am J Kidney Dis 2000;35:845.

were improved in employed recipients compared with their counterparts ($P<0.05$). The authors concluded that vocational rehabilitation after renal transplantation is crucial and is associated best with improved healthcare quality of life. In a 6-year study of 102 kidney transplant recipients, Griva et al. reported that, while emotional quality of life improves over time, physical quality of life, such as pain and physical functioning, declines.[35]

Studies have shown that immunosuppression-related side effects can compromise quality of life. These side effects include hirsutism, gingival hyperplasia, weight gain, cushingoid facies, hand tremors, alopecia, and skin disorders.[37] A cross-sectional study of 350 kidney transplant patients by Moons and associates[62a] showed that steroid-free patients experienced better social functioning, fewer psychiatric symptoms, lower symptom occurrences, and lower levels of distress ($P<0.03$) for all of the aforementioned side effects.

A Dutch study of sexual dysfunction in kidney transplant recipients compared with dialysis patients and control subjects from the general Dutch population showed significantly less sexual dysfunction in men and women with a successful kidney transplant compared with either hemodialysis or peritoneal dialysis, yet substantially more difficulties compared with control subjects ($P<0.001$) (Table 39-9).[17,37] Strategies for improving quality of life include effective management of drug side effects, improved immunosuppressive regimens, psychotherapy, social support, exercise, and vocational assistance.

CONCLUSION

The abundance of data surrounding organ transplantation with registry data available now from each continent of the world provides a rich source of data from which to analyze clinical practices and outcomes. Transplantation is perhaps the most closely scrutinized medical specialty, and the field has benefited from careful attention to quality assessment, outcomes analysis, and standardization of protocols required by governmental and other regulatory agencies. More detailed analysis of data is now forthcoming that probes issues such as access to transplantation, influence of socioeconomic status and minority race, center influence, and infection rates. Such scrutiny will continue to drive further innovation and improvements in outcomes.

Dialysis and transplantation are costly treatments, and every country, faced with rapidly increasing medical costs, has reflected on the cost-effectiveness of expensive therapies. Inevitably, the spotlight falls on dialysis and transplantation: Is this cost justified? Unquestionably, the treatments are expensive, and costs vary from nation to nation. Assuming that one considers treatment of patients with end-stage renal failure justified, transplantation is the cheaper option available. In developing countries, renal transplantation is almost the only available option because often long-term dialysis is unavailable. Of patients with the potential for full-time work, most are restored to full-time work after living donor and deceased donor transplantations. In such situations, a productive member of society is re-established, with the consequent saving in pensions or benefits to surviving family members. The demonstration that survival is enhanced by transplantation compared with dialysis in nearly all patient groups, as discussed earlier, provides more objective evidence of the key role that transplantation should play in the management of end-stage renal failure.

The justification for the treatment of end-stage renal failure by an integrated program of dialysis and transplantation seems self-evident. The primary aim is to achieve a successful transplant, using dialysis to maintain patients while awaiting a transplant, or to treat patients who are unsuitable for transplant for medical or immunological reasons. Because a large proportion of patients with end-stage renal failure who are suitable for transplantation are relatively young, achievement of a successful renal transplant in these patients is one of the more satisfying areas of medical practice today. No-one would have predicted at the time of the first successful renal transplant in 1954 that so much would have been achieved over the next 60 years.[63]

REFERENCES

1. Alexander JW, Goodman HR, Gersin K, et al. Gastric bypass in morbidly obese patients with chronic renal failure and kidney transplant. Transplantation 2004;78(3):469–74.
2. Arsan A, Guest G, Gagnadoux MF, et al. Pregnancy in renal transplantation: a pediatric unit report. Transplant Proc 1997;29(5):2479.
3. Arthur T. The role of social networks: a novel hypothesis to explain the phenomenon of racial disparity in kidney transplantation. Am J Kidney Dis 2002;40(4):678–81.
4. Ashby VB, Port FK, Wolfe RA, et al. Transplanting kidneys without points for HLA-B matching: consequences of the policy change. Am J Transplant 2011;11(8):1712–8.
5. Ayanian JZ, Cleary PD, Keogh JH, et al. Physicians' beliefs about racial differences in referral for renal transplantation. Am J Kidney Dis 2004;43(2):350–7.
6. Ayanian JZ, Cleary PD, Weissman JS, et al. The effect of patients' preferences on racial differences in access to renal transplantation. N Engl J Med 1999;341(22):1661–9.
7. Bar J, Wittenberg C, Hod M, et al. Pregnancy outcome in renal allograft recipients in Israel. Isr J Med Sci 1996;32(12):1183–5.
8. Butler JA, Roderick P, Mullee M, et al. Frequency and impact of nonadherence to immunosuppressants after renal transplantation: a systematic review. Transplantation 2004;77(5):769–76.
9. Cecka JM. The OPTN/UNOS renal transplant registry. Clin Transpl 2005;1–16.
10. Cooper JT, Chin LT, Krieger NR, et al. Donation after cardiac death: the University of Wisconsin experience with renal transplantation. Am J Transplant 2004;4(9):1490–4.
11. Cuende N, Cuende JI, Fajardo J, et al. Effect of population aging on the international organ donation rates and the effectiveness of the donation process. Am J Transplant 2007;7(6):1526–35.

12. D'Alessandro AM, Fernandez LA, Chin LT, et al. Donation after cardiac death: the University of Wisconsin experience. Ann Transplant 2004;9(1):68–71.
13. Davison JM. The effect of pregnancy on kidney function in renal allograft recipients. Kidney Int 1985;27(1):74–9.
14. Davison JM, Bailey DJ. Pregnancy following renal transplantation. J Obstet Gynaecol Res 2003;29(4):227–33.
15. Deshpande NA, James NT, Kucirka LM, et al. Pregnancy outcomes in kidney transplant recipients: a systematic review and meta-analysis. Am J Transplant 2011;11(11):2388–404.
16. Dew MA, DiMartini AF, De Vito Dabbs A, et al. Rates and risk factors for nonadherence to the medical regimen after adult solid organ transplantation. Transplantation 2007;83(7):858–73.
17. Diemont WL, Vruggink PA, Meuleman EJ, et al. Sexual dysfunction after renal replacement therapy. Am J Kidney Dis 2000;35(5):845–51.
18. Di Paolo S, Schena A, Morrone LF, et al. Immunologic evaluation during the first year of life of infants born to cyclosporine-treated female kidney transplant recipients: analysis of lymphocyte subpopulations and immunoglobulin serum levels. Transplantation 2000;69(10):2049–54.
19. Dobbels F, Van Damme-Lombaert R, Vanhaecke J, et al. Growing pains: non-adherence with the immunosuppressive regimen in adolescent transplant recipients. Pediatr Transplant 2005;9(3):381–90.
20. Doshi MD, Hunsicker LG. Short- and long-term outcomes with the use of kidneys and livers donated after cardiac death. Am J Transplant 2007;7(1):122–9.
21. Eckhoff DE, Young CJ, Gaston RS, et al. Racial disparities in renal allograft survival: a public health issue? J Am Coll Surg 2007;204(5):894–902, discussion 902–893.
22. Edwards EB, Bennett LE, Cecka JM. Effect of HLA matching on the relative risk of mortality for kidney recipients: a comparison of the mortality risk after transplant to the mortality risk of remaining on the waiting list. Transplantation 1997;64(9):1274–7.
23. Engels EA, Pfeiffer RM, Fraumeni Jr. JF, et al. Spectrum of cancer risk among US solid organ transplant recipients. JAMA 2011;306(17):1891–901.
24. Evans RW, Applegate WH, Briscoe DM, et al. Cost-related immunosuppressive medication nonadherence among kidney transplant recipients. Clin J Am Soc Nephrol 2010;5(12):2323–8.
25. Evans RW, Manninen DL, Garrison Jr. LP, et al. The quality of life of patients with end-stage renal disease. N Engl J Med 1985;312(9):553–9.
26. Fine RN, Becker Y, De Geest S, et al. Nonadherence consensus conference summary report. Am J Transplant 2009;9(1):35–41.
27. Flegal KM, Carroll MD, Ogden CL, et al. Prevalence and trends in obesity among US adults, 1999–2008. JAMA 2010;303(3):235–41.
28. Fort J. Chronic renal failure: a cardiovascular risk factor. Kidney Int Suppl 2005;(99)S25–9.
29. Friedman AN, Miskulin DC, Rosenberg IH, et al. Demographics and trends in overweight and obesity in patients at time of kidney transplantation. Am J Kidney Dis 2003;41(2):480–7.
30. Ghahramani N, Attaipour Y, Ghods AJ. Chromosomal aberrations among offspring of female renal transplant recipients. Transplant Proc 1993;25(3):2190.
31. Gjertson DW. Explainable variation in renal transplant outcomes: a comparison of standard and expanded criteria donors. Clin Transpl 2004;303–14.
32. Gore JL, Pham PT, Danovitch GM, et al. Obesity and outcome following renal transplantation. Am J Transplant 2006;6(2):357–63.
33. Grams ME, Massie AB, Coresh J, et al. Trends in the timing of pre-emptive kidney transplantation. J Am Soc Nephrol 2011;22(9):1615–20.
34. Gris JC, Branger B, Vecina F, et al. Increased cardiovascular risk factors and features of endothelial activation and dysfunction in dialyzed uremic patients. Kidney Int 1994;46(3):807–13.
35. Griva K, Stygall J, Ng JH, et al. Prospective changes in health-related quality of life and emotional outcomes in kidney transplantation over 6 years. J Transplant 2011;2011:671571.
36. Gruessner AC, Sutherland DE, Gruessner RW. Long-term outcome after pancreas transplantation. Curr Opin Organ Transplant 2012;17(1):100–5.
37. Habwe VQ. Posttransplantation quality of life: more than graft function. Am J Kidney Dis 2006;47(4 Suppl. 2):S98–110.
38. Hall EC, Massie AB, James NT, et al. Effect of eliminating priority points for HLA-B matching on racial disparities in kidney transplant rates. Am J Kidney Dis 2011;58(5):813–6.
39. Deleted in proof.
40. Hedley AA, Ogden CL, Johnson CL, et al. Prevalence of overweight and obesity among US children, adolescents, and adults, 1999–2002. JAMA 2004;291(23):2847–50.
41. Huysmans K, Lins RL, Daelemans R, et al. Hypertension and accelerated atherosclerosis in endstage renal disease. J Nephrol 1998;11(4):185–95.
42. Jassal SV, Opelz G, Cole E. Transplantation in the elderly: a review. Geriatr Nephrol Urol 1997;7(3):157–65.
43. Jindal RM, Zawada Jr ET. Obesity and kidney transplantation. Am J Kidney Dis 2004;43(6):943–52.
44. Kayler LK, Magliocca J, Zendejas I, et al. Impact of cold ischemia time on graft survival among ECD transplant recipients: a paired kidney analysis. Am J Transplant 2011;11(12):2647–56.
45. Kerman RH, Kimball PM, Van Buren CT, et al. Possible contribution of pretransplant immune responder status to renal allograft survival differences of black versus white recipients. Transplantation 1991;51(2):338–42.
46. Kootstra G, Kievit JK, Heineman E. The non heart-beating donor. Br Med Bull 1997;53(4):844–53.
47. Kootstra G, van Heurn E. Non-heartbeating donation of kidneys for transplantation. Nat Clin Pract Nephrol 2007;3(3):154–63.
48. Koyama H, Cecka JM, Terasaki PI. Kidney transplants in black recipients. HLA matching and other factors affecting long-term graft survival. Transplantation 1994;57(7):1064–8.
49. Krakauer H, Grauman JS, McMullan MR, et al. The recent U.S. experience in the treatment of end-stage renal disease by dialysis and transplantation. N Engl J Med 1983;308(26):1558–63.
50. Lamb KE, Lodhi S, Meier-Kriesche HU. Long-term renal allograft survival in the United States: a critical reappraisal. Am J Transplant 2011;11(3):450–62.
51. Laupacis A, Keown P, Pus N, et al. A study of the quality of life and cost-utility of renal transplantation. Kidney Int 1996;50(1):235–42.
52. Locke JE, Segev DL, Warren DS, et al. Outcomes of kidneys from donors after cardiac death: implications for allocation and preservation. Am J Transplant 2007;7(7):1797–807.
53. London GM, Drueke TB. Atherosclerosis and arteriosclerosis in chronic renal failure. Kidney Int 1997;51(6):1678–95.
54. Lowrie EG. Acute-phase inflammatory process contributes to malnutrition, anemia, and possibly other abnormalities in dialysis patients. Am J Kidney Dis 1998;32(6 Suppl. 4):S105–12.
55. Lunsford SL, Simpson KS, Chavin KD, et al. Racial differences in coping with the need for kidney transplantation and willingness to ask for live organ donation. Am J Kidney Dis 2006;47(2):324–31.
56. Marroquin CE, Edwards EB, Collins BH, et al. Half-life analysis of pancreas and kidney transplants. Transplantation 2005;80(2):272–5.
57. McKay DB, Josephson MA. Pregnancy in recipients of solid organs – effects on mother and child. N Engl J Med 2006;354(12):1281–93.
58. McKay DB, Josephson MA, Armenti VT, et al. Reproduction and transplantation: report on the AST consensus conference on reproductive issues and transplantation. Am J Transplant 2005;5(7):1592–9.
59. Meier-Kriesche HU, Arndorfer JA, Kaplan B. The impact of body mass index on renal transplant outcomes: a significant independent risk factor for graft failure and patient death. Transplantation 2002;73(1):70–4.
60. Meier-Kriesche HU, Kaplan B. Waiting time on dialysis as the strongest modifiable risk factor for renal transplant outcomes: a paired donor kidney analysis. Transplantation 2002;74(10):1377–81.
61. Meier-Kriesche HU, Schold JD, Kaplan B. Long-term renal allograft survival: have we made significant progress or is it time to rethink our analytic and therapeutic strategies? Am J Transplant 2004;4(8):1289–95.
62. Molnar MZ, Kovesdy CP, Mucsi I, et al. Higher recipient body mass index is associated with post-transplant delayed kidney graft function. Kidney Int 2011;80(2):218–24.
62a. Moons P, Vanrenterghem Y, Van Hooff JP, et al. Steroids may compromise quality of life of renal transplant recipients on a tacrolimus-based regimen. Transplant Proc 2002;34:1691.
63. Morris PJ. Transplantation – a medical miracle of the 20th century. N Engl J Med 2004;351(26):2678–80.

64. Morris PJ, Johnson RJ, Fuggle SV, et al. Analysis of factors that affect outcome of primary cadaveric renal transplantation in the UK. HLA Task Force of the Kidney Advisory Group of the United Kingdom Transplant Support Service Authority (UKTSSA). Lancet 1999;354(9185):1147–52.
65. Neipp M, Karavul B, Jackobs S, et al. Quality of life in adult transplant recipients more than 15 years after kidney transplantation. Transplantation 2006;81(12):1640–4.
66. Noppakun K, Cosio FG, Dean PG, et al. Living donor age and kidney transplant outcomes. Am J Transplant 2011;11(6):1279–86.
67. Nyberg G, Nilsson B, Norden G, et al. Outcome of renal transplantation in patients over the age of 60: a case-control study. Nephrol Dial Transplant 1995;10(1):91–4.
68. Ojo A, Wolfe RA, Agodoa LY, et al. Prognosis after primary renal transplant failure and the beneficial effects of repeat transplantation: multivariate analyses from the United States Renal Data System. Transplantation 1998;66(12):1651–9.
69. Opelz G, Dohler B. Multicenter analysis of kidney preservation. Transplantation 2007;83(3):247–53.
70. Organ Procurement and Transplantation Network. Policies. 2011. Available online at: http://optn.transplant.hrsa.gov/PoliciesandBylaws2/policies/pdfs/policy_7.pdf [accessed 29.11.11].
71. Ost L, Groth CG, Lindholm B, et al. Cadaveric renal transplantation in patients of 60 years and above. Transplantation 1980;30(5):339–40.
72. Pahl MV, Vaziri ND, Kaufman DJ, et al. Childbirth after renal transplantation. Transplant Proc 1993;25(4):2727–31.
73. Pallet N, Thervet E, Alberti C, et al. Kidney transplant in black recipients: are African Europeans different from African Americans? Am J Transplant 2005;5(11):2682–7.
74. Pascual M, Theruvath T, Kawai T, et al. Strategies to improve long-term outcomes after renal transplantation. N Engl J Med 2002;346(8):580–90.
75. Patzer RE, Amaral S, Wasse H, et al. Neighborhood poverty and racial disparities in kidney transplant waitlisting. J Am Soc Nephrol 2009;20(6):1333–40.
76. Patzer RE, Perryman JP, Schrager JD, et al. The role of race and poverty on steps to kidney transplantation in the southeastern United States. Am J Transplant 2012;12(2):358–68.
77. Pelletier SJ, Norman SP, Christensen LL, et al. Review of transplantation in HIV patients during the HAART era. Clin Transpl 2004;63–82.
78. Pirsch JD, Armbrust MJ, Knechtle SJ, et al. Obesity as a risk factor following renal transplantation. Transplantation 1995;59(4):631–3.
79. Port FK, Wolfe RA, Mauger EA, et al. Comparison of survival probabilities for dialysis patients vs cadaveric renal transplant recipients. JAMA 1993;270(11):1339–43.
80. Press R, Carrasquillo O, Nickolas T, et al. Race/ethnicity, poverty status, and renal transplant outcomes. Transplantation 2005;80(7):917–24.
81. Rao PS, Merion RM, Ashby VB, et al. Renal transplantation in elderly patients older than 70 years of age: results from the Scientific Registry of Transplant Recipients. Transplantation 2007;83(8):1069–74.
82. Reeves-Daniel AM, DePalma JA, Bleyer AJ, et al. The APOL1 gene and allograft survival after kidney transplantation. Am J Transplant 2011;11(5):1025–30.
83. Rianthavorn P, Ettenger RB. Medication non-adherence in the adolescent renal transplant recipient: a clinician's viewpoint. Pediatr Transplant 2005;9(3):398–407.
84. Rithalia A, McDaid C, Suekarran S, et al. Impact of presumed consent for organ donation on donation rates: a systematic review. BMJ 2009;338:a3162.
85. Roake JA, Cahill AP, Gray CM, et al. Preemptive cadaveric renal transplantation – clinical outcome. Transplantation 1996;62(10):1411–6.
85a. Robson R, Cecka JM, Opelz G, et al. Prospective registry-based observational cohort study of the long-term risk of malignancies in renal transplant patients treated with mycophenolate mofetil. Am J Transplant 2005;5:2954.
86. Roland M, Carlson L, Stock P. Solid organ transplantation in HIV-infected individuals. AIDS Clin Care 2002;14(7):59–63.
87. Roodnat JI, Zietse R, Mulder PG, et al. The vanishing importance of age in renal transplantation. Transplantation 1999;67(4):576–80.
88. Rudich SM, Kaplan B, Magee JC, et al. Renal transplantations performed using non-heart-beating organ donors: going back to the future? Transplantation 2002;74(12):1715–20.
89. Russell JD, Beecroft ML, Ludwin D, et al. The quality of life in renal transplantation – a prospective study. Transplantation 1992;54(4):656–60.
90. Santiago Delpin EA, Gonzalez Z, Morales-Otero LA, et al. Transplantation in Hispanics: the Puerto Rico experience. Transplant Proc 1989;21(6):3958–60.
91. Saunders MR, Cagney KA, Ross LF, et al. Neighborhood poverty, racial composition and renal transplant waitlist. Am J Transplant 2010;10(8):1912–7.
92. Schafer-Keller P, Steiger J, Bock A, et al. Diagnostic accuracy of measurement methods to assess non-adherence to immunosuppressive drugs in kidney transplant recipients. Am J Transplant 2008;8(3):616–26.
93. Schaubel D, Desmeules M, Mao Y, et al. Survival experience among elderly end-stage renal disease patients. A controlled comparison of transplantation and dialysis. Transplantation 1995;60(12):1389–94.
94. Schnuelle P, Lorenz D, Trede M, et al. Impact of renal cadaveric transplantation on survival in end-stage renal failure: evidence for reduced mortality risk compared with hemodialysis during long-term follow-up. J Am Soc Nephrol 1998;9(11):2135–41.
95. Schulak JA, Mayes JT, Johnston KH, et al. Kidney transplantation in patients aged sixty years and older. Surgery 1990;108(4):726–31, discussion 731–723.
96. Schweizer RT, Rovelli M, Palmeri D, et al. Noncompliance in organ transplant recipients. Transplantation 1990;49(2):374–7.
97. Scientific Registry of Transplant Recipients. OPTN / SRTR 2010 annual data report. Rockville, MD: Department of Health and Human Services, Health Resources and Services Administration, Healthcare Systems Bureau, Division of Transplantation; 2011.
98. Segev DL. Innovative strategies in living donor kidney transplantation. Nat Rev Nephrol 2012;.
99. Sibanda N, Briggs JD, Davison JM, et al. Pregnancy after organ transplantation: a report from the UK Transplant pregnancy registry. Transplantation 2007;83(10):1301–7.
100. Stegall MD, Ploeg RJ, Pirsch JD, et al. Living-related kidney transplant or simultaneous pancreas-kidney for diabetic renal failure? Transplant Proc 1993;25(1 Pt 1):230–2.
101. Stock PG, Barin B, Murphy B, et al. Outcomes of kidney transplantation in HIV-infected recipients. N Engl J Med 2010;363(21):2004–14.
102. Stock PG, Roland ME, Carlson L, et al. Kidney and liver transplantation in human immunodeficiency virus-infected patients: a pilot safety and efficacy study. Transplantation 2003;76(2):370–5.
103. Su X, Zenios SA, Chakkera H, et al. Diminishing significance of HLA matching in kidney transplantation. Am J Transplant 2004;4(9):1501–8.
104. Takahashi N, Nishida H, Hoshi J. Severe B cell depletion in newborns from renal transplant mothers taking immunosuppressive agents. Transplantation 1994;57(11):1617–21.
105. Thompson BC, Kingdon EJ, Tuck SM, et al. Pregnancy in renal transplant recipients: the Royal Free Hospital experience. QJM 2003;96(11):837–44.
106. Tilney NL. Renal transplantation between identical twins: a review. World J Surg 1986;10(3):381–8.
107. Tilney NL, Hager EB, Boyden CM, et al. Treatment of chronic renal failure by transplantation and dialysis: two decades of cooperation. Ann Surg 1975;182(2):108–15.
108. Tonelli M, Wiebe N, Knoll G, et al. Systematic review: kidney transplantation compared with dialysis in clinically relevant outcomes. Am J Transplant 2011;11(10):2093–109.
109. US Renal Data System. USRDS 2011 annual data report: atlas of chronic kidney disease and end-stage renal disease in the United States. Bethesda, MD: National Institutes of Health, National Institute of Diabetes and Digestive and Kidney Diseases; 2011.
110. Vaziri ND, Gonzales EC, Wang J, et al. Blood coagulation, fibrinolytic, and inhibitory proteins in end-stage renal disease: effect of hemodialysis. Am J Kidney Dis 1994;23(6):828–35.
111. Vital signs: state-specific obesity prevalence among adults – United States, 2009. MMWR Morb Mortal Wkly Rep 2010;59(30):951–5.
112. Vollmer WM, Wahl PW, Blagg CR. Survival with dialysis and transplantation in patients with end-stage renal disease. N Engl J Med 1983;308(26):1553–8.

113. Wanner C, Zimmermann J, Quaschning T, et al. Inflammation, dyslipidemia and vascular risk factors in hemodialysis patients. Kidney Int Suppl 1997;62:S53–5.
114. Watnick S, Rueda J. Reproduction and contraception after kidney transplantation. Curr Opin Obstet Gynecol 2008;20(3):308–12.
115. Watson CJ, Johnson RJ, Birch R, et al. A simplified donor risk index for predicting outcome after deceased donor kidney transplantation. Transplantation 2012;93(3):314–8.
116. Weng FL, Joffe MM, Feldman HI, et al. Rates of completion of the medical evaluation for renal transplantation. Am J Kidney Dis 2005;46(4):734–45.
117. Wheeler DC. Cardiovascular disease in patients with chronic renal failure. Lancet 1996;348(9043):1673–4.
118. Willis FR, Findlay CA, Gorrie MJ, et al. Children of renal transplant recipient mothers. J Paediatr Child Health 2000;36(3):230–5.
119. Wolfe RA, Ashby VB, Milford EL, et al. Comparison of mortality in all patients on dialysis, patients on dialysis awaiting transplantation, and recipients of a first cadaveric transplant. N Engl J Med 1999;341(23):1725–30.
120. Zimmermann J, Herrlinger S, Pruy A, et al. Inflammation enhances cardiovascular risk and mortality in hemodialysis patients. Kidney Int 1999;55(2):648–58.

CHAPTER 40

PSYCHOLOGICAL ASPECTS OF KIDNEY TRANSPLANTATION AND ORGAN DONATION

Patricia M. Franklin

CHAPTER OUTLINE

INTRODUCTION

End-stage renal disease is a psychologically debilitating illness with emotional morbidity. End-stage renal disease can have a major impact on patient and family lifestyles, blocking future life goals and resulting in a cycle of anger, mood swings, depression, and unfulfilled hopes. All forms of renal replacement therapy have been studied to elicit the psychological impacts of treatments and the particular stressors encountered by patients and their caregivers. These studies show that the treatment of renal failure through dialysis or transplantation creates stress and psychological difficulties for patients. The negative themes reported from study groups include loss of freedom, loss of personal control, loss of independence, blocking of hope and future dreams, and loss of normality.[24,33]

Kidney transplantation is the treatment of choice for patients with end-stage renal disease. Studies have shown that renal transplant recipients are surviving longer and have a better quality of life than patients receiving other renal replacement therapies.[37] A successful renal transplant does not render the patient free of the chronic illness or subsequent psychological problems, however. The transplant enables recipients to enjoy an improved quality of life with freedom from a machine or a dialysis exchange, but it often presents a different set of psychological stressors and challenges to overcome. Understanding of the psychological aspects of transplantation has increased in recent years, and this increased understanding has resulted in the opportunity to offer informed psychological support as an integral part of transplantation care. This chapter discusses the major psychological studies and their findings and provides brief personal experiences reported by patients to the author during 35 years of experience as a nurse psychologist working in transplant centers.

QUALITY OF LIFE AND PSYCHOLOGICAL WELLBEING FOR RENAL TRANSPLANT PATIENTS

Individual quality of life is difficult to assess because it is affected by a wide range of independent and personal variables. A large study by Evans and colleagues in the 1980s,[15] which comprised 800 patients in all treatment modalities in 11 treatment centers, concluded that "Transplant recipients generally have a higher level of functional ability, are more likely to return to work, are in better health, and have higher levels of well being, life satisfaction, psychological affect, and happiness than do patients on any form of dialysis."[14] Since this study was reported, there have been major advances in dialysis treatments, particularly in home hemodialysis, and in renal transplant immunosuppression regimens. There also have been advances in scientific techniques to evaluate issues of life satisfaction and quality of life.

However, the more recent studies incorporating these new treatments and research techniques continue to support the earlier studies. A meta-analytical review by Landreneau and colleagues undertaken in 2010[29] concluded that: "Compared to haemodialysis, renal transplantation was significantly more effective in improving quality of life in the three domains of general quality of life, physical functioning, and psychosocial functioning." Also, studies by Maglakelidze et al.,[38] which investigated quality of life of patients on hemodialysis, peritoneal dialysis and those with renal transplants concluded that "for patients on hemodialysis and peritoneal dialysis health related quality of life was similar and lower than that of the general population whereas renal transplantation significantly improves health-related quality of life to the level of healthy individuals."[38] Renal transplantation has also been shown to improve the quality of life significantly for the patients' partners.[42,50]

Although quality of life is improved dramatically in various aspects of life satisfaction after transplantation, even life with the best-functioning transplanted kidney can be negatively affected by perpetual uncertainty with the possibility of rejection and failure. Also, continuous immunosuppressive therapy can create psychological difficulties, such as bodily changes and other major challenges, which need to be negotiated successfully by transplant recipients.

RENAL DISEASE – DIALYSIS AND PREOPERATIVE ADJUSTMENTS

Although kidney transplantation is the treatment of choice for most end-stage renal disease patients, with demand for grafts far exceeding supply, many have to wait months or years before this treatment is available to them. A few patients may receive a transplant during the predialysis stage, but for most, the waiting period involves emotional adjustments to the physical, psychological, marital, and dialysis-related changes imposed by the disease. The shock of the initial diagnosis, sexual dysfunction, marital friction, changes in body image, and subsequent lower self-esteem and dependence on a machine, fluid bag, or partner can produce profound stress, adjustment anxiety, and depression. Various psychological coping strategies may be used during this time to help the patient and family members negotiate this period of disease and dialysis adjustment.

Coping strategies are psychological patterns that individuals use to manage thoughts, feelings, and actions encountered during various stages of ill health and treatments. The fundamental need to have an overall sense of control over one's life is paramount throughout chronic sickness, and research has shown that interventions designed to increase an individual's perception of control are likely to have a positive impact on patient wellbeing. Presenting treatment options with information so that realistic choices can be made helps patients maintain a sense of control.

During the early phase of ill health, denial and suppression are the most frequent avoidance strategies used. Denial as a psychological defense has been prominent in hemodialysis patients. Later, more positive coping strategies include problem solving, actively seeking information, enhancement of spiritual life, and hope of a transplant. These coping strategies are similar to ones used by end-stage cardiac disease patients.

Many younger patients find such adjustment extremely difficult, particularly young males, who find dependence on dialysis particularly frustrating. These patients may express more dissatisfaction and are more likely to show this dissatisfaction in non-compliant, self-destructive, and despairing behavior. One young male hemodialysis patient described his life as a series of frustrating "can't do's": "can't drink beer with friends, can't enjoy meals with friends, can't go on vacation with friends, can't work, and can't make love to a girlfriend."

Reasonably fit elderly patients are in some ways the most satisfied dialysis group. Many elderly patients feel satisfied with their lives and welcome the chance of a further few years resulting from treatment. Even though older patients are more satisfied with their dialysis lifestyle than younger patients, many older patients seek the better quality of life that a transplant can provide. A study that examined the differences in pretransplant and posttransplant quality of life in kidney recipients in five age groups (range 18–60 years old) reported that quality of life outcomes did not seem to favor one age group over another.[5]

The initial dialysis adjustment phases are difficult. For some patients, these adjustment phases can be traumatic. Professional, practical, and psychological support is desirable at this time.

Health beliefs and attitudes toward illness and treatments differ between individuals and among cultures, as do responses to pain and reactions to a new graft. Many patients find that peritoneal dialysis offers a moderate to good quality of life, but at Oxford a Muslim patient with a strict religious hygiene code found this treatment impossible because she felt "unclean – like a dustbin, always filling up with rubbish." Such feelings made prayer difficult and life unbearable for her. Cultural attitudes may influence the recipient's response to transplantation. A young female Asian patient at this transplant center refused the idea of a cadaver transplant because she was reluctant to accept a kidney from an anonymous donor who might be male.

Many authors have discussed health and illness beliefs and have outlined the need for staff to consider the meaning that patients attach to their illness and treatment therapies. It is important for staff members to be aware of individual perceptions and beliefs with regard to transplantation. Each belief must be recognized and validated, and, if required, appropriate support must be provided.

Many units provide predialysis information sessions for patients and family members. Bradley and McGee[2] suggest that the "most effective sessions seem to be run on a multidisciplinary basis, with input from medical, nursing, dietetic and social work staff, and include information from dialysis and transplant patients themselves." In this unit, such sessions are valuable because they provide an opportunity to give information concerning all treatment options. The sessions also provide a forum to encourage active patient and caregiver participation with regard to treatment issues and initial treatment anxieties.

Meeting other patients who have negotiated various forms of treatment successfully offers a positive image and role model and gives greater credibility to information given. Honesty is an important part of such sessions, and information givers strive to present a realistic assessment of experiences without being overprotective regarding problems or overly optimistic. Such sessions help to develop a close supportive relationship between staff members and patients at the predialysis stage.

Psychological studies have reported moderate levels of clinical depression in predialysis and hemodialysis groups,[10,28] and many units are now offering psychological therapies, such as cognitive behavioral therapy, to patients if clinical levels of depression are noted. In October 2009 the National Institute for Health and Clinical Excellence (NICE)[44] in the United Kingdom published guidelines which detailed the treatment and management of depression in adults with chronic physical health problems. They reported that "depression is approximately two to three times more common in patients with a chronic physical health problem than in people who have good physical health" and they recommended that practitioners should be alert to possible depression and should consider asking patients who may have depression two questions: "During the last month have you been bothered by feeling down, depressed, or hopeless? During the last month, have you often been bothered by having little interest or pleasure in doing things?" NICE recommends behavioral and/or cognitive therapy for patients with mild to moderate depression and cognitive behavioral therapy with antidepressant medication for more severe depression.[44]

In this Oxford transplant center, we are currently introducing a pilot study of psychological assessment questionnaires to evaluate levels of depression and anxiety in the predialysis stage and at regular stages throughout treatment so that we might offer therapies if felt necessary. The introduction of these questionnaires seems to encourage patients to feel more able to discuss elements of low mood and to ask for psychological support at times of stress and have also appeared to assist staff in discussing the difficult aspect of psychological wellbeing with patients. This study will be fully evaluated in a year's time.

HOPE OF A TRANSPLANT

Peretz[47] defined hope "as the capacity to anticipate that even though one feels uncomfortable now, one may feel better in the future." When a transplant is suggested, many patients make an immediate decision to proceed, whereas others agonize over the decision. Some patients may deny the possibility of posttransplant difficulties and may have unrealistic expectations for their future quality of life. Such denial may predispose patients to depression if major complications occur after the transplant. It is essential that indepth realistic and honest information is given at this stage so that patients may proceed in an informed manner.

In the past, renal programs often required formal pretransplant psychiatric assessment. These assessments are no longer considered necessary, but the experience at Oxford suggests that it is valuable to have a pretransplant meeting at which specific medical, social, and psychological issues are explored with the patient and family members. Individual fears raised at such a meeting include fear of changes in body image resulting from immunosuppression, fear of loss of identity when accepting a foreign organ, and fear of surgery, particularly for older patients. These concerns are similar to concerns reported by other authors. A pretransplant meeting is an opportunity to dispel myths or hearsay that may have been gleaned from other patients. Issues raised in this unit that have required careful explanation include the idea that dialysis is only a short-term treatment, and that the patient may die unless he or she receives a transplant; that it is possible to be infected with other diseases from a cadaver organ; that a male receiving a female kidney may become feminized, and vice versa; and that the donor persona may be implanted with the transplant, and that the recipient "will become a different person."

The pretransplant meeting offers the opportunity to explore, examine, and resolve individual fears and helps to initiate a trusting and supportive relationship with a member of the transplant team. The meeting is a time to offer specific information and advice concerning coping skills and responses to the profound and conflicting emotions that may be experienced. The knowledge gained by staff members during these meetings concerning individual fears and difficulties alerts the professionals to vulnerabilities that may require help postoperatively. A brief period of counseling may be in order for patients who experience the most difficulty with the decision regarding transplant.

Renal patients must temper their hope for a transplant and subsequent enhanced quality of life with the knowledge that there can be no guarantee that a suitable graft will become available or that the transplant will be successful. These uncertainties increase ambivalence toward transplantation and increase psychological stress. Most patients and family members describe the waiting time as the most difficult phase.

Patient fears that they have been forgotten, that they may miss the call, or that their chance may never come are reported frequently. Ongoing contact with the transplant center is helpful and is vital at times of additional stress when a fellow dialysis patient receives or rejects a kidney, when an abortive call occurs, or when the waiting period becomes particularly lengthy. These instances may upset the usual coping strategies, and psychological stress and depression may result. In our center, a transplant nurse specialist is assigned to each patient at the pretransplant meeting so that a supportive bond can develop, and the nurse can offer information and support during the waiting time.

IMMEDIATE POSTOPERATIVE PSYCHOLOGICAL ISSUES

Many kidney transplant recipients report an immediate feeling of rebirth after the transplant; such feelings are linked to a perceived promise of extended and enhanced quality of life. Studies suggest that psychological stress persists throughout the initial recovery period and during the early rehabilitation process. Many recipients report that, although the renal transplant is an opportunity for renewed health, it did not eliminate health-related stress from their lives. The major causes of psychological stress during the early postoperative phase include possibility of rejection and lack of control regarding the body's acceptance or rejection of the kidney, fear of infection, uncertainty about the future, and concern about long-term side effects of immunosuppressive therapy.

The fear of graft rejection is the most frequently reported, and anxiety has been shown to precede the first rejection experience. Such anticipatory anxiety is lessened if the rejection is treated successfully. Although recipients are more at ease if faced with future rejection episodes, uncertainty about future health persists for many months.

One of the most difficult aspects for recipients at this stage is the sudden removal of conscious control. The dialysis patient has become conditioned to be in control of health through adherence to diet and fluid restrictions and regular treatment regimens. After the transplant, the situation changes radically, and recipients are "at the mercy" of factors beyond conscious control: for example, "their own immune response and the effects of the foreign organ which now needs to become accepted as part of the self." Such loss of control can increase anxiety levels, and some patients report panic attacks. It is vital at this stage to discuss progress in detail with the patient and to answer all questions because many recipients seek to regain conscious control by information seeking and by planning daily psychological and activity goals. It is helpful to encourage patient participation in care with self-medication and self-observation so that partial control is achieved. Recipients should be included in discussion regarding medication options, as such choice also offers an element of control at this difficult stage.

Some recipients may have difficulty in accepting the new graft as part of self. Castelnuovo-Tedesco[4] wrote that "the graft is not psychologically inert and that the recipient may develop a prominent identification with the donor." One young female patient at Oxford who was depressed posttransplant stated, "before my transplant I had a broken body and a healthy mind – now, after my transplant, I have a healthy body and a broken mind." During gentle exploration, it was discovered that this patient found it profoundly difficult to accept that she had the kidney of a middle-aged man "inside her," fearing that her femininity was at risk.

In the past there have been reports in the media suggesting that following transplantation the recipient may experience "personality changes" from the donor.[61] Studies regarding perceived changes in personality were first reported, in the main, by heart transplant recipients and were usually linked to the belief that the heart is seen "as the source of love, emotions and, for some, the focus of personality traits." There have been several articles in the national and international press in which such "personality changes" have been reported by individual live donor and recipient pairs. These articles have hypothesized that some form of cellular memory may be responsible for these perceived changes. Such publicity has led to patients at our center becoming anxious that the transplanted kidney may result in a personality change for them. Indeed, a male recipient who had received a kidney from his wife recently expressed concerns that he may have been feminized by his wife's kidney as he now preferred more female domestic tasks. In our experience, these anxieties can be resolved by discussion and reassurance that the graft does not carry the persona of the donor and cannot alter the integrity of the recipient's personality.

Feelings of guilt and sadness concerning the donor and donor family are frequent. An adult receiving a pediatric graft may view the death as a special tragedy and experience profound guilt and grief. Recipients and caregivers report dreams in which they may see a distressed family without a father or mother, and they may relate such dreams to the donor family. Some recipients report also the need to offer prayers for the donor and the family and may experience feelings of unworthiness in receiving such a precious, life-enhancing gift. The opportunity to discuss such feelings and to give thanks through an anonymous letter usually aids resolution so that the recipient may move forward toward positive rehabilitation. Recipients in our center are now routinely sent a letter, at 6 months posttransplant, if progress is good, asking if they would like to write an anonymous letter of thanks to the donor family. They are also offered help to write such a letter if that is their wish. It is becoming more common, however, for recipients or donor families to request a meeting with each other. Many transplantation units are now facilitating such meetings, and initial reports suggest successful outcomes for the recipient and the donor family. However, there is still a need to stress caution because the donor family may be "disappointed in the recipient" or may become "intrusive into the recipient's life." Recipients may face the dilemma of wanting to refuse such a meeting, but may fear that they would be seen as ungrateful, and they may be distressed or disturbed at trying to meet the perceived needs of the donor family. It has been stated that it is paternalistic of professionals to discourage such meetings; however, professionals have a duty of care to recipients and donor families. Thorough discussion and planning must precede such meetings, and fully trained professionals must be available to offer debriefing sessions and to help if problems arise.

Depression may occur in the posttransplant period and may be linked to infection because it is especially prevalent among patients with cytomegalovirus infection or cytomegalovirus mononucleosis syndrome. Also, patients who have unrealistically high expectations preoperatively are susceptible to postoperative depressive symptoms. Such patients may have difficulty accepting that transplantation is an alternative treatment rather than a cure for end-stage renal disease. The most appropriate psychiatric diagnosis for many of these patients is an adjustment disorder. Studies report that the degree of distress often is correlated with the severity of physical symptoms and the occurrence of postoperative complications. In this center, we now offer a psychological support service to patients experiencing posttransplant low mood and/or anxiety, which can include short psychological therapy if required.

IMMUNOSUPPRESSION REGIMENS AND PSYCHOLOGICAL REACTIONS

The introduction of newer immunosuppression regimens has resulted in fewer reports of psychological reactions. Studies show, however, that patients still report that low-dose corticosteroids are responsible for mood changes and irritability in the early posttransplant period. Sometimes these emotional responses are less obvious to the patient, but are reported by friends or family members. Transient disruption of sleep, altered perception, and lability of mood often occur in patients receiving pulses of corticosteroids as antirejection therapy. A study in 2003 by Prasad and associates[49] examined the attitudes of recipients toward steroid use and other therapies. When asked which drug they would like to discontiue, 65% of patients responded and cited prednisolone. Steroid therapy is now reduced more quickly than in the past and often stopped at 3 months but many patients still fear these drugs and remember fellow patients experiencing side effects in the past and many request steroid-free treatment when discussing immunosuppresion therapies.[49]

Studies demonstrate that patients report fewer side effects with the newer regimens, but the hand trembling and hair thinning or loss resultant from tacrolimus medication and the gastrointestinal problems resultant from the mycophenolate medication can be very distressing for transplant recipients, as is the concern that skin cancer and other cancers have an increased risk for this group. Patients must be fully informed regarding the various issues pertinent to each therapy and, if possible, transplant centers should consider patients' opinions and needs and should tailor the immunosuppressive strategies and regimens to take these opinions and needs into account.

Medication Side Effects: Self-Esteem, Quality of Life, and Body Image

People in renal failure may experience negative reactions toward their bodies because of the invasive nature of the treatment. The cessation of dialysis after renal transplantation does not abolish this stress. Immunosuppression and its side effects can present a major problem related to self-esteem, confidence, and quality of life after transplantation. A transplant recipient returning to work as a senior health service manager was referred to the psychology service in this center suffering panic attacks and depression due to obvious hand trembling which she felt had vastly reduced her self-confidence, and also gastrointestinal problems which were interfering with her work. She had become so depressed by these issues that she was seriously considering resigning from her employment and had reduced most of her social life due to acute embarrassment, thus reducing her satisfaction with life.

Body image change may be particularly distressing for adolescent recipients. Adolescents are in a period of structural ego alteration with conflict about identity, psychosexual development, dependency, and authority, and the additional stress of a transplant may become a focus of derangement of their defenses. Hair loss or hair thinning can cause considerable distress, with one female patient recently refusing to meet peers and preferring social isolation. Many adolescent recipients may require additional support and understanding. For some adolescents, the side effects of immunosuppressive therapies and their perceived effects on social interaction are more unacceptable than graft failure and possible death from voluntary discontinuation of medications.

Psychological Distress and Adherence to Immunosuppression Regimens

Adherence or concordance has been defined as the extent to which a patient's behavior coincides with the prescribed regimen.[6] Poor adherence is a risk factor for morbidity and mortality after transplantation and has been the subject of much research over many years. The more recent introduction of new immunosuppression regimens was thought to decrease the level of non-adherence and improve concordance but studies show that non-adherence remains a major concern to clinicians.

Various explanations have been given for non-adherence, including inability to accept the lifestyle limitations and, in the United States, the cost of medication. A large study by Chisholm-Burns et al.[7] collected data from 525 adult kidney transplant recipients and examined the factors influencing adherence to antirejection therapy. A total of 177 patients were non-adherent, most frequently citing the reason as carelessness. Younger patients (18–29 years) were more likely to be non-adherent than patients aged 46–64 years. Adherence was not associated with time since transplant, or type of immunosuppressant regimen. However, there were significant differences between adherent and non-adherent patients in their held beliefs regarding the necessity to take their medications and the level of concern if medications were missed. Non-adherent patients scored significantly lower than adherent patients on every question of the Life Satisfaction Index indicating lower quality of life. Conclusions from this study were that non-adherence is related to patients' beliefs about their immunosuppression medications and perceived barriers, and is associated with lower quality of life. The results from this study indicate the need for ongoing monitoring and education for transplant recipients in the importance of their medications and the dangers of non-adherence and the need to offer extra support to the younger patient group, as well as education on how to assimilate medications successfully into lifestyle.[7]

Haferkamp[23] et al. developed a questionnaire to measure compliance in kidney transplant patients and to identify screening criteria for non-compliance. In this study a third of patients were perfectly compliant, another third of patients showed moderate compliance, and the last third demonstrated low compliance. Older patients were more likely to be compliant than younger patients. Patients taking mycophenolate showed better compliance than patients not taking mycophenolate.[23] As with the Chisholm study, this study demonstrated the need to support younger patients but also reported other factors involved in non-compliance, such as type of immunosupprssion regimen and aspects of life satisfaction and social support. Surman[60] noted in the late 1980s that non-adherence may occur in major depression or as part of an adjustment reaction, especially in adolescent recipients; recent studies suggest that this observation continues to be relevant today.

A study from the United Kingdom examined adherence in 58 adult renal transplant recipients. Results showed that 7 (12%) subjects missed at least 20% of days of medication, and 15 (26%) missed at least 10% of days of medication. Lower belief in the need for medication and having a transplant from a live donor were major factors associated with non-adherence. Depression also was common, although not strongly associated with non-adherence. Further research is required to examine beliefs with regard to live donation, but it seems that some recipients may believe that, because a familial graft is a good immunological match, there is less need for immunosuppression.

Valid and reliable predictors of non-adherence are unavailable, although a strong history of poor dialysis adherence in patients with non-adherence after transplantation seems to be an important predisposing factor. Non-adherence may develop postoperatively, however, in patients who had adhered with dialysis and pretransplant medical care. Some studies suggest that patients identified as high risk with regard to medication adherence should receive extensive pretransplant psychosocial evaluation and psychological counseling, to facilitate posttransplant follow-up, to strengthen the nurse–patient relationship, and to ensure patient adherence to the immunosuppressive regimen. It is vital to explore and respect the underlying motives and feelings of the recipient and to offer support to enable adherence to medication regimens. Russell and colleagues[51] noted that "the clinical nurse specialist is paramount in assisting both younger and older renal transplant recipients with immunosuppressive medication taking and, consequently, in fostering better adherence and outcomes."

FAMILY INTERACTIONS

End-stage renal disease and its treatments cause shifts within the dynamics of family interactions. Chronic ill health and subsequent medical treatments may have engendered a sense of helplessness in the patient. Family roles change as the patient is placed into a state of chronic illness and treatment-induced dependency. The spouse may have to accept greater family responsibilities and may have to assist with dialysis treatments. Many caregivers report feelings of being "unsupported, invisible and unappreciated." Individuals trying to come to terms with their own feelings find it hard to spare extra energy to cope with the feelings of those close to them.

One of the important posttransplant psychosocial tasks that the patient needs to accomplish is the gradual relinquishing of the sick role and the eventual return to non-patient status. After transplantation, recipients may be reluctant to give up the security of the patient role, resulting in the spouse resenting the continued dependence. Wilkins and associates[65] reported a study in which targeted education and specific psychosocial supports were given to transplant recipients to aid their return to normalcy. Normalcy is defined as age-appropriate and socially appropriate activities of the patient, such as employment, homemaker, and student. The researchers reported that "a programme of education and psychosocial support that emphasizes return to normalcy and non-disability, beginning with the first exposure to transplant and continuing throughout the first six months post transplant, yielded high rates of return to normality of kidney transplant recipients."[65]

An Australian[63] study entitled "When i had my transplant, i became normal," which examined adolescent perspectives on life after kidney transplantation, reported five enablers and five barriers to achieving a sense of normality. The enablers were: (1) developing their own identity; (2) peer acceptance; (3) making medications routine; (4) freedom and energy; and (5) support structures. The barriers included: "identity crisis, peer rejection, aversion to medications, lifestyle limitations, and fear and uncertainty." Study conclusions were that "Adolescent kidney transplant recipients value normality and have specific information needs about the effect of transplantation on their physical appearance and the tolerance of drugs and alcohol. Novel approaches are needed to foster self-confidence and the sense of normality, and to provide comprehensive information on the patient following kidney transplantation."[63] Experience at this center suggests that the findings of this study and its conclusions replicate much of the thoughts and needs of adult transplant recipients with regard to return to "normalcy." In fact, a recipient recently stated that she had been "sick and on dialysis for so long that she had no idea what normal was."

The return to employment can present another hurdle for some transplant recipients, particularly if they have been unable to work for several years. At this time of high unemployment in the United Kingdom it is proving extremely difficult for transplant recipients to gain employment. Employers do not always view transplant recipients as reliable and healthy employees. Healthcare personnel need to create a proactive employment atmosphere and to encourage and assist recipients in their posttransplant quest for work. They should ensure that they do not unconsciously encourage recipient dependence, but strive to support independence from the beginning of the posttransplant phase. In this center we have introduced the role of kidney patient advisors who offer advocacy and support to recipients in negotiations with employers to facilitate new employment and return to previous employment.

Marital difficulties may ensue if the transplant recipient is eager to resume his or her pre-illness position within the family. The partner or children may be disinclined to forfeit any roles that they have assumed during the pretransplant dialysis phase. Such issues usually can be resolved with the help of an empathetic counselor and honest family discussions. Particular difficulties may occur if a child or adolescent who had been chronically ill returns to the family with new mobility and vigor. Families may tend to regard the child or adolescent as fragile and may be excessively restrictive or permissive. Adolescent recipients may not be required to follow the usual family rules, causing disruption and psychological difficulties for the other siblings. These and other family issues can be treated with brief cognitive behavioral therapy.

Sexual problems may develop with incompatible sexual desires between partners, erectile dysfunction, or other sexual difficulties. Progress in the field of renal transplantation has considerably improved the quality of life of patients with chronic renal failure; however, quality-of-life studies do not always include assessment of the patient's sex life. The main causes of sexual problems are many and varied and may be psychological, physical, or related to medications; it is important to explore individual difficulties with the recipient and partner to try to elicit the most suitable interventions. A study by Darabi et al.[11] investigated the sexual function of male recipients before and after renal transplantation. The study included 100 males aged 18–61 years. Results showed that before transplantation the libido was good in 22 cases, in 52 cases it was intermediate, and in 26 cases it was poor. Potency was good in 30 cases, intermediate in 52, and poor in 18 cases (impotent). After transplantation the libido improved: 80 cases became good, and libido in 16 cases was intermediate and poor in 4 cases. Potency became good in 76 cases, intermediate in 18 cases, and in 6 cases remained poor.[11]

Lerda[30] and colleagues examined female sexual function and quality of life in dialysis and renal transplant patients. The conclusions from this study were that "Female sexual dysfunction is common in renal failure but that a successful transplant is the most effective way to retain good sexual function in women with chronic renal failure."[30] Studies conclude that assessment of and education regarding sexual functioning must be a routine component of psychosocial intervention.

GRAFT FUNCTION

Delayed or Poor Graft Function

In most cases, the new transplant begins working well almost immediately; however, some recipients may have to wait weeks or months for the graft to function. During this time, the recipient must balance hope for a successful outcome with the fear of graft loss. Recipients respond in different ways: some may become overanxious, continually seeking information and reassurance; others may become angry and depressed, continually asking "why me?" In contrast, some recipients may seem unconcerned, using denial to cover their underlying feelings of desperation. Staff members may conclude that such recipients are unaware of the true situation. In reality, the patient is aware of the issues, but is psychologically unable to face the possibility of graft failure. The fantasy that all is and will be well is more bearable during the waiting time. In this instance, denial can be a useful defense mechanism, helping to make the period of delayed function sustainable. Perceived personal control is vital during this time, and empowering patients to take control over exercise regimens, health observations, and medications lessens anxiety and increases self-confidence. Offering regular, honest information within an empathetic setting helps aid emotional stability for the recipient.

In some cases, the recipient may endure months or years of unsatisfactory graft function – a level of function that enables the recipient to be free of dialysis, but not able to obtain the desired quality of life or the expected level of rehabilitation. Many patients expect a great deal from their posttransplant lifestyle: a dramatic improvement in physical health; a return to work, study, or parental role; an improvement in self-image; an improvement in family relationships; and freedom from the sick role. Such expectations may be unrealistic and may not be fulfilled. It can be difficult for recipients to admit failure to achieve such ideals and disappointment in their new health status.

If such disappointment is expressed, the recipient may become anxious that he or she appears ungrateful for the gift of life or the medical and nursing care given. Recipients also express guilt that they are not achieving enough or are in some way letting down the donor family or the transplant team. A young Oxford patient felt that she was not "living up to the right standard" and that she "had been given a special opportunity in which she had failed." Her conversation was littered with shoulds and oughts: "I should be making more of a success of my life … I ought to be more happy and grateful."

These feelings of guilt may be enhanced by family and friends who previously offered sympathy at the rigors of dialysis, but now expect gratitude and full recovery. Partners may find the continuing need to support and care difficult, and marital problems can ensue, especially if there also is sexual friction. Recipients may experience emotional lability and depression, increasing their guilt, and with the additional physical debility resulting from heavy immunosuppression regimens, the psychological impact may be intense, resulting in low mood and clinical depression.

Psychological support should be offered to recipients and caregivers. In our institution, recipients have been found to benefit from therapies aimed at changing individual beliefs, such as cognitive and behavioral therapies. Caregivers found the opportunity to express feelings and recognize and fulfill their own needs beneficial. Marital therapies help in some cases, and if sexual difficulties are present, referral to a specialist team is required.

Graft Failure

Most recipients experience feelings of profound loss if their kidney transplant fails, although some also may feel relief if the graft has had unsatisfactory function over a protracted period. Relief may be linked to the return to dialysis and perceived control. Occasionally, denial may be used in the initial graft failure stage, but as the reality of the situation becomes apparent, sadness, anger, and depression frequently are reported. Hudson and Hiott[25] noted that recipients displayed a variety of behavior and reactions to graft loss, including bereavement reactions: "At this time patients must be helped to understand that the loss of the graft is not the end and there is still hope for the future through subsequent transplants." Gill and Lowes[21] reported that graft loss was devastating, causing feelings of grief, loss, suicide, and depression in a recipient in their study; however, depression lessened as physical health and a sense of personal control improved. In our experience, the return to dialysis is negotiated gradually and successfully by most recipients, and as the disappointment of the graft failure subsides, most quickly request the chance for another transplant.

PSYCHOLOGICAL ASPECTS OF LIVING DONATION

The first successful renal transplants performed were mostly from living related donors. The psychological reactions of donor and recipient were monitored closely in many psychiatric studies and are outlined in this section.

Early Psychological Findings in Living Related Transplantation (1960s to 1970s)

Many of the initial studies conducted in the 1960s and early 1970s questioned the fundamental willingness of relatives to make this type of sacrifice. Donor altruism – the supreme act of unselfishness and of giving freely without thought of reward – was much debated. Some researchers postulated that, although donors were "consciously altruistic," there was considerable "unconscious resentment" toward the recipient and toward hospital personnel who requested or encouraged donation.[7] Other studies concluded that donors may be "victims of family blackmail" and donated because of family pressure or integral guilt. Such pressure could be subtle or direct with a fear of family rejection if the prospective donor decided not to donate. Investigators also reported that in some situations "the black sheep" of the family offered to donate in an attempt to win family approval and become reinstated within the family.[17,56]

There were reports of postsurgical depression for some donors, with a suspected grief reaction linked to the loss of a body part and donor hostility expressed as anger that the recipient had been perceived to receive a greater amount of care and attention. Several studies also reported difficulties in the donor and recipient postsurgical relationship, with donors becoming overprotective and intrusive into recipients' lifestyle and the recipients having difficulty with the obligation of the gift.[17,56] Although many of these early studies involved small numbers of donors and recipients, the negative psychiatric findings were much reported, and some observers suggested that cadaver organs were psychologically preferable because there could be no continuing obligation for the recipient. In contrast, several studies also reported that donors described the act as positive and as one of the most meaningful experiences of their lives.

Later Psychological Studies in Living Related Transplantation (Late 1980s, and 1990s)

During the late 1970s and the 1980s, studies began to report more positive psychological findings. Simmons and colleagues[55] interviewed 230 living related donors and reported that "donors view themselves as more worthwhile because of the donation." In this study, only 5% of donors reported negative feelings about the transplant. Smith and coworkers[57] found that 97% of donors reaffirmed their decisions, and less than 15% said that they felt pressured to donate. With regard to recipient reactions, Simmons and colleagues[55] reported that, "although recipients did feel guilt about the gift that they could not reciprocate, most recipients and donors reported that there were no major problems in their relationship 1 year post-transplantation."

Following the positive results of the published studies – in particular, the large Simmons study[55] – the late 1980s saw a change in the way that transplant centers viewed living donor kidney transplants. Although some centers continued a strong stance against living donor transplants, mainly because of the physical risks to the donor, many other centers increased living donor transplant. A study by Levey and colleagues[31] noted that the physical risks to the donor were minimal, and that the benefits to the donor were considerable with regard to self-esteem and self-worth. Later studies reported that "to deny the donor the right to donate could do psychological harm."[32] Surman[60] wrote that "kidney donation has a favorable outcome for both donor and recipient and the participation of living related donors in kidney transplantation is now widely accepted."

During the early 1990s, studies again reported psychological difficulties for donor and recipient. Russell and Jacob[52] postulated that "results indicate that while psychological side effects have been reported, including depression and family conflict, these risks are generally underemphasized … health professionals should be aware that merely raising the issue of live organ donation may instigate powerful psychological processes beyond the potential donor's voluntary control and leave little room for refusal without psychological cost." A sibling donor in our own center expressed similar sentiments by saying that she wished that "The topic of live donation had never been thrown into the family circle as it caused enormous friction and sibling conflict which could only be solved by agreeing to donation."

Fox and Swazey[18] examined the concept of the recipient's obligation to repay the "gift of life" and postulated that "in the case of a live kidney transplant, the donor may exhibit a great deal of proprietary interest in the health, work and private life of the close relative who has received his or her organ, on the emotional grounds that, after all, it's my kidney … that's me in there." The great indebtedness recipients may feel to the parent, sibling, or child whose life-saving kidney they carry may make it difficult for them to maintain a reasonable amount of psychic difference and independence from the donor. These authors reported that it was common for a recipient who needs freedom from the donor but feels too beholden to him or her to negotiate it to take the drastic step of breaking the relationship completely. These authors stressed the need for careful donor selection and ongoing psychological support for donor and recipient as important aspects of care throughout the living donor and recipient experience.

More Recent Studies and Developments in Living Related Donation

The Scandinavian countries incorporated live donation into their transplantation programs in the 1960s, and the level of live donation has increased over the years. Such large numbers of live donors have enabled extensive research to occur.

Jakobsen[27] reported that nearly 500 living donors in Norway were asked: "If you could turn the clock back, would you do the same again?" Eighty-three percent said "definitely yes," and another 11% said "probably yes." Many donors were deeply grateful for having been given the opportunity to become a donor. A study from Stockholm[16] reported follow-up of 370 living kidney donors; this study concluded that less than 1% of donors regretted the donation, although several donors experienced the first few months after the donation as troublesome from a physical perspective.

Centers in the United States also have published results from studies of follow-up in large numbers of living donors. A study by Schover and colleagues[53] from the Cleveland Clinic examined 167 donors with regard to psychological aspects of the decision to donate, impact of donation on family relationships, donor reactions to graft failure, and overall satisfaction of donors. The study findings suggest that "the majority of donors make the decision to donate with little ambivalence, express comfort with the choice at long term follow up and do not experience negative consequences regarding health … or family relationships." Jacobs and coworkers[26] published a report from the University of Minnesota with follow-up of 529 living donors who had donated in the period 1985 to 1996. Study conclusions were that "donors scored higher than the general population with regard to quality of life issues. The overall donor experience was stressful for 12%, with donors more likely to say experiences were stressful if they had postoperative complications. If given the opportunity, only 4% of the donors said that they would not donate again, and 9% were unsure."

More recent studies report that most donors enjoy a high quality of life, with a boost in self-esteem and an increased sense of wellbeing.[43] Butt[3] and colleagues investigated the quality of life impact of living donor nephrectomy using a meta-analysis. Results concluded that, in the first month after donation, donors reported clinically significant decreases in physical function; however, within 3–6 months and persisting for a year postdonation, donors reported quality of life scores similar to their baseline scores.[3] Maglakelidze et al.[39] noted that the health-related quality of life of living donors was not different from that of healthy subjects and a study of 106 live kidney donors in a single German[1] transplantation center examining renal, physical, and psychological follow-up concluded that: "this cohort of live kidney donors showed good renal outcomes and superior scores in both physical and psychological health compared with the German population."[1]

The advent of laparoscopic donor surgery has resulted in a shorter hospital stay, a quicker recovery time, and minimal scarring, and these benefits seem to be encouraging more live donors to consent to surgery. A study by Nicholson et al.,[45] "Health-related quality of life after living donor nephrectomy: a randomized controlled trial of laproscopic versus open nephrectomy" concluded that: "donors undergoing laparoscopic nephrectomy reported less bodily pain in the first 6 weeks postdonation, and this was associated with an improved mental health component of quality of life compared with open donor nephrectomy." Indeed, live renal donation has increased and is now providing a large percentage of kidney transpants in many major transplanting countries.

Although quality of life studies which, in the main, depend upon quantitative methodology report high scores in live kidney donors, few studies use indepth qualitative methodology to delve more deeply into donor decision making, donor and recipient relationships, and donor postsurgery regrets. Indepth studies do suggest that some donors experience covert familial pressure to donate and find it impossible to refuse, even though they do not wish to proceed. Some also report conflict between the family of birth and the family of marriage, encounter some difficulties in the postoperative relationship with the recipient, have anxieties concerning their future health, and regret giving. Similarly, some recipients report difficulties in the postsurgery relationship with the donor and with reciprocity and feelings of obligation.[9,19] Research has shown that psychosocial risks are still apparent within the live donation process, that these risks should be recognized within transplant programs, and that professional care should be provided to ensure confidential presurgery donor and recipient advocacy combined with continuing psychosocial support for the family unit after donation.

Psychological support is crucial for the live donor should the subsequent transplant fail or the transplant recipient die. Fortunately, such occurrences are rare but in such circumstances donors report feelings of guilt, anger, and depression. All these comments have been made to myself, the author, in circumstances where the transplant has failed. Furthermore, a donor in our center became very depressed after the death of the recipient and required antidepressant medication and bereavement counseling and was unable to work for 6 months following the recipient's death.

LIVING UNRELATED DONORS

The successes achieved in living unrelated transplantation have been widely published and most transplantation centers now believe that emotionally related living donors represent a valuable option for kidney transplantation. Recipient and graft outcomes have been reported as superior to cadaver kidney transplantation and studies of psychological outcomes for living unrelated donors show an increase in life satisfaction scores. Some spouses have commented that their desire to donate is directed by both altruistic and selfish reasons as they know that the transplant will enhance the quality of life for the recipient and thus their quality of life also.

A decrease in cadaver organ donation has been reported in recent years in the United Kingdom, continental Europe, and the United States, and, as numbers of patients on the waiting lists have increased, it has become apparent that the full potential of renal transplantation will be realized only if other donor sources are developed. Therefore many units have introduced paired kidney exchange programs and altruistic donation programs.

Paired Kidney Exchange

Transplantation units throughout the world have introduced paired kidney exchange programs, with the United States leading the way. These programs enable recipients with incompatible living donors to receive a kidney from a compatible donor from another pair whilst their donor donates to a compatible recipient from another pair. These complex programs, which require skillfull and very efficient management, have become highly successful and have increased the numbers of live donor transplants and enabled recipients with incompatible donors to receive a graft.

A study by de Zuidema et al.[12] reports on a paired exchange program which operated between 2004 and 2010: 422 pairs were registered. In the 7 years of the program 313/422 (74%) of the participating patients were transplanted. Approximately half of them (167/313, 53%) received a kidney through the exchange program, while 47 (15%) received a cadaveric donor kidney and 99 (32%) were tranplanted through other living donation programs. Conclusions state that the exchange program proved to be highly successful not only in its direct results but also indirectly by triggering alternative solutions. Interestingly, there is no report of the psychological issues for donors and recipients in this study or in other transplantation literature.[12]

It may be that these programs do not appear to result in any additional psychological issues than those already reported in living donation studies. The program in our center is too small as yet to evaluate psychological outcomes but postsurgery comments from donors and recipients discussed, thus far, have been very positive, although one donor did report that she felt enormous pressure not to drop out of the program as not only would she be "letting down her recipient but all the other pairs which she felt were depending on her." It will be interesting to evaluate these programs from a psychological perspective as they develop.

Altruistic (Non-Directed) Donation

Altruistic donation – the act of living kidney donation to a stranger – has also been introduced into many transplantation centers. In the United Kingdom altruistic donation was refused in the past as living donors were required to be able to demonstrate a genetic or emotional relationship with the recipient. However, altruistic donation is now permitted and altruistic donors are now accepted to donate anonymously to a stranger in the United Kingdom. The reluctance to introduce and expand such programs in the past was due, in part, to fears that donation may engender psychological distress and/or regrets after surgery and also that donors not thought physically or psychologically suitable to donate might suffer extreme reactions of rejection if their offer was refused. However, such fears appear to have been unfounded, thus far, as early reports suggest excellent outcomes for donors and recipients. Massey et al.[40] report a study in which 24 altruistic donors were interviewed on average 2 years after donation. They conclude that "living kidney donation to a stranger does not appear to exacerbate psychological complaints. Moreover, altruistic donors report considerable satisfaction and personal benefit."

PRE-EMPTIVE TRANSPLANTATION

Many transplant centers are now reporting the advantages of pre-emptive transplantation (transplantation before start of dialysis). Several studies have reported that pre-emptive transplantation can result in better rehabilitation and lower risk of loss of employment.[59,66] Transplantation without prior dialysis resulted in less physical and psychological impact for patients and their spouses.[54] Previous anxieties that there would be poorer patient adherence if the transplant is pre-emptive have not been supported by more recent research.[54] Most centers undertaking pre-emptive transplantation favor the use of living donors because of the shortage of cadaver donors. Given the beneficial effects of pre-emptive transplantation, the emphasis has fallen again on increasing the donor pool, especially from within the live donation arena.

PSYCHOLOGICAL ISSUES AND IMPLICATIONS FOR PRACTICE FOR LIVING DONOR PROGRAMS

The psychological issues cited in this chapter and the results of our own psychological study have formed the basis for the structure of the Live Donor Programme in Oxford. This program offers early concise information to the donor and recipient and preoperative and postoperative psychological evaluation and support. It is hoped that this approach will help the donor and recipient with decision making, avoid adverse psychological outcomes, reduce psychological morbidity, and aid full donor and recipient emotional rehabilitation.

Informed Consent

The decisions confronting the potential donor and recipient generate significant stress because they are considering life-threatening, irreversible, and high-risk surgery. It is imperative that the donor and recipient are informed fully regarding the advantages and risks involved and can make the decision to give or receive freely without overt or covert coercion.

Donor Informed Consent: Anxieties and Fears

Several studies suggest that, despite the seriousness of the decision to donate, only a few potential donors deliberated before agreeing to donor assessment. Most donors in these studies regarded their choice as instantaneous and made without conscious evaluation. Conversely, studies in Oxford and London, reported together by Franklin and Crombie,[9,19] concluded that the mothers in both studies acted altruistically and offered as soon as the possibility of a transplant was suggested. In contrast, some of the fathers in the studies expressed some ambivalence about donation and found the decision making complex. Sibling decision making also was complex and difficult for some subjects in both studies, and within this group, motivational factors involved altruism, manipulation of family dynamics, coercion, and covert pressure. In these studies, the siblings seemed to have the most difficulty with the decision to donate. These sibling responses support the findings of Russell and Jacob,[52] who postulated that "by merely presenting the option, the individual is immediately placed under an unwarranted moral burden, a no win situation." Such a situation is graphically described by a sibling who felt like a "fish on a hook."[52] These results show the need for strict donor confidentiality and for the donor to have a third-party advocate who is outside the renal and transplant programs. The advocate can support the donor during the decision making process and can give the donor the confidence and support to refuse to donate if that is his or her wish.

Initial information must be detailed, and the initial approach to the donor must come at an early stage to ensure time to deliberate and to make an informed decision. In Norway, the initial approach to the donor often is made in a letter from the recipient's nephrologist. Ideally, recipients should not be asked to make the approach themselves because a refusal can be devastating, and donors may find it impossible to refuse such a request from an obviously sick relative.

The Norwegian approach of writing to relatives has been rejected in our unit because it was thought that donors may feel unable to refuse a formal medical request. In this center, we believe that information about living kidney donation should be made widely available in predialysis and dialysis outpatient areas through written leaflets and newsletters. Detailed information is given at predialysis and transplantation seminars for recipients and their families, and in most cases, the donors requested further information without the need for additional approaches.

Donor fears and anxieties reported preoperatively involve donor death, fear of rejection, and length of life of the graft, fear that the donor kidney may prove unsuitable, and concerns for long-term health. Such issues can be explored throughout the donor preoperative course, and information and appropriate support can be offered. At this time, it is possible to explore donor partner and family attitudes toward the donation. In some situations, the donor partner of a sibling may be unhappy with the donation and may believe that loyalty to the marriage should supersede loyalty to a birth relative.

Donors must be encouraged to make their own informed decisions, but if conflict ensues, appropriate support should be offered. In one case, in our center, a foster mother desperately wished to donate to her foster child, but her husband was adamantly against this decision. The outcome was that the wife withdrew the offer, but conflict within the marriage continued, and marital therapy was offered. In another case, an adult sister offered to donate to her brother, but the sister's husband objected, saying "that he would divorce his wife if she went ahead with the donation." The sister decided to proceed, and after the surgery her husband left the marital home. The donor stated that she did not regret the decision to proceed, however.

Some donors may have specific dilemmas to resolve. A partner with a spouse and daughter with polycystic disease decided to donate to the daughter because the tissue match was superior. The spouse joined the cadaver waiting list. Another partner with a spouse and daughter with polycystic disease decided to donate to the spouse, who was unwell and unable to work, with the hope that an unaffected sibling would donate to the daughter at a later date. These and other dilemmas need to be discussed fully and decisions made with further information and psychological support.

Donors who are concerned by the risks involved may delay the decision making. In this center, we respect the need for a delay and resolve the issue by suggesting that the recipient may join the cadaver waiting list and the living donor be held in reserve for a later date. It is important that the donor, recipient, and family members understand that the donation evaluation process may be stopped at any stage, and that the reason for this cancellation would remain confidential between the donor and the medical team. Recipients must not be allowed to pressure or pester the donor, and psychological support must be available to the donor and the recipient. Without this strict understanding, it may be impossible for donors to make a truly honest decision, particularly if they wish to refuse to donate.

Preoperative specific anxieties and fears reported by recipients in the Oxford study included risks to the donor, fear of rejection, and guilt about asking this of the family member or partner. Such issues can be explored throughout the recipient preoperative course, and appropriate information and support can be offered.

Recipients may find themselves in a particularly difficult situation if parents are divorced and both wish to donate. The decision as to who should be the donor may need to be made with professional advice and appropriate support given to the parents and the recipient.

Psychological care and information continue into the posttransplant and rehabilitation phases. In our experience, donors and recipients who have close relationships but retain firm boundaries within those relationships achieve the greatest rehabilitation outcome. We advise donors and recipients to celebrate the transplant together on the anniversary, but to continue independent lives at other times. This arrangement facilitates recipient ability to give thanks and donor ability to receive such thanks, but prevents overprotection or intrusion into lifestyle. Any difficulties encountered can be explored with the nurse specialist or counselor, and advice and help can be offered on a continuing basis.

PSYCHOLOGICAL ASPECTS OF CADAVER ORGAN DONATION

Many potential transplant recipients are denied the chance of a life-saving or life-enhancing graft because of a shortage of donor organs. Obstacles to cadaver organ donation are many and varied; however, relative refusal rates remain high in the United Kingdom, some parts of continental Europe, and the United States. Studies show that some critical care staff still find raising the question of donation with relatives difficult. Often this is because of a fear that they may increase relatives' distress and because they lack training in approaching bereaved families to request donation. Such a request may be a rare event in smaller critical care units.

This section outlines grief patterns and discusses aspects of communicating with relatives during the crisis time, informing of death, and requesting organ donation. Personal experience at Oxford with more than 300 donor families suggests that, when relatives are approached sensitively, the subject of organ donation does not increase their distress, and organ donation brings comfort and hope through transplantation.

Grief Process

Grief generally is described as a psychological process by which people fill the gap in their lives after a large part of their world has been lost. Engel[14] described this process as grief work: "the work of mourning by which we can become emancipated from bondage to the deceased, readjust to the environment in which the deceased is missing, and begin to form new relationships." Lindermann first described the stages of bereavement in 1944. Other classic texts have supported and expanded this early theory. Most of these writers outlined three stages of grieving: (1) an immediate stage with shock, disbelief, and denial; (2) an intermediary stage with a growing awareness accompanied by anger, anxiety, and depression; and (3) a final stage of resolution, acceptance, and healing.

More recently, theorists have argued that the concept of bereavement in stages is too structured, and that such classical texts may not entirely reflect how it is to suffer loss. Each individual responds to bereavement in a unique way, and the concept of stages may negate the individual pattern of coping. The grief process is neither universal nor predictable, with no two families responding in the same way, and with individual family members reacting with different emotional responses. Generalizations and comparisons at best may be unhelpful and at worst may be damaging, particularly if clinicians try to fit individuals into a fixed model of grief. Phillips[48] stated that "grief is a profoundly idiosyncratic experience that gets over shaped and forced into moulds. There are as many ways of grieving as there are grievers. Putting people under pressure to do it properly is disabling."

Grief now is viewed as an individual experience that may contain common behavior patterns and reactions. The intensity of the reactions may be affected by other factors, such as the nature of the relationship between the patient and the bereaved, the age of the deceased, the type of death (expected or sudden), and the bereaved's responses to previous experiences and relationships. Research and clarification regarding the various individual and familial behavior patterns have been recorded, and it is possible to recognize patterns, and plan and implement appropriate support and care.

Common Behavior Patterns in the Early Phase of the Grief Process

Common behavior patterns in the early phase of the grief process include numbness, panic, shock, denial, inability to concentrate and make decisions, inability to absorb information and use it effectively, demanding and irrational behavior, aggressive and abusive behavior, withdrawal, and passivity. An understanding of these early patterns of behavior is important to clinicians because such behavior may occur soon after the death and at the time the bereaved are meeting with health professionals in the hospital environment.

The phase of stunned numbness is described by a bereaved relative in Speck's book as a "cotton wool time when there seems to be an invisible blanket between you and the world."[58] Others speak of being "frozen in disbelief" and like a "zombie." There is a safety in this numbness in that it denies the more frightening reactions of helplessness, utter despair, and intense fear. Denial can be interpreted as a psychological defense mechanism that prevents too much emotional pain at any one moment. Numbness, denial, shock, and disbelief are increased in cases of sudden and traumatic death in which there has been no preparation for the terrible news and no possibility of anticipatory grieving. Numbness, shock, and disbelief may last for hours, days, or weeks and may damage and impede the exchange of information and all forms of communication. Denial may play a role throughout the grief process, emerging and subsiding at different times. Extended denial lengthens the grief process and may result in the bereaved feeling the reality of the death at a time when others seem to have "forgotten."

Anger, Anxiety, Depression, and Isolation

The gradual awareness of the reality of the situation often is accompanied by anger and anxiety. Such anger may be directed towards God, the deceased, or members of the caring professions, or it may be internalized and used inwardly against the bereaved individual. Internalized anger often is linked with feelings of guilt and is most apparent after sudden and traumatic death or the death of a child.

Yearning and searching for the deceased may occur and often are accompanied by feelings of emptiness and intense isolation. The loneliness may become extreme, with thoughts of not being understood by family and friends. Such intense responses may engender a fear in the bereaved that he or she is going insane and may result in the bereaved becoming absorbed with his or her own feelings to the exclusion of partners and family, increasing feelings of alienation. Sadness, depression, and exhaustion may develop gradually and may continue for many months.

Healing Behaviors to Enable the Bereaved to Continue with Their Lives

Gradual readjustment and reintegration may occur as the intensity of the emotional pain lessens, and bereaved individuals may start to look forward and find some new purpose in living or new ways of behaving that enable them to continue with their lives. Phrases such as "letting go of the deceased" and "moving on" have been used in the past, but it is widely recognized now that many relatives may wish to find ways of sustaining the bond with the deceased and integrating this bond into future life.

High-Risk Groups – Intense Bereavement Reactions

Several researchers have outlined factors that may indicate a high risk of an intense bereavement reaction requiring additional or specific support as follows: unexpected loss (the deceased was young with no previous history of illness); suicide; sudden loss with no preparation for the death; lack of social support network with the bereaved feeling isolated; the death of a child (parental grief is more severe, complex, protracted, and traumatic than grief following any other bereavement); and a death where the relationship between the deceased and the bereaved is perceived as ambivalent. Research has shown that professional counseling can reduce morbidity significantly in the cases of an intense bereavement reaction. The effect of the counseling is to reduce the risk in high-risk individuals to that of low-risk individuals without counseling.

Sudden or Traumatic Death

Sudden or traumatic death robs family members of preparatory grieving, and the shock, numbness, and disbelief are more intense in such situations. During the initial period, the bereaved often feel disoriented, powerless, and vulnerable. Breaking bad news in such circumstances requires empathy, clear communication, and support to help the relatives emerge from the acute state of shock.

Following sudden loss, family members are likely to have many questions that need to be answered with honesty because this information can help them to make some sense of meaning from the death. Open-ended questions (e.g., "How can we help you?" and "What other information would you like?") help to develop rapport and trust, ease the conversation, and encourage relatives to seek the answers that they need. Acknowledging the family's feelings and emotions (e.g., "You must be very shocked") helps family members to discuss their feelings and influences the grief process in a positive way. The aim must be to support, inform, and offer choices because helping the bereaved to make decisions themselves also helps them to regain their coping skills. Active decision making stimulates a healthy grief process.

Many relatives benefit from a further meeting with the clinician at a later stage so that unanswered questions may be asked and discussed when the numbness and shock have passed. As mentioned earlier, psychological morbidity can be reduced with early counseling, particularly for relatives who have no supportive social networks or who are unable to support each other.

Brainstem Death

One of the most difficult deaths to understand and accept is the situation in which the patient has had a major brain insult and is subsequently found to be brainstem-dead. In the case of brainstem death, it is especially important to consider the content and the timing of the information to be given to the family members. In this situation, the relatives have to understand and accept a new concept of death. Traditional acceptable images of death involve a lifeless body that is cold and asystolic. Brainstem death presents an image of life in a setting of high technology and hope where the victim is warm and has a heart beat and is breathing, albeit on a machine. The situation and setting suggest life and hope to the family, in sharp contrast to the message of death that is given to them by the clinician.

Long et al.,[35,36] in their paper, "Conflict rationalization: how family members cope with the diagnosis of brain stem death," postulate a theory of paradoxical death: "A process whereby family members and health professionals engage in a series of practical and psychological activities aimed at rationalising real or potential emotional and cognitive conflict resulting from a brain-based diagnosis of death, whilst faced with the physical image of a functioning body."

Ormrod et al.[46] interviewed 27 relatives 12 months after bereavement following certification by brainstem testing to investigate their understanding of brainstem death. They concluded that "most relatives understood that the brainstem death tests indicated that survival was not possible, although three relatives had not fully understood this and valued the opportunity to discuss it again. Five relatives chose to observe the tests, all were pleased that they had done so as this confirmed their understanding that death had occurred; however, these relatives had more evidence of psychological distress."[46]

When communicating with family members, it is helpful to use two people: an informer and a supporter. The clinician is often the informer; the supporter often is a nurse, a religious advisor, or another member of the health team. The roles of the informer and the supporter should be kept separate. The family members may blame or reject the informer; if this happens, the supporter can offer physical comfort, repeat information, and offer further support. The informer must not take such rejection personally. The family members are not rejecting the informer, but rather the information that he or she has given. The informer and supporter must understand and accept the brainstem death concept themselves, and they must use language that the family members can understand. Any hesitation or fudging of the explanation can confuse the relatives and may introduce hope that recovery is possible. The message to be given must stress that irreparable damage to the brain has occurred, and that there is no hope of recovery, that death of the brainstem is evident, and death of the brainstem is death of the person. The family members must be allowed time to assimilate and accept this information. The central facts may need to be repeated at several meetings before the relatives can understand the diagnosis and its implications.

Lloyd-Williams et al.[34] investigated the end-of-life care experiences of relatives of brain-dead intensive care patients. Participants valued the physical care their relatives had received, but communication and breaking bad news were causes of concern. They also reported difficulties with cramped relatives' rooms and little privacy to be with the patients or to say a final goodbye. They conclude that families living through the period of brain death in a loved one may have particular needs in terms of end-of-life care and may benefit from the additional support of the palliative care team.

Haddow,[22] who conducted a qualitative study with semistructured interviews with donor and non-donor families, explored the respondents' understanding of brainstem death. She concluded that "most felt that the explanation given to them was sufficient, however for some, there was an inability to understand the terms." Another study[43] quoted a donor husband: "I was all mixed up, you see, and my head was spinning around." This man later described how he had come to understand: "The best way that one of the doctors said to me was like you've got a jigsaw [puzzle] and one piece of the jigsaw [puzzle] is missing and you take it away and all the rest of the pieces are trying to, but it doesn't work. It's like that with the brain."[43]

Option of Organ Donation

As stated earlier, it is helpful wherever possible to offer hope to the family members. If death has occurred, all hope of recovery for their loved one is lost, but the bereaved can be offered an option of hope and life for others through organ and tissue donation. Tissue donation (i.e., corneal, heart valves, and skin) can be offered in most cases of asystolic death. Kidney donation can follow asystolic death in certain circumstances and, indeed, donation from "non-heart-beating donors" is increasing and these organs are valuable additions to the donor pool. Clinicians should consider the possibility of donation in every case of death and should seek specific advice from the local transplant coordinator service.

Multiple Organ Donation

Brainstem death can offer the family the option of multiple organ donation. Reports suggest that many clinicians are reluctant to introduce the option of donation because they fear that such a suggestion may increase the grief of the bereaved. Research studies have shown, however, that families gain enormous comfort from the knowledge that their tragedy has resulted in life for others. Merchant et al.[41] reported that "donation has a beneficial effect on the bereavement process." Tavakoli and colleagues[62] concluded that "organ donors' relatives reported the effectiveness of organ donation to alleviate their grief: 66% completely and 32% partially." A Dutch study supported the previous surveys and noted that some families who had refused donation regretted their decision at a later stage. Also, a study by Ormrod et al.[46] reported that "no relatives who agreed to organ donation regretted this but three who did not allow donation subsequently expressed regret." Such research conclusions are supported further by the positive feedback from donor families that is reported by the transplant coordinator teams.

Organ donation can provide something positive in an otherwise negative situation. Offering the choice to donate, if performed with empathy, does not increase the distress of the bereaved. The bereaved should not be denied this choice or this chance of comfort. A letter from a donor mother reads: "It is certainly a source of comfort to me and indeed to all our family to know that our son has been able to touch and enrich the lives of others."

When to Offer the Option of Donation

Several studies have reported that the timing of the approach may be the crucial factor in the potential family's ability to give permission for organ donation.[13,20] These studies suggest that several factors influence the consent process. First, the longer the patient is in the hospital, the more time the family members have to appreciate the fact that the patient is critically ill and will not survive. It seems to follow that family members who have had more time to absorb and accept the prognosis are better able to move beyond the denial phase and become more receptive to options. Second, the timing of the approach for organ donation has significant consequences. Research suggests that if the request for donation is made after notification of death, as opposed to before or simultaneously with the notification of death, the family members are more likely to grant consent for donation, and this trend seems to hold true regardless of whoever makes the request. Ehrle and coworkers[13] stated that one must allow time for the family members to accept death before the approach for organ donation is made.

Who Should Approach Family Members

There is no one person who is ideal to approach the family members because of the enormous variety of individuals and situations. It is most appropriate for the person who has formed a close and trusting relationship with the family members to introduce the option of donation. It is essential that this person has a positive commitment to donation and introduces donation in a positive way. Cohen and colleagues[8] examined the attitudes of healthcare professionals to brain death and the influence of their attitudes on the organ donation process. They found that "overall 78.9% of respondents had a positive attitude to brain death and that these respondents felt significantly more comfortable informing the transplant co-ordinator of a potential donor, explaining brain death to the family, raising the subject of organ donation, approaching the family about donation and providing support to the grieving family."[8]

A UK study[64] reported that clinicians working in the crisis areas thought that a lack of training and a lack of experience in offering the option of donation inhibited them in making the request. Many countries now recognize that clinicians require special communication skills to deal adequately with the bereaved and the request for donation and have introduced training programs to enhance these skills. A Canadian study showed that each experience of making the donation request built confidence. Every clinician who was experienced in talking to family members about organ donation felt positively about the experience and believed that requesting donation was easier than seeking permission for a postmortem examination.

It is helpful to remember that the family members are being asked to relate the wishes of their relative and whether objections to donation had been expressed, freeing the family members from accepting responsibility for the decision. Many family members may have discussed the idea of organ donation previously, perhaps at a time of national publicity. This knowledge of their loved one's wishes helps them with their response. It is reported widely that bereaved family members strive to fulfill the wishes of their relative at the time of death, and the presence of an organ donor card, registration on a donor registry, or a living will may help the family members toward a positive response. The bereaved may inquire about the possibility of donation before a formal approach is made.

However, Sque et al.[59] report that four main categories were identified that illustrated issues that influenced families' ability to agree or decline donation: (1) knowledge of the deceased's donation wish; (2) views held by the extended family about donation; (3) giving meaning to the death; and (4) events that occurred in the hospital that were perceived as positive or negative. This study and other studies stress the need for care in the way information is given and in the way that donation is introduced and offered to families.

How to Approach Family Members

Staff members often are reluctant to raise the question of donation because they fear that they may increase the family members' distress by saying the wrong thing. There are no right words, however; each situation is unique, and family members have their own individual responses. Requests for organ donation cannot be preplanned, although anxiety can be reduced for the person making the request if suitable phrases are considered before meeting with the family members. An example follows:

> Family member: He was a lovely man; he didn't deserve to die.
>
> Response: He sounds like a lovely man; do you think his generosity would extend to helping others through his death?

Family members respond to the option of donation in a variety of ways. Whatever the response, the caregiver should show empathy and understanding. Some family members require time to consider their response and should be offered privacy. Many relatives have additional questions concerning the process of donation and its implications. It is helpful to use open-ended questions, beginning with how, where, or what (i.e., "What further information would you like?"), at this time. Such questions offer the bereaved the opportunity to make choices and to gain the information that is important to them.

Research suggests that at this time it may be helpful for the bereaved to meet with a member of the transplant team, usually the transplant coordinator, who can answer specific questions and start to develop a rapport with the bereaved. Family members require reassurance that their loved one will be treated with dignity and respect throughout the donor surgery, that the body will not be mutilated or grossly disfigured, that the surgical wound will be sutured, that they can view the body after surgery, and that the funeral will not be delayed. The transplant coordinator works closely with other healthcare professionals to answer such questions and to facilitate the wishes of the family members. It often is comforting for the family members to know that the transplant coordinator will be present throughout the donor surgery and will perform the final care in accordance with their wishes.

There will always be family members, regardless of the manner in which the request is offered, who refuse the option of organ donation, and healthcare professionals must accept this decision. If the family members seem undecided or if the immediate response is an angry "no," it is acceptable, after a short period of reflection, to explore gently the reasons for such a response. It is found frequently that the family members may have specific concerns or unfounded ideas and fears that can be allayed by further information, removing the barriers to permission.

Research suggests that the most commonly quoted reasons for refusal include the following: the deceased had stated that he or she did not wish to donate; a fear of gross mutilation; a difference of opinion between family members; problems understanding brainstem death; and religious reasons. Regarding the last-mentioned reason, however, all the major religions support the act of donation.

If the family members agree to organ donation, many relatives may wish to spend time alone with their loved one so that they might say goodbye before the scheduled surgery. The opportunity to touch or kiss is especially appreciated. Family members should be offered privacy and should never be hurried.

Information after the donation is provided to the family members, unless they express otherwise. This feedback contains general anonymous information about the recipients and offers further contact and support. Some transplant coordinating teams offer postdonation home visits so that ongoing support is activated and any subsequent anxieties or concerns can be addressed. In some areas, donor family support groups are available.

Most centers facilitate the exchange of letters between recipients and donor families, believing that the bereaved gain comfort from the personal gratitude and wellbeing of the recipient, and that recipients need to express their thanks to adapt psychologically and to assimilate the new organ into their body and their new life. A few centers help to arrange meetings between the donor family and the recipient; however, such meetings are controversial (see discussion in earlier section).

Staff Support

The care of individuals who grieve is an important part of clinical practice; however, dealing with the dying and their family members is stressful for staff, and if this stress is unresolved, the individual staff member may become depressed and burned out. A supportive environment can reduce this stress; such an environment requires that staff members care about each other, listening to each other's problems, and offering support across all levels. Healthcare professionals have individual coping strategies, but also they should have the opportunity to discuss issues of death and dying together formally or informally as required. Clinicians who do not have this opportunity to replenish their own emotional reserves may find that they do not have anything left to give to future patients and their families.

Viewing the Body after Death

All family members should be offered the opportunity to view the patient after death. If they are reluctant, they should be encouraged gently because it is an important step in accepting the reality of the situation. The body should be prepared carefully, and the bereaved should be given privacy and permission to touch, hold, and kiss as desired. The loss of a young child is particularly distressing, and parents may appreciate a lock of hair or a photograph or handprints.

Further Care

Before family members return home, it is important that they are aware of follow-up arrangements. In most cases, this follow-up involves an appointment with the bereavement officer, who offers help and information concerning the tasks that lie ahead. In some cases, it may be appropriate to arrange a further meeting with medical staff so that additional questions may be answered.

Advice concerning expected grief reactions may be helpful; relatives can be overwhelmed by the enormity and intensity of their distress. It is important that local support is available, and the clinician should alert the family physician or other support person to the needs of the bereaved. Some relatives may request medication, but in most cases the request should be denied gently because sedation dulls reality and response and inhibits the process of grief. Most families recover from the death through the normal phases of grief. If a family member experiences specific problems, further help should be offered. Information about local bereavement organizations that can offer practical advice and experienced counseling should be made available.

Death and bereavement are an integral part of human life, and the care of individuals who grieve is an important part of clinical practice. All professionals approach the tasks of "breaking bad news" and "informing of death" with trepidation. With a knowledge of grief patterns and appropriate communication skills, it is possible to feel more comfortable with the situation and to offer empathetic and understanding care. Experience suggests that when relatives are approached sensitively, the subject of organ donation does not increase their distress. Many families gain comfort through donation and transplantation – something positive from a totally negative situation.

CONCLUSION

Kidney transplantation is the treatment of choice for most patients with end-stage renal disease. Life with the best-functioning transplanted kidney is a life with uncertainty, however. The fear and possibility of rejection are constant. Immunosuppressive therapy can lead to psychiatric and psychological morbidity, and necessary shifts in family dynamics and readjustment into society can cause emotional difficulties.

Publius Syrus (first century BC) wrote that "pain of mind is worse than pain of body." Understanding of the psychological aspects of transplantation has grown in recent years, and this increased understanding has resulted in the opportunity to offer informed psychological support as an integral part of transplantation care, reducing psychological morbidity, and enhancing rehabilitation and quality of life.

REFERENCES

1. Albertsmeyer S, Renner FC, Yildiz S, et al. One hundred six live kidney donors in a single German transplantation center: renal, physical, and psychological follow-up. Transplant Proc 2010;42(10):3992–3.
2. Bradley C, McGee H. Improving quality of life in renal failure: ways forward. In: McGee H, Bradley C, editors. Quality of life following renal failure. Chur, Switzerland: Harwood Academic Publishers; 1994.
3. Butt Z, Jensen SE, Daud A, et al. What is the quality of life impact of living donor nephrectomy? Clin Transl Sci 2010;3(2).
4. Castelnuovo-Tedesco P. Transplantation: psychological implications of changes in body image. In: Levy NB, editor. Psychonephrology, vol 1: psychological factors in haemodialysis and transplantation. New York: Plenum; 1981.
5. Cetingol M, Winsett R, Hathaway D. A comparative study of quality of life among the age groups of kidney transplant recipients. Prog Transplant 2004;14:33–8.
6. Chisholm MA. Enhancing transplant patients' adherence to medication therapy. Clin Transplant 2002;16:30–8.
7. Chisholm-Burns M, Pinsky B, Rehfeld R, et al. Patient reported factors influencing adherence to antirejection medications. Am J Transplant 2010;10:204.

8. Cohen J, Ami SB, Ashkenazi T, et al. Attitude of health care professionals to brain death: influence on the organ donation process. Clin Transplant 2008;22(2):211–5.
9. Crombie AK, Franklin PM. Family issues implicit in living donation. Mortality 2006;11:196–210.
10. Cukor D, Peterson RA, Cohen SD. Depression in end-stage renal disease hemodialysis patients. Nat Clin Pract Nephrol 2006;2:678–87.
11. Darabi M, Shakibi M. Evaluation of patient's sexual function before and after renal transplantation. J Sex Med 2010;7 (suppl. 6):397.
12. De Klerka M, De Zuidema M, Izermans JN, et al. Alternatives for unsuccessful living donor kidney exchange pairs. Clin Transpl 2010;327–32.
13. Ehrle RN, Schafer TJ, Nelson KR. Referral, request, and consent for organ donation: best practice – a blue print for success. Crit Care Nurse 1999;19:21.
14. Engel G. Psychological development in health and disease. Philadelphia: WB Saunders; 1962.
15. Evans RW, Manninen DL, Garrison Jr LP, et al. The quality of life of patients with end stage renal disease. N Engl J Med 1985;312:553.
16. Fehrman-Ekholm I, Brink B, Ericsson C, et al. Kidney donors don't regret. Transplantation 2000;69:2067.
17. Fellner CH, Marshall JR. Kidney donors: the myth of informed consent. Am J Psychiatry 1970;126:1245.
18. Fox RC, Swazey JP. Spare parts: organ replacement in American Society. New York: Oxford University Press; 1992.
19. Franklin PM, Crombie AK. Live related renal transplantation: psychological, social, and cultural issues. Transplantation 2003;76:1247–51.
20. Garrison RN, Bentley FR, Reyne GH, et al. There is an answer to the shortage of organ donors. Surg Gynaecol Obstet 1991;173:391.
21. Gill P, Lowes L. The kidney transplant failure experience: a longitudinal case study. Prog Transplant 2009;19(2):114–21.
22. Haddow G. Donor and nondonor families' accounts of communication and relations with health care professionals. Prog Transplant 2004;14:41.
23. Haferkamp L, Trk T, Franke GH, et al. Registration of medication compliance in kidney transplant recipients by using the Essen Compliance Score (ECS). NDT Plus 2010;3.
24. Harwood L, Locking-Cusolito H, Spittal J, et al. Preparing for haemodialysis: patient stressors and responses. Nephrol Nurs J 2005;32:295–303.
25. Hudson K, Hiott K. Coping with pediatric renal transplant rejection. Am Nephrol Nurs Assoc J 1986;13:261.
26. Jacobs C, Johnson E, Anderson K, et al. Kidney transplants from living donors: how donation affects family dynamics. Adv Renal Ther 1998;5:89.
27. Jakobsen A. Living renal transplantation: the Oslo experience. Nephrol Dial Transplant 1997;12:1825.
28. Kimmel P, Peterson R, Weihs K. Multiple measurements of depression predict mortality in a longitudinal study of chronic hemodialysis out-patients. Kidney Int 2000;57:2093–8.
29. Landreneau K, Lee K, Landreneau MD, et al. Quality of life in patients undergoing hemodialysis and renal transplantation. Nephrol Nurs J 2010;37(1):37–46.
30. Lerda S, Lasaponara F, Zullo G, et al. Female sexual function and quality of life in dialysis and renal transplant patients. J Psychosom Res 2010;68(6).
31. Levey AS, Hon S, Bush Jr. HL. Kidney transplantation from unrelated living donors: time to reclaim a discarded opportunity. N Engl J Med 1986;314:914.
32. Levy NB. Renal transplantation and the new medical era. Adv Psychosom Med 1986;15:167.
33. Lindgvisit R, Carlsson M, Sjod N. Perceived consequences of being a renal failure patient. Nephrol Nurs J 2000;27:291–8.
34. Lloyd-Williams M, Morton J, Peters S, et al. The end-of-life care experiences of relatives of brain dead intensive care patients. J Pain Symptom Manage 2009;37(4):659–64.
35. Long T, Sque M, Addington-Hall J, et al. Conflict rationalization: how family members cope with a diagnosis of brain stem death. Soc Sci Med 2008;67(2):253–61.
36. Long T, Sque M, Addington-Hall J, et al. What does a diagnosis of brain death mean to family members approached about organ donation? A review of the literature. Prog Transplant 2008;18(2):118–25, quiz 126.
37. McDonald SP, Russ GR. Survival of recipients of cadaveric kidney transplants compared with those receiving dialysis treatment in Australia and New Zealand. Nephrol Dial Transplant 2002;17(12):2212–9.
38. Maglakelidze N, Pantsulaia T, Mangadze L, et al. Assessment of health-related quality of life in renal transplant recipients and dialysis patients. Transplant Proc 2011;43(1):376–9.
39. Maglakelidze N, Pantsulaia T, Managadze L, et al. Assessment of health-related quality of life in living kidney donors. Transplant Proc 2011;43(1):373–5.
40. Massey E, Kranenburg L, Zuidema WC, et al. Favourable psychological outcomes among good samaritan donors: a follow-up study. Am J Transplant 2010;10:.
41. Merchant SJ, Yoshida EM, Lee TK, et al. Exploring the psychological effects of deceased organ donation on the families of organ donors. Clin Transplant 2008;22(3):341–7.
42. Morelon E, Berthoux F, Brun-Strang C, et al. Partners' concerns, needs and expectations in ESRD: results of the CODIT Study. Nephrol Dial Transplant 2004;20(8):1670–5.
43. Najarian JS. Living donor kidney transplants personal reflections. Transplant Proc 2005;37:3592–4.
44. National Institute for Health and Clinical Excellence (NICE). Depression in adults with chronic physical health problems. Treatment and Management 91. London: NICE; 2009.
45. Nicholson M, Elwell R, Kaushik M, et al. Health-related quality of life after living donor nephrectomy: a randomized controlled trial of laparoscopic versus open nephrectomy. Transplantation 2011;91(4):457–61.
46. Ormrod JA, Ryder T, Chadwick RJ, et al. Experiences of families when a relative is diagnosed brain stem dead: understanding of death, observation of brain stem death testing and attitudes to organ donation. Anaesthesia 2005;60(10):1002–8.
47. Peretz D. Development, object relations and loss. In: Schuengberg B, Carr AC, Peretz D, editors. Loss and grief: psychological management in medical practice. New York: Columbia University Press; 1970.
48. Phillips A. Can you take the pain out of death? An interview by Catherine O'Brien. Times November 10, 1999.
49. Prasad GVR, Nash M, McFarlane P, et al. Renal transplant recipient attitudes toward steroid use and steroid withdrawal. Clin Transplant 2003;17:135–9.
50. Rodrique J, Dimitri N, Reed A, et al. Spouse caregivers of kidney transplant patients: quality of life and psychosocial outcomes. Prog Transplant 2010;20(4):335–44.
51. Russell CL, Kilburn E, Conn VN, et al. Medication-taking beliefs of adult renal transplant recipients. Clin Nurse Spec 2003;17:200–10.
52. Russell S, Jacob RG. Living related organ donation: the donor's dilemma. Patient Educ Couns 1994;21:89.
53. Schover LR, Streem SB, Boparai N, et al. The psychological impact of donating a kidney: long-term follow up from a urology based center. J Urol 1997;157:1596.
54. Segoloni GP, Piccoli GB, Leonardi G. Kidney transplantation before starting dialysis therapy. G Ital Nefrol 2002;19:168–77.
55. Simmons RG, Anderson C, Kamstra L. Comparison of quality of life on continuous ambulatory peritoneal dialysis, hemodialysis and after transplantation. Am J Kidney Dis 1984;4:253.
56. Simmons RG, Klein SD, Simmons RL. The gift of life: the social and psychological impact of organ transplantation. New York: John Wiley; 1977.
57. Smith MD, Cappell DF, Province MA, et al. Living related kidney donors: a multi-centre study of donor education, socio-economic adjustment and rehabilitation. Am J Kidney Dis 1986;8:223.
58. Speck P. Loss and grief in medicine. London: Bailliere Tindall; 1978.
59. Sque M, Long T, Payne S, et al. Organ donation: key factors influencing families' decision-making. Transplant Proc 2005;37(2):543–6.
60. Surman OS. Psychiatric aspects of organ transplantation. Am J Psychiatry 1989;146:972.
61. Sylvia C. A change of heart. New York: Little, Brown; 1997.
62. Tavakoli SA, Shabanzadeh SP, Arjmand B, et al. Comparative study of depression and consent among brain death families in donor and non-donor groups from March 2001 to December 2002 in Tehran. Transplant Proc 2008;40(10):3299–302.
63. Tong A, Morton R, Howard K, et al. When i had my transplant, i became normal. Adolescent perspectives on life after kidney transplantation. Nephrology 2010;15:285–93.
64. Wakeford RE, Stepney R. Obstacles to organ donation. Br J Surg 1989;76:436.
65. Wilkins F, Bozik K, Bennett K. The impact of patient education and psychosocial supports on return to normalcy 36 months post-kidney transplant. Clin Transplant 2003;17(Suppl. 9):78–80.

CHAPTER 41

ETHICAL AND LEGAL ASPECTS OF KIDNEY DONATION

Frederike Ambagtsheer • Willem Weimar

CHAPTER OUTLINE

DEFINITIONS

Altruism: A moral act intended to promote the happiness of others

Biomedicine Convention: Legally binding treaty, drafted by the Council of Europe for the Protection of Human Rights and Dignity of the Human Being with Regard to the Application of Biology and Medicine

Black market of organs: Illegal market that coexists to meet the demand that altruistic systems fail to fulfill

Conditional donation: When a donor organ is offered to a specific class of recipient

Hippocratic oath: Requires doctors to do what they consider beneficial for their patients and to "abstain from whatever is deleterious and mischievous"

Home-based education programs: Patient and family education on transplantation and donation in the patient's own environment

Informed consent: Medical doctors provide a patient with all relevant information about a proposed procedure or treatment prior to obtaining the consent of the patient to carry out the procedure. This ensures that the autonomy of the individual is respected

Justice: Requires a fair opportunity for everyone in need of an organ transplant

Monopsonistic market: A regulated market of organ sales confined to a self-governing geopolitical area such as a nation state or the European Union

Organ trafficking: The recruitment, transport, transfer, harboring, or receipt of living or deceased persons or their organs by means of the threat or use of force or other forms of coercion, of abduction, of fraud, of deception, of the abuse of power or of a position of vulnerability, or of the giving to, or the receiving by, a third party of payments or benefits to achieve the transfer of control over the potential donor, for the purpose of exploitation by the removal of organs for transplantation

Paternalism: Neglecting a competent person's will or even acting against it

Pre-emptive transplantation: Transplantation that takes place prior to commencement of dialysis

Principle of non-maleficence: This principle stems from the Latin phrase *primum non nocere*, which means "first (or above all) do no harm"

Specified direct donation: When a person donates directly to his or her intended recipient

Specified indirect donation: When a person donates indirectly to his or her intended recipient or donates to a specified recipient through an exchange program

Subsidiarity: Removal of organs or tissue from a living person may be carried out where there is no suitable organ or tissue available from a deceased person

Transplant commercialism: A policy or practice in which an organ is treated as a commodity, including by being bought or sold or used for material gain

Transplant tourism: Travel for transplantation that involves organ trafficking and/or transplant commercialism or if the resources (organs, professionals, and transplant centers) devoted to providing transplants to patients from outside a country undermine the country's ability to provide transplant services for its own population

Travel for transplantation: The movement of organs, donors, recipients or transplant professionals across jurisdictional borders for transplantation purposes

Unspecified donation: Donation to an anonymous and unspecified recipient such as donation to the waiting list or to the recipient of an exchange couple in the case of domino-paired exchange

Utility: Each organ should be transplanted into a recipient in whom it will survive the longest

Volenti non fit iniuria: When the person concerned consents, no injury is done

World Health Organization (WHO): The United Nations specialized agency that coordinates international public health

INTRODUCTION

In organ transplantation an increasing amount of emphasis is given to ethical and legal aspects. The main reason for this is, of course, the increasing organ scarcity.[90] The range of ethical and legal considerations in relation to organ donation that is focused on in scholarly literature is considerable. This chapter aims to provide a snapshot of important ethical and legal principles that arise in contemporary, everyday medical practice concerning both deceased and living organ donation (LOD) and transplantation. The focus will primarily be on kidneys. This chapter presents ethical and legal considerations that arise in: (1) deceased donor organ allocation; (2) the expansion and encouragement of living kidney donation (LKD); and (3) commercialization of organs.

DECEASED DONOR ORGAN ALLOCATION

In general, three key principles govern the allocation of deceased donor organs[11]:

1. Impartial equitable allocation according to the principles of justice and equity
2. The requirement of informed consent
3. The absence of conditionality.

Each principle is addressed below.

Justice Versus Utility

Perhaps the greatest challenge faced by transplant professionals is how, according to what criteria, organs should be allocated. A range of options exist when considering the distribution of scarce resources. These include distribution on the basis of social worth or merit, according to the ability to pay, by queue (first come, first served), by lottery (chance), and by maximum benefit (greatest good to the greatest number). The last method is considered most appropriate by the international transplant community.[10]

However, maximizing the benefit of this scarce resource raises ethical issues about the utility of transplantation versus equitable access. The utilitarian argument proclaims that each organ should be transplanted into a recipient in whom it will survive the longest (optimal benefit from each organ). The principle of equity or justice requires a fair opportunity for everyone in need of an organ transplant.[10]

Which of the two is the better way to allocate organs? According to Courtney and Maxwell, transplant doctors must always find a compromise between both potentially conflicting ethical principles.[10] Veatch argues that the conflict between both principles is inevitable. In order to resolve the conflict, one must be aware of the problems caused by each principle.[87]

Problems Caused by Utility

Organ allocation networks were for a long time driven by utilitarian considerations. The US United Network for Organ Sharing, for instance, used to allocate livers in a way it believed would produce the most benefit. That meant giving livers to healthier and to local patients first. Giving organs to those who are sickest was not favored, because it meant decreased survival rates. It was believed that local allocation would encourage more people to donate. Local priority also meant shorter cold ischemia times and better graft and patient survival rates.

The same considerations were applied to kidney allocation. In the 1980s, transplant doctors gave priority to recipients who had the best human leukocyte antigen (HLA)–antigen match. The problem was that allocating on the basis of HLA-matching criteria may favor more healthy patients at the expense of sicker patients. Allocating organs on the basis of utility only excludes patients that have an older age, are diabetic or obese, or carry other comorbidities. Maximizing medical utility also requires relying on social data to identify groups that do better statistically, regarding for instance race, income, and gender. Defenders of the principle of justice or equity thus began to claim that allocating on the basis of utility was unfair.[87]

Problems Caused by Justice or Equity

In the 21st century, more allocation policies arose that were based on justice. Justice is considered synonymous with the concept of equity and associated with the idea of equal treatment or non-discrimination.[63]

The problem with justice as a criterion, however, is that it is not exactly clear what is meant by justice. One interpretation is to allocate organs to those on the wait list that are the "worst off." But what is meant by saying that justice requires giving priority to the worst-off patients? Similarly to those who endorse utility, a group could be selected who are socially worst off, but may not have a serious medical disease. And even if we do focus on those who are medically worst off, it still remains unclear which candidates on the wait list should be labeled worst off. The Model for End-Stage Liver Disease formula, to allocate liver grafts, implies that the worst off are those in most urgent need, and who will die the soonest. However, one could also argue that the organs should go to the person with the most severe complaints, even if he or she is not predicted to die very soon.

Who Decides Between Justice and Utility?

Who decides what the morally acceptable way of allocation is?

Most countries have no explicit legal provisions governing the manner of organ allocation.[63] Most laws state or imply that the allocation criteria should be medical only, thus leaving the question open on what ethical criterion the allocation should be based.[42]

The Council of Europe Convention for the Protection of Human Rights and Dignity of the Human Being with Regard to the Application of Biology and Medicine (1996) (Biomedicine Convention) states that "Parties, taking into account health needs and available resources, shall take appropriate measures with a view to providing, within their jurisdiction, equitable access to health care of appropriate quality" (Article 3).[8] This is proclaimed in accordance with the purpose of the Convention (Article 1) that states that the treatment of persons shall be "without discrimination."[8]

The Additional Protocol to the Biomedicine Convention concerning Transplantation of Organs and Tissues of Human Origin states that "Parties shall guarantee that a system exists to provide equitable access to transplantation services for patients ... organs and, where appropriate, tissues shall be allocated only among patients on an official waiting list, in conformity with transparent, objective and duly justified rules according to medical criteria."[9] The World Health Organization (WHO) states that "in the light of the principles of distributive justice and equity, donated organs should be made available to patients on the basis of medical need and not on the basis of financial or other considerations."[93]

The aforementioned provisions illustrate the legal intention that access and allocation cannot rely on non-medical factors. But these laws do not answer the question of who is allowed to "pick and choose" between utility and justice.

Transplant professionals, driven by the Hippocratic oath to do as much good as possible for the patient, commonly tend to lean towards the efficiency side of the calculus (local allocation). The general public,[63] philosophers, and lawyers[87] lean towards justice (national or regional allocation). During a debate about the issue between doctors and non-doctors in 1992, a political compromise was made where justice and utility were considered to count equally in organ allocation.[87]

David Price has stated that both principles are not necessarily in conflict.[63] Both are possible criteria for allocating organs. Veatch says that balancing the competing claims is a process for public debate "by the entire moral community."[87]

Allocation of Marginal Donors

Extended Donor Criteria

Due to the increasing organ scarcity, an increasing number of organs are now donated that would have been considered unsuitable for transplantation 20 years ago. This includes, for example, organs from donors older than 70 years, from non-heart-beating donors, from donors with hypertension or diabetes, and organs that suffered a long cold ischemia time.[34] The clinical outcome of a proportion of these transplants is poorer than that of donor organs of better quality.

Informed Consent

Based on the informed consent doctrine, potential recipients need to be informed of a possible poorer outcome.[34] However, they should also be made aware of what might happen if they are not transplanted. Informed consent means that "medical doctors provide a patient with all relevant information about a proposed procedure or treatment prior to obtaining the consent of the patient to carry out the procedure."[34]

This doctrine aims to promote individual autonomy, respect human dignity, and avoid deceit and coercion. Although legal standards of disclosure differ between countries, these principles apply to all western legal systems.

Allocation of marginal donor organs raises questions of justice and utility: Who should receive them? From a utilitarian perspective, patients who are not expected to be appropriate recipients will likely be disadvantaged.

Consistent application of this principle would violate the principle of equal respect and the principle that the person in greatest need has special claims to be helped.[34] This applies for instance to the concept of age. Age is taken as evidence that the benefit of the intervention will last shorter. To place older donor kidneys in older patients is common practice in the United States. In Europe this practice has been implemented in the Eurotransplant Senior Program.[25]

Absence of Conditionality

The third principle that governs the allocation of deceased donor organs is the absence of conditionality.[11] For instance, the UK Department of Health states that "it is a fundamental principle of the UK donation program, that organs are freely and unconditionally given. It is therefore not acceptable, to attach any conditions to the donation of organs, other than by specifying the organ/s for which consent/authorisation has been given."[1]

Thus, although an individual is the only person who is entitled to consent to donation of his or her organs, the moment they are donated, and enter the stage of allocation, principles of fairness and equity govern distribution, and not the authority of the individual donor.[11]

Conditional donation challenges these principles. Conditional donation is when a donor organ is offered to a specific class of recipient.[11] Directed donation (further discussed below), when a donor organ is directed towards a specific person, also challenges the principles of fairness and equity. Both forms of donation are considered unacceptable based on current allocation regimes.

Yet one can think of scenarios that may render directed donation acceptable. Take the example of a planned living donation procecure that is underway in accordance with legal and medical requirements. Prior to the procedure, the potential living donor suddenly dies and becomes a deceased organ donor. At a workshop held during the Ethical, Legal, and Psychosocial Aspects of Organ Transplantation (ELPAT) conference, the majority of participants claimed that such deceased directed donation should be allowed. However, most agreed that others in desperate urgent clinical need should not be harmed by the request for the organ by the designated recipient.[11]

EXPANSION AND ENCOURAGEMENT OF LIVING KIDNEY DONATION

New Donor–Recipient Relationships

Due to the shortage of deceased donor kidneys, LKD has become the most important alternative to fulfill the need of the increasing amount of patients with end-stage renal disease in need of transplantation.

World Health Organization

In 1991, the WHO, which is the United Nations (UN) specialized agency that coordinates international public health, drew up guiding principles on human organ transplantation. The aim of the guiding principles was to provide "an orderly, ethical and acceptable framework for regulation of the acquisition and transplantation of human organs."[93] Principle 3 stated that organs for transplantation "should be removed preferably from the bodies of deceased persons." Adult living persons "may donate organs, but in general should be genetically related to the recipient.".[93] Thus, for many years living donation was commonly restricted to genetically related adults.

Expansion of the Donor Pool

However, due to the organ scarcity, strong advancements in transplant technology and excellent results in LKD, the donor pool has expanded over the last three decades from genetically related donors to spouses,[80] friends, acquaintances, and even anonymous donors.[53] The need to expand the living donor pool has been recognized by transplant professionals and international organizations worldwide. By 2010, genetically unrelated donors accounted for 2990/6277 (48%) of LKD in the United States,[85] 574/1262 (45%) in the Eurotransplant area,[25] and 246/473 (52%) in the Netherlands.[16] In 2008 the WHO updated its guiding principles. Principle 3 now states, "living donors should be genetically, legally or emotionally related to their recipients."[94]

Spouses, friends, acquaintances, and other non-genetically related donors are often referred to as "unrelated" donors, to distinguish them from genetically related donors. Yet, many of these genetically unrelated donors have an emotional relationship with their recipient. The use of the term "unrelated" thus seems "inappropriate."[20] The introduction of new schemes, such as paired exchange programs, have contributed to the complexity of donor–recipient relationships.

Ethical, Legal, and Psychosocial Aspects of Organ Transplantation

For this reason, a Working Group of the European Platform on ELPAT developed a new classification for LOD.[20] The group distinguishes between specified and unspecified donation. Specified donation, in turn, can consist of direct and indirect donation through an exchange program. This classification is presented in Table 41-1.

Alternative Living Donation Programs

Examples of successful alternative living donation programs[67] are national kidney-exchange programs,[17,18,61] ABO-incompatible programs,[78] desensitization in HLA-incompatible recipients,[57] and domino-paired anonymous donation.[56,89] National kidney exchange enables incompatible couples to donate and receive a kidney indirectly through exchange with another incompatible couple. This is also referred to as indirect specified donation (Table 41-1). ABO-incompatible programs make it possible to transplant patients despite ABO incompatibility when, after adequate immunoabsorbent and immunomodulating treatment, an adequate decrease in anti-ABO titer can be realized. Desensitization involves the use of preconditioning, either with high-dose intravenous immune globulin

TABLE 41-1 New Ethical, Legal, and Psychosocial Aspects of Organ Transplantation (ELPAT) Classification for Living Organ Donation

Specified Donation
Direct Donation
When a person donates directly to his or her intended recipient
Donation to genetically and emotionally related recipient (e.g., to one's child, parent, or sibling)
Donation to genetically unrelated but emotionally related recipient (e.g., to one's spouse, friend, or acquaintance)
Donation to genetically related but emotionally unrelated recipient (e.g., to an estranged child, parent, or sibling)
Donation to genetically and emotionally unrelated recipient, but the recipient (or the group to which he/she should belong) is specified (e.g., to persons younger than 18 years or a specific person in need of a transplantation, who was interviewed by the media)
Indirect Donation
When a person donates indirectly to his or her intended recipient
Donation to a specified recipient through an exchange program
Unspecified Donation
Donation to an anonymous and unspecified recipient (e.g., donation to the waiting list or to the recipient of an exchange couple in the case of domino-paired exchange)

From Dor F, Massey E, Frunza M, et al. New classification of ELPAT for living organ donation. Transplantation 2011;91:935–8.

or with plasmapheresis plus low-dose intravenous immune globulin to enable transplantation across HLA barriers.[57] In a domino-paired anonymous donation, the anonymous donor donates to the recipient of an incompatible couple, while the potential donor of this couple donates to a patient on the waiting list (domino donor).[67] This is referred to as unspecified donation (Table 41-1).

The contribution of exchange programs to the overall number of LKDs has been significant. In the Netherlands, for example, by 2010, almost 30% of LKDs were performed through alternative living donation programs.[21]

The Welfare and Protection of the Live Donor

The Principle of Non-Maleficence

The expansion of specified and unspecified LKD raises ethical and legal considerations. One of the most frequently mentioned considerations is that LOD violates the principle of non-maleficence. This principle stems from the Latin phrase, *primum non nocere*, which means "first (or above all) do no harm".[4] The origins of this phrase however are unknown. It is not a literal translation of any part of the Hippocratic oath,[30] which requires doctors to do what they consider beneficial for their patients and to "abstain from whatever is deleterious and mischievous." The oath does not mention anything about "first or 'above all' do no harm".[30]

The Hippocratic oath, although a prominent principle in medical practice,[4] is not absolute.[31] It is a prima facie obligation – one that can be overridden if there are compelling counterobligations. Indeed, many medical procedures cause harm even as they benefit the patient.[31,68]

Risks Versus Benefits

In LOD, the health of one individual is put at risk in order to benefit another.[31] The justification for LOD, especially LKD, thus lies in the expectance that the benefits outweigh the harms.[68] Thus, if the benefits to the donor (psychological and moral) outweigh the risks to the donor (physical and possibly psychological), then LOD is morally permissible.[53,68] Therefore, arguments given against LOD on the claim that it violates the physician's responsibility not to do harm are not convincing.[68]

Donor Risks in Living Kidney Donation

The foregoing implies a need to understand the physical and psychological risks for the donor. The protection of live donors from these possible harms is emphasized in various national and international (legal) rules and regulations. The EU Directive on Standards of Quality and Safety of Human Organs intended for Transplantation states that "the highest possible protection of living donors should be ensured."[19] The WHO underpins that "live donations are acceptable when the donor's informed and voluntary consent is obtained, when professional care of donors is ensured and follow-up is well organized."[94]

Even though LKD transplantation has acquired an outstanding record worldwide, LKD involves risks, including morbidity and mortality, for the live donor. Nevertheless, these risks are very low. The risk of death is cited as 1 in 3000 (0.03%) and the risk of postoperative morbidity is 2–4%.[12,52] It is conceivable that the more widespread use of laparoscopic nephrectomy techniques will decrease morbidity in the coming years.[41]

Psychological harms of the donor may involve coercion. Arguably, there is always coercion in LKD, especially when the person suffering is a loved one. Pressure may be put on people to donate, leading those who are reluctant to do so to feel coerced.[81]

Elliott has argued that, to minimize the likelihood of coercion or other psychological harms of the live donor, LKD should be restricted to relatives.[22] This belief is shared by Glannon, who also states that the risk in nephrectomy is justified because of shared emotions amongst family members, but that these factors are lacking when the donor is not a relative.[35] The argument here is that the suffering of another person is perceived to be felt more intensively if the person concerned is a relative. If, for example a mother offers to donate her organ to her daughter, her explanation that her donation occurs for the sake of her child will be deemed sufficient. In contrast, if an altruistic or Samaritan donor offers to donate his or her organ to a stranger, the motivation is often not well understood.[77] Furthermore, these donors do not have the opportunity to witness and enjoy the benefits from the donation. Hence, it is perceived to be more acceptable to benefit from the donor's selflessness when he or she is a relative rather than a stranger.[22]

Coercion may also arise as a result of the expansion of alternative living donation programs. With the increased reliance on exchange programs, for example, comes the increased number of potential, suitable organ donors. In the past, when persons were eventually reluctant to donate, transplant doctors were willing to identify a plausible medical excuse, so that the person could "bow out gracefully."[81] In alternative LKD programs the possibility of a medical excuse for unwilling donors no longer exists.[44] In a study performed by Kranenburg et al. amongst 48 donors and recipients, the question was asked whether they felt additional pressure or coerciuon into donating within the exchange donation program. All but two responded that this was not the case.[44]

Legal Restrictions in Europe

The possible physical and psychological risks underlie the justifications given for restrictions in law regarding donor–recipient relationships. In Estonia, for instance, LOD is allowed only for the benefit of the donor's descendant, spouse, cohabitee, parent, grandparent, or their descendants. In the Czech Republic, Finland, Germany, Hungary, Italy, Poland, and Sweden, in addition to the listed relationships, additional donor–recipient relationships are possible due to an open clause. Denmark, the Netherlands, and Switzerland, by contrast, do not have any regulations addressing whether donor and recipient have to be related, or whether any specific procedure must be followed.[48]

National kidney exchange problems are legal in the countries that do not require a defined donor–recipient relationship (Belgium, Denmark, Latvia, the Netherlands, Portugal, Scotland, Spain, Switzerland, and the United Kingdom). In contrast, in Germany, Bulgaria, Estonia, Finland, Hungary, and Lithuania, cross-over LOD is illegal.[48]

Indeed, the differences in these national legal regulations are reflected in the wide disparity in numbers of LKD across Europe.[46]

Equal Donor Risks in Direct, Indirect, and Unspecified Living Organ Donation

Lopp,[47] Hilhorst,[39] and others[12,26,53,68] argue that none of the arguments used to justify restrictions in donor–recipient relationships (based on possible harm inflicted on the donor) are convincing.

First of all they point out that the donor's risks are equally high in direct, indirect, and unspecified LOD.[37,68] Practice and research show that there is no important difference between specified and unspecified LKD in terms of motivations and outcomes.[43,51] Motivations and reasons to donate to strangers, for instance, are found to be equally understandable as donations to relatives. Medical evaluations of unspecified donors have shown these donors to be truly generous and selfless.[51,59]

In fact, when comparing the donation to benefit a stranger to the donation to benefit a relative, the unspecified donation could be regarded as the highest expression of altruism.[47] Indeed, altruism may "receive its highest expression in the absence of personal relationships".[26] The special relationship between a donor and recipient, according to Hilhorst et al., is "not the morally relevant key feature that provides a justification for LKD."[39] Both specified and unspecified donation, Lopp argues, should be treated equally.[47]

Donor Autonomy

The same authors claim that these restrictions violate the donor's right to autonomy. When donors voluntarily decide to take part in the surgery, they exercise their right of autonomy and thus cannot be considered to be harmed. This argument is also referred to as the *volenti non fit iniuria* principle.[13] This principle means that, when the person concerned consents, no injury is done.[13,47]

The concept of informed consent is closely related to the right of autonomy.[47] Informed consent ensures that the autonomy of the individual is respected.[47] Deception and coercion are mitigated by consent procedures, which is why such procedures have become standard requirements in most countries. Reasons to refuse the donation that refer to the donor's best interests can be called paternalistic, that is, "neglecting a competent person's will or even acting against it."[39]

The principle of autonomy is applicable to all donors, be they specified or unspecified. From this perspective it has been argued that, if a competent adult wants to act altruistically and offers to donate his or her organ to a stranger unconditionally, and the adult understands the risks and benefits of the procedure, and gives informed consent to the procurement, then his or her wishes should be respected.[68]

Besides moral arguments to support organ donation by indirect or unspecified donors, there is also a pragmatic reason. Indeed, as illustrated above, there is increasing support for unspecified and indirect donation to relieve the ever-increasing demand for organs.[53,77]

Subsidiarity

Considering the excellent results in LKD, some transplant professionals have raised the question whether "health care professionals should encourage LKD."[12,37] This question touches upon the question whether LKD should be "subsidiary" to deceased donation.

The Additional Protocol to the Biomedicine Convention concerning Transplantation of Organs and Tissues of Human Origin (Article 9) declares that "Removal of organs or tissue from a living person may be carried out ... where there is no suitable organ or tissue available from a deceased person."[9] Many countries, such as Austria, the Czech Republic, Estonia, Finland, Germany, Hungary, Lithuania, Moldova, Portugal, and Slovakia, follow this proclamation and prohibit the performance of LOD when an organ from a deceased person is available.[48]

Other countries, such as Italy, Latvia, the Netherlands, Norway, Poland, Scotland, Slovenia, Spain, Sweden, and Switzerland, and the United Kingdom, do not regulate the relationship between LOD and postmortem donation. In these countries both deceased and living donation are considered equal.[48]

Encouraging Live Kidney Donation

Hilhorst et al. write that good medical and ethical reasons exist to promote the many options of LKD.[37] The advantages of LKD over cadaveric donation are manifold: LKD helps patients to circumvent the waiting list and relieves them of the burden of dialysis. Furthermore, the kidney survival rates for living kidneys are significantly better (50% still functioning after 20 years; for postmortem organs this is only 10 years). Many patients prefer living to cadaveric donation.[45] Transplant care professionals may therefore feel an obligation to bring these facts to the attention of patients and their relatives.[37]

Cronin argues that, given the low risks for the donor, it is not unethical for doctors to encourage healthy adults to donate their kidneys, even to strangers. Demonstrating that such encouragement is unethical requires a powerful argument against it.[12]

Home-Based Education Programs

There are a number of approaches to patient and family education on living donation. One is the "Norwegian approach," where the doctor discusses potential living donors with the patient and then personally contacts these individuals and invites them for evaluation.[36] Another approach (done in the United States) is home-based, where a psychologist gives transplant education to the (pre)dialysis patient and family and friends in the patient's home.[66] This program has proved successful in increasing knowledge and willingness to communicate about living donation and in decreasing living donor transplant concerns.[50]

The home-based program by Massey et al. (the Netherlands) is similar to the US "house call" but offers the educational meeting earlier in the clinical course to include the option of pre-emptive transplantation.[50] Pre-emptive transplantation, that takes place prior to commencement of dialysis, offers optimal graft and patient survival when compared to transplantation after dialysis.[40] Massey et al. state that the "interference in people's lives" is justified if a number of criteria are fulfilled. The criteria that they propose include that the patient decides whom to invite, the invitees have the right to withdraw at any point, and confidentiality should be maintained at all times.[50]

In the foregoing section, we addressed the ethical and legal issues that arise in expanding LKD. The following section focuses on the various considerations that arise in the debate on commercialization of organs.

COMMERCIALIZATION OF ORGANS

The Rise of Organ Trade

Organ Scarcity

Transplantation is becoming a victim of its own success, with demand for organs far outpacing supply.[3] With the aging of populations and growth in heart and vascular diseases, demand for transplantation is increasing exponentially.[27] In the United States, in 2007, 21 489 deceased donors were reported to the Global Database on Donation and Transplantation.[27] As of the end of February 2010, 105 966 patients were on waiting lists for transplantation.[27] According to figures by the European Commission, 40 000 people were on the waiting list for transplants in European Union countries in 2007.[7] In the Eurotransplant region, 15 605 patients were waiting for an organ on January 1, 2011. In this region, a total of 6683 transplants took place in 2010.[25]

Organ Markets

Despite strategies to enlarge the donor organ pool, such as adopting presumed consent systems, widening deceased donor criteria, and increasing the number of living (mainly kidney) donations, the worldwide organ shortage persists. Under these circumstances desperate patients seek strategies to obtain organs from outside their home countries. With organs' increased value comes their increased potential profitability, fueling desire with some people to trade and sell. Hence, next to altruistic procurement systems of organ supply, black markets coexist to meet the demand that altruistic systems fail to fulfill.[32]

The first accounts of organ trade date from the late 1980s by transplant doctors in the Gulf States[72] who were confronted with patients for follow-up who had received transplants of kidneys purchased in India. Around the same time, Scheper-Hughes wrote about "body snatching rumours" that she picked up during her research in Brazil.[74] Most accounts of organ trade in the 1990s were not regarded very seriously. Actual cases were never verified.[6]

Trends and Patterns

From the beginning of the 21st century cases of more verifiable nature came to light. Researchers began to report on negative outcomes of people selling their kidneys in countries such as India,[33] Pakistan,[58] Egypt,[5] and the Philippines.[60] An increasing number of physicians publish articles on the medical outcomes of transplant tourism.[71]

Recurring trends and patterns of organ trafficking generally evolve around a group of "donor-exporting" countries (Egypt, China, India, Pakistan, and the Philippines), "demand" countries (United States, Canada, Israel, United Kingdom, and some other European countries), and countries where the transplants take place, including the United States, Israel, and South Africa.[1,75]

Organ trade does not only involve organized, cross-border trafficking networks. It may also involve milder, more voluntary forms. In a survey performed by Van Buren et al. amongst 250 living kidney donors in Rotterdam, the Netherlands, some donors reported that they had received "rewards" or "gifts" from their recipients. Examples were weekly meals, exotic vacations, a race car, jewelry, a racehorse, and a painting.[86]

The Condemnation of Organ Trafficking, Transplant Commercialism, and Transplant Tourism

Universal Prohibition

Organ trade is prohibited worldwide. The UN Protocol to Prevent, Suppress and Punish Trafficking in Persons, Especially Women and Children, supplementing the UN Convention against Transnational Organized Crime, is the first international legal instrument to define and prohibit trafficking in human beings for the purpose of organ removal (often referred to as organ trafficking). In this definition, organ trafficking is regarded as a form of organized crime and defined in the context of trafficking in human beings.[83]

The WHO first prohibited transplant commercialism in 1987, claiming that such trade is inconsistent with the most basic human values and contravenes the Universal Declaration of Human Rights.[92] Its guiding principles declare that organs should be "donated freely, without any monetary payment or other reward of monetary value".[94] The reason given is that "payment for organs is likely to take unfair advantage of the poorest and most vulnerable groups, undermines altruistic donation, and leads to profiteering and human trafficking. Such payment conveys the idea that some persons lack dignity, that they are mere objects to be used by others."[94] The belief is that altruism rules out any financial motivation for donation. Although organ trafficking and transplant commercialism are separate crimes, commercialism is perceived to lead to trafficking.

Next to the UN and WHO, transplant commercialism and organ trafficking are also forbidden by the Council of Europe in the Protocol concerning transplantation of organs to the Convention on Human Rights and Biomedicine.[9] Article 21 declares that "the human body and its parts shall not, as such, give rise to financial gain or comparable advantage." It also states that "advertising the need for, or availability of, organs or tissues, with a view to offering or seeking financial gain or comparable advantage, shall be prohibited."[9] Article 22 states that "organ trafficking shall be prohibited."[9]

The Declaration of Istanbul

In 2008 the Transplantation Society and International Society of Nephrology convened in Istanbul to establish the Declaration of Istanbul on Organ Trafficking and Transplant Tourism (the Declaration).[62] This is the first document, drawn up by transplant professionals, that defines and condemns organ trafficking, transplant commercialism, and transplant tourism (Table 41-2).

The Declaration, by nature non-binding, has proven to have significant influence. Over 100 transplant organizations endorse its principles. Whereas the Declaration is intended to influence transplant professionals and societies, the WHO intends to influence governments. Both act in concert to address growing problems of transplant commercialism, transplant tourism, and trafficking by strict prohibition and penalization. As a result of the universal prohibition of organ commercialism and trafficking, almost all countries have implemented the prohibition into their domestic laws.

TABLE 41-2 **The Declaration of Istanbul on Organ Trafficking and Transplant Tourism**

Definitions
Organ trafficking is the recruitment, transport, transfer, harboring, or receipt of living or deceased persons or their organs by means of the threat or use of force or other forms of coercion, of abduction, of fraud, of deception, of the abuse of power or of a position of vulnerability, or of the giving to, or the receiving by, a third party of payments or benefits to achieve the transfer of control over the potential donor, for the purpose of exploitation by the removal of organs for transplantation.
Transplant commercialism is a policy or practice in which an organ is treated as a commodity, including by being bought or sold or used for material gain.
Travel for transplantation is the movement of organs, donors, recipients, or transplant professionals across jurisdictional borders for transplantation purposes. Travel for transplantation becomes transplant tourism if it involves organ trafficking and/or transplant commercialism or if the resources (organs, professionals, and transplant centers) devoted to providing transplants to patients from outside a country undermine the country's ability to provide transplant services for its own population.

From Participants in the International Summit on Transplant Tourism and Organ Trafficking Convened by the Transplantation Society and International Society of Nephrology in Istanbul, Turkey, April 30–May 2, 2008. The Declaration of Istanbul on organ trafficking and transplant tourism. Transplantation 2008;86:1013–8.

Rewarded Gifting

The Iranian Model

Iran is the only exception. Iran legally permits transplant commercialism through a government-related, regulated organ procurement system. Confronted with very low deceased donation rates, the government in 1988 introduced a model of "rewarded gifting" to promote live kidney transplantation.[29,76] People who wish to donate can refer to a government institution which matches them to a prospective recipient. Middlemen and brokers, it is claimed, remain uninvolved.[29] All donors receive a payment (the equivalent of $1200) and health insurance from the government. A large number of donors also receive an award or gift from the recipient. This reward is considered a private matter that is not interfered with.[76]

The "Iranian model" is critically scrutinized by some authors,[35] yet others claim that incentives for donation could – and should – be explored in other countries to increase the number of donations.[91] Rewards or incentives can be applied to deceased organ donation and to LKD. A "reward" is defined as a "gesture of gratitude for someone's trouble."[38]

Rewards for Deceased Organ Donation

In 2007 Hilhorst and Van Dijk submitted an advisory report on incentives for donation to the Dutch Health Minister. The report presents two ways of encouraging deceased organ donation by allowing rewards.

The first is rewarding someone for registering as a donor.[38] The report suggests rewards including small gifts (e.g., a discount card or a free first-aid kit), a small sum of money, a free passport, discount on health insurance premiums, and priority on the wait list, if the registree were to need an organ.[38]

The second way of encouraging deceased organ donation is by rewarding surviving relatives. This can occur by giving them a sum of money or by paying the funeral expenses.[38]

The authors conclude that, although these measures may have some impact, financial incentives to stimulate deceased donation are unlikely to produce a really significant effect because the number of organs available is limited and continues to fall.

Rewards for Living Kidney Donation

Already back in 1997, about 10 years after the prohibition of organ sales was first proclaimed,[92] the Bellagio Taskforce wrote that international declarations against commercialism are "put forward in one or two terse sentences with no supporting arguments."[69] Its authors continued to write that "the grounds for condemnation are not as obvious as declarations imply." For that reason it could not find an unarguable ethical principle that justified the ban on organ sales under all circumstances.[69]

The debate over rewarded gifting for live kidney donors has been ongoing since the 1980s and has not achieved consensus.[95] It is conducted from various perspectives, which are outlined below.

Ownership

The concept of ownership addresses the question of who is the owner of the organs. Answers vary from God, the government, to the individual, depending on legal, historic, religious, and medical contexts.[47,95]

In most (western) states, the principle of autonomy is dominant, meaning that (living) individuals are considered to be the owner of their organs.[47] This is why we have full autonomy for dangerous activities such as hang gliding, smoking, bungee jumping, and eating to excess.[28] Governments restrict autonomy if it harms others (e.g., speeding, drunk driving, firearms possession). That is why organ donation is permitted but sale is prohibited).[38,65] Payment is presumed to harm the poor and vulnerable.[94] According to Radcliffe-Richards, this prohibition means that people are unable "to enter freely into contract from which both sides expect to benefit, and with no obvious harm to anyone else."[64]

Indeed, the degree of harm perceived to be inflicted upon organ sellers is not without controversy. Some authors point out that it is a matter of social perception and acceptance of norms. Societal norms differ over time. Issues that used to be considered shocking, such as women's equality, interracial marriage, children born out of wedlock, necropsies, and cadaver organ transplants, are now accepted aspects of western society. Societal norms also vary across countries. Whereas euthanasia, prostitution, abortion, and drug sales are prohibited in many countries, they are accepted phenomena in some others.[28]

According to authors such as Radcliffe-Richards, the prohibition of organ sale violates our right to ownership over our bodies.[64] She argues that individuals should be free to trade organs between themselves and that the burden of proof lies with the government to put forward arguments that justify this prohibition. Friedlaender argues that a future in which people have autonomy in selling their own body parts is not unimaginable.[28]

Payment is Repugnant

Some people believe that the idea of paying for an organ is "repugnant."[73] Yet others do not agree with this argument. They point out that people who buy and sell organs clearly do not feel this repugnance. They argue that something may arouse repugnance without being immoral or being banned. Prostitution, pornography, and the drugs trade can also be repugnant, but that is not a good enough reason to ban them.[38]

Payment Undermines Human Dignity and Integrity

Another reason why payment for organs is prohibited is because it is presumed to "convey the idea that organ sellers lack dignity."[94] An organ is not something for which you should be able to pay. Against this, people claim that it has never been empirically verified whether those selling organs, eggs, or sperm indeed felt diminished self-dignity.[14,55]

It is also claimed that this argument would be a reason to prohibit all living donation, even unpaid ones. The very fact that transplants are possible does actually turn an organ into a commodity, something that has value also outside the body, and that can even be bartered through exchange programs. The organ becomes a (potentially) tradable good.[38] Why are we permitted (in some countries) to barter organs in exchange programs, but not to trade or exchange them to benefit financially the individuals involved?

Payment Undermines Altruism

One of the most widely used arguments against payment is that payment for organs "undermines altruistic donation."[94] Against this, authors claim that altruism as a value is overestimated. They believe that we set ethical standards far too high as a result. In practice, people donate for many different reasons. Why is it an act of altruism for a father in the Philippines to donate his kidney to his daughter who is suffering from a serious kidney disease, but morally reprehensible for the same father to sell his kidney to a third party to raise money to pay for a lifesaving operation for his daughter?[38,64]

The sale of an organ can take place for many different reasons, some of which are altruistic. Several motivations can coexist. As Radcliffe-Richards points out, "Selling in itself is not in itself at odds with altruism, it all depends on what the money is wanted for."[64]

Altruism also plays another part in the debate regarding rewards for organ donation. Why should you as a relative still donate if your intended recipient can obtain a kidney from an anonymous, paid donor instead?

Against this it has been argued that this effect should not necessarily be regarded as a problem. Anyone who thinks that transplants between people who know each other are more desirable than those between strangers would see a decline in related donations as a drawback. But anyone who prefers anonymous donations, for example because they have less impact on family relationships, would see this effect as a benefit. In short, the view that living donation is or should always be an act of altruism is incorrect in both empirical and moral terms. People can have many different reasons in practice for donating an organ without payment.[38]

Payment Jeopardizes Free Will

Prohibition of organ sales exists to protect those (the vulnerable poor) most prone to sell.[94] The argument is that payment jeopardizes their free will, because the poor will feel pressured to sell.

Against this, authors have put forward several counterarguments. First, the question must be raised how money affects the behavior of potential sellers. If a very large sum of money is offered, this might be attractive, even irresistible, to some people. But there is an important distinction between "irresistible" and "forced": putting a gun against a man's head to make him donate is force; offering someone a load of money in return for an organ is an attractive offer.[88] The statement that the donor's free will might be jeopardized is not an argument against payment, but against involuntary donation. Absence of free will is a risk that is associated not only with paid donations, but also with unpaid ones. If vendors can be forced to sell a kidney, then arguably they can also be forced by circumstances such as family pressure or the unbearable sight of seeing a loved one suffer.

In addition, it is said that money is only one factor among many others that determines decisions. Not all people will sell their organs for the sole purpose of payment. Indeed, in a study by Rouchi et al., performed among 600 kidney sellers in Iran, 60% reported their motivations to be partly emotional/altruistic and partly financial.[70] This shows that payment and free will are not mutually exclusive.

Payment Exploits the Poor

Prohibition of organ sales also exists because payment is expected to exploit or traffic the poor. Against this argument various counterarguments have also been given. The first is that prohibition of payment utterly fails to protect the poor and vulnerable. Prohibition does not prevent victimization. On the contrary, prohibition of organ trade has the paradox of increasing the likelihood of commercialism and trafficking. Prohibition of organ payment keeps organ supply low, thus increasing their scarcity. If organs are scarce, they become valuable, and ultimately, profitable to buy, trade, and sell.[2] This has the unintended consequence of driving illegal trade underground where victimization (as illustrated above) of the vulnerable is far more likely to occur than in regulated markets. Furthermore, criminalization of sellers makes it more difficult to identify and help potential victims of trafficking.[2,65] Concern over exploitation of the poor should lead to regulation of a market, not its continued prohibition.[79] Indeed, this argument (prevention of abuses in the black market) was one of the main reasons why prostitution, pornography, abortion, and soft drugs were legalized in the Netherlands. Evidence-based studies have illustrated that legalization has significantly reduced the abuses of the black market.[49]

The second counterargument is related to free will. To justify the prohibition of kidney sales by poor vendors, it is necessary to illustrate that organ selling must always be against the interests of potential vendors. Removing their option to sell leaves them poor, and makes their range of options smaller still. The poorer the potential seller, the more plausible it is that the sale of the organ will be worth whatever risk there is. "If a living donor can do without an organ, why shouldn't the donor profit and medical science benefit?"[65]

To Die or Let Buy?

Some people argue that perhaps it is a good thing that money persuades people to donate. Not only may it more effectively deal with the abuses in current illegal markets; it may also relieve the shortage of organs.[91] Matas states: "organ sale simply does not feel right; but letting candidates die on the waiting list (when this could be prevented) also does not feel right".[55] Are doctors "failing their patients"[28] as long as the ban on payments is maintained?

This may not be applicable in all countries. In some jurisdictions, such as the Netherlands, the number of LKDs is now so high that the waiting list has decreased substantially. Models of rewarded gifting may not be necessary in countries with high LKD rates.

The Live Kidney Donor Contributes Financially to Society

Proponents of financial rewards or incentives for live kidney donors say that the ban on payment is "hypocritical."[23] In contemporary transplant medicine, everyone profits, except the donor: society benefits, the hospital benefits, the surgeon and the medical team are paid, the transplant coordinator gets paid, and the recipient receives an enormous benefit.

Donors, if they are lucky, will be compensated for costs made as a (direct) result of the donation. Compensating live organ donors for certain costs is legitimate, but is not common practice in transplant centres.[46] WHO Guiding Principle 5 states:

> *The prohibition on sale or purchase of cells, tissues and organs does not preclude reimbursing reasonable and verifiable expenses incurred by the donor, including loss of income, or paying the costs of recovering, processing, preserving and supplying human cells, tissues or organs for transplantation.*[94]

The WHO thus permits compensation for the costs of making donations, lest they operate as a disincentive to donation. The need to cover legitimate costs of procurement and of ensuring the safety is acceptable as long as the human body and its parts are not a source of financial gain.[94]

Yet, opponents of the ban on payment say that donors deserve much more than mere compensation or reimbursement of costs. Organ transplants are expensive procedures, yet the long-term care needed while waiting for the transplant (kidney dialysis, for instance), is more expensive than the transplant procedure itself. Transplantation of kidney patients saves the costs patients would otherwise have had on dialysis.

Thus, one live kidney donor makes a significant contribution to society. How much does this contribution entail? De Charro et al.[15] and Matas and Schnitzler[54] illustrate the enormous economic benefit gained with one (live) kidney transplantation. Combining information about quality-adjusted life-years, De Charro et al.[15] estimated that the total benefit to society of one live kidney transplantation equals €80 000 annually (for western countries). Matas and Schnitzler,[54] using the same analysis in the United States, calculate an amount of $100 000 each year.

The authors of these studies suggest that giving such large payments to donors in return for their organs is not impossible. Furthermore, they illustrate that, if a regulated vending system were established for kidney donors, a significant payment could be made to them without increasing the overall costs to the healthcare system.[54]

Hilhorst and Van Dijk on the other hand say that the risk of offering too large a sum of money is that the wrong people, or people with wrong or dubious motives, may register as donors. These may be people who are medically unsuitable or who are not acting freely. It would be better to stay on the safe side and offer small amounts or "indirect" rewards, such as lifelong exemption from medical insurance premiums.[38]

De Charro et al.[15] claim that, given the high amounts, trade is inevitable, whether legal or illegal. Therefore conditions should be implemented, based on regulation, that are favorable from the suppliers'/vendors' and patients' perspectives.

What Works?

An effective approach to organ trade acknowledges that it takes on a wide variety of forms. Only after we agree on the definition of commercialism and trafficking, and on what we find condemnable, can we agree on their prohibition. Putting a price on organs (commercialism) is different from coercing someone into selling one (trafficking).[2,3]

International instruments, such as the Declaration of Istanbul, correctly define and differentiate trafficking from commercialism and tourism, yet they do not mention how both acts should be approached by policy. They wrongly conflate organ trafficking and transplant commercialism to constitute one and the same problem that warrants equally repressive, punitive responses for both. Policies aimed to suppress or reshape an illegal market work differently from policies addressing coercion and other harms associated with trafficking.[2]

Conditions for Regulation

Some authors say that an effective and appropriate response is regulation or a monopsonistic market.[24] They propose the following standards or conditions:

1. The market should be confined to a self-governing geopolitical area such as a nation state or the European Union.
2. Only citizens resident within the union or state could sell into the system and they and their families would be equally eligible to receive organs. Thus organ vendors would know they were contributing to a system which would benefit them and their families and friends since their chances of receiving an organ in case of need would be increased by the existence of the market. (If this were not the case, the main justification for the market would be defeated.)
3. There would be only one purchaser, an agency like the UK National Health Service, which would buy all organs and distribute according to some fair conception of medical priority.
4. There would be no direct sales or purchases, no exploitation of low-income countries and their populations (no buying in Turkey or India to sell in Harley Street).
5. The organs would be tested for human immunodeficiency virus (HIV), etc., their provenance known, and there would be strict controls and penalties to prevent abuse.
6. Prices would have to be high enough to attract people into the marketplace but dialysis, and other alternative care, does not come cheap.
7. Sellers of organs would know they had saved a life and would be reasonably compensated for their risk, time, and altruism.[24,38]

Matas et al. add the following critical elements that such a system would need to comply with[91]:

1. Protection. Risk to the donor should be in accord with currently accepted standards as defined for current donors. The donor benefit (in addition to helping another person) must be an opportunity to improve their own (or their family's) life. Therefore, the donor must be fully informed, understand the risks, understand the nature of the incentive and how it will be distributed, and receive the benefit. There must be follow-up and an opportunity to redress any wrongdoing.
2. Regulation and oversight. Each country will need to enact guidelines for evaluation and selection of donors, institution of the program of incentives and oversight. Regulations and oversight processes must be clearly defined and available for outside review, whether national or international. There must be clearly defined policies for follow-up, outcome determination, and for detection and correction of irregularities. There should be defined consequences for entities within the system that do not adhere to policies.
3. Transparency. Although, for political and legislative reasons, regulation and oversight are only possible at a national level, there must be transparency so that international observation is possible.

Organ Trafficking: Improving the Non-Legislative Response

In contrast to transplant commercialism, there is little doubt that organ trafficking should remain universally prohibited.[3] However, the prohibition of trafficking largely remains a paper exercise. Organ trafficking prosecutions are practically non-existent. Legislative prohibitionist efforts, no matter how sophisticated, are fruitless if they are not accompanied by enforcement by local, national, and international policing agencies.

In 2010 in Vienna, the UN Office on Drugs and Crime organized an expert meeting about the incidence of trafficking in persons for the removal of organs.[84] At this meeting three issues became evident: first, organ-trafficking researchers may have information about organ trafficking, but this information is hardly shared amongst them. Doctors also do not share information about organ trafficking. Second, there are no partnerships between researchers, transplant doctors, and judicial/law enforcers. Third, there is no awareness of the crime among judicial/law enforcement authorities. Organ trafficking is not on the "enforcement agenda" of these authorities. The lack of multinational partnerships hampers effective, non-legislative response to organ trafficking.

Therefore, awareness about the crime should be raised with local, national, and international law enforcement institutions. Partnerships should be established between various groups. Target groups are, for instance, judicial and law enforcement authorities, transplant professionals, international organizations, and human rights organizations involved in the protection of trafficking in human being victims.

Enhanced collaboration between these partnerships can be encouraged by EU funding mechanisms for research projects and cooperation actions, such as by the European Commission Home Affairs program. Other platforms with opportunities for enhanced collaboration lie with the Council of Europe, the WHO, and the Organization for Security and Cooperation in Europe. These organizations are known to have written organ-trafficking reports, yet little collaboration exists between these organizations and law enforcement institutions. Toolkits for member states and competent authorities should be developed that provide indicators for police personnel to identify organ-trafficking activities. Training of police investigators should be encouraged regarding evidence gathering of organ-trafficking cases and know-how about the modus operandi of the actors involved, and training of prosecutors and judges. Bilateral and/or multilateral cooperation in cross-border criminal procedures should be encouraged and established.

CONCLUSION

The aim of this chapter was to illustrate that, with the growth of organ demand, ethical, legal, and psychosocial aspects become more important. Transplant doctors and other professionals are increasingly confronted with these considerations. In contemporary transplant medicine, considerations of an ethical, legal, and psychosocial nature can no longer be ignored.

Acknowledgments

The authors wish to thank Leonie Lopp, Gert van Dijk, Medard Hilhorst, and the ELPAT Working Group on Living Organ Donation (led by Annette Lennerling and Frank Dor) for allowing us to use and refer to their materials.

REFERENCES

1. Allain J. Commentary trafficking of persons for the removal of organs and the admission of guilt of a South African hospital. Med Law Rev 2011;19:117–22.
2. Ambagtsheer F, Weimar W. A criminological perspective: why prohibition of organ trade is not effective and how the declaration of Istanbul can move forward. Am J Transplant 2012;12(3):571–5.
3. Ambagtsheer F, Zaitch D, Willem W. The battle for human organs. Organ trafficking and transplant tourism in a global context. Global Crime 2013. Available online at: http://dx.doi.org/10.1080/17440572.2012.753323.
4. Beauchamp T, Childress J. Principles of biomedical ethics. 5th ed. Oxford: Oxford University Press; 2001.
5. Budiani D. Facilitating organ transplants in Egypt: an analysis of doctors' discourse. Body Soc 2007;13(3):125–49.
6. Campion Vincent V, Scheper-Hughes N. On organ theft narratives. Curr Anthropol 2001;42(4):555–8.
7. Communication from the Commission to the European Parliament and the Council. Organ donation and transplantation: policy actions at EU level. Brussels: European Commission; 2007. Contract no.: COM(2007) 275 final.
8. Council of Europe. Convention for the protection of human rights and dignity of the human being with regard to the application of biology and medicine: convention on human rights and biomedicine. European treaty series no. 164, Oviedo: Council of Europe; 1997.
9. Council of Europe. Additional protocol to the convention on human rights and biomedicine, on transplantation of organs and tissues of human origin. Strasbourg: Council of Europe; 2009.
10. Courtney AE, Maxwell AP. The challenge of doing what is right in renal transplantation: balancing equity and utility. Nephron Clin Pract 2009;111(1):c62–8.
11. Cronin AJ. Directed and conditional donation: reflections on principles and practice. In: Weimar W, Busschbach J, Bos MA, editors. Organ transplantation: ethical, legal and psychosocial aspects expanding the European platform. Munich: Pabst; 2011. p. 180–9.
12. Cronin AJ. Is it unethical for doctors to encourage healthy adults to donate a kidney to a stranger? No. BMJ 2011;343:d7140.
13. Daar AS, Land W, Yahya TM, et al. Living-donor renal transplantation: evidence-based justification for an ethical option. Transplant Rev 1997;11(2):95–109.
14. de Castro LD. Commodification and exploitation: arguments in favour of compensated organ donation. J Med Ethics 2003;29(3):142–6.
15. De Charro F, Oppe M, Bos MA, et al. A regulated organ market? In: Weimar W, Bos MA, Busschbach J, editors. Organ transplantation: ethical, legal and psychosocial aspects towards a common European policy. Lengerich: Pabst; 2008. p. 43–8.
16. de Klerk M, Weimar W. Ingredients for a successful living donor kidney exchange program. Transplantation 2008;86(4):511–2.
17. De Klerk M. The Dutch living donor kidney exchange programme. Rotterdam: Erasmus Medical Center University Hospital; 2010.
18. Delmonico FL. Exchanging kidneys – advances in living-donor transplantation. N Engl J Med 2004;350(18):1812–4.
19. Directive 2010/45EU of the European Parliament and of the Council of 13 July 2010 on standards of quality and safety of human organs intended for transplantation. EUR LEX 32010L0045(01). Official Journal L 207 2010; P 0014.
20. Dor F, Massey EK, Frunza M, et al. New classification of ELPAT for living organ donation. Transplantation 2011;91(9):935–8.
21. Dutch Transplant Foundation (Nederlandse Transplantatie Stichting) Annual report (NTS Jaarverslag 2010). Leiden: Dutch Transplant Foundation; 2010. p. 1–20.
22. Elliott C. Doing harm: living organ donors, clinical research and the tenth man. J Med Ethics 1995;21(2):91–6.
23. Erin CA, Harris J. A monopsonistic market: or how to buy and sell human organs, tissues and cells ethically. In: Robinson I, editor. Life and death under high technology medicine. New York: Manchester University Press; 1994. p. 134–56.
24. Erin CA, Harris J. An ethical market in human organs. J Med Ethics 2003;29(3):137–8.
25. Eurotransplant International Foundation. Annual report 2010. Leiden: Eurotransplant International Foundation; 2010.
26. Evans M. Organ donations should not be restricted to relatives. J Med Ethics 1989;15:17–20.

27. Francis LP, Francis JG. Stateless crimes, legitimacy, and international criminal law: the case of organ trafficking. Crim Law Philos 2010;4:283–95.
28. Friedlaender MM. The right to sell or buy a kidney: are we failing our patients? Lancet 2002;359(9310):971–3.
29. Ghods AJ, Savaj S. Iranian model of paid and regulated living-unrelated kidney donation. Clin J Am Soc Nephrol 2006;1(6):1136–45.
30. Gillon R. "Primum non nocere" and the principle of non-maleficence. BMJ 1985;291:130–1.
31. Glannon W. Is it unethical for doctors to encourage healthy adults to donate a kidney to a stranger? Yes. BMJ 2011;343:d7179.
32. Goodwin M. Black markets. The supply and demand of body parts. Cambridge: Cambridge University Press; 2006.
33. Goyal M, Mehta RL, Schneiderman LJ, et al. Economic and health consequences of selling a kidney in India. JAMA 2002;288.
34. Gutmann T. Allocation and transplantation of "marginal" donor organs – ethical and legal questions. In: Gutmann T, Daar AS, Sells RA, et al., editors. Ethical, legal and social issues in organ transplantation. Munich: Pabst; 2004. p. 49–56.
35. Harmon W, Delmonico F. Payment for kidneys: a government-regulated system is not ethically achievable. Clin J Am Soc Nephrol 2006;1(6):1146–7.
36. Hartmann A. Managing a living donor program: the Oslo experience. In: 11th Conference of the European Society for Organ Transplantation Venice, Italy; 2003.
37. Hilhorst MT, Kranenburg L, Busschbach J. Should health care professionals encourage living kidney donation? Med Health Care Philos 2007;10(1):81–90.
38. Hilhorst MT, Van Dijk G. Financial incentives for organ donation. An investigation of the ethical issues. The Hague: Centre for Ethics and Health; 2007.
39. Hilhorst M, Wijsbek H, Erdman R, et al. Can we turn down autonomous wishes to donate anonymously? Transpl Int 2011;24(12):1164–9.
40. Kasiske BL, Snyder JJ, Matas AJ, et al. Preemptive kidney transplantation: the advantage and the advantaged. J Am Soc Nephrol 2002;13(5):1358–64.
41. Kok NF, IJzermans JN, Alwayn IP. Laparoscopic versus open live donor nephrectomy in renal transplantation: a meta-analysis. Ann Surg 2008;248(4):691–2.
42. Kostka U. Organ allocation and justice. In: Gutmann T, Daar AS, Sells RA, et al., editors. Ethical, legal and social issues in organ transplantation. Munich: Pabst; 2004. p. 79–88.
43. Kranenburg L, Zuidema W, Erdman R, et al. The psychological evaluation of Samaritan kidney donors: a systematic review. Psychol Med 2008;38(02):177–85.
44. Kranenburg L, Zuidema W, Vanderkroft P, et al. The implementation of a kidney exchange program does not induce a need for additional psychosocial support. Transpl Int 2007;20(5):432–9.
45. Kranenburg L, Zuidema W, Weimar W, et al. Postmortal or living related donor: preferences of kidney patients. Transpl Int 2005;18(5):519–23.
46. Lennerling A, Lovén C, Dobbels F, et al. Living organ donation practices in Europe – results from an online survey [forthcoming]. Gothenburg: University of Gothenburg; 2012.
47. Lopp L. Analysing the normative arguments that dominate the policy arena about necessity and legitimacy of legal restrictions in living donor transplantation. Muenster: Westfaelische Wilhelms-Universitat; 2012.
48. Lopp L. Comparative analysis of European transplant laws regarding living organ donation: an overview. Muenster: Westfaelische Wilhelms-Universitat; 2012.
49. MacCoun RJ, Reuter P. Drug War heresies. Cambridge: Cambridge University Press; 2001.
50. Massey EK, Hilhorst MT, Nette RW, et al. Justification for a home-based education programme for kidney patients and their social network prior to initiation of renal replacement therapy. J Med Ethics 2011;37(11):677–81.
51. Massey EK, Kranenburg LW, Zuidema WC, et al. Encouraging psychological outcomes after altruistic donation to a stranger. Am J Transplant 2010;10(6):1445–52.
52. Matas AJ, Bartlett ST, Leichtman AB, et al. Morbidity and mortality after living kidney donation, 1999–2001: survey of United States transplant centers. Am J Transplant 2003;3(7):830–4.
53. Matas AJ, Garvey CA, Jacobs CL, et al. Nondirected donation of kidneys from living donors. N Engl J Med 2000;343(6):433–6.
54. Matas AJ, Schnitzler M. Payment for living donor (vendor) kidneys: a cost-effectiveness analysis. Am J Transplant 2004;4(2): 216–21.
55. Matas AJ. The case for living kidney sales: rationale, objections and concerns. Am J Transplant 2004;4(12):2007–17.
56. Montgomery RA, Gentry SE, Marks WH, et al. Domino paired kidney donation: a strategy to make best use of live non-directed donation. Lancet 2006;368(9533):419-421.
57. Montgomery RA, Lonze BE, King KE, et al. Desensitization in HLA-incompatible kidney recipients and survival. N Engl J Med 2011;365(4):318–26.
58. Nacqvi A. A socio-economic survey of kidney vendors in Pakistan. Transpl Int 2007;20:924–5.
59. Neuberger J. Making an offer you can't refuse? A challenge of altruistic donation. Transpl Int 2011;24(12):1159–61.
60. Padilla BS. Regulated compensation for kidney donors in the Philippines. Curr Opin Organ Transplant 2009;14:120–3.
61. Park K, Moon JII, Kim SII, et al. Exchange-donor program in kidney transplantation. Transplant Proc 1999;31(1–2):356–7.
62. Participants in the International Summit on Transplant Tourism and Organ Trafficking Convened by the Transplantation Society and International Society of Nephrology. The declaration of Istanbul on organ trafficking and transplant tourism. Transplantation 2008;88(8):1013–8.
63. Price DPT. Legal systems for organ distribution in Europe: justice in allocation. In: Weimar W, Bos MA, Busschbach JJV, editors. Organ transplantation: ethical, legal and psychosocial aspects towards a common European policy. Munich: Pabst; 2008. p. 163–74.
64. Radcliffe-Richards J. Nephrarious goings on. J Med Philos 1996;21(4):375–416.
65. Radcliffe-Richards J, Daar AS, Guttmann RD, et al. The case for allowing kidney sales. Lancet 1998;351(9120):1950–2.
66. Rodrigue JR, Cornell DL, Lin JK, et al. Increasing live donor kidney transplantation: a randomized controlled trial of a home-based educational intervention. Am J Transplant 2007;7(2):394–401.
67. Roodnat JI, Kal-van Gestel JA, Zuidema W, et al. Successful expansion of the living donor pool by alternative living donation programs. Am J Transplant 2009 Sep;9(9):2150–6.
68. Ross LF. Solid organ donation between strangers. J Law Med Ethics 2002;30(3):440–5.
69. Rothman DJ, Rose E, Awaya T, et al. The Bellagio task force report on transplantation, bodily integrity, and the international traffic in organs. Transplant Proc 1997;29(6):2739–45.
70. Rouchi AH, Mahdavi-Mazdeh M, Zamyadi M. Compensated living kidney donation in Iran: donor's attitude and short-term follow-up. Iran J Kidney Dis 2009;3(1):34–9.
71. Sajjad I, Baines LS, Patel P, et al. Commercialization of kidney transplants: a systematic review of outcomes in recipients and donors. Am J Nephrol 2008;28(5):744–54.
72. Salahudeen AK, Woods HF, Pingle A, et al. High mortality among recipients of bought living-unrelated donor kidneys. Lancet 1990;336(8717):725–8.
73. Scheper-Hughes N. Parts unknown. Ethnography 2004;5(1): 29–73.
74. Scheper-Hughes N. Theft of life. Society 1990;27(6):57–62.
75. Shimazono Y. The state of the international organ trade: a provisional picture based on integration of available information. Bull WHO 2007;85:955–62.
76. Simforoosh N. Kidney donation and rewarded gifting: an Iranian model. Nat Clin Pract Urol 2007;4(6):292–3.
77. Spital A. Unrelated living kidney donors: an update of attitudes use among U.S. transplant centers. Transplantation 1994;57(12):1722–6.
78. Tanabe K. Japanese experience of ABO-incompatible living kidney transplantation. Transplantation 2007;84(12S):S4–7.
79. Taylor J. Why the 'black market' arguments against legalizing organ sales fail. Res Publica 2006;12(2):163–78.
80. Terasaki PI, Cecka JM, Gjertson DW, et al. High survival rates of kidney transplants from spousal and living unrelated donors. N Engl J Med 1995;333(6):333–6.
81. Truog RD. The ethics of organ donation by living donors. N Engl J Med 2005;353(5):444–6.
82. UK Health Departments. Requested allocation of a deceased donor organ; 29 March 2010. Available online at: www.dh.gov.uk/en/publicationsandstatistics/publications/publicationspolicyandguidance/DH_114800.

83. United Nations. Protocol to prevent, suppress and punish trafficking in persons, especially women and children, supplementing the United Nations convention against transnational organized crime. Vienna: United Nations; 2004.
84. United Nations Office on Drugs and Crime. Experts meet in Vienna to address the trafficking of persons for the removal of organs, 28 to 30 June 2010. 2013. Vienna, Austria. Available online at: http://www.unodc.org/unodc/en/human-trafficking/2010/egm-vienna-organ-trafficking.html.
85. United Network for Organ Sharing (UNOS). Available online at: www.unos.org; 2012 [accessed 25.04.12].
86. Van Buren MC, Massey EK, Maasdam L, et al. For love or money? Attitudes toward financial incentives among actual living kidney donors. Am J Transplant 2010;10(11):2488–92.
87. Veatch RM. Justice, utility, and organ allocation. In: Gutmann T, Daar AS, Sells RA, et al., editors. Ethical, legal and social issues in organ transplantation. Munich: Pabst; 2004. p. 57–67.
88. Veatch RM. Why liberals should accept financial incentives for organ procurement. Kennedy Inst Ethics J 2003;13(1):19–36.
89. Weimar W, Zuidema W, de Klerk M, et al. Altruistic kidney donation. Lancet 2006;368(9540):987.
90. Weimar W. ELPAT, the European platform on ethical, legal and psychosocial aspects of organ transplantation. In: Weimar W, Busschbach J, Bos MA, editors. Organ transplantation: ethical, legal and psychosocial aspects. Towards a common European policy. Munich: Pabst; 2008. p. 15–6.
91. Working Group on Incentives for Living Donation. Incentives for organ donation: proposed standards for an internationally acceptable system. Am J Transplant 2012;12(2):306–12.
92. World Health Organization. Development of guiding principles for human organ transplants. Fortieth world health assembly Geneva 4–15 May 1987. WHA40.13. Available online at: http://www.who.int/transplantation/en/WHA40.13.pdf.
93. World Health Organization. Human organ transplantation. A report on developments under the auspices of the WHO. Geneva: WHO; 1991.
94. World Health Organization. Guiding principles on human cell, tissue and organ transplantation. Geneva: World Health Organization; 2008.
95. Wright L, Campbell M, Daar A. Ethics in transplantation: allotransplantation and xenotransplantation. In: Morris P, Knechtle S, editors. Kidney transplantation: principles and practice. Philadelphia: Saunders Elsevier; 2008. p. 694–708.

CHAPTER 42

EVIDENCE IN TRANSPLANTATION

Simon R. Knight • Liset H.M. Pengel • Sir Peter J. Morris 

CHAPTER OUTLINE

INTRODUCTION

As every day goes by the medical literature expands almost exponentially and the literature in organ transplantation is no different. Some 20 million medical articles have been listed on PubMed and there are well over 200 000 articles on organ transplantation alone. Thus the problem of seeking evidence for our practice in organ transplantation, be it the value of a particular immunosuppressive drug or a surgical intervention such as the prophylactic use of a stent in the ureter in kidney transplantation, is not easily found by an inexperienced literature searcher.

There are a number of levels of evidence, as shown in Table 42-1 and Figure 42-1. It is level 1 and level 2 evidence that we are seeking in trying to arrive at a management decision of our patient population during and after organ transplantation or indeed of the individual patient. Systematic reviews and meta-analyses of randomized controlled trials (RCTs) comprise level 1 evidence and RCTs comprise level 2 evidence. Later on in this chapter there is a description of RCTs and also of systematic reviews and meta-analyses. Other levels of evidence exist and one such level is transplant registry data, as in our specialty we do have a number of national, regional and international registries for organ transplantation, e.g., United Network for Organ Sharing (UNOS) in the United States (http://www.unos.org), the Collaborative Transplant Study in Europe and North America (http://www.ctstransplant.org/), the ANZDATA registry for Australia and New Zealand (http://www.anzdata.org.au/), and the Eurotransplant registry (http://www.eurotransplant.org/cms/), to name but a few. National registries exist such as that maintained by National Health Service Blood and Transplantation (NHSBT) for the United Kingdom.

RCTs are the most desirable form of evidence to answer a question about an intervention but there are advantages and disadvantages, as listed in Table 42-2. RCTs are designed to eliminate bias but they do have strict inclusion and exclusion criteria. A good trial will tick all the boxes in the CONSORT statement (see later). However on the negative side in organ transplantation, trials usually have small numbers of patients, the inclusion and exclusion criteria do limit the generalizability of the results, and, of course, the length of follow-up in most trials is less than 3 years. Another potential defect is the methodological quality of trials as there is considerable variation here. In a relatively recent analysis of the methodology of reporting of trials in organ transplantation by Pengel and colleagues, just over a third of trials were considered by the authors to be of good quality.[14] This then will have an impact on the quality of a systematic review in that it is dependent on the quality of the RCTs that are used in the systematic review. If there are many poor-quality trials, this impacts on any meta-analysis, which is likely to have high levels of heterogeneity, and this reduces the value of the evidence.

TABLE 42-1 Levels of Evidence for Interventions

Level I	Systematic review and meta-analysis of randomized controlled trials
Level II	Randomized controlled trials
Level III	1. Transplant registry data 2. Non-randomized comparative studies with a concurrent control group, e.g., cohort study or case control study 3. Non-randomized comparative studies with a historical control group
Level IV	Case series

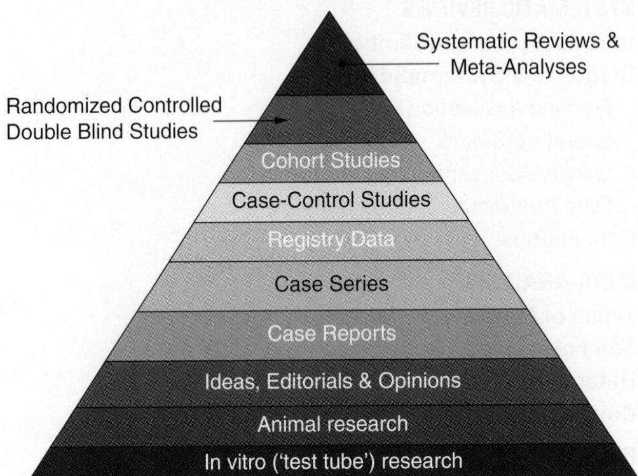

FIGURE 42-1 ■ The evidence hierarchy in clinical practice.

TABLE 42-2 Randomized Controlled Trials

Advantages	Disadvantages
Elimination of bias	Small numbers
Strict inclusion	Generalizability of results
Strict exclusion	Short follow-up
CONSORT statement	Quality of trials

CONSORT, Consolidated Standards of Reporting Trials.

On the other hand, transplant registry data have the advantage, as shown in Table 42-3, of large numbers, results are applicable to the whole population, there is a long follow-up and they not only identify current practice but also will identify rare adverse events which may not be seen in an RCT. They also provide the facility for following up long-term patients in RCTs. On the negative side, one cannot exclude a selection bias and there is no validation of data entered into a registry.

However the debate over the role of RCTs versus registry data should not be regarded as a contest. They both supply very useful data and should be regarded as complementary, and used together they can provide more robust evidence for interventions in transplantation. We think that we need to try and plan better-quality and larger RCTs in organ transplantation. There needs to be some way of making the return of all data to registries mandatory and national registries should be able to achieve that. This would also make possible the long-term follow-up of patients who

TABLE 42-3 Transplant Registry Data

Advantages	Disadvantages
Large numbers	Selection bias
Results generalizable to whole population	No validation of data entry into registry
Long follow-up	
Identify useful interventions	
Identify rare adverse events	
Identify current practice	
Facilitating long-term follow-up of RCT patients	

RCT, randomized controlled trial.

have participated in RCTs. For example, in the large ongoing 3C study in the UK of alemtuzumab versus basiliximab induction with subsequent randomization to sirolimus or tacrolimus at 6 months, all recipients have been registered with the national registry at NHSBT. This will enable long-term follow-up to be achieved relatively painlessly.

SEARCHING THE LITERATURE

Searching the literature can be a challenging task. There is an abundance of resources available and a rapidly increasing number of citations. This section provides a brief introduction of how to search for evidence in commonly used resources.

Developing a Search

A search for evidence starts with a well-constructed, answerable question.[21] Evidence-based medicine researchers often define the question to be answered across four domains: population, intervention, comparator, and outcomes of interest (PICO). An example is given in Table 42-4.

Once a clinical question has been defined a search including a number of search terms needs to be developed. The initial search should be broad, including only two or three elements of the PICO question. Combining too many search terms in the first instance increases the risk of overdefining the search, which can result in eliminating relevant search results.

Searching

Keywords Versus Thesaurus

There are two approaches to identify relevant articles. Firstly, one can search using keywords, which involves selecting words or terms to describe the key elements of the clinical question. Secondly, one can search using the thesaurus or controlled vocabulary of a database. The thesaurus is used to index articles according to standardized terminology, ensuring that articles on the same topic are indexed under the same standardized terms, which ensures greater precision when searching. MEDLINE's thesaurus is called Medical Subject Headings (MeSH), while Embase's thesaurus is called Emtree.

TABLE 42-4 **Formulation of a Question. Examples are Given for a Review Investigating the Role of Steroid Withdrawal or Avoidance Following Renal Transplantation**

	Considerations	Example
Population	Age, sex, underlying condition/pathology, comorbidities	Adult renal transplant recipients at the time of transplantation
Intervention	Drug or procedure, dose or duration	Complete steroid avoidance or withdrawal at any time posttransplantation
Comparator	No intervention, current gold standard, placebo	Maintenance steroids
Outcomes	Efficacy (acute rejection, graft/patient survival, graft function) and safety (infection, malignancy, specific side effects)	Acute rejection, graft function, graft and patient survival Steroid-related side effects (serum lipids, hypertension, new-onset diabetes, leukopenia, infection, cataracts)

Limits

To refine search results most databases allow inclusion of limits such as date of publication, language, publication type, or patient age.

Boolean Operators

Boolean operators "AND," "OR," and "NOT" can be used to combine concepts, find synonymous terms, or exclude words from the search results. Care must be taken when using the Boolean operators as inappropriate use could exclude relevant search results.

Available Resources

There are an increasing number of resources available when undertaking searches for evidence and below follows a brief description of the most commonly used resources.

Google Scholar

Google Scholar (http://scholar.google.com) is a subset of Google. It is a popular resource as it is easy to search and gives quick results, especially by using its "cited by" feature, which lists all other references that cited an article. The web search engine has simple and advanced search options, the latter allowing to search by keywords, author name, source name, date of publication, and subject areas.[2] Google Scholar summarizes only electronic references, including peer-reviewed articles, books, theses, and other publications from societies and universities.[1] Users should note that Google Scholar displays its results according to the number of citations received for an article with the most cited references listed at the top, which tends to be the older literature. Google Scholar has been criticized for a number of issues, such the inability to search MeSH terms, partial inclusion of MEDLINE records, and using infrequent updates.[1]

PubMed

PubMed is a free database of the US National Library of Medicine (www.pubmed.gov). It is the most comprehensive biomedical database and contains over 21 million fully indexed or in process articles ahead of print from MEDLINE, life science journals, and online books.[17] PubMed has the following features:

- The basic search allows one to search by word or phrase, author or journal.
- Searches can be combined using the Boolean operators.
- Limits include searching by date, type of article, language, subsets, ages, species (humans or animals), sex, and full text options.
- The advanced search allows one to use the search "Builder" and "History." Using the search Builder one can design a search using the Boolean operators.
- A very useful feature of PubMed is that by default PubMed will try to map a search term to a MeSH term (automatic term mapping).
- Search details can be found on the search results pages in the right-hand column. It shows which search and/or MeSH terms were used and users can directly add or omit terms in the search details box.
- Single citation matcher. This is a useful feature to find an article when only part of the citation details are known.
- Clinical queries. These are highly sensitive, built-in search filters to easily retrieve articles on clinical study categories (etiology, diagnosis, therapy, prognosis, and guidelines), systematic reviews, and medical genetics.

Helpful tutorials are available on the PubMed website explaining the above search options in more detail.

Embase

The Excerpta Medica database is a comprehensive biomedical and pharmacological database that provides access to medical and drug-related information. Indexing of articles is based on the Emtree thesaurus. Access to Embase is by subscription.

Cochrane Library

The Cochrane Library consists of six databases that include high-quality evidence-based information: (1) Cochrane Database of Systematic Reviews; (2) Database of Abstracts of Reviews of Effects (DARE); (3) Cochrane Central Register of Controlled Trials (CENTRAL); (4) Cochrane Methodology Register; (5) Health Technology Assessment Database; and (6) the NHS Economic Evaluation Database. CENTRAL is the largest of the six databases and includes citation to trials, most of which come from MEDLINE and Embase, with the remaining references identified from hand searches and other resources. There is a basic search which allows one to search by words in the title and/or abstract, keywords, author, or publication type. The advanced search allows searching using Boolean operators and there are several options to limit a search. It is also possible to identify and search by MeSH terms. The Cochrane Library can be searched freely but access to the citation records or full text is by subscription. The Cochrane Library has been made freely available in low-income countries or by national licenses in other countries. A detailed user guide is available from the Cochrane Library website (www.cochranelibrary.com).

The Transplant Library

The Transplant Library was developed by the Centre for Evidence in Transplantation (CET) to be the definitive resource of high-level evidence-based information on all aspects of solid-organ transplantation.[15] It is a specialist database that contains all RCTs from the earliest record to the present, including abstracts from conference proceedings of RCTs and selected, good-quality systematic reviews from 2008. Access to the Transplant Library is by subscription.

Features of the Transplant Library include the following:

- RCTs published from 2004 onwards have been given a methodological quality rating. The methodological quality items evaluated are allocation concealment, intention-to-treat analysis and the Jadad scale, which assesses whether randomization, blinding, and description of dropouts and withdrawals were adequately described.
- Includes references to abstracts from conference proceedings (not available on MEDLINE).
- Limits specific to organs transplanted, pediatric patients, and publication type to make searching faster and more effective.
- Updated with new RCTs every 2 weeks, many of which are ahead of print publication. Good-quality systematic reviews are updated every month. References are sourced from MEDLINE, the Cochrane Library (with permission) and hand searches of conference proceedings.

More information regarding the selection of records and quality assessment can be found on the CET website (www.transplantevidence.com).

RANDOMIZED CONTROLLED TRIALS

A randomized, double-blind, controlled trial is generally considered the gold-standard design to establish the efficacy of interventions. Randomization aims to balance the known and unknown prognostic factors between the different groups in a trial and minimizes the risk that trial results are influenced by factors other than the effect of the intervention(s) under investigation. Randomization should be based on the principle of tossing a coin, and appropriate methods of randomization include a computer-generated random sequence or a table of random numbers.[21] Unreliable methods of randomization or quasi-randomization are predictable sequences and include randomization based on alternation, date of birth, or hospital record number. To ensure that the randomization is adequately implemented it is crucial that the upcoming allocation code is concealed from the study investigators who enrol the study participants. Appropriate methods of concealed allocation are central randomization, coded drug containers, or sequentially numbered, opaque sealed envelopes.[8] There is great variability in the interpretation of the term double-blind, but in general trials are considered double-blind when study participants and investigators, and outcome assessors are unaware of the allocated intervention throughout the trial, for example by using identical placebos.[3,12] Allocation concealment is not the same as blinding and this is often a source of confusion.

Sources of Bias

Evaluation of the validity of trial results can be described in terms of external or internal validity. External validity refers to whether results can be generalized to a certain group of patients in a particular clinical setting.[18] Internal validity on the other hand refers to the extent to which bias is minimized in trials.[5] There are a number of different bias domains that can influence the internal validity of trials. Selection bias refers to biased allocation to the comparison groups. Both adequate generation of the randomization sequence and adequate allocation concealment can prevent selection bias. Performance bias refers to systematic differences in the care apart from the intervention being evaluated. It can be minimized by blinding of participants as awareness of the allocated intervention may influence their compliance with the intervention, tendency to drop out or seek additional treatments, or response to the intervention. Blinding of investigators is also important as unblinded investigators may behave differently in terms of care and attention given to the participants. Detection bias refers to systematic differences between groups in how outcomes are determined. Blinded outcome assessment may reduce the risk of detection bias and is particularly important when subjective outcomes are used. Attrition bias refers to systematic differences between groups in terms of withdrawals, dropouts, or exclusions of participants. Lastly, reporting bias refers to systematic differences between reported and unreported findings, where an outcome is recorded and analyzed but not reported on the basis of the result.

Assessment of Risk of Bias

The assessment of the risk of bias or methodological quality helps to assess whether the results of a particular trial or meta-analysis of several trials are valid. It has been found that some aspects of bias can influence effect estimates, for example inadequate means of allocation concealment or blinding generate larger estimates of intervention effects.[13,20]

There are different approaches to assess the extent of bias when interpreting the validity of a trial. Numerous tools to assess the quality have been developed but there is still no consensus on the most appropriate tool. A systematic review of 121 critical appraisal tools concluded that there is great variability in the items included in the tools, with only 12% of tools being based on empirical research and only few providing evidence on the reliability and validity.[9] A commonly used scale is the Jadad scale, which was developed to assess trials on pain relief but has since been used in many other disciplines.[7] It provides a composite score out of 5, assessing whether randomization, blinding, and withdrawals and/or dropouts have been adequately reported. However one of its limitations is that it does not include an assessment of allocation concealment.

One of the criticisms of using a summary scale is that weights are being given to the individual items of the scale but that there is no evidence supporting this strategy. For this reason the Cochrane Collaboration strongly advocates against the use of quality scales as a mean of judging the internal validity of a trial. Instead, they have developed the Cochrane Collaboration tool for assessing the risk of bias in RCTs.[4] The tool is based on the bias domains described above, most of which have empirical evidence showing an association with biased results. Each item is assigned a judgment of high, low, or unclear risk and in addition the assessors describe which information in the trial report their judgment is based on to ensure transparency of how they have come to their judgment.

It is generally recommended that judgments about the risk of bias should be made independently by two assessors.

CONSORT Statement

The CONSORT statement, which is short for Consolidated Standards of Reporting Trials, was first published in 1996 by the CONSORT group to provide a framework for improving the reporting of RCTs (www.consort-statement.org). The most recent version of the CONSORT statement was published in 2010 and an extensive explanation and elaboration paper have been published in a number of leading biomedical journals.[19] The CONSORT statement is a checklist of 25 items and a recommended participant flow diagram (Figure 42-2). It provides a standardization of how reports of RCTs should be prepared to ensure transparent and complete reports. The CONSORT statement has been endorsed by many

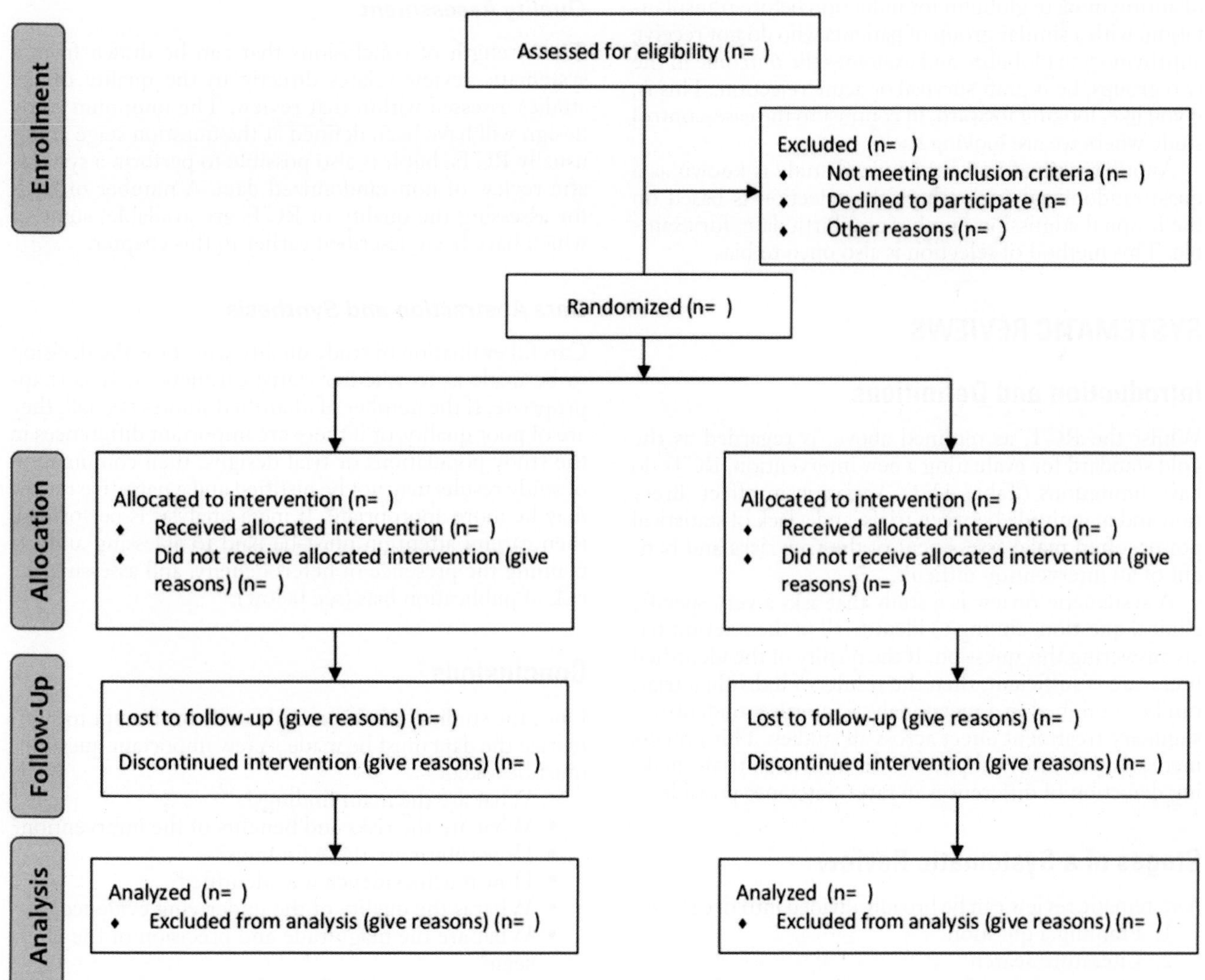

FIGURE 42-2 ■ A template Consolidated Standards of Reporting Trials (CONSORT) flow diagram. (From Schulz KF, Altman DG, Moher D, for the CONSORT Group. CONSORT 2010 statement: updated guidelines for reporting parallel group randomised trials. BMJ 2010;340:c332.)

biomedical journals and it has been shown that reports of RCTs in solid-organ transplantation published in journals that endorse the CONSORT statement do report more items of the CONSORT statement and in addition are of higher methodological quality than RCTs published in journals that do not endorse the CONSORT statement.[11]

Non-Randomized or Observational Studies

These are comparative studies but of course there are many possibilities of the introduction of bias in the comparison. The two types of study that are used most commonly are case-control studies and cohort studies.

A case-control study is a retrospective study where one examines a particular outcome of interest, for example acute rejection, and takes two cohorts of patients, one who have had acute rejection and another group who have not had acute rejection, matching them as far as possible for other confounding factors to see whether there is any difference to be identified in the two groups. This is looking back, if you like.

In a cohort study one compares a group of patients who are receiving a particular intervention, e.g., the use of antithymocyte globulin for induction before transplantation, with a similar group of patients who do not receive antithymocyte globulin, and examines the outcome in the two groups, be it graft survival or acute rejection. This is, if you like, looking forward, in contrast to the case-control study where we are looking back.

Another type of non-randomized study is known as a quasi-randomized trial, where the selection is based on the hospital admission number or a birth date, for example. This method of selection is also open to bias.

SYSTEMATIC REVIEWS

Introduction and Definitions

Whilst the RCT, as outlined above, is regarded as the gold standard for evaluating a new intervention, RCTs do have limitations (Table 42-1). Variation in effect direction and magnitude between trials, and a lack of statistical power, often make assessment of the true risks and benefit of an intervention difficult.

A systematic review is a study that asks a very specific clinical question, aiming to identify all of the relevant trials answering this question. If the quality of the identified literature is sufficient, then the results of individual trials can be combined in a meta-analysis in order to identify a summary treatment effect across all studies. This process increases the statistical power over individual trials, making detection of differences in rarer outcomes possible.

Stages of a Systematic Review

A systematic review can be broadly divided into five stages:

1. Framing a question
2. Literature search
3. Quality assessment
4. Data abstraction/synthesis
5. Conclusions.

Framing a Question

The specific question asked at the beginning of a review can have a large impact on the studies included, and therefore the results seen. The question should be formulated using the population, intervention, comparison, and outcomes or PICO framework described earlier in this chapter. The inclusion and exclusion criteria for a review are directly defined from this question, and once set, there should be resistance to changing these criteria during the review process so as to reduce the risk of introducing bias.

Literature Search

The literature search aims to identify all studies, both published and unpublished, that attempt to answer the question posed. The various resources that are available for searching the literature have been described earlier in this chapter. Identification of unpublished literature is an important way of reducing publication bias, and can include steps such as searching trial registries and contacting pharmaceutical companies and device manufacturers.

Quality Assessment

The strength of conclusions that can be drawn from a systematic review relates directly to the quality of the studies assessed within that review. The minimum study design will have been defined at the question stage and is usually RCTs, but it is also possible to perform a systematic review of non-randomized data. A number of tools for assessing the quality of RCTs are available, some of which have been described earlier in this chapter.

Data Abstraction and Synthesis

Careful evaluation of study quality will allow the decision to be made as to whether statistical meta-analysis is appropriate. If the number of identified studies is small, they are of poor quality, or if there are important differences in the study populations or trial designs, then combination of study results may not be justified and a narrative review may be more appropriate. If meta-analysis is performed, then careful attention must be paid to assessing and explaining the presence of heterogeneity, and assessing the risk of publication bias (see below).

Conclusions

Once the studies have been evaluated, an attempt to summarize the data must be made. A few important questions must be asked:

- What are the main findings?
- What are the risks and benefits of the intervention?
- How robust are these findings?
- How much evidence was identified?
- What is the quality of the underlying evidence?
- What are the magnitude and precision of the effect seen?
- Was any evidence of heterogeneity identified, and if so, could it be explained?
- Is there any evidence of publication or reporting bias?

- Are these findings generalizable and important to our population of interest?
- How similar are the patients in the included studies to our patient population?
- Are the effects seen of clinical as well as statistical significance?
- Can clear guidelines be drawn from the results of the review?
- If there is uncertainty, what further studies are required in order to clarify the impact of the treatment?

META-ANALYSIS

A meta-analysis describes the use of statistical models to combine the results of individual trials. A meta-analysis is therefore only a small part of a systematic review.

The steps of a meta-analysis are as follows.

- Comparable studies reporting each outcome of interest are identified.
- A summary effect for each study is calculated, along with a confidence interval. In the case of a binary outcome (e.g., acute rejection), this will take the form of a relative risk, odds ratio, or risk difference. In the case of a continuous outcome (e.g., serum creatinine), this will be a mean difference or standardized mean difference.
- The individual study effects are combined to provide a weighted overall summary effect and confidence interval.
- The effect seen is examined for the presence of heterogeneity, and if found, an explanation must be sought.

Types of Meta-Analysis

The two most commonly used types of meta-analysis are the fixed- and random-effects models. These differ in their underlying assumptions.

Fixed-effects meta-analysis assumes a single "true" underlying effect in all studies. Studies are weighted according to the inverse of their variance, meaning that larger studies generally have more weight in the overall analysis.

Random-effects meta-analysis allows for random variation in the effect sizes between the included studies resulting from differences in the study population or characteristics. Weighting is again based upon the inverse of variance, but the overall weighting is reduced by a factor proportional to the heterogeneity in the studies included.

In practice this means that a random-effects meta-analysis gives a more conservative estimate of the summary effect, with a wider confidence interval. Use of the fixed-effects model is reserved for homogeneous data with very little between-study variability.

The Forest Plot

The forest plot is the standard method for graphically displaying the results of a meta-analysis. It allows visual inspection of the data and summary effect. An example is shown in Figure 42-3.

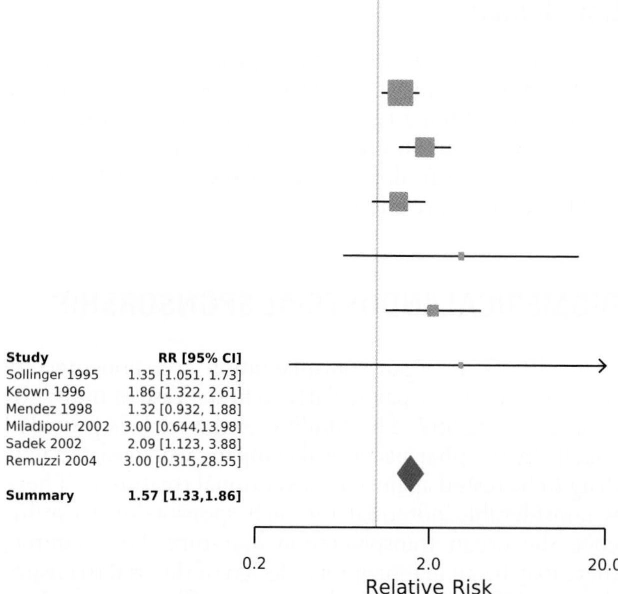

FIGURE 42-3 ■ Forest plot to show the risk of diarrhea in mycophenolate mofetil (MMF)- and azathioprine (AZA)-treated renal transplant recipients. Each blue box represents the point estimate of relative risk (RR) for the individual study, with the horizontal line representing the 95% confidence interval (CI). The size of the blue box represents the weight given to that study in meta-analysis. The vertical line represents no difference (relative risk of 1). The red diamond represents the overall summary effect from meta-analysis, with the width of the diamond representing the 95% CI for this outcome. The plot demonstrates a significantly higher risk of diarrhea in MMF-treated recipients. (Adapted from Knight SR, Russell NK, Barcena L, et al. Mycophenolate mofetil decreases acute rejection and may improve graft survival in renal transplant recipients when compared with azathioprine: a systematic review. Transplantation 2009; 87:785–794.)

Heterogeneity

Heterogeneity is the term used to describe the variation between study effect sizes in a meta-analysis. A large amount of heterogeneity suggests a great deal of variation in the studies included, which can result from either differences in study methodology and quality (methodological heterogeneity) or patient and intervention characteristics (clinical heterogeneity). If a large amount of heterogeneity is found, then these factors should be explored in order to attempt to explain it. If an explanation is not found, then one has to question whether the combination of the studies in a meta-analysis is appropriate.

Heterogeneity can be quantified in one of two ways:

1. The Cochran Q test assesses whether differences in the effect size between studies is likely to be due to chance alone. A significant test result (usually taken as $P<0.1$) suggests significant heterogeneity which is unlikely due to chance.
2. The I^2 statistic describes the percentage of the variability in effect estimates that is due to heterogeneity rather than sampling error (chance). The higher the percentage, the greater the true heterogeneity; e.g., >40% suggests a significant level of heterogeneity.

Conclusions

A systematic review is a scientific process that uses robust methodology to answer a specific question, reducing the risk of bias. Often a review will result in more questions than answers, but an important role of the systematic review is to identify deficiencies in the current literature and to guide future clinical studies.

BIOMEDICAL/INDUSTRIAL SPONSORSHIP

Many RCTs in organ transplantation are sponsored by industry and this is particularly so in the case of immunosuppressive agents. The funding of the trials is provided usually by the pharmaceutical company who wishes a new drug to be tested against a conventional treatment. There is considerable potential for such sponsorship to influence the organ transplantation literature. For example, there may be an inappropriate design of the trial to ensure the possibility of a favorable outcome. There may be failure to report trials where the outcome is not satisfactory from the point of view of the sponsoring company and there may be selective reporting of outcomes with respect to both safety and efficacy. The reporting of safety in RCTs in organ transplantation is an area that is generally not well done. Finally we have the phenomenon of ghost writing of reports which has existed for years but has only really come to light in recent years and there have been major campaigns against ghost writing by PLoS in particular.[10,16] Payment to the investigators obviously also can have an impact on the reporting of outcomes in trials and there is good evidence in the literature to support that. However it should be pointed out that industry-sponsored trials are generally of better methodological quality than non-industry-sponsored trials.[14]

CONCLUSION

Thus evidence in transplantation must be based on robust evidence and the best source of evidence is RCTs and systematic reviews. However good transplant registry data are invaluable, especially with respect to long-term follow-up and everyday practice. There are major deficiencies in the quality of evidence available at this point in time and for this reason one should have a healthy cynicism about data presented as evidence.

It is worth recording a quote from an article by John Ioannidis published in PLoS Medicine in 2005 which says: "Simulations show that for most study designs and settings it is more likely for a research claim to be false than true. Moreover, for many current scientific fields, claimed research findings may often be simply accurate measures of the prevailing bias."[6] We feel that one needs to continually bear those words in mind.

REFERENCES

1. Anders ME, Evans DP. Comparison of PubMed and Google Scholar literature searches. Respir Care 2010;55:578–83.
2. Falagas ME, Pitsouni EI, Malietzis GA, et al. Comparison of PubMed, Scopus, Web of Science, and Google Scholar: strengths and weaknesses. FASEB J 2008;22:338–42.
3. Haahr MT, Hrobjartsson A. Who is blinded in randomized clinical trials? A study of 200 trials and a survey of authors. Clin Trials 2006;3:360–5.
4. Higgins JP, Altman DG, Gotzsche PC, et al. The Cochrane Collaboration's tool for assessing risk of bias in randomised trials. BMJ 2011;343:d5928.
5. Higgins JPT, Green S. Cochrane handbook for systematic reviews of interventions. Chichester: John Wiley; 2008.
6. Ioannidis JP. Why most published research findings are false. PLoS Med 2005;2(8):e124.
7. Jadad AR, Moore RA, Carroll D, et al. Assessing the quality of reports of randomized clinical trials: is blinding necessary? Control Clin Trials 1996;17:1–12.
8. Juni P, Altman DG, Egger M. Systematic reviews in health care: assessing the quality of controlled clinical trials. Br Med J 2001;323:42–6.
9. Katrak P, Bialocerkowski AE, Massy-Westropp N, et al. A systematic review of the content of critical appraisal tools. BMC Med Res Methodol 2004;4:22.
10. Lacasse JR, Leo J. Ghostwriting at elite academic medical centers in the United States. PLoS Med 2010;7:e1000230.
11. Liang LQ, Pengel L, Morris P. Do reports of randomised controlled trials in solid organ transplantation adhere to the 2010 CONSORT statement? A 3-year overview (abstract). Glasgow: British Transplantation Society; 22-24 February 2012.
12. Miller LE, Stewart ME. The blind leading the blind: use and misuse of blinding in randomized controlled trials. Contemp Clin Trials 2011;32:240–3.
13. Moher D, Pham B, Jones A, et al. Does quality of reports of randomised trials affect estimates of intervention efficacy reported in meta-analyses? Lancet 1998;352:609–13.
14. Pengel LHM, Barcena L, Morris PJ. The quality of reporting of randomized controlled trials in solid organ transplantation. Transpl Int 2009;22:377–84.
15. Pengel L, Morris P. The transplant library of randomized controlled trials and systematic reviews. Transplantation 2011;92:613–6.
16. PLoS Medicine Editors. Ghostwriting revisited: new perspectives but few solutions in sight. PLoS Med 2011;8:e1001084.
17. PubMed (database on the internet). Available online at: http://www.ncbi.nlm.nih.gov/pubmed/; 2012.
18. Rothwell PM. External validity of randomised controlled trials: "to whom do the results of this trial apply?". Lancet 2005;365:82–93.
19. Schulz KF, Altman DG, Moher D. CONSORT 2010 statement: updated guidelines for reporting parallel group randomised trials. BMJ 2010;340:c332.
20. Schulz KF, Chalmers I, Hayes RJ, et al. Empirical evidence of bias. Dimensions of methodological quality associated with estimates of treatment effects in controlled trials. JAMA 1995;273:408–12.
21. Straus SE, Richardson WS, Glasziou P, et al. Evidence-based medicine. How to practice and teach EBM. 3rd ed. Edinburgh: Elsevier; 2005.

Index

Note
Page numbers followed by *f* indicate figures and *t* indicate tables.

B

C

D

G

H

I

N

T

U

V